PRINCIPLES AND PRACTICE OF LUNG CANCER

THE OFFICIAL REFERENCE TEXT OF THE IASLC

FOURTH EDITION

PRINCIPLES AND PRACTICE OF

LUNG CANCER

THE OFFICIAL REFERENCE TEXT OF THE IASLC

FOURTH EDITION

EDITORS

HARVEY I. PASS, MD

Professor of Surgery and Cardiothoracic Surgery
Director, Division of Thoracic Surgery and Thoracic Oncology
Department of Cardiothoracic Surgery
New York University Langone Medical Center
New York, New York

DAVID P. CARBONE, MD, PhD

Harold Moses Professor of Cancer Research
Director
Thoracic Oncology Center
Director
Thoracic/Head and Neck Cancer Program
Vanderbilt-Ingram Cancer Center
Departments of Medicine and Cancer Biology
Vanderbilt University School of Medicine
Nashville, Tennessee

JOHN D. MINNA, MD

Sarah M. and Charles E. Seay Distinguished Chair in Cancer Research
Max L. Thomas Distinguished Chair in Molecular Pulmonary Oncology
Professor and Director
Hamon Center for Therapeutic Oncology Research
Departments of Internal Medicine and Pharmacology
University of Texas Southwestern Medical Center
Dallas, Texas

DAVID H. JOHNSON, MD

Cornelius A. Craig Professor of Medical and Surgical Oncology
Director
Division of Hematology/Oncology
Department of Medicine
Vanderbilt University School of Medicine
Deputy Director
Vanderbilt-Ingram Cancer Center
Nashville, Tennessee

GIORGIO V. SCAGLIOTTI, MD

Professor of Respiratory Medicine
Department of Clinical and Biological Sciences
School of Medicine S. Luigi
University of Torino
Orbassano (Torino), Italy

ANDREW T. TURRISI III, MD

Radiation Oncologist-in-Chief
Detroit Medical Center
Sinai Grace Hospital
Detroit, Michigan

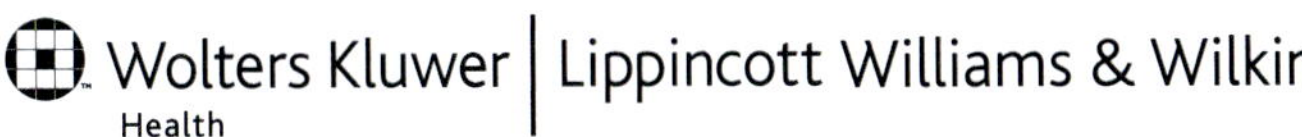

Philadelphia • Baltimore • New York • London
Buenos Aires • Hong Kong • Sydney • Tokyo

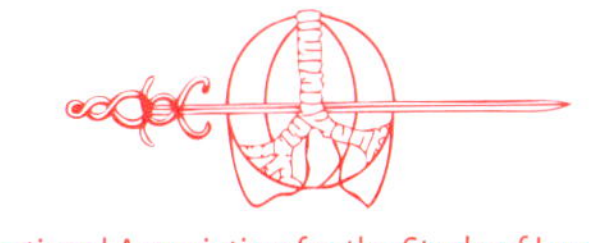

International Association for the Study of Lung Cancer

Senior Executive Editor: Jonathan W. Pine, Jr.
Senior Product Managers: Keith Donnellan, Emilie Moyer
Senior Manufacturing Manager: Benjamin Rivera
Senior Marketing Manager: Angela Panetta
Creative Services Director: Doug Smock
Production Service: Absolute Service, Inc./Maryland Composition

530 Walnut Street
Philadelphia, PA 19106 USA
LWW.com

Printed in The People's Republic of China

Library of Congress Cataloging-in-Publication Data

Principles and practice of lung cancer : the official reference text of the IASLC / editors, Harvey I. Pass ... [et al.].—4th ed.
p. ; cm.
Rev. ed. of: Lung cancer / editors, Harvey I. Pass ... [et al.], c2005.
Includes bibliographical references and index.
ISBN 978-0-7817-7365-2
1. Lungs—Cancer. I. Pass, Harvey I. II. Pass, Harvey I. Lung cancer. III. International Association for the Study of Lung Cancer.
[DNLM: 1. Lung Neoplasms. WF 658 P957 2010]
RC280.L8L8237 2010
616.99'424—dc22

2009051246

Care has been taken to confirm the accuracy of the information presented and to describe generally accepted practices. However, the authors, editors, and publisher are not responsible for errors or omissions or for any consequences from application of the information in this book and make no warranty, expressed or implied, with respect to the currency, completeness, or accuracy of the contents of the publication. Application of the information in a particular situation remains the professional responsibility of the practitioner.

The authors, editors, and publisher have exerted every effort to ensure that drug selection and dosage set forth in this text are in accordance with current recommendations and practice at the time of publication. However, in view of ongoing research, changes in government regulations, and the constant flow of information relating to drug therapy and drug reactions, the reader is urged to check the package insert for each drug for any change in indications and dosage and for added warnings and precautions. This is particularly important when the recommended agent is a new or an infrequently employed drug.

Some drugs and medical devices presented in the publication have Food and Drug Administration (FDA) clearance for limited use in restricted research settings. It is the responsibility of the healthcare provider to ascertain the FDA status of each drug or device planned for use in their clinical practice.

To purchase additional copies of this book, call our customer service department at (800) 638-3030 or fax orders to (301) 223-2320. International customers should call (301) 223-2300.

Visit Lippincott Williams & Wilkins on the Internet: http://www.lww.com. Lippincott Williams & Wilkins customer service representatives are available from 8:30 AM to 6 PM, EST.

10 9 8 7 6 5 4 3 2 1

RRS1001

This book is dedicated to our families. There are no substitutes for their patience, encouragement, love, and support.

To Helen, Ally, and Eric Pass

To Beverly and Mary-Michael Johnson for their unwavering support and love

To Kazel Carbone, Daniel, Elizabeth, Beatrice, and Anna Carbone

To Lynn, Laura, and Leslie Minna

To Silvia and to the memory of my parents, Rosa and Luigi Scagliotti

To Kathy, Richard, Casey, Harmon, Katie, Carolyn, and mostly, little Emilia Turrisi

The inspiration for this endeavor, as always, came from our patients, students, and residents as well as from our colleagues and mentors. These sources of incredible wisdom and diversity force us to grapple with our limitations and help us to recognize how we can best utilize our strengths.

CONTENTS

PREFACE

It is truly amazing how things can change in 4 years. Speculation about the use of molecular strategies has become reality in such a short time. The whole approach to the management of lung cancer at presentation and recurrence has changed. Genomic and proteomic profiles, dismissed as fishing expeditions in earlier times, are now used in validation studies, not only as prognostic, but also as predictive markers. Who would have thought that a rebirth of the idea of minimalist surgery involving sublobar resections for the management of primary lung cancer would become one of the prime questions for the disease, and that we are actually planning and performing trials, which compare surgical resection to stereotactic radiation therapy? Adjuvant studies for lung cancer have matured, and the use of preoperative therapy remains as controversial as ever. We now have to be precise in our histologic classifications of non–small cell lung cancer in order to define best treatment strategies and to avoid therapeutic complications. Finally, for the first time since 1987, a new internationally based staging system involving more than 100,000 individuals is ready for prime time and will serve as the foundation for future editions, which may incorporate clinical, pathologic, as well as molecular parameters.

This fourth edition of *Principles and Practice of Lung Cancer* is meant to serve as a foundation. Although we attempt to keep up with the newest concepts in all aspects of the disease, it is pretty clear that with the pace of discovery as it is, it will not have every detail available to the reader. The book is meant to educate about new concepts and point the reader to other sources of knowledge—including the web, journals, CME courses, and conferences—to expand on the basics presented in the book. The editors have realized also that the complexity of the disease is not geographically limited. Lung cancer is an international problem, and the book, therefore, has become an international production with the addition of Dr. Giorgio V. Scagliotti as an international editor. *Principles and Practice of Lung Cancer* has now officially become an international reference text as the textbook of the International Association for the Study of Lung Cancer (IASLC). We want this book to be available for readers in all parts of the world, just as the IASLC has attempted to bring together all international disciplines that are attempting to decrease the lethality of the disease. Just as we added mesothelioma and thymoma with the last edition, the editors felt that we should expand into other areas of thoracic malignancies, including mediastinal and carcinoid tumors.

The editors are again indebted to our publishing colleagues who helped produce this edition. Particular thanks are due to Keith Donnellan, Emilie Moyer, and Gil Rafanan for keeping things organized and on track, to Angela Panetta for marketing expertise, and to Senior Executive Editor Jonathan W. Pine, Jr.

CONTRIBUTORS

Alex A. Adjei, MD, PhD, FACP
Professor and Chairman
Department of Medicine
Katherine Anne Gioia Chair in Cancer Medicine
Roswell Park Cancer Institute
Buffalo, New York

Naveed Alam, MD, FRCSC
Lecturer
Department of Surgery
University of Melbourne
Consultant Thoracic Surgeon
Department of Surgery
St. Vincent's Hospital
Melbourne, Australia

Kathy S. Albain, MD
Professor
Medicine, Hematology/Oncology
Loyola University Health System
Maywood, Illinois

Nasser K. Altorki, MD
Professor
Department of Cardiothoracic Surgery
Weill Cornell Medical College
Attending Surgeon
Department of Cardiothoracic Surgery
New York Presbyterian Hospital
New York, New York

Christopher I. Amos, PhD
Professor
Department of Epidemiology
The University of Texas MD Anderson Cancer Center
Houston, Texas

Hisao Asamura, MD
Chief
Division of Thoracic Surgery
National Cancer Center Hospital
Tokyo, Japan

Paul Baas, MD
Head
Department of Thoracic Oncology
The Netherlands Cancer Institute
Amsterdam, The Netherlands

Joan E. Bailey-Wilson, PhD
Senior Investigator and Co-Branch Chief
Inherited Disease Research Branch
National Human Genome Research Institute
National Institutes of Health
Baltimore, Maryland

Jair Bar, MD, PhD
Clinical Fellow
Division of Medical Oncology
The Ottawa Hospital Cancer Center
Ottawa, Canada

José Belderbos, MD, PhD
Radiation Oncologist
Department of Radiation Oncology
The Netherlands Cancer Institute–Antoni van Leeuwenhoek Hospital (NKI–AVL)
Amsterdam, The Netherlands

Søren M. Bentzen, PhD, DSc
Professor
Departments of Human Oncology, Medical Physics, and Biostatistics and Medical Informatics
School of Medicine and Public Health
University of Wisconsin
Director of Research and Education
Department of Human Oncology
Paul P. Carbone Comprehensive Cancer Center
Madison, Wisconsin

Costas Bizekis, MD
Assistant Professor
Department of Cardiothoracic Surgery
New York University
Attending Surgeon
Director of Esophageal Surgery
Department of Cardiothoracic Surgery
New York University Langone Medical Center
New York, New York

Naama R. Bogot, MD
Clinical Lecturer
Division of Cardiothoracic Radiology
Department of Radiology
University of Michigan Health System
Ann Arbor, Michigan

Julie R. Brahmer, MD, MSc
Assistant Professor
Department of Oncology
The Sidney Kimmel Comprehensive Cancer Center
Johns Hopkins University School of Medicine
Baltimore, Maryland

Jacques Cadranel, MD, PhD
Professor
Chest Department
AP-HP – Tenon Hospital
Pierre and Marie Curie University
Paris, France

David P. Carbone, MD, PhD
Harold Moses Professor of Cancer Research
Director
Thoracic Oncology Center
Director
Thoracic/Head and Neck Cancer Program
Vanderbilt-Ingram Cancer Center
Departments of Medicine and Cancer Biology
Vanderbilt University School of Medicine
Nashville, Tennessee

Yvonne M. Carter, MD
Assistant Professor
Department of Surgery
Georgetown University
Division of Thoracic Surgery
Georgetown University Medical Center
Washington, District of Columbia

Tze-Ming Benson Chen, MD
Associate Program Director, Pulmonary and Critical Care Fellowship
Division of Pulmonary and Critical Care
Department of Internal Medicine
California Pacific Medical Center
San Francisco, California

Traves D. Crabtree, MD
Assistant Professor
Department of Cardiothoracic Surgery
Washington University
Barnes Hospital
St. Louis, Missouri

Walter Curran, Jr., MD
Professor and Chair
Department of Radiation Oncology
Emory University School of Medicine
Atlanta, Georgia

Stephen J. Curtis, BS
PhD Candidate
Department of Genetics
Harvard Medical School
Graduate Student
Stem Cell Program
Children's Hospital Boston
Boston, Massachusetts

Harry J. de Koning, MD, PhD
Professor
Department of Public Health
Erasmus MC, University Medical Center Rotterdam
Rotterdam, The Netherlands

Dirk De Ruysscher, MD, PhD
Professor of Respiratory Oncology
GROW Research Institute
Radiation Oncologist
Department of Radiation Oncology (Maastro Clinic)
Maastricht University Medical Center
Maastricht, The Netherlands

Chadrick E. Denlinger, MD
Assistant Professor
Department of Surgery
Medical University of South Carolina
Charleston, South Carolina

Frank C. Detterbeck, MD
Professor and Section Chief
Thoracic Surgery
Yale University School of Medicine
Attending and Section Chief
Thoracic Surgery
Yale New Haven Hospital
New Haven, Connecticut

Jessica S. Donington, MD
Assistant Professor
Department of Cardiothoracic Surgery
New York University School of Medicine
Chief, Thoracic Surgery
Department of Cardiothoracic Surgery
Bellevue Hospital
New York, New York

Christophe Dooms, MD, PhD
University Hospitals Leuven
Department of Pulmonology
Leuven, Belgium

Carolyn Dresler, MD, MPA
Director
Tobacco Prevention and Cessation Program
Arkansas Department of Health
Little Rock, Arkansas

Damian E. Dupuy, MD, FACR
Professor
Department of Diagnostic Imaging
The Warren Alpert Medical School of Brown University
Director of Tumor Ablation
Department of Diagnostic Imaging
Rhode Island Hospital
Providence, Rhode Island

Robert Eager, MD
Department of Internal Medicine
John A. Burns School of Medicine
Queens Medical Center
Honolulu, Hawaii

Wilfried E. E. Eberhardt, MD
University of Essen Medical School
Consultant
West German Cancer Center
Essen, Germany

Peter M. Ellis, MBBS, MMed, PhD, FRACP, FRCPC
Associate Professor
Departments of Oncology and Clinical Epidemiology and Biostatistics
McMaster University
Staff Medical Oncologist
Department of Medical Oncology
Juravinski Cancer Centre
Ontario, Canada

Sara Erridge, MBBS, MD, FRCR, FRCP(Edin)
Honorary Senior Lecturer
University of Edinburgh
Consultant Clinical Oncologist
Edinburgh Cancer Centre
Western General Hospital
Edinburgh, United Kingdom

Hiran C. Fernando, MBBS, FRCS
Associate Professor
Department of Cardiothoracic Surgery
Boston University
Director
Minimally Invasive Thoracic Surgery Program
Department of Cardiothoracic Surgery
Boston Medical Center
Boston, Massachusetts

Raja Flores, MD
Associate Professor of Cardiothoracic Surgery
Department of Thoracic Surgery
Cornell University Medical College
Department of Surgery
Memorial Sloan-Kettering Cancer Center
New York, New York

Wilbur A. Franklin, MD
Professor
Department of Pathology
University of Colorado Denver
Director, Colorado Molecular Correlates Laboratory
University Hospital
Aurora, Colorado

Shirish M. Gadgeel, MD
Associate Professor
Department of Internal Medicine
Karmanos Cancer Institute/Wayne State University
Karmanos Cancer Hospital
Detroit, Michigan

David R. Gandara, MD
Professor
Associate Director of Clinical Research
Department of Internal Medicine
University of California Davis Cancer Center
Sacramento, California

Marileila Varella Garcia, PhD
Professor
Departments of Medicine and Pathology
University of Colorado Denver
Anschutz Medical Center
Aurora, Colorado

Oliver Gautschi, MD
Research Group Leader
Department of Clinical Research
University of Bern
Attending Oncologist
Department of Medical Oncology
University Hospital Bern
Bern, Switzerland

Adi F. Gazdar, MD
Professor
Department of Pathology and Hamon Center for Therapeutic Oncology Research
University of Texas Southwestern Medical Center
Dallas, Texas

Peter Goldstraw, MB, FRCS
Professor of Thoracic Surgery
Imperial College
Consultant Thoracic Surgeon
Department of Thoracic Surgery
Royal Brompton Hospital
London, United Kingdom

Adriana Gonzalez, MD
Assistant Professor of Pathology
Vanderbilt-Ingram Cancer Center Member
Researcher
Vanderbilt University Medical Center
Nashville, Tennessee

Elizabeth Gore, MD
Associate Professor
Department of Radiation Oncology
Medical College of Wisconsin
Froedtert Memorial Lutheran Hospital
Milwaukee, Wisconsin

Cesare Gridelli, MD
Director
Department of Medical Oncology
S.G. Moscati Hospital
Avellino, Italy

Shawn Haji-Momenian, MD
Fellow
Department of Radiology
Feinberg School of Medicine
Northwestern University
Northwestern Memorial Hospital
Chicago, Illinois

Dennis E. Hallahan, MD
Elizabeth H. and James S. McDonnell Distinguished Professor
Department of Radiation Oncology
Washington University
Radiation Oncologist-in-Chief
Department of Radiation Oncology
Barnes-Jewish Hospital
St. Louis, Missouri

David H. Harpole, Jr., MD
Professor of Surgery
Vice-Chairman for Faculty Affairs
Department of Surgery
Duke University Medical Center
Durham, North Carolina

John Henley, MD
Staff Pathologist
Department of Pathology
Columbus Regional Hospital
Columbus, Indiana

Claudia I. Henschke, MD
Professor of Radiology
Department of Radiology and Cardiothoracic Surgery
Weill Cornell Medical College
Attending Radiologist and Division Chief
Division of Chest Imaging
Department of Radiology
The New York Presbyterian Hospital
New York, New York

Roy S. Herbst, MD, PhD
Professor of Medicine
Chief, Section of Thoracic Medical Oncology
Department of Thoracic/Head and Neck Medical Oncology
Barnhart Family Distinguished Professor in Targeted Therapies
The University of Texas MD Anderson Cancer Center
Houston, Texas

Felix J.F. Herth, MD
Heidelberg University Thorax Clinic
Chief Physician
Department of Pneumology and Internal Medicine
Thorax Clinic
University Clinic of Heidelberg
Heidelberg, Germany

Fred R. Hirsch, MD, PhD
Professor of Medicine and Pathology
Division of Medical Oncology
Department of Medicine
University of Colorado Cancer Center
Aurora, Colorado

Leora Horn, MD, MSc
Assistant Professor
Department of Medicine
Vanderbilt University Medical Center
Vanderbilt University
Nashville, Tennessee

Chao H. Huang, MD
Associate Professor
Division of Hematology/Oncology
Department of Internal Medicine
University of Kansas Medical Center
Medical Oncologist and Hematologist
Division of Medical Oncology and Hematology
Department of Internal Medicine
University of Kansas Hospital
Kansas City, Kansas

David M. Jablons, MD
Professor of Surgery
Ada Distinguished Professor
Department of Surgery
University of California, San Francisco
Chief
Section of General Thoracic Surgery
Department of Surgery
University of California–San Francisco Moffitt Long Hospital
San Francisco, California

Pasi A. Jänne, MD, PhD
Associate Professor of Medicine
Harvard Medical School
Department of Medical Oncology
Dana Farber Cancer Institute
Boston, Massachusetts

David H. Johnson, MD
Cornelius A. Craig Professor of Medical and Surgical Oncology
Director, Division of Hematology/Oncology
Department of Medicine
Vanderbilt University School of Medicine
Deputy Director, Vanderbilt-Ingram Cancer Center
Vanderbilt-Ingram Cancer Center
Nashville, Tennessee

Brian D. Kavanagh, MD
Professor
Department of Radiation Oncology
University of Colorado Denver
Vice-Chair and Clinical Practice Director
Department of Radiation Oncology
University of Colorado Hospital
Aurora, Colorado

Paul Keall, PhD
Associate Professor
Department of Radiation Oncology
Stanford University
Stanford, California

Karen Kelly, MD
Professor of Medicine
Division of Hematology/Oncology
Department of Internal Medicine
University of Kansas Medical Center
Kansas City, Kansas

Kenneth Kesler, MD
Professor of Surgery
Division of Cardiothoracic Surgery
Indiana University
Indianapolis, Indiana

Vincent S. Khoo, MB, BS, FRACR, FRCR, MD
Honorary Associate Professor
Department of Medicine, Austin Health
University of Melbourne
Melbourne, Victoria
Consultant Clinical Oncologist
Department of Clinical Oncology
Royal Marsden NHS Foundation Trust
London, United Kingdom

Fadlo Khuri, MD
Professor and Chair
Department of Hematology and Medical Oncology
Emory-Winship Cancer Institute
Attending Physician
Department of Medical Oncology
Emory University Hospital
Atlanta, Georgia

Carla F. Kim, PhD
Assistant Professor
Department of Genetics
Harvard Medical School
Assistant Professor
Stem Cell Program
Children's Hospital Boston
Boston, Massachusetts

Anthony W. Kim, MD
Assistant Professor
Department of Surgery
Section of Thoracic Surgery
Yale University School of Medicine
Attending Surgeon
Department of Surgery
Yale-New Haven Hospital
New Haven, Connecticut

Hedy Lee Kindler, MD
Associate Professor
Section of Hematology/Oncology
University of Chicago Medical Center
University of Chicago
Chicago, Illinois

Ritsuko Komaki, MD, FACR, FASTRO
Professor Tenured of University of Texas
Department of Radiation Oncology
The University of Texas MD Anderson Cancer Center
Houston, Texas

Feng-Ming (Spring) Kong, MD, PhD
Associate Professor
Department of Radiation Oncology
University of Michigan Medical School
Chief, Veterans Administration
Department of Radiation Oncology
University of Michigan Health System
Ann Arbor, Michigan

Paris A. Kosmidis, MD
Chief
Department of Medical Oncology
Hygeia Hospital
Athens, Greece

Jonathan M. Kurie, MD
Professor
Department of Thoracic/Head and Neck Medical Oncology
The University of Texas MD Anderson Cancer Center
Houston, Texas

Ware G. Kuschner, MD
Associate Professor
Department of Medicine
Division of Pulmonary and Critical Care Medicine
Stanford University School of Medicine
Staff Physician
Medical Service, Pulmonary Section
U.S. Department of Veterans Affairs Palo Alto Health Care System
Palo Alto, California

Young Kwok, MD
Assistant Professor
Department of Radiation Oncology
University of Maryland School of Medicine
Associate Director of Clinical Research
Department of Radiation Oncology
University of Maryland Medical Center
Baltimore, Maryland

Ite A. Laird-Offringa, PhD
Associate Professor
Department of Surgery and Department of Biochemistry and Molecular Biology
Keck School of Medicine
University of Southern California/Norris Comprehensive Cancer Center
Los Angeles, California

Brian E. Lally, MD
Assistant Professor
Department of Radiation Oncology
University of Miami
Miami, Florida

Stephen Lam, MD, FRCPC
Professor
Department of Medicine
University of British Columbia
Chair
Lung Tumor Group
BC Cancer Agency
Vancouver, British Columbia, Canada

Corey Langer, MD
Director of Thoracic Oncology
Abramson Cancer Center
Professor of Medicine
Hematology-Oncology Division
Department of Medicine
University of Pennsylvania
Philadelphia, Pennsylvania

Jill E. Larsen, PhD
Postdoctoral Fellow
Hamon Center for Therapeutic Oncology Research
University of Texas Southwestern Medical Center
Dallas, Texas

Cécile Le Péchoux, MD
Department of Radiation Oncology
Gustave Roussy Institute (Comprehensive Cancer Center)
Villejuif, France

Paul C. Lee, MD
Associate Professor of Cardiothoracic Surgery
Department of Cardiothoracic Surgery
Weill Cornell Medical College
Attending Surgeon
Department of Cardiothoracic Surgery
New York Presbyterian Hospital
New York, New York

Zhongxing Liao, MD
Professor
Center Medical Director
Department of Radiation Oncology
The University of Texas MD Anderson Cancer Center
Houston, Texas

Michael J. Liptay, MD
Associate Professor
Department of Cardiovascular and Thoracic Surgery
Rush University Medical School
Chief
Division of Thoracic Surgery
Rush University Medical Center
Chicago, Illinois

Simon S. Lo, MD
Associate Professor of Radiation Oncology and Neurosurgery
Department of Radiation Oncology
Arthur G. James Cancer Hospital
Ohio State University Medical Center
Columbus, Ohio

Patrick J. Loehrer, Sr., MD
Interim Director
Melvin and Bren Simon Cancer Center
Director and Bruce Kenneth Wiseman Professor of Medicine
Division of Hematology/Oncology
Department of Medicine
Indiana University School of Medicine
Indianapolis, Indiana

Bo Lu, MD, PhD
Associate Professor
Department of Radiation Oncology
Vanderbilt-Ingram Cancer Center
Vanderbilt University Medical Center
Vanderbilt University
Nashville, Tennessee

Philip C. Mack, PhD
Associate Adjunct Professor
Division of Hematology/Oncology
Department of Internal Medicine
University of California, Davis
Sacramento, California

Christian Manegold, MD
Head of Interdisciplinary Thoracic Oncology
Department of Surgery
University Medical Center Mannheim
University of Heidelberg
Mannheim, Germany

Linda W. Martin, MD, MPH
Thoracic Surgeon
The Cancer Institute
Department of Surgery
St. Joseph Medical Center
Towson, Maryland

Pierre P. Massion, MD
Associate Professor of Medicine
Department of Medicine
Associate Professor of Cancer Biology
Department of Cancer Biology
Vanderbilt University School of Medicine
Section Chief
Department of Pulmonary and Critical Care Medicine
Veterans Affairs Medical Center
Nashville, Tennessee

Gregory A. Masters, MD
Associate Professor
Department of Medicine
Thomas Jefferson University
Philadelphia, Pennsylvania
Thoracic Oncology Team
Medical Oncology Hematology Consultants
Helen F. Graham Cancer Center
Christiana Care Health System
Newark, Delaware

Robert J. McKenna, Jr., MD
Clinical Chief, Thoracic Surgery
Cedars-Sinai Medical Center
Los Angeles, California

Annette McWilliams, MD, FRCPC
Clinical Assistant Professor
Department of Medicine
University of British Columbia
Active Staff/Respiratory Physician
Systemic Therapy
British Columbia Cancer Agency
Vancouver, British Columbia, Canada

Olli S. Miettinen, MD, PhD
Professor
Departments of Epidemiology, Biostatistics, and Occupational Health and Medicine
McGill University
Montreal, Quebec

John D. Minna, MD
Sarah M. and Charles E. Seay Distinguished Chair in Cancer Research
Max L. Thomas Distinguished Chair in Molecular Pulmonary Oncology
Professor and Director
Hamon Center for Therapeutic Oncology Research
Departments of Internal Medicine and Pharmacology
University of Texas Southwestern Medical Center
Dallas, Texas

Tetsuya Mitsudomi, MD
Deputy Director and Chief
Department of Thoracic Surgery
Aichi Cancer Center Hospital
Nagoya, Japan

Luigi Moretti, MD, MPH
Clinical Fellow in Radiation Oncology
Department of Radiation Oncology
Vanderbilt-Ingram Cancer Center
Vanderbilt University
Vanderbilt University Medical Center
Nashville, Tennessee

James L. Mulshine, MD
Professor
Department of Internal Medicine
Division of Hematology and Oncology
Vice President, Research
Research Affairs
Rush University Medical Center
Chicago, Illinois

Nevin Murray, MD, FRCPC
Clinical Professor of Medicine
Department of Medicine
University of British Columbia
Medical Oncologist
Department of Medical Oncology
British Columbia Cancer Agency
Vancouver, British Columbia, Canada

John Nemunaitis, MD
Executive Medical Director
Mary Crowley Cancer Research Centers
Oncologist
Texas Oncology, PA
Dallas, Texas

Francis Nichols, MD
Associate Professor of Surgery
Chair, Division of General Thoracic Surgery
Department of Surgery
Mayo Clinic
Rochester, Minnesota

Masayuki Noguchi, MD
Department of Pathology
Institute of Basic Medical Sciences
Graduate School of Comprehensive Human Sciences
University of Tsukuba
Ibaraki, Japan

Silvia Novello, MD, PhD
Respiratory Physician
Thoracic Oncology Unit
University of Turin
Department of Clinical and Biological Sciences
San Luigi Hospital
Orbassano, Italy

Sebahat Ocak, MD
Research Fellow in Pulmonology
Division of Allergy, Pulmonary and Critical Care Medicine
Department of Internal Medicine
Vanderbilt-Ingram Cancer Center
Vanderbilt University
Nashville, Tennessee

Amir Onn, MD
Chief
Section of Pulmonary Oncology
Division of Oncology
Sheba Medical Center
Tel Hashomer, Israel

Jason R. Pantarotto, MD, FRCPC
Assistant Professor
Department of Radiology
University of Ottawa
Consultant
Division of Radiation Oncology
The Ottawa Hospital
Ottawa, Ontario, Canada

Harvey I. Pass, MD
Professor of Surgery and Cardiothoracic Surgery
Director, Division of Thoracic Surgery and Thoracic Oncology
Department of Cardiothoracic Surgery
New York University Langone Medical Center
New York, New York

Roy A. Patchell, MD
Chairman
Department of Neurology
Barrow Neurological Institute
St. Joseph's Hospital
Phoenix, Arizona

Ashish Patel, MD
Thoracic Surgeon
Department of Surgery
Kaiser Permanente
Oakland, California

Katherine M. Pisters, MD
Professor
Department of Thoracic/Head and Neck Medical Oncology
The University of Texas MD Anderson Cancer Center
Houston, Texas

Ambra Pozzi, PhD
Associate Professor
Departments of Medicine (Nephrology) and Cancer Biology
Vanderbilt University
Medical Center North
Nashville, Tennessee

Theolyn Price, MD
Resident in Thoracic and Cardiovascular Surgery
Department of Surgery
Mayo Clinic
Rochester, Minnesota

Leslie E. Quint, MD
Professor
Department of Radiology
University of Michigan Health System
Ann Arbor, Michigan

David Raben, MD
Professor and Associate Scientist
Department of Radiation Oncology
University of Colorado Denver
University of Colorado Hospital
Aurora, Colorado

Sheila C. Rankin, FRCR
Consultant Radiologist
Radiology Department
Guy's and St. Thomas NHS Foundation Trust
London, United Kingdom

Dan J. Raz, MD
Division of Thoracic Surgery
University of California, San Francisco
San Francisco, California

William F. Regine, MD
Professor
Department of Radiation Oncology
University of Maryland School of Medicine
Chairman
Department of Radiation Oncology
University of Maryland Medical Center
Baltimore, Maryland

Bruce W.S. Robinson, MD, PhD
Professor of Medicine
School of Medicine and Pharmacology
The University of Western Australia
Consultant Respiratory Physician
Department of Respiratory Medicine
Sir Charles Gairdner Hospital
Perth, Western Australia

William Rom, MD, MPH
Sol and Judith Bergstein Professor of Medicine
Departments of Medicine and Environmental Medicine
Director, Division of Pulmonary and Critical Care Medicine
Department of Medicine
New York University School of Medicine
New York, New York

Rafael Rosell, MD, PhD
Professor
School of Medicine
Autonomous University of Barcelona
Chief
Medical Oncology Service
Catalan Institute of Oncology
Hospital Germans Trias i Pujol
Badalona, Spain

Alan Sandler, MD
Professor of Medicine
Oregon Health and Science University
Portland, Oregon

Thomas J. Santo, BS
AATS Research Fellow
School of Medicine
Stony Brook University
Stony Brook, New York

Ricardo S. Santos, MD
Instructor of Surgery
Department of Cardiothoracic Surgery
Boston University School of Medicine
Head
Minimally Invasive Thoracic Surgery
Department of Cardiothoracic Surgery
Albert Einstein Israeli Hospital
São Paulo, Brazil

Anjali Saqi, MD
Associate Professor of Clinical Pathology
Department of Pathology and Cell Biology
Columbia University Medical Center
Associate Attending Director of Cytopathology
Department of Pathology and Cell Biology
New York Presbyterian Hospital
New York, New York

Giorgio V. Scagliotti, MD
Professor of Respiratory Medicine
Department of Clinical and Biological Sciences
School of Medicine S. Luigi
University of Torino
Orbassano (Torino), Italy

David Schottenfeld, MD, MSc
Professor (Emeritus)
Department of Epidemiology and Internal Medicine
University of Michigan School of Public Health
Ann Arbor, Michigan

Amanda Schwer, MD
Department of Radiation Oncology
University of Colorado Denver
University of Colorado Hospital
Aurora, Colorado

Suresh Senan, MRCP, FRCR, PhD
Professor of Clinical Experimental Radiotherapy
Department of Radiation Oncology
VU University Medical Center
Amsterdam, The Netherlands

Frances A. Shepherd, MD, FRCPC
Professor of Medicine
Department of Medicine
University of Toronto
Scott Taylor Chair in Lung Cancer Research
Department on Medical Oncology and Hematology
Princess Margaret Hospital
Toronto, Ontario, Canada

Jill M. Siegfried, PhD
Professor
Department of Pharmacology and Chemical Biology
University of Pittsburgh
Co-Director
Lung and Thoracic Malignancies Program
University of Pittsburgh Cancer Institute
Pittsburgh, Pennsylvania

Kerstin W. Sinkevicius, PhD
Postdoctoral Fellow
Department of Genetics
Harvard Medical School
Department of Hematology/Oncology
Children's Hospital Boston
Boston, Massachusetts

Mark A. Socinski, MD
Associate Professor
Clinical Research
Hematology/Oncology
University of North Carolina
Lineberger Comprehensive Cancer Center
NC Cancer Hospital
Chapel Hill, North Carolina

Timothy D. Solberg, PhD
Professor
Department of Radiation Oncology
UT Southwestern Medical Center at Dallas
Dallas, Texas

Monica Spinola, PhD
Postdoctoral Fellow
University of Texas Southwestern Medical Center
Dallas, Texas

Simon D. Spivack, MD, MPH
Associate Professor
Departments of Medicine, Epidemiology, and Genetics
Chief, Division of Pulmonary Medicine
Department of Medicine
Montefiore Medical Center
Albert Einstein College of Medicine of Yeshiva University
Bronx, New York

Laura P. Stabile, PhD
Research Assistant Professor
Department of Pharmacology and Chemical Biology
University of Pittsburgh
Pittsburgh, Pennsylvania

Matthew Steliga, MD
Assistant Professor of Surgery
Division of Cardiothoracic Surgery
Department of Surgery
University of Arkansas for Medical Sciences
Little Rock, Arkansas

Sigrid Stroobants, MD, PhD
Associate Professor
Department of Nuclear Medicine
Catholic University Leuven
Head of Clinic
Department of Nuclear Medicine
University Hospitals Leuven
Leuven, Belgium

Thomas G. Sutedja, MD, FCCP
Academic Hospital Free University
Amsterdam, The Netherlands

Robert D. Timmerman, MD
Professor
Departments of Radiation Oncology and Neurosurgery
Vice Chairman
Department of Radiation Oncology
University of Texas Southwestern
Dallas, Texas

Betty C. Tong, MD, MHS
Assistant Professor
Department of Surgery
Duke University Medical Center
Durham, North Carolina

Elizabeth L. Travis, PhD
Mattie Allen Fair Professor in Cancer Research
Department of Experimental Radiation Oncology
Department of Pulmonary Medicine
The University of Texas MD Anderson Cancer Center
Houston, Texas

Andrew T. Turrisi III, MD
Radiation Oncologist-in-Chief
Detroit Medical Center
Sinai Grace Hospital
Detroit, Michigan

Paul Van Houtte, MD
Professor
Université Libre de Bruxelles
Chairman
Department of Radiation Oncology
Institut Jules Bordet
Brussels, Belgium

Rob J. van Klaveren, MD, PhD
Associate Professor
Department of Pulmonology
Erasmus Medical Center-Daniel Den Hoed Cancer Center
Rotterdam, The Netherlands

Jan P. van Meerbeeck, MD, PhD
Professor of Thoracic Oncology
Department of Internal Medicine
University of Ghent
Head
Division of Blood, Respiration, and Digestion
Ghent University Hospital
Ghent, Belgium

Paul E. Van Schil, MD
Professor and Chair
Antwerp Surgical Training and Research Center
University of Antwerp
Chief
Department of Thoracic and Vascular Surgery
Antwerp University Hospital
Antwerp, Belgium

Nico Van Zandwijk, MD
Professor of Medicine
Director, Asbestos Diseases Research Institute
University of Sydney
New South Wales, Australia

Johan Vansteenkiste, MD, PhD
Professor
Department of Internal Medicine
Catholic University Leuven
Head of Clinic
Pneumology/Respiratory Oncology Unit
University Hospital Leuven
Leuven, Belgium

Ara Vaporciyan, MD
Associate Professor
Department of Thoracic and Cardiovascular Surgery
The University of Texas MD Anderson Cancer Center
Houston, Texas

Madeline F. Vazquez, MD
Associate Director, Manhattan Facility
Departments of Cytopathology/Surgical Pathology
CBLPath, Inc.
Rye Brook, New York

Everett E. Vokes, MD
Interim Dean and Chief Executive Officer
University of Chicago Medical Center
Chicago, Illinois

Garrett L. Walsh, MD
Professor
Department of Thoracic and Cardiovascular Surgery
Division of Surgery
The University of Texas MD Anderson Cancer Center
Houston, Texas

Marie Wislez, MD, PhD
Professor
Chest Department
AP-HP – Tenon Hospital
Pierre and Marie Curie University
Paris, France

Aaron H. Wolfson, MD
Professor and Vice Chair
Department of Radiation Oncology
University of Miami Miller School of Medicine
Miami, Florida

Antoinette J. Wozniak, MD
Professor
Division of Hematology and Oncology
Department of Medicine
Karmanos Cancer Institute
Wayne State University
Detroit, Michigan

David F. Yankelevitz, MD
Professor of Radiology
Department of Radiology and Cardiothoracic Surgery
Weill Cornell Medical College
Attending Radiologist
Department of Radiology
The New York Presbyterian Hospital
New York, New York

Mark A. Yoder, MD
Assistant Professor
Medical College
Rush University
Department of Medicine
Rush University Medical Center
Chicago, Illinois

Michael Zervos, MD
Assistant Professor
Department of Cardiothoracic Surgery
New York University
Attending Surgeon
Department of Cardiothoracic Surgery
New York University Langone Medical Center
New York, New York

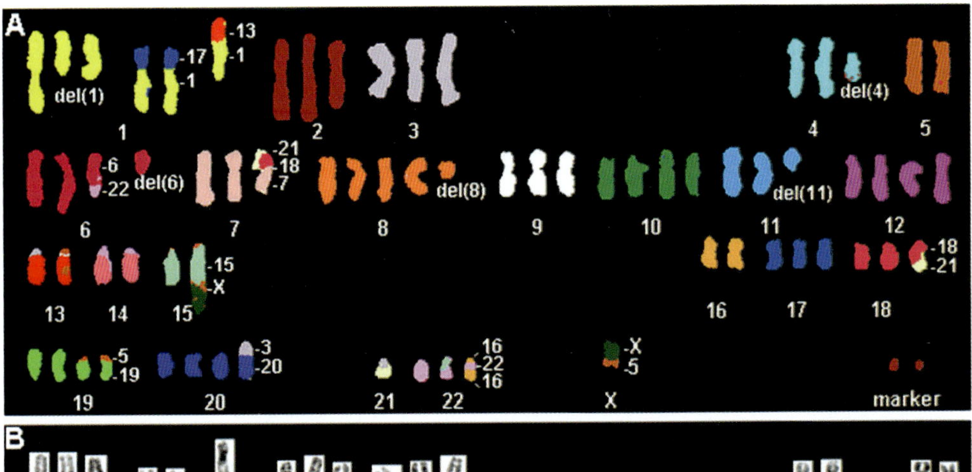

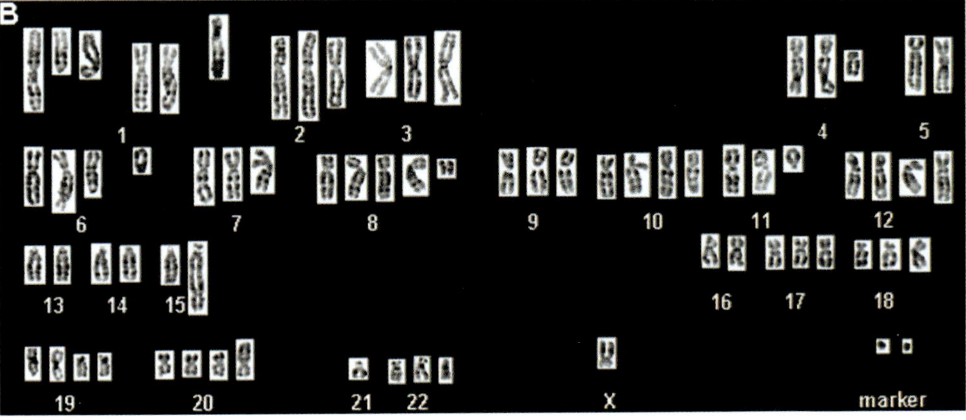

FIGURE 6.1 SKY of a primary lung adenocarcinoma showing numerous numerical and structural chromosome changes. The classified image with the pseudocolors is shown in **(A)** and the inverted DAPI image is shown in **(B)**. The specimen was near triploid, with extra copies of chromosomes 1, 10, 12, 19, and 20 and deletions of segments of chromosomes 1, 4, 5, 6, and 11. Translocations were found involving chromosomes 1 and 13, 1 and 17, 3 and 20, 5 and 19, 5 and X, 6 and 22, 7, 15, and X, 18 and 21, 16 and 22, and 18 and 21. Two very small marker chromosomes were found carrying chromosome 2 sequences.

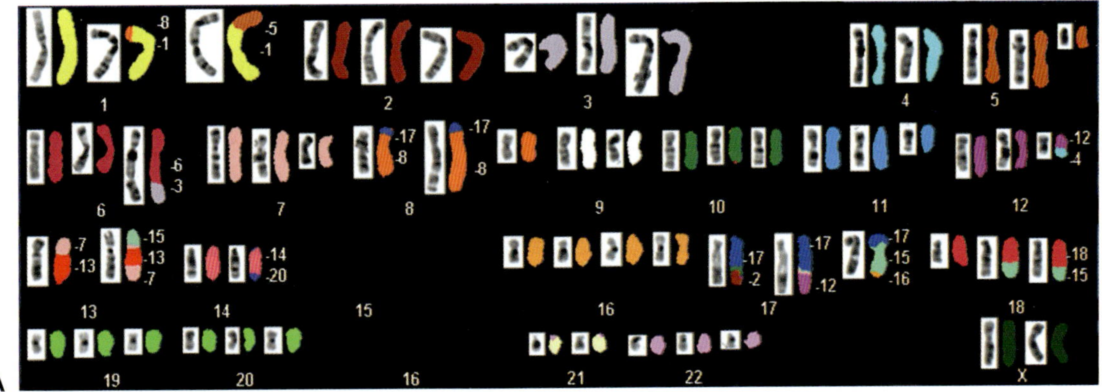

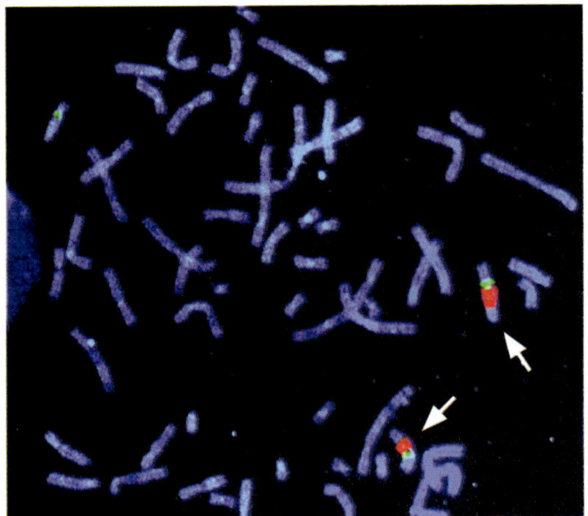

FIGURE 6.2 **A:** SKY of the non–small cell lung cancer cell line Calu 3 showing multiple abnormalities and two copies of abnormal chromosome 17, derivatives from the translocations between chromosomes 17 and 2 and chromosomes 17 and 12. In addition, the chromosome 17 material identified by SKY in the long arm (q-arm) of these derivative chromosomes was larger than expected if that arm was normal. **B:** FISH analyses with a probe set including ERBB2 and CEP 17 sequences demonstrated that there was ERBB2 gene amplification in both derivatives (indicated by the *arrows*). In the FISH assays, ERBB2 probe is highlighted by *red color* and CEP 17 by *green color*.

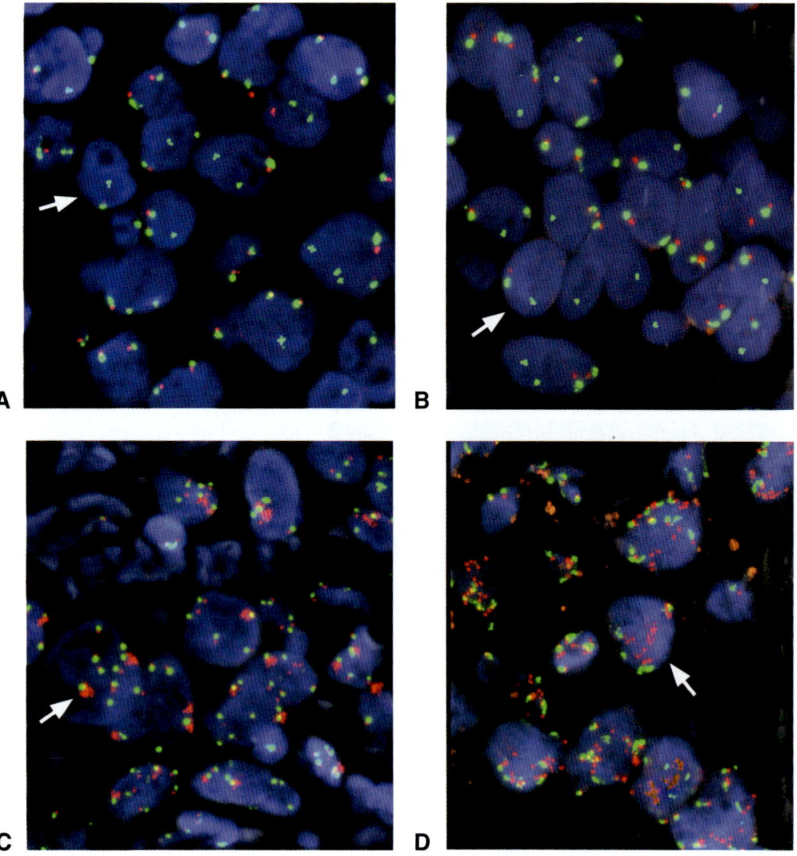

FIGURE 6.3 FISH of sections of non–small cell lung cancer with *CDKN2*-CEP9 **(A)**, *FHIT*-CEP3 **(B)**, *EGFR*-CEP7 **(C)** and *KRAS*-CEP12 **(D)** probe sets. Hybridization spots with the gene probes fluoresce in *red color* and with the centromere control probes fluoresce in *green color*. All the CEP probes and the *EGFR* probe are commercially available (Abbott Molecular). Probes for the genes *CDKN2*, *FHIT*, and *KRAS* were developed using BAC clones from the RP11 library. Panels **A** and **B** show loss of the gene sequences, respectively *CDKN2* and *FHIT*, compared with the controls used. Arrows indicate one of the nuclei with loss. Panels **C** and **D** show gene amplification, for *EGFR* and *KRAS*, respectively. It is noticeable that the clusters of *EGFR* signals are much more tightly packed than the clusters of *KRAS* signals. Arrows indicate one nucleus displaying gene amplification in each panel.

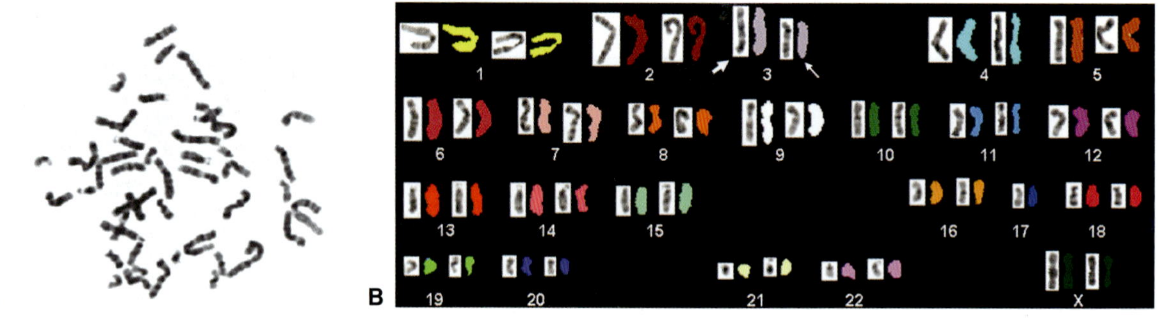

FIGURE 6.4 SKY of a bronchial epithelium cell from a heavy smoking individual showing deletion of the short arm of chromosome 3, with breakpoint at 3p21.1. **A:** Inverted DAPI image. **B:** Karyotype, including both the inverted DAPI and the classified images.

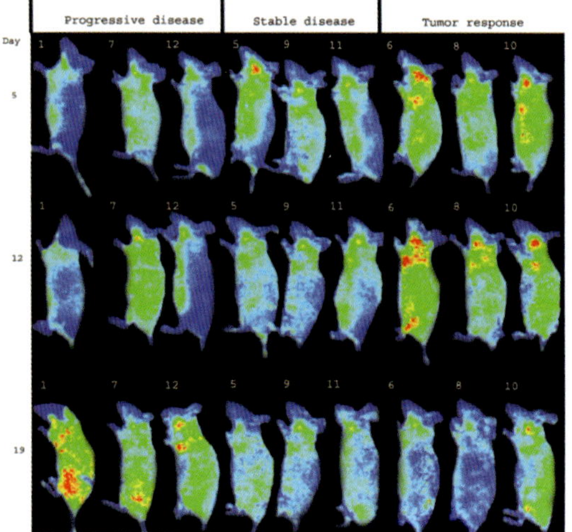

FIGURE 13.2 Noninvasive imaging reveals individual variation in mice treated with conditionally replicating oncolytic adenoviruses (CRAds). Examples of treatment results in mice treated with Ad5-Δ24RGD. The labels at left indicate the day of imaging, and each mouse is identified with a number. Mice *1*, *7*, and *12* had progressive disease; mice *5*, *9*, and *11* had stable disease; and mice *6*, *8*, and *10* achieved tumor response. (From Sarkioja M, Kanerva A, Salo J, et al. Noninvasive imaging for evaluation of the systemic delivery of capsid-modified adenoviruses in an orthotopic model of advanced lung cancer. *Cancer* 2006;107:1578–1588.)

FIGURE 13.3 Increased survival and reduced tumor development in KrasLA2 mice crossed with integrin α1-null mice. **A:** KrasLA2 mice crossed with the integrin α1-null mice (KrasLA2/α1KO) showed significantly increased survival compared to KrasLA2 mice crossed with integrin α1 wild-type mice (KrasLA2/α1WT). **B:** Top: Photograph of the lungs of KrasLA2/α1WT and KrasLA2/α1KO male mice sacrificed 120 days after birth. *Scale bar*, 5 mm. Bottom: Hematoxylin and eosin staining of lungs of KrasLA2/α1WT and KrasLA2/α1KO mice. Magnification, ×200. **C,D:** KrasLA2/α1WT and KrasLA2/α1KO mice were sacrificed 120 days after birth and tumor number (**C**) and size (**D**) were evaluated. The number of tumors visible on the lung surface was evaluated and expressed as average number of tumors per lung (**C**). Tumor diameter was measured with a caliper in 170 tumors from KrasLA2/α1WT and 102 tumors from KrasLA2/α1KO mice, and tumors were divided into three groups as indicated (**D**). (Data from Macias-Perez I, Borza C, Chen X, et al. Loss of integrin alpha1beta1 ameliorates Kras-induced lung cancer. *Cancer Res* 2008;68(15):6127–6135.)

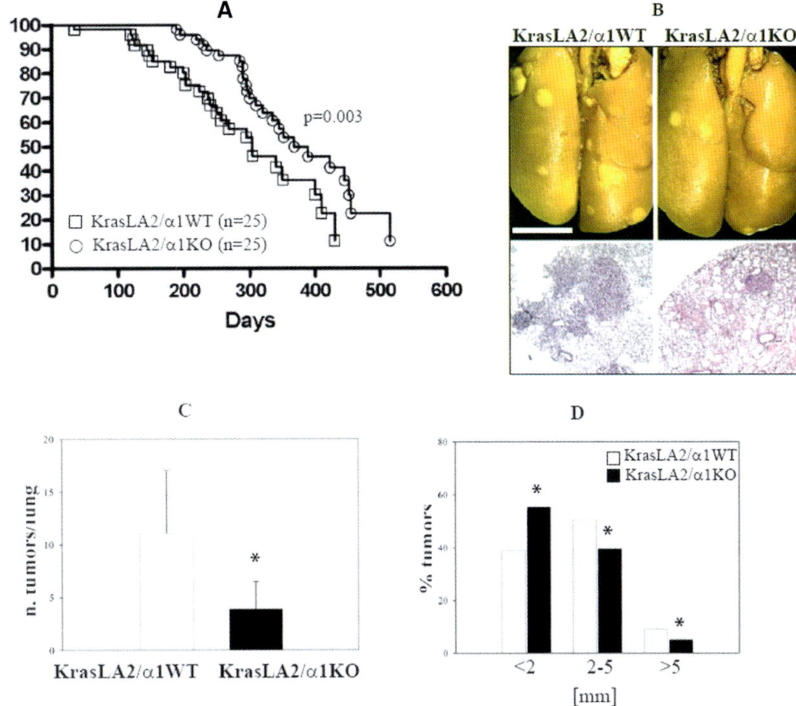

FIGURE 18.1 Squamous cell carcinoma. **A:** A syncytial cluster and rare single cells with high nuclear:cytoplasmic ratios and irregular nuclear borders (Diff-Quik, 40×). **B:** Orangeophilic cells present as clusters and singly with hyperchromatic nuclei and relatively low nuclear:cytoplasmic ratios; anucleate squames are also present (Papanicolaou stain, 20×). **C:** Cell block with intercellular bridges and keratinizing cells (cell block, hematoxylin and eosin [H&E], 40×). **D:** Polygonal-, spindle-, and bizarre-shaped squamous cells (Papanicolaou stain, 40×).

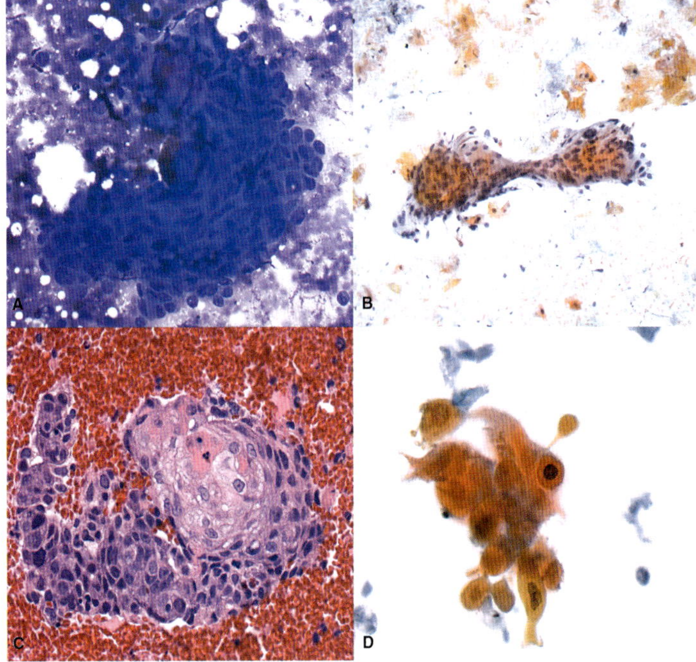

FIGURE 18.2 Squamous cell carcinoma. **A:** Atypical tadpole-shaped cell with hyperchromatic nucleus (Papanicolaou stain, ThinPrep, 40×) **B:** Marked acute inflammation and necrotic debris associated with squamous cells. *Inset:* malignant cells are also present (Papanicolaou stain, ThinPrep, 40× [*inset* 60×]).

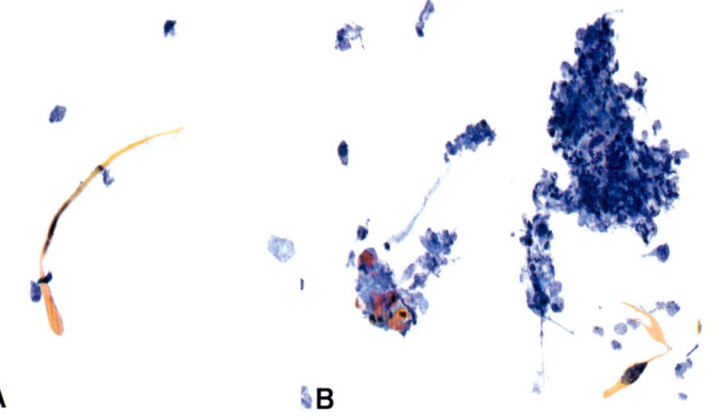

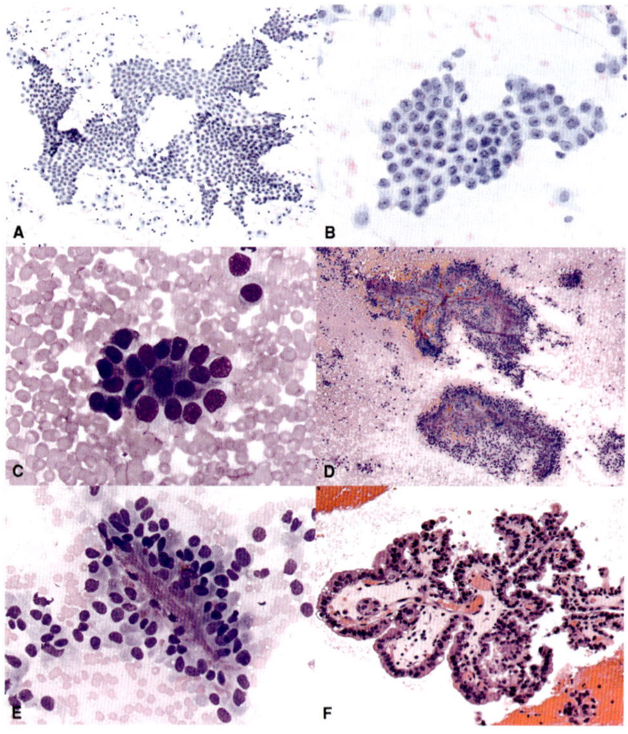

FIGURE 18.3 Adenocarcinoma. **A:** Monolayer sheets of relatively monotonous epithelial cells with pale chromatin and no significant nuclear overlap suggestive of BAC features (Papanicolaou stain, 20×). **B:** Two-dimensional sheet with bland nuclei containing pinpoint nucleoli and nuclear grooves often associated with BAC differentiation (Papanicolaou stain, 60×). **C:** Acinar formation (Diff-Quik, 20×). **D:** Fibrovascular cores surrounded by epithelial cells suggestive of papillary features (Diff-Quik, 10×). **E:** Epithelial cells enveloping delicate core in carcinoma with papillary architecture (Diff-Quik, 60×). **F:** Columnar cells line a fibrovascular core consistent with papillary features (cell block, H&E section, 20×).

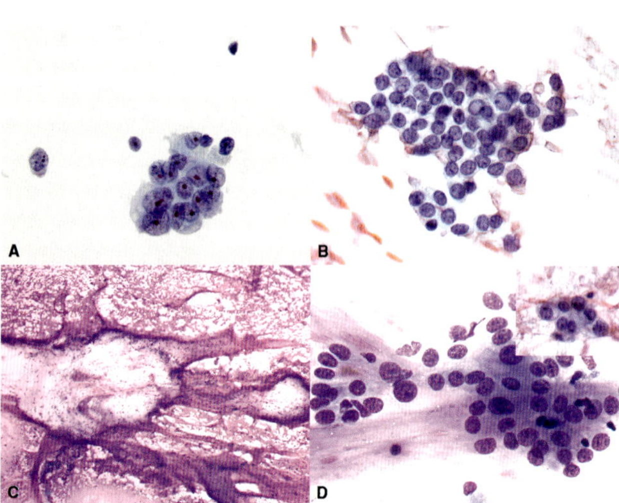

FIGURE 18.4 Adenocarcinoma. **A:** Three-dimensional cluster with nuclear pleomorphism, conspicuous nucleoli, and vacuolated cytoplasm (Papanicolaou stain, ThinPrep 60×). **B:** Cluster of epithelial cells with fine chromatin, inconspicuous nucleoli, intranuclear grooves, and inclusion (Papanicolaou stain, 60×). **C:** Adenocarcinoma with mucin: abundant mucin with scattered clusters of epithelial cells (Diff-Quik, 4×). **D:** Adenocarcinoma with mucin: malignant epithelial cells with conspicuous nucleoli and relatively abundant cytoplasm associated with mucin. *Inset:* Cells have vacuolated cytoplasm and nuclear membrane irregularities (Diff-Quik, 40×; *inset:* Papanicolaou stain 60×).

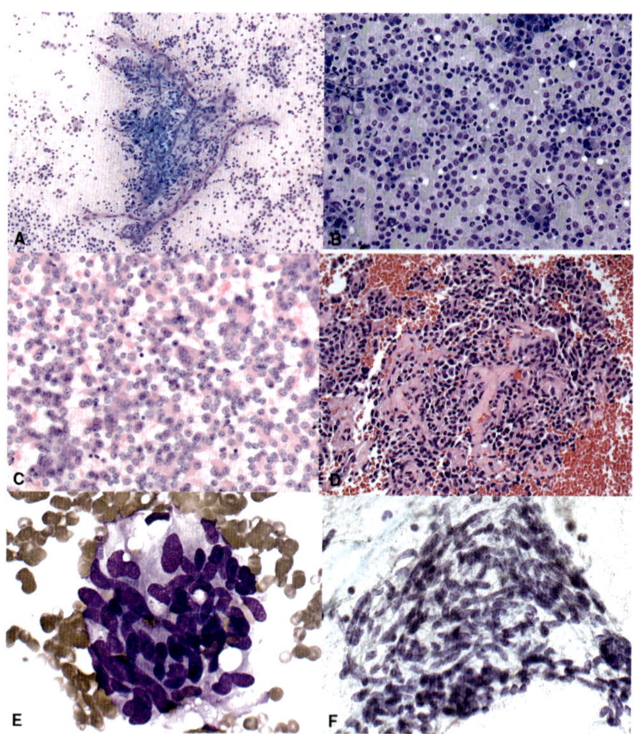

FIGURE 18.5 Typical carcinoid. **A:** Arborizing capillary network associated with monomorphic, loosely cohesive epithelial cells (touch prep, Diff-Quik, 20×). **B:** Loosely cohesive monotonous cells with eccentric nuclei and *plasmacytoid* features (touch prep, Diff-Quik, 40×). **C:** Bland cells with speckled chromatin (touch prep, H&E, 60×). **D:** Carcinoid with hyalinized stroma (cell block, H&E, 40×). **E,F:** Spindle cell carcinoid (Diff-Quik and Papanicolaou stains, 100×).

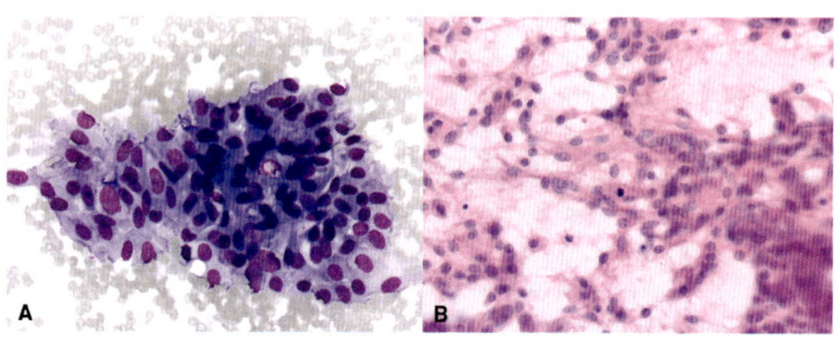

FIGURE 18.6 Atypical carcinoid. **A:** Epithelial cells with mild pleomorphism (Diff-Quik, 60×). **B:** Loose cell clusters with speckled chromatin and rare mitotic figure (touch prep, H&E, 60×).

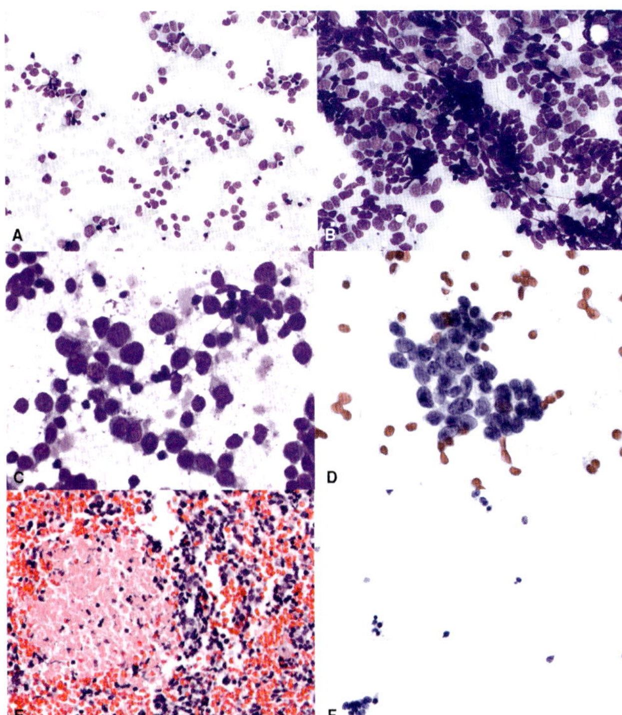

FIGURE 18.7 Small cell carcinoma. **A:** Clusters and single cells with scant cytoplasm and focal nuclear molding (Diff-Quik, 40×). **B:** Small cell carcinoma with rosettes, nuclear molding, and crush/smearing artifact (Diff-Quik, 40×). **C:** Small cell carcinoma with a dirty background and scattered apoptotic cells (Diff-Quik, 60×). **D:** Cells with high nuclear:cytoplasmic ratios, fine chromatin, and inconspicuous nucleoli (Papanicolaou stain, 60×) **E:** Eosinophilic necrotic areas and malignant small cells (cell block, H&E, 40×) **F:** Rare cell clusters and scattered single cells in small cell carcinoma mimicking lymphoma (ThinPrep, Papanicolaou stain, 60×).

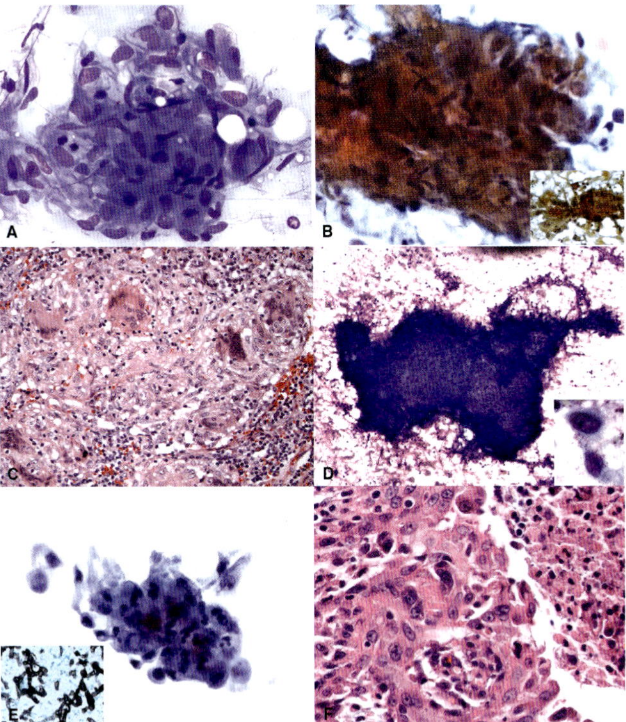

FIGURE 18.8 **A:** Granuloma: enlarged spindle-shaped and epithelioid histiocytes (Diff-Quik, 40×). **B,C:** Granuloma with atypia. **B:** Atypical spindle-shaped and epithelioid histiocytes in clusters. *Inset:* areas with streaming pattern associated with reactive changes (Papanicolaou stain, bronchial brush, 40×; *inset* 40×). **C:** Histological section from same case demonstrating histiocytes and giant cells without evidence of malignancy (H&E, 40×). **D–F:** Aspergillus with atypical squamous cells. **D:** Sheet of atypical squamous cells in an inflammatory/dirty background. *Inset:* high magnification of rare single cells with dense cytoplasm and high nuclear: cytoplasmic ratio (Diff-Quik, 10×; *inset* 40×). **E:** Atypical cells with dense cytoplasm and high nuclear:cytoplasmic ratios associated with rare fungal form and neutrophils. *Inset:* silver stain demonstrating fungal organisms. (ThinPrep, Papanicolaou stain, 60×; *inset:* Gomori methanamine stain, 40×) **F:** Histological section demonstrating atypical squamous cells and intraluminal necrotic debris (H&E, 40×)

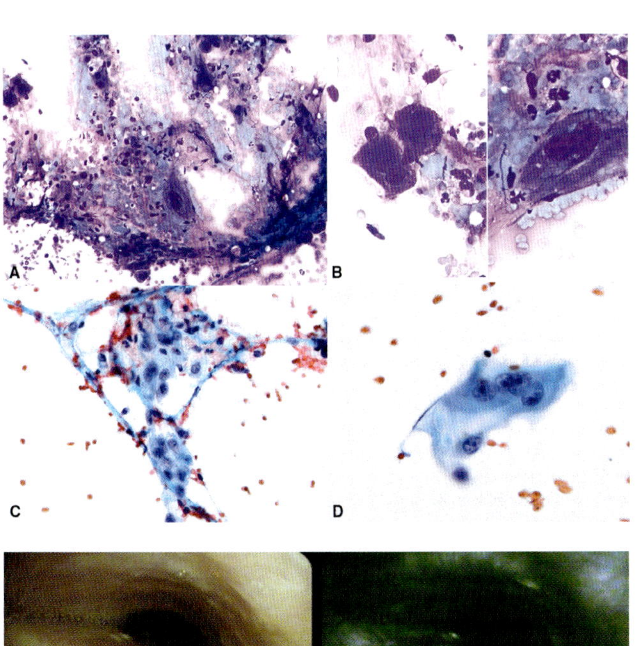

FIGURE 18.9 Therapy-related changes. **A:** Markedly atypical cells (postchemotherapy and stem cell transplant) (Diff-Quik- 20×). **B:** Cytomegaly with prominent nucleoli and relatively preserved nuclear:cytoplasmic ratios in an inflammatory background (postchemotherapy and stem cell transplant) (Diff-Quik, 60×). **C:** Atypical cells in cohesive cluster with vague *streaming pattern* without significant population of single atypical cells (postchemotherapy and stem cell transplant) (Papanicolaou stain, 60×). **D:** Multinucleated cell with prominent nucleoli and cytoplasmic vacuolization (postchemotherapy and stem cell transplant) (Papanicolaou stain, 60×).

FIGURE 19.1 White-light (*left*) and autofluorescence bronchoscopy (*right*) images of a carcinoma in situ (CIS) lesion in the left main bronchus. No abnormality was seen under white-light examination. Under fluorescence imaging, the CIS lesion as an area of decreased fluorescence.

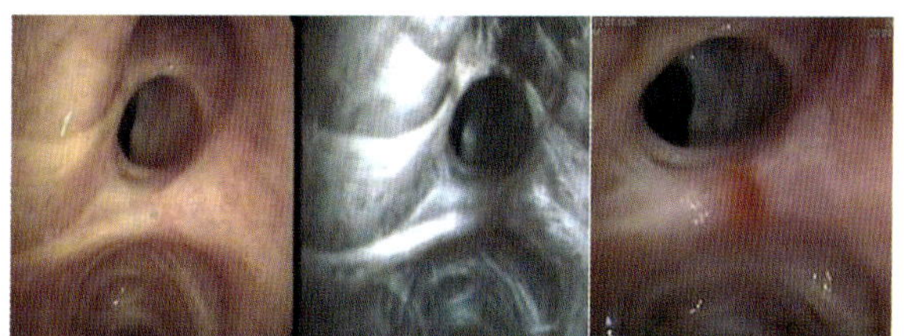

FIGURE 19.2 Real-time dual simultaneous imaging of digital video autofluroescence bronchoscope images (SAFE 3000, Pentax, Japan). Previous biopsy site over right upper lobe carina with small scarring on conventional image (*left*), abnormal but nonsuspicious digital autofluorescence (*center*), and hybrid image to enhance contrast of the localization (*right*) with histology normal biopsy.

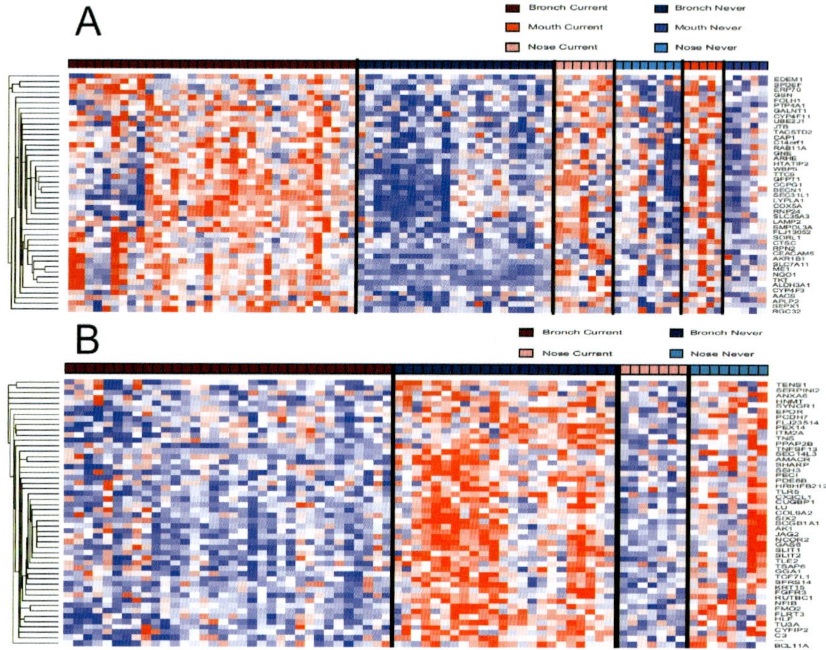

FIGURE 20.1 Hierarchical clustering of genes commonly perturbed by smoking across intrathoracic and extrathoracic airway epithelium. **A:** Supervised hierarchical clustering of the expression of 45 genes induced by smoking in the bronchial airway that are present in both the nasal and buccal "leading edge subsets" in samples from smokers and nonsmokers. These represent genes upregulated by smoking in bronchial, nasal, and buccal epithelium. **B:** Supervised hierarchical clustering of the expression of 50 genes repressed by smoking in the bronchial airway that are present in the nasal leading edge subset in samples from smokers and nonsmokers. High expression (*red*), average expression (*white*), low expression (*blue*). (From Sridhar S, Schembri F, Zeskind J, et al. Smoking-induced gene expression changes in the bronchial airway are reflected in nasal and buccal epithelium. *BMC Genomics* 2008;9:259.)

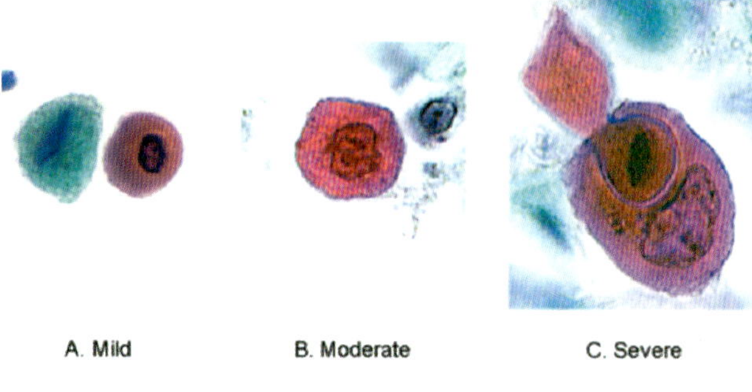

FIGURE 22.1 Dysplastic squamous cells in sputum. **A:** Mild dysplasia on the right consists of small rounded red cell with condensed nucleus and low N/C ratio. **B:** Moderately dysplastic orangophilic cell with large irregular nucleus and visible nucleolus. **C:** Carcinoma with large nucleus, high N/C ratio, and visible nucleolus. Large cell appears to be ingesting smaller one.

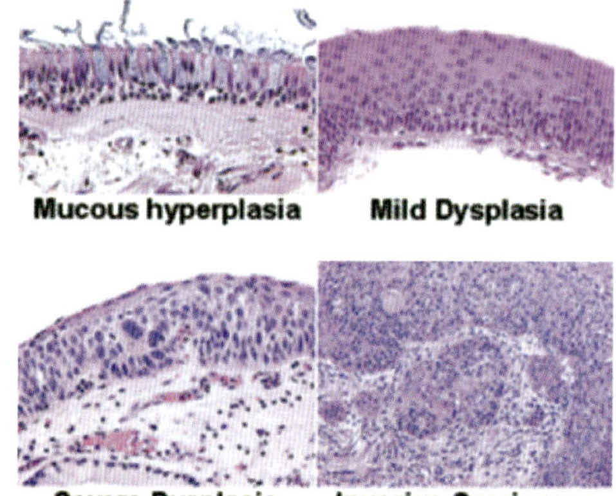

FIGURE 22.2 Chronological sequences of cellular and molecular changes that may occur during central airway carcinogenesis. Although this sequence is rarely observed in a single individual, these changes are well described in the high-risk population and the sequence provides a useful way to conceptualize multistep carcinogenesis in the lung. At the cellular level, the earliest smoking-related changes may consist of mucous gland hyperplasia (shown), basal cell hyperplasia, or squamous metaplasia, which are not recognizably premalignant changes. The earliest cellular abnormalities that suggest premalignancy are squamous dysplastic changes that may range from mild-to-severe carcinoma in situ. The appearance of stromal invasion marks progression to fully established malignancy.

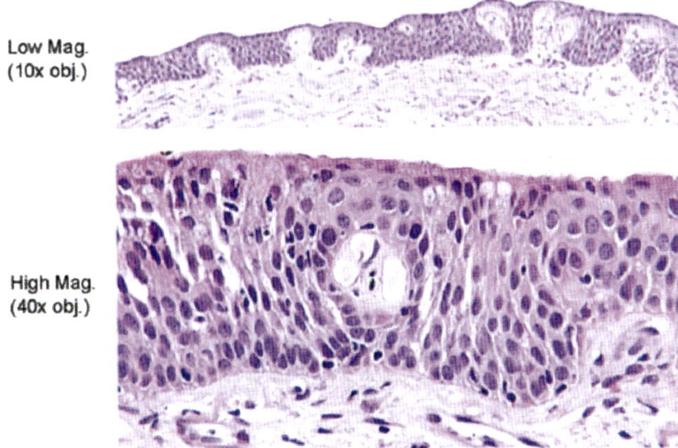

FIGURE 22.3 Premalignant changes in the bronchial epithelium. Mucociliary cells are converted to squamous cells and may elicit and angiogenic stromal response shown at low maginfication (**top**) and high magnification (**bottom**). Nuclear irregularity with clearly visible nucleoli is present in the cells surrounding the vascular loop in the lower frame.

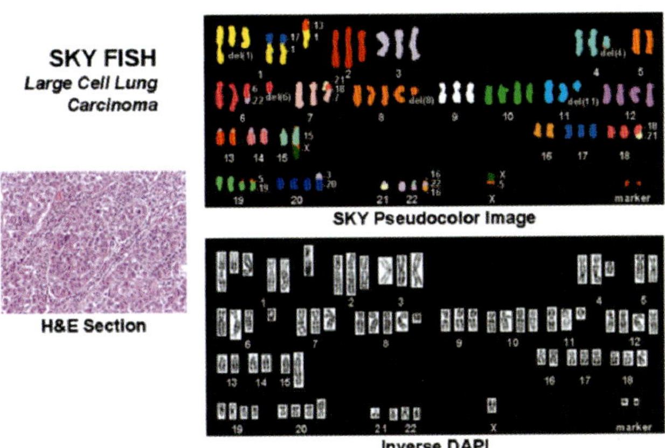

FIGURE 22.5 Chromosomal heterogeneity and instability. The high degree of chromosomal instability in lung carcinoma is reflected in numerous structural abnormalities that are visible through chromosomal imaging methods. Shown here is a spectral karyotype of a large cell undifferentiated carcinoma (H&E section). The SKY pseudocolor image of the karyotype provides a color code for each chromosome. In this figure, extra chromosomes 1, 2, 3, 4, 6, 7, 8, 9, 10, 11, 12, 18, 19, 20, and 22 are visible. A reciprocal translocation, several nonreciprocal translocations, deletions, and marker chromosomes are also present. *FISH*, fluorescence in situ hybridization; *H&E*, hematoxylin and eosin; *SKY*, spectral karyotyping.

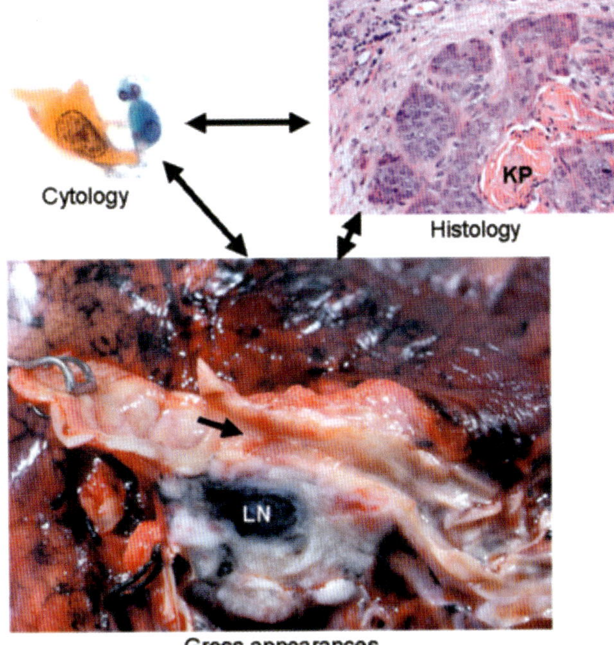

FIGURE 22.6 Various morphological appearances of squamous carcinoma. Cytological examination reveals bright orange, irregularly cells with conspicuous nucleolus. Histology of squamous cancers visible in both biopsy and resection specimens are characterized by irregular nests of cells, often with central KP. Early stage resected tumors are frequently ulcerated as indicated by the area of mucosal roughening and erythema (*arrow*). The ulcer overlies white invasive tumor tissue that surrounds a black anthrocotic LN. *KP*, keratin pearl; *LN*, lymph node.

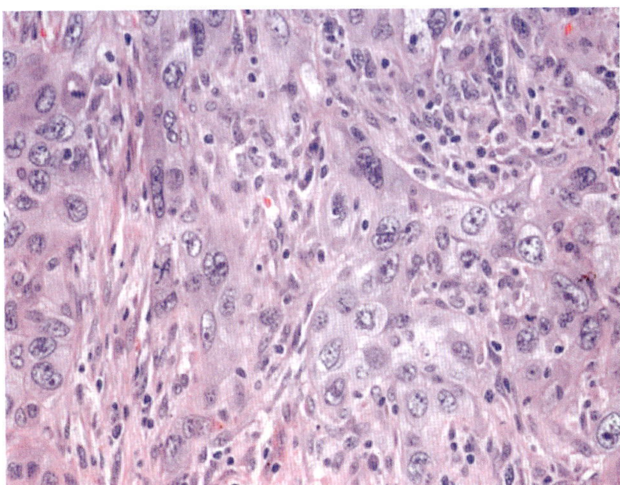

FIGURE 22.7 Large cell undifferentiated lung carcinoma exhibits no differentiating features and is composed of large cells with coarsely clumped nuclei and prominent nucleoli. Mitoses are abundant.

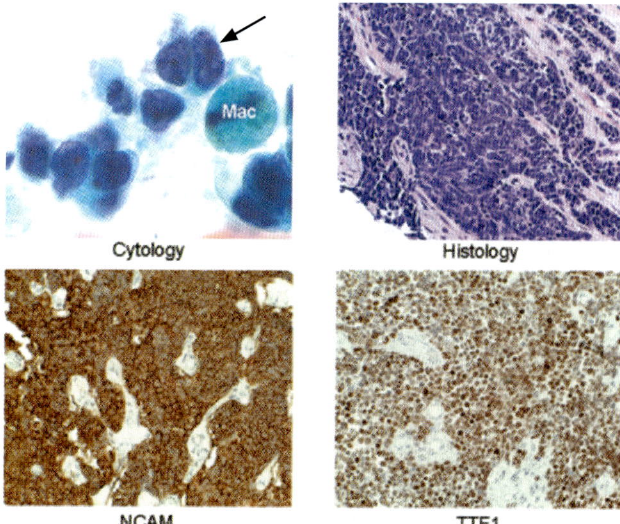

FIGURE 22.8 SCLC as found on cytology, histology, and IHC. On the upper left are clusters of small cells with scant cytoplasm, nuclear molding (*arrow*), and finely granular nuclei with inconspicuous nucleoli. Macrophage (*Mac*) provides size comparison. The frame on the upper right shows the histology of SCLC with closely packed cells with scanting cytoplasm with streaming nuclei. NCAM and TTF-1 stains are strongly positive along plasma membranes and in the nuclei. *Mac*, macrophage; *NCAM*, neural cell adhesion molecule; *TTF-1*, thyroid transcription factor-1.

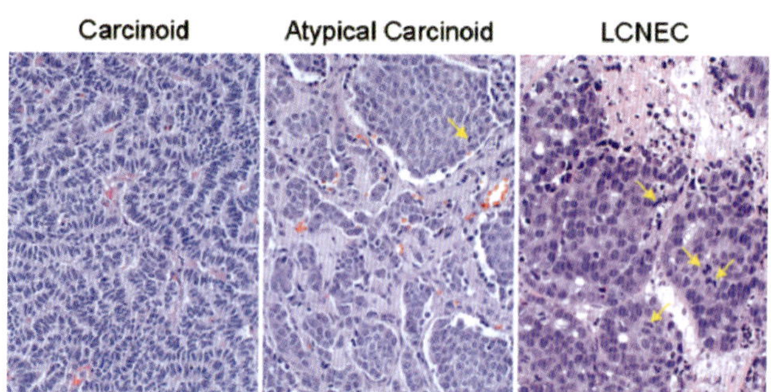

FIGURE 22.9 Histological comparison of various forms of neuroendocrine tumor of the lung. On the left is a classical carcinoid tumor with a ribbonlike pattern of growth. The central image shows more sheetlike tumor growth with occasional mitotic figures (see text). This tumor type also is defined by the presence of focal areas of necrosis. The figure on the right shows the high level of mitotic activity (*arrows*) and areas of necrosis that characterize LCNEC. *LCNEC*, large cell neuroendocrine carcinoma.

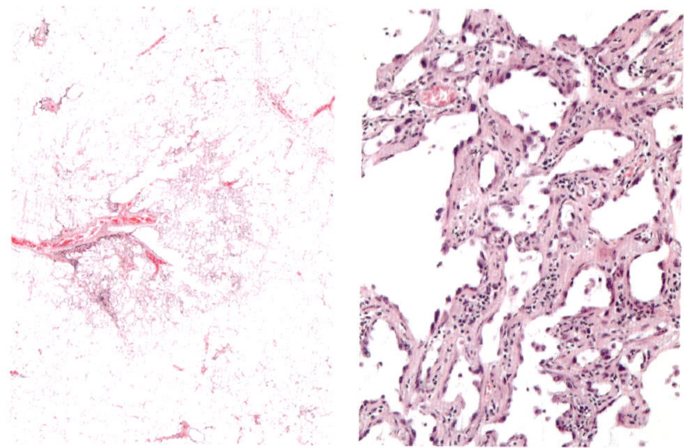

FIGURE 22.10 Atypical adenomatous hyperplasia. On the left is a low magnification view showing the small overall size of the lesion. At higher magnification (*right*), a single layer of cuboidal cells covers the alveolar septae with minimal associated inflammation.

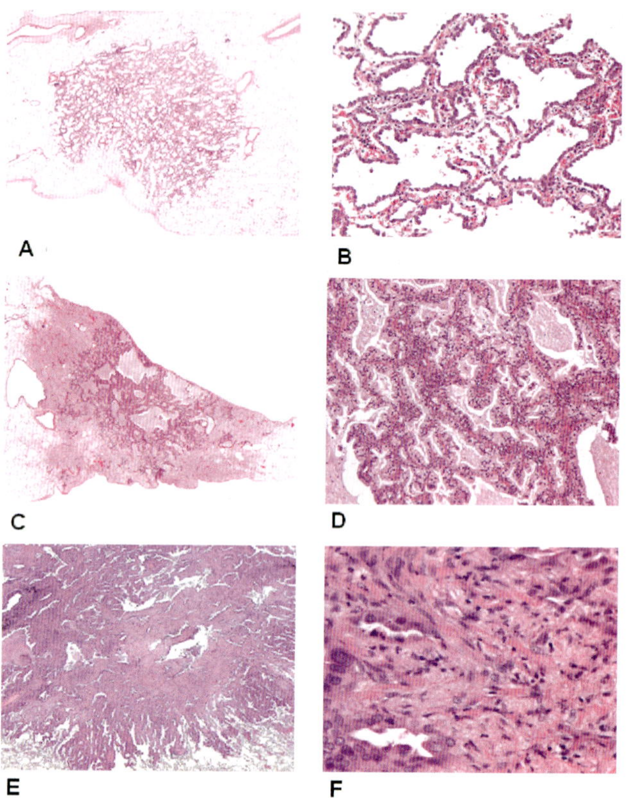

FIGURE 22.11 Histology of various forms of BAC, BAC mixed with invasive carcinoma, and pure invasive carcinoma. **A:** Small nonmucinous BAC at low magnification without evidence of stromal invasion. **B:** High magnification of **A** shows lepidic spread of well-differentiated malignant pneumocytes along alveolar septae. **C:** Pink acellular mucus fills the alveoli of this mucinous BAC photographed at low magnification. **D:** At higher magnification of **C**, mucous vacuoles are present in apex of columnar cells lining alveoli. **E:** In this invasive adenocarcinoma, there is fibrosis at the center of a tumor that exhibits extension of tumor cells. **F:** High magnification of this tumor (**E**) reveals a sclerotic response to tumor cells with pink fibers aligned parallel to the elongated fibroblastic nuclei.

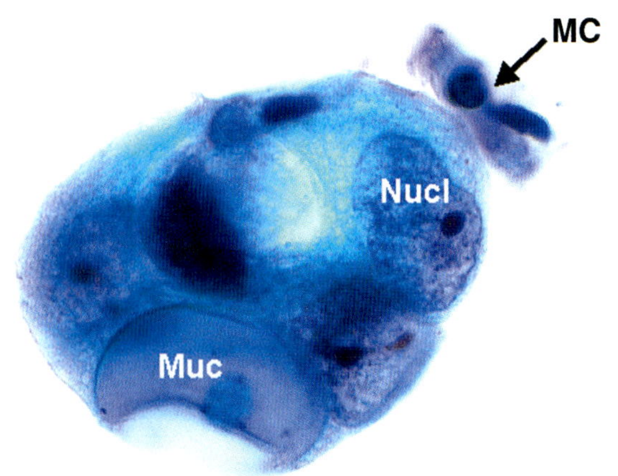

FIGURE 22.12 Cytology of adenocarcinoma showing Papanicolaou-stained cluster of adenocarcinoma cells. These are large cells with high N/C ratio and prominent nucleoli (dark circular structure in nucleus [Nucl]). Under the microscope, the cell cluster has a three-dimensional structure and a mucus vacuole (Muc) is present at one margin of the cluster. *MC* indicates smaller mucociliary cell.

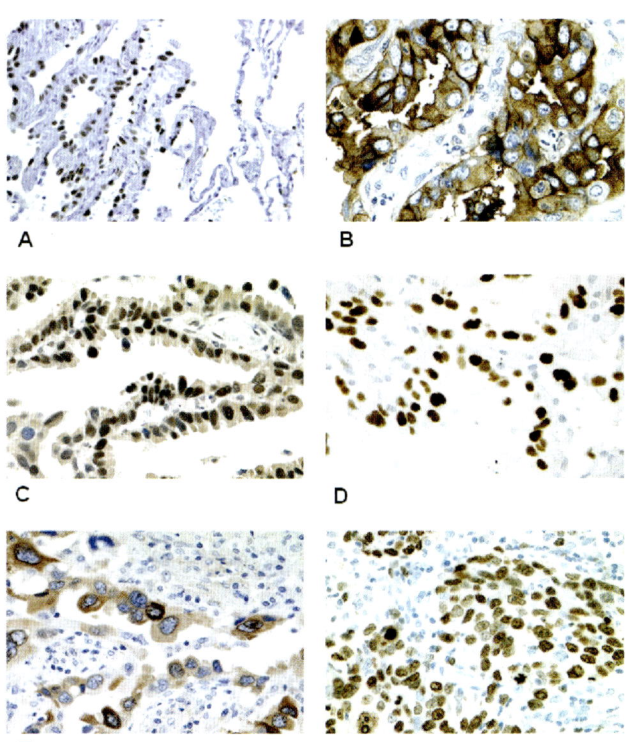

FIGURE 22.13 Immunohistochemical staining patterns for several biomarkers reported to be of diagnostic and prognostic significance in adenocarcinoma (see text). **A:** TTF-1, nuclear staining; **B:** CEA, cytoplasmic staining; **C:** p27, nuclear staining; **D:** p53; strong nuclear staining (mutant pattern); **E:** COX-2, cytoplasmic staining; **F:** MIB-1 (Ki67); nuclear staining.

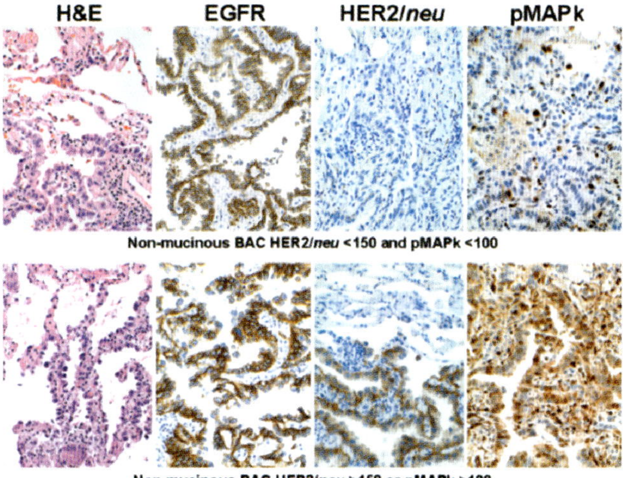

FIGURE 22.14 Immunohistochemical stains of two morphologically similar BAC. Both tumors strongly express EGFR but on the upper tumor sufficient levels of HER-2/*neu* to be visible in immunostains. Activation of intracellular signaling through the mitogen-activated protein (MAP) kinase pathway as reflected in phosphorylated MAPK (pMAPk) immunostaining levels is strongest in the lower tumor. *BAC*, bronchioloalveolar carcinoma; *EGFR*, epidermal growth factor receptor; *H&E*, hematoxylin and eosin; *pMAPk*, phosphorylated MAPK.

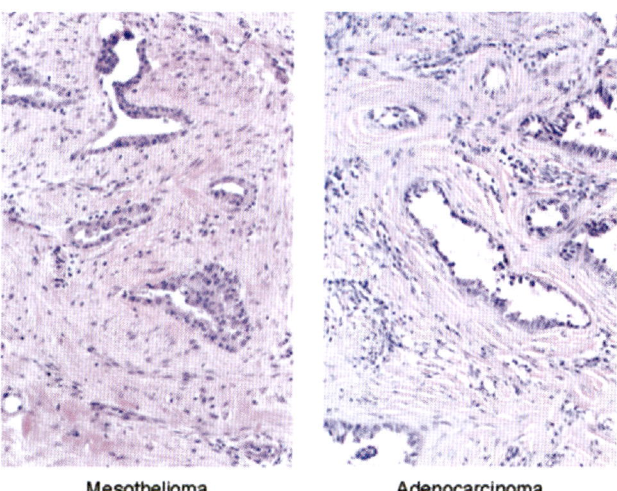

FIGURE 22.15 Histological sections showing similarity between epithelial type mesothelioma and adenocarcinoma.

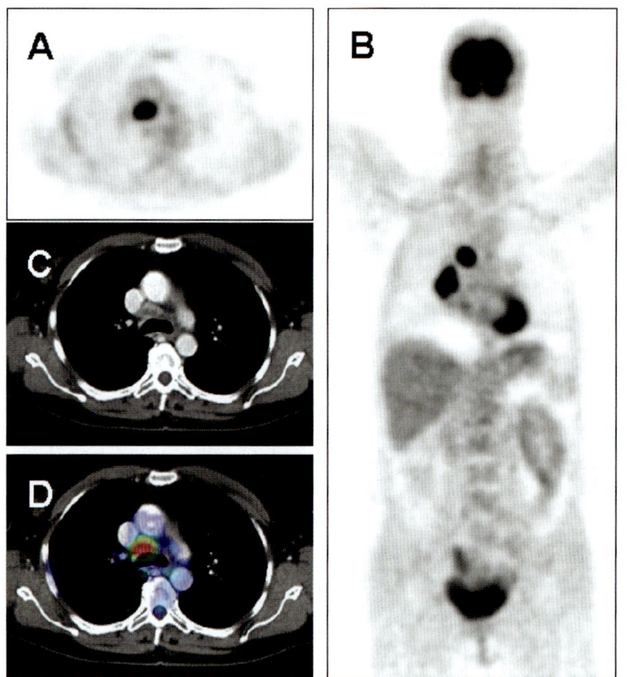

FIGURE 27.4 Transaxial **(A)** and coronal **(B)** PET images with a right lung tumor and accompanying adenopathy, either in the right hilar or mediastinal station. On CT, there is a suspect LN **(C)**, on integrated PET/CT, right paratracheal adenopathy is confirmed **(D)**.

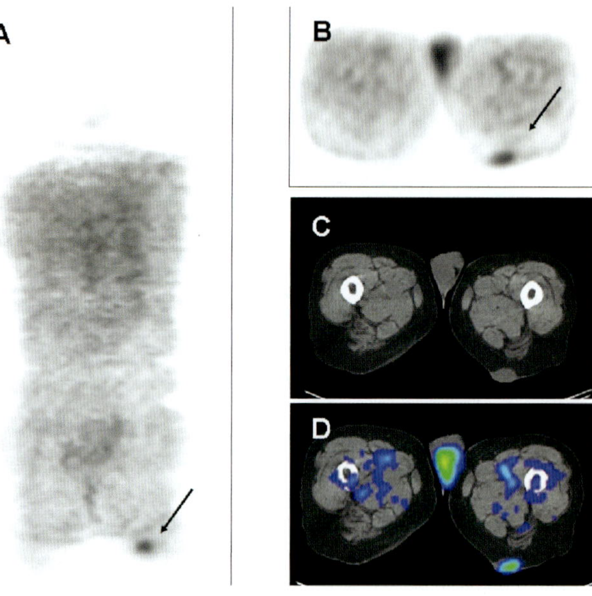

FIGURE 27.6 Patient with limited disease SCLC on conventional staging, with unexpected lesion in the left thigh on PET **(A,B)**, and on accompanying CT and PET/CT images **(C,D)**. Biopsy confirmed subcutaneous SCLC metastasis.

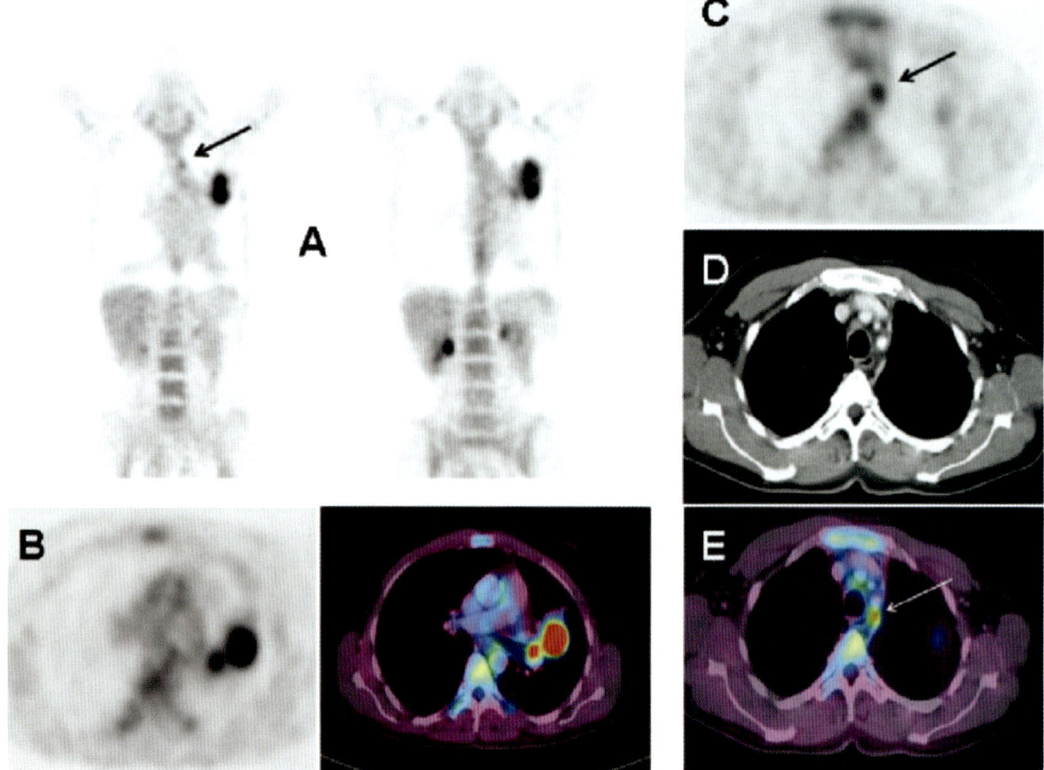

FIGURE 27.5 PET/CT in a patient with squamous cell carcinoma of the left upper lobe. FDG uptake is present in the primary tumor and an adjacent hilar LN **(A,B)**. PET also shows a focal hot spot suspected for N2 disease in level 2L (**A,C** *arrow*). PET/CT fusion images project the hot spot in brown fat tissue **(D,E)**. At thoracotomy with LN, dissection confirmed the absence of mediastinal involvement (pT2N1).

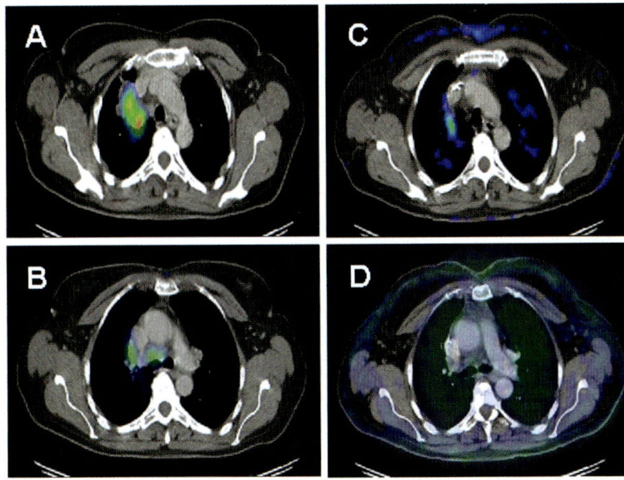

FIGURE 27.7 Right upper lobe large cell carcinoma **(A)** with right hilar and paratracheal adenopathy **(B)**, both clearly FDG avid on PET/CT fusion images. After induction chemotherapy, a major decrease in the metabolic activity of the primary tumor **(C)** and absence of FDG uptake in the mediastinum **(D)** is noted. Patient underwent complete resection, pT1N0.

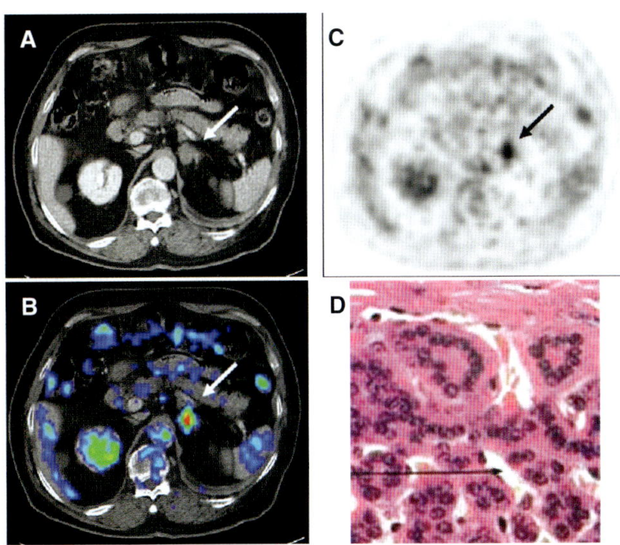

FIGURE 27.10 Patient with left upper lobe adenocarcinoma (not shown) and abnormal left adrenal gland on CT **(A)**, PET **(B)**, and fusion image **(C)**. Needle aspiration biopsy revealed normal cortical adrenal tissue **(D)**. No change in the adrenal gland during follow-up postlobectomy.

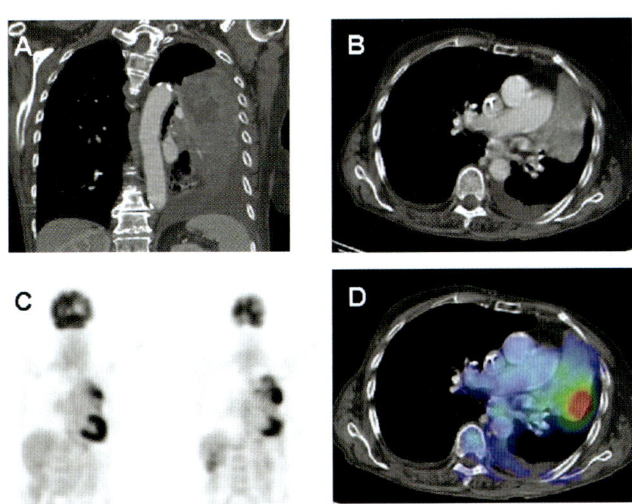

FIGURE 27.8 Patient with a squamous cell carcinoma in the left hilum (cT3N3) with atelectasis of the left upper lobe resulting in a shift of heart and mediastinum **(A,B)**. For a better discrimination of atelectasis and tumor, PET/CT was performed to optimize radiation treatment planning **(C,D)**.

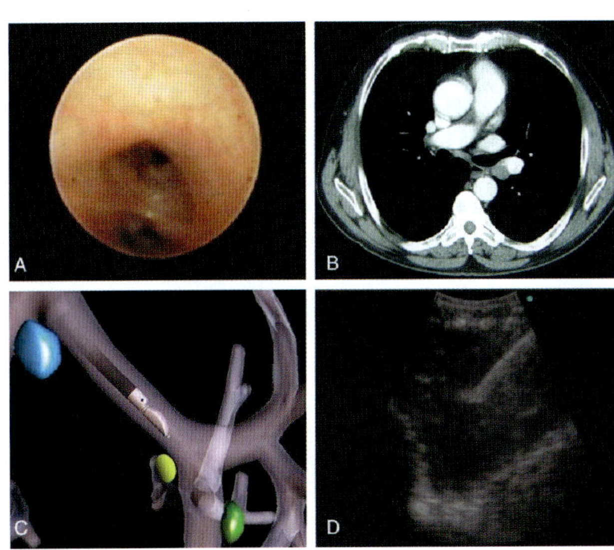

FIGURE 28.3 **A:** Intraluminal view of the carina left upper and lower lobe. **B:** CT image of node station 10 L. **C:** Position of the bronchoscope. **D:** EBUS image of the puncture procedure, the needle is visible. (Photo courtesy of Felix Herth.)

FIGURE 28.4 Optical coherence tomography (OCT) of an intraluminal squamous cell cancer in the tracheal wall. **A:** Bronchoscopic image showing nodular tumor (*T*) and normal tracheal wall (*W*). **B:** OCT showing tumor (*T*) infiltrating beyond the cartilage. **C:** Normal OCT. (From Tsuboi M, Hayashi A, Ikeda N, et al. Optical coherence tomography in the diagnosis of bronchial lesions. *Lung Cancer* 2005;49:387–394; courtesy of N. Ikeda, Mita Hospital, Japan.)

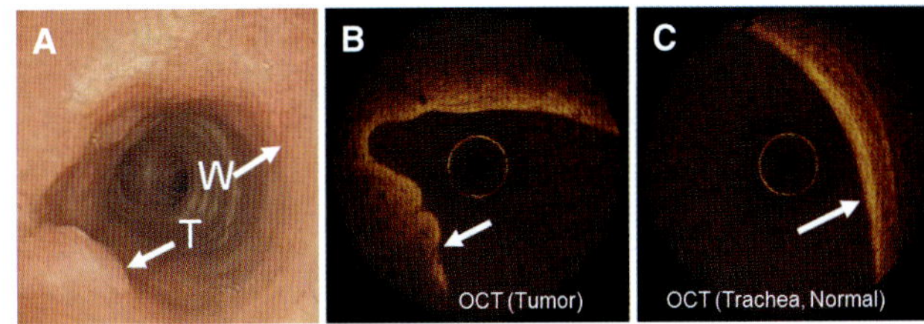

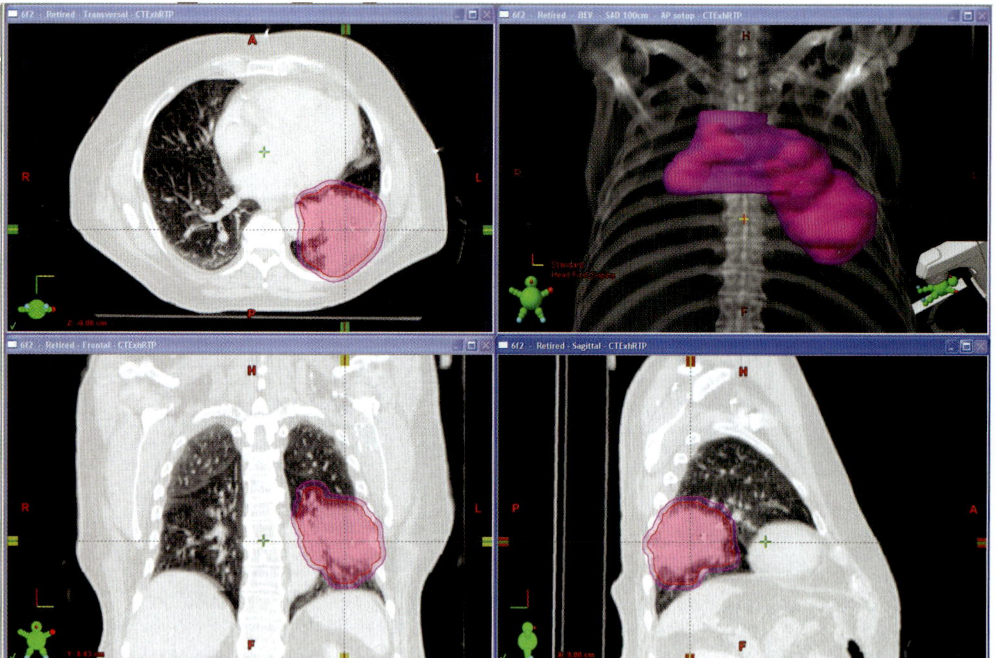

FIGURE 40.1 Views from a planning CT scan. Note the flat tabletop used for radiation therapy imaging, the absence of the patient's arms as they are above their head to avoid being radiated during treatment, and the foam mold surrounding the patient to assist with immobilization. The gross tumor volume (*red*) and planning target volume (*pink*) are shown.

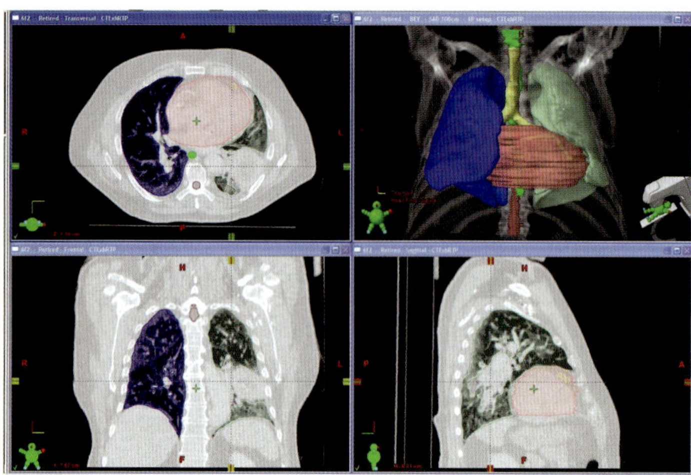

FIGURE 40.3 Dose-limiting normal tissues to avoid and/or limit radiation dose. Target volume delineation is performed on the entire 3D (or 4D) data set. Right lung: *blue*; left lung: *green*; heart: *pink*; esophagus: *green*; spinal cord: *brown*; main airways: *yellow*. The target volumes can be seen in Figure 40.1.

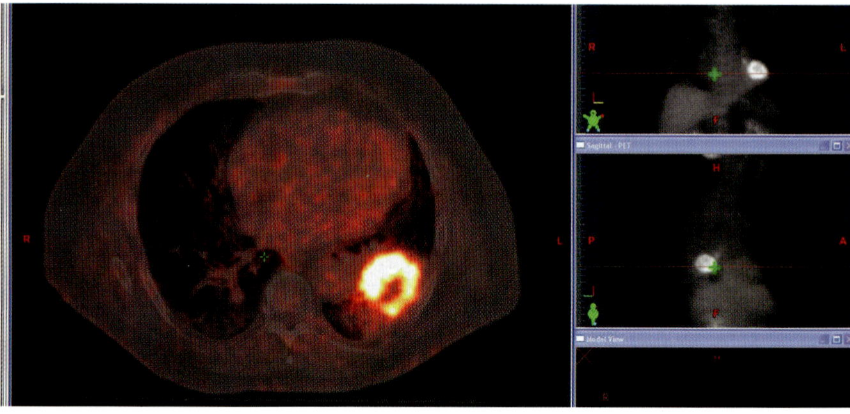

FIGURE 40.4 PET images overlaid on the CT scan from a treatment planning PET-CT simulation session. For radiation oncology, a critical step is the delineation of the tumor boundaries that are necessary for determining the shape of the radiation treatment beams.

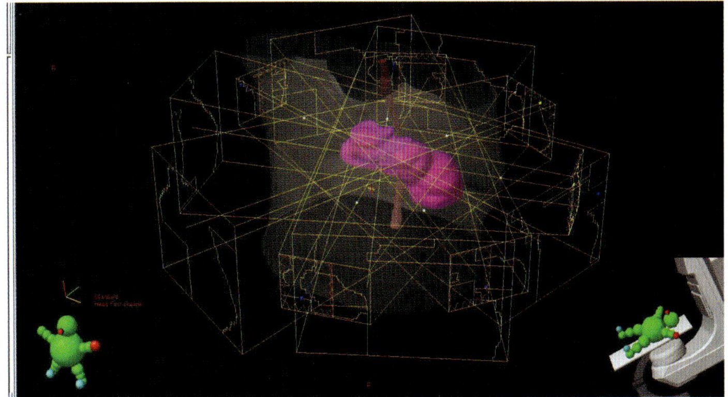

FIGURE 40.5 The beam arrangement for an intensity-modulated radiotherapy (IMRT) treatment of lung cancer.

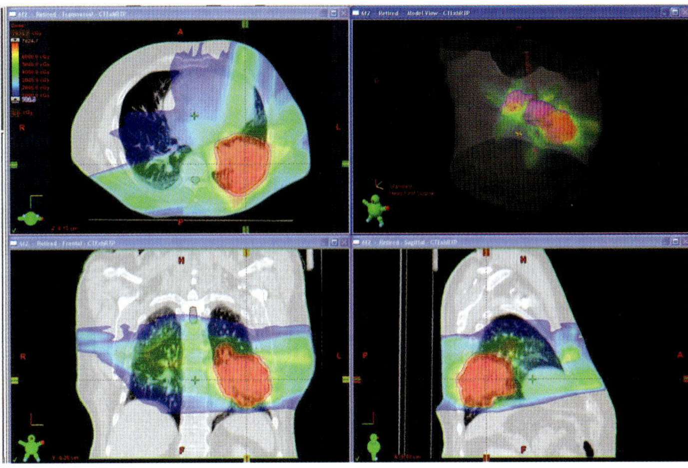

FIGURE 40.6 The dose distribution for an intensity-modulated radiotherapy (IMRT) treatment of lung cancer.

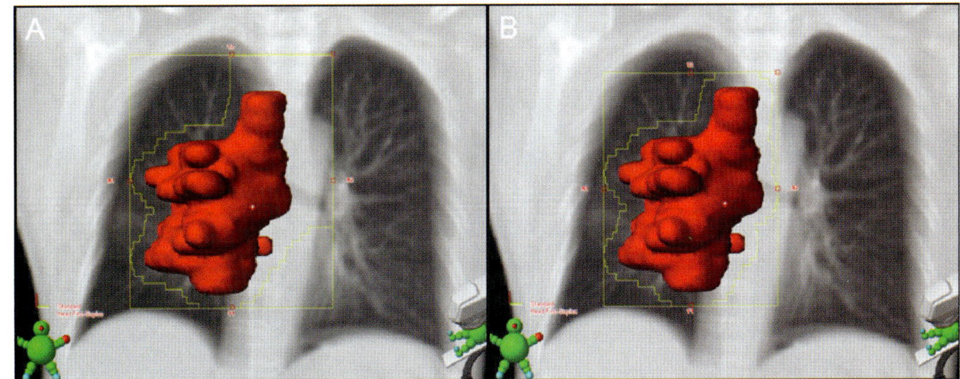

FIGURE 42.1 Treatment portals (*in yellow*) for an anterior field used in elective nodal irradiation **(A)** and involved-field radiotherapy **(B)** in the same patient. Uninvolved nodal regions, including the contralateral upper mediastinum, are routinely treated with the first approach, leading to higher doses to the contralateral lung and esophagus.

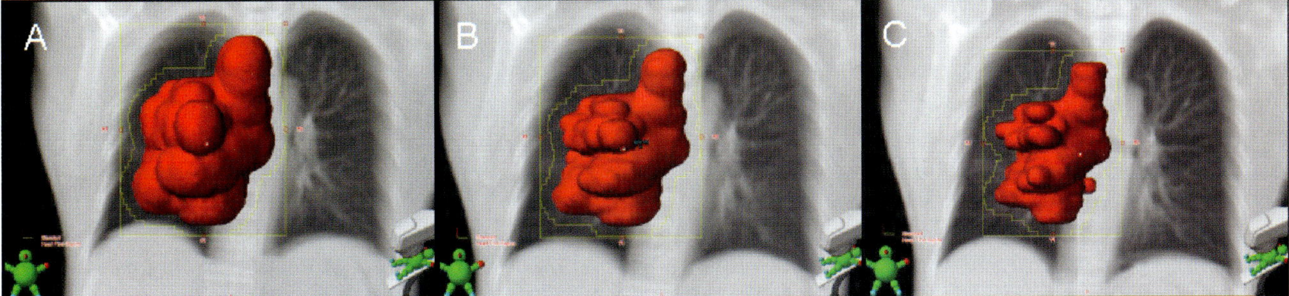

FIGURE 42.2 Planning target volumes (*red*) and corresponding treatment portals (*yellow*) for a patient with stage III NSCLC. **(A)** is derived from a single 3DCT scan with the addition of standard planning margins,[98] **(B)** is an internal target volume (ITV) encompassing all motion observed on 4DCT scan acquired during quiet respiration, and **(C)** is the ITV from motion in three phases at end inspiration for audio-coached gated radiotherapy. The amount of right lung tissue outside the portal is maximal with approach **C**.

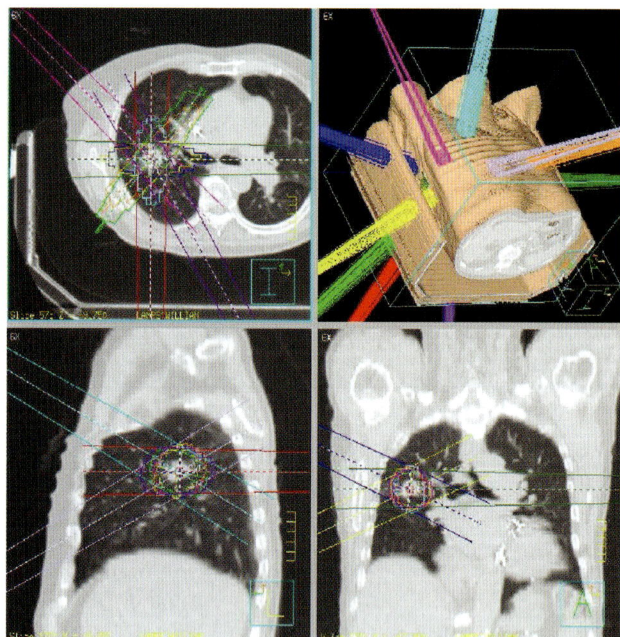

FIGURE 43.1 Typical beam arrangement for SBRT for primary early stage lung cancer. Ten nonopposing and noncoplanar beams coming from various incident directions converge on the demarcated tumor target.

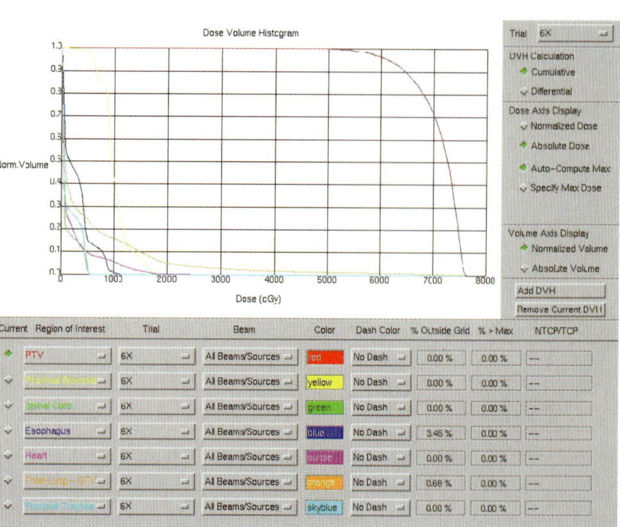

FIGURE 43.2 Dose–volume histogram for an optimized dosimetry plan using the beam arrangements from Figure 43.1. The *red line* is for the PTV, the *yellow* for the proximal bronchial tree, the *green* for the spinal cord, the *dark blue* for the esophagus, the *purple* for the heart, the *orange* for the total lung minus GTV, and the *light blue* for the proximal trachea.

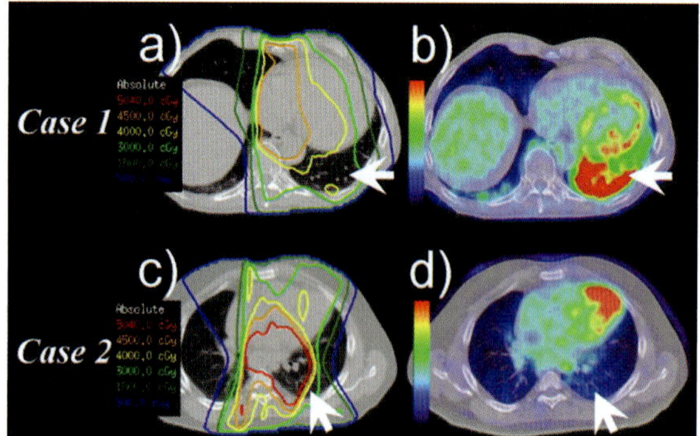

FIGURE 44.13 Radiation pneumonitis: local dose versus [18F]2-fluoro-2-deoxyglucose (FDG) uptake response in irradiated lung.[14] Radiation dose and FDG positron emission tomography (PET) response are illustrated for examples of high (case 1) and low (case 2) response. Case 1: **(A)** isodose distribution for patient with esophageal cancer shown overlaying single transaxial section from treatment planning computed tomography (CT scan; **(B)** corresponding restaging FDG–PET scan (high response), after image registration, shown overlaying transaxial treatment planning CT scan. The pulmonary region with high FDG uptake is indicated by horizontal arrows. Case 2: **(C)** isodose distribution shown overlaying transaxial section from treatment planning CT scan; **(D)** corresponding restaging FDG–PET scan shown overlaying transaxial treatment planning CT scan. The pulmonary region of high dose and its corresponding PET region are indicated by diagonal arrows. These two cases represent the range of FDG uptake response found in all 36 cases evaluated.[14] (From Guerrero T, Johnson V, Hart J, et al. Radiation pneumonitis: local dose versus [18F]-fluorodeoxyglucose uptake response in irradiated lung. *Int J Radiat Oncol Biol Phys* 2007 Jul 15;68[4]:1030–1035.)

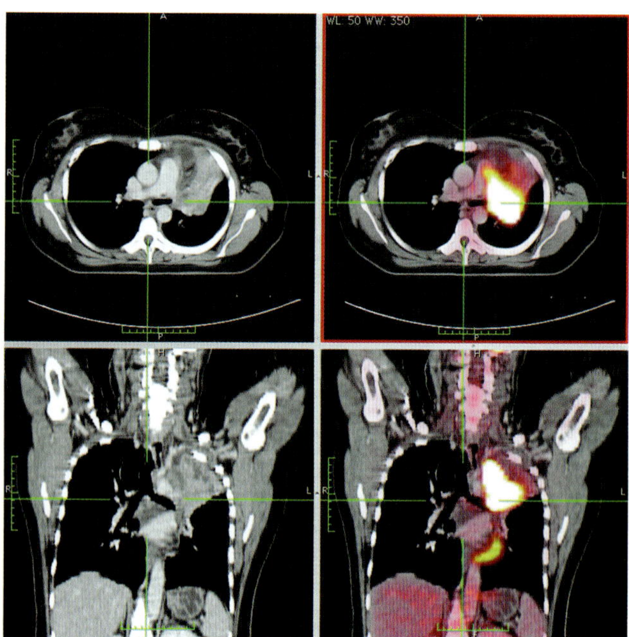

A

FIGURE 56.1 T4 disease with multimodality treatment including surgery. CT and PET/CT images of a patient with pathologically proven T4 disease at parasternal mediastinoscopy/thoracoscopy prior to induction treatment **(A)** and following an induction therapy **(B)** with induction chemotherapy (three cycles cisplatin and paclitaxel) followed by induction chemoradiotherapy (one cycle cisplatin and vinorelbine) with 45 Gy hyperfractionated accelerated radiotherapy (2 × 1.5 Gy bid). *(continued)*

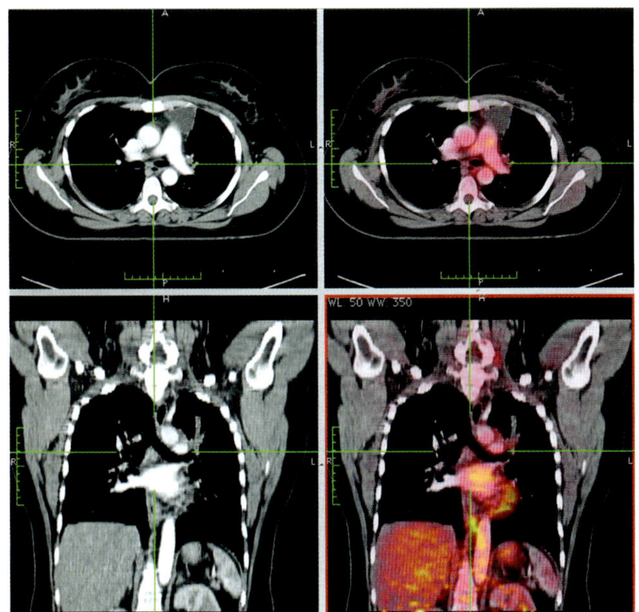

FIGURE 56.1 *(Continued)*

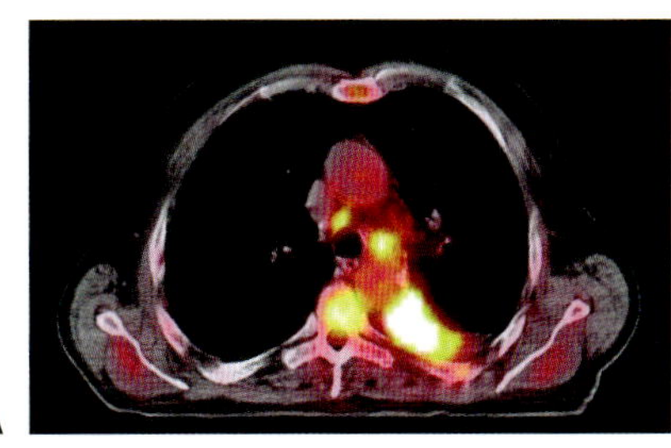

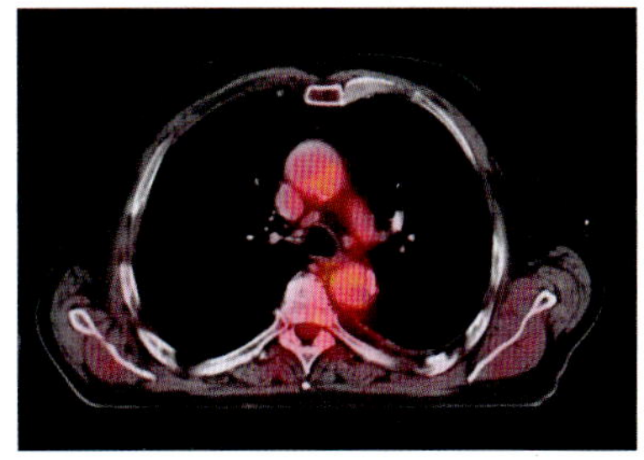

FIGURE 56.2 N3 disease with multimodality treatment including surgery. PET/CT images of a patient with mediastinoscopically proven N3 disease prior to induction treatment **(A)** and following an induction treatment **(B)** with chemotherapy (three cycles cisplatin and paclitaxel) followed by induction chemoradiotherapy (one cycle cisplatin and vinorelbine) with 45 Gy hyperfractionated accelerated radiotherapy (2 × 1.5 Gy bid).

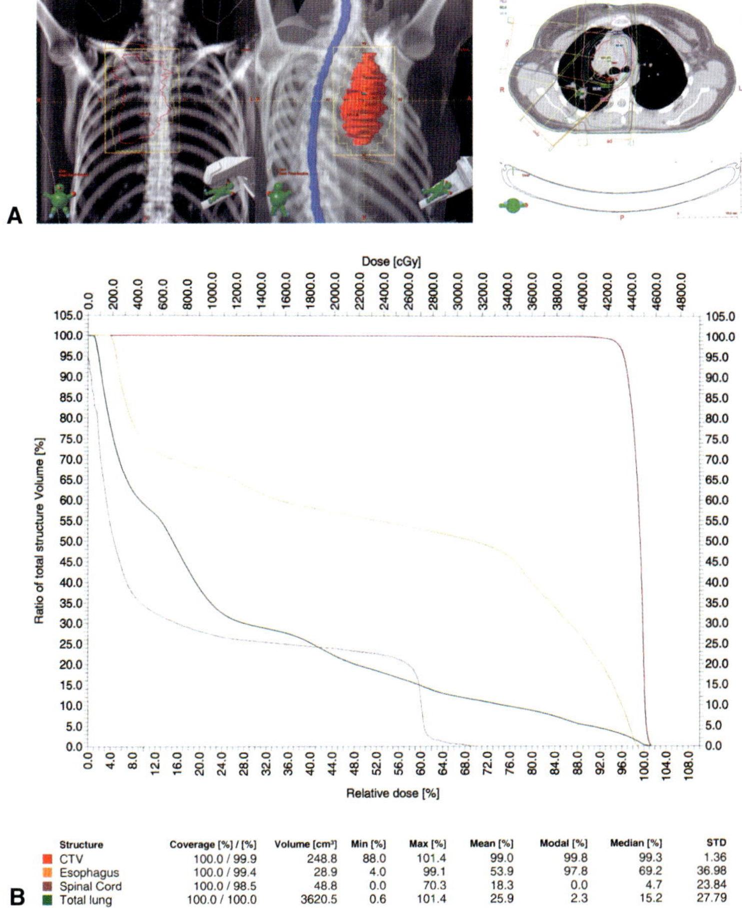

Structure	Coverage [%] / [%]	Volume [cm³]	Min [%]	Max [%]	Mean [%]	Modal [%]	Median [%]	STD
CTV	100.0 / 99.9	248.8	88.0	101.4	99.0	99.8	99.3	1.36
Esophagus	100.0 / 99.4	28.9	4.0	99.1	53.9	97.8	69.2	36.98
Spinal Cord	100.0 / 98.5	48.8	0.0	70.3	18.3	0.0	4.7	23.84
Total lung	100.0 / 100.0	3620.5	0.6	101.4	25.9	2.3	15.2	27.79

C

FIGURE 59.1 **A:** Anterior and oblique digital reconstructed radiograph (DRR). The **left panel** shows anterior port with saw-toothed edges of a multileaf collimator portal, with the physician-defined target outlined *in red*. The **right panel** displays an oblique portal *in red-pink* color wash, demonstrating the facility of avoiding the spinal cord. **B:** Dose-volume histogram (DVH): note the uniform dose coverage to the defined target (tumor) by the *red line*; the marked reduction in dose to the esophagus dose (*orange*) showing about 50% dose to only two thirds the esophageal volume, and the relatively lesser volumes of total lung irradiated. **C:** Dose distribution: these show isodose distributions in the (**left**) axial, (**middle**) coronal, and (**right**) sagittal plane. This patient was treated with four wedged fields for the entirety of the course without interruption and demonstrated a complete response by the second cycle of chemotherapy despite presenting with superior vena cava syndrome.

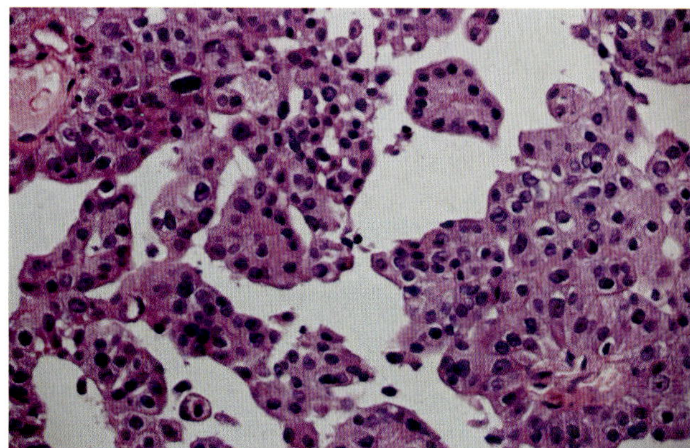

FIGURE 65.1 Reactive mesothelium. Superficial biopsy of the parietal pleura. There is no sign of infiltration, and a reactive mesothelial proliferation is the preferred diagnosis.

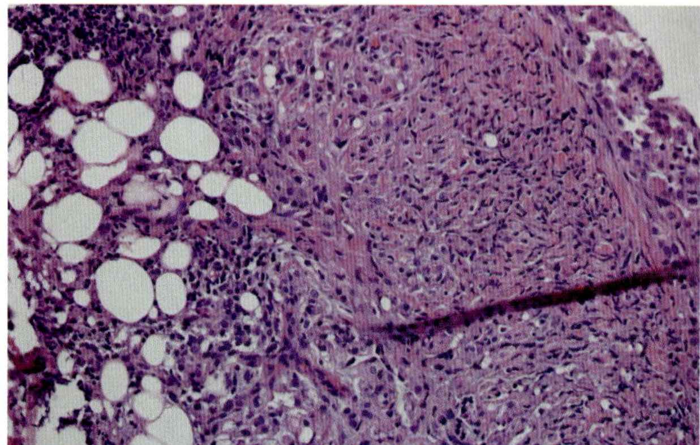

FIGURE 65.2 Deep biopsy showing invasion indicating MM. Deep biopsy from the parietal pleura in the same patient. Tumor cells show infiltration of the muscular layer and fat. The diagnosis of mesothelioma can now be confirmed.

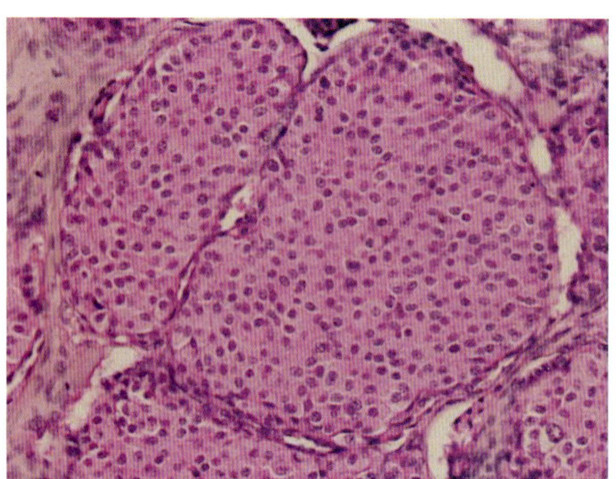

FIGURE 67.1 Typical carcinoid: endobronchial tumor of the upper lobe of the left lung in a 35-year-old woman. Well-differentiated neuroendocrine tumor without atypia, necrosis, or mitosis (hematoxylin and eosin [H&E] ×40). (Courtesy of Dr. Savvas Papadopoulos, Pathology Department, Hygeia Hospital, Athens, Greece.)

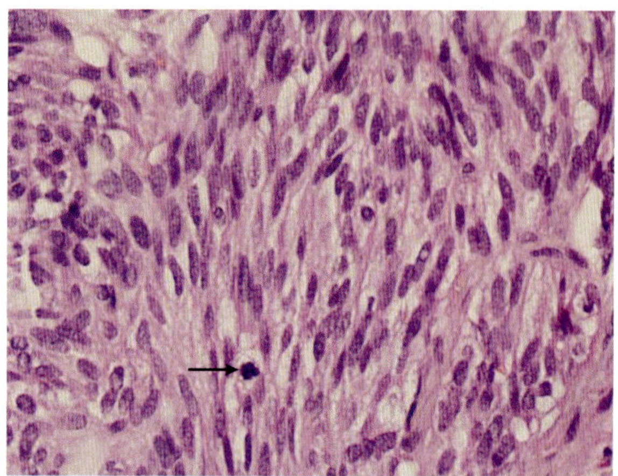

FIGURE 67.2 Spindle cell peripheral carcinoid tumor of the middle lobe of the right lung in a 46-year-old woman. *Black arrow* indicates a mitosis (hematoxylin and eosin [H&E] ×40). (Courtesy of Dr. Savvas Papadopoulos, Pathology Department, Hygeia Hospital, Athens, Greece.)

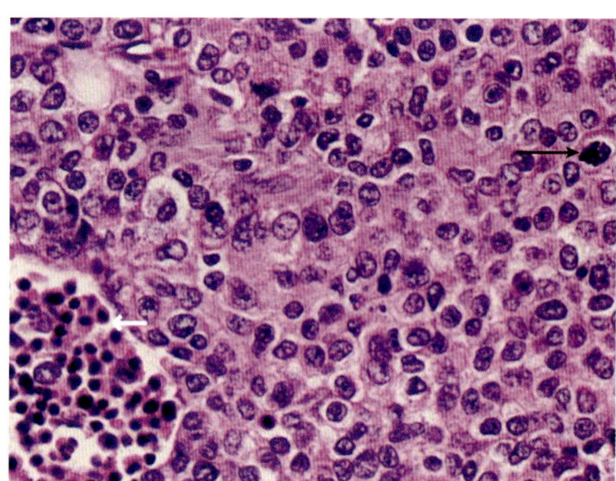

FIGURE 67.3 Atypical carcinoid tumor of the lower lobe of the right lung in a 50-year-old woman. Neuroendocrine tumor with atypia, necrosis (*white arrow*) and 9 mitoses (*black arrow*) per 10 hpf (hematoxylin and eosin [H&E] ×40). (Courtesy of Dr. Savvas Papadopoulos, Pathology Department, Hygeia Hospital, Athens, Greece.)

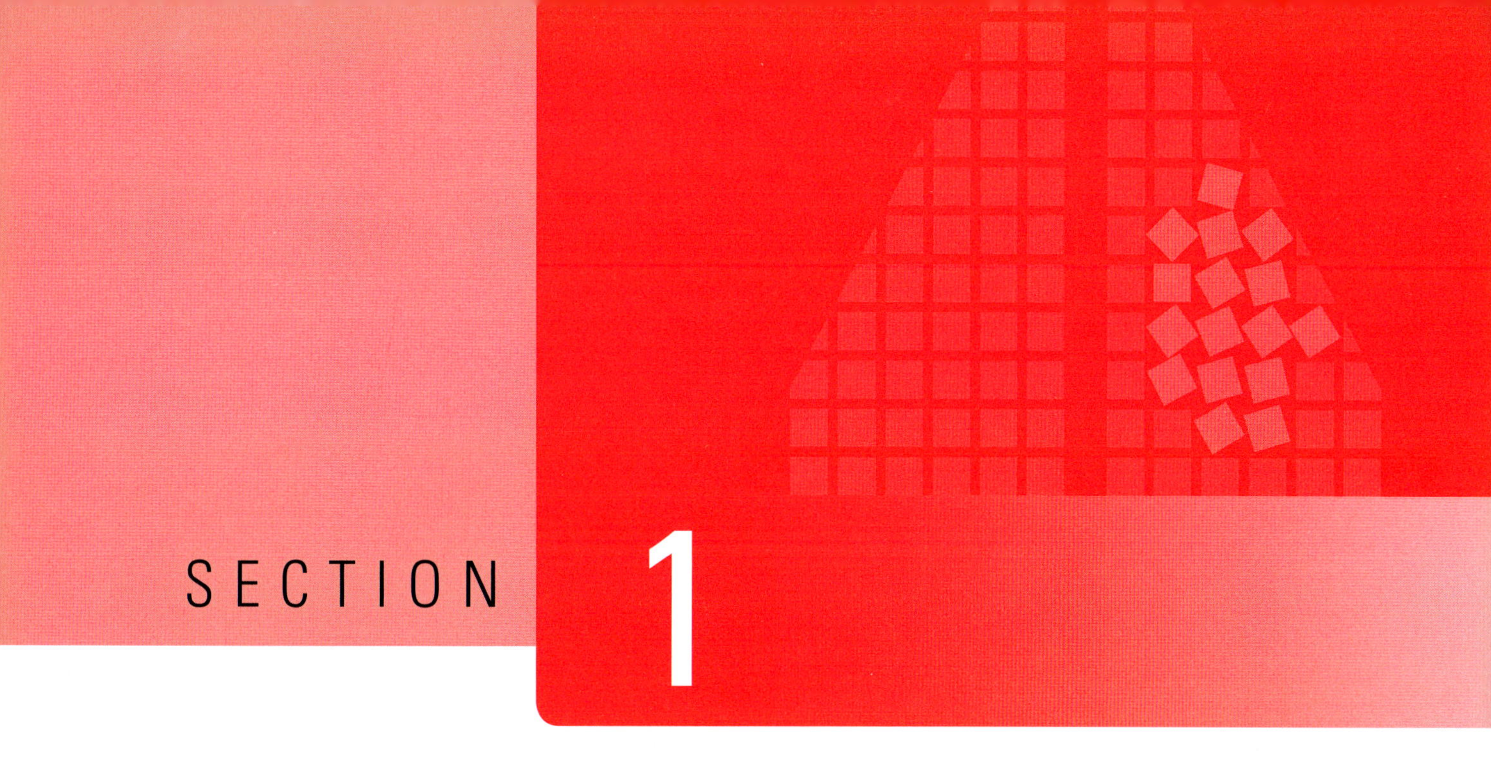

SECTION 1

Lung Cancer Epidemiology

CHAPTER 1

David Schottenfeld

The Etiology and Epidemiology of Lung Cancer

Lung cancer is the leading cause of cancer mortality in men and women in the United States, accounting for an estimated 161,840 deaths in 2008. Whereas lung cancer accounted for only 3% of all cancer deaths in women in 1950, in the year 2008 it accounted for an estimated 28% of cancer deaths. In 1990, the average annual mortality rate per 100,000 (standardized to the U.S. 2000 population) was 90.6 in men and 37.6 in women compared to 70.3 in men and 40.9 in women in 2004. Lung cancer incidence in men peaked in the 1980s and subsequently decreased after 1992 by 2.3% per year; mortality decreased 1.8% per year after having peaked around 1990. The age-adjusted lung cancer death rates in the United States surpassed those of breast cancer in white women in 1986 and in black women in 1990. It was estimated that in the year 2008, 30,550 more women will die of lung cancer (71,030) than of breast cancer (40,480).[1]

The incidence patterns, because of persistently poor survival rates, closely parallel the mortality rates. From 1992 to 2000, the average annual age-adjusted lung cancer incidence per 100,000 in men was 82.4, which was exceeded only by prostate cancer (180.6); the average annual lung cancer incidence in women was 49.4, which was second to that of breast cancer (132.5). In 2008, it was estimated that there were 215,020 new lung cancer cases diagnosed in the United States, and approximately 1.35 million cases were diagnosed worldwide with 1.18 million deaths in 2002.[2]

Lung cancer incidence and mortality patterns follow, after a latency interval of 20 or more years, the temporal patterns of cigarette smoking. In older men in the United States, lung cancer has displaced coronary heart disease as the leading cause of excess mortality among smokers. The risk of dying from lung cancer is associated with age of initiation and duration of cigarette smoking, and with the number and tar concentration of cigarettes smoked each day or as a regular pattern. The cumulative probability of lung cancer in the general population for individuals up to 74 years of age is 10% to 15% in those who smoke one or more packs of cigarettes per day. Exposure to other environmental and occupational respiratory carcinogens may be interactive with cigarette smoking and may influence trends of lung cancer incidence and mortality.[3]

DESCRIPTIVE EPIDEMIOLOGY

Age and Gender Whereas lung cancer incidence in men in the United States declined after peaking in the mid-1980s, the pattern in women differed significantly. In women, lung cancer incidence more than doubled between 1975 and 2000. Age-adjusted incidence in women increased on average by 4.1% per year between 1973 and 1990, but from 1990 to 2000, the average annual increase was only 0.2% (Fig. 1.1).

Among men and women, the rates declined in the past 10 years particularly among those younger than the age of 60 but continued to increase among those older than the age of 70. Only 5% to 10% of lung cancer cases are diagnosed in individuals younger than 50 years of age. Epidemiologic studies of lung cancer in young adults emphasize the predominance of adenocarcinomas and the importance of a positive family history. The current smoking prevalence and magnitude of estimates of relative risk (RR) caused by the average intensity and duration of smoking in women in the United States appear to be converging on the patterns in similarly exposed and aged men. Among whites, the male to female age-standardized lung cancer incidence ratio of rates is about 1:6, or 60% higher in men.[4,5]

Compared with women, men generally began smoking cigarettes at an earlier age, smoked more cigarettes per day and for a longer duration, inhaled more deeply, and consumed cigarettes with higher tar content. With increasing prevalence and duration of tobacco smoking in women after World War II, lung cancer mortality increased substantially in North America and Western Europe.

Several case-control studies have suggested that female smokers have a higher RR of lung cancer than male smokers, after adjusting for age and average daily intensity of smoking

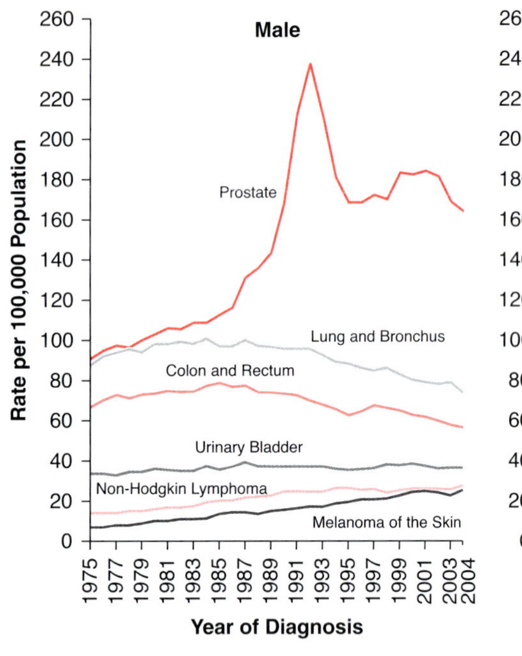

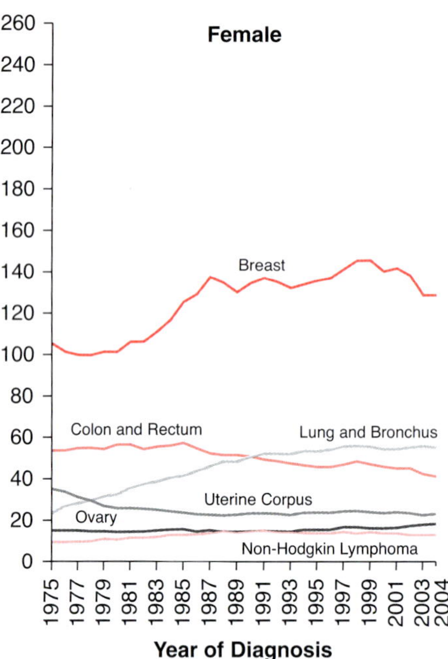

FIGURE 1.1 Annual age-adjusted cancer incidence rates for selected cancers by sex, United States, 1975 to 2004. Rates are age-adjusted to the 2000 U.S. standard population and adjusted for delays in reporting. Source: Surveillance, Epidemiology, and End Results (SEER) Program (http://www.seer.cancer.gov). Delay-Adjust Incidence database: Statistical Research and Applications Branch, released April 2007, based on the November 2006 SEER data submission. (From Jemal A, Siegel R, Ward E, et al. Cancer statistics, 2008. *CA Cancer J Clin* 2008;58:71–96.)

exposure.[6–8] The case-control design and the method of estimation of odds ratios in women may have been susceptible to recall bias, underreporting of amount smoked by the cases, and differences in baseline confounding risk factors for lung cancer between male and female nonsmoking controls (e.g., occupational risk factors, nutritional risk factors, unmeasured exposure to environmental tobacco smoke, history of non-neoplastic lung diseases, etc.). Prospective studies are required to derive unconfounded incidence measures of absolute or attributable risk that may be compared in smoking and nonsmoking men and women. In an analysis of former and current smokers in the Nurses' Health Study of women and the Health Professionals Follow-up Study in men, Bain et al.[9] reported that the hazard ratio in women ever smokers compared with men was 1.11 (95% confidence interval, 0.95 to 1.31). The analytic model controlled for the number of cigarettes smoked per day, age at starting smoking, and time since stopping smoking. Freedman et al.[10] compared the age-standardized incidence rates of lung cancer in men and women participating in the National Institutes of Health American Association of Retired Persons (AARP) cohort. In current smokers, in a model adjusted for lifetime smoking exposure, the hazard ratio was 0.9 (95% confidence interval, 0.8 to 1.0) for women compared with men. Both studies concluded that women were not more susceptible than men to the carcinogenic effects of cigarette smoking. Future studies should continue to monitor lung cancer incidence in women and men who have never smoked.

Race and Ethnicity

In the United States, the risk of lung cancer in black men has been about 50% higher than that in white men in the past 10 to 15 years, but the annual rate of decline after 1990 in black men (–2.5%) was about equal to that in white men (–2.3%) (Table 1.1). Among black men, lung cancer mortality was the second leading cause of death, ranking below coronary heart disease. The excess mortality from lung cancer among black men, compared with white men, was greatest for the age interval of 35 to 64 years. Cohorts of white men born before 1900 had higher (50%) age-specific rates than black men; however, this pattern reversed after 1915.

In the United States from 1975 to 1990, the age-adjusted lung cancer incidence in black women was 10% to 20% higher than that in white women; in the past 10 years, the average annual rate in black women (39.3 per 100,000) was slightly less than that in white women (40.9 per 100,000). After 1990, the incidence rates have continued to increase at an average annual rate of 0.7% to 0.8% for black and white women.

The Surveillance, Epidemiology, and End Results (SEER) program of the National Cancer Institute enables a comparison

TABLE 1.1 Age-Adjusted (1970 U.S. Standard) Lung Cancer Incidence per 100,000 in SEER Registry Areas by Race and Gender

Year of Diagnosis	White		Black	
	Men	Women	Men	Women
1975	75.9	21.8	101.2	20.6
1980	82.2	28.2	131	33.8
1985	82.1	35.9	131.3	40.2
1990	80.7	42.5	118.7	47
1994	72.6	43.3	110.6	48
1999*	84.4	53.3	125.6	54.4

*Rates are age-adjusted (2000 U.S. standard population). Black:white rate ratio was 1:5 (men) and 1:0 (women).

TABLE 1.2 Age-Adjusted Lung Cancer Incidence Rates per 100,000*

	White	African American	Asian American and Pacific Islander	American Indian and Alaska Native†	Hispanic/Latino‡§¶
Incidence					
Men	81.0	110.6	55.1	53.7	44.7
Women	54.6	53.7	27.7	36.7	25.2
Mortality					
Men	72.6	95.8	38.3	49.6	36.0
Women	42.1	39.8	18.5	32.7	14.6

*Per 100,000 population, age-adjusted to the 2000 U.S. standard population.

†Data based on Contract Health Service Delivery Areas (CHSDA), 624 counties comprising 54% of the U.S. American Indian/Alaska Native population; for more information, please see Espey DK, Wu XC, Swan J, et al. Annual report to the nation on the status of cancer, 1975–2004, featuring cancer in American Indians and Alaska natives. *Cancer* 2007 Nov 15;110(10):2119–2152.

‡Persons of Hispanic/Latino origin may be of any race.

§Incidence data unavailable from the Alaska Native Registry and Kentucky.

¶Mortality data unavailable from Minnesota, New Hampshire, and North Dakota.

Adapted from Ries LAG, Melbert D, Krapcho M, et al., eds. SEER Cancer Statistics Review, 1975–2004, National Cancer Institute. Bethesda, MD, http://seer.cancer.gov/csr/1975_2004/, based on November 2006 SEER data submission, posted to the SEER Web site, 2007.

of risks among various racial and ethnic groups in the United States (Table 1.2). The lowest age-adjusted lung cancer incidence rates in men and women, 50% to 70% of the rates among non-Hispanic whites, were registered for Native Americans, Hispanics, and Asian-Pacific Islanders; the highest rates were reported in blacks, native Hawaiians, and non-Hispanic whites. The ratio of male to female incidence rates reflected elevated risks in men that were 2.5 to 3.5 times the rates in women from the various racial and ethnic groups. Although the age-adjusted lung cancer incidence rates varied substantially by ethnicity, the percentage of all cancer deaths attributed to lung cancer in men and women combined was as high in Native Americans (27.7%) as in African Americans (26.1%). Lung cancer is the leading cause of cancer mortality among Hispanic men and the second leading cause among Hispanic women.

It is generally assumed that the differences in rates of lung cancer can be partially explained by different lifetime patterns of cigarette smoking. Compared with non-Hispanic white men, a higher percentage of non-Hispanic blacks were current smokers, smoked cigarettes with greater yield of tar and nicotine, and preferred to smoke mentholated cigarettes, which may stimulate deeper inhalation of cigarette smoke. However, in surveys of current smokers, black men were reported to smoke fewer cigarettes per day than white men. Molecular and biochemical studies, when controlling for differences in smoking habits, described higher serum cotinine levels and 4-aminobiphenyl-hemoglobin adduct levels in black smokers when compared with white smokers, suggesting that there may also be differences in susceptibility between blacks and whites as expressed in the metabolism of tobacco smoke.[11–14]

Socioeconomic Status Various studies have reported an inverse association between lung cancer mortality and socioeconomic status (Table 1.3). A twofold gradient in mortality was observed between low and high social class, as measured by occupation, income, or education. Smoking patterns accounted for part of the differential risk by social class, with smoking prevalence increased among blue-collar workers and among those with lower levels of education. Socioeconomic status may also serve as a surrogate measure for other risk factors such as occupation, diet, and ambient air pollutants, and may influence the quality, access, and utilization of healthcare services.[15,16]

International Patterns Global lung cancer incidence is increasing at a rate of 0.5% per year, and as a consequence, lung cancer is the leading cause of cancer incidence and mortality in European countries, accounting for about 21% of all cancer cases in men.[17–20] In less industrialized, developing countries, the proportion of all cancer deaths attributed to lung cancer is about 15%. In most parts of the world, rates were higher in urban than in rural areas and two to six times higher in men than in women. The areas with the highest incidence and mortality were in Eastern Europe, North America, Australia and New Zealand, and South America. The rates in China, Japan, and Southeast Asia were moderately high, whereas the lowest rates were observed in southern Asia, and in India and Pakistan, as well as in most countries in sub-Saharan Africa. Worldwide, in the year 2000, it was estimated that 47% to 52% of men and 10% to 12% of women smoked tobacco. In the United States, 25% of non-Hispanic white men and 23% of non-Hispanic white women were smoking tobacco. The prevalence of smoking men and women, the

TABLE 1.3 Lung Cancer Death Rates* by Educational Attainment, Race, and Sex, United States, 2001

	Male			Female		
	African American	Non-Hispanic White	Absolute Difference	African American	Non-Hispanic White	Absolute Difference
≤12 years of education	73.23	60.99	12.24	30.82	37.06	−6.24
>2 years of education	25.78	18.13	7.65	17.92	14.20	3.72
RR (95% CI)	2.84 (2.69–3.00)	3.36 (3.30–3.43)		1.72 (1.61–1.84)	2.6 (2.53–2.67)	
Absolute Difference	47.45	42.86		12.90	22.86	

*Rates are for individuals aged 25–64 years at death, per 100,000, and age-adjusted to the 2000 U.S. standard population.

CI, confidence interval; RR, relative risk.

Adapted from Albano JD, Ward E, Jemal A, et al. Cancer mortality in the United States by education level and race. *J Natl Cancer Inst* 2007;99:1384–1394.

types of cigarettes and amounts smoked, ages at initiation and duration of smoking exposure, and proportions of heavy smokers in the population, were important determinants of geocultural variations in lung cancer incidence. Recent trends in lung cancer mortality in men exhibited declining rates in all European countries except in France, Greece, Portugal, and Spain. Cigarette smoking in China has followed a pattern similar to that among adults in the United States although the significant pattern of increase, particularly among men, occurred 40 years later. Of the Chinese deaths attributed to tobacco, 15% were due to lung cancer and 45% to chronic obstructive lung disease. The relatively elevated rates of adenocarcinoma of the lung among Chinese women in China and Singapore were attributed to exposures to smoking tobacco and to environmental pollutants other than smoking tobacco (e.g., fossil fuel combustion products and cooking oils in the home).[21,22]

LIFESTYLE AND ENVIRONMENTAL RISK FACTORS

Tobacco The causal relationship between tobacco smoking and lung cancer was established by epidemiologic studies conducted in the 1950s and 1960s. The complexity of tobacco smoke, with over 3000 different chemicals, has made it difficult to identify the contribution of more than 50 putative carcinogenic agents. The carcinogens in tobacco smoke include the polynuclear aromatic hydrocarbons (PAHs), N-nitrosamines, aromatic amines, other organic (e.g., benzene, acrylonitrile) and inorganic (e.g., arsenic, acetaldehyde) compounds, and polonium-210. The composition of the smoke depends on the ambient conditions of smoking, the blend of tobacco leaf, filtration, additives, and paper wrapping. Tobacco smoke produced by the tobaccos in pipes and cigars is both harsher and more alkaline than that produced by cigarettes. Most of the compounds in tobacco are produced in an oxygen-deficient, hydrogen-rich environment, arising from pyrolysis and distillation, in the region immediately behind the burning tip of the cigarette. The nicotine concentration is addictive and toxic but not carcinogenic.[23,24]

As mainstream cigarette smoke emerges from the cigarette, it has approximately 10^9 to 10^{10} particles per mL. The aerodynamic diameters of the particles, ranging in size from 0.1 to 1.0 μm, determine the sites of deposition in the airways and alveolar regions of the lung. The fraction of smoke retained varies markedly with the pattern of inhalation. The chemical analysis of tobacco smoke is separated into particulate or "tar," and gaseous phases. Filter tips of cellulose acetate remove volatile nitrosamines and phenols selectively. The neutral fraction of the particulate phase contains potentially important tumor initiators such as the PAHs.[25]

In 1964, the first surgeon general's report on smoking summarized existing evidence and declared cigarette smoking to be the major cause of lung cancer among American men.[26] In the ensuing 30 years, epidemiologic studies have established that there were increasing risks in women and underscored the relationships with onset, duration, intensity, and cessation of smoking. Prospective studies demonstrated a rising trend in lung cancer death rates with increasing average amounts smoked per day in current smokers. The initial emphasis of epidemiologic studies of lung cancer and smoking was on men who, in almost all countries, began smoking earlier, consumed greater quantities of tobacco, and exhibited higher RRs than women.[27–29]

In the past 20 years, the prevalence of cigarette smoking in many countries, including the United States, has increased significantly among women; concomitantly, changes in smoking practices have been accompanied by increasing relative and attributable risks for lung cancer.[30–32] In a follow-up study of approximately 600,000 women conducted in 1980s by the American Cancer Society, the RR of dying of lung cancer in current smokers was 12.7; for those who smoked 30 or more cigarettes per day, the RR was increased 22.3 times compared with the never-smoker. In 1985, cigarette smoking accounted for an estimated 82% of lung cancer deaths, or 31,600 deaths.[33] The International

Agency for Research on Cancer (IARC) estimated that the smoking-attributable fraction of lung cancer deaths occurring in the United States and in England and Wales was 92% in men and 78% in women.[25] In 2001, the U.S. Health Interview Survey estimated that 46.2 million adults were current smokers and that 44.7 million adults were former smokers. Current smoking prevalence was highest among persons aged 18 to 24 years (26.9%), and among those aged 25 to 44 years (25.8%), and lowest among those aged older than 65 years (10.1%). From 2000 to 2001, current smoking prevalence, for the first time, was similar in non-Hispanic white (25.4%) and black (27.7%) men; in contrast, the prevalence in non-Hispanic black women (17.9%) was less than that in non-Hispanic white women (22.8%).[32]

Lower tar content and the use of filters are factors that may result in reduced lung cancer risks in those who smoke. In the earlier American Cancer Society (ACS) Twenty-five–State Study, men who smoked low-tar (<22 mg) cigarettes experienced 20% lower risk of dying of lung cancer when compared with men who continued to smoke high-tar cigarettes. The excess lung cancer risk for current smokers was directly proportional to the estimated milligrams of tar consumed daily. In the more recent ACS Fifty-State Study, Garfinkel and Stellman concluded that doubling the cigarette tar yield would result in a 40% increase in the RR of dying of lung cancer, independently of the amount smoked or depth of inhalation. The Federal Trade Commission estimated that the current average sales-weighted tar content of cigarettes manufactured in the United States was about 12 to 13 mg of tar per cigarette, compared with nearly 40 mg in the early 1950s. Lifelong filter cigarette smokers have experienced 20% to 40% lower risk of lung cancer than lifelong nonfilter smokers, after adjusting for differences in the amount smoked. Presumably, larger reductions in risk have not been observed because of alternations in smoking behavior in response to low-nicotine yield of manufactured cigarettes. Namely, it has been shown that in maintaining addiction, the smoker will inhale larger volumes of mainstream smoke and at more frequent intervals.[34–37]

Although these studies suggested that switching to filtered or low-tar cigarettes may modestly reduce the risk of lung cancer, the more significant reduction in risk would be derived from cessation of smoking. Whereas approximately 25% of smoking adults in the United States continue to smoke, an additional 40% to 50% have become former smokers. The RR of lung cancer among ex-smokers decreases significantly after 5 years of smoking cessation. In the initial 1 to 4 years after quitting smoking, however, the RR of lung cancer among ex-smokers may appear to be higher than among current smokers, presumably because a proportion of individuals may have stopped smoking because of illness or premonitory symptoms of lung cancer.[38,39]

It has been suggested that the risk of lung cancer in former smokers will approximate but never equal that of lifelong nonsmokers. The baseline risk of lung cancer in lifelong nonsmokers increases in relation to age raised to the fourth or fifth power. In the British Physicians Study, Doll and Peto[38] showed that the incidence of lung cancer in cigarette smokers increased approximately in proportion to the fourth power of duration of smoking, and was multiplicative with the previously described exponential increase with age among never-smokers. The percentage reduction in risk after quitting depended on the prior duration and average amount smoked each day, being more readily demonstrable among lighter smokers and smokers of lesser duration or those who quit at a younger age. Lung cancer results from a multistep process in which persistent genetic lesions accumulate at specific chromosomal loci. Most current or former smokers, in contrast to never-smokers, exhibit loss of heterozygosity at multiple allelic sites (e.g., 3p14, 9p21, p16, p53) in both normal and metaplastic or dysplastic bronchial epithelium.[40,41]

Pipe and cigar smoking have been linked to lung cancer, particularly squamous cell and small cell carcinomas, but the estimated RRs, compared with people who never smoked, who are assigned an RR of 1.0, were considerably lower than the risks reported among cigarette smokers; the risks among exclusively pipe or cigar smokers in the United States or Europe have been estimated to range from 2.0 to 9.0. In countries such as Sweden, Switzerland, and Holland, where pipe or cigar smoking was nearly as common as cigarette smoking, the RRs of lung cancer, when controlling for cumulative exposure levels, were equally high for all forms of smoked tobacco. Differences in the manner in which pipes and cigars were smoked in different countries, (i.e., depth of inhalation or average daily or cumulative amount smoked) may provide an explanation for differences in the estimated risks. Cigars are products made of tobacco, wrapped in tobacco leaves rather than in paper. Cigars smoked in Europe weigh 2 to 8 g and are similar to American "small cigars." Cigarillos are smaller than cigars weighing 1.5 to 3 g and are described as "little cigars" in the United States. Risks of lung cancer also varied with the type of tobacco used. Dark tobaccos were associated with greater risk of lung cancer than light tobaccos, and with formation of higher levels of 4-aminobiphenyl-hemoglobin adducts.[42–45]

Environmental Tobacco Smoke Environmental tobacco smoke (ETS) is comprised of sidestream smoke (about 80% released from burning tobacco in between puffs), and from the exhaled smoke (about 20% of the smoke). The smoke that the smoker inhales is known as mainstream smoke. Other minor contributors to ETS include the smoke that escapes during puffing from the burning cone, and gaseous components that diffuse through the cigarette paper. These components are diluted by the ambient air and when inhaled, in particular by nonsmokers, are referred to as "passive" or "involuntary" smoking. ETS contains various toxic agents, including mutagens and carcinogens, which, for some chemicals (e.g., nitrosamines, 4-aminobiphenyl, benzo[a]pyrene), have been measured at higher concentrations than in mainstream smoke. Estimates of ETS exposure, based on serum or urinary measurements of cotinine, the metabolite of nicotine, suggest that involuntary smokers absorb about 0.5% to 1% of the nicotine that active smokers absorb, or smoke the equivalent of about one-half cigarette a day. Studies of 4-aminobiphenyl-hemoglobin adduct levels indicate that passive smokers have approximately 14% of the concentration of active smokers.[46]

Many scientific consensus committees have concluded that exposure to ETS causes lung cancer in humans. Table 1.4 lists the RRs of lung cancer among nonsmoking women based on a review of epidemiologic studies in various countries, which have evaluated dose–response trends.[47–64] The risks increased with amounts smoked by husbands, with about 30% to 150% increases in RR experienced in general among those women most heavily exposed. A weighted analysis of 37 published epidemiological studies resulted in the conclusion that there was an elevated risk of 24% (95% confidence interval [CI], 13% to 36%) among nonsmoking wives of *smoking* husbands, when compared with nonsmoking wives of *nonsmoking* husbands. Workplace exposures to ETS are measured with less precision than spousal exposures; however, some studies have suggested that there is a dose–response relationship when combining workplace and spousal sources of ETS. It has been suggested that when using biological markers of nicotine exposure in studies of ETS and lung cancer, about 5% of female respondents, who were in fact smokers, may have reported that they were nonsmokers. Correcting for this bias, however, would result in an adjusted RR in nonsmoking women who were living with smokers of about 1.15 to 1.20. The report of the National Research Council concluded that about 20% of lung cancers occurring in nonsmoking women and men, or 3000 cases per year, may be attributable to exposure to ETS; in the context of lung cancer cases diagnosed each year in smokers and nonsmokers, 2% to 3% may be attributable to ETS.[65,66]

Air Pollution Pollutants in the urban air other than from tobacco have been investigated as potential causal agents in the epidemic rise of lung cancer in industrialized nations. The products of fossil fuel combustion, principally polycyclic hydrocarbons, have been of particular concern. Other sources of ambient air pollution have been motor vehicle and diesel engine exhausts, power plants, and industrial and residential emissions. The ratio of urban to rural age-adjusted lung cancer mortality rates in many industrialized nations have varied between 1.1 and 2.0. It has been suggested that the net attributable risk effect of protracted exposure to urban air pollutants in men with average smoking habits would be 10 cases of lung cancer per 100,000 per year. In most countries, however, a major fraction (i.e., 80% or greater) would be attributable to cigarette smoking, and the independent association with urban residence, or the "urban factor," could not be assessed without controlling for the confounding effect of differences in smoking practices, or exposures to environmental tobacco smoke, between urban and rural residents. In addition, the urban factor has yet to be defined, but is undoubtedly a complex mixture of interacting chemical compounds and elements that vary by geographic area and over time. Exposure to combustion-source ambient air pollution has been associated with declining pulmonary function, increased rates of hospitalization for respiratory illnesses, and increased rates of cardiopulmonary diseases mortality.[67–69]

Evidence in support of the potential association of air pollution with lung cancer may be provided by occupational studies of workers exposed to combustion products from fos-

TABLE 1.4 Relative Risk of Lung Cancer among Nonsmoking Women According to Level of Husband's Smoking

Author	No. of Lung Cancers	Husband's Smoking Status	
		Light	Heavy*
Hirayama[47]	201	1.4	1.9
Trichopoulos et al.[48,49]	77	1.9	2.5
Garfinkel[50]	153	1.3	1.1
Correa et al.[51]	22	1.2	3.5
Koo et al.[52]	88	1.9	1.2
Wu et al.[53]	28	1.2	2.0
Garfinkel et al.[54]	134	1.1	2.0
Akiba et al.[55]	94	1.4	2.1
Pershagen et al.[56]	67	1.0	3.2
Lam et al.[57]	199	1.9	2.1
Gao et al.[58]	406	1.2	1.7
Janerich et al.[59]	191	0.8	1.1
Fontham et al.[60]	420	1.1	1.3
Brownson et al.[62]	432	0.9	1.3
Stockwell et al.[63]	210	1.5	2.4
Fontham et al.[61]	651	1.1	1.8
Boffetta et al.[64]	509	0.6	1.3

*Definitions of heavy smokers varied by study, but typically included those who smoked 20 or more cigarettes per day.

sil fuels. Workers exposed to emissions from retort coal gas plants manifested smoking-adjusted RR of lung cancer that was approximately twice that in unexposed workers. Roofers exposed to coal tar fumes while working outdoors had an approximately 50% increase in lung cancer risk after 20 years of exposure, and 150% increase after 40 years.[70,71]

Benzo(a)pyrene has been used as a surrogate index of ambient urban air exposure produced by fossil fuel combustion and correlated with lung cancer mortality rates. However, putative carcinogenic agents present in ambient urban air may include inorganic particles or fibers (e.g., arsenic, asbestos, chromium, nickel, uranium); radionuclides (e.g., ^{210}Pb, ^{212}Pb, ^{222}Ra); and organic gaseous and particulate combustion products (e.g., dimethylnitrosamine, benzene, benzo[a]pyrene, 1,2-benzanthracene). In a longitudinal study by the ACS, age-, occupational-, and smoking-standardized rates for lung cancer were computed according to residence. Minimal differences in mortality were observed between urban and rural residential areas, or among cities categorized by indices of pollution.[72] The World Health Organization (WHO) IARC has declared diesel engine exhaust a "probable carcinogen." In studies of railroad workers exposed to diesel exhaust, Garshick et al. described a 40% increase in the smoking-adjusted RR of lung cancer.[73,74]

In a rural area in Yunan Province, China, an excess risk of lung cancer among men and women was attributed to indoor pollution because of burning soft, "smoky" coal in unvented firepits inside the home. Replacing the firepits with stoves vented with chimneys was reported to reduce lung cancer incidence by about 40% to 45%.[75] In Shanghai, the elevated risk of lung cancer was hypothesized to be a result of prolonged exposure to oil vapors, particularly from rapeseed oil that was used in high-temperature wok cooking. Condensates of the volatile emissions from rapeseed and soybean oil have been found to be mutagenic. In urban Shenyang in northeastern China, indoor pollution from coal-burning heating devices gave rise to an age-, education-, and tobacco smoking-adjusted RR of 2.3 for lung cancer in the highest exposure group.[76–78]

Indoor Radon Radon (^{222}Ra), with a half-life of 3.8 days, is an inert, radioactive, colorless, and odorless gas at usual environmental temperatures that can percolate through the earth's crust and accumulate in residential dwellings. At sufficiently high concentrations, radon and its α-particle–emitting decay products, polonium-214 and polonium-218, have been shown to cause lung cancer in cigarette smoking and nonsmoking uranium, tin, and iron-ore miners. These observations have been replicated by conducting experimental studies in rats.[79] Indoor radon exposure accounts for about 50% to 80% of the total radiation received on average in the United States. It has been estimated, based on extrapolations from high-risk miner studies, that indoor radon may cause between 6000 and 36,000 lung cancer deaths per year in the United States. Joint exposures to tobacco smoke and radon gas have been interpreted to yield risks of lung cancer that were greater than linear and additive and approximated multiplicative or log linear effects.[80–82]

Case-control studies of lung cancer have been conducted in various countries based on estimated lifetime exposures to residential radon and tobacco smoke. Axelson et al.[83] noted an increased risk of lung cancer among persons living in stone compared to wood houses in Sweden. In a later study by Pershagen et al.,[84] it was concluded that the smoking-adjusted risk of lung cancer increased in relation to the cumulative and time-weighted exposure to radon. The RR was 1.3 (95% CI, 1.1 to 1.6) for average radon concentrations, over a period of about 30 years, of 3.8 to 10.8 pCi per liter; for exposure in excess of 10.8 pCi/L, the RR was 1.8 (95% CI, 1.1 to 2.9). Moreover, there was evidence that the joint effect of radon exposure and tobacco smoking was multiplicative rather than additive. In a study conducted in New Jersey, the risk of lung cancer was increased more than twofold among women living in homes with radon levels exceeding 4 pCi/L.[85] However, in a case-control study of women who were recently diagnosed with lung cancer in China, no association was demonstrated between increasing residential radon exposure and lung cancer; 20% of the yearlong radon measurements exceeded 4 pCi/L, the level above which remedial action is recommended in the United States.[86] Conclusions that were similar to those from the study in China were presented based on a study by Létourneau et al.[87] in Canada. Thus, although radon and its α-particle–emitting decay products are classified as a human lung carcinogen, there has been uncertainty expressed about whether or to what extent residential radon exposure levels contributed to the lung cancer burden and how accurate were predictions based on extrapolations from studies of underground miners. Epidemiologic studies of indoor radon in the United States must be interpreted with caution because of limitations in estimating lifetime exposures based on current exposure measurements. Exposure reconstruction is complicated because persons reside in many homes throughout life, and the time actually spent in each home may be only approximated. Average prior residential exposure levels were generally low, exceeding remedial action levels in 5% of United States homes. Extrapolated RR estimates of less than 1.2, which was associated with average residential exposures, would have been potentially confounded by effects of active and environmental tobacco smoke inhalation. Notwithstanding these caveats, recent publications were supportive of risks of lung cancer associated with residential radon exposure that were consistent with extrapolations of risk using underground mining-based models.[88,89]

Occupational Respiratory Carcinogens Although smoking is the major cause of lung cancer, other respiratory tract carcinogens have been identified, or are suspect, and may enhance the carcinogenic effects of tobacco smoke. Notable among these independent determinants of lung cancer are chemical and physical agents that have been identified in the workplace. An example of an occupational lung cancer was described in central Europe in the latter part of the 19th century in underground metal miners. The likely cause of what was described historically as "mountain disease" has been attributed to the miners' inhalation of radon and α-emitting radon daughters. At that time, lung cancer was a rare disease, and the prevalence of cigarette smoking was low. Other occupational agents classified as group 1 carcinogens by the IARC include inorganic arsenic, asbestos, bis(chloromethyl)ether, chromium (hexavalent), nickel and nickel compounds, polycyclic aromatic compounds (PAHs), radon, and vinyl chloride (Table 1.5). Group 2A probable carcinogens included acrylonitrile, beryllium, cadmium, formaldehyde, acetaldehyde, synthetic fibers, silica, and welding fumes. Currently, occupational exposures have been estimated to account for 5% to 15% of lung cancers occurring among men and women of different cultures and nations.[90]

Asbestos The association between asbestos exposure and lung cancer has been established by epidemiological and animal experimental studies. It has been estimated that since the beginning of World War II, up to 8 million persons in the United States have been exposed to asbestos in the workplace. In the United States, more than 90% of the production and consumption of asbestos is represented by the serpentine or curly form of fiber known as chrysotile ("white asbestos"). The bronchopulmonary neoplasms of various cell types induced by asbestos tend to originate peripherally and in the lower lobes, accompanied frequently by the fibrosis of asbestosis.[91–93]

Asbestos is a general term used to describe a variety of naturally occurring hydrated silicates that produce mineral fibers upon mechanical processing. In addition to the serpentine group, there are the amphiboles, a larger family of straight, needlelike fibers that includes anthophyllite, tremolite, and amosite ("brown asbestos"), and crocidolite ("blue asbestos"). Most mesotheliomas are associated with exposure to crocidolite asbestos. Because of unique physical and chemical properties, such as noncombustibility, withstanding temperatures of over 5000°C, resistance to acids, high tensile strength, and use in thermal and acoustic insulation, asbestos has had wide applications in commercial products. Such products include textiles, cement, paper, wicks, ropes, floor and roofing tiles, water pipes, wallboard, fireproof clothing, gaskets, brake linings, etc.[94]

Various morphologic, biochemical, and molecular techniques have been utilized to document events that might be associated with asbestos toxicity at the cellular level. Prolonged exposure to asbestos results in the accumulation of macrophages and inflammatory cells in the alveoli, which is accompanied by the release of oxygen free radicals, the peroxidation of cell membranes, and damage to DNA and other macromolecules. Asbestos fibers that cross the alveolar epithelium may be translocated to the pleura by macrophages. The shape, length, and persistence of fibers may be important in eliciting cellular responses intrinsic to carcinogenesis. Longer, rodlike fibers (i.e., >5 to 10 μm in length and <0.25 μm in diameter) appear to be more cytotoxic than shorter, coarse fibers. Electrostatic charge on the fiber surface may enhance deposition in lung tissue, and the surface biochemistry may also impact the inflammatory response. Experimentally, in tracheobronchial epithelial culture systems, asbestos exhibits the characteristics of a tumor promoter; chronic exposure to asbestos, subsequent to the introduction of subcarcinogenic amounts of dimethyl benzanthracene (DMBA), has resulted in increased DNA synthesis, basal cell hyperplasia, squamous metaplasia, and squamous cell carcinoma. In the induction of mesotheliomas and pleural sarcomas, asbestos is a complete carcinogen.

The risk of lung carcinoma in cigarette smokers has been examined in several asbestos-exposed populations. In 1968, Selikoff et al.[93] reported on the effects of combined exposures to cigarette smoking and asbestos in insulation workers; the RR for lung cancer significantly exceeded the level of risk expected if each exposure were to have acted only independently (noninteractively). The synergy resulting from combined exposures to tobacco and asbestos has been demonstrated in asbestos factory workers, Quebec miners and millers, amosite asbestos factory workers, and Finnish anthophyllite miners and millers. Although most studies have concluded that the RRs were close to multiplicative, as in exposures to smoking and radon combined, a study among Canadian chrysotile miners and millers concluded that the effect of each agent was independent and additive. Various sources have concluded that asbestos exposure, in the absence of tobacco smoking, increases the risk of both squamous cell carcinoma and adenocarcinoma of the lung. It is assumed in risk assessment models that the dose–response relationship may be linear or exponential, and without an apparent threshold. On the assumption of synergy between asbestos exposure and tobacco smoking, it has been emphasized that it is especially important for asbestos-exposed persons to quit smoking as a cost-effective preventive measure.[95]

Mesothelioma has a protracted latency period averaging 35 to 40 years. Unlike carcinoma of the lung, smoking does not contribute to the development of mesothelioma in asbestos workers. Statistics on the incidence and mortality of mesothelioma are not reported routinely because of problems in histopathologic classification of mesothelial cell hyperplasia and malignant neoplasia and the distinction from metastatic sarcomas or adenocarcinomas. A combination of histochemistry, immunocytochemistry, and electron microscopy may be necessary to achieve a precise and valid diagnosis. In the SEER program consisting of various state, county and metropolitan population-based cancer registries that cover currently about 14% of the total U.S. population, the average annual age-adjusted incidence of mesothelioma (per 100,000 population) in white men nearly doubled from 1978 to 1992 (from 1.3 to 2.5), whereas the rates among white women remained stable at about 0.4. Rates in men aged 75 to 84 years increased from 6.3 to 18.2. In developed countries, approximately one mesothelioma case occurs concurrently with 100 lung carcinoma cases. The rates in nonwhites were too low to yield reliable estimates during this period of time. As reported in other countries, pleural exceeded peritoneal mesotheliomas by a ratio of 9:1 in men and 3:1 in women. The incidence rates appeared to have peaked among those born around 1910 and have declined among cohorts born subsequently.[96]

There are well-documented areas of elevated incidence of mesothelioma, such as the coastal area of Virginia, San Francisco-Oakland, Hawaii, and Seattle in the United States; England and Wales; and Japan, where there were shipbuilding centers; among women in areas where, during World War II,

TABLE 1.5 Chemicals and Industrial Processes Associated with Human Lung Cancer*

Agent	Human Target Organs	Epidemiology	Toxicology
Arsenic	Lung Skin Urinary tract	Over 95% of arsenic produced in the United States is byproduct of copper, lead, zinc, and tin ore smelting. Excess lung cancer reported in association with use and production of inorganic trivalent arsenic-containing pesticides. Dose–response trends have been validated by measuring concentrations in air and urine. In a review of published studies, combined relative risk reported as 3.69 (95% CI, 3.06–4.46).[170] Joint action with tobacco smoking appears to be more than additive and less than multiplicative. Latency of 10–35 years.	No satisfactory animal model. In tissue culture systems: Chromosomal aberrations, inhibition of DNA repair, and increased sister chromatid exchanges. The current OSHA standard for airborne inorganic arsenic is 10 μg/m^3.
Asbestos	Lung Mesothelium or serosa of pleura, pericardium, and peritoneum GI tract Larynx	Various workers in asbestos industries at increased risk: miners, millers, textile, insulation, shipyard, cement. Average latency period of 25–30 years for carcinoma of lung. Length of interval varies with type of fiber, exposure intensity and duration, host factors. Dose–response relationship that is approximately linear in form across mid to upper levels of exposure. Relative risk of lung cancer appears to decrease following cessation of exposure. Synergistic relationship with cigarette smoking, which is more than additive and close to multiplicative. Asbestos exposure in the United States accounts for approximately 5% of lung cancer deaths in men.	Asbestos minerals are divided into: a) the amphiboles, including amosite, crocidolite, anthophyllite, and tremolite; b) serpentine class, which is represented by chrysotile. All types of commercial asbestos fibers are carcinogenic in mice, rats, hamsters, and rabbits; after inhalation, or intrapleural and intraperitoneal administration, cancers of the lung and bronchus, and/or mesotheliomas have been induced. The current OSHA standard is 0.1 fibers per mL for fibers greater than 5 μm in length.
BCME and CMME	Lung	Used in manufacture of ion-exchange resins, polymers, plastics. Tumor cell type was primarily (85%) small cell (oat-cell) carcinoma. Changes in industrial process from open-kettle to closed hermetically isolated systems in 1971 have markedly reduced exposure and were accompanied by declining risk of lung cancer. Increasing risk with increasing intensity and duration of exposure.	Highly carcinogenic in rodents by inhalation, skin application, or subcutaneous injection. BCME is a more potent carcinogen than CMME.
Chromium and compounds	Lung Nasal and paranasal sinuses	Used in metal alloys, electroplating, lithography magnetic tapes, paint pigments, cement, rubber, photoengraving, composition floor covering, and as oxidant in synthesis of organic chemicals. Excess risk, threefold and higher, was demonstrated for all cell types of lung cancer in the chromate-producing industry, producers of chromate paints, and chromate plating workers, particularly from 1930–1945. Risks in other occupational settings, with lower intensity exposures, have not been consistently or substantially increased.	Epidemiologic and experimental data implicate hexavalent and not trivalent chromium compounds. The OSHA standard for chromic acid and hexavalent chromates is 0.1 mg/m^3.
Nickel and compounds	Lung Nasal and paranasal sinuses Larynx	Used in electroplating, manufacturing of stainless steel and other alloys, ceramics, storage batteries, electric circuits, petroleum refining, and oil hydrogenation.	Animal studies indicate that nickel compounds can produce local sarcomas by injection, and pulmonary tumors by inhalation and intratracheal instillation.

(continues)

TABLE 1.5 Chemicals and Industrial Processes Associated with Human Lung Cancer* *(continued)*

Agent	Human Target Organs	Epidemiology	Toxicology
		Risk associated with earliest stage of refining, involving heavy exposure to dust from relatively crude ore. In some nickel refineries, high levels of PAHs, arsenic, or other agents may have contributed to increased risks. In mining for nickel, workers may be exposed to asbestos.	Several forms of nickel may be carcinogenic, and include oxides, sulfites, and soluble nickel. The OHSA standard is 0.1 mg/m^3 for soluble compounds, and 1 mg/m^3 for nickel metal and insoluble nickel compounds.
PAHs	Lung Skin and scrotum Urinary bladder	These chemicals may result from ferrochromium production and smelting of nickel-containing ores; aluminum production, iron and steel founding, coke production, and coal gasification; coal tars, coal tar pitches, untreated mineral oils; soot from combustion and diesel engine exhausts. In relation to coke oven emissions, risk of lung cancer highest in workers on the topside of coke ovens. Among the most heavily exposed, lifetime risk could reach 40%. Combined relative risk, based on six studies, of 1.31 (95% CI, 1.13–1.44) for diesel-exposed workers.[171]	PAHs result from pyrolysis or incomplete combustion of organic compounds. Benzo(a)pyrene-DNA adducts, a marker of PAH exposure, have been detected in the blood samples of coke oven workers. Diesel exhaust, the particulate phase, has been demonstrated to be a lung carcinogen in animals.
Radon	Lung	Increased risks of lung cancer have been observed among underground miners in North America, Europe, and Asia, and quantitatively related to the inhalation of radon daughter products. Although small cell cancers predominate, all cell types are affected. Radiation and cigarette smoking are interactive with relative risks somewhat less than multiplicative. Exposure levels in miners associated with elevated risks generally exceeded 100 working-level months (about 0.5 Gy). Linear nonthreshold dose response. For the same cumulative dose, prolonged exposures at low dose rates appear more hazardous than shorter exposures at higher dose rates.	Dose of high-LET alpha particles to individual cells will vary with respiratory dynamics, thickness of the epithelial cell and overlapping mucous layers, and the clearance rate of absorbed radioactive particles. Cellular DNA damage depends on the type of radiation, amount of energy deposited per volume of tissue, the rate at which the energy is deposited, and the time over which a given dose is accumulated.
Vinyl chloride	Liver (angiosarcoma) Lung Brain Lymphoreticular	Principal use is in production of plastics, packaging materials, and vinyl asbestos floor tiles. A review of 12 cohort studies of men employed at synthetic plastics or polyvinyl chloride polymerization plants reported SMRs for lung cancer indicating an overall observed to expected lung cancer ratio of 1:12 (95% CI, 1.0–1.2).[172]	Inhalation of vinyl chloride monomer and polyvinyl chloride in experimental animals causes pulmonary fibrosis and adenomas, skin appendage tumors, and osteochondromas.

*Agents are those classified as known carcinogens (group 1) by the International Agency for Research on Cancer.

BCME, Bis(chloromethyl) ether; CMME, chloromethyl methyl ether; GI, gastrointestinal; LET, linear energy transfer; OSHA, Occupational Safety and Health Administration; PAHs, Polycyclic aromatic hydrocarbons; SMR, standardized mortality ratios.

gas masks with asbestos filters were manufactured; or in South Africa, where excess mesothelioma incidence was concentrated in mining districts. Mesotheliomas may result from neighborhood or environmental (nonoccupational) exposures to asbestos industries and from household contact with asbestos dust, primarily through the laundering of work clothing.[97–101]

All types of asbestos have the potential for causing mesothelioma, although the risks in humans are two to four times more significant for amphibole fibers, such as crocidolite and amosite, than for the serpentine fibers of chrysotile. The mechanisms of induction appear related to the physical properties of fiber size and dimension. The amphibole straight rodlike fibers can more readily be transported or penetrate to peripheral segments of the lung. The pathogenesis in mesothelial cells is accompanied by induced proto-oncogene expression and the formation of oxygen radical species.

The association between the physical structure of asbestos fibers and carcinogenicity has raised concerns regarding possible hazards of other fibers, whether natural or synthetic. Inorganic synthetic vitreous substances derived from glass, rock, slag, or clay are used primarily in the manufacture of thermal and acoustic insulation materials. Intrapleural injection of such fibers is associated with mesothelioma or sarcoma of the pleura of laboratory animals. In 1987, the WHO declared that glass wool, rock wool, slag wool, and ceramic fibers were to be classified as 2B agents, namely, agents possibly carcinogenic to humans. This category is generally used for agents for which there is limited evidence in humans and where there is the absence of sufficient evidence in experimental animals. Epidemiologic studies of the association of occupational exposures to synthetic vitreous fibers and the risk of lung cancer have not shown a consistent pattern of risk in relation to duration of employment, average intensity and cumulative exposure dose levels, or latency interval. Further, many of the studies have not controlled adequately for confounding by cigarette smoking habits or exposure to other workplace respiratory carcinogens.[102–108]

Nutrition: Antioxidants and Fat Epidemiologic studies have provided evidence about the nature of dietary deficiencies and excesses that have influenced the risk of lung cancer. The most consistent association, gathered from case-control and cohort studies, was that increased consumption of fresh vegetables and fruits lowered the risk in men and women, in current or former smokers, or particularly among never-smokers, and for all histologic types. The higher levels of consumption, when compared with the lowest reference level, tended to be associated with 40% to 50% reduction in the smoking-, age-, and gender-adjusted RR of lung cancer of various cell types. Various antioxidants were considered as putative chemopreventive nutrients, but a major focus has been on the provitamin A carotenoids, particularly β-carotene. Some investigators have reported that β-carotene was most protective in current or heavy smokers, whereas others have found that β-carotene or carotenoids were most protective in former smokers or in nonsmokers.[109–113] In a population-based case-control study of lung cancer in nonsmokers conducted in New York State, Holick et al.[114] concluded that the increased consumption of raw (not cooked) fruits and vegetables was associated with a significantly reduced risk for lung cancer. Dietary β-carotene (odds ratio = 0.70; 95% CI, 0.50 to 0.99), but not dietary retinol (vitamin A), was significantly associated with risk reduction for lung cancer in nonsmoking men and women.

By the mid-1980s, large-scale randomized clinical trials of β-carotene, β-carotene plus retinol, or β-carotene and/or vitamin E were initiated in subjects at increased risk of lung cancer. The α-tocopherol/β-carotene trial (ATBC) in Finland was a primary prevention trial among over 29,000 male smokers of 50 to 69 years of age. The 2×2 factorial design evaluated 20-mg β-carotene and/or 50-IU α-tocopherol (vitamin E) daily for 6.5 years. These doses represented a fivefold excess over the median intake of α-tocopherol and a 10-fold excess over the median intake of β-carotene in the general population. When compared with placebo groups, supplementation with vitamin E did not alter lung cancer incidence; however, participants receiving β-carotene alone or in combination with α-tocopherol had significantly higher lung cancer incidence (RR = 1.18; 95% CI, 1.03 to 1.36). The excess lung cancer incidence was demonstrable after the initial 18 months. The randomized design and analysis controlled for cigarette smoking history.[115]

The Carotene and Retinol Efficacy Trial (CARET) was a multicenter randomized trial to test whether oral administration of the combination of β-carotene (30 mg/day) and retinyl palmitate (25,000 IU/day) would decrease lung cancer incidence in high-risk populations of female smokers and male smokers and/or exposed asbestos workers. In the treatment group, when compared with the placebo group, the RR, after an average follow-up of 4 years, of death from lung cancer was 1.46 (95% CI, 1.07 to 2.00). The RRs were elevated in current smokers.[116,117] After 12 years of follow-up in the placebo arm of CARET, a significant protective effect was observed with total fruit or cruciferous vegetable consumption. The RR for highest versus lowest quintile of total fruit consumption in the placebo arm was 0.56 (95% CI, 0.39 to 0.81); for cruciferous vegetables, the RR was 0.68 (95% CI, 0.45 to 1.04).[118]

The Physicians' Health Study was a long-term randomized trial organized to test the effect of aspirin on cardiovascular disease incidence. β-Carotene (50 mg) was added in a 2×2 factorial design. In this healthy male population with 11% current cigarette smokers, and after an average follow-up of 12.5 years, the investigators concluded that the intervention did not reduce or increase the incidence of lung cancer (RR = 0.93).[119,120]

It is disconcerting and challenging to reflect about the lack of demonstrable benefit or even an adverse outcome of increased risk of lung cancer in smoking men and women participating in various chemoprevention clinical trials. The results of these clinical trials would appear to contradict the epidemiologic observational studies. β-Carotene is only one of many carotenoids ingested in vegetables and fruits and, under conditions of increased oxidative stress as in exposure to cigarette smoke or asbestos, β-carotene can be oxidized to an epoxide or reactive electrophilic derivative that would be mitogenic rather than inhibitory of cell proliferation. Handelman et al.[121]

exposed human plasma to the gas phase of cigarette smoke and observed oxidative disruption of carotenoids and α-tocopherol. In addition to carotenoids, fresh fruits and vegetables contain other micronutrients including vitamin C, folic acid, flavones, isoflavonoids (e.g., soy products), protease inhibitors, thiocyanates, and indoles (e.g., indole-3-carbinol in *Brassica* vegetables). Methyl-deficient diets result from low consumption of fruits and vegetables (folate) and of poultry, fish, and dairy products (methionine). Folic acid, methionine, and choline are interrelated in methyl group metabolism. Selective growth and transformation of cells can result from DNA hypomethylation and overexpression of proto-oncogenes or hypermethylation of CpG islands in promoter regions that may attenuate the expression of tumor suppressor genes. In the cohort study of health professionals by Feskanich et al.,[122] both fruits and vegetables, consumed with regular frequency were protective for lung cancer in women and men who never smoked (RR = 0.63; 95% CI, 0.35 to 1.12). In the study by Shen et al.,[123] the association with folate was most apparent among former heavy smokers.

Various chemopreventive mechanisms of action by micronutrients and nonnutritive phytochemicals in fruits and vegetables have been suggested by in vitro and animal feeding experimental studies. Chemoprevention refers to the use of natural or synthetic agents to reverse, prevent, or delay the progression of preneoplastic or preinvasive neoplastic disease. The complex interrelated mechanisms by which substances in vegetables and fruits may inhibit carcinogenesis include regulation of cell differentiation, "quenching" or "trapping" of oxygen or hydroxyl free radicals, preventing the formation of electrophilic metabolites from precursor compounds by inhibiting the enzymatic activation pathway (e.g., cytochrome P450) or by inducing the detoxification pathway (e.g., glutathione S-transferase [GST]), enhancing DNA methylation, inhibiting the expression of oncogenes, and stimulating immune function.[124]

Lung cancer mortality is significantly positively correlated in various countries with per capita fat availability and consumption. An increased risk of lung cancer has been reported in association with high dietary intake of foods rich in fat and cholesterol, or with elevated indices of abdominal adiposity. However, the positive association of dietary cholesterol and lung cancer risk has not been reflected in studies of serum cholesterol levels. Shekelle et al.[125] have hypothesized that a low, not elevated, serum cholesterol is predictive of increased risk of lung cancer, particularly in the subgroup of the population with low intake of β-carotene. Studies of the effects of dietary cholesterol and total and saturated fat have attempted to control for the confounding effects of gender, smoking status, and total intake of energy, fruits, vegetables, and carotenoids. In the study by Alavanja et al.[126] in female smokers in Missouri, a significant association was noted between intake of saturated fat and lung cancer. Despite the positive association with dietary fat, lung cancer risk was not associated with increasing body mass; indeed, several studies have described elevated risks in subgroups in the lowest categories of body mass index, which were not explained by confounding from cigarette smoking.[127,128] Although the potential association of specific histologic types of lung cancer with body fat distribution should be investigated further as suggested by Olson et al.,[129] the considerable inconsistencies in the associations with cholesterol and fat do not suggest that dietary fat intake has a major etiologic role.

Nonneoplastic Lung Diseases: Chronic Inflammation, Chronic Obstructive Pulmonary Disease, and Pulmonary Fibrosis Lung cancer risk has been reported to be increased among persons with a history of tuberculosis, pulmonary fibrosis as in silicosis, or chronic bronchitis and emphysema. An increased risk of lung cancer following the diagnosis of tuberculosis has been reported in cohort and case-control studies. For example, in a population-based case-control study of lung cancer that was conducted in Shanghai, Zheng et al.[130] reported that the age-, sex-, and smoking-adjusted odds ratio or RR of lung cancer was increased by 50% (95% CI, 1.2 to 1.8) among all survivors of tuberculosis, and by 100% among those diagnosed with tuberculosis within the previous 20 years. Among men, prior infection was reported by 26% of the cases and by 20% of the controls. The RR of lung cancer was higher for adenocarcinoma than for squamous or oat-cell carcinoma, and the locations of the granulomatous fibrotic lesions were highly correlated with that of the lung cancers. Based on the estimation of RR and the proportion of the population in Shanghai exposed to pulmonary tuberculosis, 9% of lung cancer cases were attributed to prior infection. In a case-control study by Hinds et al.,[131] the RR of lung cancer in never-smoking women in Hawaii with prior tuberculosis was increased significantly (OR = 8.2; 95% CI, 1.3 to 54.4).

The IARC has classified silica as a "probable" lung carcinogen (2A). Inhalation of silica causes both lung fibrosis and cancer in rats, but fibrosis in the absence of cancer has been observed in mice. For workers exposed to crystalline silica, with clinical indication of pneumoconiosis, as reported in 12 cohort and 3 case-control studies, the combined RR of lung cancer was 1.33 (95% CI, 1.12 to 1.45).[132] In a metaanalysis of lung cancer mortality among patients with silicosis, Smith et al.[133] reported a pooled estimated RR of 2.2 (95% CI, 2.1 to 2.4). RRs have been elevated in workers with increased exposure to silica dust that is incurred in mining and quarrying, and in the granite, ceramics and glass, and foundry industries. In underground mining, exposure to silicon dioxide or crystalline silica may be confounded by exposure to radon and its α-particle progeny, diesel fumes, asbestos, and other occupational carcinogens, and/or to tobacco smoke. Increased risk appears to vary with the severity of pulmonary fibrosis or with clinical signs of obstructive lung disease that accompanies chronic silicosis. The excess risk of lung cancer reported in previous studies has persisted after adjusting for smoking or has not been associated with excess risks for other smoking-related cancers, as in the upper digestive or urinary tract organs.[134]

Cigarette smoking may result in COPD and/or emphysema, and/or lung cancer. In the early 1960s, Passey[135] hypothesized that it was the irritating properties of tobacco smoke, resulting in chronic bronchitis and inflammatory destruction of lung tissue, which was of pathogenic significance in the causal pathway of lung cancer, rather than any direct action by volatile and particulate carcinogens in tobacco smoke. The experiments of Kuschner,[136] however, suggested an alternative explanation; namely that bronchial and bronchiolar inflammation, accompanied by reactive proliferation, squamous metaplasia, and dysplasia in basal epithelial cells, provided a cocarcinogenic mechanism for neoplastic cell transformation upon exposure to polycyclic aromatic hydrocarbons. Continued smoking in association with COPD, when accompanied by moderate or marked cytological atypia in exfoliated cells in the sputum, was significantly predictive of lung cancer in the Colorado Cancer Center Sputum Screening Cohort Study.[137]

Although cigarette smoking is the predominant cause of COPD, with an estimated attributable (etiologic) risk fraction exceeding 80% in smoking affected individuals, perhaps only 10% to 15% of current smokers will eventually develop clinically significant sequellae of productive cough, exertional dyspnea, and cardiovascular disease.[138,139] There are at least 10 cohort studies indicating that chronic obstructive airway disease is an independent predictor of lung cancer risk, and numerous studies reporting an increased risk of lung cancer among adults with asthma (Table 1.6).[140–149]

Chronic cigarette smoking retards mucociliary clearance of foreign particulates and respiratory tract secretions, evokes an inflammatory response accompanied by fibrosis and thickening in the membranous and respiratory bronchioles, and causes mucus gland hypertrophy, hyperplasia, and dysplasia in the proximal airways.[150] The manifestations of COPD signal the extent of bronchopulmonary structural and functional damage arising from the interaction of sustained exposure to toxic products of tobacco combustion and host susceptibility. In this context, COPD is both a biomarker of both exposure dose level and tissue susceptibility. A more controversial issue would be that of how COPD impacts the development of lung cancer. A conceptual model is proposed that incorporates the potential cocarcinogenic effects of chronic obstructive inflammatory disease in the causal pathway of cigarette smoke and lung cancer. The molecular events in the natural history of lung cancer comprise multiple genetic mutations that are determinants of neoplastic transformation and tumor progression, and the elaboration of autocrine growth factors that influence the clonal behavior and morphologic features of neoplastic cells. Chronic inflammation in the proximal and distal bronchial airways is an important cause of obstructive symptoms and provides the dynamic setting for oxidative stress and the formation of free radicals that accompany the reparative proliferative response. Increased proliferation kinetics and the interaction of hydroxyl radicals with DNA augment the likelihood of DNA structural and transcriptional errors.

GENE–ENVIRONMENT INTERACTIONS

Both genetic and environmental factors affect lung cancer risks, but the molecular pathophysiology of gene–environment interactions is complex. The genes influencing cancer susceptibility may consist of heterogeneous alleles at one locus or a combination of alleles at multiple loci. In a study of familial aggregation of lung cancer, Tokuhata and Lilienfeld[151] reported a significantly increased risk of lung cancer mortality among nonsmoking relatives of lung cancer cases when compared with nonsmoking relatives of age-, race-, and sex-matched controls. Kreuzer et al.[5] concluded that lung cancer in a first-degree relative was associated with a 2.6-fold increase in risk of lung cancer in cases diagnosed in patients younger than 50 years of age. A similar pattern of familial aggregation limited to probands with lung cancer diagnosed at a younger age than the median age in the general population was reported by Bromen et al.[152] In a segregation analysis involving 337 high-risk families with lung cancer, Sellers et al.[153] described a pattern of autosomal codominant inheritance, and hypothesized that segregation at the putative gene locus would account for 69% of the lung cancer cases diagnosed in persons up to age 50 years. Samet et al.[154] concluded that the personal risk of lung cancer was increased more than fivefold if at least one parent had lung cancer. In a study of families of women with lung cancer, an odds ratio gradient was noted: never-smoker with a positive family history (5.7), smoker with a negative family history (15.1), and smoker with a positive family history (30.0).[155] Familial aggregation of lung cancer may be attributed to shared exposures to tobacco smoking or other environmental and/or heritable determinants. On the assumption that a lung cancer susceptibility gene with a frequency of 0.3 to 0.5 would increase the risk of lung cancer in carriers, then an autosomal recessive model of inheritance would predict that siblings of cases would manifest a twofold to fourfold increased RR of lung cancer.[156]

Multiple inherited and acquired mechanisms of susceptibility to lung cancer have been proposed. Individual susceptibility to tobacco-induced lung cancer may be dependent on competitive gene–enzyme interactions that affect activation or detoxification of procarcinogens and levels of DNA adduct formation, or on the integrity of endogenous mechanisms for repairing lesions in DNA.[157] Nicotine is converted to cotinine in a two-step enzymatic process for which the rate-limiting step is the drug-metabolizing enzyme, cytochrome P450, a genetically polymorphic enzyme. Glucuronyl transferase enzymes conjugate and inactivate carcinogenic compounds, including 4-(methylnitrosamino)-1-(3-pyridyl)-1-butanone (NNK), the tobacco-specific methylnitrosamino metabolite, a potent procarcinogen in tobacco smoke. In a case-control study by Nakachi et al.[158] in which they assessed DNA polymorphisms in the cytochrome P4501A1 gene in relationship to squamous cell lung carcinoma, persons with the susceptible genotype had a RR of 7.31 after adjusting for cigarette smoking history. DNA polymorphisms in the cytochrome P450 gene (CYP1A1), or aromatic hydrocarbon hydroxylase, which is responsible for the metabolic activation of benzo(a)pyrene and other polyaromatic hydrocarbons, may represent a locus of a susceptibility gene for lung cancer. Increased activity of CYP1A1 has been demonstrated in lung cancer cells when compared with normal tissue in the same patient, suggesting that dysregulation of the gene may occur in carcinogenesis. However, no association between lung cancer and CYP1A1

TABLE 1.6 Review of Cohort Studies of Chronic Obstructive Pulmonary Disease and Lung Cancer

Author	Sources of Exposed and Nonexposed	Person-Years and Interval of Follow-up	Index of Risk	Age, Smoking-Adjusted Relative Risk (95% CI)	Commentary
Peto et al.[140]	2718 British men 25–64 years of age identified in random surveys conducted in 1954–1961.	20–25 years of follow-up.	Maximal value for: FEV_1 ÷ standing height^3 (Ht^3) chronic phlegm production by questionnaire.	When index of airway obstruction exceeded 2 SD below average (108 men) risk of lung cancer mortality increased, 1.3. Mucus hypersecretion was predictive of 40% increased risk of lung cancer, after adjustment for FEV_1/Ht^3.	Mucus hypersecretion was not predictive of COPD mortality, but was correlated with lung cancer mortality.
Skillrud et al.[141]	93 men, 20 women, 45–59 years of age from rural area of SE Minnesota; 123 controls treated for fractures, dental extractions; Matched on age, sex, occupation, smoking history.	1973–1974 until 1984.	% predicted FEV_1 ≤70% compared with FEV_1 ≥85%.	10-year cumulative probability in men: 0.108/0.025 = 4.32 (0.93, 19.99).	No lung cancer cases in women.
Tockman et al.[142]	Screening and early detection for lung cancer clinical trial at John Hopkins: 3728 white men, 45 years and older, who smoked at least 1 pack of cigarettes per day. Intermittent positive-pressure breathing trial (IPPB), 667 white men, 30–74 years of age, with COPD.	Lung cancer screening: 4436 pack-years or <2 years IPPB trial: 2001 pack-year or 3 years followed.	FEV_1 > 60% of predicted value compared with ≤60%. FEV_1/FVC ≤60% chronic cough and shortness of breath.	Lung cancer screening trial: 2.72 (0.98, 7.55) IPPB trial: 4.85.	Presence of symptoms of chronic cough or shortness of breath did not contribute significantly to lung cancer risk after adjustment for FEV_1 % predicted.
Tenkanen et al.[143]	Three urban and three rural areas in Finland; 4452 men, selected by sampling birth cohorts, 1898–1902, 1903–1907, 1908–1917, from electoral lists.	Follow-up period, 1964–1980.	Phlegm, all day for at least 3 months each year. Shortness of breath when walking. Wheezing.	Phlegm = 1.9 ($p < 0.001$) Shortness of breath = 1.6 ($0.05 < p < 0.10$) controlling for other symptoms, smoking, age Severe wheezing alone was not associated with significant increase in risk of lung cancer.	Significant lung cancer risk was associated with severe level of phlegm production, even after controlling for smoking, shortness of breath, and wheezing.

TABLE 1.6 Review of Cohort Studies of Chronic Obstructive Pulmonary Disease and Lung Cancer *(continued)*

Author	Sources of Exposed and Nonexposed	Person-Years and Interval of Follow-up	Index of Risk	Age, Smoking-Adjusted Relative Risk (95% CI)	Commentary
Kuller et al.[144]	Cigarette-smoking men (N = 8194) participating in the Multiple Risk Factor Intervention Trial. Of the above, 6075 (75%) had satisfactory pulmonary function measurements. Aged 35–57 years of age at entry.	Average follow-up, 10.5 years (1973–1984); However, the FEV_1 measurements were obtained at year 3, thus allowing for 0.5 years of follow-up.	FEV_1 levels distributed into quintiles. For example, lowest quintile included ≤2670 mL, highest quintile, ≥3749 mL.	FEV_1 (lowest) ÷ FEV_1 (highest) = 3.57 (0.94, 12.5) Proportional hazards model was compatible with 40% reduction in risk with increase in FEV_1 of 1000 mL.	Production of phlegm for >3 months in a year was a significant predictor of lung cancer, after adjusting for age, smoking, and FEV_1. There was no relation between baseline shortness of breath and subsequent lung cancer mortality.
Lange et al.[145]	Population-based sample of 7573 women and 6373 men who were participants in the Copenhagen City Heart Study.	Average follow-up period of about 10 years.	% predicted FEV_1, FEV_1/FVC%, chronic phlegm (3 months each year for >1 year).	Cox regression model controlling for age, sex, cigarette smoking. % predicted FEV_1: 40–79 = 2.1 (1.3, 3.4) <40 = 3.9 (2.2, 7.2) FEV_1 ÷ FVC <0.6 = 2.6	
Vestbo et al.[146]	Random sample (6.6%) of all men (N = 876), 46–69 years of age, living in city in Denmark, 1973.	1974–1985, 12,134 pack-years Cancer incidence was based on the Danish Cancer Registry.	Chronic phlegm (lasting ≥3 months), cough, or shortness of breath. FEV_1 per liter, under the expected FEV_1 given the height. Chronic bronchitis (defined as cough and phlegm lasting ≥3 months for ≥2 years).	Cox regression model using age as the underlying time scale: FEV_1 = 2.1 (1.3, 3.4) cough = 2.5 (1.3, 5.0) dyspnea = 2.2 (1.0, 4.9) phlegm = 1.2 (0.5, 3.0) chronic bronchitis = 0.8 (0.3, 2.7)	Regression coefficients did not differ between women and men. Among subjects who reported chronic phlegm at enrollment, only 54% reported it on reexamination 5 years later. Dyspnea was significant predictor of COPD and overall mortality.
Nomura et al.[147]	6317 Japanese-American men residing on Hawaiian island of Oahu, who were 45–68 years of age at entry.	19-year follow-up survey subsequent to examination in 1965–1968.	% predicted FEV_1, quartile distribution. Highest quartile category (>103.5%) was baseline in estimating relative risk.	Lowest quartile % predicted FEV_1 = 2.1 (1.3, 3.5) (<84.5%)	Only 2% of the cohort had % predicted FEV_1 of <60%. The data suggested that subjects with % predicted FEV_1 below 94.5%, after controlling for age and smoking, were at increased risk of lung cancer (95% CI, 1.3–4.1).

(continues)

TABLE 1.6 Review of Cohort Studies of Chronic Obstructive Pulmonary Disease and Lung Cancer *(continued)*

Author	Sources of Exposed and Nonexposed	Person-Years and Interval of Follow-up	Index of Risk	Age, Smoking-Adjusted Relative Risk (95% CI)	Commentary
Islam and Schottenfeld[148]	2099 women and 1857 men, 25 years of age or older when first examined from 1962–1965 in Tecumseh, Michigan.	Minimum of 15 years of follow-up.	Lung cancer incidence in relation to baseline ventilatory lung function and cigarette smoking status; average annual decline in FEV_1 (mL/yr); Cox proportional hazards regression model with % predicted FEV_1.	Among smoking men and women, those in lowest quartile % FEV_1 were at 2.7 times the risk of lung cancer compared with highest quartile. With each 10% decrease in % FEV_1, the risk of lung cancer increased 1.17 times, after controlling for age, sex, and cigarette smoking intensity.	Rapidly declining ventilatory function in conjunction with persistent symptoms of chronic bronchitis in current smokers is predictive of increased risk of lung cancer.
Hole et al.[149]	7058 men and 8353 women, aged 45–64 years at baseline screening 1972–1976, as part of a general population study in Renfrew and Paisley, Scotland.	25-year prospective study with 36,270 pack-years in men and 42,907 pack-years in women.	FEV_1 relative to the predicted value, in relation to cause-specific mortality, adjusted for age, sex, social class, cigarette smoking. Cox proportional hazards regression model, with hazard ratios relative to highest quintile of FEV_1.	Hazard ratios for lung cancer in subjects in the lowest quintile of FEV_1 distribution: Men: 2.53 (1.69, 3.79) Women: 4.37 (1.84, 10.42)	Significant trends were observed among lifetime never-smokers with impaired FEV_1 for ischemic heart disease, stroke, and lung cancer. The gradients of risk of dying for a nonsmoker with a low % FEV_1 were similar to the relative risks for heavy smokers but with high quintile levels of pulmonary expiratory function.

polymorphisms was reported in studies in Finland conducted by Hirvonen and coworkers.[159,160]

The genetically controlled ability to metabolize the antihypertensive agent debrisoquine has been linked to the risk of lung cancer. The P450 gene (CYP2D6) that regulates debrisoquine metabolism appears to influence the metabolism of nicotine to cotinine and metabolic activation of NNK, which is a potent carcinogen in experimental animals. Those who are extensive metabolizers in the hydroxylation of a 10-mg test dose of debrisoquine, a dominant trait affecting up to 90% of the U.S. white population, have been characterized as being at increased risk of lung cancer. Caporaso et al.[161] had initially estimated the smoking-adjusted RR to be increased sixfold, but more recently, studies have suggested more modest increases that are twofold or have failed to demonstrate an association using either the debrisoquine metabolic phenotype or polymerase chain reaction assays for detecting the genotype.[162] Various phase II detoxification systems serve to modulate risk in relation to cumulative levels of exposure to chemical metabolites. GST alleles encode a family of enzymes that catalyze the conjugation of electrophilic substrates.[163,164]

Inherited genetic traits can influence an individual's smoking addictive behavior. The candidate genes affecting smoking behavior include the dopamine receptors, dopamine and serotonin transporter alleles, and the cytochrome P450 alleles (e.g., CYP2A6). These genetic factors collectively influence binding and metabolism of nicotine and other neurotransmitters.[165] Several case-control studies have suggested that subjects with deficiency of the GST-μ isoenzyme or the GSTM1 null genotype, may have a 10% to 60% increase in lung cancer risk. Metabolites of constituents of cigarette smoke, including polycyclic aromatic hydrocarbons, aryl amines, and nitrosamines are potential substrates for GSTM1. Some studies have also evaluated potential interactions between CYP1A1 and GSTM1 genotypes.[166] Studies in Japan have reported that subjects with the combined GSTM1 null genotype and CYP1A1 polymorphisms were at increased risk.[167] The risk appears to be greater than additive in cigarette smokers with homozygous deletions of GSTM1 and CYP1A1 polymorphisms. Alexandrov et al.[168] noted that with both variant genes, the concentration levels of benzo(a)pyrene diol epoxide adducts of DNA were increased in lung parenchyma.

It is now clear that human tumors result from a complex sequence of mutational events. The bronchial epithelium of sustained smokers progresses from squamous metaplasia, to dysplasia, to invasive carcinoma, which is accompanied by progressive genomic instability. Many of the genetic defects that have been described in somatic cells of lung neoplasms are acquired during adult life and are related to exposures to environmental carcinogens. Some genetic events, however, are inherited and are present in all somatic cells. Mechanistic interactions of genes and exogenous agents may result from environmental agents altering the expression of genes involved in the regulation of the cell cycle, intercellular signaling, cell cycle arrest, and apoptosis. Susceptibility genes, in addition, include those concerned with the fidelity of DNA repair, DNA replication, and genomic stability. Individuals with combinations of alleles that dysfunctionally controlled enzyme systems regulating activation or detoxification pathways may be at increased risk of lung cancer when exposed to even low dose levels of tobacco smoke or other mutagens. However, the validity and efficiency of screening for carcinogenic metabolites in predicting human lung cancer risk is questionable in the context of a population. Strategic targeting of phenotypic or genotypic testing as a cancer control measure in high-risk families, in conjunction with behavioral counseling, may be more cost-effective. In a cohort study of monozygotic and dizygotic twin pairs followed in the National Academy of Sciences/National Research Council Twin Registry, it was concluded that inherited predisposition was not demonstrable in relationship to smoking-induced lung cancer diagnosed in men older than 50 years.[169] If one were to assume that 50% of lung cancer deaths before the age of 50 result from genetic predispositions, this would represent only 5% of lung cancer deaths.

REFERENCES

1. Jemal A, Siegel R, Ward E, et al. Cancer statistics, 2008. *CA Cancer J Clin* 2008;58(2):71–96.
2. Shopland DR, Eyre HJ, Pechacek TF. Smoking-attributable cancer mortality in 1991: is lung cancer now the leading cause of death among smokers in the United States? *J Natl Cancer Inst* 1991;83:1142–1148.
3. *A Report of the Surgeon General: The Health Benefits of Smoking Cessation.* DHSS Pub. No. (CDC) 90-8416. U.S. Department of Health and Human Services, Public Health Service, Center for Chronic Disease Prevention and Health Promotion, 1990.
4. *A Report of the Surgeon General: Women and Smoking.* Washington, DC, U.S. Department of Health and Human Services: U.S. Government Printing Office, 2001.
5. Kreuzer M, Kreienbrock L, Gerken M, et al. Risk factors for lung cancer in young adults. *Am J Epidemiol* 1998;147:1028–1037.
6. Brownson RC, Chang JC, Davis JR. Gender and histologic type variations in smoking-related risk of lung cancer. *Epidemiology* 1992;3:61–64.
7. Risch HA, Howe GR, Jain M, et al. Are female smokers at higher risk for lung cancer than male smokers? A case-control analysis by histologic type. *Am J Epidemiol* 1993;138:281–293.
8. Zang EA, Wynder EL. Differences in lung cancer risk between men and women: examination of the evidence. *J Natl Cancer Inst* 1996;88:183–192.
9. Bain C, Feskanich D, Speizer FE, et al. Lung cancer rates in men and women with comparable histories of smoking. *J Natl Cancer Inst* 2004;96:826–834.
10. Freedman ND, Leitzmann MF, Hollenbeck AR, et al. Cigarette smoking and subsequent risk of lung cancer in men and women: analysis of a prospective cohort study. *Lancet Oncol* 2008;9:649–656.
11. Wagenknecht LE, Cutter GR, Haley NJ, et al. Racial differences in serum cotinine levels among smokers in the Coronary Artery Risk Development in (Young) Adults study. *Am J Public Health* 1990; 80:1053–156.
12. Markides KS, Coreil J, Ray LA. Smoking among Mexican Americans: a three-generation study. *Am J Public Health* 1987;77:708–711.
13. Marin G, Perez-Stable EJ, Marin BV. Cigarette smoking among San Francisco Hispanics: the role of acculturation and gender. *Am J Public Health* 1989;79:196–198.
14. Novotny TE, Warner KE, Kendrick JS, et al. Smoking by blacks and whites: socioeconomic and demographic differences. *Am J Public Health* 1988;78:1187–1189.
15. Pierce JP, Fiore MC, Novotny TE, et al. Trends in cigarette smoking in the United States. Educational differences are increasing. *JAMA* 1989;261:56–60.
16. Stellman SD, Resnicow K. Tobacco smoking, cancer and social class. In: Kogevinas M, Pearce N, Susser M, et al., eds. *Social Inequalities and Cancer.* Lyon, France IARC Scientific Publications No. 138,1997:229.
17. Parkin DM, Pisani P, Ferlay J. Global cancer statistics. *CA Cancer J Clin* 1999;49:33–64.
18. Magrath I, Litvak J. Cancer in developing countries: opportunity and challenge. *J Natl Cancer Inst* 1993;85:862–874.
19. Borras JM, Fernandez E, Gonzalez JR, et al. Lung cancer mortality in European regions (1955–1997). *Ann Oncol* 2003;14:159–161.
20. Bray F, Tyczynski JE, Parkin DM. Going up or coming down? The changing phases of the lung cancer epidemic from 1967 to 1999 in the 15 European Union countries. *Eur J Cancer* 2004;40:96–125.
21. Law CH, Day NE, Shanmugaratnam K. Incidence rates of specific histological types of lung cancer in Singapore Chinese dialect groups, and their aetiological significance. *Int J Cancer* 1976;17:304–309.
22. MacLennan R, Da Costa J, Day NE, et al. Risk factors for lung cancer in Singapore Chinese, a population with high female incidence rates. *Int J Cancer* 1977;20:854–860.
23. Hecht SS. Cigarette smoking and lung cancer: chemical mechanisms and approaches to prevention. *Lancet Oncol* 2002;3:461–469.
24. Hecht SS. Tobacco smoke carcinogens and lung cancer. *J Natl Cancer Inst* 1999;91:1194–1120.
25. *Tobacco Smoking.* IARC Monographs on the Evaluation of Carcinogenic Risk of Chemicals to Humans. Vol. 38. Lyon, France, International Agency for Research on Cancer (IARC), 1986.
26. Advisory Committee to the Surgeon General of the U.S. Public Health Service. *Smoking and Health.* PHS Pub. No. 1103. Washington, DC: U.S. Government Printing Office, 1964.
27. Hammond EC. Smoking in relation to the death rates of one million men and women. *Natl Cancer Inst Monogr* 1966;19:127–204.
28. Doll R, Peto R. Mortality in relation to smoking: 20 years' observations on male British doctors. *Br Med J* 1976;2:1525–1536.
29. Rogot E, Murray JL. Smoking and causes of death among U.S. veterans: 16 years of observation. *Public Health Rep* 1980;15:213–222.

30. Harris JE. Cigarette smoking among successive birth cohorts of men and women in the United States during 1900–80. *J Natl Cancer Inst* 1983;71:473–479.
31. Fiore MC, Novotny TE, Pierce JP, et al. Trends in cigarette smoking in the United States. The changing influence of gender and race. *JAMA* 1989;261:49–55.
32. *Morbidity and Mortality Weekly Report.* Cigarette smoking among young adults—United States, 2000. Vol. 51. Massachusetts Medical Society, 2002.
33. Garfinkel L, Stellman SD. Smoking and lung cancer in women: findings in a prospective study. *Cancer Res* 1988;48:6951–6955.
34. Stellman SD, Garfinkel L. Lung cancer risk is proportional to cigarette tar yield: evidence from a prospective study. *Prev Med* 1989;18:518–525.
35. Stellman SD, Garfinkel L. Smoking habits and tar levels in a new American Cancer Society prospective study of 1.2 million men and women. *J Natl Cancer Inst* 1986;76:1057–1063.
36. Lubin JH, Blot WJ, Berrino F, et al. Patterns of lung cancer risk according to type of cigarette smoked. *Int J Cancer* 1984;33:569–576.
37. Wilcox HB, Schoenberg JB, Mason TJ, et al. Smoking and lung cancer: risk as a function of cigarette tar content. *Prev Med* 1988;17:263–272.
38. Doll R, Peto R. Cigarette smoking and bronchial carcinoma: dose and time relationships among regular smokers and lifelong non-smokers. *J Epidemiol Community Health* 1978;32:303–313.
39. Halpern MT, Gillespie BW, Warner KE. Patterns of absolute risk of lung cancer mortality in former smokers. *J Natl Cancer Inst* 1993;85:457–464.
40. Mao L, Lee JS, Kurie JM, et al. Clonal genetic alterations in the lungs of current and former smokers. *J Natl Cancer Inst* 1997;89:857–862.
41. Aoyagi Y, Yokose T, Minami Y, et al. Accumulation of losses of heterozygosity and multistep carcinogenesis in pulmonary adenocarcinoma. *Cancer Res* 2001;61:7950–7954.
42. Abelin T, Gsell OR. Relative risk of pulmonary cancer in cigar and pipe smokers. *Cancer* 1967;20:1288–1296.
43. Shapiro JA, Jacobs EJ, Thun MJ. Cigar smoking in men and risk of death from tobacco-related cancers. *J Natl Cancer Inst* 2000;92:333–337.
44. Boffetta P, Pershagen G, Jöckel KH, et al. Cigar and pipe smoking and lung cancer risk: a multicenter study from Europe. *J Natl Cancer Inst* 1999;91:697–701.
45. Bryant MS, Vineis P, Skipper PL, et al. Hemoglobin adducts of aromatic amines: associations with smoking status and type of tobacco. *Proc Natl Acad Sci U S A* 1988;85:9788–9791.
46. U.S. Surgeon General. *The Health Consequences of Involuntary Smoking.* CDC Pub No. 87-8398. Washington, DC: U.S. Department of Health and Human Services, 1986.
47. Hirayama T. Non-smoking wives of heavy smokers have a higher risk of lung cancer: a study from Japan. *Br Med J (Clin Res Ed)* 1981;282:183–185.
48. Trichopoulos D, Kalandidi A, Sparros L. Lung cancer and passive smoking: conclusion of Greek study. *Lancet* 1983;2:677–678.
49. Trichopoulos D, Kalandidi A, Sparros L, et al. Lung cancer and passive smoking. *Int J Cancer* 1981;27:1–4.
50. Garfinkel L. Time trends in lung cancer mortality among nonsmokers and a note on passive smoking. *J Natl Cancer Inst* 1981;66:1061–1066.
51. Correa P, Pickle LW, Fontham E, et al. Passive smoking and lung cancer. *Lancet* 1983;2:595–597.
52. Koo LC, Ho JH, Saw D. Is passive smoking an added risk factor for lung cancer in Chinese women? *J Exp Clin Cancer Res* 1984;3:277–284.
53. Wu AH, Henderson BE, Pike MC, et al. Smoking and other risk factors for lung cancer in women. *J Natl Cancer Inst* 1985;74:747–751.
54. Garfinkel L, Auerbach O, Joubert L. Involuntary smoking and lung cancer: a case-control study. *J Natl Cancer Inst* 1985;75:463–469.
55. Akiba S, Kato H, Blot WJ. Passive smoking and lung cancer among Japanese women. *Cancer Res* 1986;46:4804–4807.
56. Pershagen G, Hrubec Z, Svensson C. Passive smoking and lung cancer in Swedish women. *Am J Epidemiol* 1987;125:17–24.
57. Lam TH, Kung IT, Wong CM, et al. Smoking, passive smoking and histological types in lung cancer in Hong Kong Chinese women. *Br J Cancer* 1987;56:673–678.
58. Gao YT, Blot WJ, Zheng W, et al. Lung cancer among Chinese women. *Int J Cancer* 1987;40:604–609.
59. Janerich DT, Thompson WD, Varela LR, et al. Lung cancer and exposure to tobacco smoke in the household. *N Engl J Med* 1990;323:632–636.
60. Fontham ET, Correa P, WuWilliams A, et al. Lung cancer in nonsmoking women: a multicenter case-control study. *Cancer Epidemiol Biomarkers Prev* 1991;1:35–43.
61. Fontham ET, Correa P, Reynolds P, et al. Environmental tobacco smoke and lung cancer in nonsmoking women. A multicenter study. *JAMA* 1994;271:1752–1759.
62. Brownson RC, Alavanja MC, Hock ET, et al. Passive smoking and lung cancer in nonsmoking women. *Am J Public Health* 1992;82:1525–1530.
63. Stockwell HG, Goldman AL, Lyman GH, et al. Environmental tobacco smoke and lung cancer risk in nonsmoking women. *J Natl Cancer Inst* 1992;84:1417–1422.
64. Boffetta P, Agudo A, Ahrens W, et al. Multicenter case-control study of exposure to environmental tobacco smoke and lung cancer in Europe. *J Natl Cancer Inst* 1998;90:1440–1450.
65. Besaratinia A, Pfeifer GP. Second-hand smoke and human lung cancer. *Lancet Oncol* 2008;9:657–666.
66. National Research Council. *Environmental Tobacco Smoke.* Washington, DC: National Academy Press, 1986.
67. Doll R. Atmospheric pollution and lung cancer. *Environ Health Perspect* 1978;22:23–31.
68. Friberg L, Cederlöf R. Late effects of air pollution with special reference to lung cancer. *Environ Health Perspect* 1978;22:45–66.
69. Pope CA, III, Dockery DW, Schwartz J. Review of epidemiological evidence of health effects of particulate air pollution. *Inhal Toxicol* 1995;7:1–18.
70. Hammond EC, Selikoff IJ, Lawther PL, et al. Inhalation of benzpyrene and cancer in man. *Ann N Y Acad Sci* 1976;271:116–124.
71. Doll R, Vessey MB, Beasley RWR, et al. Mortality of gas workers—final report of a prospective study. *Br J Ind Med* 1972;29:394–406.
72. Hammond EC, Garfinkel L. General air pollution and cancer in the United States. *Prev Med* 1980;9:206–211.
73. *Diesel and Gasoline Exhausts and Some Nitroarenes: Evaluation of Carcinogenic Risk of Chemicals to Man.* Vol. 46. Lyon, France: International Agency for Research on Cancer (IARC), 1989.
74. Garshick E, Schenker MB, Muñoz A, et al. A retrospective cohort study of lung cancer and diesel exhaust exposure in railroad workers. *Am Rev Respir Dis* 1988;137:820–825.
75. Lan Q, Chapman RS, Schreinemachers DM, et al. Household stove improvement and risk of lung cancer in Xuanwei, China. *J Natl Cancer Inst* 2002;94:826–835.
76. Gao YT, Blot WJ, Zheng W, et al. Lung cancer and smoking in Shanghai. *Int J Epidemiol* 1988;17:277–280.
77. Xu ZY, Blot WJ, Xiao HP, et al. Smoking, air pollution, and the high rates of lung cancer in Shenyang, China. *J Natl Cancer Inst* 1989;81:1800–1806.
78. Wu-Williams AH, Dai XD, Blot W, et al. Lung cancer among women in north-east China. *Br J Cancer* 1990;62:982–987.
79. Cross FT. Invited commentary: residential radon risks from the perspective of experimental animal studies. *Am J Epidemiol* 1994;140:333–339.
80. Lagarde F, Axelsson G, Damber L, et al. Residential radon and lung cancer among never-smokers in Sweden. *Epidemiology* 2001;12:396–404.
81. Lubin JH, Boice JD Jr, Edling C, et al. Lung cancer in radon-exposed miners and estimation of risk from indoor exposure. *J Natl Cancer Inst* 1995;87:817–827.
82. Lubin JH, Boice JD Jr. Lung cancer risk from residential radon: meta-analysis of eight epidemiologic studies. *J Natl Cancer Inst* 1997;89:49–57.
83. Axelson O, Andersson K, Desai G, et al. Indoor radon exposure and active and passive smoking in relation to the occurrence of lung cancer. *Scand J Work Environ Health* 1988;14:286–292.
84. Pershagen G, Akerblom G, Axelson O, et al. Residential radon exposure and lung cancer in Sweden. *N Engl J Med* 1994;330:159–164.

85. Schoenberg JB, Klotz JB, Wilcox HB, et al. Case-control study of residential radon and lung cancer among New Jersey women. *Cancer Res* 1990;50:6520–6524.
86. Blot WJ, Xu ZY, Boice JD Jr, et al. Indoor radon and lung cancer in China. *J Natl Cancer Inst* 1990;82:1025–1030.
87. Létourneau EG, Krewski D, Choi NW, et al. Case-control study of residential radon and lung cancer in Winnipeg, Manitoba, Canada. *Am J Epidemiol* 1994;140:310–322.
88. Darby S, Whitley E, Silcocks P, et al. Risk of lung cancer associated with residential radon exposure in south-west England: a case-control study. *Br J Cancer* 1998;78:394–408.
89. Darby SC, Whitley E, Howe GR, et al. Radon and cancers other than lung cancer in underground miners: a collaborative analysis of 11 studies. *J Natl Cancer Inst* 1995;87:378–384.
90. Samet JM, Lerchen ML. Proportion of lung cancer caused by occupation: a critical review. In: Gee JB, Morgan WK, Brooks SM, eds. *Occupational Lung Disease.* New York: Raven Press, 1984:55.
91. Hughes JM, Weill H. Asbestos and man-made fibers. In: Samet JM, ed. *Epidemiology of Lung Cancer.* New York: Marcel Dekker, Inc., 1994:185.
92. Mossman BT. Carcinogenic potential of asbestos and nonasbestos fibers. *J Environ Sci Health* 1988;6:151–195.
93. Selikoff IJ, Hammond EC, Churg J. Asbestos exposure, smoking, and neoplasia. *JAMA* 1968;204:106–1012.
94. Saracci R. The interactions of tobacco smoking and other agents in cancer etiology. *Epidemiol Rev* 1987;9:175–193.
95. McDonald JC, Liddell FD, Gibbs GW, et al. Dust exposure and mortality in chrysotile mining, 1910–75. *Br J Ind Med* 1980;37:11–24.
96. Zwi AB, Reid G, Landau SP, et al. Mesothelioma in South Africa, 1976–84: incidence and case characteristics. *Int J Epidemiol* 1989;18:320–329.
97. Tagnon I, Blot WJ, Stroube RB, et al. Mesothelioma associated with the shipbuilding industry in coastal Virginia. *Cancer Res* 1980; 40:3875–3879.
98. Mossman BT, Gee JB. Asbestos-related diseases. *N Engl J Med* 1989;320:1721–1730.
99. Churg A. Lung asbestos content in long-term residents of a chrysotile mining town. *Am Rev Respir Dis* 1986;134:125–127.
100. Asbestos removal, health hazards, and the EPA. Council on Scientific Affairs, American Medical Association. *JAMA* 1991;266:696–697.
101. Acheson ED, Gardner MJ, Pippard EC, et al. Mortality of two groups of women who manufactured gas masks from chrysotile and crocidolite asbestos: a 40-year follow-up. *Br J Ind Med* 1982;39:344–348.
102. BéruBé KA, Quinlan TR, Moulton G, et al. Comparative proliferative and histopathologic changes in rat lungs after inhalation of chrysotile or crocidolite asbestos. *Toxicol Appl Pharmacol* 1996;137:67–74.
103. Goodman M, Morgan RW, Ray R, et al. Cancer in asbestos-exposed occupational cohorts: a meta-analysis. *Cancer Causes Control* 1999; 10:453–465.
104. Brody AR. Asbestos-induced lung disease. *Environ Health Perspect* 1993;100:21–30.
105. Gustavsson P, Nyberg F, Pershagen G, et al. Low-dose exposure to asbestos and lung cancer: dose-response relations and interaction with smoking in a population-based case-referent study in Stockholm, Sweden. *Am J Epidemiol* 2002;155:1016–1022.
106. *Man-made Mineral Fibers and Radon.* Vol. 43. Lyon, France: International Agency for Research on Cancer (IARC), 1988.
107. Marsh GM, Enterline PE, Stone RA, et al. Mortality among a cohort of US man-made mineral fiber workers: 1985 follow-up. *J Occup Med* 1990;32:594–604.
108. Lee IM, Hennekens CH, Trichopoulos D, et al. Man-made vitreous fibers and risk of respiratory system cancer: a review of the epidemiologic evidence. *J Occup Environ Med* 1995;37:725–738.
109. Bjelke E. Dietary vitamin A and human lung cancer. *Int J Cancer* 1975;15:561–565.
110. Mettlin C, Graham S, Swanson M. Vitamin A and lung cancer. *J Natl Cancer Inst* 1979;62:1435–1438.
111. World Cancer Research Fund/American Institute for Cancer Research. Food, Nutrition, Physical Activity, and the Prevention of Cancer: A Global Perspective. Lung cancer, Washington D.C., 2007:259–264.
112. Kvåle G, Bjelke E, Gart JJ. Dietary habits and lung cancer risk. *Int J Cancer* 1983;31:397–405.
113. Samet JM, Skipper BJ, Humble CG, et al. Lung cancer risk and vitamin A consumption in New Mexico. *Am Rev Respir Dis* 1985;131:198–202.
114. Holick CN, Michaud DS, Stolzenberg-Solomon R, et al. Dietary carotenoids, serum beta-carotene, and retinol and risk of lung cancer in the alpha-tocopherol, beta-carotene cohort study. *Am J Epidemiol* 2002;156:536–547.
115. The effect of vitamin E and beta carotene on the incidence of lung cancer and other cancers in male smokers. The Alpha-Tocopherol, Beta Carotene Cancer Prevention Study Group. *N Engl J Med* 1994; 330:1029–1035.
116. Omenn GS, Goodman GE, Thornquist MD, et al. Risk factors for lung cancer and for intervention effects in CARET, the Beta-Carotene and Retinol Efficacy Trial. *J Natl Cancer Inst* 1996;88:1550–1959.
117. Omenn GS. Chemoprevention of lung cancer: the rise and demise of beta-carotene. *Annu Rev Public Health* 1998;19:73–99.
118. Neuhouser ML, Patterson RE, Thornquist MD, et al. Fruits and vegetables are associated with lower lung cancer risk only in the placebo arm of the beta-carotene and retinol efficacy trial (CARET). *Cancer Epidemiol Biomarkers Prev* 2003;12:350–358.
119. Final report on the aspirin component of the ongoing Physicians' Health Study. Steering Committee of the Physicians' Health Study Research Group. *N Engl J Med* 1989;321:129–135.
120. Hennekens CH, Buring JE, Manson JE, et al. Lack of effect of long-term supplementation with beta carotene on the incidence of malignant neoplasms and cardiovascular disease. *N Engl J Med* 1996;334:1145–1149.
121. Handelman GJ, Packer L, Cross CE. Destruction of tocopherols, carotenoids, and retinol in human plasma by cigarette smoke. *Am J Clin Nutr* 1996;63:559–565.
122. Feskanich D, Ziegler RG, Michaud DS, et al. Prospective study of fruit and vegetable consumption and risk of lung cancer among men and women. *J Natl Cancer Inst* 2000;92:1812–1823.
123. Shen H, Wei Q, Pillow PC, et al. Dietary folate intake and lung cancer risk in former smokers:a case-control analysis. *Cancer Epidemiol Biomarkers Prev* 2003;12:980–986.
124. Soria JC, Kim ES, Fayette J, et al. Chemoprevention of lung cancer. *Lancet Oncol* 2003;4:659–669.
125. Shekelle RB, Tangney CC, Rossof AH, et al. Serum cholesterol, beta-carotene, and risk of lung cancer. *Epidemiology* 1992;3:282–287.
126. Alavanja MC, Brown CC, Swanson C, et al. Saturated fat intake and lung cancer risk among nonsmoking women in Missouri. *J Natl Cancer Inst* 1993;85:1906–1916.
127. Goodman MT, Wilkens LR. Relation of body size and risk of lung cancer. *Nutr Cancer* 1993;20:179–186.
128. Chyou PH, Nomura A, Stemmermann GN, et al. A prospective study of weight, body mass index and other anthropometric measurements in relation to site-specific cancers. *Int J Cancer* 1994;57:313–317.
129. Olson JE, Yang P, Schmitz K, et al. Differential association of body mass index and fat distribution with three major histologic types of lung cancer: evidence from a cohort of older women. *Am J Epidemiol* 2002;156:606–615.
130. Zheng W, Blot WJ, Liao ML, et al. Lung cancer and prior tuberculosis infection in Shanghai. *Br J Cancer* 1987;56:501–504.
131. Hinds MW, Cohen HI, Kolonel LN. Tuberculosis and lung cancer risk in nonsmoking women. *Am Rev Respir Dis* 1982;125:776–778.
132. Steenland K, Loomis D, Shy C, et al. Review of occupational lung carcinogens. *Am J Ind Med* 1996;29:474–490.
133. Smith AH, Lopipero PA, Barroga VR. Meta-analysis of studies of lung cancer among silicotics. *Epidemiology* 1995;6:617–624.
134. Pairon JC, Brochard P, Jaurand MC, et al. Silica and lung cancer: a controversial issue. *Eur Respir J* 1991;4:730–744.
135. Passey RD. Some problems of lung cancer. *Lancet* 1962;2:107–112.

136. Kuschner M. The causes of lung cancer. *Am Rev Respir Dis* 1968; 98:573–590.
137. Prindiville SA, Byers T, Hirsch FR, et al. Sputum cytological atypia as a predictor of incident lung cancer in a cohort of heavy smokers with airflow obstruction. *Cancer Epidemiol Biomarkers Prev* 2003;12: 987–993.
138. *The Health Consequences of Smoking: Chronic Obstructive Lung Disease. A Report of the Surgeon General.* DHHS Pub No. 84-50205. Washington, DC: U.S. Department of Health and Human Services, Office of Smoking and Health, 1984.
139. Calverley PM, Walker P. Chronic obstructive pulmonary disease. *Lancet* 2003;362:1053–1061.
140. Peto R, Speizer FE, Cochrane AL, et al. The relevance in adults of airflow obstruction, but not of mucus hypersecretion, to mortality from chronic lung disease. Results from 20 years of prospective observation. *Am Rev Respir Dis* 1983;128:491–500.
141. Skillrud DM, Offord KP, Miller RD. Higher risk of lung cancer in chronic obstructive pulmonary disease. A prospective, matched, controlled study. *Ann Intern Med* 1986;105:503–507.
142. Tockman MS, Anthonisen NR, Wright EC, et al. Airways obstruction and the risk for lung cancer. *Ann Intern Med* 1987;106:512–518.
143. Tenkanen L, Hakulinen T, Teppo L. The joint effect of smoking and respiratory symptoms on risk of lung cancer. *Int J Epidemiol* 1987;16:509–515.
144. Kuller LH, Ockene J, Meilahn E, et al. Relation of forced expiratory volume in one second (FEV1) to lung cancer mortality in the Multiple Risk Factor Intervention Trial (MRFIT). *Am J Epidemiol* 1990;132:265–274.
145. Lange P, Nyboe J, Appleyard M, et al. Ventilatory function and chronic mucus hypersecretion as predictors of death from lung cancer. *Am Rev Respir Dis* 1990;141:613–617.
146. Vestbo J, Knudsen KM, Rasmussen FV. Are respiratory symptoms and chronic airflow limitation really associated with an increased risk of respiratory cancer? *Int J Epidemiol* 1991;20:375–378.
147. Nomura A, Stemmermann GN, Chyou PH, et al. Prospective study of pulmonary function and lung cancer. *Am Rev Respir Dis* 1991;144:307–311.
148. Islam SS, Schottenfeld D. Declining FEV1 and chronic productive cough in cigarette smokers: a 25-year prospective study of lung cancer incidence in Tecumseh, Michigan. *Cancer Epidemiol Biomarkers Prev* 1994;3:289–298.
149. Hole DJ, Watt GC, Davey-Smith G, et al. Impaired lung function and mortality risk in men and women: findings from the Renfrew and Paisley prospective population study. *BMJ* 1996;313:711–715.
150. Wanner A, Salathé M, O'Riordan TG. Mucociliary clearance in the airways. *Am J Respir Crit Care Med* 1996;154:1868–1902.
151. Tokuhata GK, Lilienfeld AM. Familial aggregation of lung cancer among hospital patients. *Public Health Rep* 1963;78:277–283.
152. Bromen K, Pohlabeln H, Jahn I, et al. Aggregation of lung cancer in families: results from a population-based case-control study in Germany. *Am J Epidemiol* 2000;152:497–505.
153. Sellers TA, Bailey-Wilson JE, Elston RC, et al. Evidence for mendelian inheritance in the pathogenesis of lung cancer. *J Natl Cancer Inst* 1990; 82:1272–1279.
154. Samet JM, Humble CG, Pathak DR. Personal and family history of respiratory disease and lung cancer risk. *Am Rev Respir Dis* 1986; 134:466–470.
155. Horwitz RI, Smaldone LF, Viscoli CM. An ecogenetic hypothesis for lung cancer in women. *Arch Intern Med* 1988;148:2609–2612.
156. Peto J. Genetic predisposition to cancer. In: Cairns J, Lyon J, Skolnick M, eds. *Cancer Incidence in Defined Populations.* Cold Spring Harbor, NY: Cold Spring Harbor Laboratory, 1980:203.
157. Herbst RS, Heymach JV, Lippman SM. Molecular origins of cancer: lung cancer. *N Engl J Med* 2008;359:1367–1380.
158. Nakachi K, Imai K, Hayashi S, et al. Genetic susceptibility to squamous cell carcinoma of the lung in relation to cigarette smoking dose. *Cancer Res 1*991;51:5177–5180.
159. Hirvonen A, Husgafvel-Pursiainen K, Karjalainen A, et al. Point-mutational MspI and Ile-Val polymorphisms closely linked in the CYP1A1 gene: lack of association with susceptibility to lung cancer in a Finnish study population. *Cancer Epidemiol Biomarkers Prev* 1992;1:485–489.
160. Hirvonen A, Husgafvel-Pursiainen K, Anttila S, et al. PCR-based CYP2D6 genotyping for Finnish lung cancer patients. *Pharmacogenetics* 1993;3:19–27.
161. Caporaso NE, Tucker MA, Hoover RN, et al. Lung cancer and the debrisoquine metabolic phenotype. *J Natl Cancer Inst* 1990;82:1264–1272.
162. Shaw GL, Falk RT, Deslauriers J, et al. Debrisoquine metabolism and lung cancer risk. *Cancer Epidemiol Biomarkers Prev* 1995;4:41–48.
163. Shaw GL, Falk RT, Frame JN, et al. Genetic polymorphism of CYP2D6 and lung cancer risk. *Cancer Epidemiol Biomarkers Prev* 1998;7:215–219.
164. Nazar-Stewart V, Motulsky AG, Eaton DL, et al. The glutathione S-transferase mu polymorphism as a marker for susceptibility to lung carcinoma. *Cancer Res* 1993;53:2313–2318.
165. Arinami T, Ishiguro H, Onaivi ES. Polymorphisms in genes involved in neurotransmission in relation to smoking. *Eur J Pharmacol* 2000; 410:215–226.
166. Garcia-Closas M, Kelsey KT, Wiencke JK, et al. A case-control study of cytochrome P450 1A1, glutathione S-transferase M1, cigarette smoking and lung cancer susceptibility (Massachusetts, United States). *Cancer Causes Control* 1997;8:544–553.
167. Hayashi S, Watanabe J, Kawajiri K. High susceptibility to lung cancer analyzed in terms of combined genotypes of P450IA1 and Mu-class glutathione S-transferase genes. *Jpn J Cancer Res* 1992;83:866–870.
168. Alexandrov K, Cascorbi I, Rojas M, et al. CYP1A1 and GSTM1 genotypes affect benzo[a]pyrene DNA adducts in smokers' lung: comparison with aromatic/hydrophobic adduct formation. *Carcinogenesis* 2002;23:1969–1977.
169. Braun MM, Caporaso NE, Page WF, et al. Genetic component of lung cancer: cohort study of twins. *Lancet* 1994;344:440–443.
170. Hayes RB. The carcinogenicity of metals in humans. *Cancer Causes Control* 1997;8:371–385.
171. Boffetta P, Jourenkova N, Gustavsson P. Cancer risk from occupational and environmental exposure to polycyclic aromatic hydrocarbons. *Cancer Causes Control* 1997;8:444–472.
172. Bosetti C, La Vecchia C, Lipworth L, et al. Occupational exposure to vinyl chloride and cancer risk: a review of the epidemiologic literature. *Eur J Cancer Prev* 2003;12:427–430.

CHAPTER 2

Carolyn Dresler

The Tobacco Epidemic

Tobacco has a fascinating history. Tobacco is native only to the Americas and its scientific names include *Nicotiana rustica* and *Nicotiana tabacum*.[1] Tobacco was first experienced by Europeans when Columbus discovered the Americas in 1492 when they saw natives smoking "a kind of plant" while exploring what is now Cuba. The first two Europeans to see this smoking, Rodrigo de Jerez and interpreter Luis de Torres, even tried it themselves, becoming the first Europeans to experience tobacco.[1] Tobacco was brought back to the European countries where it rapidly spread in usage. Reportedly within 3 months after Columbus returned to Spain, the two Europeans to first experience tobacco were perpetual users of the plant. Quite quickly, the addictive nature of tobacco was noted by the Spanish, which was a novel experience for Europeans—this habitual use was felt to be un-Christian, and therefore declared a "sin."[1]

However, there was no turning back. Tobacco rapidly became a cash crop, with the product flowing from the New World to support the growing number of users in the Old World. Jamestown, much to the dismay of King James, was able to become solvent as a result of tobacco production from 1610 to 1620.[2] When King James could no longer prevent Jamestown from shipping tobacco, he placed the first New World tax—on tobacco![2] In many places in the new colonies, tobacco was used as a form of currency.[2] Tobacco cultivation spread throughout many of the colonies, and with the patent of the new Bonsack machine in 1881, which more efficiently mechanized production, the manufacturing of cigarettes began.[2] With the increasing widespread marketing of cigarettes, the death toll also began to increase.

Globally, in high-income countries, tobacco is the major causative agent for three of the top five causes of death for 2005: heart disease, stroke, lung cancer, lower respiratory infections, and chronic obstructive pulmonary disease (COPD).[3] It is predicted that by 2030, 8.3 million people globally will die from tobacco-induced disease, and tobacco will be responsible for 10% of all deaths globally.[4] Smokers will lose on average 10 years of life and 50% of people who smoke will die of a tobacco-related disease.[5] At present, globally there are a total of 848,132 lung cancer deaths in men (age-standardized rate [ASR]: 31.2) and 330,786 deaths in women (ASR: 10.3).[6] Overall, lung cancer is the number one cause of cancer deaths, accounting for 17.6% of the total number of deaths. Lung cancer is the leading cause of cancer death in men worldwide; however, the picture is a little more complicated with either breast or lung cancer being the number one cause of cancer deaths in women. The relationship of breast to lung cancer deaths often reflects the prevalence of smoking among women. Figure 2.1 illustrates the age-standardized incidence of lung cancer for regions around the world, which reflects the regions' historical use of tobacco.[6]

The tobacco epidemic is rapidly changing around the world, and it varies from country to country, mostly according to the state of economic development. Figure 2.2 illustrates the Lopez curve of the tobacco epidemic.[7] This model was developed from the 100-plus year history of smoking, particularly in the developed world. As demonstrated in Figure 2.2, a few decades after the peak in smoking prevalence, a country experiences a peak in lung cancer deaths. This model is even more powerful when gender is considered. When comparing gender-related prevalence and rate of deaths, the tobacco epidemic may then be divided into four stages. Stage I is one of quite low male and female prevalence of smoking and few smoking-related deaths. Many low-income countries, such as in sub-Saharan Africa, are in this stage. Stage II consists of a rapid rise in the number of male smokers to its peak, a start in the rise in female smokers, an upswing in the number of male deaths, but still few deaths in women. In stage III, the prevalence of male smoking begins to decline, female smoking is still increasing, and the rate of smoking-attributed male deaths is at its peak (around 30% of all deaths) with the rates for women beginning to sharply increase. In stage IV, female smoking peaks and then declines as male smoking continues

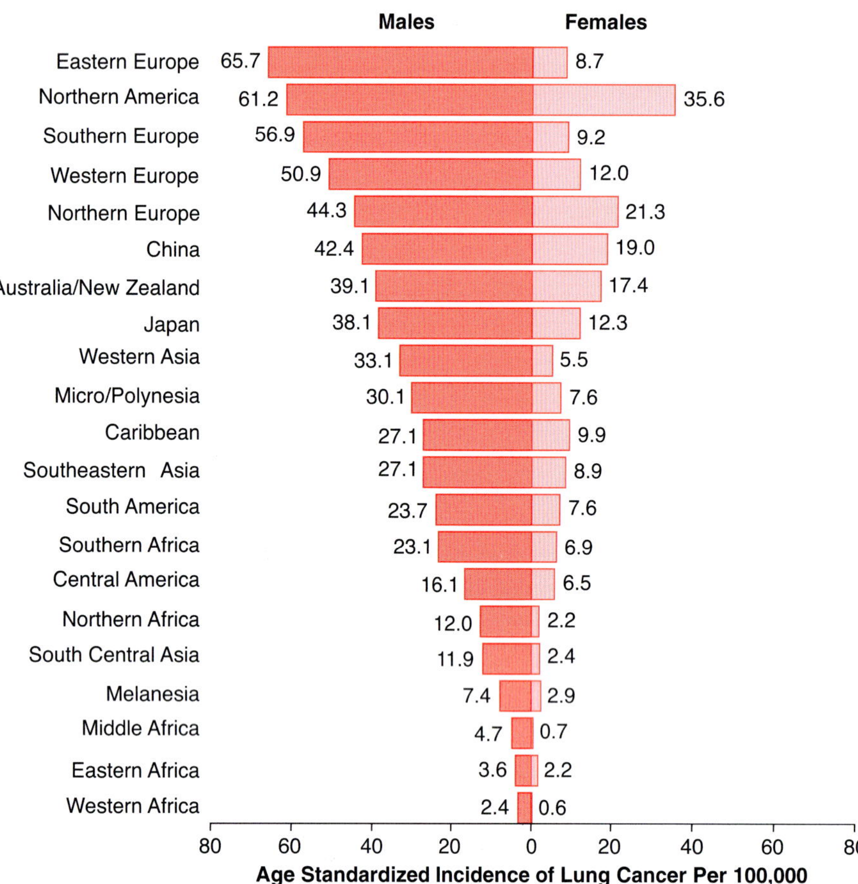

FIGURE 2.1 Age-standardized incidence of lung cancer for regions around the world. Data shown per 100,000 by sex. (From Parkin DM, Bray F, Ferlay J, et al. Global cancer statistics, 2002. *CA Cancer J Clin* 2005;55:74–108.)

to decline and smoking-attributable death for men and women decreases. Countries such as the United States and United Kingdom would be characteristic of stage IV, where the rates of female smoking–attributable deaths are just reaching their peaks, while the males rates have already started their decline.

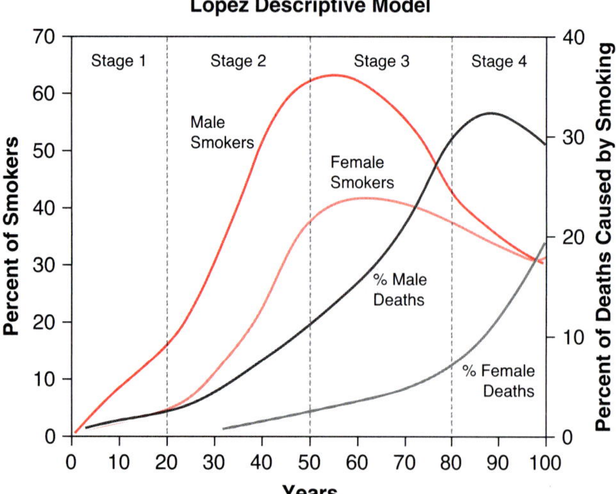

FIGURE 2.2 Stages of the tobacco epidemic—the Lopez Descriptive Model. (From Lopez AD, Collishaw NE, Piha T. A descriptive model of the cigarette epidemic in developed countries. *Tob Control* 1994;3:242–247.)

In the United States, cigarettes are by far the predominant form of tobacco consumption, as seen in Figure 2.3.[8] This pattern is seen around the world as the tobacco industry increasingly focuses outside of the more developed economies and into the more developing economies. The leading tobacco leaf importers are the Russian Federation, United States, Germany, Netherlands, Japan, United Kingdom, France, Belgium, Ukraine, and China. However, the top tobacco leaf exporters are very different: Brazil, China, United States, Zimbabwe, Italy, India, Turkey, Malawi, Greece, Argentina.[9] (China, Brazil, India, and the United States produce over two thirds of the 2004 global tobacco crop. India uses a significant proportion of their tobacco for smokeless use.)[9] Thus, the developing countries are more likely to grow and export the tobacco to the richer countries who then manufacture the finished cigarettes. In fact, Altria (the new name for Philip Morris) is the largest transnational tobacco manufacturer, and it is located in the United States. Philip Morris also has the number one global brand of cigarettes: Marlboro, and they sell them in 160 countries of the world.[9] The second largest company is British American Tobacco, located in the United Kingdom, and they have one seventh of the global market. Number three is Japan Tobacco and number four is Imperial Tobacco located in United Kingdom, and these four companies comprise 43% of the market. The largest tobacco manufacturer is the China National Tobacco Corporation, which controls 34% of the market—most of which is still within China. This, of course,

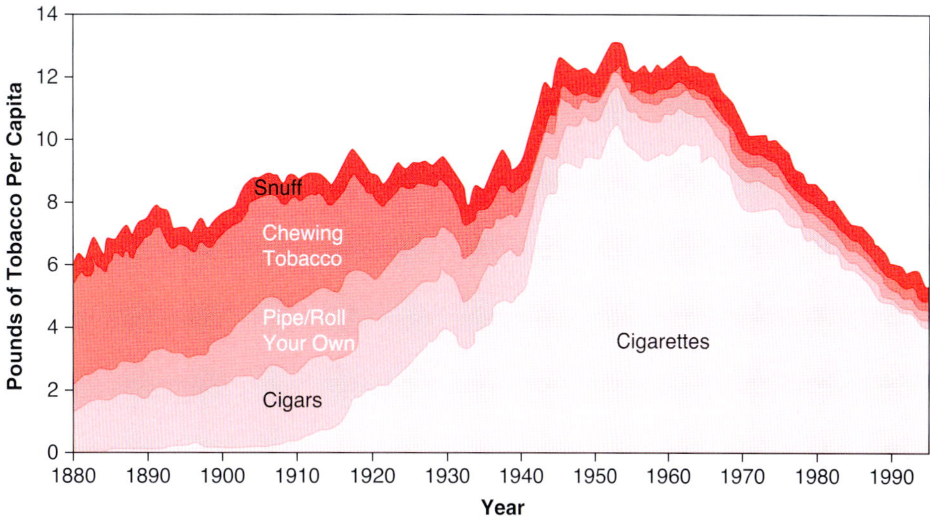

FIGURE 2.3 Per capita consumption of different forms of tobacco in the United States, 1880 to 1995. (From Burns DM, Lee L, Zhen LA, et al. Cigarette smoking behavior in the United States. In: Burns D, Garfinkel L, Samet J, eds. *Changes in Cigarette-Related Disease Risks and Their Implication for Prevention and Control; Monograph 8.* Bethesda, MD: National Institutes of Health, 1997:13.)

speaks to the size of the Chinese population and the approximately 60% of men who smoke.[9]

Global cigarette consumption has grown dramatically over the past few decades. The global cigarette consumption has gone from 10 billion sticks to 2150 billion sticks in 1960, to 5604 billion sticks in 2002, with an estimated 9 trillion cigarettes in 2025. The top five consumers of cigarettes are China, United States, Russian Federation, Japan and Indonesia.[9]

It is no wonder that the trends for tobacco-related deaths have steadily climbed as cigarette consumption increases. For example, the smoking-related mortality in men in the United Kingdom went from 27% in 1955 to 34% in 1985 and dropped to 27% in 1995, whereas in former socialist countries, the smoking-related mortality in men went from 1.3% in 1955 to 3.7% in 1985 to 5.2% in 1995.[10] This may seem like a low number in former socialist countries; however, in 2001, the smoking prevalence in Belarusian men was 56%, Georgian men 53%, Kazakhstan men 65%, and Russian men 60%.[11] The smoking prevalence rates in women, as of 2001, were relatively low (<10%); however, the tobacco industry is undoubtably targeting this potentially growing market. Evidence has already demonstrated the significant increases in cigarette production in parallel with increased consumption in the countries of the former Soviet Union who have had outside investments from the transnational tobacco industries.[12] There is enough experience to predict the tremendous death toll that these smoking prevalences will have in future years. In China, two thirds of men start smoking before the age of 25, and with projections, 100 million of the current 300 million Chinese men younger than the age of 30 will be killed by tobacco.[10]

Figure 2.4 demonstrates the comparison of cigarette consumption between the United States and Japan from 1990 to the present.[5] With these curves in mind, Figures 2.5 and 2.6[5] demonstrate the trends in lung cancer mortality in six different countries, including the United States and Japan—all are considered industrialized, "western" economies. It is striking to observe the differences between even these "westernized" economies and between the sexes. It is clear that the United Kingdom, followed by the United States had the earliest and most dramatic decline in male lung cancer death rates, whereas the picture for the women—as predicted by the Lopez curves, lags significantly behind.

It is also very important to consider the state of tobacco control within each country and how this impacts the smoking prevalence rates. Western countries have been at the forefront of tobacco control, with the resultant decrease in the number of people starting smoking, but also importantly, the number of people quitting smoking. Figures 2.7 and 2.8 demonstrate the age-specific prevalence of current and former smokers by birth cohort in U.S. men and Japanese men.[5] It is striking to observe the differences in age of onset of smoking and the numbers of former smokers (those who have quit). These differences explain the differences in the lung cancer mortality age-specific curves in Figure 2.5.

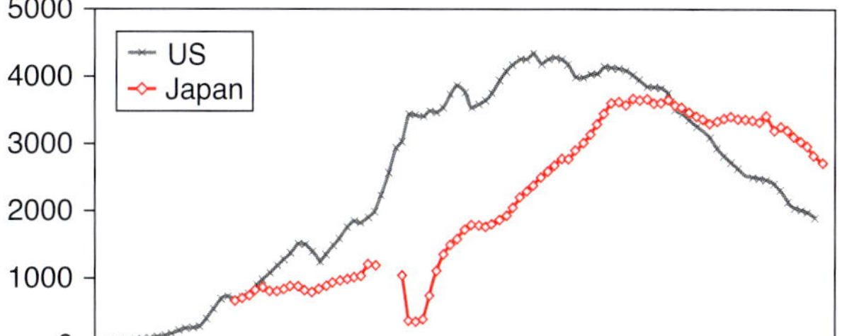

FIGURE 2.4 Trends of cigarette consumption per capita (18 years old or older) in the United States and Japan. Data are not available for 1941 to 1943 in Japan because of World War II. (From Dresler C, Leon M. *IARC Handbooks of Cancer Prevention, Tobacco Control, Vol. 11. Reversal of Risk after Quitting Smoking.* Lyon, France: International Agency for Research on Cancer, 2007.)

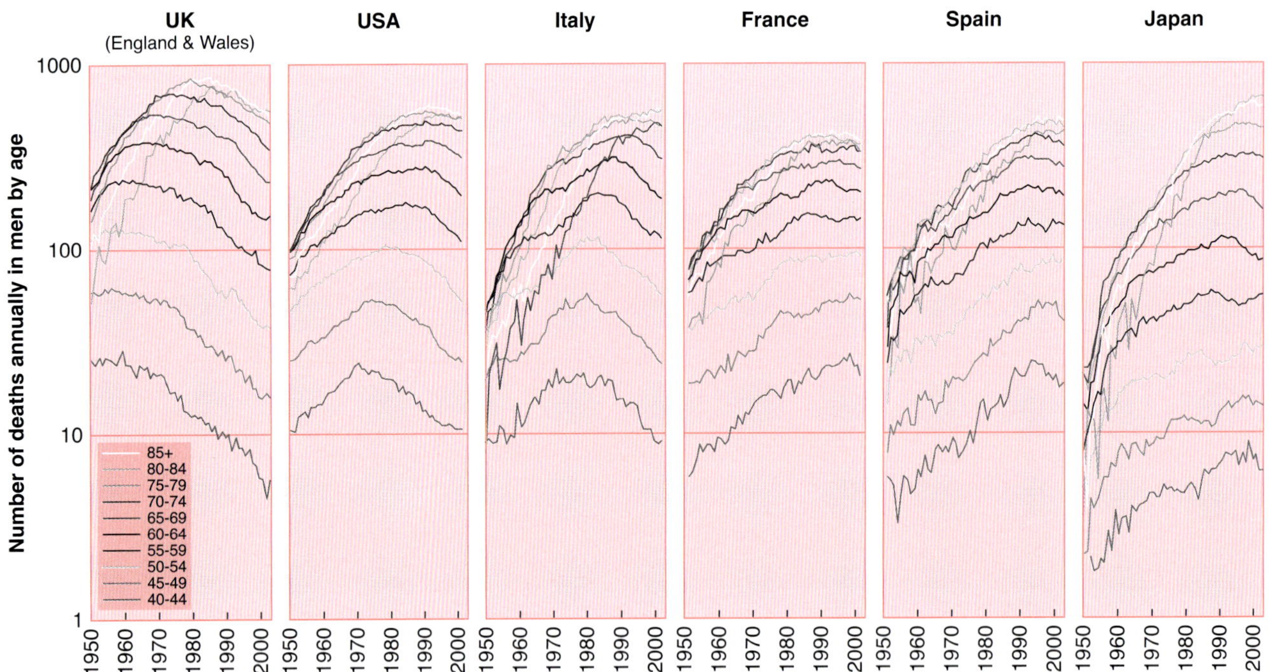

FIGURE 2.5 Trends in lung cancer mortality in six countries in men. (From Dresler C, Leon M. *IARC Handbooks of Cancer Prevention, Tobacco Control, Vol. 11. Reversal of Risk after Quitting Smoking.* Lyon, France: International Agency for Research on Cancer, 2007.)

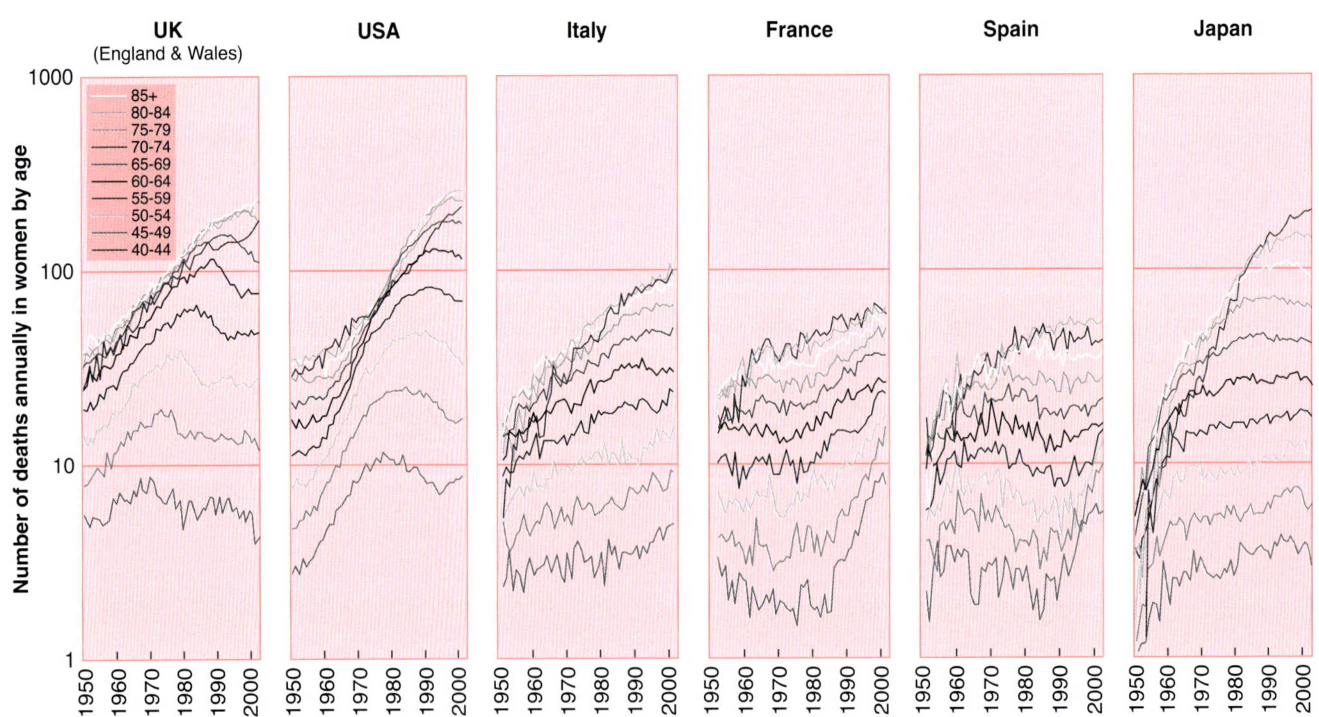

FIGURE 2.6 Trends in lung cancer mortality in six countries in women. (From Dresler C, Leon M. *IARC Handbooks of Cancer Prevention, Tobacco Control, Vol. 11. Reversal of Risk after Quitting Smoking.* Lyon, France: International Agency for Research on Cancer, 2007.)

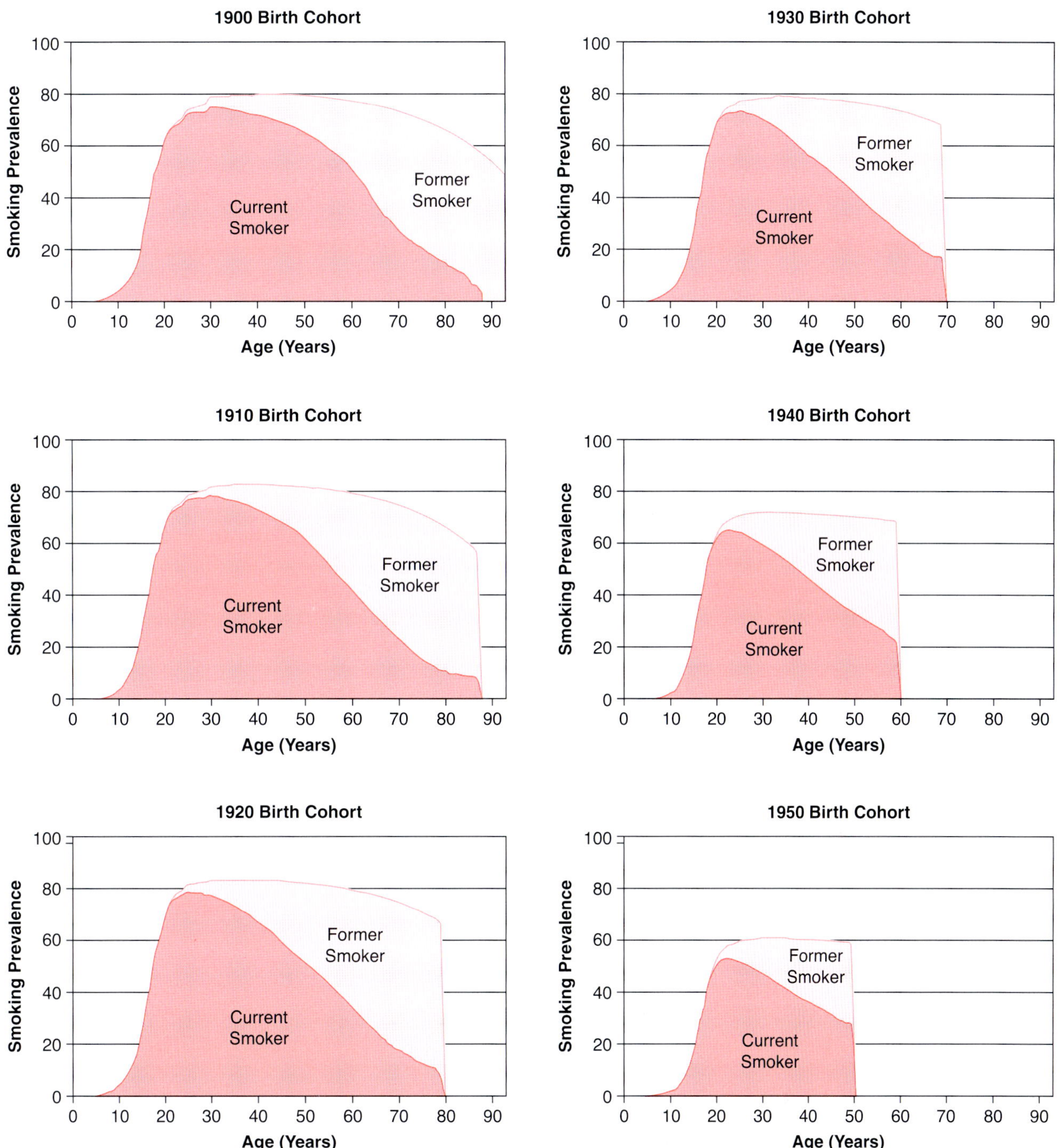

FIGURE 2.7 Age-specific prevalence of current and former smokers by birth cohort in U.S. white men. (From Dresler C, Leon M. *IARC Handbooks of Cancer Prevention, Tobacco Control, Vol. 11. Reversal of Risk after Quitting Smoking.* Lyon, France: International Agency for Research on Cancer, 2007.)

It is already well established that smoking causes lung cancer—at least for the past 50 or more years.[13,14] What is interesting is how the lung cancer epidemic is changing around the world, depending on the changes in the prevalence of cigarette smoking in the specific country. As approximately 10% to 20% of smokers will develop lung cancer—to radically decrease the number of lung cancer deaths, the prevalence of smoking must significantly decrease.

Lung cancers attributable to smoking vary around the world—particularly in women. In more developed countries, smoking causes 90% to 95% of lung cancers in men. For women, the highest rate of smoking-attributable lung cancer occurs in North America (85%), northern Europe (74%), and Australia/New Zealand (72%). In these regions, women have the longest duration of smoking. For other regions, the attributable fraction

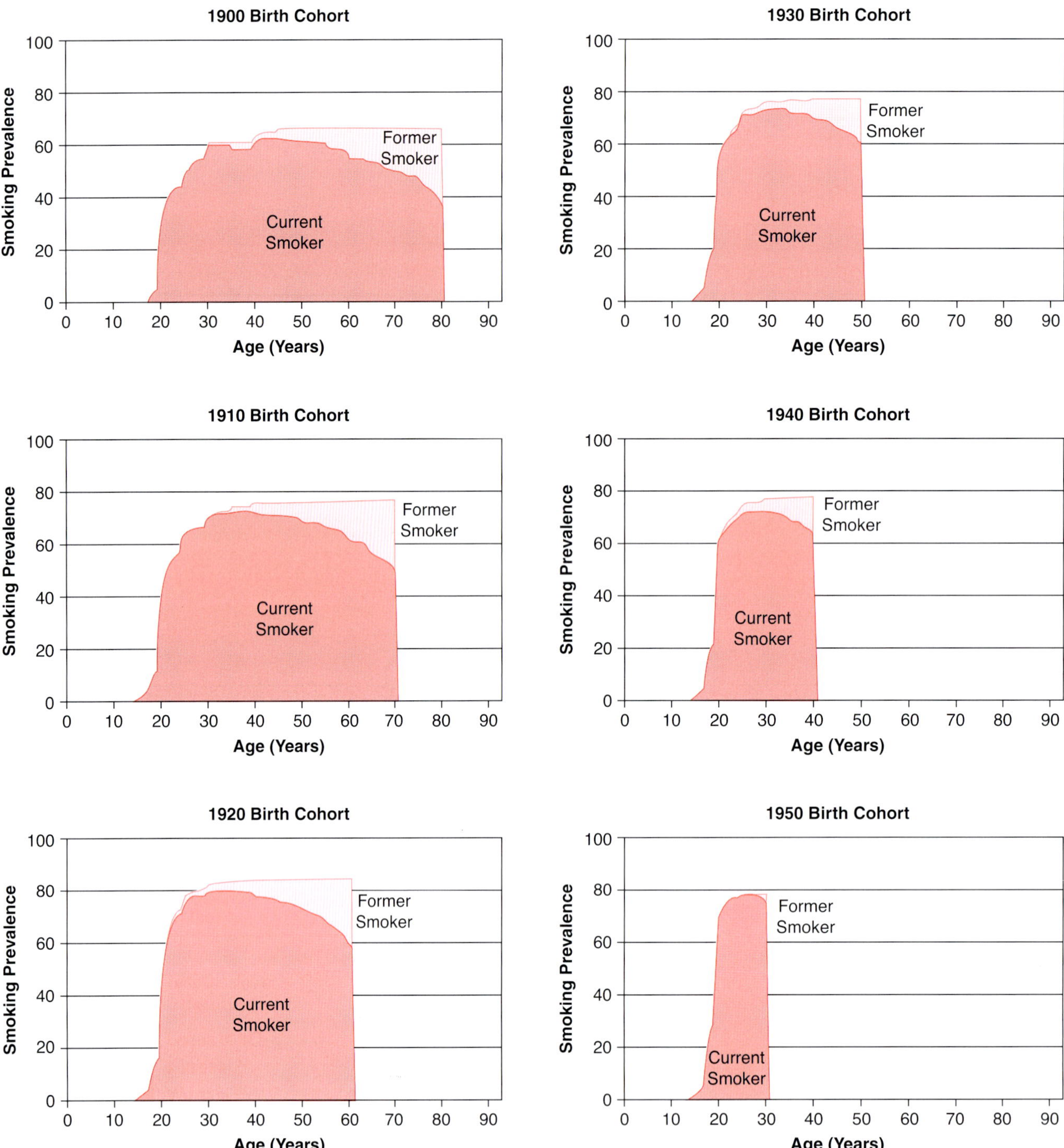

FIGURE 2.8 Age-specific prevalence of current and former smokers by birth cohort in Japanese men. (From Drester C, Leon M. *IARC Handbooks of Cancer Prevention, Tobacco Control, Vol. 11. Reversal of Risk after Quitting Smoking.* Lyon, France: International Agency for Research on Cancer, 2007.)

is lower and more highly related to exposure to indoor cooking fuels.[6] As the rate of smoking increases in women, the attributable rate necessarily will similarly increase.

The determinants of the risk of smoking to the development of lung cancer depends on the duration of smoking, the number of cigarettes smoked per day, the age of smoking initiation, the type of cigarette smoked, the depth of inhalation, underlying susceptibility, and family history. Additional risks include exposure to environmental factors (especially radon), secondhand smoke, or occupational risks. What has been changing over time is the increasing exposure to both mainstream and secondhand smoke, particularly in developing

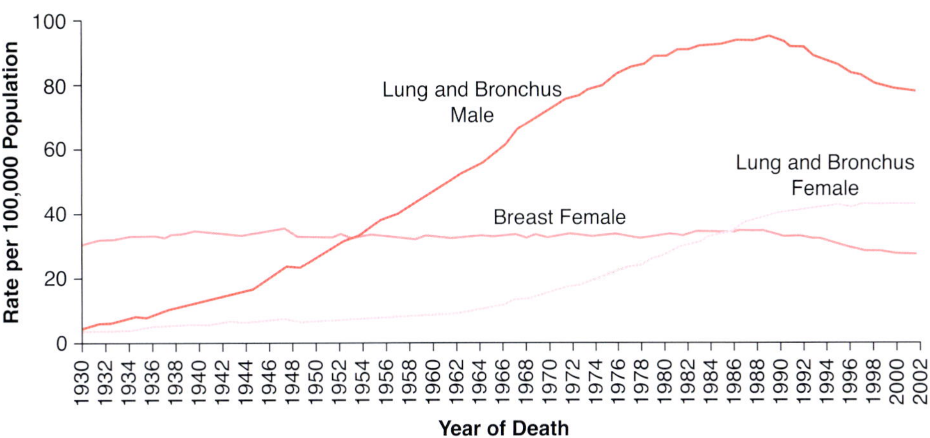

FIGURE 2.9 Annual age-adjusted lung death rates for men and women; and breast cancer deaths in women, 1930 to 2001. Rates are age-adjusted to the 2000 U.S. standard population. (From Jemal A, Murray T, Ward E, et al. Cancer statistics, 2005. *CA Clin J Clin* 2005;55:10–30.)

economies and women, whereas the other causes have remained fairly stable.

In the United States, the relative risk for developing lung cancer has been determined in two large, sequential cohort studies from the American Cancer Society. These relative risks increased between these studies, from 11.9 to 23.2 in men and 2.7 to 12.8 for women, and this reflected the changes in smoking prevalence.[15] A review of the global literature from over 130 studies showed similar relative risks for lung cancer from tobacco ranging from 15 to 30.[16] Figure 2.3 from the U.S. Surgeon General Report, 1997, demonstrates the changes in U.S. tobacco consumption[8] and Figure 2.9[17] shows the changes in male and female lung cancer rates, and for comparison, the breast cancer rates in women over the same time period. From these American data, it was calculated that the cumulative probability of dying from lung cancer is 14.6% for men and 8.3% for women from smoking, versus only 1.1% in men and 0.9% in women lifelong never-smokers.[18]

How can we now relate this information to the rest of the world? We can examine some of the countries around the world to see how the lung cancer mortality rates have changed over time.[19,20] Unfortunately, most countries do not have well-documented smoking histories for the past several decades, but their historical prevalence can be approximated from the current lung cancer death rates. Figure 2.10 demonstrates the changes over the years in the lung cancer death rates in a few representative countries from Europe. The rates from men can be contrasted with the rates for women. The similarities between how these data relate to the Lopez curves are striking. It simply demonstrates that we can readily predict the death toll from lung cancer if we do not decrease the smoking rates—particularly among women. Figure 2.11 illustrates some of the smoking prevalence rates around the world—where we need to be concerned about the lung cancer epidemic that is occurring in these countries.[21]

HISTOLOGICAL VARIABILITY

The relative risk of smoking for the development of the different histologies for lung cancer has been confirmed many times.[22–26] Figure 2.12 demonstrates these changes in the United States. However, there is considerable variation between the different histological types of lung cancer over time between genders and between countries. Figure 2.13 illustrate the various proportion of squamous cell versus adenocarcinoma lung cancer in several

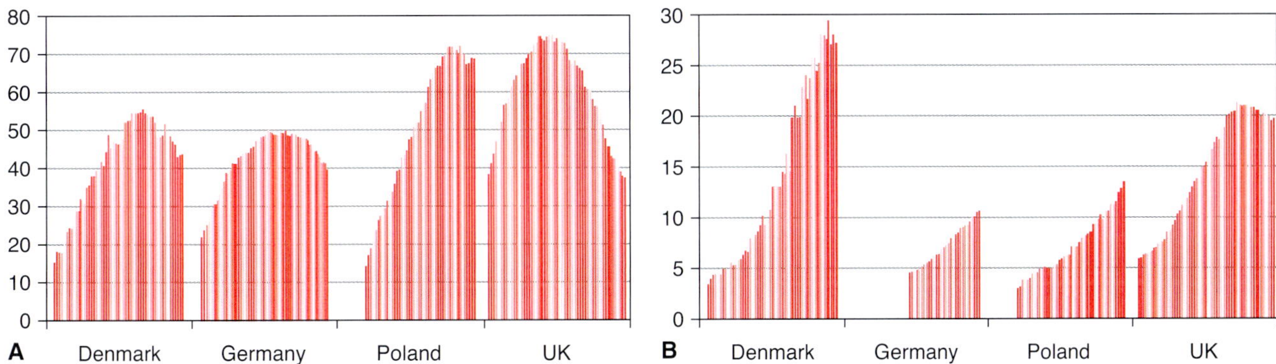

FIGURE 2.10 **A:** Age-standardized death rate (weighted) (ASR-w) for men in Denmark, Germany, Poland, and United Kingdom, 1950 to 2002.[20] **B:** Age-standardized death rate (weighted) (ASR-w) for women in Denmark, Germany, Poland, and United Kingdom, 1950 to 2002. (From Ferlay J, Bray J, Pisani P, et al. *GLOBOCAN 2002: Cancer Incidence, Mortality, and Prevalence Worldwide. IARC CancerBase No. 5, version 2.0.* Lyon, France: IARCPress, 2004.)

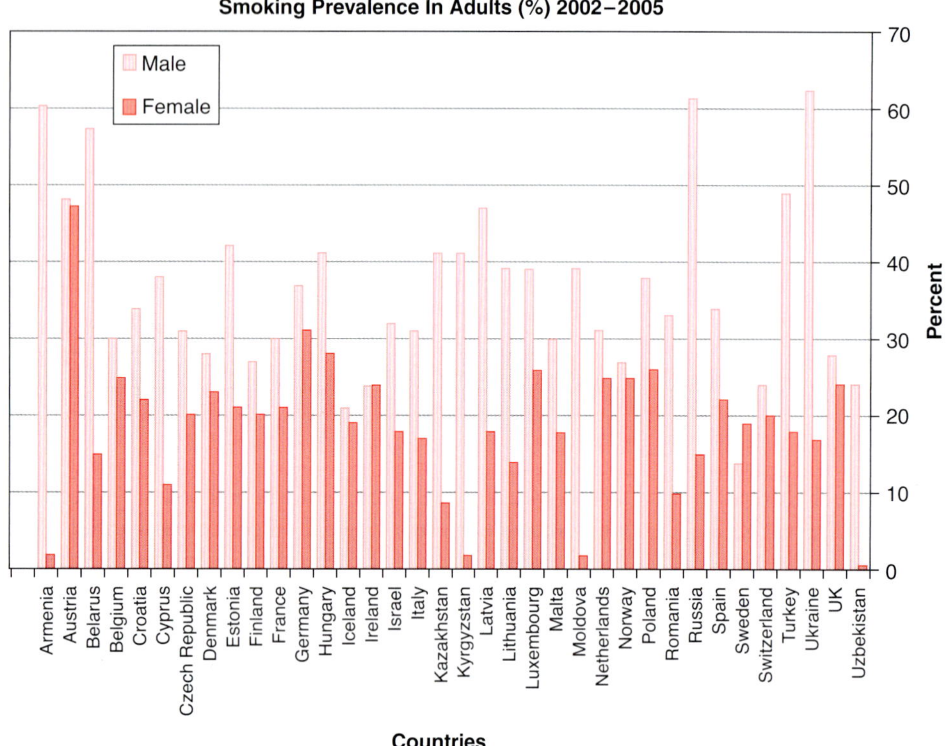

FIGURE 2.11 Adult smoking prevalence, WHO country profiles, data from 2002 to 2005. (From Cross-country profile: Tobacco Control Database; World Health Organization, Regional office for Europe. Accessed December 15, 2006.)

countries in Asia and Europe.[27] This has been attributed to several factors, including genetic susceptibility, but is more likely to be the result of differences in the smoke chemistry of the cigarettes smoked, which has changed substantially over time.[28]

Although smoking patterns vary greatly worldwide, men started smoking before women and smoked the cigarettes of earlier times, whereas women predominantly smoked the cigarettes of several decades later.[29] These latter cigarettes, particularly in many Western countries, are lower in tar, more likely to have ventilated filters, less polycyclic hydrocarbons, and more tobacco-specific nitrosamines.[29–31] It is therefore not surprising that women are more likely to develop adenocarcinoma than the predominantly squamous carcinoma seen previously in men. The histologic swing to adenocarcinoma seen in men in recent decades is consistent with this concept as they too smoke more of the lower tar and filtered cigarettes. It has also has been demonstrated that nitrosamines vary considerably around the world, even though they may have a common manufacturer.[32]

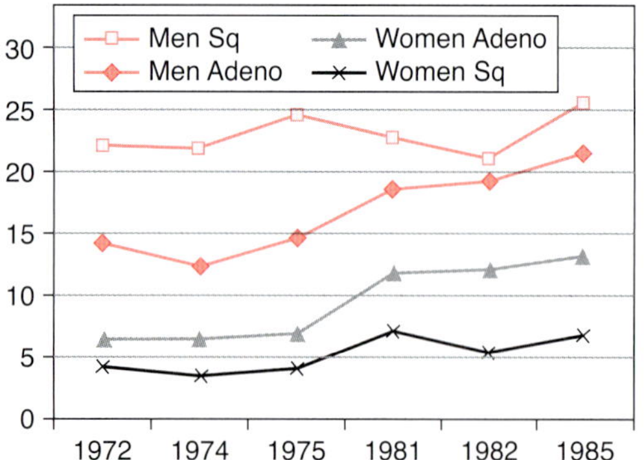

FIGURE 2.12 Changes in age-adjusted incidence rates per 100,000 for squamous cell and adenocarcinoma in the United States. (From Charloux A, Quoix E, Wolkove N, et al. The increasing incidence of lung adenocarcinoma: reality or artefact? A review of the epidemiology of lung adenocarcinoma. *Int J Epidemiol* 1997;261:14–23.)

The occurrence of adenocarcinoma among Asian women, many of whom do not smoke yet have a relatively high rate of lung cancer, requires an alternative explanation.

The literature suggests that the increased risk for lung cancer in Chinese women has been related to indoor air pollution from cooking with oil, especially rapeseed oil,[33,34] biomass fuel, and secondhand smoke.[35,36] Chinese women, and Asian women in general, have low smoking rates; however, in most areas they are increasing. Undoubtedly, these raising rates of cigarette smoking will increase the rates of tobacco-related lung cancers. However, how it will impact the ratios of squamous cell to adenocarcinoma will need to be assessed over time. Presently, there has already been a shift in the rates from predominance of squamous cell to adenocarcinoma in Japan, Israel, and countries in Europe where the prevalence of male smoking is still high.[37–40] As discussed previously, this shift in histologies is probably related to the changing cigarette in the various environments in addition to the increasing prevalence of smoking-related cancer in women. These trends should be followed closely—in addition to following how the cigarette is changing over time in each of these environments. This is a daunting task.

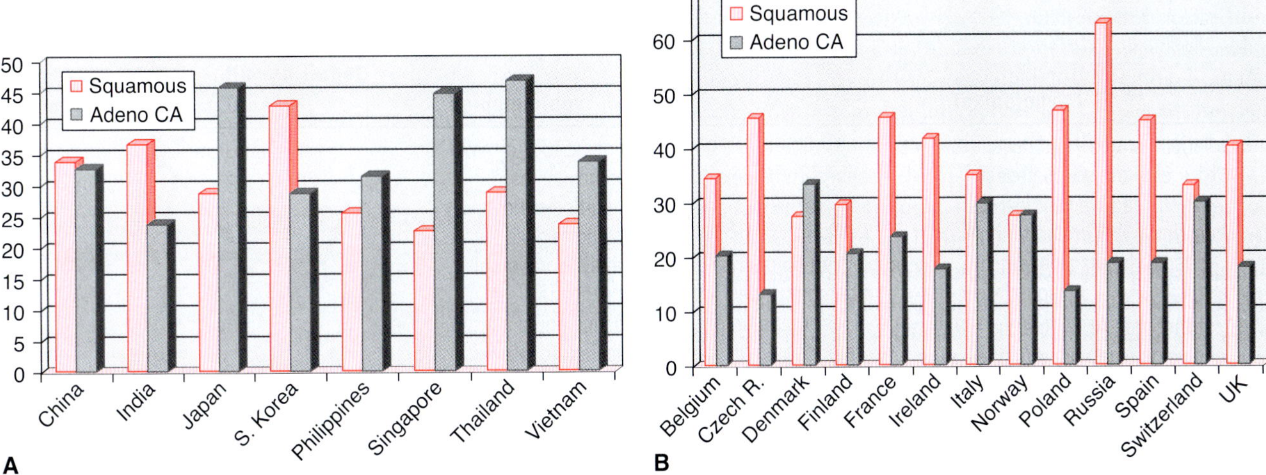

FIGURE 2.13 **A:** Age-standardized death rate (weighted) (ASR-w) for squamous cell and adenocarcinoma from 1993 to 1997 in Asian countries. **B:** Age-standardized death rate (weighted) (ASR-w) for squamous cell and adenocarcinoma from 1993 to 1997 in European countries. (From Parkin DM, Whelan SL, Ferlay J, et al., eds. *Cancer Incidence in Five Continents, Vol. VIII, IARC Scientific Publications No. 15.* Lyon, France: IARC Press, 2002.)

What might be easier would be to decrease the number of people smoking, and therefore, more rapidly decrease the deaths from lung cancer. This decrease can be obtained from tobacco control efforts.[41] Figure 2.14 demonstrates the 6% decrease in lung cancer incidence observed in California caused by the efforts in decreasing initiation and increased cessation through tobacco control efforts since 1988.[42] Peto et al.[43] have concluded that people who stop smoking in middle age can avoid 90% of their tobacco-attributable risk for lung cancer. In the United States, the data suggested that the decline in smoking over the past 50 years, accounted for 40% of the decline in overall male cancer deaths and prevented 146,000 male lung cancer deaths in the time period from 1991 to 2003.[44] Certainly, initiatives of tobacco control, screening, and improved treatment modalities should be pursued simultaneously. Even with strong tobacco control policies, we will need the research to see how best to identify and treat those that continue to be diagnosed with lung cancer—tobacco related or otherwise.

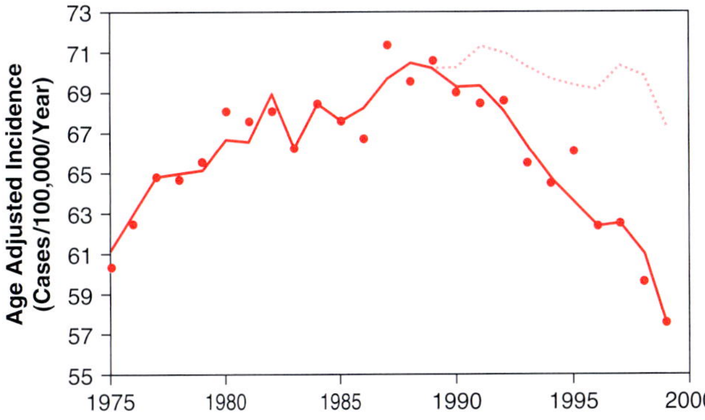

FIGURE 2.14 Decline in lung cancer incidence in California following increased tobacco control efforts: predicted (*solid line*); without tobacco control (*dotted line*). (From Barnoya J, Glantz S. Association of the California tobacco program with declines in lung cancer incidence. *Canc Causes Contr* 2004;14:689–695.)

REFERENCES

1. Gately I. *Tobacco: A Cultural History of How an Exotic Plant Seduced Civilization*. London: Simon & Schuster, 2001.
2. Burns E. *The Smoke of the Gods: A Social History of Tobacco*. Philadelphia: Temple University Press, 2007.
3. World Health Organization (WHO) Fact Sheet: The top 10 causes of death. Available at: http://www.who.int/mediacentre/factsheets/fs310/en/index.html. Accessed November 25, 2007.
4. Mathers CD, Loncar D. Projections of global mortality and burden of disease from 2002 to 2030. *PLOS Medicine* 2006;3(11):2011–b2030. Available at: http://www.plosmedicine.org. Accessed October 27, 2009.
5. Dresler C, Leon M. *IARC Handbooks of Cancer Prevention, Tobacco Control, Vol. 11. Reversal of Risk after Quitting Smoking*. Lyon, France: International Agency for Research on Cancer, 2007.
6. Parkin DM, Bray F, Ferlay J, et al. Global Cancer Statistics, 2002. *CA Cancer J Clin* 2005;55:74–108.
7. Lopez AD, Collishaw NE, Piha T. A descriptive model of the cigarette epidemic in developed countries. *Tob Control* 1994;3:242–247.
8. Burns DM, Lee L, Zhen LA, et al. Cigarette smoking behavior in the United States. In: Burns D, Garfinkel L, Samet J, eds. *Changes in Cigarette-Related Disease Risks and Their Implication for Prevention and Control; Monograph 8*. Bethesda, MD: National Institutes of Health, 1997:13.
9. Mackay J, Eriksen M, Shafey O, eds. *The Tobacco Atlas*. 2nd Ed. Atlanta, GA: American Cancer Society, 2006.
10. Boyle P, Gray N, Henningfield J, et al., eds. *Tobacco: Science, Policy and Public Health*. Oxford, UK: Oxford University Press, 2004.
11. Gilmore A, Pomerleau J, McKee M, et al. Prevalence of smoking in 8 countries of the former Soviet Union: results from the living conditions, lifestyles and health study. *Am J Public Health* 2004;94(12):2177–2187.

12. Gilmore AB, McKee M. Exploring the impact of foreign direct investment of tobacco consumption in the former Soviet Union. *Tob Control* 2005;14:13–21.
13. Doll R, Hill AB. Smoking and carcinoma of the lung: preliminary report. *Br Med J* 1950:2:739–748.
14. Mills CA, Porter MM. Tobacco smoking habits and cancer of the mouth and respiratory system. *Cancer Res* 1950;10:539–542.
15. Thun MJ, Day-Lally C, Myers DG, et al., eds. Trends in tobacco smoking and mortality from cigarette use in Cancer Prevention Studies I (1959–1965) and II (1982–1988). In: Burns D, Garfinkel L, Samet J, eds. *Changes in Cigarette-Related Disease Risks and Their Implication for Prevention and Control; Smoking and Tobacco Control Monograph 8.* Bethesda, MD: National Institutes of Health, 1997, Chapter 4.
16. Vineis P, Alavanja M, Buffler P, et al. Tobacco and cancer: recent epidemiological evidence. *J Natl Cancer Inst* 2004;96(2):99–106.
17. Jemal A, Murray T, Ward E, et al. Cancer Statistics, 2005. *CA Cancer J Clin* 2005;55:10–30.
18. Thun MJ, Henley SJ, Calle EE. Tobacco use and cancer: an epidemiologic perspective for geneticists. *Oncogene* 2002;21:7307–7325.
19. Brennan P, Bray I. Recent trends and future directions for lung cancer mortality in Europe. *Br J Cancer* 2002;87:43–48.
20. Ferlay J, Bray J, Pisani P, et al. *GLOBOCAN 2002: Cancer Incidence, Mortality and Prevalence Worldwide, IARC CancerBase No. 5, version 2.0.* Lyon, France: IARCPress, 2004.
21. Cross-country profile: Tobacco Control Database; World Health Organization, Regional office for Europe. Available at: http://data.euro.who.int/tobacco/default.aspx?TabID=2444. Accessed December 15, 2006.
22. Charloux A, Quoix E, Wolkove N, et al. The increasing incidence of lung adenocarcinoma. *Int J Epidemiol* 1997;26(1):14–23.
23. Simonato L, Agudo A, Ahrens W, et al. Lung cancer and cigarette smoking in Europe: an update on risk estimates and an assessment of inter-country heterogeneity. *Int J Cancer* 2001;91(6):876–887.
24. Lubin JH, Blot WJ. Assessment of lung cancer risk factors by histologic category *J Natl Cancer Inst* 1984;73:383–389.
25. Wu AH, Henderson BE, Pike MC, et al. Smoking and other risk factors for lung cancer in females. *J Natl Cancer Inst* 1985;74:747–751.
26. Brownson RC, Reif JF, Keefe TJ, et al. Risk factors for adenocarcinoma of the lung. *Am J Epidemiol* 1987;125:25–34.
27. Parkin DM, Whelan SL, Ferlay J, et al., eds. *Cancer Incidence in Five Continents, Vol. VIII, IARC Scientific Publications No. 15.* Lyon, France: IARC Press, 2002.
28. Gray N. The consequences of the unregulated cigarette. *Tob Control* 2006;15(5):405–408.
29. Wynder EL, Hoffman D. Smoking and lung cancer: scientific challenges and opportunities. *Cancer Res* 1994:54:5284–5295.
30. Morabia A, Wynder EL. Cigarette smoking and lung cancer cell types. *Cancer* 1991;68:2074–2078.
31. Zheng T, Holford TR, Boyle P, et al. Time trend and the age-period cohort effect on the incidence of histologic types of lung cancer in Connecticut, 1960–1989. *Cancer* 1994;74(5):1556–1567.
32. Counts ME, Morton MJ, Laffon SW, et al. Smoke composition and predicting relationships for international commercial cigarettes smoked with three machine-smoking conditions. *Regul Toxicol Pharmacol* 2005;41:185–227.
33. Yu IT, Chiu YL, Au JS, et al. Dose-response relationship between cooking fumes exposures and lung cancer among Chinese nonsmoking women. *Cancer Res* 2006;66(9):4961–4967.
34. Zhong L, Goldberg MS, Gao YT, et al. Lung cancer and indoor air pollution arising from Chinese-style cooking among nonsmoking women living in Shanghai, China. *Epidemiology* 2000;11(4):481–482.
35. Wen W, Shu XO, Gao YT, et al. Environmental tobacco smoke and mortality in Chinese women who have never smoked: prospective cohort study. *BMJ* 2006;333(7564):376.
36. Chen BH, Hong CJ, Pandey MR, et al. Indoor pollution in developing countries. *World Health Stat Q* 1990;43(3):127–138.
37. Yoshimi I, Ohshima A, Ajiki W, et al. A comparison of trends in the incidence rate of lung cancer by histological type in the Osaka Cancer Registry, Japan and in the Surveillance, Epidemiology and End Results Program, USA. *Jpn J Clin Oncol* 2003;33(2):98–104.
38. Baron-Epel O, Andreev H, Barhana M, et al. Differences in trends of lung carcinoma by histology type in Israeli Jews and Arabs, 1981–1995. *Eur J Epidemiol* 2001;17(1):11–18.
39. Harkness EF, Brewster DH, Kerr KM, et al. Changing trends in incidence of lung cancer by histologic type in Scotland. *Int J Cancer* 2002;102(2):179–183.
40. Levi F, Franceschi S, LaVecchia C, et al. Lung carcinoma trends by histologic type in Vaud and Neuchatel, Switzerland, 1974–1994. *Cancer* 1997;79(5):906–914.
41. Wingo PA, Ries LAG, Giovino GA, et al. Annual report to the nation on the status of cancer, 1973–1996, with a special section on lung cancer and tobacco smoking. *J Natl Cancer Inst* 1999;91:675–690.
42. Barnoya J, Glantz S. Association of the California tobacco program with declines in lung cancer incidence. *Cancer Causes Control* 2004;15:689–695.
43. Peto R, Darby S, Doe H, et al. Smoking, smoking cessation, and lung cancer in the UK since 1950: combination of national statistics with two case-control studies. *BMJ* 2000;321:323–329.
44. Thun MJ, Jemal A. How much of the decrease in cancer death rates in the United States is attributable to reductions in tobacco smoking? *Tob Control* 2006;15:345–347.

CHAPTER 3

Tze-Ming Benson Chen
Ware G. Kuschner

Nontobacco-Related Lung Carcinogenesis

Lung cancer is estimated to cause 17,000 to 26,000 deaths among *nonsmokers* annually in the United States.[1] Secondhand smoke exposure explains some deaths among nonsmokers, but many deaths are unrelated to tobacco smoke. Occupational and environmental exposures and genetic characteristics have been identified as risk factors for the development of lung cancer in both smokers and nonsmokers. In this chapter, we review important toxicants, other than tobacco, for which the evidence for pulmonary carcinogenic potential is strong and the population health effects data support a causal relationship between exposure and lung cancer. These toxicants share the common feature of being respirable carcinogens, but otherwise have widely different physicochemical characteristics. The substances include minerals (asbestos and silica), radioactive gas (radon), and products of fossil fuel combustion (diesel-exhaust particles).

Historically, occupational settings have been among the most important sources of exposure to the nontobacco pulmonary carcinogens. Accordingly, many cases of lung cancer attributable to nontobacco carcinogens are work related and, in turn, preventable. Moreover, we review data on some exposures mainly encountered in industrial settings, which are most persuasively linked with lung cancer. It is important to note, however, that since the beginning of the 20th century, an estimated 85,000 chemicals have been introduced into industrial applications, many of which may be encountered in respirable states.[2] Data on the carcinogenic potential of most of these chemicals are limited or nonexistent. Some cases of lung cancer may be attributable to occupational or environmental exposures yet to be recognized as carcinogenic. However, such speculation should not alter the fact that strategies to reduce the total burden of lung cancer worldwide must remain sharply focused on preventing exposure to established pulmonary carcinogens, including tobacco and nontobacco exposures.

ARSENIC

Arsenic is a naturally occurring element found throughout the earth's crust. Inorganic arsenic complexes are used predominantly to preserve wood, whereas organic arsenic is used in pesticides. In addition, arsenic trioxide (arsenite) is used in the treatment of promyelocytic leukemia.

Concerns over the potential carcinogenicity of arsenic were first raised as early as 1820 when Paris[3] first described its association with skin cancer. In 1930, Saupe[4] described two cases of lung cancer in association with arsenic exposure. Since then, a large amount of data has been published linking arsenic and lung cancer in humans. Blot and Fraumeni Jr[5] uncovered an increased risk of lung cancer–related mortality in smelter workers exposed to arsenic trioxide between 1938 and 1963. Tokudome and Kuratsune[6] found a significantly increased mortality rate from lung cancer in copper smelters employed at a metal refinery in Japan between 1949 and 1971. The average latency period for lung cancer was 37.6 years and was unrelated to the estimated levels of arsenic exposure. Rencher et al.[6a] conducted a retrospective mortality study at a copper smelter in Utah and demonstrated that 7% of all worker deaths were caused by lung cancer compared to 2.7% in the state of Utah and 2.2% at the smelter's associated mine and concentrator. Other investigators have confirmed the association between lung cancer and working directly with copper smelters.[7–11] Other studies have found increased risks of lung cancer in association with exposure to pesticides containing inorganic arsenic[12,13] and even the use of arsenic as a medicinal.[14] Of note, Guo et al.[15] concluded arsenic exposure is most strongly associated with the development of either squamous cell or small cell lung cancer.

Most studies assumed that only inhalational exposures are associated with arsenic-related lung cancer. However, along the southwest and northeast coasts of Taiwan, in the Niigata Prefecture of Japan, in Northern Chile, and in Bangladesh, ground water is heavily contaminated by arsenic, and its ingestion has been associated with increased incidences of lung cancer.[16–20] Chen et al.[21] evaluated the dose–response relationship between ingested arsenic and lung cancer risk as it relates to smoking. They found an increase in the relative risk of lung cancer of 3.29 (95% confidence interval [CI], 1.60, 2.78) among populations exposed to the highest (700 μg/L) relative to the lowest (<10 μg/L) arsenic levels in drinking water. In addition, after the instillation of a tap-water system in southwestern Taiwan, lung cancer mortality declined, further bolstering the likely relationship between ingested arsenic and lung cancer.[22]

The most significant confounding factor in these studies of arsenic and lung cancer is the contribution of smoking. Some more recent studies have tried to adjust for the effect of smoking and have demonstrated a persistent carcinogenic effect of arsenic.[23] In addition, a synergistic interaction between arsenic and smoking likely exists as suggested by Pershagen et al.[24] This study evaluated Swedish copper smelter workers and found that the age-standardized rate ratio for lung cancer death in arsenic-exposed nonsmokers was 3.0. Among those smokers without occupational arsenic exposure, the ratio was 4.9. In arsenic-exposed smokers, the age-standardized rate ratio for lung cancer was 14.6.[24] A metaanalysis by Hertz-Picciotto et al.[25] and the previously described study by Chen et al.[21] also support a synergistic effect.

Nonoccupational exposure to copper smelters (i.e., residential proximity) may also pose a carcinogenic risk. However, most studies failed to establish a statistically significant link within this setting suggesting that arsenic alone may either be a weak carcinogen or may require a cocarcinogen to induce the development of cancer.[26–28]

Reviews of the literature suggest that the average latency for lung cancer diagnosis after exposure to arsenic is about 30 years. In addition, arsenic-related pulmonary malignancies appear to have a predilection for the upper lobes.[29] All histologic cell types are represented in arsenic-related lung cancer and the relative frequencies of each cell type seem to mimic that of the general nonexposed population.[30,31]

Animal data supporting a carcinogenic role for arsenic are limited. Ishinishi et al.[32] found that intratracheal instillation of three forms of arsenic (copper ore, flue dust, and arsenic trioxide) to Wistar-King rats was associated with the formation of lung adenomas and/or adenocarcinomas. In another publication, Ishinishi et al.[33] demonstrated a 10% to 30% lifetime risk of lung adenocarcinoma in Syrian golden hamsters after weekly intratracheal instillation of 3.75 or 5.25 mg of arsenic trioxide. Ivankovic et al.[34] demonstrated the induction of multifocal bronchogenic adenocarcinomas and bronchoalveolar cell carcinomas in 9 of 15 (60%) rats after intratracheal instillation of 0.1 mL of a vineyard pesticide containing calcium arsenate. Soucy et al.[35] found dose-dependent effects of arsenic trioxide on animal models of angiogenesis, as well as melanoma tumor growth and metastasis. Interestingly, the form of arsenic appears to influence the risk of lung cancer in animal studies. Specifically, calcium arsenate appears to have the strongest tumorigenic potential, whereas arsenic trioxide is of questionable carcinogenicity.[36,37]

Arsenic has been shown to induce preneoplastic changes in human fetal lung tissue.[38] The mechanism behind such changes may lie in arsenic-induced overmethylation of DNA. Mass and Wang[39] found that exposure of human lung adenocarcinoma A549 cells to sodium arsenite or sodium arsenate resulted in a significant level of methylation of a fragment of p53, a tumor suppressor gene. This may alter the function of p53 as a checkpoint in the cell cycle permitting eventual transformation into an immortal cell line. Other mouse studies have suggested that arsenic augments the ability of the tobacco-derived carcinogen, benzo(a)pyrene, to increase the number of DNA adducts in both skin and lung, the initiation step in mutagenesis.[40]

In 1980, the International Agency for Research on Cancer (IARC) concluded that the available human data were sufficient to implicate arsenic as a pulmonary carcinogen. In October 2001, the U.S. Environmental Protection Agency (EPA) announced that on January 2006, a permissible exposure limit (PEL) of 10 ppb in drinking water would be enforced.[41]

The National Institute for Occupational Safety and Health (NIOSH) has established a PEL of 2 $\mu g/m^3$ during a 15-minute ceiling, whereas the Occupational Safety and Health Administration (OSHA) has established a PEL of 10 $\mu g/m^3$ during any 8-hour period for a 40-hour workweek. Potential household exposures to arsenic through ant pesticides containing sodium arsenate and arsenic-treated pressurized wood prompted the EPA to begin phasing out these products in 1989.

ASBESTOS

Asbestos, derived from a Greek adjective meaning inextinguishable or unquenchable, is a naturally occurring mineral used widely in the 20th century for its insulating and corrosion- and fire-resistant properties. In the late 1800s, the British discovered that asbestos fibers could be woven into textiles permitting its use in everything from brake pads to ship boiler insulators.[42] Asbestos had already been in use for centuries, and its associated adverse health effects had been recognized since at least the time of the Roman Empire when Pliny the Elder, a Roman citizen, noticed that slaves working in asbestos mines succumbed early to lung diseases. It was not until the United Kingdom Annual Report of the Chief Inspector of Factories in 1898 that the potential deleterious effects of asbestos were recognized again.[43]

Doll[44] published the landmark epidemiologic study linking lung cancer and asbestos exposure when he evaluated the autopsy results of 105 employees of an asbestos factory. Selikoff[45] provided further supportive epidemiologic evidence after reviewing the medical records of 1522 members of the asbestos workers unions in New York City and New Jersey. Wagner et al.[46] and Newhouse et al.[47] determined that even casual nonoccupational exposure to asbestos was sufficient to cause lung cancer by recognizing epidemics of mesothelioma among communities surrounding asbestos mines and neighborhoods located near asbestos textile mills.

Recent reports suggest that the mutagenic effect of asbestos involves proto-oncogenes, such as k-ras[48] and c-ras,[49] as well as tumor suppressor genes, such as p53. Nelson et al.[50] found a fivefold increase in the presence of k-ras mutations in patients diagnosed with lung adenocarcinoma who had occupational asbestos-exposure history compared to those patients with lung cancer without exposure history. Panduri et al.[51] found that p53 induces alveolar epithelial cell apoptosis in cells damaged by asbestos exposure. Supporting the important protective role of p53, Morris et al.[52] demonstrated a fivefold increase in the incidence of asbestos-associated lung cancer in mice after disrupting intrinsic p53 function. Additional findings include alterations in the insulin receptor pathway and associated downregulation of deleted in colorectal cancer (DCC) gene, KU70, and heat shock protein 27.[53] The effects of these gene alterations are the constitutive expression of proteins promoting cell division and the downregulation or removal of proteins involved in checkpoints during the cell cycle.

Possible mechanisms by which asbestos damages DNA appear to involve the production of reactive oxygen species and the activation of mitogen-activated protein kinases. Iwata et al.[54] detected the generation of reactive oxygen species by polymorphonuclear lymphocytes after exposure to anthophyllite asbestos fibers. Schabath et al.[55] demonstrated that homozygotes for the G-myeloperoxidase allele (G/G) exhibited an increased risk of asbestos-related lung cancer (odds ratio [OR] 1.72, 95% CI, 1.09 to 2.66) compared to those subjects with G/A and A/A genotypes. Another possible mechanism proposed by MacCorkle et al.[56] involves the interaction of asbestos fibers with cell's cytoskeletal proteins or proteins involved in cell division resulting in an increase in aneuploid cells.

Another theory regarding the carcinogenicity of asbestos hypothesizes that the asbestos fiber's role is to facilitate the introduction of other carcinogens like those in cigarette smoke to cells. The fibers do so by adhering to surfactant, which then creates a lipid bilayer permitting solubilization of hydrophobic carcinogens such as polycyclic hydrocarbons. This would then permit long-term high concentration exposure of the lung epithelium to carcinogenic substances.[57–59]

The latency period for the development of asbestos-related lung cancer is in excess of 20 years.[60] Asbestos has been linked to all cell types of lung cancer.[61] The risk of lung cancer in persons exposed to asbestos seems to depend on the fiber type (greater with nonchrysotile fibers even though chrysotile exposure is associated with lung cancer),[62] fiber size (greater with longer fibers),[63] exposure environment (greater in textile than in cement industries), and evidence of asbestosis on chest radiograph (greater in patients with opacities).[64–66] The estimated risk of lung cancer in some studies is about fivefold compared to the nonexposed general population. Smoking acts synergistically with asbestos and increases the risk of lung cancer almost 50-fold.[45,67]

The Asbestos Regulations of 1931 were the first attempt to regulate asbestos exposure in the workplace. Unfortunately, the permitted exposure levels were based on a study of workers at a North Carolina asbestos factory, all of whom had been employed for less than 10 years. Another methodologic problem occurred when about 150 workers were fired prior to the initiation of the study because of concerns that they may have had asbestosis. The Asbestos Regulations of 1969 decreased the permitted exposure level 15-fold to 2 fibers/mL of air. However, a company physician untrained in epidemiology based this "safe" level of exposure on an industry-sponsored study. In 1994, the United States lowered the "safe" exposure level to 0.1 fibers/mL of air, whereas Great Britain banned the use of the substance altogether in 1999. In 2001, the World Trade Organization stated that no safe level of asbestos exposure existed.[68] In 1973, the IARC concluded that asbestos was a human lung carcinogen.[69]

As of year 2000, based on data obtained from death certificates in the United Kingdom, deaths from asbestos-related lung cancer and mesothelioma continue to rise. The implication is that those exposed to the substance over the preceding 20 to 40 years will continue to be at risk for developing lung and/or pleural cancers despite cessation of exposure.[42]

Recognition that asbestos is the underlying etiology of a patient's illness should prompt physicians to make the appropriate notifications. In addition, it would be prudent to instruct the patient on the importance of avoiding further exposure to asbestos preferably by changing jobs or using protective respiratory equipment.

Asbestos-Related Mesothelioma Asbestos is the predominant cause of mesothelioma worldwide. In about two thirds of cases, an asbestos-exposure history is present. The risk of mesothelioma varies with the duration and intensity of exposure, as well as the type of asbestos fiber inhaled (highest with amosite and crocidolite). The latency period for mesothelioma is at least 25 to 30 years, and there have been reports of cases occurring more than 40 years after exposure.[70] Diagnosis often requires open-lung biopsy and unfortunately, mesotheliomas are notorious for growing along needle tracts and through surgical incisions. The most important step in evaluating a possible mesothelioma involves distinguishing it from benign mesothelioma, primary bronchogenic adenocarcinomas, and metastatic disease given the potentially different treatment options and outcomes.

BERYLLIUM

Beryllium is a naturally occurring element found in soil, rocks, coal, and oil. It was first discovered more than 2 centuries ago but was not widely used in industry until the 1940s and 1950s. Beryllium can withstand extreme heat, remain stable over a wide range of temperatures, and act as an excellent thermal conductor. It also enhances other metals when combined with them as alloys. It is essential for numerous items used in our day-to-day activities. Electrical connections in our cell phones, battery contacts, high-definition and cable television, power steering, electronic ignition systems, and air bag sensors are all modern-day systems and/or appliances that rely on beryllium to function. Mancuso et al.[71–76] first reported a potential link between beryllium and human lung cancer followed by other reports. However, other reports found no such relationship.[77–82]

Early animal studies suggested the possible role of beryllium in lung cancer; however, the mechanism is still unknown.[83] Studies have attempted to demonstrate a genotoxic event but have been mostly unsuccessful.[80–82] One study suggests a potential role for overmethylation of p16, a tumor suppressor gene; however, further work is needed to clarify its possible contribution.[84]

The varying results of beryllium studies have prompted four IARC meetings regarding the element's classification as a pulmonary carcinogen. In 1993, the working group of the IARC concluded that the evidence in human studies is sufficient to implicate beryllium as a carcinogen. The EPA has established that industries may release a total of 0.01 μg of beryllium per cubic meter averaged over 30 days. The OSHA has set a PEL of 2 μg of beryllium per cubic meter of air over an 8-hour workday.[85]

CHLOROMETHYL ETHER AND BIS(CHLOROMETHYL) ETHER

Used predominantly in industries to synthesize plastics, organic chemicals, and exchange resins, chloromethyl methyl ether (CMME) and an associated impurity, bis(chloromethyl) ether (BCME) were initially produced and used in this country soon after the end of World War II. Their potential role as carcinogen was not realized until 1968 when van Duuren[86] demonstrated the development of skin cancers in mice after exposing them to CMME. Leong et al.[87] found that BCME and CMME were pulmonary carcinogens after exposing A/Heston mice to vapors of each chemical 6 hours a day, 5 days a week, for a total of 82 to 130 exposure days. Laskin et al.[88] confirmed this inhalation effect of BCME on rats and hamsters.

The results of these initial animal studies prompted further human investigation. Albert et al.[89] evaluated lung cancer mortality at six of the seven U.S. companies that used CMME at that time. They found a 2.5-fold increase in lung cancer–related mortality among workers exposed to CMME choosing nonexposed employees at those same plants as controls. They also revealed an increase in lung cancer risk with increasing duration and intensity of exposure. DeFonso et al.[90] found that CMME with 0.5% to 4% BCME resulted in a 3.8-fold increase in lung cancer risk at a Philadelphia chemical plant, again using employees without an exposure history from the same plant as controls. Numerous studies have provided additional evidence supporting CMME and BCME's role as pulmonary carcinogens.[91–99]

The literature suggests that the latency period for lung cancer after exposure to BCME and CMME is between 21 to 25 years and is inversely related to exposure intensity and duration. A predominance of small cell carcinomas (80% to 90% of cases) is apparent in most studies.

In the 1970s, restrictions in the use of and safer handling techniques for CMME and BCME were instituted with an apparent decline in the incidence of associated cases of lung cancer.[99] Currently, the use of these substances is highly restricted, thereby minimizing potential exposure. BCME breaks down easily and quickly when exposed to sunlight or water and fortunately, does not build up in the food chain. Consequently, the only likely sources of exposure today are living near and/or working in industries that still use BCME and CMME.

The IARC officially recognized CMME and BCME as carcinogens in 1987. At this time, the EPA has set a tolerable limit of 0.0000038 parts of BCME per billion parts of water (0.0000038 ppb) in lakes and streams. Any release of more than 10 lb of BCME into the environment must be reported to the EPA. The OSHA has mandated that no more than 1 ppb of BCME be present in the air of a work environment.[100]

CHROMIUM

Chromium is a naturally occurring mineral found throughout the environment. It is present in multiple forms and is used in wood preserving, dyes, chrome plating, leather tanning, and steel production.

In the United States, recognition of chromium as a potential pulmonary carcinogen began when the chromate industry acknowledged a concern over the incidence of lung cancer among their employees. This prompted Machle and Gregorius[101] to perform a retrospective mortality study encompassing the years 1933 through 1946 of employees at seven different plants located in New Jersey, New York, Maryland, and Ohio. They compared their findings with mortality data for industrial policyholders of the Metropolitan Life Insurance Company for the first 10 months of 1947. They found a 16-fold increase in the risk of lung cancer mortality among employees (range 18 to 50). Several ensuing studies have confirmed the increased risk of lung cancer associated with chromium exposure in occupations ranging from chromate production to the use of chromate-based pigments and/or spray paints.[102–113] Masonry,[114,115] hard-chrome plating,[116–118] and stainless steel production[119] are other occupations associated with chromium exposure and increased risks of lung cancer.

Regarding oral ingestion of chromium, a systematic review of the available data does not support a carcinogenic role for chromium (VI), especially at the current mandated maximal contamination level in drinking water.[120] No data exists supporting any increase in lung cancer among residents in communities surrounding industries, which primarily produce or utilize chromium.[121]

The mean latency period for development of chromium-related lung cancer varies between 13 and 30 years with a duration-of-exposure dependent increase in the risk of cancer. The predominant histologic cell types are small cell and squamous cell carcinoma, but all cell types have been reported in the literature.

Animal studies demonstrated a mild increase in lung cancer risk after exposure to inhaled forms of chromium. Levy et al.[122] found that intrabronchial implantation of two different samples of strontium chromate in rats resulted in a significant number of lung cancers (43 of 99 and 62 of 99), almost all of which were squamous cell carcinomas. Implantation of zinc chromate resulted in a significant increase in lung cancer development as well, but with many fewer malignancies (5 of 100).

The molecular mechanisms underlying the carcinogenicity of chromium carcinogen are still being investigated, but the preponderance of evidence points toward oxidative DNA damage. Cheng et al.[123] found that chromium (VI) in the form of potassium chromate administered to Big Blue transgenic mice by intratracheal instillation resulted in a dose- and glutathione-dependent mutation frequency within 2 weeks of initial exposure. This group suggested that the potential carcinogenic mechanism is mediated through oxidative damage of DNA.

Additional support for an oxidative DNA damage mechanism was provided by Hodges et al.[124] They found that exposing human lung epithelial cells (A549) to sodium dichromate for 1 hour resulted in a significant number of DNA-strand breaks. Immunohistochemistry analysis found that levels of a DNA-repair glycosylase 8-oxodeoxyguanosine (OGG1), were increased in treated cells. In a follow-up study, Hodges et al.[125] found that treating A549 cells with sodium dichromate for 16 hours resulted in a concentration-dependent decrease in levels of OGG1 mRNA expression and OGG1 protein in nuclear extracts. The authors found that these findings demonstrated that sodium dichromate carcinogenesis may be in part mediated by suppression of DNA-repair mechanisms performed by OGG1.

One study offered a potential cocarcinogenic mechanism for chromium exposure and smoking. Feng et al.[126] noted that preexposure of normal human lung fibroblasts to chromium (VI) enhances the binding of benzo(a)pyrene diol epoxide to mutational hotspots in the p53 gene, specifically codons 248, 273, and 282.

In the 1950s and 1960s, several steps were taken to decrease worker exposure to chromium—removal of calcium chromate by changing to lime-free processes and better environmental controls. Studies attempting to evaluate these modifications have not found any significant change in lung cancer-associated mortality but were often underpowered.[127]

In 1990, the IARC[128] concluded that chromium was a human pulmonary carcinogen. The OSHA currently mandates a PEL for chromate or chromic acid of 100-μg CrO_3/m^3. The NIOSH recommends a 10-hour time-weighted average exposure limit of 1-μg $Cr(VI)/m^3$. With respect to drinking water, the EPA[129] has established a maximum contamination level of 100 μg/mL (100 ppb).

DIESEL EXHAUST

Diesel particulate matter is composed of a core of elemental carbon and adsorbed organic compounds, including polycyclic aromatic hydrocarbons and nitrate, metals, sulfate, and other trace elements. Diesel particulates consist largely of respirable range particulates that have a large surface area where organic substances can adsorb easily. Lung cancer risk has been shown to be elevated among workers in occupations where diesel engines have been used.[130] Concerns over the potential carcinogenicity of diesel exhaust arose as a result of studies demonstrating the development of different carcinomas after exposure to diesel particle extracts[131] and other studies showing mutagenic effects of diesel particulate matter.[132–137]

Garshick et al.[138] performed a case-control study of U.S. railroad workers with at least 10 years of service and born in or after 1900. Using deaths between March 1, 1981 and February 28, 1982 and work history data available from the U.S. Railroad Retirement Board (RRB), they demonstrated an OR for lung cancer of 1.41 (95% CI, 1.06, 1.88) for railroad workers younger than age 65 at death exposed to diesel exhaust for more than 20 years after adjustment for cigarette smoking and asbestos exposure. However, another study published by Garshick[139] in 2004 failed to find an association between the lung cancer mortality and the duration of time that subjects spent as railroad workers. In this study, the increase in lung cancer mortality was restricted to those subjects who worked specifically on locomotives powered by diesel engines.

Swanson et al.[140] demonstrated significantly increased risks of lung cancer after adjustment for age at diagnosis, smoking, and race among truck drivers and railroad workers employed for more than or equal to 20 and 10 years. Their adjusted ORs were 2.5 (95% CI, 1.1, 4.4) and 2.4 (95% CI, 1.1, 5.1), respectively. They also found statistically significant trends for lung cancer in farmers. They are the first investigators to document this group as being at risk. In 2003, Jarvholm et al.[141] confirmed these findings in truck drivers.

Brüske-Hohlfeld et al.[142] described an elevated risk in farmers and found an OR of 6.81 (95% CI, 1.17, 39.51) for exposures of greater than 30 years. The increase in the OR has been attributed to the repeated exposure of farmers to exhaust as they drive tractors back and forth through their fields, thereby possibly increasing the concentration of exhaust and consequently their exposure.

With the amount of evidence linking diesel exhaust to lung cancer, in 2002, the EPA[143] concluded that diesel exhaust is a potential causative agent of lung cancer. By 2007, they required that the sulfur content of diesel fuel be less than 15 ppm.[144]

MINERAL OIL

Mineral oil has been in use in the textile and metalworking industries since the latter half of the 19th century. Initial concerns over its potential role as a carcinogen were raised after an epidemic of scrotal cancers among mule spinners in the cotton industry.

Jones[144a] was the first to describe abnormalities on chest radiographs of workers exposed to mineral oil aerosols.[145] Several case reports of lung cancer in association with a mineral oil-exposure history appeared between 1940 and 1970 prompting epidemiologic studies to clarify this apparent connection.[146–148]

Other case-control studies in the 1980s found significant associations between lung cancer and mineral oil exposure in workers in the metal industry and in workers using rotary letterpress printing machines.[149] More recently, an association has also been found in aerospace workers.[150] Mineral oil contains varying amounts of polycyclic aromatic hydrocarbons, known carcinogens. These molecules are the presumed carcinogenic component of mineral oil.

In 1984, the IARC[151] concluded that there was sufficient evidence from human studies that mineral oil is a human carcinogen. Currently, OSHA has set a PEL for mineral oil of 5 mg/m^3 of air as a time-weighted average concentration over an 8-hour period. The NIOSH has established similar exposure standards.[152]

NICKEL

Nickel is a naturally occurring element found in the environment in combination with sulfur or arsenic. It is a silvery white metal initially prized for its ability to color glass green. Nickel is hard yet malleable, magnetic, and inert; consequently, it has multiple uses. Presently, most mined nickel is used to produce austenitic stainless steel, whereas the remainder is used for the production of different alloys, rechargeable batteries, catalysts, plating, coins, chemicals, and foundry products.

The carcinogenicity of nickel only became apparent in Europe after case reports of cancer among nickel-refinery workers. Doll[153] provided the first epidemiologic evidence for lung and nose cancer after occupational exposure to nickel; however, his study did not have adequate data on duration of nickel exposure or information on exposure to other potential pulmonary carcinogens such as smoking. Studies of nickel workers continued to demonstrate increased risks for lung cancer, the largest of which was conducted by the International Committee on Nickel Carcinogenesis in Man (ICNCM) in 1990.[154–157] This study evaluated 140,888 nickel workers with a minimum employment period ranging between 6 months and 5 years. The committee concluded that most of the lung cancer risk was associated with exposure to oxidic and sulfidic nickel at high concentration or to a high concentration of the oxidic form alone. Soluble-nickel exposure at low levels was associated with high risks of lung cancer, and metallic nickel had no appreciable associated risk. However, Grimsrud et al.[158] evaluated a group of Norwegian nickel-refinery workers and found that a dose-related effect was evident for lung cancer risk, as well as exposure to water-soluble nickel species but not to sulfidic, oxidic, or metallic forms. In additional studies, Grimsrud et al.[159,160] continued to demonstrate an increase in lung cancer mortality associated with process work at nickel factories. At this time, the controversy over the risks of each specific type of nickel persists.[161,162]

As in all occupational lung cancer studies, smoking has presented a problem in ascertaining the true role of nickel exposure in lung cancer risk. Attempts to tease out the contribution of smoking in lung cancer risk among nickel workers have suggested an additive effect.[163]

The latency period for nickel-related lung cancer is about 15 years. A review of the literature did not reveal any predominance of a particular histologic cell type.

Animal data have not been entirely consistent in supporting the hypothesis that nickel is a pulmonary carcinogen. Ottolenghi et al.[164] were able to induce lung cancers in rats after inhalation of nickel subsulfide. However, Dunnick et al.[165] failed to demonstrate such a response. They also evaluated the inhalational effects of oxidic nickel and again, failed to demonstrate an increase in the development of lung cancer in rats. At higher doses, an increase was found but not statistically significant. Soluble nickel inhalational studies had not been conducted prior to the National Toxicology Program 2-year inhalation study. Again, no significant increase in lung cancer incidence was found after exposure to soluble nickel.[166] Exposing animals to metallic forms of nickel have not demonstrated the development of lung cancer either, except for one study, which did produce lung cancer after intratracheal instillation of elemental nickel in rats.[167] On a molecular level, nickel has been shown to damage and mutate DNA while also preventing DNA repair.[168,169]

In 1990, the IARC concluded that nickel compounds were carcinogenic to humans. The EPA has set a long-term PEL of 0.2 mg of nickel per kilogram of body weight per day in food and drinking water. The OSHA has established an occupational level of exposure to be 1 mg on nickel per cubic meter over an 8-hour workday, 40-hour workweek. The NIOSH has set a recommended exposure level of 0.015 mg/m^3.[170]

RADON

Radon is an odorless, colorless gas, which is derived from the radioactive decay of uranium. Radon itself undergoes radioactive decay with a half-life of about 4 hours and generates two progeny or radon daughters. Radon daughters, with a half-life of about one-half hours, attach easily to dust and other airborne particles, permitting their inhalation and deposition along the respiratory airways. The daughters continue to decay until they become nonradioactive particles. During each decay cycle, release of alpha, beta, and gamma radiation occurs, thereby predisposing nearby living cells to potential DNA damage and/or mutation and subsequent development of malignancy. Numerous studies have demonstrated the mutagenic effects of radiation on cellular DNA[171–173] and the generation of lung cancers in Sprague-Dawley rats[174,175] and A/J mice.[176]

In the 1800s, uranium was used primarily as a dye, and uranium miners in Schneeberg, Germany and Joachimsthal, Czechoslovakia were known to develop lung disease and lung cancer.[177] In fact, the relationship was significant enough that by 1932, both Germany and Czechoslovakia had designated lung cancer in these miners as a compensatable disease.[178]

Studies conducted by the U.S. Public Health Service in the 1950s raised concerns about the possibility of increased risks of lung cancer among uranium miners.[179] By 1964, reports were circulating about the high concentrations of radon in uranium mines,[180] and there were concerns regarding the risk of lung cancer being related to the amount of exposure to radon daughters.[181] However, controversy existed over the influence of smoking on the risk of lung cancer.

Numerous studies among Navajo men were performed to evaluate the effects of uranium/radon on lung cancer. Mining around the Navajo Nation began in 1948, peaked around 1956, and declined to zero by 1967.[182] Several studies demonstrated an excess in lung cancer–related mortality among Navajo Indians. Archer et al.[183] found 11 lung cancer–related deaths in a follow-up study of 780 predominantly Navajo Native American Indians compared to an expected number of 2.6. Gottlieb et al.[184] documented that between February 1965 and May 1979, 16 of 17 male Navajo patients admitted with lung cancer were uranium miners (94.1%). Samet et al.[185] were able to demonstrate a significantly elevated risk of lung cancer in predominantly nonsmoking Navajo Indians. Of the 32 Navajo men with documented lung cancer between 1969 and 1981, 23 had been uranium miners. Information regarding smoking status was available for 21 of these 23 miners: 8 were nonsmokers; 2 smoked less than one cigarette per day; 6 smoked between one to three cigarettes daily; and 5 smoked between four and eight cigarettes per day. In the same issue of the *New England Journal of Medicine*, Radford et al.[186] also demonstrated an increased incidence of lung cancer in Swedish iron miners who had been exposed to low doses of radon daughters, not affected by smoking status.

In an editorial, Harley[187] discussed the potential implication of environmental exposure to radon. The average environmental radon exposure has been estimated to be about 0.2 working-level months (WLM) per year.[188] A working level is equivalent to 100 pCi/L of air at equilibrium. A WLM is the exposure derived from spending 170 hours (1 month's working hours) exposed to a working level. Based on a risk projection generated by Radford et al.,[186] this level of exposure translates into a lung cancer risk of 15 cases per 1000 persons. Lubin et al.[189] pooled the results from two case-control studies of residential radon exposure in China and found increased ORs for the risk of lung cancer. Specifically, for subjects living in the same home for 30 years or more exposed to 100 Bq/m^3 of radon, the OR for lung cancer was 1.32 (95% CI, 1.07, 1.91) where 1 Ci is equivalent to 3.7×10^{10} Bq. In 2005, Darby et al.[190] and Krewski et al.[191] also found increases in the risk of lung cancer after pooling 13 European and 7 North American case-control studies, respectively.

The highest recorded environmental radon-related exposure occurred in Pennsylvania at the home of Stanley Watras. His home level of radon was 2700 pCi/L. Geologic surveys of his home revealed that the structure was located on the Reading Prong, a large naturally occurring granite deposit. Other natural soil sources of radon include shale, phosphate, and pitchblende. It has been estimated that 1 in 15 homes have higher than acceptable radon levels as determined by the EPA (4 pCi/L). The average level in the U.S. homes is about 1 pCi/L.

Commercial kits are available to measure radon levels in homes, but consumers should be aware that only certain testing devices are certified as "meeting EPA requirements." Testing should be performed if the home is located over large deposits of granite, shale, phosphate, or pitchblende, as well as if a young patient without a significant smoke-exposure history or significant family history presents with a lung cancer. Removing radon sources from the home requires professional certified contractors. Options include sealing cracks in floors and walls, installing pipes and fans to ventilate the ground below home foundations (subslab depressurization), and/or soil depressurization. One of the most important interventions is smoking cessation, especially inside the dwelling.

SILICA

Crystalline silica is the cause of silicosis, an inhalational occupational disease. The list of occupations associated with crystalline silica exposure is extensive and includes any occupation that aerosolizes crystal dusts. Mining, sandblasting, ceramic production, and stone working are a few examples.

Hippocrates recognized the development of pulmonary disease in the setting of occupational exposure to crystalline silica dust as early as 400 BC. Silica was not thought of as a carcinogen until the 1980s after several investigators noted the development of lung and pleural cancers in rats after exposure to crystalline silica. Wagner[192–194] demonstrated an increase in the development of lymphosarcomas after intrapleural injection of crystalline silica in Wistar rats, injection of alkaline-washed quartz, cristobalite, and Min-U-Sil in Wistar rats, and injection of six different forms of crystalline silica in three different rat strains. Stenbäck and Rowland[195] demonstrated an increased incidence of respiratory tumors (44%) with intratracheal instillation of silica in combination with benzo(a)pyrene in Syrian golden hamsters compared with benzo(a)pyrene alone (10%). Holland et al.[196] also showed an increased incidence of respiratory tumors (16.7%) in Sprague-Dawley rats after intratracheal administration of silica. His group also showed that Fischer-344 rats, after inhalational exposure to silica, had an increased incidence of respiratory cancers (66.7%) compared to none in the controls.[197]

The potential role of silica in human lung cancer was brought to light with the work of several epidemiologists. In the 1500s, miners from Schneeberg and Joachimsthal had a high mortality rate, and it was recognized only later that the likely cause of this increase was lung cancer.[198] Milham Jr[199] found a threefold increase in the risk of bronchial and lung cancers in metal molders from Washington State based on death certificates between 1950 and 1971. Westerholm[200] examined the Swedish Pneumoconiosis Register and found that those who developed silicosis had a significantly elevated risk of lung cancer–related mortality. The relationship between silicosis and lung cancer has been supported by additional studies.[201–203] Finkelstein et al.[204] also demonstrated a twofold increase in lung cancer–related deaths in patients receiving workmen's compensation for silicosis between 1940 and 1975 from data obtained from the Ontario Ministry of Labor. Attfield et al.[205] found a dose–response relationship between silica exposure and lung cancer in Vermont granite workers. These case-control studies did not document the prevalence of smoking in the study population, but it was presumed to be significantly higher than that of the control population, which was the general public. In addition, demonstration of pneumoconiosis or silicosis was required in the studies by Westerholm and Finkelstein, respectively, thereby preventing conclusions regarding the risk of lung cancer in workers exposed to silica without evidence of disease on radiographs.

The controversy over the potential role of silica in lung cancer pathogenesis stems from numerous studies, which failed to find an increase in cancer risk after attempting to account for smoking and exposure to radon daughters, arsenic, and other occupational carcinogens.[206,207] Becker and Chatgidakis[208] did not find a significant difference in the incidence of bronchogenic carcinoma in white male gold miners compared to nonminers. Other studies found that the degree of silicosis did not correlate with the incidence of bronchogenic carcinoma.[209,210] In response to this controversy, Checkoway et al.[211] evaluated the incidence of lung cancer in diatomaceous earth mining and processing facility employees. They found that lung cancer incidence was associated with cumulative crystalline silica exposure and was not dependent on the presence of radiographically evident silicosis. They attempted to further bolster their findings by reviewing the available literature, but found that the design of most studies attempting to better describe the link between silica and lung cancer were potentially confounded by the use of compensation claims to identify patients with silicosis and the lack of adequate quantification of exposure.[212] A recent study concluded that silica exposure in North American industrial sand workers was associated with an increase in lung cancer after controlling for smoking.[213]

Despite these contradictory studies, in 1996, the IARC concluded that the available literature provided sufficient evidence implicating the inhalation of crystalline silica as a carcinogen. The American Thoracic Society (ATS) followed that same year with a statement describing the potential adverse effects of inhaled silica exposure, including lung cancer. However, ATS qualified the statement by questioning the carcinogenicity of silica dust in nonsmokers and in those exposed to silica dust without evidence of silicosis. In 1989, the NIOSH concurred with the findings of the IARC and ATS after conducting their own review of the literature and recommended that crystalline silica be listed as a potential occupational carcinogen.

Occupational exposure controls have been established by government agencies for silica but as part of a group of fibers labeled as synthetic vitreous fibers. The PEL set by OSHA is 5 mg/m^3 for the inhalable fraction and 15 mg/m^3 for the total dust exposure. The NIOSH has set a recommended exposure limit (REL) of 3 fibers per cubic centimeter for fibrous glass dust over a 10-hour time-weighted average.[214]

VINYL CHLORIDE

Vinyl chloride (VC) has been used for various applications as early as the 1920s, but techniques to produce a stable form of polyvinyl chloride (PVC) did not arise until the 1930s. The polymerization process required to produce PVC involves the use of a reactor. After completion of the reaction, the tank would need cleaning to remove a layer of PVC that had formed on the walls of the reactor. Currently, high-pressure jets and solvents are used for this purpose but originally, workers would climb into the reactors with spatulas or hammers and chisels. Consequently, they were exposed to high levels of VC, which was associated with an acute illness manifesting as headaches, dizziness, visual disturbances, anorexia, abdominal pains, and dyspnea.[215]

Initial concerns regarding potential carcinogenicity were raised in animal studies.[216] Soon afterward, Creech et al.[217] published a report on the increased incidence of hepatic angiosarcomas in PVC workers. Based on the results of animal studies and the demonstration of an increase in hepatic angiosarcoma in PVC workers, Tabershaw et al.[218] decided to conduct a historical prospective mortality study of 8384 men who had had at least 1 year of occupational exposure to VC. They found 13 respiratory cancers compared with 10.28 expected suggesting a potential role for VC as a pulmonary carcinogen. The first human study to show a significant increase in lung cancer was conducted by Waxweiler et al.[219] They performed a retrospective cohort study on workers exposed to VC at four plants in the United States and found an excess of respiratory cancers at plant number four (9 compared with 4.6) and 12 cases of respiratory malignancies compared with an expected 7.7 at all plants. Of note, plant 4 contributed more than two thirds of person-years to the study, which was the reasoning provided by the authors for conducting a separate analysis at that particular plant. However, a review of studies of VC and lung cancer has generated conflicting conclusions regarding the potential of VC to act as a pulmonary carcinogen.[220–222] There is little doubt about the role that VC plays in hepatic angiosarcoma, but its contribution to the development of human lung cancer is still under debate today.[222]

Regardless, the IARC concluded that VC is a human pulmonary carcinogen as a result of sufficient evidence on the carcinogenicity in humans. The EPA has mandated that human exposure be no more than 0.002 mg of VC per liter of water. The OSHA has set a PEL of 1 ppm of air during an 8-hour workday during a 40-hour workweek.[223]

WHERE TO FIND MORE INFORMATION

This chapter provides an overview on the topic of nontobacco-related lung carcinogenesis. More information is available on the Internet. Details about proportionate mortality ratios (PMR) for lung cancer in higher-risk industries may be found through the NIOSH at http://www.cdc.gov/niosh/topics/surveillance/ords/NationalStatistics/Highlights/table13-01(LC01).html. Details about PMR for lung cancer in specific occupations may be found at http://www.cdc.gov/niosh/topics/surveillance/ords/NationalStatistics/Highlights/table13-02(LC01).html. The lists of substances NIOSH has determined are potential occupational carcinogens may be found at http://www.cdc.gov/niosh/npotocca.html. Information about the NIOSH Health Hazard Evaluation program and how to request an evaluation may be found at http://www.cdc.gov/niosh/hhe/.

Other excellent sources of information about pulmonary carcinogens encountered in occupational and environmental settings may be found through Web sites sponsored by the Centers for Disease Control and Prevention (http://www.cdc.gov/), NIOSH (http://www.cdc.gov/niosh/), the U.S. EPA (http://www.epa.gov/), and the IARC (http://www.iarc.fr/).

CONCLUSION

Lung cancer among nonsmokers is an important cause of morbidity and mortality. Multiple carcinogens have been identified as contributing to the total public health burden of lung cancer. No single carcinogenic exposure accounts for a significant burden of lung cancer among individuals who have not been exposed to tobacco smoke. Although a large body of literature has identified a spectrum of respirable exposures significantly associated with the development of lung cancer in exposed populations, proving a causal link between an exposure and a case of lung cancer in an individual nonsmoker is challenging.

Reducing exposure to carcinogens through engineering controls, production substitution, and personal respiratory protection remains the principal mechanism for reducing occupational lung cancer risk. Environmental controls are relevant in any setting where pulmonary carcinogens may be encountered. If ongoing exposures are of concern, an investigation of the workplace or home environment is critical. If a potential carcinogen is discovered in either setting, trained contractors may be required to assist with clean up. Claims of past or ongoing occupational exposure to pulmonary carcinogens, such as asbestos or uranium, among individuals with lung cancer may be compensable.

REFERENCES

1. Thun MJ, Henley SJ, Burns D, et al. Lung cancer death rates in lifelong nonsmokers. *J Natl Cancer Inst* 2006;98:691–699.
2. Kuschner WG, Blanc PD. Gases and other inhalants. In: LaDou J. *Current Occupational and Environmental Medicine*. 3rd Ed. Norwalk, CT: Appleton and Lange, 2004.
3. Paris JA. *Pharmacologia*. 3rd Ed. London: Phillips, 1820.
4. Saupe E. Carcinoma of the lung in arsenic miners; two cases. *Arch Gewerbepathol* 1930;1:582.
5. Blot WJ, Fraumeni JF Jr. Arsenical air pollution and lung cancer. *Lancet* 1975;2:142–144.
6. Tokudome S, Kuratsune M. A cohort study on mortality from cancer and other causes among workers at a metal refinery. *Int J Cancer* 1976;17:310–317.

6a. Rencher AC, Carter MW, McKee DW. A retrospective epidemiological study of mortality at a large western copper smelter. *J Occup Med* 1977;19(11):754–758.

7. Axelson O, Dahlgren E, Jansson CD, et al. Arsenic exposure and mortality: a case-referent study from a Swedish copper smelter. *Br J Ind Med* 1978;35:8–15.
8. Enterline PE, Marsh GM. Mortality studies of smelter workers. *Am J Ind Med* 1980;1:251–259.
9. Wall S. Survival and mortality pattern among Swedish smelter workers. *Int J Epidemiol* 1980;9:73–87.
10. Jarup L, Pershagen G, Wall S. Cumulative arsenic exposure and lung cancer in smelter workers: a dose-response study. *Am J Ind Med* 1989;15:31–41.
11. Jarup L, Pershagen G. Arsenic exposure, smoking, and lung cancer in smelter workers—a case-control study. *Am J Epidemiol* 1991;134:545–551.
12. Barthel E. Increased risk of lung cancer in pesticide-exposed male agricultural workers. *J Toxicol Environ Health* 1981;8:1027–1040.
13. Lüchtrath H. The consequences of chronic arsenic poisoning among Moselle wine growers: pathoanatomical investigations of postmortem examinations performed between 1960 and 1977. *J Cancer Res Clin Oncol* 1983;105:173–182.
14. Heddle R, Bryant GD. Small cell lung carcinoma and Bowen's disease 40 years after arsenic ingestion. *Chest* 1983;84:776–777.
15. Guo HR, Wang NS, Hu H, et al. Cell type specificity of lung cancer associated with arsenic ingestion. *Cancer Epidemiol Biomarkers Prev* 2004;13:638–643.
16. Chen CJ, Chen CW, Wu MM, et al. Cancer potential in liver, lung, bladder, and kidney due to ingested inorganic arsenic in drinking water. *Br J Cancer* 1992;66:888–892.
17. Tsuda T, Babazono A, Yamamoto E, et al. Ingested arsenic and internal cancer: a historical cohort study followed for 33 years. *Am J Epidemiol* 1995;141:198–209.
18. Chiou HY, Hsueh YM, Liaw KF, et al. Incidence of internal cancers and ingested inorganic arsenic: a seven-year follow-up study in Taiwan. *Cancer Res* 1995;55:1296–1300.
19. Smith A, Goycolea M, Haque R, et al. Marked increase in bladder and lung cancer mortality in a region of Northern Chile due to arsenic in drinking water. *Am J Epidemiol* 1998;147:660–669.
20. Chen Y, Ahsan H. Cancer burden from arsenic in drinking water in Bangladesh. *Am J Public Health* 2004;94:741–744.
21. Chen CL, Hsu LI, Chiou HY, et al. Ingested arsenic, cigarette smoking, and lung cancer risk: a follow-up study in arseniasis-endemic areas in Taiwan. *JAMA* 2004;292:2984–2990.
22. Chiu HF, Ho SC, Yang CY. Lung cancer mortality reduction after installation of tap-water supply system in an arseniasis-endemic area in Southwestern Taiwan. *Lung Cancer* 2004;46:265–270.
23. Enterline PE, Marsh GM, Esmen NA, et al. Some effects of cigarette smoking, arsenic, and SO2 on mortality among U.S. copper smelter workers. *J Occup Med* 1987;29:831–838.
24. Pershagen G, Wall S, Taube A, et al. On the interaction between occupational arsenic exposure and smoking and its relationship to lung cancer. *Scand J Work Environ Health* 1981;7:302–309.
25. Hertz–Picciotto I, Smith AH, Holtzman D, et al. Synergism between occupational arsenic exposure and smoking in the induction of lung cancer. *Epidemiology* 1992;3:23–31.
26. Greaves WW, Rom WN, Lyon JL, et al. Relationship between lung cancer and distance of residence from nonferrous smelter stack effluent. *Am J Ind Med* 1981;2:15–23.
27. Rom WN, Varley G, Lyon JL, et al. Lung cancer mortality among residents living near the El Paso smelter. *Br J Ind Med* 1982;39:269–272.
28. Frost F, Harter L, Milham S, et al. Lung cancer among women residing close to an arsenic emitting copper smelter. *Arch Environ Health* 1987;42:148–152.
29. Frank AL. The epidemiology and etiology of lung cancer. *Clin Chest Med* 1982;3:219–228.
30. Wicks MJ, Archer VE, Auerbach O, et al. Arsenic exposure in a copper smelter as related to histological type of lung cancer. *Am J Ind Med* 1981;2:25–31.
31. Pershagen G, Bergman F, Klominek J, et al. Histological types of lung cancer among smelter workers exposed to arsenic. *Br J Ind Med* 1987;44:454–458.
32. Ishinishi N, Kodama Y, Nobutomo K, et al. Preliminary experimental study on carcinogenicity of arsenic trioxide in rat lung. *Environ Health Perspect* 1977;19:191–196.

33. Ishinishi N, Yamamoto A, Hisanaga A, et al. Tumorigenicity of arsenic trioxide to the lung in Syrian golden hamsters by intermittent instillations. *Cancer Lett* 1983;21:141–147.
34. Ivankovic S, Eisenbrand G, Preussmann R. Lung carcinoma induction in BD rats after a single intratracheal instillation of an arsenic-containing pesticide mixture formerly used in vineyards. *Int J Cancer* 1979;24: 786–788.
35. Soucy NV, Ihnat MA, Kamat CD, et al. Arsenic stimulates angiogenesis and tumorigenesis in vivo. *Toxicol Sci* 2003;76:271–279.
36. Pershagen G, Bjorklund NE. On the pulmonary tumorigenicity of arsenic trisulfide and calcium arsenate in hamsters. *Cancer Lett* 1985;27:99–104.
37. Yamamoto A, Hisanaga A, Ishinishi N. Tumorigenicity of inorganic arsenic compounds following intratracheal instillations to the lungs of hamsters. *Int J Cancer* 1987;40:220–223.
38. Dong JT, Zhou CN, Luo XM. Induction of preneoplastic lesions by sodium arsenite in human fetal respiratory epithelia in organ culture. *Environ Res* 1995;68:39–43.
39. Mass MJ, Wang L. Arsenic alters cytosine methylation patterns of the promoter of the tumor suppressor gene p53 in human lung cells: a model for a mechanism of carcinogenesis. *Mutat Res* 1997;386:263–277.
40. Evans CD, LaDow K, Schumann BL, et al. Effect of arsenic on benzo[a]pyrene DNA adduct levels in mouse skin and lung. *Carcinogenesis* 2004;25:493–497.
41. Agency for Toxic Substances and Disease Registry, U.S. Department of Health and Human Services, Public Health Service. *Toxicological Profile for Arsenic*. 2000.
42. Tweedale G. Asbestos and its lethal legacy. *Nat Rev Cancer* 2002; 2:311–315.
43. Merewether ER. Asbestosis and carcinoma of the lung. In: *Annual Report for the Chief Inspector of Factories for the Year 1947*. London: Her Majesty's Stationery Office, 1949.
44. Doll R. Mortality from lung cancer in asbestos workers. *Brit J Industr Med* 1955;12:81–86.
45. Selikoff IJ, Churg J, Hammond EC. Asbestos exposure and neoplasia. *JAMA* 1964;188:142–146.
46. Wagner JC, Sieggs CA, Marchand P. Diffuse pleural mesotheliomas and asbestos exposure in the Northwestern Cape Province. *Br J Indust Med* 1960;17:260–271.
47. Newhouse ML, Thompson H. Mesothelioma of pleura and peritoneum following exposure to asbestos in the London area. *Br J Indust Med* 1965;22:261–269.
48. Huang B, Liu B, Xu M, et al. k-ras gene mutations of asbestos and welding-fumes related human lung cancer. *Wei Sheng Yan Jiu* 2000;29:7–9.
49. Wang Q, Fan J, Wang H, et al. DNA damage and activation of c-ras in human embryo lung cells exposed to chrysotile and smoking solution. *J Environ Pathol Toxicol Oncol* 2000;19:13–19.
50. Nelson HH, Christiani DC, Wiencke JK, et al. k-ras mutation and occupational asbestos exposure in lung adenocarcinoma: asbestos-related cancer without asbestosis. *Cancer Res* 1999;59:4570–4573.
51. Panduri V, Surapureddi S, Soberanes S, et al. P53 mediates amosite asbestos-induced alveolar epithelial cell mitochondria-regulated apoptosis. *Am J Respir Cell Mol Biol* 2006;34:443–452.
52. Morris GF, Notwick AR, David O, et al. Development of lung tumors in mutant p53-expressing mice after inhalation exposure to asbestos. *Chest* 2004;125:S85–S86.
53. Zhao YL, Piao CQ, Wu LJ, et al. Differentially expressed genes in asbestos-induced tumorigenic human bronchial epithelial cells: implication for mechanism. *Carcinogenesis* 2000;21:2005–2010.
54. Iwata T, Kohyama N, Yano E. Chemiluminescent detection of induced reactive oxygen metabolite production of human polymorphonuclear leucocytes by anthophyllite asbestos. *Environ Res* 2002;88:36–40.
55. Schabath MB, Spitz MR, Delclos GL, et al. Association between asbestos exposure, cigarette smoking, myeloperoxidase (MPO) genotypes, and lung cancer risk. *Am J Ind Med* 2002;42:29–37.
56. MacCorkle RA, Slattery SD, Nash DR, et al. Intracellular protein binding to asbestos induces aneuploidy in human lung fibroblasts. *Cell Motil Cytoskeleton* 2006;63:646–657.
57. Brown RC, Fleming GTA, Knight AI. Asbestos affects the in vitro uptake and detoxification of aromatic coumpounds. *Environ Health Perspect* 1983;51:315–318.
58. Gerde P, Scholander P. Adsorption of benzo(a)pyrene on to asbestos and manmade mineral fibres in an aqueous solution and in a biological model solution. *Br J Ind Med* 1988;45:682–688.
59. Lacowicz J, Bevan DR, Riemer SC. Transport of a carcinogen, benzo[a]pyrene, from particulates to lipid bilayers: a model for the fate of particle-adsorbed polynuclear aromatic hydrocarbons, which are retained in the lungs. *Biochem Biophys Acta* 1980;629:243–258.
60. Martischnig KM, Newall DJ, Barnsley WC, et al. Unsuspected exposure to asbestos and bronchogenic carcinoma. *Br Med J* 1977;1:746–749.
61. Whitwell F, Newhouse ML, Bennett DR. A study of the histological cell types of lung cancer in workers suffering from asbestosis in the United Kingdom. *Br J Ind Med* 1974;31:398–403.
62. Hein MJ, Stayner LT, Lehman E, et al. Follow-up study of chrysotile textile workers: cohort mortality and exposure response. *Occup Environ Med* 2007;64:616–625.
63. Berman DW, Crump KS, Chatfield EJ, et al. The sizes, shapes, and mineralogy of asbestos structures that induce lung tumors or mesothelioma in AF/HAN rats following inhalation. *Risk Anal* 1995;15:181–195.
64. McDonald JC, McDonald AD. Chrysotile, tremolite, and carcinogenicity. *Ann Occup Hyg* 1997;41:699–705.
65. Hughes JM, Weill H. Asbestosis as a precursor of asbestos related lung cancer: results of a prospective mortality study. *Br J Ind Med* 1991;48:229–233.
66. Szeszenia–Dabrowska N, Urszula W, et al. Mortality study of workers compensated for asbestosis in Poland, 1970–1997. *Int J Occup Med Environ Health* 2002;15:267–278.
67. Hammond EC, Selikoff IJ, Seidman H. Asbestos exposure, cigarette smoking, and death rates. *Ann NY Acad Sci* 1979;330:473–490.
68. World Trade Organization, European Community. *Report of the Appelate Body: Measures Affecting Asbestos and Asbestos-Containing Products*. 2001. Report No. WT/DS135/AB/R.
69. International Agency for Research on Cancer (IARC). Summaries & Evaluations. *Asbestos*. Vol. 2, 1973:17.
70. Kannerstein M, Churg J, McCaughey WTE. Asbestos and mesothelioma: a review. *Pathol Annu* 1978;13:81–129.
71. Mancuso T. Relation of duration of employment and prior respiratory disease among beryllium workers. *Environ Res* 1970;3:251–275.
72. Mancuso T. Mortality study of beryllium industry workers' occupational lung cancer. *Environ Res* 1980;21:48–55.
73. Mancuso TF, El-Attar AA. Epidemiologic study of the beryllium industry: cohort methodology and mortality studies. *J Occup Med* 1969;11:422–434.
74. Steenland K, Ward E. Lung cancer incidence among patients with beryllium disease: a cohort mortality study. *J Natl Cancer Inst* 1991;83:1380–1385.
75. Ward E, Okun A, Ruder A, et al. A mortality study of workers at seven beryllium processing plants. *Am J Ind Med* 1992;22:885–904.
76. Sanderson WT, Ward E, Steenland K, et al. Lung cancer case-control study of beryllium workers. *Am J Ind Med* 2001;39:133–144.
77. MacMahon B. The epidemiological evidence on the carcinogenicity of beryllium in humans. *J Occup Med* 1994;36:15–24.
78. Hardy HL. Beryllium disease: a clinical perspective. *Environ Res* 1980;21:1–9.
79. Williams WJ. United Kingdom beryllium registry: mortality and autopsy study. *Environ Health Perspect* 1996;104(Suppl 5):949–951.
80. Nickell–Brady C, Hahn FF, Finch GL, et al. Analysis of k-ras, p53, and c-Raf-1 mutations in beryllium-induced rat lung tumors. *Carcinogenesis* 1994;15:257–262.
81. Belinsky SA, Swafford DS, Finch GL, et al. Alterations in the k-ras and p53 genes in rat lung tumors. *Environ Health Perspect* 1997;105 (Suppl 4):901–906.

82. Finch GL, March TH, Hahn FF, et al. Carcinogenic responses of transgenic heterozygous p53 knockout mice to inhaled 239PuO2 or metallic beryllium. *Toxicol Pathol* 1998;26:484–491.
83. Reeves AL, Deitch D, Vorwald AJ. Beryllium carcinogenesis. I. Inhalational exposure of rats to beryllium sulfate aerosol. *Cancer Res* 1967;27:439–445.
84. Belinsky SA, Snow SS, Nikula KJ, et al. Aberrant CpG island methylation of the p16(INK4a) and estrogen receptor genes in rat lung tumors induced by particulate carcinogens. *Carcinogenesis* 2002;23:335–359.
85. Agency for Toxic Substances and Disease Registry: U.S. Department of Health and Human Services, Public Health Service. *Toxicological Profile for Beryllium*. 2002.
86. van Duuren BL, Goldschmidt BM, Langseth L, et al. Alpha-haloethers: a new type of alkylating carcinogen. *Arch Environ Health* 1968;16: 472–476.
87. Leong BKJ, Macfarland HN, Reese WH. Induction of lung adenomas by chronic inhalation of bis (chloromethyl) ether. *Arch Environ Health* 1971;22:663–666.
88. Laskin S, Kuschner J, Drew RT, et al. Tumors of the respiratory tract induced by inhalation of bis(chloromethyl) ether. *Arch Environ Health* 1971;23:135–136.
89. Albert RE, Pasternack BS, Shore RE, et al. Mortality patterns among workers exposed to chloromethyl ethers: a preliminary report. *Environ Health Perspect* 1975;11:209–214.
90. DeFonso LR, Kelton SC. Lung cancer following exposure to chloromethyl methyl ether: An epidemiological study. *Archiv Environ Health* 1976;31:125–130.
91. Figueroa WG, Raszowski R, Weiss W. Lung cancer in chloromethyl methyl ether workers. *New Engl J Med* 1973;228:1096–1097.
92. Lemen RA, Johnson WM, Wagoner JK, et al. Cytologic observations and cancer incidence following exposure to BCME. *Ann N Y Acad Sci* 1976;271:71–80.
93. Nelson N. The chloroethers-occupational carcinogens: a summary of laboratory and epidemiology studies. *Ann N Y Acad Sci* 1976;271:81–90.
94. Weiss W, Figueroa WG. The characteristics of lung cancer due to chloromethyl ethers. *J Occup Med* 1976;18:623–627.
95. Weiss W, Moser RL, Auerbach O. Lung cancer in chloromethyl ether workers. *Am Rev Respir Dis* 1979;120:1031–1037.
96. Weiss W. Epidemic curve of respiratory cancer due to chloromethyl ethers. *J Natl Cancer Inst* 1982;69:1265–1270.
97. Maher KV, DeFonso LR. Respiratory cancer among chloromethyl ether workers. *J Natl Cancer Inst* 1987;78:839–843.
98. Collingwood KW, Pasternack BS, Shore RE. An industry-wide study of respiratory cancer in chemical workers exposed to chloromethyl ethers. *J Natl Cancer Inst* 1987;78:1127–1136.
99. Weiss W, Nash D. An epidemic of lung cancer due to chloromethyl ethers. *J Occup Environ Med* 1997;39:1003–1009.
100. Agency for Toxic Substances and Disease Registry: U.S. Department of Health and Human Services, Public Health Service. *Toxicological Profile for Bis(chloromethyl) Ether*. 1989.
101. Machle W, Gregorius F. Cancer of the respiratory system in the United States chromate-producing industry. *Public Health Reports* 1948;63:114–127.
102. Baetjer AM. Pulmonary carcinoma in chromate workers: II. Incidence of basis of hospital records. *A M A Arch Ind Hyg Occup Med* 1950;2:505–516.
103. Mancuso TF, Hueper WC. Occupational cancer and other health hazards in a chromate plant: a medical appraisal. I. Lung cancers in chromate workers. *Ind Med Surg* 1951;20:358–363.
104. Bidstrup PL, Case RAM. Carcinoma of the lung in workmen in the bichromates-producing industry in Great Britain. *Brit J Industr Med* 1956;13:260–264.
105. Taylor FH. The relationship of mortality and duration of employment as reflected by a cohort of chromate workers. *Am J Public Health Nations Health* 1966;56:218–229.
106. Enterline P. Respiratory cancer among chromate workers. *J Occup Med* 1974;16:523–536.
107. Langård S, Norseth T. A cohort study of bronchial carcinomas in workers producing chromate pigments. *Br J Ind Med* 1975;32:62–65.
108. Hayes RB, Lilienfeld AM, Snell LM. Mortality in chromium chemical production workers: a prospective study. *Int J Epidemiol* 1979;8:365–374.
109. Dalager NA, Mason TJ, Fraumeni JF Jr, et al. Cancer mortality among workers exposed to zinc chromate paints. *J Occup Med* 1980;22:25–29.
110. Sheffet A, Thind I, Miller AM, et al. Cancer mortality in a pigment plant utilizing lead and zinc chromates. *Arch Environ Health* 1982;37:44–52.
111. Langard S, Vigander T. Occurrence of lung cancer in workers producing chromium pigments. *Br J Ind Med* 1983;40:71–74.
112. Hayes RB, Sheffet A, Spirtas R. Cancer mortality among a cohort of chromium pigment workers. *Am J Ind Med* 1989;16:127–133.
113. Rosenman KD, Stanbury M. Risk of lung cancer among former chromium smelter workers. *Am J Ind Med* 1996;29:491–500.
114. Rafnsson V, Gunnarsdottir H, Kiilunen M. Risk of lung cancer among masons in Iceland. *Occup Environ Med* 1997;54:184–188.
115. Rafnsson V, Johannesdottir SG. Mortality among masons in Iceland. *Br J Ind Med* 1986;43:522–525.
116. Franchini I, Magnani F, Mutti A. Mortality experience among chromeplating workers. Initial findings. *Scand J Work Environ Health* 1983;9:247–252.
117. Sorahan T, Burges D, Hamilton L, et al. Lung cancer mortality in nickel/chromium platers, 1946–1995. *Occup Environ Med* 1998;55:236–242.
118. Sorahan T, Harrington JM. Lung cancer in Yorkshire chrome platers, 1972–97. *Occup Environ Med* 2000;57:385–389.
119. Moulin JJ, Wild P, Mantout B, et al. Mortality from lung cancer and cardiovascular diseases among stainless-steel producing workers. *Cancer Causes Control* 1993;4:75–81.
120. Proctor DM, Otani JM, Finley BL, et al. Is hexavalent chromium carcinogenic via ingestion? A weight-of-evidence review. *J Toxicol Environ Health A* 2002;65:701–746.
121. Fryzek JP, Mumma MT, McLaughlin JK, et al. Cancer mortality in relation to environmental chromium exposure. *J Occup Environ Med* 2001;43:635–640.
122. Levy LS, Martin PA, Bidstrup PL. Investigation of the potential carcinogenicity of a range of chromium containing materials on rat lung. *Br J Ind Med* 1986;43:243–256.
123. Cheng L, Sonntag DM, de Boer J, et al. Chromium (VI)-induced mutagenesis in the lungs of big blue transgenic mice. *J Environ Pathol Toxicol Oncol* 2000;19:239–249.
124. Hodges NJ, Adam B, Lee AJ, et al. Induction of DNA-strand breaks in human peripheral blood lymphocytes and A549 lung cells by sodium dichromate: association with 8-oxo-2-deoxyguanosine formation and inter-individual variability. *Mutagenesis* 2001; 16:467–474.
125. Hodges NJ, Chipman JK. Down-regulation of the DNA-repair endonuclease 8-oxo-guanine DNA glycosylase 1 (hOGG1) by sodium dichromate in cultured human A549 lung carcinoma cells. *Carcinogenesis* 2002;23:55–60.
126. Feng Z, Hu W, Rom WN, et al. Chromium (VI) exposure enhances polycyclic aromatic hydrocarbon-DNA binding at the p53 gene in human lung cells. *Carcinogenesis* 2003;24:771–778.
127. Paddle GM. Meta-analysis as an epidemiological tool and its application to studies of chromium. *Reg Toxicol Pharmacol* 1997;26:S42–S50.
128. IARC. Chromium and chromium compounds: Chromium[VI] (Group 1) Metallic chromium and chromium[III] compounds (Group 3). *International Agency for Research on Cancer: Summaries & Evaluations.* 1990;49:49.
129. Kapil V. (Agency for Toxic Substances and Disease Registry: U.S. Department of Health and Human Services, Division of Health Education and Promotion). *Case Studies in Environmental Medicine: Chromium Toxicity*. 1992. October 1992. Report No.: ATSDR-HE-CS-2001-0005.

130. Wichmann HE. Diesel exhaust particles. *Inhal Toxicol* 2007;19(Suppl 1):241–244.
131. Kotin P, Falk H, Thomas M. Aromatic hydrocarbons. III. Presence in the particulate phase of diesel engine exhausts and the carcinogenicity of exhaust extracts. *Arch Ind Health* 1955;11:113–120.
132. Huisingh J, Bradow R, Jungers R, et al. Application of bioassay to the characterization of diesel particle emissions. In: Application of short-term bioassays in the fractionation and analysis of complex environmental mixtures: [proceedings of a symposium; February; Williamsburg, VA]. In: Waters M, Nesnow S, Huisingh JL, et al., eds. *Environmental Science Research*. New York: Plenum Press, 1978.
133. Siak JS, Chan TL, Lees PS. Diesel particulate extracts in bacterial test systems. *Environ Int* 1981;5:243–248.
134. Claxton L. Mutagenic and carcinogenic potency of diesel and related environmental emissions: Salmonella bioassay. *Environ Int* 1981;5:389–391.
135. Crebelli R, Conti L, Crochi B, et al. The effect of fuel composition on the mutagenicity of diesel engine exhaust. *Mutat Res* 1995;346:167–172.
136. Mitchell AD, Evans EL, Jotz MM, et al. Mutagenic and carcinogenic potency of extracts of diesel and related environmental emissions: in vitro mutagenesis and DNA damage. *Environ Int* 1981;5:393–401.
137. Brooks A, Li A, Dutcher JS, et al. A comparison of genotoxicity of automobile exhaust particles from laboratory and environmental sources. *Environ Mutagen* 1984;6:651–668.
138. Garshick E, Schenker MB, Munoz A, et al. A case-control study of lung cancer and diesel exhaust exposure in railroad workers. *Am Rev Respir Dis* 1987;135:1242–1248.
139. Garshick E, Laden F, Hart JE, et al. Lung cancer in railroad workers exposed to diesel exhaust. *Environ Health Perspect* 2004;112:1539–1543.
140. Swanson GM, Lin CS, Curns PB. Diversity in the association between occupation and lung cancer among black and white men. *Cancer Epidemiol Biomarkers Prev* 1993;2:313–320.
141. Jarvholm B, Silverman D. Lung cancer in heavy equipment operators and truck drivers with diesel exhaust exposure in the construction industry. *Occup Environ Med* 2003;60:516–520.
142. Brüske–Hohlfeld I, Mohner M, Ahrens W, et al. Lung cancer risk in male workers occupationally exposed to diesel motor emissions in Germany. *Am J Ind Med* 1999;36:405–414.
143. Office of Transportation and Air Quality: U.S. Environmental Protection Agency. *Health Assessment Document for Diesel Engine Exhaust*. 2002. EPA/600/8-90/057F.
144. Occupational Safety & Health Administration. *Safety and Health Topics: Diesel Exhaust*. 2003. 09 July 2003.
144a. Graham Jones J. An investigation into the effects of exposure to an oil mist on workers in a mill for the cold reduction of steel strip. *Ann Occup Hyg* 1961;3:264–271.
145. Hazard of mineral-oil mist? *Lancet* 1970;2:967–968.
146. Bryan CS, Boitnott JK. Adenocarcinoma of the lung with chronic mineral oil pneumonia. *Am Rev Respir Dis* 1969;99:272–274.
147. Holmes JG, Kipling MD, Waterhouse JA. Subsequent malignancies in men with scrotal epithelioma. *Lancet* 1970;2:214–215.
148. Järvholm B. Mortality and cancer morbidity in workers exposed to cutting fluids. *Archiv Environ Health* 1987;42:361–366.
149. Leon DA, Thomas P, Hutchings S. Lung cancer among newspaper printers exposed to ink mist: a study of trade union members in Manchester, England. *Occup Environ Med* 1994;51:87–94.
150. Zhao Y, Krishnadasan A, Kennedy N, et al. Estimated effects of solvents and mineral oils on cancer incidence and mortality in a cohort of aerospace workers. *Am J Ind Med* 2005;48:249–258.
151. Tolbert PE. Oils and cancer. *Cancer Causes and Control* 1997;8:386–405.
152. Occupational Safety and Health Administration. *Occupational Safety and Health Guideline for Oil Mist: Mineral Oil*. Washington D.C., 1996.
153. Doll R. Cancer of the lung and nose in nickel workers. *Br J Ind Med* 1958;15:217–223.
154. Doll R, Matthews JD, Morgan LG. Cancers of the lung and nasal sinuses in nickel workers: a reassessment of the period of risk. *Br J Ind Med* 1977;34:102–105.
155. Enterline PE, Marsh GM. Mortality among workers in a nickel refinery and alloy manufacturing plant in West Virginia. *J Natl Cancer Inst* 1982;68:925–933.
156. Shannon HS, Julian JA, Roberts RS. Mortality study of 11,500 nickel workers. *J Natl Cancer Inst* 1984;73:1251–1258.
157. International Committee on Nickel Carcinogenesis in Man. Report of the International Committee on Nickel Carcinogenesis in Man. *Scand J Work Environ Health* 1990;16:1–82.
158. Grimsrud TK, Berge SR, Haldorsen T, et al. Exposure to different forms of nickel and risk of lung cancer. *Am J Epidemiol* 2002;156:1123–1132.
159. Grimsrud TK, Berge SR, Martinsen JI, et al. Lung cancer incidence among Norwegian nickel-refinery workers 1953–2000. *J Environ Monit* 2003;5:190–197.
160. Grimsrud TK, Peto J. Persisting risk of nickel related lung cancer and nasal cancer among Clydach refiners. *Occup Environ Med* 2006;63:365–366.
161. Sorahan T. Mortality of workers at a plant manufacturing nickel alloys, 1958–2000. *Occup Med (Lond)* 2004;54:28–34.
162. Sorahan T, Williams SP. Mortality of workers at a nickel carbonyl refinery, 1958–2000. *Occup Environ Med* 2005;62:80–85.
163. Magnus K, Anderson A, Hogetveit AC. Cancer of respiratory organs among workers at a nickel refinery in Norway, second report. *Int J Cancer* 1982;30:681–685.
164. Ottolenghi AD, Haseman JK, Payne WW, et al. Inhalation studies of nickel sulfide in pulmonary carcinogenesis of rats. *J Natl Cancer Inst* 1975;54:1165–1172.
165. Dunnick JK, Elwell MR, Radovsky AE, et al. Comparative carcinogenic effects of nickel subsulfide, nickel oxide, or nickel sulfate hexahydrate chronic exposures in the lung. *Cancer Res* 1995;55:5251–5256.
166. National Toxicology Program. NTP Toxicology and Carcinogenesis Studies of Nickel Subsulfide (CAS No. 12035-72-2) in F344 Rats and B6C3F1 Mice (Inhalation Studies). *Natl Toxicol Program Tech Rep Ser* 1996;453:1–365.
167. Pott F, Ziem U, Reiffer FJ, et al. Carcinogenicity studies on fibres, metal compounds, and some other dusts in rats. *Exp Pathol* 1987;32:129–152.
168. Maehle L, Metcalf RA, Ryberg D, et al. Altered p53 gene structure and expression in human epithelial cells after exposure to nickel. *Cancer Res* 1992;52:218–221.
169. Dally H, Hartwig A. Induction and repair inhibition of oxidative DNA damage by nickel (II) and cadmium (II) in mammalian cells. *Carcinogenesis* 1997;18:1021–1026.
170. Agency for Toxic Substances and Disease Registry: U.S. Department of Health and Human Services, Public Health Service. *Toxicological Profile for Nickel*. 1997.
171. Elkind MM. Enhanced tumorigenesis by small, protracted doses of densely ionizing radiation. *Chin Med J* 1994;107:414–419.
172. Tierney LA, Hahn FF, Lechner JF. P53, *erB*-2, and K-*ras* gene alterations are rare in spontaneous and plutonium-239-induced canine lung neoplasia. *Radiat Res* 1996;145:181–187.
173. Hei TK, Wu LJ, Liu SX, et al. Mutagenic effects of a single and an exact number of alpha particles in mammalian cells. *Proc Natl Acad Sci U S A* 1997;94:3765–3770.
174. Bignon J, Monchaux G, Chameaud J, et al. Incidence of various types of thoracic malignancy induced in rats by intrapleural injection of 2 mg of various mineral dusts after inhalation of 222Ra. *Carcinogenesis* 1983;4:621–628.
175. Lafuma J, Chmelevsky D, Chameaud J, et al. Lung carcinomas in Sprague–Dawley rats after exposure to low doses of radon daughters, fission neutrons, or gamma rays. *Radiat Res* 1989;118:230–245.
176. Groch KM, Khan MA, Brooks AL, et al. Lung cancer response following inhaled radon in the A/J and C57BL/6J mouse. *Int J Radiat Biol* 1997;71:301–308.
177. Lorenz E. Radioactivity and lung cancer: a critical review of lung cancer in the miners of Schneeberg and Joachimsthal. *J Natl Cancer Inst* 1944;5:1–15.

178. Advisory Committee on Human Radiation Experiments: U.S. Government Printing Office. *Final Report: Advisory Committee on Human Radiation Experiments*. 1995.
179. Donaldson AW. The epidemiology of lung cancer among uranium miners. *Health Physics* 1969;16:563–569.
180. Holaday DA, Doyle HN. Environmental studies in the uranium mines, radiological health, and safety in mining and milling of nuclear materials. *Vienna: International Atomic Energy Agency.* 1964;1:9–20.
181. Archer VE, Wagoner JK, Lundin FE. Lung cancer among uranium miners in the United States. *Health Physics* 1973;25:351–371.
182. Brugge D, Goble R. The history of uranium mining and the Navajo people. *Am J Pub Health* 2002;92:1410–1419.
183. Archer VE, Gillam JD, Wagoner JK. Respiratory disease mortality among uranium miners. *Ann NY Acad Sci* 1976;271:280–293.
184. Gottlieb LS, Husen LA. Lung cancer among Navajo uranium miners. *Chest* 1982;81:449–452.
185. Samet JM, Kutvirt DM, Waxweiler RJ, et al. Uranium mining and lung cancer in Navajo men. *New Engl J Med* 1984;310:1481–1484.
186. Radford E, St Clair Renard KG. Lung cancer in Swedish iron miners exposed to low doses of radon daughters. *New Engl J Med* 1984;310:1485–1494.
187. Harley NH. Radon and lung cancer in mines and homes. *N Engl J Med* 1984;310:1525–1527.
188. National Council on Radiation Protection and Measurements. *Exposures from the Uranium Series with Emphasis on Radon and Its Daughters*. 1984; NCRP Report No. 77.
189. Lubin JH, Wang ZY, Boice JD Jr, et al. Risk of lung cancer and residential radon in China: pooled results of two studies. *Int J Cancer* 2004;109:132–137.
190. Darby S, Hill D, Auvinen A, et al. Radon in homes and risk of lung cancer: collaborative analysis of individual data from 13 European case-control studies. *BMJ* 2005;330:223.
191. Krewski D, Lubin JH, Zielinski JM, et al. Residential radon and risk of lung cancer: a combined analysis of 7 North American case-control studies. *Epidemiology* 2005;16:137–145.
192. Wagner MMF, Wagner JC. Lymphomas in the Wistar rat after intrapleural inoculation of silica. *J Natl Cancer Inst* 1972;49:81–91.
193. Wagner MMF. Pathogenesis of malignant histiocytic lymphoma induced by silica in a colony of specific-pathogen-free Wistar rats. *J Natl Cancer Inst* 1976;57:509–518.
194. Wagner MM, Wagner JC, Davies R, et al. Silica-induced malignant histiocytic lymphoma: Incidence linked with strain of rat and type of silica. *Br J Cancer* 1980;41:908–917.
195. Stenbäck F, Rowland J. Experimental respiratory carcinogenesis in hamsters: environmental, physicochemical, and biological aspects. *Oncology* 1979;36:63–71.
196. Holland LM, Gonzales M, Wilson JS, et al. Pulmonary effects of shale dusts in experimental animals. In: Wagner WL, Rom WN, Merchant JA, Eds. *Health Issues Related to Metal and Nonmetallic Mining*. Boston, MA: Butterworth Publishers, 1983:485–496.
197. Holland LM, Wilson JS, Tillery MI, et al. Lung cancer in rats exposed to fibrogenic dusts. In: Goldsmith DF, Winn DM, Shy CM, Eds. *Silica, Silicosis, and Cancer: Controversy in Occupational Medicine (Cancer Research Monographs. Vol. 2)*. New York: Praeger, 1986:267–279.
198. Thiele A, Rostoski O, Saupe E, et al. Ueber den Schneeberger Lungenkrebs. *München Med Wchnschr* 1924;71:24–25.
199. Milham S Jr. Cancer mortality pattern associated with exposure to metals. *Ann N Y Acad Sci.* 1976;271:243–249.
200. Westerholm P. Silicosis: observation on a case register. *Scand J Work Environ Health* 1980;6(Suppl 2):1–86.
201. Ulm K, Gerein P, Eigenthaler J, et al. Silica, silicosis, and lung cancer: results from a cohort study in the stone and quarry industry. *Int Arch Occup Environ Health* 2004;77:313–318.
202. Kurihara N, Wada O. Silicosis and smoking strongly increase lung cancer risk in silica-exposed workers. *Ind Health* 2004;42:303–314.
203. Marinaccio A, Scarselli A, Gorini G, et al. Retrospective mortality cohort study of Italian workers compensated for silicosis. *Occup Environ Med* 2006;63:762–765.
204. Finkelstein M, Kusiak R, Suranyi G. Mortality among miners receiving workmen's compensation for silicosis in Ontario, 1940–1975. *J Occup Med* 1982;24:663–667.
205. Attfield MD, Costello J. Quantitative exposure response for silica dust and lung cancer in Vermont granite workers. *Am J Ind Med* 2004;45:129–138.
206. Heppleston AG. Silica, pneumoconiosis, and carcinoma of the lung. *Am J Ind Med* 1985;7:285–294.
207. Chen W, Bochmann F, Sun Y. Effects of work related confounders on the association between silica exposure and lung cancer: a nested case-control study among Chinese miners and pottery workers. *Int Arch Occup Environ Health* 2007;80:320–326.
208. Becker BJP, Chatgidakis CB. The heart in silicosis.In: *Proc Int Conf on Silicosis. Johannesburg: Churchill,* 1959.
209. Rüttner JR. Kann der silikose eine ätiologische Bedeutung für die Geschwulstbildung zugesprochen warden? *Oncologia* 1949;2:115–122.
210. Chatgidakis CB. Silicosis in South African white gold miners. *S African J Adv Med Sci* 1963;9:383–392.
211. Checkoway H, Hughes JM, Weill H, et al. Crystalline silica exposure, radiological silicosis, and lung cancer mortality in diatomaceous earth industry workers. *Thorax* 1999;54:56–59.
212. Checkoway H, Franzblau A. Is silicosis required for silica-associated lung cancer. *Am J Ind Med* 2000;37:252–259.
213. McDonald JC, McDonald AD, Hughes JM, et al. Mortality from lung and kidney disease in a cohort of North American industrial sand workers: an update. *Ann Occup Hyg* 2005;49:367–373.
214. Agency for Toxic Substances and Disease Registry: U.S. Department of Health and Human Services, Public Health Service. *Toxicological Profile for Synthetic Vitreous Fibers*. 2002.
215. Kielhorn J, Melber C, Wahnschaffe U, et al. Vinyl chloride: still a cause for concern. *Environ Health Perspect* 2000;108:579–588.
216. Viola PL, Bigotti A, Caputo A. Oncogenic response of rat skin, lungs, and bones to vinyl chloride. *Cancer Res* 1971;31:516–522.
217. Creech JL Jr, Johnson MN. Angiosarcoma of liver in the manufacture of polyvinyl chloride. *J Occup Med* 1974;16:150–151.
218. Tabershaw IR, Gaffey WR. Mortality study of workers in the manufacture of vinyl chloride and its polymers. *J Occup Med* 1974;16:509–518.
219. Waxweiler RJ, Stringer W, Wagoner JK, et al. Neoplastic risk among workers exposed to vinyl chloride. *Ann N Y Acad Sci* 1976;271: 40–48.
220. Heath CW Jr, Falk H, Creech JL Jr. Characteristics of cases of angiosarcoma of the liver among vinyl chloride workers in the United States. *Ann N Y Acad Sci* 1975;246:231–236.
221. Duck BW, Carter JT, Coombes EJ. Mortality study of workers in a polyvinyl-chloride production plant. *Lancet* 1975;2:1197–1199.
222. Boffetta P, Matisane L, Mundt KA, et al. Meta-analysis of studies of occupational exposure to vinyl chloride in relation to cancer mortality. *Scand J Work Environ Health* 2003;29:220–229.
223. Agency for Toxic Substances and Disease Registry: U.S. Department of Health and Human Services, Public Health Service. *Toxicological Profile for Vinyl Chloride*. 1997.

CHAPTER 4

Christopher I. Amos
Joan E. Bailey-Wilson

Genetic Susceptibility to Lung Cancer

Lung cancer is the most common cause of cancer death in the United States[1] with 162,000 deaths estimated for 2008 among 215,000 incident cases. Lung cancer became the leading cause of cancer death in men in the early 1950s and in women in 1987. From 1950 to 1988, lung cancer experienced the largest increase in mortality rate of all the cancers,[2] reflecting increases in smoking behavior. Lung cancer prognosis often remains poor because it is usually detected as a stage III or IV malignancy. Identifying genetic factors that influence lung cancer risk could help in identifying subsets of individuals at particularly high risk, in whom early detection strategies could be adopted. In addition, a better understanding of the genetic influences that increase lung cancer risk may lead to the development of novel approaches for chemoprevention and therapy.

Cancer of the lung has frequently been cited as an example of a malignancy that is solely determined by the environment[3] and the risks associated with cigarette smoking[3–6] and certain occupations, such as mining,[7] asbestos exposure, shipbuilding, and petroleum refining,[8–12] are well established. About 85% to 90% of lung cancer risk can be associated with cigarette smoking.[13–15] Environmental tobacco smoke (ETS, passive smoking) has also been shown to be associated with a mild increase in risk for lung cancer in North America and Europe.[6,16–18] A recent prospective European study estimating that between 16% to 24% of lung cancers in nonsmokers and long-term ex-smokers were attributable to ETS.[19] A metaanalysis of 22 studies showed that exposure to workplace ETS increased risk of lung cancer in workers by 24%, and that this risk was highly correlated with duration of exposure.[20]

Dietary studies have found reduction in risk associated with high compared with low consumption of carotene-containing fruits and vegetables.[21–27] Subsequent chemoprevention trials among high-risk subjects with a history of smoking and/or occupation exposure showed a surprising increase in lung cancer risk in these populations associated with beta-carotene supplementation.[28–30] At least one very large metaanalysis[31] found significant protective effects of increased levels of dietary β-cryptoxanthin, another carotenoid.

There is little doubt that most lung cancer cases are attributable to (i.e., would not occur in the absence of) cigarette smoking and other behavioral and environmental risk factors,[2,6,16,32,33] and most studies indicate that duration of cigarette smoke is a more important risk factor than intensity or number of cigarettes smoked per day.[34–36] However, it was conjectured long ago that individuals differ in their susceptibility to these environmental insults.[37–39] Mutations and loss of heterozygosity at genetic loci such as oncogenes and tumor suppressor genes (TSGs) are involved in lung carcinogenesis,[40–42] but most of these changes are thought to accumulate in individual somatic cells over time, as opposed to the inherited risk to all cells that will result from mutations or risk-increasing polymorphisms occurring in transmission from germ cells. However, numerous studies show that certain allelic variants at some genetic loci affect inherited susceptibility to lung cancer. Furthermore, mounting epidemiologic evidence has suggested that lung cancer shows familial aggregation after adjusting for cigarette smoking and other risk factors, and that differential susceptibility to lung cancer is inherited in some families. This chapter describes inherited major susceptibility loci and findings from well-replicated studies of loci for lung cancer risk that have less pronounced effects. We also relate these risks to the well-known risks as a result of environmental risk factors, particularly personal cigarette smoking.

INHALATION OF TOBACCO SMOKE

The association between cigarette smoking and lung cancer is strong and well established.[3–5,43–47] The incidence of lung cancer is correlated with the cumulative amount and duration of cigarettes smoked in a dose–response relationship,[6,44,48] and smoking cessation results in a leveling off of risk for lung cancer at the time of smoking cessation.[6,49,50] Lung cancer rates and smoking rates are also highly correlated in different geographic regions.[51] In 1991, Shopland et al.[52] showed that the relative risk (RR) of lung cancer for male smokers versus nonsmokers is

22.36 and that for female smokers versus female nonsmokers is 11.94. They also estimated that 90% of lung cancers in men and 78% in women were directly attributable to tobacco smoking. Kondo et al.[53] showed a significant (p <0.001) dose–response relationship between number of cigarettes smoked and the frequency of p53 mutations in tumors of lung cancer patients, suggesting that somatic p53 mutations may be caused by exposure to a carcinogen/mutagen in tobacco smoke or its metabolites.

BIOLOGIC RISK FACTORS

In general, all studies suggesting genetic susceptibility have also shown strong risk resulting from cigarette smoking and often have shown an interaction of high-risk genotype and smoking on lung cancer risk. When trying to determine whether a complex disease or trait such as lung cancer has a genetic susceptibility, one asks three major questions:

1. Does the disease (lung cancer) cluster in families? If some risk for lung cancer is inherited, then one would expect to see clustering of that cancer in some families above what would be expected by chance.
2. If the aggregation of lung cancer does occur in some families, can the observation be explained by shared environmental/cultural risk factors? In the study of lung cancer, one needs to assess whether the familial clustering of lung cancer is solely a result of clustering of smoking behaviors or other environmental exposures within families.
3. If the excess clustering in families is not explained by measured environmental risk factors, is the pattern of disease consistent with Mendelian transmission of a major gene (i.e., of transmission through some families of a moderately high penetrance risk allele) and can this gene(s) be localized and identified in the human genome?

In addition, inherited susceptibility factors for lung cancer can also be identified by conducting large-scale case control studies, just as these approaches have been successful for other complex diseases that often result from a complex interplay of genetic and environmental factors.

EVIDENCE FOR FAMILIAL AGGREGATION OF LUNG CANCER

Epidemiologic Cohort Studies

Tokuhata and Lilienfeld[54,55] showed familial aggregation of lung cancer over 40 years ago. After accounting for personal smoking, their results suggested the possible interaction of genes, shared environment, and common lifestyle factors in the etiology of lung cancer. In their study of 270 lung cancer patients and 270 age-, sex-, race-, and location-matched controls and their relatives, they found an RR of 2.0 to 2.5 for mortality because of lung cancer in cigarette-smoking relatives of cases compared with smoking relatives of controls. Nonsmoking relatives of lung cancer cases were also at higher risk when compared with nonsmoking relatives of controls. Smoking was a more important risk factor for men, but family history was the more important risk factor for women. They also noted a synergistic interaction between familial and smoking factors on the risk of lung cancer in relatives, with smoking relatives of lung cancer patients having much higher risk of lung cancer than either nonsmoking relatives of patients or smoking relatives of controls. They observed a substantial increase in mortality resulting from noncancerous respiratory diseases in relatives of patients compared with relatives of controls, suggesting that the case relatives have a common susceptibility to respiratory diseases. However, they found no significant differences between the spouses of the lung cancer cases and controls for lung cancer mortality, mortality from noncancerous respiratory diseases, or smoking habits.

The major weakness of this study was that smoking status alone was used. Therefore, some of the familial aggregation could be a result of familial correlation in smoking levels or age at smoking initiation. However, nonsmoking relatives of cases were at higher risk than nonsmoking relatives of controls.

At present, many other studies have shown evidence of familial aggregation of lung cancer. In 1975, Fraumeni et al.[56] reported an increased risk of lung cancer mortality in siblings of lung cancer probands. In 1982, Goffman et al.[57] reported families with excess lung cancer of diverse histologic types. Lynch et al.[58] reported evidence for increased risk of cancer at all anatomic sites for relatives of lung cancer patients but no significant increased risk for lung cancer alone in these relatives.

In southern Louisiana, case-control studies reported an increased familial risk for lung cancer[59] and smoking-related non–lung cancers[60] among relatives of lung cancer probands (the index case leading the family to be studied) after allowing for the effects of age, sex, occupation, and smoking. In these two studies, familial aggregation analyses were performed on a set of 337 lung cancer probands (cases), their spouse controls, and the parents, siblings, half-siblings, and offspring of both the probands and the controls. The probands were male and female whites who died from lung cancer during the period 1976 to 1979 in a 10-parish (county) area of southern Louisiana, a region noted for its high lung cancer mortality rates. There were about 3.5 male probands to every female lung cancer proband in the data set. A strong excess risk for lung cancer was detected among first-degree relatives of probands compared with relatives of spouse controls, after adjusting for age, sex, smoking status, total duration of smoking, cigarette pack-years, and a cumulative index of occupational/industrial exposures. Parents of probands had a fourfold risk of having developed lung cancer compared with parents of spouses, after adjusting for the effects of age, sex, smoking, and occupational exposures. Women greater than 40 years old who were relatives of probands were at nine times higher risk than similar female relatives of spouses, even among nonsmokers who had not reported excessive exposure to hazardous occupations. Among female heavy smokers who were relatives of probands, the risk was increased from fourfold to sixfold. Overall, male relatives of probands had a greater risk of lung cancer than their female counterparts. After controlling for the confounding effects of the measured environmental risk factors, relationship to a proband remained a significant determinant of lung cancer, with a 2.4 odds in favor of relatives of probands.

These same families were reanalyzed[60] to determine if non–lung cancers exhibited similar familial aggregation. When analyzing the number of cancers at any site that occurred in a family, proband families were found to be 1.7 times more likely than spouse families to have one family member (other than the proband) with cancer, and 2.2 times more likely to have two family members with cancer. Comparing case relatives and control relatives, families that had three and four or more cancers occurred with RRs of 3.7 and 5.0, respectively. Each risk estimate was significant at the 0.01 level. The most striking differences in cancer prevalence between proband and control families were noted for cancer of the nasal cavity/sinus, mid-ear, and larynx (odds ratio [OR] = 4.6); trachea, bronchus, and lung (OR = 3.0); skin (OR = 2.8); and uterus, placenta, ovary, and other female organs (OR = 2.1). After controlling for age, sex, cigarette smoking, and occupational/industrial exposures, relatives of lung cancer probands maintained an increased risk of non–lung cancer ($p < 0.05$) when compared with relatives of spouse controls.

A family case-control study, drawn from a population-based registry in Saskatchewan, Canada was reported by McDuffie.[61] A total of 359 cases and 234 age- and gender-matched community controls were included in the study. Most families reported at least one member with a history of neoplastic disease exclusive of the proband (62% of patients' families and 57% of control families). However, the families of the lung cancer cases were more likely (30%) to have two or more family members affected with any cancer than the families of the controls. The case families were also significantly more likely to have two or more relatives with lung cancer than were the control families. In addition, a higher percentage of all primary tumors were lung tumors (16.5%) in patients' relatives compared with controls' relatives (10%). The progression of increased risks for observing 1, 2, 3, and 4+ affected relatives in case families versus control families was less than that observed by Sellers et al.'s[60] study but showed the same type of progression.

Family history data from an incident case-control study in Texas were analyzed for evidence of familial aggregation by Shaw et al.[62] A total of 943 histologically confirmed lung cancer cases and 955 age-, gender-, vital status-, and ethnicity-matched controls were interviewed regarding smoking, alcohol use, cancer in first-degree relatives, medical history, and demographic characteristics. After adjusting for personal smoking status, passive smoking exposure (ever/never), and gender, there was a 1.8-fold OR associating lung cancer with having one or more first-degree relatives with lung cancer. Lung cancer risk increased as the number of relatives with cancer increased and was highest when only relatives with lung cancer were considered (ORs of 1.7 and 2.8 for one and two or more relatives with lung cancer, respectively). Lung cancer was diagnosed at a significantly younger age among cases who had first-degree relatives with lung cancer than among those who had no relatives with lung cancer. However, no such age difference was seen between cases who had first-degree relatives with any cancer versus those who had no relatives with cancer. This study also examined histologic subtypes of lung cancer cases and found that for each histologic type, there were significant risks associated with having any relatives with lung cancer, with ORs of 2.1 for adenocarcinoma, 1.9 for squamous cell carcinoma, and 1.7 for small cell lung cancer. Finally, in this study, only current and former smokers had an increased lung cancer risk associated with lung cancer in relatives.

Cannon-Albright et al.[63] examined the degree of relatedness of all pairs of lung cancer patients in the Utah Population Database (UPD). By comparing this with the degree of relatedness in sets of matched controls, they showed that lung cancer exhibited excess familiality, and three of four histological tumor types still showed excess familiality when considered separately. In the same population, but using different methodology, Goldgar et al.[64] studied lung cancer probands and controls who had died in Utah and their first-degree relatives. They found that 2.55 times more lung cancers occurred in first-degree relatives of lung cancer probands than expected (computing a familial relative risk or FRR) based on rates in control relatives. When they stratified by gender, they observed higher relative risks for female relatives of female probands (FRR = 4.02) versus male relatives of male probands (FRR = 2.5). No adjustment was made in these analyses for personal smoking or other environmental risk factors, so these results may partly reflect the familiality of smoking behaviors. However, the UPD is derived from the Church of Latter-Day Saints records, which is largely a nonsmoking population and Utah has the lowest smoking rates of any state in the United States.

In 2000, Bromen et al.,[65] in a population-based case-control study in Germany, showed that lung cancer in parents or siblings was significantly associated with an increased risk of lung cancer and that this risk was much stronger in younger participants. In 2003, Etzel et al.[66] evaluated whether first-degree relatives of lung cancer cases were at increased risk for lung cancer and for other smoking-related cancers (bladder, head and neck, kidney, and pancreas). They studied 806 hospital-based lung cancer patients and 663 controls matched on age, sex, ethnicity, and smoking history, all from the Houston, Texas area. After adjustment for smoking history of patients and their relatives, there was significant evidence for familial aggregation of lung cancer and of smoking-related cancers. However, they did not find increased aggregation in the families of young onset (less than or equal to age 55) lung cancer cases or in families of never-smokers.

Two studies in China[67,68] both found, after adjusting for age, sex, birth order, residence, family size, chronic obstructive pulmonary disease (COPD), smoking, and cumulative index of smoky coal exposure or occupational/industrial exposure index, that first-degree relatives of lung cancer patients were at significantly increased risk for lung cancer compared with the same relatives of controls. They also observed that families of the lung cancer patients were significantly more likely to have three or more affected relatives than were control families.

A series of studies using the Swedish Family-Cancer Database,[69–72] which totals over 10.2 million individuals, found that a high proportion of lung cancers diagnosed before the age of 50 appear to be heritable, and that lung cancer patients with a family history of lung cancer were at a significantly increased risk of subsequent primary lung cancers. A recent study[73] utilizing the Icelandic Cancer Registry calculated risk ratios of lung cancer in first-, second-, and third-degree relatives of 2756 lung cancer patients diagnosed between 1955 and 2002. RRs were significantly elevated for all three classes of relatives, and this increased risk was stronger in relatives of early onset lung cancer patients (age at onset less than or equal to 60 years). The effect did not appear to be solely a result of the effects of smoking in all relative types, except for cousins and spouses.

In the United Kingdom, a case-control study of lung cancer prevalence in first-degree relatives of 1482 female lung cancer cases and 1079 female controls,[74] adjusting for age and tobacco exposure (pack-years) in the cases and controls. They found that lung cancer in any first-degree relative was associated with a significant increase in lung cancer risk, and that the increase in risk was stronger in relatives of cases with onset less than 60 years or cases with three or more affected relatives. However, data on personal smoking in relatives were not available.

A study of early onset white and African American lung cancer cases and of 773 frequency-matched controls in Detroit, Michigan,[75] showed that smokers with a family history of early onset lung cancer had a higher risk of lung cancer with increasing age than smokers without a family history, and that relatives of African American cases were at higher risk than relatives of white cases, after adjusting for age, sex, pack-years of cigarette smoking, pneumonia, and COPD.

Studies of familial risk of lung cancer in nonsmokers[65,76–78] have also shown increased risk of lung cancer associated with a family history of lung cancer. Schwartz et al.[76] found increased risk of lung cancer among relatives of younger, nonsmoking lung cancer cases compared with relatives of younger controls after adjusting for smoking, occupational, and medical histories of each family member, suggesting increased susceptibility to lung cancer among relatives of early onset nonsmoking lung cancer patients. Wu et al.[77] found an increased risk of lung cancer in persons with a history of lung or aerodigestive tract cancer in first-degree relatives after adjustment for ETS exposure, which was significant for affected mothers and sisters. Mayne et al.[78] in a population-based study of nonsmokers (45% never-smokers and 55% former smokers who had quit at least 10 years prior to diagnosis or interview; 437 lung cancer cases and 437 matched population controls) in New York State, found that after adjusting for age and smoking status (yes, no) in the relatives, a positive history in first-degree relatives of any cancer including lung cancer, aerodigestive tract cancer, or breast cancer were each associated with significantly increased risk of lung cancer.

Studies in Twins The number of lung cancers observed in some twin studies have been too small to draw conclusions regarding familiality of lung cancer,[79] although possible aggregation of bronchoalveolar carcinoma has been suggested in twins and family studies.[80,81] However, this effect may be a result of aggregation of cigarette smoking because risk of this cancer is linked to tobacco consumption.[82] In 1995, in a study using a large twin registry, the National Academy of Sciences–National Research Council Twin Registry, Braun et al.[83] reported that the observed concordance rates of monozygous (MZ) twins for death from lung cancer compared with that of dizygous (DZ) twins was 1.1 (95% CI, 0.6 to 1.9), although this did not adjust for smoking behaviors in the twins. These results suggest that, as expected, on a population level, smoking behavior is probably a much stronger risk factor than inherited genetic susceptibility. Lichtenstein et al.[84] studied nearly 45,000 twins to identify clustering of excess risk in cotwins of MZ versus DZ twins. Results showed a 7.7-fold increased risk to MZ cotwins and a 6.7-fold increased risk to cotwins of DZ twins. These risks reflect combined effects of environmental and genetic determinants. Further modeling suggested that 26% of excess risk to MZ cotwins was attributed to heritable factors, whereas 12% was attributed to shared environment in the twins, and the remaining 62% was attributed to individual environmental factors. Although a very large sample size of twins was studied, the estimates still had very wide confidence intervals reflecting the study of only 608 index twins who had developed a lung cancer.

A review in 2005 by Matakidou et al.[85] of 28 case-control, 17 cohort, and seven twin studies of the relationship between family history and risk of lung cancer and a metaanalysis of risk estimates, concluded that the case-control and cohort studies consistently show an increased risk of lung cancer given a family history of lung cancer, and that risk appears to be increased given a history of early onset lung cancer or of multiple affected relatives. However, the results of the twin studies and the observed increased risk of disease in spouses highlighted the importance of environmental risk factors, such as smoking, in this disease.

HIGH-RISK SYNDROMES CONFERRING AN INCREASED RISK FOR LUNG CANCERS

Leonard et al.[86] reported that survivors of familial retinoblastoma may also be at increased risk for small cell lung cancer. The standard mortality ratio for small cell lung cancer is estimated to be 15-fold increased.[87,88] Kleinerman[89] reported that lung cancer developing among those with germline retinoblastoma mutations had the heaviest smoking histories. Retinoblastoma survivors smoke less than the general population, suggesting that targeted counseling to avoid this risky behavior in this high-risk population may be effective.[90] The RB gene is inactivated in 90% of small cell lung cancers, indicating the relevance of this gene to small cell lung cancer etiology.[91]

Mutations in the p53 gene cause Li-Fraumeni syndrome. Individuals with this syndrome are at greatly increased risks for many cancers, including breast and lung cancers, sarcomas, leukemias and lymphomas, and adrenocortical tumors. The standard incidence ratio for lung cancer was estimated to be 38, using a prospectively followed cohort of carriers of p53 mutations.[92] Cigarette smoking further increased risk threefold.

Mutations in the epidermal growth factor receptor (EGFR) locus are often found in adenocarcinomas of the lung arising in nonsmoking women, particularly among Asian populations[93] (see Chapter 49). One family with multiple adenocarcinomas was found to be segregating a mutation in the EGFR, indicating that rarely inherited mutations of this locus can increase the risk for lung cancer.[94] However, a study[95] of 237 familial lung cancer cases occurring in individuals with three or more relatives affected by lung cancer including 45 bronchoalveolar lung cancers failed to find any mutations of EGFR, suggesting that mutations of this gene are uncommon in the general North American population.

SEGREGATION ANALYSES OF LUNG AND SMOKING-ASSOCIATED CANCERS

Given the evidence for familial aggregation of lung and other smoking-associated cancers, after accounting for personal tobacco use and occupational/industrial risk factors, segregation analyses have been performed to determine whether patterns of transmission consistent with at least one major, high-penetrance genetic locus may be involved in lung cancer risk.

Sellers et al.[96] performed genetic segregation analyses on the lung cancer proband families of Ooi et al.[59] described previously. The trait was expressed as a dichotomy, affected or unaffected with lung cancer. The analyses used the general transmission probability model,[97] which allows for variable age of onset of the lung cancer.[98–100] The likelihood of the models was calculated using a correction factor appropriate for single ascertainment,[101,102] that is, conditioning the likelihood of each pedigree on the probands being affected by their ages at examination or death.

Age of onset of lung cancer was assumed to follow a logistic distribution that depended on pack-years of cigarette consumption and its square, an age coefficient and a baseline parameter. Results indicated compatibility of the data with Mendelian codominant inheritance of a rare major autosomal gene that produces earlier age of onset of the cancer. Segregation at this putative locus could account for 69% and 47% of the cumulative incidence of lung cancer in individuals up to ages 50 and 60, respectively. The gene was predicted to be involved in only 22% of all lung cancers in persons up to age 70, a reflection of an increasing proportion of noncarriers succumbing to the effects of long-term exposure to tobacco.[97,103]

Gaudermann et al.[104] reanalyzed these same data using a Gibbs sampler method to examine gene by environment interactions and found evidence for a major dominant susceptibility locus that acts in conjunction with cigarette smoking to increase risk; this model was very similar to the previous results, because the codominant Mendelian models predicted very small numbers of homozygous susceptibility allele carriers.

Yang and coworkers[105] performed complex segregation analysis on the families of nonsmoking lung cancer probands in metropolitan Detroit. Evidence was found for Mendelian codominant inheritance with modifying effects of smoking and chronic bronchitis in families of nonsmoking cases diagnosed at ages.[40–59] The estimated risk allele frequency was 0.004. Although homozygous individuals with the risk allele are rare in the study population, penetrance was very high for early onset lung cancer (85% in men and 74% in women by age 60). The probability of developing lung cancer by age 60 in individuals heterozygous for the rare allele was low in the absence of smoking and chronic bronchitis (7% in men and 4% in women), but in the presence of these risk factors it increased to 85% in men and 74% in women, which was the same level predicted for homozygotes. The attributable risk associated with the high-risk allele declines with age, when the role of tobacco smoking and chronic bronchitis become more important.

Wu et al.[106] performed segregation analysis of families of 125 women, nonsmoking lung cancer probands in Taiwan. These lung cancer probands were diagnosed with lung cancer between 1992 and 2002 at two hospitals in Taiwan. Complete data on patients, spouses, and first-degree relatives were collected for 108 families. Data collected on the patients and their relatives included demographic, lifestyle, and medical history variables. Complex segregation analysis using logistic models for age at onset, including pack-years of cigarette smoking in the model was performed on 58 of these families. An ascertainment correction was made using the phenotype of the probands, but this may have been inadequate because the 58 families were a subset of the 108 families where there was at least one additional affected relative in the family. The Mendelian codominant model that included risk caused by personal smoking fit the data best, significantly better than the sporadic or purely environmental models. This model was not rejected against the general model in an early onset (less than 60 years) subset of the families but was rejected in the later-onset families and the total dataset.

Taken together, the Taiwan, Detroit, and Louisiana studies share remarkably similar results and demonstrate statistical evidence for at least one major gene that acts in conjunction with personal smoking and possibly chronic bronchitis to increase risk of lung cancer.

Although most of these studies included measures of personal smoking on the cases (or probands) and controls in the models, some of the aggregation studies did not include measures of amount of cigarette smoking in the relatives, and only one included measures of passive smoking. The segregation analyses did not include passive smoking or occupational risk factors in the models, and only one of these three studies collected data on history of chronic bronchitis. Furthermore, segregation analyses are not sufficient to prove the existence of a major locus because only a subset of all possible models can be tested. However, tracking the inheritance of lung cancer with genetic markers in a family (linkage analysis) can provide definitive evidence for genetic susceptibility to disease. Segregation analyses are useful because they provide a model that can be used for these subsequent analyses, and they provide insights into the best designs for identifying genes that have a high risk for disease.

ONCOGENES AND TUMOR SUPPRESSOR GENES

In addition to epidemiological evidence, experimental evidence of the role of genes in lung cancer causation has been accumulating. First, it seems probable that genetic changes are responsible for the pathogenesis of most, if not all, human malignancies.[107] In particular, lung carcinogenesis is the result of a series of genetic mutations that accumulate progressively in the bronchial epithelium, first generating histologically identifiable premalignant lesions and finally resulting in an invasive carcinoma (see Chapter 5). The premalignant genetic changes may occur many years before the appearance of invasive carcinoma.

Cytogenetic and molecular studies have shown that mutations in proto-oncogenes and TSGs are critical in the multistep development and progression of lung tumors. Allele loss analyses have implicated the presence of other TSGs involved in lung tumorigenesis. These studies revealed frequent occurrences of chromosomal deletions including regions of 3p, 5q, 8p, 9p, 9q, 11p, 11q, and 17q. These studies are outside the scope of this chapter (see Chapter 6).[108–110] A recent genome-wide analysis found common amplifications of the human telomerase gene on chromosome 5p and in NK2 homeobox 1 (also known as thyroid transcription factor-1 [TITF-1]) on chromosome 14q13.3.[111]

These data have been further explored by genomic profiling of 128 lung cancer cell lines and tumors that revealed frequent focal DNA amplification at cytoband 14q13.3. The smallest region of recurrent amplification spanned TITF-1. When amplified, TITF-1 exhibited increased expression at both the RNA and protein levels. Small interfering RNA (siRNA)-mediated knockdown of TITF-1 in lung cancer cell lines with amplification led to reduced cell proliferation, manifested by both decreased cell cycle progression and increased apoptosis. These findings indicate that TITF-1 amplification and overexpression contribute to lung cancer cell proliferation rates and survival and implicate TITF-1 as a lineage-specific oncogene in lung cancer.[112]

LINKAGE ANALYSIS OF LUNG CANCER

Linkage analysis is a statistical analysis of pedigree data that looks for evidence of cosegregation through the generations in human pedigrees of alleles at a genetic "susceptibility" locus and some known genetic "marker" locus (usually a DNA polymorphism). Linkage analysis is a very powerful method for detecting genetic loci that are highly penetrant (after adjusting for environmental risk factors). However, power decreases as the susceptibility allele becomes more common and less penetrant. Because cigarette smoking is an extremely strong risk factor for lung cancer,[4] it is appropriate to seek models that incorporate effects from this risk factor.

Bailey-Wilson et al.[113] published the first evidence of linkage of a lung cancer susceptibility locus to a region of chromosome 6q. Data were collected at eight recruitment sites by the Genetic Epidemiology of Lung Cancer Consortium (GELCC): the University of Cincinnati, University of Colorado, Johns Hopkins School of Public Health, Karmanos Cancer Institute, Saccomanno Research Institute, Louisiana State University Health Sciences Center, Mayo Clinic, and Medical College of Ohio. Of the 26,108 lung cancer cases screened at GELCC sites for this study, 13.7% had at least one first-degree relative with lung cancer. Following the initial family history screening process, additional information was collected from the 3541 families with at least one first-degree relative with lung cancer. Probands and/or their family representatives were contacted to collect data regarding additional persons affected with any cancers in the extended family, vital status of affected individuals, availability of archival tissue, and willingness of family members to participate in the study. Further pedigree development and biospecimen collection (blood, buccal cells, or fixed tissue) were performed on 771 families with three or more first-degree relatives affected with lung cancer. Cancers were verified by medical records, pathology reports, cancer registry records, or death certificates for 69% of individuals affected with either lung or throat (LT) cancer, and by reports of multiple family members for the other 31% of family members affected with LT. Of these families, only 52 had enough biospecimens available to make them informative for linkage analyses. DNA isolated from blood was genotyped at the Center for Inherited Disease Research (CIDR, a National Institutes of Health [NIH]-supported core research facility), and DNA from buccal cells and archival tissue and sputum were genotyped at the University of Cincinnati, for a panel of 392 microsatellite (short tandem repeat polymorphism, STRP) marker loci. The data were checked for errors and then analyzed using parametric and nonparametric linkage methods. Marker allele frequencies were calculated separately, and linkage analyses were performed separately for the white American and African American families, with the results combined in overall tests of linkage.

The primary analytical approach assumed a model with 10% penetrance in carriers and 1% penetrance in the noncarriers. This analytical approach weights information only from the affected subjects. This linkage model was used as the primary analytical approach because of uncertainty about the strength of relationship between smoking behavior and lung cancer risk in the high-risk families that were studied, and because the complex "gene+environment" models from the published segregation analyses were not currently available in any multipoint linkage analysis program. In addition, because about 90% of the affected family members smoked, weighting only the affected individuals in the simple dominant, low-penetrance model has the effect of jointly allowing for smoking status, while ignoring information from unaffected subjects. Genetic heterogeneity (different families having different genetic causation) was allowed for during the analysis. Secondary analyses used more complex models that included age and pack-years of cigarette smoking to modify the penetrances. A genetic regressive model obtained from segregation analyses by Sellers et al.[96] was used. Nonparametric analyses were also performed as secondary analyses with variance

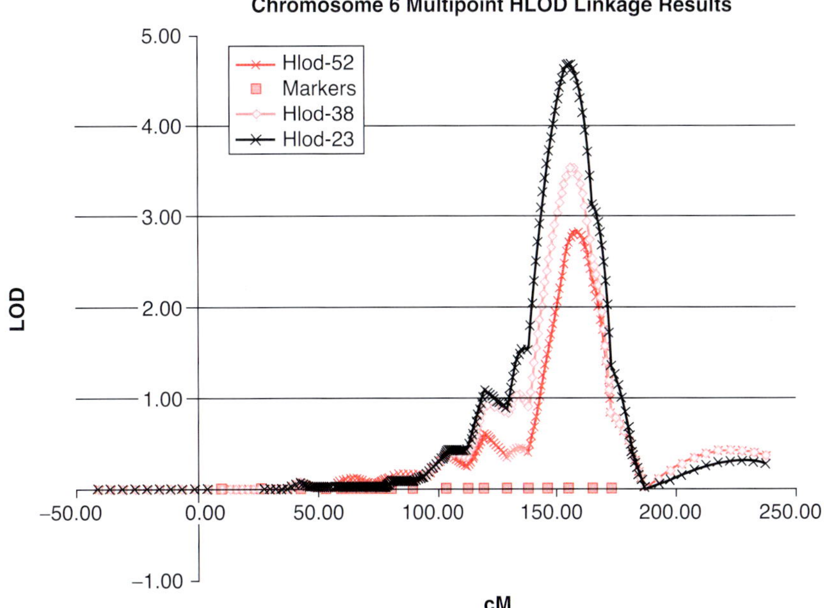

FIGURE 4.1 Plot of chromosome 6 parametric multipoint HLOD scores (lung cancer affected only analysis) from SIMWALK2 in all 52 families, in the 38 families with four or more affected individuals, and in the 23 multigenerational families with five or more affected individuals. *HLOD*, heterogeneity lod score.

components models using SOLAR (binary trait option) and mixed effects Cox regression models, in which time to onset of disease is modeled as a quantitative trait.

Multipoint parametric linkage under the simple dominant low-penetrance affected-only model (Fig. 4.1) yielded a maximum heterogeneity lod (HLOD) score of 2.79 at 155 cM (marker D6S2436) on chromosome 6q23–25 in the 52 families, with 67% of families estimated to be linked. Multipoint analysis of a subset of 38 families with four affected relatives gave an HLOD of 3.47 at this same location, with 78% of families estimated to be linked, whereas for the 23 highest-risk families (five or more affected in two or more generations), the multipoint HLOD score was 4.26, with 94% of these families estimated to be linked to this region. Nonparametric analyses and the two-point parametric analyses that used the Sellers et al. model[60,96] all provided additional support for linkage to this region.

Additional families have been collected by the GELCC to confirm this linkage result in an independent sample and to narrow the critical region that may contain a susceptibility gene. In addition, several other regions showed suggestive evidence of linkage and these are being pursued.

ASSOCIATION OF COMMON ALLELES OF SMALL EFFECT (POLYMORPHISMS) WITH LUNG CANCER RISK

Results of hundreds of studies using association analysis to evaluate the effects of various polymorphisms, in metabolic genes, growth factors, growth factor receptors, markers of DNA damage and repair and genomic instability, and in oncogenes and tumor suppressor loci have been published. Many of these studies have yielded inconsistent results. The effects of risk alleles at these loci are expected to be individually small, and they may interact with smoking and/or other loci to increase lung cancer risk. Two recent reviews[114,115] can help the reader obtain an overview of these studies. On account of the relatively weak effects of these polymorphisms, relatively few consistent replications of effects have been provided, but more recent genome-wide association studies of very large collections of samples have provided some highly significant and reproducible results.

Three manuscripts jointly appeared in *Nature*[116,117] and *Nature Genetics*[118] identifying the same region of chromosome 15q as associating highly significantly with lung cancer risk. The region that was implicated by these studies includes a neuronal nicotinic acetylcholine receptor gene cluster comprising the CHRNA3, CHRNA5, and CHRNB4 subunits. Nicotinic receptors are comprised of pentamers that include alpha and beta units, and are ubiquitously expressed, but have higher levels in the brain. The manuscript of Thorgeirsson initially scanned a population of 14,000 individuals who had provided information about their smoking histories. This study identified the 15q region as associated with smoking quantity and then further explored the regions effects on smoking dependence and lung cancer risk. The other two studies[116,118] started with large collections of lung cancer cases and control samples. Results of all studies reached a surprisingly homogeneous conclusion with increased lung cancer risks of about 1.29 among individuals carrying a heterozygous mutation (44.2% of controls for rs8034191) in the region and about 1.80 among individuals with homozygous variants (10.7% of controls). Because of strong linkage disequilibrium among the markers studied, the specific gene causing increased risks for three studies drew conflicting conclusions about the relevance of this region on smoking behavior and its influence on lung cancer risk. Thorgeirsson[117] claimed that all of the risk for lung cancer in this region appeared likely to be explained by the regions effects on smoking behavior. Amos[118] found an association of this region with both lung cancer risk and smoking behavior but found stronger effects on lung cancer risk that remained highly significant after adjusting for smoking behavior. Finally, Hung[116] did not find any association of this region on lung cancer risk. None of the studies had enough nonsmoking lung cancer cases to draw strong conclusions, but a subsequent study focusing on nonsmokers[118] fails to find any risk associated with variants in this region and lung cancer risk in this population. Comparing models of the risks of lung cancer among current smokers, Hung[116] found that carriers of the common less susceptible allele had a 14% cumulative risk of lung cancer death compared with a 23% cumulative risk of lung cancer death among those homozygous for the higher-risk variant.

Additional genetic factors are being identified and replicated by using very large collections of lung cancer cases and controls. Polymorphisms in DNA repair genes are repeatedly associated with lung cancer risk, and these are reviewed,[119–121] but many of the individual studies reporting these associations are of moderate size. A rare variant of CHEK2 (I157T) that had previously been associated with increased risk for breast cancer was found in a study of 4015 tobacco-associated cancer cases and 3052 controls to be strongly protective for the development of lung or head and neck cancers (RR = 0.44), but a risk factor for kidney cancer (RR = 1.44). Functional studies of biomarkers of DNA repair and mutagen sensitivity following exposure to clastogens repeatedly show that these are reliable predictors of lung cancer risk,[119] but applying them for patient populations is problematic because of a lack of reference laboratories and the need to study viable cells.

CONCLUSION

All of these lines of evidence suggest that there may be one or several genes causing inherited increased risk to lung cancer in the general population. Although association studies have given evidence that alleles at various genetic loci may influence lung cancer risk, there has frequently been disagreement between studies. The first linkage study of lung cancer has given significant evidence of linkage to a region on chromosome 6q. If a susceptibility locus is identified in this region, it will be of major public health importance because it will allow identification of individuals at especially high risk who can then be targeted for intensive efforts at environmental risk reduction. In addition, identification of such a gene will lead to better understanding of the mechanism of carcinogenesis in general, perhaps eventually leading to better methods of prevention and treatment. The recent identification of polymorphisms associated with lung cancer risk provides new targets for potential interventions for chemoprevention, but further study is needed to evaluate these new findings and to identify particularly high-risk subjects who might benefit most from such interventions.

Confirmation of a genetic predisposition for lung cancer can be obtained by finding evidence for linkage of the putative susceptibility gene(s) to genetic marker loci in a specific chromosomal region(s). One potential problem in the search for such a linkage is heterogeneity. There are different types of heterogeneity of this disease and of its etiological factors: (a) there is heterogeneity at the level of histological types of lung cancer; (b) there is heterogeneity at the level of exposure to various environmental risk factors; and (c) there could be heterogeneity at the level of inherited susceptibility loci, that is, there could be one locus involved in susceptibility for one family and a different locus involved in susceptibility for another family. All of these types of heterogeneity could possibly confound the identification of a susceptibility locus (or loci) for lung cancer. The suggestive evidence in the published linkage study[113] for susceptibility loci at several other regions of the genome support the possibility of locus heterogeneity in lung cancer.

If, through linkage and positional cloning techniques, a genetic locus or loci that contributes to inheritable risk for lung cancer can be identified, or one of the candidate loci suggested to modify risk by association studies can be confirmed as a susceptibility locus, then the effects of the alleles at this locus and its interaction with cigarette smoking and the other well-known environmental risk factors for lung cancer can be elucidated with much more accuracy than presently possible, and our understanding of lung carcinogenesis in general may be increased.

ACKNOWLEDGMENTS: *This work was supported by the intramural program of the National Human Genome Research Institute, NIH.*

REFERENCES

1. American Cancer Society. *Cancer Facts and Figures, 2008.* Atlanta: American Cancer Society, 2008.
2. Beckett WS. Epidemiology and etiology of lung cancer. *Clin Chest Med* 1993;14:1–15.
3. Doll R, Peto R. The causes of cancer quantitative estimates of avoidable risks of cancer in the United States today. *J Natl Cancer Inst* 1981; 66(6):1191–1308.
4. Burch PR. Smoking and lung cancer. Tests of a causal hypothesis. *J Chronic Dis* 1980;33:221–238.
5. Carbone D. Smoking and cancer. *Am J Med* 1992;93:13S–17S.
6. Doll R, Peto R, Wheatley K, et al. Mortality in relation to smoking: 40 years' observations on male British doctors. *BMJ* 1994;309:901–911.
7. Morgan WK, Seaton A. *Occupational Lung Diseases.* Philadelphia: Saunders; 1975.
8. Morgan WK, Seaton A. *Occupational Lung Diseases.* Philadelphia: W.B. Saunders; 1984.
9. Blot WJ, Fraumeni JF Jr. Geographic patterns of lung cancer: industrial correlations. *Am J Epidemiol* 1976;103: 539–550.
10. Blot WJ, Harrington JM, Toledo A, et al. Lung cancer after employment in shipyards during World War II. *N Engl J Med* 1978;299:620–624.
11. Cullen MR, Barnett MJ, Balmes JR et al. Predictors of lung cancer among asbestos-exposed men in the β-carotene and retinol efficacy trial. *Am J Epidemiol* 2005;161:260–270.
12. Gottlieb MS, Stedman RB. Lung cancer in shipbuilding and related industries in Louisiana. *South Med J* 1979;72:1099–1101.
13. Mattson ME, Pollack ES, Cullen JW. What are the odds that smoking will kill you? *Am J Public Health* 1987;77:425–431.
14. Flanders WD, Lally CA, Zhu BP, et al. Lung cancer mortality in relation to age, duration of smoking, and daily cigarette consumption: results from Cancer Prevention Study II. *Cancer Res* 2003;63:6556–6562.

15. Peto R, Darby S, Deo H, et al. Smoking, smoking cessation, and lung cancer in the UK since 1950: combination of national statistics with two case-control studies. *BMJ* 2000;321:323–329.
16. Davila DG, Williams DE. The etiology of lung cancer. *Mayo Clin Proc* 1993;68:170–182.
17. Fontham ET, Correa P, Chen VW. Passive smoking and lung cancer. *J La State Med Soc* 1993;145(4):132–136.
18. Subramanian J, Govindan R. Lung cancer in never smokers: a review. *J Clin Oncol* 2007;25:561–570.
19. Vineis P, Hoek G, Krzyzanowski M, et al. Lung cancers attributable to environmental tobacco smoke and air pollution in non-smokers in different European countries: a prospective study. *Environ Health* 2007;6:7.
20. Stayner L, Bena J, Sasco AJ, et al. Lung cancer risk and workplace exposure to environmental tobacco smoke. *Am J Public Health* 2007; 97:545–551.
21. Le ML, Hankin JH, Kolonel LN, et al. Intake of specific carotenoids and lung cancer risk. *Cancer Epidemiol Biomarkers Prev* 1993;2:183–187.
22. Comstock GW, Alberg AJ, Huang HY et al. The risk of developing lung cancer associated with antioxidants in the blood: ascorbic acid, carotenoids, alpha-tocopherol, selenium, and total peroxyl radical absorbing capacity. *Cancer Epidemiol Biomarkers Prev* 1997;6:907–916.
23. Menkes MS, Comstock GW, Vuilleumier JP, et al. Serum beta-carotene, vitamins A and E, selenium, and the risk of lung cancer. *N Engl J Med* 1986;315:1250–1254.
24. Fontham ET. Protective dietary factors and lung cancer. *Int J Epidemiol* 1990;19(Suppl 1):S32–S42.
25. Donaldson MS. Nutrition and cancer: a review of the evidence for an anti-cancer diet. *Nutr J* 2004;3:19.
26. Gonzalez CA. Nutrition and cancer: the current epidemiological evidence. *Br J Nutr* 2006;96(Suppl 1):S42–S45.
27. Divisi D, Di TS, Salvemini S, et al. Diet and cancer. *Acta Biomed* 2006;77:118–123.
28. Omenn GS, Goodman G, Thornquist M, et al. The beta-carotene and retinol efficacy trial (CARET) for chemoprevention of lung cancer in high risk populations: smokers and asbestos-exposed workers. *Cancer Res* 1994;54:2038s–43s.
29. Marwick C. Trials reveal no benefit, possible harm of beta carotene and vitamin A for lung cancer prevention. *JAMA* 1996;275:422–423.
30. Smigel K. Beta carotene fails to prevent cancer in two major studies; CARET intervention stopped. *J Natl Cancer Inst* 1996;88:145.
31. Mannisto S, Smith-Warner SA, Spiegelman D, et al. Dietary carotenoids and risk of lung cancer in a pooled analysis of seven cohort studies. *Cancer Epidemiol Biomarkers Prev* 2004;13:40–48.
32. Anberg A, Samet J. Epidemiology of lung cancer. In: Kane M, Kelly K, Miller Y, et al, eds. *The Biology of Lung Cancer. Volume 122 of the Lung Biology in Health and Disease Series.* New York: Marcel Dekker, Inc., 1998.
33. Peto R, Darby S, Deo H, et al. Smoking, smoking cessation, and lung cancer in the UK since 1950: combination of national statistics with two case-control studies. *BMJ* 2000;321:323–329.
34. Flanders WD, Lally CA, Zhu BP, et al. Lung cancer mortality in relation to age, duration of smoking, and daily cigarette consumption: results from Cancer Prevention Study II. *Cancer Res* 2003;63:6556–6562.
35. Lubin JH, Caporaso NE. Cigarette smoking and lung cancer: modeling total exposure and intensity. *Cancer Epidemiol Biomarkers Prev* 2006;15:517–523.
36. Knoke JD, Shanks TG, Vaughn JW, et al. Lung cancer mortality is related to age in addition to duration and intensity of cigarette smoking: an analysis of CPS-I data. *Cancer Epidemiol Biomarkers Prev* 2004; 13:949–957.
37. Parnell RW. Smoking and cancer [letter]. *Lancet* 1951;1:963.
38. HEATH CW. Differences between smokers and nonsmokers. *AMA Arch Intern Med* 1958;101:377–388.
39. Motulsky AG. Drug reactions enzymes, and biochemical genetics. *J Am Med Assoc* 1957;165:835–837.
40. Weir BA, Woo MS, Getz G, et al. Characterizing the cancer genome in lung adenocarcinoma. *Nature* 2007;450:893–898.
41. Niklinski J, Niklinska W, Chyczewski L, et al. Molecular genetic abnormalities in premalignant lung lesions: biological and clinical implications. *Eur J Cancer Prev* 2001;10:213–226.
42. Panani AD, Roussos C. Cytogenetic and molecular aspects of lung cancer. *Cancer Lett* 2006;239:1–9.
43. Hammond EC. Smoking in relation to the death rates of one million men and women. *Natl Cancer Inst Monogr* 1966;19:127–204.
44. Doll R, Peto R. Cigarette smoking and bronchial carcinoma: dose and time relationships among regular smokers and lifelong non-smokers. *J Epidemiol Community Health* 1978;32:303–313.
45. Garfinkel L. Selection, follow-up, and analysis in the American Cancer Society prospective studies. *Natl Cancer Inst Monogr* 1985;67:49–52.
46. Department of Health and Human Services, Public Health Service. *Reducing the Health Consequences of Smoking: 25 Years of Progress; A Report of the Surgeon General.* Washington, DC: U.S. Government Printing Office, 1989.
47. International Agency for Research on Cancer. *Tobacco Smoking.* Author 1986;15–395.
48. Damber LA, Larsson LG. Smoking and lung cancer with special regard to type of smoking and type of cancer. A case-control study in north Sweden. *Br J Cancer* 1986;53:673–681.
49. Anonymous. *Centers for Disease Control, Office on Smoking and Health. Health Benefits of Smoking Cessation: A Report of the Surgeon General, 1990.* Washington, DC: U.S. Government Printing Office, 1990.
50. Peto R, Darby S, Deo H, et al. Smoking, smoking cessation, and lung cancer in the UK since 1950: combination of national statistics with two case-control studies. *BMJ* 2000;321:323–329.
51. Silverberg E. Cancer statistics, 1980. *CA Cancer J Clin* 1980;30:23–38.
52. Shopland DR, Eyre HJ, Pechacek TF. Smoking-attributable cancer mortality in 1991: is lung cancer now the leading cause of death among smokers in the United States? *J Natl Cancer Inst* 1991;83:1142–1148.
53. Kondo K, Tsuzuki H, Sasa M, et al. A dose-response relationship between the frequency of p53 mutations and tobacco consumption in lung cancer patients. *J Surg Oncol* 1996;61:20–26.
54. Tokuhata GK, Lilienfeld AM. Familial aggregation of lung cancer in humans. *J Natl Cancer Inst* 1963;30:289–312.
55. Tokuhata GK, Lilienfeld AM. Familial aggregation of lung cancer among hospital patients. *Public Health Rep* 1963;78:277–283.
56. Fraumeni JF, Wertelecki W, Blattner WA, et al. Varied manifestations of a familial lymphoproliferative disorder. *Am J Med* 1975;59:145–151.
57. Goffman TE, Hassinger DD, Mulvihill JJ. Familial respiratory tract cancer. Opportunities for research and prevention. *JAMA* 1982;247:1020–1023.
58. Lynch HT, Kimberling WJ, Markvicka SE, et al. Genetics and smoking-associated cancers. A study of 485 families. *Cancer* 1986;57:1640–1646.
59. Ooi WL, Elston RC, Chen VW, et al. Increased familial risk for lung cancer. *J Natl Cancer Inst* 1986;76:217–222.
60. Sellers TA, Ooi WL, Elston RC, et al. Increased familial risk for non-lung cancer among relatives of lung cancer patients. *Am J Epidemiol* 1987;126:237–246.
61. McDuffie HH. Clustering of cancer in families of patients with primary lung cancer. *J Clin Epidemiol* 1991;44:69–76.
62. Shaw GL, Falk RT, Pickle LW, et al. Lung cancer risk associated with cancer in relatives. *J Clin Epidemiol* 1991;44:429–437.
63. Cannon-Albright LA, Thomas A, Goldgar DE, et al. Familiality of cancer in Utah. *Cancer Res* 1994;54:2378–2385.
64. Goldgar DE, Easton DF, Cannon-Albright LA, et al. Systematic population-based assessment of cancer risk in first-degree relatives of cancer probands. *J Natl Cancer Inst* 1994;86:1600–1608.
65. Bromen K, Pohlabeln H, Jahn I, et al. Aggregation of lung cancer in families: results from a population-based case-control study in Germany. *Am J Epidemiol* 2000;152:497–505.
66. Etzel CJ, Amos CI, Spitz MR. Risk for smoking-related cancer among relatives of lung cancer patients. *Cancer Res* 2003;63:8531–8535.
67. Jin YT, Xu YC, Yang RD, et al. Familial aggregation of lung cancer in a high incidence area in China. *Br J Cancer* 2005;92:1321–1325.
68. Jin Y, Xu Y, Xu M, et al. Increased risk of cancer among relatives of patients with lung cancer in China. *BMC Cancer* 2005;5:146.

69. Li X, Hemminki K. Familial and second lung cancers: a nation-wide epidemiologic study from Sweden. *Lung Cancer* 2003;39:255–263.
70. Li X, Hemminki K. Inherited predisposition to early onset lung cancer according to histological type. *Int J Cancer* 2004;112:451–457.
71. Li X, Hemminki K. Familial multiple primary lung cancers: a population-based analysis from Sweden. *Lung Cancer* 2005;47:301–307.
72. Hemminki K, Li X. Familial risk for lung cancer by histology and age of onset: evidence for recessive inheritance. *Exp Lung Res* 2005;31:205–215.
73. Jonsson S, Thorsteinsdottir U, Gudbjartsson DF, et al. Familial risk of lung carcinoma in the Icelandic population. *JAMA* 2004;292:2977–2983.
74. Matakidou A, Eisen T, Bridle H, et al. Case-control study of familial lung cancer risks in UK women. *Int J Cancer* 2005;116:445–450.
75. Cote ML, Kardia SL, Wenzlaff AS, et al. Risk of lung cancer among white and black relatives of individuals with early-onset lung cancer. *JAMA* 2005;293:3036–3042.
76. Schwartz AG, Yang P, Swanson GM. Familial risk of lung cancer among nonsmokers and their relatives. *Am J Epidemiol* 1996;144:554–562.
77. Wu AH, Fontham ET, Reynolds P, et al. Family history of cancer and risk of lung cancer among lifetime nonsmoking women in the United States. *Am J Epidemiol* 1996;143:535–542.
78. Mayne ST, Buenconsejo J, Janerich DT. Familial cancer history and lung cancer risk in United States nonsmoking men and women. *Cancer Epidemiol Biomarkers Prev* 1999;8:1065–1069.
79. Hrubec Z, Neel JV. Contribution of familial factors to the occurrence of cancer before old age in twin veterans. *Am J Hum Genet* 1982; 34:658–671.
80. Joishy SK, Cooper RA, Rowley PT. Alveolar cell carcinoma in identical twins. Similarity in time of onset, histochemistry, and site of metastasis. *Ann Intern Med* 1977;87:447–450.
81. Paul SM, Bacharach B, Goepp C. A genetic influence on alveolar cell carcinoma. *J Surg Oncol* 1987;36:249–252.
82. Falk RT, Pickle LW, Fontham ET, et al. Epidemiology of bronchioloalveolar carcinoma. *Cancer Epidemiol Biomarkers Prev* 1992;1:339–344.
83. Braun MM, Caporaso NE, Page WF, et al. A cohort study of twins and cancer. *Cancer Epidemiol Biomarkers Prev* 1995;4:469–473.
84. Lichtenstein P, Holm NV, Verkasalo PK, et al. Environmental and heritable factors in the causation of cancer—analyses of cohorts of twins from Sweden, Denmark, and Finland. *N Engl J Med* 2000;343:78–85.
85. Matakidou A, Eisen T, Houlston RS. Systematic review of the relationship between family history and lung cancer risk. *Br J Cancer* 2005;93:825–833.
86. Leonard RC, MacKay T, Brown A, et al. Small-cell lung cancer after retinoblastoma. *Lancet* 1988;2:1503.
87. Sanders BM, Jay M, Draper GJ, et al. Non-ocular cancer in relatives of retinoblastoma patients. *Br J Cancer* 1989;60:358–365.
88. Kleinerman RA, Tarone RE, Abramson DH, et al. Hereditary retinoblastoma and risk of lung cancer. *J Natl Cancer Inst* 2000;92:2037–2039.
89. Kleinerman RA, Tarone RE, Abramson DH, et al. Hereditary retinoblastoma and risk of lung cancer. *J Natl Cancer Inst* 2000;92:2037–2039.
90. Foster MC, Kleinerman RA, Abramson DH, et al. Tobacco use in adult long-term survivors of retinoblastoma. *Cancer Epidemiol Biomarkers Prev* 2006;15:1464–1468.
91. Wistuba II, Gazdar AF, Minna JD. Molecular genetics of small cell lung carcinoma. *Semin Oncol* 2001;28:3–13.
92. Hwang SJ, Cheng LS, Lozano G, et al. Lung cancer risk in germline p53 mutation carriers: association between an inherited cancer predisposition, cigarette smoking, and cancer risk. *Hum Genet* 2003;113:238–243.
93. Bonomi PD, Buckingham L, Coon J. Selecting patients for treatment with epidermal growth factor tyrosine kinase inhibitors. *Clin Cancer Res* 2007;13:s4606–s4612.
94. Bell DW, Gore I, Okimoto RA, et al. Inherited susceptibility to lung cancer may be associated with the T790M drug resistance mutation in EGFR. *Nat Genet* 2005;37:1315–1316.
95. Vikis H, Sato M, James M, et al. EGFR-T790M is a rare lung cancer susceptibility allele with enhanced kinase activity. *Cancer Res* 2007;67:4665–4670.
96. Sellers TA, Bailey-Wilson JE, Elston RC, et al. Evidence for mendelian inheritance in the pathogenesis of lung cancer. *J Natl Cancer Inst* 1990;82:1272–1279.
97. Elston RC, Stewart J. A general model for the genetic analysis of pedigree data. *Hum Hered* 1971;21:523–542.
98. Elston RC, Yelverton KC. General models for segregation analysis. *Am J Hum Genet* 1975;27:31–45.
99. Bonney GE. Regressive logistic models for familial disease and other binary traits. *Biometrics* 1986;42:611–625.
100. Elston RC, George VT. Age of onset, age at examination, and other covariates in the analysis of family data. *Genet Epidemiol* 1989;6:217–220.
101. Cannings C, Thompson EA. Ascertainment in the sequential sampling of pedigrees. *Clin Genet* 1977;12:208–212.
102. Elston RC, Sobel E. Sampling considerations in the gathering and analysis of pedigree data. *Am J Hum Genet* 1979;31:62–69.
103. Chen PL, Sellers TA, Bailey-Wilson JE, et al. Segregation analysis of smoking-associated malignancies: evidence for Mendelian inheritance. *Am J Med Genet* 1994;52(3):308–314.
104. Gauderman WJ, Morrison JL, Carpenter CL, et al. Analysis of gene-smoking interaction in lung cancer. *Genet Epidemiol* 1997;14:199–214.
105. Yang P, Schwartz AG, McAllister AE, et al. Lung cancer risk in families of nonsmoking probands: heterogeneity by age at diagnosis. *Genet Epidemiol* 1999;17:253–273.
106. Wu PF, Lee CH, Wang MJ, et al. Cancer aggregation and complex segregation analysis of families with female non-smoking lung cancer probands in Taiwan. *Eur J Cancer* 2004;40:260–266.
107. Croce CM. Genetic approaches to the study of the molecular basis of human cancer. *Cancer Res* 1991;51:5015s–5018s.
108. Breuer RH, Postmus PE, Smit EF. Molecular pathology of non-small-cell lung cancer. *Respiration* 2005;72:313–330.
109. Bunn PA, Jr. Molecular biology and early diagnosis in lung cancer. *Lung Cancer* 2002;38:S5–S8.
110. Thomas RK, Weir B, Meyerson M. Genomic approaches to lung cancer. *Clin Cancer Res* 2006;12:4384s–491s.
111. Kendall J, Liu Q, Bakleh A, et al. Oncogenic cooperation and coamplification of developmental transcription factor genes in lung cancer. *Proc Natl Acad Sci U S A* 2007:104;16663–16668.
112. Kwei KA, Kim YH, Girard L, et al. Genomic profiling identifies TITF1 as a lineage-specific oncogene amplified in lung cancer. *Oncogene* 2008;27(25):3635–3640.
113. Bailey-Wilson JE, Amos CI, Pinney SM, et al. A major lung cancer susceptibility locus maps to chromosome 6q23–25. *Am J Hum Genet* 2004;75:460–474.
114. Schwartz AG, Prysak GM, Bock CH, et al. The molecular epidemiology of lung cancer. *Carcinogenesis* 2007;28:507–518.
115. Kiyohara C, Otsu A, Shirakawa T, et al. Genetic polymorphisms and lung cancer susceptibility: a review. *Lung Cancer* 2002;37:241–256.
116. Hung RJ, McKay JD, Gaborieau V, et al. A susceptibility locus for lung cancer maps to nicotinic acetylcholine receptor subunit genes on 15q25. *Nature* 2008;452:633–637.
117. Thorgeirsson TE, Geller F, Sulem P, et al. A variant associated with nicotine dependence, lung cancer and peripheral arterial disease. *Nature* 2008;452:638–642.
118. Amos CI, Wu X, Broderick P, et al. Genome-wide association scan of tag SNPs identifies a susceptibility locus for lung cancer at 15q25.1. *Nat Genet* 2008;40:616–622.
119. Spitz MR, Wei Q, Dong Q, et al. Genetic susceptibility to lung cancer: the role of DNA damage and repair. *Cancer Epidemiol Biomarkers Prev* 2003;12:689–698.
120. Bartsch H, Dally H, Popanda O, et al. Genetic risk profiles for cancer susceptibility and therapy response. *Recent Results Cancer Res* 2007;174:19–36.
121. Brennan P, McKay J, Moore L, et al. Uncommon CHEK2 mis-sense variant and reduced risk of tobacco-related cancers: case control study. *Hum Mol Genet* 2007;16:1794–1801.

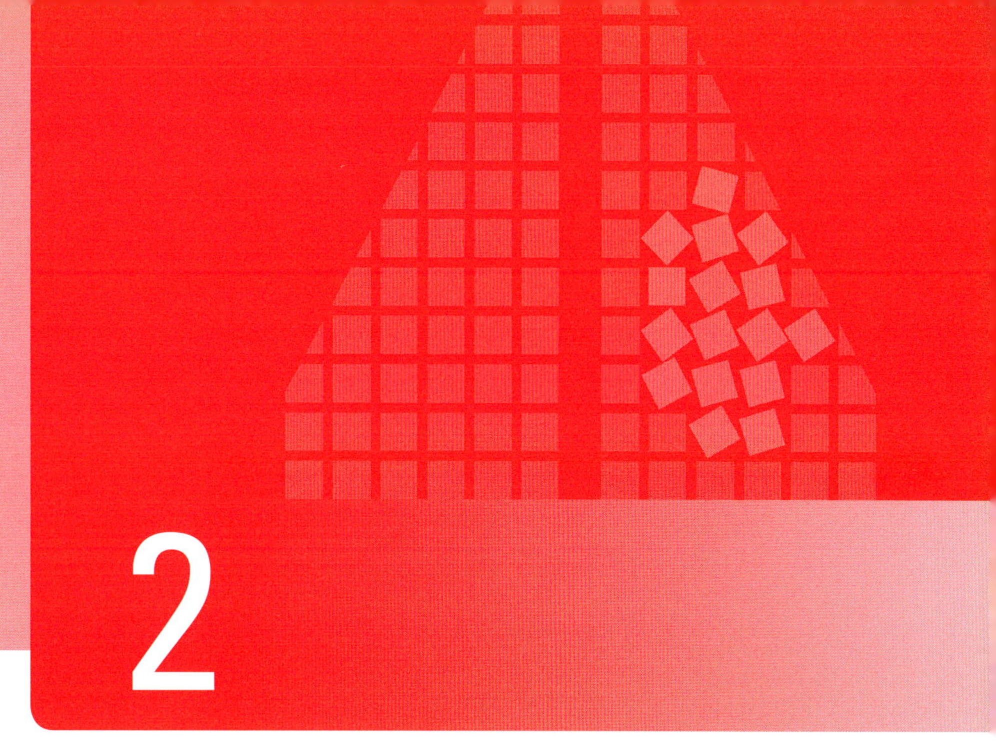

SECTION 2

Lung Cancer Biology

CHAPTER 5

Jill E. Larsen
Monica Spinola
Adi F. Gazdar
John D. Minna

An Overview of the Molecular Biology of Lung Cancer

Lung cancer cells have defects in the regulatory circuits that govern normal cell proliferation and homeostasis. Hanahan and Weinberg[1] described the "hallmarks of cancer" as six essential alterations in cell physiology that collectively dictate malignant growth. These acquired capabilities found in lung cancers are self-sufficiency of growth signals, insensitivity to growth-inhibitory (antigrowth) signals, evasion of programmed cell death (apoptosis), limitless replicative potential, sustained angiogenesis, and tissue invasion and metastasis. Transformation from a normal to malignant lung cancer phenotype is thought to arise in a multistep fashion, through a series of genetic and epigenetic alterations, ultimately evolving into invasive cancer by clonal expansion.[2] These progressive pathological changes in the bronchial epithelium—known as preneoplastic or premalignant lesions—occur primarily as one of three distinct morphological forms: squamous dysplasia, atypical adenomatous hyperplasia, and diffuse idiopathic pulmonary neuroendocrine cell hyperplasia.[3] Bronchial squamous dysplasia and carcinoma in situ (CIS) are the recognized preneoplastic lesions for squamous cell carcinoma; atypical adenomatous hyperplasia (AAH), a putative preneoplastic lesion, for a subset of adenocarcinomas; and neuroendocrine cell hyperplasia for neuroendocrine lung carcinomas.[3] These preneoplastic lesions, however, account for the development of only a subset of lung cancers; for example, the precursor lesion for the most common neuroendocrine carcinoma of the lung, small cell lung carcinoma (SCLC), is unknown. Tumors are believed to become increasingly malignant with time, initiating tumorigenesis from possibly only a handful of mutations followed by additional (and different) mutations and epigenetic changes acquired during clonal expansion, where cells possessing in vivo growth advantage become dominant.[2]

The identification and characterization of these molecular changes in lung cancer is of fundamental importance for improving the prevention, early detection, treatment, and palliation of this disease. The overall goal is to translate these findings to the clinic by using molecular alterations as (a) biomarkers for early detection, (b) targets for prevention, (c) tools for new molecular approaches, (d) signatures for personalizing prognosis and therapy selection for each patient, and (e) targets to specifically kill or inhibit the growth of lung cancer in patients.

Lung cancer arises from neoplastic changes to epithelial cells in the lung. However, it is not known whether all lung epithelial cells are susceptible to malignant transformation or only a subset of these cells; specifically, a major question is whether the changes need to take place in lung epithelial cells with stem cell–like properties. Lung cancer is a heterogeneous disease clinically, biologically, histologically, and molecularly. The underlying causes of this heterogeneity are unknown and could reflect changes occurring in cells with various potential for differentiation (e.g., squamous or adenomatous) or represent different molecular changes occurring in the same target lung epithelial cells. This heterogeneity and molecular complexity contributes to the difficulty in unraveling the pathogenesis of lung cancer. Multiple oncogenes, tumor suppressor genes (TSGs), signaling pathway components, and other cellular processes are involved in the molecular pathogenesis of lung cancer. This chapter will review molecular aberrations in lung cancer and the multiple pathways through which it develops.

The two main disease categories of lung cancer, non–small cell lung cancer (NSCLC) (representing 80% to 85% of cases) and SCLC (representing 15% to 20%), are generally classified based on differences in histological, clinical, and neuroendocrine characteristics. NSCLC and SCLC can also differ molecularly with many genetic alterations exhibiting subtype specificity (summarized in Table 5.1). Additionally, molecular studies of NSCLC have also revealed considerable differences between the subtypes of NSCLC, particularly the two most common subtypes: adenocarcinoma and squamous cell carcinoma.

TABLE 5.1 Common Genetic Alterations Found in Lung Cancer[a]

Gene	SCLC (%)	NSCLC (%)			References
		All	Adenocarcinoma	Squamous Cell	
Oncogenic Alterations					
Mutation					
BRAF	Rare	1–3	1–5	3	177,178
EGFR	Rare	~20	10–40	Rare	177,179–182
ErbB2 (HER-2)	Rare	2	4	Rare	177,183
KRAS	Rare	10–30	15–35	<5	177,184–186
MET	13	21	14	12	6
PIK3CA	Rare	1–5	2–3	2–7	56,187–189
Amplification					
EGFR	Rare	20–30	15	30	6
ErbB2 (HER-2)	5–30	2–23	6	2	6,183,190,191
MDM2		6–24	14	22	192
MET		7–21	20	21	193,194
MYC	18–30	8–22			195–198
NKX2-1 (TITF-1)	Rare	12–30	10–15	3–15	6,14,15
PIK3CA	~5	9–17	6	33–36	6,56
Increase in protein expression					
CRK		8–30	8–30		199
BCL2	75–95	10–35			186,200,201
CCND1	0	43	35–55	30–35	85,202
CD44	Rare	Common	3	48	203
c-KIT	46–91	Rare			204–210
EGFR	Rare	50–90	40–65	60–85	29–32,186
ErbB2 (HER-2)	<10	20–35	16–38	6–16	183,186,207,211–213
MYC	10–45	<10			50,214–216
PDGFRA	65	2–100	100	89	217–220
Tumor-Suppressing Alterations					
Mutation					
CDKN2A (p16)	<1	10–40			186
LKB1	Rare	30	34	19	6,186
p53	75–90	50–60	50–70	60–70	186,221–223
PTEN	15–20	<10			186
Rb	80–100	20–40			186,224–226
Deletion/LOH[b]					
CDKN2A (p16)	37	75–80			84,227,228
FHIT	100	55–75			227–229
p53	86–93	74–86			227,228
Rb	93	62			227,228
Loss of protein expression					
CAV1	95	24			230
CDKN2A ($p14^{ARF}$)	65	40–50			84,231
CDKN2A (p16)	3–37	30–79	~55	60–75	227,228
FHIT	80–95	40–70			186,227,228
PTEN		25–74	77	70	60,231
Rb	90	15–60	23–57	6–14	228
TUSC2 (FUS1)	100	82	79	87	232

TABLE 5.1 Common Genetic Alterations Found in Lung Cancer[a] *(continued)*

Gene	SCLC (%)	NSCLC (%)			References
		All	Adenocarcinoma	Squamous Cell	
Tumor-acquired DNA Methylation					
APC	15–26	24–96			93,94,233
CAV1	93	9			230
CDH1	60 40	20–35			94,233–235
CDH13	15–20	45			93,94
CDKN2A ($p14^{ARF}$)	nd[b]	6–8			94
CDKN2A (p16)	5, 0	15–41	21–36	24–33	236–238
DAPK1	nd	16–45			94,233,239
FHIT	64	37			93,94
GSTP1	16	7–12, 15			94,240
MGMT	16	16–27, 10			94,233
PTEN		26	24	30	60
RARβ	45–70	40–43			93,94,241
RASSF1A	72–85	15–45	31	43	90,94,96,233, 242,243
SEMA3B	nd	41–50	46	47	90,91
TIMP3	nd	19–26			94
Telomeres					
Telomerase activity	75–100	50–80	65–85	80–90	11–13,186,244
Chromosomal Aberrations					
Large-scale loss	1p, 3p, 4p, 4q, 5q, 8p, 10q, 13q, 17p	3p, 5q, 8p, 9p, 13q, 17p, 18q, 19p, 19q, 21q, 22q	2q, 3p, 4q, 8p, 9p, 9q, 10p, 10q, 13q, 15q, 18, 20	3p, 4q, 9p, 10p, 10q, 18, 20	24,25,55,227, 245–248
Focal deletions		2q22.1, 3p14.2, 3q25.1, 5q11.2, 7q11.22, 9p23, 9p21.3, 10q23.31, 11q11, 13q12.11, 13q14.2, 13q32.2, 18q23, 21p11.2			15,171,172
Large-scale gain	3q, 5p, 8q, 18q	1q, 3q, 5p, 6p, 7p, 7q, 8q, 20p, 20q	5p, 7p, 7q, 8q, 11q, 19, 20q	2q, 3q, 5p, 7, 8q, 11q, 13q, 19, 20q	24,25,55,227, 245–248
Focal amplifications		1p36.32, 1p34.3, 1q32.2, 1q21.2, 2p24.3, 2q11.2, 2q31.1, 3q26.31, 5p15.33, 5p15.31, 5p14.3, 5q31.3, 6p21.1, 7p11.2, 8p12, 8q21.13, 8q24.21, 10q24.1, 10q26.3, 11q13.3, 12p12.1, 12q13.2, 12q14.1, 12q15, 14q13.3, 14q32.13, 16q22.2, 17q12, 18q12.1, 19q12, 19q13.33, 20q13.32, 22q11.21			15,171,172

[a]nd, not determined.

[b]LOH, loss of heterozygosity.

EPIDEMIOLOGY AND SUSCEPTIBILITY IN LUNG CANCER

Eighty-five percent of lung cancers are caused by tobacco smoke, where exposure to carcinogens present in tobacco smoke leads to the acquisition of genetic mutations that may eventually initiate carcinogenesis. However, not all lung cancers arise in smokers, and not all smokers will develop lung cancer. Thus, inherited factors must be involved that may predispose an individual to develop lung cancer—either by increasing susceptibility to the damaging effects of carcinogen exposure or by increasing susceptibility regardless of smoking history. Worldwide, approximately 25% of lung cancer cases are not attributable to smoking.[4] These cases occur more frequently in women, especially in Asian countries, target the distal airways, and are commonly adenocarcinomas. Coupled with molecular data that indicates strikingly different mutation patterns between known lung cancer genes such as *KRAS*, epidermal growth factor receptor *(EGFR),* and *TP53* and clinical data in relation to response to targeted therapies, it has now been suggested that lung cancer in never-smokers be considered a distinct disease from the more common tobacco smoke–related lung cancer.[4]

Many studies have examined the effect of single nucleotide polymorphisms (SNPs) on the risk of developing lung cancer.[5,6] The reported risk effect in these studies is generally modest and often inconsistent, explaining why none are in routine use. However, metaanalyses as well as use of whole-genome SNP microarrays may hold the key to identifying robust and possible synergistic interactions between the modest affect of multiple SNPs. Lung cancer risk was recently associated with genomic variation at 15q24/q25.1 by three separate studies simultaneously that used whole-genome SNP microarrays.[7–9] Although the conclusions of the three studies differed in whether the risk is conferred directly with cancer or through nicotine addiction, the genes within this locus—which include several genes encoding nicotinic acetylcholine receptor subunits—represent important targets for further functional analyses.

GENOMIC INSTABILITY, TELOMERES, AND DNA DAMAGE IN LUNG CANCER

Malignant transformation is characterized by genetic instability that can exist at the chromosomal level (with loss or gain of genomic material, translocations, and microsatellite instability); at the nucleotide level (with single or several nucleotide base changes); or in the transcriptome (with altered gene expression). Abnormalities are typically targeted to proto-oncogenes, TSGs, DNA repair genes, and other genes that can promote outgrowth of affected cells.[10] The erosion of telomeres at the end of chromosomes is also associated with genomic instability leading to chromosomal abnormalities. Telomere length regulates the replicative capacity of a cell, where progressive telomere shortening occurs with each replication. Once the telomere becomes too short, the cell will undergo cellular senescence or apoptosis. Activation of telomerase, the telomere-lengthening enzyme, in premalignant cells prevents loss of telomere ends beyond critical points and is essential for cell immortality. Although silenced in normal cells, telomerase is activated in >80% of NSCLCs and almost uniformly in SCLCs.[11–13] In normal cells, the presence of DNA damage engenders a DNA repair response, and if this is not successful, the apoptosis program is activated to remove the damaged cell. However, in premalignant and cancer cells the apoptosis program is often itself damaged, thus allowing unrepaired or misrepaired DNA damage to persist in clones of cells.

ONCOGENES AND GROWTH-STIMULATORY PATHWAYS

Many oncogenes and TSGs have been identified by mapping of copy number changes throughout the cancer genome.[14–23] Earlier genomic analysis technology such as karyotyping and comparative genomic hybridization (CGH) enabled low-resolution characterization of the lung cancer genome identifying whole-arm or large-scale gain or loss on nearly every chromosomal arm, but most commonly 3p, 4q, 9p, and 17p loss and 1q, 3q, 5p, and 17q gain[24,25] (Table 5.1). However, high-resolution microarray analyses can now narrow in on these aberrant regions to detect focal amplifications and deletions often spanning only a handful of genes (Table 5.1).

Oncogenic activation typically occurs by gene amplification, point mutation, rearrangement, or through gene overexpression by other mechanisms including those mediated by microRNAs (miRNAs). These changes can result in persistent upregulation of mitogenic growth signals that induce cell growth. Although promoting the malignant transformation of a cell, persistent upregulation of a particular growth signal or pathway can also result in "oncogenic addiction"—whereby the cell becomes dependent on this aberrant oncogenic signaling for survival.[26] This presents an obvious target for therapeutics; remove or inhibit the oncogenic signal and an addicted tumor cell will die, whereas normal "nonaddicted" cells will be unaffected. Signaling pathways commonly involved in lung cancer are shown in Figure 5.1.

Epidermal Growth Factor Receptor Signaling The ErbB family of tyrosine kinase receptors includes four members—EGFR, ErbB-2 (HER-2), ErbB-3, and ErbB-4.[27] Although the intracellular tyrosine kinase domains of the four receptors are highly conserved, the extracellular domain is not so conserved, enabling the receptors to bind different ligands. Following ligand binding, the ErbB receptors form homodimers or heterodimers that results in receptor activation and subsequent activation of various signaling pathways.

Activation of EGFR through the binding of EGF and EGF-like binding growth factors such as transforming growth factor-α (TGF-α) enables the regulation of epithelial cell behavior and the initiation of tumors from epithelial cell origin through multiple signaling pathways. These include the RAS/RAF/MEK/MAPK pathway (cell proliferation), the PI3K/AKT pathway, and signal transduction and activator of transcription (STAT) 3 and STAT5 pathways (cell survival through the evasion of apoptosis)[28] (Fig. 5.1). EGFR exhibits

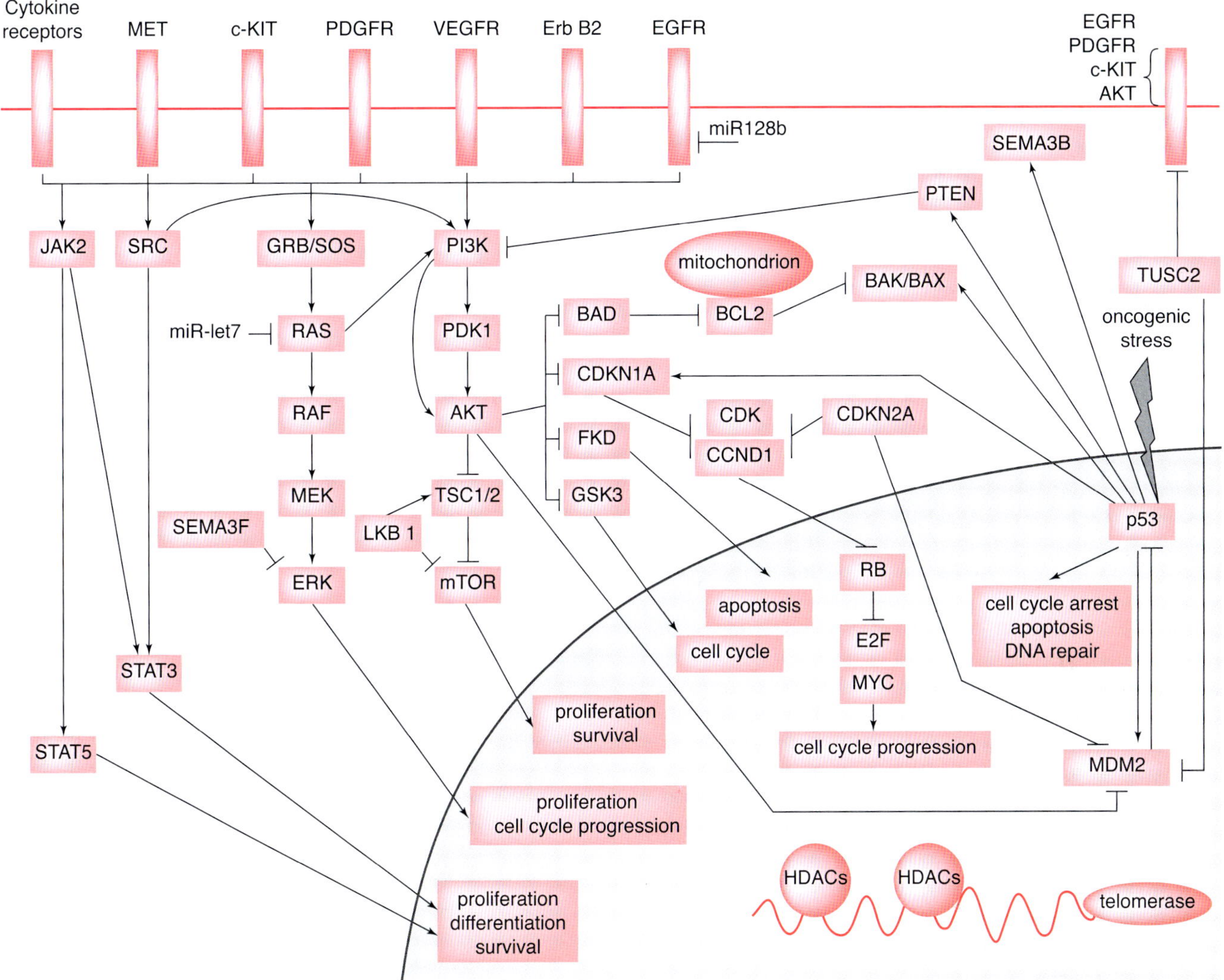

FIGURE 5.1 Signaling pathways involved in NSCLC and SCLC. Aberrant signaling resulting in activation of growth-stimulatory pathways or interference of growth inhibitory pathways has been implicated in lung cancer pathogenesis. Oncogenic activation typically occurs through amplification, mutation, rearrangement, or overexpression. In lung cancer, commonly activated oncogenes include *EGFR*, *ERBB2*, *MYC*, *KRAS*, *MET*, *CCND1*, *CDK4*, and *BCL2*. In contrast to oncogene activation, loss of TSG function is thought to require inactivation of both alleles—generally, LOH of one allele, and point mutation, epigenetic, or transcriptional silencing will inactivate the second allele. In lung cancer, commonly inactivated TSGs include *TP53*, *RB1*, *CDKN2A*, *FHIT*, and *PTEN*. Although EGFR plays a major role in lung cancer pathogenesis, several other receptor tyrosine kinases have been implicated such as members of the platelet-derived growth factor receptor (PDGFR) family c-KIT (expression is common in SCLC but rare in NSCLC[175,176]) and MET (potentially associated with acquired resistance to EGFR TKIs). Table 5.2 lists targeted therapeutic agents that have been developed against many components of these signaling pathways. *AKT*, v-akt murine thymoma viral oncogene homologue; *BAD*, Bcl2-antagonist of cell death; *BAK/BAX*, BCL2-antagonist/killer / BCL2-associated X protein; *BCL2*, B-cell CLL/lymphoma 2; *CCND1*, cyclin D1; *CDK*, cyclin-dependent kinase; *CDKN1A*, cyclin-dependent kinase inhibitor 1A; *CDKN2A*, cyclin-dependent kinase inhibitor 2A; *c-KIT*, v-kit Hardy-Zuckerman 4 feline sarcoma viral oncogene homologue; *E2F*, E2F transcription factor; *EGFR*, epidermal growth factor receptor; *Erb B2*, v-erb-b2 erythroblastic leukemia viral oncogene homologue 2; *ERK*, extracellular signal regulated kinase; *FKD*, forkhead domain; *GRB/SOS*, growth factor receptor-bound protein/son of sevenless; *GSK3*, glycogen synthase kinase 3; *HDACs*, histone deacetylase; *JAK2*, Janus kinase 2; *LKB 1*, serine/threonine kinase 11; *MDM2*, Mouse Double Minute 2; *MEK*, MAP kinse-ERK kinase; *MET*, mesenchymal–epithelial transition factor; *miR128b*, microRNA 128 b; *mTOR*, mechanistic target of rapamycin; *MYC*, v-myc myelocytomatosis viral oncogene homologue; *p53*, TP53 gene product; *PDGFR*, platelet-derived growth factor receptor; *PDK1*, pyruvate dehydrogenase kinase, isozyme 1; *PI3K*, phosphatidylinositol 3 kinase; *PTEN*, phosphatase and tensin homologue; *RAF*, v-raf-1 murine leukemia viral oncogene homolog 1; *RAS*, rat sarcoma virus oncogene 1; *RB*, retinoblastoma; *SEMA3B*, sema domain, immunoglobulin domain (Ig), short basic domain, secreted, (semaphorin) 3B; *SEMA3F*, sema domain, immunoglobulin domain (Ig), short basic domain, secreted, (semaphorin) 3F; *SRC*, rous sarcoma oncogene cellular; *STAT3*, signal transducer and activator of transcription 3; *STAT5*, signal transducer and activator of transcription 5; *TSC1/2*, Tuberosclerosis 1/2; *TUSC2*, tumor suppressor candidate 2; *VEGFR*, vascular endothelial growth factor receptor.

overexpression or aberrant activation in approximately 50% to 90% of NSCLCs with activating mutations occurring with or without amplification.[29–32] Activating mutations, which are found with increased frequency in certain subsets of lung cancer patients, occur as three different types of somatic mutations—deletions, insertions, and missense point mutations—and are located in exons 19 to 21 that code for the tyrosine kinase domain of EGFR.[17–19] Mutant EGFRs (either by exon 19 deletion or exon 21 L858R mutation) show an increased amount and duration of EGFR activation compared with wild-type receptors,[17] and have preferential activation of the PI3K/AKT and STAT3/STAT5 pathways rather than the RAS/RAF/MEK/MAPK pathway.[33] EGFR mutant tumors (primarily adenocarcinomas) are initially highly sensitive to EGFR tyrosine kinase inhibitors (TKIs).[17–19] This represents an example of oncogene addiction in lung cancer where tumors initiated through EGFR mutation-activation of EGF signaling rely on continued EGF signaling for survival. However, despite an initial response, patients treated with EGFR TKIs eventually develop resistance to TKIs, which is linked (in approximately 50% tumors) to the acquiring of a second mutation at T790M in exon 20.[34–39] The presence of the T790M mutation in a primary lung cancer that had not been treated with EGFR TKIs, however, suggests that this resistance mutation may develop with tumor progression and not necessarily as a response to treatment.[40] Recently, amplification of the mesenchymal–epithelial transition (MET) proto-oncogene has been associated with acquired resistance to EGFR TKIs in 20% of resistant cases[36,41] with MET activating the PI3K pathway through phosphorylation of ERBB3, independent of EGFR and ERBB2.[41] Importantly, inhibition of MET signaling was able to restore sensitivity to TKIs.

The RAS/RAF/MEK/MAPK/MYC Pathway The RAS proto-oncogene family (*KRAS, HRAS, NRAS,* and *RRAS*) encode four highly homologous 21kDa membrane-bound proteins involved in signal transduction. Proteins encoded by the RAS genes exist in two states: an active state, in which guanosine triphosphate (GTP) is bound to the molecule and an inactive state, where the GTP has been cleaved to guanosine diphosphate (GDP).[42] Activating point mutations can confer oncogenic potential through a loss of intrinsic GTPase activity resulting in an inability to cleave GTP to GDP. This can initiate unchecked cell proliferation through the RAS/RAF/MEK/MAPK pathway, downstream of the EGFR signaling pathway.[43] Activating *RAS* mutations occur in approximately 15% to 20% of NSCLCs and, in particular, 30% to 50% of adenocarcinomas.[44] In lung cancer, 90% of mutations are located in *KRAS* (80% in codon 12, and the remainder in codons 13 and 61) with *HRAS* and *NRAS* mutations only occasionally documented.[44] *KRAS* mutations are mutually exclusive with *EGFR* and *ERBB2* mutations, and confer resistance to EGFR TKIs and chemotherapy.[45–47] Additionally, whereas *KRAS* mutations are primarily observed in lung adenocarcinomas of smokers, *EGFR* mutations are primarily observed in lung adenocarcinomas of never-smokers.[4] These data demonstrate how lung adenocarcinoma can develop through different pathways, and it is likely, given the importance of EGFR targeted therapy that determination of *EGFR* and *KRAS* mutations in tumors will soon become part of standard care.

BRAF mutations occur in 1% to 5% of lung cancers, and mutant BRAF mouse models can develop lung adenocarcinomas.[48] The MYC proto-oncogene members are targets of RAS signaling and key regulators of numerous downstream pathways such as cell proliferation.[49] Activation of MYC members often occurs through gene amplification. MYC is most frequently activated in NSCLC,[50] with the other two members, MYCN and MYCL along with MYC, usually activated in SCLC.[24,51]

The PI3K/AKT Pathway The PI3K/AKT pathway that lies downstream of several receptor tyrosine kinases (RTKs; such as EGFR) is a key regulator of cell proliferation, cell growth, and cell survival and is commonly activated in lung cancer through changes in several of its components, including PI3K, PTEN, AKT, or EGFR or KRAS. In lung tumorigenesis, activation of the PI3K/AKT pathway is thought to occur early[52] and results in cell survival through inhibition of apoptosis. Activation can occur through the binding of the SH2-domains of p85, the regulatory subunit of PI3K, to phosphotyrosine residues of activated RTKs.[53] Alternatively, activation can occur via binding of PI3K to activated RAS. Mutation and more commonly amplification of *PIK3CA*, which encodes the catalytic subunit of phosphatidylinositol 3-kinase (PI3K), occur most commonly in squamous cell carcinomas.[20,54–56] AKT, a serine/threonine kinase that acts downstream from PI3K can also have mutations that lead to pathway activation. One of the primary effectors of AKT is mTOR, a serine/threonine kinase involved in regulating proliferation, cell cycle progression, mRNA translation, cytoskeletal organization, and survival.[57] The tumor suppressor PTEN, which negatively regulates the PI3K/AKT pathway via phosphatase activity on phosphatidylinositol 3,4,5-trisphosphate (PIP3), a product of PI3K,[58] is commonly suppressed in lung cancer by inactivating mutations or loss of expression.[59,60]

NKX2-1 (TITF1): A Lung Cancer Lineage–Dependent Oncogene Genome-wide screens for DNA copy number changes in primary NSCLCs found multiple examples of amplification at 14q13.3—and subsequent functional analysis (siRNA knockdowns in NSCLCs) identified *NKX2-1* (also termed *TITF1*) as the most likely target of amplification in lung cancer.[14,15,61] *NKX2-1* encodes a lineage-specific transcription factor essential for branching morphogenesis in lung development and the formation of type II pneumocytes, the cells lining lung alveoli.[62,63] Amplification of tissue-specific transcription factors in cancer has been observed in *AR* in prostate cancer,[64] *MITF* in melanoma,[65] and *ESR1* in breast cancer.[66] These findings have led to the development of a "lineage-dependency" concept in tumors[67] whose survival and progression of a tumor is dependent upon continued signaling through a specific lineage pathways (i.e., abnormal expression of pathways involved in normal cell development) rather than continued signaling through the pathway of oncogenic transformation as seen with oncogene addiction.[26]

EML4-ALK Fusion Proteins Oncogenic fusion proteins created by recurrent chromosomal translocations are generally not common in solid tumors such as lung cancer; however, recent studies indicate that this infrequency may be attributable to the difficulties in detection. The fusion of PTK echinoderm microtubule-associated protein like-4 (EML4)-anaplastic lymphoma kinase (ALK) was recently associated with lung cancer[68] and occurs in approximately 7% of NSCLCs.[68–70] Fusing with EML4 induces a significant transforming potential in ALK. Whereas wild-type ALK is thought to undergo transient homodimerization in response with specific ligand binding, EML4-ALK is constitutively oligomerized resulting in persistent mitogenic signaling and ultimately malignant transformation.[71] Additionally, EML4-ALK generally appears to be mutually exclusive to that of EGFR or KRAS mutations in NSCLC and is more common in never or former smokers.[72]

TUMOR SUPPRESSOR GENES AND GROWTH INHIBITORY PATHWAYS

Loss of TSG function is an important step in lung carcinogenesis process and usually both alleles need to be inactivated. Generally, loss of heterozygosity (LOH) inactivates one allele through chromosomal deletion or translocation, and point mutation, epigenetic or transcriptional silencing inactivates the second allele.[73,74] In lung cancer, commonly inactivated TSGs include *TP53*, *RB1*, *CDKN2A*, *FHIT*, *RASSF1A*, and *PTEN*.

The p53 Pathway *TP53* (17p13) encodes a phosphoprotein that prevents accumulation of genetic damage in daughter cells. In response to cellular stress, p53 induces the expression of downstream genes such as cyclin-dependent kinase (CDK) inhibitors that regulate cell cycle checkpoint signals, causing the cell to undergo G1 arrest and allowing DNA repair or apoptosis.[74] p53 inactivating mutations are the most common alterations in cancer, especially lung cancer, where 17p13 frequently demonstrates hemizygous deletion and mutational inactivation in the remaining allele.[75–77] Regulation of p53 can occur through the oncogene MDM2, which reduces p53 levels through degradation, and the $p14^{ARF}$ isoform of CDKN2A, which acts as a tumor suppressor by inhibiting MDM2. As such, the genes that encode MDM2 and $p14^{ARF}$ are altered in lung cancer with amplification of MDM2 seen in 6% of NSCLCs[78] and loss of $p14^{ARF}$ expression in approximately 40% and 65% of NSCLCs and SCLCs, respectively.[79,80] Restoration of p53 expression in vivo has been achieved with p53 gene therapy of lung cancer patients in a subpopulation of tumor cells.[81]

The CDKN2A/RB Pathway The CDKN2A-RB1 pathway controls G1- to S-phase cell cycle progression. Hypophosphorylated retinoblastoma (RB) protein, encoded by RB1, halts the G1/S-phase transition by binding to the transcription factor E2F1. This tumor-suppressing effect can be inhibited by hyperphosphorylation of RB by CDK-CCND1 complexes (complexes between CDK4 or CDK6 and CCND1), and in turn, formation of CDK-CCND1 complexes can be inhibited by CDNK2A.[82] Nearly all constituents of the CDKN2A/RB pathway have been shown to be altered in lung cancer through mutations (CDK4 and CDKN2A), deletions (RB1 and CDKN2A), amplifications (CDK4 and CCDN1), methylation silencing (CDKN2*A* and RB1), and phosphorylation (RB).[83–88]

Chromosome 3p TSGs Loss of one copy of chromosome 3p is one of the most frequent and early events in human cancer, found in 96% of lung tumors and 78% of lung preneoplastic lesions.[89] Mapping of this loss identified several genes with functional tumor-suppressing capacity including FHIT (3p14.2), RASSF1A, TUSC2 (also called FUS1), and semaphorin family members SEMA3B and SEMA3F (all at 3p21.3), and RARβ (3p24). In addition to LOH or allele loss, some of these 3p genes (FHIT, RASSF1A, SEMA3B, and RARβ) often exhibit decreased expression in lung cancer cells by means of epigenetic mechanisms such as promoter hypermethylation.[90–94] Additionally, FHIT, RASSF1A, TUSC2, and SEMA3B will reduce growth when reintroduced into lung cancer cells. FHIT, located in the most common fragile site in the human genome (FRA3B), has been shown to induce apoptosis in lung cancer.[95] RASSF1A can induce apoptosis, as well as stabilize microtubules, and affect cell cycle regulation.[96] The tumor-suppressing effect of *TUSC2* is thought to occur through inhibition of protein tyrosine kinases such as EGFR, PDGFR, *c-Abl*, c-Kit, and AKT[97] as well as inhibition of MDM2-mediated degradation of p53.[98] The candidate TSG SEMA3B encodes a secreted protein that can decrease cell proliferation and induce apoptosis when reexpressed in lung, breast, and ovarian cancer cells[90,91,99,100] in part, by inhibiting the AKT pathway.[101] Another family member, SEMA3F may inhibit vascularization and tumorigenesis by acting on VEGF and ERK1/2 activation,[102,103] and RARβ exerts its tumor-suppressing function by binding retinoic acid, thereby limiting cell growth and differentiation.

LKB1 The serine/threonine kinase LKB1 (also called STK11) is inactivated in approximately 30% of lung cancers and often correlates with KRAS activation,[104] resulting in the promotion of cell growth. It functions as a TSG by regulating cell polarity, differentiation, and metastasis and can regulate cell metabolism.[105] It has also been reported to inhibit the mTOR pathway.[106]

EPIGENETIC REGULATION

Genetic abnormalities are associated with changes in DNA sequence; however, epigenetic events may lead to changes in gene expression without any changes in DNA sequence and therefore, the latter are potentially reversible.[107] Aberrant promoter hypermethylation is an epigenetic change that occurs early in lung tumorigenesis and is found both in genes that normally undergo methylation in response to aging, as well as in genes that normally remain unmethylated regardless of age.[108] Gains of DNA methylation in a normally unmethylated promoter region of a gene results in silencing of gene transcription and is therefore a common method for the inactivation of TSGs. In lung cancer, many genes have been found to be silenced by promoter hypermethylation (summarized in Table 5.1). They include genes involved in tumor suppression, tissue invasion, DNA repair, detoxification of tobacco carcinogens, and differentiation. Recent advances in whole-genome microarray profiling have allowed researchers to globally study DNA methylation patterns in lung cancer, the results of which have led to suggestions that the role of methylation in lung tumorigenesis has been underestimated.[109–112] Restoration of expression of epigenetically silenced genes is a new targeted therapeutic approach. Histone deacetylation is an example of epigenetic change that can inhibit gene expression. Histone deacetylase (HDAC) inhibitors are being studied for the treatment of lung cancer and function by reversing gene silencing through inhibiting histone deacetylation (Fig. 5.1 and Table 5.2).

MICRORNA-MEDIATED REGULATION OF LUNG CANCER

miRNAs are a recently identified class of non–protein encoding small RNAs present in the genomes of plants and animals. Ranging in size from 20 to 25 nucleotides, miRNAs are small RNA molecules that are capable of regulating gene expression by either direct cleavage of a targeted mRNA or inhibiting translation by interacting with the 3' untranslated region (UTR) of a target mRNA. They are considered to play an important role in the pathogenesis of cancer—as either oncogenes or TSGs—because of abnormal expression found in several types of cancer, including lung cancer.[113–121] Additionally, more than 50% of miRNAs are located in cancer-associated genomic regions or fragile sites.[122,123]

As observed for analyses on mRNA, protein and methylation patterns in lung cancer, miRNA microarrays have enabled the identification of many lung cancer-associated miRNAs.[120,121,124–132] One of the most widely studied miRNAs in lung cancer is the lethal-7 (*let-7*) miRNA family. Functioning as a tumor suppressor, it has been shown to regulate NRAS, KRAS, and HMGA2[133,134] via binding to the *let-7* binding sites in their respective 3' UTRs.[133,135] It is frequently underexpressed in lung tumors, particularly NSCLC, compared with normal lung, and decreased expression has also been associated with poor prognosis.[120,125] Induction of *let-7* miRNA expression has been found to inhibit growth in vitro[120,134,136,137] and reduce tumor development in a murine model of lung cancer.[137,138] In addition to *let*-7, other miRNAs with suggested tumor-suppressing effects in lung cancer include *miR-126*, *miR-29a/b/c*, *miR-1*,[125–128] and recently, *miR-128b* was reported to be a direct regulator of EGFR with frequent LOH occurring in NSCLC cell lines.[129] Oncogenic miRNAs found to be overexpressed in lung cancer include the *miR-17-92* cluster of seven miRNAs (with suggested targets that include PTEN and RB), *miR-205*, *miR-21*, and *miR-155*.[121,130]

LUNG CANCER STEM CELLS AND HEDGEHOG, NOTCH, AND WNT SIGNALING

The Hedgehog (HH), Wnt, and Notch signaling pathways are important in normal lung development—specifically, progenitor cell development and pulmonary organogenesis—however, they are now also being studied in regard to their role in tumor development (Fig. 5.2). These signaling pathways are thought to be involved in the regulation on stem/progenitor cell self-renewal and maintenance, and although this process is normally a tightly regulated process, genes that comprise these pathways are often mutated in human cancers,[139–141] leading to abnormal activation of downstream effectors. In relation to cancer treatment, cancer stem cells are of great importance because they are thought to be resistant to cytotoxic therapies. If correct, this presents a need for effective therapies against these self-renewal signaling pathways.

In the HH pathway, increased signaling results in activation of the GLI oncogenes (GLI1, GLI2, and GLI3) that can regulate gene transcription.[142–144] The HH signaling pathway was originally shown to have persistent activation in SCLC with high expression of SHH, PTCH, and GLI1,[145] but an important role in NSCLC was also recently demonstrated.[146] The Notch signaling pathway is important in cell fate determination and can also promote and maintain survival in many human cancers.[147–150] A recent study in mammary stem cells suggests that the cytokine IL-6 may function as a regulator of self-renewal in normal and tumor mammary stem cells through the Notch pathway through upregulation of the Notch-3 receptor,[151] which is expressed in approximately 40% of resected lung cancers.[152] The multifunctional cytokine IL-6 is involved in activation of JAK family of tyrosine kinases,[153] which in turn activate multiple pathways through signaling molecules such as STAT3, MAPK, and PI3K.[154] In lung adenocarcinomas, activated mutant EGFR has also been shown to induce levels of IL-6 leading to activation of STAT3.[155] The Wnt pathway has critical roles in organogenesis, cancer initiation and progression, and maintenance of stem cell pluripotency. In NSCLC, studies have found dysregulation of Wnt pathway members such as Wnt1, Wnt2, and Wnt7a, as well as upregulation of Wnt pathway agonists (Dvl proteins, LEF1, and Ruvb11) and underexpression or silencing of antagonists (WIF-1, sFRP1, CTNNBIP1, and WISP2).[156–162]

HUMAN PAPILLOMAVIRUS–MEDIATED LUNG CANCER

Human papillomavirus (HPV) has been identified in tumors from many organs, not just gynecological tumors. Nearly 30 years ago, it was suggested to be a risk factor for lung cancer, particularly squamous cell carcinoma,[163] and since then, many studies have investigated the role of HPV in lung cancer

TABLE 5.2 Targeted Therapies against Oncogenic Pathways in Lung Cancer and Their Development in Clinical Trials

Gene	Drug	NSCLC[a]	SCLC[a]
EGFR	Cetuximab	II/III	I[b]
EGFR	Panitumumab	II	nct
EGFR	Matuzumab	II	nct
EGFR	Gefitinib	Approved	II
EGFR	Erlotinib	Approved	nct
EGFR, ErbB2	Lapatinib	II	nct
EGFR, ErbB2	HKI-272	II	nct
EGFR, ErbB2	CI-1033	II	nct
ErbB2	Trastuzumab	II	I[b]
VEGF	Bevacizumab	Approved	II
VEGFR	Cediranib	II/III	II
VEGFR, EGFR	Vandetanib	II/III	II
VEGFR, PDGFR, c-KIT	Sunitinib	II/III	II
VEGFR, PDGFR, c-KIT	Vatalanib	II	nct
VEGFR, PDGFR, c-KIT	Axitinib	II	nct
VEGFR, PDGFR, c-KIT	AMG-706	II/III	nct
c-KIT, PDGFR	Imatinib	II	II
RAS	Tipifarnib	II	II
RAS	Lonafarnib	III	nct
RAF, VEGFR, PDGFR, c-KIT	Sorafenib	II/III	II
MEK	CI-1040	II	nct
MEK	PD-325901	II	nct
MEK	AZD6244	II	nct
PI3K	LY294002	nct	nct
mTOR	Sirolimus	I/II	nct
mTOR	Temsirolimus	II	II
mTOR	Everolimus	I/II	I/II
mTOR	AP23573/deforolimus	I[b]	I[b]
BCL2	Oblimersen	II/III	I/II
BCL2	ABT-737	nct	nct
SRC	Dasatinib	II	II
Proteasome	Bortezomib	II	II
Proteasome	NPI-0052	I	nct
p53	p53 peptide vaccine	II	I[b]
FUS1	Fus1 liposome complex	I	nct
HDACs	Vorinostat	II	I/II
HDACs	Romidepsin	II	II
Telomerase	GRN163L	I	I[b]

[a]I, phase I clinical trial; II, phase II clinical trial; III, phase III clinical trial; approved, approved by the FDA; nct, not in a clinical trial at the time of manuscript preparation.

[b]In phase I clinical trial for solid tumors, not specific to NSCLC/SCLC.

and have reported considerable geographical variation. A recent metaanalysis of 53 publications, comprising 4508 cases, found that the mean incidence of HPV in lung cancer was 25% and was detected in all subtypes of lung cancer, not just squamous cell.[164] Studies from Europe and America had a lower incidence of 15% to 17%, whereas Asian lung cancer cases reported a mean incidence of 38%. This observed high penetrance of HPV in lung cancer suggests more research is required to elucidate its role in lung cancer pathogenesis; however, considering the significant variation observed between studies of cases from the same geographical location, subsequent studies will need to have large sample and a detailed study design.

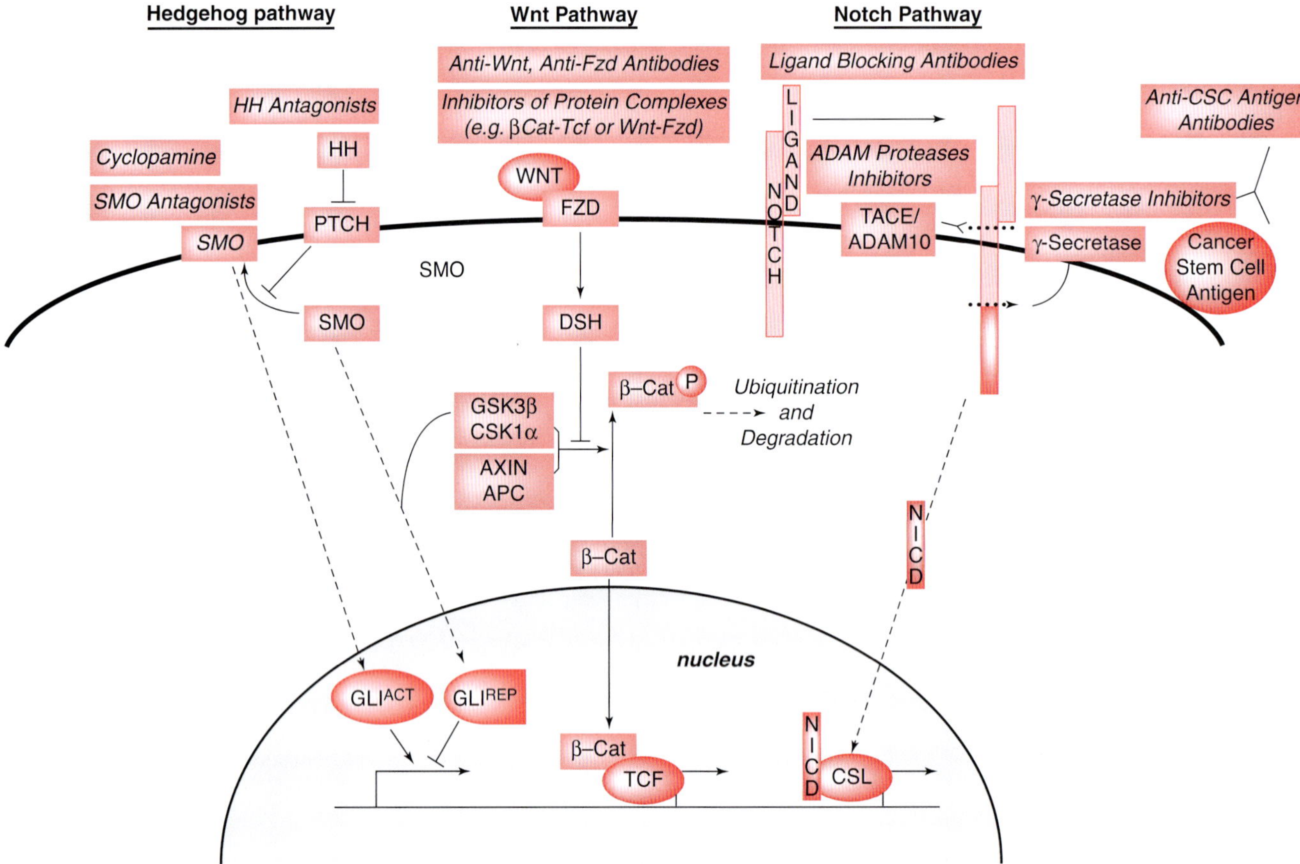

FIGURE 5.2 Stem cell self-renewal pathways and therapeutic strategies to block these pathways in cancer. Notch, Wnt, and Hedgehog (HH) are stem cell self-renewal pathways that are often deregulated and aberrantly activated in lung cancer, thus representing key therapeutic targets. Modulation of these pathways can be achieved at different levels. In general, it is possible to interfere with ligand–receptor interactions by using ligand antagonists or receptor decoys, by blocking ligand-induced conformational changes, or disrupting protein–protein interaction of complexes involved in the activation of nuclear transcription. More specifically, strategies targeting the HH pathway include the use of antagonists for ligands (HH) or receptors (Smoothened, SMO) as well as cyclopamine, a naturally occurring compound that inhibits SMO. Antibodies against Wnt ligands or the receptor FZD and inhibitors of protein complex formation can be used to inhibit the Wnt pathway. Antiligand antibodies are used as potential agents to block the Notch pathway. Cleavage of Notch receptors by ADAM proteases and γ-secretase is required to activate this pathway, and inhibitors of these enzymes are being tested for their possible therapeutic implications. At present, two drugs targeting these pathways are in early clinical trials for treatment of some cancer types: phase I trials are studying the effects of an HH antagonist (GDC-0449) on solid tumors and MK-0752, a γ-secretase inhibitor, is being tested in patients with T-cell acute lymphoblastic leukemia, breast cancer, and central nervous system tumors. Pathways are depicted schematically, and some components were omitted (*dashed lines*) for simplicity. *ADAM*, a disintegrin and metalloprotease domain; *APC*, adenomatous polyposis coli; *AXIN*, axis inhibition protein; *β-Cat*, β-catenin; *CSK1-α*, cyclin-suppressing kinase 1α; *CSL*, C-promoter binding factor 1, suppressor of hairless, and Lag1 protein complex; *DSH*, disheveled; *FZD*, frizzled; *GLI*, glioma-associated oncogene; GLI^{ACT}, active form of GLI; GLI^{REP}, repressor form of GLI; *GSK3-β*, glycogen synthase kinase 3β; *HH*, hedgehog; *NICD*, Notch intracellular domain; *P*, phosphorylation; *PTCH*, patched; *SMO*, smoothened; *TACE*, TNF-α–converting enzyme; *TCF/HNF4A*, transcription factor; *WNT*, wingless-type MMTV integration site family.

CONCLUSION

Genetic and epigenetic mechanisms underlying lung cancer development and progression continue to emerge. Over the past decade, research into the biology of many diseases has been spearheaded by the development of whole-genome microarray technology, allowing the simultaneous analysis of expression, copy number, and SNPs across thousands of genes. In lung cancer, gene expression studies have uncovered novel genes and pathways, as well as identified gene signatures that can better predict patient prognosis, response to treatment, and histology [165–168] reviewed.[169,170] High-resolution mapping of alterations in the lung cancer genome has been able to identify single genes as targets of genomic gain or loss through improved definition of known aberrant regions or by identification of focal alterations undetectable with earlier technology.[15,171–173] Large-scale sequencing and SNP analyses have also led to the identification of novel somatic mutations or SNPs in the lung cancer genome.[7–9,174] Although such genome-wide screens have the capacity of identifying novel genes or interactions in relation to lung cancer, the functional relevance of these findings still need to be elucidated using in vitro model systems such as tumor cell lines or immortalized human bronchial epithelial cells. These systems allow the characterization of single or sequential genetic alterations in relation to the development, maintenance, and progression of lung cancer and represent a crucial contribution in the understanding of the molecular biology of lung cancer. Functional characterization of genetic alterations and the signaling pathways with which they interact has enabled the development of targeted therapies for the treatment of lung cancer (Table 5.2). Ranging from drugs in clinical use to those in clinical trial, they are directed against all known pathways of lung cancer initiation and progression such as proliferation, inhibition of apoptosis, angiogenesis, and invasion. This chapter has outlined some of the significant molecular alterations known to be involved in the initiation and/or progression of lung cancer. By characterizing these aberrations, researchers endeavor to improve the detection, diagnosis, treatment, and prognosis of lung cancer through the integration of clinical and biological factors—to achieve personalized medicine.

ACKNOWLEDGMENT: *This research was supported by the National Cancer Institute Lung Cancer Specialized Program of Research Excellence (SPORE) (P50CA70907), Department of Defense VITAL and PROSPECT, NASA NSCOR (NNJ05HD36G), and by the Office of Science (BER) U.S. Department of Energy, Grant Number DE-AI02-05ER64068. JEL supported by TSANZ/Allen and Hanburys Respiratory Research Fellowship.*

REFERENCES

1. Hanahan D, Weinberg RA. The hallmarks of cancer. *Cell* 2000;100:57–70.
2. Nowell PC. The clonal evolution of tumor cell populations. *Science* 1976;194:23–28.
3. Wistuba II, Gazdar AF. Lung cancer preneoplasia. *Annu Rev Pathol* 2006;1:331–348.
4. Sun S, Schiller JH, Gazdar AF. Lung cancer in never smokers—a different disease. *Nat Rev Cancer* 2007;7:778–790.
5. Risch A, Plass C. Lung cancer epigenetics and genetics. *Int J Cancer* 2008;123:1–7.
6. Herbst RS, Heymach JV, Lippman SM. Lung cancer. *N Engl J Med* 2008;359:1367–1380.
7. Amos CI, Wu X, Broderick P, et al. Genome-wide association scan of tag SNPs identifies a susceptibility locus for lung cancer at 15q25.1. *Nat Genet* 2008;40:616–622.
8. Hung RJ, McKay JD, Gaborieau V, et al. A susceptibility locus for lung cancer maps to nicotinic acetylcholine receptor subunit genes on 15q25. *Nature* 2008;452:633–637.
9. Thorgeirsson TE, Geller F, Sulem P, et al. A variant associated with nicotine dependence, lung cancer and peripheral arterial disease. *Nature* 2008;452:638–642.
10. Sekido Y, Fong KM, Minna JD. Progress in understanding the molecular pathogenesis of human lung cancer. *Biochim Biophys Acta* 1998;1378:F21–F59.
11. Albanell J, Lonardo F, Rusch V, et al. High telomerase activity in primary lung cancers: association with increased cell proliferation rates and advanced pathologic stage. *J Natl Cancer Inst* 1997;89:1609–1615.
12. Hiyama K, Hiyama E, Ishioka S, et al. Telomerase activity in small-cell and non-small-cell lung cancers. *J Natl Cancer Inst* 1995;87:895–902.
13. Frias C, Garcia-Aranda C, De Juan C, et al. Telomere shortening is associated with poor prognosis and telomerase activity correlates with DNA repair impairment in non-small cell lung cancer. *Lung Cancer* 2008;60:416–425.
14. Kwei KA, Kim YH, Girard L, et al. Genomic profiling identifies TITF1 as a lineage-specific oncogene amplified in lung cancer. *Oncogene* 2008; 27(25):3635–3640.
15. Weir BA, Woo MS, Getz G, et al. Characterizing the cancer genome in lung adenocarcinoma. *Nature* 2007;450:893–898.
16. Merlino GT, Xu YH, Ishii S, et al. Amplification and enhanced expression of the epidermal growth factor receptor gene in A431 human carcinoma cells. *Science* 1984;224:417–419.
17. Lynch TJ, Bell DW, Sordella R, et al. Activating mutations in the epidermal growth factor receptor underlying responsiveness of non-small-cell lung cancer to gefitinib. *N Engl J Med* 2004;350:2129–2139.
18. Pao W, Miller V, Zakowski M, et al. EGF receptor gene mutations are common in lung cancers from "never smokers" and are associated with sensitivity of tumors to gefitinib and erlotinib. *Proc Natl Acad Sci U S A* 2004;101:13306–13311.
19. Paez JG, Janne PA, Lee JC, et al. EGFR mutations in lung cancer: correlation with clinical response to gefitinib therapy. *Science* 2004;304:1497–1500.
20. Massion PP, Kuo WL, Stokoe D, et al. Genomic copy number analysis of non-small cell lung cancer using array comparative genomic hybridization: implications of the phosphatidylinositol 3-kinase pathway. *Cancer Res* 2002;62:3636–3640.
21. Friend SH, Bernards R, Rogelj S, et al. A human DNA segment with properties of the gene that predisposes to retinoblastoma and osteosarcoma. *Nature* 1986;323:643–646.
22. Nobori T, Miura K, Wu DJ, et al. Deletions of the cyclin-dependent kinase-4 inhibitor gene in multiple human cancers. *Nature* 1994; 368:753–756.
23. Steck PA, Pershouse MA, Jasser SA, et al. Identification of a candidate tumour suppressor gene, MMAC1, at chromosome 10q23.3 that is mutated in multiple advanced cancers. *Nat Genet* 1997;15:356–362.
24. Fong, KM, Sekido, Y, Minna, JD. Molecular pathogenesis of lung cancer. *J Thorac Cardiovasc Surg* 1999;118:1136–1152.
25. Fong KM, Kida Y, Zimmerman PV, et al. Loss of heterozygosity frequently affects chromosome 17q in non-small cell lung cancer. *Cancer Res* 1995;55:4268–4272.
26. Weinstein IB. Cancer. Addiction to oncogenes—the Achilles heal of cancer. *Science* 2002;297:63–64.
27. Normanno N, Bianco C, Strizzi L, et al. The ErbB receptors and their ligands in cancer: an overview. *Curr Drug Targets* 2005;6:243–257.
28. Arteaga CL. Overview of epidermal growth factor receptor biology and its role as a therapeutic target in human neoplasia. *Semin Oncol* 2002;29:3–9.
29. Rusch V, Baselga J, Cordon-Cardo C, et al. Differential expression of the epidermal growth factor receptor and its ligands in primary non-small cell lung cancers and adjacent benign lung. *Cancer Res* 1993;53:2379–2385.
30. Franklin WA, Veve R, Hirsch FR, et al. Epidermal growth factor receptor family in lung cancer and premalignancy. *Semin Oncol* 2002;29:3–14.
31. Herbst, RS. Review of epidermal growth factor receptor biology. *Int J Radiat Oncol Biol Phys* 2004;59:21–26.
32. Fujino S, Enokibori T, Tezuka N, et al. A comparison of epidermal growth factor receptor levels and other prognostic parameters in non-small cell lung cancer. *Eur J Cancer* 1996;32A:2070–2074.
33. Sordella R, Bell DW, Haber DA, Settleman J. Gefitinib-sensitizing EGFR mutations in lung cancer activate anti-apoptotic pathways. *Science* 2004;305:1163–1167.
34. Pao W, Miller VA, Politi KA, et al. Acquired resistance of lung adenocarcinomas to gefitinib or erlotinib is associated with a second mutation in the EGFR kinase domain. *PLoS Med* 2005;2:E73.

35. Kobayashi S, Boggon TJ, Dayaram T, et al. EGFR mutation and resistance of non-small-cell lung cancer to gefitinib. *N Engl J Med* 2005;352:786–792.
36. Bean J, Brennan C, Shih JY, et al. MET amplification occurs with or without T790M mutations in EGFR mutant lung tumors with acquired resistance to gefitinib or erlotinib. *Proc Natl Acad Sci U S A* 2007;104:20932–20937.
37. Balak MN, Gong Y, Riely GJ, et al. Novel D761Y and common secondary T790M mutations in epidermal growth factor receptor-mutant lung adenocarcinomas with acquired resistance to kinase inhibitors. *Clin Cancer Res* 2006;12:6494–6501.
38. Kosaka T, Yatabe Y, Endoh H, et al. Analysis of epidermal growth factor receptor gene mutation in patients with non-small cell lung cancer and acquired resistance to gefitinib. *Clin Cancer Res* 2006;12:5764–5769.
39. Kwak EL, Sordella R, Bell DW, et al. Irreversible inhibitors of the EGF receptor may circumvent acquired resistance to gefitinib. *Proc Natl Acad Sci U S A* 2005;102:7665–7670.
40. Kosaka T, Yatabe Y, Endoh H, et al. Mutations of the epidermal growth factor receptor gene in lung cancer: biological and clinical implications. *Cancer Res* 2004;64:8919–8923.
41. Engelman JA, Zejnullahu K, Mitsudomi T, et al. MET amplification leads to gefitinib resistance in lung cancer by activating ERBB3 signaling. *Science* 2007;316:1039–1043.
42. Mascaux C, Iannino N, Martin B, et al. The role of RAS oncogene in survival of patients with lung cancer: a systematic review of the literature with meta-analysis. *Br J Cancer* 2005;92:131–139.
43. Shields JM, Pruitt K, McFall A, et al. Understanding Ras: 'it ain't over 'til it's over'. *Trends Cell Biol* 2000;10:147–154.
44. Rodenhuis S, Slebos RJ. Clinical significance of ras oncogene activation in human lung cancer. *Cancer Res* 1992;52:S2665–S2669.
45. Pao W, Wang TY, Riely GJ, et al. KRAS mutations and primary resistance of lung adenocarcinomas to gefitinib or erlotinib. *PLoS Med* 2005;2:E17.
46. Eberhard DA, Johnson BE, Amler LC, et al. Mutations in the epidermal growth factor receptor and in KRAS are predictive and prognostic indicators in patients with non-small-cell lung cancer treated with chemotherapy alone and in combination with erlotinib. *J Clin Oncol* 2005;23:5900–5909.
47. Riely GJ, Kris MG, Rosenbaum D, et al. Frequency and distinctive spectrum of KRAS mutations in never smokers with lung adenocarcinoma. *Clin Cancer Res* 2008;14:5731–5734.
48. Ji H, Wang Z, Perera SA, et al. Mutations in BRAF and KRAS converge on activation of the mitogen-activated protein kinase pathway in lung cancer mouse models. *Cancer Res* 2007;67:4933–4939.
49. Adhikary S, Eilers, M. Transcriptional regulation and transformation by Myc proteins. *Nat Rev Mol Cell Biol* 2005;6:635–645.
50. Nau MM, Brooks BJ Jr, Carney DN, et al. Human small-cell lung cancers show amplification and expression of the N-myc gene. *Proc Natl Acad Sci U S A* 1986;83:1092–1096.
51. Broers JL, Viallet J, Jensen SM, et al. Expression of c-myc in progenitor cells of the bronchopulmonary epithelium and in a large number of non-small cell lung cancers. *Am J Respir Cell Mol Biol* 1993;9:33–43.
52. West KA, Linnoila IR, Belinsky SA, et al. Tobacco carcinogen-induced cellular transformation increases activation of the phosphatidylinositol 3'-kinase/Akt pathway in vitro and in vivo. *Cancer Res* 2004;64:446–451.
53. Vivanco I, Sawyers CL. The phosphatidylinositol 3-Kinase AKT pathway in human cancer. *Nat Rev Cancer* 2002;2:489–501.
54. Kawano O, Sasaki H, Endo K, et al. PIK3CA mutation status in Japanese lung cancer patients. *Lung Cancer* 2006;54:209–215.
55. Garnis C, Lockwood WW, Vucic E, et al. High resolution analysis of non-small cell lung cancer cell lines by whole genome tiling path array CGH. *Int J Cancer* 2006;118:1556–1564.
56. Yamamoto H, Shigematsu H, Nomura M, et al. PIK3CA mutations and copy number gains in human lung cancers. *Cancer Res* 2008; 68:6913–6921.
57. Guertin DA, Sabatini DM. Defining the role of mTOR in cancer. *Cancer Cell* 2007;12:9–22.
58. Maehama T, Dixon JE. The tumor suppressor, PTEN/MMAC1, dephosphorylates the lipid second messenger, phosphatidylinositol 3,4,5-trisphosphate. *J Biol Chem* 1998;273:13375–13378.
59. Soria JC, Lee HY, Lee JI, et al. Lack of PTEN expression in non-small cell lung cancer could be related to promoter methylation. *Clin Cancer Res* 2002;8:1178–1184.
60. Marsit CJ, Zheng S, Aldape K, et al. PTEN expression in non-small-cell lung cancer: evaluating its relation to tumor characteristics, allelic loss, and epigenetic alteration. *Hum Pathol* 2005;36:768–776.
61. Kendall J, Liu Q, Bakleh A, et al. Oncogenic cooperation and coamplification of developmental transcription factor genes in lung cancer. *Proc Natl Acad Sci U S A* 2007;104:16663–16668.
62. Bingle CD. Thyroid transcription factor-1. *Int J Biochem Cell Biol* 1997;29:1471–1473.
63. Ikeda K, Clark JC, Shaw-White JR, et al. Gene structure and expression of human thyroid transcription factor-1 in respiratory epithelial cells. *J Biol Chem* 1995;270:8108–8114.
64. Visakorpi T, Hyytinen E, Koivisto P, et al. In vivo amplification of the androgen receptor gene and progression of human prostate cancer. *Nat Genet* 1995;9:401–406.
65. Garraway LA, Widlund HR, Rubin MA, et al. Integrative genomic analyses identify MITF as a lineage survival oncogene amplified in malignant melanoma. *Nature* 2005;436:117–122.
66. Holst F, Stahl PR, Ruiz C, et al. Estrogen receptor alpha (ESR1) gene amplification is frequent in breast cancer. *Nat Genet* 2007;39:655–660.
67. Garraway LA, Sellers WR. Lineage dependency and lineage-survival oncogenes in human cancer. *Nat Rev Cancer* 2006;6:593–602.
68. Soda M, Choi YL, Enomoto M, et al. Identification of the transforming EML4-ALK fusion gene in non-small-cell lung cancer. *Nature* 2007;448:561–566.
69. Meyerson M. Cancer: broken genes in solid tumours. *Nature* 2007;448:545–546.
70. Inamura K, Takeuchi K, Togashi Y, et al. EML4-ALK fusion is linked to histological characteristics in a subset of lung cancers. *J Thorac Oncol* 2008;3:13–17.
71. Mano H. Non-solid oncogenes in solid tumors: EML4-ALK fusion genes in lung cancer. *Cancer Sci* 2008;99:2349–2355.
72. Koivunen JP, Mermel C, Zejnullahu K, et al. EML4-ALK fusion gene and efficacy of an ALK kinase inhibitor in lung cancer. *Clin Cancer Res* 2008;14:4275–4283.
73. Knudson AG, Jr. The ninth Gordon Hamilton-Fairley memorial lecture. Hereditary cancers: clues to mechanisms of carcinogenesis. *Br J Cancer* 1989;59:661–666.
74. Breuer RH, Postmus PE, Smit EF. Molecular pathology of non-small-cell lung cancer. *Respiration* 2005;72:313–330.
75. Takahashi T, Nau MM, Chiba I, et al. p53: a frequent target for genetic abnormalities in lung cancer. *Science* 1989;246:491–494.
76. Hollstein M, Sidransky D, Vogelstein B, Harris CC. p53 mutations in human cancers. *Science* 1991;253:49–53.
77. Greenblatt MS, Bennett WP, Hollstein M, Harris CC. Mutations in the p53 tumor suppressor gene: clues to cancer etiology and molecular pathogenesis. *Cancer Res* 1994;54:4855–4878.
78. Higashiyama M, Doi O, Kodama K, et al. MDM2 gene amplification and expression in non-small-cell lung cancer: immunohistochemical expression of its protein is a favourable prognostic marker in patients without p53 protein accumulation. *Br J Cancer* 1997;75:1302–1308.
79. Gazzeri S, Della Valle V, Chaussade L, et al. The human p19ARF protein encoded by the beta transcript of the p16INK4a gene is frequently lost in small cell lung cancer. *Cancer Res* 1998;58:3926–3931.
80. Vonlanthen S, Heighway J, Tschan MP, et al. Expression of p16INK4a/p16alpha and p19ARF/p16beta is frequently altered in non-small cell lung cancer and correlates with p53 overexpression. *Oncogene* 1998;17:2779–2785.
81. Ventura A, Kirsch DG, McLaughlin ME, et al. Restoration of p53 function leads to tumour regression in vivo. *Nature* 2007;445:661–665.

82. Ohtani N, Yamakoshi K, Takahashi A, et al. The p16INK4a-RB pathway: molecular link between cellular senescence and tumor suppression. *J Med Invest* 2004;51:146–153.
83. Reissmann PT, Koga H, Takahashi R, et al. Inactivation of the retinoblastoma susceptibility gene in non-small-cell lung cancer. The Lung Cancer Study Group. *Oncogene* 1993;8:1913–1919.
84. Merlo A, Gabrielson E, Askin F, et al. Frequent loss of chromosome 9 in human primary non-small cell lung cancer. *Cancer Res* 1994;54: 640–642.
85. Brambilla E, Moro D, Gazzeri S, et al. Alterations of expression of Rb, p16(INK4A) and cyclin D1 in non-small cell lung carcinoma and their clinical significance. *J Pathol* 1999;188:351–360.
86. Sato M, Takahashi K, Nagayama K, et al. Identification of chromosome arm 9p as the most frequent target of homozygous deletions in lung cancer. *Genes Chromosomes Cancer* 2005;44:405–414.
87. Esteller M. Cancer epigenetics: DNA methylation and chromatin alterations in human cancer. *Adv Exp Med Biol* 2003;532:39–49.
88. Kotake Y, Cao R, Viatour P, et al. pRB family proteins are required for H3K27 trimethylation and Polycomb repression complexes binding to and silencing p16INK4alpha tumor suppressor gene. *Genes Dev* 2007;21:49–54.
89. Wistuba II, Behrens C, Virmani AK, et al. High resolution chromosome 3p allelotyping of human lung cancer and preneoplastic/preinvasive bronchial epithelium reveals multiple, discontinuous sites of 3p allele loss and three regions of frequent breakpoints. *Cancer Res* 2000;60:1949–1960.
90. Ito M, Ito G, Kondo M, et al. Frequent inactivation of RASSF1A, BLU, and SEMA3B on 3p21.3 by promoter hypermethylation and allele loss in non-small cell lung cancer. *Cancer Lett* 2005;225:131–139.
91. Kuroki T, Trapasso F, Yendamuri S, et al. Allelic loss on chromosome 3p21.3 and promoter hypermethylation of semaphorin 3B in non-small cell lung cancer. *Cancer Res* 2003;63:3352–3355.
92. Feng Q, Hawes SE, Stern JE, et al. DNA methylation in tumor and matched normal tissues from non-small cell lung cancer patients. *Cancer Epidemiol Biomarkers Prev* 2008;17:645–654.
93. Wistuba II, Gazdar AF, Minna JD. Molecular genetics of small cell lung carcinoma. *Semin Oncol* 2001;28:3–13.
94. Zochbauer-Muller S, Minna JD, Gazdar AF. Aberrant DNA methylation in lung cancer: biological and clinical implications. *Oncologist* 2002;7:451–457.
95. Siprashvili Z, Sozzi G, Barnes LD, et al. Replacement of Fhit in cancer cells suppresses tumorigenicity. *Proc Natl Acad Sci U S A* 1997; 94:13771–13776.
96. Agathanggelou A, Cooper WN, Latif F. Role of the Ras-association domain family 1 tumor suppressor gene in human cancers. *Cancer Res* 2005;65:3497–508.
97. Ji L, Roth JA. Tumor suppressor FUS1 signaling pathway. *J Thorac Oncol* 2008;3:327–330.
98. Deng WG, Kawashima H, Wu G, et al. Synergistic tumor suppression by coexpression of FUS1 and p53 is associated with down-regulation of murine double minute-2 and activation of the apoptotic protease-activating factor 1-dependent apoptotic pathway in human non-small cell lung cancer cells. *Cancer Res* 2007;67:709–717.
99. Tomizawa Y, Sekido Y, Kondo M, et al. Inhibition of lung cancer cell growth and induction of apoptosis after reexpression of 3p21.3 candidate tumor suppressor gene SEMA3B. *Proc Natl Acad Sci U S A* 2001; 98:13954–13959.
100. Ochi K, Mori T, Toyama Y, et al. Identification of semaphorin3B as a direct target of p53. *Neoplasia* 2002;4:82–87.
101. Castro-Rivera E, Ran S, Brekken RA, et al. Semaphorin 3B inhibits the phosphatidylinositol 3-kinase/Akt pathway through neuropilin-1 in lung and breast cancer cells. *Cancer Res* 2008;68:8295–8303.
102. Brambilla E, Constantin B, Drabkin H, et al. Semaphorin SEMA3F localization in malignant human lung and cell lines: a suggested role in cell adhesion and cell migration. *Am J Pathol* 2000;156:939–950.
103. Kessler O, Shraga-Heled N, Lange T, et al. Semaphorin-3F is an inhibitor of tumor angiogenesis. *Cancer Res* 2004;64:1008–1015.
104. Matsumoto S, Iwakawa R, Takahashi K, et al. Prevalence and specificity of LKB1 genetic alterations in lung cancers. *Oncogene* 2007;26:5911–5918.
105. Alessi DR, Sakamoto K, Bayascas JR. LKB1-dependent signaling pathways. *Annu Rev Biochem* 2006;75:137–163.
106. Shaw RJ, Bardeesy N, Manning BD, et al. The LKB1 tumor suppressor negatively regulates mTOR signaling. *Cancer Cell* 2004;6:91–99.
107. Bird A. DNA methylation patterns and epigenetic memory. *Genes Dev* 2002;16:6–21.
108. Baylin SB, Esteller M, Rountree MR, et al. Aberrant patterns of DNA methylation, chromatin formation and gene expression in cancer. *Hum Mol Genet* 2001;10:687–692.
109. Rauch TA, Zhong X, Wu X, et al. High-resolution mapping of DNA hypermethylation and hypomethylation in lung cancer. *Proc Natl Acad Sci U S A* 2008;105:252–257.
110. Shames DS, Girard L, Gao B, et al. A genome-wide screen for promoter methylation in lung cancer identifies novel methylation markers for multiple malignancies. *PLoS Med* 2006;3:E486.
111. Zhong S, Fields CR, Su N, et al. Pharmacologic inhibition of epigenetic modifications, coupled with gene expression profiling, reveals novel targets of aberrant DNA methylation and histone deacetylation in lung cancer. *Oncogene* 2007;26:2621–2634.
112. Brena RM, Morrison C, Liyanarachchi S, et al. Aberrant DNA methylation of OLIG1, a novel prognostic factor in non-small cell lung cancer. *PLoS Med* 2007;4:E108.
113. Metzler M, Wilda M, Busch K, et al. High expression of precursor microRNA-155/BIC RNA in children with Burkitt lymphoma. *Genes Chromosomes Cancer* 2004;39:167–169.
114. Michael, MZ, O'Connor SM, van Holst Pellekaan NG, et al. Reduced accumulation of specific microRNAs in colorectal neoplasia. *Mol Cancer Res* 2003;1:882–891.
115. Calin GA, Dumitru CD, Shimizu M, et al. Frequent deletions and down-regulation of micro-RNA genes miR15 and miR16 at 13q14 in chronic lymphocytic leukemia. *Proc Natl Acad Sci U S A* 2002; 99:15524–15529.
116. Eis PS, Tam W, Sun L, et al. Accumulation of miR-155 and BIC RNA in human B cell lymphomas. *Proc Natl Acad Sci U S A* 2005; 102:3627–3632.
117. He L, Thomson JM, Hemann MT, et al. A microRNA polycistron as a potential human oncogene. *Nature* 2005;435:828–833.
118. Ota A, Tagawa H, Karnan S, et al. Identification and characterization of a novel gene, C13orf25, as a target for 13q31-q32 amplification in malignant lymphoma. *Cancer Res* 2004;64:3087–3095.
119. Voorhoeve PM, le Sage C, Schrier M, et al. A genetic screen implicates miRNA-372 and miRNA-373 as oncogenes in testicular germ cell tumors. *Cell* 2006;124:1169–1181.
120. Takamizawa J, Konishi H, Yanagisawa K, et al. Reduced expression of the let-7 microRNAs in human lung cancers in association with shortened postoperative survival. *Cancer Res* 2004;64:3753–3756.
121. Hayashita Y, Osada H, Tatematsu Y, et al. A polycistronic microRNA cluster, miR-17-92, is overexpressed in human lung cancers and enhances cell proliferation. *Cancer Res* 2005;65:9628–9632.
122. Calin GA, Sevignani C, Dumitru CD, et al. Human microRNA genes are frequently located at fragile sites and genomic regions involved in cancers. *Proc Natl Acad Sci U S A* 2004;101:2999–3004.
123. Sevignani C, Calin GA, Nnadi SC, et al. MicroRNA genes are frequently located near mouse cancer susceptibility loci. *Proc Natl Acad Sci U S A* 2007;104:8017–8022.
124. Yu SL, Chen HY, Chang GC, et al. MicroRNA signature predicts survival and relapse in lung cancer. *Cancer Cell* 2008;13:48–57.
125. Yanaihara N, Caplen N, Bowman E, et al. Unique microRNA molecular profiles in lung cancer diagnosis and prognosis. *Cancer Cell* 2006; 9:189–198.
126. Fabbri M, Garzon R, Cimmino A, et al. MicroRNA-29 family reverts aberrant methylation in lung cancer by targeting DNA methyltransferases 3A and 3B. *Proc Natl Acad Sci U S A* 2007;104:15805–15810.
127. Crawford M, Brawner E, Batte K, et al. MicroRNA-126 inhibits invasion in non-small cell lung carcinoma cell lines. *Biochem Biophys Res Commun* 2008;373:607–612.

128. Nasser MW, Datta J, Nuovo G, et al. Downregulation of microRNA-1 (miR-1) in lung cancer: suppression of tumorigenic property of lung cancer cells and their sensitization to doxorubicin induced apoptosis bymiR-1. *J Biol Chem* 2008;283(48):33394–33405.
129. Weiss GJ, Bemis LT, Nakajima E, et al. EGFR regulation by microRNA in lung cancer: correlation with clinical response and survival to gefitinib and EGFR expression in cell lines. *Ann Oncol* 2008;19:1053–1059.
130. Markou A, Tsaroucha EG, Kaklamanis L, et al. Prognostic value of mature microRNA-21 and microRNA-205 overexpression in non-small cell lung cancer by quantitative real-time RT-PCR. *Clin Chem* 2008;54(10):1696–1704.
131. Garofalo M, Quintavalle C, Di Leva G, et al. MicroRNA signatures of TRAIL resistance in human non-small cell lung cancer. *Oncogene* 2008;27:3845–3855.
132. Volinia S, Calin GA, Liu CG, et al. A microRNA expression signature of human solid tumors defines cancer gene targets. *Proc Natl Acad Sci U S A* 2006;103:2257–2261.
133. Johnson SM, Grosshans H, Shingara J, et al. RAS is regulated by the let-7 microRNA family. *Cell* 2005;120:635–647.
134. Lee YS, Dutta, A. The tumor suppressor microRNA let-7 represses the HMGA2 oncogene. *Genes Dev* 2007;21:1025–1030.
135. Mayr C, Hemann MT, Bartel DP. Disrupting the pairing between let-7 and Hmga2 enhances oncogenic transformation. *Science* 2007; 315:1576–1579.
136. Johnson CD, Esquela-Kerscher A, Stefani G, et al. The let-7 microRNA represses cell proliferation pathways in human cells. *Cancer Res* 2007;67:7713–7722.
137. Esquela-Kerscher A, Trang P, Wiggins JF, et al. The let-7 microRNA reduces tumor growth in mouse models of lung cancer. *Cell Cycle* 2008;7:759–764.
138. Kumar MS, Erkeland SJ, Pester RE, et al. Suppression of non-small cell lung tumor development by the let-7 microRNA family. *Proc Natl Acad Sci U S A* 2008;105:3903–3908.
139. Daniel VC, Peacock CD, Watkins DN. Developmental signalling pathways in lung cancer. *Respirology* 2006;11:234–240.
140. Olsen CL, Hsu PP, Glienke J, et al. Hedgehog-interacting protein is highly expressed in endothelial cells but down-regulated during angiogenesis and in several human tumors. *BMC Cancer* 2004;4:43.
141. Nickoloff BJ, Osborne BA, Miele L. Notch signaling as a therapeutic target in cancer: a new approach to the development of cell fate modifying agents. *Oncogene* 2003;22:6598–6608.
142. Rubin LL, de Sauvage FJ. Targeting the Hedgehog pathway in cancer. *Nat Rev Drug Discov* 2006;5:1026–1033.
143. Riobo NA, Lu K, Emerson CP Jr. Hedgehog signal transduction: signal integration and cross talk in development and cancer. *Cell Cycle* 2006;5:1612–1615.
144. Lauth M, Toftgard R. Non-canonical activation of GLI transcription factors: implications for targeted anti-cancer therapy. *Cell Cycle* 2007;6:2458–2463.
145. Watkins DN, Berman DM, Burkholder SG, et al. Hedgehog signalling within airway epithelial progenitors and in small-cell lung cancer. *Nature* 2003;422:313–317.
146. Yuan Z, Goetz JA, Singh S, et al. Frequent requirement of hedgehog signaling in non-small cell lung carcinoma. *Oncogene* 2007;26:1046–1055.
147. Dang TP, Eichenberger S, Gonzalez A, et al. Constitutive activation of Notch3 inhibits terminal epithelial differentiation in lungs of transgenic mice. *Oncogene* 2003;22:1988–1997.
148. Politi K, Feirt N, Kitajewski J. Notch in mammary gland development and breast cancer. *Semin Cancer Biol* 2004;14:341–347.
149. Parr C, Watkins G, Jiang WG. The possible correlation of Notch-1 and Notch-2 with clinical outcome and tumour clinicopathological parameters in human breast cancer. *Int J Mol Med* 2004;14:779–786.
150. Hainaud P, Contreres JO, Villemain A, et al. The role of the vascular endothelial growth factor-Delta-like 4 ligand/Notch4-ephrin B2 cascade in tumor vessel remodeling and endothelial cell functions. *Cancer Res* 2006;66:8501–8510.
151. Sansone P, Storci G, Tavolari S, et al. IL-6 triggers malignant features in mammospheres from human ductal breast carcinoma and normal mammary gland. *J Clin Invest* 2007;117:3988–4002.
152. Haruki N, Kawaguchi KS, Eichenberger S, et al. Dominant-negative Notch3 receptor inhibits mitogen-activated protein kinase pathway and the growth of human lung cancers. *Cancer Res* 2005;65:3555–3561.
153. Ishihara K, Hirano T. Molecular basis of the cell specificity of cytokine action. *Biochim Biophys Acta* 2002;1592:281–296.
154. Hong DS, Angelo LS, Kurzrock R. Interleukin-6 and its receptor in cancer: implications for Translational Therapeutics. *Cancer* 2007;110:1911–1928.
155. Gao SP, Mark KG, Leslie K, et al. Mutations in the EGFR kinase domain mediate STAT3 activation via IL-6 production in human lung adenocarcinomas. *J Clin Invest* 2007;117:3846–3856.
156. He B, You L, Uematsu K, et al. A monoclonal antibody against Wnt-1 induces apoptosis in human cancer cells. *Neoplasia* 2004;6:7–14.
157. You L, He B, Xu Z, et al. Inhibition of Wnt-2-mediated signaling induces programmed cell death in non-small-cell lung cancer cells. *Oncogene* 2004;23:6170–6174.
158. Winn RA, Van Scoyk M, Hammond M, et al. Antitumorigenic effect of Wnt 7a and Fzd 9 in non-small cell lung cancer cells is mediated through ERK-5-dependent activation of peroxisome proliferator-activated receptor gamma. *J Biol Chem* 2006;281:26943–26950.
159. Fukui T, Kondo M, Ito G, et al. Transcriptional silencing of secreted frizzled related protein 1 (SFRP 1) by promoter hypermethylation in non-small-cell lung cancer. *Oncogene* 2005;24:6323–6327.
160. Mazieres J, He B, You L, et al. Wnt inhibitory factor-1 is silenced by promoter hypermethylation in human lung cancer. *Cancer Res* 2004; 64:4717–4720.
161. Uematsu K, He B, You L, et al. Activation of the Wnt pathway in non small cell lung cancer: evidence of dishevelled overexpression. *Oncogene* 2003;22:7218–7221.
162. Wissmann C, Wild PJ, Kaiser S, et al. WIF1, a component of the Wnt pathway, is down-regulated in prostate, breast, lung, and bladder cancer. *J Pathol* 2003;201:204–212.
163. Syrjanen KJ. Condylomatous changes in neoplastic bronchial epithelium. Report of a case. *Respiration* 1979;38:299–304.
164. Klein F, Kotb WF, Petersen I. Incidence of human papilloma virus in lung cancer. *Lung Cancer* 2008.
165. Beer DG, Kardia SL, Huang CC, et al. Gene-expression profiles predict survival of patients with lung adenocarcinoma. *Nat Med* 2002; 8:816–824.
166. Bild AH, Yao G, Chang JT, et al. Oncogenic pathway signatures in human cancers as a guide to targeted therapies. *Nature* 2006;439:353–357.
167. Potti A, Dressman HK, Bild A, et al. Genomic signatures to guide the use of chemotherapeutics. *Nat Med* 2006;12:1294–1300.
168. Shedden K, Taylor JM, Enkemann SA, et al. Gene expression-based survival prediction in lung adenocarcinoma: a multi-site, blinded validation study. *Nat Med* 2008;14:822–827.
169. Anguiano A, Nevins JR, Potti A. Toward the individualization of lung cancer therapy. *Cancer* 2008;113:1760–1767.
170. Xie Y, Minna JD. Predicting the future for people with lung cancer. *Nat Med* 2008;14:812–813.
171. Tonon G, Wong KK, Maulik G, et al. High-resolution genomic profiles of human lung cancer. *Proc Natl Acad Sci U S A* 2005; 102:9625–9630.
172. Zhao X, Weir BA, LaFramboise T, et al. Homozygous deletions and chromosome amplifications in human lung carcinomas revealed by single nucleotide polymorphism array analysis. *Cancer Res* 2005; 65:5561–5570.
173. Shibata T, Uryu S, Kokubu A, et al. Genetic classification of lung adenocarcinoma based on array-based comparative genomic hybridization analysis: its association with clinicopathologic features. *Clin Cancer Res* 2005;11:6177–6185.
174. Ding L, Getz G, Wheeler DA, et al. Somatic mutations affect key pathways in lung adenocarcinoma. *Nature* 2008;455:1069–1075.

175. Sekido Y, Obata Y, Ueda R, et al. Preferential expression of c-kit protooncogene transcripts in small cell lung cancer. *Cancer Res* 1991; 51:2416–2419.
176. Boldrini L, Ursino S, Gisfredi S, et al. Expression and mutational status of c-kit in small-cell lung cancer: prognostic relevance. *Clin Cancer Res* 2004;10:4101–4108.
177. Shigematsu H, Gazdar AF. Somatic mutations of epidermal growth factor receptor signaling pathway in lung cancers. *Int J Cancer* 2006; 118:257–262.
178. Yousem SA, Nikiforova M, Nikiforov Y. The histopathology of BRAF-V600E-mutated lung adenocarcinoma. *Am J Surg Pathol* 2008; 32:1317–1321.
179. Hirsch FR, Varella-Garcia M, Bunn PA, Jr, et al. Epidermal growth factor receptor in non-small-cell lung carcinomas: correlation between gene copy number and protein expression and impact on prognosis. *J Clin Oncol* 2003;21:3798–3807.
180. Nakamura H, Saji H, Ogata A, et al. Correlation between encoded protein overexpression and copy number of the HER2 gene with survival in non-small cell lung cancer. *Int J Cancer* 2003;103:61–66.
181. Hirashima N, Takahashi W, Yoshii S, et al. Protein overexpression and gene amplification of c-erb B-2 in pulmonary carcinomas: a comparative immunohistochemical and fluorescence in situ hybridization study. *Mod Pathol* 2001;14:556–562.
182. Tatematsu A, Shimizu J, Murakami Y, et al. Epidermal growth factor receptor mutations in small cell lung cancer. *Clin Cancer Res* 2008; 14:6092–6096.
183. Swanton C, Futreal A, Eisen T. Her2-targeted therapies in non-small cell lung cancer. *Clin Cancer Res* 2006;12:4377s–4383s.
184. Rodenhuis S, van de Wetering ML, Mooi WJ, et al. Mutational activation of the K-ras oncogene. A possible pathogenetic factor in adenocarcinoma of the lung. *N Engl J Med* 1987;317:929–935.
185. De Biasi F, Del Sal G, Hand PH. Evidence of enhancement of the ras oncogene protein product (p21) in a spectrum of human tumors. *Int J Cancer* 1989;43:431–435.
186. Potiron VA, Roche J, Drabkin HA. Semaphorins and their receptors in lung cancer. *Cancer Lett* 2009;273(1):1–14.
187. Samuels Y, Wang Z, Bardelli A, et al. High frequency of mutations of the PIK3CA gene in human cancers. *Science* 2004;304:554.
188. Lee JW, Soung YH, Kim SY, et al. PIK3CA gene is frequently mutated in breast carcinomas and hepatocellular carcinomas. *Oncogene* 2005; 24:1477–1480.
189. Davies H, Hunter C, Smith R, et al. Somatic mutations of the protein kinase gene family in human lung cancer. *Cancer Res* 2005;65:7591–7595.
190. Micke P, Hengstler JG, Ros R, et al. c-erbB-2 expression in small-cell lung cancer is associated with poor prognosis. *Int J Cancer* 2001; 92:474–479.
191. Potti A, Willardson J, Forseen C, et al. Predictive role of HER-2/neu overexpression and clinical features at initial presentation in patients with extensive stage small cell lung carcinoma. *Lung Cancer* 2002;36:257–261.
192. Dworakowska D, Jassem E, Jassem J, et al. MDM2 gene amplification: a new independent factor of adverse prognosis in non-small cell lung cancer (NSCLC). *Lung Cancer* 2004;43:285–295.
193. Cappuzzo F, Jänne PA, Skokan M, et al. MET increased gene copy number and primary resistance to gefitinib therapy in non-small-cell lung cancer patients. *Ann Oncol* 2009;20(2):298–304.
194. Beau-Faller M, Ruppert AM, Voegeli AC, et al. MET gene copy number in non-small cell lung cancer: molecular analysis in a targeted tyrosine kinase inhibitor naive cohort. *J Thorac Oncol* 2008;3:331–339.
195. Richardson GE, Johnson BE. The biology of lung cancer. *Semin Oncol* 1993;20:105–127.
196. Johnson BE, Russell E, Simmons AM, et al. MYC family DNA amplification in 126 tumor cell lines from patients with small cell lung cancer. *J Cell Biochem Suppl* 1996;24:210–217.
197. Ibson JM, Waters JJ, Twentyman PR, et al. Oncogene amplification and chromosomal abnormalities in small cell lung cancer. *J Cell Biochem* 1987;33:267–288.
198. Shiraishi M, Noguchi M, Shimosato Y, et al. Amplification of protooncogenes in surgical specimens of human lung carcinomas. *Cancer Res* 1989;49:6474–6479.
199. Miller CT, Chen G, Gharib TG, et al. Increased C-CRK protooncogene expression is associated with an aggressive phenotype in lung adenocarcinomas. *Oncogene* 2003;22:7950–7957.
200. Pezzella F, Turley H, Kuzu I, et al. bcl-2 protein in non-small-cell lung carcinoma. *N Engl J Med* 1993;329:690–694.
201. Kaiser U, Schilli M, Haag U, et al. Expression of bcl-2—protein in small cell lung cancer. *Lung Cancer* 1996;15:31–40.
202. Reissmann PT, Koga H, Figlin RA, et al. Amplification and overexpression of the cyclin D1 and epidermal growth factor receptor genes in non-small-cell lung cancer. Lung Cancer Study Group. *J Cancer Res Clin Oncol* 1999;125:61–70.
203. Eren B, Sar M, Oz B, et al. MMP-2, TIMP-2 and CD44v6 expression in non-small-cell lung carcinomas. *Ann Acad Med Singapore* 2008; 37:32–39.
204. Junker K, Wiethege T, Muller KM. Pathology of small-cell lung cancer. *J Cancer Res Clin Oncol* 2000;126:361–368.
205. Micke P, Basrai M, Faldum A, et al. Characterization of c-kit expression in small cell lung cancer: prognostic and therapeutic implications. *Clin Cancer Res* 2003;9:188–194.
206. Cook RM, Miller YE, Bunn PA, Jr. Small cell lung cancer: etiology, biology, clinical features, staging, and treatment. *Curr Probl Cancer* 1993;17:69–141.
207. Araki K, Ishii G, Yokose T, et al. Frequent overexpression of the c-kit protein in large cell neuroendocrine carcinoma of the lung. *Lung Cancer* 2003;40:173–180.
208. Rygaard K, Nakamura T, Spang-Thomsen M. Expression of the protooncogenes c-met and c-kit and their ligands, hepatocyte growth factor/scatter factor and stem cell factor, in SCLC cell lines and xenografts. *Br J Cancer* 1993;67:37–46.
209. Plummer H 3rd, Catlett J, Leftwich J, et al. c-myc expression correlates with suppression of c-kit protooncogene expression in small cell lung cancer cell lines. *Cancer Res* 1993;53:4337–4342.
210. Hibi K, Takahashi T, Sekido Y, et al. Coexpression of the stem cell factor and the c-kit genes in small-cell lung cancer. *Oncogene* 1991;6:2291–2296.
211. Weiner DB, Nordberg J, Robinson R, et al. Expression of the neu gene-encoded protein (P185neu) in human non-small cell carcinomas of the lung. *Cancer Res* 1990;50:421–425.
212. Schneider PM, Hung MC, Chiocca SM, et al. Differential expression of the c-erbB-2 gene in human small cell and non-small cell lung cancer. *Cancer Res* 1989;49:4968–4971.
213. Fernandes A, Hamburger AW, Gerwin BI. ErbB-2 kinase is required for constitutive stat 3 activation in malignant human lung epithelial cells. *Int J Cancer* 1999;83:564–570.
214. Rygaard K, Vindelov LL, Spang-Thomsen M. Expression of myc family oncoproteins in small-cell lung-cancer cell lines and xenografts. *Int J Cancer* 1993;54:144–152.
215. Takahashi T, Obata Y, Sekido Y, et al. Expression and amplification of myc gene family in small cell lung cancer and its relation to biological characteristics. *Cancer Res* 1989;49:2683–2688.
216. Spencer CA, Groudine M. Control of c-myc regulation in normal and neoplastic cells. *Adv Cancer Res* 1991;56:1–48.
217. Zhang P, Gao WY, Turner S, et al. Gleevec (STI-571) inhibits lung cancer cell growth (A549) and potentiates the cisplatin effect in vitro. *Mol Cancer* 2003;2:1.
218. Rikova K, Guo A, Zeng Q, et al. Global survey of phosphotyrosine signaling identifies oncogenic kinases in lung cancer. *Cell* 2007; 131:1190–1203.
219. Johnson FM, Krug LM, Tran HT, et al. Phase I studies of imatinib mesylate combined with cisplatin and irinotecan in patients with small cell lung carcinoma. *Cancer* 2006;106:366–374.
220. Rossi G, Cavazza A, Marchioni A, et al. Role of chemotherapy and the receptor tyrosine kinases KIT, PDGFRalpha, PDGFRbeta, and

Met in large-cell neuroendocrine carcinoma of the lung. *J Clin Oncol* 2005;23:8774–8785.
221. Carbone DP, Mitsudomi T, Chiba I, et al. p53 immunostaining positivity is associated with reduced survival and is imperfectly correlated with gene mutations in resected non-small cell lung cancer. A preliminary report of LCSG 871. *Chest* 1994;106:S377–S381.
222. Wistuba II, Berry J, Behrens C, et al. Molecular changes in the bronchial epithelium of patients with small cell lung cancer. *Clin Cancer Res* 2000;6:2604–2610.
223. Chiba I, Takahashi T, Nau MM, et al. Mutations in the p53 gene are frequent in primary, resected non-small cell lung cancer. Lung Cancer Study Group. *Oncogene* 1990;5:1603–1610.
224. Shimizu E, Zhao M, Shinohara A, et al. Differential expressions of cyclin A and the retinoblastoma gene product in histological subtypes of lung cancer cell lines. *J Cancer Res Clin Oncol* 1997;123:533–538.
225. Salgia R, Skarin AT. Molecular abnormalities in lung cancer. *J Clin Oncol* 1998;16:1207–1217.
226. Hensel CH, Hsieh CL, Gazdar AF, et al. Altered structure and expression of the human retinoblastoma susceptibility gene in small cell lung cancer. *Cancer Res* 1990;50:3067–3072.
227. Girard L, Zochbauer-Muller S, Virmani AK, et al. Genome-wide allelotyping of lung cancer identifies new regions of allelic loss, differences between small cell lung cancer and non-small cell lung cancer, and loci clustering. *Cancer Res* 2000;60:4894–4906.
228. Virmani AK, Fong KM, Kodagoda D, et al. Allelotyping demonstrates common and distinct patterns of chromosomal loss in human lung cancer types. *Genes Chromosomes Cancer* 1998;21:308–319.
229. Thiberville L, Payne P, Vielkinds J, et al. Evidence of cumulative gene losses with progression of premalignant epithelial lesions to carcinoma of the bronchus. *Cancer Res* 1995;55:5133–5139.
230. Sunaga N, Miyajima K, Suzuki M, et al. Different roles for caveolin-1 in the development of non-small cell lung cancer versus small cell lung cancer. *Cancer Res* 2004;64:4277–4285.
231. Mori S, Ito G, Usami N, et al. p53 apoptotic pathway molecules are frequently and simultaneously altered in nonsmall cell lung carcinoma. *Cancer* 2004;100:1673–1682.
232. Prudkin L, Behrens C, Liu DD, et al. Loss and reduction of FUS1 protein expression is a frequent phenomenon in the pathogenesis of lung cancer. *Clin Cancer Res* 2008;14:41–47.
233. Safar AM, Spencer H 3rd, Su X, et al. Methylation profiling of archived non-small cell lung cancer: a promising prognostic system. *Clin Cancer Res* 2005;11:4400–4405.
234. Toyooka S, Toyooka KO, Maruyama R, et al. DNA methylation profiles of lung tumors. *Mol Cancer Ther* 2001;1:61–67.
235. Shimamoto T, Ohyashiki JH, Hirano T, et al. Hypermethylation of E-cadherin gene is frequent and independent of p16INK4A methylation in non-small cell lung cancer: potential prognostic implication. *Oncol Rep* 2004;12:389–395.
236. Jarmalaite S, Kannio A, Anttila S, et al. Aberrant p16 promoter methylation in smokers and former smokers with nonsmall cell lung cancer. *Int J Cancer* 2003;106:913–918.
237. Esteller M, Sanchez-Cespedes M, Rosell R, et al. Detection of aberrant promoter hypermethylation of tumor suppressor genes in serum DNA from non-small cell lung cancer patients. *Cancer Res* 1999;59:67–70.
238. Kim DH, Nelson HH, Wiencke JK, et al. p16(INK4a) and histology-specific methylation of CpG islands by exposure to tobacco smoke in non-small cell lung cancer. *Cancer Res* 2001;61:3419–3424.
239. Tang X, Khuri FR, Lee JJ, et al. Hypermethylation of the death-associated protein (DAP) kinase promoter and aggressiveness in stage I non-small-cell lung cancer. *J Natl Cancer Inst* 2000;92:1511–1516.
240. Kim DS, Cha SI, Lee JH, et al. Aberrant DNA methylation profiles of non-small cell lung cancers in a Korean population. *Lung Cancer* 2007; 58:1–6.
241. Suh YA, Lee HY, Virmani A, et al. Loss of retinoic acid receptor beta gene expression is linked to aberrant histone H3 acetylation in lung cancer cell lines. *Cancer Res* 2002;62:3945–3949.
242. Burbee DG, Forgacs E, Zochbauer-Muller S, et al. Epigenetic inactivation of RASSF1A in lung and breast cancers and malignant phenotype suppression. *J Natl Cancer Inst* 2001;93:691–699.
243. Dammann R, Li C, Yoon JH, et al. Epigenetic inactivation of a RAS association domain family protein from the lung tumour suppressor locus 3p21.3. *Nat Genet* 2000;25:315–319.
244. Speicher MR, Gwyn Ballard S, Ward DC. Karyotyping human chromosomes by combinatorial multi-fluor FISH. *Nat Genet* 1996;12:368–375.
245. Balsara BR, Testa JR. Chromosomal imbalances in human lung cancer. *Oncogene* 2002;21:6877–6883.
246. Luk C, Tsao MS, Bayani J, et al. Molecular cytogenetic analysis of non-small cell lung carcinoma by spectral karyotyping and comparative genomic hybridization. *Cancer Genet Cytogenet* 2001;125:87–99.
247. Petersen I, Bujard M, Petersen S, et al. Patterns of chromosomal imbalances in adenocarcinoma and squamous cell carcinoma of the lung. *Cancer Res* 1997;57:2331–2335.
248. Petersen I, Langreck H, Wolf G, et al. Small-cell lung cancer is characterized by a high incidence of deletions on chromosomes 3p, 4q, 5q, 10q, 13q and 17p. *Br J Cancer* 1997;75:79–86.

CHAPTER 6

Marileila Varella Garcia

Genomic Alterations in Lung Cancer

Lung cancer has been the leading cause of cancer-related morbidity and mortality worldwide.[1] These tumors are classified into two major clinicopathological categories, small cell lung carcinoma (SCLC) and non–small cell lung carcinoma (NSCLC). SCLC, accounting for 15% to 20% of lung cancers, displays neuroendocrine features and a propensity for rapid growth and early metastasis. NSCLC, accounting for the balance of approximately 80% of lung tumors, includes adenocarcinoma and squamous cell carcinoma, the two most common histological subtypes. Lung cancers, as other carcinomas, display numerous alterations in gene expression patterns resulting from acquired genetic and epigenetic mechanisms, including DNA methylation or histone modification across large chromosomal regions. Conventional and high-throughput technologies have detected scores of genomic changes occurring in individual specimens. However, few of those are recurrent changes among a large number of tumors, a characteristic that poses a challenge for the precise definition of molecular subtypes.

It is well-known that lung cancers show genetic instability, a persistent state that causes several mutational events leading to gross genetic alterations. This genomic instability is reflected in the heterogeneity of karyotypes and molecular profiles within a given tumor type and among different foci of the same tumor. Genomic changes in cancer may occur at different levels, ranging from the single nucleotide to an entire chromosome. Changes at one or few nucleotides, the mutations, may be completely innocuous or may be responsible for dramatic functional changes depending on the specific mutated site. Changes at the chromosomal level are usually detrimental since most likely affect large number of genes. Characterization of the genomic changes and identification of which molecular events contribute to the mechanisms that are central to tumorigenesis and to the multistep tumor progression are critical needs. Ultimately, the genomic discoveries will be translated into clinical tools that may impact the practice of cancer medicine.

In this chapter, we will review the most important genomic alterations detected in lung cancers. We will also discuss recent findings that have contributed to the better understanding of the molecular features of these tumors and to the development of strategies for earlier diagnosis and more efficient therapies.

CHROMOSOMAL STRUCTURAL ALTERATIONS AND GENOMIC IMBALANCES: METHODOLOGICAL STRATEGIES FOR DETECTION

Chromosomal alterations in cancer have been detected by classical cytogenetics methods, mainly banding karyotyping (G-, R-, or Q-banding). Solid tumors frequently exhibit numerous changes in chromosome numbers, including gain of whole-genome complement and gains and losses of specific chromosomes. Tumors also have structural intrachromosomal and interchromosomal rearrangements, which change the copy numbers of genes when deletions, duplications, or amplifications occur, and affect the transcription of genes when positioning changes are introduced by insertions, inversions, and translocations. Although conventional cytogenetic methods were fundamental for important discoveries on molecular mechanisms of hematological diseases, they failed to provide similar contribution on solid tumors. Typically, rearrangements in solid tumors are numerous and complex, and the resolution of 5 to 10 megabase (Mb) of the banding karyotype is not satisfactory for identifying the spectrum of genomic changes responsible for most of the specific biological characteristics of the cancer cell.

The development of molecular cytogenetic strategies such as multiplex fluorescence in situ hybridization (M-FISH)[2] and spectral karyotyping (SKY)[3] have facilitated the identification of extranumerary chromosomes and increased the accuracy of identification of chromosomal origins of complexly rearranged chromosomal (Fig. 6.1). M-FISH and SKY, which paint genomic material from each of the 24 human chromosomes in specific fluorescent colors, are technologies especially tailored

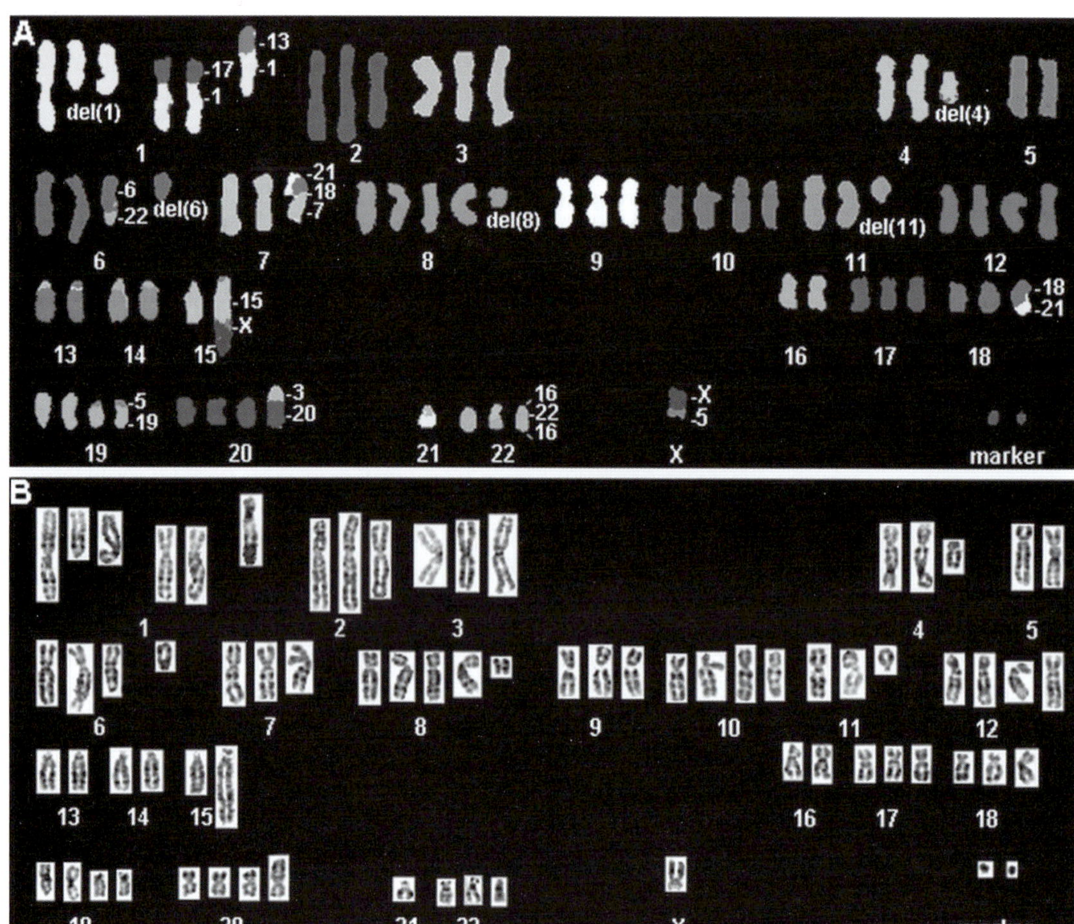

FIGURE 6.1 SKY of a primary lung adenocarcinoma showing numerous numerical and structural chromosome changes. The classified image with the pseudocolors is shown in **(A)** and the inverted-DAPI image is shown in **(B)**. The specimen was near triploid, with extra copies of chromosomes 1, 10, 12, 19, and 20 and deletions of segments of chromosomes 1, 4, 5, 6, and 11. Translocations were found involving chromosomes 1 and 13, 1 and 17, 3 and 20, 5 and 19, 5 and X, 6 and 22, 7, 15, and X, 18 and 21, 16 and 22, and 18 and 21. Two very small marker chromosomes were found carrying chromosome 2 sequences. (See color plate.)

to uncover interchromosomal rearrangements and have been successful in revealing subtle karyotypic alterations, which would be otherwise overlooked.

For detection of genomic imbalances, the cornerstone technology was the comparative genomic hybridization (CGH), which was introduced in the early 1990s.[4] As proposed initially, CGH involved hybridization of differentially labeled DNA from two genomes, the genome to be tested and a normal genome used as a reference against a normal metaphase template. This approach is called metaphase CGH (mCGH) or chromosomal-based CGH (cCGH). Measuring the fluorescent intensity that dominates each given chromosome region in the template allows the identification of regions in the tested genome carrying normal copy numbers or gains and losses relative to the normal reference. Although mCGH proved to be useful for detection of genomic imbalances in solid tumors, the analysis is performed in metaphases and the high level of chromatin condensation at that cell cycle stage also limit the resolution of genomic changes to 5 to 10 Mb. Importantly, several studies have shown that the expression of genes located in chromosomal regions of gains or losses varies consistently with the DNA copy number.[5–10] The availability of genomic resources and technological advances has fostered a major improvement in the last decade, represented by the shift from cCGH to microarray-based platforms. In their first generation, called matrix-CGH and array CGH,[11,12] these arrays included only few hundreds of DNA clones. Soon after, two microarray platforms were launched using bacterial artificial chromosome (BAC) clones as DNA probes. These instruments, the tiling BAC array[13] and the 1-Mb resolution whole-genome BAC array[14] were able to mine the entire genome for copy number variants. Despite the fact that the BAC arrays cannot reliably detect aberrations smaller than the BAC insert (100 to 200 kilobase [kb]), these new tools granted a significantly higher detection rate for copy number abnormalities than any of the metaphase-based cytogenetic techniques.

More recently, oligonucleotide-based arrays have emerged as the platform of choice for genome-wide analysis of copy number alterations because of their high-throughput and high-resolution characteristics. Some of the commercially available oligonucleotide arrays have probes specifically developed for detection of copy number variation (NimbleGen Systems and Agilent Technologies), whereas others were developed as genotyping arrays designed to identify single-nucleotide polymorphisms (SNPs) and later modified to uncover copy number variations (Affymetrix and Illumina). The NimbleGen CGH microarrays contain 45- to 85-mer oligonucleotide probes that are directly synthesized on a silica surface using light-directed photochemistry. A whole-genome tiling array is available with 2.1 million probes (HG18 WG Tiling 2.1M CGH v2.0D) and custom tiling arrays are also available. The Agilent Human Genome CGH Microarray (G2519A) contains 60-mer oligonucleotide probes printed onto glass slides through an industrial inkjet printing process. This microarray includes 40,000 probes spanning the human genome with an average spatial resolution of 75 kb, including coding and noncoding sequences, and has an emphasis on the most common cancer-related genes. Agilent arrays may also be customized from more than 8 million predesigned and validated probes. With the NimbleGen Systems and Agilent Technologies platforms, the test and reference genomes are labeled with different fluorophores (usually Cy3 and Cy5), and cohybridized to the same array, similarly to the mCGH technology. The signal intensity ratio of the test sample versus the reference sample is calculated for each probe across the entire genome.

The Affymetrix GeneChip arrays contain 25-mer SNP-based oligonucleotide markers or probes directly synthesized on the array surface. The Genome-Wide Human SNP Array 6.0 features 1.8 million genetic markers designed to uniformly cover the entire genome, including approximately half in SNPs and half in non-SNP probes for the detection of copy number variation. For the evaluation of copy number changes, the test genome is labeled and hybridized to the array and the signal intensity from the probes is computationally compared with a control set (HapMap individuals). The Illumina BeadChip arrays are made from silica beads that are self-assembled on silica slide microwells and each bead is covered with specific 50-mer SNP-based, oligonucleotide probes. The HumanCNV370-quad DNA Analysis Beadchip platform covers approximately 380,000 SNP and non–SNP-based probes. The test specimen is hybridized with the array and the copy number variations are determined by computationally comparing the signal intensity from probes with a control set provided by the platform manufacturer.

These high-resolution platforms have been successfully used to identify copy number changes in lung cancer and other solid tumors. However, two major characteristics of the solid tumors, the largely abnormal number of chromosomes and the intratumor heterogeneity, make copy number analyses difficult in these platforms. Current array CGH platforms were designed under the assumption that the natural ploidy state of the test DNA specimen is diploid, which is rarely the case in solid tumors. Therefore, the detection of a single-copy gain may represent a gain if the specimen is diploid or actually represent a loss if the specimen is tetraploid, a condition that is most common in solid tumors. Additionally, tumors are often mixtures of distinct types of cells, each of them potentially carrying different copy number changes. Because the DNA from the test specimen is extracted from the cell mixture, the results reflect an average change across the different cell types. Changes occurring in cell-specific compartments are likely to be diluted and remain undetected.

For the genome-wide high-resolution arrays, another perceived limitation is the detection of copy number variations that may not be involved in the disease. Recent studies have shown that normal, healthy individuals carry a large number of copy number variations detected by more than one consecutive probe in BAC and oligonucleotide arrays.[15,16] Thus, a more detailed characterization of the variation in the normal genome is necessary before an accurate detection of pathogenic copy number aberrations can be reached in tumors.

Chromosomal abnormalities detected by conventional and molecular technologies and genomic imbalances detected by mCGH or array platforms have been validated by independent laboratory approaches, such as fluorescence in situ hybridization (FISH) or polymerase chain reaction (PCR)–based techniques. FISH is a high-resolution technique able to identify specific regions involved in rearrangements and define them accurately (Fig. 6.2). FISH, as opposed to the PCR-based techniques, has among its critical advantages the ability to investigate the target phenomenon in single cells and to preserve the original tissue architecture. However, FISH is not a high-throughput technology and is unable to answer genome-wide questions. Nevertheless, the development of FISH methods has significantly improved the accuracy of solid tumor cytogenetics. Ultimately, it is the combination of multiple technical approaches that provides the most powerful strategy for understanding the molecular pathways underlying the lung tumor development.

CHROMOSOMAL ABNORMALITIES AND GENOMIC IMBALANCES IN LUNG CANCER: THE PUZZLING PICTURE

Alterations in the DNA content have been well documented in lung carcinomas by flow cytometry and static tissue morphometry. A metaanalysis including data from 4033 NSCLC patients from 35 published studies has shown that the majority of NSCLC were aneuploidy and patients with aneuploid tumors had a significantly shorter survival duration than those with normal DNA content reflecting both diploid and pseudodiploid chromosome NSCLC.[17] However, the aneuploid chromosomal complement in the tumor cells included great variety of structural and numerical changes, many of which could be random events.

The search for recurrent abnormalities in lung cancer, the ones most likely to play specific roles in cancer development,

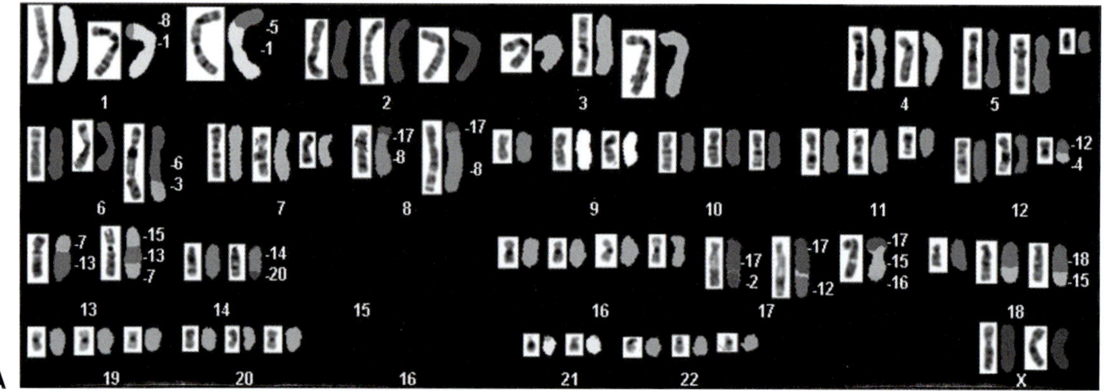

A

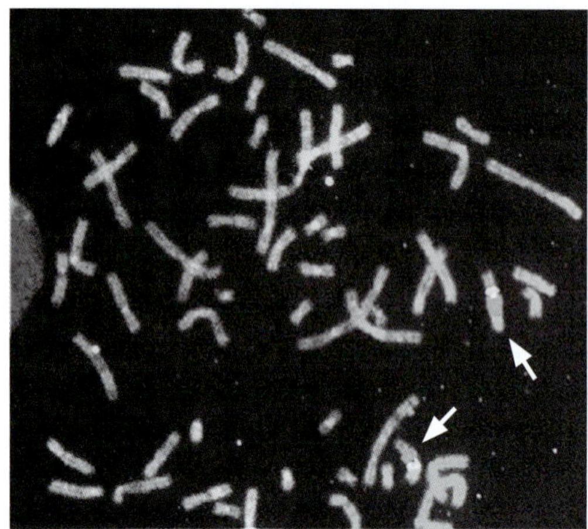

B

FIGURE 6.2 **A:** SKY of the non–small cell lung cancer cell line Calu 3 showing multiple abnormalities and two copies of abnormal chromosome 17, derivatives from the translocations between chromosomes 17 and 2 and chromosomes 17 and 12. In addition, the chromosome 17 material identified by SKY in the long arm (q-arm) of these derivative chromosomes was larger than expected if that arm was normal. **B:** FISH analyses with a probe set including ERBB2 and CEP 17 sequences demonstrated that there was ERBB2 gene amplification in both derivatives (indicated by the *arrows*). In the FISH assays, ERBB2 probe is highlighted by *red color* and CEP 17 by *green color*. (See color plate.)

has started long ago. The first recurrent changes in lung cancer, the deletions of 3p in SCLC, were identified by classical karyotypic analysis.[18] However, probably because of the complexity of the chromosomal alterations and the limitations of the conventional techniques, few karyotype reports of primary lung tumors or cell lines were published in the 2 decades following that seminal publication.[19–26] Loss of large chromosomal segments in 3p and 8p, gain of whole chromosomal arms, such as 5p, and amplification by homogeneously staining regions (HSR) and double minutes (DM) were reported. However, the conclusions of all those studies were by and large limited, often yielding incomplete karyotypes.

The advent of the CGH technology brought new momentum to the cancer field and has also impacted discoveries. Novel and histological type-specific gains and losses of chromosome segments in lung cancers were revealed in addition to those previously reported by conventional cytogenetic approaches. Chromosomal gains were detected in the long arms of chromosomes 8, 17, and 19 in NSCLC and chromosome arms 3q, 8p, and Xq in SCLC. Chromosome losses were frequent in 1p, 4q, 5q, 6q, 8p, 9p, 13q, and 17p in NSCLC and in 5q, 13q, and 17p in SCLC.[21,22,27–31]

In the end of the 1990s, studies using M-FISH and SKY were performed in lung carcinoma cell lines that had been established previously at the National Cancer Institute laboratories or were newly established by other investigators, and from resected tumors. Those studies have resulted in the identification of a greater degree of chromosomal rearrangements than it been detected by previous G-banding and mCGH analyses.[32–43] Chromosomal abnormalities were also detected in nonmalignant bronchial epithelium of heavy smokers.[44] M-FISH and SKY technologies enabled the disclosure of cryptic translocations, enhanced the ability to delineate chromosomal breakpoints when integrating information from conventional banding analysis, and clarified the chromosomal composition of unrecognized marker chromosomes. Important similarities were noticed between karyotypic changes in established cell lines and primary tumors. The vast majority of translocations were unbalanced but a significant number of balanced translocations were also detected. These studies have provided a basis for the search of genes mapped at the breakpoints that were potentially deregulated and associated with tumorigenesis.

Despite all these efforts, discovery of recurrent gene fusions generated by structural rearrangements based on cytogenetics approaches has been quite rare. One such example was the identification of a translocation between the chromosomes 15 and 19 [t(15;19)(q11;p13)] in an aggressive lung cancer metastatic to mediastinum and bone arising in a young woman without a history of smoking or a family history of cancer.[45] The breakpoint on chromosome 19 was mapped to the 5' region of the highly overexpressed *NOTCH3* gene, which led to further investigations of the role of this gene in lung cancer.

Notch3 expression was detected in approximately 40% of resected lung tumors and positively correlated with epidermal growth factor receptor (EGFR) expression. Notch inhibition was shown to increase sensitivity to EGFR tyrosine kinase inhibitors (TKIs) and decrease mitogen-activated protein kinase (*MAPK*) phosphorylation, observations that support a role for NOTCH3 signaling in lung cancer through EGFR-related pathways.[46] The translocation breakpoints were later refined to 15q13.2 and 19p13.1 and the cloning of these regions identified a novel fusion transcript in which the 3' end of the *BRD4* gene on chromosome 19p was fused to the 5' end of the *NUT* gene on chromosome 15q. The *BRD4–NUT* fusion was demonstrated to alter the cell cycle kinetics, augmenting the inhibition of the progression G1 to S phase compared with the wild type *BRD4* gene. However, the exact role of the *BRD4–NUT* fusion in the pathogenesis of lung cancers remains unclear and the t(15;19) has not been found in large lung cancer cohorts tested, which suggest that it is not common in lung cancer.[47] Gene fusions detected using other strategies are going to be discussed later. The detection of the intracellular targets of these fusions is expected to bring new insights into molecular pathways that trigger tumor development.

A much more detailed picture of genomic copy number variations has been achieved in the last years with the array analyses. A summary of detected focal gain and losses is presented in Table 6.1 for five studies focusing on SCLC specimens[19,48–51] and in Table 6.2 for 13 studies focusing on NSCLC specimens.[19,51–62] Although data are available for over 70 SCLC and close to 800 NSCLC specimens, including cell lines and primary tumors, it is difficult to compare those results. Different platforms had different probes, and it is not always possible to confirm equivalencies. Despite these limitations, it is evident that there are important recurrent genomic changes in lung cancer. The most frequently occurring high-amplitude focal amplicons in lung cancer determined by at least two studies are listed in Table 6.3. Among those, are members of the MYC family (*MYCL1*, *MYCN*, and *MYC*), participants in the EGFR pathways (*EGFR*, *PIK3CA*, *KRAS*), and other genes, such as *FGFR1*, *TP63*, *TERT*, and the cyclins *CCND1* and *CCNE1*. Some are potentially novel oncogenes in lung (*NKX2-1*, for instance) that cooperate to promote lung cancer cell proliferation.

The consolidation of the available data contributes to a growing body of evidence that multiple cooperating oncogenes participate in these amplification events in an apparently nonrandom frequency. These findings have important implications for the design of functional genomic studies projects aimed at identifying cancer-relevant genes because single-gene assays will not uncover activities that rely on interaction among multiple collaborating genes.

ABNORMALITIES IN GROWTH-INHIBITORY PATHWAYS: THE TUMOR SUPPRESSOR GENES

The chromosomal, genomic, and epigenomic studies addressed previously have revealed multiple changes involving tumor suppressor genes and oncogenes in clinically evident lung cancers.

TABLE 6.1 Genomic Regions Showing Gains and Losses in Small Cell Lung Carcinoma Primary Tumors and Cell Lines Detected by Comparative Genomic Hybridization

Reference		Technique	Specimen	Genomic Gain	Genomic Loss
Balsara and Testa[19]	*Oncogen*	mCGH		3q26–29, 5p12–13, 8q23–24	3p13–14, 4p32–35, 5q32–35, 8p21–22, 10q25, 13q13–14, 17p12–13
Peng et al.[50]	*Cancer Sci*	Array CGH	10 primary tumors	1q,2q31–33, 3q21–29, 5p12–14, 7q21–33, 8q21–24, 12q13–23, 18q11–2	1p35–36, 3p14–26, 4q21–31, 5q21–35, 10q, 13q33–34, 16q21–24, 17p11–13, 22q11–13
Zhao et al.[51]	*Cancer Res*	SNP array	19 primary tumors, 5 cell lines	1p34.2, 2q24.3–p24.2, 8q24.13–q24.21, 19q12	3q25.1, 9p23, 10q23.31
Coe et al.[48]	*Genes Chromosomes Cancer*	32K BAC array CGH	14 cell lines	1p34–36, 2p16–25, 3q21–29, 5p, 6p21, 7p22, 7q11.23, 8q24, 9q34, 11q13–14, 12p13, 12q22–24, 13q32–34, 14q, 16p, 17q, 19p, 19q, 20q, 21q22	3p, 4q, 5q, 8p, 10p, 10q, 13q, 17p,
Kim et al.[49]	*Oncogen*	BAC array CGH	24 cell lines	1p36.33, 1p34.2, 2p24.3, 2q22.3, 6p22.3, 8q12.3, 8q22, 8q24.21, 9p24.1, 11q14.2, 11q23.1, 12p13.31, 12p12.1, 12p11.22, 12p11.21, 12q24.33, 13q14.3, 14q11.2, 14q11.2, 14q22.3, 20q11.21, Xq22.2	2q24.3, 3p21.31, 4q21.23, 5q14.3, 5q23.2, 10q22.2, 16q23.1, 16p13.3, 16q23.1

TABLE 6.2 Genomic Regions Showing Gains and Losses in Non–Small Cell Lung Carcinoma Primary Tumors and Cell Lines Detected by Comparative Genomic Hybridization

Reference		Technique	Specimen	Feature	Genomic Gain	Genomic Loss
Balsara and Testa[19]	*Oncogene*	mCGH			1q31, 3q25–27, 5p13–14, 8q23–24	3p21, 8p22, 9p21–22, 13q22, 17q12–13
Jiang et al.[56]	*Neoplasia*	mCGH and cDNA arrays	6 SqCC, 14 ADC	Amplif, deletion common to both hystologies	1p36.3, 1q21, 1q21.3, 1q32, 2p12, 3q25.1, 5p15.2, 5p15.1, 5q35.3, 6p21.31, 7p22.3, 7q22.1, 8q22.1, 8q23.1, 11q13.3, 16p13.3, 17q23, 20q13.3, 22q11.23, Xp11.23, Xq13.1, Xq28	1p36, 1p35, 1p33, 1p32, 2p12, 2p12, 3p22, 3p21.3, 3p21.1, 4p15.2, 4p15.2, 4q22.1, 4q21, 5q23, 5q34, 6q23, 6p21.3, 8p22, 8p21, 9p21, 9q34.1, 10q21, 10q22.2, 10q23.2, 10q23.3, 12q24.3, 13q34, 15q21, 17q21, 18p11.3, 18p11.2, 18q21, Xq21.3, Xq26.1
Kim et al.[57]	*Clin Cancer Res*	1Mb BAC array Sanger	29 scc, 21 adc	Minimal recurrent	1p36.31–p34.1, 1p32.3, 1q21.1–q23.3, 2p16.1–p12, 3q26.1–q28, 5p15.2–p15.1, 6p21.31–p21.1, 8p12, 8q11.21–q12.1, 8q24.11–q24.3, 19p13.2–p13.11, 19q13.12, 20q13.33	5p21.2–q31.1, 13q21.1, 13q34, 20q13.2
Tonon et al.[59]	*Proc Natl Acad Sci USA*	aCGH			1p36.32, 1p34.3, 1q32.2, 2q11.2, 2q31.2, 5p15.33, 5q31.3, 8p12–8p11.22, 10q24.1, 10q26.3, 12q13.2, 14q32.13, 16q22.2, 18q12.1, 19q13.33, 20q11.21	7q34, 11q11, 13q12–11, 13q32.2, 21p11.2–21p11.1
Zhao et al.[51]	*Cancer Res*	CentXba and CentHind SNP Affy	51 primary tumors, 26 cell lines	Recurrent regions	3q26.31–q27.1, 7p12.1–q11.22, 8p12–p11.22, 8q24.13–q24.21, 12p11.21, 12q13.3–q14.1, 19q12, 22q11.21–q11.22	2q22.1, 3p14.2, 3q25.1, 9p23, p921.3
Choi et al.[52]	*Lung*	1.4K BAC aCGH Macrogen, Korea	15 ADC	Most frequent regions	1p36.33, 2q35, 5q35.3, 7p15.2, 7q35, 8q24.3, 11p15.4, 116p13.3, 17q25.3. 19q13.42, 20113.33, 21q22.3, 22q13.33	1q31.2, 2p16.3–p16.2, 4q35.1, 5q13.1, 7p12.3, 9p11.2, 11p15.1, 11q12.2, 13q33.1, 14q32.33, 19p13.2
Garnis et al.[55]	*Int J Cancer*	32,433 BAC aCGH Lam	28 cell lines	>75% for gain, >50% for loss	5p15.33, 7p22.3–7p22.1, 7p15.3–7p11.2, 7q11, 7q11.23, 8q24,21, 11q13.3, 17q25.3, 20q11.21–11.23, 20q13.33	1q21.1, 3p24.2–24.2, 3p24.1, 3p14.2–14.1, 4q13.5–q31.23, 4q33–q35.2, 6p15–q23.1, 6q24.1–q27, 8p23.3–p11.22, 9p23, 9p22.1–p21.1, 9p13–p11.2, 9p13–q21.33, 10p, 10q23.1–q26.3, 13q, 15q13.1–q15.2, 15q22.2, 18q11.2–23, 19p13.11–p12, 21q11.2–q21.3, 22q13.1
Ma et al.[58]	*J Pathol*	mCGH after DOP PCR amplification	23 tu	Most frequent regions	3q22–29, 12q23–qter, 16q23–24, 17q12–22, 17q23–25, 19q13, 20q12–13, 21q22, 22q	3p22–24, 4q32–qter, 5q21–23
Yakut et al.[61]	*Lung Cancer*	mCGH	21 SqCC, 24 nSQCC	Focal amplifications	3q21–29, 5p, 7p11, 7q21–31, 8q24, 12p, 12q13–15, 18p	

TABLE 6.2 Genomic Regions Showing Gains and Losses in Non–Small Cell Lung Carcinoma Primary Tumors and Cell Lines Detected by Comparative Genomic Hybridization *(continued)*

Reference		Technique	Specimen	Feature	Genomic Gain	Genomic Loss
Choi et al.[53]	*Lung Cancer*	MACArray Karyo 1.4K BAC Macrogen, Korea	14 SqCC	Most frequent regions	1p36.33, 2p22.1, 2q33.2, 3q28, 5p12, 6q21, 7p14.2, 7q33–35, 13q34–qter, 21q22.3, 22q11.2	1p13.3, 5q34, 8p23.3, 10q26.12, 13q14.2, 14q23.33, 15q14, 17q11.2, 19q13.11
Dehan et al.[54]	*Lung Cancer*	mCGH and 11K cDNA Agilent	23 NSCLC	Common aberrations	1q22–32.1, 2p21.2–p14, 2q11.2–q32.2, 3p14.3–q26.33, 4p16.1–q34.3, 5p15.33–13.3, 7q22.3–q31.32, 8q11.21–q24.3, 11q14.1–q22.3, 12p13.2–p11.22	1p36.33–32.3, 3p25.3, 5q23.3–q35.3, 6p22.1–p21.1, 9q33.3–q34.3, 10q22.1–26.3, 11p11.2, 11q12.2–13.4, 12q24.11–24.33, 12q13.12–14.1, 15q24.1–24.2, 16p13.3–22.2, 17p13.3–25.3, 19p13.3–13.43, 22q11.1–13.33
Kendall et al.[62]	*Proc Natl Acad Sci USA*	85K oligoarray Nimblegen Systems	77 lines, 184 lung tumors	Focal amplifications	1p34.2, 1q21.2, 2p24.3, 5p15.33, 7p11.2, 8p12, 8p11.21, 8q24.21, 11q13.3, 12p12.1, 12q15, 14q13.2	
Weir et al.[60]	*Nature*	500K SNP HMA Aff	371 ADC	Focal amplification	1q21.2, 2p15, 3q26.2, 5p15.33, 5p15.31, 5p14.3, 6p21.33, 6p21.1, 7p11.2, 7q21.2, 8p11.23, 8q21.13, 8q24.21, 11q13.3, 12p12.1, 12q14.1, 12q15, 14q13.3, 17q12, 18q11.2, 19q12, 19q13.12, 20q13.32, 22q11.21	5q11.2, 7q11.22, 9p23, 9p21.3, 10q23.31, 13q14.2, 18q23

The tumor suppressor genes, also known as recessive oncogenes, are inactivated by genetic mechanisms such as point mutations, chromosomal rearrangements, and mitotic recombinations, and by epigenetic events like hypomethylation or hypermethylation of gene promoter regions. It is largely accepted that the inactivation of tumor suppressor genes commonly occurs through a combination of two or more events, the Knudson hypothesis. Still, it is also recognized that the phenomenon in carcinomas is more complex because of mutational instability and chromosomal instability.[63] The major tumor suppressor genes involved in lung cancer are *TP53* (17p13.1), *RB1* (13q14.11), *CDKN2* (*p16*^{INK4a} or *MST1*, 9p21), and several genes located at the short arm of chromosome 3. The incidence of abnormalities in each of these genes in lung cancer, their main role in the development of the disease, and their contribution as prognostic or predictive markers will be briefly summarized.

The *TP53* gene is well-known for playing a key role on the negative regulation of G1/S-phase transition of the cell cycle[64] and for being the gatekeeper for apoptosis.[65] Mutations and overexpression of *TP53* are present almost universally in SCLC and in approximately 50% of NSCLC.[66–69] Mutations in *TP53* have been associated with smoking[70] and more aggressive tumors[66,71]; nevertheless, some studies have failed to show a prognostic role for this abnormality.[72] Physical and functional loss of *TP53* and p53 protein overexpression have been identified in dysplastic bronchial epithelium as a highly predictive marker for lung cancer.[65,73–76] *TP53* is regulated upstream by the oncogene *MDM2* (12q13–q14), which is overexpressed in 25% of NSCLCs.[77] The p53 protein also interacts with *BCL2*, which is a negative regulator of cell death prolonging survival of noncycling cells and inhibiting apoptosis.[78] Positive immunostaining for *BCL2* was found in approximately 20% of NSCLC patients and 80% of SCLC.[78–80]

The G1/S transition checkpoint is also deregulated in lung cancer cells by changes in *RB1*, *CDKN2*, *CCND*, and *CDK4*. The retinoblastoma gene (*RB1*) controls the G1/S transition through E2.[81,82] Loss of *RB1* function by deletion and nonsense mutation or splicing abnormalities, together with loss of the wild-type *RB1* allele, are very common phenomena in SCLC while occurs in less than 30% of NSCL.[82–86] In NSCLC, a strong correlation between altered *RB1* protein expression and early stage has been documented.[87] However, correlation between loss of *RB1* and clinical outcome is still controversial, with earlier findings of negative prognostic impact on survival in early stage NSCLC[88] not confirmed in later studies.[89,90]

TABLE 6.3 Genomic Regions Exhibiting Focal Amplification in Lung Cancers, Detected by at Least Two Independent Studies Using Comparative Genomic Hybridization Analyses

Cytoband	Potential Genes	Kim et al.[57] 50 NSCLC	Zhao et al.[51] 101 NSCLC	Choi et al.[52] 15 ADC	Yakut et al.[61] 45 NSCLC	Choi et al.[53] 14 SqCC	Kendall et al.[62] 184 Lung Tumors	Weir et al.[60] 371 ADC
1p34.3	MYCL1		X				X	
1q21.2–q22	ARNT	X					X	X
2p24.3	MYCN		X				X	
3q26.3	PIK3CA	X	X			X		
3q27–3q29	TP63	X				X		
5p15.33	TERT			X	X		X	X
5p15.31					X			X
5p14.3	CDH12				X			X
6p21.3							X	X
7p14.2–14.3				X		X		
7p11.2–12	EGFR		X	X	X		X	X
7q21.2–21.3	HGF, CDK6		X		X			X
8p11.23	FGFR1		X				X	X
8q24.21	MYC		X		X		X	X
11p15.4				X				X
11q13.3–13.4	CCND1		X	X			X	
12p11.2	KRAG, others		X		X			
12p12.1–12p11.2	KRAS, PTHLH					X	X	X
12q13.3–14.1	CDK4		X		X			X
12q15	MDM2			X		X	X	X
14q13	TITF1, FKHL1						X	X
18q11.2	SYT				X			X
19q12	CCNE1		X					X
19q13.1–13.3				X		X		X
22q11.21	CRKL		X	X				X

The *CDKN2* gene encodes an inhibitor of the cyclin-dependent kinase 4 and its inactivation occurs through homozygous deletion, or hemizygous deletion coupled with inactivation of the second allele by point mutation or promoter hypermethylation.[91] Loss of 9p has been detected frequently in NSCLC (16% to 100%) (Fig. 6.3A) but not in SCLC.[92–96] Loss of 9p21 is also relatively frequent in very early epithelial lesions such as hyperplasia or dysplasia[70,73,97–99] and hypermethylation at this site was found to increase during disease progression, from 17% in hyperplasia to 50% in CIS.[97] *CDKN2* hypermethylation has been reported to predict poor 5-year survival rate in resectable NSCLC,[100] and early recurrence in resected stage I NSCLC.[101]

In lung cancer, partial deletion of the short arm of chromosome 3 (3p) has been one of the earliest and most common genetic changes (Fig. 6.4). Chromosome 3p deletion occurs in almost 100% of SCLC and 90% of NSCLC.[102,103] Searches for tumor suppressor genes in this large region identified several targets at multiple sites, including *FHIT* (3p14.2), *RASSF1* (3p21.3), *TUSC2* (*FUS1*, 3p21.3), *SEMA3B* (3p21.3), *SEMA3F* (3p21.3), *MLH1* (3p22.3), and *RARB* (3p24). *FHIT* is one of the most extensively investigated suppressor genes in lung cancer[104–106]; allelic imbalance at *FHIT* was observed in 64% of NSCLC patients and loss of protein expression in 50% of lung cancers.[105–107] Allelic imbalance is associated with physical loss of the chromosomal region (Fig. 6.3B). *RASSF1* is inactivated by promoter hypermethylation in the large majority of SCLC and almost half of the NSCLC,[108–111] while not methylated in noncancerous tissues.[112] Expression of TUSC2 protein is absent or reduced in the majority of lung cancers

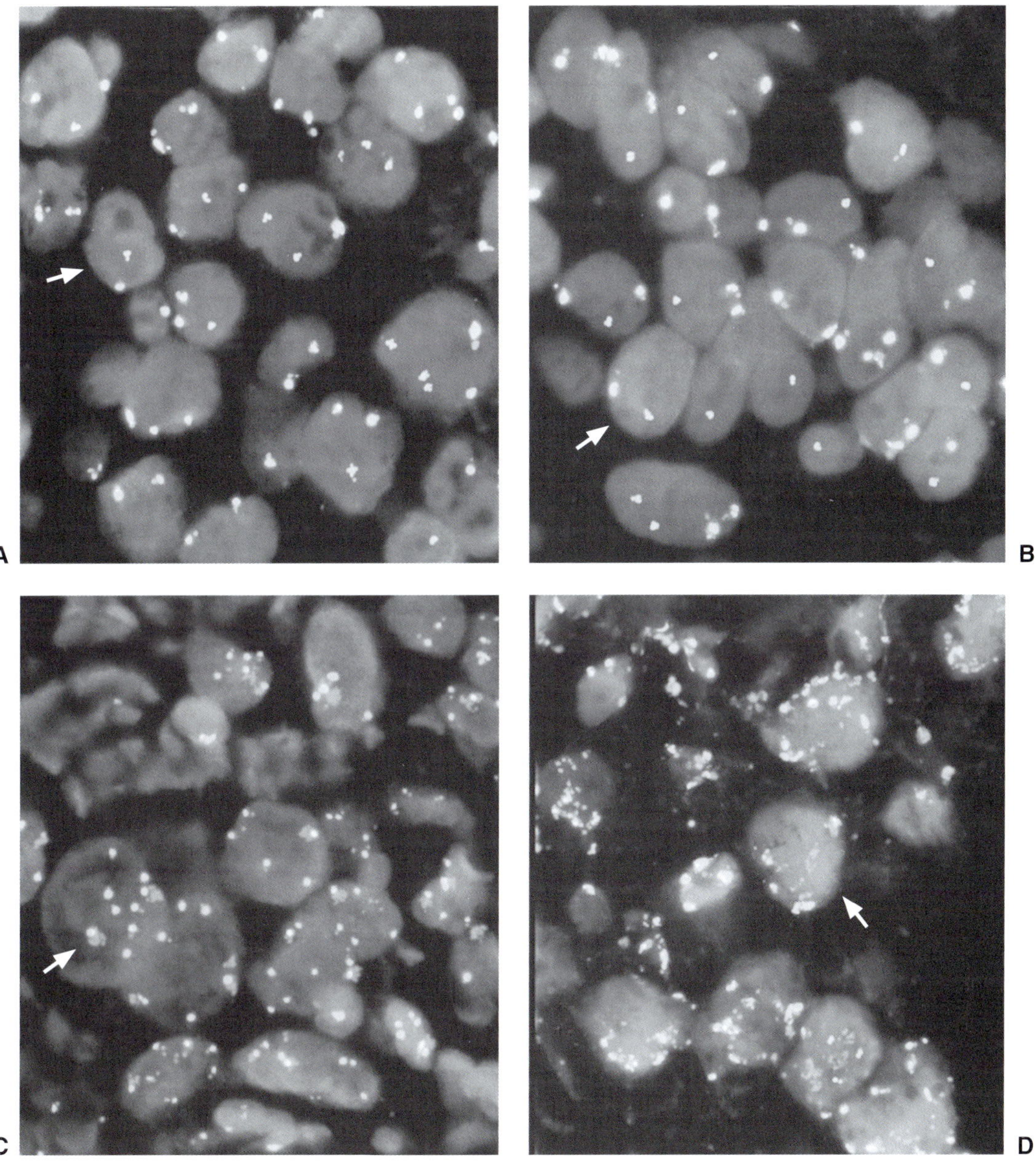

FIGURE 6.3 FISH of sections of non–small cell lung cancer with *CDKN2*-CEP9 **(A)**, *FHIT*-CEP3 **(B)**, *EGFR*-CEP7 **(C)** and *KRAS*-CEP12 **(D)** probe sets. Hybridization spots with the gene probes fluoresce in red color and with the centromere control probes fluoresce in green color. All the CEP probes and the *EGFR* probe are commercially available (Abbott Molecular). Probes for the genes *CDKN2*, *FHIT*, and *KRAS* were developed using BAC clones from the RP11 library. Panels A and B show loss of the gene sequences, respectively, *CDKN2* and *FHIT*, compared with the controls used. Arrows indicate one of the nuclei with loss. Panels C and D show gene amplification, for *EGFR* and *KRAS*, respectively. It is noticeable that the clusters of *EGFR* signals are much more tightly packed than the clusters of *KRAS* signals. Arrows indicate one nucleus displaying gene amplification in each panel. (See color plate.)

and premalignant lung lesions and restoration of its function in 3p21.3-deficient NSCLC cells significantly inhibits tumor cell growth by induction of apoptosis and alteration of cell cycle kinetics.[113] Both *SEMA3F* and *SEMA3B* transcripts are underrepresented in lung cancers, mainly squamous cell carcinomas. A recent review[114] indicated that downregulation of *SEMA3B* and *SEMA3F* is sustained by gene hypermethylation in lung cancer cell lines.[115,116] Moreover, the loss of function of these genes correlates inversely with grade and stage of lung cancer.[98,117] Additionally, the *SEMA3B* and *SEMA3F* genes were found to be targets of *TP53*,[118,119] which suggests that they could be activated during DNA damage or other stress responses. Deregulation in *MLH1*, a mismatch repair gene, was detected in up to 78% of NSCLC specimens, predominantly

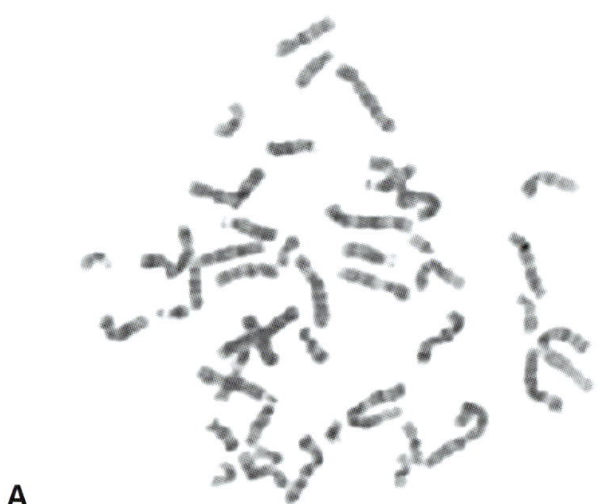

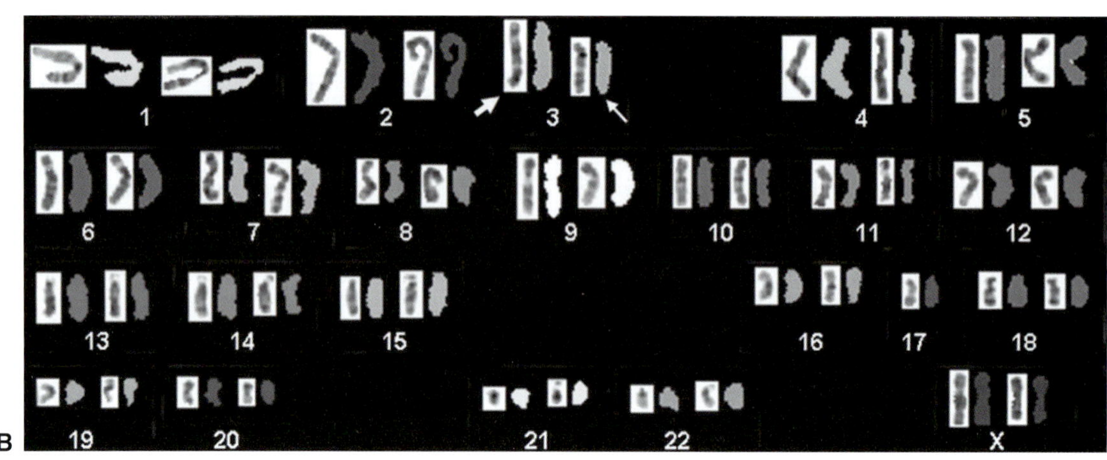

FIGURE 6.4 SKY of a bronchial epithelium cell from a heavy-smoking individual showing deletion of the short arm of chromosome 3, with breakpoint at 3p21.1. **A:** Inverted DAPI image. **B:** Karyotype, including both the inverted DAPI and the classified images. (See color plate.)

by promoter hypermethylation[120] and more recently has been associated with poor prognosis in NSCLC.[121] *RARB* mediates growth control responses[122,123] and its expression was found reduced in about 50% of NSCLC and 70% of SCLC.[124] Promoter hypermethylation is the leading cause of silencing of this gene. Conclusions have been controversial regarding the prognostic role of RARB suppression in lung cancer[125,126] as well as regarding the efficacy of retinoids as chemopreventive agents for this disease.[127,128]

ABNORMALITIES IN GROWTH-STIMULATORY SIGNALLING PATHWAYS: THE PROTO-ONCOGENES

The molecular events that lead to the cancer-initiating cell involve critical mutations in genes regulating normal cell growth and differentiation. There are numerous families of proto-oncogenes that contribute to the tumorigenesis process when constitutively activated. The most relevant molecular pathways to lung cancer pathogenesis include members of the EGFR,[129] MYC,[130] RAS,[131] and STAT[132] families, and other related genes such as *PIK3CA*,[133,134] *CCND1*,[135] and *BCL2*.[136,137] Proto-oncogenes are frequently activated by genetic mutations (*KRAS*, *EGFR*, and *PIK3CA*) and chromosomal rearrangements, such as translocations and inversions that place these genes under the regulation of constitutively activated genes (*MYC*, *BCL2*) or create chimeric proteins (*EML4-ALK*). Other mechanism of proto-oncogene activation in solid tumors is gene amplification, which recently was shown to occur more commonly in solid tumors than previously acknowledged.[138] Examples of genes found amplified in significant subsets of lung cancers are *MYC*, *EGFR*, *HER2*, *CCND1*, *PIK3CA*, and *NKX2-1* (*TITF-1*), and a summary of their incidence, role in disease initiation and progression, and prognostic and predictive impact in lung cancer will be presented.

Among the most important growth factors for lung tumor growth and proliferation are the tyrosine kinase receptors of the ERBB family, which are coded by *EGFR* (erbB1 at 7p12), *ERBB2* (HER-2/neu, 17q12), *ERBB3* (12q13), and *ERBB4* (2q33.3). The EGFR protein is frequently overexpressed in lung carcinomas (50% to 80%)[139,140] and also in metaplastic lung tissue adjacent to malignant tumors and normal-appearing bronchial epithelium of patients with lung cancer.[141,142] Phosphorylation of EGFR can activate signaling to cell proliferation and survival via RAS/MAPK and PIK3CA/AKT pathways.[143] The *EGFR* gene has been proved a relevant marker in lung cancer. Activating somatic mutations in its tyrosine kinase domain have been identified, and prevail in lung cancer patients of East Asian ethnicity, of whom 25% to 40% have mutations,[144–148] when compared to American or European patients, of whom only 8% to 15% of patients carry mutations.[146,147,149–152] *EGFR* mutations also occurs more frequently in never-smokers, women, and NSCLC with adenocarcinoma histology.[147] The *EGFR* gene is amplified in approximately 10% to 15% of advanced NSCLC (Fig. 6.3C).[139,152–156] Besides, there is a significant copy number gain for the EGFR gene in lung cancer as consequence of chromosomal aneusomy and nonbalanced translocation or other rearrangements.[157]

Results are still controversial regarding the prognostic characteristic of EGFR protein overexpression and gene amplification. Recent data support no significant impact of these factors despite a trend toward poor prognosis.[139,140,158] The activating mutations have been associated with a better prognosis and indolent disease but, thus far, there is no definitive support for this role.[159–161] Moreover, the status of the EGFR gene has proved a powerful predictive marker for target therapy agents. Not surprisingly, patients with EGFR high copy numbers and activating mutations are more sensitive to EGFR TKIs such as gefitinib and erlotinib.[143,146,149,151,152,155,162–165] NSCLC patients with EGFR gene amplification or high level of genomic gain by chromosomal aneusomy have also shown higher sensitivity to the monoclonal antibody anti-EGFR cetuximab.[154]

Overexpression of ERBB2 in lung cancer is less common than EGFR overexpression, ranging from 10% to 30% in NSCLC.[166] ERBB2 overexpression was detected in early stages of lung cancer[167] and is associated with poor survival.[168–170] FISH analysis documented occurrence of *ERBB2* gene amplification in 6% to 20% of NSCLC patients.[51,171–175] Activating mutations in *ERBB2* are very rare in lung cancer[176–178] and have been associated with resistance to EGFR TKI in cases with all clinical and biological features of sensitivity to such treatment.[178]

ERBB3 is unique within the EGFR family because of its catalytically deficient kinase domain and its signaling relies on heterodimerization with other EGFR family member, preferentially HER-2.[179] ERBB3 expression was less investigated in lung cancers but between 19% and 58% of tumor specimens revealed an increased level of expression with the highest percentages seen in squamous cell carcinomas[180]; increased expression was also found in association with shorter survival.[181] *ERBB3* gene amplification investigated by FISH was detected in approximately 5% of patients and there was no association with histology subtype.[182] The other member of the family, *ERBB4*, is activated by binding with neuregulins, betacellulin, and heparin-binding epidermal growth factor (EGF)–like growth factor. Its activation leads to cellular proliferation, chemotaxis, or differentiation via activation of specific signal transduction proteins, such as PI3-kinase and Shc.[183] The status of *ERBB4* in lung cancers is still poorly known and this gene seems to infrequently harbor mutations (<3%) in NSCLC.[184]

The genes of the *RAS* family (*HRAS* at 11p15.1, *KRAS* at 12p12.1, and *NRAS* at 1p13.2) encode for highly homologous G-proteins located at the inner surface of the cell membrane that play an essential role in the signal transduction pathways involved in differentiation, proliferation, and survival. The inactive RAS proteins are bound to guanosine diphosphate (GDP) and upon activation release GDP and bind to guanosine triphosphate (GTP). Activated RAS transduces the EGFR activation signal to multiple downstream pathways, including BRAF, MAPK, and PI3K/AKT.[131,185] The intrinsic GTPase activity of RAS terminates signaling by hydrolyzing GTP to GDP, a reaction that is accelerated by the GTPase-activating proteins (GAPs). In lung cancer, *KRAS* is more frequently mutated than *HRAS* and *NRAS*.[186] Point mutations in *KRAS* codon 12, which is prevalent in NSCLC, and in codon 13 result in an increased affinity for GTP, while mutations in codon 61 confer resistance to GAPs. The mutant proteins permanently switch to the active position and constitutively activate the downstream signaling pathways. *KRAS* mutations occur with variable frequency in the major types of lung tumors. They are very scarce in SCLC and prevail in large cell carcinomas and adenocarcinomas, of which 20% to 30% carry a *KRAS* mutation.[187–189] *KRAS* and *EGFR* mutations are almost completely exclusive.[147,176,190,191] *KRAS* mutation has been reported as a negative prognostic factor in terms of survival in NSCLC, especially in adenocarcinoma, in a metaanalysis including 28 studies with NSCLC patients and in more recent studies.[188,192] *KRAS* mutation is also a negative predictor in NSCLC for response to EGFR TKIs.[193–196] The *KRAS* gene was found amplified in lung cancer specimens (Fig. 6.3D), although the frequency in which this phenomenon occurs is unknown at this time. Other downstream effecters of the RAS pathway, such as the *BRAF* gene, which encodes a serine–threonine kinase activated by point mutation, are infrequently (<5%) mutated in lung cancers and likely to have a lesser relevant role in the pathogenesis of those carcinomas.[197,198]

The *MYC* family of genes (*MYC* or c-MYC at 8q24.1, *MYCN* at 2p24, and *MYCL1* at 1p34) encodes basic–helix-loop-helix zipper (bHLHz) transcription factors that, after dimerization with MYC-associated factor X (Max), binds to E-box motifs (CACGTG, CANNTG) and stimulates the transcription of various target genes relevant for cell growth, differentiation, and apoptosis.[130,199] One of these target genes is E2F and, interestingly, it was reported that cMYC activates expression of a cluster of six microRNAs on chromosome 13, two of which (*MIRN17-5p* and *MIRN20A*) negatively regulate *E2F*.[200] These findings reveal a tightly controlled mechanism for activation of transcription and limitation of translation exert by *MYC* on *E2F*. Additionally, there is increasing evidence that the *MYC* genes bind very ubiquitously throughout the genome, apparently to genomic sites of up to 15% of all cellular genes, which hints at a potential nontranscriptional function for them.[201] The alternative model for MYC role in cell growth and tumorigenesis is corroborated by studies showing that MYC promotes DNA replication via nontranscriptional mechanisms and its deregulation causes DNA damage predominantly during the S phase.[202] Amplification and overexpression of the MYC family of oncogenes occurs in 18% to 54% of SCLCs, being more common in chemorefractory disease.[126,203] In advanced NSCLC, from

20% to more than 50% of tumors were found to have *MYC* gene amplification and this phenomenon was associated with tumor progression and worse prognosis.[204,205] A recent investigation using high-resolution array platform showed that *MYC* was the most frequently amplified oncogene in lung cancer cell lines,[138] which 28% of the 53 investigated lung carcinoma cell lines showing amplified levels of its genomic region.

The PI3K–PTEN-AKT signaling pathway overcomes mechanisms that promote apoptosis by transmitting a strong cell survival signal. Interactions between cell surface receptors, such as IGF1R, PDGF, and EGFR, and extracellular ligands, such as EGF and TGF-α, result in activation of tyrosine kinases and recruitment of class I PI3Ks, a family of heterodimeric complexes composed of a p110 catalytic and a p85 regulatory subunit.[206] PI3K phosphorylates phosphatidylinositol, which recruits specific intracellular proteins, such as phosphoinositide-dependent kinase-1 (PDK-1) and Akt/PKB, to the cytoplasmic membrane, through mechanisms regulated by the *PTEN* gene.[207] Akt is a serine/threonine kinase that acts downstream of EGFR to regulate numerous other proteins involved in growth, survival, and movement of cells, and angiogenesis. Akt activation results in inactivation of pro-apoptotic proteins, including members of the Bcl2 and caspase families[208,209] and other proteins that indirectly inhibit apoptosis, such as mdm-2 and the forkhead transcription factors.[210] The p110-α catalytic subunit of PI3Ks is coded by the *PI3KCA* gene (3q26) and there is increasing evidence that constitutive activation of the PI3K pathways in lung cancer occur as a consequence of mutation or amplification of the *PIK3CA* gene. *PIK3CA* genomic gain detected by FISH was reported in 43% of lung cancers with prevalence in squamous cell carcinoma.[133,134] High level of phosphorylated Akt expression has been observed in premalignant and malignant human bronchial epithelial cells[134,211,212] and in approximately 50% of advanced NSCLC.[152,213]

High-resolution genomic profiling of lung cancer cell lines and tumors revealed new genes frequently involved in amplifications. One of them is the homeobox transcription factor *NKX2-1* (*TTF-1* or *TITF-1*) mapped at 14q13.3.[60,62] *NKX2-1* plays a master role in induction and maintenance of lung and thyroid morphogenesis and in the differentiation of epithelial cell lineages.[214] *NKX2-1* gene amplification is accompanied by increased expression at both the RNA and protein levels, and knockdown with small interfering RNA (siRNA) in lung cancer cell lines led to reduced cell cycle progression and increased apoptosis. Gain at 14q13.3 was present in 7% to 33% of cell lines and tumors and was significantly more frequent in adenocarcinomas than squamous cell carcinomas.[215] Interestingly, the *NKX2-1* amplification was associated with the presence of *EGFR*-activating mutations but not *KRAS* or *TP53* mutations, and its overexpression was highlighted as a good prognostic factor in a metaanalysis.[216] The oncogenic role of a tissue-specific transcription factor linked to lineage proliferation and survival may look somewhat peculiar but it reflects the principle of the oncology recapitulating ontogeny. This phenomenon has been detected involving other genes and solid tumor combinations, such as breast cancer and *ESR1*, melanoma and *MITF*, prostate cancer and *AR*, and was also detected previously in lung cancer with the *TP63* gene.[62,217,218] It has been postulated that genetic alterations that directly interfere with transcriptional networks normally regulating lung development may be a more common feature of lung cancer than previously realized.[62]

Genomic changes in proto-oncogenes may occur in association with therapeutic strategies applied to the patients. An interesting example of this phenomenon in lung cancer implicates mesenchymal–epithelial transition (*MET*) (7q31.2), the receptor for the hepatocyte growth factor (*HGF*). *MET* is frequently deregulated in cancers via constitutive kinase activation, paracrine/autocrine activation, mutation, gene amplification, and epigenetic mechanisms.[219] Enhanced *MET* regulation leads to oncogenic changes including cell proliferation, reduced apoptosis, angiogenesis, altered cytoskeletal function, and metastasis. MET overexpression occurs in a varied lung cancer histologies, with stronger expression in NSCLC.[219] Mutations in the tyrosine kinase domain of *MET* were detected in SCLC and NSCLC[220,221] but are uncommon. *MET* gene amplification was relatively frequent (20%) in few NSCLC cell lines tested,[222] but appears to be infrequent (<5%) in unselected clinical NSCLC specimens.[223] Recently, amplification of *MET* was identified in in vitro studies as a major mechanism by which lung tumors overcome therapeutic inhibition of EGFR growth signals.[224] In addition, assessment of tumor tissue from gefitinib or erlotinib resistant NSCLC patients demonstrated *MET* amplification in 21% to 22% of patients,[223,224] a much higher frequency than in the unselected patients. Mechanistically, it was shown that MET protein regulates ERBB3-dependent activation of PI3K at the same time that signals through ERBB3 in amplified cancers, and this redundant activation of ERBB3 supports the downstream signaling even in the presence of EGFR inhibitors.[223,224]

The increased knowledge about the mechanisms leading and maintaining oncogene activation in lung cancer has already provided a striking contribution toward development of new therapeutic approaches. It has also sustained the better understanding of the complex signaling network in normal and cancer cells. Observations that the inactivation of few or even a single oncogene was sufficient to induce a sustained tumor regression have supported the *oncogene addiction* hypothesis by which tumors may become irrevocably addicted to the oncogene that initiated tumorigenesis and a sudden interruption of its activity balances toward proliferative arrest and apoptosis.[225–227] More recently, a compelling alternative has been raised to explain those observations, the "oncogene amnesia" hypothesis. The premise of this hypothesis is that the oncogene activation initiates tumorigenesis by overriding essential mechanisms for cellular mortality, self-renewal, and genomic integrity, thus inducing a state of cellular amnesia.[228] The rationale behind the oncogenic amnesia hypothesis is that the inactivation of a single oncogene in a tumor that has acquired all oncogenic lesions required to overcome the cellular safety mechanisms can restore pathways leading to proliferative arrest, differentiation, cellular senescence, and apoptosis. In this way, the oncogenes initiate cancer inducing a cellular state of enforced amnesia in which, only upon oncogene inactivation, the tumor becomes aware of its transgression.[228] Oncogene addiction and oncogene amnesia are not necessarily exclusive mechanisms, as the hypotheses are proposed, they may coexist in complex tumors as carcinomas.

GENE FUSIONS IN LUNG CANCER: RARE OR UNDETECTED?

Gene fusions encoding chimeric oncoproteins usually result from chromosomal structural rearrangements such as translocations, inversions, and insertions. When the coding regions of two genes are juxtaposed, the chimeric transcript produces a novel protein with an altered function. Despite the numerous chromosomal rearrangements detected by karyotyping techniques, only occasional activation of oncogenes has been found as recurrent event in carcinomas through fusions.[229,230] Thyroid carcinomas exhibit the largest number of reported gene fusions, most of them involving the *RET* and *BRAF* genes. Aggressive midline and mucoepidermoid carcinomas have one described gene fusion each (*BRD4-NUT* and *MECT1-MAML2*, respectively), while fusions involving the *TFE3* gene in kidney carcinoma and *ETV6-NTRK3* and *ODZ4-NRG1* in breast carcinoma were reported in very rare patients (<1%). The recent discovery of gene fusions in a large proportion of prostate carcinomas brought new excitement to the field. These fusions are generated by translocations or interstitial deletions, but were identified by advanced technical bioinformatics approaches for analyses of gene expression rather than by cytogenetic approaches.[231] The prostate cancer fusions occur between *TMPRSS2*, a prostate-specific, strongly androgen-regulated gene, and the genes of the ETS transcription factor family (*ERG*, *ETV1*, and *ETV4*)[232,233] or between *ETV1* and other partners.[234] The fusion of the five prime untranslated region (5′ UTR) of *TMPRSS2* to ERG through an intronic deletion is the prevalent event in prostate cancer.[231] Investigation of the prognostic impact of the presence of *TMPRSS2-ERG* fusion in prostate carcinoma has generated conflicting results. A significant association with specific death or development of metastases is supported by some studies,[235,236] whereas longer progression-free survival in patients treated by prostatectomy was reported by other.[237]

More recently, the fusion of the *ALK* (anaplastic lymphoma kinase) and *EML4* (echinoderm microtubule-associated proteinlike 4) genes, separated by 12 Mb in the short arm of chromosome 2 and oriented in opposite 5′ to 3′ directions, has been identified in NSCLC patients of Japanese origin.[238] Soon after that publication, other reports have confirmed the occurrence of the *EML4-ALK* gene fusion, in four distinct variant forms, in Asian and white lung cancer patients.[239–243] All variant forms of the *EML4-ALK* fusion gene possess prominent transforming activity. The fusion creates a chimeric protein with sequences of *EML4* replacing the extracellular and transmembrane domains of *ALK*, which results in constitutive dimerization of the ALK kinase domain and consequent increase in its catalytic activity.[238] The frequency of NSCLC carrying this fusion is reportedly low, ranging from 1.5% to 2.6% in whites[242,244] and from 2.6% to 6.7% in Asians.[238,241–243,245] The frequency of *EML4-ALK* was associated with adenocarcinoma histology and limited smoking history (<10 pack-years).[242] The *EML4-ALK* fusion was found in patients who had exon 19 deletion in the EGFR gene but not in patients with *KRAS* or *BRAF* mutations.[242] The prognostic implication of this fusion in lung cancer is not explored yet, but the overexpression of ALK in the tumors carrying the fusion may qualify them for treatment with inhibitors of ALK kinase, as demonstrated in in vitro models.[242]

The detection of gene fusions with relevant role in cancer causation and progression has been hampered by the challenge of molecularly identifying cytogenetically cryptic rearrangements. The *TMPRSS2* and *ETV* gene fusions in prostate cancer and *EML4-ALK* in lung cancer were identified by cutting-edge investigative tools. The ongoing advances in the development of more sophisticated tools for analyses of the molecular data already available are expected to substantially increase the detection of intracellular targets of fusions in a near future.

MICRORNAS IN LUNG CANCER

MicroRNAs are a recently identified class of highly conserved, endogenous, short noncoding RNAs of 21 to 25 nucleotides that regulate gene expression in a sequence-specific manner. These molecules work posttranscriptionally by binding to complementary sequences in the three prime untranslated region (3'UTR) of target messenger RNAs (mRNAs), which may lead to repression of protein translation and downregulation of protein expression.[246–248] Expression patterns and function of microRNAs in normal cells are not completely understood. Some microRNAs are located within introns of pre-mRNAs and are likely transcribed together with the cognate protein-coding genes,[246,249,250] whereas others are clustered and transcribed as multicistronic primary transcripts.[251,252] Although the precise functions have not yet been characterized for most of the detected microRNAs, it is known that each individual microRNA can target numerous transcripts,[253,254] whereas each single gene can be targeted by numerous microRNAs.[250,255–258] This new mechanism of gene regulation provides an alternative biologic explanation for the impact of chromosomal loss or gain in one area of the genome on the expression of genes mapped in another part of the genome.

Expression of microRNAs is emerging as an important area in cancer biology because of the evidence that they are essential regulators of various physiologic and developmental processes[249] and are altered in human cancer.[259,260] Most importantly, signatures of microRNA expression can define molecular subsets of tumors[259,261] and predict outcome.[260,262,263]

There are already scores of studies in microRNAs and lung cancer with relevant results. For instance, they have been shown to hold a prognostic effect. Lung adenocarcinoma patients with high expression of either *MIRN155* (21q21.3), *MIRN1*, *MIRN106A*, *MIRN 93*, or *MIRN21* and low expression of either *MIRNLET7A2*, *MIRNLET7A*, or *MIRN145* were found to have a significantly worse prognosis[262] and shortened postoperative survival in NSCLC.[263] Interestingly, underexpression of two microRNAs mapped at 3p was recently found to be associated with overexpression of RAS and EGFR in lung cancer. Loss of these microRNAs would be equivalent to the loss of a tumor suppressor gene because they downregulate the expression of the target genes. RAS was determined to be downregulated by the *MIRNLET7G* (miRNA let-7g) gene, which resides on chromosome 3p21.2.[264,265] Expression levels of *MIRNLET7G* were on average 30% lower in NSCLC samples than in normal adjacent tissues[264] and reduction of tumor growth was observed in tumor xenographs when overexpression of *MIRNLET7G* was induced from lentiviral vectors.[265] The gene *MIRN128-2* (miRNA 128b) mapped at 3p22 was predicted to target EGFR, which is frequently overexpressed in lung cancer. This finding was hypothesized to provide a functional link between two common molecular phenomena in lung cancer, the loss of 3p, and the deregulation of EGFR.[266] Further exploration of this potential link led to molecular evidence that *MIRN128-2* directly regulates EGFR and, most importantly, studies in clinical specimens showed that loss of this miRNA gene was associated with significantly better disease control and longer survival in NSCLC treated with gefitinib, an EGFR TKI. In short, *MIRN128-1* loss had similar impact in the sensitivity to the EGFR inhibitors as EGFR gene gain.

Under the same premises, overexpressed microRNAs are expected to serve as oncogenes and there are examples of this role in lung cancer, one of which involves the *MIRN17-92* cluster. This gene cluster comprises seven distinct microRNAs residing in intron 3 of the *MIRHG1* gene at 13q31.3 and was shown to be markedly overexpressed and occasionally amplified in lung cancer.[267] The predicted targets for the microRNA cluster comprise a large number of genes, including the tumor suppressors *PTEN* and *RB2*.[255] Therefore, amplification of the *MIRN17-92* cluster offers the molecular conditions for suppression of *PTEN* and *RB2*.

Studies focusing on the functional role of microRNA in cancer, including lung cancer, have been expanded dramatically lately. Ultimately this knowledge is expected to contribute not only to the better understanding of cell growth and differentiation but also to the development of novel therapeutics and translational tools such as biomarkers for assessment of risk for disease, early diagnosis, and selection of patients for treatment with specific agents.

CONCLUSION

Lung cancer is a challenging disease to patients and their families, to physicians, and researchers. Lung cancers are characterized by an extremely diverse collection of genomic alterations, of which a proportion of unknown dimension is still concealed. However, numerous pathogenetically important changes have already been detected in substantial fraction of patients and translated into a system for detection and determination of the prognosis of the disease. Specific genomic profiles have supported the development of new treatment strategies and a growing use of customized therapy regimens using molecular targeted or chemotherapeutic agents. These aspects will be discussed in more details in other chapters. Despite the apparent caveat that each of the customized therapies is likely to benefit only a small subset of lung cancer patients, the high incidence of this disease worldwide ultimately guarantees that the benefit will impact a large number of patients. Therefore, it remains critical to improve the characterization of emerging genomic profiles and to discover new subsets of lung cancer patients. The achievement of these goals is dependent on new and important insights into the molecular pathways that underlie lung tumor development.

REFERENCES

1. Jemal A, Siegel R, Ward E, et al. Cancer statistics, 2008. *CA Cancer J Clin* 2008;58(2):71–96.
2. Speicher MR, Gwyn Ballard S, Ward DC. Karyotyping human chromosomes by combinatorial multi-fluor FISH. *Nat Genet* 1996;12(4):368–375.
3. Schröck E, du Manoir S, Veldman T, et al. Multicolor spectral karyotyping of human chromosomes. *Science* 1996;273(5274):494–497.
4. Kallioniemi A, Kallioniemi OP, Sudar D, et al. Comparative genomic hybridization for molecular cytogenetic analysis of solid tumors. *Science* 1992;258(5083):818–821.
5. Heidenblad M, Lindgren D, Veltman JA, et al. Microarray analyses reveal strong influence of DNA copy number alterations on the transcriptional patterns in pancreatic cancer: implications for the interpretation of genomic amplifications. *Oncogene* 2005;24(10):1794–7801.
6. Hertzberg L, Betts DR, Raimondi SC, et al. Prediction of chromosomal aneuploidy from gene expression data. *Genes Chromosomes Cancer* 2007;46(1):75–86.
7. Hyman E, Kauraniemi P, Hautaniemi S, et al. Impact of DNA amplification on gene expression patterns in breast cancer. *Cancer Res* 2002;62(21):6240–6245.
8. Masayesva BG, Ha P, Garrett-Mayer E, et al. Gene expression alterations over large chromosomal regions in cancers include multiple genes unrelated to malignant progression. *Proc Natl Acad Sci U S A* 2004;101(23):8715–8720.
9. Pollack JR, Sørlie T, Perou CM, et al. Microarray analysis reveals a major direct role of DNA copy number alteration in the transcriptional program of human breast tumors. *Proc Natl Acad Sci U S A* 2002;99(20):12963–12968.
10. Wang Q, Diskin S, Rappaport E, et al. Integrative genomics identifies distinct molecular classes of neuroblastoma and shows that multiple genes are targeted by regional alterations in DNA copy number. *Cancer Res* 2006;66(12):6050–6062.
11. Pinkel D, Segraves R, Sudar D, et al. High resolution analysis of DNA copy number variation using comparative genomic hybridization to microarrays. *Nat Genet* 1998;20(2):207–211.
12. Solinas-Toldo S, Lampel S, Stilgenbauer S, et al. Matrix-based comparative genomic hybridization: biochips to screen for genomic imbalances. *Genes Chromosomes Cancer* 1997;20(4):399–407.
13. Ishkanian AS, Malloff CA, Watson SK, et al. A tiling resolution DNA microarray with complete coverage of the human genome. *Nat Genet* 2004;36(3):299–303.
14. Chung YJ, Jonkers J, Kitson H, et al. A whole-genome mouse BAC microarray with 1-Mb resolution for analysis of DNA copy number changes by array comparative genomic hybridization. *Genome Res* 2004;14(1):188–196.

15. de Smith AJ, Tsalenko A, Sampas N, et al. Array CGH analysis of copy number variation identifies 1284 new genes variant in healthy white males: implications for association studies of complex diseases. *Hum Mol Genet* 2007;16(23):2783–2794.
16. de Ståhl TD, Sandgren J, Piotrowski A, et al. Profiling of copy number variations (CNVs) in healthy individuals from three ethnic groups using a human genome 32 K BAC-clone-based array. *Hum Mutat* 2008;29(3):398–408.
17. Choma D, Daurès JP, Quantin X, et al. Aneuploidy and prognosis of non-small-cell lung cancer: a meta-analysis of published data. *Br J Cancer* 2001;85(1):14–22.
18. Whang-Peng J, Kao-Shan CS, Lee EC, et al. Specific chromosome defect associated with human small-cell lung cancer; deletion 3p(14–23). *Science* 1982;215(4529):181–182.
19. Balsara BR, Testa JR. Chromosomal imbalances in human lung cancer. *Oncogene* 2002;21(45):6877–6883.
20. Berker-Karaüzüm S, Lüleci G, Ozbilim G, et al. Cytogenetic findings in thirty lung carcinoma patients. *Cancer Genet Cytogenet* 1998; 100(2):114–123.
21. Petersen I, Bujard M, Petersen S, et al. Patterns of chromosomal imbalances in adenocarcinoma and squamous cell carcinoma of the lung. *Cancer Res* 1997;57(12):2331–2335.
22. Petersen I, Langreck H, Wolf G, et al. Small-cell lung cancer is characterized by a high incidence of deletions on chromosomes 3p, 4q, 5q, 10q, 13q and 17p. *Br J Cancer* 1997;75(1):79–86.
23. Testa JR, Siegfried JM. Chromosome abnormalities in human non-small cell lung cancer. *Cancer Res* 1992;52(9 Suppl):2702s–2706s.
24. Testa JR, Siegfried JM, Liu Z, et al. Cytogenetic analysis of 63 non-small cell lung carcinomas: recurrent chromosome alterations amid frequent and widespread genomic upheaval. *Genes Chromosomes Cancer* 1994;11(3):178–194.
25. Testa JR, Liu Z, Feder M, et al. Advances in the analysis of chromosome alterations in human lung carcinomas. *Cancer Genet Cytogenet* 1997;95(1):20–32.
26. Feder M, Siegfried JM, Balshem A, et al. Clinical relevance of chromosome abnormalities in non-small cell lung cancer. *Cancer Genet Cytogenet* 1998;102(1):25–31.
27. Levin NA, Brzoska P, Gupta N, et al. Identification of frequent novel genetic alterations in small cell lung carcinoma. *Cancer Res* 1994;54(19):5086–5091.
28. Levin NA, Brzoska PM, Warnock ML, et al. Identification of novel regions of altered DNA copy number in small cell lung tumors. *Genes Chromosomes Cancer* 1995;13(3):175–185.
29. Michelland S, Gazzeri S, Brambilla E, et al. Comparison of chromosomal imbalances in neuroendocrine and non-small-cell lung carcinomas. *Cancer Genet Cytogenet* 1999;114(1):22–30.
30. Ried T, Petersen I, Holtgreve-Grez H, et al. Mapping of multiple DNA gains and losses in primary small cell lung carcinomas by comparative genomic hybridization. *Cancer Res* 1994;54(7):1801–1806.
31. Schwendel A, Langreck H, Reichel M, et al. Primary small-cell lung carcinomas and their metastases are characterized by a recurrent pattern of genetic alterations. *Int J Cancer* 1997;74(1):86–93.
32. Dennis TR, Stock AD. A molecular cytogenetic study of chromosome 3 rearrangements in small cell lung cancer: consistent involvement of chromosome band 3q13.2. *Cancer Genet Cytogenet* 1999;113(2):134–140.
33. Grigorova M, Lyman RC, Caldas C, et al. Chromosome abnormalities in 10 lung cancer cell lines of the NCI-H series analyzed with spectral karyotyping. *Cancer Genet Cytogenet* 2005;162(1):1–9.
34. Luk C, Tsao MS, Bayani J, et al. Molecular cytogenetic analysis of non-small cell lung carcinoma by spectral karyotyping and comparative genomic hybridization. *Cancer Genet Cytogenet* 2001;125(2):87–99.
35. Sy SM, Fan B, Lee TW, et al. Spectral karyotyping indicates complex rearrangements in lung adenocarcinoma of nonsmokers. *Cancer Genet Cytogenet* 2004;153(1):57–59.
36. Sy SM, Wong N, Lee TW, et al. Distinct patterns of genetic alterations in adenocarcinoma and squamous cell carcinoma of the lung. *Eur J Cancer* 2004;40(7):1082–1094.
37. Tai AL, Fang Y, Sham JS, et al. Establishment and characterization of a human non-small cell lung cancer cell line. *Oncol Rep* 2005;13(6): 1029–1032.
38. Harada R, Uemura Y, Kobayashi M, et al. Establishment and characterization of a new lung cancer cell line (MI-4) producing high levels of granulocyte colony stimulating factor. *Jpn J Cancer Res* 2002;93(6):667–676.
39. Ashman JN, Brigham J, Cowen ME, et al. Chromosomal alterations in small cell lung cancer revealed by multicolour fluorescence in situ hybridization. *Int J Cancer* 2002;102(3):230–236.
40. Berrieman HK, Ashman JN, Cowen ME, et al. Chromosomal analysis of non-small-cell lung cancer by multicolour fluorescent in situ hybridisation. *Br J Cancer* 2004;90(4):900–905.
41. Gunawan B, Mirzaie M, Schulten HJ, et al. Molecular cytogenetic analysis of two primary squamous cell carcinomas of the lung using multicolor fluorescence in situ hybridization. *Virchows Arch* 2001;439(1):85–89.
42. Roschke AV, Tonon G, Gehlhaus KS, et al. Karyotypic complexity of the NCI-60 drug-screening panel. *Cancer Res* 2003;63(24):8634–8647.
43. Speicher MR, Petersen S, Uhrig S, et al. Analysis of chromosomal alterations in non-small cell lung cancer by multiplex-FISH, comparative genomic hybridization, and multicolor bar coding. *Lab Invest* 2000;80(7):1031–1041.
44. Varella-Garcia M, Chen L, Powell RL, et al. Spectral karyotyping detects chromosome damage in bronchial cells of smokers and patients with cancer. *Am J Respir Crit Care Med* 2007;176(5):505–512.
45. Dang TP, Gazdar AF, Virmani AK, et al. Chromosome 19 translocation, overexpression of Notch3, and human lung cancer. *J Natl Cancer Inst* 2000;92(16):1355–1357.
46. Haruki N, Kawaguchi KS, Eichenberger S, et al. Dominant-negative Notch3 receptor inhibits mitogen-activated protein kinase pathway and the growth of human lung cancers. *Cancer Res* 2005;65(9):3555–3561.
47. Haruki N, Kawaguchi KS, Eichenberger S, et al. Cloned fusion product from a rare t(15;19)(q13.2;p13.1) inhibit S phase in vitro. *J Med Genet* 2005;42(7):558–564.
48. Coe BP, Lee EH, Chi B, et al. Gain of a region on 7p22.3, containing MAD1L1, is the most frequent event in small-cell lung cancer cell lines. *Genes Chromosomes Cancer* 2006;45(1):11–19.
49. Kim YH, Girard L, Giacomini CP, et al. Combined microarray analysis of small cell lung cancer reveals altered apoptotic balance and distinct expression signatures of MYC family gene amplification. *Oncogene* 2006;25(1):130–138.
50. Peng WX, Shibata T, Katoh H, et al. Array-based comparative genomic hybridization analysis of high-grade neuroendocrine tumors of the lung. *Cancer Sci* 2005;96(10):661–667.
51. Zhao X, Weir BA, LaFramboise T, et al. Homozygous deletions and chromosome amplifications in human lung carcinomas revealed by single nucleotide polymorphism array analysis. *Cancer Res* 2005;65(13):5561–5570.
52. Choi JS, Zheng LT, Ha E, et al. Comparative genomic hybridization array analysis and real-time PCR reveals genomic copy number alteration for lung adenocarcinomas. *Lung* 2006;184(6):355–362.
53. Choi YW, Choi JS, Zheng LT, et al. Comparative genomic hybridization array analysis and real time PCR reveals genomic alterations in squamous cell carcinomas of the lung. *Lung Cancer* 2007;55(1):43–51.
54. Dehan E, Ben-Dor A, Liao W, et al. Chromosomal aberrations and gene expression profiles in non-small cell lung cancer. *Lung Cancer* 2007;56(2):175–184.
55. Garnis C, Lockwood WW, Vucic E, et al. High resolution analysis of non-small cell lung cancer cell lines by whole genome tiling path array CGH. *Int J Cancer* 2006;118(6):1556–1564.
56. Jiang F, Yin Z, Caraway NP, et al. Genomic profiles in stage I primary non small cell lung cancer using comparative genomic hybridization analysis of cDNA microarrays. *Neoplasia* 2004;6(5):623–635.
57. Kim TM, Yim SH, Lee JS, et al. Genome-wide screening of genomic alterations and their clinicopathologic implications in non-small cell lung cancers. *Clin Cancer Res* 2005;11(23):8235–8242.

58. Ma J, Gao M, Lu Y, et al. Gain of 1q25–32, 12q23–24.3, and 17q12–22 facilitates tumorigenesis and progression of human squamous cell lung cancer. *J Pathol* 2006;210(2):205–213.
59. Tonon G, Wong KK, Maulik G, et al. High-resolution genomic profiles of human lung cancer. *Proc Natl Acad Sci U S A* 2005;102(27):9625–9630.
60. Weir BA, Woo MS, Getz G, et al. Characterizing the cancer genome in lung adenocarcinoma. *Nature* 2007;450(7171):893–898.
61. Yakut T, Schulten HJ, Demir A, et al. Assessment of molecular events in squamous and non-squamous cell lung carcinoma. *Lung Cancer* 2006;54(3):293–301.
62. Kendall J, Liu Q, Bakleh A, et al. Oncogenic cooperation and coamplification of developmental transcription factor genes in lung cancer. *Proc Natl Acad Sci U S A* 2007;104(42):16663–16668.
63. Knudson AG. Chasing the cancer demon. *Annu Rev Genet* 2000;34:1–19.
64. Levine AJ, Momand J, Finlay CA. The p53 tumour suppressor gene. *Nature* 1991;351(6326):453–546.
65. Kishimoto Y, Murakami Y, Shiraishi M, et al. Aberrations of the p53 tumor suppressor gene in human non-small cell carcinomas of the lung. *Cancer Res* 1992;52(17):4799–4804.
66. Takahashi T, Nau MM, Chiba I, et al. p53: a frequent target for genetic abnormalities in lung cancer. *Science* 1989;246(4929):491–944.
67. Huang CL, Yokomise H, Miyatake A. Clinical significance of the p53 pathway and associated gene therapy in non-small cell lung cancers. *Future Oncol* 2007;3(1):83–93.
68. Subramanian J, Govindan R. Lung cancer in never smokers: a review. *J Clin Oncol* 2007;25(5):561–570.
69. Toyooka S, Tsuda T, Gazdar AF. The TP53 gene, tobacco exposure, and lung cancer. *Hum Mutat* 2003;21(3):229–239.
70. Breuer RH, Snijders PJ, Sutedja GT, et al. Expression of the p16(INK4a) gene product, methylation of the p16(INK4a) promoter region and expression of the polycomb-group gene BMI-1 in squamous cell lung carcinoma and premalignant endobronchial lesions. *Lung Cancer* 2005;48(3):299–306.
71. Vega FJ, Iniesta P, Caldes T, et al. p53 exon 5 mutations as a prognostic indicator of shortened survival in non-small-cell lung cancer. *Br J Cancer* 1997;76(1):44–51.
72. Berghmans T, Mascaux C, Martin B, et al. Prognostic role of p53 in stage III non-small cell lung cancer. *Anticancer Res* 2005;25(3c):2385–2389.
73. Breuer RH, Snijders PJ, Sutedja TG, et al. Suprabasal p53 immunostaining in premalignant endobronchial lesions in combination with histology is associated with bronchial cancer. *Lung Cancer* 2003;40(2):165–172.
74. Mitsudomi T, Lam S, Shirakusa T, et al. Detection and sequencing of p53 gene mutations in bronchial biopsy samples in patients with lung cancer. *Chest* 1993;104(2):362–365.
75. Mitsudomi T, Oyama T, Kusano T, et al. Mutations of the p53 gene as a predictor of poor prognosis in patients with non-small-cell lung cancer. *J Natl Cancer Inst* 1993;85(24):2018–2023.
76. Ponticiello A, Barra E, Giani U, et al. P53 immunohistochemistry can identify bronchial dysplastic lesions proceeding to lung cancer: a prospective study. *Eur Respir J* 2000;15(3):547–552.
77. Higashiyama M, Doi O, Kodama K, et al. MDM2 gene amplification and expression in non-small-cell lung cancer: immunohistochemical expression of its protein is a favourable prognostic marker in patients without p53 protein accumulation. *Br J Cancer* 1997;75(9):1302–1308.
78. Mori S, Ito G, Usami N, et al. p53 apoptotic pathway molecules are frequently and simultaneously altered in nonsmall cell lung carcinoma. *Cancer* 2004;100(8):1673–1682.
79. Stefanaki K, Rontogiannis D, Vamvouka C, et al. Immunohistochemical detection of bcl2, p53, mdm2 and p21/waf1 proteins in small-cell lung carcinomas. *Anticancer Res* 1998;18(2A):1167–1173.
80. Daniel JC, Smythe WR. The role of Bcl-2 family members in non-small cell lung cancer. *Semin Thorac Cardiovasc Surg* 2004;16(1):19–27.
81. Ewen ME. The cell cycle and the retinoblastoma protein family. *Cancer Metastasis Rev* 1994;13(1):45–66.
82. Sherr CJ. The INK4a/ARF network in tumour suppression. *Nat Rev Mol Cell Biol* 2001;2(10):731–737.
83. Dosaka-Akita H, Cagle PT, Hiroumi H, et al. Differential retinoblastoma and p16(INK4A) protein expression in neuroendocrine tumors of the lung. *Cancer* 2000;88(3):550–556.
84. Cagle PT, el-Naggar AK, Xu HJ, et al. Differential retinoblastoma protein expression in neuroendocrine tumors of the lung. Potential diagnostic implications. *Am J Pathol* 1997;150(2):393–400.
85. Xu HJ, Hu SX, Cagle PT, et al. Absence of retinoblastoma protein expression in primary non-small cell lung carcinomas. *Cancer Res* 1991;51(10):2735–2739.
86. Wikenheiser-Brokamp KA. Retinoblastoma regulatory pathway in lung cancer. *Curr Mol Med* 2006;6(7):783–793.
87. Goldstein NS. Analysis of stage I lung carcinoma patients including p53 and Rb protein. *Ann Thorac Surg* 2000;69(5):1648–1649.
88. Xu HJ, Quinlan DC, Davidson AG, et al. Altered retinoblastoma protein expression and prognosis in early-stage non-small-cell lung carcinoma. *J Natl Cancer Inst* 1994;86(9):695–699.
89. Chen JT, Chen YC, Chen CY, et al. Loss of p16 and/or pRb protein expression in NSCLC. An immunohistochemical and prognostic study. *Lung Cancer* 2001;31(2–3):163–170.
90. Hommura F, aka-Akita H, Kinoshita I, et al. Predictive value of expression of p16INK4A, retinoblastoma and p53 proteins for the prognosis of non-small-cell lung cancers. *Br J Cancer* 1999;81(4):696–701.
91. Gazzeri S, Gouyer V, Vour'ch C, et al. Mechanisms of p16INK4A inactivation in non small-cell lung cancers. *Oncogene* 1998;16(4):497–504.
92. Gorgoulis VG, Zacharatos P, Kotsinas A, et al. Alterations of the p16-pRb pathway and the chromosome locus 9p21–22 in non-small-cell lung carcinomas: relationship with p53 and MDM2 protein expression. *Am J Pathol* 1998;153(6):1749–1765.
93. Sanchez-Cespedes M, Decker PA, et al. Increased loss of chromosome 9p21 but not p16 inactivation in primary non-small cell lung cancer from smokers. *Cancer Res* 2001;61(5):2092–2096.
94. Singhal S, Vachani A, ntin-Ozerkis D, et al. Prognostic implications of cell cycle, apoptosis, and angiogenesis biomarkers in non-small cell lung cancer: a review. *Clin Cancer Res* 2005;11(11):3974–3986.
95. Wiest JS, Franklin WA, Drabkin H, et al. Genetic markers for early detection of lung cancer and outcome measures for response to chemoprevention. *J Cell Biochem Suppl* 1997;28–29:64–73.
96. Yanagawa N, Tamura G, Oizumi H, et al. Frequent epigenetic silencing of the p16 gene in non-small cell lung cancers of tobacco smokers. *Jpn J Cancer Res* 2002;93(10):1107–1113.
97. Belinsky SA, Nikula KJ, Palmisano WA, et al. Aberrant methylation of p16(INK4a) is an early event in lung cancer and a potential biomarker for early diagnosis. *Proc Natl Acad Sci U S A* 1998;95(20):11891–11896.
98. Brambilla E, Constantin B, Drabkin H, et al. Semaphorin SEMA3F localization in malignant human lung and cell lines: A suggested role in cell adhesion and cell migration. *Am J Pathol* 2000;156(3):939–950.
99. Niklinski J, Niklinska W, Chyczewski L, et al. Molecular genetic abnormalities in premalignant lung lesions: biological and clinical implications. *Eur J Cancer Prev* 2001;10(3):213–226.
100. Wang J, Lee JJ, Wang L, et al. Value of p16INK4a and RASSF1A promoter hypermethylation in prognosis of patients with resectable non-small cell lung cancer. *Clin Cancer Res* 2004;10(18 Pt 1):6119–6125.
101. Brock MV, Hooker CM, Ota-Machida E, et al. DNA methylation markers and early recurrence in stage I lung cancer. *N Engl J Med* 2008;358(11):1118–1128.
102. Braithwaite KL, Rabbitts PH. Multi-step evolution of lung cancer. *Semin Cancer Biol* 1999;9(4):255–65.
103. Kok K, Naylor SL, Buys CH. Deletions of the short arm of chromosome 3 in solid tumors and the search for suppressor genes. *Adv Cancer Res* 1997;71:27–92.
104. Croce CM, Sozzi G, Huebner K. Role of FHIT in human cancer. *J Clin Oncol* 1999;17(5):1618–1624.
105. Garinis GA, Gorgoulis VG, Mariatos G, et al. Association of allelic loss at the FHIT locus and p53 alterations with tumour kinetics and chromosomal instability in non-small cell lung carcinomas (NSCLCs). *J Pathol* 2001;193(1):55–65.

106. Sard L, Accornero P, Tornielli S, et al. The tumor-suppressor gene FHIT is involved in the regulation of apoptosis and in cell cycle control. *Proc Natl Acad Sci U S A* 1999;96(15):8489–8492.
107. Sozzi G, Pastorino U, Moiraghi L, et al. Loss of FHIT function in lung cancer and preinvasive bronchial lesions. *Cancer Res* 1998;58(22):5032–5037.
108. Burbee DG, Forgacs E, Zochbauer-Muller S, et al. Epigenetic inactivation of RASSF1A in lung and breast cancers and malignant phenotype suppression. *J Natl Cancer Inst* 2001;93(9):691–699.
109. Chen H, Suzuki M, Nakamura Y, et al. Aberrant methylation of RASGRF2 and RASSF1A in human non-small cell lung cancer. *Oncol Rep* 2006;15(5):1281–1285.
110. Dammann R, Schagdarsurengin U, Seidel C, et al. The tumor suppressor RASSF1A in human carcinogenesis: an update. *Histol Histopathol* 2005;20(2):645–663.
111. Kaira K, Sunaga N, Tomizawa Y, et al. Epigenetic inactivation of the RAS-effector gene RASSF2 in lung cancers. *Int J Oncol* 2007;31(1):169–173.
112. Feng Q, Hawes SE, Stern JE, et al. DNA methylation in tumor and matched normal tissues from non-small cell lung cancer patients. *Cancer Epidemiol Biomarkers Prev* 2008;17(3):645–654.
113. Ji L, Roth JA. Tumor suppressor FUS1 signaling pathway. *J Thorac Oncol* 2008;3(4):327–330.
114. Potiron VA, Roche J, Drabkin HA. Semaphorins and their receptors in lung cancer. *Cancer Lett* 2009;273(1):1–14.
115. Ito M, Ito G, Kondo M, Uchiyama M, et al. Frequent inactivation of RASSF1A, BLU, and SEMA3B on 3p21.3 by promoter hypermethylation and allele loss in non-small cell lung cancer. *Cancer Lett* 2005;225(1):131–139.
116. Kuroki T, Trapasso F, Yendamuri S, et al. Allelic loss on chromosome 3p21.3 and promoter hypermethylation of semaphorin 3B in non-small cell lung cancer. *Cancer Res* 2003;63(12):3352–3355.
117. Lantuejoul S, Constantin B, Drabkin H, et al. Expression of VEGF, semaphorin SEMA3F, and their common receptors neuropilins NP1 and NP2 in preinvasive bronchial lesions, lung tumours, and cell lines. *J Pathol* 2003;200(3):336–347.
118. Futamura M, Kamino H, Miyamoto Y, et al. Possible role of semaphorin 3F, a candidate tumor suppressor gene at 3p21.3, in p53-regulated tumor angiogenesis suppression. *Cancer Res* 2007;67(4):1451–1460.
119. Ochi K, Mori T, Toyama Y, et al. Identification of semaphorin3B as a direct target of p53. *Neoplasia* 2002;4(1):82–87.
120. Wang YC, Lu YP, Tseng RC, et al. Inactivation of hMLH1 and hMSH2 by promoter methylation in primary non-small cell lung tumors and matched sputum samples. *J Clin Invest* 2003;111(6):887–95.
121. Seng TJ, Currey N, Cooper WA, et al. DLEC1 and MLH1 promoter methylation are associated with poor prognosis in non-small cell lung carcinoma. *Br J Cancer* 2008;99(2):375–382.
122. Alvarez S, Germain P, Alvarez R, et al. Structure, function and modulation of retinoic acid receptor beta, a tumor suppressor. *Int J Biochem Cell Biol* 2007;39(7–8):1406–1415.
123. Xu XC. Tumor-suppressive activity of retinoic acid receptor-beta in cancer. *Cancer Lett* 2007;253(1):14–24.
124. Virmani AK, Rathi A, Zöchbauer-Müller S, et al. Promoter methylation and silencing of the retinoic acid receptor-beta gene in lung carcinomas. *J Natl Cancer Inst* 2000;92(16):1303–1307.
125. Katayama H, Hiraki A, Fujiwara K, et al. Aberrant promoter methylation profile in pleural fluid DNA and clinicopathological factors in patients with non-small cell lung cancer. *Asian Pac J Cancer Prev* 2007;8(2):221–224.
126. Kim YT, Park SJ, Lee SH, et al. Prognostic implication of aberrant promoter hypermethylation of CpG islands in adenocarcinoma of the lung. *J Thorac Cardiovasc Surg* 2005;130(5):1378.
127. Bogos K, Renyi-Vamos F, Kovacs G, et al. Role of retinoic receptors in lung carcinogenesis. *J Exp Clin Cancer Res* 2008;27(1):18.
128. Kim JS, Lee H, Kim H, et al. Promoter methylation of retinoic acid receptor beta 2 and the development of second primary lung cancers in non-small-cell lung cancer. *J Clin Oncol* 2004;22(17):3443–3450.
129. Bunn PA Jr, Franklin W. Epidermal growth factor receptor expression, signal pathway, and inhibitors in non-small cell lung cancer. *Semin Oncol* 2002;29(5 Suppl 14):38–44.
130. Zajac-Kaye M. Myc oncogene: a key component in cell cycle regulation and its implication for lung cancer. *Lung Cancer* 2001;34(Suppl 2):S43–S46.
131. Molina JR, Adjei AA. The Ras/Raf/MAPK pathway. *J Thorac Oncol* 2006;1(1):7–9.
132. Karamouzis MV, Konstantinopoulos PA, Papavassiliou AG. The role of STATs in lung carcinogenesis: an emerging target for novel therapeutics. *J Mol Med* 2007;85(5):427–436.
133. Angulo B, Suarez-Gauthier A, Lopez-Rios F, et al. Expression signatures in lung cancer reveal a profile for EGFR-mutant tumours and identify selective PIK3CA overexpression by gene amplification. *J Pathol* 2008;214(3):347–356.
134. Massion PP, Taflan PM, Shyr Y, et al. Early involvement of the phosphatidylinositol 3-kinase/Akt pathway in lung cancer progression. *Am J Respir Crit Care Med* 2004;170(10):1088–1094.
135. Gautschi O, Ratschiller D, Gugger M, et al. Cyclin D1 in non-small cell lung cancer: a key driver of malignant transformation. *Lung Cancer* 2007;55(1):1–14.
136. Thomadaki H, Scorilas A. BCL2 family of apoptosis-related genes: functions and clinical implications in cancer. *Crit Rev Clin Lab Sci* 2006;43(1):1–67.
137. Zinkel S, Gross A, Yang E. BCL2 family in DNA damage and cell cycle control. *Cell Death Differ* 2006;13(8):1351–1359.
138. Lockwood WW, Chari R, Coe BP, et al. DNA amplification is a ubiquitous mechanism of oncogene activation in lung and other cancers. *Oncogene* 2008;27(33):4615–4624.
139. Hirsch FR, Varella-Garcia M, Bunn PA Jr, et al. Epidermal growth factor receptor in non-small-cell lung carcinomas: correlation between gene copy number and protein expression and impact on prognosis. *J Clin Oncol* 2003;21(20):3798–3807.
140. Hirsch FR, Varella-Garcia M, Cappuzzo F, et al. Combination of EGFR gene copy number and protein expression predicts outcome for advanced non-small-cell lung cancer patients treated with gefitinib. *Ann Oncol* 2007;18(4):752–760.
141. Franklin WA, Veve R, Hirsch FR, et al. Epidermal growth factor receptor family in lung cancer and premalignancy. *Semin Oncol* 2002;29 (1 Suppl 4):3–14.
142. Merrick DT, Kittelson J, Winterhalder R, et al. Analysis of c-ErbB1/epidermal growth factor receptor and c-ErbB2/HER-2 expression in bronchial dysplasia: evaluation of potential targets for chemoprevention of lung cancer. *Clin Cancer Res* 2006;12(7 Pt 1):2281–2288.
143. Sharma SV, Bell DW, Settleman J, et al. Epidermal growth factor receptor mutations in lung cancer. *Nat Rev Cancer* 2007;7(3):169–181.
144. Endo K, Konishi A, Sasaki H, et al. Epidermal growth factor receptor gene mutation in non-small cell lung cancer using highly sensitive and fast TaqMan PCR assay. *Lung Cancer* 2005;50(3):375–384.
145. Kosaka T, Yatabe Y, Endoh H, et al. Mutations of the epidermal growth factor receptor gene in lung cancer: biological and clinical implications. *Cancer Res* 2004;64(24):8919–8923.
146. Paez JG, Janne PA, Lee JC, et al. EGFR mutations in lung cancer: correlation with clinical response to gefitinib therapy. *Science* 2004;304(5676):1497–1500.
147. Shigematsu H, Lin L, Takahashi T, et al. Clinical and biological features associated with epidermal growth factor receptor gene mutations in lung cancers. *J Natl Cancer Inst* 2005;97(5):339–346.
148. Tokumo M, Toyooka S, Kiura K, et al. The relationship between epidermal growth factor receptor mutations and clinicopathologic features in non-small cell lung cancers. *Clin Cancer Res* 2005;11(3):1167–1173.
149. Pao W, Miller V, Zakowski M, et al. EGF receptor gene mutations are common in lung cancers from "never smokers" and are associated with sensitivity of tumors to gefitinib and erlotinib. *Proc Natl Acad Sci U S A* 2004;101(36):13306–13311.
150. Marchetti A, Martella C, Felicioni L, et al. EGFR mutations in non-small-cell lung cancer: analysis of a large series of cases and development of a rapid and sensitive method for diagnostic screening with potential implications on pharmacologic treatment. *J Clin Oncol* 2005;23(4):857–865.

151. Lynch TJ, Bell DW, Sordella R, et al. Activating mutations in the epidermal growth factor receptor underlying responsiveness of non-small-cell lung cancer to gefitinib. *N Engl J Med* 2004;350(21):2129–2139.
152. Cappuzzo F, Hirsch FR, Rossi E, et al. Epidermal growth factor receptor gene and protein and gefitinib sensitivity in non-small-cell lung cancer. *J Natl Cancer Inst* 2005;97(9):643–655.
153. Felip E, Rojo F, Reck M, et al. A phase II pharmacodynamic study of erlotinib in patients with advanced non-small cell lung cancer previously treated with platinum-based chemotherapy. *Clin Cancer Res* 2008;14(12):3867–3874.
154. Hirsch FR, Herbst RS, Olsen C, et al. Increased EGFR gene copy number detected by fluorescent in situ hybridization predicts outcome in non-small-cell lung cancer patients treated with cetuximab and chemotherapy. *J Clin Oncol* 2008;26(20):3351–3357.
155. Zhu CQ, da Cunha SG, Ding K, et al. Role of KRAS and EGFR as biomarkers of response to erlotinib in National Cancer Institute of Canada Clinical Trials Group Study BR.21. *J Clin Oncol* 2008;26(26): 4268–4275.
156. Sone T, Kasahara K, Kimura H, et al. Comparative analysis of epidermal growth factor receptor mutations and gene amplification as predictors of gefitinib efficacy in Japanese patients with nonsmall cell lung cancer. *Cancer* 2007;109(9):1836–1844.
157. Varella-Garcia M. Stratification of non-small cell lung cancer patients for therapy with epidermal growth factor receptor inhibitors: the EGFR fluorescence in situ hybridization assay. *Diagn Pathol* 2006;1:19.
158. Kanematsu T, Yano S, Uehara H, et al. Phosphorylation, but not overexpression, of epidermal growth factor receptor is associated with poor prognosis of non-small cell lung cancer patients. *Oncol Res* 2003;13(5):289–298.
159. Kobayashi N, Toyooka S, Ichimura K, et al. Non-BAC component but not epidermal growth factor receptor gene mutation is associated with poor outcomes in small adenocarcinoma of the lung. *J Thorac Oncol* 2008;3(7):704–710.
160. Shepherd FA, Tsao MS. Unraveling the mystery of prognostic and predictive factors in epidermal growth factor receptor therapy. *J Clin Oncol* 2006;24(7):1219–1220.
161. Cappuzzo F. EGFR FISH versus mutation: different tests, different end-points. *Lung Cancer* 2008;60(2):160–165.
162. Mitsudomi T, Kosaka T, Endoh H, et al. Mutations of the epidermal growth factor receptor gene predict prolonged survival after gefitinib treatment in patients with non-small-cell lung cancer with postoperative recurrence. *J Clin Oncol* 2005;23(11):2513–2520.
163. Hirsch FR, Varella-Garcia M, McCoy J, et al. Increased epidermal growth factor receptor gene copy number detected by fluorescence in situ hybridization associates with increased sensitivity to gefitinib in patients with bronchioloalveolar carcinoma subtypes: a Southwest Oncology Group Study. *J Clin Oncol* 2005;23(28):6838–6845.
164. Hirsch FR, Varella-Garcia M, Bunn PA Jr, et al. Molecular predictors of outcome with gefitinib in a phase III placebo-controlled study in advanced non-small-cell lung cancer. *J Clin Oncol* 2006;24(31):5034–5042.
165. Janne PA, Johnson BE. Effect of epidermal growth factor receptor tyrosine kinase domain mutations on the outcome of patients with non-small cell lung cancer treated with epidermal growth factor receptor tyrosine kinase inhibitors. *Clin Cancer Res* 2006;12(14 Pt 2): 4416s–4420s.
166. Mitsudomi T, Yatabe Y. Mutations of the epidermal growth factor receptor gene and related genes as determinants of epidermal growth factor receptor tyrosine kinase inhibitors sensitivity in lung cancer. *Cancer Sci* 2007;98(12):1817–1824.
167. Pastorino U, Sozzi G, Miozzo M, et al. Genetic changes in lung cancer. *J Cell Biochem Suppl* 1993;17F:237–248.
168. Korrapati V, Gaffney M, Larsson LG, et al. Effect of HER2/neu expression on survival in non-small-cell lung cancer. *Clin Lung Cancer* 2001;2(3):216–219.
169. Saad RS, Liu Y, Han H, Landreneau RJ, et al. Prognostic significance of HER2/neu, p53, and vascular endothelial growth factor expression in early stage conventional adenocarcinoma and bronchioloalveolar carcinoma of the lung. *Mod Pathol* 2004;17(10):1235–1242.
170. Szelachowska J, Jelen M, Kornafel J. Prognostic significance of intracellular laminin and Her2/neu overexpression in non-small cell lung cancer. *Anticancer Res* 2006;26(5B):3871–3876.
171. Cappuzzo F, Varella-Garcia M, Shigematsu H, et al. Increased HER2 gene copy number is associated with response to gefitinib therapy in epidermal growth factor receptor-positive non-small-cell lung cancer patients. *J Clin Oncol* 2005;23(22):5007–5018.
172. Hirsch FR, Varella-Garcia M, Franklin WA, et al. Evaluation of HER-2/neu gene amplification and protein expression in non-small cell lung carcinomas. *Br J Cancer* 2002;86(9):1449–1456.
173. Heinmoller P, Gross C, Beyser K, et al. HER2 status in non-small cell lung cancer: results from patient screening for enrollment to a phase II study of herceptin. *Clin Cancer Res* 2003;9(14):5238–5243.
174. Ugocsai K, Mandoky L, Tiszlavicz L, et al. Investigation of HER2 overexpression in non-small cell lung cancer. *Anticancer Res* 2005;25(4): 3061–3066.
175. Pellegrini C, Falleni M, Marchetti A, et al. HER-2/Neu alterations in non-small cell lung cancer: a comprehensive evaluation by real time reverse transcription-PCR, fluorescence in situ hybridization, and immunohistochemistry. *Clin Cancer Res* 2003;9(10 Pt 1):3645–3652.
176. Mounawar M, Mukeria A, Le CF, et al. Patterns of EGFR, HER2, TP53, and KRAS mutations of p14arf expression in non-small cell lung cancers in relation to smoking history. *Cancer Res* 2007;67(12):5667–5672.
177. Shigematsu H, Takahashi T, Nomura M, et al. Somatic mutations of the HER2 kinase domain in lung adenocarcinomas. *Cancer Res* 2005;65(5):1642–1646.
178. Cappuzzo F, Bemis L, Varella-Garcia M. HER2 mutation and response to trastuzumab therapy in non-small-cell lung cancer. *N Engl J Med* 2006;354(24):2619–2621.
179. Sithanandam G, Anderson LM. The ERBB3 receptor in cancer and cancer gene therapy. *Cancer Gene Ther* 2008;15(7):413–48.
180. Hilbe W, Dirnhofer S, Oberwasserlechner F, et al. Immunohistochemical typing of non-small cell lung cancer on cryostat sections: correlation with clinical parameters and prognosis. *J Clin Pathol* 2003;56(10): 736–741.
181. Lai WW, Chen FF, Wu MH, et al. Immunohistochemical analysis of epidermal growth factor receptor family members in stage I non-small cell lung cancer. *Ann Thorac Surg* 2001;72(6):1868–1876.
182. Cappuzzo F, Toschi L, Domenichini I, et al. HER3 genomic gain and sensitivity to gefitinib in advanced non-small-cell lung cancer patients. *Br J Cancer* 2005;93(12):1334–1340.
183. Carpenter G. ErbB-4: mechanism of action and biology. *Exp Cell Res* 2003;284(1):66–77.
184. Soung YH, Lee JW, Kim SY, et al. Somatic mutations of the ERBB4 kinase domain in human cancers. *Int J Cancer* 2006;118(6):1426–1429.
185. Kranenburg O. The KRAS oncogene: past, present, and future. *Biochim Biophys Acta* 2005;1756(2):81–82.
186. Aviel-Ronen S, Blackhall FH, Shepherd FA, et al. K-ras mutations in non-small-cell lung carcinoma: a review. *Clin Lung Cancer* 2006;8(1):30–38.
187. Hilbe W, Dlaska M, Duba HC, et al. Automated real-time PCR to determine K-ras codon 12 mutations in non-small cell lung cancer: comparison with immunohistochemistry and clinico-pathological features. *Int J Oncol* 2003;23(4):1121–1126.
188. Marks JL, Broderick S, Zhou Q, et al. Prognostic and therapeutic implications of EGFR and KRAS mutations in resected lung adenocarcinoma. *J Thorac Oncol* 2008;3(2):111–116.
189. Sekido Y, Fong KM, Minna JD. Molecular genetics of lung cancer. *Annu Rev Med* 2003;54:73–87.
190. Finberg KE, Sequist LV, Joshi VA, et al. Mucinous differentiation correlates with absence of EGFR mutation and presence of KRAS mutation in lung adenocarcinomas with bronchioloalveolar features. *J Mol Diagn* 2007;9(3):320–326.
191. Shibata T, Hanada S, Kokubu A, et al. Gene expression profiling of epidermal growth factor receptor/KRAS pathway activation in lung adenocarcinoma. *Cancer Sci* 2007;98(7):985–991.

192. Mascaux C, Iannino N, Martin B, et al. The role of RAS oncogene in survival of patients with lung cancer: a systematic review of the literature with meta-analysis. *Br J Cancer* 2005;92(1):131–139.
193. Bonomi PD, Buckingham L, Coon J. Selecting patients for treatment with epidermal growth factor tyrosine kinase inhibitors. *Clin Cancer Res* 2007;13(15 Pt 2):S4606–S4612.
194. Endoh H, Yatabe Y, Kosaka T, et al. PTEN and PIK3CA expression is associated with prolonged survival after gefitinib treatment in EGFR-mutated lung cancer patients. *J Thorac Oncol* 2006;1(7):629–634.
195. Massarelli E, Varella-Garcia M, Tang X, et al. KRAS mutation is an important predictor of resistance to therapy with epidermal growth factor receptor tyrosine kinase inhibitors in non-small-cell lung cancer. *Clin Cancer Res* 2007;13(10):2890–2896.
196. Pao W, Wang TY, Riely GJ, et al. KRAS mutations and primary resistance of lung adenocarcinomas to gefitinib or erlotinib. *PLoS Med* 2005;2(1):E17.
197. Shigematsu H, Gazdar AF. Somatic mutations of epidermal growth factor receptor signaling pathway in lung cancers. *Int J Cancer* 2006;118(2):257–262.
198. Ueda M, Toji E, Nunobiki O, et al. Mutational analysis of the BRAF gene in human tumor cells. *Hum Cell* 2008;21(2):13–17.
199. Dang CV, O'Donnell KA, Zeller KI, et al. The c-Myc target gene network. *Semin Cancer Biol* 2006;16(4):253–264.
200. O'Donnell KA, Wentzel EA, Zeller KI, et al. c-Myc-regulated microRNAs modulate E2F1 expression. *Nature* 2005;435(7043):839–843.
201. Knoepfler PS, Zhang XY, Cheng PF, et al. Myc influences global chromatin structure. *EMBO J* 2006;25(12):2723–2734.
202. Dominguez-Sola D, Ying CY, Grandori C, Ruggiero L, et al. Non-transcriptional control of DNA replication by c-Myc. *Nature* 2007; 448(7152):445–451.
203. Bergh JC. Gene amplification in human lung cancer. The myc family genes and other proto-oncogenes and growth factor genes. *Am Rev Respir Dis* 1990;142(6 Pt 2):S20–S26.
204. Brennan J, O'Connor T, Makuch RW, et al. Myc family DNA amplification in 107 tumors and tumor cell lines from patients with small cell lung cancer treated with different combination chemotherapy regimens. *Cancer Res* 1991;51(6):1708–1712.
205. Kubokura H, Tenjin T, Akiyama H, et al. Relations of the c-myc gene and chromosome 8 in non-small cell lung cancer: analysis by fluorescence in situ hybridization. *Ann Thorac Cardiovasc Surg* 2001;7(4):197–203.
206. Toker A, Newton AC. Cellular signaling: pivoting around PDK-1. *Cell* 2000;103(2):185–188.
207. Li J, Yen C, Liaw D, et al. PTEN, a putative protein tyrosine phosphatase gene mutated in human brain, breast, and prostate cancer. *Science* 1997;275(5308):1943–1947.
208. Cardone MH, Roy N, Stennicke HR, et al. Regulation of cell death protease caspase-9 by phosphorylation. *Science* 1998;282(5392):1318–1321.
209. Di CA, Pandolfi PP. The multiple roles of PTEN in tumor suppression. *Cell* 2000;100(4):387–390.
210. Mayo LD, Donner DB. The PTEN, Mdm2, p53 tumor suppressor-oncoprotein network. *Trends Biochem Sci* 2002;27(9):462–467.
211. Brognard J, Clark AS, Ni Y, et al. Akt/protein kinase B is constitutively active in non-small cell lung cancer cells and promotes cellular survival and resistance to chemotherapy and radiation. *Cancer Res* 2001;61(10):3986–3997.
212. Lee HY. Molecular mechanisms of deguelin-induced apoptosis in transformed human bronchial epithelial cells. *Biochem Pharmacol* 2004;68(6):1119–1124.
213. Cappuzzo F, Magrini E, Ceresoli GL, et al. Akt phosphorylation and gefitinib efficacy in patients with advanced non-small-cell lung cancer. *J Natl Cancer Inst* 2004;96(15):1133–1141.
214. Kimura S, Hara Y, Pineau T, et al. The T/ebp null mouse: thyroid-specific enhancer-binding protein is essential for the organogenesis of the thyroid, lung, ventral forebrain, and pituitary. *Genes Dev* 1996;10(1):60–69.
215. Berghmans T, Mascaux C, Haller A, et al. EGFR, TTF-1 and Mdm2 expression in stage III non-small cell lung cancer: a positive association. *Lung Cancer* 2008;62(1):35–44.
216. Berghmans T, Paesmans M, Mascaux C, et al. Thyroid transcription factor 1—a new prognostic factor in lung cancer: a meta-analysis. *Ann Oncol* 2006;17(11):1673–1676.
217. Kwei KA, Kim YH, Girard L, et al. Genomic profiling identifies TITF1 as a lineage-specific oncogene amplified in lung cancer. *Oncogene* 2008; 27(25):3635–3640.
218. Petitjean A, Hainaut P, Caron de FC. TP63 gene in stress response and carcinogenesis: a broader role than expected. *Bull Cancer* 2006;93(12): E126–E135.
219. Cipriani NA, Abidoye OO, Vokes E, et al. MET as a target for treatment of chest tumors. *Lung Cancer* 2009;63(2):169–179.
220. Ma PC, Kijima T, Maulik G, et al. c-MET mutational analysis in small cell lung cancer: novel juxtamembrane domain mutations regulating cytoskeletal functions. *Cancer Res* 2003;63(19):6272–6281.
221. Ma PC, Jagadeeswaran R, Jagadeesh S, et al. Functional expression and mutations of c-Met and its therapeutic inhibition with SU11274 and small interfering RNA in non-small cell lung cancer. *Cancer Res* 2005;65(4):1479–1488.
222. Lutterbach B, Zeng Q, Davis LJ, et al. Lung cancer cell lines harboring MET gene amplification are dependent on Met for growth and survival. *Cancer Res* 2007;67(5):2081–2088.
223. Bean J, Brennan C, Shih JY, et al. MET amplification occurs with or without T790M mutations in EGFR mutant lung tumors with acquired resistance to gefitinib or erlotinib. *Proc Natl Acad Sci U S A* 2007;104(52):20932–20937.
224. Engelman JA, Zejnullahu K, Mitsudomi T, et al. MET amplification leads to gefitinib resistance in lung cancer by activating ERBB3 signaling. *Science* 2007;316(5827):1039–1043.
225. Gazdar AF, Shigematsu H, Herz J, et al. Mutations and addiction to EGFR: the Achilles 'heal' of lung cancers? *Trends Mol Med* 2004;10(10):481–486.
226. Weinstein IB. Cancer. Addiction to oncogenes—the Achilles heal of cancer. *Science* 2002;297(5578):63–64.
227. Weinstein IB, Joe A. Oncogene addiction. *Cancer Res* 2008;68(9): 3077–3080.
228. Felsher DW. Oncogene addiction versus oncogene amnesia: perhaps more than just a bad habit? *Cancer Res* 2008;68(9):3081–3086.
229. Mitelman F, Johansson B, Mertens F. Fusion genes and rearranged genes as a linear function of chromosome aberrations in cancer. *Nat Genet* 2004;36(4):331–334.
230. Mitelman F, Johansson B, Mertens F. The impact of translocations and gene fusions on cancer causation. *Nat Rev Cancer* 2007;7(4):233–245.
231. Kumar-Sinha C, Tomlins SA, Chinnaiyan AM. Recurrent gene fusions in prostate cancer. *Nat Rev Cancer* 2008;8(7):497–511.
232. Tomlins SA, Rhodes DR, Perner S, et al. Recurrent fusion of TMPRSS2 and ETS transcription factor genes in prostate cancer. *Science* 2005;310(5748):644–648.
233. Tomlins SA, Mehra R, Rhodes DR, et al. TMPRSS2:ETV4 gene fusions define a third molecular subtype of prostate cancer. *Cancer Res* 2006;66(7):3396–3400.
234. Tomlins SA, Laxman B, Dhanasekaran SM, et al. Distinct classes of chromosomal rearrangements create oncogenic ETS gene fusions in prostate cancer. *Nature* 2007;448(7153):595–599.
235. Demichelis F, Rubin MA. TMPRSS2-ETS fusion prostate cancer: biological and clinical implications. *J Clin Pathol* 2007;60(11):1185–1186.
236. Yoshimoto M, Joshua AM, Cunha IW, et al. Absence of TMPRSS2: ERG fusions and PTEN losses in prostate cancer is associated with a favorable outcome. *Mod Pathol* 2008 21(12):1451–1460.
237. Saramaki OR, Harjula AE, Martikainen PM, et al. TMPRSS2:ERG fusion identifies a subgroup of prostate cancers with a favorable prognosis. *Clin Cancer Res* 2008;14(11):3395–3400.
238. Soda M, Choi YL, Enomoto M, et al. Identification of the transforming EML4-ALK fusion gene in non-small-cell lung cancer. *Nature* 2007;448(7153):561–566.
239. Choi YL, Takeuchi K, Soda M, et al. Identification of novel isoforms of the EML4-ALK transforming gene in non-small cell lung cancer. *Cancer Res* 2008;68(13):4971–4976.

240. Perner S, Wagner PL, Demichelis F, et al. EML4-ALK fusion lung cancer: a rare acquired event. *Neoplasia* 2008;10(3):298–302.
241. Inamura K, Takeuchi K, Togashi Y, et al. EML4-ALK fusion is linked to histological characteristics in a subset of lung cancers. *J Thorac Oncol* 2008;3(1):13–17.
242. Koivunen JP, Mermel C, Zejnullahu K, et al. EML4-ALK fusion gene and efficacy of an ALK kinase inhibitor in lung cancer. *Clin Cancer Res* 2008;14(13):4275–4283.
243. Shinmura K, Kageyama S, Tao H, et al. EML4-ALK fusion transcripts, but no NPM-, TPM3-, CLTC-, ATIC-, or TFG-ALK fusion transcripts, in non-small cell lung carcinomas. *Lung Cancer* 2008;61(2):163–169.
244. Perner S, Rubin MA. A variant TMPRSS2 isoform and ERG fusion product in prostate cancer with implications for molecular diagnosis. *Mod Pathol* 2008;21(8):1056–1057.
245. Perner S, Rubin MA. A variant TMPRSS2 isoform and ERG fusion product in prostate cancer with implications for molecular diagnosis. *Mod Pathol* 2008;21(8):1056–1057.
246. Lagos-Quintana M, Rauhut R, Lendeckel W, et al. Identification of novel genes coding for small expressed RNAs. *Science* 2001;294(5543): 853–858.
247. Lee RC, Feinbaum RL, Ambros V. The C. elegans heterochronic gene lin-4 encodes small RNAs with antisense complementarity to lin-14. *Cell* 1993;75(5):843–854.
248. Lau NC, Lim LP, Weinstein EG, et al. An abundant class of tiny RNAs with probable regulatory roles in Caenorhabditis elegans. *Science* 2001;294(5543):858–862.
249. Scott GK, Goga A, Bhaumik D, et al. Coordinate suppression of ERBB2 and ERBB3 by enforced expression of micro-RNA miR-125a or miR-125b. *J Biol Chem* 2007;282(2):1479–1486.
250. John B, Enright AJ, Aravin A, et al. Human microRNA targets. *PLoS Biol* 2004;2(11):e363.
251. He L, Hannon GJ. MicroRNAs: small RNAs with a big role in gene regulation. *Nat Rev Genet* 2004;5(7):522–531.
252. Ambros V. The functions of animal microRNAs. *Nature* 2004; 431(7006):350–355.
253. Lim LP, Lau NC, Garrett-Engele P, et al. Microarray analysis shows that some microRNAs downregulate large numbers of target mRNAs. *Nature* 2005;433(7027):769–773.
254. Bartel DP. MicroRNAs: genomics, biogenesis, mechanism, and function. *Cell* 2004;116(2):281–297.
255. Lewis BP, Shih IH, Jones-Rhoades MW, et al. Prediction of mammalian microRNA targets. *Cell* 2003;115(7):787–798.
256. Lewis BP, Burge CB, Bartel DP. Conserved seed pairing, often flanked by adenosines, indicates that thousands of human genes are microRNA targets. *Cell* 2005;120(1):15–20.
257. Krek A, Grun D, Poy MN, et al. Combinatorial microRNA target predictions. *Nat Genet* 2005;37(5):495–500.
258. Kiriakidou M, Nelson PT, Kouranov A, et al. A combined computational-experimental approach predicts human microRNA targets. *Genes Dev* 2004;18(10):1165–1178.
259. Volinia S, Calin GA, Liu CG, et al. A microRNA expression signature of human solid tumors defines cancer gene targets. *Proc Natl Acad Sci U S A* 2006;103(7):2257–2261.
260. Calin GA, Sevignani C, Dumitru CD, et al. Human microRNA genes are frequently located at fragile sites and genomic regions involved in cancers. *Proc Natl Acad Sci U S A* 2004;101(9):2999–3004.
261. Lu J, Getz G, Miska EA, et al. MicroRNA expression profiles classify human cancers. *Nature* 2005;435(7043):834–838.
262. Yanaihara N, Caplen N, Bowman E, et al. Unique microRNA molecular profiles in lung cancer diagnosis and prognosis. *Cancer Cell* 2006;9(3):189–198.
263. Takamizawa J, Konishi H, Yanagisawa K, et al. Reduced expression of the let-7 microRNAs in human lung cancers in association with shortened postoperative survival. *Cancer Res* 2004;64(11):3753–3756.
264. Johnson SM, Grosshans H, Shingara J, et al. RAS is regulated by the let-7 microRNA family. *Cell* 2005;120(5):635–647.
265. Kumar MS, Lu J, Mercer KL, et al. Impaired microRNA processing enhances cellular transformation and tumorigenesis. *Nat Genet* 2007;39(5):673–677.
266. Weiss GJ, Bemis LT, Nakajima E, et al. EGFR regulation by microRNA in lung cancer: correlation with clinical response and survival to gefitinib and EGFR expression in cell lines. *Ann Oncol* 2008;19(6): 1053–1059.
267. Hayashita Y, Osada H, Tatematsu Y, et al. A polycistronic microRNA cluster, miR-17-92, is overexpressed in human lung cancers and enhances cell proliferation. *Cancer Res* 2005;65(21):9628–9632.

CHAPTER 7

Ite A. Laird-Offringa

Epigenetic Changes in Lung Cancer: Pathobiological and Clinical Aspects

Within a decade after the publication of the first human genome sequence,[1] and even before a full understanding of all its implications has been attained, a new frontier has emerged: epigenetics.[2] The study of factors superimposed on the genes, or "epi"genetics, focuses on mitotically heritable modifications of DNA and histones, and the associated chromatin components that affect gene expression without altering gene sequence.[3] Epigenetics is one of the most exciting new frontiers in genome analysis. Two of the most widely studied epigenetic modifications are DNA methylation and histone modification. Many of the interacting proteins that bind directly or indirectly to methylated DNA or modified histones catalyze the formation or removal of other alterations, forming a complex regulatory network that is only beginning to be deciphered.[3–6] It has become clear that epigenetic deregulation contributes very importantly to cancer development and progression.[7–11] Profound epigenetic changes are seen in all cancer types, including lung cancer.[12–16] Epigenetic alterations in lung cancer show potential as molecular markers that could be applied to early detection, tumor classification, risk assessment, prognostication, and monitoring of cancer recurrence.[17–20] In addition, understanding the consequences of epigenetic changes can help dissect the molecular basis of lung cancer, providing new focal points for targeted therapies.

One of the most exciting aspects of epigenetic changes is their inherent reversibility. This has encouraged the development of novel drugs for cancer treatment, such as histone deacetylase inhibitors (HDACI) and DNA methylation inhibitors.[21,22] A number of these drugs are in clinical trials for numerous cancers, including those of the lung. With the advent of ever more powerful tools for genome-wide assessment,[23] our understanding of the lung cancer epigenome and its application to diagnosis and treatment promises to increase dramatically in the years to come.[7] Here, the basic concepts of epigenetics will be reviewed, and our current knowledge concerning epigenetic alterations in lung cancer will be discussed, including the type of changes identified and their pathological and clinical implications. Given the very large number of epigenetic alterations analyzed to date and the dramatic acceleration in acquired data, it is impossible to be comprehensive in one short chapter. Therefore, the important advances made in lung cancer research will be illustrated based on a limited number of key examples, and reviews will be cited throughout as a source of more detailed information.

GENETIC AND EPIGENETIC INTERACTIONS

Initial research into the molecular basis of lung cancer focused on genetic alterations, such as mutations, loss of heterozygosity, deletions, and gene amplification.[24,25] Examples of genetic alterations in lung cancer include mutations in KRAS and the epidermal growth factor receptor (EGFR), loss of heterozygosity at chromosome 3p, and MYC gene amplification. However, it has become abundantly clear that epigenetic alterations contribute equally importantly to lung cancer development and progression.[12–14] Epigenetic alterations seen in lung cancer consist of DNA methylation changes (both loss and gain of methylation), changes in histone modifications, and alterations in chromatin structure and chromatin-associated proteins. Interactions between genetic and epigenetic hits in cancer cells can result in further alterations,[2,11,26,27] as outlined in Figure 7.1. For example, *genetic* alterations in the genes encoding components of the epigenetic machinery (such as DNA methyltransferases and HDACs) can affect the activity of these enzymes and thereby the transcriptional activity of many additional genes. In numerous cancers, including lung cancer, somatic changes in parts of the epigenetic machinery are seen.[27] This potential for genetic alterations to affect epigenetics is underscored by the reported link between lung cancer risk and genetic polymorphisms in several genes encoding epigenetic enzymes.[27] Conversely, *epigenetic* alterations can lead to further genetic damage. For example, hypermethylation of DNA repair genes or genes encoding detoxification enzymes can affect the cell's susceptibility to mutagenesis and could result in the genetic (in)activation of additional genes.[26] DNA methylation of 6-O-methylguanine DNA methyltransferase (MGMT),

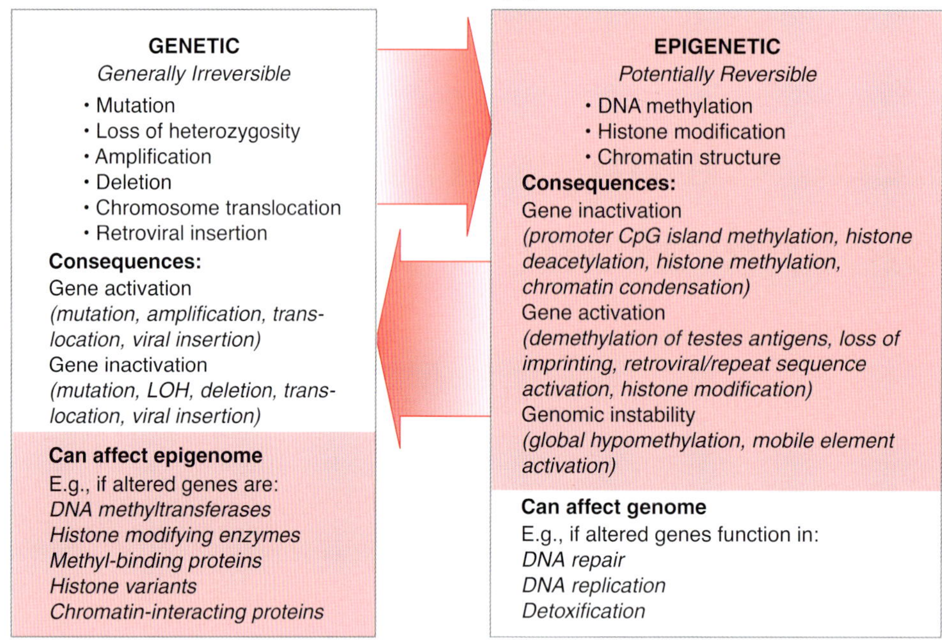

FIGURE 7.1 Interaction between genetic and epigenetic alterations in cancer. **Left panel:** Genetic "hits," which are generally irreversible and can result in activation or inactivation of the altered gene. If such a gene encodes a product involved in epigenetic regulation, like a histone methyltransferase, a DNA methyl-binding protein,[67] a histone isoform, an enzyme that adds or removes histone modifications, or a protein that interacts with such modifications (transcriptional regulators, coactivators, or corepressors), this could result in epigenetic alterations. **Right panel:** Epigenetic hits are potentially reversible, and when they occur in genes that affect the integrity of the genome, such as DNA repair genes or genes encoding proteins involved in DNA replication or detoxification, they can increase the likelihood of acquisition of additional genetic alterations.

an enzyme involved in repair of alkylated guanine, is commonly seen in lung cancer.[15] Inactivation of MGMT has been linked to an increase in RAS gene mutation frequency.[28] In support of their potential to affect cancer development, polymorphisms in MGMT and other DNA repair genes have been linked to lung cancer risk in various populations.[29–31] These examples illustrate that genetic and epigenetic changes should not be seen as independent but as components of a complex interactive network that is responsible for the development and progression of lung cancer (Fig. 7.1). Combined analysis of both types of molecular changes will accelerate the elucidation of the molecular pathways affected in lung cancer, and could be especially helpful in characterizing particular types of lung cancer (e.g., histological subtypes or lung cancer from smokers vs. nonsmokers). This holistic view of (epi)genetic alterations is also highly relevant to the clinic, as the use of certain cytotoxic drugs may potentiate or inhibit the efficacy of epigenetic drugs and vice versa.[21,22]

DNA METHYLATION

In mammals, DNA methylation occurs at the 5-position of cytosine, in the context of a mini palindrome: a cytosine-phosphate-guanine (CpG) dinucleotide. The palindromic nature of methylation allows the propagation of this modification following DNA replication. In the normal mammalian genome, some areas are heavily methylated, such as sections of the inactive X chromosome in women, pericentromeric regions, and parentally imprinted genes. Indeed, DNA methylation is essential for proper development and viability.[3] Methylation in mammals is carried out by at least three enzymes, the maintenance DNA methyltransferase DNMT1 (which methylates daughter strands following DNA replication) and de novo DNA methyltransferases DNMT3A and 3B.[32] All three genes are essential, as illustrated by mouse knockout experiments.[32] A large number of splice isoforms exists, a number of which appear to target particular genes or areas of the genome and some of which are implicated in cancer.[33,34] In lung cancer, overexpression of the deltaDNMT3B4 variant correlates strongly with RASSF1A methylation, and knockdown of this methyltransferase resulted in a rapid demethylation of the RASSF1A CpG island.[35] This effect was gene-specific, as no changes in methylation of CDKN2A were observed.

CpG dinucleotides exist in two general environments in normal cells: sparsely distributed and clustered. On the one hand, CpGs are sprinkled throughout the genome, and these CpGs are usually methylated. Spontaneous deamination of methyl-C results in thymine, which is less efficiently repaired than the uracil resulting from deamination of unmethylated cytosine. This has resulted in depletion over time of CpGs in areas that are usually methylated.[36] Thus, the remaining dense clusters of CpGs, called CpG islands,[37] are presumed to be normally unmethylated. It is estimated that 40% of human genes contain such CpG islands in their promoter regions.[1]

In cancer, a profound disruption of DNA methylation is seen (see Fig. 7.2, top).[7–11] Global hypomethylation occurs, which has been proposed to occur very early during cancer development and results in a net loss of methyl-C. This is thought to contribute to carcinogenesis in two possible ways: the transcriptional activation of previously methylated sequences and the loss of chromosome stability. In contrast, the local hypermethylation at promoter CpG islands contributes to carcinogenesis through gene inactivation, silencing a wide variety of growth control and tumor suppressor genes, such as genes involved in growth, adhesion, apoptosis, cell cycle, differentiation, signaling, and transcription.

DNA methylation is by far the best-studied epigenetic change in many cancers, including lung cancer. This is, on the one hand, because promoter CpG island hypermethylation is linked to gene silencing, and such silencing is thought to play a key role in the development and progression of cancer. On the other hand, DNA methylation has been extensively analyzed because it promises to provide powerful molecular markers for lung cancer.[14,15,38] Importantly, straightforward techniques exist to assess this modification.[39] Initially, analysis strategies were based on a target gene approach, utilizing DNA methylation-sensitive restriction enzymes and polymerase chain reaction (PCR)-based methods that rely on bisulfite conversion. Bisulfite conversion, a chemical treatment that converts unmethylated cytosine to uracil while methylated cytosine is protected,[40] allows methylation information to be incorporated into the DNA sequence (otherwise it would be lost during PCR).

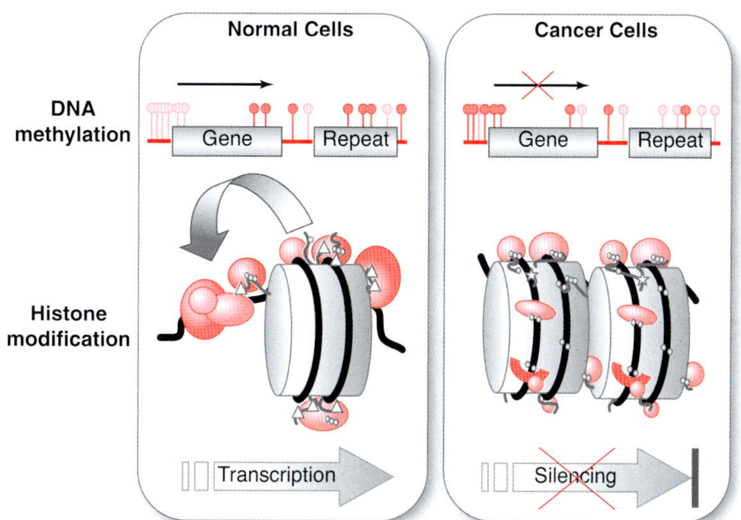

FIGURE 7.2 Epigenetic abnormalities in cancer. In nontumor cells **(left)**, CpG islands are generally unmethylated (*gray lollipops*), while sporadic CpGs are usually methylated (*black lollipops*). In actively transcribed genes, the structure of chromatin is loose, allowing access of the transcriptional machinery to the promoter region. Acetylation of lysines (*triangles*) in the N-terminal tails of histones 3 and 4 reduces positive charge and relaxes the attraction to negatively charged DNA. Acetylation, monomethylation, dimethylation, and trimethylation (*balls*) and other modifications such as phosphorylation and sumoylation (*stars*) of the histone tails can mediate interactions directly or indirectly with the transcriptional machinery and with enzymes that can add further posttranslational modifications. In cancer cells **(right)**, a genome-wide loss of DNA methylation at sporadic CpGs and previously methylated sequences such as repeats is seen. (In certain cases this can lead to gene activation, *not shown.*) Simultaneously, many promoter CpG islands become hypermethylated. This can result in silencing of tumor suppressor genes. Methyl-binding proteins interacting with methylated cytosines can recruit histone deacetylases, which can in turn lead to reduced chromatin access and transcriptional silencing. This model is a simplification; methylation, histone modification, and transcription are not always concordant—not all methylated genes are silenced, nor are all silent genes methylated.

Bisulfite-converted DNA can be analyzed by many methods, depending on the design and location of the PCR primers. The most common methods are bisulfite genomic sequencing, methylation-specific PCR (MSP), and its real-time version, MethyLight or its variation quantitative MSP (QMSP). Bisulfite genomic sequencing consists of amplification followed by cloning and sequencing and provides information on the methylation status of all the Cs on the same DNA strand in the amplified area.[41] MSP utilizes primers that cover a number of methylation sites,[42] allowing interrogation of one or more CpGs in a small area. MethyLight incorporates the inclusion of a fluorescent probe between the primers, enabling real-time PCR detection, and includes control reactions on fully methylated DNA (treated with *Sss*I enzyme), allowing quantitative measurement of methylation.[43,44] More recently, higher throughput and more genome-wide approaches have been developed, such as restriction landmark genomic scanning[45] and specific amplification/purification of methylated versus unmethylated DNA (using restriction enzymes[46] or binding enrichment)[47,48] followed by probing of microarrays. Expression profiling of cancer cell lines treated with demethylating drugs has also been used to identify DNA methylation-silenced genes (e.g., in non–small cell lung cancer [NSCLC]).[49] In the future, direct sequencing with high-throughput methods[23] using either methylation-enriched or bisulfite-treated DNA will be applied. Although reports based on these latter methods are beginning to be published,[50] these techniques are in their infancy and many technical hurdles remain. In addition, they are extremely costly. At this time, high-throughput bead-based PCR methods combine the best of both worlds in richness of data and affordability, allowing the reproducible and rapid interrogation of thousands of targeted loci (Illumina Inc., GoldenGate platform,).[51] This approach was successfully applied to lung adenocarcinoma (Table 7.1)[51] and has recently been further developed to provide close to genome-wide representation of CpG islands (Illumina Inc., Infinium platform). All of these methods have yielded a great amount of information on DNA methylation changes in many cancers including lung cancer. This knowledge, and further epigenomic profiling, promise to change the way in which lung cancer is detected and treated.

Effects of Hypomethylation in Lung Cancer Because an overall hypomethylation is observed in cancer cells, it had originally been assumed that the cancer-causing effect of methylation changes was based on loss of promoter CpG island methylation resulting in proto-oncogene activation.[52] Indeed, loss of methylation can lead to gene activation in lung cancer, although the activated genes are not necessarily considered canonical proto-oncogenes. One category of such genes is the parentally imprinted genes—genes for which either the maternally or paternally inherited allele is normally methylated. Hypomethylation can result in loss of imprinting, thereby contributing to cancer development; biallelic expression of the normally imprinted insulin-like growth factor 2, mesoderm-specific transcript and H19 genes has been seen in lung cancer and is thought to contribute to the carcinogenic phenotype.[53,54] Another type of gene that can be activated by hypomethylation is the family of testis-specific antigens—these genes are usually methylated and silent in all somatic tissues but the testes.[55] Expression of testis-specific antigens has been noted in many tumor types including lung cancer, and these antigens are seen as potential immunotherapy targets.[55–57] Loss of methylation of transposable elements and repeats is also observed in lung cancer[58] and can lead to mobility of such elements, causing further genetic damage.[11] In addition, read-through from such demethylated elements may result in the aberrant activation of neighboring genes. Hypomethylation might also play a role in the activation of microRNAs (miRNAs), many of which are deregulated in cancer.[59,60] In the lung, the normally methylated let-7a-3 miRNA was found to be hypomethylated in two out of eight lung adenocarcinomas and forced overexpression of this miRNA increased the oncogenic properties of lung cancer cell line A549.[61]

Besides contributing to carcinogenesis through gene activation, a second consequence of hypomethylation is thought to be genomic instability. Mice genetically engineered to underexpress DNA methyltransferases show an increased frequency of loss of heterozygosity and an elevated incidence of hematopoietic malignancies.[62] Inactivation of DNMT1 and DNMT3b in a human colorectal cancer cell line led to aneuploidy.[63] However, there appears to be little evidence that hypomethylation is severely deleterious in this way in lung cancer. A recent analysis of methylation of five human squamous cell lung carcinomas and normal matched tissue showed prominent hypomethylation of repetitive elements but little methylation loss in single-copy sequences.[58] This supports the notion that the effect of hypomethylation in lung cancer might be limited and that clinical benefits might be achieved with methylation-blocking therapies. Importantly, the leukemia-prone DNMT hypomorphic mice mentioned previously show a lower incidence of intestinal cancer, pointing to a protective effect of hypomethylation in certain tumor types.[64] Indeed, treatment of a mouse xenograft model for human lung cancer with DNA methylation and histone deacetylation inhibitors suppressed tumor growth without apparent toxicity.[65] A similar treatment of a murine lung cancer model cut lung tumor development in half, emphasizing the potential of epigenetic drugs for lung cancer treatment.[66]

HYPERMETHYLATION IN LUNG CANCER: APPLICATION TO MARKER DEVELOPMENT

Although it would appear that the effects of hypomethylation in lung cancer are modest, hypermethylation of promoter CpG islands is widely observed.[12–16,38] Hypermethylation is associated with transcriptional shutdown.[3] This could happen directly through steric interference of methylated cytosines with transcription factor and cofactor binding sites, or indirectly, through the attraction of methyl-binding proteins to the DNA, which in turn recruit HDAC enzymes and other epigenetic

TABLE 7.1 Epigenetic Profiling of DNA Methylation Loci in Lung Cancer

Method	Details[a]	Lung Cancer Type[b]	Promising Markers[c]	Reference
MethyLight	Examined 42 candidate loci from 304 prescreened markers. 8 show $p \leq 3 \times 10E\text{-}5$ T (n = 45) vs. AdjNTL (n = 45)	SQ	GDNF, MTHFR, OPCML, PAX8, PITX2, PTPRN2, TNFRSF25, TCF21 Top 8 marker panel shows 95.6% sensitivity and specificity on this sample population.	20
MethyLight	27 genes on 49 paired T and AdjNTL	NSCLC	BVES, CDKN2A, RARB, RASSF1, $p \leq 0.001$ T vs. AdjNTL	88
MethyLight	Out of a prescreen of over 100 loci, 28 were chosen for evaluation, 7 show $p < 0.0001$ in 51T vs. 38AdjNTL	AD	CDH13, CDKN2A EX2, CDX2, HOXA1, OPCML, RASSF1, SFPR1, TWIST1 Top 4 marker panel CDKN2A EX2, CDX2, HOXA1 and OPCML detects cancer with 94% sensitivity and 90% specificity	19
Restriction landmark genomic scanning (RLGS)	Analyzed 1184 CpG islands in 16 NSCLC	NSCLC	GNAL and IPF1 methylated in 8/16 NSCLC	86
MALDI-TOF mass spectrometry analysis of bisulfite-treated, PCRed DNA	47 gene promoter regions in 96 T with matched AdjNTL	AD, SQ	GAGED2, MGP, RASSF1, SDK2, SERPINB5, TNA, all $p < 10E\text{-}6$ in tumor vs. matched AdjNTL, identify T vs. AdjNTL with 95% sensitivity and specificity	75
Examined genes differentially expressed in fetal vs. adult lung	Studied a subset of 453 differentially expressed genes in 12 AD+3SQ vs. 5 normal adult lung samples	AD, SQ	MEOX2 is hypermethylated in 14/15 lung cancers	87
5-aza-dC/ expression microarray	132 genes induced by 5-aza-dC, 31 methylated, top 8 analyzed in 20 T vs. 20 AdjNTL lung	NSCLC	Three most promising genes: LOX, BNC1, CTSZ methylated in 19, 18, 10 of 20 tumors vs. 4, 3, 0 of 20 nontumor lung	49
Microarray-based approach	245 CpG positions in 59 candidate genes in 26 SQ, 22 AD, 26 AdjNTL	AD, SQ	SQ: ARHI, GP1BB, MGMT, RARB, and TMEFF2 AD: TMEFF2, MGMT, and CDKNIC	89
Methylation-sensitive restriction enzymes/ microarray	Lung cancer cell lines for MSRE/ microarray, chose subset of genes for testing in 22 LuCa T, 1 control lung	LuCa	ASC, PAX3 hypermethylated in 82%, 86% of lung tumors, respectively	90
Methylation-sensitive restriction enzymes/ microarray	Lung cancer cell lines, validation of two genes in 8AD, 8SQ, 5 SCLC	LuCa	CIDEB methylated in 15/21 lung cancers (71%)	91
MIRA/microarray	Purification of methylated DNA using methyl-binding domains followed by microarray hybridization	SQ	HOXA3, 5, 7, and 9 are more highly methylated in 4/4 T than AdjNTL	92
MIRA/microarray of 4 SQ vs. AdjNTL on partial genomic tiling arrays	4 SQ vs. AdjNTL on partial genomic tiling arrays, detailed analysis of gene subset on 20 SQ T and 20 AdjNTL	SQ	EVX2 (16/20), IRX2 (19/20), MEIS1 (17/20), MSX2 (19/20) NRE2E1 (20/20), OSR1 (20/20), OTX1 (20/20), PAX6 (17/20), ONECUT2 (14/20), TFAP2A (19/20), ZNF577 (18/20)	58
Illumina GoldenGate	Screened 1536 CpG sites in 371 genes, identified 55-gene panel that is 92% sensitive and 100% specific on 12 AD and 12 matched AdjNTL	AD	Eight markers examined in detail by bisulfite genomic sequencing, all hypermethylated in 4/4 tumors vs. 2 normal lung samples *ASCL2*, *CDH13*, *HOXA11*, *HOXA5*, *NPY*, *RUNX3*, *TERT*, and *TP73*	51

[a] T, tumor; AdjNTL, adjacent nontumor lung.

[b] AD, adenocarcinoma; LuCa, mix of lung cancer types or no type specified; NSCLC, non–small cell lung cancer; SQ, squamous cell lung cancer.

[c] Human Genome Organization name used unless none is available. Sensitivity and specificity numbers based on tumor tissues, not remote media.

modifiers (see Fig. 7.2).[67] In lung cancer, hundreds of studies have been devoted to the characterization of hypermethylation events. One of the driving forces behind this research is the desire to identify DNA methylation markers for early lung cancer detection.[14,15,38] DNA hypermethylation analyses could yield powerful candidate markers for lung cancer because only a small region of each gene needs to be interrogated, and DNA is a PCR-amplifiable substance that can be detected in bodily fluids.[14,15,38] Successful development of markers for cancer is a long process that should culminate in a randomized case-control study that demonstrates a reduction in mortality.[68] The process for the development of DNA methylation loci into markers for early lung cancer detection is diagrammed in the right panel of Figure 7.3.

Most DNA methylation studies in lung cancer have focused on NSCLC, which makes up about 85% of all lung cancers. Small cell lung cancer, a very aggressive cancer with poor survival, is considered by many to be a poor candidate for the development of early detection molecular makers due to the rapid progression of the disease. In contrast, NSCLC patients, which include the major groups adenocarcinoma (~40%), squamous cell carcinoma (~30%), large cell carcinoma (~10%), and miscellaneous other histological subtypes such as carcinoids and neuroendocrine cancers (~5%),[69] could benefit importantly if cancers that would normally lead to death could be detected at an early stage.[70] A comparison of methylation profiles of SCLC and NSCLC cell lines and tumors indicates that hypermethylation profiles are distinct for these two groups.[71–73] Not surprisingly, differences between hypermethylation profiles of NSCLC histological subtypes have also been observed,[15,20,72,74–77] meshing with other molecular and clinicopathological differences found in these tumor types.[78–81] This suggests that a panel of DNA methylation markers would be optimal, and that this panel should include pan-lung cancer markers as well as ones for distinct histological subtypes. Indeed, a panel of markers would be needed even for a single subtype because penetrance of molecular changes in cancer is usually less than 100%; it would be unexpected to find one marker with very high sensitivity and specificity.[20,74]

The first step in molecular marker development is the identification of promising candidate markers.[68] In the case of DNA methylation markers for lung cancer, it is of high priority to identify frequently methylated genes or loci (we refer to the CpG island section we are probing as a *locus*, because a given gene can be probed in multiple areas within a single or multiple CpG islands). These loci should also show substantially increased methylation levels over those found in healthy tissues. Thus, the initial focus should be on penetrance and DNA methylation levels. Because even noncancerous lung tissue from long-term smokers may have accumulated substantial methylation caused by age and environmental exposure,[77,82–85] many labs, including ours, have chosen to compare cancer tissues to this type of "high-background" control tissue (referred to here as adjacent nontumor lung [AdjNTL]) (Table 7.1). This ensures that identified hypermethylation markers are indeed cancer-specific and not merely indicative of environmental exposure. (Comparison to healthy lung from nonsmokers would be of use for the development of risk markers or identification

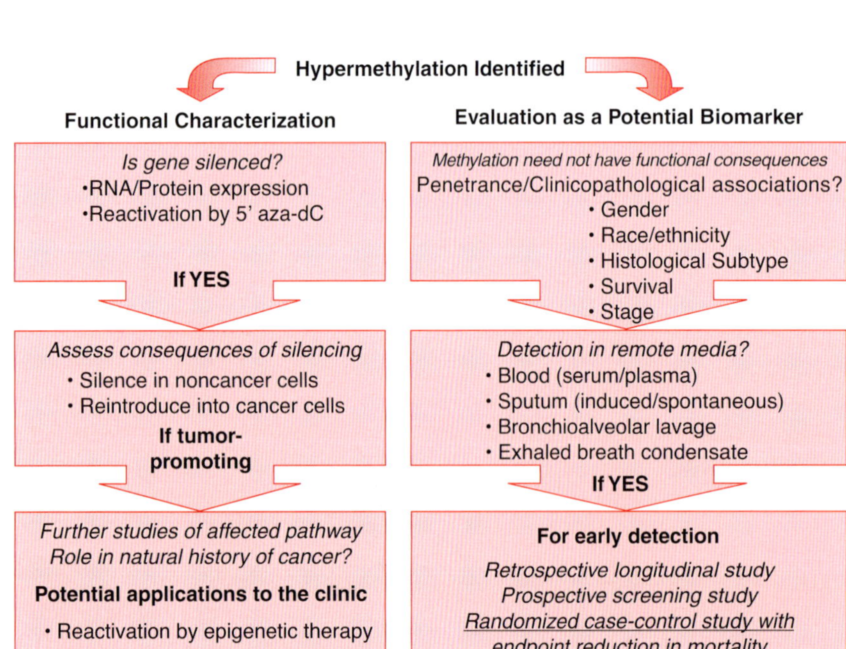

FIGURE 7.3 Schematic outlining studies for functional characterization of gene hypermethylation **(left)** or for development of hypermethylated loci into lung cancer biomarkers **(right)**.

of candidates for chemoprevention treatments [perhaps even epigenetic ones], once these become available.)

Many of the genes studied early on did not show high methylation frequencies,[15] but more recent efforts by several groups to examine much larger collections of genes have yielded a number of panels that might deliver high sensitivity and specificity, based on the examination of tissues (Table 7.1).[20,49,51,58,74,75,86–92] Some these panels contain genes that were identified early on (such as CDKN2A/p16, MGMT, and RASSF1),[74,75,88] but many new loci have been added to the repertoire, including homeotic genes involved in development, such as members of the HOX and PAX families.[19,20,51,58,90,92] The latter group of methylated loci agrees with the observation that genes occupied in embryonic stem cells by transcriptionally repressive polycomb group complexes appear to be prone to methylation in cancer.[93] The significance of methylation of these genes is unclear, since it is thought that they may already have been silent in noncancerous lung, but their involvement hints at the potential role of stem cells in lung cancer development.[93] Whether the hypermethylation of potential DNA methylation markers is functional or not (i.e., leads to transcriptional silencing) is not relevant, as long as penetrance is high and hypermethylation is associated with the presence of cancer. Many of the marker panels in Table 7.1 must still be validated on independent tumor sets, and their ability to identify lung cancer independently of gender, histological subtype, racial/ethnic group, and/or stages of cancer must be further scrutinized (Fig. 7.3, right panel). Once that is accomplished, they can be taken to the next phase of marker development: clinical assay validation.[68] For these panels to function in early lung cancer detection, they must be detectable in patient remote media: bodily fluids that could carry methylated DNA molecules from the cancer and that could be sampled relatively noninvasively.

Detection of DNA Methylation Markers in Bodily Fluids Potential remote media for lung cancer detection are coughed-up sputum (spontaneously collected from smokers or induced in never-smokers or ex-smokers), blood (plasma or serum), bronchoalveolar lavage (BAL, a saline rinse that can be collected during bronchoscopy), bronchial brushings, and exhaled breath condensate (EBC, collected as condensation from breath using a cooling device).[38] DNA methylation markers have been detected in sputum, plasma, serum and BAL, and data from a large number of studies is summarized in Table 7.2 (the table was compiled with special attention to BAL studies, which have provided the most promising results to date; key results are indicated in bold). One problem with many studies is the lack of control subjects, which makes results difficult to interpret. In addition, some studies cite frequencies based on the number of methylation-positive remote samples found in patients in which the tumor is positive. Although this is helpful to determine the experimental sensitivity of the test, it does not provide a good estimate of clinical sensitivity.

There are no published reports of detection of DNA methylation markers in EBC, but microsatellite alterations and p53 mutations have been detected in this material when collected from lung cancer patients [94,95] While the microsatellite alterations in EBC matched those of the lung tumors, the p53 mutations detected in EBC and the corresponding lung cancer did not match.[95] Thus, the DNA in EBC may not be from the tumor, but might derive from elsewhere in the lung or the throat and mouth.[96] Similar concerns apply to sputum, with the added caveat that sputum is thought to provide samples of DNA and cells from central lung areas, and thus might favor detection of squamous lung cancer over the generally more peripherally located adenocarcinoma. In one sputum study, a high fraction of samples was positive for LAMC2 and SFRP1methylation when using nested MSP (in which a pre-amplification is incorporated to increase signal).[17] However, a very large fraction of the controls was also positive, perhaps related to the many amplification cycles.

Blood (plasma or serum) would be the easiest bodily fluid to obtain for screening, but analyses to date indicate the medium is not very sensitive (Table 7.2). In addition, DNA methylation signatures observed could arise from anywhere in the body. However, the new high-throughput DNA methylation profiling technologies might make it feasible to identify *lung cancer*–specific DNA methylation signatures. This would require the profiling of DNA methylation in all other common types of cancer, something that is ongoing in different laboratories. Any identified potential lung cancer–specific markers would need to be evaluated in other cancer types using standardized methods. Alternatively, the combination of blood-based methylation signatures with high-resolution imaging (LDSCT) might be sufficient to address the issue of organ of origin. It remains a question what size the tumor must be in order to shed sufficient DNA into the blood for remote detection.

Of the remote media tested, BAL appears the most promising, showing sensitivities for individual loci approaching 50% or higher. Combination of markers into panels will help boost sensitivity, as exemplified by studies of Grote and coworkers.[97,98] The finding that combined methylation analysis of CDKN2A and RARB detects lung cancer cases with a sensitivity of 69% and a specificity of 87% is highly encouraging.[98] Combination of APC, CDKN2A, and RASSF1 also showed promise, detecting 63% of central and 44% of peripheral cancers and exhibiting a very low background of 1/102 cases with benign lung disease.[97] Based on the detection of methylation in BAL from noncancer patients in a number of studies, it would be important to use quantitative measurements and to set a cutoff value for positive methylation.[97–100] The fact that the collection of lavage fluid can be directed to a particular area of the lung makes it especially suited to combine with imaging approaches. This, in addition to the promising results obtained to date, suggest that analysis of DNA methylation in BAL might be the key to early lung cancer detection.

Besides their use for early detection, DNA methylation markers identified in bodily fluids could be utilized for risk assessment and monitoring of recurrence. In the case of quantitative markers, cutoff values could be stratified to distinguish

TABLE 7.2 Detection of DNA Methylation Markers in Remote Media

Locus[a]	Remote Medium[b]	Fraction Methylated in Cases[c]	Fraction Methylated in Controls[d]	Method[e]	Reference
APC	Sputum	3/13	1/25	QMSP	138
	BAL	**89/155 (57%);** 14/85; 5/17[f]	**28/67 (42%);** 1/102; 0/10	All QMSP	97, 99, 139
	BAL	1/24	n.a.	MSP; QMSP	140
	Blood	42/89	n.a.	QMSP	141
ARF	BAL	0/31	0/10	QMSP	99
BHLHB5	Sputum	12/98	11/92	neMSP	17
CDH1	BAL	**13/27[f]**	**0/10** (with cutoff value)	QMSP	99
CDH13	Sputum	7/53 (survivors); 27/98	34/118; 23/92	All neMSP	142, 143
	Sputum	19/72		neMSP	143
	BAL	11/85	n.a.	MSP	144
	Blood	14/61; 21/63; 3/52	n.a.	QMSP;MSP;MSP	143, 145, 146
CDKN2A/p16	Sputum	39/98; 3/13; 1/29; 26/51; 19/53	25/92; 2/25; 20/112; 7/25; 30/118	neMSP;QMSP; MSP; MSSNuPE; neMSP	17, 101, 138, 142, 147
	Sputum	71/95; 11/11; 6/22; 29/72	n.a.	neMSP; neMSP; MSP; MSP	143, 148–150
	BAL	**18/75 (25%); 10/85 (12%); 26/51 (51%);** 1/7[f]	**0/64; 0/102; 7/25 (28%);** 0/10	QMSP; QMSP; MSSNuPE; QMSP	97–99, 101
	BAL	14/68; 4/17; 12/19[g]; 4/24; 14/85; 4/20; 4/14[h]	n.a.	MSP; MSP; MSP; MSP; QMSP; MSP; MSP; MSP	140, 144, 151–155
	Blood	11/44 Lung cancer survivors	16/121 (healthy smokers), 7/74 (nonsmokers)	neMSP	142
	Blood	1/10; 103/136; 16/61; 14/100; 3/9; 12/35; 77/105; 15/72; 24/63; 2/14[f]	n.a.	MSP: neMSP; QMSP; MSP; MSP; QMSP; neMSP; MSP; MSP	143, 145, 146, 148, 152, 155–158
COX2	BAL	6/20	n.a.	MSP	154
DAPK	Sputum	42/98; 25/53	30/92; 21/118	All neMSP	17, 142
	Sputum	22/72	n.a.	MSP	143
	BAL	14/68; 3/24; 3/20	n.a.	All MSP	140, 144, 151, 154
	Blood	10/100; 4/5; 7/72	n.a.	All MSP	143, 156, 157
FHIT	BAL	7/24; 19/85	n.a.	All MSP	140, 144
GATA4; GATA5	Sputum	48/98; 34/98	42/92; 26/92	neMSP	17, 14
	Sputum	31/72	n.a.	MSP	143
	BAL	19/85	n.a.	MSP	144
	Blood	20/63; 10/45	n.a.	Both MSP	143, 146
GSTP1	BAL	1/3[f]	0/10	QMSP	99
	Blood	1/2	n.a.	MSP	157
HLHP	Sputum	42/98	36/92	neMSP	17
HOXA9	Sputum	14/22	n.a.	MSP	150

TABLE 7.2 Detection of DNA Methylation Markers in Remote Media *(continued)*

Locus[a]	Remote Medium[b]	Fraction Methylated in Cases[c]	Fraction Methylated in Controls[d]	Method[e]	Reference
HS3ST2(3-OST-2)	Sputum	5/13	3/25	QMSP	138
IGFBP3	Sputum	25/98	30/92	neMSP	17
LAMC2	Sputum	72/98	70/92	neMSP	17
MAGEA1; MAGEB2	Sputum	11/22; 9/22	n.a.	MSP	150
MGMT	Sputum	19/53 (survivors); 23/98	17/118 (healthy smokers); 22/92	neMSP; neMSP	17, 142
	Sputum	7/11; 23/72;	n.a.	neMSP; MSP	143, 149
	BAL	7/12[f]	0/10 (with cutoff)	QMSP	99
	BAL	6/68; 3/24; 11/20	n.a.	All MSP	140, 151, 154
	Blood	17/100; 4/6; 4/72	n.a.	All MSP	143, 156, 157
MLH1	Sputum	9/21	n.a.	MSP	159
PAX5 alpha/beta	Sputum	Alpha: 21/53 (survivors); 29/98	Alpha: 14/118 (healthy smokers); 24/92	All neMSP	17, 142
		Beta: 13/53 (survivors); 41/98	Beta: 11/118 (healthy smokers); 32/92		
RARB	Sputum	8/29	58/118	MSP	147
	BAL	**42/75 (56%); 40/84 (48%)**; 0/3[f]	**8/64 (13%); 21/102 (21%)**; 0/10	All QMSP	97–99
	BAL	48/68; 13/85; 3/20	n.a.	All MSP	144, 151, 154
	Blood	6/100; 23/63	n.a.	MSP	146, 156
RASSF1	Sputum	13/53; 12/98; 5/13; 1/29	8/118; 6/92; 2/25; 1/112	neMSP; neMSP; neMSP; QMSP	17, 138, 142, 147
	Sputum	19/72	n.a.	MSP	143
	BAL	**72/157 (45%); 35/85 (41%)**; 4/14[f]	**0/46; 0/102**; 0/10	All QMSP	97, 99, 160
	BAL	15/85; 6/20	n.a.	All MSP	144, 154
	Blood	10/12; 11/100; 7/72; 23/75; 24/63	n.a.	All MSP	143, 146, 156, 161, 162
SEMA3B	BAL	0/75	0/64	QMSP	98
SFRP1	Sputum	68/98	71/92	neMSP	17
SOCS1	BAL	6/20	n.a.	MSP	154
TCF21	Sputum	7/13	0/25	QMSP	163

[a]Human genome organization name used unless none available, the 5′ CpG island of RASSF1 was analyzed, referred to as RASSF1A in the literature.

[b]Blood includes serum and plasma. Bronchial brushing studies, which are very rare and not especially informative, are not listed. There are no reports of DNA methylation detection in EBC. This table lists many studies of blood and sputum but may not be comprehensive; however, due to its highly promising nature, all published BAL studies are included. Separate rows are listed for each locus for studies with and without controls.

[c]Compelling data are highlighted in bold, % methylation is listed only in a few very promising cases.

[d]Order of data matches that in previous column. Compelling data are highlighted in bold, % methylation is listed only in a few very promising cases. n.a. indicates no controls are available.

[e]Order of data matches that of data in previous two columns, *all* indicates that the same procedure was used in all cases. MSP, methylation-specific PCR; QMSP, any form of quantitative MSP; neMSP, nested MSP preceded by a preamplification step; MSSNuPE, methylation-specific single nucleotide primer extension.

[f]In this report, only BAL from tumors positive for methylation was assessed, the total number of tumor cases was 31.

[g]Out of the 19/50 patients with methylation in their tumors.

[h]Out of the 14 of 33 patients with methylation in their tumors.

between methylation detected in normal tissue from nonsmokers, histologically normal tissue of cases prior to diagnosis, lung cancer, or recurring lung cancer. Several studies have shown that methylation can be detected long before the cancer becomes clinically apparent.[101–103] However, as noted previously, the sensitivity of the least invasive approaches (sputum, blood) has not been high, and use of BAL would require bronchoscopy, a semi-invasive procedure.

Functional Implications of DNA Hypermethylation

For the purposes of early detection, the functional consequences of hypermethylation are not important. However, for the purposes of prognostication or providing tailored therapies, whether observed DNA methylation events have functional consequences could be of highly relevant. This idea is supported by the prognostic utility of expression arrays.[104] Figure 7.3 (left panel) outlines the approach to determine whether promoter CpG island hypermethylation of a gene is functionally significant. After lack of expression has been verified by mRNA and/or protein analysis, 5′aza-deoxycytidine treatment of cell lines can be used to determine if the gene can be reactivated by demethylation. A potential caveat of such experiments is that reactivation could be the indirect consequence of demethylation of other genes. Next, reexpression of the gene in cancer cells in which the gene was silenced, and silencing (e.g., through targeted RNAi transfection) of the gene in cells in which the gene is still expressed will help determine the role of the gene in cancer development and progression. In the silencing experiment, the choice of cells is important (primary, immortalized, transformed) and should be influenced by the perceived stage of cancer development at which the gene of interest is thought to play a role. Experiments such as these have implicated a variety of hypermethylated genes in lung cancer.[12,13,15,38,105] It should be noted that methylation of genes that were already silent in lung tissue might not be a functional event per se, but might still be informative, as it could provide hints to the origin of the cancer or the involvement of stem cells.[93]

Genes that appear to be silenced by methylation and that limit any aspect of the transformed phenotype when reactivated can be excellent tools for prognostication or targets for therapy; the testing of associations between clinical data and DNA methylation status in patient populations could provide markers for survival or response to therapy. In addition, the silenced genes could point to the involvement of molecular pathways that might be targeted by new drug therapies. An important caveat of studies of associations between DNA methylation and clinicopathological variables is that a correction should be applied for multiple hypothesis testing when multiple new loci and clinical parameters are examined.[106]

Although many genes/loci silenced in lung cancer by DNA methylation have been studied to date, only a handful have been analyzed in depth. The most intensive focus has been on CDKN2A/p16, a gene encoding an inhibitor of cyclin-dependent kinases 4 and 6, which in turn bind to cyclin D1 and promote the phosphorylation and inactivation of the retinoblastoma gene product, RB. RB is a key cell cycle regulator that is frequently inactivated in SCLC.[25] In contrast in NSCLC, it is CDKN2A that is inactivated in the majority of tumors, and in many cases, this occurs through promoter hypermethylation.[14,15,107,108] Methylation of the CDKN2A promoter CpG island appears to be a very early change in the development of squamous cell lung cancer as well as adenocarinoma.[16,102,109] In a cohort of high-risk long-term smokers from whom sputum was examined for seven DNA methylation markers, hypermethylation of CDKN2A was most strongly associated with lung cancer risk.[17] These observations are consistent with the idea that disruption of cell cycle regulation is an important early event in the transition from normalcy to cancer, an observation that is emphasized by the fact that human bronchial epithelial (HBE) cells can be immortalized through CDK4 activation in combination with overexpression of telomerase.[110] It is intriguing that in NSCLC, the CDKN2A promoter CpG island appears to be the weak link in the regulatory pathway, and it is tempting to speculate that this might be linked to occupancy of this region by polycomb complexes in stem cells.[111] Methylation of the gene appears to become more pronounced during progression[109] and is associated with an unfavorable prognosis in lung adenocarcinoma.[112] These observations fit well with a recent report exploring the potential link between methylation of several genes and risk of progression in stage I NSCLC.[18] In this study, 51 patients with stage I NSCLC who had a recurrence within 40 months after surgery were matched for age, sex, surgery date, and stage with 116 patients who did not have a recurrence. The odds ratio for recurrence was found to be significantly elevated when CDKN2A was methylated in the tumor, regional nodes (N1) or mediastinal (N2) nodes of the patients, or when CDH13 was methylated in the mediastinal nodes. Combination of CDKN2A and CDH13 methylation in the tumor and mediastinal lymph nodes was associated with an odds ratio of recurrent cancer of 15. In a separate validation set of 20 cases, the authors observed an association between methylation of CDKN2A and CDH13 (individually as well as together) in regional nodes, with an odds ratio for recurrence of 8 for methylation of each gene alone, and of 19 when both genes were methylated. These compelling results indicate that methylation profiling may have important applications in prognostication (Fig. 7.4).

One caveat with the design of studies of this kind is potential confounding factors, such as tumor size. If a range is used to categorize tumor size (e.g., $\leq$3 cm), the distribution of tumor sizes within this range may not be equal for cases (showing recurrence) and controls (no recurrence). Since the actual size of the tumor may be a key factor in progression, it would be important to examine this variable closely in relation to methylation.

A second gene that has been extensively studied in DNA methylation analysis is MGMT.[14,15] Mentioned previously as a target of epigenetic regulation that could promote further genetic changes, this DNA repair gene appears to be another hot spot for early methylation, showing increasing methylation as cells progress from a field defect to hyperplasia, and

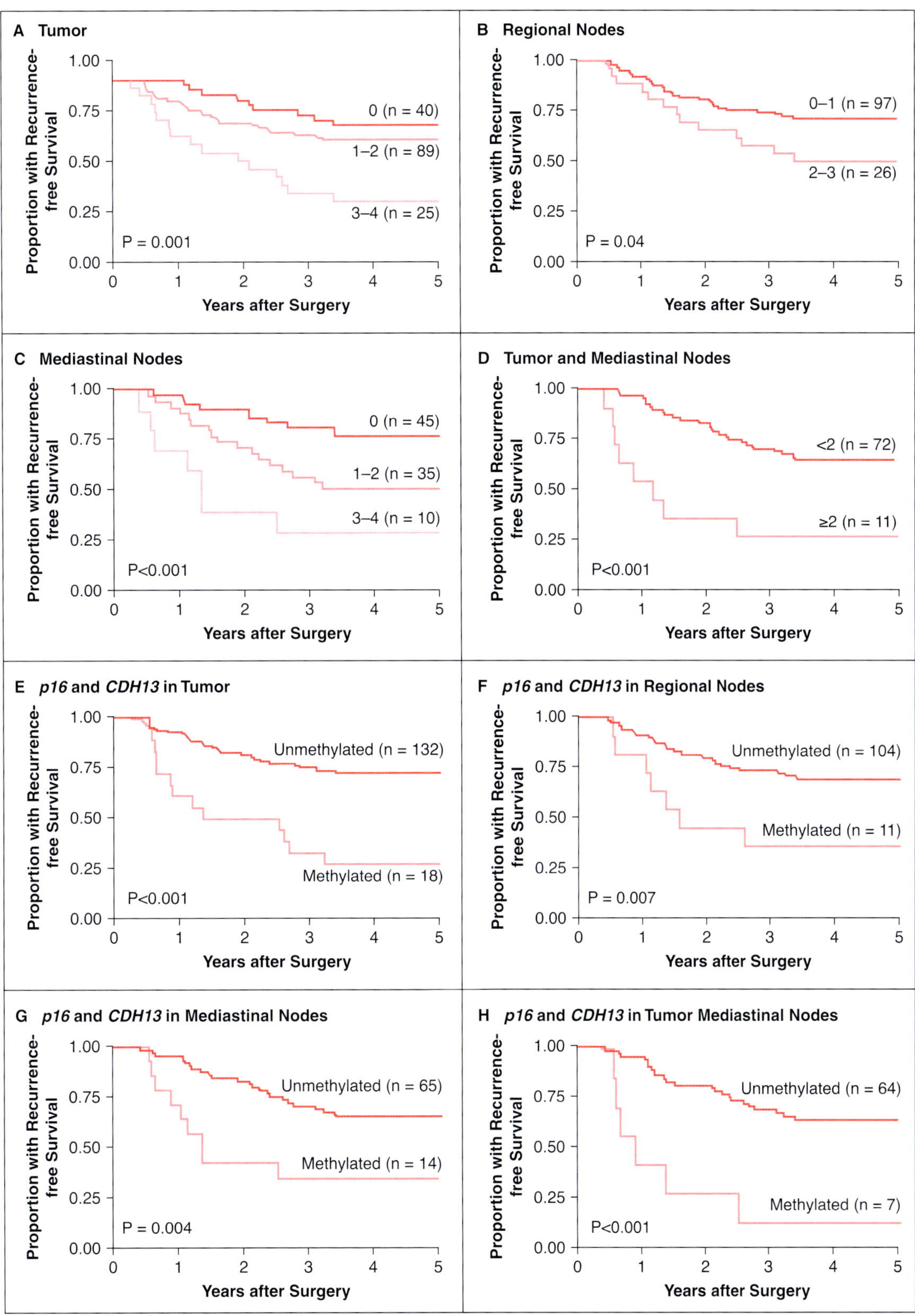

FIGURE 7.4 Kaplan-Meier estimates of recurrence-free survival among 167 case patients and controls with stage I non–small cell lung cancer from the original cohort, according to the site and number or presence or absence of methylated genes. Data are reported for a four-gene panel consisting of the cyclin-dependent kinase inhibitor 2A gene p16, the H-cadherin gene CDH13, the Ras association domain family 1 gene RASSF1A, and the adenomatous polyposis coli gene APC. In all three types of tissue, the recurrence-free survival rates decrease with an increasing number of methylated genes (**A,B,C**) and when certain genes are methylated (**E,F,G**). This same effect on recurrence-free survival is evident when the tumor and mediastinal lymph nodes are considered together (**D,H**). (From Brock MV, Hooker CM, Ota-Machida E, et al. DNA methylation markers and early recurrence in stage I lung cancer. *N Engl J Med* 2008;358:1118–1128.)

further to adenocarcinoma.[16,109] Interestingly, methylation was also found to be associated with tumor progression and poor survival.[113,114] Conflicting reports about the preferential methylation of MGMT in smokers[115] versus nonsmokers have been made.[113]

Of the genes listed in Table 7.2 as potential DNA methylation markers in lung cancer, RARB is one of the two most promising because it is frequently detected in BAL of cancer cases. This gene encodes the retinoic acid receptor beta. Retinoids, vitamin A, and its analogs, play important roles in development, differentiation, proliferation, and apoptosis.[116] Retinoids have been considered strong candidates for chemoprevention of lung cancer,[116] an idea that makes sense considering the hypermethylation of RARB (Table 7.1). Unfortunately, the outcome of retinoid chemoprevention clinical trials was an increase rather than decrease in the risk of lung cancer.[117] Nevertheless, in vitro experiments suggest that retinoic acid can prevent the oncogenic transformation of immortalized HBE cells.[118] Hypermethylation of RARB was linked with retinoic acid resistance in an HBE cell line and treatment with DNA methylation inhibitor azacitidine restored the cells' ability to respond to retinoic acid.[119] Like methylation of MGMT, RARB hypermethylation appears to be an early event in lung adenocarcinoma development, showing low but detectable levels in adjacent lung and increasing methylation in hyperplasia and adenocarcinoma.[109,120]

Similarly to MGMT and RARB, RASSF1 methylation occurs early, showing a progression in frequency of methylation from the surrounding histologically normal tissue of a tumor, to hyperplasia and to lung adenocarcinoma.[109] RASSF1 methylation is frequently detectable in BAL and appears to be the most specific marker examined in BAL to date (Table 7.2). The gene encodes a putative RAS effector protein.[121] It lies on chromosome 3p21, in an area of common loss of heterozygosity in lung cancer, and is frequently methylated in human malignancies including lung cancer (Table 7.2).[14,15,121] The gene has alternative first exons, alpha and gamma, each with a CpG island. The upstream island (RASSF1A) is hypermethylated in lung cancer, and its methylation is strongly correlated with expression of the delta subfamily of the DNA methyltransferase 3B.[35] This DNMT3B subfamily consists of at least seven splice variants. Knockdown of DNMT3B4 in lung cancer cell lines resulted in reactivation of the RASSF1A but not the CDKN2A promoter, implying that DNMT3B isoforms could be involved in initiating promoter-specific DNA methylation. RASSF1A methylation is suggested to correlate with a poor prognosis, although this observation should be confirmed by an independent study.[122]

Besides CDKN2A, MGMT, RARB, and RASSF1, there are many other genes that could be of interest, functionally or therapeutically. Three genes worth mentioning briefly are CDH13, OPCML, and miRNA-29 (miR-29). As mentioned previously, hypermethylation of CDH13, encoding the cell adhesion molecule heart cadherin, was associated with increased risk of recurrence.[18] OPCML, encoding an opioid-binding cell adhesion molecule-like, had been pegged as a suspected tumor suppressor gene many years ago by Maneckjee and Minna[123] based on the apoptotic response of lung cancer cell lines to opioids, which antagonized the growth stimulatory effect of nicotine. The frequent and high methylation of OPCML in both adenocarcinoma and squamous cell lung cancer suggests that it might function as a pan-lung cancer marker.[19,20] The miR-29 family of three RNAs is an example of miRNAs that are silenced by hypermethylation in lung cancer (in contrast to the activated let-7a-3 mentioned earlier).[124] Expression of these RNAs is inversely correlated with DNMT3a and 3b in lung cancer, which appears to be mediated by targeting of miR-29 to the 3′ untranslated regions of the methyltransferase mRNAs. Reactivation of miR-29 could be one way in which methyltransferase expression and tumorigenic potential of lung cancer cells could be mitigated, as illustrated by the reduced tumor growth in nude mice of A549 lung cancer cells transfected with miR-29.[124]

From the data described previously, it is clear that progress is being made in understanding the functional consequences and clinical implications of DNA hypermethylation. However, much work remains to be done to independently verify observations before they can lead to clinical implementation (such as treatment decisions based on methylation profiles). The general reversal of methylation is already a clinical target though, with numerous drugs that counteract DNA methylation under development and a number of them in clinical trials (see later in this chapter).[21]

Histone Modifications and Their Role in Lung Cancer The link between DNA methylation and chromatin structure is formed by proteins that bind directly or indirectly to methylated DNA and modify the flexible histone N-termini (Fig. 7.2). The nucleosomal core around which DNA is coiled is composed of two molecules each of histones 2A, 2B, 3, and 4. The lysine and arginine-rich N-terminal regions extend from the core and can be heavily decorated with monomethylation, dimethylation, and trimethylation, acetylation, ubiquitination, phosphorylation, and other modifications.[5,125] These modifications do not exist in isolation; functional and physical cross talk ensures a complex web of epigenetic signals, in which DNA methyltransferases, methyl-binding proteins, histone variants, histone-modifying enzymes, and other chromatin and transcriptional components play a role (Fig. 7.2).[126] Many of the enzymes that modify histones recognize other modifications on the same or different histone tails, or on DNA. For example, proteins that bind to methylated DNA frequently carry additional domains that interact directly or indirectly with histone-modifying proteins, such as deacetylases.[67] Acetylation of histones on lysine promotes active transcription. On the one hand, this modification reduces positive charge and minimizes the electrostatic attraction of the histone tails for the DNA phosphate backbone, thereby relaxing chromatin structure. In addition, acetylated histone N-terminal tails are landing pads for bromodomain-containing proteins, such as transcriptional coactivator p300/CBP associated factor and TAF1, a component of the transcription initiation complex.[5] Multiple enzymes that add or remove acetyl groups exist in the cell. In contrast to acetylation, methylation does not affect histone tail charge, functioning by altering protein/protein interactions. One or two methyl groups can be added to arginine and up to three to lysine; the effects depend on the modified position and the number of added methyl groups. For example, histone 3 lysine 9 and lysine 27 trimethylation (H3K9me3, H3K27me3) are repressive marks, while histone 3 lysine 4 trimethylation is found in transcribed regions.

In contrast to the abundance of information about DNA methylation in lung cancer, relatively little is known about how histone modification is affected; molecular changes on the histone N-terminal regions are much more difficult to interrogate in comparison to DNA methylation. The most commonly used technique is formaldehyde cross-linking followed by specific immunoprecipitation of particular histone modifications and PCR-based or global (e.g., microarray, high-throughput sequencing) characterization of the coprecipitated DNA sequences. One recent study classified NSCLC patients into seven distinct groups based on differential histone modifications and observed differences in survival depending on histology and histone 3 modifications.[127] This early study hints at the potential use of this kind of epigenetic characterization to guide treatment.

EPIGENETIC THERAPY FOR LUNG CANCER

Much more widely studied than the modifications themselves are the enzymes that mediate the decorations of histone tails. The ability to inhibit HDACs, enzymes that are thought to be involved in inappropriate gene repression in cancer, has given rise to a flurry of drug development and preclinical studies using lung cancer cell lines.[21,128] Many studies report inhibition of growth and induction of apoptosis by HDACI, and these drugs are being used in phase I and II in clinical trials.[129,130] Although gene reactivation is observed in many cases, it is not clear whether this is an effect of deacetylase inhibitors on histone tails or on other proteins that are acetylated, such as heat shock protein 90 (HSP90).[129] HDACI LBH589 increased HSP90 acetylation in lung cancer cells, thereby decreasing HSP90 protein chaperone ability, an activity that helps EGFR mutant proteins maintain functionality.[131] The exciting link in lung cancer between EGFR signaling and histone deacetylation has been confirmed by several studies[132–134] and supports the evaluation of combinations of drugs that target deacetylation and tyrosine kinases in clinical trials. Of additional interest is the profiling of lung cancer cells to identify genes that modulate sensitivity to HDACIs[135] and the combination of standard therapies such as radiation treatment with HDACIs—approaches that show promise in preclinical models.[136]

One type of drug that forms a logical combination with HDACIs is DNA methylation inhibitors. A variety of different DNA methyltransferase inhibitors that work through different mechanisms is available.[21] Because some of these DNA methyltransferase inhibitors, such as 5-aza-deoxycytidine work through incorporation into the DNA (where DNA methyltransferases are consequently trapped), their efficacy may be partially related to DNA damage.[21] One study of human lung cancer cells treated with 5-axa-deoxycytidine and HDACI indicated that the synergy with HDACIs was related to DNA damage rather than inhibition of DNA methylation.[137] Despite our incomplete understanding of the mechanism of epigenetic therapy, its clinical promise is high, and phase I and II trials in lung cancer are ongoing (see http://www.clinicaltrials.gov/).[22,129,130]

CONCLUSION

Powerful tools are being honed for the (epi)genomic analysis of lung cancer, and these will rapidly increase our understanding of its molecular underpinnings, as well as provide molecular markers for detection, diagnosis, prognostication, and monitoring of recurrence. A key area that will require rapid development to make the most of these technologies is bioinformatics, since the staggering amount of data generated must be analyzed and interpreted. The combination of new (epi)genetic insights, novel epigenetic drugs, and an emerging understanding of how these and other drugs function has generated an aura of hope and excitement in the lung cancer field. The possibility to build on existing therapies such as EGFR inhibitors or radiation treatment by combining them with HDACI and DNA methylation inhibitors opens many new therapeutic avenues. With progress looming on the fronts of early detection as well as treatment, it can truly be said that epigenetics has given new breath to the fight against lung cancer.

ACKNOWLEDGMENTS: *I am grateful to M. Kazarian and P. P. Anglim for reviewing the manuscript. Work in the Laird-Offringa lab is supported by NIH/NCI grants R21 102247, R01 CA120689, R01 CA119029; the Whittier Foundation; the Kazan, McClain, Abrams, Fernandez, Lyons & Farrise Foundation; Paul and Michelle Zygielbaum; Joan's Legacy; the Hoag Family Foundation; the Canary Foundation; and the Thomas G. Labrecque Foundation. The Laird-Offringa lab does not accept any money from the tobacco industry. The content of this chapter is solely the responsibility of the author and does not necessarily represent the official views of the funding agencies. I have no conflicts of interest to declare.*

REFERENCES

1. Lander ES, Linton LM, Birren B, et al. Initial sequencing and analysis of the human genome. *Nature* 2001;409:860–921.
2. Gosden RG, Feinberg AP. Genetics and epigenetics—nature's pen-and-pencil set. *N Engl J Med* 2007;356:731–733.
3. Jaenisch R, Bird A. Epigenetic regulation of gene expression: how the genome integrates intrinsic and environmental signals. *Nat Genet* 2003;33(suppl):245–54.
4. Wang Z, Zang C, Rosenfeld JA, et al. Combinatorial patterns of histone acetylations and methylations in the human genome. *Nat Genet* 2008;40:897–903.
5. Taverna SD, Li H, Ruthenburg AJ, et al. How chromatin-binding modules interpret histone modifications: Lessons from professional pocket pickers. *Nat Struct Mol Biol* 2007;14:1025–1040.

6. Klose RJ, Bird AP. Genomic DNA methylation: the mark and its mediators. *Trends Biochem Sci* 2006;31:89–97.
7. Jones PA, Baylin SB. The epigenomics of cancer. *Cell* 2007;128:683–692.
8. Gal-Yam EN, Saito Y, Egger G, et al. Cancer epigenetics: modifications, screening, and therapy. *Annu Rev Med* 2008;59:267–280.
9. Laird PW. Cancer epigenetics. *Hum Mol Genet* 2005;14 Spec No 1: R65–R76.
10. Grønbaek K, Hother C, Jones PA. Epigenetic changes in cancer. *APMIS* 2007;115:1039–1059.
11. Esteller M. Epigenetics in cancer. *N Engl J Med* 2008;358:1148–1159.
12. Bowman RV, Yang IA, Semmler AB, et al. Epigenetics of lung cancer. *Respirology* 2006;11:355–365.
13. Risch A, Plass C. Lung cancer epigenetics and genetics. *Int J Cancer* 2008;123:1–7.
14. Belinsky SA. Gene-promoter hypermethylation as a biomarker in lung cancer. *Nat Rev Cancer* 2004;4:707–717.
15. Tsou JA, Hagen JA, Carpenter CL, et al. DNA methylation analysis: a powerful new tool for lung cancer diagnosis. *Oncogene* 2002;21:5450–5461.
16. Kerr KM, Galler JS, Hagen JA, et al. The role of DNA methylation in the development and progression of lung adenocarcinoma. *Dis Markers* 2007;23:5–30.
17. Belinsky SA, Liechty KC, Gentry FD, et al. Promoter hypermethylation of multiple genes in sputum precedes lung cancer incidence in a high-risk cohort. *Cancer Res* 2006;66:3338–3344.
18. Brock MV, Hooker CM, Ota-Machida E, et al. DNA methylation markers and early recurrence in stage I lung cancer. *N Engl J Med* 2008;358:1118–1128.
19. Tsou JA, Galler JS, Siegmund KD, et al. Identification of a panel of sensitive and specific DNA methylation markers for lung adenocarcinoma. *Mol Cancer* 2007;6:70.
20. Anglim PA, Galler JS, Koss MN, et al. Identification of a panel of sensitive and specific DNA methylation markers for squamous cell lung cancer. *Mol Cancer* 2008;7:62.
21. Yoo CB, Jones PA. Epigenetic therapy of cancer: past, present, and future. *Nat Rev Drug Discov* 2006;5:37–50.
22. Smith LT, Otterson GA, Plass C. Unraveling the epigenetic code of cancer for therapy. *Trends Genet* 2007;23:449–456.
23. Wold B, Myers RM. Sequence census methods for functional genomics. *Nat Methods* 2008;5:19–21.
24. Sekido Y, Fong KM, Minna JD. Molecular genetics of lung cancer. *Annu Rev Med* 2003;54:73–87.
25. Zochbauer-Muller S, Gazdar AF, Minna JD. Molecular pathogenesis of lung cancer. *Annu Rev Physiol* 2002;64:681–708.
26. Brena RM, Costello JF. Genome-epigenome interactions in cancer. *Hum Mol Genet* 2007;16 Spec No 1:R96–R105.
27. Miremadi A, Oestergaard MZ, Pharoah PD, et al. Cancer genetics of epigenetic genes. *Hum Mol Genet* 2007;16 Spec No 1:R28–R49.
28. Patra SK. Ras regulation of DNA-methylation and cancer. *Exp Cell Res* 2008;314:1193–1201.
29. Povey AC, Margison GP, Santibáñez-Koref MF. Lung cancer risk and variation in MGMT activity and sequence. *DNA Repair* (Amst) 2007;6:1134–1144.
30. Crosbie PA, McGown G, Thorncroft MR, et al. Association between lung cancer risk and single nucleotide polymorphisms in the first intron and codon 178 of the DNA repair gene, o6-alkylguanine-DNA alkyltransferase. *Int J Cancer* 2008;122:791–795.
31. Zienolddiny S, Campa D, Lind H, et al. Polymorphisms of DNA repair genes and risk of non-small cell lung cancer. *Carcinogenesis* 2006;27:560–567.
32. Chen T, Li E. Establishment and maintenance of DNA methylation patterns in mammals. *Curr Top Microbiol Immunol* 2006;301:179–201.
33. Chen T, Li E. Structure and function of eukaryotic DNA methyltransferases. *Curr Top Dev Biol* 2004;60:55–89.
34. Linhart HG, Lin H, Yamada Y, et al. DNMT3B promotes tumorigenesis in vivo by gene-specific de novo methylation and transcriptional silencing. *Genes Dev* 2007;21:3110–3122.
35. Wang J, Bhutani M, Pathak AK, et al. Delta DNMT3B variants regulate DNA methylation in a promoter-specific manner. *Cancer Res* 2007;67:10647–10652.
36. Pfeifer GP. Mutagenesis at methylated CpG sequences. *Curr Top Microbiol Immunol* 2006;301:259–281.
37. Takai D, Jones PA. Comprehensive analysis of CpG islands in the human chromosomes 21 and 22. *Proc Natl Acad Sci USA* 2002;99:3740–3745.
38. Anglim PP, Alonzo TT, Laird-Offringa IA. DNA methylation-based biomarkers for early detection of non-small cell lung cancer: An update. *Mol Cancer* 2008;23:81.
39. Laird PW. The power and the promise of DNA methylation markers. *Nat Rev Cancer* 2003;3:253–266.
40. Olek A, Oswald J, Walter J. A modified and improved method for bisulphite based cytosine methylation analysis. *Nucleic Acids Res* 1996;24:5064–5066.
41. Frommer M, McDonald LE, Millar DS, et al. A genomic sequencing protocol that yields a positive display of 5-methylcytosine residues in individual DNA strands. *Proc Natl Acad Sci USA* 1992;89:1827–1831.
42. Herman JG, Graff JR, Myöhänen S, Nelkin BD, et al. Methylation-specific pcr: a novel pcr assay for methylation status of CpG islands. *Proc Natl Acad Sci USA* 1996;93:9821–9826.
43. Trinh BN, Long TI, Laird PW. DNA methylation analysis by MethyLight technology. *Methods* 2001;25:456–462.
44. Eads CA, Danenberg KD, Kawakami K, et al. Methylight: a high-throughput assay to measure DNA methylation. *Nucleic Acids Res* 2000;28:E32.
45. Costello JC, Fruhwald MC, Smiraglia DJ, et al. Aberrant CpG-island methylation has non-random and tumor-type-specific patterns. *Nature Genet* 2000;25:132–138.
46. Huang TH, Perry MR, Laux DE. Methylation profiling of CpG islands in human breast cancer cells. *Hum Mol Genet* 1999;8:459–470.
47. Rauch T, Li H, Wu X, et al. Mira-assisted microarray analysis, a new technology for the determination of DNA methylation patterns, identifies frequent methylation of homeodomain-containing genes in lung cancer cells. *Cancer Res* 2006;66:7939–7947.
48. Weber M, Davies JJ, Wittig D, et al. Chromosome-wide and promoter-specific analyses identify sites of differential DNA methylation in normal and transformed human cells. *Nat Genet* 2005;37:853–862.
49. Shames DS, Girard L, Gao B, et al. A genome-wide screen for promoter methylation in lung cancer identifies novel methylation markers for multiple malignancies. *PLoS Med* 2006;3:E486.
50. Meissner A, Mikkelsen TS, Gu H, et al. Genome-scale DNA methylation maps of pluripotent and differentiated cells. *Nature* 2008;454:766–770.
51. Bibikova M, Lin Z, Zhou L, et al. High-throughput DNA methylation profiling using universal bead arrays. *Genome Res* 2006;16:383–393.
52. Feinberg AP, Vogelstein B. Hypomethylation distinguishes genes of some human cancers from their normal counterparts. *Nature* 1983;301:89–92.
53. Kohda M, Hoshiya H, Katoh M, et al. Frequent loss of imprinting of IGF2 and MEST in lung adenocarcinoma. *Mol Carcinog* 2001;31:184–191.
54. Kondo M, Suzuki H, Ueda R, et al. Frequent loss of imprinting of the H19 gene is often associated with its overexpression in human lung cancers. *Oncogene* 1995;10:1193–1198.
55. Simpson AJ, Caballero OL, Jungbluth A, et al. Cancer/testis antigens, gametogenesis and cancer. *Nat Rev Cancer* 2005;5:615–625.
56. Scanlan MJ, Altorki NK, Gure AO, et al. Expression of cancer-testis antigens in lung cancer: definition of bromodomain testis-specific gene (BRDT) as a new CT gene, CT9. *Cancer Lett* 2000;150:155–164.
57. Jang SJ, Soria JC, Wang L, et al. Activation of melanoma antigen tumor antigens occurs early in lung carcinogenesis. *Cancer Res* 2001;61:7959–7963.
58. Rauch TA, Zhong X, Wu X, et al. High-resolution mapping of DNA hypermethylation and hypomethylation in lung cancer. *Proc Natl Acad Sci USA* 2008;105:252–257.
59. Cowland JB, Hother C, Grønbaek K. Micrornas and cancer. *APMIS* 2007;115:1090–1106.
60. Saito Y, Jones PA. Epigenetic activation of tumor suppressor microRNAs in human cancer cells. *Cell Cycle* 2006;5:2220–2222.

61. Brueckner B, Stresemann C, Kuner R, et al. The human let-7a-3 locus contains an epigenetically regulated microRNA gene with oncogenic function. *Cancer Res* 2007;67:1419–1423.
62. Eden A, Gaudet F, Waghmare A, et al. Chromosomal instability and tumors promoted by DNA hypomethylation. *Science* 2003;300:455.
63. Karpf AR, Matsui S. Genetic disruption of cytosine DNA methyltransferase enzymes induces chromosomal instability in human cancer cells. *Cancer Res* 2005;65:8635–8639.
64. Trinh BN, Long TI, Nickel AE, et al. DNA methyltransferase deficiency modifies cancer susceptibility in mice lacking DNA mismatch repair. *Mol Cell Biol* 2002;22:2906–2917.
65. Cantor JP, Iliopoulos D, Rao AS, et al. Epigenetic modulation of endogenous tumor suppressor expression in lung cancer xenografts suppresses tumorigenicity. *Int J Cancer* 2007;120:24–31.
66. Belinsky SA, Klinge DM, Stidley CA, et al. Inhibition of DNA methylation and histone deacetylation prevents murine lung cancer. *Cancer Res* 2003;63:7089–7093.
67. Clouaire T, Stancheva I. Methyl-CpG binding proteins: specialized transcriptional repressors or structural components of chromatin? *Cell Mol Life Sci* 2008;65:1509–1522.
68. Pepe MS, Etzioni R, Feng Z, et al. Phases of biomarker development for early detection of cancer. *J Natl Cancer Inst* 2001;93:1054–1061.
69. Travis WD. Pathology of lung cancer. *Clin Chest Med* 2002;23:65–81.
70. Bach PB. Is our natural-history model of lung cancer wrong? *Lancet Oncol* 2008;9:693–697.
71. Virmani AK, Tsou JA, Siegmund KD, et al. Hierarchical clustering of lung cancer cell lines using DNA methylation markers. *Cancer Epid Biom Prev* 2002;11:291–297.
72. Toyooka S, Toyooka KO, Maruyama R, et al. DNA methylation profiles of lung tumors. *Mol Cancer Therap* 2001;1:61–67.
73. Sathyanarayana UG, Toyooka S, Padar A, et al. Epigenetic inactivation of laminin-5-encoding genes in lung cancers. *Clin Cancer Res* 2003;9:2665–2672.
74. Tsou JA, Galler JS, Siegmund KD, et al. Identification of a panel of highly sensitive and specific DNA methylation markers for lung adenocarcinoma. *Mol Cancer* 2007;6:70.
75. Ehrich M, Field JK, Liloglou T, et al. Cytosine methylation profiles as a molecular marker in non-small cell lung cancer. *Cancer Res* 2006;66:10911–10918.
76. Brena RM, Morrison C, Liyanarachchi S, et al. Aberrant DNA methylation of OLIG1, a novel prognostic factor in non-small cell lung cancer. *PLoS Med* 2007;4:E108.
77. Toyooka S, Maruyama R, Toyooka KO, et al. Smoke exposure, histologic type and geography-related differences in the methylation profiles of non-small cell lung cancer. *Int J Cancer* 2003;103:153–160.
78. Hofmann HS, Bartling B, Simm A, et al. Identification and classification of differentially expressed genes in non-small cell lung cancer by expression profiling on a global human 59.620-element oligonucleotide array. *Oncol Rep* 2006;16:587–595.
79. Zhou W, Heist RS, Liu G, et al. Polymorphisms of vitamin D receptor and survival in early-stage non-small cell lung cancer patients. *Cancer Epidemiol Biomarkers Prev* 2006;15:2239–2245.
80. Raponi M, Zhang Y, Yu J, et al. Gene expression signatures for predicting prognosis of squamous cell and adenocarcinomas of the lung. *Cancer Res* 2006;66:7466–7472.
81. Tam IY, Chung LP, Suen WS, et al. Distinct epidermal growth factor receptor and KRAS mutation patterns in non-small cell lung cancer patients with different tobacco exposure and clinicopathologic features. *Clin Cancer Res* 2006;12:1647–1653.
82. Vineis P, Husgafvel-Pursiainen K. Air pollution and cancer: biomarker studies in human populations. *Carcinogenesis* 2005;26:1846–1855.
83. Issa JP. CpG-island methylation in aging and cancer. *Curr Top Microbiol Immunol* 2000;249:101–118.
84. Belinsky SA, Snow SS, Nikula KJ, et al. Aberrant CpG island methylation of the p16(ink4a) and estrogen receptor genes in rat lung tumors induced by particulate carcinogens. *Carcinogenesis* 2002;23:335–339.
85. Marsit CJ, Kim DH, Liu M, et al. Hypermethylation of RASSF1A and BLU tumor suppressor genes in non-small cell lung cancer: implications for tobacco smoking during adolescence. *Int J Cancer* 2005;114:219–223.
86. Dai Z, Lakshmanan RR, Zhu WG, et al. Global methylation profiling of lung cancer identifies novel methylated genes. *Neoplasia* 2001;3:314–323.
87. Cortese R, Hartmann O, Berlin K, et al. Correlative gene expression and DNA methylation profiling in lung development nominate new biomarkers in lung cancer. *Int J Biochem Cell Biol* 2008;40:1494–1508.
88. Feng Q, Hawes SE, Stern JE, et al. DNA methylation in tumor and matched normal tissues from non-small cell lung cancer patients. *Cancer Epidemiol Biomarkers Prev* 2008;17:645–654.
89. Field JK, Liloglou T, Warrak S, et al. Methylation discriminators in NSCLC identified by a microarray based approach. *Int J Oncol* 2005;27:105–111.
90. Fukasawa M, Kimura M, Morita S, et al. Microarray analysis of promoter methylation in lung cancers. *J Hum Genet* 2006;51:368–374.
91. Hatada I, Fukasawa M, Kimura M, et al. Genome-wide profiling of promoter methylation in human. *Oncogene* 2006;25:3059–3064.
92. Rauch T, Wang Z, Zhang X, et al. Homeobox gene methylation in lung cancer studied by genome-wide analysis with a microarray-based methylated CpG island recovery assay. *Proc Natl Acad Sci U S A* 2007;104:5527–5532.
93. Widschwendter M, Fiegl H, Egle D, et al. Epigenetic stem cell signature in cancer. *Nat Genet* 2007;39:157–158.
94. Carpagnano GE, Foschino-Barbaro MP, Spanevello A, et al. 3p microsatellite signature in exhaled breath condensate and tumor tissue of patients with lung cancer. *Am J Respir Crit Care Med* 2008;177:337–341.
95. Gessner C, Kuhn H, Toepfer K, et al. Detection of p53 gene mutations in exhaled breath condensate of non-small cell lung cancer patients. *Lung Cancer* 2004;43:215–222.
96. Powell CA. Waiting to exhale. *Am J Respir Crit Care Med* 2008;177: 246–247.
97. Schmiemann V, Bocking A, Kazimirek M, et al. Methylation assay for the diagnosis of lung cancer on bronchial aspirates: A cohort study. *Clin Cancer Res* 2005;11:7728–7734.
98. Grote HJ, Schmiemann V, Geddert H, et al. Aberrant promoter methylation of p16(ink4a), RARB2 and SEMA3B in bronchial aspirates from patients with suspected lung cancer. *Int J Cancer* 2005;116:720–725.
99. Topaloglu O, Hoque MO, Tokumaru Y, et al. Detection of promoter hypermethylation of multiple genes in the tumor and bronchoalveolar lavage of patients with lung cancer. *Clin Cancer Res* 2004;10:2284–2288.
100. Zöchbauer-Müller S, Fong KM, et al. Aberrant promoter methylation of multiple genes in non-small cell lung cancers. *Cancer Res* 2001;61:249–255.
101. Kersting M, Friedl C, Kraus A, et al. Differential frequencies of p16ink4a promoter hypermethylation, p53 mutation, and K-ras mutation in exfoliative material mark the development of lung cancer in symptomatic chronic smokers. *J Clin Oncol* 2000;18:3221–3229.
102. Belinsky SA, Nikula KJ, Palmisano WA, et al. Aberrant methylation of p16 ink4a is an early event in lung cancer and potential biomarker for early diagnosis. *Proc Natl Acad Sci USA* 1998;95:11891–11896.
103. Palmisano WA, Crume KP, Grimes MJ, et al. Aberrant promoter methylation of the transcription factor genes PAX5 alpha and beta in human cancers. *Cancer Res* 2003;63:4620–4625.
104. Gordon GJ, Jensen RV, Hsiao LL, et al. Using gene expression ratios to predict outcome among patients with mesothelioma. *J Natl Cancer Inst* 2003;95:598–605.
105. Belinsky SA. Role of the cytosine DNA-methyltransferase and p16/ink4a genes in the development of mouse lung tumors. *Exp Lung Res* 1998;24:463–479.
106. Benjamini Y, Hochberg Y. Controlling the false discovery rate: A practical and powerful approach to multiple testing. *J R Statist Soc B* 1995;57:289–300.
107. Tanaka H, Fujii Y, Hirabayashi H, et al. Disruption of the RB pathway and cell-proliferative activity in non-small cell lung cancers. *Int J Cancer* 1998;79:111–115.

108. Kashiwabara K, Oyama T, Sano T, et al. Correlation between the methylation status of the p16/CDKN2A gene and the expression of the p16 and RB proteins in primary non-small cell lung cancer. *Int J Cancer* 1998;79:215–220.
109. Licchesi JD, Westra WH, Hooker CM, et al. Promoter hypermethylation of hallmark cancer genes in atypical adenomatous hyperplasia of the lung. *Clin Cancer Res* 2008;14:2570–2578.
110. Ramirez RD, Sheridan S, Girard L, et al. Immortalization of human bronchial epithelial cells in the absence of viral oncoproteins. *Cancer Res* 2004;64:9027–9034.
111. Valk-Lingbeek ME, Bruggeman SW, van Lohuizen M. Stem cells and cancer; the polycomb connection. *Cell* 2004;118:409–418.
112. Toyooka S, Suzuki M, Maruyama R, et al. The relationship between aberrant methylation and survival in non-small cell lung cancers. *Br J Cancer Res* 2004;91:771–774.
113. Pulling LC, Divine KK, Klinge DM, et al. Promoter hypermethylation of the o6-methylguanine-DNA methyltransferase gene: more common in lung adenocarcinomas from never-smokers than smokers and associated with tumor progression. *Cancer Res* 2003;63:4842–4848.
114. Brabender J, Usadel H, Metzger R, et al. Quantitative o(6)-methylguanine DNA methyltransferase methylation analysis in curatively resected non-small cell lung cancer: associations with clinical outcome. *Clin Cancer Res* 2003;9:223–227.
115. Liu Y, Lan Q, Siegfried JM, et al. Aberrant promoter methylation of p16 and MGMT genes in lung tumors from smoking and never-smoking lung cancer patients. *Neoplasia* 2006;8:46–51.
116. Bogos K, Renyi-Vamos F, Kovacs G, et al. Role of retinoic receptors in lung carcinogenesis. *J Exp Clin Cancer Res* 2008;27:18.
117. Omenn GS. Chemoprevention of lung cancers: lessons from CARET, the beta-carotene and retinol efficacy trial, and prospects for the future. *Eur J Cancer Prev* 2007;16:184–191.
118. Langenfeld J, Lonardo F, Kiyokawa H, et al. Inhibited transformation of immortalized human bronchial epithelial cells by retinoic acid is linked to cyclin E down-regulation. *Oncogene* 1996;13:1983–1990.
119. Petty WJ, Li N, Biddle A, et al. A novel retinoic acid receptor beta isoform and retinoid resistance in lung carcinogenesis. *J Natl Cancer Inst* 2005;97:1645–1651.
120. Licchesi JD, Westra WH, Hooker CM, et al. Epigenetic alteration of Wnt pathway antagonists in progressive glandular neoplasia of the lung. *Carcinogenesis* 2008;29:895–904.
121. Pfeifer GP, Dammann R. Methylation of the tumor suppressor gene RASSF1A in human tumors. *Biochemistry (Mosc)* 2005;70:576–583.
122. Yanagawa N, Tamura G, Oizumi H, et al. Promoter hypermethylation of RASSF1A and RUX3 genes as an independent prognostic prediction marker in surgically resected non-small cell lung cancers. *Lung Cancer* 2007;58:131–138.
123. Maneckjee R, Minna JD. Opioids induce while nicotine suppresses apoptosis in human lung cancer cells. *Cell Growth Differ* 1994;5:1033–1040.
124. Fabbri M, Garzon R, Cimmino A, et al. MicroRNA-29 family reverts aberrant methylation in lung cancer by targeting DNA methyltransferases 3A and 3B. *Proc Natl Acad Sci U S A* 2007;104:15805–15810.
125. Bhaumik SR, Smith E, Shilatifard A. Covalent modifications of histones during development and disease pathogenesis. *Nat Struct Mol Biol* 2007;14:1008–1016.
126. Adcock IM, Ford P, Ito K, et al. Epigenetics and airways disease. *Respir Res* 2006;7:21.
127. Barlési F, Giaccone G, Gallegos-Ruiz MI, et al. Global histone modifications predict prognosis of resected non small-cell lung cancer. *J Clin Oncol* 2007;25:4358–4364.
128. Schrump DS, Hong JA, Nguyen DM. Utilization of chromatin remodeling agents for lung cancer therapy. *Cancer J* 2007;13:56–64.
129. Aparicio A. The potential of histone deacetylase inhibitors in lung cancer. *Clin Lung Cancer* 2006;7:309–312.
130. Gridelli C, Rossi A, Maione P. The potential role of histone deacetylase inhibitors in the treatment of non-small-cell lung cancer. *Crit Rev Oncol Hematol* 2008;68:29–36.
131. Edwards A, Li J, Atadja P, et al. Effect of the histone deacetylase inhibitor LBH589 against epidermal growth factor receptor-dependent human lung cancer cells. *Mol Cancer Ther* 2007;6:2515–2524.
132. Kamemura K, Ito A, Shimazu T, et al. Effects of downregulated HDAC6 expression on the proliferation of lung cancer cells. *Biochem Biophys Res Commun* 2008; 74:84–89.
133. Shimamura T, Shapiro GI. Heat shock protein 90 inhibition in lung cancer. *J Thorac Oncol* 2008;3:S152–S159.
134. Yu XD, Wang SY, Chen GA, et al. Apoptosis induced by depsipeptide FK228 coincides with inhibition of survival signaling in lung cancer cells. *Cancer J* 2007;13:105–113.
135. Chen G, Li A, Zhao M, et al. Proteomic analysis identifies protein targets responsible for depsipeptide sensitivity in tumor cells. *J Proteome Res* 2008;7:2733–2742.
136. Geng L, Cuneo KC, Fu A, et al. Histone deacetylase (HDAC) inhibitor LBH589 increases duration of gamma-H2AX foci and confines HDAC4 to the cytoplasm in irradiated non-small cell lung cancer. *Cancer Res* 2006;66:11298–11304.
137. Chai G, Li L, Zhou W, et al. HDAC inhibitors act with 5-aza-2′-deoxycytidine to inhibit cell proliferation by suppressing removal of incorporated abases in lung cancer cells. *PLoS ONE* 2008;3:e2445.
138. Shivapurkar N, Stastny V, Suzuki M, et al. Application of a methylation gene panel by quantitative pcr for lung cancers. *Cancer Lett* 2007;247:56–71.
139. Grote HJ, Schmiemann V, Kiel S, et al. Aberrant methylation of the adenomatous polyposis coli promoter 1A in bronchial aspirates from patients with suspected lung cancer. *Int J Cancer* 2004;110:751–755.
140. de Fraipont F, Moro-Sibilot D, Michelland S, et al. Promoter methylation of genes in bronchial lavages: a marker for early diagnosis of primary and relapsing non-small cell lung cancer? *Lung Cancer* 2005;50:199–209.
141. Usadel H, Brabender J, Danenberg KD, et al. Quantitative adenomatous polyposis coli promoter methylation analysis in tumor tissue, serum, and plasma DNA of patients with lung cancer. *Cancer Res* 2002;62:371–375.
142. Belinsky SA, Klinge DM, Dekker JD, et al. Gene promoter methylation in plasma and sputum increases with lung cancer risk. *Clin Cancer Res* 2005;11:6505–6511.
143. Belinsky SA, Grimes MJ, Casas E, et al. Predicting gene promoter methylation in non-small-cell lung cancer by evaluating sputum and serum. *Br J Cancer* 2007;96:1278–1283.
144. Kim H, Kwon YM, Kim JS, et al. Tumor-specific methylation in bronchial lavage for the early detection of non-small-cell lung cancer. *J Clin Oncol* 2004;22:2363–2370.
145. Ulivi P, Zoli W, Calistri D, et al. p16INK4A and CDH13 hypermethylation in tumor and serum of non-small cell lung cancer patients. *J Cell Physiol* 2006;206:611–615.
146. Hsu HS, Chen TP, Hung CH, et al. Characterization of a multiple epigenetic marker panel for lung cancer detection and risk assessment in plasma. *Cancer* 2007;110:2019–2026.
147. Cirincione R, Lintas C, Conte D, et al. Methylation profile in tumor and sputum samples of lung cancer patients detected by spiral computed tomography: a nested case-control study. *Int J Cancer* 2006;118:1248–1253.
148. Liu Y, An Q, Li L, et al. Hypermethylation of p16INK4A in Chinese lung cancer patients: Biological and clinical implications. *Carcinogenesis* 2003;24:1897–1901.
149. Palmisano WA, Divine KK, Saccomanno G, et al. Predicting lung cancer by detecting aberrant promoter methylation in sputum. *Cancer Res* 2000;60:5954–5958.
150. Olaussen KA, Soria JC, Park YW, et al. Assessing abnormal gene promoter methylation in paraffin-embedded sputum from patients with NSCLC. *Eur J Cancer* 2005;41:2112–2119.
151. Chan EC, Lam SY, Tsang KW, et al. Aberrant promoter methylation in Chinese patients with non-small cell lung cancer: Patterns in primary tumors and potential diagnostic application in bronchoalevolar lavage. *Clin Cancer Res* 2002;8:3741–3746.

152. Kurakawa E, Shimamoto T, Utsumi K, et al. Hypermethylation of p16(INK4A) and p15(INK4B) genes in non-small cell lung cancer. *Int J Oncol* 2001;19:277–281.
153. Ahrendt SA, Chow JT, Xu LH, et al. Molecular detection of tumor cells in bronchoalveolar lavage fluid from patients with early stage lung cancer. *J Natl Cancer Inst* 1999;91:332–339.
154. Guo M, House MG, Hooker C, et al. Promoter hypermethylation of resected bronchial margins: a field defect of changes? *Clin Cancer Res* 2004;10:5131–5136.
155. Ng CSH, Zhang J, Wan S, et al. Tumor p16M is a possible marker of advanced stage in non-small cell lung cancer. *J Surg Oncol* 2002;79: 101–106.
156. Fujiwara K, Fujimoto N, Tabata M, et al. Identification of epigenetic aberrant promoter methylation in serum DNA is useful for early detection of lung cancer. *Clin Cancer Res* 2005;11:1219–1225.
157. Esteller M, Sanchez-Cespedes M, Rosell R, et al. Detection of aberrant promoter hypermethylation of tumor suppressor genes in serum DNA from non-small cell lung cancer patients. *Cancer Res* 1999;59:67–70.
158. Bearzatto A, Conte D, Frattini M, et al. P16(INK4A) hypermethylation detected by fluorescent methylation-specific PCR in plasmas from non-small cell lung cancer. *Clin Cancer Res* 2002;8:3782–3787.
159. Wang YC, Lu YP, Tseng RC, et al. Inactivation of HMLH1 and HMSH2 by promoter methylation in primary non-small cell lung tumors and matched sputum samples. *J Clin Invest* 2003;111:887–895.
160. Grote HJ, Schmiemann V, Geddert H, et al. Methylation of Ras association domain family protein 1A as a biomarker of lung cancer. *Cancer* 2006;108:129–134.
161. Sozzi G, Musso K, Ratcliffe C, et al. Detection of microsatellite alterations in plasma DNA of non-small cell lung cancer patients: a prospect for early diagnosis. *Clin Cancer Res* 1999;5:2689–2692.
162. Wang Y, Yu Z, Wang T, et al. Identification of epigenetic aberrant promoter methylation of RASSF1A in serum DNA and its clinicopathological significance in lung cancer. *Lung Cancer* 2007;56:289–294.
163. Shivapurkar N, Stastny V, Xie Y, et al. Differential methylation of a short CpG-rich sequence within exon 1 of TCF21 gene: a promising cancer biomarker assay. *Cancer Epidemiol Biomarkers Prev* 2008;17:995–1000.

CHAPTER 8

Jair Bar
Amir Onn
Roy S. Herbst

Molecular Events Surrounding the Angiogenic Switch of Lung Cancer

Multicellular organisms such as humans require a complex vascular system to supply cells with oxygen and glucose and to dispose of waste products. During embryonic development and at the main phases of organ growth, the vascular system evolves with the growing organism. However, in adulthood, the vascular system is quiescent. A well-controlled angiogenic response (production of blood vessels from existing blood vessels) to specific transient cues may occur. Other than the changes that occur in the female reproductive system or in wound healing, endothelial cells rarely proliferate in adults. This tight control is the result of a continuous balance between angiogenic signaling and inhibition. Several proangiogenic and antiangiogenic molecules have been identified, many of which are potentially active in creating this balance (Table 8.1). The exceptions to this balance include pathologic conditions such as wound healing, inflammation, and cancer, in which the formation of new blood vessels is vital.[1] The abnormal state of cancer, in which proangiogenic signaling does not abate, is reminiscent of what happens in wounds; however, it occurs in a perpetual manner. In this sense, cancer can be regarded as a "wound that never heals."[2]

Blood supply is delivered by a highly organized conduit network that is spread out, designed to reach most cells. The exchange of nutrients and waste molecules between the blood and cells occurs through capillary walls, the thinnest vessels, those that connect the arterial tree to the venous tree. Vascular capillaries are formed from endothelial cells, which create the tubal conduit for blood, surrounded by a basement membrane. Pericytes (mural vascular cells) are embedded in the basement membrane. These cells provide physical support for the blood vessel and provide communication ports with endothelial cells, thus controlling capillary function. Unlike vascular smooth muscle cells, which are found in the media layer of large blood vessels, most pericytes are in direct contact with endothelial cells; cell–cell communications take place between these cell types.[3]

As a malignant growth exceeds the size of a few hundred microns, nutrient diffusion becomes a growth-limiting factor. Hypoxia and various cancer-specific genetic abnormalities drive the secretion of proangiogenic factors and suppression of antiangiogenic factors. In this manner, the tumor microenvironment becomes proangiogenic. New blood vessels are formed, and existing blood vessels are modified to provide a better blood supply to the tumor. The production of blood vessels from existing blood vessels is called *angiogenesis*, whereas production of de novo blood vessels is termed *vasculogenesis*. Both of these processes are controlled by the counteracting effects of proangiogenic and antiangiogenic factors. The tipping of the balance toward a proangiogenic state is called the *angiogenic switch*. This switch seems to be essential to cancer progression. Accordingly, tumoral angiogenesis was suggested as a therapeutic target more than 35 years ago.[4] Only in recent years has this idea entered clinical practice; antiangiogenesis is used to treat colon, kidney, breast, and other cancers. The clinical importance of angiogenesis inhibition in the treatment of non–small cell lung cancer (NSCLC) was demonstrated by an improved outcome after treatment with an antiangiogenic agent and classic chemotherapy.[5,6]

In this chapter, we will discuss the importance of the angiogenic switch in cancer, as demonstrated in studies of whole organs and the major cell types and mechanisms that supply nutrients to cancer. In vitro studies and the major molecular players will be presented. The role of vasculogenesis in tumor perfusion is controversial and sometimes difficult to distinguish from that of angiogenesis. Thus, both are discussed in this chapter. We conclude with the available data on the angiogenic switch and alternative modes of lung cancer vascularization, and a note about the clinical implications of this information.

ANGIOGENIC SWITCH IN CANCER: WHOLE-ORGAN STUDIES

A milestone of molecular biology and cancer research is the development of specific gene silencing and upregulation techniques in in vivo mouse models. Several mouse models of the angiogenic switch are described in the succeeding discussion.

TABLE 8.1 Proangiogenic and Antiangiogenic Factors

Factor Type	Proangiogenic	Antiangiogenic
Physical and biochemical factors	Hypoxia, hypoglycemia (VHL→HIF, VEGF)	Normoxia, normoglycemia
Transcription factors	HIF-1α[133]	p53[136]
Coagulation system components	Plasmin[133]	Angiostatin[100]
MMP-mediated ECM degradation	MMP9→VEGF release[51]	MMP→endostatin, arrestin, canstatin, tumstatin
Immune system effects	TAMs,[216] mast cells[163]	Macrophage-derived methalloelastase (produces angiostatin from plasminogen),[132] NK cells[118]
Stromal fibroblast derived	SDF-1,[70] VEGF,[161] HGF[229]	
Basement membrane–derived molecules	MMP9, VEGF, fragments of collagen IV	Endostatin, arrestin, canstatin, tumstatin
Chemokines	IL-8/CXCL8[253]	PF-4/CXCL4, variant PF-4/CXCL4[254]
Cell–cell adhesion molecules	ICAM-2[103]	Membranous E-cadherin
Context dependent	Ang-2 (if high VEGF), pericytes (stabilizing blood vessels, allowing better functionality)	Ang-2 (if low VEGF), pericytes (stabilizing blood vessels and preventing their evolvement)

ECM, extra-cellular matrix; HGF, hepatocyte growth factor; HIF, hypoxia inducible factor; ICAM, inter-cellular adhesion factor; IL-8, interleukin-8; MMP, matrix metalloprotease; PF, platelet factor; SDF, stromal cell derived factor; TAM, tumor-associated macrophages; VEGF, vascular endothelial growth factor; VHL, Von Hippel-Lindau.

Mouse Models The RIP-Tag mouse model was created by genetically manipulating mouse pancreatic β-cells to express the SV40 large T antigen; a hyperproliferative stage arises in about half the pancreatic islets, and in a minority of those, pancreatic islet cell carcinoma develops. The induction of angiogenic activity demarcates an angiogenic stage, which is found in islets that have progressed past the proliferative stage and apparently precedes carcinoma.[7] The isolation and examination of these islets revealed that an angiogenic phenotype is not a direct outcome of oncogene expression, nor is it the inevitable effect of a proliferative mass that requires an increased blood supply. The RIP-Tag model demonstrated discrete stages of tumor progression in which additional genetic manipulation can be used to determine the roles of various molecules in each phase. Thus, this model was used to evaluate the roles of vascular endothelial growth factor (VEGF) in the angiogenic switch,[8] matrix metalloproteases (MMP9) in the release of VEGF from the extracellular matrix (ECM),[9] and VEGF receptor 2 (VEGFR-2) expression on vascular endothelial cells[10] (see succeeding discussion).

Tumor fragments transplanted onto the irises of rabbits were used in a classic model that demonstrated the importance of the angiogenic switch.[11] In some cases, the tumor fragments induced angiogenesis and progressed; in others, they remained clinically dormant. Active proliferation and apoptosis were found at the cellular level in clinically dormant tumors. Similar apparent dormancy has also been described in other conditions in which angiogenesis was inhibited.[12]

The angiogenic switch is required not only for the progression of primary tumors but also for the growth of metastatic deposits. In a mouse model of metastatic disease, removal of the primary tumor induced rapid growth in previously dormant metastatic deposits. An angiogenesis inhibitor produced by the primary tumor was later identified. The rapid growth of the micrometastasis was accompanied by angiogenesis induction and a concomitant apoptosis reduction, with no change in the proliferative rate.[12] Both activators and inhibitors of angiogenesis are produced in intact organisms, and the balance between them determines the vascularity of the tumor and its metastasis and progression.

Angiogenesis Evaluation in Human Cancer In clinical studies, the most useful method for evaluating tumor vascularity is counting microvessel density (MVD) in tumor sections by immunohistochemically staining for one of several molecular markers of endothelial cells, namely factor VIII, von Willebrand factor, CD31, or CD34. Under low magnification, areas of high MVD can be observed, usually at the tumor periphery. The actual MVD is determined in those areas by counting the number of capillaries per high-power field. Various protocols for counting or subjective visual evaluation exist.[13] MVD has been correlated with imaging-determined tumor perfusion[14] and clinical outcome in many tumor types. However, many vessels visualized by immunohistochemical staining may not be functional. CD105 staining was recently suggested to be specific for active blood vessels as opposed to general endothelial markers that stain also nonfunctional vessels.[15] Proliferating endothelial cells can also be assessed by immunohistochemical analysis, because they are a more reliable marker of ongoing angiogenesis than MVD. Double-staining for endothelial-specific proteins and Ki-67 is used to estimate the proportion of proliferating cells; this method was better correlated with stage than counting MVD in colorectal cancer.[16] An important caveat of these methods is the high variability within tumors[17]; thus, sampling errors may be significant. Although highly useful and clinically prognostic in many studies (see later), these methods provide no information about tumor perfusion, which is the biologically relevant end point of the angiogenic switch. For this, other approaches must be used.

An indirect method of evaluating tumor angiogenesis is the assessment of tumor hypoxia. Carbonic anhydrase IX, a transcriptional target of hypoxia-inducible factor 1 (HIF-1), may be a surrogate marker of tumor hypoxia. High levels are found in hypoxic areas in several cancer types, including NSCLC, and its expression is associated with a poor prognosis.[18] Pimonidazole is an exogenous marker of hypoxia[19] that can be used in immunohistochemical analyses of biopsy samples[20]; however, this method is not commonly used, because it requires pimonidazole to be intravenously infused to patients prior to biopsy. Interestingly, tumor cell necrosis, a plausible indicator of tumor hypoxia, has not been reported to be a prognostic factor in lung cancer. Nuclear medicine allows molecular imaging, including the ability to detect hypoxia. The positron emission tomography tracer 18F-misonidazole[21] and other tracers are being assessed as prognostic or predictive markers in several cancer types. However, such tools require further validation and are not yet available in most cancer centers.

Major inducers and inhibitors of angiogenesis can be used as surrogate markers for angiogenesis in cancer. The levels of VEGF, its receptors, and various endogenous facilitators and inhibitors of angiogenesis can be evaluated in patients' tumor tissues or serum. Importantly, such studies can be performed in large-scale setups and may be useful clinically. Alternatively, immunohistochemical analyses of protein expression in tumors can be performed, but these have the same potential sampling bias of MVD studies.

Additional parameters of angiogenic activity that can be assessed from a blood sample include circulating endothelial cells (CECs) and circulating endothelial progenitor cells (circulating EPC; CEPs). CECs were first reported more than 30 years ago by Hladovec and Rossmann.[22,23] Mature CECs probably originate from cells shed from vessel walls. Some of such cells possess progenitor characteristics and are referred to as CEPs; they are thought to originate from the bone marrow. Both CECs and CEPs may be useful surrogate markers for angiogenic activity and for tumors' response to antiangiogenic treatment.[24] However, the assessment of CECs or CEPs in patients' blood is technically challenging, and no consensus exists about assessment methods or even CEPs' significance (see discussion later).

Tumor perfusion can be assessed in vivo using various imaging studies. Most of these methods are investigational, although promising. Microscopic bubbles can be used as contrast material in sonography studies to demonstrate blood flow in vivo. Computed tomography and magnetic resonance imaging using intravenous contrast material can also be used to measure blood flow and volume. Positron emission tomography nuclear imaging using ^{11}C- or ^{15}O-marked carbon monoxide can be used for the same purpose. Molecular imaging, in which the contrast material is conjugated to a molecule that binds to a cancer endothelial-specific epitope, is currently being evaluated.[25]

Angiogenic Switch in Human Cancer Stepwise progression is evident in several cancer types, and discrete stages can be differentiated in pathologic specimens. For example, breast cancer is preceded by carcinoma in situ, in which vessel density is correlated with several poor prognostic factors.[26] Additional indicators of angiogenic activity, such as messenger RNA (mRNA) expression levels of VEGF and its receptors, were upregulated in breast in situ carcinoma, similar to what was found in invasive breast cancer.[27] Cervical squamous cell intraepithelial neoplasia is the precursor of cervical carcinoma and is graded according to the proportion of dysplasia. Vessel density in the stroma below the basement membrane of the dysplastic epithelium was correlated with the grade of epithelial dysplasia.[28] Evaluation of dysplastic bronchial epithelium, lung premalignant lesions, revealed increased MVD and increased levels of VEGF levels compared with normal controls. A characteristic pattern of VEGFR and VEGF isoform expression comparable to invasive lung cancer was found. Apparently normal lungs of heavy smokers harbored enhanced VEGF mRNA levels.[29] Abnormal microvasculature structure was described to appear near dysplastic squamous bronchial epithelium.[30] The results of these studies suggest that, similar to what was demonstrated in mouse models, human cancer must acquire a vascular supply in order to progress. At least in some types of cancer, including lung cancer, the angiogenic switch occurs prior to the invasive phase of cancer progression.

Angiogenic Signaling in Response to Hypoperfusion Oncogene activation and tumor suppressor gene inactivation can activate the angiogenesis switch (see later). However, hypoperfusion is an alternative, and conceptually antagonizing, source of proangiogenic signals. Tumors that outgrow their blood supply experience reduced oxygen and glucose levels. Hypoxic regions are commonly found in several cancer types. These regions may indicate highly dysregulated cell growth; they are associated with a poor prognosis.[31,32] Hypoxia may select for more aggressive tumor cells[33] or activate signaling pathways that lead to increased invasion and metastasis. For example, in NSCLC cells, hypoxia induced in a HIF-1α-dependent manner CXCR4 expression.[34] CXCR4 is a cytokine receptor involved in invasion and metastasis.[35] A direct consequence of hypoxia and hypoglycemia is HIF-dependent induction of VEGF expression in malignant cells.[36] VEGF activates an angiogenic response, which results in new blood vessels, improved tumor vascularization, and potentially relief of hypoxia and hypoglycemia. VEGF induction by hypoxia or hypoglycemia involves an apparently normal feedback mechanism, in which reduced perfusion activates a corrective mechanism. Normally, once perfusion has improved, VEGF secretion is reduced.[36] Hypoperfusion-induced signaling is not perpetual, unlike the angiogenic switch. However, newly formed blood vessels of tumors are not as functional as mature vessels of normal tissues: They are only partially covered by pericytes and are highly permeable, torturous, and chaotic.[25] The inefficiency of the newly formed tumor blood supply causes the hypoxia-induced signaling to prevail and paradoxically contributes to cancerous growth.

CELLULAR PLAYERS AND MECHANISMS IN TUMOR VASCULARIZATION

Endothelial Sprouting and Pericyte Coverage

Tumor blood vessels form and develop with tumors by several mechanisms, the most studied of which is endothelial sprouting, whereby new capillaries bud from nearby existing ones. Sprouting can proceed through a phase of a vascular network that is superfluous and undergoes pruning, or it can be guided to hypoperfused regions as it is created, mostly by VEGF gradients.[37] The phases of endothelial sprouting have been carefully described.[38] The basement membrane of postcapillary venules is degraded at the location of the future endothelial sprout. Through the resultant opening in the basement membrane, endothelial cells migrate and form a cord of cells; this is followed by the appearance of a lumen. According to another report, the sprouting vessel sustains a lumen and continuous intracellular junctions as it is produced, rather than going through a stage of dedifferentiated cord of cells as commonly thought.[39]

Endothelial cell migration is a major process in angiogenesis. It is regulated by chemotaxis toward VEGF, basic fibroblast growth factor (bFGF), and other angiogenic factors. It is also controlled by haptotaxis, the migration toward a gradient of immobilized ligands, which is dependent on integrin-ECM interactions. Mechanotaxis is the sensing of sheer stress of blood flow by cytoskeletal elements and migration in its direction and is another mechanism that controls endothelial migration.[40,41]

The last phase of the angiogenesis process is the recruitment of pericytes and deposition of new basement membrane.[42] Pericytes of the parent blood vessel proliferate and migrate to envelop the new vessel.[39] The platelet-derived growth factor (PDGF) pathway is the major regulator of pericyte recruitment and maintenance. PDGF-B is secreted mostly by endothelial cells. Acting on PDGF receptor-β (PDGFR-β) on pericytes, it facilitates their recruitment to new blood vessels. Pericytes, in turn, contribute to the stability and functionality of blood vessels, partly through the secretion of VEGF.[43] Importantly, tumor blood vessels that lack pericyte coverage are the first to regress after VEGF pathway inhibition.[44] Tumor blood vessels contain more than one subtype of pericytes, which vary in their molecular marker expression and dependence on PDGF signaling for tight adhesion to endothelial cells.[45]

The origin of tumor vascular pericytes is thought to be mesenchymal progenitor cells,[43] which are characterized by Tie2 expression,[46] or bone marrow–derived hematopoietic stem cells.[47] Some models indicate that endothelial cells and pericytes share a common angioblast progenitor cell.[48] The differences between vascular smooth muscle cells and pericytes are not clear, suggesting that they are similar cell types in different phases of phenotypic change.[3] Regardless of the origin of these cells, the clinical activity of PDGFR inhibition in the treatment of cancer indicates that pericytes are important in the maturation and modulation of tumor angiogenesis[43] (see Fig. 8.1 for a schematic representation of the major cell types and niches that modulate tumor angiogenesis).

Vasculogenesis: Cells from the Bone Marrow

Vasculogenesis is the de novo formation of blood vessels from vascular progenitor cells. Circulating bone marrow–originating cells travel to specific foci and undergo in situ differentiation

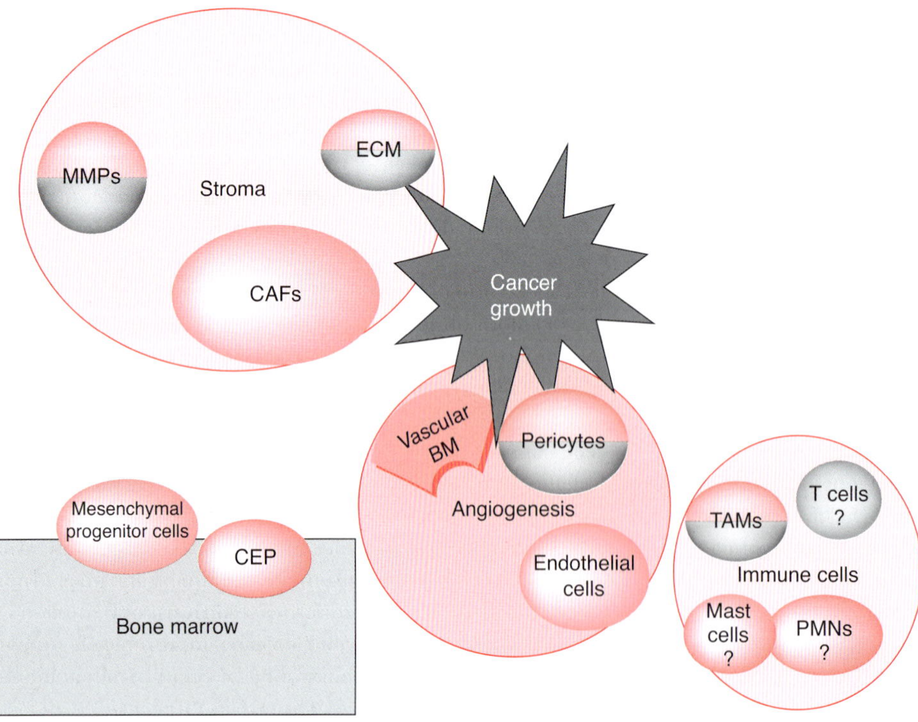

FIGURE 8.1 The major cell types and niches that play a role in angiogenesis. Red marks factors that positively regulate cancer angiogenesis, blue marks antiangiogenic factors. Half-red and half-black indicates different effects in different circumstances. ? indicates equivocal evidence. *BM*, basement membrane; *CAFs*, Cancer-associated fibroblasts; *CEP*, circulating endothelial progenitor cells; *ECM*, extracellular matrix; *MMPs*, matrix metalloproteases; *PMNs*, polymorphonuclear neutrophils; *TAMs*, tumor-associated macrophages

to form mature components of blood vessels. Vasculogenesis was initially thought to occur only in embryonic tissues, but it has been found to occur in adults as well. Bone marrow–derived endothelial progenitor cells (EPC) were found to be mobilized (thus becoming CEPs) by GM-CSFs or ischemia in experimental animals and travel to areas of ischemia.[49] Studies in which mice underwent bone marrow transplantation from mice that expressed a unique marker demonstrated that bone marrow–derived cells contribute directly to blood vessel formation.[49,50] VEGFR-2 is critical for vasculogenesis in embryos[51] and adult tissues.[52] In addition, increased expression of stromal cell–derived factor-1 (SDF-1, also called CXCL12)-in peripheral blood and ischemic tissues, in parallel to reduced SDF-1/CXCL12 expression in bone marrow, may enhance the recruitment of CEPs to ischemic tissues. SDF-1/CXCL12 enhanced the number of EPC in ischemic vessels by promoting their adhesion through $\alpha 2$, $\alpha 4$, and $\alpha 5$ integrins to fibronectin and collagen I.[53] CEPs have also been found in patients, in numbers that were correlated with plasma levels of VEGF 165.[54]

CEPs were also shown to contribute to the formation of blood vessels in cancer. Id knockout mice display defective angiogenesis, not allowing them to support the growth of implanted tumors.[55] This phenotype was saved by transplantation with wild-type bone marrow. Donor-derived, VEGFR-2-positive CEPs formed most of the tumor blood vessels in this model. Donor-derived, VEGFR-1-positive myeloid precursors were also recruited to the tumors, where they were thought to have secreted angiogenic cytokines.[52] The role of inflammatory cells in angiogenesis will be discussed later. The expression of the transcription factor Id1 in CEPs was essential for their contribution to lung metastasis in another mouse model.[56] Systemic 17-β estradiol administration contributed to the recruitment of CEPs to tumors in a mouse model of breast cancer.[57] Blood counts of CEPs may be a promising surrogate marker for angiogenesis or vasculogenesis, possibly useful in the real-time assessment of the efficiency of treatment targeting tumor blood vessels.[24] For example, vascular-disrupting agents induced a surge in the CEP blood concentration in a mouse cancer model. Treatment with anti-VEGFR-2 antibody disrupted this surge and augmented the efficacy of cancer eradication. Blocking the CEP surge prevented the regrowth of tumor from the rim of viable cells that typically remain when most of the tumor necrotizes.[58] Cancer-associated fibroblasts (CAFs), a prominent component of the stromal reaction to cancer, contributed to the recruitment of CEPs.[59] SDF-1/CXCL12 release by CAFs is critical to this recruitment.[59] CEPs were found in the blood of cancer patients and were demonstrated to respond to effective systemic therapy.[60] Therefore, bone marrow–derived EPCs may be one of the important manners by which tumors develop their vascular supply.

The importance of EPCs is controversial, spurring disputes in the scientific literature.[61,62] Estimations of their contributions to tumor endothelium vary from significant (10% to 50%) to negligible.[24,63] Studies finding no evidence of EPC contribution to tumor endothelium were also reported.[61] A plausible explanation for this variability was suggested when time-dependent changes in EPC contribution were evaluated. Using high-resolution microscopy, aided by flow cytometry, bone marrow–originating cells can be located in inoculated tumors in mice that have undergone bone marrow transplantations of GFP-positive cells. In this model, the proportion of EPCs among endothelial cells was about 30% in the first 4 to 6 days of tumor growth but dropped to less than 1% after 4 weeks. This study also demonstrated bone marrow–derived cells close to endothelial cells, suggesting that they are a source of EPC overestimation in tumor vessels.[64] A study of cancers that developed in bone marrow transplant recipients that are gender mismatched with their donor revealed that about 5% of their tumor endothelial cells are donor-originated.[63] Importantly, almost all of the CEC that had a significant proliferative capacity, were donor-originated.[65] This study suggests that even very low numbers of EPC might contribute significantly to tumor vasculature.

The evaluation of CEPs in blood samples of cancer patients is hampered by the low numbers of these cells in circulation and the technical difficulties of their positive identification. Identification methods include enrichment by cell sorting and immunomagnetic beads. However, these methods depend on specific surface markers, which are lacking. For example, CD146 may be a specific marker of CEPs or CECs and may be measurable in the serum of cancer patients. CD146 mRNA levels in serum were correlated with CECs in breast cancer patients.[66] However, a fluorescence-activated cell sorting analysis of blood mononuclear cells demonstrated that CD146 was expressed mainly on a subpopulation of T cells.[67] Recently, tumor endothelial marker 1/endosialin/CD248 was reported to be highly expressed in CEPs, suggesting a new method of measuring or potentially eradicating blood CEPs.[68] An important property of CEPs that may be useful in their identification is their ability to proliferate, but this would not differentiate CEPs from hematopoietic progenitor cells. The technical difficulties of detecting a minute subpopulation of cells in the blood have not been satisfactorily solved.[24] The results of studies of CEPs and CECs in the blood of cancer patients must be interpreted cautiously.

Alternative Mechanisms of Enhanced Vascularization In vessel co-option, tumors or metastatic foci develop along existing blood vessels. In this way, tumors become vascularized with no need for blood vessel formation.[69] Vessel co-option occurs in the initial growth phase of tumors. As cancer cells proliferate, the tumor outgrows its blood supply. The co-opted host blood vessels then undergo regression, possibly as a host defense mechanism. The endothelial cells of these vessels are detached from their supporting cells, at which point they undergo apoptosis. Angiopoietin 2 (Ang-2) expression is induced in the co-opted vessels prior to their regression. Ang-2 is involved in physiologic vessel remodeling in a VEGF-dependent manner (see succeeding discussion). Co-option of existing vessels may be an important method for obtaining a vascular supply in early tumors. Its extent is controlled by the local production of VEGF, Ang-1, and Ang-2.

Intussusceptive microvascular growth, the longitudinal separation of existing vessels into daughter vessels, is another mechanism of enhancing blood supply to tumors. In this way, the network's complexity and efficiency improves, with no need for endothelial cell proliferation.

Vasculogenic mimicry, which has been observed mostly in melanomas, is the ability of cancer cells to transform into endothelial-like cells in specific sites, thus forming blood vessels made of cancer cells.[38] The importance of these alternative mechanisms of vascular supply in cancer growth is not known.

Role of Immune System Cells in Angiogenesis

The stroma of cancer is infiltrated by immune system cells in varying proportions. The role of the immune system in the progression of cancer is not obvious but seems to be context dependent. The immune system has a cancer-inhibitory effect, as evidenced by the high risk of cancer in immunocompromised patients. In addition, a correlation was found between increased effector memory T-cell infiltration of the tumor and a good prognosis in colon cancer patients.[70] However, in many other settings, the immune system apparently contributes to cancer progression. The adaptive immune system can mount an antitumor response in some conditions. In contrast, innate immune system cells may be more commonly recruited by cancer cells and function in a pro-cancer manner.[71] Neutrophilic infiltration of tumors is common, but its clinical significance is not clear. In bronchoalveolar carcinoma, it has been associated with a poor prognosis,[72] but data on its importance in other cancers are limited. Lung cancer–infiltrating lymphocytes exert an anticancerous effect, as in colon cancer. High densities of $CD4^+$ and $CD8^+$ lymphocytes in the stroma of NSCLC tumors have been found to be associated with a good prognosis.[73,74]

Monocytes circulate in the blood; once recruited to sites of tissue inflammation, they differentiate into macrophages. Various chemoattractants play a role in the chemotaxis of monocytes into tumors, possibly mostly to hypoxic areas of tumors.[75] Macrophages constitute a major subset of the immune system cells that populate the tumor stroma: tumor-associated macrophages (TAMs). TAMs seem to promote the progression of cancer.[76] Unlike classically activated macrophages (M1 macrophages), TAMs have a poor antigen-presenting ability and produce factors that suppress T-cell proliferation and activity. The chemokines and chemokine receptors profile they express is adapted for scavenging for debris, promoting cell migration and angiogenesis, and repairing and remodeling wounded or damaged tissues. Cancer microenvironment exposure to interleukin (IL)-4 and IL-10 can induce monocytes to develop into TAMs (otherwise known as polarized type II [alternatively activated] or M2 macrophages).[77] Proangiogenic monocytes that localize in tumors are also characterized as Tie-2 expressors.[46] Macrophage infiltration was found to be associated with vessel density in several types of cancer. In a mouse model of breast cancer, depletion of macrophages inhibited the angiogenic switch and cancer progression. Increased macrophage infiltration was correlated with earlier tumor progression.[78]

IL-1β is a proangiogenic cytokine that depends on macrophage recruitment to tumor sites for its angiogenic effect.[79] MMP9 release by macrophages, leading to mobilization of VEGF,[80] is a mechanism in which the infiltration of macrophages or other myelomonocytes[81] induces angiogenesis. In addition, IL-8/CXCL8, another proangiogenic factor, was upregulated in both cancer cells and macrophages when these two cell types were cultured together, and IL-8/CXCL8 mRNA levels in lung cancer specimens were correlated with MVD and poor patient prognosis.[82] Relating an angiogenic response to inflammation, which is common in cancer, IL-1α was shown to recruit VEGF-expressing inflammatory cells. VEGFR-2 blockage prevented this angiogenic response.[83] Regardless of the available data on the contribution of macrophages to angiogenesis, tumor islet infiltration by macrophages was a good prognostic factor in a study of 175 NSCLC patients. On the other hand, stromal macrophage infiltration was associated with a poor prognosis.[84] These results were reproduced in a study of 199 NSCLC patients.[85] Importantly, the studies that showed a positive prognostic effect of macrophages in lung tumors differed from earlier studies by differentiating between stromal and tumoral macrophages.

Natural killer (NK) cells are another part of the innate immune system that have important interactions with cancer and cancer-induced angiogenesis. NK cells recognize and lyse cancer cells and are thought to have important roles in immune surveillance against cancer. IL-12 is an antiangiogenic agent that depends on NK cell recruitment to affect cancer angiogenesis.[86] NK cells secrete interferon-γ, causing inhibition of endothelial cell proliferation; this is probably the major mechanism of NK cells' antiangiogenic effects.[87]

Mast cells were found to be essential for tumor progression in a mouse model of squamous cell carcinoma and were required for neoangiogenesis.[88] Mast cell infiltration was correlated with MVD in a study of NSCLC specimens.[89] However, mast cell tumor infiltration was associated with a good prognosis in NSCLC specimens.[84] More detailed studies of the role of mast cells in lung cancer are required. In light of the inhibitory effect of most anticancer treatments on the immune system, further insight is required into the effect of immune system cells on angiogenesis and cancer progression.

Tumor Stroma–Dependent Effects

The stroma of tumors is more than a mechanical scaffold; stromal cells seem to be reprogrammed by cancer cells to participate in cancer progression. A mouse model demonstrated activation of the VEGF gene promoter in tumor stroma fibroblasts.[90] CAFs also contribute to cancer progression,[91] apparently by activating angiogenesis. Activation of hepatocyte growth factor (HGF)–c-Met signaling is another role of the stroma in tumor angiogenesis (see succeeding discussion).[92]

MMPs are a family of Zn2++ proteases that are produced mostly by stromal fibroblasts and by cancer and endothelial cells. These proteases have important roles in angiogenesis. MMP2 and MMP9, for example, mediate the breakdown of collagen type IV, a major component of the vascular basement membrane. The mobilization of growth factors, including

VEGF[80] and additional angiogenic molecules from the ECM, is another angiogenic activity of MMP. This mobilization may be essential in the initial stages of cancer, becoming less important as the tumor progresses and alternative sources of VEGF become available. MMP9 was also shown to be required for the recruitment of bone marrow–derived cells into the tumor microenvironment, for the maturation of tumor vasculature, and for pericyte coverage.[93] In contrast, at later stages of tumor growth and MMP activity, the dominant end products of MMP protein cleavage are antiangiogenic factors.[94] Although MMPs are correlated with angiogenic activity in lung cancer, general MMPs inhibition did not improve the clinical outcome of NSCLC patients.[95] Modification of specific MMP(s) might be required for impacting clinical end points.

Vascular Basement Membrane The ECM that envelops endothelial cells, and within which pericytes are embedded, is called the *vascular basement membrane*. The major collagen that constitutes the basement membrane is collagen IV, which has the unique ability to self-assemble into sheets. Additional components are laminins, which bind cell membrane anchors such as integrins on one side and ECM collagen on the other side. The mature basement membrane signals differentiation and reduced proliferation to adjacent endothelial cells. The same protein constituents, while being deposited as a new basement membrane, present different molecular moieties to the cells around them. Through integrins, they provide proliferation and migration signals. The ECM structural components also include molecular messengers, such as endostatin, that can be proteolytically released from collagen XVIII and functions as an antiangiogenic effector. Arrestin, canstatin, and tumstatin are also collagen-derived antiangiogenic molecules. On the other hand, triple-helix fragments of collagen IV activate endothelial cell migration. Therefore, specific molecules in the ECM/basement membrane can convey different messages at different phases of tumor growth. Deposited by the resident cells, the ECM/basement membrane is an important manner of cell–cell indirect communication. This adds another level of complexity to the cellular events occurring in the process of new blood vessel formation.

IN VITRO ASSAYS OF ANGIOGENIC AND ANTIANGIOGENIC FACTORS

The search for proangiogenic and antiangiogenic molecules has been made possible by methods that enable the measurement of angiogenesis activity. Unlike cell proliferation or death, which can be easily evaluated in convenient in vitro assays, angiogenesis involves complex interactions between endothelial cells and their surroundings. Because of this, angiogenesis measurements are subject to substantial assay-dependent biases. Several angiogenesis bioassays that represent various in vivo phases of angiogenesis have been developed. The assays used most often are those of endothelial cell proliferation and migration, two biologic events that are critical to the formation of new blood vessels. Proliferation is evaluated by measuring cell number changes, cell cycle alterations, or DNA incorporation, whereas migration assays usually involve scoring cells that migrate across a porous membrane toward a putative chemoattractant (Boyden chamber assay).

Additional assays include the tube formation assay, aortic ring assay, and chick-embryo chorioallantoic-membrane bioassay. The tube formation assay involves visualizing tubelike structures that form when endothelial cells are cultured on an artificial ECM, and the aortic ring assay evaluates similar structures that grow from a slice of rat aorta in culture. The chick-embryo chorioallantoic-membrane bioassay uses the vascular structures in a fertilized chick egg, either in uvo or in vitro.[96] The rabbit cornea implant assay involves placing a pellet of sustained-release polymers in a normally avascular cornea and examining the evolving blood vessels.[97] The matrigel-plug assay is a simpler version of the cornea implant assay. It involves the subcutaneous injection of a matrigel plug into a mouse and evaluation of its vascularization. None of these assays is flawless; thus, caution must be exercised when interpreting results from a single type of angiogenesis assay.

MAJOR MOLECULAR PLAYERS

VEGF Signal Transduction Pathway

VEGF Family Members VEGF, also called VEGF-A, increases endothelial permeability[98]; therefore, it was initially named vascular permeability factor. This protein was found to function as a mitogenic and survival factor, specific to endothelial cells.[99] VEGF is a heparin-binding glycoprotein with at least five family members, VEGF-A to -D and placental growth factor (PlGF). VEGF binds mostly Flt-1(fms-like tyrosine kinase-1)/VEGFR-1 and Flk-1(fetal liver kinase-1)/VEGFR-2/KDR (kinase domain region), parts of a family of tyrosine kinase receptors. VEGFR-1 and -2 are mainly expressed by vascular endothelial cells[100] but are also expressed by monocytes,[101] hematopoietic stem cells,[102] and some cancer cells.[103] VEGFR-2 is a major positive regulator of the vascular system. Its ligands are VEGF, VEGF-D, and VEGF-C. It activates the proliferation and migration of endothelial cells and acts as a survival factor for these cells. The role of VEGFR-1 in angiogenesis is less clear, demonstrating a higher binding affinity of VEGF than for VEGFR-2 but lower kinase activity and no mitogenic response. Mice manipulated not to express VEGFR-1 have an abnormal vascular system because of an increased number of hemangioblasts.[104] Interestingly, mice expressing a VEGFR-1 that lacks the kinase domain developed normally, suggesting that this protein functions as a negative regulator of the VEGF pathway by trapping ligand molecules.[105] The ligands of VEGFR-1 include VEGF, VEGF-B, and PlGF. The differences between VEGFR-1 and VEGFR-2 lie mostly in the intra-cellular C-terminal domain of these receptors.[106] VEGF-C and VEGF-D mainly regulate lymph vessel formation through activation of VEGFR-3,[107] although VEGFR-3 activity seems to be required also for blood vessel angiogenesis.[108] Interestingly, LKB-1, a serine/threonine kinase that is mutated in almost a third of lung cancers, was found to repress VEGF-C, among other targets[109] (see Fig. 8.2 for a scheme of the VEGF pathway).

The induction of VEGF production can result from various signals. Physiologically, it is controlled by the HIF-1 pathway in response to hypoxia. Mitogenic signals, including phosphatidylinositol 3-kinase (PI3K) and Ras, also increase VEGF mRNA levels.[110,111] Various isoforms of protein kinase C (PKC) have also been shown to induce VEGF.[112] EGFR inhibition reduced VEGF levels in a HIF-1–dependent and in a HIF-1–independent manner.[113] In addition, activated oncogenes and deregulated tumor suppressor genes contribute to VEGF's activation in tumors. Src kinase was found to be induced by hypoxia and to activate the VEGF promoter.[114,115] Wild-type p53 suppressed VEGF promoter activity, whereas mutant p53 had no effect or activated it.[115,116] HIF-1α degradation induced by p53 was also demonstrated, secondary to p53-dependent activation of Mdm2.[117]

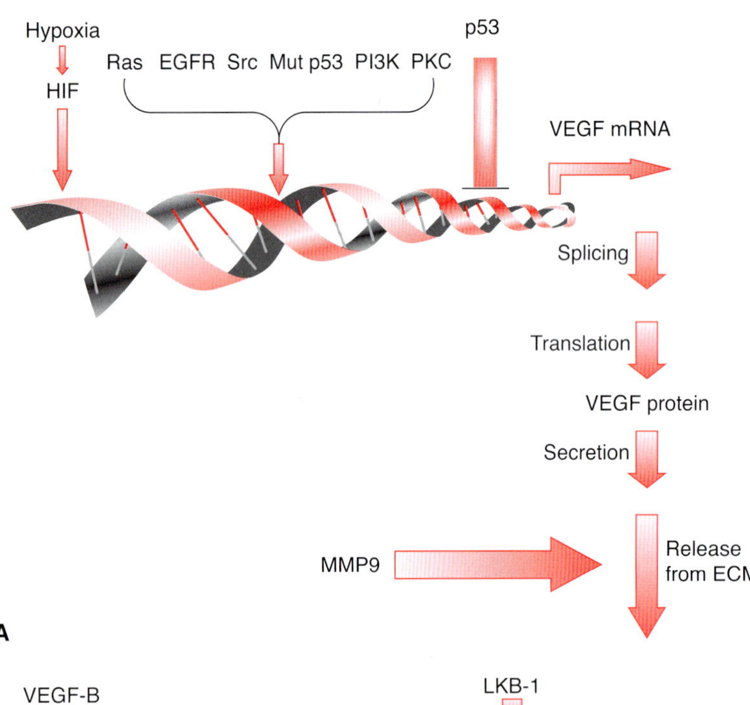

FIGURE 8.2 **A:** Control of VEGF transcription and posttranscriptional control. **B:** Major signaling activated by the VEGF pathway. For simplicity, only the major interactions and pathways are delineated. *AKT*, AKT8 virus oncogene homologue; *Cdc*, cell division control protein; *ECM*, extracellular matrix; *EGFR*, epidermal growth factor receptor; *ERK*, extracellular signal regulated kinase; *FAK*, focal adhesion kinase; *HIF*, hypoxia-inducible factor; *MAPK*, mitogen acturated protein kinase; *MEK*, MAPK/Erk kinase; *MMP9*, matrix metallopeptidase 9; *mRNA*, microRNA; *Mut*, methylmalonyl Coenzyme A mutase; *NP1*, Neuropilin1; *PI3K*, phosphatidylinositol 3 kinase; *PIGF*, placental growth factor; *PKC*, protein kinase C; *PLC*, phospholipase C; *RhoA*, ras homolog gene family, member A; *Src*, rous sarcoma oncogene cellular; *VEGF*, vascular endothelial growth factor.

VEGF receptors are activated by receptor dimerization induced by binding of the ligand dimer. This dimerization allows cross-phosphorylation of specific tyrosine residues of the receptors, creating docking sites for adapter molecules. The phosphorylation map and site-specific adapter proteins of VEGFR-2 have been delineated.[118] Various signaling pathways are activated downstream of VEGF receptors. VEGFR-2 is a survival factor for endothelial cells through PI3K and AKT.[119] VEGFR-2 also activates phospholyphase Cγ (PLCγ), which is not activated by VEGFR-1, EGF, or FGF. Signaling through VEGFR-2 independently activated phospholyphase Cγ, PKCε, and PI3K.[120] VEGFR-2 activates mitogen-activated protein kinase (MAPK) through mitogen-activated protein kinase kinase (MEK) and phospholyphase Cγ. Blockage of PKC reduced DNA replication induced by VEGF but had no effect on DNA replication induced by FGF or EGF.[120] Therefore, the signaling pathways used by VEGFR-2 are different from those used by other mitogens, although the end points of these cascades overlap. The MEK-ERK, PKC, and PI3K control DNA replication, cell proliferation, and survival signals in response to VEGF.

Some modulation of the VEGF pathway occurs through regulation of the receptor. For example, vascular endothelial (VE)-cadherin, a cell–cell adhesion molecule that is specifically expressed by endothelial cells, modulates signaling relayed by VEGFR-2. By blocking the internalization of this receptor, VE-cadherin inhibits its downstream signaling in confluent endothelial cells.[121] Downregulation of VEGFR-2 may occur in a PKC-regulated manner.[122] Another important modulator of VEGF receptor activity is neuropilin-1, a coreceptor of VEGF, originally recognized as a semophorin coreceptor that participates in neuronal guidance. Neuropilin-1 enhances the activation of VEGFR-2 by VEGF and the mitogenic and chemotactic response it evokes. It functions in an isoform-specific manner, binding VEGF165 but not VEGF121 (see below).[123] VEGFR-1 can also bind neuropilin-1, possibly as a negative regulator of its activity.[124] Neuropilin-1 is expressed by endothelial cells and cancer cells and contributes to their migration and in vivo progression. Neuropilin-1 mRNA levels were measured in the tumors of 60 NSCLC patients and were found to be an independent negative prognostic factor.[125]

New blood vessel formation requires endothelial cell migration, a biologic phenomena that involves complex modifications of cell–cell and cell–matrix adhesions. VEGF activates actin cytoskeleton remodeling and motility. These phenomena are mediated through VEGFR-2 and various adapter proteins, including src family kinase proteins such as Fyn and the small GTPases Cdc42, RhoA, and Rac-1. SAPK2/p38 activation modulates actin fiber polymerization, and focal adhesion kinase controls the formation of focal adhesion.[126,127] These molecular events are critical for the motility and migration of endothelial cells in response to VEGF signaling.

VEGF signaling apparently affects not only the cells that surround the tumor but also distant tissues. Activation of VEGFR-1 in the lungs of mice, in a premetastatic phase, was required for the induction of MMP9. This induction was evident only in the lungs of tumor-bearing mice; thus, it was the result of a tumor-originated influence. Lung endothelial cells and lung macrophages had elevated MMP9 levels in tumor-bearing mice, and this increase was essential for the formation of lung metastasis.[128] VEGFR-1 bearing hematopoietic progenitor cells localized to a premetastatic niche and were followed by metastasis formation in another mouse model.[129]

Five isoforms of VEGF are expressed by human cells, all of which are produced from the same VEGF gene through alternative splicing. These isoforms are named VEGF121, VEGF145, VEGF165, VEGF189, and VEGF206, according to the number of amino acids of the produced protein.[130] VEGF121 is the only isoform that does not bind heparin and is thus freely diffusible. The other four isoforms bind heparin; the two shortest, VEGF145 and VEGF165, are also secreted. VEGF145 binds ECM in a heparin-independent manner.[131] VEGF189 and VEGF206 are basic large proteins that are associated with the cell surface through their high affinity to proteoglycans or bound to the ECM, where they can activate VEGF signaling and be released to a soluble form.[132] Interestingly, VEGF189 was found to be prognostically important in NSCLC,[133] whereas VEGF165 had prognostic implications in osteosarcoma patients.[134] Thus, the various isoforms of VEGF exert different biologic activities in different tissues.

The RIP-Tag mice model offers insight into the activation of the VEGF pathway during the angiogenic switch. Targeted knockout of VEGF or inhibition of VEGFR-2 by small molecule inhibitors in the RIP-Tag mice, reduced tumor initiation and progression, demonstrating the critical role of this molecule.[8] Progression of carcinomas in this model was accompanied by an increased release of VEGF from the tumor mass and increased binding of the ligand to VEGFR-2. Interestingly, no increase in the expression of this protein or its receptors was found. MMP9 expression was found to be increased in stromal cells in progressing tumors. It was shown to increase the release of ECM-bound VEGF and thus its ability to activate the receptor.[9] Therefore, nontumorigenic cells in the tumor stroma can control the angiogenic switch by producing MMP and modulating the release of VEGF from the ECM.

Angiopoietins and Tie Receptors Angiopoietins are a family of angiogenesis modulators composed of four ligands that bind the Tie-2 tyrosine kinase receptor. Ang-1 and Ang-4 function mostly as positive regulators, whereas Ang-2 and Ang-3 are mostly antiangiogenic. However, these roles are context dependent. Knockout Ang-1 mice do not form a normal vascular network in utero, at least partly because of reduced pericyte coverage. Ang-2 overexpression has a similar phenotype to that of Ang-1 knockout, indicating that Ang-2 has an antagonistic role in Tie-2 activity. Ang-2 antagonizes the Ang-1-dependent recruitment of pericytes to new blood vessels, thus preventing their stabilization. However, Ang-2 knockout mice have defects in adult vascular sprouting. This finding suggests that destabilization of the vessel structure is needed for angiogenesis to progress. Ang-2 seems to have a proangiogenic role when VEGF is abundant but an antiangiogenic role when VEGF levels are low.[135] The Tie-2 receptor is expressed by endothelial cells and by pericytes and smooth muscle cells. Its expression by blood monocytes might be important for their recruitment to tumor tissues.[136] Importantly, Ang-2 expression has negative prognostic implications in lung cancer patients, especially when VEGF expression is high[137] (see succeeding discussion). Ang-2 and Tie-2 apparently regulate the survival of vessels co-opted by cancer[138] (see previous discussion). Interestingly, Ang-1 has a negative role in tumor angiogenesis, probably secondary to enhanced pericyte vessel coverage and reduced vessel permeability.[139] The resultant vessels do not allow extravasation of plasma proteins and a less proangiogenic environment is formed.

Unexpected Outcomes of VEGF Inhibition In studies in which the VEGF pathway was effectively attenuated, rebound angiogenesis was observed despite persistent inhibition of the VEGF pathway. Alternative angiogenic mechanisms were upregulated when the VEGF pathway was suppressed, including induction of FGF family members, angiopoietins, and vessel co-option.[10] The activation of additional proangiogenic pathways may be triggered by hypoxia in tumors subjected to VEGF inhibition. However, increased levels of some of these factors persist when no hypoxia is apparent. Therefore, pathologic angiogenesis is controlled by various signaling pathways that may be important therapeutic targets.[97]

The other important finding in models of VEGF-dependent tumor growth treated with VEGF inhibitors is increased invasiveness of tumors that thrive in these conditions.[9,10] This phenomenon could be secondary to hypoxia-induced activation of the HGF-Met pathway,[140] urokinase-type plasminogen activator,[141] or other survival pathways. Hypoxia may select for tumor cells with increased aggressiveness, such as through loss of p53[142,143] or other genetic events.[144] As VEGF pathway inhibition is assayed as a cancer therapeutic strategy, further understanding about cancer escape mechanisms is needed.

HIF HIF-1 is the major transcription factor that regulates the response of tissues to oxygen deprivation.[145] It is expressed ubiquitously in humans, where it upregulates erythropoiesis and blood vessel formation and controls metabolic pathways. HIF-1α subunits are tightly regulated by hypoxia through control of their degradation, in addition to hypoxia-independent regulation by growth factor signaling.[146] Under normoxia, they are marked for degradation via the 26S proteosome by its E3-ubiquitin ligase von Hippel-Lindau (VHL), a tumor suppressor gene.[147] Oxygen levels are sensed by prolyl hydoxylase, an enzyme that hydroxylates specific prolyl residues of HIF-1α when oxygen is available. This modified domain of HIF-1α is the binding site of VHL, which activates its rapid degradation. Lack of oxygen thus prevents VHL-dependent degradation of HIF-1α, causing an accumulation of this protein.[148,149]

HIF-1β is expressed constitutively, forming a heterodimer with a HIF α subunit, thus activating more than 70 genes whose products carry out the complex regulation mastered by HIF-1. HIF-1α and HIF-2α are the products of two different genes, regulated similarly by hypoxia, both of which can heterodimerize with HIF-1β and activate each a distinct set of genes.[150] Both α subunits are produced by various cell types, including endothelial cells.[151,152] The relative contributions of HIF-1 or -2α differ under different conditions.[153] HIF-1α expression by tumor cells was found to contribute to tumor progression.[154] HIF-2α is highly expressed in tumor-infiltrating macrophages, and this expression was correlated with tumor angiogenesis in a series of breast carcinomas.[155] Thus, HIF-2α may participate in the contribution of the tumor microenvironment to tumor vascularity.[152] In addition, the role of HIF-3α has yet to be defined. A splice variant of HIF-3α was found to antagonize the transactivation of hypoxia-inducible genes by HIF.[156]

Endogenous Antiangiogenic Factors Some antiangiogenic factors are produced by cleavage of larger proteins. For example, angiostatin, a potent angiogenesis inhibitor, is the cleavage product of plasminogen, a component of the coagulation control mechanism.[157] Macrophage-derived methalloelastase is thought to be responsible for the in vivo conversion of plasminogen to angiostatin.[158] Thus, tumor-infiltrating macrophages may determine the production of antiangiogenic factors. In addition, cancer cells may secrete enzymes that can produce angiostatin.[159] The conversion of plasminogen to the proangiogenic plasmin is essential for the production of angiostatin.[159] Angiostatin's mechanism of action might be through inhibition of plasmin production.[160] This cross-talk between an angiogenic molecule and an antiangiogenic factor is consistent with the continuous balancing mechanisms between these effects.

Endostatin is an antiangiogenic factor that was shown to be generated by tumor cell lines. A biochemical analysis indicated that it is a fragment of collagen XVIII.[161] Recently, α(II) collagen prolyl-4-hydroxylase [α(II)PH] was found to catalyze a rate-limiting step in collagen synthesis that is apparently required in endostatin production. Importantly, α(II)PH was found to be a direct transcriptional target of p53, a well-recognized tumor suppressor gene, in tumor cells. p53 expression was found to increase the expression of α(II)PH, leading to enhanced endostatin production. By an apparently similar mechanism, p53 led to the production of tumstatin from collagen IV.[143] Thrombospondin-1 is another antiangiogenic molecule induced by p53, through transcriptional activation.[33] Thrombospondin-1 secretion decreases with malignant progression,[162] possibly a reflection of the common loss of p53 transcriptional activity in tumor cells. Endostatin and tumstatin function through binding of integrins and modulating various signaling pathways,[163,164] whereas the mechanism of action of thrombosponsdin-1 involves inhibition of MMP9 activation[165] and activating endothelial cell apoptosis through CD36.[166]

Additional potent antiangiogenic factors are produced by the cleavage of common proteins,[167] suggesting a paradigm. C-terminal fragments of various collagens are cryptic antiangiogenic agents, becoming active once released from the parent collagen.[168] The control of angiogenesis seems to require reserves of antiangiogenic factors available for rapid mobilization.

PDGF Platelet-derived growth factor beta polypeptide (PDGF-BB) and PDGF-β receptor are the major molecules involved in regulating the pericytes perivascular envelope.[169,170] PDGF-B is secreted by tumor endothelial cells, and tumor cells in some cases, and forms the active dimer of PDGF-BB. PDGF-β receptor is expressed mainly by pericytes, although it has also been found on tumor endothelial cells. The activation of the PDGF-β receptor results in the recruitment of pericytes to the developing tumor vessel, as in physiologic angiogenesis.[171] Pericytes have a supportive and modulating role in the evolving vessel. Abnormal pericyte coverage in PDGF-B null mice resulted in vessel dilatation, leakage, aneurism formation, and hemorrhage in late gestation.[172] Interestingly, the retention of PDGF-B on the surface of the secreting cell is important for correct pericyte deposition, at least during embryonic development. Local retention of growth factors is a mechanism whereby extracellular matrix and proteases affect biologic phenomena. The retention of PDGF-B is mediated by its C-terminal motif of positively charged amino acids, which bind negatively charged heparan sulphate proteoglycans.[173] Blood vessels of tumors inoculated into mice that expressed an ECM retention-defective mutant PDGF-B had defects in pericyte coverage. PDGF-B expression by tumor cells only partially compensated for this defect, suggesting that PDGF-B must be expressed by endothelial cells[174] to facilitate the correct homing of pericytes to blood vessels.

bFGF bFGF is a potent angiogenic factor that stimulates the proliferation and migration of endothelial cells as well as the production of MMPs. However, unlike VEGF, bFGF affects various cell types, including endothelial cells, smooth muscle cells, fibroblasts, and epithelial cells.[175,176] bFGF can be found in high levels in some low-proliferation tissues, indicating tight control of its activity after its production. bFGF is at least partly regulated by its extracellular export.[177,178] In addition, binding of the FGF receptor by bFGF requires the presence of an ECM/basement membrane proteoglycan such as perlecan.[179] Capillary endothelial cells express and secrete bFGF and thus induce their own proliferation and migration.[180] bFGF signaling cross-talks with additional angiogenic pathways. Hypoxic induction of HIF-1α in endothelial cells is bFGF dependent.[181] bFGF signaling has been shown to activate transcription of the PDGF receptor, whereas PDGF-BB amplified bFGF receptor expression.[182] bFGF has a major role in angiogenesis, but its involvement in many other pathologic and normal processes makes it a problematic therapeutic target.

The overexpression of FGF-10 in respiratory epithelial lung cells in mice induced multifocal pulmonary adenomas within 1 to 4 weeks. Interestingly, all these tumors regressed shortly after withdrawal of the transgene-activating agent, indicating that no irreversible carcinogenic change occurred and that the tumors were dependent on FGF-10 expression. Angiogenesis measures were not reported for this model, but given the importance of the FGF pathway in tumor angiogenesis, an angiogenic switch was plausibly involved.[183]

Chemokines Chemokines are small (8–10 kDa) proteins that regulate mainly leukocyte trafficking. Various chemokines also influence angiogenesis, both negatively and positively. The C-X-C chemokine family can be divided to two subfamilies. Those that contain a Glu-Leu-Arg motif at the NH3-terminus (ELR+), activate the CXCR2 receptor, and are mostly angiogenic. CXC chemokines that lack this motif (ELR−), act through CXCR3 and are angiostatic. Platelet factor-4 (PF-4, also called CXCL4) is an example of an ELR− chemokine, which is a strong inhibitor of angiogenesis. A variant of PF-4/CXCL4 exists, which is a stronger inhibitor of angiogenesis than PF-4/CXCL4.[184] IL-8/CXCL8 is an ELR+ chemokine and is indeed a potent angiogenic factor.[82] SDF-1/CXCL12 is an exception to the aforementioned rule, being an ELR− chemokine, but activating the CXCR4 receptor, and thought to have an angiogenic effect.[185] In a mouse model of lung cancer, inhibition of SDF1/CXCL12 abrogated metastasis formation but did not affect angiogenesis,[35] suggesting it might not have a major angiogenic role in lung cancer. The C-X-C chemokines act through the activation of G-protein–coupled serpentine (seven-transmembrane spanning) receptors.

Cell–Cell Adhesion Molecules The various cellular events that occur during the formation of new blood vessels involve interactions among endothelial cells, pericytes, smooth muscle cells, inflammatory cells, and epithelial cells that are governed mainly by cell–cell adhesion molecules. Several of these molecules have a role in modulating angiogenesis.

Platelet endothelial cell–cell adhesion molecule-1 (PECAM-1 or CD31) is commonly used as a marker of endothelial cells in immunohistochemical studies.[186] Binding of this molecule by an inhibitory antibody suppresses angiogenic activity.[187] PECAM-1 is expressed also by platelets and inflammatory cells. It plays a role in leukocyte migration, and is involved in several signaling pathways.[186] PECAM-1 might contribute to endothelial cells function. It can also be speculated that the contribution of this molecule to angiogenesis might be through recruitment of inflammatory cells, or through the anchoring of platelets in angiogenic sites. Platelets seem to have an important role in storing and delivering angiogenic and antiangiogenic factors.[97,188]

Intercellular adhesion molecule 2 (ICAM-2), a member of the immunoglobulin superfamily, is a transmembrane protein that is involved in binding various integrins and other molecules. In addition, through homophilic interactions (binding the same protein expressed on another cell), ICAM-2 is involved in endothelial cell survival and migration. It is commonly expressed in endothelial cell–cell junctions[189] and was found in a mouse model to be involved in angiogenesis. Mice that did not express this protein were defective in angiogenesis in in vivo assays, and endothelial cells from these mice demonstrated defective migration and increased apoptosis.[190] Importantly, plasma ICAM levels were found to be prognostic in a clinical study of lung cancer patients treated with an anti-VEGF antibody (see later).[191]

Cadherins are transmembrane proteins that populate adherence junctions. The extracellular domains of cadherins form calcium-dependent, homophilic transdimers when they bind similar proteins on neighboring cells, mediating cell–cell adhesions. The cytoplasmic tails of cadherins bind to several potential signaling proteins, most notably β-catenin, a transcriptional cofactor in Wnt signaling. β-catenin bound to a cadherin intracellular domain participates in cell–cell interactions and does not function as a transcription factor. When cadherin membranous localization is disrupted, β-catenin is released from the cytoskeleton and can enter the nucleus, where it functions as a transcription factor with oncogenic features. Membranous E-cadherin expression in NSCLC tumor specimens was found to be prognostic.[192–194] Tumors that expressed low levels of membranous E-cadherin were more likely to metastasize to regional lymph nodes, accompanied by reduced survival. It can be speculated that low membranous localization of E-cadherin allows enhanced oncogenic transcriptional activity of β-catenin, and an angiogenic switch (see succeeding discussion).

TGF-β and EGFR Pathway Transforming growth factor (TGF)-β is a pleiotropic factor that can have different effects on different cells. It is required for endothelial differentiation[195] and induces angiogenesis in vivo[196]; however, in a different experimental setup, disruption of TGF-β signaling induced angiogenesis and tumor formation.[197] TGF-β was shown to cause endothelial cell apoptosis, which appears to be essential for angiogenesis.[198]

This apparent correlation between endothelial cell apoptosis and enhanced angiogenesis underscores the complexity of angiogenesis and the potential biases of studies that use endothelial cell proliferation or survival as a surrogate for the in vivo end point. Importantly, TGF-β levels in adenocarcinoma NSCLC tumor samples were correlated positively with MVD and negatively with prognosis.[199] Tumor endothelial cell survival involves also the EGFR pathway, demonstrated to depend on EGF secretion by tumor cells.[200] ERK activation downstream of EGFR was found to activate a crosstalk between cancer cells and endothelial cells that promotes angiogenesis.[201] Some prostaglandins (a large group of signal mediators) also induce angiogenesis; the most notable of these is prostaglandin E2. The angiogenic effect of prostaglandin E2 is dependent on TGF-β and MMPs.[202]

Nitric Oxide Nitric oxide is a small signaling molecule that is involved in many biologic phenomena. It affects angiogenesis both negatively and positively, depending on its concentration.[203] For example, nitric oxide regulates thrombospondin 1 levels in a triphasic manner.[204] It participates in the biologic response to both angiogenic and antiangiogenic factors, possibly through their effects on nitric oxide synthase. The nitric oxide synthase 2 isoform was found to be correlated with VEGF levels and MVD in 106 NSCLC tissue specimens.[205] Treatment with nitric oxide donors combined with chemotherapy given to NSCLC patients, improved their outcome in a large randomized phase II trial.[206] The complex and dosage-dependent effects of nitric oxide on various aspects of cancer biology makes it difficult to predict the possible effect it might have had on angiogenesis in those lung cancers.

ROLE OF ANGIOGENIC SIGNALS IN LUNG CANCER

Prognostic Markers of Angiogenesis MVD is commonly used as an immunohistochemically derived indication of angiogenesis in tumors. MVD was found to be correlated with prognosis in NSCLC in several studies.[207–215] However, MVD has not been found to be correlated with prognosis in other studies.[205,216,217] In one of the larger studies that reported no correlation of MVD with prognosis,[216] MVD was assessed in tissue microarrays, which are comprised of small cores taken from each tumor. The manner in which tumor areas were chosen for the tissue microarray probably differed from those normally chosen for MVD scoring (see previous discussion). This difference might explain the discordant results regarding the prognostic value of MVD. In another study of 106 NSCLC patients,[205] MVD was correlated with clinical disease stage, but not with survival.

MVD, as assessed immunohistochemically with CD105, is suggested to mark only active blood vessels. MVD assessed by CD105 was more strongly correlated with VEGF tumor levels than was MVD assessed by CD34 (panendothelial marker). MVD by CD105 was also more strongly correlated with clinical outcome in a study of 236 NSCLC patients.[15] CD34 apparently marks all blood vessels, including vessels that are not functional. Overall, the evidence suggests that angiogenic activity as assessed by tumor MVD is prognostically important in lung cancer. Fine tuning and standardization of the MVD measurement methods is needed.

Tumor expression of VEGF, as evaluated by immunohistochemical analysis, was found to have a negative prognostic value in NSCLC patients,[216,218–221] although a lack of correlation has also been reported[103] (see Table 8.2 for a summary of the prognostic angiogenic factors in lung cancer). Regarding a different type of lung cancer, small cell lung cancer (SCLC), tumor VEGF expression was also found here to be a poor prognostic factor in a study of 75 surgically resected patients.[222] In another study of SCLC, serum levels of VEGF of 69 patients were found to be associated with poor outcome and poor survival,[223] attesting to the importance of angiogenesis also for this type of lung cancer.

Levels of VEGF (and bFGF) in NSCLC tissue extracts, including both tumor and stromal components, have prognostic implications.[224] Interestingly, VEGF-C expression in stromal cells of NSCLC was found to have a positive prognostic value.[216] Given the important role of the stroma in tumor progression and regression, this finding entails further investigation.

TABLE 8.2 Angiogenic Factors and Importance in NSCLC

Angiogenic Factor	Poor Prognostic Factor by Immunohistochemical Analysis (N of Patients in the Study Cited)	Poor Prognostic Factor by Levels in Tumor Extract (N of Patients in the Study Cited)	Poor Prognostic Factor by Blood Levels (N of Patients in the Study Cited)	Predictive Value	Targeted Therapy	Clinically Effective (N of Patients in the Study Cited)
VEGF	Y (105),[209] (109 SCCa),[219] (85, Stg I),[220] (120, Stg I and II)[221]; N (69, Stg I and II)[103]	Y (71)[224] (57, only VEGF189 mRNA isoform)[133]	Equivocal	Y: Plasma levels Predictive of response to bevacizumab[191]	Bevacizumab	Y (878)[5]
bFGF	Y[229]	Y (71)[224]	Equivocal[229]			
PDGF					Multikinase inhibitors	Phase III trials
IL-8/CXCL8		Y: mRNA levels[82]				
HGF		Y (53)[244]				
VEGFR	Y: VEGFR3 (335)[216]		Y: mRNA levels of VEGFR2 higher in nonresponders (53)[226]		Multikinase inhibitors	Phase III trials
Ang-2	Y: only with high VEGF (236)[137]					
PIGF	Y (91)[233]	Y (91)[233]				
BNIP	Y (105)[237]					
HIF-1α	Y (172)[238]	N: (54, Stg IIb–III)[239]				
Trx-1	Y (102)[243]					
CEP			Y: (CD34$^+$VEGFR2$^+$, FACS)[226]			

FACS, fluorescence-activated cell sorting; N, no; SCCa, squamous cell carcinoma; Stg, stage; Y, yes.

VEGF mRNA levels were investigated in NSCLC tissue specimens and were found to be associated with a grim prognosis.[225] An in-depth study of VEGF splice variants in tumor tissues revealed that the 189 isoform was associated with a poor prognosis in resected NSCLC patients.[133] Other VEGF splice variants were not associated with prognosis in that cohort of patients, suggesting that VEGF levels in tissues studies should differentiate between the various VEGF splice variants.

Serum VEGF levels have been found to be prognostic in some studies[227,228] but not others.[229,230] E4599, a study of 878 NSCLC patients with advanced disease, was retrospectively analyzed to determine the prognostic and predictive significance of VEGF plasma levels. All patients had received carboplatin and paclitaxel, and some were randomly assigned to bevacizumab. VEGF plasma levels were predictive of response to bevacizumab but were not prognostic of survival.[191] Another study evaluated 462 early stage lung cancer patients for polymorphisms in the VEGF gene, and reported them to be prognostically important. The examined polymorphisms are expected to correlate with reduced VEGF serum levels,[231] but actual serum level evaluations were not available. It can be speculated that VEGF levels within a cancer are important whereas serum levels are modulated by additional mechanisms, irrelevant for tumor biology.

VEGF receptor levels have also been evaluated. One large study evaluated VEGF and VEGFR isoform levels by immunohistochemical analysis in 335 NSCLC patients (stages I to IIIa).[216] These levels were evaluated separately in tumor and adjacent stroma tissue. Although several factors were found to be associated with poor prognosis in univariate analysis, this association was found only for VEGFR-3 tumor expression in multivariate analysis.[216] In another study of NSCLC patients, real-time RT-PCR analysis revealed that VEGFR-2 mRNA blood levels were correlated with response to treatments and with clinical outcome.[226]

Tumor expression of Ang-2, a context-dependent modulator of angiogenesis, was found to have a negative effect on survival in a study of 236 resectable NSCLC patients. This effect was evident only among tumors that expressed high levels of VEGF and was not significant in those with low VEGF levels.[137] This result is consistent with the known molecular mechanisms involved; Ang-2 positively controls angiogenesis only when VEGF is abundant (see previous discussion).

bFGF is considered an important angiogenesis inducer and prognostic factor in tumors: Its expression in NSCLC tissue is associated with a poor prognosis. However, data on the prognostic value of bFGF blood levels vary.[229]

Interleukin-8 (IL-8, also called CXCL8) was shown to be highly expressed in bronchiogenic lung carcinomas. Its expression in lung cancer cells was significantly induced by coculturing with macrophages. Tumor-infiltrating macrophages and IL-8/CXCL8 mRNA levels in NSCLC tumors were found to be correlated with microvascular density and patient survival.[82] A study of specific neutralizing antibodies demonstrated that IL-8/CXCL8 was responsible for endothelial cell migration and for the angiogenic response elicited by NSCLC tumor extracts in a corneal neovascularization assay.[232]

PlGF, a VEGFR-1 ligand was also found to be correlated with stage in NSCLC. PlGF protein levels (as measured by immunostaining) and gene transcript levels (as measured by RT-PCR) were correlated with poor prognosis.[233] Because VEGFR-1 is a negative regulator of the VEGF pathway, PlGF's correlation with poor prognosis might be through a different pathway. Possibly related is an in vitro study of NSCLC cell lines, where PlGF was found to influence cell motility, through ROCK1, a major regulator of the cytoskeleton.[234]

Aberrant expression of p53, commonly used as an indicator of mutant p53, was correlated with increased mRNA levels of VEGF, IL-8/CXCL8, and MVD and poor prognosis in 65 NSCLC patients.[235] A larger study reported poor prognosis for patients with an aberrant p53 expression, after tumor resection with no further treatment. However, such patients gained significant benefit when given adjuvant chemotherapy.[236] It can be speculated that tumors with an aberrant p53 have higher levels of angiogenic factors in their microenvironment; chemotherapy agents might thus be better delivered to micrometastasis disease.

A transcriptional target of HIF-1, BNIP3, was evaluated in 105 NSCLC patients. BNIP3 is a pro-apoptotic mitochondrial protein that can activate necrosis-like cell death and may be important in the necrotic response to hypoxia in tumors. BNIP3 levels were found to be highly correlated with poor prognosis in patients with resectable disease.[237] HIF-1α protein levels, as assessed by immunohistochemical analysis, were correlated with poor prognosis in 172 NSCLC tumors (stages I to IIIa).[238] On the other hand, HIF-1α mRNA levels, as measured by RT-PCR, were not correlated with clinical outcome in a study of 54 NSCLC patients.[239] Therefore, HIF-1α regulation at a posttranslational level, by VHL-mediated degradation, might be its dominant regulatory mechanism in NSCLC. Regarding another surrogate marker of hypoxia, carbonic anhydrase IX was also found to be associated with poor prognosis in early NSCLC.[18]

A more direct method of quantifying hypoxia in NSCLC is with the use of nuclear medicine tracers. An 18F-misonidazole evaluation of 14 NSCLC patients predicted recurrence after curative radiotherapy in those patients that had evidence of significant tumor hypoxia.[240] Additional hypoxia tracers exist, such as copper-60 derivate ([60]Cu-ATSM), which also has prognostic value in NSCLC.[241]

Trx-1 is a small redox protein that modulates the activity of various enzymes, including DNA binding and transactivation by transcription factors. Trx-1 was shown to increase the protein level and activity of HIF-1α in cancer cells.[242] Interestingly, Trx-1 levels were found to be correlated with lymph node invasion and a poor prognosis in a study of 102 early stage NSCLC patients.[243] Although possibly related to several other pathways, Trx increased levels could have activated the HIF pathway and thus disease progression.

HGF-Met signaling is also implicated in the progression of lung cancer. HGF levels, as quantified in lung tumor tissue, were associated with a poor prognosis.[244] Recently, somatic mutations were discovered in the c-Met receptor of NSCLC specimens. The mutations were concentrated in a region close to a splice junction and led to an alternatively spliced protein. This protein was defective in Cbl-mediated degradation, demonstrating prolonged ligand-induced activation.[245] The HGF-Met pathway affects multiple cellular pathways, including tumor angiogenesis.[92] In many cases, HGF production is enhanced in tumor-associated fibroblasts, demonstrating another tumor-stroma interaction that promotes cancer progression.

Blood levels of CEPs were investigated in 53 patients with various stages and histologic subtypes of NSCLC. CEPs were detected in this study by a flow cytometric $CD34^{+}VEGFR2^{+}$ analysis. In the multivariate analysis, the CEP count was a statistically significant prognostic marker, whereas surprisingly, disease stage had no prognostic value.[226] The blood mRNA transcript levels of several possible CEPs' molecular markers (CD34, CD-133, and VE-cadherin) were not correlated with prognosis or with the CEP count, whereas high mRNA levels of VEGFR2 were correlated with a lack of response to therapy.[226] Another small study reported the feasibility of magnetic bead separation for CEP identification in lung cancer.[246] The lack of consensus in the field about the importance of CEP and the lack of reliable methods for CEP detection hinder our understanding of their role in lung cancer.

Immune system cell infiltration affects angiogenesis and prognosis in NSCLC. In bronchoalveolar carcinoma pathologic specimens, neutrophil accumulation in the alveolar lumen was associated with a poor prognosis. Neutrophil count was correlated with IL-8/CXCL8 levels in the BAL fluid of these patients. The origin of the secreted IL-8/CXCL8 seemed to be the cancer cells.[72] Thus, IL-8/CXCL8 can function as an angiogenic factor either by directly activating endothelial cells[247] or indirectly by recruiting immune system cells to tumor sites. IL-8/CXCL8 also has a direct mitogenic effect on lung cancer cells.[248]

Nonangiogenesis Variant of NSCLC In contrast to the data implicating vascular angiogenesis as a critical requirement to tumor growth, notable exceptions have been observed.

In NSCLC, a nonangiogenic histologic pattern with a higher incidence of lymph node metastasis and a poorer prognosis was described.[249,250] Histologically, it had a nondestructive, alveolar pattern of malignant cell spread. A detailed analysis of the tumor vessels suggested that the tumor had co-opted existing blood vessels and possibly even lymphatic vessels.[251] Although suggestive to be a subtype of bronchoalveolar carcinoma, analysis of squamous cell lung cancers revealed also a subgroup of low-vascularity squamous cell tumors.[252] These squamous cell carcinomas were characterized by a high proliferation rate, low apoptotic activity, high VEGF expression, and low bFGF expression, and were associated with a poor prognosis. In another study, c-ErbB2 overexpression was correlated with a poor prognosis in a low-angiogenesis subgroup of NSCLC tumors.[253] These findings indicate that lung cancer can grow without neoangiogenesis. A lack of new vessel formation does not necessarily hinder tumor progression, although it dictates a specific growth pattern. More data is required about the molecular mechanisms involved in the progression of low-angiogenic tumors and about potential therapeutic targets in this subgroup.

Lymphangiogenic Switch in Lung Cancer Most research on cancerous vascularization has focused on angiogenesis and blood vessels' connections to the tumor. The tumor's vascular supply is essential to its growth; thus, angiogenesis induction is a critical turning point. However, the lymphatic network is also being recognized as important in later stages of lung cancer progression. Lymphangiogenesis is correlated with lymph node metastasis and prognosis.[251] VEGF-C controls lymphangiogenesis and lymph node metastasis in mouse models of lung cancer.[254] Accordingly, VEGF-C protein levels in the serum of 116 NSCLC patients were correlated with the risk of lymph node metastasis.[255] Targeting in parallel VEGF-A and VEGF-C might be pharmacologically applicable and could be therapeutically advantageous.

Mouse Models of Lung Cancer Angiogenic Switch

K-Ras is activated by a somatic mutation in 20% to 30% of NSCLCs.[256] A correlation was found between K-Ras mutation and high VEGF expression in a group of 181 NSCLC tumors.[257] Another report did not find a correlation between K-Ras mutations and vascularity or VEGF levels.[258] Mice manipulated to express active K-Ras in lung epithelium (KRas^{LA1} mice) developed atypical adenomatous hyperplasia and adenomas, which progressed to adenocarcinoma.[259,260] The oncogenic effect of K-Ras in this model was shown to be Rac1 dependent.[261] PI3K activation and increased phophatidyleinositole[3–5] triphosphate levels probably also mediated the oncogenic effect of K-Ras, as PTEN deletion accelerated K-Ras–induced lung cancer formation.[262] c-Met-HGF signaling contributes to tumor progression in this model, at least partly through enhanced angiogenesis.[263] Accordingly, an inhibitor of c-Met led to reduced VEGF production and enhanced thrombospondin-1 expression in lung cancer cells.[264] In addition, Ras signaling activated expression of CXCR2 ligands, causing accumulation of inflammatory cells and vascular endothelial cells in the premalignant lesions of the KRas^{LA1} mice. Blockage of CXCR2 signaling prevented the progression of these lung lesions and caused apoptosis of vascular endothelial cells within them.[265] CXCR2 inhibition had a tumor-inhibitory effect in a microenvironment-dependent manner. This suggests that KRas activation in lung cancer is proangiogenic and tumorigenic through recruitment of inflammatory cells and vascular endothelial cells.

A mouse model of lung cancer involving the targeting of either a wild-type c-Raf kinase or a constitutively active c-Raf kinase to lung epithelial cells was reported.[266] After a relative long latency period, isolated foci of lung adenomas developed, with no evidence of invasion or metastasis.[266] Additional genetic events are assumed to take place in some of the primed cells to explain these observations, making this model suitable for studies of lung cancer progression. In a study using the c-Raf mouse lung cancer model, disruption of intercellular adhesions through the downregulation of E-cadherin promoted an angiogenic switch.[267] E-cadherin disruption led to nuclear localization of β-catenin and secondary upregulation of VEGF-A, VEGF-C, and VEGFR-3. Phenotypically, this resulted in a marked increase in MVD, and evidence of increased permeability, typically seen when the VEGF pathway is activated. Lymphatic vessel density was also increased, accompanied by micrometastasis in draining lymph nodes.[267] Loss of E-cadherin–mediated cell–cell contacts might be a major regulator of the angiogenic switch in lung cancer.

CLINICAL IMPLICATIONS OF ANGIOGENESIS INHIBITION IN LUNG CANCER

Although beyond the scope of this chapter, we will mention briefly a few of the major angiogenesis inhibitors that are in clinical use or are being studied in lung cancer patients. This issue is discussed comprehensively later in this manuscript by Christian Manegold and Alan Sandler.

Bevacizumab (Avastin, Roche) is a monoclonal antibody that is directed against the VEGF ligand. It was the first antiangiogenic treatment to be approved for cancer. Bevacizumab was evaluated in a phase III study of 878 patients with advanced disease who received paclitaxel and carboplatin and was found to result in an increased survival duration, from 10.3 to 12.3 months.[5] Bevacizumab treatment was also evaluated in combination with cisplatinum and gemcitabine and was shown to increase progression-free survival (http://meeting.ascopubs.org/cgi/content/abstract/25/18_suppl/LBA7514, 2007).

Recombinant endostatin was evaluated as a treatment for 42 neuroendocrine cancer patients, with no documented responses.[268] Endostar, (YH-16, Medgenn Co.) is a recombinant human endostatin modified by the addition of nine amino acids. In a study of 493 advanced NSCLC patients, addition of endostatin to chemotherapy led to increased time to progression, from 3.6 to 6.3 months (http://meeting.ascopubs.org/cgi/content/abstract/23/16_suppl/7138, 2005). These findings suggest that endostatin has an important role in lung cancer treatment. Endostar was recently approved for the treatment of NSCLC patients in China. It remains to be seen if this drug will be reevaluated in other countries.

Vandetanib (ZD6474) is a multikinase inhibitor that targets VEGFR, EGFR, and Ret. It is being studied in several phase II trials as a treatment for NSCLC.

Many other phase I and II studies of multikinase inhibitors are ongoing, many of them targeting VEGFR and PDGFR. This active clinical research is a result of the studies cited previously that demonstrated VEGF as a major regulator of angiogenesis. PDGFR is being evaluated as a clinical target, reflecting the understanding that pericyte coverage is an essential part of vascular small vessels. Many other targeted therapies are being studied as potential antiangiogenic or vascularization-disrupting agents. The bench-to-bedside transition of angiogenesis and vasculogenesis inhibition is among the shortest in cancer research. Hopefully, the combination of preclinical research and antiangiogenic treatment development will evolve to result in effective treatments for lung cancer patients.

REFERENCES

1. Carmeliet P. Angiogenesis in life, disease and medicine. *Nature* 2005;438(7070):932–936.
2. Dvorak HF. Tumors: wounds that do not heal. Similarities between tumor stroma generation and wound healing. *N Engl J Med* 1986;315(26):1650–1659.
3. Armulik A, Abramsson A, Betsholtz C. Endothelial/pericyte interactions. *Circ Res* 2005;97(6):512–523.
4. Folkman J. Tumor angiogenesis: therapeutic implications. *N Engl J Med* 1971;285(21):1182–1186.
5. Sandler A, Gray R, Perry MC, et al. Paclitaxel-carboplatin alone or with bevacizumab for non-small-cell lung cancer. *N Engl J Med* 2006;355(24):2542–2550.
6. Jain RK, Duda DG, Clark JW, et al. Lessons from phase III clinical trials on anti-VEGF therapy for cancer. *Nat Clin Pract Oncol* 2006;3(1):24–40.
7. Folkman J, Watson K, Ingber D, et al. Induction of angiogenesis during the transition from hyperplasia to neoplasia. *Nature* 1989;339(6219):58–61.
8. Inoue M, Hager JH, Ferrara N, et al. VEGF-A has a critical, nonredundant role in angiogenic switching and pancreatic beta cell carcinogenesis. *Cancer Cell* 2002;1(2):193–202.
9. Bergers G, Brekken R, McMahon G, et al. Matrix metalloproteinase-9 triggers the angiogenic switch during carcinogenesis. *Nat Cell Biol* 2000;2(10):737–744.
10. Casanovas O, Hicklin DJ, Bergers G, et al. Drug resistance by evasion of antiangiogenic targeting of VEGF signaling in late-stage pancreatic islet tumors. *Cancer Cell* 2005;8(4):299–309.
11. Gimbrone MA Jr, Leapman SB, Cotran RS, et al. Tumor dormancy in vivo by prevention of neovascularization. *J Exp Med* 1972;136(2):261–276.
12. Holmgren L, O'Reilly MS, Folkman J. Dormancy of micrometastases: balanced proliferation and apoptosis in the presence of angiogenesis suppression. *Nat Med* 1995;1(2):149–153.
13. Fox SB, Leek RD, Weekes MP, et al. Quantitation and prognostic value of breast cancer angiogenesis: comparison of microvessel density, Chalkley count, and computer image analysis. *J Pathol* 1995;177(3):275–283.
14. Buadu LD, Murakami J, Murayama S, et al. Breast lesions: correlation of contrast medium enhancement patterns on MR images with histopathologic findings and tumor angiogenesis. *Radiology* 1996;200(3):639–649.
15. Tanaka F, Otake Y, Yanagihara K, et al. Evaluation of angiogenesis in non-small cell lung cancer: comparison between anti-CD34 antibody and anti-CD105 antibody. *Clin Cancer Res* 2001;7(11):3410–3415.
16. Baeten CI, Castermans K, Hillen HF, et al. Proliferating endothelial cells and leukocyte infiltration as prognostic markers in colorectal cancer. *Clin Gastroenterol Hepatol* 2006;4(11):1351–1357.
17. Schor AM, Pazouki S, Morris J, et al. Heterogeneity in microvascular density in lung tumours: comparison with normal bronchus. *Br J Cancer* 1998;77(6):946–951.
18. Swinson DE, Jones JL, Richardson D, et al. Carbonic anhydrase IX expression, a novel surrogate marker of tumor hypoxia, is associated with a poor prognosis in non-small-cell lung cancer. *J Clin Oncol* 2003;21(3):473–482.
19. Raleigh JA, Chou SC, Arteel GE, et al. Comparisons among pimonidazole binding, oxygen electrode measurements, and radiation response in C3H mouse tumors. *Radiat Res* 1999;151(5):580–589.
20. Varia MA, Calkins-Adams DP, Rinker LH, et al. Pimonidazole: a novel hypoxia marker for complementary study of tumor hypoxia and cell proliferation in cervical carcinoma. *Gynecol Oncol* 1998;71(2):270–277.
21. Mathias CJ, Welch MJ, Kilbourn MR, et al. Radiolabeled hypoxic cell sensitizers: tracers for assessment of ischemia. *Life Sci* 1987;41(2):199–206.
22. Hladovec J, Rossmann P. Circulating endothelial cells isolated together with platelets and the experimental modification of their counts in rats. *Thromb Res* 1973;3:665–674.
23. Hladovec J, Prerovsky I, Stanek V, et al. Circulating endothelial cells in acute myocardial infarction and angina pectoris. *Klin Wochenschr* 1978;56(20):1033–1036.
24. Bertolini F, Shaked Y, Mancuso P, et al. The multifaceted circulating endothelial cell in cancer: towards marker and target identification. *Nat Rev Cancer* 2006;6(11):835–845.
25. McDonald DM, Choyke PL. Imaging of angiogenesis: from microscope to clinic. *Nat Med* 2003;9(6):713–725.
26. Guidi AJ, Fischer L, Harris JR, et al. Microvessel density and distribution in ductal carcinoma in situ of the breast. *J Natl Cancer Inst* 1994;86(8):614–619.
27. Brown LF, Guidi AJ, Schnitt SJ, et al. Vascular stroma formation in carcinoma in situ, invasive carcinoma, and metastatic carcinoma of the breast. *Clin Cancer Res* 1999;5(5):1041–1056.
28. Smith-McCune KK, Weidner N. Demonstration and characterization of the angiogenic properties of cervical dysplasia. *Cancer Res* 1994;54(3):800–804.
29. Merrick DT, Haney J, Petrunich S, et al. Overexpression of vascular endothelial growth factor and its receptors in bronchial dypslasia demonstrated by quantitative RT-PCR analysis. *Lung Cancer* 2005;48(1):31–45.
30. Keith RL, Miller YE, Gemmill RM, et al. Angiogenic squamous dysplasia in bronchi of individuals at high risk for lung cancer. *Clin Cancer Res* 2000;6(5):1616–1625.
31. Hockel M, Knoop C, Schlenger K, et al. Intratumoral pO2 predicts survival in advanced cancer of the uterine cervix. *Radiother Oncol* 1993;26(1):45–50.
32. Brizel DM, Scully SP, Harrelson JM, et al. Tumor oxygenation predicts for the likelihood of distant metastases in human soft tissue sarcoma. *Cancer Res* 1996;56(5):941–943.
33. Dameron KM, Volpert OV, Tainsky MA, et al. Control of angiogenesis in fibroblasts by p53 regulation of thrombospondin-1. *Science* 1994;265(5178):1582–1584.
34. Phillips RJ, Mestas J, Gharaee-Kermani M, et al. Epidermal growth factor and hypoxia-induced expression of CXC chemokine receptor 4 on non-small cell lung cancer cells is regulated by the phosphatidylinositol 3-kinase/PTEN/AKT/mammalian target of rapamycin signaling pathway and activation of hypoxia inducible factor-1alpha. *J Biol Chem* 2005;280(23):22473–22481.
35. Phillips RJ, Burdick MD, Lutz M, et al. The stromal derived factor-1/CXCL12-CXC chemokine receptor 4 biological axis in non-small cell lung cancer metastases. *Am J Respir Crit Care Med* 2003;167(12):1676–1686.

36. Shweiki D, Neeman M, Itin A, et al. Induction of vascular endothelial growth factor expression by hypoxia and by glucose deficiency in multicell spheroids: implications for tumor angiogenesis. *Proc Natl Acad Sci U S A* 1995;92(3):768–772.
37. Gerhardt H, Golding M, Fruttiger M, et al. VEGF guides angiogenic sprouting utilizing endothelial tip cell filopodia. *J Cell Biol* 2003; 161(6):1163–1177.
38. Dome B, Hendrix MJ, Paku S, et al. Alternative vascularization mechanisms in cancer: pathology and therapeutic implications. *Am J Pathol* 2007;170(1):1–15.
39. Paku S, Paweletz N. First steps of tumor-related angiogenesis. *Lab Invest* 1991;65(3):334–346.
40. Lamalice L, Le Boeuf F, Huot J. Endothelial cell migration during angiogenesis. *Circ Res* 2007;100(6):782–794.
41. Wels J, Kaplan RN, Rafii S, et al. Migratory neighbors and distant invaders: tumor-associated niche cells. *Genes Dev* 2008;22(5):559–574.
42. Ausprunk DH, Folkman J. Migration and proliferation of endothelial cells in preformed and newly formed blood vessels during tumor angiogenesis. *Microvasc Res* 1977;14(1):53–65.
43. Lamagna C, Bergers G. The bone marrow constitutes a reservoir of pericyte progenitors. *J Leukoc Biol* 2006;80(4):677–681.
44. Benjamin LE, Golijanin D, Itin A, et al. Selective ablation of immature blood vessels in established human tumors follows vascular endothelial growth factor withdrawal. *J Clin Invest* 1999;103(2):159–65.
45. Hasumi Y, Klosowska-Wardega A, Furuhashi M, et al. Identification of a subset of pericytes that respond to combination therapy targeting PDGF and VEGF signaling. *Int J Cancer* 2007;121(12):2606–2614.
46. De Palma M, Venneri MA, Galli R, et al. Tie2 identifies a hematopoietic lineage of proangiogenic monocytes required for tumor vessel formation and a mesenchymal population of pericyte progenitors. *Cancer Cell* 2005;8(3):211–226.
47. Bababeygy SR, Cheshier SH, Hou LC, et al. Hematopoietic stem cell-derived pericytic cells in brain tumor angio-architecture. *Stem Cells Dev* 2008;17(1):11–18.
48. Yamashita J, Itoh H, Hirashima M, et al. Flk1-positive cells derived from embryonic stem cells serve as vascular progenitors. *Nature* 2000; 408(6808):92–96.
49. Takahashi T, Kalka C, Masuda H, et al. Ischemia- and cytokine-induced mobilization of bone marrow-derived endothelial progenitor cells for neovascularization. *Nat Med* 1999;5(4):434–438.
50. Li B, Sharpe EE, Maupin AB, et al. VEGF and PlGF promote adult vasculogenesis by enhancing EPC recruitment and vessel formation at the site of tumor neovascularization. *Faseb J* 2006;20(9):1495–1497.
51. Shalaby F, Rossant J, Yamaguchi TP, et al. Failure of blood-island formation and vasculogenesis in Flk-1-deficient mice. *Nature* 1995; 376(6535):62–66.
52. Lyden D, Hattori K, Dias S, et al. Impaired recruitment of bone-marrow-derived endothelial and hematopoietic precursor cells blocks tumor angiogenesis and growth. *Nat Med* 2001;7(11):1194–1201.
53. De Falco E, Porcelli D, Torella AR, et al. SDF-1 involvement in endothelial phenotype and ischemia-induced recruitment of bone marrow progenitor cells. *Blood* 2004;104(12):3472–3482.
54. Kalka C, Tehrani H, Laudenberg B, et al. VEGF gene transfer mobilizes endothelial progenitor cells in patients with inoperable coronary disease. *Ann Thorac Surg* 2000;70(3):829–834.
55. Lyden D, Young AZ, Zagzag D, et al. Id1 and Id3 are required for neurogenesis, angiogenesis and vascularization of tumour xenografts. *Nature* 1999;401(6754):670–677.
56. Gao D, Nolan DJ, Mellick AS, et al. Endothelial progenitor cells control the angiogenic switch in mouse lung metastasis. *Science* 2008; 319(5860):195–198.
57. Suriano R, Chaudhuri D, Johnson RS, et al. 17Beta-estradiol mobilizes bone marrow-derived endothelial progenitor cells to tumors. *Cancer Res* 2008;68(15):6038–6042.
58. Shaked Y, Ciarrocchi A, Franco M, et al. Therapy-induced acute recruitment of circulating endothelial progenitor cells to tumors. *Science* 2006;313(5794):1785–1787.
59. Orimo A, Gupta PB, Sgroi DC, et al. Stromal fibroblasts present in invasive human breast carcinomas promote tumor growth and angiogenesis through elevated SDF-1/CXCL12 secretion. *Cell* 2005;121(3):335–348.
60. Willett CG, Boucher Y, di Tomaso E, et al. Direct evidence that the VEGF-specific antibody bevacizumab has antivascular effects in human rectal cancer. *Nat Med* 2004;10(2):145–147.
61. Purhonen S, Palm J, Rossi D, et al. Bone marrow-derived circulating endothelial precursors do not contribute to vascular endothelium and are not needed for tumor growth. *Proc Natl Acad Sci U S A* 2008; 105(18):6620–6625.
62. Kerbel RS, Benezra R, Lyden DC, et al. Endothelial progenitor cells are cellular hubs essential for neoangiogenesis of certain aggressive adenocarcinomas and metastatic transition but not adenomas. *Proc Natl Acad Sci U S A* 2008;105(34):E54; author reply E55.
63. Peters BA, Diaz LA, Polyak K, et al. Contribution of bone marrow-derived endothelial cells to human tumor vasculature. *Nat Med* 2005; 11(3):261–262.
64. Nolan DJ, Ciarrocchi A, Mellick AS, et al. Bone marrow-derived endothelial progenitor cells are a major determinant of nascent tumor neovascularization. *Genes Dev* 2007;21(12):1546–1558.
65. Lin Y, Weisdorf DJ, Solovey A, et al. Origins of circulating endothelial cells and endothelial outgrowth from blood. *J Clin Invest* 2000; 105(1):71–77.
66. Furstenberger G, von Moos R, Senn HJ, et al. Real-time PCR of CD146 mRNA in peripheral blood enables the relative quantification of circulating endothelial cells and is an indicator of angiogenesis. *Br J Cancer* 2005;93(7):793–798.
67. Duda DG, Cohen KS, di Tomaso E, et al. Differential CD146 expression on circulating versus tissue endothelial cells in rectal cancer patients: implications for circulating endothelial and progenitor cells as biomarkers for antiangiogenic therapy. *J Clin Oncol* 2006;24(9): 1449–1453.
68. Bagley RG, Rouleau C, St Martin T, et al. Human endothelial precursor cells express tumor endothelial marker 1/endosialin/CD248. *Mol Cancer Ther* 2008;7(8):2536–2546.
69. Nagano N, Sasaki H, Aoyagi M, et al. Invasion of experimental rat brain tumor: early morphological changes following microinjection of C6 glioma cells. *Acta Neuropathol* 1993;86(2):117–125.
70. Pages F, Berger A, Camus M, et al. Effector memory T cells, early metastasis, and survival in colorectal cancer. *N Engl J Med* 2005; 353(25):2654–2666.
71. de Visser KE, Eichten A, Coussens LM. Paradoxical roles of the immune system during cancer development. *Nat Rev Cancer* 2006;6(1):24–37.
72. Bellocq A, Antoine M, Flahault A, et al. Neutrophil alveolitis in bronchioloalveolar carcinoma: induction by tumor-derived interleukin-8 and relation to clinical outcome. *Am J Pathol* 1998;152(1):83–92.
73. Al-Shibli KI, Donnem T, Al-Saad S, et al. Prognostic effect of epithelial and stromal lymphocyte infiltration in non-small cell lung cancer. *Clin Cancer Res* 2008;14(16):5220–5227.
74. Kawai O, Ishii G, Kubota K, et al. Predominant infiltration of macrophages and CD8(+) T Cells in cancer nests is a significant predictor of survival in stage IV nonsmall cell lung cancer. *Cancer* 2008;113(6):1387–1395.
75. Lewis C, Murdoch C. Macrophage responses to hypoxia: implications for tumor progression and anti-cancer therapies. *Am J Pathol* 2005;167(3):627–635.
76. Pollard JW. Tumour-educated macrophages promote tumour progression and metastasis. *Nat Rev Cancer* 2004;4(1):71–78.
77. Mantovani A, Sozzani S, Locati M, et al. Macrophage polarization: tumor-associated macrophages as a paradigm for polarized M2 mononuclear phagocytes. *Trends Immunol* 2002;23(11):549–555.
78. Lin EY, Li JF, Gnatovskiy L, et al. Macrophages regulate the angiogenic switch in a mouse model of breast cancer. *Cancer Res* 2006; 66(23):11238–11246.
79. Nakao S, Kuwano T, Tsutsumi-Miyahara C, et al. Infiltration of COX-2-expressing macrophages is a prerequisite for IL-1 beta-induced neovascularization and tumor growth. *J Clin Invest* 2005;115(11):2979–2991.

80. Giraudo E, Inoue M, Hanahan D. An amino-bisphosphonate targets MMP-9-expressing macrophages and angiogenesis to impair cervical carcinogenesis. *J Clin Invest* 2004;114(5):623–633.
81. Ahn GO, Brown JM. Matrix metalloproteinase-9 is required for tumor vasculogenesis but not for angiogenesis: role of bone marrow-derived myelomonocytic cells. *Cancer Cell* 2008;13(3):193–205.
82. Chen JJ, Yao PL, Yuan A, et al. Up-regulation of tumor interleukin-8 expression by infiltrating macrophages: its correlation with tumor angiogenesis and patient survival in non-small cell lung cancer. *Clin Cancer Res* 2003;9(2):729–737.
83. Salven P, Hattori K, Heissig B, et al. Interleukin-1alpha promotes angiogenesis in vivo via VEGFR-2 pathway by inducing inflammatory cell VEGF synthesis and secretion. *Faseb J* 2002;16(11):1471–1473.
84. Welsh TJ, Green RH, Richardson D, et al. Macrophage and mast-cell invasion of tumor cell islets confers a marked survival advantage in non-small-cell lung cancer. *J Clin Oncol* 2005;23(35):8959–8967.
85. Kawai O, Ishii G, Kubota K, et al. Predominant infiltration of macrophages and CD8(+) T Cells in cancer nests is a significant predictor of survival in stage IV nonsmall cell lung cancer. *Cancer* 2008; 113(6):1387–1395.
86. Yao L, Sgadari C, Furuke K, et al. Contribution of natural killer cells to inhibition of angiogenesis by interleukin-12. *Blood* 1999;93(5): 1612–1621.
87. Hayakawa Y, Takeda K, Yagita H, et al. IFN-gamma-mediated inhibition of tumor angiogenesis by natural killer T-cell ligand, alpha-galactosylceramide. *Blood* 2002;100(5):1728–1733.
88. Coussens LM, Raymond WW, Bergers G, et al. Inflammatory mast cells up-regulate angiogenesis during squamous epithelial carcinogenesis. *Genes Dev* 1999;13(11):1382–1397.
89. Ibaraki T, Muramatsu M, Takai S, et al. The relationship of tryptase- and chymase-positive mast cells to angiogenesis in stage I non-small cell lung cancer. *Eur J Cardiothorac Surg* 2005;28(4):617–621.
90. Fukumura D, Xavier R, Sugiura T, et al. Tumor induction of VEGF promoter activity in stromal cells. *Cell* 1998;94(6):715–725.
91. Kalluri R, Zeisberg M. Fibroblasts in cancer. *Nat Rev Cancer* 2006; 6(5):392–401.
92. Matsumoto K, Nakamura T. Hepatocyte growth factor and the Met system as a mediator of tumor-stromal interactions. *Int J Cancer* 2006;119(3):477–483.
93. Jodele S, Chantrain CF, Blavier L, et al. The contribution of bone marrow-derived cells to the tumor vasculature in neuroblastoma is matrix metalloproteinase-9 dependent. *Cancer Res* 2005;65(8):3200–3208.
94. Kalluri R. Basement membranes: structure, assembly and role in tumour angiogenesis. *Nat Rev Cancer* 2003;3(6):422–433.
95. Leighl NB, Paz-Ares L, Douillard JY, et al. Randomized phase III study of matrix metalloproteinase inhibitor BMS-275291 in combination with paclitaxel and carboplatin in advanced non-small-cell lung cancer: National Cancer Institute of Canada-Clinical Trials Group Study BR.18. *J Clin Oncol* 2005;23(12):2831–2839.
96. Ribatti D, Vacca A, Roncali L, et al. The chick embryo chorioallantoic membrane as a model for in vivo research on angiogenesis. *Int J Dev Biol* 1996;40(6):1189–1197.
97. Folkman J. Angiogenesis: an organizing principle for drug discovery? *Nat Rev Drug Discov* 2007;6(4):273–286.
98. Dvorak HF, Orenstein NS, Carvalho AC, et al. Induction of a fibrin-gel investment: an early event in line 10 hepatocarcinoma growth mediated by tumor-secreted products. *J Immunol* 1979;122(1):166–174.
99. Connolly DT, Heuvelman DM, Nelson R, et al. Tumor vascular permeability factor stimulates endothelial cell growth and angiogenesis. *J Clin Invest* 1989;84(5):1470–1478.
100. Quinn TP, Peters KG, De Vries C, et al. Fetal liver kinase 1 is a receptor for vascular endothelial growth factor and is selectively expressed in vascular endothelium. *Proc Natl Acad Sci U S A* 1993;90(16):7533–7537.
101. Barleon B, Sozzani S, Zhou D, et al. Migration of human monocytes in response to vascular endothelial growth factor (VEGF) is mediated via the VEGF receptor flt-1. *Blood* 1996;87(8):3336–3343.
102. Hattori K, Heissig B, Wu Y, et al. Placental growth factor reconstitutes hematopoiesis by recruiting VEGFR1(+) stem cells from bone-marrow microenvironment. *Nat Med* 2002;8(8):841–849.
103. Decaussin M, Sartelet H, Robert C, et al. Expression of vascular endothelial growth factor (VEGF) and its two receptors (VEGF-R1-Flt1 and VEGF-R2-Flk1/KDR) in non-small cell lung carcinomas (NSCLCs): correlation with angiogenesis and survival. *J Pathol* 1999;188(4):369–377.
104. Fong GH, Zhang L, Bryce DM, et al. Increased hemangioblast commitment, not vascular disorganization, is the primary defect in flt-1 knock-out mice. *Development* 1999;126(13):3015–3025.
105. Hiratsuka S, Minowa O, Kuno J, et al. Flt-1 lacking the tyrosine kinase domain is sufficient for normal development and angiogenesis in mice. *Proc Natl Acad Sci U S A* 1998;95(16):9349–9354.
106. Rahimi N. VEGFR-1 and VEGFR-2: two non-identical twins with a unique physiognomy. *Front Biosci* 2006;11:818–829.
107. Alitalo K, Carmeliet P. Molecular mechanisms of lymphangiogenesis in health and disease. *Cancer Cell* 2002;1(3):219–227.
108. Laakkonen P, Waltari M, Holopainen T, et al. Vascular endothelial growth factor receptor 3 is involved in tumor angiogenesis and growth. *Cancer Res* 2007;67(2):593–599.
109. Ji H, Ramsey MR, Hayes DN, et al. LKB1 modulates lung cancer differentiation and metastasis. *Nature* 2007;448(7155):807–810.
110. Maity A, Pore N, Lee J, et al. Epidermal growth factor receptor transcriptionally up-regulates vascular endothelial growth factor expression in human glioblastoma cells via a pathway involving phosphatidylinositol 3′-kinase and distinct from that induced by hypoxia. *Cancer Res* 2000;60(20):5879–5886.
111. Arbiser JL, Moses MA, Fernandez CA, et al. Oncogenic H-ras stimulates tumor angiogenesis by two distinct pathways. *Proc Natl Acad Sci U S A* 1997;94(3):861–866.
112. Xu H, Czerwinski P, Hortmann M, et al. Protein kinase C alpha promotes angiogenic activity of human endothelial cells via induction of vascular endothelial growth factor. *Cardiovasc Res* 2008;78(2):349–355.
113. Pore N, Jiang Z, Gupta A, et al. EGFR tyrosine kinase inhibitors decrease VEGF expression by both hypoxia-inducible factor (HIF)-1-independent and HIF-1-dependent mechanisms. *Cancer Res* 2006; 66(6):3197–3204.
114. Mukhopadhyay D, Tsiokas L, Zhou XM, et al. Hypoxic induction of human vascular endothelial growth factor expression through c-Src activation. *Nature* 1995;375(6532):577–581.
115. Mukhopadhyay D, Tsiokas L, Sukhatme VP. Wild-type p53 and v-Src exert opposing influences on human vascular endothelial growth factor gene expression. *Cancer Res* 1995;55(24):6161–6165.
116. Kieser A, Weich HA, Brandner G, et al. Mutant p53 potentiates protein kinase C induction of vascular endothelial growth factor expression. *Oncogene* 1994;9(3):963–969.
117. Ravi R, Mookerjee B, Bhujwalla ZM, et al. Regulation of tumor angiogenesis by p53-induced degradation of hypoxia-inducible factor 1alpha. *Genes Dev* 2000;14(1):34–44.
118. Matsumoto T, Bohman S, Dixelius J, et al. VEGF receptor-2 Y951 signaling and a role for the adapter molecule TSAd in tumor angiogenesis. *Embo J* 2005;24(13):2342–2353.
119. Gerber HP, McMurtrey A, Kowalski J, et al. Vascular endothelial growth factor regulates endothelial cell survival through the phosphatidylinositol 3′-kinase/Akt signal transduction pathway. Requirement for Flk-1/KDR activation. *J Biol Chem* 1998;273(46):30336–30343.
120. Wu LW, Mayo LD, Dunbar JD, et al. Utilization of distinct signaling pathways by receptors for vascular endothelial cell growth factor and other mitogens in the induction of endothelial cell proliferation. *J Biol Chem* 2000;275(7):5096–5103.
121. Lampugnani MG, Orsenigo F, Gagliani MC, et al. Vascular endothelial cadherin controls VEGFR-2 internalization and signaling from intracellular compartments. *J Cell Biol* 2006;174(4):593–604.
122. Singh AJ, Meyer RD, Band H, et al. The carboxyl terminus of VEGFR-2 is required for PKC-mediated down-regulation. *Mol Biol Cell* 2005; 16(4):2106–2118.

123. Soker S, Takashima S, Miao HQ, et al. Neuropilin-1 is expressed by endothelial and tumor cells as an isoform-specific receptor for vascular endothelial growth factor. *Cell* 1998;92(6):735–745.
124. Fuh G, Garcia KC, de Vos AM. The interaction of neuropilin-1 with vascular endothelial growth factor and its receptor flt-1. *J Biol Chem* 2000;275(35):26690–26695.
125. Hong TM, Chen YL, Wu YY, et al. Targeting neuropilin 1 as an antitumor strategy in lung cancer. *Clin Cancer Res* 2007;13(16):4759–4768.
126. Lamalice L, Houle F, Jourdan G, et al. Phosphorylation of tyrosine 1214 on VEGFR2 is required for VEGF-induced activation of Cdc42 upstream of SAPK2/p38. *Oncogene* 2004;23(2):434–445.
127. Lamalice L, Houle F, Huot J. Phosphorylation of Tyr1214 within VEGFR-2 triggers the recruitment of Nck and activation of Fyn leading to SAPK2/p38 activation and endothelial cell migration in response to VEGF. *J Biol Chem* 2006;281(45):34009–34020.
128. Hiratsuka S, Nakamura K, Iwai S, et al. MMP9 induction by vascular endothelial growth factor receptor-1 is involved in lung-specific metastasis. *Cancer Cell* 2002;2(4):289–300.
129. Kaplan RN, Riba RD, Zacharoulis S, et al. VEGFR1-positive haematopoietic bone marrow progenitors initiate the pre-metastatic niche. *Nature* 2005;438(7069):820–827.
130. Robinson CJ, Stringer SE. The splice variants of vascular endothelial growth factor (VEGF) and their receptors. *J Cell Sci* 2001;114(Pt 5):853–865.
131. Poltorak Z, Cohen T, Sivan R, et al. VEGF145, a secreted vascular endothelial growth factor isoform that binds to extracellular matrix. *J Biol Chem* 1997;272(11):7151–7158.
132. Park JE, Keller GA, Ferrara N. The vascular endothelial growth factor (VEGF) isoforms: differential deposition into the subepithelial extracellular matrix and bioactivity of extracellular matrix-bound VEGF. *Mol Biol Cell* 1993;4(12):1317–1326.
133. Yuan A, Yu CJ, Kuo SH, et al. Vascular endothelial growth factor 189 mRNA isoform expression specifically correlates with tumor angiogenesis, patient survival, and postoperative relapse in non-small-cell lung cancer. *J Clin Oncol* 2001;19(2):432–441.
134. Lee YH, Tokunaga T, Oshika Y, et al. Cell-retained isoforms of vascular endothelial growth factor (VEGF) are correlated with poor prognosis in osteosarcoma. *Eur J Cancer* 1999;35(7):1089–1093.
135. Lobov IB, Brooks PC, Lang RA. Angiopoietin-2 displays VEGF-dependent modulation of capillary structure and endothelial cell survival in vivo. *Proc Natl Acad Sci U S A* 2002;99(17):11205–11210.
136. Murdoch C, Tazzyman S, Webster S, et al. Expression of Tie-2 by human monocytes and their responses to angiopoietin-2. *J Immunol* 2007;178(11):7405–7411.
137. Tanaka F, Ishikawa S, Yanagihara K, et al. Expression of angiopoietins and its clinical significance in non-small cell lung cancer. *Cancer Res* 2002;62(23):7124–7129.
138. Holash J, Maisonpierre PC, Compton D, et al. Vessel cooption, regression, and growth in tumors mediated by angiopoietins and VEGF. *Science* 1999;284(5422):1994–1998.
139. Metheny-Barlow LJ, Li LY. The enigmatic role of angiopoietin-1 in tumor angiogenesis. *Cell Res* 2003;13(5):309–317.
140. Pennacchietti S, Michieli P, Galluzzo M, et al. Hypoxia promotes invasive growth by transcriptional activation of the met protooncogene. *Cancer Cell* 2003;3(4):347–361.
141. Rofstad EK, Rasmussen H, Galappathi K, et al. Hypoxia promotes lymph node metastasis in human melanoma xenografts by up-regulating the urokinase-type plasminogen activator receptor. *Cancer Res* 2002;62(6):1847–1853.
142. Graeber TG, Osmanian C, Jacks T, et al. Hypoxia-mediated selection of cells with diminished apoptotic potential in solid tumours [see comments]. *Nature* 1996;379(6560):88–91.
143. Teodoro JG, Parker AE, Zhu X, et al. p53-mediated inhibition of angiogenesis through up-regulation of a collagen prolyl hydroxylase. *Science* 2006;313(5789):968–971.
144. Steeg PS. Angiogenesis inhibitors: motivators of metastasis? *Nat Med* 2003;9(7):822–823.
145. Semenza GL. Hydroxylation of HIF-1: oxygen sensing at the molecular level. *Physiology (Bethesda)* 2004;19:176–182.
146. Zelzer E, Levy Y, Kahana C, et al. Insulin induces transcription of target genes through the hypoxia-inducible factor HIF-1alpha/ARNT. *Embo J* 1998;17(17):5085–5094.
147. Yu AY, Frid MG, Shimoda LA, et al. Temporal, spatial, and oxygen-regulated expression of hypoxia-inducible factor-1 in the lung. *Am J Physiol* 1998;275(4 Pt 1):L818–826.
148. Epstein AC, Gleadle JM, McNeill LA, et al. C. elegans EGL-9 and mammalian homologs define a family of dioxygenases that regulate HIF by prolyl hydroxylation. *Cell* 2001;107(1):43–54.
149. Yasuda H. Solid tumor physiology and hypoxia-induced chemo/radio-resistance: novel strategy for cancer therapy: nitric oxide donor as a therapeutic enhancer. *Nitric Oxide* 2008;19(2):205–216
150. Hu CJ, Wang LY, Chodosh LA, et al. Differential roles of hypoxia-inducible factor 1alpha (HIF-1alpha) and HIF-2alpha in hypoxic gene regulation. *Mol Cell Biol* 2003;23(24):9361–9374.
151. Tian H, Hammer RE, Matsumoto AM, et al. The hypoxia-responsive transcription factor EPAS1 is essential for catecholamine homeostasis and protection against heart failure during embryonic development. *Genes Dev* 1998;12(21):3320–3324.
152. Patel SA, Simon MC. Biology of hypoxia-inducible factor-2alpha in development and disease. *Cell Death Differ* 2008;15(4):628–634.
153. Carroll VA, Ashcroft M. Role of hypoxia-inducible factor (HIF)-1alpha versus HIF-2alpha in the regulation of HIF target genes in response to hypoxia, insulin-like growth factor-I, or loss of von Hippel-Lindau function: implications for targeting the HIF pathway. *Cancer Res* 2006;66(12):6264–6270.
154. Ryan HE, Lo J, Johnson RS. HIF-1 alpha is required for solid tumor formation and embryonic vascularization. *Embo J* 1998;17(11): 3005–3015.
155. Leek RD, Talks KL, Pezzella F, et al. Relation of hypoxia-inducible factor-2 alpha (HIF-2 alpha) expression in tumor-infiltrative macrophages to tumor angiogenesis and the oxidative thymidine phosphorylase pathway in Human breast cancer. *Cancer Res* 2002;62(5): 1326–1329.
156. Makino Y, Cao R, Svensson K, et al. Inhibitory PAS domain protein is a negative regulator of hypoxia-inducible gene expression. *Nature* 2001;414(6863):550–554.
157. O'Reilly MS, Holmgren L, Shing Y, et al. Angiostatin: a novel angiogenesis inhibitor that mediates the suppression of metastases by a Lewis lung carcinoma. *Cell* 1994;79(2):315–328.
158. Dong Z, Kumar R, Yang X, et al. Macrophage-derived metalloelastase is responsible for the generation of angiostatin in Lewis lung carcinoma. *Cell* 1997;88(6):801–810.
159. Gately S, Twardowski P, Stack MS, et al. The mechanism of cancer-mediated conversion of plasminogen to the angiogenesis inhibitor angiostatin. *Proc Natl Acad Sci U S A* 1997;94(20):10868–10872.
160. Sharma MR, Rothman V, Tuszynski GP, et al. Antibody-directed targeting of angiostatin's receptor annexin II inhibits Lewis Lung Carcinoma tumor growth via blocking of plasminogen activation: possible biochemical mechanism of angiostatin's action. *Exp Mol Pathol* 2006;81(2): 136–145.
161. O'Reilly MS, Boehm T, Shing Y, et al. Endostatin: an endogenous inhibitor of angiogenesis and tumor growth. *Cell* 1997;88(2):277–285.
162. Good DJ, Polverini PJ, Rastinejad F, et al. A tumor suppressor-dependent inhibitor of angiogenesis is immunologically and functionally indistinguishable from a fragment of thrombospondin. *Proc Natl Acad Sci U S A* 1990;87(17):6624–6628.
163. Digtyar AV, Pozdnyakova NV, Feldman NB, et al. Endostatin: current concepts about its biological role and mechanisms of action. *Biochemistry (Mosc)* 2007;72(3):235–246.
164. Hamano Y, Kalluri R. Tumstatin, the NC1 domain of alpha3 chain of type IV collagen, is an endogenous inhibitor of pathological angiogenesis and suppresses tumor growth. *Biochem Biophys Res Commun* 2005;333(2):292–298.

165. Rodriguez-Manzaneque JC, Lane TF, Ortega MA, et al. Thrombospondin-1 suppresses spontaneous tumor growth and inhibits activation of matrix metalloproteinase-9 and mobilization of vascular endothelial growth factor. *Proc Natl Acad Sci U S A* 2001;98(22):12485–12490.
166. Jimenez B, Volpert OV, Crawford SE, et al. Signals leading to apoptosis-dependent inhibition of neovascularization by thrombospondin-1. *Nat Med* 2000;6(1):41–48.
167. Petitclerc E, Boutaud A, Prestayko A, et al. New functions for non-collagenous domains of human collagen type IV. Novel integrin ligands inhibiting angiogenesis and tumor growth in vivo. *J Biol Chem* 2000;275(11):8051–8061.
168. Marneros AG, Olsen BR. The role of collagen-derived proteolytic fragments in angiogenesis. *Matrix Biol* 2001;20(5–6):337–345.
169. Ostman A. PDGF receptors-mediators of autocrine tumor growth and regulators of tumor vasculature and stroma. *Cytokine Growth Factor Rev* 2004;15(4):275–286.
170. Furuhashi M, Sjoblom T, Abramsson A, et al. Platelet-derived growth factor production by B16 melanoma cells leads to increased pericyte abundance in tumors and an associated increase in tumor growth rate. *Cancer Res* 2004;64(8):2725–2733.
171. Abramsson A, Lindblom P, Betsholtz C. Endothelial and nonendothelial sources of PDGF-B regulate pericyte recruitment and influence vascular pattern formation in tumors. *J Clin Invest* 2003;112(8):1142–1151.
172. Lindahl P, Johansson BR, Leveen P, et al. Pericyte loss and microaneurysm formation in PDGF-B-deficient mice. *Science* 1997;277(5323): 242–245.
173. Lindblom P, Gerhardt H, Liebner S, et al. Endothelial PDGF-B retention is required for proper investment of pericytes in the microvessel wall. *Genes Dev* 2003;17(15):1835–1840.
174. Hellström M, Kalén M, Lindahl P, et al. Role of PDGF-B and PDGFR-beta in recruitment of vascular smooth muscle cells and pericytes during embryonic blood vessel formation in the mouse. *Development* 1999;126(14):3047–3055.
175. Montesano R, Vassalli JD, Baird A, et al. Basic fibroblast growth factor induces angiogenesis in vitro. *Proc Natl Acad Sci U S A* 1986;83(19): 7297–7301.
176. Folkman J, Shing Y. Angiogenesis. *J Biol Chem* 1992;267(16):10931–10934.
177. Rogelj S, Weinberg RA, Fanning P, et al. Basic fibroblast growth factor fused to a signal peptide transforms cells. *Nature* 1988;331(6152):173–175.
178. Kandel J, Bossy-Wetzel E, Radvanyi F, et al. Neovascularization is associated with a switch to the export of bFGF in the multistep development of fibrosarcoma. *Cell* 1991;66(6):1095–1104.
179. Aviezer D, Hecht D, Safran M, et al. Perlecan, basal lamina proteoglycan, promotes basic fibroblast growth factor-receptor binding, mitogenesis, and angiogenesis. *Cell* 1994;79(6):1005–1013.
180. Schweigerer L, Neufeld G, Friedman J, et al. Capillary endothelial cells express basic fibroblast growth factor, a mitogen that promotes their own growth. *Nature* 1987;325(6101):257–259.
181. Calvani M, Rapisarda A, Uranchimeg B, et al. Hypoxic induction of an HIF-1alpha-dependent bFGF autocrine loop drives angiogenesis in human endothelial cells. *Blood* 2006;107(7):2705–2712.
182. Cao Y, Cao R, Hedlund EM. Regulation of tumor angiogenesis and metastasis by FGF and PDGF signaling pathways. *J Mol Med* 2008;86(7):785–789.
183. Clark JC, Tichelaar JW, Wert SE, et al. FGF-10 disrupts lung morphogenesis and causes pulmonary adenomas in vivo. *Am J Physiol Lung Cell Mol Physiol* 2001;280(4):L705–L715.
184. Struyf S, Burdick MD, Peeters E, et al. Platelet factor-4 variant chemokine CXCL4L1 inhibits melanoma and lung carcinoma growth and metastasis by preventing angiogenesis. *Cancer Res* 2007;67(12):5940–5948.
185. Kryczek I, Wei S, Keller E, et al. Stroma-derived factor (SDF-1/CXCL12) and human tumor pathogenesis. *Am J Physiol Cell Physiol* 2007;292(3): C987–C995.
186. Woodfin A, Voisin MB, Nourshargh S. PECAM-1: a multi-functional molecule in inflammation and vascular biology. *Arterioscler Thromb Vasc Biol* 2007;27(12):2514–2523.
187. DeLisser HM, Christofidou-Solomidou M, Strieter RM, et al. Involvement of endothelial PECAM-1/CD31 in angiogenesis. *Am J Pathol* 1997;151(3):671–677.
188. Janowska-Wieczorek A, Wysoczynski M, Kijowski J, et al. Microvesicles derived from activated platelets induce metastasis and angiogenesis in lung cancer. *Int J Cancer* 2005;113(5):752–760.
189. McLaughlin F, Hayes BP, Horgan CM, et al. Tumor necrosis factor (TNF)-alpha and interleukin (IL)-1beta down-regulate intercellular adhesion molecule (ICAM)-2 expression on the endothelium. *Cell Adhes Commun* 1998;6(5):381–400.
190. Huang MT, Mason JC, Birdsey GM, et al. Endothelial intercellular adhesion molecule (ICAM)-2 regulates angiogenesis. *Blood* 2005; 106(5):1636–1643.
191. Dowlati A, Gray R, Sandler AB, et al. Cell adhesion molecules, vascular endothelial growth factor, and basic fibroblast growth factor in patients with non-small cell lung cancer treated with chemotherapy with or without bevacizumab—an Eastern Cooperative Oncology Group Study. *Clin Cancer Res* 2008;14(5):1407–1412.
192. Liu D, Huang C, Kameyama K, et al. E-cadherin expression associated with differentiation and prognosis in patients with non-small cell lung cancer. *Ann Thorac Surg* 2001;71(3):949–954; discussion 954–955.
193. Bremnes RM, Veve R, Gabrielson E, et al. High-throughput tissue microarray analysis used to evaluate biology and prognostic significance of the E-cadherin pathway in non-small-cell lung cancer. *J Clin Oncol* 2002;20(10):2417–2428.
194. Huang C, Liu D, Masuya D, et al. Clinical application of biological markers for treatments of resectable non-small-cell lung cancers. *Br J Cancer* 2005;92(7):1231–1239.
195. Dickson MC, Martin JS, Cousins FM, et al. Defective haematopoiesis and vasculogenesis in transforming growth factor-beta 1 knock out mice. *Development* 1995;121(6):1845–1854.
196. Roberts AB, Sporn MB, Assoian RK, et al. Transforming growth factor type beta: rapid induction of fibrosis and angiogenesis in vivo and stimulation of collagen formation in vitro. *Proc Natl Acad Sci U S A* 1986;83(12):4167–4171.
197. Baek HJ, Lim SC, Kitisin K, et al. Hepatocellular cancer arises from loss of transforming growth factor beta signaling adaptor protein embryonic liver fodrin through abnormal angiogenesis. *Hepatology* 2008;48(4):1128–1137.
198. Ferrari G, Cook B, Terushkin V, et al. Transforming growth factor-beta 1 (tgf-β1) induces angiogenesis through vascular endothelial growth factor (vegf)-mediated apoptosis. Available from *Nature Precedings* <http://dx.doi.org/10.1038/npre.2008.1758.1> (2008).
199. Hasegawa Y, Takanashi S, Kanehira Y, et al. Transforming growth factor-beta1 level correlates with angiogenesis, tumor progression, and prognosis in patients with nonsmall cell lung carcinoma. *Cancer* 2001; 91(5):964–971.
200. Kim SJ, Uehara H, Karashima T, et al. Blockade of epidermal growth factor receptor signaling in tumor cells and tumor-associated endothelial cells for therapy of androgen-independent human prostate cancer growing in the bone of nude mice. *Clin Cancer Res* 2003;9(3): 1200–1210.
201. Zeng Q, Li S, Chepeha DB, et al. Crosstalk between tumor and endothelial cells promotes tumor angiogenesis by MAPK activation of Notch signaling. *Cancer Cell* 2005;8(1):13–23.
202. Alfranca A, Lopez-Oliva JM, Genis L, et al. PGE2 induces angiogenesis via MT1-MMP-mediated activation of the TGFbeta/Alk5 signaling pathway. *Blood* 2008;112(4):1120–1128.
203. Ridnour LA, Thomas DD, Donzelli S, et al. The biphasic nature of nitric oxide responses in tumor biology. *Antioxid Redox Signal* 2006; 8(7–8):1329–1337.
204. Ridnour LA, Isenberg JS, Espey MG, et al. Nitric oxide regulates angiogenesis through a functional switch involving thrombospondin-1. *Proc Natl Acad Sci U S A* 2005;102(37):13147–13152.
205. Marrogi AJ, Travis WD, Welsh JA, et al. Nitric oxide synthase, cyclooxygenase 2, and vascular endothelial growth factor in the angiogenesis of non-small cell lung carcinoma. *Clin Cancer Res* 2000;6(12):4739–4744.

206. Yasuda H, Yamaya M, Nakayama K, et al. Randomized phase II trial comparing nitroglycerin plus vinorelbine and cisplatin with vinorelbine and cisplatin alone in previously untreated stage IIIB/IV non-small-cell lung cancer. *J Clin Oncol* 2006;24(4):688–694.
207. Macchiarini P, Fontanini G, Dulmet E, et al. Angiogenesis: an indicator of metastasis in non-small cell lung cancer invading the thoracic inlet. *Ann Thorac Surg* 1994;57(6):1534–1539.
208. Giatromanolaki A, Koukourakis M, O'Byrne K, et al. Prognostic value of angiogenesis in operable non-small cell lung cancer. *J Pathol* 1996;179(1):80–88.
209. Fontanini G, Lucchi M, Vignati S, et al. Angiogenesis as a prognostic indicator of survival in non-small-cell lung carcinoma: a prospective study. *J Natl Cancer Inst* 1997;89(12):881–886.
210. Duarte IG, Bufkin BL, Pennington MF, et al. Angiogenesis as a predictor of survival after surgical resection for stage I non-small-cell lung cancer. *J Thorac Cardiovasc Surg* 1998;115(3):652–658; discussion 658–659.
211. D'Amico TA, Massey M, Herndon JE 2nd, et al. A biologic risk model for stage I lung cancer: immunohistochemical analysis of 408 patients with the use of ten molecular markers. *J Thorac Cardiovasc Surg* 1999;117(4):736–743.
212. Yano T, Tanikawa S, Fujie T, et al. Vascular endothelial growth factor expression and neovascularisation in non-small cell lung cancer. *Eur J Cancer* 2000;36(5):601–609.
213. Cox G, Walker RA, Andi A, et al. Prognostic significance of platelet and microvessel counts in operable non-small cell lung cancer. *Lung Cancer* 2000;29(3):169–177.
214. O'Byrne KJ, Koukourakis MI, Giatromanolaki A, et al. Vascular endothelial growth factor, platelet-derived endothelial cell growth factor and angiogenesis in non-small-cell lung cancer. *Br J Cancer* 2000;82(8):1427–1432.
215. Herbst RS, Onn A, Sandler A. Angiogenesis and lung cancer: prognostic and therapeutic implications. *J Clin Oncol* 2005;23(14):3243–3256.
216. Donnem T, Al-Saad S, Al-Shibli K, et al. Inverse prognostic impact of angiogenic marker expression in tumor cells versus stromal cells in non small cell lung cancer. *Clin Cancer Res* 2007;13(22 Pt 1):6649–6657.
217. Chandrachud LM, Pendleton N, Chisholm DM, et al. Relationship between vascularity, age and survival in non-small-cell lung cancer. *Br J Cancer* 1997;76(10):1367–1375.
218. Fontanini G, Vignati S, Boldrini L, et al. Vascular endothelial growth factor is associated with neovascularization and influences progression of non-small cell lung carcinoma. *Clin Cancer Res* 1997;3(6):861–865.
219. Volm M, Koomagi R, Mattern J. Prognostic value of vascular endothelial growth factor and its receptor Flt-1 in squamous cell lung cancer. *Int J Cancer* 1997;74(1):64–68.
220. Han H, Silverman JF, Santucci TS, et al. Vascular endothelial growth factor expression in stage I non-small cell lung cancer correlates with neoangiogenesis and a poor prognosis. *Ann Surg Oncol* 2001;8(1):72–79.
221. Giatromanolaki A, Koukourakis MI, Kakolyris S, et al. Vascular endothelial growth factor, wild-type p53, and angiogenesis in early operable non-small cell lung cancer. *Clin Cancer Res* 1998;4(12):3017–3024.
222. Fontanini G, Faviana P, Lucchi M, et al. A high vascular count and overexpression of vascular endothelial growth factor are associated with unfavourable prognosis in operated small cell lung carcinoma. *Br J Cancer* 2002;86(4):558–563.
223. Salven P, Ruotsalainen T, Mattson K, et al. High pre-treatment serum level of vascular endothelial growth factor (VEGF) is associated with poor outcome in small-cell lung cancer. *Int J Cancer* 1998;79(2):144–146.
224. Iwasaki A, Kuwahara M, Yoshinaga Y, et al. Basic fibroblast growth factor (bFGF) and vascular endothelial growth factor (VEGF) levels, as prognostic indicators in NSCLC. *Eur J Cardiothorac Surg* 2004; 25(3):443–448.
225. Yuan A, Yu CJ, Shun CT, et al. Total cyclooxygenase-2 mRNA levels correlate with vascular endothelial growth factor mRNA levels, tumor angiogenesis and prognosis in non-small cell lung cancer patients. *Int J Cancer* 2005;115(4):545–555.
226. Dome B, Timar J, Dobos J, et al. Identification and clinical significance of circulating endothelial progenitor cells in human non-small cell lung cancer. *Cancer Res* 2006;66(14):7341–7347.
227. Kaya A, Ciledag A, Gulbay BE, et al. The prognostic significance of vascular endothelial growth factor levels in sera of non-small cell lung cancer patients. *Respir Med* 2004;98(7):632–636.
228. Laack E, Scheffler A, Burkholder I, et al. Pretreatment vascular endothelial growth factor (VEGF) and matrix metalloproteinase-9 (MMP-9) serum levels in patients with metastatic non-small cell lung cancer (NSCLC). *Lung Cancer* 2005;50(1):51–58.
229. Bremnes RM, Camps C, Sirera R. Angiogenesis in non-small cell lung cancer: the prognostic impact of neoangiogenesis and the cytokines VEGF and bFGF in tumours and blood. *Lung Cancer* 2006;51(2):143–158.
230. Mack PC, Redman MW, Chansky K, et al. Lower osteopontin plasma levels are associated with superior outcomes in advanced non-small-cell lung cancer patients receiving platinum-based chemotherapy: SWOG Study S0003. *J Clin Oncol* 2008;26(29):4771–4776.
231. Heist RS, Zhai R, Liu G, et al. VEGF polymorphisms and survival in early-stage non-small-cell lung cancer. *J Clin Oncol* 2008;26(6):856–862.
232. Smith DR, Polverini PJ, Kunkel SL, et al. Inhibition of interleukin 8 attenuates angiogenesis in bronchogenic carcinoma. *J Exp Med* 1994;179(5):1409–1415.
233. Zhang L, Chen J, Ke Y, et al. Expression of Placenta growth factor (PlGF) in non-small cell lung cancer (NSCLC) and the clinical and prognostic significance. *World J Surg Oncol* 2005;3:68.
234. Chen J, Ye L, Zhang L, et al. Placenta growth factor, PLGF, influences the motility of lung cancer cells, the role of Rho associated kinase, Rock1. *J Cell Biochem* 2008;105(1):313–320.
235. Yuan A, Yu CJ, Luh KT, et al. Aberrant p53 expression correlates with expression of vascular endothelial growth factor mRNA and interleukin-8 mRNA and neoangiogenesis in non-small-cell lung cancer. *J Clin Oncol* 2002;20(4):900–910.
236. Tsao MS, Aviel-Ronen S, Ding K, et al. Prognostic and predictive importance of p53 and RAS for adjuvant chemotherapy in non small-cell lung cancer. *J Clin Oncol* 2007;25(33):5240–5247.
237. Giatromanolaki A, Koukourakis MI, Sowter HM, et al. BNIP3 expression is linked with hypoxia-regulated protein expression and with poor prognosis in non-small cell lung cancer. *Clin Cancer Res* 2004; 10(16):5566–5571.
238. Swinson DE, Jones JL, Cox G, et al. Hypoxia-inducible factor-1 alpha in non small cell lung cancer: relation to growth factor, protease and apoptosis pathways. *Int J Cancer* 2004;111(1):43–50.
239. Felip E, Taron M, Rosell R, et al. Clinical significance of hypoxia-inducible factor-1a messenger RNA expression in locally advanced non-small-cell lung cancer after platinum agent and gemcitabine chemotherapy followed by surgery. *Clin Lung Cancer* 2005;6(5):299–303.
240. Eschmann SM, Paulsen F, Reimold M, et al. Prognostic impact of hypoxia imaging with 18F-misonidazole PET in non-small cell lung cancer and head and neck cancer before radiotherapy. *J Nucl Med* 2005;46(2):253–260.
241. Dehdashti F, Mintun MA, Lewis JS, et al. In vivo assessment of tumor hypoxia in lung cancer with 60Cu-ATSM. *Eur J Nucl Med Mol Imaging* 2003;30(6):844–850.
242. Welsh SJ, Bellamy WT, Briehl MM, et al. The redox protein thioredoxin-1 (Trx-1) increases hypoxia-inducible factor 1alpha protein expression: Trx-1 overexpression results in increased vascular endothelial growth factor production and enhanced tumor angiogenesis. *Cancer Res* 2002;62(17):5089–5095.
243. Kakolyris S, Giatromanolaki A, Koukourakis M, et al. Thioredoxin expression is associated with lymph node status and prognosis in early operable non-small cell lung cancer. *Clin Cancer Res* 2001;7(10):3087–3091.
244. Siegfried JM, Weissfeld LA, Luketich JD, et al. The clinical significance of hepatocyte growth factor for non-small cell lung cancer. *Ann Thorac Surg* 1998;66(6):1915–1918.
245. Kong-Beltran M, Seshagiri S, Zha J,et al. Somatic mutations lead to an oncogenic deletion of met in lung cancer. *Cancer Res* 2006;66(1):283–289.
246. Pircher A, Kähler CM, Skvortsov S, et al. Increased numbers of endothelial progenitor cells in peripheral blood and tumor specimens in non-small cell lung cancer: a methodological challenge and an ongoing debate on the clinical relevance. *Oncol Rep* 2008;19(2):345–352.

247. Li A, Dubey S, Varney ML, et al. IL-8 directly enhanced endothelial cell survival, proliferation, and matrix metalloproteinases production and regulated angiogenesis. *J Immunol* 2003;170(6):3369–3376.
248. Zhu YM, Webster SJ, Flower D, et al. Interleukin-8/CXCL8 is a growth factor for human lung cancer cells. *Br J Cancer* 2004;91(11):1970–1976.
249. Pastorino U, Andreola S, Tagliabue E, et al. Immunocytochemical markers in stage I lung cancer: relevance to prognosis. *J Clin Oncol* 1997; 15(8):2858–2865.
250. Pezzella F, Pastorino U, Tagliabue E, et al. Non-small-cell lung carcinoma tumor growth without morphological evidence of neo-angiogenesis. *Am J Pathol* 1997;151(5):1417–1423.
251. Renyi-Vamos F, Tovari J, Fillinger J, et al. Lymphangiogenesis correlates with lymph node metastasis, prognosis, and angiogenic phenotype in human non-small cell lung cancer. *Clin Cancer Res* 2005;11(20): 7344–7353.
252. Mattern J, Koomägi R, Volm M. Biological characterization of subgroups of squamous cell lung carcinomas. *Clin Cancer Res* 1999;5(6):1459–1463.
253. Giatromanolaki A, Koukourakis MI, O'Byrne K, et al. Non-small cell lung cancer: c-erbB-2 overexpression correlates with low angiogenesis and poor prognosis. *Anticancer Res* 1996;16(6B):3819–3825.
254. He Y, Kozaki K, Karpanen T, et al. Suppression of tumor lymphangiogenesis and lymph node metastasis by blocking vascular endothelial growth factor receptor 3 signaling. *J Natl Cancer Inst* 2002;94(11):819–825.
255. Tamura M, Oda M, Tsunezuka Y, et al. Chest CT and serum vascular endothelial growth factor-C level to diagnose lymph node metastasis in patients with primary non-small cell lung cancer. *Chest* 2004; 126(2):342–346.
256. Fisher GH, Wellen SL, Klimstra D, et al. Induction and apoptotic regression of lung adenocarcinomas by regulation of a K-Ras transgene in the presence and absence of tumor suppressor genes. *Genes Dev* 2001; 15(24):3249–3262.
257. Konishi T, Huang CL, Adachi M, et al. The K-ras gene regulates vascular endothelial growth factor gene expression in non-small cell lung cancers. *Int J Oncol* 2000;16(3):501–511.
258. Tsao MS, Liu N, Nicklee T, et al. Angiogenesis correlates with vascular endothelial growth factor expression but not with Ki-ras oncogene activation in non-small cell lung carcinoma. *Clin Cancer Res* 1997; 3(10):1807–1814.
259. Johnson L, Mercer K, Greenbaum D, et al. Somatic activation of the K-ras oncogene causes early onset lung cancer in mice. *Nature* 2001; 410(6832):1111–1116.
260. Jackson EL, Willis N, Mercer K, et al. Analysis of lung tumor initiation and progression using conditional expression of oncogenic K-ras. *Genes Dev* 2001;15(24):3243–3248.
261. Kissil JL, Walmsley MJ, Hanlon L, et al. Requirement for Rac1 in a K-ras induced lung cancer in the mouse. *Cancer Res* 2007;67(17):8089–8094.
262. Iwanaga K, Yang Y, Raso MG, et al. Pten inactivation accelerates oncogenic K-ras-initiated tumorigenesis in a mouse model of lung cancer. *Cancer Res* 2008;68(4):1119–1127.
263. Yang Y, Wislez M, Fujimoto N, et al. A selective small molecule inhibitor of c-Met, PHA-665752, reverses lung premalignancy induced by mutant K-ras. *Mol Cancer Ther* 2008;7(4):952–960.
264. Puri N, Khramtsov A, Ahmed S, et al. A selective small molecule inhibitor of c-Met, PHA665752, inhibits tumorigenicity and angiogenesis in mouse lung cancer xenografts. *Cancer Res* 2007;67(8):3529–3534.
265. Wislez M, Fujimoto N, Izzo JG, et al. High expression of ligands for chemokine receptor CXCR2 in alveolar epithelial neoplasia induced by oncogenic kras. *Cancer Res* 2006;66(8):4198–4207.
266. Kerkhoff E, Fedorov LM, Siefken R, et al. Lung-targeted expression of the c-Raf-1 kinase in transgenic mice exposes a novel oncogenic character of the wild-type protein. *Cell Growth Differ* 2000;11(4): 185–190.
267. Ceteci F, Ceteci S, Karreman C, et al. Disruption of tumor cell adhesion promotes angiogenic switch and progression to micrometastasis in RAF-driven murine lung cancer. *Cancer Cell* 2007;12(2):145–159.
268. Kulke MH, Bergsland EK, Ryan DP, et al. Phase II study of recombinant human endostatin in patients with advanced neuroendocrine tumors. *J Clin Oncol* 2006;24(22):3555–3561.

CHAPTER 9

Pierre P. Massion
David P. Carbone

Applications of Proteomics to the Management of Lung Cancer

Lung cancer is the third most common cancer in the United States, yet it causes more deaths than breast, colon, pancreas, and prostate cancer combined.[1] Attempts to alter these statistics have been challenging in all respects. From risk assessment to diagnosis, staging, assessment of response to therapy, and prognostication, there is much room for improvement in this disease (Fig. 9.1). Rapid developments in technology have allowed the direct analysis of patterns of protein expression in tumors and blood samples, and these proteomic analyses promise to assist in making progress in each of these areas.

Proteins are ultimately responsible for the function of the vast majority of biological systems, and it is clear that many of the crucial proteins in a cell are primarily regulated by post-translational modifications such as proteolytic processing, phosphorylation, or acetylation. Thus, a full knowledge of the derangement in the expression, modification, and function of proteins in cancer cells is likely to be more informative than study of DNA or RNA alone. The aim of proteomics is therefore the characterization of proteins to obtain a more integrated view of the biology. In order to further understand the molecular biology of lung cancer, we need to probe these tissues and related biological materials with tools that address the molecular complexity of the proteome in lung cancer. New technologies are being rapidly developed to allow the increasingly thorough, systematic, and simultaneous analyses of thousands of proteins in cancer cells. In particular, these studies give us a unique insight into the biology of cancer, can yield important new therapeutic targets, and may enable the identification of novel biomarkers to differentiate tumor from normal cells and predict individuals likely to develop lung cancer.

In this chapter, we will review the progress made in clinical proteomics as it applies to the management of lung cancer. We will focus our discussion on how this approach may advance the areas of early detection, response to therapy, and prognostic evaluation.

PROTEOMICS TECHNOLOGIES

Sample Preparation With proteomics strategies, one strives to identify novel proteins and understand their structure, function, interaction with proteins and other molecules, and to bring this knowledge to the clinic by means of new diagnostic and predictive biomarkers and well as identification of therapeutic targets. The rapid advance of mass spectrometry (MS) and related technologies offers powerful new tools to analyze the proteome. In contrast to standard protein biochemistry, proteomics is defined as the study of the proteome, the complete set of proteins produced by a species, using the technologies of large-scale protein separation and identification (Table 9.1).[2]

Protein biochemistry has long been exploited to understand how biological systems function and lead to a cancer phenotype. Early efforts were geared to study primarily one protein at a time with biochemical methods of increasing power and sensitivity. The world of immunoassays brought and continues to bring major contributions to the field alone or in combination with MS.

In proteomic analysis, the isolation and preparation of samples for analysis is of critical importance, and the precise technique chosen depends on the scientific question being addressed, whether it may be a comprehensive expression analysis, evaluation of secreted proteins, nuclear proteins, proteins with a particular modification (e.g., phosphorylation), or those that bind to other proteins. Many approaches are available: some gel-based, some based on separation by reverse phase chromatography, affinity, size exclusion, ion exchange, and isoelectric focusing. The separation/purification strategies all have the advantage of separating the targets of interest from very abundant proteins in the milieu. The trade-off is between the addition of complexity and variability to the analysis and increased sensitivity. For example, proteomics of blood samples is complicated by the fact that the vast majority of the proteins in blood are made up of albumin and immunoglobulin, but the proteins of interest may be 7 to 10 orders of magnitude less abundant, and much more readily found if the abundant proteins are removed. An example of successful

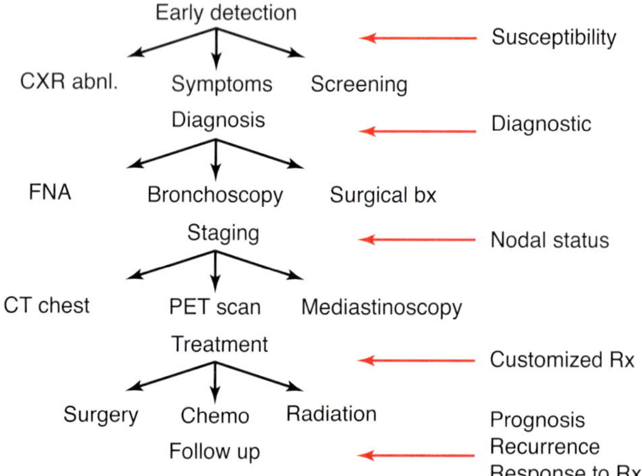

FIGURE 9.1 Schematic representation of major areas of management of lung cancer in the clinical context and potential applications of proteomic approaches to address questions of susceptibility, diagnosis, staging, and therapeutics. *abnl*, abnormal; *bx*, biopsy; *CT*, computed tomography; *CXR*, chest x-ray; *FNA*, fine-needle aspiration.

TABLE 9.1 Analytical Approaches to the Proteome

Protein biochemistry
Immunoblotting
Immunohistochemistry
ELISA
Flow cytometry
Protein chemical analysis
Antibody production
Proteomics
Sample preparation for isolation of proteins
Gel-based separation followed by MS
LC-HPLC
Affinity columns
Affinity tags
Mass spectrometry–based protein identification
MALDI MS/MS
ESI MS
Electron transfer dissociation MS
Protein arrays including reverse phase arrays

separation strategy is immunoaffinity phosphoproteomics, which combines immunoaffinity purification with tandem MS. Using this approach, Rikova et al.[3] discovered oncogenic kinases such as platelet-derived growth factor receptor (PDGFR)-alpha and discoidin domain receptor family, member 1 (DDR1) that had not been implicated in the pathogenesis of lung cancer.

The Mass Spectrometer A mass spectrometer analyzes proteins after their conversion to gaseous ions, based on their mass to charge ratio. It is essentially made of three basic elements: an ion source for converting them to gaseous ions, a mass analyzer for separating the ions by mass, and a detector for detecting the ionized proteins (Fig. 9.2).

Tandem mass spectrometry (MS/MS) is a major analytic tool used for evaluating proteins and protein complexes. With this approach, protein samples are first digested with proteases into a mixture of peptides and analyzed. Peptide ions are separated in the first stage, then each peptide is fragmented in the collision cell, and the fragments are then separated again to identify them. The precise measurement of the mass of these fragments allows the reconstruction of the identity and composition of the original peptide (Fig. 9.3). There are many modes of MS/MS. Different mass analyzers currently used for MS/MS analysis are quadrupole ion trap (QIT), triple quadrupole (TQ), quadrupole time of flight (QTOF), or Fourier transform ion-cyclotron resonance (FTICR).

Specific mass spectrometers have specific applications. For example, electron transfer dissociation (ETD) MS allows detailed analysis of phosphorylated peptides that is of optimal

Samples ▶	Ion sources ▶	Mass analyzers ▶	Detectors ▶	Data analysis
Tissue	Electron spray	Time-of-flight MS	Current produced	Mass spectrum
Blood	MALDI	Quadrupole MS		Mass chromatogram
Urine		Ion Trap MS		Contour maps
Sputum		FTICR MS		
BAL		Orbitrap		
Exhaled Breath				

FIGURE 9.2 Principles of mass spectrometry analysis. The time-of-flight (TOF) analyzer uses an electric field to accelerate the ions, and then measures the time they take to reach the detector. A quadrupole mass analyzer acts as a mass-selective filter. The quadrupole ion trap works on the same physical principles as the quadrupole mass analyzer, but the ions are trapped and sequentially ejected. *BAL*, bronchoalveolar lavage; *FTICR*, Fourier transform ion-cyclotron resonance; *LTQ*, linear quadrupole ion trap; *MALDI*, matrix-assisted laser desorption ionization; *MS*, spectometry. The Orbitrap is a novel form of MS instrumentation with 60 to 100 k resolution and <2 ppm mass accuracy.

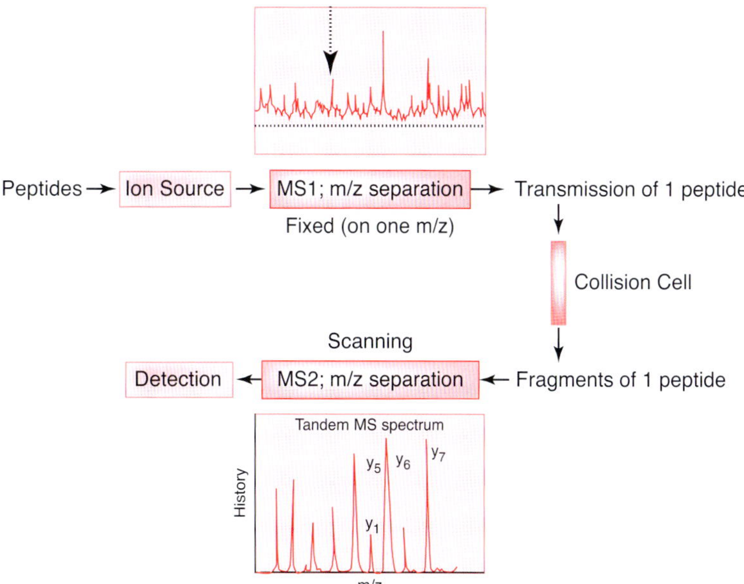

FIGURE 9.3 Principle of tandem mass spectrometry. A peptide mixture is injected into the MS. Unlike the single-stage mass spectrometer that scans the entire range of masses, the first analyzer is set up to transmit only one peptide—therefore, one mass over charge (m/z). This peptide is then broken apart in a collision cell to generate peptide fragments. The m/z of these peptides is then determined by another mass analyzer. The amino acid sequence of the peptide is determined by subtracting fragment ion masses from each other, yielding the residue mass of a particular amino acid. The process is repeated until the sequence has been resolved.

quality.[4] The LTQ integrates the steps of mass analyzer, collision cell, and then another mass analyzer actually does it tandem in time, meaning that three steps occur in the same location—in an ion trap. An LTQ tandem MS is particularly well equipped for excellent throughput, good sensitivity, MSn capabilities, and a robust instrument. Each clinical question needs to be addressed separately and proteomics may provide tools to address them. The suite of technologies available to researchers is ever increasing and their selection very much depends on the goals and the type of samples to analyze.

Analysis of Complex Protein Mixtures The proteome has multiple layers of complexity. The composition of the proteome is not static like DNA. The structure is at least an order of magnitude more complex than the genome, the dynamic range in protein concentrations in given biological specimens is huge (10^{12}), we have no target amplification method such as PCR for genomic analysis, and the methods used still have limitations in sensitivity primarily because of our ability to separate protein complexes in subgroups pure enough for analysis. Quantitative analysis is also challenging, but new methodologies are being developed to address this challenge. High-throughput analysis of the proteome without compromising reproducibility is difficult as well.

The analysis of the complex mixture can be conceptualized in two major ways, the *top-down* and the *bottom-up* approaches. In the top-down approach, one starts with a specific protein candidate; it is then separated, purified, and its structure is identified. Recent technologies, such as FITRC MS, increase the resolution and allow the analysis of larger peptide fragments. However, the bottom-up approach takes the challenge of embracing complexity from the start and directly analyzes complex mixtures with a large number of proteins, and uses computational peptidomics to reconstruct the identities of the proteins in the mixture. This later approach is less intuitive and may benefit from higher throughput. It is recently being facilitated by modern bioinformatics tools, enabling the analysis of proteomic digestion with different enzymes than trypsin and therefore increasing the likelihood of detecting increasing number of peptides mapping to the same protein therefore improving the confidence of identification.

Biomarkers The assumption underlying the concept of proteomic biomarkers is that certain characteristics of proteomes are highly correlated with specific clinically relevant biological states. These characteristics include changes in expression levels of proteins and the presence of specific modified protein forms (Table 9.2). Specific effort has been exerted in cancer proteomics to develop biomarkers for the early detection of disease by analysis of plasma or serum proteins. Detection of cancers at early stages maximizes survival, and identification of blood-borne markers would lead to minimally invasive tests.

The best biomarkers are those that are reproducibly measured, related to the disease process, and trigger a clinical decision

TABLE 9.2 Characteristics of a Biomarker and the Process Selection of Candidates

Characteristics of a Biomarker
1. Should be an indicator or surrogate marker of clinical end point
2. Should be measurable, quantifiable, reproducible
3. Should evaluate a biological process and predict the outcome
Process of Selection of Candidates
1. Demonstrate that marker appears in accessible material
2. Establish quantitative criteria for the presence of the marker
3. Validate marker against accepted end points
4. Confirm its predictive value in prospective study

resulting in improved clinical outcomes. Despite an intense search for such biomarkers in the last 20 years, there are none currently available for early diagnosis of lung cancer.[5] One reason for such a lack of success thus far is the enormous challenge offered by lung cancer development. The onset of the disease process is extremely slow (months to years) and we have no means of evaluating the rate of progression. Therefore, there is a critical need for new biomarkers that are related to the disease process and that can be measured early, easily, and repeatedly to assess progression of the process.

Approaches to Biomarker Discovery Using Proteomics Biomarker identification has been addressed by multiple proteomic technologies (Fig. 9.4). MALDI profiling is rapid, high throughput, but detects only the most abundant proteins of relatively low molecular weight, and does not enable direct identification when applied to complex proteomes. Two-dimensional (2D) gel-based analysis suffers problems of interlaboratory reproducibility and throughput. More recent in-depth proteomic analyses are trying to overcome these limitations and are summarized here.

High-Throughput Profiling Techniques The rapid proteomic profiling of blood, tissue, or urine with minimal sample preparation, using the peak pattern as a diagnostic tool, has generated great enthusiasm and yet has been minimally successful at providing robust signatures to translate to the clinic. In this approach, the focus is on the use of MS peak patterns of abundant proteins or peptide fragments that correlate with an early disease stage but are usually not part of the disease mechanism. MALDI TOF MS is capable for very high throughput where a sample can be analyzed in seconds and has higher tolerance for salts, buffers, and other biological contaminants. Because of these qualities, MALDI MS has been utilized to study proteins/peptides in serum,[6–10] urine,[11] tissue extracts,[12,13] whole cells,[14] and laser-captured microdissected cells.[15]

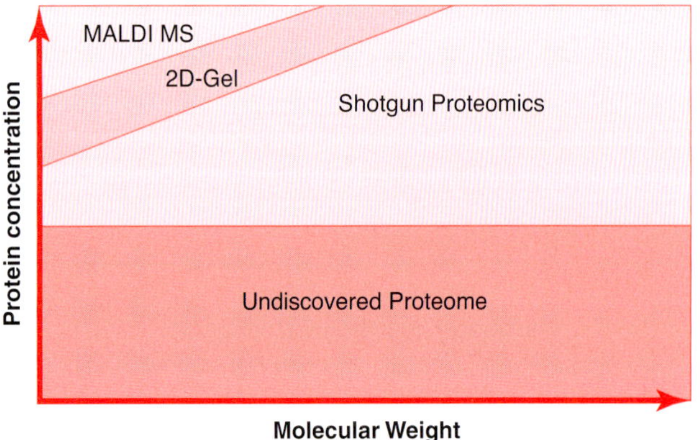

FIGURE 9.4 Proteome and analytical coverage of its complexity by current technologies according to protein concentration (depth) and molecular weight (breath). *MALDI MS*, matrix-assisted laser desorption ionization mass spectometry.

Profiling using this technology in biological fluids or tissue samples is not without challenges. The enormous complexity of the sample composition, the large dominance of few proteins in the sample, and their ability to mask lower abundance limits the informativity of this approach. Truly tumor-derived markers are likely to be present at low levels in blood, similar to levels of the thousands of other proteins in blood that derive from normal tissue leakage. Thus, the dynamic range of protein concentrations adds a new dimension of technical considerations to successful analysis of the serum/plasma proteome.[16] These profiling experiments have been applied to a series of biological specimens. Yet, reproducibility between platforms and institutions remains a problem such that none of the profiling experiments have yet made an impact in clinical medicine. This is in contrast with greater early steps in the translation of genomic signatures to the clinic.[17,18]

Finally, protein arrays have recently been developed and offer a series of targets printed onto different surfaces. Proteins,[19] peptides, antibodies,[20,21] or lysates[22] will then be detected by antibodies, serum, or multicolor detection systems. The Swedish Human Protein Atlas (HPA) program proposes a systematic analysis of the human proteome using antibody-based proteomics combining affinity-purified antibodies with protein profiling assembled in tissue microarrays.[23]

In-Depth Proteomics Analysis The analysis of the plasma proteome has made great progress in the last few years. http://www.hupo.org/research/hppp/. This is largely a consequence of novel methods of serum fractionation and MS-based protein identification techniques; the number of plasma proteins now includes major categories of proteins in the human proteome.[24] The list confirms the presence of a number of interesting candidate marker proteins in plasma and serum.[25] The detection of low-abundance proteins in the plasma requires combinations of powerful technologies. The identification of proteins whose expression levels are altered with the disease state progression (2DE, MS, shotgun proteomics) requires methodological improvements over the profiling experiments. Methods related to separation of ions and ionization have moved the field forward.

Two technology platforms have been developed to enable unbiased discovery of candidate markers from tissues and biofluids and verification of candidate markers by targeted analysis. Unbiased discovery employs a shotgun proteomics platform based on isoelectric focusing of peptides from tissue protein digests, followed by reverse phase LC-MS-MS on Thermo LTQ or LTQ-Orbitrap instruments. Verification is done by targeted quantitation of peptides derived from biomarker candidate proteins using liquid chromatography–multiple-reaction monitoring MS (LC-MRM-MS).[26–28]

In shotgun analyses, protein mixtures are digested to peptides, which then are analyzed, most commonly by multidimensional LC-MS-MS. MS-MS spectra encode the sequences of peptides, as well as the masses and sequence positions of any modifications (Fig. 9.5). Matching of MS-MS spectra to database sequences enables identification of the peptides and the

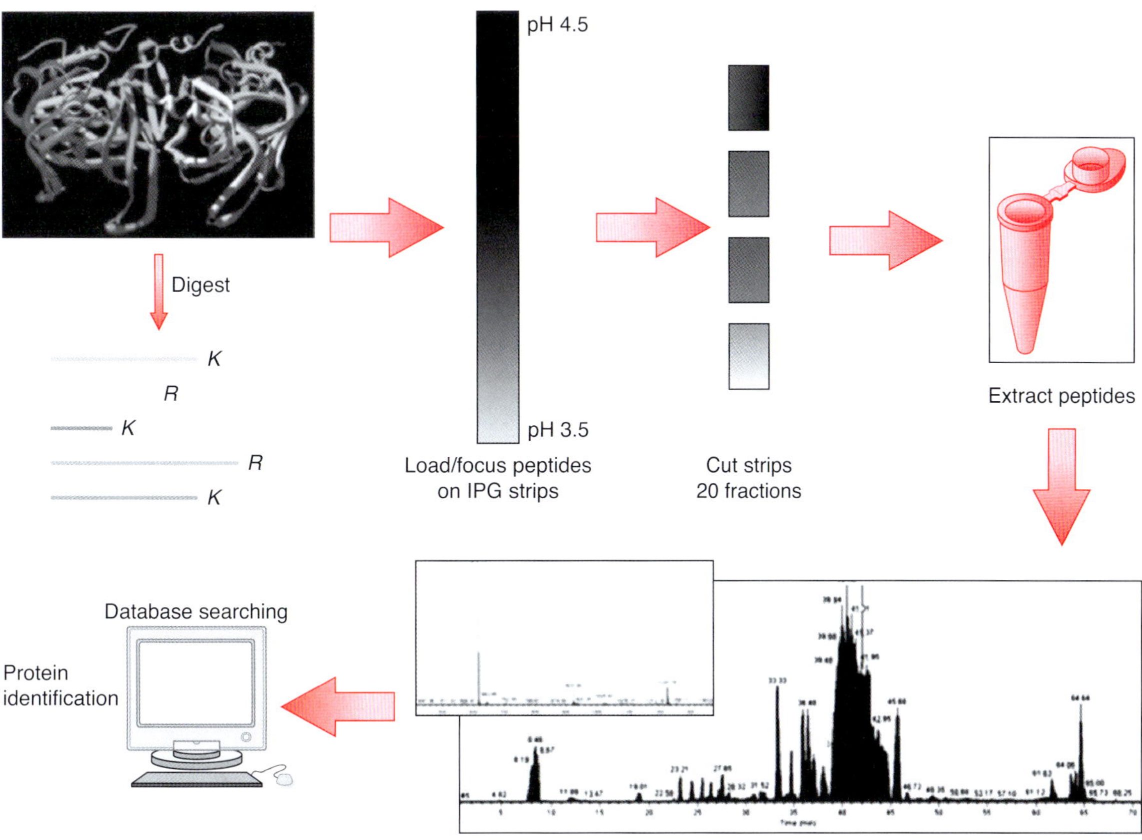

FIGURE 9.5 Overview of tissue shotgun proteomics.

proteins from which they were derived. Shotgun analyses by LC-MS-MS also result in direct identification of the peptides detected and provide for quantitative analysis of protein components. Shotgun proteomics has proven the most versatile and effective method for dissecting multiprotein complexes, signaling networks, and complex subcellular proteomes.[29] Shotgun analyses can confidently identify 3000 to 5000 proteins from a 200-μg protein sample. Shotgun analyses have generated the most complete proteomic inventories to date of major eukaryotic subcellular organelles, whole cell and tissue proteomes, and proteomes of human biofluids, including plasma and serum.[28,30–33]

Targeted quantitative analysis of top candidates can be done by LC-MRM-MS analysis, as a first level of verification of the shotgun results. Briefly, tissue lysates are run on a NuPAGE gel and peptides are extracted, then injected in a TSQ Quantum Ultra mass spectrometer. Peptides are loaded and desalted and resolved in reverse phase chromatography, eluted with a linear gradient. For MRM, four transitions are recorded, and chromatographic peak areas for the transitions are summed and compared to summed peak areas for beta actin. Differences between peaks are evaluated for statistical significance. Targeted LC-MRM-MS analyses can analyze up to 100 candidates per run in individual tissue or plasma specimens. Moreover, the application of both stable isotope tagging and label-free quantitation has enabled the application of shotgun proteomics to quantitative comparisons of complex proteome samples.[34–39]

Proteomic Data Analysis Analysis and interpretation of the data derived from MS-based proteomic technologies represents unique challenges as well. From MALDI MS experiments, Spectra are generated in the mass-to-charge (m/z) 3000 to 50,000. Internal calibration is performed using internal or external calibrants. The data processing consists of internal calibration, smoothing, baseline correction, normalization to the total ion current, feature selection with a signal-to-noise ratio, and binning of features. This processing results in 100 to 300 m/z peaks per spectrum on average, using conservative parameters. Statistical analyses of these data for biomarkers focus on the selection of MS features and differential expression levels between the study groups and on building class prediction models based on the selected features.[40–44] The misclassification rate is typically estimated using the leave one out cross-validation.

From tandem MS analysis, raw data is extracted for individual spectra with filters applied to remove obvious background ions and low-quality spectra. These spectra yield a list of peptide sequences and the frequency that each peptide is detected. These sequences are searched against the NCBI protein database to generate candidate proteins from which they may have come. This list is filtered in various ways to reduce

TABLE 9.3 Advantages and Difficulties in Proteomics

Advantages of a Proteomic Approach	Difficulties in Proteomics
• Most nucleic acid sequences have their effect via translation into proteins. • Protein expression is often not tightly associated with RNA expression. • Ability to detect posttranslational modifications (e.g., phosphorylation, lipidation, ubiquitination, glycosylation).	• Composition of the proteome • Structure is complex • Dynamic range is large • No amplification method • Sensitivity of methods • Quantitation • Throughput

the likelihood of false matches, and the protein and hit count lists from different study groups are compared to generated candidate biomarkers.

In summary, while genes carry the genetic information, proteins are principal actors of vital regulatory processes. Proteomics has many theoretical advantages over the more established genomic and transcriptomic approaches to these questions, but has been hampered by a number of technical problems (Table 9.3). Another major challenge is the need for extensive validation in using these novel global proteomics research platforms prior to routine clinical applications. Once interested in applying any new technology, one should remember to carefully frame a biological question, understand the literature, consider the limitations of each approach, and use the most appropriate technology to answer the question.

EARLY DETECTION

Biomarker discovery for early detection of disease is made challenging by the fact that patients are often identified late in the course of disease, while it is abundantly clear that those treated during early disease stages have a much better prognosis. Access to samples before diagnosis is very difficult. Another major challenge is the target sample to be analyzed. Complex samples such as serum or urine although readily accessible add to the complexity of the task. Tumor biomarkers for lung cancer can be categorically classified into serum biomarkers, tissue biomarkers, and sputum. Exhaled breath condensate is an interesting source of material, but has not proven feasible yet. Serum biomarkers stand out as being the most attractive at this time because of their easy and routine accessibility. See also Chapter 22.

Biomarkers of early detection of lung cancer are still at an early stage of development.[45] The Early Detection Research Network (National Cancer Institute, division of cancer prevention) has proposed a stepwise method for evaluating biomarkers, and to identify people at risk (http://www.cancer.gov/edrn).[46] None of current biomarkers for the early detection of lung cancer have passed the early validation (phase II). While genetics has provided considerable insights into the molecular biology of lung cancer,[47] the overall correlation between level of expression of the messenger RNA molecules and protein expression is relatively poor.[48] It is possible that proteomic technologies offer a new avenue for biomarker discovery.

Proteomics-based early detection strategies for cancer diagnosis include the analysis of complex mixtures such as tissue samples, serum, plasma, sputum, and exhaled breath condensate. The inherent analytical advantages of MS, including sensitivity and speed, promise to make MS a mainstay of biomarker discovery. The optimal use of these technologies depends on the desired goal, such as protein identification, identification of posttranslation modification, or determination of protein–protein interactions.

The direct analysis of serum proteomes to detect disease markers has attracted widespread interest and intense scrutiny. Early work using either MALDI or a proprietary MALDI variant termed surface-enhanced laser desorption ionization (SELDI) demonstrated that spectra of crude serum protein mixtures or subfractions displayed differences in spectral features that appeared to correlate with disease status.[49–51] The application of multivariate analytical methods generated models that correlated spectral features with disease status.

To determine the diagnostic accuracy of MALDI mass spectrometric analysis of serum in lung cancer, we used MALDI-MS to analyze undepleted and unfractionated serum from a total of 288 NSCLC patients and matched controls divided into training (92 cases and 92 controls) and test (50 cases and 56 controls) sets.[10] In the training set, they defined a seven-signal proteomic signature distinguishing lung cancer serum from matched controls with an overall accuracy of 78%, a sensitivity of 67.4%, and a specificity of 88.9%. In the test set, the signature reached an overall accuracy of 72.6%, a sensitivity of 58%, and a specificity of 85.7%. As diagnosis of early stage lung cancer is important, authors searched for a protein signature discriminating stage I lung cancers from controls and found a six-signal signature reaching 70.8% sensitivity and 84.4% specificity in the training set, and 57.1% sensitivity and 71.4% specificity in the test set (Fig. 9.6).

With a multivariate logistic regression model applied on a total of 223 cases and controls, they showed that the serum signature was associated with lung cancer diagnosis independently of gender, smoking status, smoking pack-years, and C-reactive protein levels, and had the strongest association with lung cancer diagnosis among all the covariates in the model. Using SELDI-TOF-MS on serum samples from 158 lung cancer patients and 50 controls, Yang et al.[52] reported a five-signal protein signature distinguishing lung cancer cases from controls with 86.9% sensitivity and 80.0% specificity in the validation set.

Initial reports suggesting that these features comprise new families of biomarkers were followed by considerable critical analysis, which pointed out several problems.[53–55] First, MALDI and SELDI analyses were subject to systematic bias due to inconsistent sample collection, processing, and poor instrument calibration. Second, the analyses of small numbers of samples displaying large numbers of spectral features led to

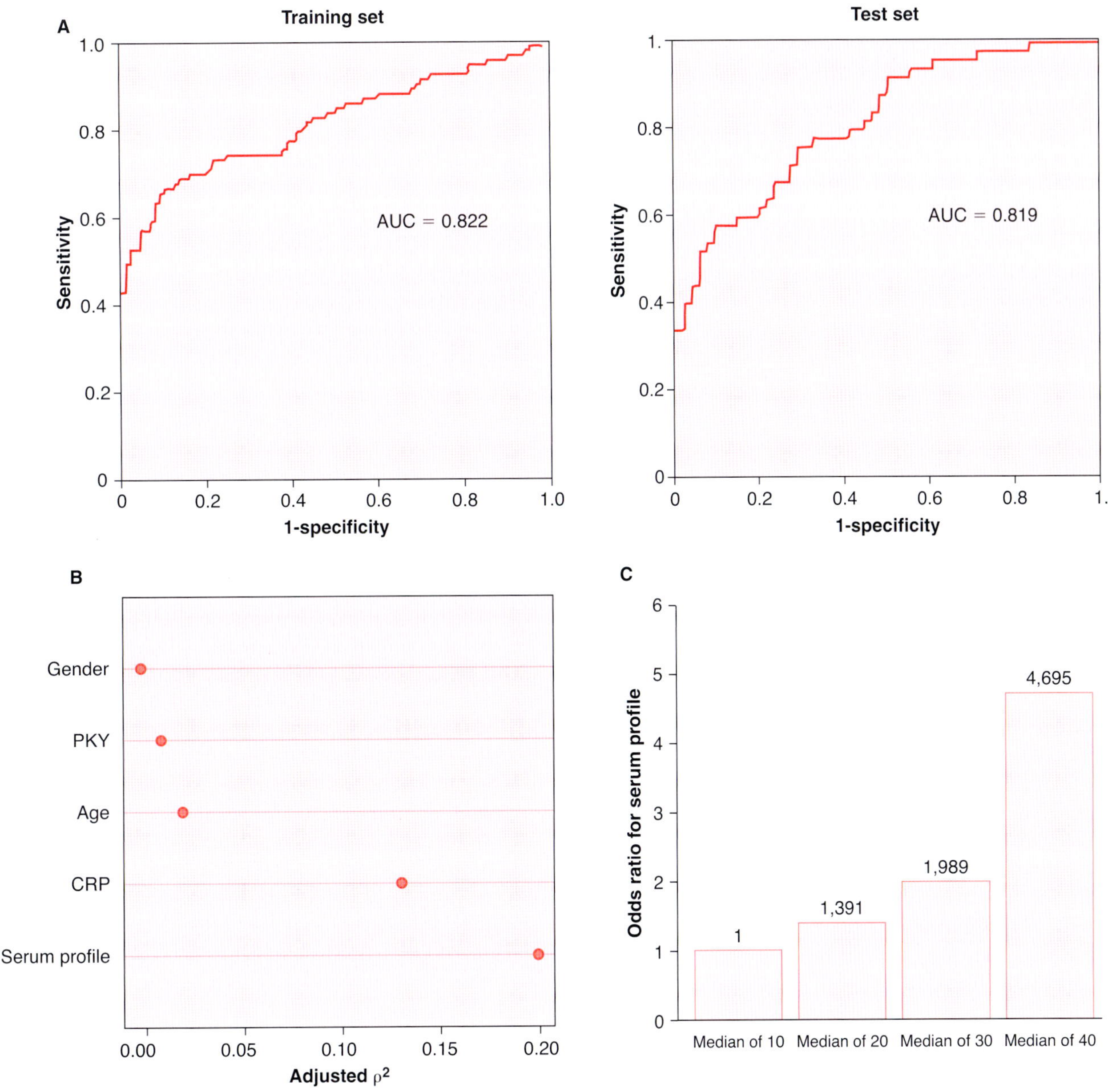

FIGURE 9.6 **A:** Receiver operating characteristic curves addressing diagnostic efficacy of cases and controls in the two datasets (182 training sample set, 106 matched test set). **B:** Nonmonotonic (quadratic in ranks) generalization of the Spearman rank–correlation coefficient, for each of these five predictors. The generalized Spearman coefficient helps to describe the strength of marginal relationships between each of these predictor variables and the response (being with lung cancer or not). This plot shows that the serum profile has the strongest correlation with the response among these five predictors. **C:** Odds ratio of being diagnosed with lung cancer according to serum profile quantile distribution. *AUC*, area under the curve; *CRP*, C-reactive protein; *PKY*, Smoking Pack Years. (From Yildiz PB, Shyr Y, Rahman JS, et al. Diagnostic accuracy of MALDI mass spectrometric analysis of unfractionated serum in lung cancer. *J Thorac Oncol* 2007;2:893–901.)

models that "overfit" the data and did not scale effectively to larger sample numbers. Third, spectral features that correlated to disease state were found to be poorly reproducible between different laboratories. Finally, MALDI- and SELDI-based methods did not enable direct identification of the protein and peptide species that constituted putative markers. Eventual identification of some of the species associated with spectral signals revealed that they were all abundant blood proteins or their proteolysis products, many of which were produced ex vivo during sample handling or serum preparation.[56,57]

Moreover, some of the most characteristic markers (e.g., serum amyloid A) were associated with multiple cancers.[10,58] Recent work by Villanueva et al.[59] demonstrated that blood from patients with different cancer types yielded characteristic

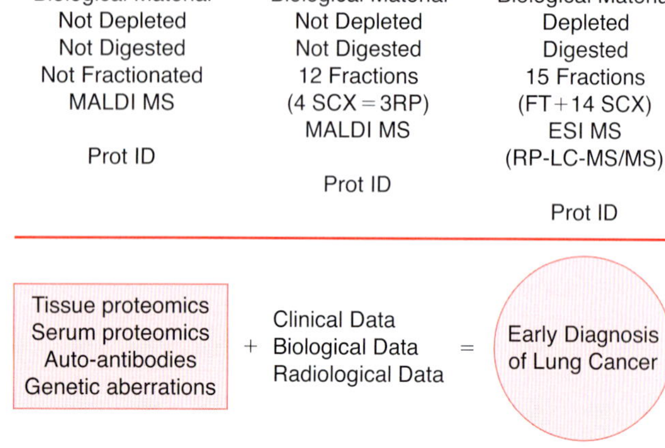

FIGURE 9.7 MS approaches and integration in a multivariable model for the early diagnosis of lung cancer. *ESI MS*, electrospray ionization mass spectometry; *FT*, Flow Through; *LC*, liquid chromatography; *MALDI MS*, matrix-assisted laser desorption ionization mass spectometry; *Prot ID*, Protein Identification; *RP*, Reverse Phase; *SCX*, Strong Cation Exchange.

sets of proteolysis products of abundant blood proteins during serum preparation.

The proteomic characteristics observed in MALDI and SELDI analyses are interesting but may ultimately be of questionable value in the detection and diagnosis of cancer in human populations. Clearly, the majority of identified species do not arise from cancers themselves, but rather from systemic responses to disease. The distribution of protein proteolysis products is exquisitely sensitive to sampling methods and processing, and the different proteolysis products can only be distinguished by MS instruments. Most importantly, the relationship of these putative markers to cancer is unclear, as is their ability to distinguish different cancers.

Ultimately, the early diagnosis of lung cancer will be addressed in an integrated way after gathering information from clinical, biological, imaging, and molecular data (Fig. 9.7).

PROTEOMICS FOR CLASSIFICATION OF PROGNOSIS

The clinical behavior of individual patients with lung cancer is extremely diverse. Some tumors progress rapidly with widespread metastases, and some grow only very slowly over the course of years and never result in clinical symptoms. Knowledge of this propensity when selecting initial therapy would be extremely useful in determining whether treatment is needed at all and how aggressive an approach is indicated. Deciding on the need for adjuvant chemotherapy is an example. Presumably, this diversity results from variability in the precise molecular makeup of individual tumors, and a pattern of molecular features associated with clinical course, independent of therapy, is referred to as a prognostic signature. Features associated with the benefit or lack of benefit from a specific intervention are considered to make up a predictive signature, and will be addressed in the next section.

As discussed previously, many of the functionally important molecules in the development of cancer are regulated by posttranslational modifications, implying that direct assessment of the proteins themselves might be more informative than RNA or DNA. Attempts have been made to apply proteomic technologies to uncovering an accurate prognostic signature for lung cancer. Gharib et al.[60] used 2D gels to study the differences in protein expression patterns for 93 resected lung adenocarcinomas and 10 normal lung samples, and assessed their association with survival. In this study, they found that two of the five cytokeratin 7 isoforms, one of eight CK8 isoforms, and one of three CK19 isoforms were associated with survival. One of these, CK19, had independently been found to be a useful tumor marker for lung cancer. Also uncovered in this dataset was the significant downregulation of selenium-binding protein 1, also strongly associated with survival.[61] Another study used 2D gels to study 20 squamous cell lung cancers with matched normal tissues[62] and identified tumor/normal differential expression of mdm2, c-jun, and EGFR, and found 26 proteins reactive to patient autoantibodies, but no survival analysis was done. The finding that not all of the CK19 isoforms conveyed prognostic significance underscores the power of proteomic technologies to uncover these associations. Unfortunately, because specific antibodies for individual isoforms are rarely available, it also underscores a problem with this approach in the practical clinical measurement of these features.

MALDI-TOF has also been applied to this problem, and in a study of 79 tumors and 14 normal lung tissues, classifiers were defined that were able to discriminate tumor from normal, and lung cancer from metastatic disease.[40] A 15-protein classifier was constructed that was able to predict survival after resection (Fig. 9.8).

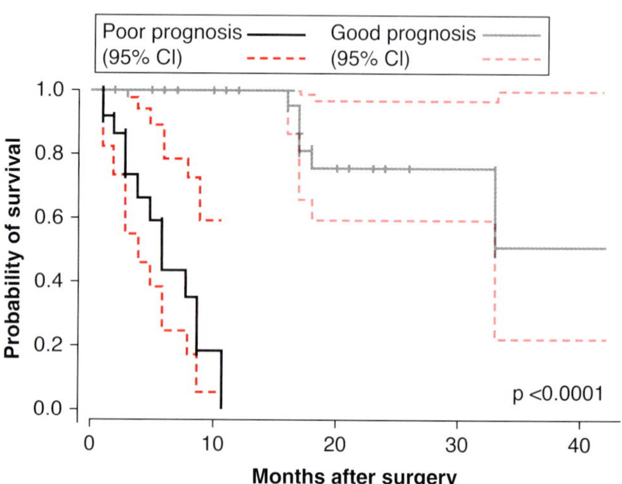

FIGURE 9.8 Kaplan-Meier survival curves for groups with poor and good prognosis according to proteomic pattern compromised of 15 distinct MS peaks. $p < 0.0001$ according to log-rank test. *CI*, confidence interval. (From Yanagisawa K, Shyr Y, Xu BJ, et al. Proteomic patterns of tumour subsets in non-small-cell lung cancer. *Lancet* 2003;362:433–439.)

These proteins included thymosin beta4 and SUMO-2, both with interesting biological implications. Thymosin beta4 has been associated with inhibition of caspase-3 in taxol-induced tumor cell death,[63] as well as stabilization of HIF-1 alpha,[64] and its expression is regulated by hMLH1.[65] SUMO-2 is also associated with multiple important cancer pathways.[66–70] A subsequent study of a larger cohort of 174 NSCLC tumors with a longer follow-up derived a 25 signal classifier overlapping with the previous classifier, and also able to divide patients into high- and low-risk groups.[71] However, MALDI-TOF is limited by nonstandardized or transportable analytic platforms and its low sensitivity and selectivity for low–molecular-weight proteins. It is also difficult to identify the precise protein detected, making translation to clinical practice difficult.

Analysis of serum by SELDI-TOF has also uncovered an unidentified 4628 Da protein associated with survival in 87 advanced stage NSCLC patients.[72] However, this was evaluated only in a cross-validation approach and not an independent test set, and needs additional validation.

LC-MS/MS analysis of lung cancer tumors has great promise for the discovery of tumor signatures, as it is capable of detecting many more proteins than MALDI-TOF and gives the identity of the observed protein features. In one very preliminary study,[73] 24 surgically resected adenocarcinomas were analyzed by SDS-page gel followed by in-gel digestion and C-18 LC separation and MS/MS analysis. They identified 51 candidate signals and selected two of the corresponding proteins, myosin IIA and vimentin, as biomarkers. When evaluated by immunohistochemistry, they were able to use these two markers to classify good and poor prognosis groups (Fig. 9.9).

None of these markers have reached routine clinical practice to date, at least partly due to the difficult steps of taking a research lab–based assay for large numbers of candidate markers and translating that into a reproducible and accurate high-throughput commercial product capable of validating them in a prospective fashion in large enough cohorts of patients. Work continues in this direction, however.

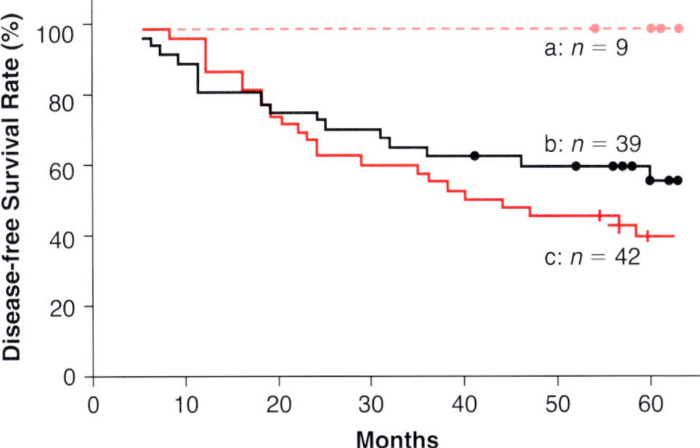

FIGURE 9.9 Kaplan-Meier curves for disease-free survival after complete resection in patients with stage I lung adenocarcinoma. **A:** Cases lacking both myosin IIA and vimentin expression (nonrelapse survival rate at 5 years: 100%). **B:** Cases negative for myosin IIA and positive for vimentin, or positive for myosin IIA and negative for vimentin (nonprelapse survival rate at 5 years: 58.0%). **C:** Cases positive for both myosin IIA and vimentin (nonrelapse survival rate at 5 years: 42.0%). Group a showed significantly higher survival than group b, and significantly higher survival than group c (a, b: $p = 0.029$; a–c: $p = 0.006$). (From Maeda J, Hirano T, Ogiwara A, et al. Proteomic analysis of stage I primary lung adenocarcinoma aimed at individualisation of postoperative therapy. *Br J Cancer* 2008;98:596–603.)

RESPONSE TO THERAPY

More important than simple prognostic classification is predicting response to therapy. Identification of patients destined to do poorly regardless of therapy is much less interesting than identification of specific therapies capable of assisting in the selection of the optimal intervention able to alter a patient's outcome.

Several proteomic studies have attempted to define protein signatures capable of predicting benefit from specific interventions. In its simplest form, single immunohistochemical marker studies are being tested for their utility in defining patients who will benefit from specific therapies. For example, immunohistochemical expression of excision repair cross-complementing rodent repair deficiency, complementation group 1 (ERCC1) is associated with lack of benefit from platinum-based therapy,[74] and high thymidylate synthase expression in squamous cell lung cancer predicts lack of benefit from pemetrexed.[75] Some studies are attempting to use proteomic technologies to measure the levels of several candidate markers and cytokines in the blood and correlate these with response. One such study[76] looked at biomarkers associated with benefit from bevacizumab, and antibody against VEGF, and found that baseline intercellular adhesion molecule (ICAM) levels were prognostic for survival and predictive of response to chemotherapy with or without bevacizumab, and that VEGF levels were predictive of response to bevacizumab but not survival. Other studies have attempted to find blood-based biomarkers of response to VEGFR tyrosine kinase inhibitors.[77] Using high-throughput platforms, several groups are now studying the utility of measuring 100 or more such markers simultaneously.[78,79]

2D gel analysis of squamous cell lung cancer has identified candidate proteins associated with resistance to mitoxantrone,[80] and taxanes,[81] but no clinical candidate markers have been identified in these datasets. A study of H322 and H1299 lung cancer cells using 2D gels identified thioredoxin reductase to be associated with resistance to the histone deacetylase inhibitor depsipeptide.[82] 2D differential in-gel electrophoresis (DIGE) technology also identified nine proteins associated with response to the EGFR tyrosine kinase inhibitor gefitinib.[83] These proteins included fatty acid binding protein and glutathione-S-transferase P, and application of this signature to an external sample set confirmed the predictive ability, but only involved 14 patients.

To date, MS/MS proteomic analysis of lung cancer tumors has also failed to find markers predictive of response to uracil-tegafur,[73] but other studies looking at other chemotherapies are in progress. The potential power of tandem MS not only for identification of markers predictive of benefit from therapy, but also new targets for therapy in specific tumors is demonstrated in a recent study of the phosphoproteome of lung cancer cells.[3] This study evaluated tyrosine phosphorylated peptides in 41 NSCLC cell lines and over 150 tumors and found known therapeutic target phosphorylation as well as activation of potential but not previously identified kinases such as DDR1. In spite of this progress, to date, none of the markers from 2D gels or mass spectrometric analysis of lung tumors has advanced to careful clinical testing.

Probably most surprising is the report that a serum protein signature has been reported that could accurately define patients with good or poor survival after treatment with gefitinib or erlotinib.[84] It is more intuitive that an accurate predictive signature is more likely to be defined from tumor protein expression patterns than from patterns in the blood, but this group defined a signature of eight proteins that was capable of classifying good and poor outcomes in a training cohort of 139 second-plus line patients treated with gefitinib and applied this classifier in a blinded way to two independent test cohorts, one second-plus line treated with gefitinib, and one a cooperative group trial of erlotinib in first-line therapy (E3503) (Fig. 9.10).

Remarkably, highly statistically significant classification was achieved for both progression-free survival and overall survival

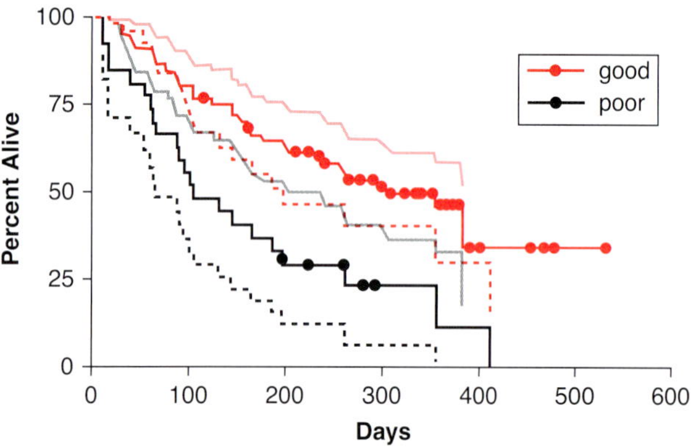

Number of Patients at Risk:

Time [Days]	0	50	100	150	200	250	300	350	400
Good	69	64	56	51	43	37	26	18	6
Poor	27	22	16	12	8	7	3	3	2

FIGURE 9.10 Kaplan-Meier analysis of overall survival in the Eastern Cooperative Oncology Group validation cohort (n = 96). These patients had advanced non–small-cell lung cancer and had been treated first line with erlotinib alone. *Solid lines*, event-free fraction; *dashed lines*, 95% confidence intervals; *tick marks*, censored patients. (From Taguchi F, Solomon B, Gregorc V, et al. Mass spectrometry to classify non-small-cell lung cancer patients for clinical outcome after treatment with epidermal growth factor receptor tyrosine kinase inhibitors: a multicohort cross-institutional study. *J Natl Cancer Inst* 2007;99:838–846.)

in these cohorts, and not in three control cohorts treated with chemotherapy or surgery alone. None of these patient cohorts was from a randomized trial, however, so it is impossible to determine if this classifier is truly specifically predictive of benefit from erlotinib. This test has been commercialized and prospective testing is in progress.

CONCLUSION

The rapid development of proteomic technologies has provided a large amount of novel information leading to the assembly of large protein inventories and a better understanding of how they interact, the role of specific posttranslational modifications, and advances in biology. Proteomic analysis has the potential to profile differences between lung tumor and no tumor, between different stages and histology of cancer, and between different cancer samples at the same stage of progression. The ability to identify important proteins involved in the transformation process may lead to early markers for detection of specific types of cancers and treatments based on the molecular profile of lung cancer. Molecular profiling may assist in identifying high-risk populations and offers a unique opportunity to study early carcinogenesis and potentially to reduce cancer mortality through its integration with genomics. The importance of clinical proteomics comes from the fact that it will have a fundamental impact on our understanding into complex disease processes, such as lung cancer, and will offer new opportunities in the diagnosis, prognosis, and therapy of disease. The development of specific and sensitive diagnostic biomarkers using biological fluids, such as sputum and serum, should improve screening, early detection, monitoring of disease progression, treatment response, and surveillance for recurrence. Proteomic biomarker discovery analysis is still early in this process and will benefit from these technologies to detect, identify, and specifically quantify protein markers. The biological amplification of protein signals through the immune system may also claim autoantibodies as potential biomarkers. The development of immunoaffinity assays to validate candidate biomarkers is required. Finally, a major challenge is the need for extensive validation in using these novel global proteomics research platforms prior to routine clinical applications.

REFERENCES

1. Jemal A, Siegel R, Ward E, et al. Cancer statistics, 2008. *CA Cancer J Clin* 2008;58:71–96.
2. Wilkins MR, Appel RD, Van Eyk JE, et al. Guidelines for the next 10 years of proteomics. *Proteomics* 2006;6:4–8.
3. Rikova K, Guo A, Zeng Q, et al. Global survey of phosphotyrosine signaling identifies oncogenic kinases in lung cancer. *Cell* 2007;131:1190–1203.
4. Syka JE, Coon JJ, Schroeder MJ, et al. Peptide and protein sequence analysis by electron transfer dissociation mass spectrometry. *Proc Natl Acad Sci U S A* 2004;101:9528–9533.
5. Ludwig JA, Weinstein JN. Biomarkers in cancer staging, prognosis and treatment selection. *Nat Rev Cancer* 2005;5:845–856.

6. Sidransky D, Irizarry R, Califano JA, et al. Serum protein maldi profiling to distinguish upper aerodigestive tract cancer patients from control subjects. *J Natl Cancer Inst* 2003;95:1711–1717.
7. Villanueva J, Philip J, Entenberg D, et al. Serum peptide profiling by magnetic particle-assisted, automated sample processing and maldi-tof mass spectrometry. *Anal Chem* 2004;76:1560–1570.
8. Zimmerman LJ, Wernke GR, Caprioli RM, et al. Identification of protein fragments as pattern features in maldi-ms analyses of serum. *J Proteome Res* 2005;4(5):1672–1680.
9. Mobley JA, Lam YW, Lau KM, et al. Monitoring the serological proteome: The latest modality in prostate cancer detection. *J Urol* 2004; 172:331–337.
10. Yildiz PB, Shyr Y, Rahman JS, et al. Diagnostic accuracy of maldi mass spectrometric analysis of unfractionated serum in lung cancer. *J Thorac Oncol* 2007;2:893–901.
11. M'Koma AE, Blum DL, Norris JL, et al. Detection of pre-neoplastic and neoplastic prostate disease by maldi profiling of urine. *Biochem Biophys Res Commun* 2007;353:829–834.
12. Rahman SM, Shyr Y, Yildiz PB, et al. Proteomic patterns of preinvasive bronchial lesions. *Am J Respir Crit Care Med* 2005;172:1556–1562.
13. Yanagisawa K, Xu BJ, Carbone DP, et al. Molecular fingerprinting in human lung cancer. *Clin Lung Cancer* 2003;5:113–118.
14. Amann JM, Chaurand P, Gonzalez A, et al. Selective profiling of proteins in lung cancer cells from fine-needle aspirates by matrix-assisted laser desorption ionization time-of-flight mass spectrometry. *Clin Cancer Res* 2006;12:5142–5150.
15. Xu BJ, Caprioli RM, Sanders ME, et al. Direct analysis of laser capture microdissected cells by maldi mass spectrometry. *J Am Soc Mass Spectrom* 2002;13:1292–1297.
16. Anderson NL, Anderson NG. The human plasma proteome: history, character, and diagnostic prospects. *Mol Cell Proteomics* 2002;1:845–867.
17. Paik S, Shak S, Tang G, et al. A multigene assay to predict recurrence of tamoxifen-treated, node-negative breast cancer. *N Engl J Med* 2004;351:2817–2826.
18. van de Vijver MJ, He YD, van't Veer LJ, et al. A gene-expression signature as a predictor of survival in breast cancer. *N Engl J Med* 2002; 347:1999–2009.
19. Zhu H, Snyder M. Protein arrays and microarrays. *Curr Opin Chem Biol* 2001;5:40–45.
20. Madoz-Gurpide J, Wang H, Misek DE, et al. Protein based microarrays: a tool for probing the proteome of cancer cells and tissues. *Proteomics* 2001;1:1279–1287.
21. Zhong L, Hidalgo GE, Stromberg AJ, et al. Using protein microarray as a diagnostic assay for non-small cell lung cancer. *Am J Respir Crit Care Med* 2005;172:1308–1314.
22. Paweletz CP, Charboneau L, Bichsel VE, et al. Reverse phase protein microarrays which capture disease progression show activation of pro-survival pathways at the cancer invasion front. *Oncogene* 2001;20: 1981–1989.
23. Bjorling E, Lindskog C, Oksvold P, et al. A web-based tool for in silico biomarker discovery based on tissue-specific protein profiles in normal and cancer tissues. *Mol Cell Proteomics* 2008;7:825–844.
24. Omenn GS. Strategies for plasma proteomic profiling of cancers. *Proteomics* 2006;6:5662–5673.
25. Anderson NL, Polanski M, Pieper R, et al. The human plasma proteome: A nonredundant list developed by combination of four separate sources. *Mol Cell Proteomics* 2004;3:311–326.
26. Keshishian H, Addona T, Burgess M, et al. Quantitative, multiplexed assays for low abundance proteins in plasma by targeted mass spectrometry and stable isotope dilution. *Mol Cell Proteomics* 2007;6: 2212–2229.
27. Stahl-Zeng J, Lange V, Ossola R, et al. High sensitivity detection of plasma proteins by multiple reaction monitoring of n-glycosites. *Mol Cell Proteomics* 2007;6:1809–1817.
28. Anderson L, Hunter CL. Quantitative mass spectrometric multiple reaction monitoring assays for major plasma proteins. *Mol Cell Proteomics* 2006;5:573–588.
29. Yates JR III, Gilchrist A, Howell KE, et al. Proteomics of organelles and large cellular structures. *Nat Rev Mol Cell Biol* 2005;6:702–714.
30. Forner F, Foster LJ, Campanaro S, et al. Quantitative proteomic comparison of rat mitochondria from muscle, heart, and liver. *Mol Cell Proteomics* 2006;5:608–619.
31. Omenn GS, States DJ, Adamski M, et al. Overview of the hupo plasma proteome project: results from the pilot phase with 35 collaborating laboratories and multiple analytical groups, generating a core dataset of 3020 proteins and a publicly-available database. *Proteomics* 2005;5:3226–3245.
32. Peng J, Elias JE, Thoreen CC, et al. Evaluation of multidimensional chromatography coupled with tandem mass spectrometry (lc/lc-ms/ms) for large-scale protein analysis: the yeast proteome. *J Proteome Res* 2003;2:43–50.
33. Yi EC, Marelli M, Lee H, et al. Approaching complete peroxisome characterization by gas-phase fractionation. *Electrophoresis* 2002;23: 3205–3216.
34. Blonder J, Yu LR, Radeva G, et al. Combined chemical and enzymatic stable isotope labeling for quantitative profiling of detergent-insoluble membrane proteins isolated using triton x-100 and brij-96. *J Proteome Res* 2006;5:349–360.
35. Tian Q, Stepaniants SB, Mao M, et al. Integrated genomic and proteomic analyses of gene expression in mammalian cells. *Mol Cell Proteomics* 2004;3:960–969.
36. Yan W, Lee H, Deutsch EW, et al. A dataset of human liver proteins identified by protein profiling via isotope-coded affinity tag (icat) and tandem mass spectrometry. *Mol Cell Proteomics* 2004;3:1039–1041.
37. Brand M, Ranish JA, Kummer NT, et al. Dynamic changes in transcription factor complexes during erythroid differentiation revealed by quantitative proteomics. *Nat Struct Mol Biol* 2004;11:73–80.
38. Old WM, Meyer-Arendt K, Aveline-Wolf L, et al. Comparison of label-free methods for quantifying human proteins by shotgun proteomics. *Mol Cell Proteomics* 2005;4:1487–1502.
39. Ono M, Shitashige M, Honda K, et al. Label-free quantitative proteomics using large peptide data sets generated by nano-flow liquid chromatography and mass spectrometry. *Mol Cell Proteomics* 2006;5:1338–1347.
40. Yanagisawa K, Shyr Y, Xu BJ, et al. Proteomic patterns of tumour subsets in non–small-cell lung cancer. *Lancet* 2003;362:433–439.
41. Yamagata N, Shyr Y, Yanagisawa K, et al. A training-testing approach to the molecular classification of resected non-small cell lung cancer. *Clin Cancer Res* 2003;9:4695–4704.
42. Tukey JW. Tightening the clinical trial. *Control Clin Trials* 1993;14: 266–285.
43. Shyr Y, Kim K. Weighted flexible compound covariate method for classifying microarray data. In: Berrar D, ed. *A Practical Approach to Microarray Data Analysis*. New York: Kluwer Academic, 2003:186–200.
44. Hedenfalk I, Duggan D, Chen Y, et al. Gene-expression profiles in hereditary breast cancer. *N Engl J Med* 2001;344:539–548.
45. Wardwell NR, Massion PP. Novel strategies for the early detection and prevention of lung cancer. *Semin Oncol* 2005;32:259–268.
46. Sullivan PM, Etzioni R, Feng Z, et al. Phases of biomarker development for early detection of cancer. *J Natl Cancer Inst* 2001;93:1054–1061.
47. Chanin TD, Merrick DT, Franklin WA, et al. Recent developments in biomarkers for the early detection of lung cancer: perspectives based on publications 2003 to present. *Curr Opin Pulm Med* 2004;10:242–247.
48. Chen G, Gharib TG, Huang CC, et al. Proteomic analysis of lung adenocarcinoma: Identification of a highly expressed set of proteins in tumors. *Clin Cancer Res* 2002;8:2298–2305.
49. Adam BL, Qu Y, Davis JW, et al. Serum protein fingerprinting coupled with a pattern-matching algorithm distinguishes prostate cancer from benign prostate hyperplasia and healthy men. *Cancer Res* 2002;62: 3609–3614.
50. Petricoin EF, Ardekani AM, Hitt BA, et al. Use of proteomic patterns in serum to identify ovarian cancer. *Lancet* 2002;359:572–577.
51. Petricoin EF, 3rd, Ornstein DK, Paweletz CP, et al. Serum proteomic patterns for detection of prostate cancer. *J Natl Cancer Inst* 2002;94: 1576–1578.

52. Yang SY, Xiao XY, Zhang WG, et al. Application of serum seldi proteomic patterns in diagnosis of lung cancer. *BMC Cancer* 2005;5:83.
53. Baggerly KA, Morris JS, Coombes KR. Reproducibility of seldi-tof protein patterns in serum: Comparing datasets from different experiments. *Bioinformatics* 2004;20:777–785.
54. Baggerly KA, Morris JS, Edmonson SR, et al. Signal in noise: evaluating reported reproducibility of serum proteomic tests for ovarian cancer. *J Natl Cancer Inst* 2005;97:307–309.
55. Coombes KR, Morris JS, Hu J, et al. Serum proteomics profiling—a young technology begins to mature. *Nat Biotechnol* 2005;23:291–292.
56. Koomen JM, Li D, Xiao LC, et al. Direct tandem mass spectrometry reveals limitations in protein profiling experiments for plasma biomarker discovery. *J Proteome Res* 2005;4:972–981.
57. Marshall J, Kupchak P, Zhu W, et al. Processing of serum proteins underlies the mass spectral fingerprinting of myocardial infarction. *J Proteome Res* 2003;2:361–372.
58. Howard BA, Wang MZ, Campa MJ, et al. Identification and validation of a potential lung cancer serum biomarker detected by matrix-assisted laser desorption/ionization-time of flight spectra analysis. *Proteomics* 2003;3:1720–1724.
59. Villanueva J, Shaffer DR, Philip J, et al. Differential exoprotease activities confer tumor-specific serum peptidome patterns. *J Clin Invest* 2006;116:271–284.
60. Gharib TG, Chen G, Wang H, et al. Proteomic analysis of cytokeratin isoforms uncovers association with survival in lung adenocarcinoma. *Neoplasia* 2002;4:440–448.
61. Chen G, Wang H, Miller CT, et al. Reduced selenium-binding protein 1 expression is associated with poor outcome in lung adenocarcinomas. *J Pathol* 2004;202:321–329.
62. Li C, Xiao Z, Chen Z, et al. Proteome analysis of human lung squamous carcinoma. *Proteomics* 2006;6:547–558.
63. Moon EY, Song JH, Yang KH. Actin-sequestering protein, thymosin-beta-4 (tb4), inhibits caspase-3 activation in paclitaxel-induced tumor cell death. *Oncol Res* 2007;16:507–516.
64. Oh JM, Ryoo IJ, Yang Y, et al. Hypoxia-inducible transcription factor (hif)-1 alpha stabilization by actin-sequestering protein, thymosin beta-4 (tb4) in hela cervical tumor cells. *Cancer Lett* 2008;264:29–35.
65. Brieger A, Plotz G, Zeuzem S, et al. Thymosin beta 4 expression and nuclear transport are regulated by hmlh1. *Biochem Biophys Res Commun* 2007;364:731–736.
66. Anderson DD, Woeller CF, Stover PJ. Small ubiquitin-like modifier-1 (sumo-1) modification of thymidylate synthase and dihydrofolate reductase. *Clin Chem Lab Med* 2007;45:1760–1763.
67. Chung V, Zhou B, Liu X, et al. Sumoylation plays a role in gemcitabine- and bortezomib-induced cytotoxicity in human oropharyngeal carcinoma kb gemcitabine-resistant clone. *Mol Cancer Ther* 2006;5: 533–540.
68. Kang JS, Saunier EF, Akhurst RJ, et al. The type i tgf-beta receptor is covalently modified and regulated by sumoylation. *Nat Cell Biol* 2008; 10:654–664.
69. Miyazono K, Kamiya Y, Miyazawa K. Sumo amplifies tgf-beta signalling. *Nat Cell Biol* 2008;10:635–637.
70. Seeler JS, Bischof O, Nacerddine K, et al. Sumo, the three rs and cancer. *Curr Top Microbiol Immunol* 2007;313:49–71.
71. Yanagisawa K, Tomida S, Shimada Y, et al. A 25-signal proteomic signature and outcome for patients with resected non-small-cell lung cancer. *J Natl Cancer Inst* 2007;99:858–867.
72. Jacot W, Lhermitte L, Dossat N, et al. Serum proteomic profiling of lung cancer in high-risk groups and determination of clinical outcomes. *J Thorac Oncol* 2008;3:840–850.
73. Maeda J, Hirano T, Ogiwara A, et al. Proteomic analysis of stage I primary lung adenocarcinoma aimed at individualisation of postoperative therapy. *Br J Cancer* 2008;98:596–603.
74. Fujii T, Toyooka S, Ichimura K, et al. Ercc1 protein expression predicts the response of cisplatin-based neoadjuvant chemotherapy in non-small-cell lung cancer. *Lung Cancer* 2008;59:377–384.
75. Scagliotti GV, Parikh P, von Pawel J, et al. Phase iii study comparing cisplatin plus gemcitabine with cisplatin plus pemetrexed in chemotherapy-naive patients with advanced-stage non-small-cell lung cancer. *J Clin Oncol* 2008;26:3543–3551.
76. Dowlati A, Gray R, Sandler AB, et al. Cell adhesion molecules, vascular endothelial growth factor, and basic fibroblast growth factor in patients with non-small cell lung cancer treated with chemotherapy with or without bevacizumab—an eastern cooperative oncology group study. *Clin Cancer Res* 2008;14:1407–1412.
77. Norden-Zfoni A, Desai J, Manola J, et al. Blood-based biomarkers of su11248 activity and clinical outcome in patients with metastatic imatinib-resistant gastrointestinal stromal tumor. *Clin Cancer Res* 2007;13: 2643–2650.
78. Tran HT, Kim ES, Lee JJ, et al. Correlation between plasma cytokine/angiogenic factors (c/af) and signaling pathways activation from baseline tumor biopsy specimens in patients with advanced non small cell lung cancer (nsclc): preliminary analysis from the biomarker-based approaches of targeted therapy for lung cancer elimination (battle) clinical study. *2008 ASCO Annual Meeting*. Chicago, IL, 2008. abstract 8010.
79. Grote T, Siwak DR, Fritsche HA, et al. Validation of reverse phase protein array for practical screening of potential biomarkers in serum and plasma: accurate detection of ca19-9 levels in pancreatic cancer. *Proteomics* 2008;8:3051–3060.
80. Murphy L, Clynes M, Keenan J. Proteomic analysis to dissect mitoxantrone resistance-associated proteins in a squamous lung carcinoma. *Anticancer Res* 2007;27:1277–1284.
81. Murphy L, Henry M, Meleady P, et al. Proteomic investigation of taxol and taxotere resistance and invasiveness in a squamous lung carcinoma cell line. *Biochim Biophys Acta* 2008;1784(9):1184–1191.
82. Chen G, Li A, Zhao M, et al. Proteomic analysis identifies protein targets responsible for depsipeptide sensitivity in tumor cells. *J Proteome Res* 2008;7:2733–2742.
83. Okano T, Kondo T, Fujii K, et al. Proteomic signature corresponding to the response to gefitinib (iressa, zd1839), an epidermal growth factor receptor tyrosine kinase inhibitor in lung adenocarcinoma. *Clin Cancer Res* 2007;13:799–805.
84. Taguchi F, Solomon B, Gregorc V, et al. Mass spectrometry to classify non-small-cell lung cancer patients for clinical outcome after treatment with epidermal growth factor receptor tyrosine kinase inhibitors: a multicohort cross-institutional study. *J Natl Cancer Inst* 2007;99: 838–846.

CHAPTER 10

Betty C. Tong
David H. Harpole, Jr.

Molecular Prognostication of Lung Cancer

At present, the best prognostic indicator of long-term survival for patients with lung cancer is tumor stage. The recent proposed revisions to the *TNM Classification of Malignant Tumours* by the International Association for the Study of Lung Cancer (IASLC) are an analysis of 67,725 cases of non–small cell lung cancer (NSCLC) to further refine the prognostic accuracy of tumor staging (see Chapter 30).[1] Regrettably, however, up to 30% of patients who undergo curative resection for stage I lung cancer will have recurrence of their disease. Present conventional wisdom is that the long-term survival in many cancers may be increased if clinicians had the means to identify and treat patients who would benefit from adjuvant therapy that might not otherwise be indicated based on their initial tumor stage. To this end, many investigators have examined molecular and genetic factors that may influence tumor behavior and therefore long-term prognosis.

A number of genetic alterations and abnormal expression of several regulatory genes have been detected and described for lung cancer. These alterations are caused by gene mutation, chromosomal modification, epigenetic silencing, and deregulated messenger RNA (mRNA). In addition, several studies have correlated specific molecular genetic changes with clinical prognosis and survival for patients with lung cancer. Currently, several clinical trials are underway to further define patients' molecular "signatures" in an effort to predict both overall prognosis as well as response to therapy for lung cancer (http://www.clinicaltrials.gov).

Early studies attemping to comment on prognostic variables in lung cancer are summarized in a comprehensive and systematic review of 887 studies, which identified 169 host- and tumor-related molecular factors associated with prognosis in lung cancer.[2] Several factors were significantly associated with survival, independent of stage and reported in more than three studies: p53, p21, Ki-67, and p185 gene status; serum cytokeratin 19 fragments; agryophilic nucleolar organizer region; and markers of angiogenesis such as vascular endothelial growth factor (VEGF) expression and vessel invasion. Other studies have used molecular, immunohistochemical, and clinical–pathologic markers to predict patient prognosis and outcomes.[3–5]

The subsequent development of oligonucleotide and complementary DNA (cDNA) arrays to analyze gene expression on a larger scale has contributed significantly to the understanding of molecular and genetic alterations in lung cancer. These tools allow for the simultaneous analysis of literally thousands of genes such that a genetic profile or signature can be constructed for a particular patient or tumor. In addition to genetic profiling, investigators have identified several proteomic (see Chapter 9) and microRNA (miRNA) profiles for lung tumors. These profiles are correlated to clinical behavior, thereby providing prognostic information for patients with lung cancer.

INDIVIDUAL GENE ALTERATIONS AND PATIENT SURVIVAL

K-ras Members of the *ras* gene family encode cell membrane-associated G-proteins, which serve as mediators of signal transduction for cellular proliferation (also reviewed in Chapter 5). Up to 30% of NSCLCs are characterized by mutations in the *k-ras* gene[6,7]; most of these mutations are found in adenocarcinomas and are associated with a history of tobacco use.[8] The most common mutation of *k-ras* is a G→T transversion in codon 12 that results in constitutive activation and continuous transmission of growth signals to the nucleus. Alterations in *k-ras* appear to be early events in lung carcinogenesis, having been observed in atypical alveolar hyperplasia lesions that are thought by many to be precursors of lung adenocarcinomas.[9] The prognostic significance of *k-ras* mutations in lung cancer remains controversial. Although many studies report an association between decreased survival and worse prognosis in patients whose tumors exhibit *k-ras* mutations, others, including a metaanalysis of 881 cases, report no significant link between ras mutation status and prognosis.[10–13]

p53 The p53 tumor suppressor gene is mutated in more than half of all human malignancies, and alterations in the p53 gene are the most frequently found in human cancer (also reviewed in Chapter 5). Approximately 50% of NSCLCs and over 90% of small cell lung cancers (SCLC) harbor mutations or deletions of the p53 gene.[10,14] Inactivation of p53 results in diminished efficiency of DNA repair, derangements of cell cycle regulation, and overall increased genomic instability.[15] In the normal state, the p53 network is quiet and senescent. In times of cellular injury or stress, however, the p53 network is activated and its downstream effects include cell cycle regulation, induction of apoptosis and DNA repair mechanisms.

A prospective study by Ahrendt et al.[16] demonstrated that p53 gene mutations were independently predictive of decreased survival in stage I tumors but not in stage II or III tumors. Missense mutations were not significant for patient outcome. However, p53 mutations that were truncating, structural, or those abolishing DNA contact were associated with a poorer overall patient outcome among all samples. The relationship between p53 mutational status and adverse survival outcomes has been corroborated by several other studies incorporating NSCLC samples from all tumor stages.[17–25]

Immunohistochemical studies of p53 have been less consistent. In the largest studies examining p53 expression levels, some authors have reported a correlation between abnormal p53 expression and poor prognosis; however, others report no statistically significant relationship.[3,26–33] Carbognani et al.[34] examined the role of p53 status in long-term survival following resection of NSCLC. Using immunohistochemical analysis of several prognostic markers, p53 status was the only independent predictor of 10-year survival following resection of adenocarcinoma. In another study, Tsao et al.[13] observed that p53 protein overexpression was a marker of poor prognosis and shorter overall survival. In addition, patients with tumors containing wild-type p53 had a survival benefit from adjuvant chemotherapy as compared to those with functionally aberrant p53 status. Despite the mixed evidence from immunohistochemical studies, however, a metaanalysis of 56 studies was conducted to further investigate the role of p53 alterations and lung cancer.[35] Abnormal p53 status was associated with decreased overall survival in patients with NSCLC across all stages and in both squamous cell and adenocarcinoma histologies.

Cell Cycle Regulation

Rb and p16 The retinoblastoma (*Rb*) susceptibility gene is a tumor suppressor gene with a key role in human carcinogenesis (also reviewed in Chapter 5). The *Rb* gene is inactivated in 20% to 30% of NSCLCs and up to 90% of SCLC.[10] Despite this, the effect of *Rb* mutation or abnormal expression on patient prognosis is controversial, with most studies demonstrating no significant relationship between *Rb* abnormalities and survival.[27,36–38]

However, Burke et al.[39] recently demonstrated that the additive effect of concurrent abnormalities in either or both of the *Rb* and p53 pathways was predictive of patient prognosis in NSCLC. In this study, there was no association between patient survival and isolated abnormalities of the Rb pathway proteins pRb, cyclin D1, and p16^{INK4A} and p53 pathway proteins p53 and p21^{Waf1}. However, certain combinations of abnormalities were predictive of poor prognosis. These included concurrent pRb negative status and cyclin D1 overexpression; concurrent pRb negative, cyclin D1 overexpression, and p53 mutation; concurrent cyclin D1 overexpression and p53 mutation.

The p16^{INK4A} gene, located on chromosome 9p21, is a tumor suppressor gene that encodes a cyclin-dependent kinase (CDK) inhibitor (see also Chapter 14). Normally, p16 binds to the cyclin D/CDK4/6 complexes to inhibit phosphorylation of the Rb protein, thereby inhibiting G1→S progression. In a recent analysis of tumors from patients with histologically proven N2 NSCLCs, the immunohistologic presence of both p16 and p21 protein correlated with improved long-term survival.[40]

Similarly, dysfunctional or absent p16 expression can result in unchecked progression through the cell cycle. p16 plays a prominent role in NSCLC; inactivation is present in 40% to 70% of NSCLCs. Mechanisms of p16 inactivation include point mutations or deletions in coding regions, as well as epigenetic silencing by hypermethylation of the gene promoter cytosine-guanine-phosphate (CpG) island. Alteration and inactivation of p16 are associated with a number of clinical correlates in NSCLC, including metastases, poor prognosis and overall decreased survival.[41–44]

The cyclins, p21$^{WAF1/CIP1}$, and p27 Other cell cycle regulatory genes of interest include cyclin D1, cyclin E, cyclin B1, p21$^{WAF1/CIP1}$, and p27. Cyclin D1 plays a role in cell cycle regulation by allowing transition from G1 to S phase. Although overexpression of cyclin D1 occurs in 25% to 47% of NSCLC, its prognostic effects are somewhat controversial. In some studies, overexpression has been correlated with the presence of lymph node metastasis, advanced pathologic stage, and shorter overall survival.[38,45] However, other investigators have reported favorable outcomes associated overexpression of cyclin D1.[5,46]

Cyclin E helps to regulate entry into the S phase of the cell cycle by formation of a complex with CDK2 and subsequent phosphorylation of pRb. High levels of cyclin E expression in NSCLC are found in up to 53% of NSCLCs, and have been correlated with tumor invasion, unfavorable prognosis, and decreased patient survival.[47,48] The cyclin B1/CDC2 complex regulates the G2-M phase checkpoint of the cell cycle. In early stage NSCLCs, overexpression of cyclin B1 occurs more commonly in tumors of squamous histology, and high levels of expression have been linked to shorter survival.[49]

p21 and p27 belong to the Cip/Kip family of CDK inhibitors, which bind to and inactivate CDKs in times of cellular stress, hypoxia, DNA damage, and in response to growth inhibitory signals (also reviewed in Chapters 5 and 14). p21$^{WAF1/CIP1}$ can inhibit cell cycle progression at multiple sites. Early in G1, p21$^{WAF1/CIP1}$ binds to the cyclin D/CDK4 and cyclin E/CDK2 complexes. Prior to transition from S phase to G2, p21$^{WAF1/CIP1}$ can inhibit the cyclin A/CDK2 complex. Although some authors determined that p21 expression was associated with improved survival, others found no relationship.[50–52] p27^{Kip1} interacts with both cyclin D1 and cyclin E to regulate the cell cycle. Several studies have employed immunohistochemical techniques to determine p27 expression; decreased levels of p27 expression have been uniformly correlated with poor prognosis in NSCLC.[53–55]

Protein Kinases

EGFR The epidermal growth factor receptor (EGFR) family (also reviewed in Chapters 5 and 49) includes a group of tyrosine kinases whose activation results in a cascade of downstream signals that ultimately enhance cellular proliferation, tumor cell motility and angiogenesis, and decrease apoptosis.[56] Although EGFR is overexpressed in many epithelial cancers, including 40% to 80% of all NSCLCs, these aberrations are rare in SCLC.[57] Downstream targets of EGFR activation include the *ras* and *raf* pathways that directly regulate gene transcription and cellular proliferation. Another gene targeted by EGFR activation is the serine threonine kinase *Akt*, which acts as a key regulator of cellular survival through suppression of apoptosis.[58]

EGFR mutations in lung cancer are associated with nonsmokers, women, patients from East Asian countries, adenocarcinoma histology, and, specifically, bronchoalveolar subtype.[59–63] In addition, tumors with *k-ras* mutations (associated with tobacco exposure) and those with EGFR mutations appear to be mutually exclusive.[60,63] It was initially thought that EGFR tyrosine kinase inhibitors such as erlotinib and gefitinib might revolutionize the treatment of patients with overexpression of EGFR in NSCLC. However, clinical studies have demonstrated significant responses in only specific subsets of patients, limiting gefitinib to use as a second- or third-line agent and erlotinib as a first-line agent specifically for elderly patients and those with EGFR mutations.[64,65]

The impact of EGFR mutation and overexpression on lymph node metastasis, patient prognosis, and overall survival is controversial. Gene amplification often occurs with EGFR overexpression (as opposed to transcriptional or translational modification), and this has been associated with lymph node metastasis and advanced pathologic stage.[66] Although many have found that EGFR mutation and overexpression correlates with worse survival in NSCLC, other studies report no significant association between the two.[59,63] A recent metaanalysis of 16 studies found that immunohistologic expression of EGFR does not correlate with overall prognosis in patients with NSCLC.[67]

ErbB2/HER-2/neu Another member of the protein kinase gene family is *ErbB2/Her2/neu*. Screening studies for mutations in the kinase domain of *ErbB2/Her2/neu* in NSCLCs have revealed that mutations in squamous cell carcinomas are rare, but found in approximately 10% to 30% of adenocarcinomas.[68–70] As with mutations of EGFR, mutations of *ErbB2/Her2/neu* are more common in nonsmokers than in smokers.[63] *ErbB2/Her2/neu* overexpression has been associated with early tumor recurrence, chemotherapeutic drug resistance, poorer prognosis, and overall shorter survival time.[71–74]

Angiogenesis and Growth Factors

(see also Chapters 8 and 48) For tumors to grow, they must obtain oxygen and nutrients. Tumors greater than ~1 mm in size cannot depend on simple diffusion and therefore must create a vascular supply to meet these metabolic demands. VEGF is a potent growth factor for endothelial cells, promoting angiogenesis by increasing vascular permeability and stimulating endothelial cell proliferation. The VEGF receptors, VEGFR-1, -2, and -3, are tyrosine kinases. VEGF expression has been demonstrated in NSCLCs and is stimulated by tissue hypoxia, other growth factors, and cytokines.[75,76]

The presence of VEGF in NSCLC tumors of all stages has been uniformly correlated with poorer prognosis and impaired survival.[77] Bevacizumab (Avastin) is a humanized monoclonal antibody that binds to circulating VEGF and inhibits its interaction with the VEGF receptors. The Eastern Cooperative Oncology Group (ECOG) phase III trial E4599 demonstrated an overall survival benefit for patients with advanced stage adenocarcinoma who received bevacizumab in addition to paclitaxel and carboplatin.[78] Another phase III trial, the European AVAstin in Lung cancer (AVAiL) trial, demonstrated a favorable progression-free survival for patients with nonsquamous NSCLC receiving bevacizumab in addition to cisplantin and gemcitabine.[79] In addition to other studies of bevacizumab in NSCLC, several multitargeted tyrosine kinase inhibitors are under clinical investigation. Targets of interest include several VEGF receptors, EGFR, platelet-derived growth factor (PDGF), raf, and kit.

Interleukin-8 (IL-8) also has angiogenic properties in NSCLC.[80] IL-8 expression in tumors has been correlated not only with angiogenesis and microvessel density, but also with advanced stage, lymph node metastasis and overall patient prognosis.[81] Other growth factors of interest include PDGF and basic fibroblast growth factor (bFGF). PDGF increases DNA synthesis, tumor growth, and endothelial cell migration; it has been correlated with decreased 5-year survival for patients with resected primary lung adenocarcinomas.[77,82] FGF2 stimulates tumor growth and angiogenesis, and in vitro studies have established a synergistic effect of FGF2 and PDGF.[83]

The Matrix Metalloproteinase Family

The matrix metalloproteinase (MMP) family is a group of proteolytic enzymes associated with degradation of extracellular matrix and penetration of basement membranes, two key elements in the metastasis of tumors. MMP-2 (also known as gelatinase A) has been associated with lymphatic and vascular invasion of NSCLC.[84] Overexpression of MMP-2, as measured by immunohistochemical analysis, has been identified as a negative prognostic factor in lung cancer survival.[85] Similarly, differential levels of MMP-7 expression were found between resected squamous cell carcinomas and adenocarcinomas, with higher levels in the squamous cell carcinomas.[86] MMP-7-positive status was significantly associated with poor prognosis and shorter overall survival. In contrast, the data regarding MMP-9 are controversial. Although some studies suggest a negative prognostic influence of MMP-9, others have found no significant relationship between the two.[87–89]

Recently, Sienel et al.[90] described a role for the extracellular matrix metalloproteinase inducer (EMMPRIN) in determining prognosis for lung adenocarcinoma. EMMPRIN is a transmembrane glycoprotein that has been shown to stimulate synthesis of several MMPs, including MMP-1, -2, -3, and -9. EMMPRIN expression was determined in a cohort of NSCLCs using immunohistochemical staining, and a score was assigned to each specimen. Furthermore, investigators recorded either a membranous or cytoplasmic pattern of staining. For patients with adenocarcinoma, a membranous staining pattern was independently associated with poor prognosis, defined as either local recurrence or distant metastasis. These relationships were not significant for other histologic subtypes.

Maspin is a member of the serpin (serine protease inhibitor) family and has been shown to be a suppressor of tumor growth and metastasis in several types of tumors. Maspin can inhibit invasion and metastasis of malignancies, although direct evidence of the clinicopathologic significance of cytoplasmic relative to nuclear expression is limited. Cytoplasmic and nuclear expression patterns of maspin are involved in the cellular differentiation of normal lung tissue and the histogenesis of different lung carcinomas. The cytoplasmic maspin may play an important role in lung carcinomas by regulating apoptosis and thus is a favorable prognostic marker for AD patients, whereas the nuclear location may be linked to promotion of angiogenesis. Immunohistochemistry reveals that maspin expression is virtually universal in NSCLC, but squamous cell carcinoma show almost exclusively a combined nuclear-cytosolic stain. In contrast, nuclear maspin, but not combined nuclear-cytoplasmic maspin, significantly correlates with low histological grade, lower proliferative rate, absence of invasion, and negative p53 stain in ACa. Nuclear localization of maspin may thus stratify subtypes of NSCLC with favorable clinical–pathological features.[91–95]

GENE EXPRESSION ARRAYS

The development of gene expression microarrays has enabled investigators to move beyond analysis of single genes and not only explore patterns or profiles of gene expression in tissues but also compare these patterns between tissue types. These gene expression profiles have been shown to be consistent between institutions, with good comparability of sample characteristics.[96,97] Examining the expression profiles of tumors allows for novel identification of genes previously not associated with malignancy. In addition, comparing expression profiles between groups of patients has enabled investigators to perform molecular phenotyping and classification of tumors. Unique and characteristic profiles have been identified not only for the histologic types of NSCLC, but also for subgroups within these histologic classes.[98–101]

There are other potential uses for data acquired from microarray-derived gene expression profiles. Correlating these profiles with defined tumor behavior may help to elucidate specific processes or pathways involved in carcinogenesis. For example, profiling invasive and metastatic tumors may reveal novel genes or pathways of interest that could subsequently be targeted for anticancer therapeutics. Also, these methods may be used to investigate a tumor's response (or nonresponse) to therapy, elucidating possible mechanisms of drug resistance and providing a basis for predicting future clinical behavior (see Chapter 47).

Gene expression profiles have also been used to refine and predict prognosis and survival among patients with identical TNM staging but differing clinical outcome,[102,103] and is the focus of this chapter. Other uses include identification of novel biomarkers associated with and specific to lung tissue and/or NSCLC.[104] In the current era of molecular therapeutics, there is potential to use these gene expression profiles and biomarkers not only to classify tumors with molecular staging techniques, but also to identify targets for therapy and treatment. As these techniques continue to develop, it is possible that lung cancer staging, and therefore treatment, will depend not only on TNM status but also on the genetic profiles generated by these methods.

Lung Cancer Heterogeneity Clinically, lung cancer is classified as small cell (SCLC) and non–small cell (NSCLC), with NSCLC accounting for approximately 80% of all lung cancers. Within each histologic subtype, there is significant heterogeneity such that NSCLCs are further classified as adenocarcinoma, squamous cell carcinoma, large cell carcinoma, and neuroendocrine carcinoma as well as tumors with mixed histology such as adenosquamous tumors.[105] Among adenocarcinomas, further variation is present in acinar, papillary, bronchoalveolar carcinoma (BAC), and mucinous carcinoma subtypes. For example, BAC appears to arise from type II pneumocytes and is generally associated with better prognosis compared with invasive adenocarcinomas.[106]

The heterogeneity among primary lung tumor subtypes likely reflects the potential cell derivation, and these differences may be further increased by the diverse genetic alterations observed in lung cancers.[107–110] Additional tumor heterogeneity may be a result of alterations in gene expression that affect diverse processes such as proliferation, apoptosis, and cellular differentiation, among others.[111,112] To this end, gene expression profiling methods have been employed to better understand this heterogeneity and to identify specific pathways or genes that might distinguish tumors of different cellular origin or clinical behavior.

One of the first studies of gene profiling for lung cancer was performed by Petersen et al.[113] Comparing a metastatic lung adenocarcinoma with human small airway epithelial cells, cDNA libraries of upregulated and downregulated genes were constructed. DNA sequencing of over 500 clones revealed 315 unknown and 205 known cDNA fragments. Gene expression analysis of 167 of these clones was performed using northern blot techniques, confirming differential expression in 58% of the clones. In addition, an expression pattern similar to that of the metastatic adenocarcinoma was observed in lung cancer cell lines. No primary lung tumors were examined in this study.

Garber et al.[114] performed a more global analysis of gene expression using 23,100 element cDNA arrays and 12,600 transcript containing oligonucleotide arrays. Samples in this study included 41 adenocarcinomas, 16 squamous cell carcinomas, 5 large cell carcinomas, and 5 small cell lung tumors. In addition, there were 11 tumors with corresponding lymph node or intrapulmonary metastasis as well as 5 normal lung samples. Hierarchical clustering was performed on a subset of genes representing only 918 of the 23,100 transcripts. These methods distinguished relatively distinct groups of squamous cell, small cell, and large cell carcinomas; in addition, three groups of adenocarcinomas were recognized. These results suggested that the histologic origin of these tumors was reflected in the expression patterns determined by these 918 genes. Furthermore, the authors suggested that the division of adenocarcinomas into three groups reflects tumor heterogeneity within this subgroup of NSCLC and that cumulative patient survival differed between these clusters. It should be noted, however, that clinical factors such as differentiation, grade, or tumor stage were not used in determining the three groups. In addition, most of the paired samples of primary and metastatic tumors demonstrated relatively similar gene expression patterns. Specific genes differentially expressed in the three adenocarcinoma clusters included VEGFc (highly expressed in the poor outcome group) and thyroid transcription factor (highly expressed in the good outcome group). These results are consistent with known information regarding VEGF expression, differentiation status, and prognosis for patients with lung adenocarcinoma.[2,76,99]

Bhattacharjee et al.[99] also utilized gene expression profiling to classify lung tumors into histologic subtypes. Using oligonucleotide arrays, they examined 125 adenocarcinomas, 21 SCCs, 20 carcinoid tumors, 6 SCLC tumors, and 17 normal lung samples. Hierarchical and probabilistic clustering of the 3312 most variably expressed transcripts separated the tumors into distinct clusters, which reflected their histologic subtype. In addition, primary lung tumors were distinguished from adenocarcinomas of colonic origin metastatic to the lung based on their expression profiles.

Specific genes with high expression levels in each histologic group were identified. Marker genes such as TGF-β receptor type II, tetranectin, and ficolin 3 characterized normal lung samples. Both carcinoid tumors and small cell tumors expressed high levels of neuroendocrine genes such as insulinoma-associated gene 1, gastrin-releasing peptide, and chromogranin A. However, few other markers were common between SCLC and carcinoid tumors. For SCLC, high expression of cell proliferation-associated genes such as PCNA, thymidylate synthase, MCM2, and MCM6 was demonstrated. Similarly, carcinoid tumors were defined by a distinct expression profile. A separate clustering of the adenocarcinoma expression profiles defined four subclasses, C1 to C4. Consistent with the Garber et al.[114] study, many of the genes associated with each of the four clusters appeared to reflect tumor differentiation status or stage-related differences. In addition, Kaplan-Meier analysis revealed a significantly worse median overall survival for patients in the C2 subgroup, comprised of tumors with high expression levels of neuroendocrine genes.

Nacht et al.[114a] investigated patterns of gene expression in NSCLC using serial analysis of gene expression (SAGE). Libraries were established from normal human bronchiole epithelial cells, small airway epithelial cells, two squamous cell carcinomas, two adenocarcinomas, and the A549 lung adenocarcinoma cell line. From these samples, 18,300 independent clones were sequenced and 574,634 tags were generated, representing 66,502 distinct transcripts. Adenocarcinomas demonstrated high levels of the CD74 antigen, major histocompatibility complex (MHC) class II, and immunoglobulin (Ig) heavy constant $\gamma 3$, whereas genes highly expressed in squamous cell tumors included glutathione peroxidase 2 (GPX2) and tumor necrosis factor receptor subfamily member 18. Consistent with other studies, high levels of surfactants A and B were observed in adenocarcinoma; however, this likely reflects the differences in the cell type derivation of these tumors.[99,114] Additional investigation was performed on 10 NSCLCs, 4 normal controls and a larger panel of 32 normal lung and lung tumors using both real-time reverse transcription polymerase chain reaction (RT-PCR), and 12,600-element containing (U95) oligonucleotide arrays. Although only a small number of genes were compared by both approaches, 21 of 23 exhibited similar expression patterns as determined by both SAGE and the oligonucleotide-based techniques. Although the basic molecular features of adenocarcinoma and squamous cell carcinoma can be distinguished by gene expression profiling, the authors suggested that the histological and clinical behavior of the tumors may depend on more subtle changes in expression levels for a variety of genes and pathways.

Several studies have used gene expression arrays to determine differences between matched tumor and normal samples. Using differential cDNA library screening, McDoniels-Silvers et al.[115] examined differentially expressed genes between primary lung adenocarcinoma, SCC, and corresponding normal lung tissues. Dot-blot hybridization techniques confirmed that 1163 clones were differentially expressed between the normal and tumor tissues. Using RT-PCR methods, the authors confirmed that 113 genes were differentially expressed between normal and tumor tissues, some of them underexpressed or overexpressed in tumors relative to normal lung, or selectively expressed in adenocarcinoma versus squamous cell carcinoma. With this approach, genes that were highly overexpressed were selected with the greatest frequency. In addition to some genes with unknown functions, the gene identified as highly overexpressed included genes involved in glycolysis, cell respiratory complex, inflammation, and cell adhesion.

Nakamura et al.[116] used 425 element cDNA arrays to examine stage I tumors, including both adenocarcinoma and squamous cell carcinoma, for genes that are differentially expressed between tumors and corresponding noncancerous lung tissue. In the tumor samples, 74 genes were underexpressed and 40 genes were overexpressed when compared to normal controls. Elevated expression of plasminogen activator, MMPs 1, 3, 7, and 10 and keratins 4, 6B, 8, 13, 14, 19, and 20 were observed in the carcinoma group. Conversely, several cell adhesion–related genes including cadherin 5, cadherin 6, protocadherin 2, catenin beta 1, integrin beta 1, and CD31 had decreased expression in the tumor group.

Wikman et al.[117] described the use of arrays containing 1176 genes to compare fourteen lung adenocarcinomas with normal lung tissue as well as lung tissue from four normal references. Two statistical methods, principal component analysis and permutation tests, were used to identify the most differentially expressed genes between the tumors and normal tissues. Three main groups of genes were identified to be dysregulated most frequently: those involved in cell motility and structure, matrix maintenance and degradation, and cell cycle regulation. Genes upregulated in tumors relative to normal samples included known tumor markers such as *topoisomerase 2A (TOP2A), KRT19, KRT8, tenascin, polo-like kinase (PLK) 1,* and *cyclin B1 (CCNB1).* In addition, *MMP11, MMP12,* and tissue inhibitor of metalloproteinase 1 *(TIMP1)* were upregulated in the tumors, whereas *TIMP3* was downregulated. For lung cancer, previous reports have demonstrated high levels of expression of MMP genes, whereas TIMP3 is subject to epigenetic silencing by methylation.[118–120] In addition, the elevated mRNA expression of cytokeratins *(KRT8, 18,* and *19)* was consistent with the gene profiling studies of others.[102,121] Other genes elevated in the adenocarcinoma group included *CCNB1,* macrophage migration inhibitory factor *(MIF),* high-mobility–group protein Y (HMGI) and hepatocyte-derived growth factor *(HDGF).* Genes that were downregulated in the tumors included *SOCS2* and *SOCS3,* caveolins 1 and 2, gravin, and the mitogen-responsive phosphoprotein *DOC2/DAB2.*

Gene Expression Arrays and Prognostication

Several studies have correlated results from gene expression arrays with patient prognosis. In a study of 19 stage I and II adenocarcinomas, Miura et al.[122] used cDNA microarrays to examine tumors from 14 smokers versus 5 nonsmokers; among these patients, 6 were 5-year survivors and 12 died of lung cancer recurrence. Gene expression patterns differed between the smokers and nonsmokers. Several genes exhibiting lower levels of expression in smokers were those located in known regions of genomic imbalance for NSCLC such as chromosome 3p21.3.[123] Other genes with lower expression among smokers were located in chromosomal regions 4q, 11q23–24, 19p, and19q. The authors suggested that inactivation of these genes was related to tobacco carcinogenesis. In addition, tobacco-related carcinoma was associated with high expression levels of RAB4, DJ1, MCT, and ribosomal protein L22. Of the genes examined, 27 genes were differentially expressed between nonsurvivors and survivors. Fourteen genes had high expression levels in nonsurvivors, including anaphase-promoting complex 2 (APC2). In contrast, expression levels of the mitotic spindle checkpoint regulatory genes hBUB3 and hZW10 were lower in tumors from nonsurvivors, highlighting the importance of cell cycle regulation in human carcinogenesis.

Wigle et al.[124] utilized 19,200 element-containing cDNA arrays and examined 39 NSCLCs that showed either cancer recurrence or no recurrence. The cohort included adenocarcinoma and squamous cell carcinoma as well as other histologic subtypes; stage I, II, and III lung cancers were included. Based on unsupervised hierarchical clustering of a subset of 2899 genes, two groups differed significantly in disease-free survival. Genes associated with a more aggressive NSCLC behavior included ataxia telengiectasia mutated (ATM), upregulation of the flt1 VEGF receptor, and phosphoinositide-3-kinase regulatory subunit (*PIK3R2*). Using Cox proportional hazards model testing, investigators determined 22 genes that were significant for disease-free survival.

Beer et al.[102] examined 86 lung adenocarcinomas using oligonucleotide arrays (HuGeneFL) containing 6800 transcripts. Sixty-seven of the samples were stage I tumors, whereas 19 were stage III; 10 samples of normal lung tissue were also examined. Three clusters of tumors were identified using hierarchical clustering and other supervised analytical approaches. Significant relationships were observed between cluster and tumor differentiation as well as cluster and tumor stage. Suggesting that the gene expression profile of some early stage tumors is similar to that of more clinically aggressive tumors, the authors noted that some of the stage I adenocarcinomas clustered with higher stage tumors. To help determine which genes were best related to patient prognosis, a 50-gene "risk index" based on the top 50 survival-related genes was devised. Using this approach, low- and high-risk stage I adenocarcinomas that differed significantly with regard to survival were correctly identified.

The survival-related genes identified in this study were broadly grouped into the following categories: cell cycle and cell signaling related; apoptosis related; transcription and translation; cell adhesion and structure; genes encoding chaperones, receptors, enzymes, and transcription factors; and those with unknown function. Genes of particular interest included VEGF, keratin 7, cathepsin L, and the CRK oncogene. Other lung cancer profiling studies had reported elevated expression of cathepsin L and keratin 7 genes in aggressive tumors.[99,114] In addition, VEGF has been previously identified as being associated with poor prognosis lung cancer.[2,76]

Kikuchi et al.[125] and Inamura et al.[126] identified genes associated with lymph node metastasis among primary lung ADs, and Hoang et al.[127] identified genes associated with nonmetastatic tumors, those with micrometastases, and those with overt metastasis. Xi et al.[128] used the Bhattacharjee et al.[99] (see previous discussion) and the Beer et al.[102] (see discussion on prognosis later) datasets to examine whether gene expression in primary AD tumors was indicative of lymph node metastases. A 318-gene signature was able to accurately classify node positive patients in the training[102] and test[99] sets, but frequently misclassified node negative patients. The classification as node negative or positive in the node-negative patients was associated with survival. These studies suggest that the survival differences observed among stage I ADs in the Garber et al.[114] and Bhattacharjee et al.[99] datasets might be related to the presence of micrometastases or metastatic potential. The use of gene expression for "molecular staging" may enhance the sensitivity of clinical and pathologic methods for staging tumors, improving treatment decisions and ultimately outcomes for lung cancer patients.

Several studies using the primary lung tumor to predict lymph node metastases Kikuchi et al.[125] examined 37 NSCLCs using cDNA microarrays containing 23,040 genes. The initial data set was trimmed to 899 genes and investigators used hierarchical clustering methods to separate the tumors into groups based on their histologic subtypes. Next, the investigators established a predictive scoring system based on the expression profiles of selected genes. When used to calculate the predictive score, 40 genes provided the best separation of node-positive and negative adenocarcinomas. Previous studies have reported an association between tumor metastasis and several of the genes used to calculate the predictive score: ARHA, DB1, NESH, and TACSTD1.[129–132] Finally, the authors studied the expression of the metastasis-related genes after treatment with six different chemotherapeutic agents: cisplatin, docetaxel, gemcitabine, irinotecan, paclitaxel, and vinorelbine. Analysis revealed a number of genes correlating the sensitivity of the adenocarcinomas or SCC to the six drugs. In particular, YWHAQ gene expression levels correlated with the sensitivity of lung adenocarcinomas to cisplatin, docetaxel, gemcitabine, and paclitaxel. Xi et al.[133] used the Bhattacharjee et al.[99] (see previous discussion) and the Beer et al.[102] datasets to examine whether gene expression in primary adenocarcinoma tumors was indicative of lymph node metastases. A 318-gene signature was able to accurately classify node-positive patients in the training and test[99] sets, but frequently misclassified node negative patients. The classification as node negative or positive in the node-negative patients was associated with survival. These studies suggest that the survival differences observed among stage I adenocarcinomas might be related to the presence of micrometastases or metastatic potential.

In 2006, Potti et al.[134] reported the use of gene expression arrays to develop a risk model of recurrence for early stage lung cancers. Using an initial set of 89 NSCLCs, which included both squamous cell carcinoma and adenocarcinoma, investigators first established a collection of gene expression profiles, which they termed *metagenes*. Prognostic models were built from the metagenes using classification- and regression-tree analysis. In the initial training cohort, the metagene model predicted disease recurrence with an accuracy of 93%, compared with 64% as predicted by the prognostic model built with clinical data alone. These data were supported in Kaplan-Meier survival analyses. Validation of the metagene model was performed on two independent cohorts from multicenter cooperative group trials, the American College of Surgeons Oncology Groups (ACOSOG) Z0030 study and the Cancer and Leukemia Group B (CALGB) 9761 trial. With these results, investigators described a possible role for predicting disease recurrence for patients with early stage lung cancers, thereby identifying patients for whom adjuvant chemotherapy might otherwise not be indicated.

More recently, Chen et al.[135] reported the use of gene expression arrays to develop a five-gene model for prediction of relapse-free and overall survival in lung cancer. Expression arrays were used on 125 tumors. Through Cox regression analysis and calculation of hazard ratios (HR), 16 genes were correlated with death from any cause. Risk scores were calculated for these 16 genes and patients were classified as having a high- or low-risk gene signature. Expression levels of the 16 genes were confirmed by RT-PCR and further statistical analysis identified 5 genes that were significantly associated with patient survival: monocyte-to-macrophage differentiation-associated protein (MMD), dual-specificity phosphatase 6 (DUSP6), v-erb-b2 avain erythroblastic leukemia viral oncogene homologue 3 (ERBB3), signal transducer and activator of transcription 1 (STAT1), and lymphocyte-specific protein tyrosine kinase (LCK). Some of these have previously been described as playing a role in carcinogenesis: DUSP6 has been implicated in tumor suppression and apoptosis; ERBB3 is a tyrosine kinase and member of the EGFR family; STAT1 has been implicated in cell growth and apoptosis through induction of $p21^{Waf1}$ and caspase; and LCK is a member of the Src family of tyrosine kinases and has been shown to regulate mobility of cancer cells.[136–142] The predictive value of the five-gene signature was subsequently validated on an independent cohort of 60 additional patients. Compared to those with a low-risk gene signature, patients with a high-risk gene signature had a significantly shorter median survival. Results were similar when patients with stage I disease were examined separately; however, there was no correlation between gene signature and overall survival for patients with stage II disease. An insightful editorial regarding this work was published by Herbst and Lippman[143] who pointed out that since the specimens were not microdissected, the analysis could be misleading with regard to the importance of invasion-related genes, which can vary in expression throughout a tumor. Moreover future studies must analyze molecular epidemiologic, stromal, and vascular factors that are critical to the metastatic process. Finally, the choice of the cutoff of expression levels and filtering of the data could influence how the genes were selected. Nevertheless, further validation studies on a set of 86 tumors previously analyzed by another group[102] also demonstrated a significant risk for death from any cause with the high-risk gene signature as well as a trend toward significance when analyzed for survival.

Reproducibility of Data One challenge in the use of gene expression arrays for prognostication in lung cancer is the reliability of platforms across institutions and reproducibility of data or identification of candidate genes involved in prognosis across institutions. Some investigators have addressed this by validating their predictive models with cohorts from outside studies and institutions.[135,144] In an effort to investigate the variability between laboratories and across institutions, Dobbin et al.[97] reported both "within-laboratory" and between-laboratory reproducibility of microarray data across four institutions for a set of primary tumors, lung cancer cell lines and purified RNA samples. Although the between-laboratory variation was highest, the investigators concluded that the reproducibility, and therefore, the comparability of the data were adequate for the samples studied.

Hayes et al.[100] evaluated three cohorts of adenocarcinomas, each from a different institution and with its own gene array platform. Statistical analysis identified 2553 genes that were present and reliable across the three platforms. Adenocarcinoma tumor subtypes, named bronchioid, squamoid, and magnoid by the authors, were each distinguished by several hundred genes. Lists of genes characteristic of tumor subtype in one cohort were predictive of tumor subtypes in the other two cohorts. While investigators were able to analyze survival data for only one cohort of patients, patients with stage I and II tumors had significantly shorter survival times when their tumors were classified as squamoid and magnoid. In contrast, for patients with stage III and IV tumors, there was a trend toward increased survival for patients with squamoid subtype.

Sun et al.[145] used two lung cancer oligonucleotide microarray data sets of adenocarcinoma and squamous cell carcinoma as training sets to select prognostic genes independent of conventional predictors. The top 50 genes from each set were used to predict the outcomes of two independent validation data sets of 84 and 91 NSCLC cases. Adenocarcinomas with the 50-gene signature from *adenocarcinoma* in both validation data sets had a 2.4-fold (95% confidence interval [CI], 1.3 to 4.4 and 1.0 to 5.8) increased mortality after adjustment for conventional predictors. Squamous cell carcinoma with the same high-risk signature had an adjusted risk of 1.1 (95% CI, 0.4 to 3.2) in one data set and 2.5 (95% CI, 1.1 to 5.8) in another. Adenocarcinoma with the 50-gene signature from *squamous cell carcinoma* had an elevated risk of 3.5 (95% CI, 1.4 to 9.0) after adjustment for conventional predictors. Squamous cell carcinoma with this high-risk signature had an adjusted risk of 1.8 (95% CI, 0.7 to 4.6). The authors thus illustrated that two nonoverlapping but functionally related gene expression signatures provided consistently improved survival prediction for NSCLC regardless of the histologic cell type.

Skrzypski et al.[146] studied the expression of 29 progression and metastasis genes derived from previous lung cancer microarray data. Their expression was assessed by reverse transcriptase quantitative PCR in frozen primary tumor specimens obtained from 66 SCC patients who had undergone surgical resection.

In a multivariate Cox model, the genes CSF1 (HR, 3.5; $p = 0.005$), EGFR (HR, 2.7; $p = 0.02$), CA IX (HR, 0.2; $p < 0.0001$), and tumor size >4 cm (HR, 2.7; $p = 0.02$) emerged as significant markers for survival and the expression of the three genes (CSF1, EGFR, and CA IX)as risk factors was positively validated in a separate cohort of 26 patients in an independent laboratory ($p = 0.05$)

Raz et al.[147] generated a four-gene model based on expression of WNT3a, ERBB3, LCK, and RND3 that was used to generate a risk score. The Gene Risk score predicted mortality better than clinical stage or tumor size (adjusted HR, 6.7; 95% CI, 1.6 to 28.9; $p = 0.001$). Among 70 patients with stage I disease, 5-year overall survival was 87% among patients with low-risk scores, and 38% among patients with high-risk scores ($p = 0.0002$). Among all patients, 5-year overall survival was 62% and 41%, respectively ($p = 0.0054$). Disease-free survival was also significantly different among low- and high-risk score patients.

Most recently, Shedden et al.[148] reported results from a large retrospective multisite, blinded study of 442 lung adenocarcinomas designed to test the prognostic performance of gene microarray data alone versus performance with the inclusion of clinical covariates. Data were generated using a common platform, and training set data were generated at two of the participating sites. The results were validated using independent data generated from two additional sites after a blinded protocol. Eight different methods, including gene clustering, univariate testing, and mechanistic groupings, were used to provide prognostic data. Many genes were identified as important for prognosis in more than one statistical method, including those involved in cell proliferation such as cyclins, checkpoint genes, topoisomerases, and chromosomal and spindle protein genes. The most successful classifier methods incorporated both gene expression and clinical data, and the investigators stressed the importance of coordinating the collection of both clinical and pathologic data across multiple institutions for future prospective studies.

EPIGENETIC SILENCING AND GENE METHYLATION

In addition to the role of genetic alterations in the pathogenesis of lung cancer, epigenetic modification, or DNA methylation, also plays a key role in human carcinogenesis (see also Chapter 7). Gene promoter regions have CpG islands that are subject to aberrant hypermethylation by cytosine-DNA methyltransferases. When this occurs, the composition of chromatin around the island is modified, and access to the promoter region by key regulatory proteins involved in transcription is denied. Through the amplification of methylated alleles in the promoter region of specific genes, the methylation-specific PCR (MSP) assay allows for rapid detection of methylation in genes of interest. As a result, several key genes have been identified, which are altered by DNA methylation in the development of lung cancer.

Genes involved in all aspects of cellular function—regulation of cell cycle, DNA repair, *RAS* signaling and invasion, apoptosis—are affected by epigenetic silencing in the development of NSCLC. Methylation of the death-associated protein kinase (DAPK) is found in up to 48% of adenocarcinomas and approximately 25% to 33% of squamous cell carcinomas.[149] *DAPK* is a serine/threonine kinase involved in apoptosis resulting from DNA damage, through TNF-α, FAS-, or γ-interferon–associated pathways, or by downstream activation of p53. An association has been made between methylation of DAPK and increasing pathologic stage in NSCLC[150]; for those patients with resected stage I tumors, methylated DAPK has been associated with poorer disease-specific and overall survival.[151]

The family of cadherins includes cell-surface glycoproteins, which are responsible for adhesion and cell recognition. Two of these, *E-cadherin* and *H-cadherin*, are methylated in NSCLC. Methylation of *E-cadherin* ranges from 16% to 45%, whereas that of *H-cadherin* was found in approximately 43% of NSCLCs.[152,153] Impaired or absent expression of E-cadherin has been linked to poor differentiation, lymph node metastasis and poorer prognosis and survival in patients with NSCLC.[154] Metastatic potential is also regulated by the tissue inhibitor of metalloproteinases (TIMPs), which inhibit the proteolytic activity of MMPs. Methylation of TIMPs has been observed in 19% to 26% of NSCLCs.[153]

One of the best studied genes in DNA methylation and NSCLC is p16^{CDKN2A}. It is affected in up to 67% of adenocarcinomas and 70% of squamous cell carcinomas.[155] In experimental models of cancer development and progression, methylation of p16^{CDKN2A} is an early event in lung carcinogenesis, and its prevalence increases with disease progression.[156] In addition, methylation of p16^{CDKN2A} is associated with increased tobacco exposure.[157] In a large study of NSCLCs in which methylation status of five genes was examined, Toyooka et al.[158] determined that only methylation of p16^{CDKN2A} was associated with poor survival.

The *RASSF1* gene is a member of a family of genes that encode for *ras*-binding proteins; several different transcripts are produced by alternative promoter selection and splicing. mRNA expression of *RASSF1A* is often lost in NSCLCs; this led to the observation that *RASSF1* is methylated in 30% to 40% of primary NSCLCs.[159,160] However, the association between methylation of *RASSF1A* and patient survival is controversial. While Burbee et al.[159] determined that methylation of *RASSF1A* in lung cancer was associated with shorter overall survival, Toyooka et al.[158] were unable to confirm these findings in a larger study.

In 2003, Harden et al.[161] examined promoter methylation in 90 primary stage I lung cancers and their associated lymph nodes. Methylation at p16 was demonstrated in 15/90 tumors (17%); 14/90 (16%) at O^6-methylguanine-DNA-methyltransferase (MGMT); 7/90 (8%) at glutathione S-transferase P1 (GSTP1), 15/90 (17%) at the DAPK1 gene, and 65/90 (72%) at the adenomatous polyposis coli (APC) gene. Methylation of both APC and GSTP1 were more often associated with squamous morphology and a worse clinical outcome. Interestingly, data from gene expression profiles have demonstrated significantly diminished levels for *APC* in adenocarcinomas, and that tumors with lower levels of expression showed a trend toward worse outcome.[102]

Gu et al.[162] examined the methylation status in a cohort of 155 patients with stages I to III NSCLC. Nine genes were studied: p16, CDH1, TIMP3, RASSF1A, HFIT, APC, DAPK, MGMT, and GSTP1. The investigators calculated a methylation index (MI), defined as the ratio of the number of methylated genes to the number studied, nine in this case. They determined that the MI was significantly higher in adenocarcinomas relative to SCCs and in patients with >50 pack-year smoking history relative to <50 pack-years. In addition, the MI was higher in older patients (>66 years) relative to the MI of patients younger than 66 years of age. However, there was no difference between early stage tumors and late-stage tumors. Survival analysis revealed that patients with methylation of *CDH1* had a significantly longer survival than those without. In contrast, patients with p16 methylation had worse survival than those without p16 methylation. As the number of unfavorable methylation events increased, the median survival time was significantly diminished.

Recently, Brock et al.[163] demonstrated a relationship between gene methylation, specific combinations of gene methylation and tumor recurrence for patients with resected stage I NSCLC. From a cohort of 71 patients, seven genes were studied from tumor and associated mediastinal lymph nodes sampled at the time of surgery. The four genes with the largest differences in the frequency of methylation between tumors and controls were p16, the H-cadherin gene 13 (*CDH13*), *RASSF1A*, and *APC*. A higher number of methylated genes in each sample was associated with poorer survival. Specifically, patients with two or more methylated genes of interest in either the primary tumor or mediastinal lymph nodes had a 5-year recurrence-free survival rate of 27.3%, compared to 65.3% for patients with fewer than two methylated genes of interest. There was an additive effect to patients whose samples demonstrated methylation of both p16 and *CDH13*. Methylation of both genes in either the primary tumor, regional or mediastinal lymph nodes, was associated with significantly shorter recurrence-free survival. Although these results suggest a possible role for using methylation status as a means of detecting occult micrometastasis, large-scale, prospective, multi-institution studies have yet to be conducted.

PROTEOMIC ANALYSIS AND PROGNOSTICATION

Proteomic approaches involve the comprehensive investigation of proteins using high-throughput technologies such as two-dimensional (2D) polyacrylamide gel electrophoresis or mass spectrometry (see also Chapter 9). One disadvantage of genomic approaches is the ability to study posttranslational modification of proteins such as phosphorylation, glycosylation, or proteolytic processing. These processes are important not only for determining protein function, but are also dysregulated in malignancy.[164,165] Proteomic approaches may be used to profile tumors through examination of proteome expression; other possible study mechanisms include protein–protein interactions or even specific proteins and their posttranslational modification.

As with genomic strategies, investigators have demonstrated that patterns of protein expression correlate with specific histopathologic features of the primary tumors. In one study using 2D electrophoresis, a group of 52 protein spots differed in intensity between small cell carcinoma, squamous cell carcinoma and adeoncarcinoma tumor specimens.[166] Another study comparing of proteomic patterns between squamous cell carcinoma and corresponding normal tissues identified 76 proteins that were differentially expressed between tumor and normal tissues. The identified proteins were subsequently identified and classified as oncoproteins, signaling molecules, and cell cycle regulators.[167]

Other proteomic analysis of a group of NSCLC tumors with known survival and outcome data revealed a characteristic pattern comprised of 15 mass spectrometry peaks. Using this, investigators were able to distinguish between patients with favorable versus adverse outcomes.[168] In the same study, class-prediction models were able to distinguish primary lung tumors from lesions metastatic to the lungs (of other organ primary); these methods were also used to identify the presence of tumor metastatic to lymph nodes with 85% accuracy.

Differential expression of specific protein isoforms have been correlated with patient survival in NSCLC. Gharib et al.[169] determined that four cytokeratin types, CK7, CK8, CK18, and CK19, had at least one isoform that was significantly increased in lung adenocarcinoma compared to normal lung tissue. Of these, all five CK7 isoforms, one CK8 isoform and one CK19 isoform were associated with unfavorable prognosis. There was little correlation between these isoforms and other clinicopathologic characteristics. Highlighting the advantages of proteomic analysis, several isoforms were detected for each of the cytokeratin types, suggesting the presence of several levels of regulation and posttranslational modification.

Chen et al.[170] examined 682 protein spots from a cohort of adenocarcinomas. They identified 46 proteins that were significantly associated with patient survival and 33 of these were subsequently identified by mass spectrometry. Of these, increased expression was demonstrated in four proteins and seven mRNAs encoding enzymes in the glycolysis pathway. These were all associated with poor survival, potentially reflecting increased metabolic activity in these tumors. Furthermore, the authors devised a risk index based on the 20 proteins (of the original set of 46) most associated with survival. Using this index, they were able to identify a subset of patients with stage I adenocarcinoma that had significantly worse outcomes.

More recently, Yanagisawa et al.[171] described a proteomic signature of 25 mass spectrometry signals to predict prognosis for NSCLC. First comparing NSCLC tissue and normal lung tissue, they found 694 proteomic signals that were differentially expressed. Based on these 694 signals, groups with high and low risk of recurrence based on clinical data were compared. From this, a weighted voting prognosis signature using 25 proteomic signals was devised to predict patient outcomes. Validation studies demonstrated that for patients with stage I NSCLC, relapse-free and overall survival were significantly different between the high- and low-risk groups as determined by the risk score. This was also true for patients grouped together with stage II or stage III disease, thereby predicting clinical prognosis with relative accuracy.

MICRORNAS AND PROGNOSTICATION

miRNAs are regulatory RNAs found in humans, plants, and animals where they play a role in regulating important cellular processes such as cell development, proliferation, and even cell death. They are noncoding fragments of RNA that hybridize to complementary gene sequences in the 3′ untranslated region (3′ UTR) of target mRNA. Initially discovered in *Caenorhabditis elegans* miRNAs and their associated proteins are abundantly present in cells.[172] Their role in human carcinogenesis has yet to be clearly defined. However, the gene loci for many miRNAs correspond to fragile chromosomal sites and abnormal expression of miRNAs have been demonstrated in a number of human cancers including leukemias, lymphomas, colorectal cancer, and lung cancer.[173]

miRNAs are initially transcribed into long precursor RNAs called pri-miRNAs and processed by Drosha, a cellular nuclease, into pre-miRNAs.[174,175] Following transport to the cytoplasm by Exportin-5, the DICER enzyme cleaves the pre-miRNAs, resulting in a mature intermediate measuring 17 to 24 nucleotides long.[176–178] miRNAs can regulate mRNA translation or increase the stability of mRNA, thereby altering the amount of final product.[179] Through posttranscriptional regulation and subsequent alteration of gene expression, miRNAs can affect a number of cellular functions such as cellular differentiation, proliferation, or even apoptosis.[180]

Unique miRNA expression profiles have been described for NSCLC and these have been correlated with patient survival. Comparing lung tumors to noncancerous lung tissue, Yanaihara et al.[181] identified a panel of 43 miRNAs differentially expressed in the lung tumors. Six of these miRNAs were expressed differently between tumors of squamous cell carcinoma and adenocarcinoma histology. Analysis of clinical data demonstrated that high expression of *hsa-mir-155*, *hsa-mir-17-3p*, *hsa-mir-106a*, *hsa-mir-93*, and *hsa-mir-21*, along with low expression of *hsa -let-7-a-2*, *hsa -let-7b*, or *hsa-mir-145* was associated with a significantly worse prognosis for patients with adenocarcinoma. In addition, Kaplan-Meier survival analysis demonstrated that high expression of *hsa-mir-155* was an unfavorable prognostic factor for adenocarcinoma, independent of other clinicopathologic variables. Markou et al.[182] evaluated the prognostic value of mature miRNA-21 (miR-21) and mature miRNA-205 (miR-205) overexpression in NSCLC. We detected overexpression of mature miR-21 in 52% NSCLC specimens and overexpression of miR-205 in 65%. miR-21 overexpression correlated with overall survival of the patients ($p = 0.027$), whereas overexpression of mature miR-205 did not.

In another study, Yu et al.[183] identified a five-miRNA signature from a cohort of 56 NSCLC tumors, which included both squamous cell carcinoma and adenocarcinoma. Two of the miRNAs, *hsa-mir-221*, and *hsa-let-7a*, were protective, whereas *hsa-mir-137*, *hsa-mir-372*, and *hsa-mir-182* were "risky." A risk-score formula was devised based on the expression levels of these five miRNAs. Compared to those with low-risk miRNA signatures, patients whose tumors had high-risk miRNA signatures had significantly shorter median relapse-free survival times and shorter median overall survival times. These findings were validated in the same study using an independent set of samples. In addition, multivariate regression analysis demonstrated that the risk conferred by the miRNA signature was independent of tumor histology. However, when patients were classified by stage, the miRNA signature was predictive only of relapse-free survival in stage I patients. For stage II patients, no statistically significant associations were made, possibly due to small sample size. For stage III patients, the miRNA signature was predictive of both relapse-free survival and overall survival.

A specific subset of miRNA of interest in lung cancer is the *lethal-7* (*let-7*) miRNA family, which is abundantly expressed in normal human lung tissue. In a study of 143 lung cancer cases for which follow-up and survival data were available, Takamizawa et al.[184] demonstrated that reduced *let-7* miRNAs expression was associated with significantly shorter long-term survival, and that this was independent of disease stage. In addition, at least one member of the *let-7* family has been shown to negatively regulate *ras* expression in human cells.[173] These findings suggest a possible mechanism for *let-7* in the pathogenesis of lung cancer, and additional study will further elucidate the role of this and other miRNAs in the development and pathogenesis of lung cancer.

Identifying miRNAs regulators in lung cancer could also improve patient selection for targeted agents in addition to their prognostic potential. Since allelic loss in chromosome 3p is frequent and early in lung carcinogenesis, Weiss et al.[185] investigated if the loss of miRNA-128b, a miRNA located on chromosome 3p and a putative regulator of EGFR, correlated with response to targeted EGFR inhibition. Weiss et al.[185] found that miRNA-128b directly regulated EGFR and that miRNA-128b loss of heterozygosity (LOH) was frequent in tumor samples. Moreover, miRNA-128b LOH correlated significantly with clinical response and survival following gefitinib, while EGFR expression and mutation status did not correlate with survival outcome.

CLINICAL POTENTIAL AND FUTURE DIRECTIONS

Lung cancer is a complex disease that involves a number of molecular and cellular processes, several of which may be altered in the process of tumor development. In this chapter, we have reviewed a small yet pertinent number of studies demonstrating the potential of molecular biologic techniques to predict prognosis for patients with NSCLC. Currently, the most reliable prognostic method remains clinical staging. As molecular techniques continue to undergo refinement both in predictive capability and reproducibility, it is conceivable that future staging systems will incorporate genetic, proteomic, or miRNA signatures.

However, several challenges need to be addressed prior to everyday use of these molecular techniques. First, continued progress must be made toward reproducibility of testing and profiling of tumors across institutions. Recent contributions from Shedden et al.[148] have demonstrated that interlaboratory and intralaboratory variation can be minimized to provide relatively consistent gene expression profiling data for a set of tumors. To date, similar studies have not been conducted across institutions to validate methylation or proteomic profiles for primary lung tumors and associated lymph nodes.

Another challenge in bringing molecular techniques into everyday clinical use is expanding the application of these techniques beyond the laboratory of the academic medical center to the bedside and practitioner in the community hospital. Furthermore, most patients with lung cancer are diagnosed at an advanced stage and not considered to be candidates for surgery. In contrast, the vast majority of studies defining molecular profiles for lung cancer have involved patients with early stage tumors who have undergone surgical resection. While profiling techniques are being developed to predict those with resected early stage disease that may benefit from therapy not otherwise indicated, further work is underway to characterize more advanced tumors based on their gene expression profiles and response to chemotherapeutic agents. Molecular techniques may soon be used to select chemotherapeutic agents for patients based on their tumors' molecular chemoresistance profiles.[186] In that case, the challenge will be to generate an accurate molecular profile with minimally invasive sampling techniques or serum-based assays that avoid subjecting the patient to major surgery.

Finally, the heterogeneity of NSCLC tumors creates a significant challenge for the identification and development of effective treatments. Gene expression profiling and other molecular techniques have added much to our understanding of the biology of NSCLC. Targeted therapies such as bevacizumab and erlotinib have demonstrated effectiveness for many of patients with lung cancer. Similarly, an ideal application for gene expression profiling of NSCLC would be to use the expression data to better understand tumor heterogeneity and discover what may be unique properties for specific subsets of these tumors. Future studies have the potential to further enhance our understanding of NSCLC and identify novel pathways and mechanisms in the pathogenesis of this disease. Undoubtedly, this will result in the identification of additional prognostic markers as well as unique targets for development of future therapies, with their clinical application ultimately being used to benefit patients.

REFERENCES

1. Goldstraw P, Crowley J, Chansky K, et al. The IASLC Lung Cancer Staging Project: proposals for the revision of the TNM stage groupings in the forthcoming (seventh) edition of the TNM Classification of malignant tumours. *J Thorac Oncol* 2007 Aug;2(8):706–714.
2. Brundage MD, Davies D, Mackillop WJ. Prognostic factors in non-small cell lung cancer: a decade of progress. *Chest* 2002 Sep;122(3):1037–1057.
3. Harpole DH Jr, Herndon JE II, Wolfe WG, et al. A prognostic model of recurrence and death in stage I non-small cell lung cancer utilizing presentation, histopathology, and oncoprotein expression. *Cancer Res* 1995 Jan 1;55(1):51–56.
4. Nemunaitis J, Klemow S, Tong A, et al. Prognostic value of K-ras mutations, ras oncoprotein, and c-erb B-2 oncoprotein expression in adenocarcinoma of the lung. *Am J Clin Oncol* 1998 Apr;21(2):155–160.
5. Nishio M, Koshikawa T, Yatabe Y, et al. Prognostic significance of cyclin D1 and retinoblastoma expression in combination with p53 abnormalities in primary, resected non-small cell lung cancers. *Clin Cancer Res* 1997 Jul;3(7):1051–1058.
6. Breuer RH, Postmus PE, Smit EF. Molecular pathology of non-small-cell lung cancer. *Respiration* 2005 May-Jun;72(3):313–330.
7. Kaye FJ. Molecular biology of lung cancer. *Lung Cancer* 2001 Dec;34 (Suppl 2):S35–S41.
8. Ahrendt SA, Decker PA, Alawi EA, et al. Cigarette smoking is strongly associated with mutation of the K-ras gene in patients with primary adenocarcinoma of the lung. *Cancer* 2001 Sep 15;92(6):1525–1530.

9. Westra WH, Baas IO, Hruban RH, et al. K-ras oncogene activation in atypical alveolar hyperplasias of the human lung. *Cancer Res* 1996 May 1;56(9):2224–2228.
10. Fischer JR, Lahm H. Validation of molecular and immunological factors with predictive importance in lung cancer. *Lung Cancer* 2004 Aug;45(Suppl 2):S151–S161.
11. Huncharek M, Muscat J, Geschwind JF. K-ras oncogene mutation as a prognostic marker in non-small cell lung cancer: a combined analysis of 881 cases. *Carcinogenesis* 1999 Aug;20(8):1507–1510.
12. Vielh P, Spano JP, Grenier J, et al. Molecular prognostic factors in resectable non-small cell lung cancer. *Crit Rev Oncol Hematol* 2005 Mar;53(3):193–197.
13. Tsao MS, Aviel-Ronen S, Ding K, et al. Prognostic and predictive importance of p53 and RAS for adjuvant chemotherapy in non small-cell lung cancer. *J Clin Oncol* 2007 Nov 20;25(33):5240–5247.
14. Ahrendt SA, Chow JT, Yang SC, et al. Alcohol consumption and cigarette smoking increase the frequency of p53 mutations in non-small cell lung cancer. *Cancer Res* 2000 Jun 15;60(12):3155–3159.
15. Vogelstein B, Lane D, Levine AJ. Surfing the p53 network. *Nature* 2000 Nov 16;408(6810):307–310.
16. Ahrendt SA, Hu Y, Buta M, et al. p53 mutations and survival in stage I non-small-cell lung cancer: results of a prospective study. *J Natl Cancer Inst* 2003 Jul 2;95(13):961–970.
17. Fukuyama Y, Mitsudomi T, Sugio K, et al. K-ras and p53 mutations are an independent unfavourable prognostic indicator in patients with non-small-cell lung cancer. *Br J Cancer* 1997;75(8):1125–1130.
18. Hashimoto T, Tokuchi Y, Hayashi M, et al. p53 null mutations undetected by immunohistochemical staining predict a poor outcome with early-stage non-small cell lung carcinomas. *Cancer Res* 1999 Nov 1;59(21):5572–5577.
19. Horio Y, Takahashi T, Kuroishi T, et al. Prognostic significance of p53 mutations and 3p deletions in primary resected non-small cell lung cancer. *Cancer Res* 1993 Jan 1;53(1):1–4.
20. Huang CL, Taki T, Adachi M, et al. Mutations of p53 and K-ras genes as prognostic factors for non-small cell lung cancer. *Int J Oncol* 1998 Mar;12(3):553–563.
21. Laudanski J, Niklinska W, Burzykowski T, et al. Prognostic significance of p53 and bcl-2 abnormalities in operable nonsmall cell lung cancer. *Eur Respir J* 2001 Apr;17(4):660–666.
22. Mitsudomi T, Oyama T, Kusano T, et al. Mutations of the p53 gene as a predictor of poor prognosis in patients with non-small-cell lung cancer. *J Natl Cancer Inst* 1993 Dec 15;85(24):2018–2023.
23. Skaug V, Ryberg D, Kure EH, et al. p53 mutations in defined structural and functional domains are related to poor clinical outcome in non-small cell lung cancer patients. *Clin Cancer Res* 2000 Mar;6(3):1031–1037.
24. Tomizawa Y, Kohno T, Fujita T, et al. Correlation between the status of the p53 gene and survival in patients with stage I non-small cell lung carcinoma. *Oncogene* 1999 Jan 28;18(4):1007–1014.
25. Vega FJ, Iniesta P, Caldés T, et al. p53 exon 5 mutations as a prognostic indicator of shortened survival in non-small-cell lung cancer. *Br J Cancer* 1997;76(1):44–51.
26. Dalquen P, Sauter G, Torhorst J, et al. Nuclear p53 overexpression is an independent prognostic parameter in node-negative non-small cell lung carcinoma. *J Pathol* 1996 Jan;178(1):53–58.
27. D'Amico TA, Massey M, Herndon JE II, et al. A biologic risk model for stage I lung cancer: immunohistochemical analysis of 408 patients with the use of ten molecular markers. *J Thorac Cardiovasc Surg* 1999 Apr;117(4):736–743.
28. Kwiatkowski DJ, Harpole DH Jr, Godleski J, et al. Molecular pathologic substaging in 244 stage I non-small-cell lung cancer patients: clinical implications. *J Clin Oncol* 1998 Jul;16(7):2468–2477.
29. Lee YC, Chang YL, Luh SP, et al. Significance of P53 and Rb protein expression in surgically treated non-small cell lung cancers. *Ann Thorac Surg* 1999 Aug;68(2):343–347; discussion 348.
30. Moldvay J, Scheid P, Wild P, et al. Predictive survival markers in patients with surgically resected non-small cell lung carcinoma. *Clin Cancer Res* 2000 Mar;6(3):1125–1134.
31. Nishio M, Koshikawa T, Kuroishi T, et al. Prognostic significance of abnormal p53 accumulation in primary, resected non-small-cell lung cancers. *J Clin Oncol* 1996 Feb;14(2):497–502.
32. Pappot H, Francis D, Brünner N, et al. p53 protein in non-small cell lung cancer as quantitated by enzyme-linked immunosorbent assay: relation to prognosis. *Clin Cancer Res* 1996 Jan;2(1):155–160.
33. Pastorino U, Andreola S, Tagliabue E, et al. Immunocytochemical markers in stage I lung cancer: relevance to prognosis. *J Clin Oncol* 1997 Aug;15(8):2858–2865.
34. Carbognani P, Tincani G, Crafa P, et al. Biological markers in non-small cell lung cancer. Retrospective study of 10 year follow-up after surgery. *J Cardiovasc Surg (Torino)* 2002 Aug;43(4):545–548.
35. Steels E, Paesmans M, Berghmans T, et al. Role of p53 as a prognostic factor for survival in lung cancer: a systematic review of the literature with a meta-analysis. *Eur Respir J* 2001 Oct;18(4):705–719.
36. Akin H, Yilmazbayhan D, Kilicaslan Z, et al. Clinical significance of P16INK4A and retinoblastoma proteins in non-small-cell lung carcinoma. *Lung Cancer* 2002 Dec;38(3):253–260.
37. Haga Y, Hiroshima K, Iyoda A, et al. Ki-67 expression and prognosis for smokers with resected stage I non-small cell lung cancer. *Ann Thorac Surg* 2003 Jun;75(6):1727–1732; discussion 1732–1733.
38. Jin M, Inoue S, Umemura T, et al. Cyclin D1, p16 and retinoblastoma gene product expression as a predictor for prognosis in non-small cell lung cancer at stages I and II. *Lung Cancer* 2001 Nov;34(2):207–218.
39. Burke L, Flieder DB, Guinee DG, et al. Prognostic implications of molecular and immunohistochemical profiles of the Rb and p53 cell cycle regulatory pathways in primary non-small cell lung carcinoma. *Clin Cancer Res* 2005 Jan 1;11(1):232–241.
40. Mohamed S, Yasufuku K, Hiroshima K, et al. Prognostic implications of cell cycle-related proteins in primary resectable pathologic N2 nonsmall cell lung cancer. *Cancer* 2007 Jun 15;109(12):2506–2514.
41. Groeger AM, Caputi M, Esposito V, et al. Independent prognostic role of p16 expression in lung cancer. *J Thorac Cardiovasc Surg* 1999 Sep;118(3):529–535.
42. Huang CI, Taki T, Higashiyama M, et al. p16 protein expression is associated with a poor prognosis in squamous cell carcinoma of the lung. *Br J Cancer* 2000 Jan;82(2):374–380.
43. Kawabuchi B, Moriyama S, Hironaka M, et al. p16 inactivation in small-sized lung adenocarcinoma: its association with poor prognosis. *Int J Cancer* 1999 Feb 19;84(1):49–53.
44. Kratzke RA, Greatens TM, Rubins JB, et al. Rb and p16INK4a expression in resected non-small cell lung tumors. *Cancer Res* 1996 Aug 1;56(15):3415–3420.
45. Keum JS, Kong G, Yang SC, et al. Cyclin D1 overexpression is an indicator of poor prognosis in resectable non-small cell lung cancer. *Br J Cancer* 1999 Sep;81(1):127–132.
46. Gugger M, Kappeler A, Vonlanthen S, et al. Alterations of cell cycle regulators are less frequent in advanced non-small cell lung cancer than in resectable tumours. *Lung Cancer* 2001 Aug-Sep;33(2–3):229–239.
47. Fukuse T, Hirata T, Naiki H, et al. Prognostic significance of cyclin E overexpression in resected non-small cell lung cancer. *Cancer Res* 2000 Jan 15;60(2):242–244.
48. Mishina T, Dosaka-Akita H, Hommura F, et al. Cyclin E expression, a potential prognostic marker for non-small cell lung cancers. *Clin Cancer Res* 2000 Jan;6(1):11–16.
49. Soria JC, Rodriguez M, Liu DD, et al. Aberrant promoter methylation of multiple genes in bronchial brush samples from former cigarette smokers. *Cancer Res* 2002 Jan 15;62(2):351–355.
50. Esposito V, Baldi A, De Luca A, et al. Prognostic role of the cyclin-dependent kinase inhibitor p27 in non-small cell lung cancer. *Cancer Res* 1997 Aug 15;57(16):3381–3385.

51. Komiya T, Hosono Y, Hirashima T, et al. p21 expression as a predictor for favorable prognosis in squamous cell carcinoma of the lung. *Clin Cancer Res* 1997 Oct;3(10):1831–1835.
52. Shoji T, Tanaka F, Takata T, et al. Clinical significance of p21 expression in non-small-cell lung cancer. *J Clin Oncol* 2002 Sep 15;20(18):3865–3871.
53. Hayashi H, Ogawa N, Ishiwa N, et al. High cyclin E and low p27/Kip1 expressions are potentially poor prognostic factors in lung adenocarcinoma patients. *Lung Cancer* 2001 Oct;34(1):59–65.
54. Hommura F, Dosaka-Akita H, Mishina T, et al. Prognostic significance of p27KIP1 protein and ki-67 growth fraction in non-small cell lung cancers. *Clin Cancer Res* 2000 Oct;6(10):4073–4081.
55. Tsukamoto S, Sugio K, Sakada T, et al. Reduced expression of cell-cycle regulator p27(Kip1) correlates with a shortened survival in non-small cell lung cancer. *Lung Cancer* 2001 Oct;34(1):83–90.
56. Scagliotti GV, Selvaggi G, Novello S, et al. The biology of epidermal growth factor receptor in lung cancer. *Clin Cancer Res* 2004 Jun 15;10 (12 Pt 2):S4227–S4232.
57. Johnson BE, Jänne PA. Epidermal growth factor receptor mutations in patients with non-small cell lung cancer. *Cancer Res* 2005 Sep 1;65(17):7525–7529.
58. Datta SR, Brunet A, Greenberg ME. Cellular survival: a play in three Akts. *Genes Dev* 1999 Nov 15;13(22):2905–2927.
59. Jeon YK, Sung SW, Chung JH, et al. Clinicopathologic features and prognostic implications of epidermal growth factor receptor (EGFR) gene copy number and protein expression in non-small cell lung cancer. *Lung Cancer* 2006 Dec 28;54(3):387–398.
60. Murray S, Timotheadou E, Linardou H, et al. Mutations of the epidermal growth factor receptor tyrosine kinase domain and associations with clinicopathological features in non-small cell lung cancer patients. *Lung Cancer* 2006 May;52(2):225–233.
61. Paez JG, Jänne PA, Lee JC, et al. EGFR mutations in lung cancer: correlation with clinical response to gefitinib therapy. *Science* 2004 Jun 4;304(5676):1497–1500.
62. Pham D, Kris MG, Riely GJ, et al. Use of cigarette-smoking history to estimate the likelihood of mutations in epidermal growth factor receptor gene exons 19 and 21 in lung adenocarcinomas. *J Clin Oncol* 2006 Apr 10;24(11):1700–1704.
63. Sugio K, Uramoto H, Ono K, et al. Mutations within the tyrosine kinase domain of EGFR gene specifically occur in lung adenocarcinoma patients with a low exposure of tobacco smoking. *Br J Cancer* 2006 Mar 27;94(6):896–903.
64. Jackman DM, Yeap BY, Lindeman NI, et al. Phase II clinical trial of chemotherapy-naive patients > or = 70 years of age treated with erlotinib for advanced non-small-cell lung cancer. *J Clin Oncol* 2007 Mar 1;25(7):760–766.
65. Reck M, Crinò L. Advances in anti-VEGF and anti-EGFR therapy for advanced non-small cell lung cancer. *Lung Cancer* 2009 Jan;63(1):1–9.
66. Suzuki M, Shigematsu H, Hiroshima K, et al. Epidermal growth factor receptor expression status in lung cancer correlates with its mutation. *Hum Pathol* 2005 Oct;36(10):1127–1134.
67. Meert AP, Martin B, Delmotte P, et al. The role of EGF-R expression on patient survival in lung cancer: a systematic review with meta-analysis. *Eur Respir J* 2002 Oct;20(4):975–981.
68. Bunn PA Jr, Helfrich B, Soriano AF, et al. Expression of Her-2/neu in human lung cancer cell lines by immunohistochemistry and fluorescence in situ hybridization and its relationship to in vitro cytotoxicity by trastuzumab and chemotherapeutic agents. *Clin Cancer Res* 2001 Oct;7(10):3239–3250.
69. Lee JW, Soung YH, Kim SY, et al. ERBB2 kinase domain mutation in the lung squamous cell carcinoma. *Cancer Lett* 2006 Jun 8;237(1):89–94.
70. Stephens P, Hunter C, Bignell G, et al. Lung cancer: intragenic ERBB2 kinase mutations in tumours. *Nature* 2004 Sep 30;431(7008): 525–526.
71. Hsieh CC, Chow KC, Fahn HJ, et al. Prognostic significance of HER-2/neu overexpression in stage I adenocarcinoma of lung. *Ann Thorac Surg* 1998 Oct;66(4):1159–1163; discussion 1163–1164.
72. Saad RS, Liu Y, Han H, et al. Prognostic significance of HER2/neu, p53, and vascular endothelial growth factor expression in early stage conventional adenocarcinoma and bronchioloalveolar carcinoma of the lung. *Mod Pathol* 2004 Oct;17(10):1235–1242.
73. Sekido Y, Fong KM, Minna JD. Molecular genetics of lung cancer. *Annu Rev Med* 2003;54:73–87.
74. Selvaggi G, Scagliotti GV, Torri V, et al. HER-2/neu overexpression in patients with radically resected nonsmall cell lung carcinoma. Impact on long-term survival. *Cancer* 2002 May 15;94(10):2669–2674.
75. Fontanini G, Faviana P, Lucchi M, et al. A high vascular count and overexpression of vascular endothelial growth factor are associated with unfavourable prognosis in operated small cell lung carcinoma. *Br J Cancer* 2002 Feb 12;86(4):558–563.
76. Han H, Silverman JF, Santucci TS, et al. Vascular endothelial growth factor expression in stage I non-small cell lung cancer correlates with neoangiogenesis and a poor prognosis. *Ann Surg Oncol* 2001 Jan-Feb; 8(1):72–79.
77. Singhal S, Vachani A, Antin-Ozerkis D, et al. Prognostic implications of cell cycle, apoptosis, and angiogenesis biomarkers in non-small cell lung cancer: a review. *Clin Cancer Res* 2005 Jun 1;11(11): 3974–3986.
78. Azim HA Jr, Ganti AK. Targeted therapy in advanced non-small cell lung cancer (NSCLC): where do we stand? *Cancer Treat Rev* 2006 Dec;32(8):630–636.
79. Aita M, Fasola G, Defferrari C, et al. Targeting the VEGF pathway: Antiangiogenic strategies in the treatment of non-small cell lung cancer. *Crit Rev Oncol Hematol* 2008 Dec;68(3):183–196.
80. Arenberg DA, Polverini PJ, Kunkel SL, et al. The role of CXC chemokines in the regulation of angiogenesis in non-small cell lung cancer. *J Leukoc Biol* 1997 Nov;62(5):554–562.
81. Yuan A, Yang PC, Yu CJ, et al. Interleukin-8 messenger ribonucleic acid expression correlates with tumor progression, tumor angiogenesis, patient survival, and timing of relapse in non-small-cell lung cancer. *Am J Respir Crit Care Med* 2000 Nov;162(5):1957–1963.
82. Takanami I, Imamura T, Yamamoto Y, et al. Usefulness of platelet-derived growth factor as a prognostic factor in pulmonary adenocarcinoma. *J Surg Oncol* 1995 Jan;58(1):40–43.
83. Nissen LJ, Cao R, Hedlund EM, et al. Angiogenic factors FGF2 and PDGF-BB synergistically promote murine tumor neovascularization and metastasis. *J Clin Invest* 2007 Oct;117(10):2766–2777.
84. Brown PD, Bloxidge RE, Stuart NS, et al. Association between expression of activated 72-kilodalton gelatinase and tumor spread in non-small-cell lung carcinoma. *J Natl Cancer Inst* 1993 Apr 7;85(7):574–578.
85. Passlick B, Sienel W, Seen-Hibler R, et al. Overexpression of matrix metalloproteinase 2 predicts unfavorable outcome in early-stage non-small cell lung cancer. *Clin Cancer Res* 2000 Oct;6(10):3944–3948.
86. Liu D, Nakano J, Ishikawa S, et al. Overexpression of matrix metalloproteinase-7 (MMP-7) correlates with tumor proliferation, and a poor prognosis in non-small cell lung cancer. *Lung Cancer* 2007 Dec;58(3): 384–391.
87. Cox G, Jones JL, O'Byrne KJ. Matrix metalloproteinase 9 and the epidermal growth factor signal pathway in operable non-small cell lung cancer. *Clin Cancer Res* 2000 Jun;6(6):2349–2355.
88. Shou Y, Hirano T, Gong Y, et al. Influence of angiogenetic factors and matrix metalloproteinases upon tumour progression in non-small-cell lung cancer. *Br J Cancer* 2001 Nov 30;85(11):1706–1712.
89. Sienel W, Hellers J, Morresi-Hauf A, et al. Prognostic impact of matrix metalloproteinase-9 in operable non-small cell lung cancer. *Int J Cancer* 2003 Feb 20;103(5):647–651.
90. Sienel W, Polzer B, Elshawi K, et al. Cellular localization of EMMPRIN predicts prognosis of patients with operable lung adenocarcinoma independent from MMP-2 and MMP-9. *Mod Pathol* 2008 Sep;21(19):1130–1138.
91. Katakura H, Takenaka K, Nakagawa M, et al. Maspin gene expression is a significant prognostic factor in resected non-small cell lung cancer (NSCLC). Maspin in NSCLC. *Lung Cancer* 2006 Mar;51(3): 323–328.

92. Takanami I, Abiko T, Koizumi S. Expression of maspin in non-small-cell lung cancer: correlation with clinical features. *Clin Lung Cancer* 2008 Nov;9(6):361–366.
93. Zheng HC, Saito H, Masuda S, et al. Cytoplasmic and nuclear maspin expression in lung carcinomas: an immunohistochemical study using tissue microarrays. *Appl Immunohistochem Mol Morphol* 2008 Oct;16(5):459–465.
94. Nakagawa M, Katakura H, Adachi M, et al. Maspin expression and its clinical significance in non-small cell lung cancer. *Ann Surg Oncol* 2006 Nov;13(11):1517–1523.
95. Lonardo F, Li X, Siddiq F, et al. Maspin nuclear localization is linked to favorable morphological features in pulmonary adenocarcinoma. *Lung Cancer* 2006 Jan;51(1):31–39.
96. Meyerson M, Carbone D. Genomic and proteomic profiling of lung cancers: lung cancer classification in the age of targeted therapy. *J Clin Oncol* 2005 May 10;23(14):3219–3226.
97. Dobbin KK, Beer DG, Meyerson M, et al. Interlaboratory comparability study of cancer gene expression analysis using oligonucleotide microarrays. *Clin Cancer Res* 2005 Jan 15;11(2 Pt 1):565–572.
98. Granville CA, Dennis PA. An overview of lung cancer genomics and proteomics. *Am J Respir Cell Mol Biol* 2005 Mar;32(3):169–176.
99. Bhattacharjee A, Richards WG, Staunton J, et al. Classification of human lung carcinomas by mRNA expression profiling reveals distinct adenocarcinoma subclasses. *Proc Natl Acad Sci U S A* 2001 Nov 20; 98(24):13790–13795.
100. Hayes DN, Monti S, Parmigiani G, et al. Gene expression profiling reveals reproducible human lung adenocarcinoma subtypes in multiple independent patient cohorts. *J Clin Oncol* 2006 Nov 1;24(31): 5079–5090.
101. Petty RD, Nicolson MC, Kerr KM, et al. Gene expression profiling in non-small cell lung cancer: from molecular mechanisms to clinical application. *Clin Cancer Res* 2004 May 15;10(10):3237–3248.
102. Beer DG, Kardia SL, Huang CC, et al. Gene-expression profiles predict survival of patients with lung adenocarcinoma. *Nat Med* 2002 Aug;8(8):816–824.
103. Raponi M, Zhang Y, Yu J, et al. Gene expression signatures for predicting prognosis of squamous cell and adenocarcinomas of the lung. *Cancer Res* 2006 Aug 1;66(15):7466–7472.
104. Iwao K, Watanabe T, Fujiwara Y, et al. Isolation of a novel human lung-specific gene, LUNX, a potential molecular marker for detection of micrometastasis in non-small-cell lung cancer. *Int J Cancer* 2001 Feb 15;91(4):433–437.
105. Travis WD, Brambilla E, Müller-Hermelink HK, et al., eds. *World Health Organisation Classification of Tumors. Pathology and Genetics of Tumours of the Lung, Pleura, Thymus and Heart.* 4th Ed. Geneva: WHO, 2004.
106. Yousem SA, Beasley MB. Bronchioloalveolar carcinoma: a review of current concepts and evolving issues. *Arch Pathol Lab Med* 2007 Jul;131(7):1027–1032.
107. Balsara BR, Testa JR. Chromosomal imbalances in human lung cancer. *Oncogene* 2002 Oct 7;21(45):6877–6883.
108. Luk C, Tsao MS, Bayani J, et al. Molecular cytogenetic analysis of non-small cell lung carcinoma by spectral karyotyping and comparative genomic hybridization. *Cancer Genet Cytogenet* 2001 Mar;125(2): 87–99.
109. Sato S, Nakamura Y, Tsuchiya E. Difference of allelotype between squamous cell carcinoma and adenocarcinoma of the lung. *Cancer Res* 1994 Nov 1;54(21):5652–5655.
110. Shiseki M, Kohno T, Nishikawa R, et al. Frequent allelic losses on chromosomes 2q, 18q, and 22q in advanced non-small cell lung carcinoma. *Cancer Res* 1994 Nov 1;54(21):5643–5648.
111. Fong KM, Sekido Y, Minna JD. Molecular pathogenesis of lung cancer. *J Thorac Cardiovasc Surg* 1999 Dec;118(6):1136–1152.
112. Salgia R, Skarin AT. Molecular abnormalities in lung cancer. *J Clin Oncol* 1998 Mar;16(3):1207–1217.
113. Petersen S, Heckert C, Rudolf J, et al. Gene expression profiling of advanced lung cancer. *Int J Cancer* 2000 May 15;86(4):512–517.
114. Garber ME, Troyanskaya OG, Schluens K, et al. Diversity of gene expression in adenocarcinoma of the lung. *Proc Natl Acad Sci U S A* 2001 Nov 20;98(24):13784–13789.
114a. Nacht M, Dracheva T, Gao Y, et al. Molecular characteristics of non-small cell lung cancer. *Proc Natl Acad Sci U S A* 2001;98(26):15203–15208.
115. McDoniels-Silvers AL, Nimri CF, Stoner GD, et al. Differential gene expression in human lung adenocarcinomas and squamous cell carcinomas. *Clin Cancer Res* 2002 Apr;8(4):1127–1138.
116. Nakamura H, Saji H, Ogata A, et al. cDNA microarray analysis of gene expression in pathologic Stage IA nonsmall cell lung carcinomas. *Cancer* 2003 Jun 1;97(11):2798–2805.
117. Wikman H, Kettunen E, Seppänen JK, et al. Identification of differentially expressed genes in pulmonary adenocarcinoma by using cDNA array. *Oncogene* 2002 Aug 22;21(37):5804–5813.
118. Kang SH, Choi HH, Kim SG, et al. Transcriptional inactivation of the tissue inhibitor of metalloproteinase-3 gene by dna hypermethylation of the 5′-CpG island in human gastric cancer cell lines. *Int J Cancer* 2000 Jun 1;86(5):632–635.
119. Karameris A, Panagou P, Tsilalis T, et al. Association of expression of metalloproteinases and their inhibitors with the metastatic potential of squamous-cell lung carcinomas. A molecular and immunohistochemical study. *Am J Respir Crit Care Med* 1997 Dec;156(6):1930–1936.
120. Nawrocki B, Polette M, Marchand V, et al. Expression of matrix metalloproteinases and their inhibitors in human bronchopulmonary carcinomas: quantificative and morphological analyses. *Int J Cancer* 1997 Aug 7;72(4):556–564.
121. Heighway J, Knapp T, Boyce L, et al. Expression profiling of primary non-small cell lung cancer for target identification. *Oncogene* 2002 Oct 31; 21(50):7749–7763.
122. Miura K, Bowman ED, Simon R, et al. Laser capture microdissection and microarray expression analysis of lung adenocarcinoma reveals tobacco smoking- and prognosis-related molecular profiles. *Cancer Res* 2002 Jun 1;62(11):3244–3250.
123. Lerman MI, Minna JD. The 630-kb lung cancer homozygous deletion region on human chromosome 3p21.3: identification and evaluation of the resident candidate tumor suppressor genes. The International Lung Cancer Chromosome 3p21.3 Tumor Suppressor Gene Consortium. *Cancer Res* 2000 Nov 1;60(21):6116–6133.
124. Wigle DA, Jurisica I, Radulovich N, et al. Molecular profiling of non-small cell lung cancer and correlation with disease-free survival. *Cancer Res* 2002 Jun 1;62(11):3005–3008.
125. Kikuchi T, Daigo Y, Katagiri T, et al. Expression profiles of non-small cell lung cancers on cDNA microarrays: identification of genes for prediction of lymph-node metastasis and sensitivity to anti-cancer drugs. *Oncogene* 2003 Apr 10;22(14):2192–2205.
126. Inamura K, Togashi Y, Okui M, et al. HOXB2 as a novel prognostic indicator for stage I lung adenocarcinomas [erratum in: *J Thorac Oncol* 2008; 3(1):100. Ishikawa, Yuichi (added)]. *J Thorac Oncol* 2007;2(9):802–807.
127. Hoang CD, D'Cunha J, Tawfic SH, et al. Expression profiling of non-small cell lung carcinoma identifies metastatic genotypes based on lymph node tumor burden. *J Thorac Cardiovasc Surg* 2004;127(5):1332–1341; discussion 1342.
128. Xi L, Coello MC, Litle VR, et al. A combination of molecular markers accurately detects lymph node metastasis in non-small cell lung cancer patients. *Clin Cancer Res* 2006;12(8):2484–2491.
129. Fukata M, Kaibuchi K. Rho-family GTPases in cadherin-mediated cell-cell adhesion. *Nat Rev Mol Cell Biol* 2001 Dec;2(12):887–897.
130. Ichigotani Y, Yokozaki S, Fukuda Y, et al. Forced expression of NESH suppresses motility and metastatic dissemination of malignant cells. *Cancer Res* 2002 Apr 15;62(8):2215–2219.
131. Meyaard L, van der Vuurst de Vries AR, de Ruiter T, et al. The epithelial cellular adhesion molecule (Ep-CAM) is a ligand for the leukocyte-associated immunoglobulin-like receptor (LAIR). *J Exp Med* 2001 Jul 2; 194(1):107–112.
132. Wieland I, Arden KC, Michels D, et al. Isolation of DICE1: a gene frequently affected by LOH and downregulated in lung carcinomas. *Oncogene* 1999 Aug 12;18(32):4530–4537.

133. Xi L, Lyons-Weiler J, Coello MC, et al. Prediction of lymph node metastasis by analysis of gene expression profiles in primary lung adenocarcinomas. *Clin Cancer Res* 2005 Jun 1;11(11):4128–4135.
134. Potti A, Mukherjee S, Petersen R, et al. A genomic strategy to refine prognosis in early-stage non-small-cell lung cancer. *N Engl J Med* 2006 Aug 10;355(6):570–580.
135. Chen HY, Yu SL, Chen CH, et al. A five-gene signature and clinical outcome in non-small-cell lung cancer. *N Engl J Med* 2007 Jan 4;356(1):11–20.
136. Furukawa T, Sunamura M, Motoi F, et al. Potential tumor suppressive pathway involving DUSP6/MKP-3 in pancreatic cancer. *Am J Pathol* 2003 Jun;162(6):1807–1815.
137. Kumar A, Commane M, Flickinger TW, et al. Defective TNF-alpha-induced apoptosis in STAT1-null cells due to low constitutive levels of caspases. *Science* 1997 Nov 28;278(5343):1630–1632.
138. Mahabeleshwar GH, Das R, Kundu GC. Tyrosine kinase, p56lck-induced cell motility, and urokinase-type plasminogen activator secretion involve activation of epidermal growth factor receptor/extracellular signal regulated kinase pathways. *J Biol Chem* 2004 Mar 12; 279(11):9733–9742.
139. Mahabeleshwar GH, Kundu GC. Tyrosine kinase p56lck regulates cell motility and nuclear factor kappaB-mediated secretion of urokinase type plasminogen activator through tyrosine phosphorylation of IkappaBalpha following hypoxia/reoxygenation. *J Biol Chem* 2003 Dec 26;278(52):52598–52612.
140. Muller-Tidow C, Diederichs S, Bulk E, et al. Identification of metastasis-associated receptor tyrosine kinases in non-small cell lung cancer. *Cancer Res* 2005 Mar 1;65(5):1778–1782.
141. Yu H, Jove R. The STATs of cancer—new molecular targets come of age. *Nat Rev Cancer* 2004 Feb;4(2):97–105.
142. Zamoyska R, Basson A, Filby A, et al. The influence of the src-family kinases, Lck and Fyn, on T cell differentiation, survival and activation. *Immunol Rev* 2003 Feb;191:107–118.
143. Herbst RS, Lippman SM. Molecular signatures of lung cancer—toward personalized therapy. *N Engl J Med* 2007 Jan 4;356(1):76–78.
144. Potti A, Nevins JR. Utilization of genomic signatures to direct use of primary chemotherapy. *Curr Opin Genet Dev* 2008 Feb;18(1):62–67.
145. Sun Z, Wigle DA, Yang P. Non-overlapping and non-cell-type-specific gene expression signatures predict lung cancer survival. *J Clin Oncol* 2008 Feb 20;26(6):877–883.
146. Skrzypski M, Jassem E, Taron M, et al. Three-gene expression signature predicts survival in early-stage squamous cell carcinoma of the lung. *Clin Cancer Res* 2008 Aug 1;14(15):4794–4799.
147. Raz DJ, Ray MR, Kim JY, et al. A multigene assay is prognostic of survival in patients with early-stage lung adenocarcinoma. *Clin Cancer Res* 2008 Sep 1;14(17):5565–5570.
148. Director's Challenge Consortium for the Molecular Classification of Lung Adenocarcinoma, Shedden K, Taylor JM, et al. Gene expression-based survival prediction in lung adenocarcinoma: a multi-site, blinded validation study. *Nat Med* 2008 Aug;14(8):822–827.
149. Belinsky SA. Gene-promoter hypermethylation as a biomarker in lung cancer. *Nat Rev Cancer* 2004 Sep;4(9):707–717.
150. Kim DH, Nelson HH, Wiencke JK, et al. Promoter methylation of DAP-kinase: association with advanced stage in non-small cell lung cancer. *Oncogene* 2001 Mar 29;20(14):1765–1770.
151. Lu C, Soria JC, Tang X, et al. Prognostic factors in resected stage I non-small-cell lung cancer: a multivariate analysis of six molecular markers. *J Clin Oncol* 2004 Nov 15;22(22):4575–4583.
152. Toyooka KO, Toyooka S, Virmani AK, et al. Loss of expression and aberrant methylation of the CDH13 (H-cadherin) gene in breast and lung carcinomas. *Cancer Res* 2001 Jun 1;61(11):4556–4560.
153. Zöchbauer-Müller S, Fong KM, Virmani AK, et al. Aberrant promoter methylation of multiple genes in non-small cell lung cancers. *Cancer Res* 2001 Jan 1;61(1):249–255.
154. Liu D, Huang C, Kameyama K, et al. E-cadherin expression associated with differentiation and prognosis in patients with non-small cell lung cancer. *Ann Thorac Surg* 2001 Mar;71(3):949–954; discussion 954–955.
155. Bearzatto A, Conte D, Frattini M, et al. p16(INK4A) Hypermethylation detected by fluorescent methylation-specific PCR in plasmas from non-small cell lung cancer. *Clin Cancer Res* 2002 Dec;8(12):3782–3787.
156. Digel W, Lübbert M. DNA methylation disturbances as novel therapeutic target in lung cancer: preclinical and clinical results. *Crit Rev Oncol Hematol* 2005 Jul;55(1):1–11.
157. Kim DH, Nelson HH, Wiencke JK, et al. p16(INK4a) and histology-specific methylation of CpG islands by exposure to tobacco smoke in non-small cell lung cancer. *Cancer Res* 2001 Apr 15;61(8):3419–3424.
158. Toyooka S, Suzuki M, Maruyama R, et al. The relationship between aberrant methylation and survival in non-small-cell lung cancers. *Br J Cancer* 2004 Aug 16;91(4):771–774.
159. Burbee DG, Forgacs E, Zöchbauer-Müller S, et al. Epigenetic inactivation of RASSF1A in lung and breast cancers and malignant phenotype suppression. *J Natl Cancer Inst* 2001 May 2;93(9):691–699.
160. Dammann R, Li C, Yoon JH, et al. Epigenetic inactivation of a RAS association domain family protein from the lung tumour suppressor locus 3p21.3. *Nat Genet* 2000 Jul;25(3):315–319.
161. Harden SV, Tokumaru Y, Westra WH, et al. Gene promoter hypermethylation in tumors and lymph nodes of stage I lung cancer patients. *Clin Cancer Res* 2003 Apr;9(4):1370–1375.
162. Gu J, Berman D, Lu C, et al. Aberrant promoter methylation profile and association with survival in patients with non-small cell lung cancer. *Clin Cancer Res* 2006 Dec 15;12(24):7329–7338.
163. Brock MV, Hooker CM, Ota-Machida E, et al. DNA methylation markers and early recurrence in stage I lung cancer. *N Engl J Med* 2008 Mar 13;358(11):1118–1128.
164. Anderson L, Seilhamer J. A comparison of selected mRNA and protein abundances in human liver. *Electrophoresis* 1997 Mar-Apr; 18(3–4):533–537.
165. Chen G, Gharib TG, Huang CC, et al. Discordant protein and mRNA expression in lung adenocarcinomas. *Mol Cell Proteomics* 2002 Apr;1(4):304–313.
166. Oh JM, Brichory F, Puravs E, et al. A database of protein expression in lung cancer. *Proteomics* 2001 Oct;1(10):1303–1319.
167. Li C, Xiao Z, Chen Z, et al. Proteome analysis of human lung squamous carcinoma. *Proteomics* 2006 Jan;6(2):547–558.
168. Yanagisawa K, Shyr Y, Xu BJ, et al. Proteomic patterns of tumour subsets in non-small-cell lung cancer. *Lancet* 2003 Aug 9;362(9382): 433–439.
169. Gharib TG, Chen G, Wang H, et al. Proteomic analysis of cytokeratin isoforms uncovers association with survival in lung adenocarcinoma. *Neoplasia* 2002 Sep-Oct;4(5):440–448.
170. Chen G, Gharib TG, Wang H, et al. Protein profiles associated with survival in lung adenocarcinoma. *Proc Natl Acad Sci U S A* 2003 Nov 11; 100(23):13537–13542.
171. Yanagisawa K, Tomida S, Shimada Y, et al. A 25-signal proteomic signature and outcome for patients with resected non-small-cell lung cancer. *J Natl Cancer Inst* 2007 Jun 6;99(11):858–867.
172. Lau NC, Lim LP, Weinstein EG, et al. An abundant class of tiny RNAs with probable regulatory roles in Caenorhabditis elegans. *Science* 2001 Oct 26;294(5543):858–862.
173. Johnson SM, Grosshans H, Shingara J, et al. RAS is regulated by the let-7 microRNA family. *Cell* 2005 Mar 11;120(5):635–647.
174. Bartel DP. MicroRNAs: genomics, biogenesis, mechanism, and function. *Cell* 2004 Jan 23;116(2):281–297.
175. Gregory RI, Shiekhattar R. MicroRNA biogenesis and cancer. *Cancer Res* 2005 May 1;65(9):3509–3512.
176. Yi R, Qin Y, Macara IG, et al. Exportin-5 mediates the nuclear export of pre-microRNAs and short hairpin RNAs. *Genes Dev* 2003 Dec 15; 17(24):3011–3016.
177. Lee Y, Jeon K, Lee JT, et al. MicroRNA maturation: stepwise processing and subcellular localization. *Embo J* 2002 Sep 2;21(17):4663–4670.
178. Lee Y, Ahn C, Han J, et al. The nuclear RNase III Drosha initiates microRNA processing. *Nature* 2003 Sep 25;425(6956):415–419.
179. Eder M, Scherr M. MicroRNA and lung cancer. *N Engl J Med* 2005 Jun 9;352(23):2446–2448.

180. Calin GA, Croce CM. MicroRNA signatures in human cancers. *Nat Rev Cancer* 2006 Nov;6(11):857–866.
181. Yanaihara N, Caplen N, Bowman E, et al. Unique microRNA molecular profiles in lung cancer diagnosis and prognosis. *Cancer Cell* 2006 Mar;9(3):189–198.
182. Markou A, Tsaroucha EG, Kaklamanis L, et al. Prognostic value of mature microRNA-21 and microRNA-205 overexpression in non-small cell lung cancer by quantitative real-time RT-PCR. *Clin Chem* 2008 Oct;54(10):1696–1704.
183. Yu SL, Chen HY, Chang GC, et al. MicroRNA signature predicts survival and relapse in lung cancer. *Cancer Cell* 2008 Jan;13(1):48–57.
184. Takamizawa J, Konishi H, Yanagisawa K, et al. Reduced expression of the let-7 microRNAs in human lung cancers in association with shortened postoperative survival. *Cancer Res* 2004 Jun 1;64(11): 3753–3756.
185. Weiss GJ, Bemis LT, Nakajima E, et al. EGFR regulation by microRNA in lung cancer: correlation with clinical response and survival to gefitinib and EGFR expression in cell lines. *Ann Oncol* 2008 Jun; 19(6):1053–1059.
186. Anguiano A, Potti A. Genomic signatures individualize therapeutic decisions in non-small-cell lung cancer. *Expert Rev Mol Diagn* 2007 Nov; 7(6):837–844.

CHAPTER 11

Kerstin W. Sinkevicius
Stephen J. Curtis
Carla F. Kim

Examining the Cancer Stem Cell Hypothesis in Human Lung Cancers

The cancer stem cell (CSC) hypothesis, which suggests that tumors are maintained by a population of cells possessing stem cell characteristics, has emerged as an attractive explanation for tumor growth, recurrence, and metastasis. CSCs in human leukemia, breast, brain, colon, and pancreatic cancers have been identified in transplantation assays.[1–6] Whereas the incidence of oncogenic mutations, such as those in K-ras or the epidermal growth factor receptor (EGFR), in human lung cancers has been well described, the role of CSCs in lung tumors remains poorly defined. An important goal for lung cancer research is now to determine the role of CSCs in lung tumorigenesis. An improved understanding of the cellular mechanisms of lung CSC renewal should elucidate new therapeutic approaches for lung cancer.

THE CANCER STEM CELL HYPOTHESIS

Although many current cancer therapies are based on their ability to kill most cells within a tumor, it has been recognized for more than 30 years that not all cells within a tumor are alike. Studies have shown that only a fraction of cells within a tumor can be propagated in patients, mouse transplants, or cell cultures.[7–10] These rare *clonogenic* cancer cells were hypothesized to arise in a stochastic fashion: although the overall occurrence is rare, any cell within the tumor is equally likely to exhibit clonogenic activity. An alternative hypothesis to explain these findings is that a rare subpopulation exists within tumors, and that these rare tumor cells have unique biological characteristics that provide clonogenic activity. In support of the latter hypothesis, it has been recently demonstrated that several types of hematopoietic and solid tumors harbor a distinct subpopulation of cells called CSCs that can propagate the tumor phenotype in vivo.[1–6,11] These cells are called CSCs because the same molecular markers used to isolate the normal tissue stem cells could be used to isolate clonogenic tumor cells in some tissues, the cells could be passaged serially through mice (demonstrating their ability to self-renew, a hallmark property of stem cells), and the isolated tumor cell population gave rise to a heterogeneous tumor (suggesting an ability to differentiate, a second hallmark property of stem cells).[12]

The CSC hypothesis has also emerged as an attractive explanation for tumor resistance to chemotherapy, recurrence, and metastasis. It has been hypothesized that CSCs have distinct biological mechanisms that render them more resistant to chemotherapy than other cancer cells, explaining the refractory nature of many tumors to treatment.[12–14] Specifically, CSCs are hypothesized to be resistant to chemotherapy because they may be quiescent and may efficiently export drugs, like stem cells in normal tissues.[15] CSCs may also be the cells that are required to generate metastases. For example, the pathways responsible for the dissemination and homing of normal stem cells during development may be aberrantly upregulated in CSCs. Therapeutic strategies that specifically eliminate the CSC population may therefore be more effective than standard means of therapy.[16–19]

STRATEGIES FOR IDENTIFICATION OF CANCER STEM CELLS

Methods used in identification and characterization of stem cell populations from normal adult tissues have proven to be useful in uncovering CSC populations. The most widely used technique for isolating stem cells has been fluorescent-activated cell sorting (FACS) using a combination of cell-surface markers that select cells with markers of more primitive cells and exclude cells of differentiated cell lineages, followed by transplantation of sorted cancer cells into immunodeficient mice (Table 11.1). For example, CSCs were first identified in human acute myeloid leukemias as the cancer cells that had the same surface marker status as human hematopoietic stem cells (CD34+ CD38−).[1] CD133, a positive marker of hematopoietic stem cells and neural stem cells, has been used as a marker of CSCs from brain and colon cancer.[3–5] CSCs have also been shown to exhibit similarities to normal stem cells

TABLE 11.1 Summary of Cell-Surface Markers Used to Prospectively Isolate Putative Cancer Stem Cells from Multiple Tissues*

Type of Cancer	CSC Expression Pattern	Reference(s)
Leukemia	CD34+ CD38−	1,89–91
Breast	CD44+ CD24−/low	2
Brain	CD133+	92
Pancreatic	CD44+ CD24+ ESA+	44
Colon	CD133+	4,6
Head and neck	CD44+	93
Lung	CD133+	94

*The marker-expression patterns used to enrich for cells with tumor-propagating potential from multiple types of cancer are shown.

+, cells expressing this marker; −, cells not expressing this marker; CSC, cancer stem cell; ESA, epithelial-specific antigen.

with regard to their ability to self-renew in serial-plating experiments in culture[5,20–24] as well as their demonstrated activation of developmental pathways known to function in normal stem cells. For example, chronic myelogenous leukemia CSCs exhibit Wnt pathway activation as determined by elevated levels of nuclear β-catenin,[25] and mixed-lineage leukemia CSCs are granulocyte-macrophage progenitors that share a gene-expression program with hematopoietic stem cells.[24] Several pathways known to be crucial for development, such as the Wnt, Hedgehog, Notch, and Polycomb-group protein pathways, have been implicated in adult stem cell self-renewal, and dysregulation of these pathways contributes to many types of cancer.[26,27]

NON–SMALL CELL LUNG CANCER

Lung cancer remains the major cause of death from cancer worldwide,[28] and relatively little is known about the molecular heterogeneity of the cells within lung cancers. Lung cancer can be divided into two histopathological groups: 80% are non–small cell lung cancers (NSCLCs), and 20% exhibit neuroendocrine features. NSCLCs can be further subdivided into adenocarcinomas (50% to 60%), squamous cell carcinomas (20% to 25%), and large cell carcinomas. The average 5-year survival rate for NSCLC is only 16% because most lung cancers are refractory to chemotherapeutics or quickly become resistant to therapeutic response.[29] Also contributing to lung cancer morbidity, most NSCLC patients already have advanced diseases at the time of diagnosis; 21% of diagnosed cases have distant metastases in the brain, bone, liver, or adrenal glands.[29–31] Surgery or therapies that treat primary lung tumors rarely prevent metastases. For example, 72% of patients who had NSCLC tumors surgically removed eventually develop distant metastases, most commonly in the bone or brain.[32] Lung CSCs may be responsible for these observations, and an improved understanding of the cellular mechanisms operating in lung cancers should elucidate new therapeutic approaches.

Therapeutic Resistance of Lung Adenocarcinomas Harboring Epidermal Growth Factor Receptor Mutations The recent treatment success of gefitinib (Iressa) and erlotinib (Tarceva), two small molecule inhibitors of EGFR, in a fraction of patients with NSCLC has solidified the premise that EGFR is an important molecule in the pathogenesis of lung cancer (see Chapter 49). Several groups have independently identified frequent somatic mutations in the kinase domain of the EGFR gene in lung adenocarcinoma. These occurred in up to 10% of lung adenocarcinoma specimens sequenced in the United States and up to 30% of those sequenced in Asia. The mutations are associated with sensitivity to both gefitinib and erlotinib, explaining in part the rare and dramatic clinical responses to treatment with these agents.[33–35] Subsequent studies by multiple groups have now identified EGFR kinase domain mutations from more than 600 lung cancer patients. These mutations cluster in four groups or regions: exon 19 deletions, exon 20 insertions, and point mutations at G719S and L858R. Exon 19 deletions and exon 21 L858R point mutations account for more than 85% of all EGFR kinase domain gefitinib- and erlotinib-sensitizing mutations.

In the clinical setting, although these EGFR-mutant NSCLCs initially respond rapidly and dramatically to gefitinib and erlotinib, tumors eventually become refractory to treatment, and nearly all patients who initially respond to these drugs subsequently relapse.[36–38] Three studies identified EGFR T790M mutations in approximately 50% of the tumors from patients who relapsed.[39–41] These mutants, when combined with sensitizing EGFR kinase domain mutation, permit the continued growth of tumor cells in the presence of erlotinib and gefitinib. Structural studies suggest that the T790M mutation introduces a bulky methionine residue in the EGFR kinase domain, which sterically hinders tyrosine kinase inhibitor (TKI) binding.[36–38] Whereas gefitinib and erlotinib are reversible inhibitors that mimic adenosine triphosphate (ATP), irreversible inhibitors such as HKI-272 or BIBW2992 mimic ATP and covalently bind to EGFR, enabling them to inhibit EGFR kinase activity even in the presence of T790M.[42–44] Although irreversible inhibitors are currently being tested in clinical trials, animal models suggest that tumors will eventually become refractory to these treatments as well.[44] Thus, it is crucial to determine the cellular basis of lung adenocarcinoma resistance to treatment and develop new therapeutic strategies that will not be susceptible to resistance mechanisms.

Evidence for Non–Small Cell Lung Cancer Stem Cells Several pieces of evidence suggest that NSCLC tumors, including adenocarcinomas, contain a rare population of cells with stem cell characteristics. The initial sensitivity of human adenocarcinomas with activating EGFR mutations to EGFR TKIs and the acquired resistance to these treatments suggest that drug-resistant CSCs may be present in these tumors.[36–38] *Side population cells*, isolated by their ability to efflux Hoechst dye, were identified in six human NSCLC cell lines. These cells exhibit several stem cell characteristics, including increased drug-exporting transporter expression, enriched tumor-initiating capacity, and resistance to multiple chemotherapies.[45] Additionally, CD133+ cells from human lung tumors were recently shown to form self-renewing spheres in culture that could propagate tumors when transplanted subcutaneously into immunodeficient mice.[46] Importantly, although these studies support the likelihood of CSCs in lung cancers, the isolation and characterization of a population of human lung cancer cells that can serially passage the lung tumor phenotype in the lung microenvironment has not been reported, and the operation of pathways that regulate stem cells in advanced lung tumors has not been understood.

Identification of Normal Lung Stem Cells Recent identification of putative endogenous and extrinsic lung stem cell populations has added to the diversity of the respiratory system.[47–52] The pulmonary system contains various epithelial cell populations. Each population resides in a distinct anatomical location, or niche.[53] Basal cells, secretory Goblet cells, submucosal glands, and ciliated cells line the trachea and upper airways. The nonciliated columnar Clara cells that line the bronchioles and terminal bronchioles secrete surfactants to aide in oxygen exchange and provide a protective epithelial barrier in the airways. The alveolar epithelium is composed of alveolar type II (AT2) cells, the cuboidal epithelial cells that produce surfactants and the resulting surface tension required for gas exchange, as well as alveolar type I (AT1) cells, the flat epithelial cells that deliver oxygen to the blood. Human and murine lung adenocarcinomas most frequently arise in the distal lung where AT2 and Clara cells reside, and these tumors are frequently positive for molecular markers of either AT2 cells or Clara cells.

Our laboratory determined that cells expressing both the AT2 cell marker, prosurfactant protein-C (SP-C), and the Clara cell marker (CCSP [also known as CCA], CC10, uterglobin, Scgb1a1) are present in normal murine lung, and that they constitute a stem cell population in the distal lung epithelium. These cells, named bronchioalveolar stem cells (BASCs), reside in the bronchioalveolar duct junction (BADJ) in terminal bronchioles, which is the last portion of the airway before the alveolar space. BASCs can be isolated from mouse lung using a FACS methodology based on the presence of the surface markers (stem cell antigen-1 [Sca-1] and CD34) and the absence of the hematopoietic and endothelial cell markers (CD45 and CD31), respectively. BASCs self-renew over multiple passages and give rise to bronchiolar and alveolar cells in culture, providing evidence that they are a stem cell population. Further supporting the hypothesis that BASCs are stem cells, they are quiescent in normal lung and proliferate in response to lung injury.[47] Notably, Sca-1 cannot be used to isolate human cell populations; separate studies are underway in our laboratory to identify additional markers of murine BASCs that may help in identification of human BASCs and human lung CSCs.

Role of Bronchioalveolar Stem Cells in Murine Lung Tumorigenesis To examine lung stem cells and their role in cancer, we have used a mouse model that accurately recapitulates human lung adenocarcinoma. K-ras, a component of the Ras signal transduction pathway, functions in multiple aspects of growth control and is mutated to an oncogenic form in 15% to 50% of human lung adenocarcinomas.[54–56] In "Lox-Stop-Lox" *K-ras (LSL-K-ras)* mice, expression of oncogenic *K-ras* is spatially and temporally controlled by a removable transcriptional termination (stop) element. Intranasal infection with a recombinant adenovirus-carrying Cre recombinase (AdenoCre) results in deletion of the stop element, producing the *Lox-K-ras* allele that expresses oncogenic *K-ras G12D* from the endogenous *K-ras* promoter. These mice develop epithelial hyperplasia that appear to progress to adenomas and overt adenocarcinomas.[57] The tumors recapitulate the histopathological and molecular signature of human lung adenocarcinomas.[57,58] Interestingly, BASCs were also detected in these lung adenocarcinomas, indicating that they may contribute to tumor growth and progression.[57] This raises the possibility that BASCs in these murine lung cancers are the CSC population.

MOVING FORWARD IN LUNG CANCER STEM CELL BIOLOGY

Designing Experiments to Test the Cancer Stem Cell Hypothesis: Transplantation and Culture An important aim of basic lung cancer research is to determine if human lung adenocarcinomas contain a CSC population. Following the methodology that has been successful in other malignancies, one method to test this possibility would be to examine dissociated cells from human lung adenocarcinomas, sort cells by FACS, and test the ability of tumor cell subpopulations to propagate tumors with orthotopic transplantation assays.

CSCs in human leukemia, melanoma, breast, brain, colon, and pancreatic malignancies have been shown to be required for serial rounds of tumor propagation in transplantation assays that often utilize orthotopic strategies.[1–6,11] For example, the function of breast CSCs was elucidated by injecting cancer cells into the mammary gland, thereby mimicking the normal environment of the tumor cells.

A current literature search indicates that the CSC hypothesis remains largely untested for lung cancer. Experiments with human lung cancer cell lines and sphere-forming lung cancer cells have suggested that cancer cells that exhibit some properties of stem cells are present within lung cancers. These studies relied on the use of the Hoechst dye exclusion method to isolate the side population and the presence of the CD133 cell-surface marker, respectively. Importantly, fresh lung tumors were shown to contain a CD133+ cell fraction that could propagate lung tumors when injected subcutaneously in immunodeficient mice.[46]

Although the studies described previously constitute an important beginning in addressing the CSC hypothesis in lung cancer, several key experiments have not yet been reported. First, serial transplantation of lung CSCs has not been demonstrated. Because multiple rounds of propagation of tumors are typically used to show the self-renewal capacity of putative CSCs, this key property of stem cells has not been shown for human lung cancer. Second, the use of subcutaneous injection to test lung CSC activity does not reflect the normal cellular milieu in which lung cancers arise, grow, and progress. Particularly important for future work to develop therapeutic intervention of CSCs, previous studies have shown that lung tumor cells growing in subcutaneous regions do not exhibit the same physiological response to chemotherapy as do tumors growing in the lung.[59,60] Therefore, experiments to test for lung CSC activity have not yet been done in the most relevant tissue setting.

Future experiments should build upon the valuable studies described previously with human lung cancer cell lines and work in primary murine lung adenocarcinomas to determine if human lung adenocarcinomas contain a CSC population. Importantly, serial transplantations of uncultured primary tumor cells from human lung and characterization of the resulting tumors are required. Furthermore, testing the ability of cells sorted by both the putative lung CSC marker CD133 and novel cell-surface markers in serial transplantation assays will likely be helpful in learning how to prospectively identify CSCs. If CSC surface markers from other tissues are not useful for the lung, a side population of human lung adenocarcinoma cells might be isolated by their ability to efflux Hoechst dye; this technique has already been verified to work well in human lung cancer cell lines.[45] Adenocarcinoma side population cells with CSC activity could be isolated by FACS and characterized by microarray analysis to elucidate new lung CSC surface markers. Transplantation of tumor cells into the lung, where the normal microenvironment may have important roles on cancer progression, niche effects on CSCs, and cancer cell response to therapeutics,[61,62] should be done to more clearly define the role of CSCs in human lung adenocarcinomas or other types of lung cancer.

In parallel to testing for CSCs using murine transplantation assays, a culture-based method to determine if a subset of lung cancer cells exhibits the stem cell properties of self-renewal and differentiation will be valuable. Self-renewing sphere colonies were originally observed when primary tumor cells from human brain were cultured on nonadherent plates in serum-free media supplemented with EGF and basic fibroblast growth factor (bFGF),[20] and have been subsequently established from primary tumor cells of colon, breast, and melanoma in human.[5,21–23] Tumor sphere culture conditions could be used to identify human lung cancer cells that can be propagated over multiple passages, providing a surrogate assay to complement in vivo cell transplantation studies. The development of this in vitro cell culture system would likely assist in the isolation and characterization of human lung adenocarcinoma CSCs. The establishment of cultures of lung adenocarcinoma CSCs would also enhance future studies of the pathways that regulate self-renewal and differentiation of these cells, as well as for identification of small molecules that inhibit CSC activity. Importantly, culture assays should only be used if the culture conditions retain cells that exhibit the ability to propagate tumors in the lung that are indistinguishable from those arising from primary cell injections. The combination of in vivo and in vitro assays for CSCs would provide the repertoire of tools needed for functional analysis of lung CSCs.

Connecting Cancer Stem Cells and Chemotherapeutic Resistance Distinct aspects of CSC biology, such as more active DNA-damage response, may render CSCs more resistant to therapeutics than other cancer cells.[12–14] In addition, the quiescent nature of CSCs or their proposed ability to efficiently export drugs, characteristics that have both been shown in some stem cells in normal tissues,[63] may impact the response to therapy. Elucidation of a lung CSC population and therapeutic strategies that specifically eliminate lung CSCs may offer more effective means of therapy that can be combined with current clinical approaches.[12,14,64]

Resistance to chemotherapy is a major cause of the high mortality rate associated with advanced lung cancer. Chemotherapy is associated with only a 20% to 40% chance of tumor regression in advanced NSCLC, and thus, for most patients, chemotherapy is ineffective.[65] Adenocarcinomas bearing mutations in oncogenic K-ras are among the most chemorefractory lung tumors, suggesting that mutant K-ras CSCs in these tumors may be more inherently drug resistant than other lung cancer CSCs.[66,67] The initial sensitivity of human adenocarcinomas with activating EGFR mutations to EGFR TKIs and the acquired resistance to these treatments suggest that drug-resistant CSCs may be present in these tumors.[36–38] The molecular mechanisms of EGFR-inhibitor resistance have been well characterized in comparison with other forms of chemotherapy for lung cancer, yet the cellular nature of these mechanisms is poorly understood. For example, it is not yet clear whether EGFR-inhibitor resistance arises from de novo EGFR mutations after treatment or if rare preexisting chemoresistant subclones expand after initial treatment response.

CSCs may play an important role in the resistance of lung adenocarcinomas. More specifically, it is possible that CSCs are either more numerous or more chemorefractory in K-ras mutant lung adenocarcinomas than in other forms of adenocarcinoma. Second, EGFR-mutant NSCLC tumors may recur during TKI treatments because of the presence of a resistant CSC population. Evidence supports these ideas in other solid malignancies. For example, it was recently shown that the percentage of breast CSCs is significantly increased in the tumors of patients treated with chemotherapy.[22]

Future studies to connect CSCs to therapy response in lung cancer may be best done by analysis of murine lung cancers, because they currently offer several advantages over patient samples for understanding the role of CSCs in adenocarcinoma. First, the identity of human lung CSCs has not yet been established, whereas a stem cell population that appears to be important in tumorigenesis in a mouse model of adenocarcinoma has been identified (above). Second, there is typically no clinical basis for biopsy or surgical removal of recurring or chemoresistant lung adenocarcinomas from patients. In addition, with the exception of EGFR-mutant tumors, the timing of acquired chemoresistance is not known in patients. These facts make it challenging to acquire large numbers of fresh chemoresistant human lung cancer samples in which to examine CSCs, and even more difficult to have matched chemonaive and chemoresistant cancer cells from the same patient. Many mouse models of lung cancer are now available that accurately recapitulate the mutational status and chemoresistance of human lung adenocarcinomas, and one can easily obtain genetically matched tumors that arise in the absence of chemotherapy and at specific time points during or after the development of chemoresistant tumors, providing materials that are simply not available from patients in the same numbers. When possible, primary human samples should be used to validate findings in mice that establish the relationship between lung CSCs and chemotherapeutic response.

Metastasis and Cancer Stem Cells: Another Missing Link The CSC hypothesis predicts that stem cell characteristics, which allow CSCs to disseminate and colonize to new tissues, are responsible for metastatic disease. Importantly, even for known CSCs, their role in metastasis is largely unexplored, and it is possible that cells with stem cell properties cause metastases. Just as described for matched chemonaive and chemoresistant human lung cancer samples, it is challenging to obtain large numbers of matched primary and metastatic lung cancer samples from patients. In addition, although lung cancer metastases to the brain are surgically removed, most advanced stage primary and metastatic lung cancers in these patients are not surgically removed. There is no documented improvement of patient survival for operation of these advanced stage lesions. Therefore, the question of metastasis and stem cells is another setting ideal for the use of mouse models to obtain genetically matched primary and metastatic lung adenocarcinoma cells. In particular, *LSL-K-ras p53-lox/lox* mutant murine lung tumors are an ideal model to use for the study of metastatic disease because of the observed incidence of metastasis in these mice. Archived human samples could also be examined to determine if pathways identified in mouse studies are useful prognostic markers of metastatic disease in patients.

Searching for Molecular Targets in Cancer Stem Cells The CSC hypothesis predicts that the same pathways, which are essential for promoting self-renewal of normal stem cells, are also important for propagating the growth of cancer cells. In fact, many cancer mutations cause upregulation of pathways that promote self-renewal.[26] In addition, it has been shown that CSCs, which are identified by markers distinct from markers of normal tissue stem cells, can exhibit shared gene-expression signatures with stem cells.[24] Thus, stem cell pathways may be upregulated in chemoresistant lung adenocarcinomas compared to chemonaive tumors.

A logical place to start examining the importance of stem cell regulatory molecules in lung cancer are the Wnt, Hedgehog (Hh), and Bmi-1 pathways, because they have been implicated in stem cell self-renewal and lung biology. In addition, evidence suggests that dysregulation of these pathways contributes to NSCLC. Wnt pathways play a crucial role in lung embryonic development, and more specifically, in cell fate decisions and differentiation.[68–70] β-catenin levels are elevated in some NSCLCs; however, unlike many other cancers, APC and β-catenin mutations are rare in NSCLC.[70–74] The mechanisms leading to elevated β-catenin levels in primary NSCLCs, therefore, most likely occur upstream of β-catenin, for example, via overexpression of Wnt effectors or repression of Wnt antagonists.[70–75] The Hh pathways play a crucial role in lung embryonic development.[76] Most NSCLC tumors exhibit increased expression of Hh-signaling proteins compared to normal lung tissues, and 87% of lung adenocarcinomas have increased levels of GLI1.[77] Moderate-to-high levels of Bmi-1 are expressed in most NSCLC tumors, and Bmi-1 status is a useful prognosis factor of lung adenocarcinoma tumor metastasis and patient survival.[78,79] We have also recently found that Bmi-1 is required for lung tumorigenesis in the K-ras mouse model of lung cancer and is also required for BASC self-renewal, suggesting that the Bmi-1 pathway is one molecular link between stem cell function and tumorigenesis in the lung.[80] Future studies will likely elucidate the connections between these important pathways and others to test for activation in lung cancer.

In addition to the pathways discussed previously, the CSC hypothesis also predicts that the pathways responsible for the dissemination and homing of normal stem cells during development and wound healing are upregulated in metastatic tumor cells. In support of this idea, adhesion, chemokine, and cytokine receptors have been implicated in metastasis.[81] The SDF-1/chemokine (C-X-C motif) receptor 4 (CXCR4) axis plays a crucial role in hematopoietic stem cell (HSC) trafficking and has been hypothesized to be harnessed by CSCs during metastasis.[82] During embryogenesis, a chemokine SDF-1 gradient secreted by the bone marrow attracts HSCs expressing CXCR4 from the fetal liver, and in adults, the gradient is also crucial for retention of the HSCs in the adult bone marrow.[82]

The SDF-1/CXCR4 axis is crucial in CSC-driven pancreatic metastasis, whereas in CD133+ pancreatic CSCs propagated primary tumors, only CD133+ cells that were CXCR4+ were capable of producing metastases.[83] Although the role of CXCR4 in tumor metastasis is the most well defined, other chemokine receptors are also involved in invasion and migration: CCR7 is involved in the dissemination of many types of tumor cells to the lymph nodes; CCR10 is involved in homing of melanoma cells to the skin[84,85]; and chemokines such as CCL2, CCL5, and CXCL8, can stimulate the migration of some types of tumor cell lines.[84]

Lung CSCs with chemokine receptors may initiate lung cancer invasion and migration. Many types of human tumors that exhibit high CXCR4 expression levels, including NSCLCs, are prone to metastasis.[84,86] In NSCLC, recent studies have shown that high primary tumor CCR7 and CXCL8 mRNA levels are correlated with the presence of lymph node metastases.[87,88] Thus, it is likely that other chemokine receptors play a role in lung cancer metastasis and that a more global survey of chemokine receptors in adenocarcinoma could provide additional molecules to examine in lung CSC studies.

POTENTIAL CAVEATS IN THE STUDY OF LUNG CANCER STEM CELLS

Several aspects of CSC biology may limit the ability to propagate human lung cancer cells in mice or in culture, and thus make it difficult to test the CSC hypothesis in lung cancer. First, human lung CSCs may require human stromal cells or other factors from the human lung microenvironment for growth and tumor propagation. Instead of sorted cells, it is possible to implant intact pieces of tumor subcutaneously for a first round of tumor growth in mice. This technique has been performed in prior studies used to identify breast CSCs.[2] In addition, lung tumor samples that can be obtained from patients will be early stage tumors, as these are typically the only stage of lung cancer that is treatable with surgery. It is possible that these early stage tumors will not have an adequate number of CSCs for propagation. It may be necessary to use more advanced cancer samples to identify lung CSCs.

It remains possible that no unique population of cells has the ability to preferentially propagate human lung adenocarcinoma tumors, which would argue more in favor of the stochastic theory of tumor cell clonogenicity (above) in lung cancer rather than the CSC hypothesis. For example, different subsets of cancer cells may acquire CSC activity through mutation during tumor growth, and there may not be cell-intrinsic properties that separate cancer-propagating and nonpropagating populations within lung tumors beyond their genetic component. CSCs from brain tumors do not have a significantly different pattern of genetic alterations compared with the non-CSC from the same tumors,[3] indicating that genomic changes alone do not account for all observed CSC activity; yet, it will be important to compare the genomic status of cancer cell subpopulations. Second, the inherent difficulty with the CSC hypothesis is that negative results may not completely rule out the hypothesis. It may not be possible to formally exclude that the correct marker or strategy was not applied to identify the elusive lung CSC. Given the potential promise for future cancer therapy that has been associated with the CSC concept, it is imperative to perform studies such as those discussed here to begin determining if the CSC hypothesis is a valid model for understanding lung cancer biology despite these challenges.

CONCLUSION

At least three distinct, yet complementary, aspects of the CSC hypothesis remain to be addressed for human lung adenocarcinomas and all forms of lung cancer: to determine if a CSC population exists in human lung cancers, to determine how tumor-propagating frequency and activation of stem cell pathways are changed in chemoresistant lung cancer cells, and to identify molecular markers that may connect lung CSCs and metastatic cells. If CSCs are identified in human lung cancers, many important future directions will be possible. Gene-expression profiling of human lung CSCs may lead to the identification of new lung CSC markers or pathways that regulate CSCs. Furthermore, molecules identified as differentially expressed in lung CSCs, chemoresistant cancer cells, or adenocarcinoma metastases could be investigated for their causal role in these aspects of tumorigenesis and their usefulness as biomarkers for screening patients for lung cancer. Strategies such as those described here will make important inroads to future studies to use the biology of stem cells to improve the outcome of lung cancer patients.

REFERENCES

1. Bonnet D, Dick JE. Human acute myeloid leukemia is organized as a hierarchy that originates from a primitive hematopoietic cell. *Nature* 1997;3(7):730–737.
2. Al-Hajj M, Wicha MS, Benito-Hernandez A, et al. Prospective identification of tumorigenic breast cancer cells. *Proc Natl Acad Sci U S A* 2003;100(7):3983–3988.
3. Singh SK, Hawkins C, Clarke ID, et al. Identification of human brain tumour initiating cells. *Nature* 2004;432:396–401.
4. O'Brien CA, Pollett A, Gallinger S, et al. A human colon cancer cell capable of initiating tumour growth in immunodeficient mice. *Nature* 2007;445:106–110.
5. Ricci-Vitiani L, Lombardi DG, Pilozzi E, et al. Identification and expansion of human colon cancer-initiating cells. *Nature* 2007;445:111–115.
6. Dalerba P, Dylla SJ, Park IK, et al. Phenotypic characterization of human colorectal cancer stem cells. *Proc Natl Acad Sci U S A* 2007;104(24):10158–10163.
7. Hamburger A, Salmon SE. Primary bioassay of human tumor stem cells. *Science* 1977;197(4302):461–463.
8. Hamburger A, Salmon SE. Primary bioassay of human myeloma stem cells. *J Clin Invest* 1977;60(4):846–854.
9. Aye MT, Niho Y, Till JE, et al. Studies of leukemic cell populations in culture. *Blood* 1974;44(2):205–219.

10. Brunschwig A, Southam CM, Levin AG. Host resistance to cancer. Clinical experiments by homotransplants, autotransplants, and admixture of autologous leucocytes. *Ann Surg* 1965;162(3):416–425.
11. Schatton T, Murphy GF, Frank NY, et al. Identification of cells initiating human melanomas. *Nature* 2008;451(7176):345–349.
12. Reya T, Morrison SJ, Clarke MF, et al. Stem cells, cancer, and cancer stem cells. *Nature* 2001;414(6859):105–111.
13. Bao S, Wu Q, McLendon RE, et al. Glioma stem cells promote radioresistance by preferential activation of the DNA damage response. *Nature* 2006;444(7120):756–760.
14. Hirschmann-Jax C, Foster AE, Wulf GG, et al. A distinct "side population" of cells with high drug efflux capacity in human tumor cells. *Proc Natl Acad Sci U S A* 2004;101(39):14228–14233.
15. Tumbar T, Guasch G, Greco V, et al. Defining the epithelial stem cell niche in skin. *Science* 2004;303(5656):359–363.
16. Reya T, Morrison SJ, Clarke MF, et al. Stem cells, cancer, and cancer stem cells. *Nature* 2001;414(6859):105–111.
17. Huntly BJ, Gilliland DG. Leukaemia stem cells and the evolution of cancer-stem-cell research. *Nat Rev Cancer* 2005;5(4):311–321.
18. Hirschmann-Jax C, Foster AE, Wulf GG, et al. A distinct "side population" of cells with high drug efflux capacity in human tumor cells. *Proc Natl Acad Sci U S A* 2004;28;101(39):14228–14233.
19. Hirschmann-Jax C, Foster AE, Wulf GG, et al. A distinct "side population" of cells in human tumor cells: implications for tumor biology and therapy. *Cell Cycle* 2005;4(2):203–205.
20. Singh SK, Clarke ID, Terasaki M, et al. Identification of a cancer stem cell in human brain tumors. *Cancer Res* 2003;63:5821–5828.
21. Ponti D, Costa A, Zaffaroni N, et al. Isolation and in vitro propagation of tumorigenic breast cancer cells with stem/progenitor cell properties. *Cancer Res* 2005;65(13):5506–5511.
22. Yu F, Yao H, Zhu P, et al. let-7 regulates self renewal and tumorigenicity of breast cancer cells. *Cell* 2007;131:1109–1123.
23. Fang D, Nguyen TK, Leishear K, et al. A tumorigenic subpopulation with stem cell properties in melanomas. *Cancer Res* 2005;65(20): 9328–9337.
24. Krivtsov AV, Twomey D, Feng Z, et al. Transformation from committed progenitor to leukaemia stem cell initiated by MLL-AF9. *Nature* 2006;442(7104):818–822.
25. Jamieson CH, Ailles LE, Dylla SJ, et al. Granulocyte-macrophage progenitors as candidate leukemic stem cells in blast-crisis CML. *N Engl J Med* 2004;351(7):657–667.
26. Pardal R, Clarke MF, Morrison SJ. Applying the principles of stem-cell biology to cancer. *Nat Rev Cancer* 2003;3:895–902.
27. Lobo NA, Shimono Y, Qian D, et al. The biology of cancer stem cells. *Annu Rev Cell Dev Biol* 2007;23:675–99.
28. SR. ACS. *Age-Adjusted Cancer Death Rates, Females or Males by Site, US, 1930–2001 US Mortality Public Use Data Tapes 1960–2001, US Mortality Volumes 1930–1959, National Center for Health Statistics.* Centers for Disease Control and Prevention, 2004.
29. Jemal A, Siegel R, Ward E, et al. Cancer statistics, 2007. *CA Cancer J Clin* 2007;57(1):43–66.
30. De Petris L, Crino L, Scagliotti GV, et al. Treatment of advanced non-small cell lung cancer. *Anna Oncol* 2006;17(Suppl 2):II36–II41.
31. Quint LE, Tummala S, Brisson LJ, et al. Distribution of distant metastases from newly diagnosed non-small cell lung cancer. *Ann Thorac Surg* 1996;62:246–250.
32. Pisters KM, Ginsberg RJ, Giroux DJ, et al. Induction chemotherapy before surgery for early-stage lung cancer: a novel approach. Bimodality Lung Oncology Team. *J Thorac Cardiovas Surg* 2000;119(3): 429–439
33. Lynch TJ, Bell DW, Sordella R, et al. Activating mutations in the epidermal growth factor receptor underlying responsiveness of non-small cell lung cancer to gefitinib. *N Engl J Med* 2004;350(21): 2129–2139.
34. Paez JG, Janne PA, Lee JC, et al. EGFR mutations in lung cancer: correlation with clinical response to gefitinib therapy. *Science* 2004;304(5676):497–500.
35. Pao W, Miller V, Zakowski M, et al. EGF receptor gene mutations are common in lung cancers from "never smokers" and are associated with sensitivity of tumors to gefitinib and erlotinib. *Proc Natl Acad Sci U S A* 2004;101(36):13306–13311.
36. Kobayashi S, Boggon TJ, Dayaram T, et al. EGFR mutation and resistance of non-small cell lung cancer to gefitinib. *N Engl J Med* 2005;352(8):786–792.
37. Pao W, Miller VA, Politi KA, et al. Acquired resistance of lung adenocarcinomas to gefitinib or erlotinib is associated with a second mutation in the EGFR kinase domain. *PLoS Med* 2005;2:E73.
38. Kosaka T, Yatabe Y, Endoh H, et al. Analysis of epidermal growth factor receptor gene mutation in patients with non-small cell lung cancer and acquired resistance to gefitinib. *Clin Cancer Res* 2006;12(19): 5764–5769.
39. Kobayashi S, Boggon TJ, Dayaram T, et al. EGFR mutation and resistance of non-small-cell lung cancer to gefitinib. *N Engl J Med* 2005 Feb 24;352(8):786–792.
40. Kwak EL, Sordella R, Bell DW, et al. Irreversible inhibitors of the EGF receptor may circumvent acquired resistance to gefitinib. *Proc Natl Acad Sci U S A* 2005;102(21):7665–7670.
41. Pao W, Miller VA, Politi KA, et al. Acquired resistance of lung adenocarcinomas to gefitinib or erlotinib is associated with a second mutation in the EGFR kinase domain. *PLoS Med* 2005 Mar;2(3):e73.
42. Kwak EL, Sordella R, Bell DW, et al. Irreversible inhibitors of the EGF receptor may circumvent acquired resistance to gefitinib. *Proc Natl Acad Sci U S A.* 2005;102(21):7665–7670.
43. Yun CH, Mengwasser KE, Torns AV, et al. The T790M mutation in EGFR kinase causes drug resistance by increasing the affinity for ATP. *Proc Natl Acad Sci U S A* 2008;105(8):2070–2075.
44. Li D, Shimamura T, Ji H, et al. Bronchial and peripheral murine lung carcinomas induced by T790M-L858R mutant EGFR respond to HKI-272 and rapamycin combination therapy. *Cancer Cell* 2007;12:81–93.
45. Ho MM, Ng AV, Lam S, et al. Side population in human lung cancer cell lines and tumors is enriched with stem-like cancer cells. *Cancer Res* 2007;67(10):4827–4833.
46. Eramo A, Lotti F, Sette G, et al. Identification and expansion of the tumorigenic lung cancer stem cell population. *Cell Death Differ* 2007;15(3):504–514.
47. Kim CFB, Jackson EL, Woolfenden AE, et al. Identification of bronchioalveolar stem cells in normal lung and lung cancer. *Cell* 2005;121:823–835.
48. Gomperts BN, Strieter RM. Stem cells and chronic lung disease. *Ann Rev Med* 2007;58:285–298.
49. Giangreco A, Reynolds SD, Stripp BR. Terminal bronchioles harbor a unique airway stem cell population that localizes to the bronchoalveolar duct junction. *Am J Pathol* 2002;161(1):173–182.
50. Ling TY, Kuo MD, Li CL, et al. Identification of pulmonary Oct-4+ stem/progenitor cells and demonstration of their susceptibility to SARS coronavirus (SARS-CoV) infection in vitro. *Proc Natl Acad Sci U S A* 2006;103(25):9530–9535.
51. Schmidt M, Sun G, Stacey MA, et al. Identification of circulating fibrocytes as precursors of bronchial myofibroblasts in asthma. *J Immunol* 2003;171(1):380–390.
52. Phillips RJ, Burdick MD, Hong K, et al. Circulating fibrocytes traffic to the lungs in response to CXCL12 and mediate fibrosis. *J Clin Invest* 2004;114(3):438–446.
53. Parker R, Joseph J, Dussek J, et al. Respiratory system. In: Williams PL, Bannister LH, Berry MM, et al., eds. *Gray's Anatomy.* 38th Ed. New York: Churchill Livingstone, 1999:1627–1682.
54. Rodenhuis S, Slebos RJ, Boot AJ, et al. Incidence and possible clinical significance of K-ras oncogene activation in adenocarcinoma of the human lung. *Cancer Res* 1988;48(20):5738–5741.
55. Kobayashi T, Tsuda H, Noguchi M, et al. Association of point mutation in c-Ki-ras oncogene in lung adenocarcinoma with particular reference to cytologic subtypes. *Cancer* 1990;66(2):289–294.
56. Mills NE, Fishman CL, Rom WN, et al. Increased prevalence of K-ras oncogene mutations in lung adenocarcinoma. *Cancer Res* 1995;55(7): 1444–1447.

57. Jackson EL, Willis N, Mercer K, et al. Analysis of lung tumor initiation and progression using conditional expression of oncogenic K-ras. *Genes Dev* 2001;15:3243–3248.
58. Sweet-Cordero A, Mukherjee S, Subramanian A, et al. An oncogenic KRAS2 expression signature identified by cross-species gene-expression analysis. *Nat Genet* 2005;37:48–55.
59. Onn A, Isobe T, Itasaka S, et al. Development of an orthotopic model to study the biology and therapy of primary human lung cancer in nude mice. *Clin Cancer Res* 2003;9(15):5532–5539.
60. Fujino H, Kondo K, Ishikura H, et al. Matrix metalloproteinase inhibitor MMI-166 inhibits lymphogenous metastasis in an orthotopically implanted model of lung cancer. *Mol Cancer Ther* 2005;4(9):1409–1416.
61. Li L, Neaves WB. Normal stem cells and cancer stem cells: the niche matters. *Cancer Res* 2006;66(9):4553–4557.
62. Scadden DT. The stem-cell niche as an entity of action. *Nature* 2006;441:1075–1079.
63. Tumbar T, Guasch G, Greco V, et al. Defining the epithelial stem cell niche in skin. *Science* 2004;303:359–363.
64. Huntly BJ, Gilliland DG. Leukaemia stem cells and the evolution of cancer-stem-cell research. *Nat Rev Cancer* 2005;5:311–321.
65. Schiller JH, Harrington D, Belani CP, et al. Comparison of four chemotherapy regimens for advanced non-small cell lung cancer. *N Engl J Med* 2002;346(2):92–98.
66. Schiller JH, Adak S, Feins RH, et al. Lack of prognostic significance of p53 and K-ras mutations in primary resected non-small cell lung cancer on E4592: a laboratory ancillary study on an eastern cooperative oncology group prospective randomized trial of postoperative adjuvant therapy. *J Clin Oncol* 2001;19(2):448–457.
67. Winton T, Livingston R, Johnson D, et al. Vinorelbine plus cisplatin vs. observation in resected non-small cell lung cancer. *N Engl J Med* 2005;352(25):2589–2597.
68. Mucenski ML, Wert SE, Nation JM, et al. β-catenin is required for specification of proximal/distal cell fate during lung morphogenesis. *J Biol Chem* 2003;278(41):40231–40238.
69. Shu W, Guttentag S, Wang Z, et al. Wnt/β-catenin signaling acts upstream of N-myc, BMP4, and FGF signaling to regulate proximal-distal patterning in the lung. *Dev Biol* 2005;283(1):226–239.
70. Pongraca JE, Stockley RA. Wnt signaling in lung development and diseases. *Respir Res* 2006;7(15).
71. Kotsinas A, Evangelou K, Zacharatos P, et al. Proliferation, but not apoptosis, is associated with distinct β-catenin expression patterns in non-small cell lung carcinomas. *Am J Pathol* 2002;161:1619–1634.
72. Ohgaki H, Kros JM, Okamoto Y, et al. APC mutations are infrequent but present in human lung cancer. *Cancer Lett* 2004;207(2):197–203.
73. Sunaga N, Kohno T, Kolligs FT, et al. Constitutive activation of the Wnt signaling pathway by CTNNB1 (β-catenin) mutations in a subset of human lung adenocarcinoma. *Genes Chromosomes Cancer* 2001;30(3):316–321.
74. Ueda M, Gemmill RM, West J, et al. Mutations of the β- and γ-catenin genes are uncommon in human lung, breast, kidney, cervical, and ovarian carcinomas. *Br J Cancer* 2001; 85(1):64–68.
75. Mazieres J, He B, You L, et al. Wnt signaling in lung cancer. *Cancer Letters* 2005;222:1–10.
76. Pepicelli CV, Lewis PM, McMahon AP. Sonic hedgehog regulates branching morphogenesis in the mammalian lung. *Curr Biol* 1998;8(19):1083–1086.
77. Yuan Z, Goetz JA, Singh S, et al. Frequent recombination of hedgehog signaling in non-small cell lung carcinoma. *Oncogene* 2007;26: 1046–1055.
78. Vonlanthen S, Heighway J, Altermatt HJ, et al. The bmi-1 oncoprotein is differentially expressed in non-small cell lung cancer and correlates with INK4A-ARF locus expression. *Br J Cancer* 2001;84(10):1372–1376.
79. Glinsky GV, Berezovska O, Glinskii AB. Microarray analysis identifies a death-from-cancer signature predicting therapy failure in patients with multiple types of cancer. *J Clin Invest* 2005;115(6):1503–1521.
80. Dovey JS, Zacharek SJ, Kim CF, et al. Bmi1 is critical for lung tumorigenesis and bronchioalveolar stem cell expansion. *Proc Natl Acad Sci U S A* 2008;105(33):11857–11862.
81. Gupta GP, Massague J. Cancer metastasis: building a framework. *Cell* 2006;127:679–695.
82. Kucia M, Reca R, Miekus K, et al. Trafficking of normal stem cells and metastasis of cancer stem cells involve similar mechanisms: pivotal role of the SDF-1-CXCR4 axis. *Stem Cells* 2005;23:879–894.
83. Hermann PC, Huber SL, Herrler T, et al. Distinct populations of cancer stem cells determine tumor growth and metastatic activity in human pancreatic cancer. *Cell Stem Cell* 2007;1:313–323.
84. Ben-Baruch A. The multifaceted roles of chemokines in malignancy. *Cancer Metastasis Rev* 2006;25:357–371.
85. Balkwill F. Cancer and the chemokine network. *Nat Rev Cancer* 2004;4: 540–550.
86. Su L, Zhang J, Xu H, et al. Differential expression of CXCR4 is associated with the metastatic potential of human non-small cell lung cancer cells. *Clin Cancer Res* 2005;1(11):8273–8280.
87. Takanami I. Overexpression of CCR7 mRNA in non-small cell lung cancer: correlation with lymph node metastasis. *Int J Cancer* 2003; 105(2):186–189.
88. Yuan A, Yang PC, Yu CJ, et al. Interleukin-8 messenger ribonucleic acid expression correlates with tumor progression, tumor angiogenesis, patient survival, and timing of relapse in non-small cell lung cancer. *Am J Respir Crit Care Med* 2000;162(5):1957–1963.
89. McCulloch EA. Stem cells in normal and leukemic hemopoiesis (Henry Stratton Lecture, 1982). *Blood* 1983;62(1):1–13.
90. Lapidot T, Sirard C, Vormoor J, et al. A cell initiating human acute myeloid leukaemia after transplantation into SCID mice. *Nature* 1994 Feb 17;367(6464):645–648.
91. Dick JE. Normal and leukemic human stem cells assayed in SCID mice. *Semin Immunol* 1996;8(4):197–206.
92. Singh SK, Hawkins C, Clarke ID, et al. Identification of human brain tumour initiating cells. *Nature* 2004 Nov 18;432(7015):396–401.
93. Prince ME, Sivanandan R, Kaczorowski A, et al. Identification of a subpopulation of cells with cancer stem cell properties in head and neck squamous cell carcinoma. *Proc Natl Acad Sci U S A* 2007;104(3): 973–978.
94. Eramo A, Lotti F, Sette G, et al. Identification and expansion of the tumorigenic lung cancer stem cell population. *Cell Death Differ* 2008; 15(3):504–514.

CHAPTER 12

Marie Wislez
Jacques Cadranel
Jonathan M. Kurie

Lung Cancer and Its Microenvironment

The association between inflammation and cancer was identified in the 19th century. Initially, it was believed that leukocyte infiltrates in tumors represented an attempt by the host to eradicate malignant cells. It was later demonstrated that several chronic inflammatory conditions, such as inflammatory bowel disease, *Helicobacter pylori* infection, hepatitis B or C infection, and prostatitis, predisposed people to cancer of the colon, stomach, liver, and prostate, respectively. In addition, malignant tissues that contain inflammatory cells such as macrophages in breast cancer or neutrophils and mast cells in lung cancer are associated with an unfavorable outcome.

Lung cancer risk is clearly enhanced by cigarette smoking, and chronic inflammation associated with chronic obstructive pulmonary disease probably enhances this risk, although an increase is difficult to demonstrate. Some lung cancers that occur in association with scars could have no relationship with smoking habits. In patients with idiopathic fibrosis, lung cancer incidence is much higher than in the general population.[1] Oncogene activation is often associated with inflammatory response. For example, scar-associated cancers seem to more often have *KRAS* (codon 12) mutations. Further, a transgenic mouse model of lung cancer generated by *KRAS* activation showed a robust inflammatory response compared to the wild-type mice.[2,3] Lastly, in several mouse models, this inflammatory response has been demonstrated to be not only associated with but also required for tumor initiation or growth.[4,5]

The tumor microenvironment is composed of structural (extracellular matrix [ECM]), soluble (growth factors, chemokines, cytokines, proteases, and hormones, among others), and cellular components (tumor cells, fibroblasts, inflammatory cells, vascular and lymphatic endothelial cells, and vascular smooth muscle cells and pericytic cells, among others). Characterization of the inflammatory cells within tumors has revealed both the adaptive and innate arms of the immune response. For example, dendritic cells (DCs) present tumor antigens to T lymphocytes ($CD4^+$, $CD8^+$, and natural killer [NK]), promoting an antitumor cytotoxic T-cell response. This response is negated by a population of immature myeloid cells called myeloid-derived suppressor cells that promotes the development of $FOXP3^+$ $CD4^+$ T cells or Tregs, which suppress the antitumor cytotoxic T-cell response and induce polarized differentiation of monocytes into tumor-associated macrophages (TAMs or M2 macrophages). TAMs, vascular endothelial cells, and fibroblasts within the tumor stroma secrete a number of growth factors and chemokines that promote tumorigenesis. Thus, conflicting immunologic forces fight for supremacy in the tumor microenvironment. This chapter will deal with recent research on the tumorigenic and antitumorigenic effects of the immune system on the lung. The latter was discussed fully in a recent review.[6]

ANGIOGENESIS

Angiogenesis is the growth of the new blood vessels, necessary for cancerous tumors to keep growing and spreading (see Chapter 8). Many proteins and other smaller molecules have been identified as *angiogenic*, particularly vascular endothelial growth factor (VEGF), basic fibroblast growth factor (bFGF), and CXC chemokines, among others. The binding of these molecules to their appropriate receptor activates a series of relay proteins that transmits a signal into the nucleus of the endothelial cells. The nuclear signal ultimately prompts a group of genes to make products needed for new endothelial cell growth. First, the activated endothelial cells produce matrix metalloproteinases (MMPs), a class of degradative enzymes that break down the extracellular matrix, thus permitting the migration of endothelial cells that had been tethered to the matrix. As they migrate into the surrounding tissues, activated endothelial cells begin to divide. Soon they organize into hollow tubes that evolve gradually into a mature network of blood vessels. Cancer cells originating in a primary tumor can spread to another organ and form metastases that can remain dormant for years. The induction of this vasculature in primary tumor or in metastases, termed *angiogenic switch*, can occur at various stages of tumor progression, depending on the tumor type and the environment (see Chapter 8).[7] In many studies, angiogenic switch has been reported to be closely associated with malignant transition. Cancer cells themselves could release molecules to activate this process, as could cells from the tumor microenvironment. This review will describe effects of the cells from the tumor microenvironment on angiogenesis.

FIBROBLASTS

Normal stroma contains fibroblasts in association with physiological extracellular matrix. Reactive stroma is associated with an increased number of fibroblasts, enhanced capillary density, and type I collagen and fibrin deposition. In chickens that are cancer-prone because they have been infected with Rous sarcoma virus, wounding leads to invasive carcinoma, demonstrating that reactive stroma provides oncogenic signals that facilitate tumorigenesis.[8] Fibroblasts are associated with cancer cells (tumor-associated fibroblasts [TAFs], carcinoma-associated fibroblasts [CAFs]) at all stages of cancer progression. The growth factors, chemokines, and extracellular matrix—these fibroblasts produce facilitate angiogenic recruitment of endothelial cells and pericytes. They are phenotypically and functionally distinct from fibroblasts that are not in the tumor microenvironment. The modified phenotype they acquire is similar to that of fibroblasts associated with wound healing. Smooth muscle differentiation (myofibroblasts) is prominent in stromal cells of malignant breast tissue but rarely seen in normal breast tissue.[9] The signals that mediate the transition of normal fibroblasts into TAF or CAF are not fully understood, but transforming growth factor-β (TGF-β), platelet-derived growth factor (PDGF), and fibroblast growth factor 2 (FGF2) are the main mediators to induce fibroblast activation. TGF-β induces the acquisition of activated phenotype of fibroblasts in culture[10] and has been shown to be correlated with desmoplastic reaction and poor prognosis in breast cancer.[11] PDGF induces the proliferation of fibroblasts and has been shown to be associated with cancer progression in breast cancer.[12] FGF2 also stimulates proliferation of fibroblasts and is also recognized for its potential to induce angiogenesis.[13]

The fact that fibroblasts contribute to tumor initiation, growth, and metastasis have been demonstrated by both in vivo and in vitro study.[14] Whereas normal fibroblasts are required to maintain epithelial homeostasis, CAFs probably initiate and promote tumorigenic alterations in epithelial cells. Fibroblasts cultured from malignant tumors have stimulatory effects on breast tumor cell lines, whereas fibroblasts cultured from normal tissue are inhibitory.[15] If CAFs are coinoculated with prostate, breast, or bladder tumor cell lines into nude mice, tumor latency is shortened and tumor growth increased,[16] whereas normal fibroblasts do not have this effect. Increased cell proliferation and angiogenesis also result. Lastly, fibroblasts could promote metastasis by secreting growth factors that create a niche that promotes the growth of cancer cells at distant sites.[17]

CAFs could also modulate the immune response. CAFs isolated from primary non–small cell lung cancers (NSCLCs) were able to enhance or suppress tumor-associated T-cell function.[18]

The epithelial-to-mesenchymal transition (EMT) might be an additional source of fibroblast-like cells (with an altered genome). In EMT, epithelial cells lose cell–cell contacts and acquire mesenchymal properties. Cancer cells undergoing EMT develop invasive and migratory abilities and express EMT markers (E-Cadherin, Vimentin) that have been shown to be markers of tumor progression.[19–21] This phenotype has also been shown to be associated with resistance to certain therapies such as epidermal growth factor receptor (EGFR) tyrosine kinase inhibitor (TKI) in NSCLC.[21,22]

MACROPHAGES

Most solid tumors are abundantly populated with TAMs. These cells can compromise clinical outcome. Clinical studies have shown a correlation between TAM density and poor prognosis for several types of cancer, an association that is particularly strong for breast, prostate, ovarian, and cervical cancers.[23] For NSCLC, TAM density correlated significantly and negatively with overall survival or relapse-free survival in two of three published studies.[24–26]

Macrophages are recruited to tumors by a wide variety of growth factors—granulocyte colony-stimulating factor (G-CSF), granulocyte-monocyte colony-stimulating factor (GM-CSF), macrophage-stimulating protein (MSP), VEGF, TGF-β—and chemokines, which include CC chemokines, monocyte chemoattractant protein family, macrophage inflammatory protein-1 (MIP-1), and macrophage migration inhibitory factor (MIF).[27]

Tumor-derived molecules probably influence TAM phenotype. Exposure to IL-4 and IL-10 in tumors may induce TAMs to develop into M2 macrophages, which are characterized by poor antigen-presenting capacity and production of factors that suppress T-cell proliferation and activity and induce angiogenesis, whereas M1 macrophages are efficient immune cells.[28]

Macrophages induce angiogenesis. Correlations between number of macrophages and microvessel count have been observed for many tumor types including lung cancer.[24,25,29] Macrophage infiltration into tumor is not homogeneous: studies using hypoxic markers have shown that TAMs accumulate in hypoxic and necrotic areas. Hypoxia induces synthesis of macrophage chemoattractants such as VEGF by upregulating hypoxia-inducible factor (HIF), which recruits and immobilizes macrophages in such areas.[30] Here, these cells synthesize angiogenic regulators, which results in formation of new blood vessels. These regulators are angiogenic factors (VEGF, PDGF, IL-8) and angiogenesis-modulating enzymes (MMPs and cyclooxygenase-2 [COX-2]). In vitro studies, based on coculture experiences, showed that exposure of macrophage to tumor cells increases synthesis of angiogenic factors.[25,31,32] In transgenic mice susceptible to mammary cancer (PyMT mice), malignant transition was demonstrated to be regulated by infiltrated macrophages in primary mammary tumors. Inhibition of macrophage recruitment into the tumors delayed the angiogenic switch and malignant progression, while genetic restoration of the macrophage population rescued angiogenesis.[33]

Macrophages have been shown to stimulate proliferation of tumor cells. In K-ras^{LA1} mice, which develop lung adenocarcinoma through somatic activation of a K-ras allele, intraepithelial and airspace macrophage infiltration is observed beginning at the earliest stage of neoplasia and increasing with malignant progression.[3] In this model, inhibition of malignant progression by a targeted treatment directed against the mTOR pathway was accompanied by macrophage loss. Conditioned media from primary cultures of macrophages stimulated the proliferation of lung tumor cells, which was consistent with previous reports demonstrating a stimulatory effect of alveolar macrophages on the proliferation of normal and distal airway epithelial cells in other animal models.[34–36] In a transgenic mouse model of preneoplastic progression in the mammary gland, conditional depletion of macrophages inhibited epithelial cell proliferation and lateral budding.[37]

Macrophages are involved in invasion and metastasis. In the PyMT mouse model of breast cancer progression, leukocytic infiltrates were present in areas of basement membrane breakdown[38] suggesting their involvement in tumor invasion; macrophage depletion resulted in reduced formation of lung metastases.[4] In coculture experiments, interaction between macrophages and tumor cells facilitated invasion of tumor cells into a collagen matrix.[39] In a chemotaxis-based in vivo invasion assay, a paracrine loop involving macrophages and tumor cells was essential for motility and invasion of tumor cells in mammary tumor.[40] Colony-stimulating factor-1 (CSF-1) secreted by carcinoma cells leads to the activation of macrophages to secrete EGFR ligands, leading to stimulation of carcinoma cell movement.[40]

NEUTROPHILS

Neutrophil infiltration has been described in NSCLC, and particularly in the bronchioloalveolar subtype.[41,42] Recent studies support the fact that this could be induced by Ras activation, one of the most common oncogenic events in pulmonary adenocarcinoma.[5] Neutrophils could be recruited to tumors by CXC chemokines with an N-terminal Glu-Leu-Arg (ELR) motif. These chemokines are also autocrine growth factors for certain types of cancer cells.[43–45] Mutations in the proto-oncogene *KRAS* occur in 10% to 30% of lung adenocarcinomas,[46] and expression of mutant *KRAS* in the alveolar epithelium leads to the development of lung adenocarcinoma in mice.[45–50] In addition to its role in the transformation of alveolar epithelial cells, the presence of *KRAS* mutations is a predictor of shorter survival in NSCLC patients[51] and of resistance to therapy.[52] Sparmann et al.[5] demonstrated that the CXC chemokine CXCL8 (interleukin-8) is a transcriptional target of Ras signaling and is required for the initiation of tumor-associated inflammation and neovascularization in xenograft models. In this model, neutralization of CXCL8 in RasV12-expressing subcutaneous tumors attenuates neoplastic growth; CXCL8 inhibition does not affect tumor cell proliferation but leads to an increase in tumor cell death and an impairment of tumor vascularization coincident with an impairment of stromal infiltration of neutrophils. In the heterotopic and orthotopic Lewis lung cancer models, tumor growth is associated with enhanced neovascularization, neutrophil inflammation, and expression of CXC chemokines. Neutralization of CXC chemokine receptor decreases tumor size and increases tumor necrosis.[53]

In Kras^{LA1} mice, a mouse model in which lung adenocarcinoma develops through somatic activation of a *KRAS* allele carrying an activating mutation in codon 12 (G12D),[50] neutrophils, and vascular endothelial cells infiltration increased during malignant progression, and the murine functional homologues of human CXCR2 chemokines (KC, MIP-2) and their receptor CXCR2 are highly expressed.[54] CXCR2 inhibition blocks the expansion of early alveolar neoplastic lesions, but this antitumor effect does not occur outside the presence of the tumor microenvironment.

In humans, adenocarcinomas with bronchoalveolar features are also characterized by an intense inflammatory reaction, predominantly consisting of alveolar neutrophils and macrophages. Increased numbers of tumor-infiltrating neutrophils are linked to poorer outcome in these patients.[41] The tumor environment drives local neutrophil recruitment and activation via CXC chemokine release, but it also prolongs alveolar neutrophil survival through the production of soluble antiapoptotic factors GM-CSF and G-CSF.[55] The mechanisms by which neutrophils influence the prognosis of adenocarcinomas with bronchoalveolar features could be multiple. It has been postulated that the persistence of neutrophil alveolitis would result in persistent release of proinflammatory mediators such as cytokines, proteases, and reactive oxygen and nitrogen species that can damage DNA and activate oncogenes.[56,57] Among these factors released by neutrophils, hepatocyte growth factor (HGF) seems to be particularly involved in the progression of these types of tumors, especially through its mitogenic and scattering properties, favoring c-Met–expressing tumor cell migration along the alveolar basal membrane.[58] Lastly, neutrophils might be involved in luminal tumor spread by promoting tumor cell shedding,[59] which is described pathologically as the presence of micropapillary clusters that are also involved in the mechanism of aerogenous progression.[60]

MAST CELLS

Several different studies showed a significant association between mast cell density, angiogenesis, and poor prognosis in NSCLC.[61–64] Using monoclonal antibodies for tryptase—a specific marker for mast cells—and for endothelial cell surface molecules, several studies quantified mast cell and microvessel density in lung cancer tissue. Takanami et al.[61] showed a correlation between mast cell density and microvessel count in a study of 180 patients with resected pulmonary adenocarcinoma. Mast cell density was also associated with N classification and was an independent factor for survival duration. Production of angiogenic factors such as VEGF or other proinflammatory cytokines by mast cells is probably involved in this phenomenon.[64]

DENDRITIC CELLS

Effective antitumor responses require antigen-presenting cells (APCs), lymphocytes, and NK effectors. DCs are bone marrow–derived leukocytes characterized by a high level of expression of major histocompatibility complex (MHC) and costimulatory molecules. They are the most effective APCs. To initiate and maintain an effective antitumor response after antigen uptake, DC should migrate to draining lymph nodes and to prime T cells. This priming reaction is triggered by an activation-driven maturation process of DC characterized by upregulation of costimulatory molecules (CD40, CD80, and CD86), a switch in the chemokine receptor repertoire, and production of immunomodulatory cytokines (IL-12 and IFN-a) necessary for the generation of cytotoxic T lymphocytes.[65] However, immunosuppressive cytokines such as IL-10, TGF-b, prostaglandin E2 (PGE2), and VEGF interfere with DC maturation and migration, altering tumor response. To improve antitumor immunity, tumor cells have been transduced with genes encoding molecules able to attract and to activate DC but with limited efficacy in curing established tumors. To overcome tumor microenvironment-associated suppressive effect on the DC, a recent work used a strategy that incorporates ex vivo–activated DC as the delivery for chemokine expression. The authors transduced the gene of the secondary lymphoid chemokine (CCL21, CCR7 receptor ligand) into DC ex vivo and delivered the gene-modified DC (DC-AdCCL21) in a mouse model of spontaneous bronchoalveolar carcinoma.[66] A single intratracheal administration led to a marked reduction in tumor burden with extensive mononuclear cell infiltration of the tumors. The reduction of tumor burden was accompanied by the enhanced elaboration of type I cytokines (IL-12 and IFN-g and GM-CSF) and antiangiogenic cytokines and a decrease in immunosuppressive cytokines (IL-10, TGF-b, PGE2) in the tumor microenvironment.[66] Continuous administration of DC-AdCCL21 significantly prolonged survival of mice.[66] In another study, repeated treatments with a combination of a microbial stimulus (a Toll-like receptor 9 ligand, CpG oligonucleotide) and an antibody blocking the IL-10 receptor reversed the functional paralysis of DC and reestablished IL-12 production.[67] Lastly, a combination of local treatment of CCL16 and cpG together with systemic administration of antibody blocking the IL-10 receptor cured syngeneic tumors in mice.[68]

ADAPTATIVE IMMUNITY

Lung cancer cells themselves find a way to avoid activating the adaptative immune system. Although they express tumor antigens, the limited expression of MHC antigens, defective antigen processing, and lack of costimulatory molecules make them ineffective APC.[69] For example, the absence of expression of costimulatory B7 molecules renders tumors invisible to the immune system, whereas enhanced expression of inhibitory B7 molecules protects them from effective T-cell destruction.[70]

Tumor-reactive T cells accumulate in the lung tumor microenvironment but fail to respond because of suppressive tumor cell–derived factors. These factors can reduce T-cell survival. Lymphocytes exposed to lung tumor supernatant undergo enhanced apoptosis with an impairment of nuclear factor κB activation due to reduced IκB kinase (IKK) activity.[71]

A high proportion of tumor-infiltrating lymphocytes in the tumor microenvironment are regulatory T cells. The CD4+ CD25+ T regulatory cells found in lung tumors have been shown to selectively inhibit the host immune response and contribute to the progression of lung cancer. They mediate potent inhibition of autologous T-cell proliferation while they fail to inhibit the proliferation of allogeneic T cells.[72]

B cells also play a crucial role in the onset of chronic inflammation associated with epithelial cancer development.[73] In a recent study using a transgenic mouse model of skin carcinogenesis where the gene of human papillomavirus 16 (HPV-16) is expressed under control of the human keratin 14 promotor, B cells were shown to be activated peripherally—with no need to be recruited in neoplastic tissue. They were also shown to initiate immunoglobulin deposition into neoplastic tissue, paralleling the recruitment of inflammatory cells (mast cells and granulocytes) and malignant progression.[73] Antibodies mediate recruitment of innate immune cells via engagement of FcR expressed on immune cells. Other studies have reported that humoral immune responses potentiate in vivo growth and invasion of injected murine and human tumor cell lines via recruitment and activation of granulocytes and macrophages.[31] The authors suggested that pharmacological intervention attenuating B cell activation or blocking B cell–mediated recruitment of innate immune cells may be effective in preventing premalignant epithelial progression.

CLINICAL IMPLICATIONS

Ongoing biochemical processes in the tumor microenvironment create new targets for cancer therapy. One advantage of therapies targeting the microenvironment is that these nontumor cells are presumably genetically stable, whereas tumor cells are genetically unstable and thus can accumulate adaptive mutations and rapidly acquire drug resistance. Several drugs directed against nontumor cells or their soluble mediators have been developed and are now being evaluated in clinical trials.

MMPs that break down the ECM are necessary for angiogenesis and invasion of tumor cells, into both the surrounding normal tissue and the blood and lymphatic systems. ECM is also a rich source of sequestered heparin, binding progrowth and proangiogenic factors, which are made available following increased production of matrix-degrading enzymes. Clinical trials were undertaken to determine if inhibitors of MMPs (MMPI) improved overall survival in NSCLC or SCLC. Marimastat, a nonselective MMPI, has also been tested in a number of malignancies, including small cell lung cancer and breast, gastric, and pancreatic cancers; the results were negative.[74–77] Musculoskeletal toxicity was a significant problem in all studies. The failure of the broad-spectrum MMP inhibitors (MMP-I) in the clinic has been explained by the fact that some MMPs can also release antiangiogenic proteins. Prinomastat, a more targeted MMPI with activity mainly against MMP2 and MMP9, was given versus placebo in patients with advanced NSCLC in combination with gemcitabine–cisplatin chemotherapy. This study was closed after an interim analysis showed a lack of efficacy.[78] A parallel study of similar design found no benefit when prinomastat was administered in addition to paclitaxel and carboplatin in patients with advanced NSCLC.[79] Another selective MMPI, BAY 12-9566, has been evaluated in several disease settings, but after disappointing results in studies of SCLC and pancreatic cancer, its development has been suspended.

Fibroblasts might be a novel therapeutic target in cancer. The cell-surface serine protease known as fibroblast activation protein (FAP) is mostly expressed in wound healing and in tumor stroma. A phase I dose escalation study with an antibody directed to human FAP (sibrotuzumab) in patients with colorectal cancer or NSCLC has shown that the antibody bound specifically to the tumor sites.[80] Targeting CAFs as a therapeutic strategy against cancer needs further study.

A plethora of antiangiogenic agents inhibiting either angiogenic growth factors or their receptors have been developed and tested in preclinical experiments. More recent data from the clinical trials of the VEGF-specific antibody, bevacizumab (Avastin), showed that in patients with metastatic colorectal cancer, breast cancer, and NSCLC, there was a significant survival benefit when combined with chemotherapy,[81,82] leading to the Food and Drug Administration (FDA) approval of bevacizumab. Treatment with thalidomide, another antiangiogenic agent, was not associated with a significant improvement in survival of SCLC patients. However, there was pronounced heterogeneity in survival outcomes between groups of patients.[83] Some benefit was observed among patients with a performance status (PS) of 1 or 2, showing that angiogenesis deserves further study as a therapeutic target in this disease.

Epidemiological studies have demonstrated that people taking nonsteroidal anti-inflammatory drugs (NSAIDs) have a clear reduction in their risk of developing colorectal cancer,[84] and possibly other tumors. As a result, there were high expectations for the next-generation NSAIDs, the selective COX-2 inhibitors, in the prevention and treatment of cancers associated with chronic inflammation. Celecoxib had demonstrated ability to reduce the incidence of colorectal cancer.[85] The addition of rofecoxib did not improve overall survival compared with first-line treatment with cisplatin plus gemcitabine in patients with advanced NSCLC in a prospective, open-label, randomized phase III trial.[86] Most of the clinical trials have closed early because long-term high-dose COX-2 inhibitor elevates the risk of cardiovascular events[87]; alternative drugs will need to be identified.

CONCLUSION

A growing body of evidence demonstrates that cancer cells have accomplices. Quite early in tumor development, cancer cells co-opt blood vessels and recruit leukocytes and fibroblasts, reprogramming them to provide nourishment in the form of peptides that support cell proliferation and metastasis. Although their ability to dupe the host into becoming an ally provides cancer cells with a selective advantage, it may also be their Achilles heel. Initial efforts to elucidate the mechanisms by which cancer cells interact with surrounding cells within the tumor has revealed several potential therapeutic opportunities. Future research will better define these bidirectional interactions between tumor and host, and future clinical trials should be designed to capitalize on this understanding.

REFERENCES

1. Ardies CM. Inflammation as cause for scar cancers of the lung. *Integr Cancer Ther* 2003;2:238–246.
2. Ji H, Houghton AM, Mariani TJ, et al. K-ras activation generates an inflammatory response in lung tumors. *Oncogene* 2006;25:2105–2112.
3. Wislez M, Spencer ML, Izzo JG, et al. Inhibition of mammalian target of rapamycin reverses alveolar epithelial neoplasia induced by oncogenic K-ras. *Cancer Res* 2005;65:3226–3235.
4. Lin EY, Nguyen AV, Russell RG, et al. Colony-stimulating factor 1 promotes progression of mammary tumors to malignancy. *J Exp Med* 2001;193:727–740.
5. Sparmann A, Bar-Sagi D. Ras-induced interleukin-8 expression plays a critical role in tumor growth and angiogenesis. *Cancer Cell* 2004; 6:447–458.
6. Hagemann T, Balkwill F, Lawrence T. Inflammation and cancer: a double-edged sword. *Cancer Cell* 2007;12:300–301.
7. Bergers G, Benjamin LE. Tumorigenesis and the angiogenic switch. *Nat Rev Cancer* 2003;3:401–410.
8. Dolberg DS, Hollingsworth R, Hertle M, et al. Wounding and its role in RSV-mediated tumor formation. *Science* 1985;230:676–678.
9. Sappino AP, Skalli O, Jackson B, et al. Smooth-muscle differentiation in stromal cells of malignant and non-malignant breast tissues. *Int J Cancer* 1988;41:707–712.
10. Ronnov-Jessen L, Petersen OW. Induction of alpha-smooth muscle actin by transforming growth factor-beta 1 in quiescent human breast gland fibroblasts. Implications for myofibroblast generation in breast neoplasia. *Lab Invest* 1993;68:696–707.
11. Lohr M, Schmidt C, Ringel J, et al. Transforming growth factor-beta1 induces desmoplasia in an experimental model of human pancreatic carcinoma. *Cancer Res* 2001;61:550–555.
12. Bronzert DA, Pantazis P, Antoniades HN, et al. Synthesis and secretion of platelet-derived growth factor by human breast cancer cell lines. *Proc Natl Acad Sci U S A* 1987;84:5763–5767.

13. Folkman J, Klagsbrun M, Sasse J, et al. A heparin-binding angiogenic protein—basic fibroblast growth factor—is stored within basement membrane. *Am J Pathol* 1988;130:393–400.
14. Cheng JD, Weiner LM. Tumors and their microenvironments: tilling the soil. Commentary re: A. M. Scott et al., A Phase I dose-escalation study of sibrotuzumab in patients with advanced or metastatic fibroblast activation protein-positive cancer. Clin. Cancer Res., 9: 1639–1647, 2003. *Clin Cancer Res* 2003;9:1590–1595.
15. Adams EF, Newton CJ, Braunsberg H, et al. Effects of human breast fibroblasts on growth and 17 beta-estradiol dehydrogenase activity of MCF-7 cells in culture. *Breast Cancer Res Treat* 1988;11:165–172.
16. Camps JL, Chang SM, Hsu TC, et al. Fibroblast-mediated acceleration of human epithelial tumor growth in vivo. *Proc Natl Acad Sci U S A* 1990;87:75–79.
17. Olaso E, Santisteban A, Bidaurrazaga J, et al. Tumor-dependent activation of rodent hepatic stellate cells during experimental melanoma metastasis. *Hepatology* 1997;26:634–642.
18. Nazareth MR, Broderick L, Simpson-Abelson MR, et al. Characterization of human lung tumor-associated fibroblasts and their ability to modulate the activation of tumor-associated T cells. *J Immunol* 2007;178: 5552–5562.
19. Thomson S, Buck E, Petti F, et al. Epithelial to mesenchymal transition is a determinant of sensitivity of non-small-cell lung carcinoma cell lines and xenografts to epidermal growth factor receptor inhibition. *Cancer Res* 2005;65:9455–9462.
20. Witta SE, Gemmill RM, Hirsch FR, et al. Restoring E-cadherin expression increases sensitivity to epidermal growth factor receptor inhibitors in lung cancer cell lines. *Cancer Res* 2006;66:944–950.
21. Yauch RL, Januario T, Eberhard DA, et al. Epithelial versus mesenchymal phenotype determines in vitro sensitivity and predicts clinical activity of erlotinib in lung cancer patients. *Clin Cancer Res* 2005;11:8686–8698.
22. Fujimoto N, Segawa Y, Takigawa N, et al. Clinical investigation of bronchioloalveolar carcinoma: a retrospective analysis of 53 patients in a single institution. *Anticancer Res* 1999;19:1369–1373.
23. Pollard JW. Tumour-educated macrophages promote tumour progression and metastasis. *Nat Rev Cancer* 2004;4:71–78.
24. Chen JJ, Lin YC, Yao PL, et al. Tumor-associated macrophages: the double-edged sword in cancer progression. *J Clin Oncol* 2005;23:953–964.
25. Chen JJ, Yao PL, Yuan A, et al. Up-regulation of tumor interleukin-8 expression by infiltrating macrophages: its correlation with tumor angiogenesis and patient survival in non-small cell lung cancer. *Clin Cancer Res* 2003;9:729–737.
26. Welsh TJ, Green RH, Richardson D, et al. Macrophage and mast-cell invasion of tumor cell islets confers a marked survival advantage in non-small-cell lung cancer. *J Clin Oncol* 2005;23:8959–8967.
27. Lewis CE, Pollard JW. Distinct role of macrophages in different tumor microenvironments. *Cancer Res* 2006;66:605–612.
28. Mantovani A, Sozzani S, Locati M, et al. Macrophage polarization: tumor-associated macrophages as a paradigm for polarized M2 mononuclear phagocytes. *Trends Immunol* 2002;23:549–555.
29. Yuan A, Yang PC, Yu CJ, et al. Interleukin-8 messenger ribonucleic acid expression correlates with tumor progression, tumor angiogenesis, patient survival, and timing of relapse in non-small-cell lung cancer. *Am J Respir Crit Care Med* 2000;162:1957–1963.
30. Lewis JS, Landers RJ, Underwood JC, et al. Expression of vascular endothelial growth factor by macrophages is up-regulated in poorly vascularized areas of breast carcinomas. *J Pathol* 2000;192:150–158.
31. Barbera-Guillem E, Nyhus JK, Wolford CC, et al. Vascular endothelial growth factor secretion by tumor-infiltrating macrophages essentially supports tumor angiogenesis, and IgG immune complexes potentiate the process. *Cancer Res* 2002;62:7042–7049.
32. White ES, Strom SR, Wys NL, et al. Non-small cell lung cancer cells induce monocytes to increase expression of angiogenic activity. *J Immunol* 2001;166:7549–7555.
33. Lin EY, Li JF, Gnatovskiy L, et al. Macrophages regulate the angiogenic switch in a mouse model of breast cancer. *Cancer Res* 2006;66: 11238–11246.
34. Brandes ME, Finkelstein JN. Stimulated rabbit alveolar macrophages secrete a growth factor for type II pneumocytes. *Am J Respir Cell Mol Biol* 1989;1:101–109.
35. Leslie CC, McCormick-Shannon K, Cook JL, et al. Macrophages stimulate DNA synthesis in rat alveolar type II cells. *Am Rev Respir Dis* 1985;132:1246–1252.
36. Takizawa H, Beckmann JD, Shoji S, et al. Pulmonary macrophages can stimulate cell growth of bovine bronchial epithelial cells. *Am J Respir Cell Mol Biol* 1990;2:245–255.
37. Schwertfeger KL, Xian W, Kaplan AM, et al. A critical role for the inflammatory response in a mouse model of preneoplastic progression. *Cancer Res* 2006;66:5676–5685.
38. Lin EY, Gouon-Evans V, Nguyen AV, et al. The macrophage growth factor CSF-1 in mammary gland development and tumor progression. *J Mammary Gland Biol Neoplasia* 2002;7:147–162.
39. Goswami S, Sahai E, Wyckoff JB, et al. Macrophages promote the invasion of breast carcinoma cells via a colony-stimulating factor-1/epidermal growth factor paracrine loop. *Cancer Res* 2005;65:5278–5283.
40. Wyckoff J, Wang W, Lin EY, et al. A paracrine loop between tumor cells and macrophages is required for tumor cell migration in mammary tumors. *Cancer Res* 2004;64:7022–7029.
41. Bellocq A, Antoine M, Flahault A, et al. Neutrophil alveolitis in bronchioloalveolar carcinoma: induction by tumor-derived interleukin-8 and relation to clinical outcome. *Am J Pathol* 1998;152:83–92.
42. Wislez M, Massiani MA, Milleron B, et al. Clinical characteristics of pneumonic-type adenocarcinoma of the lung. *Chest* 2003;123:1868–1877.
43. Murphy C, McGurk M, Pettigrew J, et al. Nonapical and cytoplasmic expression of interleukin-8, CXCR1, and CXCR2 correlates with cell proliferation and microvessel density in prostate cancer. *Clin Cancer Res* 2005;11:4117–4127.
44. Schadendorf D, Moller A, Algermissen B, et al. M. IL-8 produced by human malignant melanoma cells in vitro is an essential autocrine growth factor. *J Immunol* 1993;151:2667–2675.
45. Zhu YM, Webster SJ, Flower D, et al. Interleukin-8/CXCL8 is a growth factor for human lung cancer cells. *Br J Cancer* 2004;91:1970–1976.
46. Shigematsu H, Lin L, Takahashi T, et al. Clinical and biological features associated with epidermal growth factor receptor gene mutations in lung cancers. *J Natl Cancer Inst* 2005;97:339–346.
47. Fisher GH, Wellen SL, Klimstra D, et al. Induction and apoptotic regression of lung adenocarcinomas by regulation of a K-ras transgene in the presence and absence of tumor suppressor genes. *Genes Dev* 2001; 15:3249–3262.
48. Guerra C, Mijimolle N, Dhawahir A, et al. Tumor induction by an endogenous K-ras oncogene is highly dependent on cellular context. *Cancer Cell* 2003;4:111–120.
49. Jackson EL, Willis N, Mercer K, et al. Analysis of lung tumor initiation and progression using conditional expression of oncogenic K-ras. *Genes Dev* 2001;15:3243–3248.
50. Johnson L, Mercer K, Greenbaum D, et al. Somatic activation of the K-ras oncogene causes early onset lung cancer in mice. *Nature* 2001; 410:1111–1116.
51. Mascaux C, Iannino N, Martin B, et al. The role of RAS oncogene in survival of patients with lung cancer: a systematic review of the literature with meta-analysis. *Br J Cancer* 2005;92:131–139.
52. Pao W, Wang TY, Riely GJ, et al. KRAS Mutations and Primary Resistance of Lung Adenocarcinomas to Gefitinib or Erlotinib. *PLoS Med* 2005;2:E17.
53. Keane MP, Belperio JA, Xue YY, et al. Depletion of CXCR2 inhibits tumor growth and angiogenesis in a murine model of lung cancer. *J Immunol* 172:2853–2860.
54. Wislez M, Fujimoto N, Izzo JG, et al. High expression of ligands for chemokine receptor CXCR2 in alveolar epithelial neoplasia induced by oncogenic kras. *Cancer Res* 2006;66:4198–4207.
55. Wislez M, Fleury-Feith J, Rabbe N, et al. Tumor-derived granulocyte-macrophage colony-stimulating factor and granulocyte colony-stimulating factor prolong the survival of neutrophils infiltrating bronchoalveolar subtype pulmonary adenocarcinoma. *Am J Pathol* 2001;159:1423–1433.

56. Jackson JH, Vollenweider M, Hill J, et al. Stimulated human leukocytes cause activating mutations in the K-ras protooncogene. *Oncogene* 12;14(23):2803–2808
57. Weitberg AB, Weitzman SA, Destrempes M, et al. Stimulated human phagocytes produce cytogenetic changes in cultured mammalian cells. *N Engl J Med* 1983;308(1):26–30.
58. Wislez M, Rabbe N, Marchal J, et al. Hepatocyte growth factor production by neutrophils infiltrating bronchioloalveolar subtype pulmonary adenocarcinoma: role in tumor progression and death. *Cancer Res* 2003;63:1405–1412.
59. Wislez M, Antoine M, Rabbe N, et al. Neutrophils promote aerogenous spread of lung adenocarcinoma with bronchioloalveolar carcinoma features. *Clin Cancer Res* 2007;13:3518–3527.
60. Hoshi R, Tsuzuku M, Horai T, et al. Micropapillary clusters in early-stage lung adenocarcinomas: a distinct cytologic sign of significantly poor prognosis. *Cancer* 2004;102:81–86.
61. Takanami I, Takeuchi K, Naruke M. Mast cell density is associated with angiogenesis and poor prognosis in pulmonary adenocarcinoma. *Cancer* 2000;88(12):2686–2692.
62. Ibaraki T, Muramatsu M, Takai S, et al. The relationship of tryptase- and chymase-positive mast cells to angiogenesis in stage I non-small cell lung cancer. *Eur J Cardiothorac Surg* 2005;28:617–621.
63. Tomita M, Matsuzaki Y, Onitsuka T. Correlation between mast cells and survival rates in patients with pulmonary adenocarcinoma. *Lung Cancer* 1999;26:103–108.
64. Imada A, Shijubo N, Kojima H, et al. Mast cells correlate with angiogenesis and poor outcome in stage I lung adenocarcinoma. *Eur Respir J* 2000;15:1087–1093.
65. Chiodoni C, Paglia P, Stoppacciaro A, et al. Dendritic cells infiltrating tumors cotransduced with granulocyte/macrophage colony-stimulating factor (GM-CSF) and CD40 ligand genes take up and present endogenous tumor-associated antigens, and prime naive mice for a cytotoxic T lymphocyte response. *J Exp Med* 1999;190(1):125–133.
66. Yang SC, Batra RK, Hillinger S, et al. Intrapulmonary administration of CCL21 gene-modified dendritic cells reduces tumor burden in spontaneous murine bronchoalveolar cell carcinoma. *Cancer Res* 2006; 66:3205–3213.
67. Vicari AP, Chiodoni C, Vaure C, et al. Reversal of tumor-induced dendritic cell paralysis by CpG immunostimulatory oligonucleotide and anti-interleukin 10 receptor antibody. *J Exp Med* 2002;196:541–549.
68. Guiducci C, Vicari AP, Sangaletti S, et al. Redirecting in vivo elicited tumor infiltrating macrophages and dendritic cells towards tumor rejection. *Cancer Res* 2005;65:3437–3446.
69. Restifo NP, Esquivel F, Kawakami Y, et al. Identification of human cancers deficient in antigen processing. *J Exp Med* 1993;177:265–272.
70. Zang X, Allison JP. The b7 family and cancer therapy: costimulation and coinhibition. *Clin Cancer Res* 2007;13:5271–5279.
71. Batra RK, Lin Y, Sharma S, et al. Non-small cell lung cancer-derived soluble mediators enhance apoptosis in activated T lymphocytes through an I kappa B kinase-dependent mechanism. *Cancer Res* 2003; 63:642–646.
72. Woo EY, Yeh H, Chu CS, et al. Cutting edge: regulatory T cells from lung cancer patients directly inhibit autologous T cell proliferation. *J Immunol* 2002;168: 4272–4276.
73. de Visser KE, Korets LV, Coussens LM. De novo carcinogenesis promoted by chronic inflammation is B lymphocyte dependent. *Cancer Cell* 2005;7:411–423.
74. Bramhall SR, Hallissey MT, Whiting J, et al. Marimastat as maintenance therapy for patients with advanced gastric cancer: a randomised trial. *Br J Cancer* 2002;86:1864–1870.
75. Bramhall SR, Schulz J, Nemunaitis J, et al. A double-blind placebo-controlled, randomised study comparing gemcitabine and marimastat with gemcitabine and placebo as first line therapy in patients with advanced pancreatic cancer. *Br J Cancer* 2002;87:161–167.
76. Miller KD, Gradishar W, Schuchter L, et al. A randomized phase II pilot trial of adjuvant marimastat in patients with early-stage breast cancer. *Ann Oncol* 2002;13:1220–1224.
77. Shepherd FA, Giaccone G, Seymour L, et al. Prospective, randomized, double-blind, placebo-controlled trial of marimastat after response to first-line chemotherapy in patients with small-cell lung cancer: a trial of the National Cancer Institute of Canada-Clinical Trials Group and the European Organization for Research and Treatment of Cancer. *J Clin Oncol* 2002;20:4434–4439.
78. Bissett D, O'Byrne KJ, von Pawel J, et al. Phase III study of matrix metalloproteinase inhibitor prinomastat in non-small-cell lung cancer. *J Clin Oncol* 2005;23:842–849.
79. Smylie M, Mercier R, Aboulafia D. Phase III study of the matrix metalloprotease (MMP) inhibitor prinomastat in patients having advanced non-small cell lung cancer. [Abstract]. *Proc Am Soc Clin Oncol* 2001;20:1226.
80. Scott AM, Wiseman G, Welt S, et al. A Phase I dose-escalation study of sibrotuzumab in patients with advanced or metastatic fibroblast activation protein-positive cancer. *Clin Cancer Res* 2003;9:1639–1647.
81. Hurwitz H, Fehrenbacher L, Novotny W, et al. Bevacizumab plus irinotecan, fluorouracil, and leucovorin for metastatic colorectal cancer. *N Engl J Med* 2004;350:2335–2342.
82. Sandler A, Gray R, Perry MC, et al. Paclitaxel-carboplatin alone or with bevacizumab for non-small-cell lung cancer. *N Engl J Med* 2006; 355:2542–2550.
83. Pujol JL, Breton JL, Gervais R, et al. Phase III double-blind, placebo-controlled study of thalidomide in extensive-disease small-cell lung cancer after response to chemotherapy: an intergroup study FNCLCC cleo04 IFCT 00–01. *J Clin Oncol* 200725:3945–3951.
84. Thun MJ, Namboodiri MM, Heath CW Jr. Aspirin use and reduced risk of fatal colon cancer. *N Engl J Med* 1991;325:1593–1596.
85. Arber N, Eagle CJ, Spicak J, et al. Celecoxib for the prevention of colorectal adenomatous polyps. *N Engl J Med* 2006;355:885–895.
86. Gridelli C, Gallo C, Ceribelli A, et al. Factorial phase III randomised trial of rofecoxib and prolonged constant infusion of gemcitabine in advanced non-small-cell lung cancer: the GEmcitabine-COxib in NSCLC (GECO) study. *Lancet Oncol* 2007;8:500–512.
87. Bresalier RS, Sandler RS, Quan H, et al. Cardiovascular events associated with rofecoxib in a colorectal adenoma chemoprevention trial. *N Engl J Med* 2005;352:1092–1102.

CHAPTER 13

Ambra Pozzi

Mouse Models of Lung Cancer

Lung cancer has increased in incidence throughout the 20th century and is now the most common cancer in the Western World. Compared to other cancers, the pathogenesis of lung cancer remains highly elusive because of its aggressive biologic nature and considerable heterogeneity. Most patients die of progressive metastatic diseases despite aggressive local and systemic therapies. To better understand the different steps in lung cancer progression and, most importantly, to devise more effective lung cancer therapies, there is considerable need for improved experimental models of lung cancer.

Currently, several animal species are widely used for experimental lung cancer research, including dogs, primates, hamsters, and mice.[1–3] Among the different animal species, mice have become the preferred model to study lung cancer development and progression because of their relative cost-effectiveness, the ease of genetic manipulation, and the large number of genetically altered mice available for experimentation. Primary lung tumors in mice have morphologic, histogenic, and molecular features similar to human lung adenocarcinoma, particularly the bronchioloalveolar carcinoma subtype. Because of this, and because of the genetic homology between man and mouse, this model system is receiving intense research attention.

Three major different models are commonly used to induce lung cancer in mice, namely chemically and/or carcinogen-induced lung cancer, orthotopic models of lung cancer, and genetic models of lung cancer. In addition, spontaneous lung cancer develops in approximately 3% of mice and has a strain-dependent incidence in inbred mice (Fig. 13.1).[4] Mice that develop spontaneous lung tumors also respond to chemicals and carcinogens, thus making them an ideal system to study chemically and/or carcinogen-induced lung cancer. Each of the mouse models available allows the analysis of different aspects of the disease, such as carcinogenesis, initiation, promotion, metastasis, as well as host–tumor interaction and angiogenesis. For example, the chemically induced lung cancer models allow the study of tumor initiation and promotion; the orthotopic model allows the analysis of primary as well as metastatic lung cancers, whereas the genetic model allows the identification of genes involved in lung cancer development and progression.

Despite the fact that these models reflect the histopathology and the steps involved in lung cancer progression, each of them has limitations. These include lack of metastasis (genetic- and chemically induced lung cancer), the development of tumors only late in their course of development (chemically induced lung cancer), and the development of only one subset of lung cancer, namely adenoma and/or adenocarcinoma. For these reasons, more than one model is used when studying the etiology, pathogenesis, and progression of lung cancer.

In this chapter, we will describe the main features of the available mouse models of lung cancer, and how these models can be used for translational research. We will mainly point out practical benefits, such as their application for identifying therapeutic strategies for the treatment and prevention of lung cancer.

CHEMICALLY INDUCED LUNG CANCER

Cigarette smoking represents the prominent cause of lung cancer. More than 20 lung carcinogens have been identified in cigarette smoke, and they can act as initiators and/or promoters of lung cancer by accelerating tumor onset and increasing tumor multiplicity.[5] Although 85% of lung cancers are thought to be as a result of cigarette smoking, individuals exposed to asbestos, arsenic, nickel, radiation, and those with pulmonary fibrosis are also at increased risk.[6] For this reason, chemically and carcinogen-induced animal models of lung cancer have been developed. They are used not only to identify possible molecules and/or environmental factors able to induce lung cancer but also to study the early stage of carcinogenesis and cancer progression. Chemically and/or carcinogen-induced lung tumors have been described in various species, including dogs, cats, ferrets, and mice.[6] The susceptibility of mice to develop chemically and/or carcinogen-induced lung cancer is strain dependent. Mouse strains have been categorized into sensitive, intermediate, and resistant,[7] based on the time of occurrence of lung tumors after

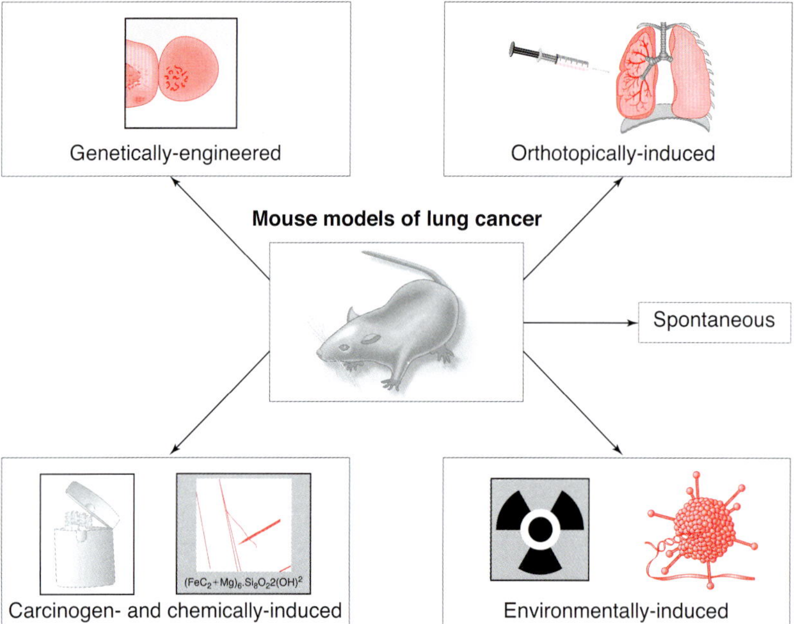

FIGURE 13.1 Examples of murine models of lung cancer. Mouse models of lung cancer include spontaneous lung tumors; carcinogen- and/or chemically induced tumors (i.e., tobacco, asbestos); environmentally induced tumors (i.e., radiation, viruses), genetically induced tumors (i.e., transgenic expression or germline disruptions of genes), and orthotopically induced tumors (i.e., injection of human tumor cells directly in the lung).

chemical exposure, and on the number of tumors. The A/J mouse strain belongs to the sensitive group with at least 20 times higher susceptibility than resistant strains like C57BL/6J and C3H/HeJ or intermediate strains like BALB/c. The propensity of these sensitive strains to develop lung tumors strongly correlates with a polymorphism in the second intron of the K-ras gene.[8] The polymorphism is a 37-nucleotide–intronic sequence that is tandemly duplicated in resistant strains and is present as a single copy in sensitive strains. This polymorphism seems to confer different nuclear protein-binding abilities that may influence gene expression.[9] In addition to the K-ras gene, the pulmonary adenoma susceptibility 1 (Pas1) locus on chromosome 6 has been implicated in the development of lung cancer in the A/J strain.[10] Based on the fact that both the Pas1 and K-ras genes map on chromosome 6,[11] it has been proposed that the Pas1 gene could be identical to the K-ras oncogene, and natural and/or chemically induced point mutation in Pas1 gene could lead to lung tumors similarly to what observed with the K-ras gene.[8] When A/J mice are exposed to urethane, mutations in either one of these polymorphic loci occur, resulting in the development of benign lung adenoma within few months from the exposure.[12] Some of these tumors can progress to adenocarcinomas with histopathology similar to that seen in humans.[13]

More recently, Stathopoulos and colleagues[14] have elegantly shown that epithelial nuclear factor (NF)-κB activation facilitates urethane-induced lung carcinogenesis. In this context, mouse strains susceptible to lung tumor formation (i.e., FVB, BALB/c) exhibited early NF-κB activation and inflammation in the lungs after urethane treatment. In contrast, the resistant strain C57B6 failed to activate NF-κB or induce lung inflammation. Interestingly, selective NF-κB inhibition resulted in increased apoptosis of airway epithelial cells after urethane exposure, highly suggesting that NF-κB signaling in airway epithelium is integral to chemically induced tumorigenesis.[14]

Another common example of carcinogen-induced lung neoplasia is the classical two-step initiation/promotion model. Injection of the initiator 3-methylcholanthrene, followed by various exposures to the promoter butylated hydroxytoluene, has been shown to induce adenocarcinoma in BALB/c mice within 16 weeks from the exposure to the initiator. The first stage in this two-stage carcinogenesis procedure (initiation) induces an irreversible lesion in the DNA of a single cell, while the second stage (promotion) initiates cell clonally expands.

Mice are also used to assess carcinogenic activity of various chemicals, including benzopyrenes, metals, nitrosamines, and polyaromatic hydrocarbons.[12] Biochemical effects of lung chemicals can be detected within hours or days of their administration. In strains susceptible to lung tumorigenesis, exposure to chemicals leads to rapid formation of hyperplastic foci in the bronchioles and alveoli. All or some of these foci then evolve into microscopic adenomas, and few months later, some of these adenomas display the nuclear atypia and invasiveness of adenocarcinomas in situ.[15] In contrast, exposure of chemicals in resistant strains only leads to the development of few adenomas and/or papillary tumors within several months from the original exposure.

Given the high incidence of cigarette-induced lung cancer, many animal models have been used to determine the effect of cigarette smoke on lung cancer incidence, formation, and progression.[3] Despite the vast research conducted, it is debatable whether the measured response to cigarette smoke in animal species for assessing carcinogenic potential in humans reflects the strong epidemiological evidence in human smokers. In a recent review article, Coggins[3] points out some of the pitfalls related to exposure of animal models to cigarette smoke. In this context, the cigarettes used in many studies were unfiltered and had very high yields; thus being very different from the cigarettes commonly smoked today. In addition, whereas some studies used nose-only smoking machines, others used whole-body exposures. Moreover, whereas certain animal models were exposed to single cigarettes, others were exposed to rotating carousels. Finally, when dogs were used for studies, invasive tracheotomy technique was used to facilitate smoke breathing. As results, often lung necrosis and/or inflammation with no apparent neoplasm were evident. Thus, these studies not only do not entirely mimic the exposure of smoke as observed in humans, but also do not recapitulate the events of lung cancer initiation/formation. Lastly, studies performed in rats and mice exposure for lifetime to cigarette smoke suggested that, although both species developed alveolar epithelial hyperplasia, alveolar adenomas, and alveolar carcinomas, the incidence of all three were more evident in the rats. Thus, mice might not represent the most suitable model for smoke-mediated lung cancer.[16]

Mice, however, have been successfully used to study susceptibility to lung cancer following exposure to environmental agents such as radiation and viruses.[17,18] Although these two nonchemical models have the advantage that they are not strain dependent, they present the major disadvantage that tumors develop in various organs, beside the lungs, making the analysis of primary versus potential metastatic lung cancer more difficult to evaluate.

The observation that sensitive mice are more susceptible to chemically induced lung cancer became the basis for quantitative carcinogenicity bioassay[12] and screening systems for chemopreventive agents.[19] Cancer chemoprevention can be defined as the use of agents able to prevent, inhibit, or reverse the process of carcinogenesis.[20] Various anti-inflammatory drugs such as indomethacin or aspirin have been used to lower chemically induced lung tumor development and multiplicity,[21] and specific cyclooxygenase-2 inhibitors have been used to reduce the growth of adenocarcinoma after treatment with carcinogens.[15] In addition, pretreatment of mice with drugs able to inhibit DNA methylation showed chemopreventive efficacy in primary mouse lung tumors induced by nitrosamines (see Chapter 7).[22] Finally, the effect of natural products can be tested for their preventive effect on carcinogen-induced lung cancer. Kohno and colleagues[23] identified chemopreventive factors (i.e., beta-cryptoxanthin and hesperidin) in commercial mandarin juice, able to suppress lung cancer initiated with nitrosamines in A/J mice. In addition, pretreatment with perillyl alcohol, a naturally occurring monoterpene found in lavender, cherries, and mint, 1 week before lung tumor initiation with nitrosamines, significantly reduced tumor incidence and tumor multiplicity, strongly suggesting that this monoterpene is an effective chemopreventive compound in mouse lung tumor bioassay.[24]

In summary, chemically and/or carcinogen-induced lung cancer models offer the major advantage that the induction of lung tumors is highly reproducible, and they can also be used to screen potential carcinogens as well as to identify chemopreventive agents. There are, however, disadvantages of these models. In particular, they are time consuming, strain dependent, lead primarily to the development of non–small cell lung carcinoma (NSCLC), allow the detection of lung tumors at late stage of progression, and lead to the development of tumors with low metastatic potential. Moreover, for study related to cigarette-smoke–induced lung cancer, mice might not represent the best animal models available. Finally, administration of chemicals or carcinogens can yield to various different tumor cell types, many of which might not be directly relevant to human lung cancer.

ORTHOTOPIC MODEL OF LUNG CANCER

Orthotopic models of cancers consist in the injection of tumor cell suspension as well as in the implantation of fresh tumor tissues directly into the appropriate organ of origin. Human tumors and/or human cancer cells can be orthotopically implanted in various organs, including stomach, colon, pancreas, prostate, mammary gland, bladder, and lung.[25] The availability of immunodeficient mouse strains such as the nude mice, the $Rag2^{-/-}$ mice, and the severe combined immunodeficient (SCID) mice facilitated the establishment of human orthotopic models of cancer because of the inefficiency of these mice to reject human cells. The injection of tumor cells in the organ of origin clearly allows a better understanding of the role of the microenvironment in the development of primary tumors. In addition, a major advantage of this model is that it allows studying and recapitulating of the entire process of tumor progression consisting of local tumor growth, vascular and lymphatic invasion at the local site, flow in the vessels and lymphatic, extravasation at the metastatic organs, and seeding and growth at relevant metastatic sites. The availability of both human NSCLC and small cell lung carcinoma (SCLC) cells make the orthotopic model an attractive assay to study lung cancer growth and development as, at present, there is only one genetic mouse model of primary SCLC available (see discussion later). In addition, based on the observation that the microenvironment profoundly affects the phenotype and progression of many tumor types,[26] the injection of lung cancer cells directly into the organ of origin may recapitulate the events of lung cancer growth and progression similar to those observed in humans. Several orthotopic injection routes have been developed for lung cancer, including intrabronchial,[27–29] intrathoracic,[30] intrapleural or intravenous,[31] and direct injection of tumor cells[32,33] as well as implantation of fragments of subcutaneously growing tumor tissues[34] into the lung parenchyma of recipient mice. Of these models, the direct injection of tumor cells into the lung parenchyma represents an exceptionally rapid procedure with limited trauma to the mice and reduced intrapleural leakage of tumor cells. In addition, this method had been successfully used to produce a solitary tumor nodule in the lung followed by metastasis to the mediastinal lymph nodes. It is well recognized that the orthotopically growing tumors will grow and metastasize to organs similarly to the human situation. Thus, the presence of tumors in the contralateral noninjected lung, as well as presence of metastases in lymph nodes, liver, brain, and bones can be used to evaluate the metastatic efficiency of different lung cancer cell lines.[33]

One of the major issues related to cancer is the detection of micrometastases (single cell or clusters of fewer than 10 cells). To improve the visualization of tumors in different organs, tumor cells can be stably labeled with different fluorescent or bioluminescent markers such as green fluorescent protein (GFP)[35] and luciferase.[36] Single GFP-labeled tumor cells can be detected in freshly isolated organs with a fluorescence microscope,[37] and the number of tumors growing on the surface and/or within the organs can be evaluated, and quantitative measurements can be obtained using computer software imaging programs.[33] Retroviral delivery of GFP has been successfully used not only to label primary human tumors, but also to analyze regional and distant metastases.[38] A significant advantage of using GFP- or luciferase-expressing cells is that tumors can be visualized and measured externally in live mice. Hoffman[37] implanted highly metastatic human cell line expressing GFP into the left lungs of nude mice and then followed primary and metastatic growth in real time by analyzing the mice under fluorescence light. Similarly, Rosol and colleagues[39] injected into the left ventricle luciferase-labeled metastatic cells and followed in real time their localization in the lungs by using in vivo bioluminescent imaging. More recently, Acuff and colleagues[29] have used luciferase-labeled human NSCLC cells to determine in real time the contribution of host-derived matrix metalloproteinases to the survival and the early establishment of tumors in the lung. Finally, noninvasive in real-time imaging has been recently employed to determine the effect of systemic delivery of capsid-modified adenoviruses in an orthotopic model of advanced lung cancer.[40] Thus, the use of labeled cells clearly facilitates in vivo imaging as well as longitudinal studies as the same mouse can be monitored over time (Fig. 13.2).

The different orthotopic models of lung cancers, in combination with the intravital imaging of GFP-expressing cells, clearly allow one to follow in real time the effects of chemopreventive and/or antimetastatic drugs. In addition, they allow to asses some critical parameters related to the use of these drugs for cancer treatment and/or prevention, such as (a) the selection of the tumor models that better resemble the phases of tumor progression in humans, (b) the route of administration of the drug, (c) the maximal dose tolerated, (d) the relationship between the desired therapeutic benefits and the length of the treatment, and (e) how long the beneficial effects of the drug last upon withdrawal. It has been observed that orthotopically transplanted human SCLC display a different chemosensitivity pattern compared with the subcutaneously transplanted model,[41] clearly suggesting a different pharmacodynamics between the orthotopic lung and the ectopic subcutaneous sites. Using an orthotopic human lung cancer model, Liu and colleagues[42] showed that KP-392, a potent selective inhibitor of integrin-linked kinase, can be used in combination with cisplatin to enhance tumor necrosis and decrease lung cancer progression. In addition, in vivo inhibition of both vascular endothelial growth factor receptor 2 (VEGFR2) and epidermal growth factor receptor (EGFR) signaling pathways by ZD6474 resulted in profound reduced angiogenesis as well as growth of human lung adenocarcinoma cells orthotopically injected in mice,[43] suggesting that blocking both EGFR and VEGFR signaling might be viewed as a valid tool for the management of locally advanced lung cancer. Finally, aerosol nonviral gene delivery system has been recently used to successfully deliver p53 gene to mice intratracheally inoculated with H358 human NSCLC cell line,[44] strongly indicating this therapeutic strategy might be viewed as an option for patients with early lung cancer.

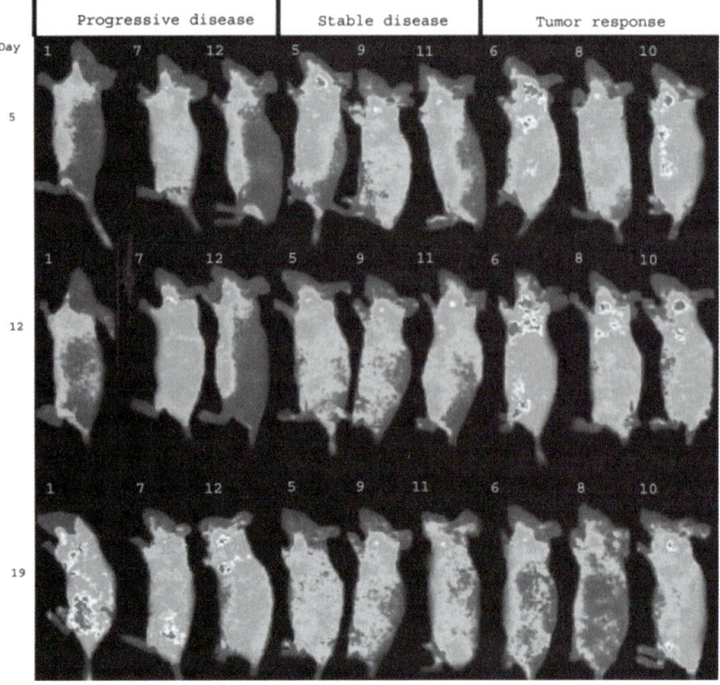

FIGURE 13.2 Noninvasive imaging reveals individual variation in mice treated with conditionally replicating oncolytic adenoviruses (CRAds). Examples of treatment results in mice treated with Ad5-Δ24RGD. The labels at left indicate the day of imaging, and each mouse is identified with a number. Mice *1*, *7*, and *12* had progressive disease; mice *5*, *9*, and *11* had stable disease; and mice *6*, *8*, and *10* achieved tumor response. (From Sarkioja M, Kanerva A, Salo J, et al. Noninvasive imaging for evaluation of the systemic delivery of capsid-modified adenoviruses in an orthotopic model of advanced lung cancer. *Cancer* 2006;107:1578–1588.) (See color plate.)

Thus, the orthotopic models of human cancer offer a tool for the discovery of new chemopreventive and antimetastatic agents, for the design of drug treatment regimes, and for investigating their mechanism of actions in a model that better resembles the phases of tumor progression observed in humans.

GENETIC MODELS OF LUNG CANCER

The generation of transgenic mouse strains able to develop lung cancer similar to the human situation enabled the identification of the genes that drive lung cancer development and progression. Multiple genetic changes are involved in the development and progression of lung cancer.[45] These genetic changes were found to inactivate tumor suppressor genes, activate oncogenes, cause loss of heterozygosity (i.e., deletion of one of two copies of allelic DNA sequences in particular chromosomal regions), or amplify specific chromosomal regions. Three major tumor suppressor genes have been identified as being inactivated in lung cancer. The p53 and retinoblastoma (Rb) genes are frequently inactivated by genetic alterations such as chromosomal deletions and loss-of-function mutations, whereas the p16 gene is inactivated by genetic alterations as well as by transcriptional silencing because of hypermethylation.[45] Among the oncogenes, K-ras represents the main member of this family involved in the development of lung cancer and up to 30% of adenocarcinomas contains activated K-ras.[46]

To recapitulate the events of lung tumor development and progression, mice harboring genetic mutations similar to that observed in human lung cancer have been generated. Most of these genetically manipulated mice are suitable for the study of genetic alteration in NSCLC as they primarily develop pulmonary adenomas and adenocarcinomas. Transgenic mice that express SV40 large T antigen, under the control of promoters specific to pulmonary epithelium, develop multiple lung tumors that cause early death.[47] Moreover, transgenic mice expressing the proto-oncogenic H-ras under control of its own promoter have a high incidence of lung tumors,[48] and transgenic mice carrying a dominant negative mutation in the p53 gene placed under the control of its own endogenous promoter[49] or under a Clara cell secretory protein promoter to target p53 expression specifically in the lung[50] are more susceptible to several potential lung carcinogens, including nitrosamines and benzo(a)pyrene. The lung adenomas generated in the dominant negative p53 transgenic mice exposed to carcinogens possess activating mutations in the K-ras proto-oncogene.[51] Thus, the dominant negative p53 transgenic mice not only offer a suitable model to study the additive effects of genetic alteration and environmental factors in the development of lung cancer, but also clearly demonstrate that the progression of lung cancer is a multiple-hit genetic event.

Besides mutations in key genes such as oncogenes or tumor suppressor genes, altered expression of various growth factors can be used as prognostic marker for lung cancer. Increased plasma levels of insulin-like growth factor-II (IGF-II), for example, are associated with a poor prognosis in human pulmonary adenocarcinoma[52] and specific transgenic overexpression of IGF-II in lung epithelium induces spontaneous lung tumors in 69% of mice older than 18 months of age.[53] These tumors display morphological characteristics of human pulmonary adenocarcinoma (i.e., epithelial origin, tubuloacinar architecture), strongly suggesting a critical role for IGF-II in NSCLC development.

In addition to transgenic mice, mice that have germline disruptions of genes involved in lung cancer have been generated. Mice heterozygous and homozygous deficient for the tumor suppressor genes p53[54] and p16INK4a[55] are viable but have shortened life span because of the predominant occurrence of lymphomas and various sarcomas. Although the incidence of lung cancer is not increased in the p53- and p16INK4a-null mice, most likely because of their short life span, bronchiolar neuroendocrine cell hyperplasia has been described in p53-null mice.[56] Interestingly, similar histological findings have been noted in some patients with benign obstructive respiratory disorders or with carcinoid tumors of the lung, an uncommon human pulmonary epithelial malignancy that rarely metastasizes.[57]

Thirty percent of human tumors carry Ras gene mutations. Of the three genes in this family, composed of K-ras, N-ras, and H-ras, K-ras is the most frequently mutated member in human tumors, including adenocarcinomas of the pancreas (~70% to 90% incidence), colon (~50%), and lung (~25% to 50%). Mice harboring the latent oncogenic mutation G12D in the endogenous K-ras gene (K-rasLA) have been generated.[58] Because early expression of oncogenic K-ras causes mice to die very early during development, the K-rasLA mice have been generated using the "hit-and-run" gene-targeting procedure that involves two distinct steps of homologous recombination. The first recombination event (insertion event) is created in embryonic stem cells ("hit" step), whereas the second recombination event (excision event) occur in vivo only upon a somatic recombination event ("run" step). All mice, carrying this latent allele of K-ras, develop multiple lung tumors, evident as early as 1 week after birth, with histological features of human NSCLC. These tumors, unlike the human situation, do not or rarely metastasize, most likely because of a significant reduced life span of the mice.[58]

The K-rasLA mice have been either crossed with various transgenic mice, or treated with selective drugs to determine the contribution of specific gene products in K-ras–mediated lung tumorigenesis (Table 13.1). In this context, treatment of K-rasLA1 mice with anti-CXCR2 neutralizing antibodies[59] or the EGFR inhibitor gefitinib[60] has resulted in inhibition of lung cancer progression and reduced number/expansion of alveolar neoplasia, respectively. Similarly, the cross of K-rasLA2 mice with mice lacking the collagen receptor integrin-$\alpha1\beta1$ resulted in prolonged survival as well as reduced number and size of NSCLC, suggesting that collagen receptors and K-ras might cooperate in lung cancer progression (Macias-Perez, Pozzi, unpublished; Table 13.1 and Fig. 13.3). In contrast, the cross of K-ras-LA with TGF-β heterozygote[61] or p53-null mice[58] led to decreased survival rate with accelerated onset and

TABLE 13.1 Examples of How Mice Expressing Oncogenic K-Ras Have Been Used for Analysis of NSCLC Progression and/or Treatment

Mouse Lung Cancer Model	Animal Model of Interest	Treatment	Results	References
KrasLA1		Anti-CXCR2 neutralizing antibodies	Inhibition of malignant lung cancer progression	59
KrasLA1		Gefitinib	Reduced number and expansion of alveolar neoplasia	60
KrasLA2	Integrin-α1 null		Prolonged survival with reduced number, size, and incidence of NSCLC	Figure 13.3
KrasLA	TGF-β heterozygotes		Decreased survival with accelerated progression of adenocarcinomas	61
KrasLA1	p53 null		Accelerated onset of cancer, resulting in significant decreased survival	58
Conditionally activatable oncogenic *K-ras*	$Rac1^{fl/fl}$	AdenoCre intranasal infection	Prolonged survival with reduced number, size, and incidence of NSCLC	64
Conditionally activatable oncogenic *K-ras*	$p53^{fl/fl}$	AdenoCre intranasal infection	Increased tumor multiplicity and decreased median survival	65
Conditionally activatable oncogenic *K-ras*	$p6^{Ink4a}$ null	AdenoCre intranasal infection	Mild increased tumor multiplicity with no changes in median survival	65
Conditionally activatable oncogenic *K-ras*	Ink4a/Arf null	AdenoCre intranasal infection	Increased tumor multiplicity with no changes in median survival	65
Conditionally activatable oncogenic *K-ras*	$Lkb1^{fl/fl/}$	AdenoCre intranasal infection	Increased tumor multiplicity and decreased median survival	65
Conditionally activatable oncogenic *K-ras*	LucRep mouse	AdenoCre intranasal infection	In vivo detection of single lesion measuring 1–2 mm in diameter	66

progression of lung cancer, suggesting that TGF-β and p53 inhibit K-ras–mediated lung cancer initiation/progression.

Clearly, the generation of transgenic mice carrying the same mutated genes observed in human lung cancer has enabled scientists to better characterize the mechanisms by which these genes drive lung cancer development. However, these genetic models of lung cancer present the major disadvantages that (a) mice develop primarily a subset of lung cancer; (b) tumors usually do not metastasize, unlike in the human situation; and (c) because of the short life span of tumor-bearing mice, it is impossible to study the progression of lung cancer. To improve mouse models of lung cancer initiation and progression, Jackson and colleagues[62] generated a Lox-Stop-Lox K-ras conditional mouse strain in which expression of oncogenic K-ras is controlled by a removable transcriptional termination *stop* element. Upon removal of the stop element, achieved by intranasal administration of AdenoCre virus, the mice develop lung cancer. Usually, tumors are visible within 2 weeks postinfection, and they evolve from adenomatous hyperplasia to adenocarcinoma within 16 weeks postinfection. Similarly, Meuwissen and colleagues[63] generated transgenic animals in which the chicken β-actin promoter drives the expression of GFP and oncogenic $K\text{-}ras^{V12}$ gene. As a polyadenylation signal behind the GFP cassette prevents read-through into the $K\text{-}ras^{V12}$ gene, expression of $K\text{-}ras^{V12}$ is dependent on Cre-lox–mediated deletion of the GFP fragment. Within up to 56 weeks postinfection, all mice developed multiple lesions that subsequently developed into larger, papillary-like tumors within 8 weeks postinfection.[63]

Without any doubt, the advances of these inducible methods over existing models are that timing of tumor initiation and location can be controlled and tumor multiplicity can be adjusted by varying the administration of AdenoCre. Recently, the K-ras–floxed mice described previously have been crossed with either the $Rac1^{fl/fl}$ mice[64] or the $Lkb1^{fl/fl}$ mice[65] and the incidence of lung cancer was followed upon AdenoCre intranasal infection. Whereas expression of oncogenic K-ras in the absence of small GTPase Rac1 led to prolonged survival with reduced number, size, and incidence of NSCLC[64] (Table 13.1), expression of oncogenic K-ras in the absence of the serine/threonine kinase 11 Lkb1 increased tumor multiplicity and metastasis, but decreased median survival[65] (Table 13.1). Thus, these studies establish Rac1 as a critical key player in lung cancer progression, whereas LKB1 can be viewed as antipulmonary tumorigenic kinase, controlling initiation, differentiation, and metastasis. Finally, Lyons and colleagues[66] have crossed the K-ras–floxed mice with the LucRep transgenic mouse that enables bioluminescence imaging only upon AdenoCre treatment. Direct imaging of the lungs from K-ras–floxed/LucRep mice treated with AdenoCre revealed the in vivo detection of single lesion measuring between 1 and 2 mm in diameter.[66] Thus, the LucRep mice can be successfully used not only for noninvasive bioluminescence

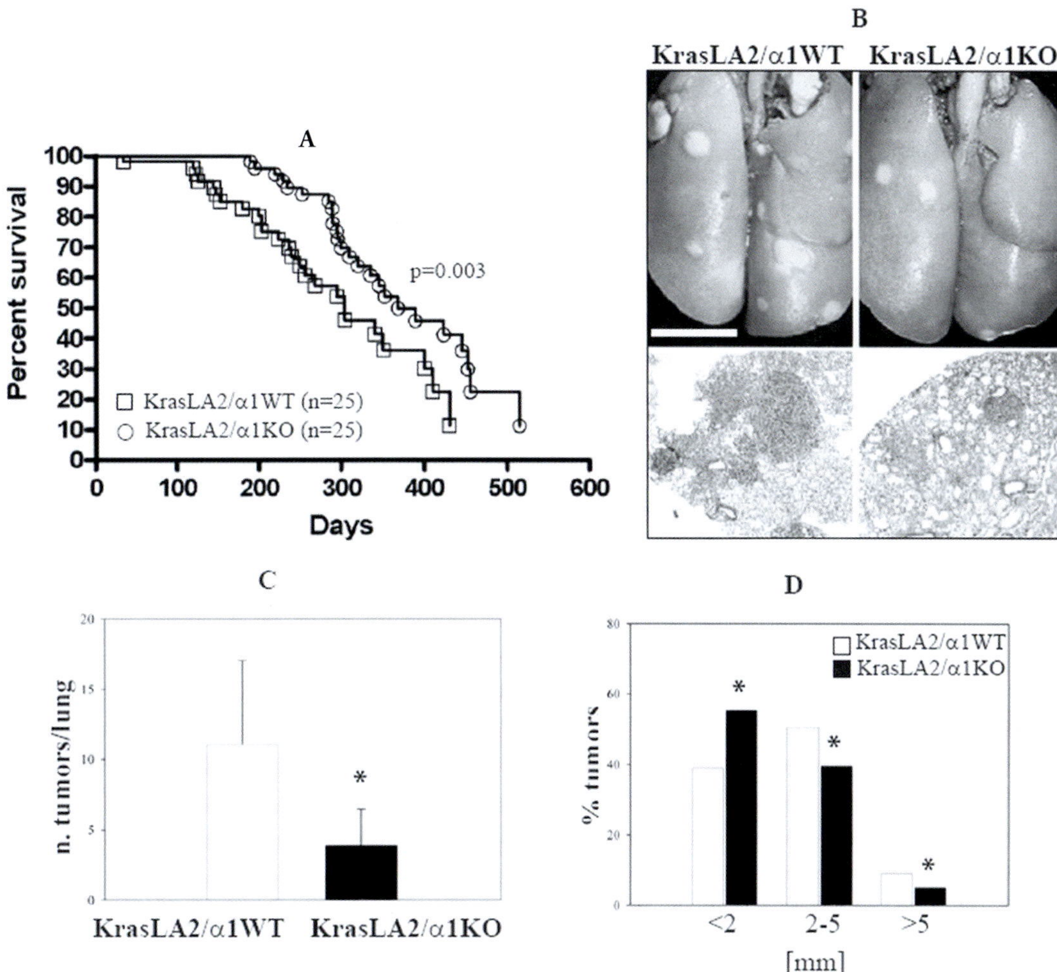

FIGURE 13.3 Increased survival and reduced tumor development in KrasLA2 mice crossed with integrin α1-null mice. **A:** KrasLA2 mice crossed with the integrin α1-null mice (KrasLA2/α1KO) showed significantly increased survival compared to KrasLA2 mice crossed with integrin α1 wild-type mice (KrasLA2/α1WT). **B:** Top: Photograph of the lungs of KrasLA2/α1WT and KrasLA2/α1KO male mice sacrificed 120 days after birth. *Scale bar*, 5 mm. Bottom: Hematoxylin and eosin staining of lungs of KrasLA2/α1WT and KrasLA2/α1KO mice. Magnification, ×200. (See color plate.) **C,D:** KrasLA2/α1WT and KrasLA2/α1KO mice were sacrificed 120 days after birth and tumor number (**C**) and size (**D**) were evaluated. The number of tumors visible on the lung surface was evaluated and expressed as average number of tumors per lung (**C**). Tumor diameter was measured with a caliper in 170 tumors from KrasLA2/α1WT and 102 tumors from K-rasLA2/α1KO mice, and tumors were divided into three groups as indicated (**D**). (Data from Macias-Perez I, Borza C, Chen X, et al. Loss of integrin alpha1beta1 ameliorates Kras-induced lung cancer. *Cancer Res* 2008;68(15):6127–6135.)

imaging, but also for the analysis of tumors that cannot be easily identified by traditional histology.

Administration of AdenoCre has also been used for the establishment of the first mouse genetic model of SCLC 9.[67,68] Meuwissen et al.[67] have produced an animal model of SCLC that closely resembles the human disease. Conditional mice carrying combined floxed Rb and p53 genes were treated with AdenoCre via intratracheal injection to delete these two tumor suppressor genes specifically in the lung. Cre-mediated deletion of all four conditional alleles resulted in the development of lung tumors with the histological and immunohistochemical characteristics of human SCLC. The originality of this model is that lung tumors not only present the typical neuroendocrine features as seen in human SCLC, but they also metastasize to sites that mimic the human disease, including adrenal gland, ovaries, and liver. Interestingly, in certain double floxed Rb and p53 mice treatment with AdenoCre led to conditional inactivation of the p53 gene only, but not Rb gene, giving rise to NSCLC-like adenocarcinomas.[67] Thus, this model suggests that whereas inactivation of a single tumor suppressor gene is sufficient for the development of NSCLC, simultaneous inactivation of at least two different tumor suppressor genes is necessary for the establishment of SCLC. In addition, this model emphasizes the importance of Rb during the development of SCLC.

The genetic models of lung cancers, similarly to the chemical and orthotopic models, appear to be particularly applicable not only for basic mechanistic studies, but also for analyzing the efficacy of chemopreventive and/or chemotherapeutic agents. This kind of study, however, is limited to primary lung cancer, as in these genetic models of lung cancer, primary tumors do not or rarely metastasize, making the comparison with human tumors, and the evaluation of potential antimetastatic drugs difficult to evaluate. Interestingly, it has been proposed that the effect of genetic mutations on the development of metastatic tumors can be influenced by the genetic background of the mouse. Using a transgene-induced mouse tumor model that exhibits a high incidence of pulmonary metastases and a breeding strategy to vary genetic background, Lifsted and colleagues[69] found significant differences in metastatic efficiency between the original strains and first-generation hybrids, without altering tumor initiation or growth kinetics. As all tumors are initiated by the same oncogenic event, differences in the metastasis are most likely because of genetic background effects, rather than different combinations of oncogenic mutations. Quantitative genetic mapping in the different backcrossing has allowed the identification of at least three loci that are associated with altered metastatic potential, strongly reinforcing the notion that tumorigenesis and metastasis are complex phenotypes involving not only cellular responses to extrinsic stimuli, but also inherent genetic components.[70] Thus, finding the ideal genetic background for the development of primary as well as metastatic lung cancers might enable researchers to study the different steps involved in lung cancer progression, to screen potential antimetastatic molecules, and to understand their mechanism of action.

CONCLUSION

Cancer susceptibility is a complex interaction of an individual's genetic composition and environmental exposures. Tremendous work has been done to understand cancer over the past 100 years, from recognition of cancer as a genetic disease to identification of specific carcinogens, isolation of oncogenes, and recognition of tumor suppressors. Lung cancer is most likely the result of an intricate interaction of polymorphic susceptibility genes with many environmental factors. Although genetic mutations in mice and humans do not always lead to the same tumor spectrum, the underlying molecular mechanisms are frequently relevant to both species. The different mouse models of lung cancers described in this chapter, mainly if used in combination with one another, will facilitate the identification of genes that modulate an individual's susceptibility to cancer after a certain environmental exposure, and will clearly allow researchers to gain important insights into lung cancer development, treatment, and, most importantly, prevention.

ACKNOWLEDGMENTS: *I thank the National Cancer Institute (NCI/NIH-CA94849) and the NIDDK (RO1-DK074359) for their support. I apologize to many colleagues performing outstanding research on mouse models of lung cancer whose work has not been cited because of space constraints.*

REFERENCES

1. Coggins CR. A review of chronic inhalation studies with mainstream cigarette smoke, in hamsters, dogs, and nonhuman primates. *Toxicol Pathol* 2001;29:550–557.
2. Liu J, Johnston MR. Animal models for studying lung cancer and evaluating novel intervention strategies. *Surg Oncol* 2002;11:217–227.
3. Coggins CR. An updated review of inhalation studies with cigarette smoke in laboratory animals. *Int J Toxicol* 2007;26:331–338.
4. Tuveson DA, Jacks T. Modeling human lung cancer in mice: similarities and shortcomings. *Oncogene* 1999;18:5318–5324.
5. Hecht SS. Tobacco smoke carcinogens and lung cancer. *J Natl Cancer Inst* 1999;91:1194–11210.
6. Beadsmoore CJ, Screaton NJ. Classification, staging and prognosis of lung cancer. *Eur J Radiol* 2003;45:8–17.
7. Malkinson AM, Beer DS. Major effect on susceptibility to urethan-induced pulmonary adenoma by a single gene in BALB/cBy mice. *J Natl Cancer Inst* 1983;70:931–936.
8. You M, Wang Y, Lineen AM, et al. Mutagenesis of the K-ras protooncogene in mouse lung tumors induced by N-ethyl-N-nitrosourea or N-nitrosodiethylamine. *Carcinogenesis* 1992;13:1583–1586.
9. Chen B, You L, Wang Y, et al. Allele-specific activation and expression of the K-ras gene in hybrid mouse lung tumors induced by chemical carcinogens. *Carcinogenesis* 1994;15:2031–2035.
10. Gariboldi M, Manenti G, Canzian F, et al. A major susceptibility locus to murine lung carcinogenesis maps on chromosome 6. *Nat Genet* 1993; 3:132–136.
11. Lin L, Festing MF, Devereux TR, et al. Additional evidence that the K-ras protooncogene is a candidate for the major mouse pulmonary adenoma susceptibility (Pas-1) gene. *Exp Lung Res* 1998;24:481–497.
12. Shimkin MB, Stoner GD. Lung tumors in mice: application to carcinogenesis bioassay. *Adv Cancer Res* 1975;21:1–58.
13. Malkinson AM. Primary lung tumors in mice: an experimentally manipulable model of human adenocarcinoma. *Cancer Res* 1992;52 (9 Suppl):S2670–S2676.
14. Stathopoulos GT, Sherrill TP, Cheng DS, et al. Epithelial NF-kappaB activation promotes urethane-induced lung carcinogenesis. *Proc Natl Acad Sci U S A* 2007;104:18514–18519.
15. Malkinson AM. Primary lung tumors in mice as an aid for understanding, preventing, and treating human adenocarcinoma of the lung. *Lung Cancer* 2001;32:265–279.
16. Hahn FF, Gigliotti AP, Hutt JA, et al. A review of the histopathology of cigarette smoke-induced lung cancer in rats and mice. *Int J Toxicol* 2007;26:307–313.
17. Szymanska H, Sitarz M, Krysiak E, et al. Genetics of susceptibility to radiation-induced lymphomas, leukemias and lung tumors studied in recombinant congenic strains. *Int J Cancer* 1999;83:674–678.
18. Todaro GJ, Fryling C, De Larco JE. Transforming growth factors produced by certain human tumor cells: polypeptides that interact with epidermal growth factor receptors. *Proc Natl Acad Sci U S A* 1980; 77:5258–5262.
19. Stoner GD, Adam–Rodwell G, Morse MA. Lung tumors in strain A mice: application for studies in cancer chemoprevention. *J Cell Biochem Suppl* 1993;17F:95–103.
20. Sporn MB, Dunlop NM, Newton DL, et al. Prevention of chemical carcinogenesis by vitamin A and its synthetic analogs (retinoids). *Fed Proc* 1976;35:1332–13328.

21. Duperron C, Castonguay A. Chemopreventive efficacies of aspirin and sulindac against lung tumorigenesis in A/J mice. *Carcinogenesis* 1997;18:1001–1006.
22. Lantry LE, Zhang Z, Crist KA, et al. 5-Aza-2′-deoxycytidine is chemopreventive in a 4-(methyl-nitrosamino)-1-(3-pyridyl)-1-butanone-induced primary mouse lung tumor model. *Carcinogenesis* 1999;20:343–346.
23. Kohno H, Taima M, Sumida T, et al. Inhibitory effect of mandarin juice rich in beta-cryptoxanthin and hesperidin on 4-(methylnitrosamino)-1-(3-pyridyl)-1-butanone-induced pulmonary tumorigenesis in mice. *Cancer Lett* 2001;174:141–150.
24. Lantry LE, Zhang Z, Gao F, et al. Chemopreventive effect of perillyl alcohol on 4-(methylnitrosamino)-1-(3-pyridyl)-1-butanone induced tumorigenesis in (C3H/HeJ X A/J)F1 mouse lung. *J Cell Biochem Suppl* 1997;27:20–25.
25. Manzotti C, Audisio RA, Pratesi G. Importance of orthotopic implantation for human tumors as model systems: relevance to metastasis and invasion. *Clin Exp Metastasis* 1993;11:5–14.
26. Fidler IJ. Host and tumour factors in cancer metastasis. *Eur J Clin Invest* 1990;20:481–486.
27. Mase K, Iijima T, Nakamura N, et al. Intrabronchial orthotopic propagation of human lung adenocarcinoma—characterizations of tumorigenicity, invasion and metastasis. *Lung Cancer* 2002;36:271–276.
28. Kozaki K, Miyaishi O, Tsukamoto T, et al. Establishment and characterization of a human lung cancer cell line NCI-H460-LNM35 with consistent lymphogenous metastasis via both subcutaneous and orthotopic propagation. *Cancer Res* 2000;60:2535–2540.
29. Acuff HB, Carter KJ, Fingleton B, et al. Matrix metalloproteinase-9 from bone marrow-derived cells contributes to survival but not growth of tumor cells in the lung microenvironment. *Cancer Res* 2006;66:259–266.
30. McLemore TL, Liu MC, Blacker PC, et al. Novel intrapulmonary model for orthotopic propagation of human lung cancers in athymic nude mice. *Cancer Res* 1987;47:5132–5140.
31. Kuo TH, Kubota T, Watanabe M, et al. Orthotopic reconstitution of human small-cell lung carcinoma after intravenous transplantation in SCID mice. *Anticancer Res* 1992;12:1407–1410.
32. Doki Y, Murakami K, Yamaura T, et al. Mediastinal lymph node metastasis model by orthotopic intrapulmonary implantation of Lewis lung carcinoma cells in mice. *Br J Cancer* 1999;79:1121–1126.
33. Chen X, Su Y, Fingleton B, et al. An orthotopic model of lung cancer to analyze primary and metastatic NSCLC growth in integrin alpha1-null mice. *Clin Exp Metastasis* 2005;22:185–193.
34. Howard RB, Mullen JB, Pagura ME, et al. Characterization of a highly metastatic, orthotopic lung cancer model in the nude rat. *Clin Exp Metastasis* 1999;17:157–162.
35. Hoffman R. Green fluorescent protein imaging of tumour growth, metastasis, and angiogenesis in mouse models. *Lancet Oncol* 2002;3:546–556.
36. El Hilali N, Rubio N, Martinez-Villacampa M, et al. Combined noninvasive imaging and luminometric quantification of luciferase-labeled human prostate tumors and metastases. *Lab Invest* 2002;82:1563–1571.
37. Hoffman RM. Visualization of GFP-expressing tumors and metastasis in vivo. *Biotechniques* 2001;30:1016–1022, 1024–1026.
38. Hasegawa S, Yang M, Chishima T, et al. In vivo tumor delivery of the green fluorescent protein gene to report future occurrence of metastasis. *Cancer Gene Ther* 2000;7:1336–1340.
39. Rosol TJ, Tannehill-Gregg SH, LeRoy BE, et al. Animal models of bone metastasis. *Cancer* 2003;97:748–757.
40. Sarkioja M, Kanerva A, Salo J, et al. Noninvasive imaging for evaluation of the systemic delivery of capsid-modified adenoviruses in an orthotopic model of advanced lung cancer. *Cancer* 2006;107:1578–1588.
41. Kubota T. Metastatic models of human cancer xenografted in the nude mouse: the importance of orthotopic transplantation. *J Cell Biochem* 1994;56:4–8.
42. Liu J, Costello PC, Pham NA, et al. Integrin-linked kinase inhibitor KP-392 demonstrates clinical benefits in an orthotopic human non-small cell lung cancer model. *J Thorac Oncol* 2006;1:771–779.
43. Wu W, Onn A, Isobe T, et al. Targeted therapy of orthotopic human lung cancer by combined vascular endothelial growth factor and epidermal growth factor receptor signaling blockade. *Mol Cancer Ther* 2007;6:471–483.
44. Zou Y, Tornos C, Qiu X, et al. P53 aerosol formulation with low toxicity and high efficiency for early lung cancer treatment. *Clin Cancer Res* 2007;13:4900–4908.
45. Kohno T, Yokota J. How many tumor suppressor genes are involved in human lung carcinogenesis? *Carcinogenesis* 1999;20:1403–1410.
46. Salgia R, Skarin AT. Molecular abnormalities in lung cancer. *J Clin Oncol* 1998;16:1207–1217.
47. Wikenheiser KA, Clark JC, Linnoila RI, et al. Simian virus 40 large T antigen directed by transcriptional elements of the human surfactant protein C gene produces pulmonary adenocarcinomas in transgenic mice. *Cancer Res* 1992;52:5342–5352.
48. Saitoh A, Kimura M, Takahashi R, et al. Most tumors in transgenic mice with human c-Ha-ras gene contained somatically activated transgenes. *Oncogene* 1990;5:1195–1200.
49. Lubet RA, Zhang Z, Wiseman RW, et al. Use of p53 transgenic mice in the development of cancer models for multiple purposes. *Exp Lung Res* 2000;26:581–593.
50. Tchou-Wong KM, Jiang Y, Yee H, et al. Lung-specific expression of dominant-negative mutant p53 in transgenic mice increases spontaneous and benzo[a]pyrene-induced lung cancer. *Am J Respir Cell Mol Biol* 2002;27:186–193.
51. Zhang Z, Liu Q, Lantry LE, et al. A germ-line p53 mutation accelerates pulmonary tumorigenesis: p53-independent efficacy of chemopreventive agents green tea or dexamethasone/myo-inositol and chemotherapeutic agents taxol or adriamycin. *Cancer Res* 2000;60:901–907.
52. Spitz MR, Barnett MJ, Goodman GE, et al. Serum insulin-like growth factor (IGF) and IGF-binding protein levels and risk of lung cancer: a case-control study nested in the beta-carotene and Retinol Efficacy Trial Cohort. *Cancer Epidemiol Biomarkers Prev* 2002;11:1413–1418.
53. Moorehead RA, Sanchez OH, Baldwin RM, et al. Transgenic overexpression of IGF-II induces spontaneous lung tumors: a model for human lung adenocarcinoma. *Oncogene* 2003;22:853–857.
54. Donehower LA, Harvey M, Slagle BL, et al. Mice deficient for p53 are developmentally normal but susceptible to spontaneous tumours. *Nature* 1992;356:215–221.
55. Serrano M, Lee H, Chin L, et al. Role of the INK4a locus in tumor suppression and cell mortality. *Cell* 1996;85:27–37.
56. Williams BO, Remington L, Albert DM, et al. Cooperative tumorigenic effects of germline mutations in Rb and p53. *Nat Genet* 1994;7:480–484.
57. Aguayo SM, Miller YE, Waldron JA Jr, et al. Brief report: idiopathic diffuse hyperplasia of pulmonary neuroendocrine cells and airways disease. *N Engl J Med* 1992;327:1285–1288.
58. Johnson L, Mercer K, Greenbaum D, et al. Somatic activation of the K-ras oncogene causes early onset lung cancer in mice. *Nature* 2001;410:1111–1116.
59. Wislez M, Fujimoto N, Izzo JG, et al. High expression of ligands for chemokine receptor CXCR2 in alveolar epithelial neoplasia induced by oncogenic kras. *Cancer Res* 2006;66:4198–4207.
60. Fujimoto N, Wislez M, Zhang J, et al. High expression of ErbB family members and their ligands in lung adenocarcinomas that are sensitive to inhibition of epidermal growth factor receptor. *Cancer Res* 2005;65:11478–11485.
61. Pandey J, Umphress SM, Kang Y, et al. Modulation of tumor induction and progression of oncogenic K-ras-positive tumors in the presence of TGF-b1 haploinsufficiency. *Carcinogenesis* 2007;28:2589–2596.
62. Jackson EL, Willis N, Mercer K, et al. Analysis of lung tumor initiation and progression using conditional expression of oncogenic K-ras. *Genes Dev* 2001;15:3243–3248.

63. Meuwissen R, Linn SC, van der Valk M, et al. Mouse model for lung tumorigenesis through Cre/lox controlled sporadic activation of the K-ras oncogene. *Oncogene* 2001;20:6551–6558.
64. Kissil JL, Walmsley MJ, Hanlon L, et al. Requirement for Rac1 in a K-ras induced lung cancer in the mouse. *Cancer Res* 2007;67:8089–8094.
65. Ji H, Ramsey MR, Hayes DN, et al. LKB1 modulates lung cancer differentiation and metastasis. *Nature* 2007;448:807–810.
66. Lyons SK, Meuwissen R, Krimpenfort P, et al. The generation of a conditional reporter that enables bioluminescence imaging of Cre/loxP-dependent tumorigenesis in mice. *Cancer Res* 2003; 63:7042–7046.
67. Meuwissen R, Linn SC, Linnoila RI, et al. Induction of small cell lung cancer by somatic inactivation of both Tr*p53* and Rb1 in a conditional mouse model. *Cancer Cell* 2003;4:181–189.
68. Meuwissen R, Berns A. Mouse models for human lung cancer. *Genes Dev* 2005;19:643–664.
69. Lifsted T, Le Voyer T, Williams M, et al. Identification of inbred mouse strains harboring genetic modifiers of mammary tumor age of onset and metastatic progression. *Int J Cancer* 1998;77:640–644.
70. Le Voyer T, Rouse J, Lu Z, et al. Three loci modify growth of a transgene-induced mammary tumor: suppression of proliferation associated with decreased microvessel density. *Genomics* 2001;74:253–261.

CHAPTER 14

Luigi Moretti
Sebahat Ocak
Dennis E. Hallahan
Bo Lu

Cell Cycle and Vascular Targets for Radiotherapy

CELL CYCLE TARGETS FOR RADIOTHERAPY

The cell cycle checkpoints ensure that cells replicate their genomes with high fidelity. In response to DNA-damaging agents such as ionizing radiation or cytotoxic chemotherapy, cell cycle checkpoints delay progression through cell cycle to allow repair before completion of mitosis. Critical parts of the cell cycle machinery are the evolutionarily conserved cyclin-dependent kinases (Cdks), which regulate the transition from one phase of the cell cycle to the next. The Cdks are activated by cyclins and inhibited by naturally occurring Cdk inhibitors (CKI). Cell cycle arrest after DNA damage is critical for maintenance of genomic integrity, and loss of normal cell cycle checkpoint signaling is common in cancers and is considered a pathologic hallmark of neoplastic transformation.[1]

The ability to manipulate cell cycle signaling has important clinical implications in lung cancer. For example, modulation of the checkpoints before the completion of DNA repair could enhance cellular sensitivity to DNA damage agents such as radiotherapy, leading to cell death.

This chapter focuses on the cell cycle dysregulation present in lung cancer, the cell cycle effects of radiotherapy, and on the role a cell cycle modulator may play in combination therapy. The knowledge of these concepts might lead to more efficient use of current anticancer therapies and to the development of novel agents.

Cell Cycle Signaling Response to Ionizing Radiation Cell proliferation results of the repeated progression through a cycle made of four phases and regulated by a defined set of protein complexes.[2,3] Molecular mediators of the cell cycle include cyclins that promote cell cycle transition; Cdks that regulate the cell cycle by forming complexes with their cyclin catalytic partners; and endogenous CKIs that inhibit cyclin–Cdk complexes (Fig. 14.1). The cellular response to DNA damage is the activation of cell cycle checkpoints that serve as natural surveillance mechanism for DNA integrity (Fig. 14.2). Irradiation induces both single- and double-stranded DNA breaks (DNA DSBs), the latter being generally considered the lethal event.[4–7] Two major systems contribute to the repair of DNA DSBs induced by radiation. Homologous recombination, during the late S and G2 stages of the cell cycle, is critical in cell signaling and is regulated by the cell cycle, whereas nonhomologous end-joining is more important during G1 and early S phases and is the predominant mechanism of DNA DSBs repair.

Central to the signal transduction pathways are two phosphatidylinositol 3-kinase–like kinases (PIKKs), ataxia telangiectasia mutated (ATM), and ATM and Rad3-related (ATR), which transmit the damage response signal through phosphorylation.[8] Radiation-induced DNA damage activates ATM, serving as proximal damage sensor, by autophosphorylation at Ser[1981] resulting in ATM dimmer dissociation.[9–12] Evidence suggests an activating role for the Mre11-Rad50-NBS1 (MRN) complex that binds independently to DNA DSBs and facilitate the signaling of ATM.[13,14] Cells with defective or lacking ATM or mutated ATM gene are extremely sensitive to irradiation, suggesting that ATM is a cornerstone in the DNA damage response.[15–17] ATM and ATR respond to single-stranded regions of DNA by replicative stress.[18] Once activated, ATM can potentially activate signaling receptors and stimulate cell cycle checkpoints, p53 activity, and DNA repair complex function.[19–21]

Cell cycle checkpoints monitor the structural integrity of chromosomes before progression through crucial cell cycle stages.[22] Checkpoints occur at entry into S phase (the G1/S checkpoint), entry into mitosis (the G2/M checkpoint), as well as during replication (intra-S checkpoints).[23,24] After irradiation, the damage response signaling pathways facilitate communication between damage recognition proteins and the checkpoint machinery to effect arrest of cell cycle progression (G1 or G2 arrest) and increase the opportunity for repair before undertaking important events such as replication or mitosis.[25]

In most solid tumor cells, G1 arrest is dependent on the activation of the tumor suppressor gene p53 and the downstream CKI p21, which also plays a role in cellular senescence, apoptosis, and DNA repair.[26,27] It is not clear whether p53

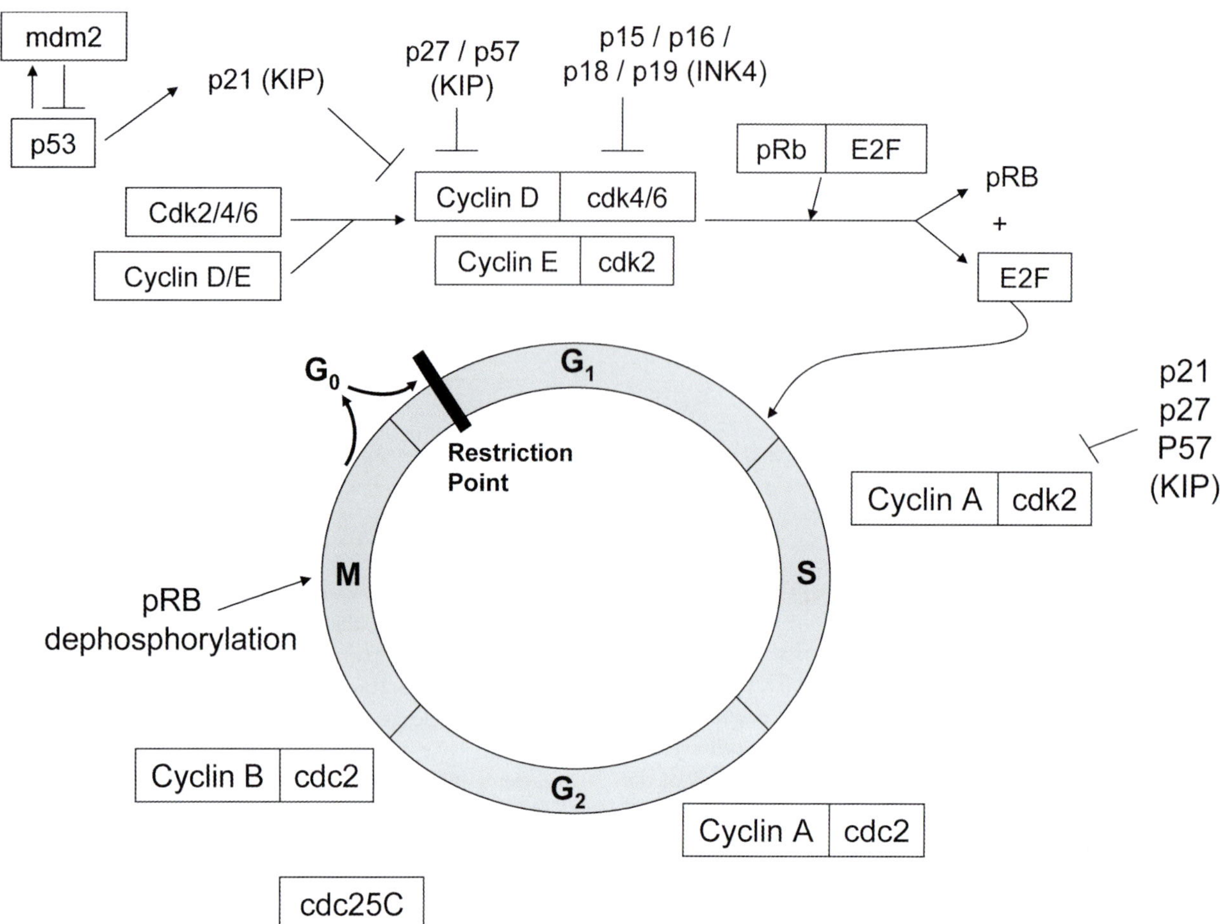

FIGURE 14.1 Schematic overview of cell cycle regulation. The cell cycle has four phases: M, G1, S, and G2, defined by the status of the genetic material. DNA replication occurs in S phase, and chromosome segregation occurs in M phase or mitosis. Two gap phases serve as checkpoints for entry into S and M (G1 and G2, respectively). These gap phases are characterized by DNA content, 2N in G1 and 4N in G2. Resting or quiescent cells are in a phase called G0. Entry into each phase of the cell cycle is strictly ordered and regulated. Passing of the cell through the restriction point is a key step in cell cycle progression. G1/S transition is promoted by the E2F transcription factor, whereas the G2/M transition can be induced by Cyclin B. Furthermore, cell cycle regulation occurs via a complex of cyclin proteins and catalytic kinases known as cyclin-dependent kinases (Cdk), which are held in an inactive state by physical interactions with endogenous Cdk-inhibitors (CKI) such as p16, p21, and p27. *cdc25C*, cell division cycle 25 homologue C; *Cdk2/4/6*, cyclin-dependent kinase 2/4/6; *E2F*, E2F transcription factor 2; *KIP*, kinase-interacting protein; *mdm2*, Mdm2 p53 binding protein homologue; *pRB*, phosphorylated-Retinoblastoma.

gene and G1 arrest have an influencing role in radioresistance in solid tumor cells.[28] In contrast, G2 arrest, which can be influenced by p53, may have a radioprotective function by providing cells time to repair DNA damage, and is controlled by the nuclear activities of the cyclin B1-CDC2 complex.[29,30] Two ATM-dependent G1/S checkpoints can be individualized. First, ATM activation in G1 leads to CHK2 phosphorylation and in turn, to phosphorylation of the phosphatase CDC25A. This increases the proteolytic degradation of CDC25A and prevents activating dephosphorylation of CDK2 and initiation of the G1/S checkpoint.[31,32] Second, ATM phosphorylates the tumor suppressor p53, either directly or indirectly through CHK2, stabilizing the protein and prolonging its half-life, which function as a transcription factor for the CKI p21. p53 serine 15/20 phosphorylation disrupts the normal binding of the oncoprotein MDM2 to p53, thereby inhibiting its degradation process and prolonging its half-life. This pathway has a role in the maintenance of the G1/S checkpoint.[33]

Two distinct G2/M checkpoints can also be identified, determined by the kind of DNA damage and by the time sequence.[34] The first checkpoint, ATM dependent, occurs rapidly after radiation-induced damage and is controlled by CHK1-mediated signaling that leads to inhibition of cyclin B1/CDC2 activity. It represents the failure of cells that had been in G2 at the time of irradiation to progress into mitosis. This G2/M checkpoint, which is dose independent, may be the transducer element linking low-dose hyperradiosensitivity to the subsequent process of resistance.[35] In contrast, the dose-dependent G2/M

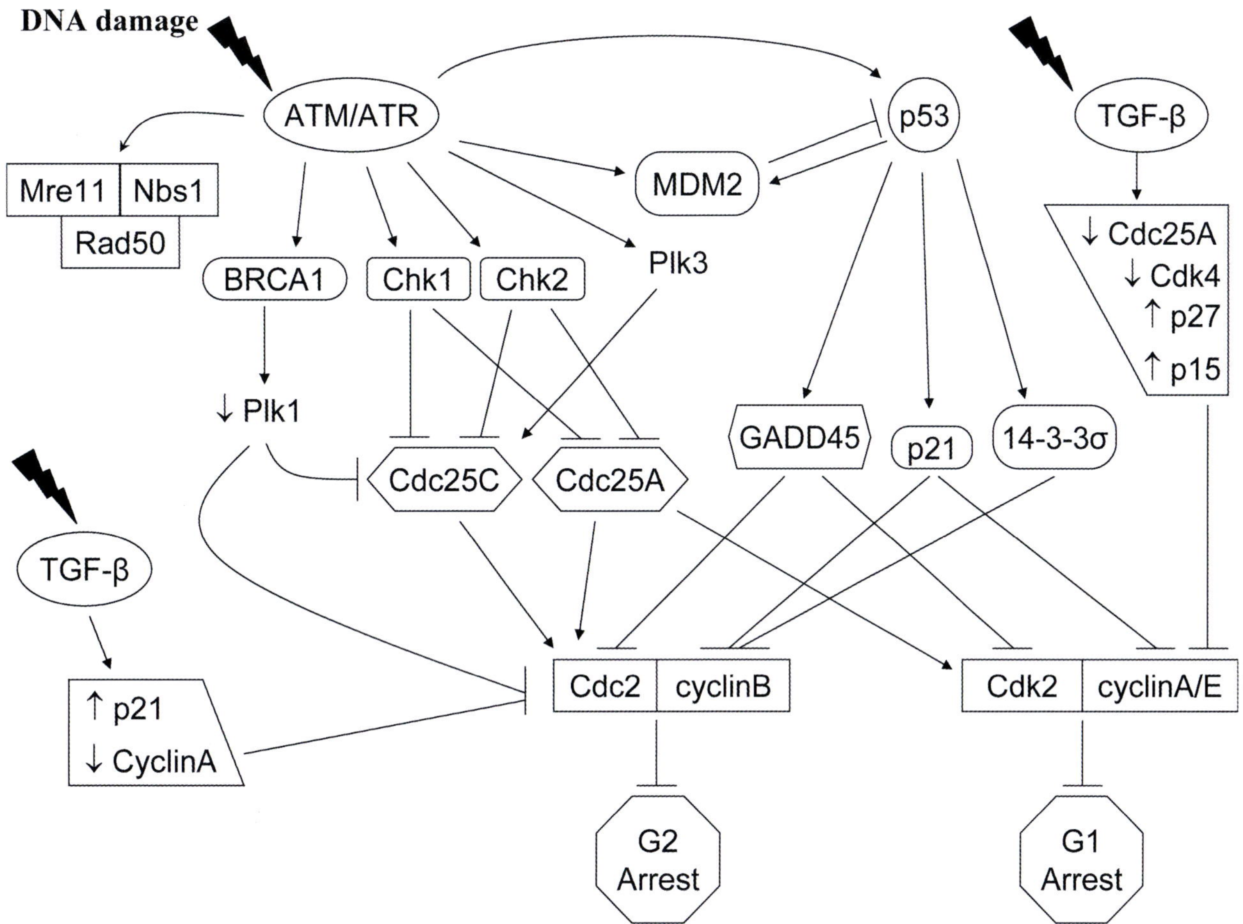

FIGURE 14.2 Schematic overview of cell cycle checkpoints after irradiation. In mammalian cells, radiation-induced DNA damage is first detected by sensor DNA-bound protein complexes. ATM and ATR are primary signal transducers that are activated by DNA damage at all points in the cell cycle. p53 is a key effector of the G1 and G2 checkpoint responses. Expression of p53 can arrest cells in the G1 phase in response to DNA damage, thereby arresting DNA replication for repair. Many cells also exhibit a G2 arrest following exposure to ionizing radiation, allowing repair before progressing through the cell cycle. However, a major mechanism underlying the G2 DNA damage checkpoint is p53 independent. It involves chk1 and chk2, which inhibit CDC25C to carry out the activating dephosphorylation of cdc2. Therefore, G2 cells accumulate inhibited cyclin B/cdc2 complexes and are incapable of entering into mitosis. CDC25A, responsible for activating dephosphorylation of cdk2, is a key target. In response to DNA damage, phosphorylation of CDC25A by chk1 or chk2 leads to its destabilization and the accumulation of inactive cdk2 phosphorylated complexes. Because ongoing DNA replication requires the activity of cdk2, DNA synthesis ceases until damage is repaired. *ATM/ATR*, ataxia telangiectasia mutated/ataxia telangiectasia and Rad3 related; *BRCA1*, breast cancer 1; *Cdc2*, cell division cycle 2; *Cdc25A*, cell division cycle 25 homologue A; *Cdc25C*, cell division cycle 25 homologue C; *Cdk2*, cyclin-dependent kinase 2; *Cdk4*, cyclin-dependent kinase 4; *Chk1*, checkpoint kinase 1; *Chk2*, cell cycle checkpoint kinase 2; *GADD45*, growth arrest and DNA damage-inducible protein 45; *MDM2*, Mdm2 p53 binding protein homologue; *Mre11*, meiotic recombination 11; *Nbs1*, Nijmegen breakage syndrome 1; *Plk1*, polo-like kinase 1; *Plk3*, polo-like kinase 3; *Rad50*, RAD50 homologue; *TGF-β*, transforming growth factor, beta.

accumulation begins to be measurable several hours after irradiation. This mechanism is ATM independent, and represents the accumulation of cells that were in earlier phases of the cell cycle at the time of exposure.[34] G2/M accumulation after exposure to radiation is not affected by the early G2/M checkpoint and is enhanced in cells lacking the radiation-induced S-phase checkpoint, such as those lacking NBS1 or BRCA1 function.[34] It is initiated by the phosphorylation of checkpoint kinases, CHK1 and CHK2, and CDC25A/C, which inactivate the enzymes, blocking activation of CDK1, and causing a G2 arrest. p53 was shown to suppress promoters of cdc2 and cyclin B, which leads to G2/M arrest, and to have a regulation role in the sustain of the G2/M arrest.[36] DNA damage by radiation blocks pRb phosphorylation through p21 to maintain the pRb-regulated cell cycle arrest to complete DNA damage repair. The further identification of cell cycle signaling elements in response to ionizing radiation will have important implication for the development of anticancer targeted strategies.

TABLE 14.1 Most Frequent Cell Cycle Genes/Proteins Presenting Mutations or Altered Expression in Lung Cancer

Gene	Protein	Function	Cycle Phase	Alteration in Lung Cancer
ATM	ATM	Checkpoints, repair	S	Mutated, deleted
AURKA	Aurora A	Mitotic kinase	M	Overexpressed
CCND1,2,3	Cyclins D	Positive regulator of cdk4/6	G1/S	Overexpressed
CCNE1	Cyclin E1	Positive regulator of cdk2	G1/S	Overexpressed, deregulated
CDK4	Cdk4	Inactivates pRb	G1/S	p16-resistant mutations
CDKN2A	p16INK4a	cdk4/6 inhibitor	G1/S	Mutated, deleted, methylated
CDKN1B	p27Kip1	cdk2 inhibitor	G1/S	Underexpressed
CDKN1C	p57Kip2	cdk2 inhibitor	G1/S	Underexpressed, methylated
CDKN2A	p14Arf	Activator of p53	G1/S	Mutated, deleted
CHK2	chk2	Checkpoints	S	Mutated
CKS1,2	cks1, cks2	cdk-binding proteins	G1/S	Overexpressed
hCDC4	hCdc4	Turnover of cyclin E	G1/S	Mutated, deleted
MTBP	MDM-2	Inhibitor of p53	G1/S	Overexpressed
NBS1	Nbs1	Checkpoints, repair	S, G2	Mutated
PLK	Plk1	Mitotic kinase	M	Overexpressed
PTTG1	Securin	Anaphase inhibitor	G1/S	Overexpressed
RB1	pRb	Represses E2F transcription	G1/S	Mutated, deleted
RB2	p130	Inhibits cdks, represses E2F	G1/S	Mutated, deleted
SKP2	Skp2	Turnover of p27	G1/S	Overexpressed
TP53	p53	Checkpoints, apoptosis	G1, G2/M	Mutated, deleted

Cell Cycle Alterations in Lung Cancer Molecular analysis demonstrates that alterations in components of the cell cycle machinery and checkpoint signaling pathways occur in most lung tumors (Table 14.1). Alterations in the cell cycle machinery that occur most frequently include overexpression of cyclins, cdks, and Cdc25 phosphatases, loss or mutation of the RB tumor suppressor, and loss of cdk expression. The most frequently altered cell cycle checkpoint signaling molecule is the p53 tumor suppressor.

Cyclins D1 Following a mitogenic signal during the G1 phase, cyclin D1 assembles with cdk4 and a CDK-interacting protein (CIP) (p21)/kinase-interacting protein (KIP) (p27) protein. This complex enters the nucleus and phosphorylates the retinoblastoma tumor suppressor protein Rb1,[37] promoting the release of E2F transcription factor from the Rb1/E2F complex[38] and thus the progression from G1 to S phase. During G1/S transition, glycogen synthase kinase (GSK)-3β enters the nucleus and phosphorylates cyclin D1, allowing its nuclear export by Crm1[39,40] and degradation by the 26S-proteasome.[40,41] Under certain conditions, the cyclin D1/cdk4 complex can also act as a mediator of programmed cell death.[42,43] Cyclin D1 can also directly interact with several nuclear receptors and transcription factors,[44–48] by repressing or inducing them. This transcriptional function links cyclin D1 not only to cell cycle and apoptosis but also to migration, invasion, differentiation, inflammation, and angiogenesis. Cyclin D1 has been identified as a proto-oncogene, PRAD1, and was found to be overexpressed relative to normal tissue in many human cancers.[3,49,50] Overexpression of cyclin D1 is associated with dysregulation of cell cycle and is reported in 25% to 60% of non–small cell lung cancer (NSCLC),[51,52] varying from 30% to 35% in squamous cell carcinoma (SCC) and 36% to 56% in adenocarcinoma (ADC) in the largest series.[53–55] Cyclin D1 overexpression is less common in neuroendocrine tumors (NE) and, among these, more frequent in atypical carcinoids (20%) and large cell neuroendocrine cancers (LCNE) (9.5%). Cyclin D1 dysregulation is frequently an early event in tumorigenesis, elevated levels being already found in bronchial[56,57] and alveolar hyperplasia.[58,59] Cyclin D1 level has also been linked to heavy smoking and said to constitute a marker of tobacco exposure.[52,60,61]

Cdk Inhibitors

p21. p21 was the first CKI to be discovered. It is a member of the KIP family of proteins that nonspecifically inhibit cyclin–cdk complexes in the nucleus.[62] It can inhibit the cyclin D/cdk4 and cyclin E/cdk2 complexes early in G1, and it can also inhibit the cyclin A/cdk2 complex later, prior to the S-phase/G2-phase transition.[63] p21 transcript is directly activated by p53 and seems to be a fundamental partner for p53. It contributes to p53-induced apoptosis[64] and blocks the G2/M transition through cdc2 inhibition, mediating the pro-apoptotic and cell cycle–arresting effects induced by p53 in response to genotoxic stimuli.[65] Recent studies have shown potential new roles for p21 and p27, as inhibitors of apoptosis and so, as potential oncogenes. These roles have been related to their relocalization to the cytoplasm,[66–70] whereas the cell cycle inhibitory activity is dependent on the nuclear localization. Although p21 is infrequently expressed in normal lung,[71] it is overexpressed in 35% to 51% of NSCLC cases, without significant differences between ADC and SCC.[71–75] p21 expression has been correlated with better differentiation in NSCLC.[71,73,74] In two studies adequately controlled for disease stage, p21 expression was associated with improved survival,[72,75] whereas another study reached slightly different conclusions.[76] In an analysis combining p21 and TGF-β, an improved survival was observed in early stage NSCLC when p21 and TGF-β were in concordance, presenting both high or both low expression.[76] Absence of p21 expression has been correlated to a worse prognosis when associated with p53 positivity[75] and absence of p16 expression.[77]

p27. p27, another member of the KIP family, blocks the activity of cyclin D1-CDK4/6 and cyclin E-CDK2 and is an important negative regulator of the G1 to S transition.[66,78] In the normal resting cell, concentration of p27 is high and declines in response to proliferative stimuli. p27 overexpression leads to cell cycle arrest, whereas its loss of expression may result in tumor development and/or progression. As described for p21, some studies have suggested p27 to be an oncogene by inhibiting apoptosis, and that this role is related to its cytoplasmic relocalization.[66,79] In vivo studies have shown that p27 expression decreases progressively during lung carcinogenesis.[80] Increased p27 proteolytic activity has been associated to low levels of p27.[77,81] Low p27 expression has been associated with higher stages of lung cancer,[82] as well as poor survival in NSCLC, either by itself[77,81–83] and/or when associated to other abnormalities like p53 mutations and/or Rb loss,[84] Ras mutations,[85] high cyclin E levels,[79] high proliferative rates[84,85] and aneuploidy.[84] A favorable response to chemotherapeutic agents, including drugs targeting EGFR and HER-2, has been correlated to increased p27 expression.[86,87]

p16. p16 is a member of the INK4 family of proteins that inhibits cdk4 and cdk6 activation through a competitive mechanism for cyclin D binding site and specifically during the G1 phase.[88] Loss of p16 has similar effects on G1 progression than overexpression of cyclin D and loss of Rb. The discovery of p16 overexpression in Rb −/− cells, which alters the relationships between cyclin D, cdk4, and cdk6, suggests the existence of a feedback mechanism between p16 and Rb.[89] Decreased p16 is one of the most frequent alterations in lung cancer. Interestingly, loss of p16 is usually found in NSCLC, whereas loss of Rb is found in SCLC. These changes in p16 and Rb seem to be mutually exclusive.[90–93] The strong inverse correlation is more evident in SCC and SCLC than in ADC.[94,95]

p14. p14 is an alternate transcription product from the INK4/ARF locus shared with p16.[96–98] By its ability to antagonize the MDM2-mediated ubiquitination and degradation of p53,[99–102] it induces apoptosis[103,104] and growth inhibition.[99] p14 is decreased in 50% of NSCLC,[97,101] where it has an inverse relationship with MDM-2 expression.[101] p14 can be lost secondary to losses at the p16 locus, and also because of the gene promoter methylation.[103,105]

p53 TUMOR SUPPRESSOR. p53, mapped on chromosomic region 17p13, is a tumor suppressor gene that, after sublethal DNA damage, mediates cell cycle arrest in the G1 phase.[106,107] In this pathway, p53 interacts with several genes. The first one is mdm2: Levels of p53 are kept low by its association with the mdm2 oncogene product, which binds p53 and shuttles it out of the nucleus for proteolytic degradation, establishing an autoregulated feedback circuit. The second gene target is gadd45, that belongs to a gene family implicated in cellular growth arrest.[108,109] The third target is the gene coding for p21, which develops inhibitory action on multiple cyclin–cdk complexes and also complexes with PCNA, a protein playing a key role in DNA reparation processes.[110] The fourth target is the gene coding for Bax, which promotes apoptotic mechanisms and forms a heterodimer with Bcl-2 gene.[111] As a key regulator of cell growth and cell death, p53 is activated by several kinases that regulate the DNA damage checkpoint following many environmental stimuli, including DNA-damaging agents such as ionizing radiation, and is crucial in preventing the propagation of mutations in normal cells.[67] Activated p53 induces cell cycle arrest ($p21^{Cip1/Waf1}$) to allow cells to repair the damage or apoptosis if the damage is too severe and/or irreparable.[112] During carcinogenesis, p53 is frequently inactivated by multiple mechanisms. The most common mechanism is mutation at the p53 gene, which occurs in more than 50% of all human cancers. In response to DNA damage, some p53 mutants show less capacity to bind and initiate transcription from their target genes, such as p21, Mdm2, Bax, and cyclin G, and so, some of the p53-mediated effects are blunted,[113] resulting in insensitivity to growth-inhibitory signals as well as evasion of apoptosis. Mouse models have confirmed cooperation between mutated p53 and mutative active K-ras in NSCLC development[114] and between p53 and Rb in SCLC development.[115]

p53 mutation is one of the most common genetic alterations in lung cancer, with about 70% of SCLC and 50% of NSCLC presenting mutations in one allele of p53, often accompanied with loss of the wild-type allele.[116] In NSCLC, p53 mutations are more frequently found in SCC than ADC.[117] The p53 mutational spectra of lung cancer are different from those of other cancers with an excess of G:C to T:A observed,[118] these ones especially linked to exposure to tobacco carcinogens such as benzopyrene.[119] Several studies investigated the association of p53 abnormalities with prognosis in lung cancer, with discordant results. Some of them showed an association of p53 overexpression (mutants form have a longer half-life and lead to the detection of high levels of protein by IHC) with shorter survival,[120–122] others failed to find such an association.[123,124] Concurrent p53 and p16 abnormalities have been associated to a worse prognosis.[125,126] Many reports have linked the presence of p53 mutations to resistance to DNA-damaging chemotherapeutics agents,[127] and this is not surprising as we know that most chemotherapeutics agents act by stimulating apoptosis.

Cell Cycle as Target for Combined Treatment with Radiotherapy Cellular radiosensitivity varies along the different phases of cell cycle. The majority of cells surviving after a first dose of radiation were most likely in a less sensitive (G1 phase) or in a resistant phase of the cell cycle (late S phase). Those cells will then progress into a more sensitive cell cycle phase, that is at or close to mitosis, which represents a more ideal time for delivering radiation therapy. Several cell cycle regulatory proteins are potential molecular targets for cancer therapy, and agents can be combined to radiation to enhance its effects on lung cancer. Efforts have been made to sensitize cancer cells to the cytotoxicity of DNA damage by anticancer agents as early as four decades ago with compounds such as caffeine, which resulted in abrogation of the G2 cell cycle checkpoint. Many malignant cells, including lung cancer, have defective G1 checkpoint mechanisms and depend far more on G2 checkpoint than normal cells. More recently, several potent agents have been studied in preclinical and clinical trials. Among them is flavopiridol, the first CKI to enter clinical trials as a potential anticancer agent that exerts both cytostatic and cytotoxic actions on cancer cells. Another well-known drug is UCN-01, a potent prototypical chk1 inhibitor, which function as a CKI at high concentrations. Such compounds seek to force cells to enter mitosis without allowing adequate time for DNA repair, increasing the likelihood that cell death will occur by accumulation of DNA lesions. Treatment strategies consisting in abrogation of G2 checkpoints can also be achieved with the use of microtubule-targeting compounds, such as taxanes and epothilones to stall cells in G2/M (by preventing mitosis, thereby trapping cells in the phase of the cell cycle where ionizing radiation have the greatest effects). Microtubule-stabilizing agents will be discussed as mitotic targets in combination with ionizing radiation. Finally, Aurora kinases, part of the spindle checkpoint, are recent agents that can also be used in combined anticancer therapy (Table 14.2).

Cyclin-Dependent Kinases (CDK) Modulators Cell cycle regulatory proteins such as CDKs are potential molecular targets for radiation therapy.[128–130] The rationale for targeting the cell cycle and the CDKs in lung cancer therapy has been based on the frequency of their perturbations in lung tumors (overexpression of cyclins, and/or absent or diminished levels of CKI).[54,55,131,132] For example, overexpression of cyclin D1 and loss of p16 gene expression has been associated with the development of lung cancer (see previous discussion). These defects in tumor cells lead to uncontrolled proliferation as a result of the loss of checkpoint integrity. In addition, cell cycle arrest by CKI has been shown to induce apoptosis.[1,133–135]

FLAVOPIRIDOL. Flavopiridol is a semisynthetic flavone that directly competes with the ATP substrate and reversibly inhibits kinase activity of multiple classes of CDKs, including cdk1, cdk2, cdk4, cdk6, cdk7, and cdk9 at submicromolar concentrations (IC50 values of 100 to 400).[136] This pancyclin inhibitor causes arrest at both G1 and G2/M phases of the cell cycle by several mechanisms: direct inhibition of cdks 1, 2, and 4, and indirect inhibition by downregulating cyclin H-cdk7,[137–140] as well as tumor growth arrest in most solid tumors and xenografts.[140–144] Flavopiridol also promotes a decrease in the level of cyclin D1,[135] which is commonly overexpressed in many cancers including lung cancer where it has been described as a poor prognosis marker.[51–55,131,145–149] However, at considerably higher concentrations than necessary to inhibit CDKs, flavopiridol inhibits the activity of several other protein kinases[150,151] including signal transducing kinases protein kinase A (PKA), PKC, and Erk-1, the receptor tyrosine kinase EGFR, and receptor-associated protein kinases such as c-Src.[152] In addition, although described as cytostatic, flavopiridol has been shown to be also cytotoxic to many lung cancer cell lines[143,144,153,154] by induction of apoptosis except in the A549 lung carcinoma cell line.[154] Normally, DNA-damaging agents induce p53, which in turn transcriptionally induces p21 and Mdm-2, the later binds p53 and targets it for degradation.[155] Although upregulating p53, flavopiridol was shown to inhibit transcription of p21 and Mdm-2 and to inhibit cell proliferation in A549 lung cancer cells.[153]

TABLE 14.2 Potential Cell Cycle Targets for Combination Therapy with Ionizing Radiation

Pathway Target	Role	Agents	Treatment Category	References
Cdks	Mitotic entrance, chromosome condensation, bipolar spindle assembly, APC/C regulation, nuclear envelope breakdown	Flavopiridol, UCN-01	CDK inhibitor	130,156
Chk1/Chk2	DNA damage checkpoint, mitotic entrance	UCN-01	Chk inhibitor	29,338,339
Tubulin	Mitotic spindle structure	Taxanes, epothilones	Microtubule-stabilizing agent	52,60–63
Aurora kinase A	Spindle formation, centrosome separation	VX-680, PHA-680632	Aurora kinase inhibitor	205
Aurora kinase B	Spindle assembly checkpoint, cytokinesis	ZM447439, VX-680, PHA-680632	Aurora kinase inhibitor	206,207
Akt/mTOR	Cell growth and proliferation	Rapamycin, RAD001, CCI-779	mTOR inhibitor	215,216, 221,222

Despite promising preclinical data, flavopiridol has not demonstrated in trial significant clinical activity as a single agent in patients with metastatic lung cancer.[129] The unexpected and significant toxicity of this agent given as single cancer therapy in all these clinical trials have so far discouraged its use in monotherapy.

Another approach for the use of flavopiridol in anticancer therapy is to take advantage of its potential to augment cytotoxic actions of chemotherapeutic agents and radiation. This strategy of combining flavopiridol with chemotherapy has been investigated in several studies showing promising results. Flavopiridol enhanced the cytotoxic effects of many chemotherapeutic agents in vitro (12, 13, 14, 15, 16, and 17) as well as in vivo (8, 13, and 15), in a sequence-dependent manner. Similar results were observed in the combined approach with ionizing radiation both in vitro,[156,157] and in vivo[130] in various human cancer types.[156,158–160] Flavopiridol sensitized human cancers to radiation in a dose-dependent manner, by cell cycle redistribution, by inhibiting cellular repair from radiation damage, and possibly by effects on angiogenic factors. In addition, studies also demonstrated the effects of flavopiridol in enhancing apoptosis and tumor regression.[160–163] The therapeutic ratio of radiotherapy in the in vivo tumor models was increased by flavopiridol.[130,156] More specifically, the radiosensitizing action of flavopiridol was recently determined in zebrafish embryos using cyclin D1 (CCND1) downregulation by antisense hydroxylprolyl-phosphono peptide nucleic acid oligomers compared to control.[164] This study demonstrated that the specific sensitizing effects of flavopiridol in response to radiation were in part caused by the inhibition of cyclin D1, one of its primary pharmacologic targets.[158] Another study analysed the sequence-dependent effects of flavopiridol when combined to radiation and showed that the maximum radiopotentiation and apoptosis were observed when the lung cancer cells were treated with the sequence of docetaxel, then radiation, and finally flavopiridol both in vitro and in vivo. Therefore, the combined, sequence-dependent strategy radiation/flavopiridol has the potential to enhance outcome in many types of cancer and needs to be further investigated in a well-designed clinical trial.

Chk1 Inhibitors

UCN-01. Staurosporine is a potent nonspecific protein and tyrosine kinase inhibitor (TKI). UCN-01 or 7-hydroxystaurosporine, an analogue of staurosporine, was found to be a nonspecific inhibitor of CDKs, protein kinase C (PKC) isoenzymes, and causes cell arrest in G1 and G2 phases in different cell types.[165] UCN-01 is a checkpoint protein kinase inhibitor that promotes cellular G1 arrest by inhibiting the activity of CDK-1 and CDK-2, thereby downregulating cyclins and increasing the expression of CKI, p21. Interestingly, UCN-01 abrogates the G2 checkpoint induced by radiation, leading irradiated cells into early mitosis and the onset of apoptotic death.[29,166] The mechanisms by which the cells enter mitosis include activation of cdc2 kinase, and a direct inhibiting effect on the G2-associated checkpoint protein kinase 1 (Chk1).[167,168] UCN-01 inhibits the cdc25C regulatory pathway and interferes with DNA damage-mediated inhibition of cdc2-cyclin B1-kinase. It targets more strongly Chkl than Chk2 (IC50 −20 nM vs. −1 pM).[29,168,169] It has been shown that Chk1 is required for the radiation-induced G2 checkpoint.[170,171] Chk1 may control the G_2 checkpoint via phosphorylation-mediated negative regulation of Cdc25A, Cdc25C, and Cdc25B.[170,172,173] Thus, the potential of Chk1 inhibitors would most likely be as sensitizer to other anticancer treatments such as radiotherapy because inhibiting Chk kinases forces the cell to enter mitosis with DNA damage accumulation. Cancer cells could likely be particularly sensitive to such treatment, since they commonly lack normal G1 checkpoint control and may rely more on the S and G2 checkpoints compared to normal cells.[174] In vitro, UCN-01 exhibits a potent radiosensitivity effect in mutated p53 carrying NSCLC cell models.[175,176] Despite encouraging preclinical results, combination studies of UCN-01 with radiotherapy have not yet been opened, whereas UCN-01 alone has undergone phase I and II clinical trials in several cancer types.[177–179]

Microtubule-Stabilizing Agents In all eukaryotic cells, microtubules are essential components of the cytoskeleton, and crucial in the successful process of mitosis and cell division, via uniquely rapid dynamics in the mitotic spindle.[180] Microtubule-stabilizing agents, which interfere with microtubule dynamics, have been particularly effective as anticancer therapy and are a well-known strategy to induce G2/M arrest.[181] These agents suppress cancer cell growth by promoting accelerated assembly of excessively stable microtubules, resulting in G2/M cell cycle arrest and cell death. The abrogation of the G2 cell cycle checkpoint will lead to the forced accumulation of tumor cells in the radiosensitive G2/M phase of the cell cycle, where irradiation could achieve a higher rate of unrepaired chromosomal aberrations during mitosis. Additionally, antimicrotubule agents have the capacity to induce apoptosis, mediated through inactivation of bcl-2 proto-oncogene, even in p53-mutated and radioresistant cells.[182–184] It has been increasingly recognized that the combined use of microtubule-stabilizing agents such as taxanes in combination with radiotherapy is a clinically interesting strategy to improve anticancer treatment.[185]

TAXANES. Taxanes, such as paclitaxel and docetaxel, have already been proved to have a potent anticancer activity against many cancer types.[186] In addition, they are able to block cells at the radiosensitive G2/M phase of the cell cycle, suggesting the rationale for the use of taxanes to enhance radiotherapy.[185] Several studies showed the effectiveness of taxanes in enhancing tumor radiosensitivity in vitro and increasing significantly tumor growth delay in vivo.[187,188] Paclitaxel mechanism of action, however, is not limited to G2/M accumulation and results from direct cytotoxic effect in addition to the cell cycle effects as well. Furthermore, taxanes showed significant clinical efficacy for several tumor types, including non–small cell lung, breast, and ovarian cancers. The specific molecular mechanisms of taxanes antitumor activity in lung cancer have been extensively reviewed.[189] The use of taxanes in cancer treatment, however, is often limited by resulting toxicities, such as neutropenia (which can be very severe), and peripheral neuropathy,[190,191] and by multidrug resistance (MDR).[192] This has lead to the development of novel microtubule-stabilizing agents, such as epothilones, with improved overall safety and broader antitumor activity, particularly in MDR.[193,194]

EPOTHILONES. Epothilones are natural products fungicidal macrolides, originally isolated from the myxobacterium *Sorangium cellulosum*. They were found to exert strong microtubule-stabilizing effects similar to that of paclitaxel, even though structurally unrelated to taxanes.[193,194] Epothilone B (Patupilone, EP0906) and epothilone A (demethylated epothilone B) are both natural products, whereas semisynthetic epothilones were developed including ixabepilone (BMS-247550, the lactam analog of epothilone B) and epothilone D (KOS-862). Epothilone and its analogs can sensitize both paclitaxel-sensitive as well as paclitaxel-resistant cells to ionizing radiation at low concentration both in vitro and in vivo.[52,60–63] BMS-247550 has been characterized for its radiosensitizing potential against human paclitaxel-sensitive lung carcinoma cells showing additive apoptosis and enhanced tumor growth delay when used in combination with ionizing radiation.[79] Similarly, epothilone B sensitized P-glycoprotein–overexpressing p53-mutated colon ADC to radiation in vitro and in vivo.[80] Kim et al.[195] reported the radiosensitizing effects of BMS-247550 in human lung carcinoma model. The study also demonstrated that the enhancement was correlated with the percentage of G2/M arrest induced by epothilone and with the induction of apoptosis. These preclinical results support the concept of combining epothilones with radiation to enhance lung cancer response to therapy. To date, only a phase I study of epothilone B administered concurrently with radiotherapy is ongoing for cancer patients presenting advanced solid tumors or recurrent disease for which there is no standard therapy or tumors have failed standard therapy. Objectives of the trial are to evaluate the safety and toxicity profile of epothilone B, and tumor response, when combined to radiation therapy.

Aurora Kinase Inhibitors Aurora kinases represent a novel family of serine/threonine kinases crucial for cell cycle control. In mammals, there are three types of Aurora kinases: Aurora A, B, and C.[196] Thus far, very limited data are reported on Aurora C, which expression is limited to the testes.[197] Despite the fact that they share >70% homology in their catalytic domain, Aurora A and Aurora B have different subcellular localization and functions during mitosis.[198] Aurora A is localized at the centrosome during duplication and to the spindle poles in mitosis. Aurora A kinase activity is regulated by TPX2, a protein required for spindle assembly. Silencing of Aurora A leads to abnormal spindle morphology in human cells.[199] Aurora A reaches the maximum activity at the G2-M transition.[200] At the G2-M transition, centrosome separation requires functional Aurora A.[199] Aurora A contributes also to transition from G2 to M phase. Suppression of Aurora A by RNA interference results in G2-M arrest of HeLa cells and promotes apoptosis.[201] It was shown that ectopic expression of Aurora A results in a bypass of the G2-M checkpoint induced by DNA damage.[202] Inhibitors of Aurora kinases were developed to take advantage of these targets to modulate the abnormal cell cycle regulation for cancer therapy and tested in cultured cells and xenograft models.[203,204]

We and others reported on the effects of combining Aurora kinase inhibition with ionizing radiation.[205–207] ZM447439 is one of such Aurora A and B inhibitors,[208] but is known to produce cellular phenotypes consistent with inhibition of Aurora B rather than A, including the Aurora B–specific inhibition of histone H3 phosphorylation on serine 10.[208,209] ZM447439 caused p53-dependent multinucleation, growth inhibition in a colony-forming assay with a marked toxicity toward proliferating cells, and increased the amount of apoptotic cells. Interestingly, expression of Aurora B and survivin, two of the proteins that constitute the chromosomal passenger complex, was increased after irradiation of mesothelioma cells, consistent with their known activity and levels peaking in G2/M that correspond to the radiation-induced cell cycle arrest.[197] We found that ZM447439 sensitized mesothelioma cells to irradiation, and that the combination of both Aurora B and survivin inhibition resulted in a deeper radiosensitization.[207] This effect can be explained by the small molecule, ATP-binding nature of ZM447439, which can disrupt cell division but not the binding to survivin and thus the localization to centromere. Tao et al.[205] demonstrated that inhibition of Aurora A either by PHA680632 or by small interfering RNA (siRNA) against Aurora A enhanced cell killing after exposure to radiation in vitro. Moreover, they also showed that PHA680632 alone were able to induce a marked tumor growth inhibition in vivo and that irradiation treatment combined with PHA680632 led to an additive tumor growth inhibition compared with each agent alone, especially in p53-deficient cells. Although it did not act as radiosensitizer, this study showed the potential of PHA680632 when used in combined-modality strategy and can serve as proof of concept for Aurora A targeting with ionizing radiation. More encouraging results were very recently reported using VX-680 with radiation.[206] VX-680, also known as MK-0457, targets the ATP-binding site of Aurora kinases for reversible inhibition, and was proven to greatly inhibit tumor growth in three xenograft models in vivo, including leukemia, colon, and pancreatic tumors.[210] In a laryngeal SCC in vitro model, VX-680 upregulated p53 and effectively sensitized tumor cells to radiotherapy, whereas overexpression of Aurora A generated radioresistance.[206] Taken together, these promising preliminary results suggest the possibility to use Aurora kinases as a target for radiation therapy.

mTOR Inhibitors The mammalian target of rapamycin (mTOR), a serine/threonine kinase, is a downstream mediator in the phosphatidylinositol 3-kinase/Akt signaling pathway, which plays a critical role in regulating basic cellular functions including cellular growth and proliferation.[211] The PI3K/Akt/mTOR signaling pathway is altered in many cancer types, including lung.[212] Rapamycin (sirolimus), and its improved analogs (rapalogs: CCI-779 - temsirolimus, RAD001 - everolimus, and AP23573 - deforolimus), the main mTOR inhibitors used in studies have shown G1-phase arrest[213] and significant antitumor activity in various radiation models. mTOR inhibition combined with radiation showed decreased tumor vascular density in murine models and sensitized vascular endothelium.[214] Moreover, RAD001 has been shown to increase the radiosensitivity of breast[215] and prostate[216] cancer cells, mainly via induction of autophagy cell death. Phosphatase and tensin homolog (PTEN)-deficient prostate cancer cells were even more sensitive to ionizing radiation as compared to PTEN-efficient cancer cells,[216] suggesting important clinical implications given the frequent presence of PTEN deletions in many types of cancer.[217–219] Interestingly, mTOR inhibitors seems to be more effective in tumor cells than in normal cells, possibly because transformed cells have increased activation of the Akt/mTOR pathway.[220] RAD001 has also been shown to further enhance the radiosensitization obtained by inhibition of apoptosis in either lung or breast cancer cells, again by increased autophagy.[221,222] These findings suggest potential autophagy targets to enhance efficacy of therapeutic strategies using mTOR inhibitors.[223] Currently, mTOR inhibitors are being evaluated in multiple clinical trials. In phase I and II trials, mTOR inhibitors appear to be well tolerated, with most common and transient adverse events being skin reactions, stomatitis, myelosuppression, and metabolic abnormalities.[224–230]

Interestingly, recent data suggest a certain antitumor activity, such as tumor regressions and prolonged stable disease, which has been reported among patients with various malignancies, including NSCLC. Based on these encouraging data, a phase I/II study of RAD001 and radiation therapy in patients with brain metastasis from NSCLC is currently ongoing at Vanderbilt University.

VASCULAR TARGETS FOR RADIOTHERAPY

One of the most important promoters of angiogenesis is the vascular endothelial growth factor (VEGF), which binds to specific receptors including VEGF-receptor 2 to stimulate blood vessel formation, growth, and permeability. Clinical correlative studies have established that tissue VEGF expression is correlated with a poorer prognosis in NSCLC.[231–235] VEGF, fibroblast growth factor (FGF), and platelet-derived growth factor (PDGF) receptors are tyrosine kinase receptors that are expressed on the surface of endothelial, stromal, and tumor cells, and play important roles during tumor angiogenesis. Studies of these factors and their receptors have led to the development of antiangiogenic agents that target the function of VEGF, FGF, and PDGF.

Radiotherapy promotes expression of angiogenic activators, VEGF, FGF, and PDGF.[236–238] Radiation-induced VEGF activation subsequently attenuates vasculature damage and lead to a reduced tumor cytotoxicity.[239] Serving as a paracrine proliferative stimulus, VEGF also instigates the growth of previously dormant microtumors located out-of-field with respect to the radiation treatment field.[240] In addition, radiation triggers phenotypic changes favorable for tumor angiogenesis.[241] Recently, the combination of radiotherapy with antiangiogenic agents has been found to ameliorate the problem of vascular radioresistance. Antiangiogenic agents act on the endothelial cells by suppressing the radiation-induced release of proangiogenic factors. Just as with radiation alone, antiangiogenic agents used as a monotherapy results in objective response rates of 10% or less[242] with a gradual loss of activity and efficacy.[243–245] This is a result of the protean nature of tumor cells in being able to activate secondary angiogenic pathways when the primary angiogenic pathway is inhibited.[246] When antiangiogenic agents and radiation are combined, however, their antitumor effects become additive or synergistic under the principles of nonoverlapping toxicities and spatial cooperation.[247] This phenomenon has been shown in most preclinical studies, suggesting that the combination of antiangiogenic agents with radiation treatment has the potential to enhance tumor cytotoxicity and prevent the development of distant metastases.

Radiotherapy also activates initiator of prosurvival signaling pathways, such as phospholipases, lipid kinases, and phosphatases, thereby increasing viability of vascular endothelial cells. Therefore, this section will focus on potential targets for radiation therapy, including VEGF inhibitors, as well as the eicosanoid, sphingolipid, and ceramide pathways. Only representative antiangiogenic agents are discussed (Table 14.3 provide a more comprehensive list).

VEGF Inhibitors VEGF is a ligand with a central role in controlling tumor blood vessel development and survival.[248–250] Numerous evidence indicate that targeting VEGF and its signaling pathway, when combined with radiation, could significantly enhance tumor toxicity in preclinical models.[238,251–255] Interestingly, VEGF inhibition does not increase the hypoxic cell fraction in tumors.[251,252] These results are encouraging because hypoxia is associated with enhanced radioresistance and malignant progression in tumors of the uterine cervix, head and neck, and sarcomas.[256] Furthermore, emerging concepts, such as the tumor vascular normalization, suggest that the combination of antiangiogenic agents and radiotherapy could engender a transient normalization of the abnormal tumor vasculature and a time period of increased oxygenation.[257] Anti-VEGFR-2 antibody can create such a time dependent enhancement of radiation-induced tumor regression.[258] Alternatively, Lee et al.[251] attributed this transient oxygenation to the capacity of radiation therapy to ablate mainly immature tumor vessels and oxygen-consuming cells. Nevertheless, the two therapeutic modalities combined are superior than either alone.

VEGF inhibitors include VEGF receptor TKI VEGF trep and anti-VEGF antibody. When combined with radiation, these inhibitors have produced promising antitumor efficacy in preclinical studies. Three of these agents, bevacizumab,

TABLE 14.3 Potential Vascular Target for Combined Treatment with Radiation Therapy

Agent	Target / Action	Growth Delay	Clinical Trial (Combined with Radiotherapy)	References
AZD2171	VEGFR TKI inhibition of PDGF and c-Kit	+	–	258–260
PTKI787/ZK222584 (Valatinib)	VEGFR TKI	+	Phase I	254,266,267
SU5416	VEGFR TKI	+	Phase I, II	253,255,340–342
SU6668	VEGFR TKI inhibition of FGFR, PDGFR, Flk-1/KDR	+	–	253,263,343,344
SU11248 (Sunitinib)	Multikinase inhibitor (inhibition of VEGFR-1, VEGFR-2, VEGFR-3, c-KIT, PDGFRα, PDGFRβ)	+	Phase I	265,345
Sorafenib (BAY 43-9006)	Multikinase inhibitor (inhibition of b-raf, c-raf, VEGFR, Flt3, PDGFR-β, c-KIT, FGF 1, p38α, RET)	+	Phase I, II	346
SU11657	Multikinase inhibitor (inhibition of PDGFR-β, VEGFR, KIT, Flt3)	+	–	347
DC101	Anti-VEGFR-2 antibody	+	–	252,258,342,348, 349
Bevacizumab (Avastin)	Anti-VEGF antibody	+	Phase I, II	350,351
Anti-VEGF$_{165}$	Anti-VEGF antibody	+	–	238,352
ZD6474 (Zactima)	VEGFR/EGFR TKI	+	Phase I, II	261,262,353
Celecoxib	COX-2 inhibitor	+	Phase I, II	277,283,289,290
SC-236	COX-2 inhibitor	+	–	281,285,354
Rofecoxib	COX-2 inhibitor	+	–	164
NS-398	COX-2 inhibitor	+	–	283,355
ZD6126	Vascular-damaging agent	+/–	–	262,356,357
Combretastatin A-4 disodium phosphate (CA4P)	Vascular-damaging agent	+	Phase I, II	358,359
Angiostatin	Endogenous inhibitor	+/–	–	238,360,361
Anginex	Designed antiangiogenic peptide	+	–	350,360
LY294002	PI3K inhibitor	+	–	302,362
IC486068	PI3K inhibitor	+	–	363

sorafenib, sunitinib, are currently in clinical trials. Many inhibitors of VEGFR TKI have proved to be potent radiosensitizers in mouse models of lung cancer. One such example is AZD2171, an orally available pan-VEGFR TKI with activity against PDGF receptor and c-Kit.[259] AZD2171 has been shown to induce a synergistic tumor growth delay when given on days 4 to 6 prior to fractionated RT.[258,260] Alternatively, the administration of ZD6474 (Zactima), an EGFR and VEGFR TKI, on xenograft models of lung cancer showed greater antitumor effects when given 30 minutes after radiotherapy (36 ± 1 days, $p < 0.001$ vs. radiation alone or the concurrent schedule).[261] The results regarding sequence optimization vary across studies, and might be dependent on many factors including the drug's intrinsic properties, total radiation dose, dose per fraction, and overall treatment time. Conversely, a recent report showed that the sequencing of ZD6474/radiotherapy had little impact on treatment outcomes in a human colorectal carcinoma model, although this combined strategy had a clear therapeutic advantage.[262] Further studies examining the sequencing of therapies are needed to ascertain the most favorable schedule of VEGF antagonist with radiation therapy.

Other VEGFR TKIs investigated to date with radiation in preclinical models include SU6668 and SU11248. With SU6668, a synergistic tumor growth delay was observed with concurrent radiation therapy, and it was found to inhibit Akt phosphorylation and activation in mouse models with Lewis lung carcinoma or glioblastoma multiforme (GL261).[263] SU11248 (sunitinib) is a low nM-selective inhibitor of multiple angiogenic RTKs including VEGFR1, VEGFR2, VEGFR3, c-KIT, PDGFR-α, and PDGFR-β.[264] When given as a maintenance dose after concurrent radiation therapy, sunitinib effectively prevented tumor regrowth and significantly prolonged local tumor control.[265]

PTK787/ZK222584 (valatinib) is a small molecule-VEGFR TKI shown to enhance tumor hypoxia in a range that is associated with enhanced radioresistance when given in monotherapy but was reverted by concurrent ionizing radiation in vivo.[266] The bimodality treatment resulted in a supra-additive growth delay of tumor allografts and was associated with the highest apoptotic rate and the lowest tumor cell proliferation index. This study suggests that the risk of treatment-induced hypoxia by antiangiogenic agents exists but is minimized by concurrent radiotherapy, thus providing a mechanistic basis for the combination of antiangiogenic agents with radiation for cancer therapy. A study by Zips et al.[267] used different combination schedules of a PTK787/ZK222584 with irradiation of human SCCs in nude mice. Short-term neoadjuvant and simultaneous administration showed no effect on tumor growth delay, whereas long-term inhibition of angiogenesis after radiotherapy significantly reduced the growth rate of local recurrences but did not improve local tumor control. These results suggest that recurrences after irradiation depend on VEGF-driven angiogenesis, whereas surviving tumor cells retain their clonogenic potential during adjuvant treatment with PTK787/ZK222584. In addition, irradiated vessels appear to be more sensitive to VEGF inhibition, which is supported by the observation that in vitro–irradiated endothelial cells show an increased VEGFR2 expression.[268] In this setting, however, the radioprotective function of VEGF will not be counteracted during radiation therapy.

The study performed by Kozin et al.[252] on human xenograft tumors treated with the anti-VEGFR-2 antibody DC101 and irradiation showed promising results. In the 54A and U87 tumor models, the combined treatment resulted in a statistically significant decrease of the dose necessary for local tumor control. Specifically, TCD_{50} (radiation dose yielding 50% tumor cure) values were decreased by 41% in 54A carcinoma and by 24% in U87 tumors. Finally, AEE788, a dual TKI of both epidermal growth factor receptor (EGFR) and VEGFR, was shown to improve tumor control when combined with radiation in prostate cancer cells, especially highly EGFR-expressing tumors.[269] These studies indicate the potential of anti-VEGF strategies to improve the outcome of curative radiotherapy.

Eicosanoid and Lysophospholipid Signaling Pathways The phospholipase A2 (PLA_2) superfamilly produces arachidonic acid, precursor of the eicosanoid metabolites and lysophosphocholine (LPC). PLA_2 is activated in irradiated endothelial cells.[270]

Eicosanoid Pathways PLA_2 catalyzes the hydrolysis of the sn-2 position of glycerophospholipids-releasing arachidonic acid, which in turn is metabolized to prostaglandins by the cyclooxygenase (COX) pathway. COX is the rate-limiting enzyme in the conversion of arachidonic acid to prostaglandins. Two isoforms of COX were described, COX-1 and COX-2. Whereas COX-1 is constituvely expressed in most tissues, COX-2 is induced in pathological states such as inflammatory processes and cancer.[271] Overexpression of COX-2 is frequently present in lung cancer and may play a significant role in carcinogenesis.[272,273] Upregulation of COX-2 and its major metabolite, prostaglandin E2 (PGE2), has been implicated in angiogenesis, tumor growth, invasion, metastasis, apoptosis resistance, and suppression of antitumor immunity.[272–275] It has also been associated with aggressive biological tumor behaviour, resistance to standard cancer treatment, and adverse patient outcome in patients with resected early stage ADC of the lung.[274,275] More precisely, COX-2 partakes in tumor angiogenesis via various mechanisms including the increased expression of VEGF, generation of prostaglandins known to stimulate endothelial cell migration, and inhibition of endothelial cell apoptosis.[276–278] Nonselective COX inhibitors, such as indomethacin, have been shown to enhance tumor radiation response in vitro,[279,280] and preclinical studies provide evidence that administration of COX-2 inhibitors with radiation increases local tumor control.[281,282] Antitumor effects may be related to the enhancement of irradiation-induced apoptosis,[283,284] although this hypothesis remains controversial.[281,285] Other mechanisms include the modulation of tumor intrinsic radiosensitivity[285] and tumor angiogenesis.[281,284] It has been suggested that COX-2 inhibition confers radiosensitivity through the suppression of prostaglandin production. Prostaglandins can play a cytoprotective role against irradiation,[286,287] and the removal of COX-2 derived PGE_2 has been demonstrated to enhance the efficacy of radiotherapy.[276] However, a recent study by Shin et al.[288] suggests that radiocytoxicity enhancement by COX-2 inhibitors is attributed to their alterations of cell cycle and is unrelated to PGE_2. In this study, the addition of PGE_2 after the administration of celecoxib, a COX-2 inhibitor, produced no significant radiation-enhancing effects in A549 and COX-2 transfected HCT-116 cells. They hypothesized that COX-2 inhibition might alter the G2-M checkpoint after noting a correlation between COX-2 overexpression and prolonged radiation-induced G2-M arrest. Most experimental data, however, do not support this hypothesis, and additional studies are needed to delineate the specific mechanism of radiation therapy enhancement by COX-2 inhibitors.

Two COX-2 inhibitors, celecoxib and SC-236, were tested in preclinical studies and showed interesting results. Celecoxib in monotherapy strongly inhibited neovascularization and reduced tumor growth and metastasis.[277,289] A possible correlation between basal COX-2 expression level and celecoxib-induced radiation sensitivity has been suggested.[283] Interestingly, celecoxib exerted an inhibitory effect on the EGFR-mediated mechanisms of radioresistance, specifically by preventing both basal and radiation-stimulated nuclear transport of EGFR.[290] SC-236 also induced significant growth delay effects when administered oraly in irradiated sarcoma FSA rodent model.[281] The enhanced radiation response was associated with decreased PGE_2 levels and markedly reduced neoangiogenesis. A greater than additive prolongation of tumor growth was achieved by a combination of radiation and SC-236 in human glioma U251.[285] Based on these observations several ongoing clinical trials are currently evaluating COX-2 inhibitors as adjuvants with radiation therapy in patients with advanced NSCLC, and preliminary results are encouraging. Further understanding of the mechanisms of COX-2 in interaction with radiation may facilitate future development of targeted strategies for lung cancer treatment.

Lysophospholipid Pathways Schematicaly, the PLA_2 superfamilly can be divided into four main types: the cytosolic ($cPLA_2$), the secretory ($sPLA_2$), platelet-activating factor acetylhydrolases (PAF-AHs), and the calcium-independent cytosolic PLA2 enzymes ($iPLA_2$).[291] Activation of $cPLA_2$ leads to the increased production of lysophospholipids, such as LPC.[292,293] LPC functions as a second messenger in the signal transduction pathways that regulate vascular proliferation,[294–296] migration, expression of adhesion molecules,[297–299] and inflammation.[292,293] LPC stimulates proliferation in endothelial cells by transactivating VEGFR-2 and activating Akt and ERK1/2.[295] Ionizing radiation activates prosurvival pathways in the vascular endothelium, including PI3K/Akt (PI3K/Akt)[300–302] and MAPK pathways,[301,303] thereby regulating the cellular response and sensitivity to radiation. Recently, Yazlovitskaya et al.[270] identified a molecular sequence involving activation of $cPLA_2$ followed by the increased production of LPC, transactivation of Flk-1, and phosphorylation of Akt and ERK1/2 in irradiated vascular endothelial cells, constituting an immediate radiation-triggered prosurvival signaling pathway. These data suggest that $cPLA_2$ signaling mediates radiation-dependent prosurvival response in vascular endothelial cells and participates in endothelial radioresistance.

Recent studies have established that autotaxin (ATX), also known as phosphodiesterase-Iα or nucleotide pyrophosphatase/phosphodiesterase 2, mediates the conversion of lysophosphatidylcholine to lysophosphatidic acid (LPA) and stimulates tumor cell motility.[304] LPA acts on specific G-protein–coupled receptors to stimulate the proliferation, migration, and survival of malignant cells.[305] ATX is also strongly implicated in tumor aggressiveness, metastasis, and angiogenesis in preclinical models,[306,307] and is overexpressed in various cancers including lung.[308,309] Therefore, the ATX-LPA pathway is an attractive target for anticancer and antiangiogenesis therapy.

Ceramide Signaling Pathway During recent years, evidence has been provided that sphingolipids including ceramide, sphingosine, and sphingosine 1-phosphate (S1P) are more than just structural components. Sphingolipids play important roles in cell growth as well as cell survival and death signaling,[310–312] and ceramide has been shown to function as a lipid second messenger.[313] The best characterized membrane signaling pathway is initiated by radiation-induced activation of enzymatic hydrolysis of the membrane sphingomyelin by sphingomyelinases (SMase), into the formation of ceramide.[312,314–317] In vitro and in vivo studies showed the crucial roles of acid sphingomyelinase enzyme activation and a rapid ceramide generation in radiation-induced endothelial cell death.[314] Ionizing radiation acts directly on bovine aortic endothelial cell membrane preparations devoid of nuclei, proving that ceramide generation after irradiation is independent of DNA damage and cell cycle regulation induced by DNA DSBs.[318] Importantly, only high radiation dose (at least 15 Gy) was shown to induce ceramide production, as opposed to low-dose irradiation that did not result in ceramide generation.[239] It has also been shown that cells deficient in sphingomyelinases are more resistant to radiation-induced apoptosis.[319,320] There are several isoforms of SMase based on required pH for their optimal activity: acid (ASMase), neutral (NSMase), or alkaline (Smase). Ceramide generation via activation of SMase precedes apoptosis in response to many different stimuli in addition to radiation, including TNF-α (tumor necrosis factor α), Fas ligand, and exposure to glucocorticoid.[321] Ceramide-mediated response to radiation has been shown to activate various protein kinase cascades, including the classical mitogen-activated protein kinase (MAPK/ERK) cascade,[322,323] and the stress-activated protein kinase/c-Jun N-terminal kinase (SAPK/JNK) signaling pathway, leading to p53-independent apoptosis.[324] This molecular cascade triggered by ceramide is mediated by MEKK1 and involves sequential phosphorylation and activation of SEK1/MKK4 and SAPK/JNK that lead to the phosphorylation of c-Jun, a transcription factor in the nuclei.[324–326] Once generated, ceramide may accumulate or be converted into ceramide 1-phosphate by ceramide kinase phosphorylation,[312] sphingosine by ceramidases deacylation, and subsequent sphingosine-1-phosphate (S1P) by further phosphorylation by sphingosine kinase.[327] Interesingly, ceramide and S1P exert opposing functions in the regulation of cell death and survival, hence the relative balance between ceramide/S1P determines the fate of cells in response to specific stimuli.[328] Modulation of sphingolipid-induced apoptosis has been proposed as a way to increase the sensitivity of tumors to various therapeutic agents.[328,329] Sphingosine kinase, ceramidase, and glycosylceramide synthase, among other enzymes important to sphingolipid metabolism, are being studied as potential new drug targets. S1P promotes cell growth and survival, angiogenesis, vascular maturation, and mediates cell migration. Using a monoclonal antibody with high affinity for S1P, Visentin et al.[330] have shown that selective absorption of S1P is sufficient to block angiogenesis and endothelial cell migration in response to VEGF and basic FGF and could thus represent a promising approach to cancer therapy. Multiple investigators have demonstrated the dependence of radiation-induced apoptosis on ceramide,[320,331–334] and that radiation sensitivity may be augmented by addition of exogenous sphingoid bases or modulators of endogenous ceramide production.[335–337] Preclinical studies of existing drugs, and the development of new drugs for novel targets in the various sphingolipid pathways, are warranted to enhance radiation therapy for lung cancer.

REFERENCES

1. Hartwell LH, Kastan MB. Cell cycle control and cancer. *Science* 1994;266:1821–1828.
2. Sanchez I, Dynlacht BD. New insights into cyclins, CDKs, and cell cycle control. *Semin Cell Dev Biol* 2005;16:311–321.
3. Sherr CJ. Cancer cell cycles. *Science* 1996;274:1672–1677.
4. Hartley KO, Gell D, Smith GC, et al. DNA-dependent protein kinase catalytic subunit: a relative of phosphatidylinositol 3-kinase and the ataxia telangiectasia gene product. *Cell* 1995;82:849–856.
5. Radford IR. p53 status, DNA double-strand break repair proficiency, and radiation response of mouse lymphoid and myeloid cell lines. *Int J Radiat Biol* 1994;66:557–560.
6. Radford IR, Murphy TK. Radiation response of mouse lymphoid and myeloid cell lines. Part III. Different signals can lead to apoptosis and may influence sensitivity to killing by DNA double-strand breakage. *Int J Radiat Biol* 1994;65:229–239.
7. Warters RL, Lyons BW. Variation in radiation-induced formation of DNA double-strand breaks as a function of chromatin structure. *Radiat Res* 1992;130:309–318.
8. Kurz EU, Lees-Miller SP. DNA damage-induced activation of ATM and ATM-dependent signaling pathways. *DNA Repair (Amst)* 2004;3: 889–900.
9. Bartkova J, Bakkenist CJ, Rajpert-De Meyts E, et al. ATM activation in normal human tissues and testicular cancer. *Cell Cycle* 2005;4:838–845.
10. Samuel T, Weber HO, Funk JO. Linking DNA damage to cell cycle checkpoints. *Cell Cycle* 2002;1:162–168.
11. Banin S, Moyal L, Shieh S, et al. Enhanced phosphorylation of p53 by ATM in response to DNA damage. *Science* 1998;281:1674–1677.
12. Canman CE, Lim DS. The role of ATM in DNA damage responses and cancer. *Oncogene* 1998;17:3301–3308.
13. Stracker TH, Theunissen JW, Morales M, et al. The Mre11 complex and the metabolism of chromosome breaks: the importance of communicating and holding things together. *DNA Repair (Amst)* 2004;3:845–854.
14. Uziel T, Lerenthal Y, Moyal L, et al. Requirement of the MRN complex for ATM activation by DNA damage. *Embo J* 2003;22:5612–5621.
15. Meyn MS. Ataxia-telangiectasia and cellular responses to DNA damage. *Cancer Res* 1995;55:5991–6001.
16. Shiloh Y. ATM and ATR: networking cellular responses to DNA damage. *Curr Opin Genet Dev* 2001;11:71–77.
17. Kastan M. Ataxia-telangiectasia—broad implications for a rare disorder. *N Engl J Med* 1995;333:662–663.
18. Hoekstra MF. Responses to DNA damage and regulation of cell cycle checkpoints by the ATM protein kinase family. *Curr Opin Genet Dev* 1997;7:170–175.
19. Barzilai A, Yamamoto K. DNA damage responses to oxidative stress. *DNA Repair (Amst)* 2004;3:1109–1115.
20. Abraham RT. Checkpoint signaling: epigenetic events sound the DNA strand-breaks alarm to the ATM protein kinase. *Bioessays* 2003;25: 627–630.
21. Amundson SA, Bittner M, Fornace AJ Jr. Functional genomics as a window on radiation stress signaling. *Oncogene* 2003;22:5828–5833.
22. Lukas J, Lukas C, Bartek J. Mammalian cell cycle checkpoints: signalling pathways and their organization in space and time. *DNA Repair (Amst)* 2004;3:997–1007.
23. Bartek J, Lukas J. Mammalian G1- and S-phase checkpoints in response to DNA damage. *Curr Opin Cell Biol* 2001;13:738–747.
24. Huang LC, Clarkin KC, Wahl GM. Sensitivity and selectivity of the DNA damage sensor responsible for activating p53-dependent G1 arrest. *Proc Natl Acad Sci U S A* 1996;93:4827–4832.
25. Linke SP, Clarkin KC, Wahl GM. p53 mediates permanent arrest over multiple cell cycles in response to gamma-irradiation. *Cancer Res* 1997;57:1171–1179.
26. Brugarolas J, Chandrasekaran C, Gordon JI, et al. Radiation-induced cell cycle arrest compromised by p21 deficiency. *Nature* 1995;377: 552–557.
27. Deng C, Zhang P, Harper JW, et al. Mice lacking p21CIP1/WAF1 undergo normal development, but are defective in G1 checkpoint control. *Cell* 1995;82:675–684.
28. Bernhard EJ, McKenna WG, Muschel RJ. Radiosensitivity and the cell cycle. *Cancer J Sci Am* 1999;5:194–204.
29. Wang Q, Fan S, Eastman A, et al. UCN-01: a potent abrogator of G2 checkpoint function in cancer cells with disrupted p53. *J Natl Cancer Inst* 1996;88:956–965.
30. Bernhard EJ, Maity A, Muschel RJ, et al. Effects of ionizing radiation on cell cycle progression. A review. *Radiat Environ Biophys* 1995;34:79–83.
31. Costanzo V, Robertson K, Ying CY, et al. Reconstitution of an ATM-dependent checkpoint that inhibits chromosomal DNA replication following DNA damage. *Mol Cell* 2000;6:649–659.
32. Mailand N, Falck J, Lukas C, et al. Rapid destruction of human Cdc25A in response to DNA damage. *Science* 2000;288:1425–1429.
33. Kuerbitz SJ, Plunkett BS, Walsh WV, et al. Wild-type p53 is a cell cycle checkpoint determinant following irradiation. *Proc Natl Acad Sci U S A* 1992;89:7491–7495.
34. Xu B, Kim ST, Lim DS, et al. Two molecularly distinct G(2)/M checkpoints are induced by ionizing irradiation. *Mol Cell Biol* 2002;22: 1049–1059.
35. Marples B, Wouters BG, Joiner MC. An association between the radiation-induced arrest of G2-phase cells and low-dose hyper-radiosensitivity: a plausible underlying mechanism? *Radiat Res* 2003;160:38–45.
36. Passalaris TM, Benanti JA, Gewin L, et al. The G(2) checkpoint is maintained by redundant pathways. *Mol Cell Biol* 1999;19:5872–5881.
37. Kato JY, Matsuoka M, Strom DK, et al. Regulation of cyclin D-dependent kinase 4 (cdk4) by cdk4-activating kinase. *Mol Cell Biol* 1994;14:2713–2721.
38. Kato J, Matsushime H, Hiebert SW, et al. Direct binding of cyclin D to the retinoblastoma gene product (pRb) and pRb phosphorylation by the cyclin D-dependent kinase CDK4. *Genes Dev* 1993;7:331–342.
39. Diehl JA, Cheng M, Roussel MF, et al. Glycogen synthase kinase-3beta regulates cyclin D1 proteolysis and subcellular localization. *Genes Dev* 1998;12:3499–3511.
40. Guo Y, Yang K, Harwalkar J, et al. Phosphorylation of cyclin D1 at Thr 286 during S phase leads to its proteasomal degradation and allows efficient DNA synthesis. *Oncogene* 2005;24:2599–2612.
41. Baldin V, Lukas J, Marcote MJ, et al. Cyclin D1 is a nuclear protein required for cell cycle progression in G1. *Genes Dev* 1993;7:812–821.
42. Kranenburg O, van der Eb AJ, Zantema A. Cyclin D1 is an essential mediator of apoptotic neuronal cell death. *Embo J* 1996;15:46–54.
43. Sumrejkanchanakij P, Tamamori-Adachi M, Matsunaga Y, et al. Role of cyclin D1 cytoplasmic sequestration in the survival of postmitotic neurons. *Oncogene* 2003;22:8723–8730.
44. Bienvenu F, Gascan H, Coqueret O. Cyclin D1 represses STAT3 activation through a Cdk4-independent mechanism. *J Biol Chem* 2001;276:16840–16847.
45. Knudsen KE, Arden KC, Cavenee WK. Multiple G1 regulatory elements control the androgen-dependent proliferation of prostatic carcinoma cells. *J Biol Chem* 1998;273:20213–20222.
46. Knudsen KE, Cavenee WK, Arden KC. D-type cyclins complex with the androgen receptor and inhibit its transcriptional transactivation ability. *Cancer Res* 1999;59:2297–2301.
47. Qin C, Burghardt R, Smith R, et al. Peroxisome proliferator-activated receptor gamma agonists induce proteasome-dependent degradation of cyclin D1 and estrogen receptor alpha in MCF-7 breast cancer cells. *Cancer Res* 2003;63:958–964.
48. Zwijsen RM, Buckle RS, Hijmans EM, et al. Ligand-independent recruitment of steroid receptor coactivators to estrogen receptor by cyclin D1. *Genes Dev* 1998;12:3488–3498.
49. Motokura T, Bloom T, Kim HG, et al. A novel cyclin encoded by a bcl1-linked candidate oncogene. *Nature* 1991;350:512–515.
50. van Diest PJ, Michalides RJ, Jannink L, et al. Cyclin D1 expression in invasive breast cancer. Correlations and prognostic value. *Am J Pathol* 1997;150:705–711.

51. Caputi M, Groeger AM, Esposito V, et al. Prognostic role of cyclin D1 in lung cancer. Relationship to proliferating cell nuclear antigen. *Am J Respir Cell Mol Biol* 1999;20:746–750.
52. Ratschiller D, Heighway J, Gugger M, et al. Cyclin D1 overexpression in bronchial epithelia of patients with lung cancer is associated with smoking and predicts survival. *J Clin Oncol* 2003;21:2085–2093.
53. Anton RC, Coffey DM, Gondo MM, et al. The expression of cyclins D1 and E in predicting short-term survival in squamous cell carcinoma of the lung. *Mod Pathol* 2000;13:1167–1172.
54. Ikehara M, Oshita F, Ito H, et al. Expression of cyclin D1 but not of cyclin E is an indicator of poor prognosis in small adenocarcinomas of the lung. *Oncol Rep* 2003;10:137–139.
55. Yamanouchi H, Furihata M, Fujita J, et al. Expression of cyclin E and cyclin D1 in non-small cell lung cancers. *Lung Cancer* 2001;31:3–8.
56. Lonardo F, Rusch V, Langenfeld J, et al. Overexpression of cyclins D1 and E is frequent in bronchial preneoplasia and precedes squamous cell carcinoma development. *Cancer Res* 1999;59:2470–2476.
57. Brambilla E, Gazzeri S, Moro D, et al. Alterations of Rb pathway (Rb-p16INK4-cyclin D1) in preinvasive bronchial lesions. *Clin Cancer Res* 1999;5:243–250.
58. Tominaga M, Sueoka N, Irie K, et al. Detection and discrimination of preneoplastic and early stages of lung adenocarcinoma using hnRNP B1 combined with the cell cycle-related markers p16, cyclin D1, and Ki-67. *Lung Cancer* 2003;40:45–53.
59. Kurasono Y, Ito T, Kameda Y, et al. Expression of cyclin D1, retinoblastoma gene protein, and p16 MTS1 protein in atypical adenomatous hyperplasia and adenocarcinoma of the lung. An immunohistochemical analysis. *Virchows Arch* 1998;432:207–215.
60. Bombi JA, Martinez A, Ramirez J, et al. Ultrastructural and molecular heterogeneity in non-small cell lung carcinomas: study of 110 cases and review of the literature. *Ultrastruct Pathol* 2002;26:211–218.
61. Volm M, Koomagi R. Association of cyclin D1 expression in lung cancer and the smoking habits of patients. *Cancer Lett* 1999;141:147–150.
62. Fero ML, Rivkin M, Tasch M, et al. A syndrome of multiorgan hyperplasia with features of gigantism, tumorigenesis, and female sterility in p27(Kip1)-deficient mice. *Cell* 1996;85:733–744.
63. Zhang H, Xiong Y, Beach D. Proliferating cell nuclear antigen and p21 are components of multiple cell cycle kinase complexes. *Mol Biol Cell* 1993;4:897–906.
64. Winters ZE. P53 pathways involving G2 checkpoint regulators and the role of their subcellular localisation. *J R Coll Surg Edinb* 2002;47:591–598.
65. Taylor WR, Stark GR. Regulation of the G2/M transition by p53. *Oncogene* 2001;20:1803–1815.
66. Coqueret O. Linking cyclins to transcriptional control. *Gene* 2002;299:35–55.
67. Weinberg WC, Denning MF. P21Waf1 control of epithelial cell cycle and cell fate. *Crit Rev Oral Biol Med* 2002;13:453–464.
68. Blagosklonny MV. Are p27 and p21 cytoplasmic oncoproteins? *Cell Cycle* 2002;1:391–393.
69. Roninson IB. Oncogenic functions of tumour suppressor p21(Waf1/Cip1/Sdi1): association with cell senescence and tumour-promoting activities of stromal fibroblasts. *Cancer Lett* 2002;179:1–14.
70. Gartel AL, Tyner AL. The role of the cyclin-dependent kinase inhibitor p21 in apoptosis. *Mol Cancer Ther* 2002;1:639–649.
71. Hayashi H, Miyamoto H, Ito T, et al. Analysis of p21Waf1/Cip1 expression in normal, premalignant, and malignant cells during the development of human lung adenocarcinoma. *Am J Pathol* 1997;151:461–470.
72. Komiya T, Hosono Y, Hirashima T, et al. p21 expression as a predictor for favorable prognosis in squamous cell carcinoma of the lung. *Clin Cancer Res* 1997;3:1831–1835.
73. Takeshima Y, Yamasaki M, Nishisaka T, et al. p21WAF1/CIP1 expression in primary lung adenocarcinomas: heterogeneous expression in tumor tissues and correlation with p53 expression and proliferative activities. *Carcinogenesis* 1998;19:1755–1761.
74. Vonlanthen S, Heighway J, Kappeler A, et al. p21 is associated with cyclin D1, p16INK4a and pRb expression in resectable non-small cell lung cancer. *Int J Oncol* 2000;16:951–957.
75. Shoji T, Tanaka F, Takata T, et al. Clinical significance of p21 expression in non-small-cell lung cancer. *J Clin Oncol* 2002;20:3865–3871.
76. Bennett WP, el-Deiry WS, Rush WL, et al. p21waf1/cip1 and transforming growth factor beta 1 protein expression correlate with survival in non-small cell lung cancer. *Clin Cancer Res* 1998;4:1499–1506.
77. Esposito V, Baldi A, Tonini G, et al. Analysis of cell cycle regulator proteins in non-small cell lung cancer. *J Clin Pathol* 2004;57:58–63.
78. Nakayama K, Ishida N, Shirane M, et al. Mice lacking p27(Kip1) display increased body size, multiple organ hyperplasia, retinal dysplasia, and pituitary tumors. *Cell* 1996;85:707–720.
79. Hayashi H, Ogawa N, Ishiwa N, et al. High cyclin E and low p27/Kip1 expressions are potentially poor prognostic factors in lung adenocarcinoma patients. *Lung Cancer* 2001;34:59–65.
80. Kang Y, Ozbun LL, Angdisen J, et al. Altered expression of G1/S regulatory genes occurs early and frequently in lung carcinogenesis in transforming growth factor-beta1 heterozygous mice. *Carcinogenesis* 2002;23:1217–1227.
81. Kawana H, Tamaru J, Tanaka T, et al. Role of p27Kip1 and cyclin-dependent kinase 2 in the proliferation of non-small cell lung cancer. *Am J Pathol* 1998;153:505–513.
82. Tsukamoto S, Sugio K, Sakada T, et al. Reduced expression of cell-cycle regulator p27(Kip1) correlates with a shortened survival in non-small cell lung cancer. *Lung Cancer* 2001;34:83–90.
83. Ishihara S, Minato K, Hoshino H, et al. The cyclin-dependent kinase inhibitor p27 as a prognostic factor in advanced non-small cell lung cancer: its immunohistochemical evaluation using biopsy specimens. *Lung Cancer* 1999;26:187–194.
84. Tsoli E, Gorgoulis VG, Zacharatos P, et al. Low levels of p27 in association with deregulated p53-pRb protein status enhance tumor proliferation and chromosomal instability in non-small cell lung carcinomas. *Mol Med* 2001;7:418–429.
85. Hommura F, Dosaka-Akita H, Mishina T, et al. Prognostic significance of p27KIP1 protein and ki-67 growth fraction in non-small cell lung cancers. *Clin Cancer Res* 2000;6:4073–4081.
86. Oshita F, Kameda Y, Nishio K, et al. Increased expression levels of cyclin-dependent kinase inhibitor p27 correlate with good responses to platinum-based chemotherapy in non-small cell lung cancer. *Oncol Rep* 2000;7:491–495.
87. Gandara DR, Lara PN, Lau DH, et al. Molecular-clinical correlative studies in non-small cell lung cancer: application of a three-tiered approach. *Lung Cancer* 2001;34(Suppl 3):S75–S80.
88. Serrano M, Hannon GJ, Beach D. A new regulatory motif in cell-cycle control causing specific inhibition of cyclin D/CDK4. *Nature* 1993;366:704–707.
89. Parry D, Bates S, Mann DJ, et al. Lack of cyclin D-Cdk complexes in Rb-negative cells correlates with high levels of p16INK4/MTS1 tumour suppressor gene product. *Embo J* 1995;14:503–511.
90. Betticher DC, White GR, Vonlanthen S, et al. G1 control gene status is frequently altered in resectable non-small cell lung cancer. *Int J Cancer* 1997;74:556–562.
91. Sakaguchi M, Fujii Y, Hirabayashi H, et al. Inversely correlated expression of p16 and Rb protein in non-small cell lung cancers: an immunohistochemical study. *Int J Cancer* 1996;65:442–445.
92. Tanaka H, Fujii Y, Hirabayashi H, et al. Disruption of the RB pathway and cell-proliferative activity in non-small-cell lung cancers. *Int J Cancer* 1998;79:111–115.
93. Kashiwabara K, Oyama T, Sano T, et al. Correlation between methylation status of the p16/CDKN2 gene and the expression of p16 and Rb proteins in primary non-small cell lung cancers. *Int J Cancer* 1998;79:215–220.
94. Burke L, Flieder DB, Guinee DG, et al. Prognostic implications of molecular and immunohistochemical profiles of the Rb and p53 cell cycle regulatory pathways in primary non-small cell lung carcinoma. *Clin Cancer Res* 2005;11:232–241.
95. Leversha MA, Fielding P, Watson S, et al. Expression of p53, pRB, and p16 in lung tumours: a validation study on tissue microarrays. *J Pathol* 2003;200:610–619.

96. Rocco JW, Sidransky D. p16(MTS-1/CDKN2/INK4a) in cancer progression. *Exp Cell Res* 2001;264:42–55.
97. Geradts J, Wilentz RE, Roberts H. Immunohistochemical [corrected] detection of the alternate INK4a-encoded tumor suppressor protein p14(ARF) in archival human cancers and cell lines using commercial antibodies: correlation with p16(INK4a) expression. *Mod Pathol* 2001;14:1162–1168.
98. Lowe SW, Sherr CJ. Tumor suppression by Ink4a-Arf: progress and puzzles. *Curr Opin Genet Dev* 2003;13:77–83.
99. Gao N, Hu YD, Cao XY, et al. The exogenous wild-type p14ARF gene induces growth arrest and promotes radiosensitivity in human lung cancer cell lines. *J Cancer Res Clin Oncol* 2001;127:359–367.
100. Weber HO, Samuel T, Rauch P, et al. Human p14(ARF)-mediated cell cycle arrest strictly depends on intact p53 signaling pathways. *Oncogene* 2002;21:3207–3212.
101. Eymin B, Gazzeri S, Brambilla C, et al. Mdm2 overexpression and p14(ARF) inactivation are two mutually exclusive events in primary human lung tumors. *Oncogene* 2002;21:2750–2761.
102. Sanchez-Cespedes M, Reed AL, Buta M, et al. Inactivation of the INK4A/ARF locus frequently coexists with TP53 mutations in non-small cell lung cancer. *Oncogene* 1999;18:5843–5849.
103. Park MJ, Shimizu K, Nakano T, et al. Pathogenetic and biologic significance of TP14ARF alterations in nonsmall cell lung carcinoma. *Cancer Genet Cytogenet* 2003;141:5–13.
104. Tango Y, Fujiwara T, Itoshima T, et al. Adenovirus-mediated p14ARF gene transfer cooperates with Ad5CMV-p53 to induce apoptosis in human cancer cells. *Hum Gene Ther* 2002;13:1373–1382.
105. Jarmalaite S, Kannio A, Anttila S, et al. Aberrant p16 promoter methylation in smokers and former smokers with nonsmall cell lung cancer. *Int J Cancer* 2003;106:913–918.
106. Oliner JD, Kinzler KW, Meltzer PS, et al. Amplification of a gene encoding a p53-associated protein in human sarcomas. *Nature* 1992;358:80–83.
107. Quinlan DC, Davidson AG, Summers CL, et al. Accumulation of p53 protein correlates with a poor prognosis in human lung cancer. *Cancer Res* 1992;52:4828–4831.
108. Fornace AJ Jr, Nebert DW, Hollander MC, et al. Mammalian genes coordinately regulated by growth arrest signals and DNA-damaging agents. *Mol Cell Biol* 1989;9:4196–4203.
109. Puisieux A, Lim S, Groopman J, et al. Selective targeting of p53 gene mutational hotspots in human cancers by etiologically defined carcinogens. *Cancer Res* 1991;51:6185–6189.
110. Waga S, Hannon GJ, Beach D, et al. The p21 inhibitor of cyclin-dependent kinases controls DNA replication by interaction with PCNA. *Nature* 1994;369:574–578.
111. Selvakumaran M, Lin HK, Miyashita T, et al. Immediate early up-regulation of bax expression by p53 but not TGF beta 1: a paradigm for distinct apoptotic pathways. *Oncogene* 1994;9:1791–1798.
112. Giaccia AJ, Kastan MB. The complexity of p53 modulation: emerging patterns from divergent signals. *Genes Dev* 1998;12:2973–2983.
113. de Vries A, Flores ER, Miranda B, et al. Targeted point mutations of p53 lead to dominant-negative inhibition of wild-type p53 function. *Proc Natl Acad Sci U S A* 2002;99:2948–2953.
114. Johnson L, Mercer K, Greenbaum D, et al. Somatic activation of the K-ras oncogene causes early onset lung cancer in mice. *Nature* 2001;410:1111–1116.
115. Meuwissen R, Linn SC, Linnoila RI, et al. Induction of small cell lung cancer by somatic inactivation of both Trp53 and Rb1 in a conditional mouse model. *Cancer Cell* 2003;4:181–189.
116. Brambilla C, Fievet F, Jeanmart M, et al. Early detection of lung cancer: role of biomarkers. *Eur Respir J Suppl* 2003;39:S36–S44.
117. Tammemagi MC, McLaughlin JR, Bull SB. Meta-analyses of p53 tumor suppressor gene alterations and clinicopathological features in resected lung cancers. *Cancer Epidemiol Biomarkers Prev* 1999;8:625–634.
118. Hainaut P, Pfeifer GP. Patterns of p53 G→T transversions in lung cancers reflect the primary mutagenic signature of DNA-damage by tobacco smoke. *Carcinogenesis* 2001;22:367–374.
119. Greenblatt MS, Bennett WP, Hollstein M, et al. Mutations in the p53 tumor suppressor gene: clues to cancer etiology and molecular pathogenesis. *Cancer Res* 1994;54:4855–4878.
120. Pollan M, Varela G, Torres A, et al. Clinical value of p53, c-erbB-2, CEA and CA125 regarding relapse, metastasis and death in resectable non-small cell lung cancer. *Int J Cancer* 2003;107:781–790.
121. Kwiatkowski DJ, Harpole DH Jr, Godleski J, et al. Molecular pathologic substaging in 244 stage I non-small-cell lung cancer patients: clinical implications. *J Clin Oncol* 1998;16:2468–2477.
122. Osaki T, Oyama T, Inoue M, et al. Molecular biological markers and micrometastasis in resected non-small-cell lung cancer. Prognostic implications. *Jpn J Thorac Cardiovasc Surg* 2001;49:545–551.
123. Zereu M, Vinholes JJ, Zettler CG. p53 and Bcl-2 protein expression and its relationship with prognosis in small-cell lung cancer. *Clin Lung Cancer* 2003;4:298–302.
124. Geradts J, Fong KM, Zimmerman PV, et al. Correlation of abnormal RB, p16ink4a, and p53 expression with 3p loss of heterozygosity, other genetic abnormalities, and clinical features in 103 primary non-small cell lung cancers. *Clin Cancer Res* 1999;5:791–800.
125. Cheng YL, Lee SC, Harn HJ, et al. Prognostic prediction of the immunohistochemical expression of p53 and p16 in resected non-small cell lung cancer. *Eur J Cardiothorac Surg* 2003;23:221–228.
126. Wang Y, Zhang Z, Kastens E, et al. Mice with alterations in both p53 and Ink4a/Arf display a striking increase in lung tumor multiplicity and progression: differential chemopreventive effect of budesonide in wild-type and mutant A/J mice. *Cancer Res* 2003;63:4389–4395.
127. El-Deiry WS. The role of p53 in chemosensitivity and radiosensitivity. *Oncogene* 2003;22:7486–7495.
128. Senderowicz AM, Sausville EA. Preclinical and clinical development of cyclin-dependent kinase modulators. *J Natl Cancer Inst* 2000;92: 376–387.
129. Shapiro GI, Supko JG, Patterson A, et al. A phase II trial of the cyclin-dependent kinase inhibitor flavopiridol in patients with previously untreated stage IV non-small cell lung cancer. *Clin Cancer Res* 2001;7:1590–1599.
130. Mason KA, Hunter NR, Raju U, et al. Flavopiridol increases therapeutic ratio of radiotherapy by preferentially enhancing tumor radioresponse. *Int J Rad Oncol Biol Phys* 2004;59:1181–1189.
131. Nguyen VN, Mirejovsky P, Mirejovsky T, et al. Expression of cyclin D1, Ki-67 and PCNA in non-small cell lung cancer: prognostic significance and comparison with p53 and bcl-2. *Acta Histochem* 2000;102: 323–338.
132. MacLachlan TK, Sang N, Giordano A. Cyclins, cyclin-dependent kinases and cdk inhibitors: implications in cell cycle control and cancer. *Crit Rev Eukaryot Gene Expr* 1995;5:127–156.
133. Harper JW, Elledge SJ. Cdk inhibitors in development and cancer. *Curr Opin Genet Dev* 1996;6:56–64.
134. Chen YN, Sharma SK, Ramsey TM, et al. Selective killing of transformed cells by cyclin/cyclin-dependent kinase 2 antagonists. *Proc Natl Acad Sci U S A* 1999;96:4325–4329.
135. Carlson B, Lahusen T, Singh S, et al. Down-regulation of cyclin D1 by transcriptional repression in MCF-7 human breast carcinoma cells induced by flavopiridol. *Cancer Res* 1999;59:4634–4641.
136. De Azevedo WF Jr, Mueller-Dieckmann HJ, Schulze-Gahmen U, et al. Structural basis for specificity and potency of a flavonoid inhibitor of human CDK2, a cell cycle kinase. *Proc Natl Acad Sci U S A* 1996;93:2735–2740.
137. Kaur G, Stetler-Stevenson M, Sebers S, et al. Growth inhibition with reversible cell cycle arrest of carcinoma cells by flavone L86-8275. *J Natl Cancer Inst* 1992;84:1736–1740.
138. Losiewicz MD, Carlson BA, Kaur G, et al. Potent inhibition of CDC2 kinase activity by the flavonoid L86-8275. *Biochem Biophys Res Commun* 1994;201:589–595.
139. Worland PJ, Kaur G, Stetler-Stevenson M, et al. Alteration of the phosphorylation state of p34cdc2 kinase by the flavone L86-8275 in breast carcinoma cells. Correlation with decreased H1 kinase activity. *Biochem Pharmacol* 1993;46:1831–1840.

140. Carlson BA, Dubay MM, Sausville EA, et al. Flavopiridol induces G1 arrest with inhibition of cyclin-dependent kinase (CDK) 2 and CDK4 in human breast carcinoma cells. *Cancer Res* 1996;56:2973–2978.
141. Drees M, Dengler WA, Roth T, et al. Flavopiridol (L86-8275): selective antitumor activity in vitro and activity in vivo for prostate carcinoma cells. *Clin Cancer Res* 1997;3:273–279.
142. Sedlacek HH, Czech J, Naik R, et al. Flavopiridol (L86 8275; NSC 649890), a new kinase inhibitor for tumor therapy. *Int J Oncol* 1996;9:1143–1168.
143. Litz J, Carlson P, Warshamana-Greene GS, et al. Flavopiridol potently induces small cell lung cancer apoptosis during S phase in a manner that involves early mitochondrial dysfunction. *Clin Cancer Res* 2003;9:4586–4594.
144. Shapiro GI, Koestner DA, Matranga CB, et al. Flavopiridol induces cell cycle arrest and p53-independent apoptosis in non-small cell lung cancer cell lines. *Clin Cancer Res* 1999;5:2925–2938.
145. Brambilla E, Moro D, Gazzeri S, et al. Alterations of expression of Rb, p16(INK4A) and cyclin D1 in non-small cell lung carcinoma and their clinical significance. *J Pathol* 1999;188:351–360.
146. Mishina T, Dosaka-Akita H, Kinoshita I, et al. Cyclin D1 expression in non-small-cell lung cancers: its association with altered p53 expression, cell proliferation and clinical outcome. *Br J Cancer* 1999;80:1289–1295.
147. Volm M, Koomagi R, Rittgen W. Clinical implications of cyclins, cyclin-dependent kinases, RB and E2F1 in squamous-cell lung carcinoma. *Int J Cancer* 1998;79:294–299.
148. Keum JS, Kong G, Yang SC, et al. Cyclin D1 overexpression is an indicator of poor prognosis in resectable non-small cell lung cancer. *Br J Cancer* 1999;81:127–132.
149. Gugger M, Kappeler A, Vonlanthen S, et al. Alterations of cell cycle regulators are less frequent in advanced non-small cell lung cancer than in resectable tumours. *Lung Cancer* 2001;33:229–239.
150. Sedlacek HH. Mechanisms of action of flavopiridol. *Crit Rev Oncol Hematol* 2001;38:139–170.
151. Dai Y, Grant S. Cyclin-dependent kinase inhibitors. *Curr Opin Pharmacol* 2003;3:362–370.
152. Grant S, Roberts JD. The use of cyclin-dependent kinase inhibitors alone or in combination with established cytotoxic drugs in cancer chemotherapy. *Drug Resist Updat* 2003;6:15–26.
153. Demidenko ZN, Blagosklonny MV. Flavopiridol induces p53 via initial inhibition of Mdm2 and p21 and, independently of p53, sensitizes apoptosis-reluctant cells to tumor necrosis factor. *Cancer Res* 2004;64:3653–3660.
154. Bible KC, Kaufmann SH. Flavopiridol: a cytotoxic flavone that induces cell death in noncycling A549 human lung carcinoma cells. *Cancer Res* 1996;56:4856–4861.
155. Hayon IL, Haupt Y. p53: an internal investigation. *Cell Cycle* 2002;1:111–116.
156. Raju U, Nakata E, Mason KA, et al. Flavopiridol, a cyclin-dependent kinase inhibitor, enhances radiosensitivity of ovarian carcinoma cells. *Cancer Res* 2003;63:3263–3267.
157. Chien M, Astumian M, Liebowitz D, et al. In vitro evaluation of flavopiridol, a novel cell cycle inhibitor, in bladder cancer. *Cancer Chemother Pharmacol* 1999;44:81–87.
158. Sato S, Kajiyama Y, Sugano M, et al. Flavopiridol as a radio-sensitizer for esophageal cancer cell lines. *Dis Esophagus* 2004;17:338–344.
159. Camphausen K, Brady KJ, Burgan WE, et al. Flavopiridol enhances human tumor cell radiosensitivity and prolongs expression of gamma-H2AX foci. *Mol Cancer Ther* 2004;3:409–416.
160. Jung C, Motwani M, Kortmansky J, et al. The cyclin-dependent kinase inhibitor flavopiridol potentiates gamma-irradiation-induced apoptosis in colon and gastric cancer cells. *Clin Cancer Res* 2003;9:6052–6061.
161. Newcomb EW, Lymberis SC, Lukyanov Y, et al. Radiation sensitivity of GL261 murine glioma model and enhanced radiation response by flavopiridol. *Cell Cycle* 2006;5:93–99.
162. Raju U, Ariga H, Koto M, et al. Improvement of esophageal adenocarcinoma cell and xenograft responses to radiation by targeting cyclin-dependent kinases. *Radiother Oncol* 2006;80:185–191.
163. Kim JC, Saha D, Cao Q, et al. Enhancement of radiation effects by combined docetaxel and flavopiridol treatment in lung cancer cells. *Radiother Oncol* 2004;71:213–221.
164. McAleer MF, Duffy KT, Davidson WR, et al. Antisense inhibition of cyclin D1 expression is equivalent to flavopiridol for radiosensitization of zebrafish embryos. *Int J Radiat Oncol Biol Phys* 2006;66:546–551.
165. Seynaeve CM, Stetler-Stevenson M, Sebers S, et al. Cell cycle arrest and growth inhibition by the protein kinase antagonist UCN-01 in human breast carcinoma cells. *Cancer Res* 1993;53:2081–2086.
166. Hui ZG, Li YX, Yang WZ, et al. [Abrogation effect of UCN-01 on radiation-induced G2 phase arrest of tumor cells and its mechanism.]. *Ai Zheng* 2005;24:1–6.
167. Playle LC, Hicks DJ, Qualtrough D, et al. Abrogation of the radiation-induced G2 checkpoint by the staurosporine derivative UCN-01 is associated with radiosensitisation in a subset of colorectal tumour cell lines. *Br J Cancer* 2002;87:352–358.
168. Busby EC, Leistritz DF, Abraham RT, et al. The radiosensitizing agent 7-hydroxystaurosporine (UCN-01) inhibits the DNA damage checkpoint kinase hChk1. *Cancer Res* 2000;60:2108–2112.
169. Graves PR, Yu L, Schwarz JK, et al. The Chk1 protein kinase and the Cdc25C regulatory pathways are targets of the anticancer agent UCN-01. *J Biol Chem* 2000;275:5600–5605.
170. Zhao H, Watkins JL, Piwnica-Worms H. Disruption of the checkpoint kinase 1/cell division cycle 25A pathway abrogates ionizing radiation-induced S and G2 checkpoints. *Proc Natl Acad Sci U S A* 2002;99:14795–14800.
171. Xiao Z, Chen Z, Gunasekera AH, et al. Chk1 mediates S and G2 arrests through Cdc25A degradation in response to DNA-damaging agents. *J Biol Chem* 2003;278:21767–21773.
172. Sanchez Y, Wong C, Thoma RS, et al. Conservation of the Chk1 checkpoint pathway in mammals: linkage of DNA damage to Cdk regulation through Cdc25. *Science* 1997;277:1497–1501.
173. Mailand N, Podtelejnikov AV, Groth A, et al. Regulation of G(2)/M events by Cdc25A through phosphorylation-dependent modulation of its stability. *Embo J* 2002;21:5911–5920.
174. Dixon H, Norbury CJ. Therapeutic exploitation of checkpoint defects in cancer cells lacking p53 function. *Cell Cycle* 2002;1:362–368.
175. Xiao HH, Makeyev Y, Butler J, et al. 7-Hydroxystaurosporine (UCN-01) preferentially sensitizes cells with a disrupted TP53 to gamma radiation in lung cancer cell lines. *Radiat Res* 2002;158:84–93.
176. Mack PC, Jones AA, Gustafsson MH, et al. Enhancement of radiation cytotoxicity by UCN-01 in non-small cell lung carcinoma cells. *Radiat Res* 2004;162:623–634.
177. Lara PN Jr, Mack PC, Synold T, et al. The cyclin-dependent kinase inhibitor UCN-01 plus cisplatin in advanced solid tumors: a California cancer consortium phase I pharmacokinetic and molecular correlative trial. *Clin Cancer Res* 2005;11:4444–4450.
178. Kortmansky J, Shah MA, Kaubisch A, et al. Phase I trial of the cyclin-dependent kinase inhibitor and protein kinase C inhibitor 7-hydroxystaurosporine in combination with Fluorouracil in patients with advanced solid tumors. *J Clin Oncol* 2005;23:1875–1884.
179. Hotte SJ, Oza A, Winquist EW, et al. Phase I trial of UCN-01 in combination with topotecan in patients with advanced solid cancers: a Princess Margaret Hospital Phase II Consortium study. *Ann Oncol* 2006;17:334–340.
180. Mitchison TJ. Microtubule dynamics and kinetochore function in mitosis. *Annu Rev Cell Biol* 1988;4:527–549.
181. Altmann KH. Microtubule-stabilizing agents: a growing class of important anticancer drugs. *Curr Opin Chem Biol* 2001;5:424–431.
182. Haldar S, Jena N, Croce CM. Inactivation of Bcl-2 by phosphorylation. *Proc Natl Acad Sci U S A* 1995;92:4507–4511.
183. Haldar S, Basu A, Croce CM. Bcl2 is the guardian of microtubule integrity. *Cancer Res* 1997;57:229–233.
184. Haldar S, Chintapalli J, Croce CM. Taxol induces bcl-2 phosphorylation and death of prostate cancer cells. *Cancer Res* 1996;56:1253–1255.
185. Hei TK, Piao CQ, Geard CR, et al. Taxol and ionizing radiation: interaction and mechanisms. *Int J Radiat Oncol Biol Phys* 1994;29:267–271.

186. Rowinsky EK. The development and clinical utility of the taxane class of antimicrotubule chemotherapy agents. *Annu Rev Med* 1997;48:353–374.
187. Mason K, Staab A, Hunter N, et al. Enhancement of tumor radioresponse by docetaxel: involvement of immune system. *Int J Oncol* 2001;18:599–606.
188. Creane M, Seymour CB, Colucci S, et al. Radiobiological effects of docetaxel (Taxotere): a potential radiation sensitizer. *Int J Radiat Biol* 1999;75:731–737.
189. Zhao J, Kim JE, Reed E, et al. Molecular mechanism of antitumor activity of taxanes in lung cancer (Review). *Int J Oncol* 2005;27: 247–256.
190. Rowinsky EK, Donehower RC. Paclitaxel (taxol). *N Engl J Med* 1995;332:1004–1014.
191. Rowinsky EK, Eisenhauer EA, Chaudhry V, et al. Clinical toxicities encountered with paclitaxel (Taxol). *Semin Oncol* 1993;20:1–15.
192. Geney R, Ungureanu M, Li D, et al. Overcoming multidrug resistance in taxane chemotherapy. *Clin Chem Lab Med* 2002;40:918–925.
193. Bollag DM, McQueney PA, Zhu J, et al. Epothilones, a new class of microtubule-stabilizing agents with a taxol-like mechanism of action. *Cancer Res* 1995;55:2325–2333.
194. Altmann KH, Wartmann M, O'Reilly T. Epothilones and related structures—a new class of microtubule inhibitors with potent in vivo antitumor activity. *Biochim Biophys Acta* 2000;1470:M79–M91.
195. Kim JC, Kim JS, Saha D, et al. Potential radiation-sensitizing effect of semisynthetic epothilone B in human lung cancer cells. *Radiother Oncol* 2003;68:305–313.
196. Andrews PD, Knatko E, Moore WJ, et al. Mitotic mechanics: the auroras come into view. *Curr Opin Cell Biol* 2003;15:672–683
197. Carmena M, Earnshaw WC. The cellular geography of aurora kinases. *Nat Rev Mol Cell Biol* 2003;4:842–854.
198. Brown JR, Koretke KK, Birkeland ML, et al. Evolutionary relationships of Aurora kinases: implications for model organism studies and the development of anti-cancer drugs. *BMC Evol Biol* 2004;4:39.
199. Marumoto T, Honda S, Hara T, et al. Aurora-A kinase maintains the fidelity of early and late mitotic events in HeLa cells. *J Biol Chem* 2003;278:51786–51795.
200. Katayama H, Brinkley WR, Sen S. The Aurora kinases: role in cell transformation and tumorigenesis. *Cancer Metastasis Rev* 2003;22:451–464.
201. Du J, Hannon GJ. Suppression of p160ROCK bypasses cell cycle arrest after Aurora-A/STK15 depletion. *Proc Natl Acad Sci U S A* 2004;101:8975–8980.
202. Cazales M, Schmitt E, Montembault E, et al. CDC25B phosphorylation by Aurora-A occurs at the G2/M transition and is inhibited by DNA damage. *Cell Cycle* 2005;4:1233–1238.
203. Hata T, Furukawa T, Sunamura M, et al. RNA interference targeting aurora kinase a suppresses tumor growth and enhances the taxane chemosensitivity in human pancreatic cancer cells. *Cancer Res* 2005;65:2899–2905.
204. Wang XX, Liu R, Jin SQ, et al. Overexpression of Aurora-A kinase promotes tumor cell proliferation and inhibits apoptosis in esophageal squamous cell carcinoma cell line. *Cell Res* 2006;16:356–366.
205. Tao Y, Zhang P, Frascogna V, et al. Enhancement of radiation response by inhibition of Aurora-A kinase using siRNA or a selective Aurora kinase inhibitor PHA680632 in p53-deficient cancer cells. *Br J Cancer* 2007;97(12):1664–1672.
206. Guan Z, Wang XR, Zhu XF, et al. Aurora-A, a negative prognostic marker, increases migration and decreases radiosensitivity in cancer cells. *Cancer Res* 2007;67:10436–10444.
207. Kim KW, Mutter RW, Willey CD, et al. Inhibition of survivin and aurora B kinase sensitizes mesothelioma cells by enhancing mitotic arrests. *Int J Radiat Oncol Biol Phys* 2007;67:1519–1525.
208. Ditchfield C, Johnson VL, Tighe A, et al. Aurora B couples chromosome alignment with anaphase by targeting BubR1, Mad2, and Cenp-E to kinetochores. *J Cell Biol* 2003;161:267–280.
209. Keen N, Taylor S. Aurora-kinase inhibitors as anticancer agents. *Nat Rev Cancer* 2004;4:927–936.
210. Harrington EA, Bebbington D, Moore J, et al. VX-680, a potent and selective small-molecule inhibitor of the Aurora kinases, suppresses tumor growth in vivo. *Nat Med* 2004;10:262–267.
211. Hwang M, Perez CA, Moretti L, et al. The mTOR signaling network: insights from its role during embryonic development. *Curr Med Chem* 2008;15:1192–1208.
212. Guertin DA, Sabatini DM. An expanding role for mTOR in cancer. *Trends Mol Med* 2005;11:353–361.
213. De Virgilio C, Loewith R. Cell growth control: little eukaryotes make big contributions. *Oncogene* 2006;25:6392–6415.
214. Shinohara ET, Cao C, Niermann K, et al. Enhanced radiation damage of tumor vasculature by mTOR inhibitors. *Oncogene* 2005;24:5414–5422.
215. Albert JM, Kim KW, Cao C, et al. Targeting the Akt/mammalian target of rapamycin pathway for radiosensitization of breast cancer. *Mol Cancer Ther* 2006;5:1183–1189.
216. Cao C, Subhawong T, Albert JM, et al. Inhibition of mammalian target of rapamycin or apoptotic pathway induces autophagy and radiosensitizes PTEN null prostate cancer cells. *Cancer Res* 2006;66:10040–10047.
217. Di Cristofano A, Pandolfi PP. The multiple roles of PTEN in tumor suppression. *Cell* 2000;100:387–390.
218. Freeman D, Lesche R, Kertesz N, et al. Genetic background controls tumor development in PTEN-deficient mice. *Cancer Res* 2006;66: 6492–6496.
219. Steck PA, Pershouse MA, Jasser SA, et al. Identification of a candidate tumour suppressor gene, MMAC1, at chromosome 10q23.3 that is mutated in multiple advanced cancers. *Nat Genet* 1997;15:356–362.
220. Aoki M, Blazek E, Vogt PK. A role of the kinase mTOR in cellular transformation induced by the oncoproteins P3k and Akt. *Proc Natl Acad Sci U S A* 2001;98:136–141.
221. Kim KW, Hwang M, Moretti L, et al. Autophagy upregulation by inhibitors of caspase-3 and mTOR enhances radiotherapy in a mouse model of lung cancer. *Autophagy* 2008;4:659–668.
222. Kim KW, Mutter RW, Cao C, et al. Autophagy for cancer therapy through inhibition of pro-apoptotic proteins and mammalian target of rapamycin signaling. *J Biol Chem* 2006;281:36883–36890.
223. Jaboin JJ, Shinohara ET, Moretti L, et al. The role of mTOR inhibition in augmenting radiation induced autophagy. *Technol Cancer Res Treat* 2007;6:443–447.
224. Forouzesh B, Buckner J, Adjei A, et al. Phase I, bioavailability, and pharmacokinetic study of oral dosage of CCl-779 administered to patients with advanced solid malignancies. *Eur J Cancer* 2002;38:S54.
225. Pandya KJ, Levy DE, Hidalgo M, et al. A randomized, phase II ECOG trial of two dose levels of temsirolimus (CCI-779) in patients with extensive stage small cell lung cancer in remission after induction chemotherapy. A preliminary report. *J Clin Oncol* 2005;23:S622.
226. Baselga J, Burris H, Judson I, et al. Molecular pharmacodynamic (MPD) phase I study with serial tumor and skin biopsies of the oral mTOR inhibitor Everolimus (E, RAD001) at different doses and schedules in patients (pts) with advanced solid tumors. *Ejc Supplements* 2005;3:419–419.
227. Mita MM, Mita AC, Chu QS, et al. Phase I trial of the novel mammalian target of rapamycin inhibitor deforolimus (AP23573; MK-8669) administered intravenously daily for 5 days every 2 weeks to patients with advanced malignancies. *J Clin Oncol* 2008;26:361–367.
228. Molina JR, Mandrekar SJ, Rowland K, et al. A phase IINCCTG "window of opportunity front-line" study of the mTOR inhibitor, CCI-779 (temsirolimus) given as a single agent in patients with advanced NSCLC. *J Thorac Oncol* 2007;2:S413–S413.
229. O'Donnell A, Faivre S, Burris HA, et al. Phase I pharmacokinetic and pharmacodynamic study of the oral mammalian target of rapamycin inhibitor everolimus in patients with advanced solid tumors. *J Clin Oncol* 2008;26:1588–1595.
230. Tabernero J, Rojo F, Burris H, et al. A phase I study with tumor molecular pharmacodynamic (MPD) evaluation of dose and schedule of the oral mTOR-inhibitor everolimus (RAD001) in patients (pts) with advanced solid tumors. *J Clin Oncol* 2005;23:193S–193S.
231. Yuan A, Yu CJ, Kuo SH, et al. Vascular endothelial growth factor 189 mRNA isoform expression specifically correlates with tumor angiogenesis, patient survival, and postoperative relapse in non-small-cell lung cancer. *J Clin Oncol* 2001;19:432–441.

232. Han H, Silverman JF, Santucci TS, et al. Vascular endothelial growth factor expression in stage I non-small cell lung cancer correlates with neoangiogenesis and a poor prognosis. *Ann Surg Oncol* 2001;8:72–79.
233. Mineo TC, Ambrogi V, Baldi A, et al. Prognostic impact of VEGF, CD31, CD34, and CD105 expression and tumour vessel invasion after radical surgery for IB-IIA non-small cell lung cancer. *J Clin Pathol* 2004;57:591–597.
234. Fontanini G, Vignati S, Boldrini L, et al. Vascular endothelial growth factor is associated with neovascularization and influences progression of non-small cell lung carcinoma. *Clin Cancer Res* 1997;3:861–865.
235. Fontanini G, Faviana P, Lucchi M, et al. A high vascular count and overexpression of vascular endothelial growth factor are associated with unfavourable prognosis in operated small cell lung carcinoma. *Br J Cancer* 2002;86:558–563.
236. Houchen CW, George RJ, Sturmoski MA, et al. FGF-2 enhances intestinal stem cell survival and its expression is induced after radiation injury. *Am J Physiol* 1999;276:G249–G258.
237. Thornton SC, Walsh BJ, Bennett S, et al. Both in vitro and in vivo irradiation are associated with induction of macrophage-derived fibroblast growth factors. *Clin Exp Immunol* 1996;103:67–73.
238. Gorski DH, Beckett MA, Jaskowiak NT, et al. Blockage of the vascular endothelial growth factor stress response increases the antitumor effects of ionizing radiation. *Cancer Res* 1999;59:3374–3378.
239. Garcia-Barros M, Paris F, Cordon-Cardo C, et al. Tumor response to radiotherapy regulated by endothelial cell apoptosis. *Science* 2003;300: 1155–1159.
240. Chung YL, Jian JJ, Cheng SH, et al. Sublethal irradiation induces vascular endothelial growth factor and promotes growth of hepatoma cells: implications for radiotherapy of hepatocellular carcinoma. *Clin Cancer Res* 2006;12:2706–2715.
241. Sonveaux P, Brouet A, Havaux X, et al. Irradiation-induced angiogenesis through the up-regulation of the nitric oxide pathway: implications for tumor radiotherapy. *Cancer Res* 2003;63:1012–1019.
242. Hicklin DJ, Ellis LM. Role of the vascular endothelial growth factor pathway in tumor growth and angiogenesis. *J Clin Oncol* 2005;23:1011–1027.
243. Liu W, Ahmad SA, Reinmuth N, et al. Endothelial cell survival and apoptosis in the tumor vasculature. *Apoptosis* 2000;5:323–328.
244. Yu JL, Rak JW, Coomber BL, et al. Effect of p53 status on tumor response to antiangiogenic therapy. *Science* 2002;295:1526–1528.
245. Yang JC, Haworth L, Sherry RM, et al. A randomized trial of bevacizumab, an anti-vascular endothelial growth factor antibody, for metastatic renal cancer. *N Engl J Med* 2003;349:427–434.
246. Moffat BA, Chen M, Kariaapper MS, et al. Inhibition of vascular endothelial growth factor (VEGF)-A causes a paradoxical increase in tumor blood flow and up-regulation of VEGF-D. *Clin Cancer Res* 2006;12:1525–1532.
247. Steel G, Peckham M. Exploitable mechanisms in combined radiotherapy-chemotherapy: the concept of additivity. *Int J Radiat Oncol Biol Phys* 1979;5:85–91.
248. Shibuya M. Structure and dual function of vascular endothelial growth factor receptor-1 (Flt-1). *Int J Biochem Cell Biol* 2001;33:409–420.
249. Achen MG, Jeltsch M, Kukk E, et al. Vascular endothelial growth factor D (VEGF-D) is a ligand for the tyrosine kinases VEGF receptor 2 (Flk1) and VEGF receptor 3 (Flt4). *Proc Natl Acad Sci U S A* 1998;95:548–553.
250. Ferrara N. VEGF: an update on biological and therapeutic aspects. *Curr Opin Biotechnol* 2000;11:617–624.
251. Lee CG, Heijn M, di Tomaso E, et al. Anti-Vascular endothelial growth factor treatment augments tumor radiation response under normoxic or hypoxic conditions. *Cancer Res* 2000;60:5565–5570.
252. Kozin SV, Boucher Y, Hicklin DJ, et al. Vascular endothelial growth factor receptor-2-blocking antibody potentiates radiation-induced long-term control of human tumor xenografts. *Cancer Res* 2001;61:39–44.
253. Ning S, Laird D, Cherrington JM, et al. The antiangiogenic agents SU5416 and SU6668 increase the antitumor effects of fractionated irradiation. *Radiat Res* 2002;157:45–51.
254. Hess C, Vuong V, Hegyi I, et al. Effect of VEGF receptor inhibitor PTK787/ZK222584 [correction of ZK222548] combined with ionizing radiation on endothelial cells and tumour growth. *Br J Cancer* 2001;85:2010–2016.
255. Geng L, Donnelly E, McMahon G, et al. Inhibition of vascular endothelial growth factor receptor signaling leads to reversal of tumor resistance to radiotherapy. *Cancer Res* 2001;61:2413–2419.
256. Hirota K, Semenza GL. Regulation of angiogenesis by hypoxia-inducible factor 1. *Crit Rev Oncol Hematol* 2006;59:15–26.
257. Jain RK. Normalization of tumor vasculature: an emerging concept in antiangiogenic therapy. *Science* 2005;307:58–62.
258. Winkler F, Kozin SV, Tong RT, et al. Kinetics of vascular normalization by VEGFR2 blockade governs brain tumor response to radiation: role of oxygenation, angiopoietin-1, and matrix metalloproteinases. *Cancer Cell* 2004;6:553–563.
259. Wedge SR, Kendrew J, Hennequin LF, et al. AZD2171: a highly potent, orally bioavailable, vascular endothelial growth factor receptor-2 tyrosine kinase inhibitor for the treatment of cancer. *Cancer Res* 2005;65:4389–4400.
260. Cao C, Albert JM, Geng L, et al. Vascular endothelial growth factor tyrosine kinase inhibitor AZD2171 and fractionated radiotherapy in mouse models of lung cancer. *Cancer Res* 2006;66:11409–11415.
261. Williams KJ, Telfer BA, Brave S, et al. ZD6474, a potent inhibitor of vascular endothelial growth factor signaling, combined with radiotherapy: schedule-dependent enhancement of antitumor activity. *Clin Cancer Res* 2004;10:8587–8593.
262. Brazelle WD, Shi W, Siemann DW. VEGF-associated tyrosine kinase inhibition increases the tumor response to single and fractionated dose radiotherapy. *Int J Radiat Oncol Biol Phys* 2006;65:836–841.
263. Lu B, Geng L, Musiek A, et al. Broad spectrum receptor tyrosine kinase inhibitor, SU6668, sensitizes radiation via targeting survival pathway of vascular endothelium. *Int J Radiat Oncol Biol Phys* 2004;58:844–850.
264. Cascone T, Gridelli C, Ciardiello F. Combined targeted therapies in non-small cell lung cancer: a winner strategy? *Curr Opin Oncol* 2007;19:98–102.
265. Schueneman AJ, Himmelfarb E, Geng L, et al. SU11248 maintenance therapy prevents tumor regrowth after fractionated irradiation of murine tumor models. *Cancer Res* 2003;63:4009–4016.
266. Riesterer O, Honer M, Jochum W, et al. Ionizing radiation antagonizes tumor hypoxia induced by antiangiogenic treatment. *Clin Cancer Res* 2006;12:3518–3524.
267. Zips D, Hessel F, Krause M, et al. Impact of adjuvant inhibition of vascular endothelial growth factor receptor tyrosine kinases on tumor growth delay and local tumor control after fractionated irradiation in human squamous cell carcinomas in nude mice. *Int J Radiat Oncol Biol Phys* 2005;61:908–914.
268. Kermani P, Leclerc G, Martel R, et al. Effect of ionizing radiation on thymidine uptake, differentiation, and VEGFR2 receptor expression in endothelial cells: the role of VEGF(165). *Int J Radiat Oncol Biol Phys* 2001;50:213–220.
269. Huamani J, Willey C, Thotala D, et al. Differential efficacy of combined therapy with radiation and AEE788 in high and low EGFR–expressing androgen-independent prostate tumor models. *Int J Radiat Oncol Biol Phys* 2008;71:237–246.
270. Yazlovitskaya EM, Linkous AG, Thotala DK, et al. Cytosolic phospholipase A(2) regulates viability of irradiated vascular endothelium. *Cell Death Differ* 2008;15(10):1641–1653.
271. Fu JY, Masferrer JL, Seibert K, et al. The induction and suppression of prostaglandin H2 synthase (cyclooxygenase) in human monocytes. *J Biol Chem* 1990;265:16737–16740.
272. Hida T, Yatabe Y, Achiwa H, et al. Increased expression of cyclooxygenase 2 occurs frequently in human lung cancers, specifically in adenocarcinomas. *Cancer Res* 1998;58:3761–3764.
273. Wolff H, Saukkonen K, Anttila S, et al. Expression of cyclooxygenase-2 in human lung carcinoma. *Cancer Res* 1998;58:4997–5001.
274. Achiwa H, Yatabe Y, Hida T, et al. Prognostic significance of elevated cyclooxygenase 2 expression in primary, resected lung adenocarcinomas. *Clin Cancer Res* 1999;5:1001–1005.
275. Khuri FR, Wu H, Lee JJ, et al. Cyclooxygenase-2 overexpression is a marker of poor prognosis in stage I non-small cell lung cancer. *Clin Cancer Res* 2001;7:861–867.
276. Davis TW, O'Neal JM, Pagel MD, et al. Synergy between celecoxib and radiotherapy results from inhibition of cyclooxygenase-2-derived

prostaglandin E2, a survival factor for tumor and associated vasculature. *Cancer Res* 2004;64:279–285.

277. Masferrer JL, Leahy KM, Koki AT, et al. Antiangiogenic and antitumor activities of cyclooxygenase-2 inhibitors. *Cancer Res* 2000;60:1306–1311.
278. Turini ME, DuBois RN. Cyclooxygenase-2: a therapeutic target. *Annu Rev Med* 2002;53:35–57.
279. Furuta Y, Hunter N, Barkley T Jr, et al. Increase in radioresponse of murine tumors by treatment with indomethacin. *Cancer Res* 1988;48:3008–3013.
280. Teicher B, Bump E, Palayoor S. Signal transduction inhibitors as modifiers of radiation therapy in human prostate carcinoma xenografts. *Radiat Oncol Invest* 1996;4:221–230.
281. Kishi K, Petersen S, Petersen C, et al. Preferential enhancement of tumor radioresponse by a cyclooxygenase-2 inhibitor. *Cancer Res* 2000;60: 1326–1331.
282. Gallo O. Re: enhancement of tumor response to gamma-radiation by an inhibitor of cyclooxygenase-2 enzyme. *J Natl Cancer Inst* 2000;92:346–347.
283. Pyo H, Choy H, Amorino GP, et al. A selective cyclooxygenase-2 inhibitor, NS-398, enhances the effect of radiation in vitro and in vivo preferentially on the cells that express cyclooxygenase-2. *Clin Cancer Res* 2001;7:2998–3005.
284. Milas L, Kishi K, Hunter N, et al. Enhancement of tumor response to gamma-radiation by an inhibitor of cyclooxygenase-2 enzyme. *J Natl Cancer Inst* 1999;91:1501–1504.
285. Petersen C, Petersen S, Milas L, et al. Enhancement of intrinsic tumor cell radiosensitivity induced by a selective cyclooxygenase-2 inhibitor. *Clin Cancer Res* 2000;6:2513–2520.
286. Milas L. Cyclooxygenase-2 (COX-2) enzyme inhibitors as potential enhancers of tumor radioresponse. *Semin Radiat Oncol* 2001;11:290–299.
287. Furuta Y, Hall ER, Sanduja S, et al. Prostaglandin production by murine tumors as a predictor for therapeutic response to indomethacin. *Cancer Res* 1988;48:3002–3007.
288. Shin YK, Park JS, Kim HS, et al. Radiosensitivity enhancement by celecoxib, a cyclooxygenase (COX)-2 selective inhibitor, via COX-2-dependent cell cycle regulation on human cancer cells expressing differential COX-2 levels. *Cancer Res* 2005;65:9501–9509.
289. Masferrer J. Approach to angiogenesis inhibition based on cyclooxygenase-2. *Cancer J* 2001;7 Suppl 3:S144–150.
290. Dittmann KH, Mayer C, Ohneseit PA, et al. Celecoxib induced tumor cell radiosensitization by inhibiting radiation induced nuclear EGFR transport and DNA-repair: a Cox-2 independent mechanism. *Int J Radiat Oncol Biol Phys* 2008;70(1):203–212.
291. Chakraborti S. Phospholipase A(2) isoforms: a perspective. *Cell Signal* 2003;15:637–665.
292. Hirabayashi T, Murayama T, Shimizu T. Regulatory mechanism and physiological role of cytosolic phospholipase A2. *Biol Pharm Bull* 2004;27:1168–1173.
293. Prokazova NV, Zvezdina ND, Korotaeva AA. Effect of lysophosphatidylcholine on transmembrane signal transduction. *Biochemistry (Mosc)* 1998;63:31–37.
294. Fujita Y, Yoshizumi M, Izawa Y, et al. Transactivation of fetal liver kinase-1/kinase-insert domain-containing receptor by lysophosphatidylcholine induces vascular endothelial cell proliferation. *Endocrinology* 2006;147:1377–1385.
295. Murugesan G, Sandhya Rani MR, Gerber CE, et al. Lysophosphatidylcholine regulates human microvascular endothelial cell expression of chemokines. *J Mol Cell Cardiol* 2003;35:1375–1384.
296. Kume N, Gimbrone MA Jr. Lysophosphatidylcholine transcriptionally induces growth factor gene expression in cultured human endothelial cells. *J Clin Invest* 1994;93:907–911.
297. Kita T, Kume N, Ochi H, et al. Induction of endothelial platelet-derived growth factor-B-chain and intercellular adhesion molecule-1 by lysophosphatidylcholine. *Ann N Y Acad Sci* 1997;811:70–75.
298. Cybulsky MI, Gimbrone MA Jr. Endothelial expression of a mononuclear leukocyte adhesion molecule during atherogenesis. *Science* 1991;251:788–791.
299. Murohara T, Scalia R, Lefer AM. Lysophosphatidylcholine promotes P-selectin expression in platelets and endothelial cells. Possible involvement of protein kinase C activation and its inhibition by nitric oxide donors. *Circ Res* 1996;78:780–789.
300. Tan J, Geng L, Yazlovitskaya EM, et al. Protein kinase B/Akt-dependent phosphorylation of glycogen synthase kinase-3beta in irradiated vascular endothelium. *Cancer Res* 2006;66:2320–2327.
301. Valerie K, Yacoub A, Hagan MP, et al. Radiation-induced cell signaling: inside-out and outside-in. *Mol Cancer Ther* 2007;6:789–801.
302. Edwards E, Geng L, Tan J, et al. Phosphatidylinositol 3-kinase/Akt signaling in the response of vascular endothelium to ionizing radiation. *Cancer Res* 2002;62:4671–4677.
303. Dent P, Yacoub A, Fisher PB, et al. MAPK pathways in radiation responses. *Oncogene* 2003;22:5885–5896.
304. Umezu-Goto M, Kishi Y, Taira A, et al. Autotaxin has lysophospholipase D activity leading to tumor cell growth and motility by lysophosphatidic acid production. *J Cell Biol* 2002;158:227–233.
305. Mills GB, Moolenaar WH. The emerging role of lysophosphatidic acid in cancer. *Nat Rev Cancer* 2003;3:582–591.
306. Nam SW, Clair T, Campo CK, et al. Autotaxin (ATX), a potent tumor motogen, augments invasive and metastatic potential of ras-transformed cells. *Oncogene* 2000;19:241–247.
307. Nam SW, Clair T, Kim YS, et al. Autotaxin (NPP-2), a metastasis-enhancing motogen, is an angiogenic factor. *Cancer Res* 2001;61:6938–6944.
308. Klominek J, Robert KH, Bergh J, et al. Production of a motility factor by a newly established lung adenocarcinoma cell line. *Anticancer Res* 1998;18:759–767.
309. Yang Y, Mou L, Liu N, et al. Autotaxin expression in non-small-cell lung cancer. *Am J Respir Cell Mol Biol* 1999;21:216–222.
310. Kolesnick RN. Sphingomyelinase action inhibits phorbol ester-induced differentiation of human promyelocytic leukemic (HL-60) cells. *J Biol Chem* 1989;264:7617–7623.
311. Kolesnick RN, Clegg S. 1,2-Diacylglycerols, but not phorbol esters, activate a potential inhibitory pathway for protein kinase C in GH3 pituitary cells. Evidence for involvement of a sphingomyelinase. *J Biol Chem* 1988;263:6534–6537.
312. Mathias S, Pena LA, Kolesnick RN. Signal transduction of stress via ceramide. *Biochem J* 1998;335(Pt 3):465–480.
313. Okazaki T, Bielawska A, Bell RM, et al. Role of ceramide as a lipid mediator of 1 alpha,25-dihydroxyvitamin D3-induced HL-60 cell differentiation. *J Biol Chem* 1990;265:15823–15831.
314. Haimovitz-Friedman A, Kan CC, Ehleiter D, et al. Ionizing radiation acts on cellular membranes to generate ceramide and initiate apoptosis. *J Exp Med* 1994;180:525–535.
315. Spiegel S, Foster D, Kolesnick R. Signal transduction through lipid second messengers. *Curr Opin Cell Biol* 1996;8:159–167.
316. Merrill AH, Jr., Schmelz EM, Dillehay DL, et al. Sphingolipids—the enigmatic lipid class: biochemistry, physiology, and pathophysiology. *Toxicol Appl Pharmacol* 1997;142:208–225.
317. Hannun YA, Luberto C, Argraves KM. Enzymes of sphingolipid metabolism: from modular to integrative signaling. *Biochemistry* 2001;40: 4893–4903.
318. Paris F, Fuks Z, Kang A, et al. Endothelial apoptosis as the primary lesion initiating intestinal radiation damage in mice. *Science* 2001;293:293–297.
319. Michael JM, Lavin MF, Watters DJ. Resistance to radiation-induced apoptosis in Burkitt's lymphoma cells is associated with defective ceramide signaling. *Cancer Res* 1997;57:3600–3605.
320. Santana P, Pena LA, Haimovitz-Friedman A, et al. Acid sphingomyelinase-deficient human lymphoblasts and mice are defective in radiation-induced apoptosis. *Cell* 1996;86:189–199.
321. Kolesnick RN, Haimovitz-Friedman A, Fuks Z. The sphingomyelin signal transduction pathway mediates apoptosis for tumor necrosis factor, Fas, and ionizing radiation. *Biochem Cell Biol* 1994;72:471–474.
322. Raines MA, Kolesnick RN, Golde DW. Sphingomyelinase and ceramide activate mitogen-activated protein kinase in myeloid HL-60 cells. *J Biol Chem* 1993;268:14572–14575.
323. Huwiler A, Brunner J, Hummel R, et al. Ceramide-binding and activation defines protein kinase c-Raf as a ceramide-activated protein kinase. *Proc Natl Acad Sci U S A* 1996;93:6959–6963.

324. Verheij M, Ruiter GA, Zerp SF, et al. The role of the stress-activated protein kinase (SAPK/JNK) signaling pathway in radiation-induced apoptosis. *Radiother Oncol* 1998;47:225–232.
325. Chen YR, Wang X, Templeton D, et al. The role of c-Jun N-terminal kinase (JNK) in apoptosis induced by ultraviolet C and gamma radiation. Duration of JNK activation may determine cell death and proliferation. *J Biol Chem* 1996;271:31929–31936.
326. Ip YT, Davis RJ. Signal transduction by the c-Jun N-terminal kinase (JNK)—from inflammation to development. *Curr Opin Cell Biol* 1998;10:205–219.
327. Li CM, Park JH, Simonaro CM, et al. Insertional mutagenesis of the mouse acid ceramidase gene leads to early embryonic lethality in homozygotes and progressive lipid storage disease in heterozygotes. *Genomics* 2002;79:218–224.
328. Kolesnick R. The therapeutic potential of modulating the ceramide/sphingomyelin pathway. *J Clin Invest* 2002;110:3–8.
329. Ogretmen B, Hannun YA. Biologically active sphingolipids in cancer pathogenesis and treatment. *Nat Rev Cancer* 2004;4:604–616.
330. Visentin B, Vekich JA, Sibbald BJ, et al. Validation of an anti-sphingosine-1-phosphate antibody as a potential therapeutic in reducing growth, invasion, and angiogenesis in multiple tumor lineages. *Cancer Cell* 2006;9:225–238.
331. Chmura SJ, Nodzenski E, Beckett MA, et al. Loss of ceramide production confers resistance to radiation-induced apoptosis. *Cancer Res* 1997;57:1270–1275.
332. Chmura SJ, Nodzenski E, Kharbanda S, et al. Down-regulation of ceramide production abrogates ionizing radiation-induced cytochrome c release and apoptosis. *Mol Pharmacol* 2000;57:792–796.
333. Garzotto M, Haimovitz-Friedman A, Liao WC, et al. Reversal of radiation resistance in LNCaP cells by targeting apoptosis through ceramide synthase. *Cancer Res* 1999;59:5194–5201.
334. Kimura K, Markowski M, Edsall LC, et al. Role of ceramide in mediating apoptosis of irradiated LNCaP prostate cancer cells. *Cell Death Differ* 2003;10:240–248.
335. Nava VE, Cuvillier O, Edsall LC, et al. Sphingosine enhances apoptosis of radiation-resistant prostate cancer cells. *Cancer Res* 2000;60:4468–4474.
336. Chmura SJ, Mauceri HJ, Advani S, et al. Decreasing the apoptotic threshold of tumor cells through protein kinase C inhibition and sphingomyelinase activation increases tumor killing by ionizing radiation. *Cancer Res* 1997;57:4340–4347.
337. Lin X, Fuks Z, Kolesnick R. Ceramide mediates radiation-induced death of endothelium. *Crit Care Med* 2000;28:N87–N93.
338. Ree AH, Bratland A, Nome RV, et al. Inhibitory targeting of checkpoint kinase signaling overrides radiation-induced cell cycle gene regulation: a therapeutic strategy in tumor cell radiosensitization? *Radiother Oncol* 2004;72:305–310.
339. Hui ZG, Li YX, Yang WZ, et al. [Abrogation of radiation-induced G2 arrest and radiosensitization by 7-hydroxystaurosporine (UCN-01) in human nasopharyngeal carcinoma cell line]. *Ai Zheng* 2003;22:6–10.
340. Schuuring J, Bussink J, Bernsen HJ, et al. Irradiation combined with SU5416: microvascular changes and growth delay in a human xenograft glioblastoma tumor line. *Int J Radiat Oncol Biol Phys* 2005;61:529–534.
341. Lund EL, Olsen MW, Lipson KE, et al. Improved effect of an antiangiogenic tyrosine kinase inhibitor (SU5416) by combinations with fractionated radiotherapy or low molecular weight heparin. *Neoplasia* 2003;5:155–160.
342. Gong H, Pottgen C, Stuben G, et al. Arginine deiminase and other antiangiogenic agents inhibit unfavorable neuroblastoma growth: potentiation by irradiation. *Int J Cancer* 2003;106:723–728.
343. Griffin RJ, Williams BW, Wild R, et al. Simultaneous inhibition of the receptor kinase activity of vascular endothelial, fibroblast, and platelet-derived growth factors suppresses tumor growth and enhances tumor radiation response. *Cancer Res* 2002;62:1702–1706.
344. Bergers G, Song S, Meyer-Morse N, et al. Benefits of targeting both pericytes and endothelial cells in the tumor vasculature with kinase inhibitors. *J Clin Invest* 2003;111:1287–1295.
345. Osusky KL, Hallahan DE, Fu A, et al. The receptor tyrosine kinase inhibitor SU11248 impedes endothelial cell migration, tubule formation, and blood vessel formation in vivo, but has little effect on existing tumor vessels. *Angiogenesis* 2004;7:225–233.
346. Plastaras JP, Kim SH, Liu YY, et al. Cell cycle dependent and schedule-dependent antitumor effects of sorafenib combined with radiation. *Cancer Res* 2007;67:9443–9454.
347. Rubin EH, Rothermel J, Tesfaye F, et al. Phase I dose-finding study of weekly single-agent patupilone in patients with advanced solid tumors. *J Clin Oncol* 2005;23:9120–9129.
348. Fenton BM, Paoni SF, Ding I. Pathophysiological effects of vascular endothelial growth factor receptor-2-blocking antibody plus fractionated radiotherapy on murine mammary tumors. *Cancer Res* 2004;64:5712–5719.
349. Li J, Huang S, Armstrong EA, et al. Angiogenesis and radiation response modulation after vascular endothelial growth factor receptor-2 (VEGFR2) blockade. *Int J Radiat Oncol Biol Phys* 2005;62:1477–1485.
350. Dings RP, Loren M, Heun H, et al. Scheduling of radiation with angiogenesis inhibitors anginex and Avastin improves therapeutic outcome via vessel normalization. *Clin Cancer Res* 2007;13:3395–3402.
351. Hoang T, Huang S, Armstrong E. Enhancement of radiation response in upper aero-digestive tract tumors with bevacizumab (Avastin). *Lung Cancer* 2005;49(Suppl 2):S370.
352. Gupta VK, Jaskowiak NT, Beckett MA, et al. Vascular endothelial growth factor enhances endothelial cell survival and tumor radioresistance. *Cancer J* 2002;8:47–54.
353. Damiano V, Melisi D, Bianco C, et al. Cooperative antitumor effect of multitargeted kinase inhibitor ZD6474 and ionizing radiation in glioblastoma. *Clin Cancer Res* 2005;11:5639–5644.
354. Raju U, Nakata E, Yang P, et al. In vitro enhancement of tumor cell radiosensitivity by a selective inhibitor of cyclooxygenase-2 enzyme: mechanistic considerations. *Int J Radiat Oncol Biol Phys* 2002;54:886–894.
355. Kuipers GK, Slotman BJ, Wedekind LE, et al. Radiosensitization of human glioma cells by cyclooxygenase-2 (COX-2) inhibition: independent on COX-2 expression and dependent on the COX-2 inhibitor and sequence of administration. *Int J Radiat Biol* 2007;83:677–685.
356. Wachsberger PR, Burd R, Marero N, et al. Effect of the tumor vascular-damaging agent, ZD6126, on the radioresponse of U87 glioblastoma. *Clin Cancer Res* 2005;11:835–842.
357. Raben D, Bianco C, Damiano V, et al. Antitumor activity of ZD6126, a novel vascular-targeting agent, is enhanced when combined with ZD1839, an epidermal growth factor receptor tyrosine kinase inhibitor, and potentiates the effects of radiation in a human non-small cell lung cancer xenograft model. *Mol Cancer Ther* 2004;3:977–983.
358. Ng QS, Goh V, Carnell D, et al. Tumor antivascular effects of radiotherapy combined with combretastatin a4 phosphate in human non-small-cell lung cancer. *Int J Radiat Oncol Biol Phys* 2007;67:1375–1380.
359. Murata R, Overgaard J, Horsman MR. Combretastatin A-4 disodium phosphate: a vascular targeting agent that improves that improves the anti-tumor effects of hyperthermia, radiation, and mild thermoradiotherapy. *Int J Radiat Oncol Biol Phys* 2001;51:1018–1024.
360. Dings RP, Williams BW, Song CW, et al. Anginex synergizes with radiation therapy to inhibit tumor growth by radiosensitizing endothelial cells. *Int J Cancer* 2005;115:312–319.
361. Griscelli F, Li H, Cheong C, et al. Combined effects of radiotherapy and angiostatin gene therapy in glioma tumor model. *Proc Natl Acad Sci U S A* 2000;97:6698–6703.
362. Kumar P, Benedict R, Urzua F, et al. Combination treatment significantly enhances the efficacy of antitumor therapy by preferentially targeting angiogenesis. *Lab Invest* 2005;85:756–767.
363. Geng L, Tan J, Himmelfarb E, et al. A specific antagonist of the p110delta catalytic component of phosphatidylinositol 3'-kinase, IC486068, enhances radiation-induced tumor vascular destruction. *Cancer Res* 2004;64:4893–4899.

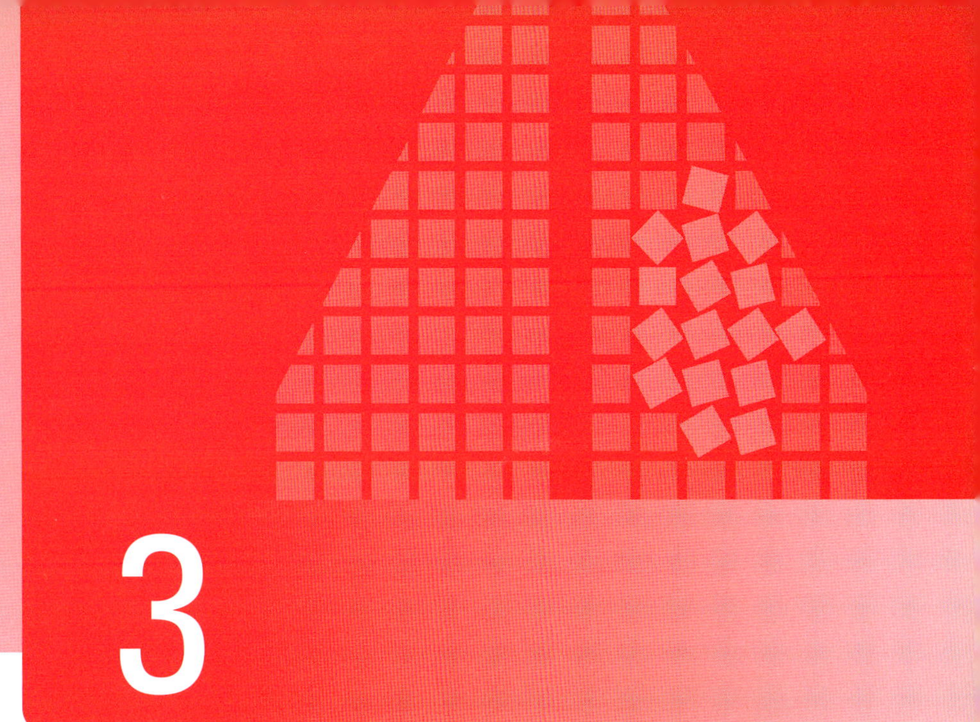

SECTION 3

Screening and Prevention

CHAPTER 15

Anthony W. Kim
Mark A. Yoder
Michael J. Liptay
James L. Mulshine

Population-Based Lung Cancer Prevention: An Overview

Lung cancer remains the leading cause of cancer-related mortality in the United States, with 160,390 deaths projected for 2007.[1] Lung cancer accounts for the largest number of cancer deaths worldwide as well, with an estimated 1.3 million deaths in 2005.[2] These dismal numbers reflect persistent national and global challenges to lung cancer control.

Cancer control in general relies upon prevention, early detection, and treatment. Advances in the treatment of lung cancer, including minimally invasive surgery and targeted molecular therapies, have a limited impact on the burden of lung cancer because of the fact that most cancers continue to be diagnosed at an advanced stage. The presence of symptoms at the time of diagnosis is associated with a high probability of advanced disease. The failure of screening with chest radiography and sputum cytopathology to impact lung cancer mortality suggests that detection of asymptomatic disease is necessary but not sufficient to achieve this goal. A resurgence of interest in early detection has followed the widespread availability of chest computed tomography (CT). Although this technology has proven superior to chest radiography in detecting early stage lung cancers, a beneficial effect on lung cancer mortality remains to be proven.[3] Smoking control programs continue to represent the most logical approach to curtailing lung cancer incidence, but economic and political forces oppose such efforts.[1] Reducing smoking prevalence decreases an individual smoker's risk of lung cancer as well as that of others through a reduction in secondhand smoke exposure. Unfortunately, an elevated risk of lung cancer persists for many years after smoking cessation.[4,5] This risk is highest among individuals who have undergone a curative resection for lung cancer, who have a 1% to 5% annual risk of developing a second primary lung cancer.[6] Chemoprevention has been studied as a mechanism to decrease lung cancer risk in these high-risk groups as well as in the general population.

A population-based approach to lung cancer prevention will be required to achieve the greatest reduction in lung cancer mortality, as many individuals lack access to the healthcare system and may not otherwise be aware of their lung cancer risk. High-risk individuals must therefore be actively selected from the general population to ensure that the majority has the opportunity to receive appropriate preventive measures. Investigators have used such an approach to identify and recruit subjects into an ongoing chest CT screening trial,[7] and we have previously reviewed the criteria for a population-based approach to early lung cancer detection.[8] In contrast to breast or colon cancer, where the major defining risk factor is age, the profound risk associated with tobacco use allows for a powerful and economical additional selection factor to enrich for lung cancer risk. Other risk factors of lung cancer exist, however, and these collectively account for about 10% of lung cancer diagnoses. Which preventive measures should be applied to which specific subgroups of the population are questions that ongoing studies will help to address, but the answers will likely be dynamic as novel approaches are developed. This chapter will review contemporary lung cancer prevention strategies with a focus on their potential for implementation at a population level.

PREVENTION OF PRIMARY DISEASE

Smoking Cessation Lung cancer initially had a humble beginning, with early case reports remarking on the rarity of the disease. Only after the tremendous increase in smoking worldwide following World War I did lung cancer begin to achieve its current level of notoriety.[9] Since the initial linkage between tobacco smoke and lung cancer in 1950,[10,11] this risk factor has been extensively investigated. Smoking currently accounts for 87% of lung cancer deaths,[12] and thus smoking cessation represents the most broadly applicable approach to primary prevention. Initiatives in the United States have only recently begun to result in a reduction in lung cancer mortality.[3] One reason for this sluggish response is that a former smoker's risk of lung cancer never returns to that of a nonsmoker.[4,5] In fact, at present, about 50% of cancer diagnoses are made among former smokers.[5,9] New medications may improve the success of individual smoking cessation attempts, but this rate remains below 10% over the long term with heavy smokers. Despite these limitations, tobacco control and smoking cessation remain key components of the primary prevention of lung cancer, with the long-term potential to banish this lethal disease back into obscurity. Lung cancer risk increases with duration of smoking. However, the increasing risk of lung cancer stops rising with smoking cessation.

Obstacles to Population-Level Smoking Cessation Initiatives Several obstacles stand in the way of smoking cessation initiatives. Smoking prevalence remains high. Worldwide smoking prevalence is 47% among men and 12% among women.[9] An estimated 45 million Americans are current smokers, with a like number of former smokers.[13] Adolescent smoking is also a persistent and serious problem. Tobacco addiction is not typically considered a pediatric disease, but data suggest that most adult smokers become addicted between age 13 and 17.[9] With this background, the fact that about 30% of high school students report the use of some form of tobacco product within the previous month[14] takes on greater significance. Secondhand smoke expands the reach of lung cancer to nonsmokers. About 126 million nonsmoking Americans are exposed to secondhand smoke in the workplace, home, vehicles, or public places,[15] and about 3000 nonsmokers die of lung cancer as a result each year.[16] Despite legally imposed limitations, the tobacco industry continues to advance its interests, with promotional expenditures exceeding tobacco control spending by a ratio of 23 to 1 in 2003. Declines in smoking cessation rates among adults and high school students appear to have stalled,[17] likely as a consequence of increased industry marketing expenditures, decreased funding for comprehensive tobacco control programs, and lack of a significant increase in tobacco prices.[18] While rates of smoking prevalence in other developed countries have largely mirrored the decline observed in the United States, increased marketing in the face of limited financial resources has resulted in increased tobacco consumption in developing countries.[19]

Recommendations for Smoking Cessation Initiatives The U.S. Surgeon General's report specified the goals of preventing tobacco use initiation among the young, promoting quitting, and eliminating nonsmokers' exposure to secondhand smoke.[1] A subcommittee of the U.S. Interagency Committee on Smoking and Health (ICSH), with public input, developed a national action plan consisting of ten recommendations for smoking cessation.[20] The Centers for Disease Control and Prevention provided recommendations for the essential components of comprehensive tobacco control programs.[21] The World Health Organization recently published its recommendations to curb the global smoking epidemic.[19] These recommendations are summarized in Table 15.1, most of which will be discussed in more detail.

Youth Access Laws Laws aimed at restricting children and adolescents from purchasing tobacco products have not been very successful. Some studies suggest that such laws have no impact on adolescent smoking,[22,23] whereas others demonstrate a decrease in the number of adolescents who experiment with smoking.[24] Regardless, most smokers become addicted before they can purchase cigarettes legally.[25] Lack of enforcement may largely explain the lack of efficacy of this approach.

TABLE 15.1 Recommendations for Tobacco Control Initiatives[1,19–21]

Intervention	Effect(s)
Monitor tobacco use and prevention policies	Assesses control program and industry compliance
Protect people from tobacco smoke -Comprehensive smoke-free laws	Decreases tobacco consumption and smoking prevalence
Offer help to quit tobacco use -National tobacco quit line -Comprehensive coverage of counseling and pharmacotherapy	Increases long-term smoking cessation rate Expands access by underserved individuals
Warn about the dangers of tobacco smoke -Antismoking media campaign	Decreases tobacco consumption and smoking prevalence
Enforce bans on advertising, promotion, and sponsorship	Decreases tobacco consumption
Raise taxes on tobacco	Decreases tobacco consumption Provides funding for control program
Smoking cessation research	Discovers better interventions
System-based improvements -Training of clinicians -Systematic implementation by health systems -Add smoking cessation as health systems quality indicator	

Smoke-Free Laws As of January 2008, 26 states, encompassing 53% of Americans, had enacted or implemented legislation that prohibits smoking in the workplace, restaurants, or bars.[26] However, only 5% of the global population is protected by smoke-free laws.[19] Comprehensive public smoking bans are the most effective, with exposure to secondhand smoke being reduced from 46% in countries without regulations to 12% in those with extensive restrictions, but only to 35% in countries with limited restrictions.[27] Additional benefits of such programs are a reduction in smoking prevalence and tobacco consumption by smokers, as well as lower rates of youth smoking specifically.[15] A metaanalysis reported a 3.8% reduction in smoking prevalence and decrease by 3.1 cigarettes per day per continuing smoker. These results equate to a 29% reduction in cigarette consumption per employee. Public smoking bans decrease youth smoking prevalence, and school bans decrease daily consumption.[22]

Greece has the highest proportion (45%) of adult smokers in Europe. Many European countries have now adopted public smoking bans. Ireland was the first European country to implement a comprehensive ban on smoking in public places in March 2004. Norway followed soon after, but allowed a smokers' corner in workplaces. Italy banned workplace smoking in January 2005 and Naples and Verona have made smoking illegal in public parks. Belgium allows smoking in cafes and bars if they have ventilation installed and are at least 50 sq m (538 sq ft) in area. In France, a law forbidding smoking in public places was extended to bars, cafes, and hotels in January 2008, with fines up to 450 euros (£332; $662). Eight German states, including Berlin, have also ushered banned smoking in 2008 declaring their pubs and restaurants smoke free. Almost a third of Germans smoke and the authorities in Berlin decided not to enforce the restrictions actively for the first 6 months.

In summary, highly restrictive smoke free laws have a tremendous potential to reduce smoking prevalence and tobacco consumption at the population level, but are underutilized even in developed countries.

Methods to Improve Individual Smoking Cessation Rates The rate of smoking cessation without any intervention is about 1% per year. This value varies by population, however, with this low rate being typical of smokers seen in a general medicine clinic. Higher baseline rates can be expected of individuals presenting to a smoking cessation clinic or following hospitalization for a smoking-related illness, such as myocardial infarction. Despite this discouraging figure, many smokers are motivated to make cessation attempts, with about 42% reporting at least one attempt in the prior 1 year.[14,28] A significant opportunity exists for healthcare providers to intervene, as 70% of smokers visit their physicians annually. Physician counseling for only 2 to 3 minutes increases the rate of smoking cessation to 3%, making this intervention more cost-effective than treatment of dyslipidemia or mild-to-moderate hypertension. Tobacco quit lines are another means of providing counseling. Smokers are four times more likely to utilize a quit line than to seek help in person, and success rates of up to 20% can be achieved.[20] Quit lines are toll free and thus expand the access of underserved populations to smoking cessation resources. Telephone counseling in more effective than mailed self-help materials,[29] and personalized correspondence is superior to standardized letters.[22] Pharmacologic therapy, in the form of nicotine replacement, bupropion, or varenicline, also improves long-term smoking cessation rates.[30] Although counseling and pharmacotherapy are cost-effective when compared to other covered services,[20] insurance coverage of smoking cessation treatments varies. Only 20% of employer-sponsored plans provide at least some coverage,[31–34] Medicaid provides no coverage in 14 states,[31] and Medicare only covers treatment of individuals with smoking-related diseases.[35] Clearly, support for at least some of these interventions is a realistic goal for any country in the world.

Antismoking Media Campaigns Many smokers are not aware of the negative health consequences of smoking. Media campaigns offer a mechanism of providing education and countering specific misconceptions about smoking. Most recently, these campaigns have successfully targeted child and adolescent smoking. A media campaign coupled with a school-based program resulted in a decrease in reported smoking and weekly smoking in children in grades 4 through 6. Twelve- to thirteen-year-old individuals who reported seeing antismoking advertisements (ads) had half the chance of becoming established smokers as those who did not see the ads.[24] A nationwide antismoking media campaign was credited with 22% of the decline in youth smoking between 1990 and 2002.[36] Additional factors in this decline were restrictions on public smoking and an increase in the price of cigarettes.[37–39] Securing the financial resources necessary to conduct large-scale antismoking media campaigns is a challenge, made more serious by expanded tobacco industry marketing in developing countries, but it can be offset or overcome in the following way.

Excise Taxes Imposing a tax on tobacco products has the potential to accomplish several goals. Currently, taxes are levied by state and local governments in the United States, resulting in striking disparities in the price of tobacco products across the country. Not surprisingly, most smokers obtain cigarettes in geographic locations with the lowest cost or employ other high-price avoidance strategies.[40] This practice is associated with a lower probability of making a cessation attempt and possibly a lower quit rate.[41] A federal tax on tobacco products would have the effect of equalizing their price, thereby preventing this evasion tactic. Imposing such a tax would have at least two other potential benefits. A 10% increase in cigarette price reduces consumption by 3% to 5%.[42] This effect is more pronounced among economically disadvantaged individuals, including children and adolescents.[20] Although smoking cessation is the preferred outcome, a reduction in consumption may decrease the risk of lung cancer. A 50% reduction in consumption among those smoking 15 or more cigarettes per day is associated with a 27% reduction in lung cancer risk.[43] The second direct benefit is the revenue that these taxes generate, which is generally sufficient to fund other components of a comprehensive tobacco control program. Tobacco companies spend about $11 billion per year to offset these taxes.[44]

Outcomes of Comprehensive Tobacco Control Programs The fundamental measures employed by comprehensive tobacco control programs are excise taxes, antismoking media campaigns, and smoke-free laws. Results from two programs, in Massachusetts and New York, have been published. The Massachusetts Tobacco Control Program (MTCP) reduced consumption from 547 million packs to 280 million from 1992 to 2004, a decline of 4% per year. Even after adjustment for unequal increases in excise taxes, this decrease exceeded that of states that did not have control programs in place over the study period. Smoking prevalence decreased from 23.5% to 19.4% over 1990 to 1999. High school smoking prevalence decreased from 30.2% to 20.9% from 1993 to 2003. Smoking bans decreased exposure to smoking in the workplace from 44% to 15% from 1993 to 2001, in the home from 28% to 16%, and in restaurants from 64% to 37% from 1993 to 2002.[24] New York City's program incorporated a tax increase, workplace smoking ban, and free nicotine patch program. These efforts resulted in an 11% reduction, from 21.6% to 19.2%, in smoking prevalence over 1 year, equating to 140,000 individuals who quit smoking. Forty-five percent of smokers reported cutting down, thinking about quitting, trying to quit, or quitting as a result of these initiatives. Forty-six percent of individuals reported less exposure to secondhand smoke following introduction of the program. The proportion of nonsmokers reporting secondhand smoke exposure at home decreased 29%, from 8.5% to 6%, equating to 105,000 fewer nonsmokers exposed. The proportion reporting workplace exposure decreased 18%, from 8.9% to 7.3%, a reduction of 67,000 nonsmokers exposed. Not surprisingly in a program implemented within a relatively narrow geographic region, purchases through alternative channels increased 89%, but nevertheless yielded a net reduction in consumption of 15%.[45] A statewide ban on public smoking decreased exposure to secondhand smoke from 19.8% to 3.1% in restaurants and from 52.4% to 13.4% in bars in New York. Salivary cotinine levels, a marker of smoke exposure, decreased from 0.078 ng/mL to 0.041 ng/mL among nonsmokers.[46] Overall findings from comprehensive tobacco control programs suggest that warning labels and advertising restrictions are less effective than increased taxes, smoking bans, and counteradvertising.[22] Concordant with the results observed in Massachusetts, per capita cigarette purchases declined 16% to 20% in states implementing tax-supported antismoking programs.[22]

Impact on Lung Cancer Mortality Smoking prevalence fell from 42.3% to 23.2% in the United States between 1965 and 1997, but lung cancer incidence increased 230% between 1965 and 1999.[9] This highlights the fact that lung cancer risk reduction is both delayed and incomplete following smoking cessation. The cumulative incidence of lung cancer through age 75 is about 16% for lifelong smokers, compared to less than 1% for lifelong nonsmokers. Smoking cessation at age 30, 40, or 50 years results in cumulative incidence rates of about 2%, 3%, and 6%, respectively.[47] These data indicate that a significant burden of lung cancer risk, and thus lung cancer mortality, can be eliminated by early smoking cessation, but that the risk never decreases to the level of a lifelong nonsmoker. This reality suggests that smoking cessation remains a critical prevention strategy; however, in an evolving situation where the number of former smokers whose significant lung cancer risk never normalizes, additional public health measures are required.[48]

Population-Based Screening Published lung cancer screening trials have generally involved current and former smokers. Family history may be an additional factor to consider when selecting the population to screen. A family history of lung cancer is an independent risk factor for lung cancer. The diagnosis of squamous cell carcinoma in a first-degree relative appears to confer the greatest risk.[49] The risk of lung cancer in secondhand smoke–exposed individuals is measurable but significantly lower than in smokers. This means the potential cost benefit ratio will not be as favorable as for the smoking cohort and no prospective information addresses this circumstance as yet. Two large ongoing trials are accruing to address this issue (Flight Attendants Medical Research Institute, [FAMRI] and the International Early Lung Cancer Action Project [I-ELCAP]). Other risk factors for lung cancer include radon, asbestosis, certain metals (chromium, cadmium, arsenic), some organic chemicals, radiation, air pollution, tuberculosis, and genetic factors.[1] Other approaches to early lung cancer detection have been reported such as with techniques to evaluate tobacco-exposed bronchial epithelial cells recovered in the sputum of smokers. An antibody against heterogeneous nuclear ribonucleoprotein A2/B1 has demonstrated high sensitivity and specificity for the detection of lung cancer in high-risk individuals.[50–52] However, scaling such a test to achieve the requisite accuracy at affordable cost is a profound challenge given the comparable cost and availability of spiral CT screening.[53]

CHEMOPREVENTION

Lung cancer, like many other cancers, appears to be the final consequence of dysregulation involving varied pathways. However, this results in a common "phenotypic" outcome. Population-based lung cancer screening has yet to evolve into an established format. Looking forward, population-based screening could evolve as a multifaceted public health strategy, including successful youth-directed tobacco control, more effective smoking cessation for existing smokers, and integrated early detection, management, and chemoprevention for current and former smoker.

The conceptual basis for chemoprevention arises from the consideration of the long evolution of an epithelial cancer. This opportunity is best demonstrated by considering the colon cancer model. Multiple steps cumulatively define a continuum at the cellular level. These steps then served as watershed points at which more aggressive histopathologic progression could be identified and thereby mark the point at which cancer had evolved. In general, it is believed that lung cancer evolves by two potential pathways. The first involves the proliferation

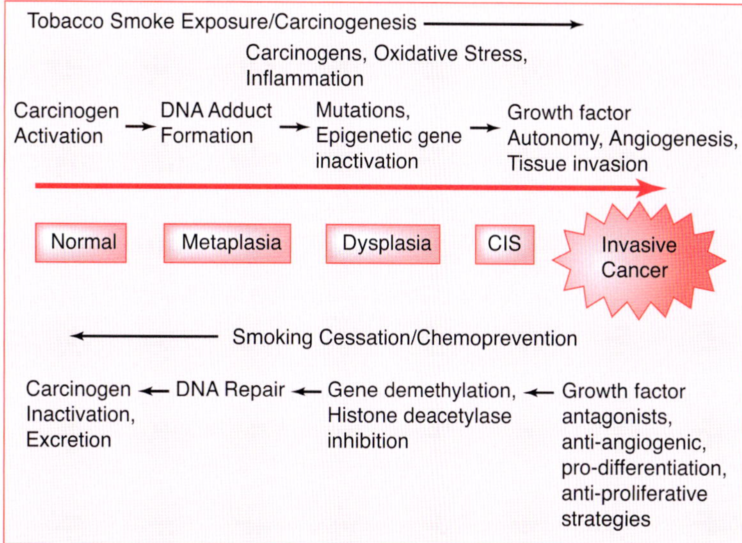

FIGURE 15.1 Schematic representation of the evolution of normal bronchial epithelium to invasive lung cancer. (Reprinted with permission from Keith RL, Miller YE. Lung cancer: genetics of risk and advances in chemoprevention. *Curr Opin Pulm Med* 2005;11:265–271.)

of aberrant cells that continue to devolve into carcinoma by sequential progression from hyperplasia through metaplasia and dysplasia. The second pathway involves "redifferentiation" or the dedifferentiation of bronchial epithelial cells that eventually redifferentiate into carcinoma.[54] It is conceivable that combinations of both pathways at various points ultimately results in the phenotypic presentation of lung cancer.

The term *chemoprevention* was introduced by Sporn et al.[55] in 1976 and was used to describe interventions used to slow or reverse progression of premalignant lesions to frank cancer. Targeting the "at-risk" population is crucial to the success of population-based chemoprevention. In lung cancer, chemoprevention strategies are targeted at the following three main groups:

1. Primary—chemoprevention among individuals at high risk who are otherwise healthy
2. Secondary—chemoprevention among individuals at high risk with premalignant conditions
3. Tertiary—chemoprevention among individuals with a known history of malignancy aimed at preventing second malignancies[56]

Chemoprevention agents encompass a tremendous number of potential natural and synthetic agents. These can be broadly subdivided into pharmaceutical, nutritional, and molecular targets. Each one of these broad categories can be further subdivided.

Chemoprevention Strategies Experimental work in rodents suggests that specific drugs can mitigate the progressive development of lung neoplasias after the exposure to specific tobacco-carcinogen exposures.[57,58] Additional impetus arises from the clinical experience with antiestrogens in the chemoprevention of breast cancer.[59,60] However, the clinical development of these drugs is fraught with a number of challenges, including the protracted time and profound monetary resources required for such commercial development efforts. Defining objective surrogates of long-term outcomes has also been an unresolved challenge.[61] As previously mentioned, it is largely held that a multistep carcinogenesis pathway exists from the normal bronchial epithelium to the frankly malignant tissue (Fig. 15.1). Along this pathway, changes from hyperplasia, atypia, metaplasia, and dysplasia are believed to occur and these changes are being utilized as surrogate end point biomarkers rather than frank carcinoma.[62–64]

Diet and Nutrition The literature is replete with articles that espouse or refute the benefits of a specific type of diet on the risk associated with lung cancer. There are no randomized controlled trials evaluating the advantages or disadvantages of the consumption of any particular food group and its putative cause of lung carcinogenesis. The conclusion that the consumption of meat and fish plays a role in the development of lung cancer is controversial at best. Some studies have demonstrated that consumption of meat defined as pork, chicken, or red meat is associated with a protective effect[65,66] whereas others have demonstrated the opposite effect.[67]

Case-control studies have shown an inverse relationship between the amount of fruits and vegetables consumed and the risk of lung cancer among both smokers and nonsmokers.[68,69] Similar results have been observed in other studies, however, with less profound findings.[70]

Vitamin supplementation, on the other hand, has yet to be associated with any significant chemopreventative impact. Its use has not been shown to positively influence lung cancer mortality.[71,72]

Pharmaceutical Interventions

CYCLOOXYGENASE INHIBITORS. The inflammatory pathway in which arachidonic acid is metabolized to prostaglandins, prostacyclins, and leukotrienes by the cyclooxygenase (COX) enzyme is one of the mechanisms by which lung cancer is thought to develop. There are two isoforms of this COX enzyme, COX-1 and COX-2, of which COX-2 is thought to involved in carcinogenesis, primarily through a variety of downstream effects.[91] Naturally, inhibition of either one or both COX enzymes is perceived as a theoretical means by which lung cancer may be prevented.

Although some case-control studies have suggested that aspirin (ASA) use is associated with a decreased risk of lung cancer,[73–76] others have either failed to demonstrate a protective effect, demonstrated only a statistically marginal benefit, or have revealed only a nonstatistically significant beneficial trend of ASA use with lung cancer.[77–82] When examining the population with a positive tobacco history, several investigators have been able to show a decreased risk of lung cancer.[74,75,83] Harris et al.[74] demonstrated a risk reduction among heavy smokers. While Moysich et al.[75] did not identify a dose-dependent relationship with ASA in smokers, they found a risk reduction with greater frequency of use.

Population-based cohort studies have demonstrated that nonsteroidal anti-inflammatory drugs (NSAIDs) for greater than 1 year in duration can be associated with a decreased relative risk in the development of lung cancer.[84] Among ever-smokers, a protective effect of NSAID use has been demonstrated.[83] Among high-risk heavy smokers, case-control studies have shown a decreased risk of lung cancer also.[74] Other studies have demonstrated that there is no protective benefit to NSAID use in the development of lung cancer, but these epidemiologic studies have been limited by the fact that confounding information is present precluding a definitive conclusion.[85,86]

The potential role of inhibiting the COX-2 pathway has been supported by successful results in the animal models that blocked this enzyme specifically.[87,88] Manipulation of the prostaglandins distal to the COX-2 pathway in other animal models further demonstrated the antineoplastic potential of manipulating this pathway.[89] Several investigators have extensively reported on the use of specific cycloxygenase-2 inhibition with celecoxib to modulate several surrogate end point biomarkers in human bronchial epithelium.[90–92] Presently, clinical trials studying the role COX-2 inhibition in lung cancer chemoprevention are ongoing.[72]

STATINS. Recent evidence has suggested that 3-hydroxy-3-methylglutaryl coenzyme A reductase inhibitors, otherwise known as *statins*, may be protective against the development of lung cancer.[93] In their retrospective case-control study, Khurana et al.[93] reported that statin use of greater than 6 months was associated with a significant reduction in lung cancer by 55%. This decrease was noted to increase to 77% among those using statins for greater than 4 years. Unfortunately, the retrospective nature of this study did not allow for the detection of any meaningful interaction between statin use and other significant factors associated with lung cancer, including smoking history.

CAROTENOIDS. However, particularly recently, a large body of evidence based on randomized controlled trials has established β-carotene at best as having a conflicting role in the prevention of lung cancer. In two large randomized control trials, the α-tocopherol β-carotene (ATBC) and the β-carotene and α-tocopherol (CARET) studies, there was no protective benefit noted among the overall population in the development of lung cancer. In fact, in both studies, β-carotene intake was found to be associated with a significantly increased lung cancer incidence and mortality.[94,95] In the ATBC trial, the participants were all male current smokers,[95] whereas the participants in the CARET trial were male and female current and former smokers.[94] In the Physician's Health Study, randomization of the participants into the β-carotene versus placebo groups was performed in an attempt to evaluate a positive effect in reducing the incidence of malignancies or cardiovascular outcomes. Of the participants, 50% were either current or former smokers. Ultimately, there was no difference in the incidence of lung cancer between the two groups.[96] Similar findings were observed in the Women's Health Study. In that study, no differences in lung cancer rates were observed among current, former, and never-smokers who took β-carotene compared to those receiving placebo, and thus no beneficial effect of β-carotene could be demonstrated.[97] This confusing situation highlights the challenge in trying to find effective chemoprevention agents.

RETINOIDS/VITAMIN A. There is a profound wealth of data supporting the role of vitamin A in the prevention, attenuation, or regression of carcinogenesis.[98–100] Since the aforementioned CARET study intimately tied together the use of β-carotene and vitamin A, the conclusion that β-carotene did not have any chemopreventative role was only half of the story. The other half reads similarly, in that the administration of vitamin A also had no beneficial effect and, in fact, was associated with a significantly increased relative risk of lung cancer.[94]

Tertiary chemoprevention trials also have not demonstrated any benefit of retinoids in the prevention of second primary lung cancers. Individuals who have been successfully treated for stage I NSCLC by operative resection, has not been shown to realize benefits in terms of recurrence, second primary tumors, or mortality rates when given oral vitamin A. In fact, secondary analysis demonstrated an earlier time to recurrence and mortality among current smokers.[101] In Europe, the European Study on Chemoprevention with Vitamin A and N-Acetylcysteine (EUROSCAN) showed similar results with retinyl palmitate having no effect on the rate of survival or second primary tumor among patients who had been treated with curative intent prior to this chemoprevention trial.[102] It was surmised that the reason for this result was that retinyl palmitate was not efficiently converted into *all*-trans retinoic acid (the active form of the drug).

The negative results of the aforementioned trials may have been due to the establishment of inadequate vitamin A levels within the lung tissue itself. In the trial by Lippman et al.,[101] only a homeopathic dose of retinyl palmitate was employed and this may have resulted in lower lung tissue concentrations. In the original work by Hong et al.[103] demonstrating a beneficial effect of vitamin A in carcinogenesis, there was also an associated increase in significant side effects associated with the administration of high doses of vitamin A. Not surprisingly, while other trials since theirs have demonstrated less toxic side effects, there has also been an absence of beneficial effects observed with lower doses of vitamin A. The benefits of increased local concentrations of vitamin A in lung tissue is further supported by experimental work with animal models and vitamin A deficiency demonstrating that only aerosolized vitamin A in animals shows a consistent beneficial effect.[58] Clinical trials in humans have yet to establish this effect with consistency, although an aerosolized trial from Germany was able to show regression of bronchial dysplasia.[104] It is believed that the aerosol form of vitamin A is successful because it functions directly at the bronchial epithelium where vitamin A exists and is depleted.

TOCOPHEROLS/VITAMIN E. In the double-blind, randomized, placebo-controlled ATBC trial mentioned earlier, there was a 2% reduction in lung cancer among the participants that were given vitamin E. This reduction however, was not significant during the 5- to 8-year follow-up period. Interestingly, during this same follow-up period the overall mortality rate among recipients receiving α-tocopherol was slightly higher than among those not receiving α-tocopherol. In the randomized, placebo-controlled Women's Health Study, women receiving vitamin E did not have a statistically significant difference in lung cancer rates than those receiving placebo.[105] In Heart Outcomes Prevention Evaluation (HOPE) trial and its continuation study, the HOPE-The Ongoing Outcomes (HOPE-TOO) trial the incidence of lung cancer was no different between the participants given vitamin E versus the placebo as identified. The median follow-up for the 7030 participants that went on to the HOPE-TOO continuation was 7 years.[106]

BUDESONIDE/FLUTICASONE. Lam et al.[107] conducted a phase II study to determine whether inhaled budesonide had a beneficial effect in smokers with known bronchial dysplasia. Ultimately, the authors showed that inhaled budesonide had no effect in causing regression of the previously identified dysplasia nor in the prevention of new lesions. In another trial, patients at risk of developing lung cancer had a decrease in the number of indeterminate pulmonary nodules on CT scan when given fluticasone.[108] Although encouraging, this was a secondary analysis of patients given fluticasone as part of a chemoprevention trial that ultimately demonstrated its administration was not associated with an alteration of the natural course of premalignant lesions. This study was not designed to look at cancer end points and as such did not look at the actual cancer rates.[109] More recent studies have demonstrated a dose-dependent decreased risk of lung cancer associated with inhaled corticosteroids in patients with COPD after adjusting for various confounding factors.[110]

SELENIUM. In 1996, the results of the Nutritional Prevention of Cancer (NPC) trial were published. The initial objective of this study was to evaluate the role of selenium in decreasing the rate of skin malignancies in 1312 high-risk participants. Although this study demonstrated that there was no decrease in skin malignancies, a secondary end point identified was a substantial, but not a significant, 26% decrease in the incidence of lung cancer.[111] Presently, there are ongoing clinical trials evaluating selenium in both secondary and tertiary chemoprevention protocols.

OTHER AGENTS. Currently, there are several other investigational agents being evaluated in their role in chemoprevention such as the organosulfurs Oltipraz and Anethole Dithiolethione (ADT).[65] Other agents may be evaluated in their role as chemopreventative agents as more information is learned from their role as biomarkers in early detection (see succeeding discussion).[56,65,112–115]

SECONDARY PREVENTION OF LUNG CANCER

Over 210,000 new cases of lung cancer will be diagnosed in 2008. Of these, only 20% are surgically resectable.[1] Of this subset, only 15% are stage I lesions, that is, lesions that have not progressed to involve the lymph nodes. While detecting early stage NSCLC is considered secondary lung cancer prevention (or prevention of metastatic cancer), it is important because the patient still has the possibility of being cured, typically with a surgical approach. In addition to being associated with an improved survival, this is crucial to the prevention of the presentation of the typical patient with lung cancer with advanced or metastatic lung cancer. Currently, the most promising approach to early lung cancer detection is with an imaging study, namely, a chest CT scan.

Radiology Screening

CT Screening Screening with chest CT has the potential to detect small lesions at an earlier stage than would occur with a conventional approach. Seventy-five percent of cancers diagnosed following the onset of symptoms are stage III or IV. In one recent study, 85% of lung cancers diagnosed in the context of screening current or former smokers were stage I, and only 5 of the 484 lung cancer diagnoses were made following the development and evaluation of symptoms. Five-year survival was estimated at 84%,[116] compared to 14% for lung cancer diagnosed conventionally.[117] Further details on the CT screening of lung cancer are seen in Chapter 16.

In 2003 based on early CT trial reports, the U.S. Preventive Services Task Force did not find the evidence strong enough to support a benefit with CT-based screening but neither did they find evidence of harm. This inconclusive recommendation is the same as their current recommendation for prostate cancer screening and surprisingly prostate cancer screening has been federally reimbursed for many years.[118]

Clinical Management for Screened Lesions One of the most challenging areas of lung cancer screening is the rapidly evolving ability of higher-resolution CT scanners to find a large number of lung nodules in the lungs of smokers. CT screening identifies nodules that have baseline features suggestive of lung cancer such a size, shape, or pattern of calcification. Newer approaches to CT-based lung cancer detection involve evaluation of features such as nodule growth.[97] In the most recent series, about 13% of individuals undergoing an initial CT screening will have findings that require further action. Of those with negative or "non-actionable" initial scans, only about 5% will have findings requiring further intervention on their annual follow-up screening CT. In both cases, this intervention is most often a repeat CT scan, with only approximately 2% to 4% of individuals being screened requiring an invasive test to achieve a definitive diagnosis.[119,120] This may involve various approaches. In the screening setting, it is critical to optimize the efficiency of this process especially through the parsimonious use of invasive procedures. At highly qualified institutions, the diagnostic workup typically involves using an aspiration needle biopsy to confirm that a growing nodule is cancer. When a biopsy is performed in the context of the specific protocol, it yields a diagnosis of cancer at least 90% of the time.[119] The frequency of complications such as pneumothorax requiring tube thoracostomy are low enough (5%) to justify its use.[121] This approach is associated with an extremely low frequency of futile thoracotomy (thoracic resection for a nonmalignant diagnosis). Other institutions include positron emission tomography (PET) scan to evaluate questionable nodules. The investigators in their screening trial reported an efficient process with an accuracy rate of CT/PET being 91%, but they did report a futile thoracotomy rate of approximately 5% (8/157).[122]

Surgical Management Issues In the large prospective experience of the I-ELCAP, postoperative mortality for earlier stage lung cancers removed by anatomic resection has been 0.5% (2/411). This mortality rate within the context of a lung cancer screening trial is similar to the mortality rate of 0.6% reported by Pastorino et al.[99] associated with lobectomy for stage IA NSCLCs identified by current conventional methods. Interestingly, these same investigators also participated in another lung cancer screening trial in the same city and reported a surgical mortality rate of 0% for early stage lung cancers.

Through the efforts of population-based screening protocols, the detection of smaller nodules and ultimately earlier stage lung cancers is occurring.[123,124] Commensurate with the lesser size of early stage lung cancers has been the advent and popularization of less invasive procedures. This has ultimately translated into a lower mortality and morbidity rates for the thoracic surgeon. In the largest video-assisted thoracoscopic surgery (VATS) lobectomy series reported from the United States, McKenna et al.[125] reported a morbidity rate of approximately 15% and a mortality rate of less than 1%. Most of the complications were non–life threatening. In the recently published ACOSOG Z0030 trial that prospectively collected data to compare outcomes of patients undergoing mediastinal lymph node dissection versus lymph node sampling, the morbidity rate after lobectomy was 37% and 1%, respectively. The majority of these tumors were early stage lesions.[126]

In addition to minimally invasive approaches to the very early stage I lung cancer, lung cancer screening with modern day CT scanners has resurrected interest in parenchymal sparing operations for small and peripheral NSCLCs. In 1995, the results of the only randomized, controlled trial comparing limited resections, including wedge resection and anatomic segmentectomy, to the formal anatomic lobectomy were reported. This study found that, while not statistically significant, there was an increased rate of recurrence and mortality in the limited resection population. Based on these findings, the investigators advised against lesser resections for known stage I NSCLCs[127]. The applicability of this study to current practice may be limited by a number of differences. The tumors included in the aforementioned study were those that were up to 3 cm in size. Asamura et al.[128] argued that the current staging system that defines T_1 tumors as less than 3 cm may be too heterogeneous. Their review of the 1994 Japanese lung cancer registry found that patient with lesions less than 2 cm actually fared better than those between 2.1 and 3.0 cm, which would still be classified as a T_1 lesion in the current staging system. Their findings suggested, and they argue, that subclassification of T_1 lesions into those that are ≤2.0 cm would be of benefit for prognostic purposes. In addition to this potential difference in tumor biology, current CT scanner technology is more advanced than when the limited resection study was performed. Furthermore, since lung cancer screening at this time was not in practice, none of the enrolled patients were those identified by lung cancer screening protocols.

A metaanalysis evaluating limited resection versus lobectomy for small (≤3 cm) peripheral NSCLCs found that survival was not significantly different. Interestingly, this finding occurred despite the fact that the most common reason for a limited resection was poor cardiopulmonary function, a condition that would suggest a more fragile patient.[129] In the context of lung cancer screening, the role of a limited resection has resurfaced as a question. Asamura et al.[123] reviewed their experience with subcentimeter lung cancers, some of which were identified by lung cancer screening protocols. The subcentimeter nodules identified were categorized into three groups based on their appearance, nonsolid ground-glass opacity (GGO), part-solid GGO, and solid-type tumor. Of the 28 GGO lesions, 15 underwent a limited resection, versus only 4 of the 20 solid-type lesions. No difference in 5-year survival differences were observed between the GGO, part-solid GGO, and solid-type tumors. Similar outstanding survival rates have been observed in studies evaluating sublobar resections for slightly larger GGOs (≤2 cm) identified by high-resolution CT scanners.[130] The findings of these studies might suggest that small nodules identified by screening CT scans, particularly GGOs, may not require an anatomic lobectomy and may be equally served with a limited resection. The question of whether a limited resection suffices for stage IA tumors, of which many will be identified by screening protocols, may not be answerable until the mature data from randomized comparisons of standard compared to more limited surgical approaches, such as with Cancer and Leukemia Group B (CALGB) Study 140503, are reported.[131]

Pennathur et al.[132] and Dupuy et al.[133] have furthered the role of minimally invasive surgery to include percutaneous ablative techniques without the use of the conventional thoracotomy or newer thoracoscopy.[134] Currently, this modality of therapy has not replaced the established role of surgery in the medically fit patient. However, it is a reasonable alternative in the medically inoperable patient that is found to have stage I disease.[132,133] With increased experience in this subset of patients, the indications for percutaneous ablation may expand to include those with subcentimeter stage I lung cancers that are identified by screening protocols. This, in fact, may be occurring as some pulmonary radiofrequency ablation studies have incorporated medically fit patients who have simply refused surgery.[134]

From a survival standpoint, it has been suggested that by virtue of detecting earlier stage lesions, 5-year survival may be improved over conventionally cited survival.[119] Some investigator argue that an increased survival following surgery for any screened lung cancer may reflect lead-time bias. Henschke et al.[135] have suggested that a lung cancer mortality reduction benefit will not ultimately be found unless there is an improved lead time. Furthermore, true lead-time bias is thought to occur when relatively short-term survivals (such as 5-year interval) are compared between groups. This may not be the case with current screening regimens that have improved long-term (10 year) survival.[136]

Other investigators have suggested that the apparent benefit of lung cancer screening relates to finding more indolent lung cancers. This is referred to as overdiagnosis bias and has been suggested as a reason why prior efforts at lung cancer screening with chest radiographs and sputum cytopathology did not result in significantly improved lung cancer–related mortality.[137,138] This has been questioned recently by Raz et al.[136] who reviewed the long-term survival of patients with completely untreated stage I NSCLC. They discovered that the median survival among patients not treated by any modality including surgery, chemotherapy, or radiation was 9 months overall and 13 months in the subset with T_1 disease. This led the authors to conclude that treatment of identified stage I NSCLC is imperative.

The medically stable patient with a lung cancer detected by screening techniques deserves an opportunity for intervention. Despite the criticisms leveled against screening for lung cancer, recent mathematical modeling has suggested benefit in the form of mortality reduction associated with screening.[139,140] Furthermore, the decreased morbidity and mortality associated with minimally invasive techniques in the proper hands makes surgical resection of the suspicious lesions that are identified by screening an attractive and effective treatment option.

While the goal of surgical resection or ablation includes the eradication of ever smaller early stage NSCLC, invariably there will be lung nodules that are removed, which will ultimately prove to be benign. The decreased mortality and morbidity associated with newer surgical approaches and other experimental intervention techniques may improve the therapeutic index with surgical intervention in screening settings.

Special Considerations

Gene Therapy in the Prevention of Primary Lung Cancer As mentioned earlier, the development of lung cancer is thought to follow a stepwise progression. The underlying mechanism of this progression is thought to be dependent on genetic alterations that occur at key points. Naturally, the earlier genetic changes that manifest as the early or precancerous changes could possibly be targets of therapy. Despite this knowledge, genetic therapy for lung cancer is well short of this desired goal. Most genetic therapy centers on the role of the tumor suppressor gene p53.[62,141] Despite its purported role in the progression of disease from either bronchial atypia or squamous metaplasia to low-grade dysplasia, much of the work on the p53 tumor suppressor gene appears to center on promoting its activity in patients with advanced malignancy.[62,141] At present, including the work regarding the p53 tumor suppressor gene, no genetic therapy is available that definitively halts the progression of normal bronchial epithelial cells down the sequence of hyperplasia to dysplasia and ultimately to carcinoma. This remains a conceptually exciting area for ongoing research.

Biomarkers in the Early Detection and Prevention of Primary Lung Cancer In terms of early detection, serum and plasma analysis of circulating DNA has been thought to be a novel biomarker. In particular, identifying free DNA that has undergone changes such as methylation, (Refer to Laird Offinga Chapter) loss of heterozygosity, allele shifts, microsatellite instability, or other mutations may allow for identification of early lung cancers.[142] These genetic changes may add to the variety of proteomic biomarkers that are forthcoming.

From a population-based lung cancer screening perspective, there are currently no established biomarkers routinely targeted in the prevention of lung cancer or used in the early detection of lung cancer. However, much work is being pursued in the field of proteomics to arrive at a point where proteins expressed in the sputum or serum of patients may be able to complement or direct image-guided screening protocols. Presently, the American Association of Cancer Research has established a task force to evaluate the possibility of identifying biomarkers of precancerous lesion along the multistep carcinogenesis pathway. Identifying and intervening at these surrogate end point biomarker milestones may potentially ultimately reduce the rates of lung cancer.[143] A detailed description of all the researched biomarkers is beyond the scope of this chapter, but presently a concerted effort in proteomic analysis is being undertaken to identify targets for lung cancer detection and/or prevention.

Within the context of chemoprevention, two pathways that have received a substantial amount of attention for their potential role in biomarker protein detection and cancer prevention include the COX pathway and epidermal growth factor receptor (EGFR) pathway. The EGFR pathway involves a tyrosine kinase receptor that results in autophosphorylation and activation of downstream pathways. One of the significant downstream pathways involves the COX-2 pathway. The products of both pathways may work to potentiate the effectiveness of the other.[144,145] Simultaneous inhibition of the COX-2 and EGFR pathways has demonstrated an augmented antiproliferative and pro-apoptotic effect in cancer cell lines in vitro. This presumed potentiation of the EGFR pathway inhibition by COX-2 is thought to be representative of a more complete blockade of both pathways.[144] Chemoprevention efforts aimed toward inhibiting the pathway or products of

COX-2 and identifying and blocking the EGFR pathway are attractive targets for chemoprevention, but in both instances approaches to manage side effects of this therapy may be needed prior to large-scale application, if sufficient efficacy data emerges.

Identification of circulating DNA released from tumor cells, genetic alterations such as microsatellite instability in addition to actual mutations, epigenetic changes such as tumor suppressor gene promoter methylation, as well as an entire host of other expressed proteins represent potential biomarkers that may be available in the future.[146] Unfortunately, these and other serum, plasma, sputum, and tissue assays are only in their investigational stages and have yet to definitively be associated with lung cancer and much less play a role in chemoprevention.

REFERENCES

1. American Cancer Society. Cancer Facts & Figures 2007. Atlanta: American Cancer Society, 2007.
2. World Health Organization. Cancer: Fact Sheet No. 297, February 2006. Available at: http://www.who.int/mediacentre/factsheets/fs297/en/index.html. Accessed February 14, 2008.
3. Espey DK, Wu XC, Swan J, et al. Annual report to the nation on the status of cancer, 1975–2004, featuring cancer in American Indians and Alaska Natives. *Cancer* 2007;110:2119–2152.
4. Peto R, Darby S, Deo H, et al. Smoking, smoking cessation, and lung cancer in the UK since 1950: combination of national statistics with two case-control studies. *BMJ* 2000;321:323–329.
5. Tong L, Spitz MR, Fueger JJ, et al. Lung carcinoma in former smokers. *Cancer* 1996;78:1004–1010.
6. Grover F, Piantadosi S. Recurrence and survival following resection of bronchioloalveolar carcinoma of the lung—The Lung Cancer Study Group experience. *Ann Surg* 1989;209:779–790.
7. van Iersel CA, de Konig HJ, Draisma G, et al. Risk-based selection from the general population in a screening trial: selection criteria, recruitment and power for the Dutch-Belgian randomized lung cancer multi-slice CT screening trial (NELSON). *Int J Cancer* 2006;120:868–874.
8. Bastarrika G, Pueyo JC, Mulshine JL. Radiologic screening for lung cancer. *Expert Rev Anticancer Ther* 2002;2:385–392.
9. Strauss GM, Dominioni L. Perception, paradox, paradigm: Alice in the wonderland of lung cancer prevention and early detection. *Cancer* 2000;89:2422–2231.
10. Doll R, Hill A. Smoking and carcinoma of the lung. *BMJ* 1950:739–748.
11. Wynder EL, Graham EA. Tobacco smoking as a possible etiologic factor in bronchiogenic carcinoma: a study of 684 proved cases. *JAMA* 1950;143:329–336.
12. U.S. Department of Health and Human Services. Reducing the health consequences of smoking: 25 years of progress. A report of the Surgeon General. In: U.S. Department of Health and Human Services, Centers for Disease Control and Prevention, National Center for Chronic Disease Prevention and Health Promotion, Office on Smoking and Health, 1989.
13. American Lung Association. Smoking 101 fact sheet, August 2008. Available at: http://www.lungusa.org/site/c.dvLUK9O0E/b.39853/. Accessed September 5, 2009.
14. Centers for Disease Control and Prevention (CDC). Youth Risk Behavior Surveillance—United States, 2005: Surveillance Summaries, June 9, 2006. *MMWR Morb Mortal Wkly Rep* 2006;55(No. SS-5):1–108.
15. U.S. Department of Health and Human Services. The health consequences of involuntary exposure to tobacco smoke: a report of the Surgeon General. Atlanta, GA: U.S. Department of Health and Human Services, Centers for Disease Control and Prevention, Coordinating Center for Health Promotion, National Center for Chronic Disease Prevention and Health Promotion, Office of Smoking and Health, 2006.
16. Centers for Disease Control and Prevention (CDC). Annual smoking-attributable mortality, years of potential life lost, and productivity losses—United States, 1997–2001. *MMWR Morb Mortal Wkly Rep* 2005;54:625–628.
17. American Lung Association. Epidemiology and Statistics Unit. Research and Program Services. Trends in tobacco use. Washington, D.C.: American Lung Association, 2007.
18. Centers for Disease Control and Prevention (CDC). Cigarette use among high school students—United States, 1991–2005. *MMWR Morb Mortal Wkly Rep* 2006;55:724–726.
19. World Health Organization. WHO Report on the Global Tobacco Epidemic, 2008: The MPOWER package. Geneva, World Health Organization, 2008.
20. Fiore MC, Croyle RT, Curry SJ, et al. Preventing 3 million premature deaths and helping 5 millions smokers quit: a national action plan for tobacco cessation. *Am J Public Health* 2004;94:205–210.
21. Centers for Disease Control and Prevention. Best practices for comprehensive tobacco control programs—2007. Atlanta: U.S. Department of Health and Human Services, Centers for Disease Control and Prevention, National Center for Chronic Disease Prevention and Health Promotion, Office on Smoking and Health, October 2007.
22. Orleans CT, Cummings KM. Population-based tobacco control: progress and prospects. *Am J Health Promot* 1999;14:83–91.
23. Fichtenberg CM, Glantz SA. Youth access interventions do not affect youth smoking. *Pediatrics* 2002;109:1088–1092.
24. Koh HK, Judge CM, Robbins H, et al. The first decade of the Massachusetts Tobacco Control Program. *Public Health Rep* 2005;120:482–495.
25. Halpern-Felsher BL, Biehl M, Kropp RY, et al. Perceived risks and benefits of smoking: differences among adolescents with different smoking experiences and intentions. *Prev Med* 2004;39:559–567.
26. American Nonsmokers' Rights Foundation. Overview list: how many smoke-free laws? Available at: http://www.no-smoke.org/pdf/mediaordlist.pdf. Updated January 2, 2008. Accessed January 4, 2008.
27. Pickett MS, Schober SE, Brody DJ et al. Smoke-free laws and secondhand smoke exposure in US non-smoking adults, 1999–2002. *Tob Control* 2006;15:302–307.
28. Centers for Disease Control and Prevention. Tobacco use among adults – United States, 2005. *MMWR Morb Mortal Wkly Rep* 2006;55:1145–1148.
29. An LC, Zhu SH, Nelson DB et al. Benefits of telephone care over primary care for smoking cessation: a randomized trial. *Arch Intern Med* 2006;166:536–542.
30. Cummings KM, Hyland A, Fix B, et al. Free nicotine patch giveaway program: 12-month follow-up of participants. *Am J Prev Med* 2006;31:181–184.
31. Curry SJ, Orleans CT, Keller P, et al. Promoting smoking cessation in the healthcare environment: 10 years later. *Am J Prev Med* 2006;31:269–272.
32. McPhillips-Tangum C, Rehm B, Carreon R, et al. Addressing tobacco in managed care: results of the 2003 survey. *Prev Chronic Dis* (serial online) 2006 Jul (1/8/08). Available at: http://www.cdc.gov/pcd/issues/2006/jul/05_0173.htm.
33. Bondi MA, Harris JR, Atkins D, et al. Employer coverage of clinical preventive services in the United States. *Am J Health Promot* 2006;20:214–222.
34. Halpin HA, Bellows NM, McMenamin SB. Medicaid coverage for tobacco-dependence treatments. *Health Aff (Millwood)* 2006;25:550–556.
35. American Cancer Society. *Cancer Prevention & Early Detection Facts & Figures 2007*. Atlanta: American Cancer Society, 2007.
36. Farrelly MC, Davis KC, Haviland ML, et al. Evidence of a dose-response relationship between "truth" antismoking ads and youth smoking prevalence. *Am J Public Health* 2005;95:425–431.
37. Ross H, Powell LM, Tauras JA, et al. New evidence on youth smoking behavior based on experimental price increases. impacTEEN (serial online) 2003 October (1/8/08). Available at: http://www.impacteen.org/generalarea_pdfs/ Ross_paperpeerelast101003.pdf.
38. Farrelly, MC, Healton, CG, Davis KC, et al. Getting to the truth: evaluating national tobacco countermarketing campaigns. *Am J Public Health* 2002;92:901–907.

39. Wakefield M, Forster J. Growing evidence for new benefit of clean indoor air laws: reduced adolescent smoking. *Tob Control* 2005;14:292–293.
40. Hyland A, Bauer JE, Li Q, et al. Higher cigarette prices influence cigarette purchase patterns. *Tob Control* 2005;14:86–92.
41. Hyland A, Higbee C, Li Q, et al. Access to low-taxed cigarettes deters smoking cessation attempts. *Am J Public Health* 2005;95:994–995.
42. U.S. Department of Health and Human Services. Reducing tobacco use: a report of the Surgeon General. Atlanta, GA: U.S. Department of Health and Human Services, Centers for Disease Control and Prevention, National Center for Chronic Disease Prevention and Health Promotion, Office on Smoking and Health, 2000.
43. Godtfredsen NS, Prescott E, Osler M. Effect of smoking reduction on lung cancer risk. *JAMA* 2005;294:1505–1510.
44. Lindblom E. Cigarette company price discounts and marketing expenditures are increasing smoking levels, especially among kids. Available at: http://www.tobaccofreekids.org/ research/factsheets/pdf/0272.pdf. Posted May 7, 2007. Accessed November 7, 2007.
45. Frieden TR, Mostashari F, Kerker BD, et al. Adult tobacco use levels after intensive tobacco control measures: New York City, 2002–2003. *Am J Public Health* 2005;95:1016–1023.
46. Centers for Disease Control and Prevention (CDC). Reduced secondhand smoke exposure after implementation of a comprehensive statewide ban—New York, June 26, 2003–June 30, 2004. *MMWR Morb Mortal Wkly Rep* 2007;56:705–708.
47. Peto R, Darby S, Deo H, et al. Smoking, smoking cessation, and lung cancer in the UK since 1950: combination of national statistics with two case-control studies. *BMJ* 2000;321:323–329.
48. Vineis P, Alavanja M, Buffler P, et al. Tobacco and cancer: recent epidemiological evidence. *J Natl Cancer Inst* 2004;96:99–106.
49. Nitadori J, Inoue M, Iwasaki M, et al. Association between lung cancer incidence and family history of lung cancer: data from a large-scale population-based cohort study, the JPHC Study. *Chest* 2006;130:968–975.
50. Tockman MS, Mulshine JL, Piantadosi S, et al. Prospective detection of preclinical lung cancer: results from two studies of heterogeneous nuclear ribonucleoprotein A2/B1 overexpression. *Clin Cancer Res* 1997;3: 2237–2246.
51. Hirsch FR, Franklin WA, Gazdar AF, et al. Early detection of lung cancer: clinical perspectives of recent advances in biology and radiology. *Clin Cancer Res* 2001;7:5–22.
52. Sueoka E, Goto Y, Sueoka N, et al. Heterogeneous nuclear ribonucleoprotein B1 as a new marker of early detection for human lung cancers. *Cancer Res* 1999;59:1404–1407.
53. Mulshine JL, De Luca LM, Dedrick RL, et al. Considerations in developing successful, population-based molecular screening and prevention of lung cancer. *Cancer* 2000;89:2465–2467.
54. Ten Have-Opbroek AA, Benfield JR, Hammond WG, et al. In favour of an oncofoetal concept of bronchogenic carcinoma development. *Histol Histopathol* 1994;9:375–384.
55. Sporn MB, Dunlop NM, Newton DL, et al. Prevention of chemical carcinogenesis by vitamin A and its synthetic analogs (retinoids). *Fed Proc* 1976;35:1332–1338.
56. van Zandwijk N. Chemoprevention in lung carcinogenesis—an overview. *Eur J Cancer* 2005;41:1990–2002.
57. Wattenberg LW, Wiedmann TS, Estensen RD, et al. Chemoprevention of pulmonary carcinogenesis by aerosolized budenoside female A/J mice. *Cancer Res* 1997;57:5489–5492.
58. Dahl AR, et al. Inhaled isoretinoin (13-cis retinoic acid) is an effective lung cancer chemopreventative agent in A/J mice at low doses: a pilot study. *Clin Cancer Res* 2000;6:3015–3024.
59. Jordan C. Historical perspective on hormonal therapy of advanced breast cancer. *Clin Ther* 2002;24(suppl):A3–A16.
60. Fisher B, Constantino JP, Wickerham DL, et al. Tamoxifen for the prevention of breast cancer: current status of the national surgical adjuvant breast and bowel project P-1 study. *J Natl Cancer Inst* 2005;97:1652–1662.
61. Kelloff GJ, O'Shaughnessy JA, Gordon GB, et al. Counterpoint: Because some surrogate end point biomarkers measure the neoplastic process they will have high utility in the development of cancer chemopreventive agents against sporadic cancers. *Cancer Epidemiol Biomarkers Prev* 2003;12:593–596.
62. Toloza EM, Morse MA, Lylerly HK. Gene therapy for lung cancer. *J Cell Biochem* 2006;99:1–22.
63. Kelloff GJ, Lippman SM, Dannenberg AJ, et al. Progress in chemopreventioin drug development: the promise of molecular biomarkers for prevention of intraepithelial neoplasia and cancer—a plan to move forward. *Clin Cancer Res* 2006;12:3661–3697.
64. Keith RL, Miller YE. Lung cancer: genetics of risk and advances in chemoprevention. *Curr Opin Pulm Med* 2005;11:265–271.
65. Swanson CA, Mao BL, Li JY, et al. Dietary determinants of lung-cancer risk: results from a case-control study in Yunnan Province, China. *Int J Cancer* 1992;50:876–880.
66. Dosil-Díaz O, Ruano-Ravina A, Gestal-Otero JJ, et al. Meat and fish consumption and risk of lung cancer: a case-control study in Galicia, Spain. *Cancer Lett* 2007;252:115–122.
67. Brennan P, Fortes C, Butler J, et al. A multicenter case-control study of diet and lung cancer among non-smokers. *Cancer Causes Control* 2000;11:49–58.
68. Galeone C, Negri E, Pelucchi C, et al. Dietary intake of fruit and vegetable and lung cancer risk: a case-control study in Harbin, northeast China. *Ann Oncol* 2007;18:388–392.
69. Nyberg F, Agrenius V, Svartengren K, et al. Dietary factors and risk of lung cancer in never-smokers. *Int J Cancer* 1998;78:430–436.
70. Feskanich D, Ziegler RG, Michaud DS, et al. Prospective study of fruit and vegetable consumption and risk of lung cancer among men and women. *J Natl Cancer Inst* 2000;92:1812–1823.
71. Gray J, Mao JT, Szabo E, et al. Lung cancer chemoprevention: ACCP evidence-based clinical practice guidelines (2nd edition). *Chest* 2007;132:S56–S68.
72. Kamangar F, Qiao YL, Yu B, et al. Lung cancer chemoprevention: a randomized, double-blind trial in Linxian, China. *Cancer Epidemiol Biomarkers Prev* 2006;15:1562–1564.
73. Akhmedkhanov A, Toniolo P, Zeleniuch-Jacquotte A, et al. Aspirin and lung cancer in women. *Br J Cancer* 2002;87:49–53.
74. Harris RE, Beebe-Donk J, Schuller HM. Chemoprevention of lung cancer by non-steroidal anti-inflammatory drugs among cigarette smokers. *Oncol Rep* 2002;9:693–695.
75. Moysich KB, Menezes RJ, Ronsani A, et al. Regular aspirin use and lung cancer risk. *BMC Cancer* 2002;2:31.
76. Schreinemachers DM, Everson RB. Aspirin use and lung, colon, and breast cancer incidence in a prospective study. *Epidemiology* 1994;5:138–146.
77. Cook NR, Lee IM, Gaziano JM, et al. Low-dose aspirin in the primary prevention of cancer: the Women's Health Study: a randomized controlled trial. *JAMA* 2005;294:47–55.
78. Friis S, Sørensen HT, McLaughlin JK, et al. A population-based cohort study of the risk of colorectal and other cancers among users of low-dose aspirin. *Br J Cancer* 2003;88:684–688.
79. Holick CN, Michaud DS, Leitzmann MF, et al. Aspirin use and lung cancer in men. *Br J Cancer* 2003;89:1705–1708.
80. Paganini-Hill A, Chao A, Ross RK, et al. Aspirin use and chronic diseases: a cohort study of the elderly. *BMJ* 1989;299:1247–1250.
81. Peto R, Gray R, Collins R, et al. Randomised trial of prophylactic daily aspirin in British male doctors. *Br Med J (Clin Res Ed)* 1988;296: 313–316.
82. Feskanich D, Bain C, Chan AT, et al. Aspirin and lung cancer risk in a cohort study of women: dosage, duration and latency. *Br J Cancer* 2007;97:1295–1299.
83. Muscat JE, Chen SQ, Richie JP Jr, et al. Risk of lung carcinoma among users of nonsteroidal antiinflammatory drugs. *Cancer* 2003;97:1732–1736.
84. Hernández-Diaz S, García Rodriguez LA. Nonsteroidal anti-inflammatory drugs and risk of lung cancer. *Int J Cancer* 2007;120:1565–1572.
85. Skriver MV, Norgaard M, Poulsen AH, et al. Use of nonaspirin NSAIDs and risk of lung cancer. *Int J Cancer* 2005;117:873–876.
86. Wall RJ, Shyr Y, Smalley W. Nonsteroidal anti-inflammatory drugs and lung cancer risk: a population-based case control study. *J Thorac Oncol* 2007;2:109–114.

87. Tanaka T, Delong PA, Amin K, et al. Treatment of lung cancer using clinically relevant oral doses of the cyclooxygenase-2 inhibitor rofecoxib: potential value as adjuvant therapy after surgery. *Ann Surg* 2005;241:168–178.
88. Rioux N, Castonguay A. Prevention of NNK-induced lung tumorigenesis in A/J mice by acetylsalicylic acid and NS-398. *Cancer Res* 1998;58:5354–5360.
89. Keith RL, Miller YE, Hudish TM, et al. Pulmonary prostacyclin synthase overexpression chemoprevents tobacco smoke lung carcinogenesis in mice. *Cancer Res* 2004;64:5897–5904.
90. Masferrer JL, Leahy KM, Koki AT, et al. Antiangiogenic and antitumor activities of cyclooxygenase-2 inhibitors. *Cancer Res* 2000; 60:1306–1311.
91. Mao JT, Tsu IH, Dubinett SM, et al. Modulation of pulmonary leukotriene B4 production by cyclooxygenase-2 inhibitors and lipopolysaccharide. *Clin Cancer Res* 2004;10:6872–6878.
92. Mao JT, Fishbein MC, Adams B, et al. Celecoxib decreases Ki-67 proliferative index in active smokers. *Clin Cancer Res* 2006;12:314–320.
93. Khurana V, Bejjanki HR, Caldito G, et al. Statins reduce the risk of lung cancer in humans: a large case-control study of US veterans. *Chest* 2007;131:1282–1288.
94. Omenn GS, Goodman GE, Thornquist MD, et al. Effects of a combination of beta carotene and vitamin A on lung cancer and cardiovascular disease. *N Engl J Med* 1996;334:1150–1155.
95. The Alpha-Tocopherol, Beta Carotene Cancer Prevention Study Group. The effect of vitamin E and beta carotene on the incidence of lung cancer and other cancers in male smokers. *N Engl J Med* 1994;330:1029–1035.
96. Lee IM, Cook NR, Manson JE, et al. Beta-carotene supplementation and incidence of cancer and cardiovascular disease: the women's health study. *J Natl Cancer Inst.* 1999;91:2102–2106.
97. Yankelevitz DF, Reeves AP, Kostis WJ, et al. Small pulmonary nodules: volumetrically determined growth rates based on CT evaluation. *Radiology* 2000;217:251–256.
98. Hong WK, Lippman SM, Itri LM, et al. Prevention of second primary tumors with isotretinoin in squamous-cell carcinoma of the head and neck. *N Engl J Med* 1990;323:795–801.
99. Pastorino U, Infante M, Maioli M, et al. Adjuvant treatment of stage I lung cancer with high-dose vitamin. *J Clin Oncol* 1993;11:1216–1222.
100. Mulshine JL, De Luca LM. Lung cancer chemoprevention: an opportunity for direct delivery. In: Kelloff GJ, Hawk ET, Sigman CC, eds. *Cancer Chemoprevention Vol. 2: Strategies for Cancer Chemoprevention.* 2nd ed. New Jersey: Human Press, 2005.
101. Lippman SM, Lee JJ, Karp DD, et al. Randomized phase III intergroup trial of isotretinoin to prevent second primary tumors in stage I non-small-cell lung cancer. *J Natl Cancer Inst* 2001;93:605–618.
102. van Zandwijk N, Dalesio O, Pastorino U, et al. EUROSCAN, a randomized trial of vitamin A and N-acetylcysteine in patients with head and neck cancer or lung cancer. For the European Organization for Research and Treatment of Cancer Head and Neck and Lung Cancer Cooperative Groups. *J Natl Cancer Inst* 2000;92:977–986.
103. Hong WK, Endicott J, Itri LM, et al. 13-cis-retinoic acid in the treatment of oral leukoplakia. *N Engl J Med* 1986;315:1501–1505.
104. Kohlhäufl M, Häussinger K, Stanzel F, et al. Inhalation of aerosolized vitamin A: reversibility of metaplasia and dysplasia of human respiratory epithelia — a prospective pilot study. *Eur J Med Res* 2002;7:72–78.
105. Lee IM, Cook NR, Gaziano JM, et al. Vitamin E in the primary prevention of cardiovascular disease and cancer: the women's health study; a randomized controlled trial. *JAMA* 2005;294:56–65.
106. Hennekens CH, Buring JE, Manson JE, et al. Lack of effect of long-term supplementation with beta carotene on the incidence of malignant neoplasms and cardiovascular disease. *N Engl J Med* 1996;334:1145–1149.
107. Lam S, leRiche JC, McWilliams A, et al. A randomized phase IIb trial of pulmicort turbuhaler (budesonide) in people with dysplasia of the bronchial epithelium. *Clin Cancer Res* 2004;10:6502–6511.
108. van den Berg RM, Teertstra HJ, van Zandwijk N, et al. CT detected indeterminate pulmonary nodules in a chemoprevention trial of fluticasone. *Lung Cancer* 2008;60:57–61.
109. van den Berg RM, van Tinteren H, van Zandwijk N, et al. The influence of fluticasone inhalation on markers of carcinogenesis in bronchial epithelium. *Am J Respir Crit Care Med* 2007;175:1061–1065.
110. Parimon T, Chien JW, Bryson CL, et al. Inhaled corticosteroids and risk of lung cancer among patients with chronic obstructive pulmonary disease. *Am J Respir Crit Care Med* 2007;175:712–719.
111. Reid ME, Duffield-Lilico AJ, Garland L, et al. Selenium supplementation and lung cancer incidence: an update of the nutritional prevention of cancer trial. *Cancer Epidemiol Biomarkers Prev* 2002;11;1285–1291.
112. Omenn GS. Chemoprevention of lung cancers: lessons from CARET, the beta-carotene and retinol efficacy trial, and prospects for the future. *Eur J Cancer Prevention* 2007;16:184–191.
113. Hirsch FR, Lippman SM. Advances in the biology of lung cancer chemoprevention. *J Clin Oncol* 2005;23:3186–3197.
114. Wardwell NR, Massion PP. Novel strategies for the early detection and prevention of lung cancer. *Semin Oncol* 2005;32:259–268.
115. Veronesi U, Bonanni B. Chemoprevention: from research to clinical oncology. *Eur J Cancer* 2005;41:1833–1841.
116. Henschke C, Yankelevitz D, Libby D, et al. Survival of patients with stage I lung cancer detected on CT screening. *N Engl J Med* 2006; 355:1763–1771.
117. SEER cancer statistics review, 1975–2003. National Cancer Institute, 2006. Available at: http://seer.cancer.gov/csr/1975_2003/results_merged/topic_lifetime_risk.pdf. Accessed November 21, 2006.
118. Humphrey LL, Teutsch S, Johnson M. Lung cancer screening with sputum cytological examination, chest radiography and computed tomography: an update for the U.S. Preventive Services Task Force. *Ann Intern Med* 2004;140:740–753.
119. Henschke C, Yankelevitz D, Libby D, et al. Survival of patients with stage I lung cancer detected on CT screening. *N Engl J Med* 2006; 355:1763–1771.
120. Swensen SJ, Jett JR, Hartman TE, et al. CT screening for lung cancer: five-year prospective experience. *Radiology* 2005;235:259–265.
121. Gould MK, Fletcher J, Iannettoni MD, et al. American College of Chest Physicians. Evaluation of patients with pulmonary nodules: when is it lung cancer?: ACCP evidence-based clinical practice guidelines (2nd edition). *Chest* 2007;132:108–130S.
122. Veronesi G, Bellomi M, Veronesi U, et al. Role of positron emission tomography scanning in the management of lung nodules detected at baseline computed tomography screening. *Ann Thorac Surg* 2007;84: 959–965.
123. Asamura H, Suzuki K, Watanabe S, et al. A clinicopathological study of resected subcentimeter lung cancers: a favorable prognosis for ground glass opacity lesions. *Ann Thorac Surg* 2003;76:1016–1022.
124. Henschke CI, McCauley DI, Yankelevitz DF, et al. Early lung cancer action project: overall design and findings from baseline screening. *Lancet* 1999;354:99–105.
125. McKenna RJ, Houck W, Fuller CB. Video-assisted thoracic surgery lobectomy: experience with 1100 cases. *Ann Thorac Surg* 2006;81: 421–426.
126. Allen MS, Darling GE, Pechet TT, et al. Morbidity and mortality of major pulmonary resections in patients with early-stage lung cancer: initial results of the randomized prospective ACOSOG Z0030 trial. *Ann Thorac Surg* 2006;81;1013–1020.
127. Ginsberg RJ, Rubinstein LV. Randomized trial of lobectomy versus limited resection for T1 N0 non-small cell lung cancer. Lung Cancer Study Group. *Ann Thorac Surg* 1995;60:615–622.
128. Asamura H, Goya T, Koshiishi Y, et al. How should the TNM staging system for lung cancer be revised? A simulation based on the Japanese Lung Cancer Registry populations. *J Thorac Cardiovasc Surg* 2006;132:316–319.
129. Nakamura H, Kawasaki N, Taguchi M, et al. Survival following lobectomy vs limited resection for stage I lung cancer: a meta-analysis. *Br J Cancer* 2005;28;92:1033–1037.
130. Nakayama H, Yamada K, Saito H, et al. Sublobar resection for patients with peripheral small adenocarcinomas of the lung: surgical outcome is associated with features on computed tomographic imaging. *Ann Thorac Surg* 2007;84:1675–1679.

131. National Cancer Institute, Clinical Trials. Phase III Randomized Study of Lobectomy Versus Sublobar Resection in Patients with Small Peripheral Stage IA Non-Small Cell Lung Cancer. Available at: http://www.cancer.gov/clinicaltrials/CALGB-140503.
132. Pennathur A, Luketich JD, Abbas G, et al. Radiofrequency ablation for the treatment of stage I non-small cell lung cancer in high-risk patients. *J Thorac Cardiovasc Surg* 2007;134:857–864.
133. Dupuy DE, DiPetrillo T, Gandhi S, et al. Radiofrequency ablation followed by conventional radiotherapy for medically inoperable stage I non-small cell lung cancer. *Chest* 2006;129:738–745.
134. Simon CJ, Dupuy DE, DiPetrillo TA, et al. Pulmonary radiofrequency ablation: long-term safety and efficacy in 153 patients. *Radiology* 2007;243:268–275.
135. Henschke CI, Yankelevitz DF, Altorki NK. The role of CT screening for lung cancer. *Thorac Surg Clin* 2007;17:137–142.
136. Raz DJ, Zell JA, Ou SH, et al. Natural history of stage I non-small cell lung cancer: implications for early detection. *Chest* 2007;132:193–199.
137. Parkin DM, Moss SM. Lung cancer screening. Improved survival but no reduction in deaths–the role of "overdiagnosis." *Cancer* 2000;89:2369–2376.
138. Hamashima C, Sobue T, Muramatsu Y, et al. Comparison of observed and expected numbers of detected cancers in the research center for cancer prevention and screening program. *Jpn J Clin Oncol* 2006;36:301–308.
139. McMahon PM, Kong CY, Johnson BE, et al. Estimating long-term effectiveness of lung cancer screening in the Mayo CT screening study. *Radiology* 2008;248:278–287.
140. Chien CR, Chen TH. Mean sojourn time and effectiveness of mortality reduction for lung cancer screening with computed tomography. *Epidemiology* 2008;122(11):2594–2599.
141. Daniel JC, Smythe WR. Gene therapy of lung cancer. *Semin Surg Oncol* 2003;21:196–204.
142. Chorostowska-Wynimko J, Szpechcinski A. The impact of genetic markers on the diagnosis of lung cancer: a current perspective. *J Thorac Oncol* 2007;2:1044–1051.
143. Kelloff GJ, Lippman SM, Dannenberg AJ, et al. AACR Task Force on Cancer Prevention. Progress in chemoprevention drug development: the promise of molecular biomarkers for prevention of intraepithelial neoplasia and cancer—a plan to move forward. *Clin Cancer Res* 2006;12:3661–3697.
144. Gadgeel SM, Ali S, Philip PA, et al. Response to dual blockade of epidermal growth factor receptor (EGFR) and cycloxygenase-2 in non-small cell lung cancer may be dependent on the EGFR mutational status of the tumor. *Cancer* 2007;110:2775–2784.
145. Lippman SM, Gibson N, Subbaramaiah K, et al. Combined targeting of the epidermal growth factor receptor and cyclooxygenase-2 pathways. *Clin Cancer Res* 2005;11:6097–6099.
146. Greenberg AK, Lee MS. Biomarkers for lung cancer: clinical uses. *Curr Opin Pulm Med* 2007;13:249–255.

CHAPTER 16

Claudia I. Henschke
David F. Yankelevitz
Olli S. Miettinen

Screening for Lung Cancer

WHY CONSIDER SCREENING

Lung cancer makes, at present, for quite a sad chapter in pulmonary medicine. In the United States, some 170,000 cases are diagnosed annually[1]; the average cost of care per patient is about $50,000[2–4]; and yet, the annual number of deaths from this disease is almost as high as the number of cases diagnosed, some 160,000.[1] This is to say that, despite the very costly care, the *case–fatality rate*—the proportion of cases that are fatal—is near 95%.

While the overall case–fatality rate remains dismal, cases diagnosed in stage I—before clinically manifest metastases—are quite commonly curable and, thus, nonfatal. Depending on the size of the tumor at diagnosis, the curability rate ranges from some 50% to more than 90%[5–8] (see Chapters 30 and 32). Thus, the problem with lung cancer now is that those stage I diagnoses remain quite uncommon, representing only some 15% of all diagnoses of lung cancer.[9]

The solution to this problem potentially is the pursuit of early, latent-state diagnosis in persons at relatively high risk for lung cancer; that is, *screening* high-risk people for lung cancer, before any overt, clinical manifestations of the disease.

That *some* increase in stage I diagnoses can be achieved by means of a suitable regimen of screening is obvious; but the question is whether the attainable increase is substantial enough to justify the screening, especially for people with only moderately elevated risk for lung cancer. It is thus important to know the *magnitude* of the stage shift, notably the increase in the proportion of stage I diagnoses, and this in reference to a well-thought-out, realistic regimen of the screening. For, the attainable rate of curability is, to a close approximation, the proportion of stage I diagnoses multiplied by the curability rate of stage I cases, specifically such stage I cases that are diagnosed in the context of the screening—asymptomatic and with the tumor typically smaller than in stage I diagnoses in the absence of screening.

Screening for lung cancer has been of interest not only because of the generally dismal prognosis in the absence of screening but also for two other reasons: highly discriminating risk assessment is possible to identify those at high risk, and the small, latent-state lung cancers tend to be relatively well identifiable against the backdrop of the airy parenchyma of the lungs in radiographic imaging, particularly in computed tomography (CT) imaging.

Interest particularly heightened when several studies demonstrated the considerable superiority of CT over traditional radiography (chest x-ray [CXR]) in the identification of small pulmonary nodules.[10–13] What is more, research on CT screening for lung cancer has already led to quite a well-established regimen for it,[14,15] and the research also has produced evidence indicating the attainability of quite a high rate of curability of this, thus far, near-uniformly fatal disease.[16–18] Thus, the time has come for physicians to consider CT screening for lung cancer of persons at high risk for the disease or for persons who are asking their doctors about it. These decisions should be made on a case by case with the individual at issue suitably informed by his or her doctor.

Research on Screening for Lung Cancer In the early 1970s, the National Cancer Institute (NCI) funded a screening trial for lung cancer.[19] In this trial, sputum cytology was the screening test and half of the 30,000 high-risk participants were to be randomly assigned to the "intervention" (sputum cytology every 4 months for 6 years) and half to the "control" (no screening). All participants were to have annual CXR. This study evolved into three separate ones, each having about 10,000 participants: the Memorial Sloan-Kettering Lung Project (MSKLP),[20,21] the Johns Hopkins Lung Project (JHLP),[22,23] and the Mayo Lung Project (MLP).[24,25] The MSKLP and JHLP performed the study as planned for 6 years. The MLP investigators, however, wanted to test both sputum cytology and the CXR and thus developed a different protocol. They first screened all of the 10,933 participants using both sputum cytology and CXR, and then assigned 9211 people with no evidence of cancer on the baseline round to either receive sputum cytology and CXR every 4 months for 6 years or to no screening; all received the usual Mayo Clinic advice of having annual screening.

At the completion of these studies in the late 1970s, none showed a reduction in lung cancer mortality because of screening using sputum cytology. Beyond this, because of the results of the MLP, CXR was also deemed not to be useful, even though the investigators themselves[26–28] as well as independent experts[29–31] judged the MLP to be inconclusive and seriously flawed. Further, the International Union Against Cancer (UICC) workshop on screening for cancer[32] in 1984 concluded that "the effectiveness of annual CXR in reducing lung cancer mortality was not evaluable in these trials. A case-control study was proposed to attempt a relatively quick evaluation, to be followed by a randomized trial if indicated. A search for new screening procedures is warranted."

Subsequently, in Japan where screening with CXR continued as a matter of national policy, five case-control studies were performed.[33–37] These five studies considered the timing of diagnosis with respect to the screening test, accumulated many more lung cancers than have been found in the randomized trials, and provided convincing evidence that deaths from lung cancer were less common if the diagnosis was achieved within 12 months of having CXR, but not when the delay was longer.

Ultimately in the United States, the NCI funded another screening trial to assess the benefit screening for prostate, lung, colorectal, and ovarian cancer, known as the PLCO trial.[38] For lung cancer, participants were randomly assigned to receive the "intervention" (baseline and two annual CXRs) or no screening. It was started in 1993, but the conclusions of this trial have not yet been reported.

Interestingly, at the same time as the lung cancer trial was being planned in the early 1970s, the NCI also funded a trial to assess the benefit of screening for colorectal cancer.[39] This trial enrolled 45,000 participants, 15,000 received annual screening, 15,000 biannual screening, and 15,000 no screening, but even with the greater number of participants, it did not show a mortality reduction after 5 years of screening and further follow-up. But for this trial, different from the lung cancer trials, the decision was made to provide another 5 years of screening and ultimately some 20 years after the trial started, it demonstrated a significant mortality reduction, improved survival rate, and a decrease in the incidence of late-stage cancers due to screening.[39,40] Since then, many advances in screening for colon cancer have been introduced, and they are accepted and reimbursed without any further evidence from randomized trials.

Research in the CT Era In 1993, we initiated the Early Lung Cancer Action Project (ELCAP) for research on CT screening for lung cancer.[10,11,41] To us, different from the prior randomized trials, screening is not a single test nor an intervention, rather it is a sequential process of pursuing early, latent-stage *diagnosis* of the cancer in order to provide for early treatment of it.[42] From this vantage, we saw it necessary to first endeavor to develop a justifiable regimen for the diagnostic process; that is, a suitable definition of the initial test, of its positive result, and of the workup that is to follow that positive result, possibly leading to diagnosis of the cancer.[42] Thereupon, the principal concern was the *diagnostic* performance properties of the regimen, and updating of this regimen based on emerging evidence and new technologies. Secondarily, there was going to be need for *prognostic* research, focusing on the curability of screen-diagnosed cases of lung cancer, stage I cases in particular.

Initially, the first version of the CT screening regimen was compared with its CXR counterpart, applying both to all participants in the study.[11] Each regimen's diagnostic performance was addressed in terms of the proportion of stage I diagnoses among all diagnoses and the proportion of screen-diagnoses among all diagnoses. In the baseline round, 29 cases of lung cancer were diagnosed, 27 of them screen-diagnosed, two interim-diagnosed. Of the 29, 25 were in clinical stage I, all of them screen diagnosed.[11] CXR screening identified only seven of the 27 cases of screen diagnosed by the CT regimen, and only 4 of the 23 stage I cases. Consequently, only CT was used in the 1184 repeat screenings.[41] In these repeat screenings, seven cases of lung cancer were diagnosed, and there were no interim diagnoses. Of the seven, six were in clinical stage I.

Subsequent studies of the expanded ELCAP in New York State[43] and then throughout the world[44] showed that the proportion of diagnoses in clinical stage I has remained high, around 85%, for both baseline and annual repeat rounds of screening, with rare interim diagnoses, confirming the initial ELCAP results.

Prognostic research as to the curability of screen-diagnosed cases of lung cancer was provided after long term follow-up of the diagnosed cases of lung cancer. This research demonstrated an estimated curability rate of 80% for all those diagnosed with lung cancer, regardless of stage and treatment. If diagnosed in clinical stage I and promptly resected, the estimated rate was 92%.[44] The high curability rates are not surprising as others previously had shown that when lung cancer is diagnosed when it is still small and in stage I, it is highly curable.[5–8]

The high proportion of stage I diagnoses and the high estimated curability rate have raised the concern by some that these may be due to "overdiagnosed" lung cancers,[45] meaning that CT screening identifies slow-growing cancers which, if not resected, would not lead to death. The I-ELCAP protocol aims to minimize "overdiagnosis"[15] by requiring documentation of growth of small nodules prior to biopsy, biopsy diagnosis prior to resection, review of the resected specimens by a panel of expert pulmonary pathologists, and by addressing the outcomes of patients diagnosed in stage I but not treated. The review by pathologists who are experts in pulmonary pathology has confirmed that all diagnosed with lung cancer had genuine lung cancers whose pathologic criteria met the World Health Organization (WHO) criteria of malignancy,[46] and patients diagnosed with stage I lung cancer who had no treatment, all died of it.[44]

Other studies had also shown that if left untreated, stage I lung cancers identified in the absence of screening, are usually fatal[47,48] and so are stage I cases diagnosed by CXR screening.[49–51] If, nevertheless, substantial concern about overdiagnosis still exists, then a randomized trial could ethically be performed by randomly assigning patients diagnosed with potential overdiagnosed lung cancers to either immediate treatment or delayed treatment. For early prostate cancer, such a trial was performed and it demonstrated that even for a cancer with a much lower fatality rate, surgical resection was significantly better.[52]

Slower-growing cancers are proportionately more common among cases diagnosed in the baseline round of screening, a phenomenon that has been termed *length bias*.[45] This bias is reflected by the pathologic subtypes of cancers diagnosed in the baseline round in which a higher proportion of adenocarcinomas and lower proportion of squamous and small cell carcinomas were identified as compared with the repeat rounds.[46] Further insight as to which cancers might be slower growing was provided by the initial 1000 ELCAP participants as we had identified a higher proportion of cancers manifesting as subsolid (nonsolid and part-solid) nodules in the baseline rounds than in the repeat rounds.[53,54] The significance of finding subsolid nodules, previously termed *ground-glass opacities*, relative to lung cancer had not been fully appreciated (see Chapter 33). Remarkably, the rate of malignancy was significantly higher for part-solid nodules than for either solid or nonsolid ones.[53] We also found that the distribution by type of malignancy was very different, with the malignancies manifesting as subsolid nodules either being adenocarcinomas with bronchioloalveolar features or adenocarcinomas-mixed subtype, whereas malignancies manifesting as solid nodules included the entire spectrum of the cell types of lung cancer with the exception of adenocarcinoma with bronchioloalveolar features.[46] Analyses of the growth rates of adenocarcinomas has allowed us to identify those manifesting as nonsolid nodules as being slower growing lung cancers.[54]

The clinical concern about slowly growing malignancies is to understand their course in the absence of treatment and then to treat them appropriately. In the lung, typical carcinoid tumors are a good example. Although considered to be benign in the 1970s, this cell type was reclassified as a malignancy in the 1980s when it was recognized that this was a neuroendocrine tumor, albeit a slowly growing one. Faster-growing neuroendocrine tumors are atypical carcinoids, and small cell carcinomas. Clinical management has taken these differences into account so that different treatment options are provided for these different subtypes. Similarly, clinical management and treatment might well be different for certain subtypes of adenocarcinoma, particularly those manifesting as nonsolid nodules.

It now is quite commonplace to think about overdiagnosis as encompassing identification not only of slowly growing cancers but also of genuinely life-threatening cancers in persons who die of some other cause. In the former case, the person is thus subjected to overtreatment, that is, treatment of a screen-detected cancer when not at risk of dying of the cancer, the cancer being effectively benign. Diagnosis of the latter type occurs when screening is performed on wrong indications (as for life expectancy) as the person has a genuine life-threatening cancer but dies of another cause. We do not view this latter type as an overdiagnosed cancer and have addressed competing causes of death in the context of CT screening separately.[55]

Important updates on the regimen of screening were based on information obtained from the initial ELCAP and its successors. With the technologic advances in CT scanners markedly reducing the image thickness, the definition of a positive result of the initial test at baseline needed to be updated to avoid unnecessary diagnostic workup. From the accumulated information on the very small noncalcified nodules less than 5.0 mm in diameter, ever more frequently detected at baseline, we found that such nodules only required a follow-up CT scan 1 year later, at the time of the first annual repeat screening.[56] We also found that short-term follow-up CT obviated the need for further evaluation of up to 75% of the newly identified nodules on repeat screenings, as they had either resolved or regressed.[57] The usefulness of growth as an indication for biospy of small nodules was tested[58–62] and was found to minimize unnecessary biopsies, so that for recommended biopsies the malignancy rate was above 90%,[43,44] while when not recommended but performed, the malignancy rate was essentially zero. The workup following other findings on the CT scans, such as mediastinal masses,[63] cardiac calcifications,[64] and emphysema[65] were formulated leading the way to combined screening of the major tobacco-related diseases in the chest, that is, lung cancer, emphysema, and coronary artery disease.

Curability Gain and Mortality Reduction As should be evident from the foregoing, screening for lung cancer is a complex topic of *diagnostic* pursuit in *clinical* medicine, not one of population-level intervention in community medicine. The proximal aim of the screening is the attainment of early diagnosis; the purpose of pursuing early diagnosis is to provide for early treatment; and the purpose of seeking to provide for early treatment is the ultimate one: to thereby enhance the probability that treatment results in *cure* of the cancer in the cared-for person. Were the screening to be provided in the framework of community medicine—as "mass" screening in the meaning of more or less indiscriminate application of a single, simple test to members of the cared-for population—"its ultimate purpose would be seen to be reduction in the rate of lung cancer mortality in the cared-for population, consequent the test-positives" referrals to clinical care—for further diagnostic workup, ultimately leading to early diagnoses of the cancer and their associated enhanced curability in individual cases.

The consequence of screening on the rate of a cancer's curability can be studied through rates of surviving the cancer, although only with attention to an important subtlety in this. A misleading way, it is generally understood, is to compare, say, 5-year survival rates between those whose cancer is diagnosed in the framework of screening (screen- and interim-diagnosed cases combined) and those in whom the cancer is diagnosed in the absence of screening. Most of the cases diagnosed under screening are diagnosed with a "lead time," earlier than they would be diagnosed in the absence of screening—pursuit of this lead time being the very essence of screening. Consequent to this, assessment of the curability gain from screening in terms of comparison of survival rates can be marred by "lead time bias": the, say, 5-year survival rate following diagnosis among the screened is prone to be higher than among the unscreened already on the basis of the lead time peculiar to the screened, even if early treatment is no more commonly curative than is treatment in the absence of screening.

Study of a cancer's curability requires a "survival analysis" in which survival over a particular, rather short span of time subsequent to diagnosis—5 years, say—is replaced by long-term survival, in a particular meaning of this. The survival rate naturally is a decreasing function of time since diagnosis; but in the absence of deaths from other, "competing" causes, this time function levels off and reaches its asymptote. This "cause-specific" asymptotic survival rate represents the rate with which the cancer has been cured. By the same token, this survival rate is the cancer's *curability rate* provided that the most effective treatment has been applied in all of the cases, without any undue delays after their diagnoses. Competing causes of death cannot be eliminated, of course; but elimination of their role can be achieved statistically, so as to address the cause-specific survival rate that refers to the cancer in the absence of other causes of death.

In the I-ELCAP, we addressed the curability of lung cancer, given its diagnosis in the framework of such screening as had been applied in that program.[44] Of all the diagnoses, 85% had been achieved in clinical stage I; and for those in whom stage I diagnosis had been followed by timely resection, the 10-year cause-specific survival rate—apparently representing the survival function's asymptote—was 92%. These results suggested the overall curability rate of 0.85 (0.92) = 78%. This may, however, be an overestimate, on the basis not only of involvement of some overdiagnosed cases but also of application of the Kaplan-Meier estimation of the survival rate to follow up well past the time of the last death from lung cancer, with very few subjects contributing to the follow-up beyond that time.

Insofar as overdiagnosis is perceived to be a possibility in ELCAP-type screening for lung cancer, the need in practice may be to refrain from routine early treatment of the types of stage I cases that are most likely to be very slowly progressing, to treat them only once follow-up shows definite further growth at a substantial rate. The frequency with which this provides for avoidance of overtreatment—of overdiagnosed cases—has not yet been assessed in the I-ELCAP, nor elsewhere. But the assessment is feasible, and it will be done, possibly leading to downward adjustment of the curability-rate estimate. Accrual of further experience with long-term survival may have the same effect.

The curability gain can, in principle, be quantitatively assessed through *mortality* reduction also. If the screening of a cohort is continued long enough, there comes a period of follow-up time in which the proportional gain in curability is manifest in the same proportional reduction in the cause-specific mortality rate. This, however, is not a practical way of assessing the curability gain from CT screening for lung cancer.

Now, there are those who take interest in quantification of the mortality reduction associated with screening of for an arbitrary, short duration, and without concern to focus on the period of follow-up time in which the curability gain takes its maximal manifestation in proportional reduction in the cause-specific mortality—addressing, instead, the reduction in the cumulative mortality from the cancer over the entire, arbitrarily long duration of follow-up. This was the case in the Mayo Lung Project originally,[24] and also upon a subsequent major extension of its duration of follow-up.[66] There is concern that the duration of screening and follow-up for the ongoing National Lung Screening Trial (NLST)[67] could be impacted by its study design and could prematurely create the impression that not much is gained from the screening—or, even, that nothing is gained.[68]

Guidelines for Screening for Lung Cancer and Needed Revisions

Prior to the late 1970s, CXR had been recommended by the American Cancer Society (ACS) for people at high risk of lung cancer, that is, heavy smokers and workers in asbestos industry.[69] Subsequently, the ACS adopted new guidelines for making the recommendations that called for good evidence of "test efficacy" in that the medical benefits were to outweigh the risks, the cost of the testing was to be in reasonable proportion to the expected benefits, and the test was to be practical and feasible. Largely as a result of the randomized trials described previously, the ACS changed its recommendation to be against screening for lung cancer in 1980.[69] Later in 2000, a nine-point protocol was introduced which placed primary importance on the results of randomized trials, less on nonrandomized studies and even less on expert opinion.[70] In 2001, the ACS clarified its recommendation against screening for lung cancer, stating that "The ACS does not recommend lung cancer screening for asymptomatic individuals at risk for lung cancer," but pointed out that the ACS distinguishes between recommendations concerning mass screening from those pertaining to clinical decisions on or by individuals. Thus the recommendation against screening expressly was not intended to discourage early-detection tests on individuals, as it was stated that "individual physicians and patients may decide that the evidence is sufficient to warrant the use of these screening tests on an individual basis."[71]

The U.S. Public Health Service convened the U.S. Preventive Services Task Force (USPSTF) in 1984 to provide guidelines for screening. Later in 1998, this task force was placed under the Agency for Healthcare Research and Quality (AHRQ). The mission of the USPSTF was to evaluate the benefit of preventive services with specificity to age, gender, and risk factors for disease; to make recommendations about which preventive services should be incorporated into primary-care routines, for which populations, and to develop a research agenda for clinical preventive care.[72,73] It has subsumed screening under preventive (rather than diagnostic) services. The recommendations are graded according to the strength of the evidence and the magnitude of the net benefit (benefits minus harms) on a scale from a strong recommendation for to recommending against, or to neither recommending for or against. The quality of the evidence is graded as being good, fair, or poor and randomized trials are considered to be superior to "cohort and case-control" studies. In 1998, the USPSTF recommended against screening for lung cancer, against use of either CXR or sputum cytology as a screening test.[73] In 2004, the USPSTF changed its recommendation to the judgement that there is insufficient evidence to recommend for or against the screening with either CT, CXR, or sputum cytology.[74] This change in recommendation by the USPSTF was stated to be primarily based on five case-control studies performed in Japan as previously reported, which demonstrated a benefit of annual CXR screening.[33–37]

The practically exclusive reliance of both the ACS and the USPSTF on randomized trials in evaluating screening for lung cancer has persisted, despite two extensive reviews having demonstrated that well-designed "cohort" and "case-control" studies on screening show little evidence of overestimation of the benefit.[75,76] And it has persisted even when both agencies have recommended screening for breast and colorectal cancers, before there was any evidence from randomized trials, and despite controversial results from these.

Both the ACS and USPSTF guidelines state that a person interested in being screened for lung cancer discuss it with his/her physician. Needed for such a discussion naturally is information on the benefit from the screening specific to the individual's risk characteristics.

The benefit from screening needs to be addressed in terms of individual's probabilities of: (a) the screening if now applied, resulting in the diagnosis of lung cancer; (b) surviving all other potential causes of death over particular periods of prospective time; and (c) cure resulting from presymptomatic treatment of lung cancer.[77] We addressed the survival benefit specific to the baseline round of screening for smokers 60 to 84 years of age. The estimated probability of survival gain was 0.4% for a 60-year-old individual with 10 pack-years of smoking who quit 20 years ago, 3.1% for a 70-year-old current smoker with 100 pack-years, and 2.0% for an 85-year-old current smoker with 150 pack-years. Clearly, the benefit increases with increasing age up to 70 years and ultimately decreases. We provided this information both for current and former smokers. Thus, when seeking counsel about initiation of screening for lung cancer, an estimate of the probability of survival gain from the first round of CT screening, specific to the person's age and history of smoking can be provided. Based on this information, we believe there is sufficient evidence for it to be reasonable for a person at high risk for lung cancer with a sufficient life expectancy to pursue screening.

CONCLUSION

There is a growing body of evidence collected over the past 12 years that CT screening for lung cancer leads to a dramatic increase in the proportion of early stage genuine (fatal in the absence of early treatment) lung cancer relative to symptom-prompted diagnosis and a marked improvement in long-term survival (Table 16.1). As lung cancer is the most common cause of cancer death in both men and women in the industrialized world, it is a major public health problem. We think that the guidelines should be revised to recognize the following points as has already been published by the Society of Thoracic Radiology in the minority report[82]:

1. It is well-accepted that the curability of Stage I lung cancers is very high relative to the curability of late-stage cancers; and within Stage I, cancers less than 3 cm in diameter (Stage IA) are more curable than those that are larger (Stage IB);
2. Studies on annual CT screening have established that the lung cancers are much more commonly diagnosed at Stage I and at smaller sizes than by chest radiography.
3. Based on the points above, it is knowable that annual CT screening for lung cancer provides for prevention of death from lung cancer by early intervention. Quantitative assessment of the actual magnitude of this benefit is being pursued by studies in the U.S. and elsewhere.
4. A person at high-risk for lung cancer yet free of suspicion-raising symptoms of it, who is interested in potentially being screened, should be fully apprized of the implications of screening and of the treatment that may result. In light of this, it is reasonable for the individual to choose to be screened by a suitably defined CT regimen.

Point 3 follows from points 1 and 2. Point 4 draws from point 3 together with the principle of Patients' Autonomy, recently enunciated by a prestigious European–U.S. Joint Commission.[83]

Editors note: The screening of lung cancer is a highly controversial topic and the results of the NLST will not be known when this edition of Lung Cancer is published. Unfortunately, there are few other organized programs in the United States or abroad besides the I-ELCAP which continue to offer "fee for service" lung cancer screening with a methodology that insures that the client as well as the referring physician is appraised of the status of the studies. The I-ELCAP group has made a strong argument for the use of lung cancer screening in high risk individuals, yet validation of benefit remains a topic for future discussion.

TABLE 16.1 Diagnostic and Prognostic Performance of Computed Temography Screening Trials

Project Name, Years Criteria for Enrollment		Enrolled Baseline Annual	Patients with Lung Cancer Baseline + Interim + Sputum Only Annual + Interim + Sputum Only	Lung Cancer Prevalence Baseline Annual	Ratio Baseline Annual	% Stage I* Baseline Annual	Lung Cancer Survival Rate
ELCAP, New York, 1993–1999[11,41]	Median age: 67 Median pack-years: 45%	1000	27 + 2 + not done	2.9%	4.9	86%	
Age >60 yrs; pack-year >10	%current smokers: 43% %male: 54%	1184	7 + 0 + not done	0.6%		86%	
Nagano, Japan, 1996–1998[13,78]	Median age: 64 Median pack-years: NR	5483	37 + 0 + 1	0.7%	3.2	100%	10-yr overall: 86%;
Age >40 yrs; pack-year not required	%current smokers: 46% %male: 55%	8303	18 + 0 + 0	0.2%		86%	path stage I: 90%
ALCA-NCC, Japan, 1993–2001[12,16]	Median age: NR Median pack-years: NR	1611	13 + 0 + 1	0.9%	3.1	79%	5-yr overall: 71%;
Age >40 yrs; pack-year not required	%current smokers: 86% %male: 88%	7891	19 + 0 + 3	0.3%		82%	Baseline: 76%; annual 65%
Hitachi, Japan, 2001–2002[79]	Median age: NR Median pack-years: NR	7956	36 + 0 + 0	0.5%	6.3	86%	
Age >40 yrs; pack-yr not required	%current smokers: 62% %male: 79%	5568	4 + 0 + 0	0.1%		100%	
Mayo Clinic, 1999–2004[80]	Median age: 59 Median pack-years: 51	1520	30 + 0 + 1	2.0%	2.6	77%[a]	
Age >50 yrs; pack-year >20;	%current smokers: 61%	4472	31 + 3 + 1	0.8%		71%[a]	Path stage I: 94%
Istituto Tumori, Italy, 2000–2001[81]	Median age: 58 Median pack-years: 40%	1035	12[b] + 6[c] + 0 + not done	1.7%	3.5	72%	
Age >50 yrs; pack-year >20	%current smokers: 86% %male: 71%	996	5[c] + 0 + not done	0.5%		100%	Path stage I: 94%
International-ELCAP, 1993–2006[44]	Median age: 61 Median pack-years: 30%	31,567	405 + 5 + not done	1.3%	4.8	85%[d]	10-yr overall: 80%;
Age >40 yrs; pack-year not required quit <10 yrs ago	%current smokers: 37% %male: 58% %male: 52%	27,456	74 + 0 + not done	0.3%		86%[d]	Timely resected stage I: 92%

[a]Included six limited small cell in stage I for consistency with other studies.
[b]One typical carcinoid included.
[c]Six had been identified at baseline low-dose CT, either <5 or >5 mm and considered benign and were identified as cancers on first annual.
[d]Clinical staging prior to surgery.
NR, no record.

Summary

1. Lung cancer prevalence rate depends on risk characteristics. It ranged from 0.1% to 0.8% per 1000 screened depending on age and smoking history.
   *Stage I diagnoses include non–small and small cell cancers without lymph node metastases and multiple adenocarcinoma without lymph node metastases (based on pathology if resected).
2. Seven studies showed consistency in finding a high proportion of stage I diagnoses ranging from 71% to 100% and the frequency depends on the regimen of screening and adherence to it.
3. Two studies reported overall long-term survival rates 71% or higher. Survival was 92% or better if in stage I and resected. Survival rate reflects proportion in stage I.
4. Few interim diagnoses of lung cancer (symptom-prompted between screenings) and few detected only by sputum cytology.
5. For comparison, a consistent definition of baseline, repeat cancers, and interim cancers is needed: (a) baseline cancer: nodule is identified on initial CT at baseline, (b) annual cancer: nodule is first identified on initial CT at annual repeat, and (c) interim cancer: symptom-prompted diagnoses between screenings.

REFERENCES

1. American Cancer Society. Statistics for 2006. Cancer Facts and Figures. Available at: http://www.cancer.org/docroot/stt/stt_0.asp. Accessed January 16, 2007.
2. Kutikova L. Bowman L, Chang S, et al. The economic burden of lung cancer and associated costs of treatment failure in the United States. *Lung Cancer* 2005;50:143–154.
3. Woodward RM, Brown ML, Stewart ST, et al. The value of medical interventions for lung cancer in the elderly: results from SEER-CMHSF. *Cancer* 2007;110:2511–2518.
4. Warren JL, Yabroff KR, Meekins A, et al. Evaluation of trends in the cost of initial cancer treatment. *J Natl Can Inst* 2008;100:888–897.
5. Martini N, Bains MS, Burt ME, et al. Incidence of local recurrence and second primary tumors in resected Stage I lung cancer. *J Thorac Cardiovasc Surg* 1995;109:120–129.
6. Buell PE. The importance of tumor size in prognosis for resected bronchogenic carcinoma. *J Surg Oncol* 1971;3:539–551.
7. Mountain CF. Revisions in the International System for Staging Lung Cancer. *Chest* 1997;111:1710–1717.
8. Inoue K, Sato M, Fujimura S, et al. Prognostic assessment of 1310 patients with non-small-cell lung cancer who underwent complete resection from 1980 to 1993. *J Thorac Cardiovasc Surg* 1998;116:407–411.
9. SEER Relative Survival Rates by Stage at Diagnosis. SEER 9 Registries for 1988–2003. Fast Stats: Lung and Bronchus Cancer. Available at: http://seer.cancer.gov/faststats/sites.php?site=Lung%20and%20Bronchus%20Cancer&stat=Survival. Accessed August 14, 2009.
10. Henschke CI, Miettinen OS, Yankelevitz DF, et al. Radiographic screening for cancer: New paradigm for its scientific basis. *Clin Imaging* 1994;18:16–20.
11. Henschke CI, McCauley DI, Yankelevitz DF, et al. Early Lung Cancer Action Project: overall design and findings from baseline screening. *Lancet* 1999;10;354:99–105.
12. Kaneko M, Eguchi K, Ohmatsu H, et al. Peripheral Lung Cancer: Screening and detection with low-dose spiral CT versus radiography. *Radiology* 1996;201:798–802.
13. Sone S, Takashima S, Li F, et al. Mass screening for lung cancer with mobile spiral computed tomography scanner. *Lancet* 1998;351:1242–1245.
14. Henschke CI, Yankelevitz DF, Smith JP, et al. Screening for lung cancer: the early lung cancer action approach. *Lung Cancer* 2002;35:143–148.
15. International Early Lung Cancer Action Program protocol. Available online at: http://www.IELCAP.org. Accessed August 14, 2009.
16. Sobue T, Moriyama N, Kaneko M, et al. Screening for lung cancer with low-dose helical computed tomography: anti-lung cancer association project. *J Clin Oncol* 2002;20:911–920.
17. International Early Lung Cancer Action Program Investigators; Henschke CI, Yankelevitz DF, Libby DM, et al. Survival of patients with stage I lung cancer detected on CT screening. *N Engl J Med* 2006;355:1763–1771.
18. Sone S, Nakayama T, Honda T, et al. Long-term follow-up study of a population-based 1996–1998 mass screening programme for lung cancer using mobile low-dose spiral computed tomography. *Lung Cancer* 2007;58:329–341.
19. Berlin NI, Buncher CR, Fontana RS, et al. The National Cancer Institute Cooperative Early Lung Cancer Detection Program. Results of the initial screen (prevalence). Early lung cancer detection: introduction. *Am Rev Respir Dis* 1984 Oct;130(4):545–549.
20. Flehinger BJ, Melamed MR, Zaman MB, et al. Early lung cancer detection: results of the initial (prevalence) radiologic and cytologic screening in the Memorial Sloan-Kettering study. *Am Rev Respir Dis* 1984 Oct;130(4):555–560.
21. Melamed MR, Flehinger BJ, Zaman MB, et al. Screening for early lung cancer. Results of the Memorial Sloan-Kettering study in New York. *Chest* 1984;86:44–53.
22. Frost JK, Ball WC Jr, Levin ML, et al. Early lung cancer detection: results of the initial (prevalence) radiologic and cytologic screening in the Johns Hopkins study. *Am Rev Respir Dis* 1984;130:549–554.
23. Tockman MS. Survival and mortality from lung cancer in a screened population. *Chest* 1986;89:S324–S326.
24. Fontana RS, Sanderson DR, Taylor WF, et al. Early lung cancer detection: results of the initial (prevalence) radiologic and cytologic screening in the Mayo Clinic study. *Am Rev Respir Dis* 1984;130:561–565.
25. Fontana RS, Sanderson DR, Woolner LB, et al. Lung cancer screening: the Mayo program. *J Occup Med* 1986;28:746–750.
26. Fontana RS, Sanderson DR, Woolner LB, et al. Screening for lung cancer. A critique of the Mayo Lung Project. *Cancer* 1991;67:1155–1164.
27. Fontana RS. The Mayo Lung Project. International Conference on Prevention and Early Diagnosis of Lung Cancer. Varese, Italy, Dec 9–10;1998:15–20.
28. Flehinger BJ, Kimmel M, Polyak T, et al. Screening for lung cancer. The Mayo Lung Project revisited. *Cancer* 1993;73:1573–1580.
29. Miettinen OS. Screening for lung cancer. *Radiol Clin North Am* 2000;38:479–486.
30. Strauss GM, Gleason RE, Sugarbaker DJ. Screening for lung cancer. Another look; a different view. *Chest* 1997;111:754–768.
31. Strauss GM. Screening for lung cancer: an evidence-based synthesis. *Surg Oncol Clin N Am* 1999;8:747–774.
32. Prorok PC, Chamberlain J, Day NE, et al. UICC workshop on the evaluation of screening programmes for cancer. *Int J Cancer* 1984;34:1–4.
33. Sobue T. A case-control study for evaluating lung cancer screening in Japan. *Cancer* 2000;89:2392–2396.
34. Sagawa M, Tsubono Y, Saito Y, et al. A case-control study for evaluating the efficacy of mass screening program for lung cancer in Miyagi Prefecture, Japan. *Cancer* 2001 Aug 1;92:588–594.
35. Tsukada H, Kurita Y, Yokoyama A, et al. An evaluation of screening for lung cancer in Niigata Prefecture, Japan: a population-based case-control study. *Br J Cancer* 2001;85:1326–1331.
36. Nishii K, Ueoka H, Kiura K, et al. A case-control study of lung cancer screening in Okayama Prefecture, Japan. *Lung Cancer* 2001;34:325–332.
37. Okamoto N, Suzuki T, Hasegawa H, et al. Evaluation of a clinic-based screening program for lung cancer with a case-control design in Kanagawa, Japan. *Lung Cancer* 1999;25:77–85.
38. Prorok PC, Andriole GL, Bresalier RS, et al. Design of the Prostate, Lung, Colorectal and Ovarian (PLCO) Cancer Screening Trial. *Control Clin Trials* 2000;21:S273–S309.
39. Mandel JS, Bond JH, Church TR, et al. Reducing mortality from colorectal cancer by screening for fecal occult blood. *N Engl J Med* 1993;328:1365–1371.
40. Mandel JS, Church TR, Bond JH, et al. The effect of fecal occult-blood screening on the incidence of colorectal cancer. *N Engl J Med* 2000;343:1603–1607.
41. Henschke CI, Naidich DP, Yankelevitz DF, et al. Early lung cancer action project: initial findings on repeat screenings. *Cancer* 2001;92:153–159.
42. Henschke CI, Yankelevitz DF, Smith JP, et al. The use of spiral CT in lung cancer screening. In: DeVita VT, Hellman S, Rosenberg SA, eds. *Progress in Oncology 2002.* Sudbury, MA: Jones and Barlett, 2002.
43. New York Early Lung Cancer Action Project Investigators. CT screening for lung cancer: diagnoses resulting from the New York Early Lung Cancer Action Project. *Radiology* 2007;243:239–249.
44. International Early Lung Cancer Action Program Investigators. Survival of patients with stage I lung cancer detected on CT screening. *N Engl J Med* 2006;355:1763–1771.
45. Henschke CI, Smith JP, Miettinen OS. Response to letters to the editor. *N Engl J Med* 2007;356:743–747.
46. Carter D, Vazquez M, Flieder DB, et al. Comparison of pathologic findings of baseline and annual repeat cancers diagnosed on CT screening. *Lung Cancer* 2007;56(2):193–199.
47. Henschke CI, Wisnivesky JP, Yankelevitz DF, et al. Small stage I cancers of the lung: genuineness and curability. *Lung Cancer* 2003;39:327–330.
48. Raz DJ, Zell JA, Ou SH, et al. Natural history of stage I non-small cell lung cancer. *Chest* 2007;132:193–199.
49. Flehinger BJ, Kimmel M, Melamed MR. Survival from early lung cancer. Implications for screening. *Chest* 1992;101:13–18.

50. Sobue T, Suzuki R, Matsuda M, et al. Survival for clinical stage I lung cancer not surgically treated. Comparison between screen-detected and symptom-detected cases. *Cancer* 1992;69:685–692.
51. Yankelevitz DF, Kostis WJ, Henschke CI, et al. Overdiagnosis in chest radiographic screening for lung carcinoma: frequency. *Cancer* 2003;97:1271–1275.
52. Bill-Axelrod A, Holmberg L, Ruutu M, et al. Radical prostatectomy versus watchful waiting in early prostate cancer. *N Eng J Med* 2005;352:1977–1984.
53. Henschke CI, Yankelevitz DF, Mirtcheva R, et al. CT screening for lung cancer: Frequency and significance of part-solid and nonsolid nodules. *AJR Am J Roentgenol* 2002;178:1053–1057.
54. Henschke CI, Shaham D, Yankelevitz DF, et al. CT screening for lung cancer: significance of diagnoses in its baseline cycle. *Clin Imaging* 2006;30:11–15.
55. Henschke CI, Yip R, Yankelevitz DF, et al. Computed tomography screening for lung cancer: competing causes of death. *Clin Lung Cancer* 2006;7:323–325.
56. Henschke CI, Yankelevitz DF, Naidich D, et al. CT screening for lung cancer: suspiciousness of nodules at baseline according to size. *Radiology* 2004;231:164–168.
57. Libby DM, Wu N, Lee IJ, et al. CT screening for lung cancer: the value of short-term CT follow-up. *Chest* 2006;129:1039–1042.
58. Yankelevitz DF, Gupta R, Zhao B, et al. Repeat CT scanning for evaluation of small pulmonary nodules: preliminary results. *Radiology* 1999;212:561–566.
59. Yankelevitz DF, Reeves AP, Kostis WJ, et al. Determination of malignancy in small pulmonary nodules based on volumetrically determined growth rates: preliminary results. *Radiology* 2000;217:251–256.
60. Kostis WJ, Reeves AP, Yankelevitz DF, et al. Three-dimensional segmentation and growth-rate estimation of small pulmonary nodules in helical CT images. *IEEE Tran Med Imaging* 2003;22: 1259–1274.
61. Reeves A, Chan A, Yankelevitz D, et al. On measuring the change in size of pulmonary nodules. *IEEE Trans Med Imaging* 2006;25:433–450.
62. Kostis WJ, Yankelevitz DF, Reeves AP, et al. Small pulmonary nodules: reproducibility of three-dimensional volumetric measurement and estimation of time to follow-up CT. *Radiology* 2004;231:446–452.
63. Henschke CI, Lee I, Wu N, et al. CT screening for lung cancer: prevalence and incidence of mediastinal masses. *Radiology* 2006;239: 581–590.
64. Shemesh J, Henschke CI, Yip R, et al. Detection of coronary artery calcification by age and gender on low-dose CT screening for lung. *Cancer Clin Imaging* 2006;30:181–185.
65. Kostis WJ, Fluture S, Yankelevitz DF, et al. Method for analysis and display of distribution of emphysema in CT scans. *SPIE Medical Imaging* 2003;5032:199–206.
66. Marcus PM, Bergstralh EJ, Fagerstrom RM, et al. Lung cancer mortality in the Mayo Lung Project: impact of extended follow-up. *J Natl Cancer Inst* 2000;92(16):1308–1316.
67. http://www.cancer.gov/nlst. Accessed December 27, 2009.
68. Henschke CI, Yankelevitz DF, Kostis WJ. CT screening for lung cancer. Semin Ultrasound, CT, and MRI. 2003;24:23–32.
69. The American Cancer Society. Cancer of the lung. *Cancer* 1980;30: 199–207.
70. Smith RA, Mettlin CJ, Davis KJ, et al. American Cancer Society guidelines for the early detection of cancer. *Cancer* 2000;50:34–49.
71. Smith RA, von Eschenbach AC, Wender R, et al. American Cancer Society guidelines for the early detection of cancer: update of early detection guidelines for prostate, colorectal, and endometrial cancers: Also: update 2001—testing for early lung cancer detection. *Cancer* 2001;51:38–75.
72. U.S. Preventive Services Task Force. Available at: http://www.ahrq.gov/clinic/uspstfab.htm. Accessed December 7, 2007.
73. U.S. Preventive Services Task Force. *Guide to Clinical Preventive Services. Screening for Lung Cancer.* Washington, D.C., 1989;45–47.
74. Humphrey LL, Johnson M, Teutsch S. Lung cancer screening with sputum cytologic examination, chest radiography, and computed tomography: an update of the U.S. Preventive Services Task Force. *Ann Intern Med* 2004:140:738–753.
75. Benson K, Hartz AJ. A comparison of observational studies and randomized, controlled trials. *N Engl J Med* 2000;342:1878–1886.
76. Concato J, Shah N, Horwitz RI. Randomized, controlled trials, observational studies, and the hierarchy of research designs. *N Engl J Med* 2000;342:1887–1892.
77. International Early Lung Cancer Action Program Investigators. CT screening for lung cancer: individualizing the benefit of the screening. *Eur Resp J* 2007;30: 843–847.
78. Sone S, Nakayama T, Honda T, et al. Long-term follow-up study of a population-based 1996–1998 mass screening programme for lung cancer using mobile low-dose spiral computed tomography scanner. *Lung Cancer* 2007;58:329–341.
79. Nawa T, Nakagawa T, Kusano S, et al. Lung cancer screening using low-dose spiral CT: results of baseline and 1-year follow-up studies. *Chest* 2002;122:15–20.
80. Swensen SJ, Jett JR, Hartman TE, et al. CT screening for lung cancer: five-year prospective experience. *Radiology* 2005;235:259–265.
81. Pastorino U, Bellomi M, Landoni C, et al. Early lung-cancer detection with spiral CT and positron emission tomography in heavy smokers: 2-year results. *Lancet* 2003;362:593–597.
82. Henschke CI, Austin JH, Bauer T, et al. Minority Report: CT screening for lung cancer. *J Thorac Imaging.* 2005;20:324–325.
83. Medical professionalism in the new millennium: a physician charter. *Ann Intern Med* 2002;136:243–246.

CHAPTER 17

Rob J. van Klaveren
Harry J. de Koning

Low-Dose Computed Tomography Screening: Experiences from the Randomized Population-Based Nelson Screening Trial

NELSON TRIAL DESIGN

The Dutch–Belgian lung cancer screening trial (NELSON) investigates whether 16-detector, low-dose, multislice computed tomography (MSCT) screening in year 1, 2, and 4 will decrease lung cancer mortality compared to a control group without screening. Secondary end points of the study are to estimate the cost-effectiveness of this screening program and to assess the impact on quality of life. The design of the NELSON trial is shown in Figure 17.1. NELSON is the only large-scale, randomized, controlled, population-based lung cancer CT-screening trial in Europe, with 15,523 participants. Recruitment started in the second half of 2003, and the first CT screenings were made in April 2004. As of October 2007, the baseline-screening round has been completed, the second round is near its completion, and the third round has recently been started. The screening part of the trial will be finished by the end of 2009, but the follow-up period will continue until the end of 2015. During the first round, lung function tests have been performed, and biosamples (blood, plasma, serum, and sputum cytology) have been taken. The blood sampling and lung function test are repeated during the last screening round.

Recruitment During the first recruitment phase (second half of 2003), addresses of all men born between January 1, 1928 and January 1, 1953 were obtained from the population registries in seven districts in the Netherlands (Groningen, Drenthe, Utrecht, Eemland, Midden-Nederland, Kennemerland, and Amstelland-de Meerlanden) (Fig. 17.1). In addition, addresses of all men and women of the same age were obtained from the population registries of 14 municipalities around Leuven in Belgium. They received a first questionnaire about general health, alcohol consumption, physical exercise, cancer history, family history of lung cancer, body weight and length, education, and their opinion on screening programs in general. The questionnaire contained 11 questions on smoking from the Minimum Common Dataset (May 2002) of the EU–U.S. Collaborative Spiral CT-working group, adapted from the National Cancer Institutes Cancer Data Standards Registry, the recommended smoking measures of the Behavior Change Consortium of the U.S. National Institutes of Health, and from Pistelli et al.[1–3] The most important questions were: "When you last smoked every day, on average, how many cigarettes (shag) do/did you smoke a day?" (<5, 5 to 10, 11 to 15, 16 to 20, 21 to 25, 26 to 30, 31 to 40, 41 to 50, 51 to 60, >60); "What is the total number of years you have smoked/smoke cigarettes or shag every day? Do not include any time you stayed off cigarettes or shag for 6 months or longer." (0 to 5, 6 to 10, 11 to 15, 16 to 20, 21 to 25, 26 to 30, 31 to 35, 36 to 40, 41 to 45, 46 to 50, >50 years) and; "If you have quit smoking, how long has it been since you quit?" (<1 month, 1 to 6 months, 7 months to 1 year, 1 to 3 years, 3 to 5 years, 6 to 10 years, 11 to 15 years, 16 to 20 years, >20 years, not applicable). The questionnaire was accompanied by brief information about the trial.

During this first recruitment phase, 106,931 of the 335,441 subjects (32%) who received the first NELSON questionnaire responded. Mean age of the respondents was 61 (standard deviation: 6.8 years). Response rates were lower in Belgium where we approached more women than in the Netherlands, but were overall equally distributed over the age categories (Table 17.1). Table 17.2 shows the number of respondents for each level of smoking duration, the number of cigarettes smoked per day, and the duration of smoking cessation. Nearly one third of the 106,931 respondents (33,909 [32%]) never smoked, 26,733 (25%) has been smoking for less than 20 years, and 24,783 (23%) quit smoking for more than 20 years.

Selection of Potential Participants In the Netherlands, at present, 23% of women smoke compared to 32% of men.[4] In the past, this difference was greater when even fewer women and more men smoked. Therefore, fewer women in the Dutch population have accrued a long-term exposure to cigarettes compared to men. Because of the lower fraction of high-risk subjects among women, we anticipated before start of the trial that recruiting an equal number of

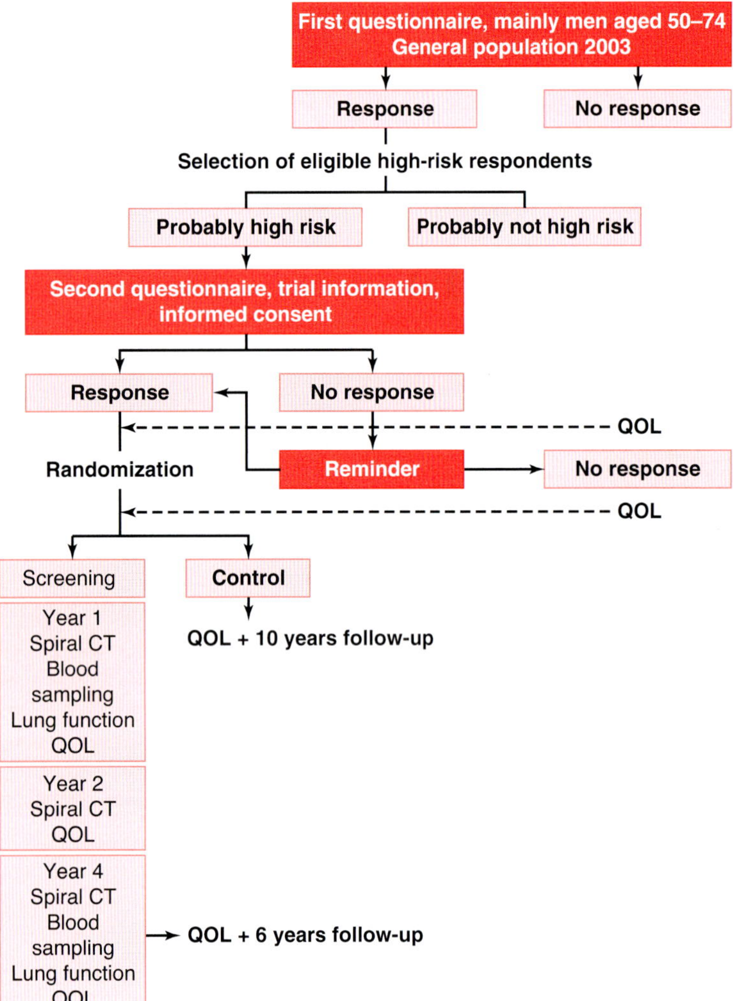

FIGURE 17.1 The different steps in the recruitment process of the Dutch–Belgian helical CT lung cancer screening trial (NELSON) and the different time point at which quality of life will be assessed. *CT*, computed tomography; *QOL*, quality of life.

high-risk women and men would require an enormous effort. Therefore, the Dutch Health Council and the Ministry of Health agreed to invite first men and only in the second phase also women. In that way, we would still be able to demonstrate possible differences in lung cancer detection between men and women, and at the same time limit our recruitment efforts.

Because the smoking exposure history of all respondents on the first NELSON questionnaire was available, a careful decision could be made on whom to invite for the trial. First, the estimated lung cancer mortality risk of the respondents was determined. Next, the required sample size to show a mortality benefit of screening of 20%, 25%, and 30%, and the corresponding number of eligible subjects was determined for various selection scenarios, and finally, the *required participation rate* was determined, defined as the required response of eligible subjects to reach the required sample size. In the optimal selection scenario, the required participation rate was as low as possible, and the required sample size was within the ranges of our capacity in the Netherlands and Belgium (±16,000 participants).

Our estimates of lung cancer mortality were based on the U.S. Cancer Prevention Study II (CPS II), a cohort study that started in 1982 and followed 508,579 men and 676,527 women, aged 30 years or older for 6 years.[5] The CPS II reports lung cancer mortality rates per 100,000 person-years (PY) for groups of men with attained ages 50 to 79 (50 to 59, 60 to 69, and 70 to 79 years), smoking duration of 20 years or more (20 to 29, 30 to 39, 40 to 49, and ≥50 years), and one or more cigarettes smoked per day (1 to 19, 20, 21 to 39, 40, and ≥41 cigarettes per day). Because the CPS II monograph included only data on current smokers, the U.S. Cancer Prevention Study I (CPS I) was used to estimate the effect of smoking cessation. This prospective cohort study started following up 456,491 men and 594,551 women older than 30 years on July 1, 1960. Follow-up was a maximum of 12 years.[6] By varying the thresholds for duration of smoking, the duration of smoking cessation, and the number of cigarettes smoked per day, the mean-estimated expected lung cancer mortality rate (per 1000 PY) for various selection scenarios was determined. Based on the most optimal selection scenario, current and former smokers with 10 years or less

TABLE 17.1 Characteristics of 335,441 Persons Who Received the First NELSON Questionnaire (First Recruitment) and Characteristics of the 106,931 Respondents

	Received Questionnaire, n	Response, n (%)
Gender		
Male	273,044	94,761 (34.7%)
Female*	4018	887 (22.1%)
Unknown†	58,379	11,283 (19.3%)
Country		
Netherlands	269,119	93,515 (34.7%)
Belgium	66,322	13,416 (20.2%)
Age‡		
mean (sd)	61.2 (7)	61 (6.8)
49 yrs	252	53 (21.0%)
50–59 yrs	151,563	49,781 (32.8%)
60–69 yrs	105,396	36,407 (34.5%)
70 yrs and older	45,496	13,363 (29.4%)
Unknown†	32,734	7327 (22.4%)
Total	335,441	106,931 (31.9%)§

*Only in Belgium women were approached in the first recruitment round.

†The population registries of some communities in Belgium did not supply us with data on gender and/or birth date, and gender was not asked in our first questionnaire.

‡Age at mean date of response, which was October 1, 2003.

§Total also includes 69 subjects who responded, but returned a blank questionnaire.

From van Iersel CA, de Koning HJ, Draisma G, et al. Risk-based selection from the general population in a screening trial: selection criteria, recruitment, and power for the Dutch–Belgian randomised lung cancer multi-slice CT screening trial (NELSON). *Int J Cancer* 2007;120:868–874.

of cessation, who smoked more than 15 cigarettes a day for more than 25 years or 10 cigarettes a day for more than 30 years, were selected.[7] Persons with a moderate or bad self-reported health who were unable to climb two flights of stairs and persons with a body weight greater than or equal to 140 kg were excluded from participation. Lung cancer patients diagnosed less than 5 years ago, subjects symptomatic for lung cancer, and persons who had a chest-CT examination less than 1 year before they filled in the first NELSON questionnaire were excluded as well.

Power and Required Sample Size The required sample sizes to demonstrate a lung cancer mortality reduction of 20%, 25%, or 30% were calculated for the various selection scenarios. A 1:1 randomization, a power of 80%, a one-sided α-significance level of 0.05, 95% compliance in the screen group, 5% contamination rate in the control group, and 10 years of follow-up after randomization were assumed.[8] With a power of 80%, enrolment of 17,300 subjects in NELSON is required to demonstrate a lung cancer mortality reduction of 25% or more and 27,900 subjects to demonstrate a lung cancer mortality reduction of 20% or more 10 years of follow-up. In Denmark, 4100 men and women, current and former smokers (quit <10 years), aged 50 to 70, with at least 20 pack-years of smoking have been recruited through the public media. It is planned to pool mortality data with the Danish trial, so that the total number of participants in the NELSON trial will be more than 20,000. NELSON will then be the only trial without screening in controls that is expected to have an 80% power to show a lung cancer mortality reduction of at least 25% 10 years after randomization. When pooling with the Danish trial data, the fraction of women, which comprises 45% of all Danish trial participants, will also increase.

Our population-based recruitment gave insight in the risk profiles of the general population and we estimated that about 15% to 25% of the general (Dutch) population, age 50 to 75 would be the target for routine screening if our eligibility criteria would be applied. We, therefore, believe that our results are generalizable to a sufficiently large part of our population. Another advantage of a population-based recruitment approach is that it is less likely that potential participants exaggerated their smoking history to increase their chance to be invited for the trial, because they were unaware of the selection criteria.

TABLE 17.2 Number of Current smokers and Former Smokers (n = 73,022) of Total Respondents (106,931) on the First NELSON Questionnaire, Grouped by Smoking History (Ages 50–75)*

Number of Respondents, n

Cigarettes per Day	Smoking Duration (yrs)	Duration of Cessation						Total of Every Smokers(%)
		Current Smokers	1 mo–5 yrs	6–10 yrs	11–15 yrs	16–20 yrs	>20 yrs	
1–20	0–20	1718	949	753	1294	2153	14,562	21,429 (29%)
	21–30	1865	1176	1299	1740	1420	3246	10,746 (15%)
	31–40	5426	2268	1347	1173	701	935	11,850 (16%)
	41–50	3683	1260	599	383	145	183	6253 (9%)
	≥51	64	14	0	0	0	0	78 (0.1%)
21–40	0–20	208	152	131	338	639	3164	4632 (6%)
	21–30	572	469	643	957	707	1384	4732 (6%)
	31–40	3035	1445	928	720	366	394	6888 (9%)
	41–50	1978	809	329	239	84	77	3516 (5%)
	≥51	37	10	3	0	0	1	51 (0.1%)
≥41	0–20	27	29	22	39	91	464	672 (1%)
	21–30	61	67	93	131	120	259	731 (1%)
	31–40	260	188	148	132	70	96	894 (1%)
	41–50	236	126	91	51	20	18	542 (1%)
	≥51	5	1	0	2	0	0	8 (0.01%)
Total	**Total of every smokers (%)**	19,175 (26%)	8963 (12%)	6386 (9%)	7199 (10%)	6516 (9%)	24,783 (34%)	73,022 (100%)

*Numbers also include respondents who later appeared to be ineligible for participation for reasons other than smoking history (exclusion criteria) (11%).
From van Iersel CA, de Koning HJ, Draisma G, et al. Risk-based selection from the general population in a screening trial: selection criteria, recruitment, and power for the Dutch–Belgian randomised lung cancer multi-slice CT screening trial (NELSON). *Int J Cancer* 2007;120:868–874.

NELSON MANAGEMENT SYSTEM

To conduct this logistically complex multicenter study, the NELSON Management System (NMS) has been developed. It is a Web-based, interactive database application used for data collection and management of all study-related processes with a completely trackable data collection, study monitoring, reporting of scan results, and scheduling of appointments for follow-up scans. Because the system works with action dates, it provides us with a complete overview and control of the planned actions, such as the planning of follow-up scans, sending of invitations to participants, test results and workup, and evaluation of suspicious nodules.

Screens The participants randomized to the screen arm were invited by an invitation letter to one of the four screening sites (University Hospital Groningen, University Hospital Utrecht and Kennemer Gasthuis Haarlem in the Netherlands, and University Hospital Gasthuisberg Leuven in Belgium). The CT scans used were all 16-detector MSCT scanners (M×8000 IDT or Brilliance 16P, Philips Medical Systems, Cleveland, OH, U.S.A., or Sensation-16, Siemens Medical Solutions, Forchheim, Germany). All scans were realized in about 12 seconds in spiral mode with 16 × 0.75-mm collimation and 15-mm table feed per rotation (pitch = 1.5), in a cranial–caudal scan direction, without contrast in low-dose setting. Depending on the body weight (<50 kg, 50 to 80 kg, and >80 kg), the kilovolt (peak) (kV[p]) settings were 80 to 90, 120, and 140 kV(p), respectively; and to achieve a volume computed tomography dose index (CTDIvol) of 0.8, 1.6, and 3.2 milligrays (mGy), respectively, the milliampere second (mAs) setting were adjusted accordingly depending on the machine used. To minimize breathing artefacts, scans were performed in inspiration after appropriate instruction of the participants.

Image Reading Images have been read on Siemens workstations using the syngo LungCARE software package (version Somaris/5 VB 10A-W) for multidimensional image processing and computer viewing. Lung windows were assessed at a width of 1500 and a level of −650 Hounsfield units. After a first reading by qualified and dedicated radiologists with on average 7 years of reading experience, the data were stored locally on the PACS system, and sent overnight via a protected internet connection to Groningen for second reading and central storage. The consensus double readings were also performed by two qualified radiologists, full time engaged with 1 and 4 years of experience after board certification, respectively. Both the first and second readers evaluated the CT scans independently and uploaded their results into the central database. The nodule management system automatically matched all nodules detected by the first and second reader based on location and size. Subsequently, the second reader checked this automatching for each individual nodule and made manual adjustments in case the matching was incorrect. During this procedure of consensus double reading, the second reader was not blinded for the results of the first reader. This procedure provided three groups of nodules: nodules detected by both readers, nodules detected only by the first reader, and nodules detected only by the second reader. The second reader also checked the consistency of the follow-up recommendations of both readers. If there was a discrepancy, the second reader informed the first reader and both readers reevaluated the CT scan to reach consensus. If no consensus was reached, an expert reader (radiologist with more than 20 years of experience) made the final decision.

During CT evaluation, for each evaluable nodule, the surface characteristics, distance to the pleura, and the aspect of the nodule (i.e., solid, partial solid, or nonsolid) were entered by the radiologist in an electronic data collection form customized for the LungCARE Siemens workstation. Nodules were classified as peripheral if the distance to the thoracic wall was less than one third of the total distance to the lung hilum. Together with the calculated sizes and volumes generated by the Siemens software, these data were automatically uploaded in NMS immediately after completion of the reading for an unlimited number of evaluated nodules per scan. In case of consecutive CT scans, nodules were matched with the same nodules documented on previous scans to determine changes in volume and to estimate the volume doubling time (VDT). After the second reading of the CT scan and after reaching consensus about the screen result and the planned actions to be taken, the NMS generated the appropriate standard letter to inform both the participant and the general practitioner within 3 weeks after the CT scan. Throughout the study, the definition of growth was kept constant and was defined as a percent volume change (PVC) of 25% or more after at least a 3-month interval according to the following formula:

(1) $$\text{PVC}\ (\%) = 100\ (V_2 - V_1)/V_2$$

TABLE 17.3 NELSON Classification of the Different Noncalcified Nodules According to Size at Baseline Screening

NODCAT Baseline	Definition
1	Benign nodule (fat or benign calcifications) or other benign characteristics
2	Any nodule, smaller than NODCAT 3, and no characteristics of NODCAT 1
3	Solid: 50–500 mm^3 Solid, pleural based: 5–10 mm d_{min} Partial solid, nonsolid component: ≥8 mm d_{mean} Partial solid, solid component: 50–500 mm^3 Nonsolid: ≥8 mm d_{mean}
4	Solid: >500 mm^3 Solid, pleural based: >10 mm d_{min} Partial solid, solid component: >500 mm^3

From Xu DM, Gietema H, de Koning H, et al. Nodule management protocol of the NELSON randomised lung cancer screening trial. *Lung Cancer* 2006;54:177–184.

Baseline Screen Protocol Noncalcified nodules (NCN) were classified in four nodules categories (NODCAT) based on size, either 3D (solid and partial solid lesions) or 2D (solid pleural lesions and nonsolid lesions), or based on growth (GROWCAT) according to formula (Table 17.3).[1] NODCAT 1 was defined as benign, NODCAT 2 as nonsignificantly small, NODCAT 3 as indeterminate, and NODCAT 4 as potentially malignant. Based on the highest nodule category found, participants with NODCAT 1 and 2 received a negative test result and were invited for an annual repeat scan (first incidence screen) 1 year later because the likelihood of malignancy in a NODCAT 2 nodule at baseline is less than 1% (Table 17.4).[9,10] NODCAT 3

TABLE 17.4 NELSON Management Protocol for Noncalcified Nodules at Baseline Screening

Nodule Type	NODCAT 1	NODCAT 2	NODCAT 3	NODCAT 4	GROWCAT C
Solid	Negative test	Negative test	Indeterminate test	Positive test	Positive test
	Annual CT	Annual CT	3-month follow-up CT	Refer to pulmonologist for workup and diagnosis	Histological diagnosis required
Partial solid	Negative test	Negative test	Indeterminate test	Positive test	Positive test
	Annual CT	Annual CT	3-month follow-up CT	Refer to pulmonologist for workup and diagnosis	Histological diagnosis required
Solid/pleural based	Negative test	Negative test	Indeterminate test	Positive test	Positive test
	Annual CT	Annual CT	3-month follow-up CT	Refer to pulmonologist for workup and diagnosis	Histological diagnosis required
Nonsolid	Negative test	Negative test	Indeterminate test	Nonexisting category	Positive test
	Annual CT	Annual CT	3-month follow-up CT		Histological diagnosis required

From Xu DM, Gietema H, de Koning H, et al. Nodule management protocol of the NELSON randomised lung cancer screening trial. *Lung Cancer* 2006;54:177–184.

was defined as an indeterminate test result that required a repeat scan 3 to 4 months later to assess growth. If there was no significant growth on the repeat scan, the test result was called negative, and participants were scheduled for an annual repeat CT scan 8 to 9 months later. If there was significant growth, the test result was positive (GROWCAT C), which means that a histological diagnosis had to be obtained (Table 17.4). NODCAT 4 was also a positive test result, which required referral to a pulmonologist for workup and diagnosis. In case of NODCAT 4 and GROWCAT C, the general practitioner was first informed by the radiologist of the screening site by phone about the test results and its consequences, followed by a letter to the participant and the general practitioner.

INCIDENCE SCREEN PROTOCOL

At annual repeat screening, there are two possibilities: either an NCN already exists, and comparison with baseline screening is possible, or the NCN is new. For the new nodules, the same classification according to size was made as for the baseline screening round. Follow-up was different, however, because at incidence screen, new nodules are supposed to have a relatively higher growth rate (Table 17.5).[9]

For all existing nodules, except for NODCAT 1, always a comparison with the baseline screening round was made. If in solid nodules or solid components of partial solid nodules the PVC was 25% or more (Table 17.5), the VDT based on changes in calculated volumes over time (VDT_v) was determined according to formula (2):[11]

(2) $$VDT_v \text{ (days)} = [\ln 2 \times \Delta t]/[\ln(V_2/V_1)]$$

In situations in which a reliable volume estimate could not be made because of software limitations and/or manual measurement was preferred in either one of the two evaluations, changes in volumes based on changes in estimated diameter over time (VDT_d) was determined according to formula (3):

(3) $$VDT_d \text{ (days)} = [\ln 2 \times \Delta t]/[3\ln (MaxDiamXY2/MaxDiamXY1]$$

where MaxDiamXY is equal to maximum diameter in X/Y-axis.

However, if *both* scans had to be evaluated by manual measurements, such as for pleural-based solid nodules or nonsolid nodules, the following formula for growth determination was applicable:

(4) $$VDT_d = [\ln 2 \times \Delta t]/[\ln((MaxDiamXY2 \times PerpDiamXY2 \times MaxDiamZ2)/(MaxDiamXY1 \times PerpDiamXY1 \times MaxDiamZ1))]$$

where MaxDiamXY is equal to maximum diameter in X/Y-axis, PerpdiamXY is equal to maximum diameter perpendicular to MaxDiamXY, and MaxDiamZ is equal to maximum diameter in Z-axis. If MaxDiamZ was missing, then MaxDiamZ equalled $0.7 \times |\text{Caudal slice number} - \text{Cranial slice number}|$.

TABLE 17.5 Follow-up Protocol for Noncalcified Nodules at Annual Repeat Screening

	Year 1	Year 2	Year 3	Year 4
Volume	V_1	V_2	V_3	V_4
Percentage volume change : PVC (%) (solid nodules only)		$100 (V_2 - V_1)/V_2$	$100 (V_3 - V_1)/V_1$	$100 (V_4 - V_1)/V_1$
Growth (%)		PVC <25%: no PVC ≥25%: yes	PVC <25%: no PVC ≥25%: yes	PVC <25%: no PVC ≥25%: yes
If growth:				
Determine volume doubling time (VDT)				
Volume (solid): VDTv (days)		$VDTv = [\ln 2 \times \Delta t]/[\ln(V_2/V_1)]$	$VDTv = [\ln 2 \times \Delta t]/[\ln(V_3/V_1)]$	$VDTv = [\ln 2 \times \Delta t]/[\ln(V_4/ V_1)]$
Diameter (part solid, nonsolid, pleural based, manual measurements): VDTd (days)		$VDTd = [\ln 2 \times \Delta t]/[3\ln(D_2/D_1)]$	$VDTd = [\ln 2 \times \Delta t]/[3\ln (D_3/D_1)]$	$VDTd = [\ln 2 \times \Delta t]/[3\ln(D_4/D_1)]$
Select lowest VDT (either VDTv or VDTd)				
VDT >600 days **GROWCAT A**		Annual CT year 4	Annual CT year 4	Stop
VDT 400–600 days **GROWCAT B**		Annual CT year 3	Annual CT year 4	Stop
VDT <400 days or new solid component in nonsolid lesion **GROWCAT C**		Refer to pulmonologist	Refer to pulmonologist	Refer to pulmonologist

From Xu DM, Gietema H, de Koning H, et al. Nodule management protocol of the NELSON randomised lung cancer screening trial. *Lung Cancer* 2006;54:177–184.

TABLE 17.6 NELSON Management Protocol for Noncalcified Nodules at Incidence Screening

Nodule type	NODCAT 1	NODCAT 2	NODCAT 3	NODCAT 4	GROWCAT C
Solid	Negative test CT in year 4	Indeterminate test CT in year 3	Indeterminate test CT after 6–8 weeks	Positive test Refer to pulmonologist for workup and diagnosis	Positive test Histological diagnosis required
Partial solid	Negative test CT in year 4	Indeterminate test CT in year 3	Indeterminate test CT after 6–8 weeks	Positive test Refer to pulmonologist for workup and diagnosis	Positive test Histological diagnosis required
Solid-pleural based	Negative test CT in year 4	Indeterminate test CT in year 3	Indeterminate test CT after 6–8 weeks	Positive test Refer to pulmonologist for workup and diagnosis	Positive test Histological diagnosis required
Nonsolid	Negative test CT in year 4	Indeterminate test CT in year 3	Indeterminate test CT after 6–8 weeks	Nonexisting category	Positive test Histological diagnosis required

From Xu DM, Gietema H, de Koning H, et al. Nodule management protocol of the NELSON randomised lung cancer screening trial. *Lung Cancer* 2006;54:177–184.

According to the VDT, growing NCNs were classified in three growth categories: GROWCAT A with a VDT more than 600 days, GROWCAT B with a VDT between 400 to 600 days, and GROWCAT C with a VDT less than 400 days. Nonsolid nodules in which a new solid component appeared were also classified GROWCAT C (Table 17.6).[9]

During incidence screening, the test result (negative, indeterminate, positive) was based on the highest GROWCAT or the highest NODCAT in case of a new nodule. Subjects with no growth or GROWCAT A received a negative test result, and they were rescheduled for a CT scan in year 4. For subjects with GROWCAT B or a new NODCAT 2, the test result was indeterminate, and a repeat scan was made 1 year later (year 3) (Table 17.4). A new NODCAT 3 was also an indeterminate test result, which however, required a repeat scan 6 to 8 weeks later. Participants with GROWCAT C or a new NODCAT 4 had a positive test result and were referred to a chest physician for workup and diagnostic evaluation.[9]

Management of NODCAT 4 and GROWCAT C Nodules

Baseline NODCAT 4 If the highest category was a NODCAT 4, the participant was referred to the chest physician of choice via the general practitioner, usually the chest physician associated with the screening center. Primary objective was to confirm the presence of malignancy by performing routine physical examinations, routine laboratory tests, and a bronchoscopy (bronchial washing for cytology and culture and transbronchial biopsy or brushing on indication). A percutaneous CT-guided fine-needle aspiration (FNA) to obtain histology or cytology of the lesion is not a routine procedure in the Netherlands and Belgium, and if the FNA technique was used, it was only for large peripheral nodules with good access. The FNA result can be malignant, specific benign, or nonspecific benign. Specific benign diagnoses include tuberculosis, mycoses, nocardia, hamartoma, or a benign lymph node. If a malignancy was proven, the patient was further staged and followed by surgical resection. A definitively specified benign diagnosis required treatment or just observation, but if no diagnosis or a nonspecific benign diagnosis was obtained, the follow-up strategy was based on the assessment of nodule growth similar as to NODCAT 3 (i.e., a repeat scan after 3 to 4 months). If at that time there was no growth, the test result was negative, and participants were scheduled for an annual repeat CT scan 8 to 9 months later. If there was growth, the test result was positive (GROWCAT C), which meant that a definitive histological diagnosis had to be obtained. Actually, this workup was according to our national CBO guidelines for the diagnosis and treatment of non–small cell lung cancer,[12] with the exception that a ^{18}F-fluorodeoxyglucose (FDG)-positron emission tomography (PET) scan was not routinely included in the workup of a NODCAT 4, primarily because our NELSON trial is a CT-screening trial, in which the presence or absence of growth of the nodule is leading, and not the outcome of the PET scan. Furthermore, the pretest probability of malignancy in this population of current and former smokers is very high, and a substantial proportion of the PET scan is false negative because of bronchioloalveolar cell carcinomas (BAC) or adenocarcinomas with BAC features, limiting the diagnostic value of the PET in the context of this CT-screening trial.[13–15]

Baseline or Incidence: GROWCAT C The workup for participants with growing lesions (GROWCAT C) was essentially the same as for NODCAT 4, except that for these nodules a final histological diagnosis had to be obtained either by FNA, video-assisted thoracoscopic surgery (VATS), or wedge resection and examination on frozen section, and that further observation by follow-up CT scans was no longer allowed. If malignant, the nodule had to be surgically removed after appropriate staging. If the outcome of the investigation was that the lesion was benign, the participant was rescheduled for the next regular annual CT scan.

REFERENCES

1. National Cancer Institute, Division of Cancer Prevention. NCI cancer Data Standards Registry (caDSR). Version 3.0.1.2 Build 20. Available at: http://cdebrowser.nci.nih.gov/ CDEBrowser/. Accessed 2005.
2. National Institutes of Health, Behavior Change Consortium. Recommended smoking measures. Available at: http://www1.od.nih.gov/behaviorchange/measures/smoking.htm. Accessed 2005.
3. Pistelli F, Viegi G, Carrozzi L, et al. Appendix compendium of respiratory standard questionnaires for adults (CORSQ). *Eur Respir Rev* 2001; 11:118–143.
4. Statistics Netherlands. Self-reported health and lifestyle, smoking, 2003 statline. Available at: http://statline.cbs.nl/StatWeb. Accessed 2005.
5. Thun MJ, Meyers DG, Day-Lally C, et al. Chapter 5: Age and the exposure–response relationships between cigarette smoking and premature death in Cancer Prevention Study II. In: Burns DM, Garfinkel L, Samet J, eds. *Smoking and Tobacco Control Monograph No. 8: Changes in Cigarette-Related Risks and Their Implications for Prevention and Control.* Bethesda, MD: US Department of Health and Human Services. Public Health Service, National Institute of Health, National Cancer Institute, 1997:383–475.
6. Burns DM, Shanks TG, Choi W, et al. The American Cancer Society Cancer Prevention Study I: 12-year follow up of 1 million men and women. In: Burns DM, Garfinkel L, Samet J, eds. *Smoking and Tobacco Control Monograph No. 8: Changes in Cigarette-Related Risks and Their Implications for Prevention and Control.* Bethesda, MD: US Department of Health and Human Services. Public Health Service, National Institute of Health, National Cancer Institute, 1997:113–304.
7. van Iersel CA, de Koning HJ, Draisma G, et al. Risk-based selection from the general population in a screening trial: selection criteria, recruitment and power for the Dutch-Belgian randomised lung cancer multislice CT screening trial (NELSON). *Int J Cancer* 2007;120:868–874.
8. Gohagan JK, Prorok PC, Kramer BS, et al. Prostate cancer screening in the prostate, lung, colorectal and ovarian cancer screening trial of the National Cancer Institute. *J Urol* 1994;152:1905–1909.
9. Xu DM, Gietema H, de Koning H, et al. Nodule management protocol of the NELSON randomised lung cancer screening trial. *Lung Cancer* 2006;54:177–184.
10. Henschke CI, Yankelevitz DF, Naidich DP, et al. CT screening for lung cancer: suspiciousness of nodules according to size on baseline scans. *Radiology* 2004;231:164–168.
11. Yankelevitz DF, Reeves AP, Kostis WJ, et al. Small pulmonary nodules: volumetrically determined growth rates, based on CT evaluation. *Radiology* 2000;217:251–256.
12. *CBO Richtlijn Niet-Kleincellig Longcarcinoom: Stadiering en Behandeling.* Van Zuiden Communications BV, Alphen aan de Rijn, the Netherlands, 2004.
13. Lindell RM, Hartman TE, Swensen SJ, et al. Lung cancer screening experience: a retrospective review of PET in 22 non-small cell lung carcinomas detected on screening chest CT in a high-risk population. *AJR Am J Roentgenol* 2005;185:126–131.
14. Pastorino U, Bellomi M, Landoni C. Early lung cancer detection with spiral CT and positron emisson tomography in heavy smokers: 2-year results. *Lancet* 2003;362:593–597.
15. Bastarrika G, García-Velloso MF, Lozano MD, et al. Early lung cancer detection using spiral computed tomography and positron emission tomography. *Am J Respir Crit Care Med* 2005;171:1378–1383.

CHAPTER 18

Anjali Saqi
Madeline F. Vazquez

Fine-Needle Aspiration Cytology of Benign and Malignant Tumors of the Lung

The cytologic diagnosis of lung cancer can be made by the evaluation of exfoliated cells in sputum and/or cells obtained by transbronchoscopic techniques including bronchial washing, bronchial brushing, bronchoalveolar lavage, and by fine-needle aspiration biopsy (FNAB), most commonly, transthoracic FNAB under computed tomography (CT) guidance. The sensitivity of a single sputum specimen for the detection of lung cancer is approximately 50% and increases with the number of specimens examined.[1] The highest sensitivity is obtained for centrally localized squamous cell carcinoma and the lowest for small cell carcinoma. For endobronchial lesions that can be directly visualized with a bronchoscope, the sensitivity of a single bronchial washing or brushing for detecting lung cancer is about 65%, similar to endobronchial or transbronchial biopsy.[2] Combining sputum cytology with bronchial brush cytology increases the sensitivity than with either method alone.[3] Bronchoalveolar lavage utilizing narrow-diameter bronchoscopes has the higher yield for the detection of lung cancer in peripheral lesions with a reported sensitivity of 35% to 65%.[4] By far, the most reliable cytologic method for diagnosing a localized peripheral lung lesion is transthoracic CT-guided FNAB, which has a sensitivity that exceeds 85% for the detection of lung cancer. Metaanalyses of transthoracic needle aspiration biopsy reports show a high sensitivity (0.88 to 0.99) and specificity (0.99 to 1.00) for the diagnosis of lung cancer.[5] Most of the work on cytology screening for lung cancer has been on sputum specimens for the diagnosis of squamous cell carcinoma and its precursors. Lung cancer is thought to arise from a series of sequential preneoplastic changes that have been well defined for centrally arising squamous cell carcinoma but not other lung cancer subtypes. There are different patterns of molecular alterations in small cell carcinoma, squamous cell carcinoma, and adenocarcinoma. For example, Wistuba and colleagues[6] found a higher incidence of deletions at 17p13 (TP53), 13q14 (RB), 9q21 (p16 INKa), 8p21–23, and several 3p regions in squamous cell carcinoma than in adenocarcinoma. On the other hand, K-RAS mutations have been detected in bronchoalveolar lavage fluids from patients with adenocarcinoma but not in patients with other lung cancer subtypes. It has been hypothesized that molecular analysis of sputum for biomarkers of lung cancer may provide an effective means of screening smokers to enable early lung cancer detection. However, the use of biomarkers for lung cancer screening is complicated by the fact that they can be detected in chronic smokers long before any clinical evidence of neoplasia. For example, p16 promotor hypermethylation and TP53 have been detected in sputum in chronic smokers without lung cancer and K-RAS mutations have been detected in atypical adenomatous hyperplasia (AAH).[7] At our institution, the focus has shifted from the use of cytology for screening for early lung cancer to the diagnosis of CT screen–detected lung cancer by transthoracic FNAB. It is minimally invasive, does not require hospitalization, and serious risks are uncommon and limited to pneumothorax and minimal hemorrhage. The FNAB is performed using a 22-gauge Westcott needle with immediate on-site assessment of air-dried smears utilizing the Diff-Quik staining method (Dade AG, Dudingen, Switzerland). Smears are also submerged in alcohol for Papanicolaou staining and blood clots are submitted directly in formalin for a cell block preparation.

SQUAMOUS CELL CARCINOMA

Squamous cell carcinoma (Figs. 18.1 and 18.2) is strongly associated with cigarette smoking. It is a malignant epithelial tumor that was the most common histological subtype, but its incidence has now been surpassed by adenocarcinoma reflecting trends in reduced tobacco exposure with introduction of filters and low tar contents.[8] Squamous cell carcinoma arises from dysplastic squamous epithelium and can present centrally or peripherally. In addition to the classic squamous cell carcinoma, the World Health Organization recognizes several additional histological patterns including papillary, clear cell, small cell, and basaloid variants.

Typically, squamous cell carcinomas are classified into well, moderately, and poorly differentiated categories, and the cytological appearance is dependent on the extent of differentiation.

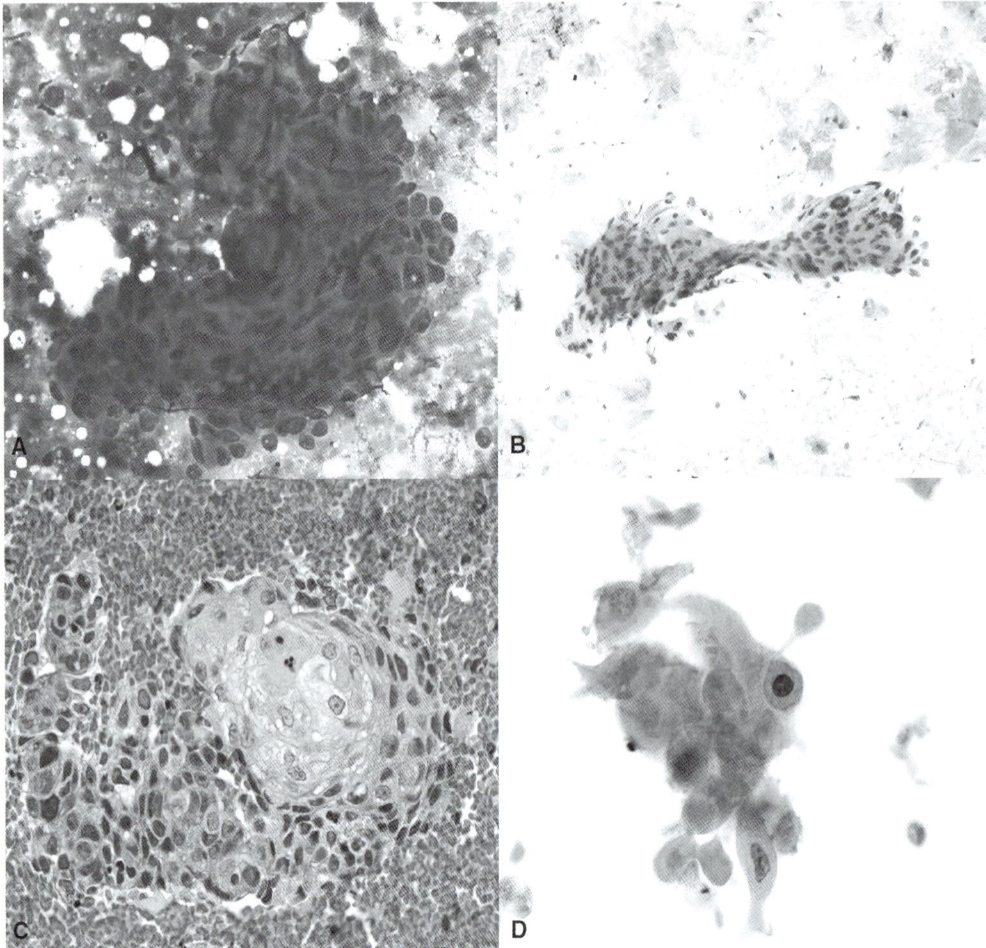

FIGURE 18.1 Squamous cell carcinoma. **A:** A syncytial cluster and rare single cells with high nuclear:cytoplasmic ratios and irregular nuclear borders (Diff-Quik, 40×). **B:** Orangeophilic cells present as clusters and singly with hyperchromatic nuclei and relatively low nuclear:cytoplasmic ratios; anucleate squames are also present (Papanicolaou stain, 20×). **C:** Cell block with intercellular bridges and keratinizing cells (cell block, hematoxylin and eosin [H&E], 40×). **D:** Polygonal-, spindle-, and bizarre-shaped squamous cells (Papanicolaou stain, 40×). (See color plate.)

In general, squamous cell carcinomas can be associated with tumor diathesis, acute inflammation, or foreign body–type giant cell reaction.[9] In cytological preparations, squamous cell carcinoma occurs as single cells or loose clusters; tissue fragments are more common in aspirates.[10] Nuclear:cytoplasmic ratios may range from low to high, with lower ratios being more frequent in the well-differentiated carcinomas.[11] The cells have sharp distinct cell borders,[11] and the nuclei are often hyperchromatic to pyknotic *India ink* with coarse chromatin.

On histological sections, squamous cell carcinoma is defined by keratinization and/or intercellular bridges. In smears and liquid-based preparations of well-differentiated squamous cell carcinoma, intact intercellular bridges and keratin pearls are uncommon,[10] but they may be readily seen in cell

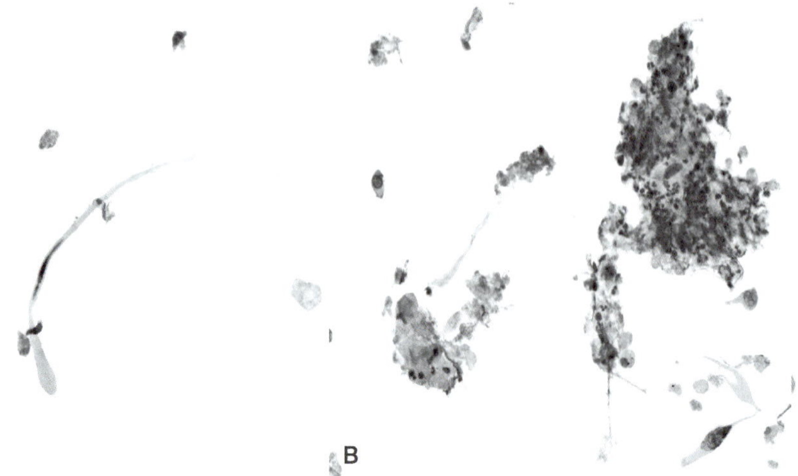

FIGURE 18.2 Squamous cell carcinoma. **A:** Atypical tadpole-shaped cell with hyperchromatic nucleus (Papanicolaou stain, ThinPrep, 40×) **B:** Marked acute inflammation and necrotic debris associated with squamous cells. *Inset:* malignant cells are also present (Papanicolaou stain, ThinPrep, 40× [*inset:* 60×]). (See color plate.)

blocks sections. Rather, squamous cells are characterized by dense dark blue cytoplasm or orangeophilia on Diff-Quik and Papanicolaou-stained specimens, respectively. Polygonal cells, bizarre cells with tadpole/caudate and spindle cell configurations,[10] and Herxheimer spirals in cytoplasmic tails are also associated with squamous differentiation. As squamous cell carcinoma becomes less differentiated, the aforementioned features become less prominent. Poorly differentiated carcinomas form syncytial groups especially in aspirates, and the cells have cyanophilic cytoplasm, higher nuclear:cytoplasmic ratios, and prominent nucleoli.[9]

The remaining relatively uncommon variants of squamous cell carcinoma have predominantly been described in surgical pathology literature but awareness of these variants is important to preclude misdiagnosis. Histologically, basaloid squamous cell carcinoma shows cells with peripheral palisading, scant cytoplasm, and hyperchromatic nuclei admixed with areas of typical squamous differentiation.[12] The small cell variant has focal squamous differentiation and small cells with morphologic traits of non–small cell carcinoma including coarse or vesicular chromatin, prominent nucleoli, and distinct cell borders.[12,13]

Carcinomas are often classified as non–small cell or small cell carcinoma for appropriate therapeutic management. An attempt to distinguish between squamous cell carcinoma and adenocarcinoma, rather than cataloging the two as poorly differentiated non–small cell carcinoma, is also becoming important as new agents for treatment are emerging. Bevacizumab, an antivascular endothelial growth factor monoclonal antibody, is being implemented for non–small cell lung cancer treatment, but it is contraindicated in patients with squamous cell carcinoma because of reports of pulmonary hemorrhage.[14] Tyrosine kinase inhibitors of epidermal growth receptors are also being used to treat adenocarcinoma with bronchioloalveolar features likely being more sensitive than other non–small cell carcinomas.[15] Given the differences in treatment options, subclassification of histological subtype can avert side effects as well as tailor appropriate therapy.

Immunohistochemistry Most squamous cell carcinomas express high–molecular weight cytokeratin, cytokeratins 5/6 and p63. Thyroid transcription factor-1 (TTF-1)[16] and cytokeratin 7 (CK7)[17] staining is present in a subset of cases.

Differential Diagnosis Cytology specimens with predominantly well-differentiated squamous cells have to be diagnosed cautiously. Such cells may represent mature keratinized superficial cells of a carcinoma without adequate sampling of smaller malignant cells, especially on exfoliative respiratory specimens,[11] or they may reflect reactive, metaplastic, or degenerative changes, even in the presence of nuclear hyperchromasia and cellular irregularities.[11] Reparative processes have atypia, but two-dimensional polarized "school of fish" sheets with enlarged nuclei, vesicular chromatin, and prominent nucleoli distinguish them from carcinoma.[9] Atypical squamous cells can accompany marked acute inflammation and necrosis, suggestive of an abscess.[11] An infectious process (e.g., aspergillosis) has to be considered, but intense orangeophilia and increased number of single cells should raise the possibility of squamous cell carcinoma.[18] A histiocytic reaction to keratin can erroneously be interpreted as *granulomatous inflammation*.[11]

Basaloid and small cell variants of squamous cell carcinoma have similarities to (combined) small cell carcinoma.[13] Cytological features, including dense cytoplasm, lack of nuclear molding, coarse chromatin, and nucleoli favor squamous cell carcinoma. Immunostains can aid in the diagnosis.

Finally, primary pulmonary squamous cell carcinoma is morphologically similar to its head and neck counterparts, and clinical history is necessary in determining the origin.

ADENOCARCINOMA

There has been a shift in the predominant histological subtype of non–small cell carcinoma. Adenocarcinoma (Figs. 18.3 and 18.4) has surpassed the incidence of squamous cell carcinoma, once the foremost culprit of lung carcinomas.[8] Like squamous cell carcinoma, adenocarcinoma is linked to smoking, but it is also prevalent among nonsmokers and women.[19,20] Adenocarcinoma, defined by glandular differentiation or mucin synthesis, tends to present peripherally. The World Health Organization classifies adenocarcinoma into acinar, papillary, bronchioloalveolar, solid with mucin production, and mixed patterns; less common variants such as fetal, mucinous cystadenocarcinoma, mucinous *colloid*, signet ring, and clear cell adenocarcinomas also comprise this category.[12] Most adenocarcinomas demonstrate pattern heterogeneity and therefore are mixed subtype,[21] whereas pure subtypes are comparatively infrequent.

The histological features of adenocarcinoma, including well, moderate, and poor differentiation, are often mirrored in cytology specimens. In general, adenocarcinoma has a clean or necrotic background,[9] and has cyanophilic yet more translucent cytoplasm than squamous cell carcinoma.[12] The cytoplasm may be foamy, granular, lacy, or vacuolated. Based on the underlying architecture and differentiation, the neoplastic cells are arranged as single cells, two-dimensional sheets, three-dimensional clusters, syncytial groups, acini, or papillae. Similarly, the cellular (cytoplasmic vacuolization) and nuclear features (intranuclear inclusions, intranuclear grooves, chromasia, chromatin pattern, and nucleoli) reflect the differentiation of the tumor.

Bronchioloalveolar Carcinoma Bronchioloalveolar carcinoma (BAC) is the in situ component of adenocarcinoma, which may be mucinous or nonmucinous. Histologically, BAC is defined as adenocarcinoma with predominantly lepidic growth along alveolar walls without stromal (desmoplastic reaction), vascular, or pleural invasion.[12,22] Pure BAC is rather uncommon,[23] but intermingling with other patterns, as in mixed subtype, is quite frequent. Among adenocarcinomas, BAC has a greater predilection among women[24] and is more prevalent in nonsmokers. Because most BACs present peripherally, they are less likely to occur in

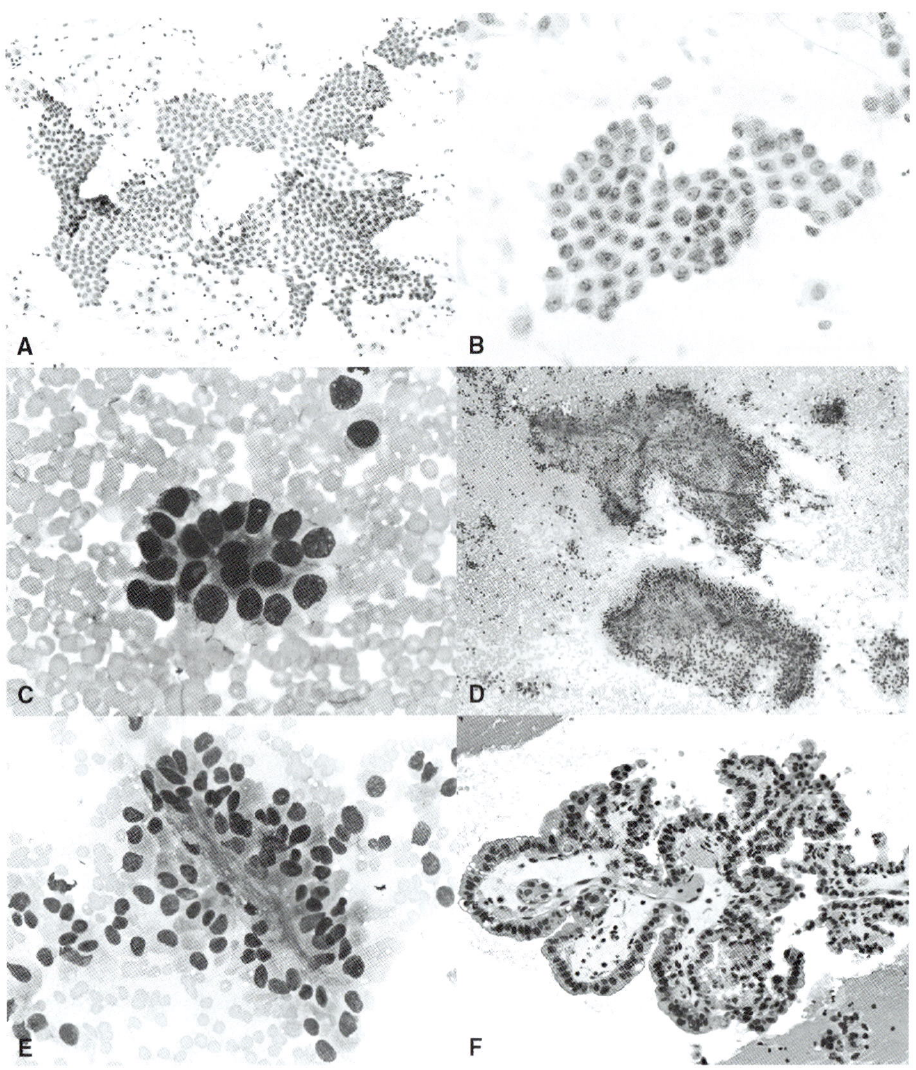

FIGURE 18.3 Adenocarcinoma. **A:** Monolayer sheets of relatively monotonous epithelial cells with pale chromatin and no significant nuclear overlap suggestive of BAC features (Papanicolaou stain, 20×). **B:** Two-dimensional sheet with bland nuclei containing pinpoint nucleoli and nuclear grooves often associated with BAC differentiation (Papanicolaou stain, 60×). **C:** Acinar formation (Diff-Quik, 20×). **D:** Fibrovascular cores surrounded by epithelial cells suggestive of papillary features (Diff-Quik, 10×). **E:** Epithelial cells enveloping delicate core in carcinoma with papillary architecture (Diff-Quik, 60×). **F:** Columnar cells line a fibrovascular core consistent with papillary features (cell block H&E section, 20×). (See color plate.)

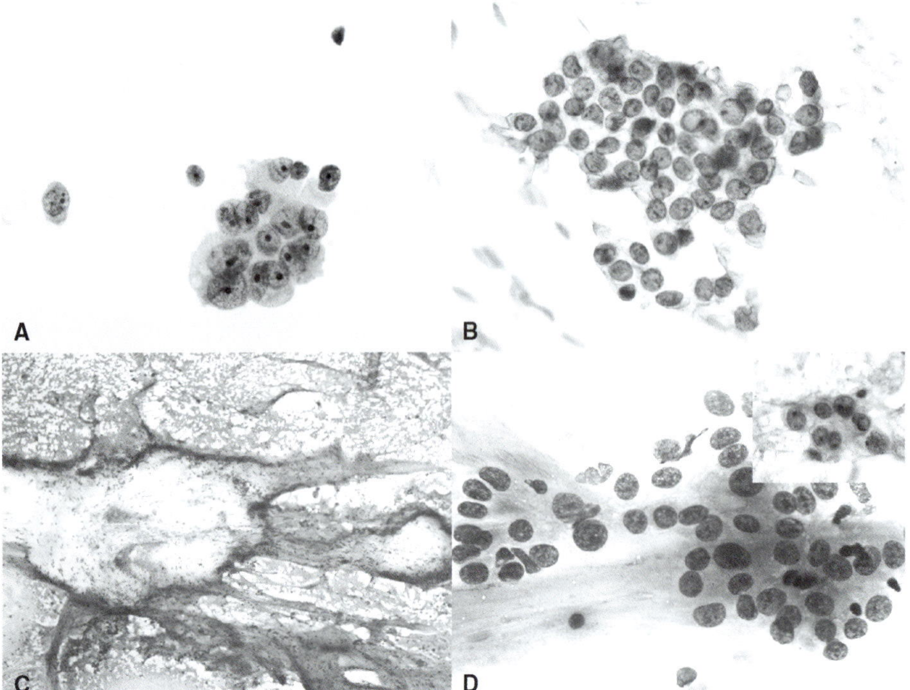

FIGURE 18.4 Adenocarcinoma. **A:** Three-dimensional cluster with nuclear pleomorphism, conspicuous nucleoli, and vacuolated cytoplasm (Papanicolaou stain, ThinPrep 60×). **B:** Cluster of epithelial cells with fine chromatin, inconspicuous nucleoli, intranuclear grooves, and inclusion (Papanicolaou stain, 60×). **C:** Adenocarcinoma with mucin: abundant mucin with scattered clusters of epithelial cells (Diff-Quik, 4×). **D:** Adenocarcinoma with mucin: malignant epithelial cells with conspicuous nucleoli and relatively abundant cytoplasm associated with mucin. *Inset:* Cells have vacuolated cytoplasm and nuclear membrane irregularities (Diff-Quik, 40×; inset Papanicolaou stain 60×). (See color plate.)

sputum, lavages, and washes and are more amenable to aspiration biopsies. Relatively benign biological behavior and propensity for multifocality[24] make identification of BAC significant rather than mere academic interest.

Several studies have demonstrated BAC cytological and histological correlation.[23,25–27] BACs tend to have a clean background, monolayered sheets[23] in orderly arrangement without nuclear overlap,[26] single relatively uniform cells containing moderate to abundant cytoplasm, pale fine chromatin, and inconspicuous nuclei; intranuclear inclusions and invaginations may also be present.[25] Most BACs are deceptively bland, but low-grade cytology should exclude neither a reactive process (over BAC) nor a well-differentiated invasive adenocarcinoma.[27] Conversely, mild cellular pleomorphism is evident in BACs[23] and does not imply invasive adenocarcinoma. Significant features distinguishing mucinous BAC from adenocarcinoma include abundant nuclear grooves, extracellular mucin,[23] and greater propensity toward three-dimensional groups than sheets.[28]

Pure BAC or predominant BAC pattern in mixed adenocarcinoma is associated with better prognosis,[26,29] so rendering a diagnosis of adenocarcinoma with BAC prominence on aspiration biopsy may guide therapeutic options. Lesions with a predominantly BAC may be amenable to relatively conservative surgical excision[30] and preoperative testing for sensitivity to specific drugs.[31,32] Detecting BAC on cytology also preoperatively alerts to the tendency of aerogenous spread and multifocal disease.[26,33]

Diagnostic accuracy of BAC is achieved by correlation with radiologic presentation (i.e., ground-glass opacity and solid component), operator expertise and adequate sampling. BAC features by cytology may yield predominantly non-BAC adenocarcinoma upon resection (or vice versa) as consequence of inadequately or peripherally sampled tumor.[27] Although cytological examination can indicate BAC features, histological examination to unequivocally exclude invasion is necessary for definitive diagnosis.[27]

Adenocarcinoma In contrast to BAC, other subtypes of adenocarcinoma tend to have greater architectural complexity with three-dimensional clusters, cell balls, and syncytia. Presence of papillary fronds (often containing intranuclear inclusions, ± psammoma bodies[34,26]) and luminal/glandular formations echo histological papillary and acinar architectures, respectively. Micropapillary morphology, associated with aggressive behavior in breast, has also been described in the cytology literature.[35] Cells of non-BAC tend to have conspicuous nucleoli,[27] chromatin ranging from finely granular to coarse and hyperchromatic and minimal to marked pleomorphism in well to poorly differentiated adenocarcinomas, respectively. In poorly differentiated carcinomas, a non–small cell carcinoma rather than either squamous cell carcinoma or adenocarcinoma[27] diagnosis is sometimes rendered. If available, material for immunostains to distinguish the two is beneficial as the tumors have different levels of sensitivity and adverse effects to therapeutic agents.

Immunohistochemistry Lung adenocarcinomas are frequently cytokeratin 7 (CK7)-positive and cytokeratin 20 (CK20)-negative. TTF-1,[36] although specific for pulmonary (and thyroid) origin, is not 100% sensitive; incorporating thyroglobulin stain into the immunohistochemical panel, especially in presence of papillary architecture, is beneficial for excluding thyroid metastasis. Surfactant apoprotein, associated with lung origin, is also expressed in a fraction of nonpulmonary adenocarcinomas.[37] Mucinous adenocarcinomas are often immunoreactive with CK7 and CK20, but not TTF-1.[36]

A CK7+, CK20−, TTF-1− immunoprofile in a lung mass is not uncommon. Because breast and upper gastrointestinal tract adenocarcinomas also exhibit this staining pattern, excluding metastatic disease is crucial. Inclusion of estrogen and progesterone receptors,[38] gross cystic disease fluid protein, mammaglobin, and caudal-type homeobox transcription factor-2 (CDX-2) in the battery of stains is prudent in such cases. Estrogen/progesterone[38] and CDX-2[39] expression have been also described in a subset of pulmonary adenocarcinomas.

Adenocarcinoma, BAC, and reactive atypia are morphological diagnosis. Although limited, evidence supporting application of p53 in discriminating BAC from non-BAC adenocarcinoma may have a role in cytology.[28]

Differential Diagnosis The main differential diagnosis problem is the distinction between peripheral adenocarcinoma of the lung and malignant pleural mesothelioma of epithelioid type. Malignant epithelioid mesothelioma has tubular and papillary architecture and CK7+/CK20−/TTF-1− profile like adenocarcinoma. Immunostains CD15, CEA, BerEP4 (for adenocarcinoma) and calretinin, CK 5/6, WT-1 (for mesothelial origin) can resolve the diagnosis of an epithelioid pleural-based lesion.

Several entities mimic adenocarcinoma including nonneoplastic lesions, metastases, mesothelial cells, and benign pulmonary neoplasms. Benign processes such as chemotherapy/radiation, pneumonia, and infarcts can mimic adenocarcinoma (see section on pitfalls). Reactive atypical pneumocytes can be challenging to differentiate from BAC on aspirates. Hyperplastic reactive cells display cilia and terminal bars. Also cellular enlargement, pleomorphism, binucleation, and nucleoli tend to be more prominent in reactive cells than BAC.[27]

Metastatic adenocarcinoma can appear histologically identical to pulmonary adenocarcinoma, and cytological features, although not unequivocally diagnostic, may steer in the distinction. Metastatic colon cancer is characterized by dirty necrosis and elongated nuclei. Primary lung adenocarcinoma often has mixed subtype with bronchioloalveolar features, whereas metastasis tends to illustrate morphological homogeneity.[12] Although these morphological features are helpful, confirmatory immunostains are necessary.

Sheets of mesothelial cells may result in misdiagnosis of BAC[25]; presence of intercellular bridges in mesothelial cells is helpful in separating the two entities.

Histologically, BAC is separated from its precursor AAH, with the latter measuring <5 mm and absence of interstitial inflammation and fibrosis.[12] In cytology, lesions that are suspicious but not diagnostic of adenocarcinoma, defined as scant clusters of bland, yet atypical bronchioloalveolar cells with uniform round nuclei, pinpoint nucleoli in a histiocytic background, are designated *atypical bronchioloalveolar cell proliferation* (ABP) and demonstrate BAC or invasive adenocarcinoma on resections,[27] the discrepancy possibly a consequence of inadequate sampling.

Sclerosing hemangioma and hamartoma are benign/low-grade pulmonary neoplastic mimickers of adenocarcinoma, and their differentiation from adenocarcinoma can alter surgical management. Sclerosing hemangioma is defined histologically by its constellation of architectural patterns including solid, papillary, hemorrhagic, and sclerotic and relatively bland stromal and surface cells.[12] The architectural patterns of sclerosing hemangioma resemble those of adenocarcinoma, and the cells with bland cytology, inconspicuous nucleoli, intranuclear inclusions, and sparse/absent mitotic activity recapitulate features of BAC.[40] Presence of hyalinized stromal tissue, foamy and/or hemosiderin-laden macrophages, two cell populations, and absence of marked pleomorphism are consistent with sclerosing hemangioma.[40]

Pulmonary hamartoma is a benign neoplasm composed of mesenchymal tissue (connective tissue, muscle, adipose tissue, and cartilage) with entrapped respiratory epithelium.[12] The undifferentiated fibromyxoid component and bronchiolar cell proliferation with intranuclear inclusions and mild atypia resemble mucin and atypical cellular proliferation, respectively, suggestive of mucinous adenocarcinoma.[41] Smears of the fibromyxoid stroma display fibrillar edges and entrapped spindle-shaped cells, whereas mucin is devoid of these characteristics; mildly atypical epithelial hyperplasia is described in hamartomas.[41] Cartilaginous fragments and "popcorn calcification" on imaging are diagnostic of hamartoma.

NEUROENDOCRINE NEOPLASMS

Pulmonary neuroendocrine tumors comprise approximately 20% of lung malignancies.[42] According to the most recent World Health Organization classification, they are histologically divided into a three-tier, four-category system including low-grade (typical carcinoid), intermediate-grade (atypical carcinoid), and high-grade (small cell carcinoma and large cell neuroendocrine carcinoma) tumors.[22] Overall, all tumors have characteristic neuroendocrine architecture including organoid, nesting, trabecular, insular, palisading, ribbon, papillary, cord, or rosettelike patterns. The distinction among the spectrum of neuroendocrine tumors is largely based on the number of mitoses and presence/absence of necrosis. Typical carcinoids have less than two mitoses per 2 mm^2 and no necrosis; atypical carcinoids have between 2 and 10 mitoses per 2 mm^2 and/or necrosis; large cell neuroendocrine carcinomas and small cell carcinomas have greater than 10 mitoses per 2 mm^2 and necrosis. Although the diagnostic criteria are primarily based on histological features, the architectural patterns and nuclear features are often reflected in cytological specimens. However, application of these criteria to neuroendocrine tumors in small biopsy specimens[42] and cytological specimens can be challenging.

Typical and Atypical Carcinoids

Typical Carcinoid Typical carcinoid (Fig. 18.5) comprises approximately 1% to 2% of pulmonary neoplasms,[42] and it is not associated with smoking. Typical carcinoid occurs at any age, with the mean age being 50 years.[42] Carcinoid aspirates are usually hypercellular and demonstrate loose cell clusters and single cells.[43] The cell groups often form syncytia, rosettes,[43] and trabeculae. Clusters may also be associated with a prominent streaming, arborizing capillary network in a hemorrhagic background,[44] a feature characteristic of typical and atypical carcinoids but not high-grade neuroendocrine carcinomas.[45–47] Papillary architecture is also seen in some carcinoids.[48,44] Single cells are also frequently seen in aspirates of carcinoids. Overall, the cells can have eccentrically placed nuclei with faint eosinophilic granular cytoplasm imparting a plasmacytoid appearance, or they may be stripped of their fragile cytoplasm and show bare nuclei.[44] Nuclei are relatively uniform/monomorphic and round with smooth contours. Spindle-shaped cells are also present in spindle cell carcinoids. Slightly larger and pleomorphic cells can also be observed in carcinoids.[47] The nuclei have fine granular chromatin and inconspicuous nucleoli. Rare intranuclear inclusions have also been described.[44] No obvious nuclear molding, necrosis, or mitoses are observed. In addition to the aforementioned characteristics, carcinoids may also have oncocytic, acinic cell, signet ring cell, and melanocytic features, but these traits have no impact on prognosis.[42]

Atypical Carcinoids Atypical carcinoid (Fig. 18.6) patients have a mean age of 54 years[42] and tend to be nonsmokers. Most of the cytology literature describing atypical carcinoid predates the current World Health Organization's classification of neuroendocrine tumors. Despite the modification, the overall cytological features of atypical carcinoid are similar to typical carcinoids with few minor exceptions. The neoplastic cells may be slightly more pleomorphic and larger. In addition, atypical carcinoids are associated with mitoses and/or necrosis, similar to their histological counterparts.

Immunohistochemistry Typical carcinoid stains with cytokeratin but a minority may be negative. Staining with neuroendocrine markers (chromogranin, synaptophysin, and CD56) is often strong. TTF-1 staining is variable with some series reporting no staining,[49] and others demonstrating expression in approximately one third of typical carcinoids.[50] Atypical carcinoid, like typical carcinoid, stains with cytokeratin. Expression of neuroendocrine markers is relatively less intense,[42] but TTF-1 staining is more common in atypical carcinoids.[50]

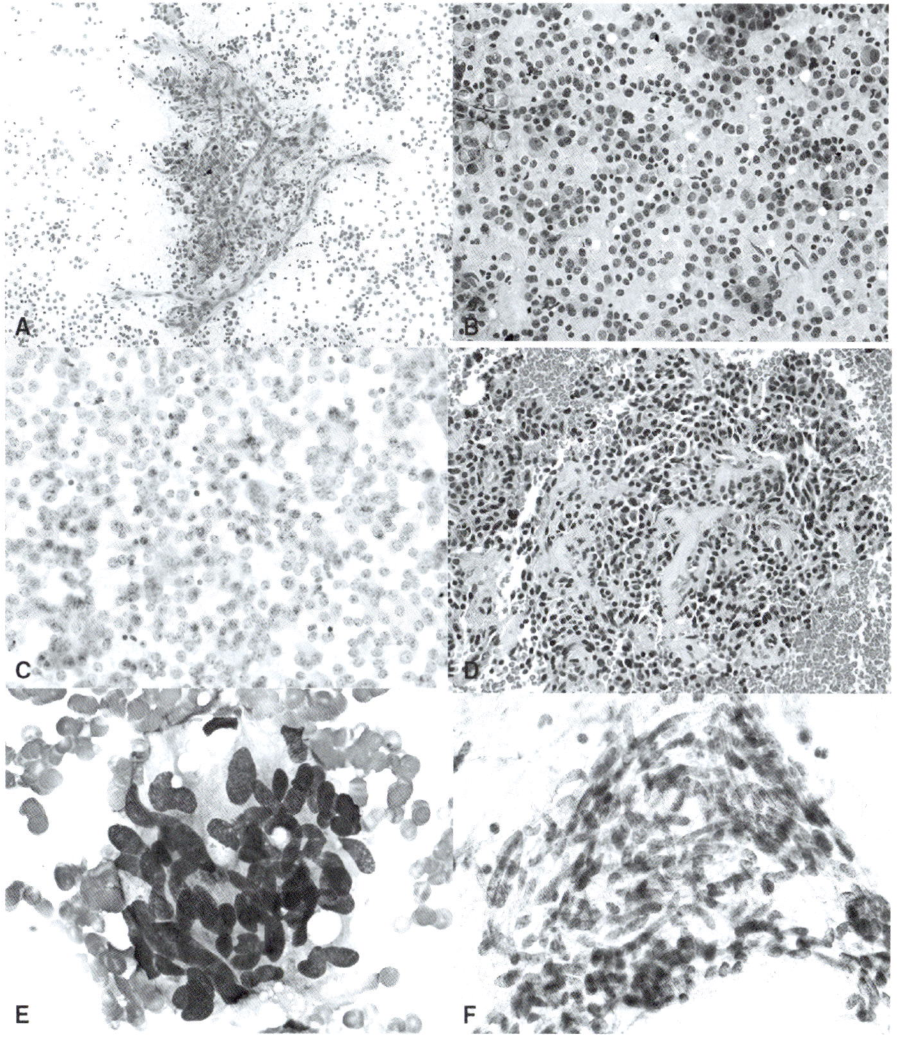

FIGURE 18.5 Typical carcinoid. **A:** Arborizing capillary network associated with monomorphic, loosely cohesive epithelial cells (touch prep, Diff-Quik, 20×). **B:** Loosely cohesive monotonous cells with eccentric nuclei and *plasmacytoid* features (touch prep, Diff-Quik, 40×). **C:** Bland cells with speckled chromatin (touch prep, H&E, 60×). **D:** Carcinoid with hyalinized stroma (cell block, H&E, 40×). **E, F:** Spindle cell carcinoid (Diff-Quik and Papanicolaou stains, 100×). (See color plate.)

Differential Diagnosis Carcinoid and atypical carcinoid can be challenging to distinguish from each other as well as other neuroendocrine neoplasms. Typical and atypical carcinoids can be difficult to differentiate from each other in a limited aspirate sample where mitoses and necrosis cannot be thoroughly assessed. A typical carcinoid may be misclassified as an atypical carcinoid following necrosis that may occur during a prior fine-needle aspiration.[42] Furthermore, presence of some large and pleomorphic cells may suggest a high-grade neuroendocrine tumor; however, a diagnosis of small cell and large cell neuroendocrine carcinoma should be avoided in the absence of necrosis and brisk mitotic activity.[47] Ki67 and Pax-5 immunostains may also be helpful; often >50% staining favors a high-grade neuroendocrine neoplasm.[51,52]

The monomorphism of carcinoid and prominent papillary pattern may be confused with sclerosing hemagioma.[48,44]

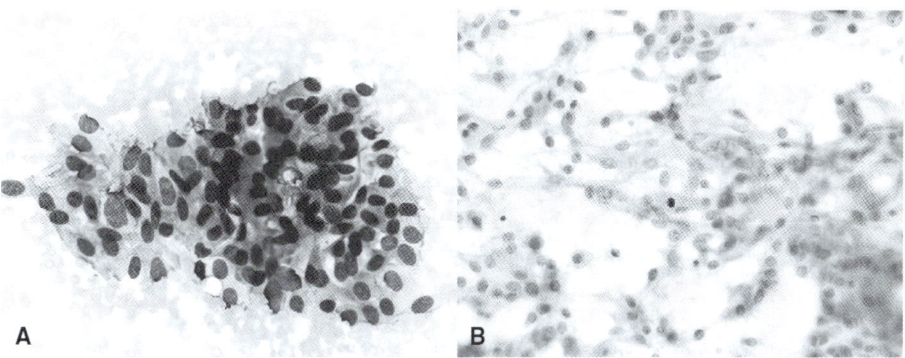

FIGURE 18.6 Atypical carcinoid. **A:** Epithelial cells with mild pleomorphism (Diff-Quik, 60×). **B:** Loose cell clusters with speckled chromatin and rare mitotic figure (touch prep, H&E, 60×). (See color plate.)

Sclerosing hemangiomas tend to have hyalinized stromal tissue, foamy and/or hemosiderin-laden macrophages, two cell populations, and stippled chromatin[40]; also, neuroendocrine markers are negative. Carcinoids can also mimic metastatic breast carcinoma,[12] especially those with neuroendocrine features.[53] Comparison with the primary breast carcinoma histology and immunostains (TTF-1, estrogen receptor and progesterone receptor, BRST-2) can be helpful in determining the primary.

Small Cell Carcinoma Small cell carcinoma (Fig. 18.7) comprises approximately 20% to 25% of lung carcinomas.[42] Small cell carcinoma, unlike carcinoid, is related to tobacco use and occurs in slightly older patients with a median age of 62 years. The significance of separating small cell carcinoma from non–small cell carcinoma is well established. Similarly, the distinction between small cell carcinoma and other pulmonary neuroendocrine tumors is also critical; this can be challenging because the diagnosis is often made on small biopsies and cytological specimens.

Aspirates of small cell carcinoma show clusters or linearly arranged cells with prominent nuclear molding and single cells with high nuclear:cytoplasmic ratios, round, ovoid, and spindle-shaped cells with scant basophilic cytoplasm. In the surgical pathology literature, the cells are typically less than the diameter of three small resting lymphocytes.[54] The nuclei have fine "salt and pepper" stippled chromatin with absent/inconspicuous nucleoli. The background demonstrates nuclear smearing/crush artifact, necrosis, and apoptosis. Paranuclear blue inclusions, which are spherical light to dark blue structures that indent the nucleus,[55] are often associated with small cell carcinomas and seen primarily on air-dried smears.[56]

Immunohistochemistry Neuroendocrine markers including chromogranin, synaptophysin, and NCAM (CD56) can also be helpful, but they stain approximately up to two third of cases.[54] TTF-1 expression has been described in up to approximately 95%[42] of small cell carcinomas of the lung; however, it also stains small cell carcinomas of extrapulmonary origin and non–small cell carcinomas.

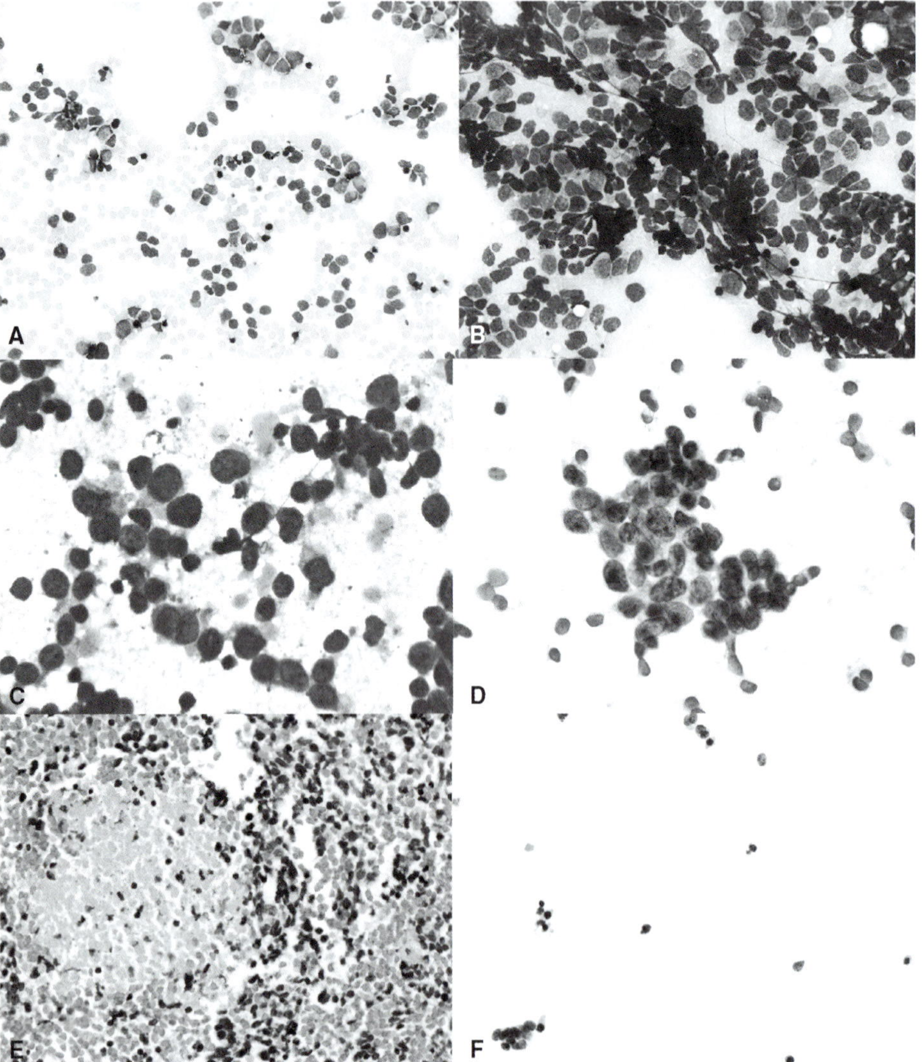

FIGURE 18.7 Small cell carcinoma. **A:** Clusters and single cells with scant cytoplasm and focal nuclear molding (Diff-Quik, 40×). **B:** Small cell carcinoma with rosettes, nuclear molding, and crush/smearing artifact (Diff-Quik, 40×). **C:** Small cell carcinoma with a dirty background and scattered apoptotic cells (Diff-Quik, 60×). **D:** Cells with high nuclear:cytoplasmic ratios, fine chromatin, and inconspicuous nucleoli (Papanicolaou stain, 60×) **E:** Eosinophilic necrotic areas and malignant small cells (cell block, H&E, 40×) **F:** Rare cell clusters and scattered single cells in small cell carcinoma mimicking lymphoma (ThinPrep, Papanicolaou stain, 60×). (See color plate.)

Differential Diagnosis In surgical specimens, cellular dyscohesion is also noted in rare cases of small cell carcinoma.[54] An aspirate from such areas as well as the small size[57] of low-grade lymphomas may lead to an erroneous diagnosis of lymphoma. Unlike carcinomas, lymphomas are associated with lymphoglandular bodies in the background. Confirmation of epithelial origin with a cytokeratin stain is valuable too. Paranuclear blue inclusions, often associated with small cell carcinoma, have also been described in minority of rhabdomyosarcomas,[56] non–small cell carcinomas,[55] and lymphomas.[55]

Large Cell Neuroendocrine Carcinoma Large cell neuroendocrine carcinomas predominate in smokers and men, and the median age of presentation is approximately 63 years.[58] Histologically, large cell neuroendocrine carcinomas have the typical neuroendocrine architecture. They also have tumor necrosis and high mitotic rate like small cell carcinomas. Unlike the latter, however, large cell neuroendocrine carcinomas on histological sections have large tumor cells with low nuclear: cytoplasmic ratio, eosinophilic cytoplasm, coarse chromatin, and frequent nucleoli.[59] These features are recapitulated in cytological specimens.[60–62] The aspirates show neoplastic cells in flattened three-dimensional sheets with peripheral palisading and single cells comprised of pleomorphic large cells with moderate to scant cytoplasm, large nuclei with thick membranes and coarse or finely granular chromatin, prominent nucleoli, focal nuclear molding, and crush artifact.[60]

Immunohistochemistry By definition, large cell neuroendocrine carcinomas should express at least one of the neuroendocrine markers (chromogranin, synaptophysin, CD56). Approximately 50% of large cell neuroendocrine tumors express TTF-1.[49] These tumors typically do not express high–molecular weight cytokeratin.[49,63]

Differential Diagnosis Given the brisk mitotic activity and necrosis, large cell neuroendocrine carcinoma could be mistaken for small cell carcinoma. The cell size (3 to 5 times the size of a red blood cell in large cell neuroendocrine carcinoma and 1 to 2.5 times the size of a red blood cell in small cell carcinoma) and distinct nucleoli (in large cell neuroendocrine carcinoma) can be used to distinguish the two entities.[61] A few prominent nucleoli can be seen in small cell carcinoma, and the diagnosis should be based on the cytological features of the predominant cell type.

Combined Small Cell Carcinoma Combined small cell carcinoma has small cell carcinoma and non–small cell carcinoma, which may constitute large cell carcinoma, adenocarcinoma, squamous cell, spindle, or giant cell carcinoma.[54]

Prognosis and Treatment The subclassification of neuroendocrine tumors is important because it impacts prognosis and treatment. Statistically significant differences in survival have been reported between typical/atypical carcinoids and large cell neuroendocrine carcinomas[22]; however, a significant difference in survival has not been identified between large cell neuroendocrine carcinoma and small cell carcinoma.[64]

Large Cell Carcinoma Large cell carcinoma is a diagnosis of exclusion of poorly differentiated carcinoma without evidence supporting squamous, glandular, or neuroendocrine components. The cells have large cells with vesicular nuclei and prominent nucleoli.[12] Ultrastructurally, there is evidence of minimal differentiation toward squamous cell carcinoma or adenocarcinoma.[12]

PRIMARY SALIVARY GLAND-TYPE NEOPLASMS

Salivary gland-type neoplasms are rare and histologically indistinguishable from their head/neck counterparts. The World Health Organization classifies adenoid cystic and mucoepidermoid carcinoma as salivary gland tumors and pleomorphic adenoma as adenoma of salivary gland type. These tumors usually present centrally and the former arise in large airways (i.e., trachea, carina, or main stem bronchus) from submucosal tracheobronchial glands.[65] Uncommon presentation, rather than salivary gland-type morphology, makes the diagnosis of this neoplastic subtype in the lung challenging. Because these tumors have equivalents in the head/neck and other organs, particularly adenoid cystic carcinoma, determining primary versus metastatic disease can be problematic. Prior clinical history, location, and multifocal pulmonary disease may favor metastasis over primary.

Adenoid Cystic Carcinoma Adenoid cystic carcinoma is rare lung tumor with predisposition for local recurrences and late distant metastasis[12] typically presenting as a central submucosal mass, therefore, usually not present on exfoliative cytology examination. As a result of its uncommonness and location, adenoid cystic descriptions are relatively more prevalent in the histological than cytological literature. The cribriform (most common), tubular, and solid architecture described in surgical pathology are recapitulated in cytological specimens. The cellular adequacy is dependent on sampling. The neoplastic cells are arranged as two-dimensional sheets, cohesive three-dimensional clusters, and singly.[66] The cells are basaloid appearing, bland, small, round to oval, and hyperchromatic with scant cytoplasm. The nuclei have finely distributed hyperchromatic chromatin and inconspicuous nucleoli.[67] Metachromatic (Diff-Quik) or light blue (Papanicolaou stain) characteristic hyaline basement membranelike globules or cylinders are intimately associated with the cells, yet sharply demarcated from them.[68] The globules also appear independent of the cellular component[66] and are scant or absent in the solid variant. Intracytoplasmic and nuclear inclusions, nuclear molding, and dual cell population of round and spindle cells may occur.[66]

Immunohistochemistry The epithelial and myoepithelial cell phenotype is reflected in the dual immunophenotype. The tumors express cytokeratin (an epithelial marker) and vimentin, smooth muscle actin, S-100, and p63, markers associated with myoepithelial origin.

Differential Diagnosis Reserve cell hyperplasia also has small cells, but the cells are even smaller than those of adenoid cystic carcinoma and cuboidal to columnar surfaced by cilia or terminal bars. The small cells of adenoid cystic carcinoma solicit a diagnosis of neuroendocrine tumors like carcinoid and small cell carcinoma. Slightly greater degree of pleomorphism, hyperchromasia, and coarse chromatin are present in carcinoid. Small cell carcinoma demonstrates necrosis, brisk mitotic activity, stippled chromatin, and nuclear molding, although the latter is described focally in adenoid cystic carcinoma.[66] Ancillary immunohistochemical studies can be highly useful for differentiating neuroendocrine tumors from adenoid cystic carcinoma. Extracellular substances such as amyloid[66] and corpora amylacia are alternative potentials for the cylindrical globules; however, lymphoplasmacytic cells as opposed to epithelial cells surround amyloid.[66]

Mucoepidermoid Carcinoma

Mucoepidermoid carcinoma is a malignant tumor spanning a broad age range but with a predilection for younger (<30 years) patients.[12] The tumor is classified as either low-grade or high-grade and has low metastatic rate or locally aggressive/metastatic potential, respectively.[69] Histologically, glandular, tubular, and cystic structures with mucin and bland nuclei predominate in low-grade subtype, whereas intermediate and squamous areas with pleomorphism and mitoses largely comprise high-grade tumors.[12]

Cytologically, mucoepidermoid carcinoma has three cell types—mucinous, squamous, and intermediate—occurring singly or as clusters, with or without associated extracellular mucin, and necrotic debris.[67] The glandular cells tend to have eccentrically placed nuclei, sometimes secondary to indentation by cytoplasmic vacuoles, indistinct cell borders, and delicate cytoplasm, in contrast to the intermediate/squamous cells that have denser cytoplasm, centrally located nuclei and sharp borders.[67] The nuclear:cytoplasmic ratio among the cell types is variable.[67]

Immunohistochemistry Immunohistochemical stains may be helpful for separating mucoepidermoid carcinoma from adenocarcinoma. Both are CK7+ and CK20−; TTF-1 is expressed by adenocarcinoma and CK 5/6 by mucoepidermoid carcinoma.[70]

Differential Diagnosis Failure to recognize the combination of cell types, may lead to an erroneous diagnosis of either adenocarcinoma or squamous cell carcinoma. Conversely, appreciation of the different cells can suggest adenosquamous carcinoma. The distinction, if it exists,[71] may only be evident histologically, with identification of an in situ component, exophytic endobronchial growth,[12] absence of single cell keratination,[21] squamous pearls,[12] transition from low- to high-grade areas,[69] and central location in mucoepidermoid carcinoma.[17]

Pleomorphic Adenoma

Pleomorphic adenomas of the lung are biphasic tumors with epithelial and myoepithelial components not sufficiently described in cytology, but likely to have similar traits as in the head and neck tumors. Unlike in the salivary gland, pulmonary pleomorphic adenomas lack significant glandular[69] and chondroid areas[12] but have branching ductules lined by epithelial and myoepithelial cells and periodic acid-Schiff material on histology.[72] Pleomorphic adenomas also have fibrillar metachromatic stroma.

Immunohistochemistry All cells stain with pancytokeratin; however, vimentin, smooth muscle actin, and glial firbrillary acidic protein is specific for the myoepithelial cells.[12]

Differential Diagnosis Like adenoid cystic carcinoma, pleomorphic adenoma has hyaline material, but it is more fibrillar, and its transition with the cells is more gradual than in adenoid cystic caricinoma.[66,68]

PITFALLS IN PULMONARY CYTOLOGY

Pulmonary cytology has sensitivity and specificity ranging from 60% to 90%.[73] Even among the experienced cytopathologists, there are equivocal cases that are diagnostic dilemmas.[74] Majority of the medicolegal pathology cases involve surgical pathology, but approximately one third comprise cytology specimens, with false-positive diagnoses on sputum cytology/bronchial washing and lung aspirates being the third leading source of errors.[75] False-positive diagnoses tend to be more common than false-negative diagnoses.[74,76,77] Although difficult to entirely avoid in an active, high-volume pulmonary cytology practice, knowledge of complete clinical history (e.g., presence of localized mass lesion versus rapid clinical course/acute pulmonary damage), radiological findings, and common origins of cytological misinterpretations can minimize errors.

False-Negative Diagnosis

Sputum, bronchoalveolar lavage, and transthoracic fine-needle aspiration cytology specimens are often used to diagnose pulmonary lesions. Sputum and bronchoalveoleolar lavage specimens may not be accessible to small peripheral lesions, so CT-guided transthoracic fine-needle aspirations are employed to target the specific pathological process. Despite image-guidance, false-negative diagnoses in pulmonary fine-needle aspirations occur and are frequently a consequence of inadequate sampling,[76,77] for which repeat aspiration is recommended.[77] The negative predictive values of fine-needle aspirations range from 53.3%[77] to 77%.[76]

In some instances, false-negative diagnoses result from interpretive errors, especially in squamous cell carcinomas associated with marked active inflammation. A *carcinomatous abscess* with few dysplastic, foreign body reaction to keratin[9] and malignant cells in a predominantly inflammatory could be dismissed as reactive epithelial changes.[78] Malignant characteristics include keratinous fragments and/or ghost cells, irregular cells, and pyknotic nuclei.[9] Metastatic breast carcinoma can appear bland and be misclassified as a benign process.[74]

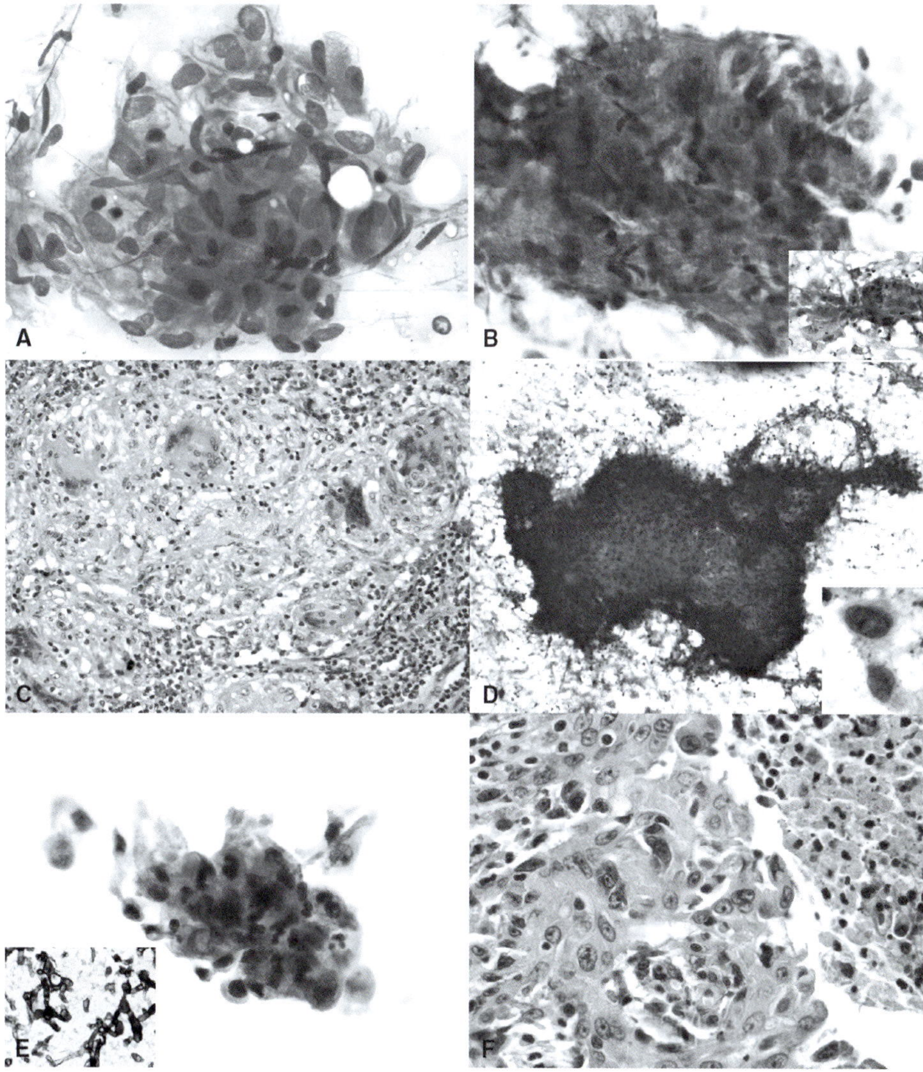

FIGURE 18.8 **A:** Granuloma: enlarged spindle-shaped and epithelioid histiocytes (Diff-Quik, 40×). **B,C:** Granuloma with atypia. **B:** Atypical spindle-shaped and epithelioid histiocytes in clusters. *Inset:* areas with streaming pattern associated with reactive changes (Papanicolaou stain, bronchial brush, 40×; *inset* 40×). **C:** Histological section from same case demonstrating histiocytes and giant cells without evidence of malignancy (H&E, 40×). **D–F:** Aspergillus with atypical squamous cells. **D:** Sheet of atypical squamous cells in an inflammatory/dirty background. *Inset:* high magnification of rare single cells with dense cytoplasm and high nuclear:cytoplasmic ratio (Diff-Quik, 10×; *inset* 40×). **E:** Atypical cells with dense cytoplasm and high nuclear: cytoplasmic ratios associated with rare fungal form and neutrophils. *Inset:* silver stain demonstrating fungal organisms. (ThinPrep, Papanicolaou stain, 60×; inset: Gomori methanamine stain, 40×) **F:** Histological section demonstrating atypical squamous cells and intraluminal necrotic debris (H&E, 40×) (See color plate.)

False-Positive Diagnosis Since the implementation of lung screening and CT scans, greater numbers of pulmonary lesions are detected. In some instances, sophisticated imaging modalities such as positron emission tomography (PET) are used. PET positivity results indicate malignant/"active" lesions, but sometimes, inflammatory processes also yield false-positive results (Figs. 18.8 and 18.9).

Similarly, in cytology, several benign processes can mimic carcinoma. Devoid of architectural clues evident in histological sections, the distinction between reactive change/atypia and malignant processes in cytology can be difficult. Some lesions have been reported more often in exfoliative specimens and others in fine-needle aspirations. Also, the various entities usually emulate squamous cell carcinoma and/or adenocarcinoma.

There are several sources of pulmonary cytological pitfalls including infectious/granulomatous disease (fungal infections, dirofilariasis, tuberculosis, *Pneumocystis carinii*, cytomegalovirus), acute lung injury (diffuse alveolar damage [DAD], thromboemboli, infarction), iatrogenic effect (chemotherapy, radiotherapy), meosthelial cell proliferation, benign neoplasms (e.g., hamartoma), prior procedure-related changes, and vegetable contaminants.[79]

Infections

Fungal Granulomas in the lung are associated with various etiologies, including infectious processes. Fungal infections (e.g., *Aspergillus*) are a source of reactive squamous atypia that mimics keratinizing squamous cell carcinoma.[18,80,81] The cytological specimens from the infections show squamous cells arranged singly and in clusters[18] with eosinophilic to orangeophilic cytoplasm, hyperchromatic nuclei, high nuclear: cytoplasmic ratio, and smudgy chromatin. In contrast, squamous cell carcinomas have more orangeophilic cytoplasm and greater numbers of single atypical cells.[18] Necrosis may be associated with both lesions[18] and cannot, therefore, be useful in discriminating between the two.

Mycobacterial Similarly, mycobacterial infections (i.e., tuberculosis) produce granulomatous inflammation, which can simulate carcinoma.[78] However, coexistence of tuberculosis and lung carcinoma including squamous cell carcinoma

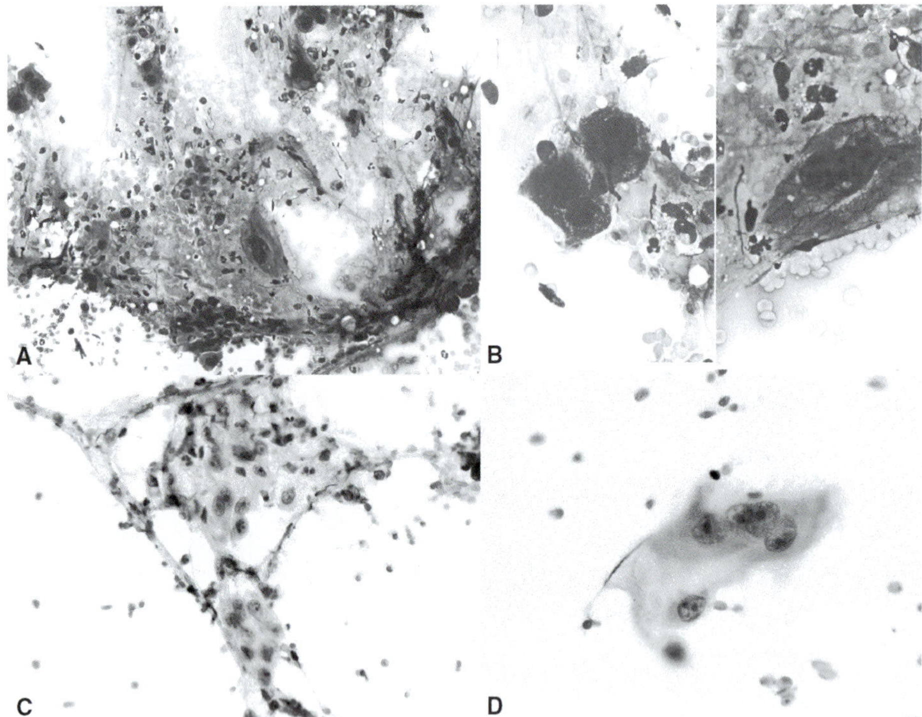

FIGURE 18.9 Therapy-related changes. **A:** Markedly atypical cells (postchemotherapy and stem cell transplant) (Diff-Quik- 20×). **B:** Cytomegaly with prominent nucleoli and relatively preserved nuclear:cytoplasmic ratios in an inflammatory background (postchemotherapy and stem cell transplant) (Diff-Quik, 60×). **C:** Atypical cells in cohesive cluster with vague *streaming pattern* without significant population of single atypical cells (postchemotherapy and stem cell transplant) (Papanicolaou stain, 60×). **D:** Multinucleated cell with prominent nucleoli and cytoplasmic vacuolization (postchemotherapy and stem cell transplant) (Papanicolaou stain, 60×). (See color plate.)

(the predominant subtype[82]), adenocarcinoma, large cell carcinoma, and small cell carcinoma has also been described.[83]

Parasitic (Dirofilariasis) *Dirofilaria immitis* is a canine heart roundworm that can infect humans. Pulmonary disease may be incidental or symptomatic, present as solitary or multiple nodule(s),[84] and suggest malignancy radiographically and clinically.[85] The infection can cause infarction secondary to pulmonary artery embolization of the parasite from the right ventricle and granulomatous reaction surrounding a thrombosed artery.[84] Some cytological cases are associated with reactive squamous metaplasia of surrounding airways, which may be erroneously diagnosed as squamous cell carcinoma,[84] whereas others demonstrate papillary clusters with cells containing high nuclear:cytoplasmic ratio, nuclear irregularity, mild hyperchromasia, and prominent nucleoli in the perilesional bronchiolar epithelium suggestive of adenocarcinoma. Scarcity of atypical cells and lack of significant hyperchromasia should favor a reparative/reactive process in pulmonary dirofilariasis.[86,87] This distinction is important because dirofilarial infection is benign and requires no surgical intervention.[85]

***Pneumocystis Pneumoniae* and Cytomegalovirus** False-positive diagnoses have been linked with cytomegalovirus[88] and *P. pneumoniae*[89] as well.

Wegener Granulomatosis Wegener granulomatosis, although not of infectious etiology, is a systemic vasculitis characterized by a triad of upper respiratory, lower respiratory, and renal involvement. Pulmonary Wegener granulomatosis has different histological appearances with the characteristic pattern demonstrating geographic necrosis, multinucleated giant cells, and mixed inflammatory infiltrate. Similar to the infectious and granulomatous entities, cytological atypia of Wegener granulomatosis may be a potential source of false-positive diagnosis.[90] Hyperchromatic atypical squamous cells in a background of necrosis, acute inflammation, and hemorrhage may be misdiagnosed as squamous cell carcinoma[90,91] and atypical bronchial cells as BAC.[92]

Acute Lung Injury Reactive type II pneumocytes, progenitors of type I pneumocytes in response to injury, are present in specimens when they are hyperplastic, thereby posing a potential diagnostic pitfall.[74,93,94] In bronchoalveolar lavage specimens, reactive type II pneumocytes have been associated with acute lung injury,[95] organizing pneumonia,[78] alveolar hemorrhage,[89] ventilator-associated pneumonia,[89] hypersensitivity pneumonitis,[89] eosinophilic pneumonia,[89] medication-induced injury,[89] DAD, and embolism/infarction. The cells tend to be large with high nuclear:cytoplasmic ratios and vacuolated cytoplasm[89] suggestive of adenocarcinoma.

Diffuse Alveolar Damage DAD has acute and organizing stages during which alveolar hyperplasia develops. Bronchoalveolar lavage specimens obtained from patients with DAD demonstrate cellular specimens with single cells, two-dimensional sheets, and three-dimensional cell clusters[96] that can occasionally form glandlike structures with scalloped edges suggestive of adenocarcinoma.[93] The cells have nuclear atypia, cytoplasmic hobnails characteristic of hyperplastic cells, ≥1 prominent nucleolus,[96] hyperchromasia, slight nuclear irregularities, high nuclear:cytoplasmic ratio,[93] and infrequently, dense cytoplasm suggestive of squamous differentiation.[96] Many of these features overlap with malignancy, but lack of uniformity among cell clusters, lack of markedly increased nuclear:cytoplasmic ratio, scalloping of cell groups with hobnails, and intercellular clearing "windows" support type II pneumocyte hyperplasia over carcinoma.[93]

Pulmonary Embolism/Infarction Pulmonary embolism with or without infarction can cause cytological atypia suggestive of adenocarcinoma.[97–100] Atypical cytological features include three-dimensional cell clusters with cytoplasmic vacuolization, enlarged nuclei with regular borders, and prominent nucleoli. Unlike malignant neoplasms, the atypia is focal and fleeting, often apparent 2 to 3 weeks postthromboembolism.[99] Single atypical cells often seen in conjunction with malignant neoplasms are lacking.[98,99,101]

Type II Pneumocytes versus Malignancy There is definite overlap between reactive type II pneumocyte hyperplasia and carcinoma, particularly BAC. Several criteria have been outlined in the literature to distinguish the lesions. First and foremost, a search for cilia and/or terminal bars is an important and simple clue to make a diagnosis oriented to a benign process. Reactive/reparative processes tend to have two-dimensional sheets, maintain uniformity and polarity,[79] and demonstrate cellular streaming.[102] Two cell populations[102] (i.e., relatively uniform and loosely cohesive benign cells and dyscohesive malignant cells with large nuclei), tissue fragments consisting of ≥2 cells with common inner or outer *community* borders and single cells, elongated or *tenacious* cytoplasmic borders, intranuclear intracytoplasmic inclusions, paucity of multinucleated giant cells, and increased nuclear area are more frequent in adenocarcinoma.[103] Other characteristics such as hyperchromasia, prominent nucleoli, nuclear membrane irregularities, elevated nucleus:cytoplasmic ratio,[103] and mitotic activity,[79] although often associated with malignancy, are also evident in reactive processes.[103]

Asthma Bronchial asthma results in excessive columnar epithelial cell shedding, sometimes as papillary formations suggestive of adenocarcinoma.[104] The cells tend to be of uniform shape and size with peripheral palisading.[104] Presence of eosinophils and Charcot-Leyden crystals is also helpful, but lacking in the acute phase.[104]

Lipoid Pneumonia Cytoplasmic vacuolization in lipid pneumonia may also resemble vacuoles of mucinous adenocarcinoma.[79] Lack of a mucinous background and histochemical/immunostains (mucicarmine, cytokeratin, CD68) can be helpful in making the distinction.

Chemotherapy and Radiotherapy Many anticancer drugs can cause atypical changes in the respiratory tract that resemble adenocarcinoma and squamous cell carcinoma.[102] Cellular changes associated with chemotherapy and/or radiation include cytomegaly with preserved nuclear:cytoplasmic ratio, multinucleation, macronucleoli, and nuclear pleomorphism.[105] The chromatin is uniform or smudgy, but a coarse chromatin pattern can be present.[102] Abnormal-appearing cells are often part of a tightly cohesive cluster or sheet without prominent single atypical cells (Fig. 18.9).

Mesothelial Cell Proliferations In transthoracic aspirates, particularly of pleural-based lesions, mesothelium is sometimes inadvertently sampled. Sheets of mesothelial cells can be misdiagnosed as squamous cell carcinoma,[80] or the honeycomb arrangement of relatively bland cells may suggest a diagnosis of BAC. Recognition of intercellular windows in mesothelial cells and, if necessary, immunohistochemical stains for mesothelial cells (calretinin, cytokeratin 5/6, WT-1) and epithelial cells (B72.3, BerEP4, CEA) are also helpful.

Pulmonary Hamartomas Pulmonary hamartomas may also be mistaken for adenocarcinoma.[74,41] The myxoid background may be interpreted as mucin, whereas bronchiolar hyperplasia, intranuclear inclusions, intranuclear invaginations, and multinucleation can suggest adenoarcinoma.[41,106,74]

Unlike mucin, fibromyxoid stroma has fibrillar edges and spindle-shaped nuclei. A cell block can also be made at time of on-site evaluation for further characterization. The mucicarmine stain would be negative, and S-100 immunostain would highlight the spindle stromal cells. In addition, when present, the chondroid/cartilaginous component may be better preserved in cell block sections but not easily visualized in smears.

Suture Granuloma and Posttracheostomy Atypia Fine-needle aspirate of a PET-active lesion in a patient with a history of multiple primary carcinomas was interpreted as non–small cell carcinoma based on presence of dysplastic cells. Surgical excision showed an inflammatory nodule at the prior suture site.[107] Posttracheostomy atypia following laryngectomy and/or tracheostomy can show cells with irregular nuclear contours and fine or coarse chromatin suggestive of squamous cell carcinoma.[108] Absence of a mass clinically should dictate caution.

Vegetable Contaminant Patients with aspiration pneumonia may have vegetable cells contaminants suggestive of pulmonary epithelial cell atypia.[109] Features suggestive of malignancy include linear arrangement of asparagus cells suggestive of metastatic lobular breast carcinoma,[109] vacuolated and swollen cytoplasm indicative of mucin,[109] and dark cytoplasm reminiscent of atypical enlarged nuclei.[109] Regular quadrangular shape, extremely large size and refractory walls favor vegetable cell contamination.[109]

Megakaryocytes Megakaryocytes are seen incidentally in histological specimens as large, hyperchromatic, irregular cells bulging from capillaries in patients with smoking history, sepsis, cardiovascular disease, and metastatic malignancy.[110] Although rare in cytology, their atypical appearance can mislead to a diagnosis of malignancy.[11] Lobulated nuclei (single or multiple), ruffled border, and variation in cytoplasm (dense centrally and pale peripherally) are clues to megakaryocytic origin.[11]

CONCLUSION

A cytological diagnosis is a synthesis of clinical, radiological, and morphological features with appropriate sampling and specimen preservation. False-positive diagnoses, particularly in sputa, are of 10 related to insufficient clinical history.[73] Adjunct studies such as immunohistochemical stains and fluorescence in situ hybridization (FISH) analysis[74] may be helpful in some cases. Despite these measures, cytology has limitations, and a definitive diagnosis cannot always be ascertained. If uncertainty remains, it is prudent to suggest additional sampling or a frozen section prior to definitive surgery.

REFERENCES

1. Risse EK, Vooijs GP, van't Hof MA. Relationship between the cellular composition of sputum and the cytologic diagnosis of lung cancer. *Acta Cytol* 1987;31(2):170–176.
2. Travis WD LJ, Mackay B. Classification, histology, cytology and electron microscopy. In: HI P, ed. *Lung Cancer*. 2nd Ed. Philadelphia: Lippincott Williams and Wilkins, 2000:453–495.
3. Sing A, Freudenberg N, Kortsik C, et al. Comparison of the sensitivity of sputum and brush cytology in the diagnosis of lung carcinomas. *Acta Cytol* 1997;41(2):399–408.
4. de Gracia J, Bravo C, Miravitlles M, et al. Diagnostic value of bronchoalveolar lavage in peripheral lung cancer. *Am Rev Respir Dis* 1993;147(3):649–652.
5. Schreiber G, McCrory DC. Performance characteristics of different modalities for diagnosis of suspected lung cancer: summary of published evidence. *Chest* 2003;123(1 Suppl):S115–S128.
6. Wistuba II, Mao L, Gazdar AF. Smoking molecular damage in bronchial epithelium. *Oncogene* 2002;21(48):7298–7306.
7. Westra WH, Slebos RJ, Offerhaus GJ, et al. K-ras oncogene activation in lung adenocarcinomas from former smokers. Evidence that K-ras mutations are an early and irreversible event in the development of adenocarcinoma of the lung. *Cancer* 1993;72(2):432–438.
8. Travis WD, Lubin J, Ries L, et al. United States lung carcinoma incidence trends: declining for most histologic types among males, increasing among females. *Cancer* 1996;77(12):2464–2470.
9. Silverman JF, Geisinger KR. Lung. In: Silverman JF, Geisinger KR, eds. *Fine Needle Aspiration Cytology of the Thorax and Abdomen*. Hong Kong: Churchill Livingstone, 1996:51.
10. Johnston WW, Elson CE. Respiratory tract. In: Bibbo M, ed. *Comprehensive Cytopathology*. 2nd Ed. Philadelphia: W.B. Saunders, 1997:325–401.
11. Geisinger KR, Stanley M, Raab SS, et al. Normal pulmonary cytology and diffuse lung diseases; localized lung diseases. *Modern Cytopathology*. Philadelphia: Churchill Livingstone, 2004:361–432.
12. Travis WD, Brambilla E, Muller-Hermelink HK, eds. *Pathology and Genetics of Tumours of the Lung, Pleura, Thymus and Heart*. 1st Ed. Lyon: International Agency for Research on Cancer, 2004:344.
13. Abe S, Ogura S, Nakajima I, et al. Small-cell-type poorly differentiated squamous cell carcinoma of the lung. Cytologic, immunohistochemical and nuclear DNA content analysis. *Anal Quant Cytol Histol* 1990;12(2):73–77.
14. Cohen MH, Gootenberg J, Keegan P, et al. FDA drug approval summary: bevacizumab (Avastin) plus Carboplatin and Paclitaxel as first-line treatment of advanced/metastatic recurrent nonsquamous non-small cell lung cancer. *Oncologist* 2007;12(6):713–718.
15. Hsieh RK, Lim KH, Kuo HT, et al. Female sex and bronchioloalveolar pathologic subtype predict EGFR mutations in non-small cell lung cancer. *Chest* 2005;128(1):317–321.
16. Tan D, Li Q, Deeb G, et al. Thyroid transcription factor-1 expression prevalence and its clinical implications in non-small cell lung cancer: a high-throughput tissue microarray and immunohistochemistry study. *Hum Pathol* 2003;34(6):597–604.
17. Ordonez NG. The diagnostic utility of immunohistochemistry in distinguishing between epithelioid mesotheliomas and squamous carcinomas of the lung: a comparative study. *Mod Pathol* 2006;19(3):417–428.
18. Crapanzano JP, Zakowski MF. Diagnostic dilemmas in pulmonary cytology. *Cancer* 2001;93(6):364–375.
19. Lubin JH, Blot WJ. Assessment of lung cancer risk factors by histologic category. *J Natl Cancer Inst* 1984;73(2):383–389.
20. Ramalingam S, Pawlish K, Gadgeel S, et al. Lung cancer in young patients: analysis of a Surveillance, Epidemiology, and End Results database. *J Clin Oncol* 1998;16(2):651–657.
21. Terasaki H, Niki T, Matsuno Y, et al. Lung adenocarcinoma with mixed bronchioloalveolar and invasive components: clinicopathological features, subclassification by extent of invasive foci, and immunohistochemical characterization. *Am J Surg Pathol* 2003;27(7):937–951.
22. Brambilla E, Travis WD, Colby TV, et al. The new World Health Organization classification of lung tumours. *Eur Respir J* 2001;18(6):1059–1068.
23. Auger M, Katz RL, Johnston DA. Differentiating cytological features of bronchioloalveolar carcinoma from adenocarcinoma of the lung in fine-needle aspirations: a statistical analysis of 27 cases. *Diagn Cytopathol* 1997;16(3):253–257.
24. Holst VA, Finkelstein S, Yousem SA. Bronchioloalveolar adenocarcinoma of lung: monoclonal origin for multifocal disease. *Am J Surg Pathol* 1998;22(11):1343–1350.
25. MacDonald LL, Yazdi HM. Fine-needle aspiration biopsy of bronchioloalveolar carcinoma. *Cancer* 2001;93(1):29–34.
26. Ohori NP, Santa Maria EL. Cytopathologic diagnosis of bronchioloalveolar carcinoma: does it correlate with the 1999 World Health Organization definition? *Am J Clin Pathol* 2004;122(1):44–50.
27. Vazquez MF, Koizumi JH, Henschke CI, et al. Reliability of cytologic diagnosis of early lung cancer. *Cancer* 2007;111(4):252–258.
28. Saleh HA, Haapaniemi J, Khatib G, et al. Bronchioloalveolar carcinoma: diagnostic pitfalls and immunocytochemical contribution. *Diagn Cytopathol* 1998;18(4):301–306.
29. Yim J, Zhu LC, Chiriboga L, et al. Histologic features are important prognostic indicators in early stages lung adenocarcinomas. *Mod Pathol* 2007;20(2):233–241.
30. Rusch VW, Tsuchiya R, Tsuboi M, et al. Surgery for bronchioloalveolar carcinoma and "very early" adenocarcinoma: an evolving standard of care? *J Thorac Oncol* 2006;1(9 Suppl):S27–S31.
31. Wei EX, Anga AA, Martin SS, et al. EGFR expression as an ancillary tool for diagnosing lung cancer in cytology specimens. *Mod Pathol* 2007;20(9):905–913.
32. Zudaire I, Lozano MD, Vazquez MF, et al. Molecular characterization of small peripheral lung tumors based on the analysis of fine needle aspirates. *Histol Histopathol* 2008;23(1):33–40.
33. Garfield DH, Cadranel JL, Wislez M, et al. The bronchioloalveolar carcinoma and peripheral adenocarcinoma spectrum of diseases. *J Thorac Oncol* 2006;1(4):344–359.
34. Chen KT. Psammoma bodies in fine-needle aspiration cytology of papillary adenocarcinoma of the lung. *Diagn Cytopathol* 1990;6(4):271–274.
35. Duncan LD, Jacob S, Atkinson S. Fine needle aspiration cytologic findings of micropapillary carcinoma in the lung: a case report. *Acta Cytol* 2007;51(4):605–609.
36. Kaufmann O, Dietel M. Thyroid transcription factor-1 is the superior immunohistochemical marker for pulmonary adenocarcinomas

and large cell carcinomas compared to surfactant proteins A and B. *Histopathology* 2000;36(1):8–16.

37. Chhieng DC, Cangiarella JF, Zakowski MF, et al. Use of thyroid transcription factor 1, PE-10, and cytokeratins 7 and 20 in discriminating between primary lung carcinomas and metastatic lesions in fine-needle aspiration biopsy specimens. *Cancer* 2001;93(5):330–336.
38. Dabbs DJ, Landreneau RJ, Liu Y, et al. Detection of estrogen receptor by immunohistochemistry in pulmonary adenocarcinoma. *Ann Thorac Surg* 2002;73(2):403–405; discussion 406.
39. Mazziotta RM, Borczuk AC, Powell CA, et al. CDX2 immunostaining as a gastrointestinal marker: expression in lung carcinomas is a potential pitfall. *Appl Immunohistochem Mol Morphol* 2005;13(1):55–60.
40. Ng WK, Fu KH, Wang E, et al. Sclerosing hemangioma of lung: a close cytologic mimicker of pulmonary adenocarcinoma. *Diagn Cytopathol* 2001;25(5):316–320.
41. Saqi A, Shaham D, Scognamiglio T, et al. Incidence and cytological features of pulmonary hamartomas indeterminate on CT scan. *Cytopathology* 2008;19(3):185–191.
42. Flieder DB. Neuroendocrine tumors of the lung: recent developments in histopathology. *Curr Opin Pulm Med* 2002;8(4):275–280.
43. Collins BT, Cramer HM. Fine needle aspiration cytology of carcinoid tumors. *Acta Cytol* 1996;40(4):695–707.
44. Anderson C, Ludwig ME, O'Donnell M, et al. Fine needle aspiration cytology of pulmonary carcinoid tumors. *Acta Cytol* 1990;34(4):505–510.
45. Yao D DR, Yankelevitz D, Vazquez MF. Prominent vascularity distinguishes typical carcinoid and atypical carcinoid from high grade neuroendocrine carcinoma on transthoracic fine needle aspirates. *Mod Pathol* 2002;15:94A.
46. Mitchell ML, Parker FP. Capillaries. A cytologic feature of pulmonary carcinoid tumors. *Acta Cytol* 1991;35(2):183–185.
47. Renshaw AA, Haja J, Lozano RL, et al. Distinguishing carcinoid tumor from small cell carcinoma of the lung: correlating cytologic features and performance in the College of American Pathologists Non-Gynecologic Cytology Program. *Arch Pathol Lab Med* 2005; 129(5):614–618.
48. Evans H, Blaney R. Pulmonary carcinoid with papillary structure: report of a case with fine-needle aspiration cytology. *Diagn Cytopathol* 1994;11(2):178–181.
49. Sturm N, Rossi G, Lantuejoul S, et al. Expression of thyroid transcription factor-1 in the spectrum of neuroendocrine cell lung proliferations with special interest in carcinoids. *Hum Pathol* 2002;33(2):175–182.
50. Folpe AL, Gown AM, Lamps LW, et al. Thyroid transcription factor-1: immunohistochemical evaluation in pulmonary neuroendocrine tumors. *Mod Pathol* 1999;12(1):5–8.
51. Rusch VW, Klimstra DS, Venkatraman ES. Molecular markers help characterize neuroendocrine lung tumors. *Ann Thorac Surg* 1996; 62(3):798–809; discussion 809–810.
52. Aslan DL, Gulbahce HE, Pambuccian SE, et al. Ki-67 immunoreactivity in the differential diagnosis of pulmonary neuroendocrine neoplasms in specimens with extensive crush artifact. *Am J Clin Pathol* 2005;123(6):874–878.
53. Saqi A, Oster MW, Vazquez MF. Metastatic mammary carcinomas with endocrine features: potential diagnostic pitfalls. *Diagn Cytopathol* 2005;33(1):49–53.
54. Nicholson SA, Beasley MB, Brambilla E, et al. Small cell lung carcinoma (SCLC): a clinicopathologic study of 100 cases with surgical specimens. *Am J Surg Pathol* 2002;26(9):1184–1197.
55. Mullins RK, Thompson SK, Coogan PS, et al. Paranuclear blue inclusions: an aid in the cytopathologic diagnosis of primary and metastatic pulmonary small-cell carcinoma. *Diagn Cytopathol* 1994; 10(4):332–335.
56. Wittchow R, Laszewski M, Walker W, et al. Paranuclear blue inclusions in metastatic undifferentiated small cell carcinoma in the bone marrow. *Mod Pathol* 1992;5(5):555–558.
57. Delgado PI, Jorda M, Ganjei-Azar P. Small cell carcinoma versus other lung malignancies: diagnosis by fine-needle aspiration cytology. *Cancer* 2000;90(5):279–285.
58. Jiang SX, Kameya T, Shoji M, et al. Large cell neuroendocrine carcinoma of the lung: a histologic and immunohistochemical study of 22 cases. *Am J Surg Pathol* 1998;22(5):526–537.
59. Travis WD, Linnoila RI, Tsokos MG, et al. Neuroendocrine tumors of the lung with proposed criteria for large-cell neuroendocrine carcinoma. An ultrastructural, immunohistochemical, and flow cytometric study of 35 cases. *Am J Surg Pathol* 1991;15(6):529–553.
60. Wiatrowska BA, Krol J, Zakowski MF. Large-cell neuroendocrine carcinoma of the lung: proposed criteria for cytologic diagnosis. *Diagn Cytopathol* 2001;24(1):58–64.
61. Yang YJ, Steele CT, Ou XL, et al. Diagnosis of high-grade pulmonary neuroendocrine carcinoma by fine-needle aspiration biopsy: nonsmall-cell or small-cell type? *Diagn Cytopathol* 2001;25(5):292–300.
62. Marmor S, Koren R, Halpern M, et al. Transthoracic needle biopsy in the diagnosis of large-cell neuroendocrine carcinoma of the lung. *Diagn Cytopathol* 2005;33(4):238–243.
63. Sturm N, Lantuéjoul S, Laverriere MH, et al. Thyroid transcription factor 1 and cytokeratins 1, 5, 10, 14 (34betaE12) expression in basaloid and large-cell neuroendocrine carcinomas of the lung. *Hum Pathol* 2001;32(9):918–925.
64. Travis WD, Rush W, Flieder DB, et al. Survival analysis of 200 pulmonary neuroendocrine tumors with clarification of criteria for atypical carcinoid and its separation from typical carcinoid. *Am J Surg Pathol* 1998;22(8):934–944.
65. Molina JR, Aubry MC, Lewis JE, etal. Primary salivary gland-type lung cancer: spectrum of clinical presentation, histopathologic and prognostic factors. *Cancer* 2007;110(10):2253–2259.
66. Daneshbod Y, Modjtahedi E, Atefi S, et al. Exfoliative cytologic findings of primary pulmonary adenoid cystic carcinom: a report of 2 cases with a review of the cytologic features. *Acta Cytol* 2007;51(4):558–562.
67. Segletes LA, Steffee CH, Geisinger KR. Cytology of primary pulmonary mucoepidermoid and adenoid cystic carcinoma. A report of four cases. *Acta Cytol* 1999;43(6):1091–1097.
68. Qiu S, Nampoothiri MM, Zaharopoulos P, et al. Primary pulmonary adenoid cystic carcinoma: report of a case diagnosed by fine-needle aspiration cytology. *Diagn Cytopathol* 2004;30(1):51–56.
69. Moran CA. Primary salivary gland-type tumors of the lung. *Semin Diagn Pathol* 1995;12(2):106–122.
70. Shilo K, Foss RD, Franks TJ, et al. Pulmonary mucoepidermoid carcinoma with prominent tumor-associated lymphoid proliferation. *Am J Surg Pathol* 2005;29(3):407–411.
71. Heitmiller RF, Mathisen DJ, Ferry JA, et al. Mucoepidermoid lung tumors. *Ann Thorac Surg* 1989;47(3):394–399.
72. Sakamoto H, Uda H, Tanaka T, et al. Pleomorphic adenoma in the periphery of the lung. Report of a case and review of the literature. *Arch Pathol Lab Med* 1991;115(4):393–396.
73. Jay SJ, Wehr K, Nicholson DP, et al. Diagnostic sensitivity and specificity of pulmonary cytology: comparison of techniques used in conjunction with flexible fiber optic bronchoscopy. *Acta Cytol* 1980;24(4):304–312.
74. Glatz K, Savic S, Glatz D, et al. An online quiz uncovers limitations of morphology in equivocal lung cytology. *Cancer* 2006;108(6): 480–487.
75. Kornstein MJ, Byrne SP. The medicolegal aspect of error in pathology: a search of jury verdicts and settlements. *Arch Pathol Lab Med* 2007;131(4):615–618.
76. Afify A, Davila RM. Pulmonary fine needle aspiration biopsy. Assessing the negative diagnosis. *Acta Cytol* 1999;43(4):601–604.
77. Zakowski MF, Gatscha RM, Zaman MB. Negative predictive value of pulmonary fine needle aspiration cytology. *Acta Cytol* 1992;36(3): 283–286.
78. Silverman JF. Inflammatory and neoplastic processes of the lung: differential diagnosis and pitfalls in FNA biopsies. *Diagn Cytopathol* 1995;13(5):448–462.
79. Policarpio-Nicolas ML, Wick MR. False-positive interpretations in respiratory cytopathology: exemplary cases and literature review. *Diagn Cytopathol* 2008;36(1):13–19.

80. Naryshkin S, Young NA. Respiratory cytology: a review of non-neoplastic mimics of malignancy. *Diagn Cytopathol* 1993;9(1):89–97.
81. Ritter JH, Wick MR, Reyes A, et al. False-positive interpretations of carcinoma in exfoliative respiratory cytology. Report of two cases and a review of underlying disorders. *Am J Clin Pathol* 1995;104(2):133–140.
82. Kobashi Y, Fukuda M, Nakata M, et al. Coexistence of metastatic lung cancer and pulmonary tuberculosis diagnosed in the same cavity. *Int J Clin Oncol* 2005;10(5):366–370.
83. Kurasawa T, Takahashi M, Kuze F, et al. A clinical study on coexistence of active pulmonary tuberculosis and lung cancer [in Japanese]. *Kekkaku* 1992;67(2):119–125.
84. Flieder DB, Moran CA. Pulmonary dirofilariasis: a clinicopathologic study of 41 lesions in 39 patients. *Hum Pathol* 1999;30(3):251–256.
85. Foroulis CN, Khaldi L, Desimonas N, et al. Pulmonary dirofilariasis mimicking lung tumor with chest wall and mediastinal invasion. *Thorac Cardiovasc Surg* 2005;53(3):173–175.
86. Akaogi E, Ishibashi O, Mitsui K, et al. Pulmonary dirofilariasis cytologically mimicking lung cancer. A case report. *Acta Cytol* 1993; 37(4):531–534.
87. Risher WH, Crocker EF Jr, Beckman EN, et al. Pulmonary dirofilariasis. The largest single-institution experience. *J Thorac Cardiovasc Surg* 1989;97(2):303–308.
88. Grunze H. Cytologic diagnosis of tumors of the chest. *Acta Cytol* 1973; 17(2):148–159.
89. Linssen KC, Jacobs JA, Poletti VE, et al. Reactive type II pneumocytes in bronchoalveolar lavage fluid. *Acta Cytol* 2004;48(4):497–504.
90. Awasthi A, Malhotra P, Gupta N, et al. Pitfalls in the diagnosis of Wegener's granulomatosis on fine needle aspiration cytology. *Cytopathology* 2007;18(1):8–12.
91. Williamson JD, Murphree SS, Wills-Frank L. Atypical squamous cells as a diagnostic pitfall in pulmonary Wegener's granulomatosis. A case report. *Acta Cytol* 2002;46(3):571–576.
92. Pitman MB, Szyfelbein WM, Niles J, et al. Clinical utility of fine needle aspiration biopsy in the diagnosis of Wegener's granulomatosis. A report of two cases. *Acta Cytol* 1992;36(2):222–229.
93. Grotte D, Stanley MW, Swanson PE, et al. Reactive type II pneumocytes in bronchoalveolar lavage fluid from adult respiratory distress syndrome can be mistaken for cells of adenocarcinoma. *Diagn Cytopathol* 1990;6(5):317–322.
94. Stanley MW, Henry-Stanley MJ, Gajl-Peczalska KJ, et al. Hyperplasia of type II pneumocytes in acute lung injury. Cytologic findings of sequential bronchoalveolar lavage. *Am J Clin Pathol* 1992;97(5):669–677.
95. McKee G, Parums DV. False-positive cytodiagnosis in fibrosing alveolitis. *Acta Cytol* 1990;34(1):105–107.
96. Beskow CO, Drachenberg CB, Bourquin PM, et al. Diffuse alveolar damage. Morphologic features in bronchoalveolar lavage fluid. *Acta Cytol* 2000;44(4):640–646.
97. Kaminsky DA, Leiman G. False-positive sputum cytology in a case of pulmonary infarction. *Respir Care* 2004;49(2):186–188.
98. Lawther RE, Graham AN, McCluggage WG, et al. Pulmonary infarct cytologically mimicking adenocarcinoma of the lung. *Ann Thorac Surg* 2002;73(6):1964–1965.
99. Bewtra C, Dewan N, O'Donahue WJ Jr. Exfoliative sputum cytology in pulmonary embolism. *Acta Cytol* 1983;27(5):489–496.
100. Scoggins WG, Smith RH, Frable WJ, et al. False-positive cytologicial diagnosis of lung carcinoma in patients with pulmonary infarcts. *Ann Thorac Surg* 1977;24(5):474–480.
101. Tanimura S, Tomoyasu H, Bamba J, et al. Three cases of pulmonary embolism incorrectly diagnosed as lung cancer [in Japanese]. *Jpn J Thorac Cardiovasc Surg* 1998;46(11):1137–1140.
102. Naryshkin S, Bedrossian CW. Selected mimics of malignancy in sputum and bronchoscopic cytology specimens. *Diagn Cytopathol* 1995; 13(5):443–447.
103. Zaman SS, van Hoeven KH, Slott S, et al. Distinction between bronchioloalveolar carcinoma and hyperplastic pulmonary proliferations: a cytologic and morphometric analysis. *Diagn Cytopathol* 1997; 16(5):396–401.
104. Naylor B, Railey C. A pitfall in the cytodiagnosis of sputum of asthmatics. *J Clin Pathol* 1964;17:84–89.
105. Koss LG SW, Wiodzimierz O. *Cytologic Interpretation and Histologic Basis*. New York: Igaku-Shoin, 1992:474–530.
106. Hughes JH, Young NA, Wilbur DC, et al. Fine-needle aspiration of pulmonary hamartoma: a common source of false-positive diagnoses in the College of American Pathologists Interlaboratory Comparison Program in Nongynecologic Cytology. *Arch Pathol Lab Med* 2005;129(1):19–22.
107. Yüksel M, Akgül AG, Evman S, et al. Suture and stapler granulomas: a word of caution. *Eur J Cardiothorac Surg* 2007;31(3):563–565.
108. Berman JJ, Murray RJ, Lopez-Plaza IM. Widespread posttracheostomy atypia simulating squamous cell carcinoma. A case report. *Acta Cytol* 1991;35(6):713–716.
109. Weaver KM, Novak PM, Naylor B. Vegetable cell contaminants in cytologic specimens: their resemblance to cells associated with various normal and pathologic states. *Acta Cytol* 1981;25(3):210–214.
110. Sharma GK, Talbot IC. Pulmonary megakaryocytes: "missing link" between cardiovascular and respiratory disease? *J Clin Pathol* 1986; 39(9):969–976.

CHAPTER 19

Annette McWilliams
Stephen Lam

Early Detection of Lung Cancer Using Bronchoscopy

Although the overall lung cancer survival is poor with only 15% of patients surviving 5 years after diagnosis,[1] patients with tumors <2 cm have a 5-year survival of 77%.[1] The survival of those with preinvasive or microinvasive bronchial cancers is even better at >90%.[2] Over the last 2 decades, the largest gain in life expectancy in lung cancer patients is among those with localized disease versus those with regional or distant metastasis.[3] Clearly, strategies to improve outcome by detecting and treating the disease in the preinvasive or localized stages is needed.

There are unique challenges to localize preneoplastic lesions or early cancers in the lung. In contrast to other epithelial organs such as the oral cavity, cervix, or colon, the lung consists of a complex branching system of conducting airways leading to alveoli with a surface area the size of a tennis court. In addition, instead of a single cell type, lung cancer consists of several cell types and they are preferentially located in different parts of the tracheobronchial tree. Squamous cell carcinoma and small cell carcinoma, accounting for approximately 45% to 50% of the lung cancers are preferentially located in the central airways (trachea, main, lobar, and segmental bronchi). Adenocarcinoma, accounting for approximately 40% to 50% of all lung cancers, is preferentially located in the peripheral airways inaccessible to standard fiberoptic/video bronchoscopes because of the size of these instruments with an outer diameter of ≥4.9 mm. Ultrathin bronchoscopes with an outer diameter of 2.9 mm are available, but they cannot reach peripheral airways ≤2 mm in diameter. Thus, there is no single method that can scan the entire bronchial epithelium and allow tissue sampling for pathological diagnosis and molecular profiling.

DETECTION OF EARLY CANCER IN CENTRAL AIRWAYS

Rapid evaluation of the central airways became possible with the development of flexible fiberoptic white-light bronchoscopy by Dr. Shigeto Ikeda in the late 1960s. There has been continuing technological advancement over the last 40 years. The development of videobronchoscopy, with better image resolution and quality, is now replacing the former fiberoptic systems. However, early central lung cancers remain difficult to detect with white-light bronchoscopy even with the improved image capability of videobronchoscopy.[4] Recent incorporation of optical zoom or magnifying lenses may enhance the examination of the bronchial mucosa and improve the detection of early vascular changes that can be associated with early malignant change.[5] Other developments that can be used in adjunct with white-light imaging for localization of preneoplastic lesions and early lung cancer include autofluorescence bronchoscopy (AFB), narrow-band imaging (NBI), and optical coherence tomography (OCT). The recent development of endobronchial ultrasound is an additional tool for the bronchoscopic assessment of central early lung cancers.

Autofluorescence Reflectance Bronchoscopy Autofluorescence reflectance bronchoscopy has been shown in multiple studies to significantly increase the detection of preneoplastic lesions and carcinoma in situ when used as an adjunct to white-light bronchoscopy[6–26] (Table 19.1). In addition, it is important in the staging of early central lung cancers prior to curative endobronchial therapy.[27,28] It enables the bronchoscopist to obtain a more accurate visualization of the margins and assessment of lesion size.[27,28]

This technique utilizes the spectral differences in fluorescence and absorption properties of normal and dysplastic bronchial epithelium and has served as the basis for the design of several autofluorescence imaging devices for localization of early lung cancer.[6,12,13] More recent versions of these devices use a combination of reflectance and fluorescence for imaging.[14,22,23,25,29,30]

AFB was first developed in the early 1990s at the British Columbia Cancer Research Centre in Vancouver, British Columbia, and became commercially available in 1998.[10] The LIFE-Lung system (Xillix Technologies, Vancouver, BC) used a helium–cadmium laser for illumination (442 nm) and detected

TABLE 19.1 Results of Multicenter Clinical Trials and Randomized Studies of Autofluorescence Bronchoscopy

	Device	No. of Subjects	Sensitivity (%)		Specificity (%)	
			WLB	AFB	WLB	AFB
Lam et al.[12]*	LIFE-Lung	173	9	66	90	66
Ernst et al.[23]*	D-Light	293	11	66	95	73
Edell 2005[14]*	Onco-LIFE	170	10	44	94	75
Hirsch et al.[24]†	LIFE-Lung	55	18	73	78	46
Häussinger et al.[25]†	D-Light	1173	58	82	62	58

*Multicenter clinical trial.

†Randomized trial.

AFB, autofluorescence bronchoscopy; WLB, white-light bronchoscopy.

the emitted red and green autofluorescent light with two image-intensified charge-coupled device (CCD) cameras. Normal areas appear green, and abnormal areas appear reddish brown because of reduced green autofluorescence in preneoplastic and neoplastic lesions.

Subsequent improvements in technology made it possible to use nonimage intensified CCDs for detection. Two second-generation devices approved by Food and Drug Administration (FDA) made use of a combination of fluorescence and reflectance to enhance contrast between normal and abnormal tissues (Table 19.2). The Onco-LIFE system (Novadq Technologies, Richmond, Canada) utilizes a combination of reflectance and fluorescence imaging. Blue light (395 to 445 nm) and small amount of red light (675 to 720 nm) from a filtered mercury arc lamp is used for illumination (Fig. 19.1). A red reflectance image is captured in combination with the green autofluorescence image to enhance the contrast between premalignant, malignant, and normal tissues as well as to correct for differences in light intensities from changes in angle and distance of the bronchoscope from the bronchial surface.[14] Using reflected near infrared red light as a reference has the theoretical advantage over reflected blue light in that it is less absorbed by hemoglobin and hence less influenced by changes in vascularity associated with inflammation. The D-Light system (Karl Storz Endoscopy of America, Culver City, California) consists of a red/green/blue (RGB) CCD camera and a filtered Xe lamp (380 to 460 nm). It combines an autofluorescence image from wavelengths >480 nm with a blue reflectance image.[25] Frame averaging is used to amplify the weak autofluorescence signal.

These earlier autofluorescence systems were developed to be used with fiberoptic bronchoscopes. With the advanced CCD sensor technology and more widespread use of videobronchoscopy, autofluorescence systems that can be used with videobronchoscopes have been developed (Table 19.2). The Pentax SAFE-3000 system (Pentax Corporation, Tokyo, Japan) uses a semiconductor laser diode that emits 408 nm wavelength light for illumination and detects autofluorescence using a single high-sensitivity color CCD sensor in the fluorescence spectrum 430 to 700 nm (Fig. 19.2). Reflected blue light is used to generate a fluorescence-reflectance image. The white-light and fluorescence images can also be made displayed simultaneously.[29] The Olympus autofluorescence imaging bronchovideoscope system (Olympus Corporation, Tokyo, Japan) uses blue light (395 to 445 nm) for illumination. An

TABLE 19.2 Autofluorescence Imaging Systems

Device	Excitation Light	Image Composition	Abnormal Lesion
Onco-LIFE	395–445 nm 675–720 nm	Green fluorescence Red reflectance	Reddish brown on green background
Storz D-light	380–460 nm	Green/red fluorescence Blue reflectance	Purple on bluish green background
SAFE 3000*	408 nm	Green/red fluorescence Blue reflectance	Purple on bluish green background
Olympus AFI*	395–445 nm 550 nm, 610 nm	Green/red fluorescence Green/red reflectance	Magenta/purple on green background

*Videobronchoscope systems.

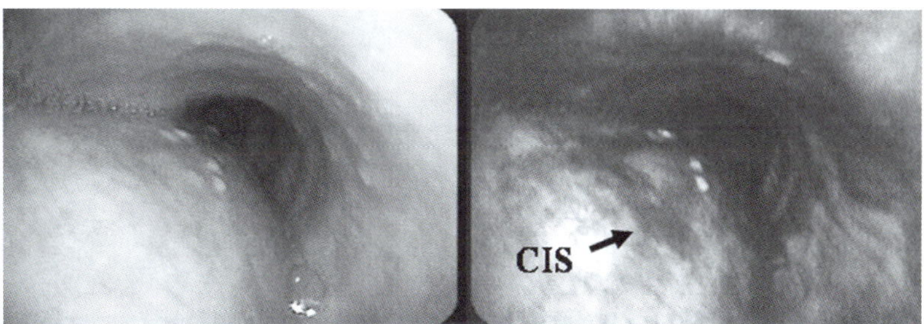

FIGURE 19.1 White-light (*left*) and autofluorescence bronchoscopy (*right*) images of a carcinoma in situ (CIS) lesion in the left main bronchus. No abnormality was seen under white-light examination. Under fluorescence imaging, the CIS lesion as an area of decreased fluorescence. (See color plate.)

autofluorescence image (490 to 700 nm) as well as two reflectance images, one green (550 nm) and one red (610 nm) are captured sequentially and integrated by a videoprocessor to produce a composite image.[30]

A reduction in specificity has been associated with the increased sensitivity for detection of early lesions. However, there is some data that shows that areas with abnormal autofluorescence contain increased chromosomal aberrations despite a benign histopathology, and that the presence of multiple areas of abnormal autofluorescence is an indicator of overall increased lung cancer risk.[31,32] Recently, the use of a quantitative score during autofluorescence examination has been shown to improve specificity.[33]

Optical Coherence Tomography

Currently, there are two imaging modalities with sufficient spatial resolution and tissue depth penetration to address the relatively high false-positive AFB results and to determine whether the tumor has already invaded through the basement membrane (Fig. 19.3). Confocal microendoscopy offers spatial resolution down to the submicron range, but epithelial cells do not autofluoresence strong enough to allow detection without application of a contrast agent.[34,35] In addition, because contact with the bronchial surface is required, fragile epithelium can be scraped off during imaging. Motion artifacts caused by cardiac pulsation and respiratory movements can also lead to suboptimal confocal imaging of cellular details. OCT is a promising micron-scale–resolution method that may be more suitable for rapid endoscopic imaging. OCT is a noncontact method that delivers near infrared light to the tissue and allows imaging of cellular and extracellular structures from analysis of the backscattered light with a spatial resolution of 3 to 15 μm and a depth penetration of approximately 2 mm to provide near-histological images in the bronchial wall.[36–39] Preliminary studies showed that invasive cancer can be distinguished from carcinoma in situ (CIS), and that dysplasia can be distinguished from metaplasia, hyperplasia, or normal.[39–41] A progressive increase in the epithelial thickness was found to parallel the severity of the histopathology grade. The nuclei of the cells also became darker and less light scattering in lesions that were moderately dysplastic or worse. The basement membrane became disrupted or disappeared with invasive carcinoma.[41] However, CIS could not be distinguished from high-grade dysplasia. Therefore, systems with higher resolution and Doppler capability and polarization sensitivity that can measure tissue microstructures in greater detail and quantify microvascular blood flow are needed.[42] Doppler OCT (DOCT) systems already exist that can detect extremely slow blood flow (<20 μm/sec in blood vessels as small as ~15 μm diameter).[43,44] DOCT's unprecedented micron-scale spatial resolution and

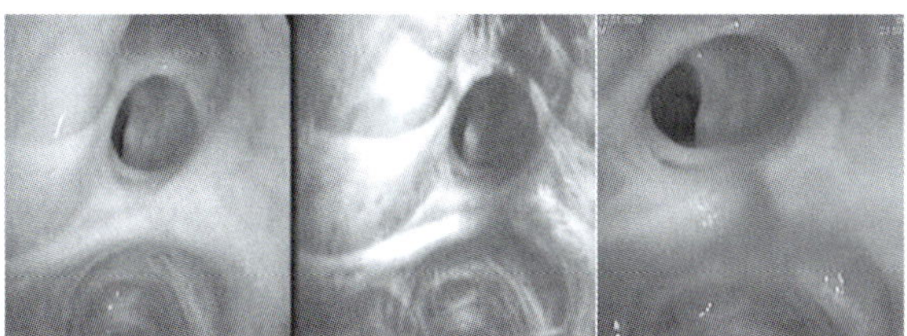

FIGURE 19.2 Real-time dual simultaneous imaging of digital video autofluroescence bronchoscope images (SAFE 3000, Pentax, Japan). Previous biopsy site over right upper lobe carina with small scarring on conventional image (*left*), abnormal but nonsuspicious digital autofluorescence (*center*), and hybrid image to enhance contrast of the localization (*right*) with histology normal biopsy. (See color plate.)

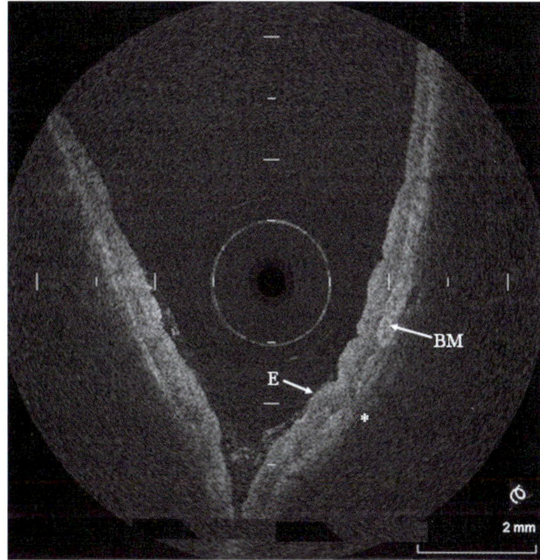

FIGURE 19.3 Optical coherence tomography image of the carcinoma in situ (CIS) lesion. There was microinvasive cancer through the basement membrane (*). *BM*, basement membrane; *E*, epithelial surface. (Bronchoscopic OCT photograph courtesy of Stephen Lam MD, copyright, British Columbia Cancer Agency.)

ability to monitor functional blood flow parameters at the microvascular level should prove valuable for (a) structural and functional lesion assessment,[45] (b) differential diagnosis/staging (invasion through the basement membrane and hence may no longer be curable by endoscopic therapy such as electrocautery treatment),[39,41] and (c) therapeutic feedback monitoring during endobronchial therapy such as photodynamic therapy.[44,46]

High-Magnification Videobronchoscopy

Increased vessel density in the bronchial submucosa is often present in squamous dysplasia and may play an early role in cancer pathogenesis.[47] Angiogenic squamous dysplasia is a specific lesion characterized by a collection of blood vessels juxtaposed to and projecting into an area of epithelial dysplasia.[47] High-magnification bronchoscopy (Olympus Optical Corporation, Tokyo, Japan) combines both fibreoptic and videobronchoscope technologies to produce 100 to 110× magnification of the bronchial wall compared with standard videobronchoscopes.[5,48] This enables the visualization of microvascular networks in the bronchial mucosa. An increase in microvessels can be seen by high-magnification imaging in most areas of abnormal autofluorescence and dysplasia, and discrimination from bronchial inflammation is possible.[5]

Narrow-Band Imaging

NBI (Olympus Optical Corporation, Tokyo, Japan) is a novel system that also utilizes the changes seen in the microvascular network of bronchial dysplasia. This technique uses a narrow-band filter rather than the conventional broad RGB filter used in standard videobronchoscopes. The conventional RGB filter uses 400 to 500 nm (blue), 500 to 600 nm (green), and 600 to 700 nm (red). NBI uses three narrow bands 400 to 430 nm (blue covers hemoglobin absorption at 410 nm), 420 to 470 nm (blue), and 560 to 590 nm (green) to create the images. Blue light has a short wavelength, reaches into the bronchial submucosa, and is absorbed by hemoglobin. On evaluation of airway lesions that were abnormal under autofluorescence imaging, this technique provides more accurate images of microvessels compared with high-magnification videobronchoscopy using broadband RGB technology.[48] Further evaluation of NBI in a small series has been performed in comparison with standard white-light videobronchoscopy. It was found to improve the detection of dysplasia/malignancy when used as an adjunct to white light compared with white-light imaging alone. The relative sensitivity was 1.63.[49] A direct comparison between NBI and AFB to determine their relative merits have not been conducted.

Endobronchial Ultrasound for Central Lesions

Endobronchial ultrasound is a new technology that is likely to have a significant contribution to the correct staging of early central lung cancer. The layers of the bronchial wall can be visualized, and detection of unsuspected invasion is improved.[50–52] The use of endobronchial ultrasound may also be used as an adjunct to AFB, where it may be used to further assess lesions with significantly abnormal autofluorescence and improve prediction of malignancy.[53]

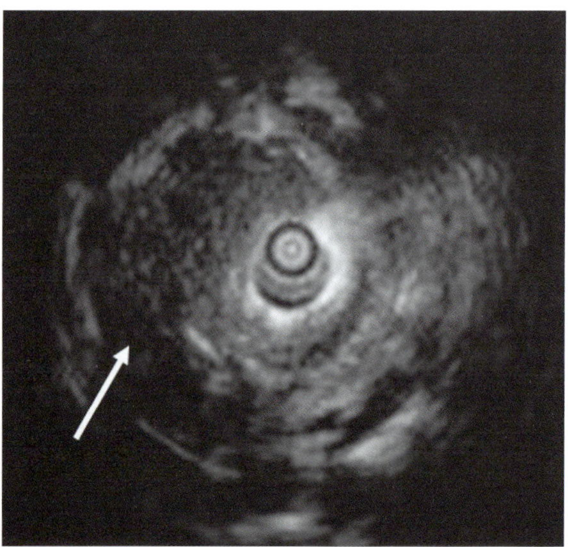

FIGURE 19.4 Endoscopic ultrasound of a central lesion referred for curative endobronchial therapy. Destruction of the bronchial wall structures can be seen on the left (*arrow*).

Evaluation of the curability of early central lung cancers with endobronchial therapies such as photodynamic therapy, electrocautery, and cryotherapy has previously relied on endobronchial characteristics. These include size, visual margins, and nodularity particularly under autofluorescence imaging. These have been correlated with risk of bronchial wall invasion and lymph node metastasis.[54–56] However, it is important to evaluate the depth of invasion and involvement of the cartilaginous layer to make the most appropriate choice of curative therapy. Thoracic computed tomography (CT) scan is not useful for small central lung cancers either for detection of the lesion or the assessment of intrabronchial wall invasion.[27,51,57] Endobronchial ultrasound using a radial probe inserted through the working channel of a flexible bronchoscope can be used to assess depth of invasion of a central cancer into or through the bronchial wall with a sensitivity of 86% and specificity of 67% (Fig. 19.4).[51,53] This will assist the physician in choosing either endobronchial therapy or immediate referral for surgery if unsuspected invasion is detected.[58]

DETECTION OF EARLY CANCER IN PERIPHERAL LUNG

The advent of multidetector row CT scanners has resulted in the detection of multiple small nodules in many patients both in a research setting, where CT scan is being investigated as a lung cancer screening tool, and in the clinical setting.[57,59,60] Although most small nodules have low risk of malignancy, persistent serial growth on CT follow-up or change in appearance of nonsolid lesions is worrisome for malignancy and requires investigation.[57,59,61] The diagnosis of these small peripheral lung lesions presents particular challenges because of invisibility on fluoroscopy and the inability of standard bronchoscopic access. Overall, the sensitivity of bronchoscopy for peripheral lesions is 78% but falls to <35% with lesions <20 mm in diameter.[62] Approach with transthoracic fine-needle aspiration is also difficult even under CT guidance because of the small size of these lesions, and it carries a significant risk of pneumothorax.

A promising approach is to use image guidance to assist the bronchoscopist in locating the lesions. Techniques that have been developed include endobronchial ultrasound or electromagnetic navigation (see Chapter 28).

Endobronchial Ultrasound for Peripheral Lesions

The use of miniaturized radial high-frequency (20 MHz) ultrasound probes through a flexible bronchoscope enables the localisation and characterisation of peripheral lung lesions. Detailed 360-degree images of lesions with spatial resolution <1 mm can be seen.[63] Different patterns of ultrasound echoes may indicate the presence of malignant or benign disease.[63–65] In general, a heterogenous internal echogenicity, absence of linear-discrete air bronchogram, and/or a continuous hyperechoic margin appears more suspicious of malignancy.[63–65] The presence of two or more of these ultrasound features increases the likelihood of malignancy to 89%, and absence of any of these features is highly likely to exclude malignancy (negative predictive value 85%).[65]

Early use of the radial probe for localization of peripheral lesions was followed by removal of the probe and insertion of sampling tools into the chosen airway. The use of a guide sheath as an extended working channel was then incorporated into the procedure. Thus, once the lesion had been localized, the probe was removed leaving the guide sheath in place, then forceps and/or a bronchial brush could be advanced through the sheath to obtain specimens. Diagnostic yields vary between 63% and 77%[66–74] (Table 19.3). Results are influenced by size of the target lesion and position of the probe within the lesion.[68,69,73,74] The diagnostic yield for lesions ≤15 mm diameter is 40% compared with 76% for lesions >15 mm diameter.[74] If the probe is able to be positioned within the lesion, the yield is higher at 83% compared with 61% if adjacent to the lesion or 4% when outside the lesion.[74] In addition, the diagnostic yield is increased with up to five cumulative sequential transbronchial biopsies.[74]

Therefore, this is an effective technique that can achieve good diagnostic yield for peripheral lung lesions without the associated radiation exposure of fluoroscopy or CT. However, small lesions <10 to 15 mm remain a challenge.

Electromagnetic Navigation

A promising approach to examine small peripheral lung lesions is to use an electromagnetic navigation guidance system to guide a small sensor-tipped catheter to the peripheral lung, using virtual CT as a road map.[75–81] Registration points are first marked in the virtual CT constructed from a spiral CT scan. During the procedure, the patient lies on top of a board that generates a weak electromagnetic field. The physician uses the sensor-tipped catheter to touch the same registration points corresponding to that marked on the virtual CT (e.g., main carina, upper-lobe entrance, middle- and lower-lobe entrance). After that, a sheathed catheter that bends in eight directions is maneuvered using virtual CT as a road map similar to a global positioning system (GPS) device. Once the target is reached, the sensor catheter is removed. Forceps

TABLE 19.3 Reported Performance of Endobronchial Ultrasound for Diagnosis of Peripheral Lung Lesions

	Number of Lesions Attempted	Mean Diameter (mm)	Positive Diagnosis	Pneumothorax Rate
Herth et al.[66]*	50	33.1 ± 9.2	80%	2%
Shirakawa et al.[67]†	50	NS	71%	NS
Kurimoto et al.[68]	150	NS	77%	0
Kikuchi et al.[69]	24	18.4 ± 6.3	67%	4.2%
Paone et al.[70]*	87	NS	76%	0
Asahina et al.[71]	30	18.9 ± 6.5	63%	0
Herth et al.[72]	54	22 ± 7	70%	2%
Yoshikawa et al.[73]	123	31 ± 15.9	62%	1%
Yamada et al.[74]	158	20.8 ± 6.1	67%	NS

*Without guide sheath.

†Half lesions without guide sheath.

NS, not stated.

TABLE 19.4 Reported Performance of Electromagnetic Navigation Bronchoscopy for Diagnosis of Peripheral Lung Lesions

	Number of Lesions Attempted	Mean Diameter (mm)	Positive Diagnosis	Pneumothorax Rate
Becker et al.[75]	30	Mean not stated	67%	3%
Hautmann et al.[76]	16	22 ± 6	69%	NS
Schwarz et al.[77]	13	33.5 ± 11	69%	0%
Gildea et al.[78]	56	23 ± 13	71%	3.5%
Wilson and Bartlett[79]	271	21 ± 14	56%	1%
Makris et al.[80]*	40	23.5 ± 15	63%	8%
Eberhardt et al.[81]*	92	24 ± 8	67%	2%

*Fluoroscopy not used.

NS, not stated.

are introduced through the sheath, and transbronchial biopsies are performed. Most of these reports used the device in combination with fluoroscopy, which is not used for bronchoscopy in all clinical centres.[75–79] Two centers achieved similar results without fluoroscopy[80,81] (Table 19.4). The diagnostic yield appears to be independent of size, but few lesions ≤10 mm have been included in these studies. Early experience showed improved diagnostic accuracy from <30% to ≥50% for tumors ≤2 cm in diameter. Accuracy is better when the geographic miss is minimized, specifically when the deviation from the target lesion is ≤4 mm.[80]

Multimodality Bronchoscopic Diagnosis Diagnostic accuracy may be improved further by the combination of endoscopic ultrasound with electromagnetic navigation. In one series without the use of fluoroscopy, an endobronchial ultrasound probe was used to verify catheter placement within the target before biopsies were performed. This technique was able to achieve a diagnostic accuracy of 88% compared with ultrasound alone (69%) or electromagnetic navigation alone (59%).[82]

Coupling electromagnetic navigation with endosocopic ultrasound or optical imaging such as OCT may allow better localization and characterization of small lung lesions, increase biopsy yield, and separate preneoplastic or early cancer lesions from benign lesions. It may also enable delivery and placement of fiducial markers to facilitate radiofrequency ablation, radiosurgery or photodynamic therapy (PDT) of peripheral lesions, and potentially allow treatment-induced changes to be monitored in real time.[44,45]

CONCLUSION

Advances in optical imaging such as AFB, NBI, OCT, and endobronchial ultrasound as well as an image-guided navigation system provide unprecedented opportunity to localize preinvasive lung cancer and preneoplastic lesions in the lung, allow biopsy to characterize these lesions better, and to study their natural history. Localization of these early central lesions enables minimally invasive endobronchial treatment without removing adjacent normal lung tissue and, in the future, may also assist with minimally invasive techniques for treatment of peripheral lesions.

REFERENCES

1. Rami-Porta R, Ball D, Crowley J, et al. The IASLC Lung cancer staging project: proposals for the revision of the T descriptors in the forthcoming (seventh) edition of the TNM classification for lung cancer. *J Thorac Oncol* 2007;2(7):593–602.
2. Saito Y, Nagamoto N, Ota S, et al. Results of surgical treatment for roentgenographically occult bronchogenic squamous cell carcinoma. *J Thorac Cardiovasc Surg* 1992;104:401–407.
3. Woodward RM, Martin ML, Cronin KA, et al. The value of medical interventions for lung cancer in the elderly. Results from SEER-CMHSF. *Cancer* 2007;110:2511–2518.
4. Chhajed PN, Shibuya K, Hoshino H, et al. A comparison of video and autofluorescence bronchoscopy in patients at high risk of lung cancer. *Eur Respir J* 2005;25(6):951–955.
5. Shibuya K, Hoshino H, Chiyo M, et al. Subepithelial vascular patterns in bronchial dysplasias using a high magnification bronchovideoscope. *Thorax* 2002;57:902–907.
6. Wagnieres G, McWilliams A, Lam S. Lung cancer imaging with fluorescence endoscopy. In: Mycek M, Pogue B, eds. *Handbook of Biomedical Fluorescence*. New York: Marcel Dekker, 2003:361–396.
7. Hung J, Lam S, LeRiche J, et al. Autofluorescence of normal and malignant bronchial tissue. *Laser Surg Med* 1991;11:99–105.
8. Qu J, MacAulay C, Lam S, et al. Laser-induced fluorescence spectroscopy at endoscopy: tissue optics, monte carlo modeling, and in vivo measurements. *Opt Eng* 1995;34:3334–3343.
9. Qu J, MacAulay C, Lam S, et al. Optical properties of normal and carcinoma bronchial tissue. *Appl Optics* 1994;33(31):7397–7405.
10. Lam S, MacAulay C, Hung J, et al. Detection of dysplasia and carcinoma in situ with a lung imaging fluorescence endoscope device. *J Thorac Cardiovasc Sug* 1993;105:1035–1040.
11. Lam S, MacAulay C, LeRiche J, et al. Early localization of bronchogenic carcinoma. *Diag Therapeu Endo* 1994;1:75–78.
12. Lam S, Kennedy T, Unger M, et al. Localization of bronchial intraepithelial neoplastic lesions by fluorescence bronchoscopy. *Chest* 1998;113:696–702.

13. Lam S, MacAulay C, LeRiche J, et al. Detection and localization of early lung cancer by fluorescence bronchoscopy. *Cancer* 2000;89(11 Suppl):2468–2473.
14. Onco-LIFE endoscopic light source and camera. P950043/S003. Available at http://www.fda.gov/cdrh/pmapage/html. Accessed June 30, 2005.
15. Venmans BJW, van Boxem AJM, Smit EF, et al. Early detection of preinvasive lesions in high-risk patients. A comparison of conventional flexible and fluorescence bronchoscopy. *J Bronchology* 1998;5:280–283.
16. Vermylen P, Pierard P, Roufosse C, et al. Detection of bronchial preneoplastic lesions and early lung cancer with fluorescence bronchoscopy: a study about its ambulatory feasibility under local anesthesis. *Lung Cancer* 1999;25(3):161–168.
17. Horvath T, Horvathova M, Salajka F, et al. Detection of bronchial neoplasia in uranium miners by autofluorescence bronchoscopy. *Diagn Ther Endosc* 1999:5:91–98.
18. Kusunoki Y, Imamura F, Uda H, et al. Early detection of lung cancer with laser-induced fluorescence endoscopy and spectrofluorometry. *Chest* 2000;118(6):1776–1782.
19. Shibuya K, Fujisawa T, Hoshino H, et al. Fluorescence bronchoscopy in the detection of preinvasive bronchial lesions in patients with sputum cytology suspicious or positive for malignancy. *Lung Cancer* 2001;32(1):19–25.
20. Sato M, Sakurada A, Sagawa M, et al. Diagnostic results before and after introduction of autofluorescence bronchoscopy in patients suspected of having lung cancer detected by sputum cytology in lung cancer mass screening. *Lung Cancer* 2001;32(3):247–253.
21. Goujon D, Zellweger M, Radu A, et al. In vivo autofluorescence imaging of early cancers in the human tracheobronchial tree with a spectrally optimized system. *J Biomed Opt* 2003;8(1):17–25.
22. Fielding D. Practical issues in autofluorescence bronchoscopy with Storz D Light bronchoscope. *Photodiagn Photodyn Ther* 2004;1(3): 247–251.
23. Ernst A, Simoff MJ, Mathur PN, et al. D-light autofluorescence in the detection of premalignant airway changes: a multicenter trial. *J Bronchol* 2005;12(3):133–138.
24. Hirsch FR, Prindiville SA, Miller YE, et al. Fluorescence versus white-light bronchoscopy for detection of preneoplastic lesions: a randomized study. *J Natl Cancer Inst* 2001;93(18):1385–1391.
25. Häussinger K, Becker H, Stanzel F, et al. Autofluorescence bronchoscopy with white light bronchoscopy compared with white light bronchoscopy alone for the detection of precancerous lesions: a European randomised controlled multicentre trial. *Thorax* 2005;60(6):496–503.
26. Kennedy TC, Franklin WA, Prindiville SA, et al. High prevalence of occult endobronchial malignancy in high risk patients with moderate sputum atypia. *Lung Cancer* 2005;49(2):187–191.
27. Sutedja TG, Codrington H, Risse EK, et al. Autofluorescence bronchoscopy improves staging of radiographically occult lung cancer and has an impact on therapeutic strategy. *Chest* 2001;120(4):1327–1332.
28. Ikeda N, Hiyoshi T, Kakihana M, et al. Histopathological evaluation of fluorescence bronchoscopy using resected lungs in cases of lung cancer. *Lung Cancer* 2003;41(3):303–309.
29. Ikeda N, Honda H, Hayashi A, et al. Early detection of bronchial lesions using newly developed videoendoscopy-based autofluorescence bronchoscopy. *Lung Cancer* 2006;52:21–27.
30. Chiyo M, Shibuya K, Hoshino H, et al. Effective detection of bronchial preinvasive lesions by a new autofluorescence imaging bronchovideoscope system. *Lung Cancer* 2005;48:307–313.
31. Helfritzsch H, Junker K, Bartel M, et al. Differentiation of positive autofluorescence bronchoscopy findings by comparative genomic hybridization. *Oncol Rep* 2002;9(4):697–701.
32. Pasic A, Vonk-Noordegraaf A, Risse EK, et al. Multiple suspicious lesions detected by autofluorescence bronchoscopy predict malignant development in the bronchial mucosa in high risk patients. *Lung Cancer* 2003;41(3):295–301.
33. Lee P, McWilliams A, Lam S, et al. Quantitative image analysis for intra-epithelial neoplasia. *J Thorac Oncol* 2007;2(8):Suppl 4:S812.
34. Thiberville L, Moreno-Swirc S, Vercauteren T, et al. In vivo imaging of the bronchial wall microsctructure using fibered confocal fluorescence microscopy. *Am J Respir Crit Care Med* 2007;175:22–31.
35. MacAulay C, Lane P, Richards-Kortum R. In vivo pathology: microendoscopy as a new endoscopic imaging modality. *Gastrointest Endosc Clin N Am* 2004;14:595–620.
36. Huang D, Swanson EA, Lin CP, et al. Optical coherence tomography. *Science* 1991:254:1178–1781.
37. Fujimoto JG, Brezinski ME, Tearney GJ, et al. Biomedical imaging and optical biopsy using optical coherence tomography. *Nat Med* 1995;1:970–972.
38. Tearney GJ, Brezinski ME, Bouma BE et al. In vivo endoscopic optical biopsy with optical coherence tomography. *Science* 1997;276:2037–2039.
39. Tsuboi M, Hayashi A, Ikeda N, et al. Optical coherence tomography in the diagnosis of bronchial lesions. *Lung Cancer* 2005;49:387–394.
40. Whiteman SC, Yang Y, van Pittius DG, et al. Optical coherence tomography: Real-time imaging of bronchial airways microstructure and detection of inflammatory/neoplastic morphological changes. *Clin Cancer Res* 2006;12:813–818.
41. Lam S, Standish B, Baldwin C, et al. In vivo optical coherence tomography imaging of pre-invasive bronchial lesions. *Clin Cancer Res* 2008;14:2006–2011
42. Yang VX, Vitkin IA. Principles of Doppler optical coherence tomography. In: Regar E, van Leeuwen T, Serruys, P. *Handbook of Optical Coherence Tomography in Cardiology*. Oxford, UK: Taylor and Francis Medical, 2006.
43. Yang VXD, Tang S, Gordon ML, et al. Endoscopic Doppler optical coherence tomography in the human GI tract: initial experience. *Gastrointest Endosc* 2005;61:879–890.
44. Standish BA, Yang VXD, Munce NR, et al. Doppler optical coherence tomography monitoring of microvascular response during photodynamic therapy in a Barrett's Esophagus rat model. *Gastrointest Endosc* 2007;66:326–333.
45. Skliarenko JV, Lunt SJ, Gordon ML, et al. Effects of the vascular disrupting agent ZD6126 on interstitial fluid pressure and cell survival in tumors. *Cancer Res* 2006;66:2074–2080.
46. Li H, Standish BA, Mariampillai A, et al. Feasibility of interstitial Doppler optical coherence tomography for in vivo detection of microvascular changes during photodynamic therapy. *Lasers Surg Med* 2006;38:754–761.
47. Keith RL, Miller YE, Gemmill RM, et al. Angiogenic squamous dysplasia in bronchi of individuals at high risk for lung cancer. *Clin Cancer Res* 2000;6:1616–1625.
48. Shibuya K, Hoshino H, Chiyo M, et al. High magnification bronchovideoscopy combined with narrow band imaging could detect capillary loos of angiogenic squamous dysplasia in heavy smokers at high risk for lung cancer. *Thorax* 2003;58:989–995.
49. Vincent B, Fraig M, Silvestri G. A Pilot study of narrow-band imaging compared to white light bronchoscopy for evaluaton of normal airways and premalignant and malignant airways disease. *Chest* 2007;131:1794–1788.
50. Kurimoto N, Murayama M, Yoshioka S, et al. Assessment of usefulness of endobronchial ultrasonography in determination of depth of tracheobronchial tumor invasion. *Chest* 1999;115:1500–1506.
51. Miyazu Y, Miyazawa T, Kurimoto N, et al. Endobronchial ultrasonography in the assessment of centrally located early-stage lung cancer before photodynamic therapy. *Am J Respir Crit Care Med* 2002;165: 832–837.
52. Takahashi H, Sagawa M, Sato M, et al. A prospective evaluation of transbronchial ultrasonography for assessment of depth of invasion in early bronchogenic squamous cell carcinoma. *Lung Cancer* 2003;42:42–49.
53. Herth F, Becker H, LoCicero J, et al. Endobronchial ultrasound improves classification of suspicious lesions detected by autofluorescence bronchoscopy. *J Bronchol* 2003;10(4):249–252.
54. Konaka C, Hirano T, Kato H, et al. Comparison of endoscopic features of early-stage squamous cell lung cancer and histological findings. *Br J Cancer* 1999;80:1435–1439.

55. Furuse K, Fukuoka M, Kato H, et al. A prospective phase II study on photodynamic therapy for centrally located early-stage lung cancer. *J Clin Oncol* 1993;11(10):1852–1857.
56. Furukawa K, Kato H, Konaka C, et al. Locally recurrent central-type early stage lung cancer <1.0 cm in diameter after complete remission by photodynamic therapy. *Chest* 2005;128:3269–3275.
57. McWilliams AM, Mayo JR, Ahn MI, et al. Lung cancer screening using multi-slice thin-section computed tomography and autofluorescence bronchoscopy. *J Thorac Oncol* 2006;1(1):61–68.
58. Kennedy T, McWilliams A, Edell E, et al. Bronchial intraepithelial neoplasia/early central airways lung cancer: ACCP evidence-based clinical practice guidelines. 2nd Ed. *Chest* 2007;132:S221–S233.
59. Swensen SJ, Jett JR, Hartman TE, et al. CT screening for lung cancer: five-year prospective experience. *Radiology* 2005:235:259–265.
60. MacMahon H, Austin J, Gamsu G, et al. Guidelines for management of small pulmonary nodules detected on CT scans: a statement from the Fleischner society. *Radiology* 2005;237:395–400.
61. Henschke CI, Naidich DP, Yankelevitz DF, et al. Early lung cancer action project: initial results of annual repeat screening. *Cancer* 2001;92:153–159.
62. Rivera M, Mehta A. Initial diagnosis of lung cancer: ACCP evidence-based clinical practice guidelines. 2nd Ed. *Chest* 2007;132(3):S131–S148.
63. Kurimoto N, Murayama M, Yoshioka S, et al. Analysis of the internal structure of peripheral pulmonary lesions using endobronchial ultrasonography. *Chest* 2002;122:1887–1894.
64. Chao TY, Lie CH, Chung YH, et al. Differentiating peripheral pulmonary lesions based on images of endobronchial ultrasonography. *Chest* 2006;130:1191–1197.
65. Kuo CH, Lin SM, Chen HC, et al. Diagnosis of peripheral lung cancer with three echoic features via endobronchial ultrasound. *Chest* 2007;132:922–929.
66. Herth F, Ernist A, Becker H. Endobronchial ultrasound-guided transbronchial lung biopsy in solitary pulmonary nodules and peripheral lesions. *Eur Respir J* 2002;20:972–974.
67. Shirakawa T, Imamura F, Hamamoto J, et al. Usefulness of endobronchial ultrasonography for transbronchial lung biopsies of peripheral lung lesions. *Respiration* 2004;71:260–268.
68. Kurimoto N, Miyazawa T, Okimasa S, et al. Endobronchial ultrasonography using a guide sheath increases the ability to diagnose peripheral pulmonary lesions endoscopically. *Chest* 2004;126:959–965.
69. Kikuchi E, Yamazaki K, Sukoh N, et al. Endobronchial ultrasonography with guide-sheath for peripheral pulmonary lesions. *Eur Respir J* 2004;24:533–537.
70. Paone G, Nicastri E, Lucantoni G, et al. Endobronchial ultrasound-driven biopsy in the diagnosis of peripheral lung lesions. *Chest* 2005;128:3551–3557.
71. Asahina H, Yamazaki K, Onodera Y, et al. Transbronchial biopsy using endobronchial ultrasonography with a guide sheath and virtual bronchoscopic navigation. *Chest* 2005;128:1761–1765.
72. Herth F, Eberhardt R, Becker H, et al. Endobronchial ultrasound-guided transbronchial lung biopsy in fluroscopically invisible solitary pulmonary nodules: a prospective trial. *Chest* 2006;129: 147–150.
73. Yoshikawa M, Sukoh N, Yamakazi K, et al. Diagnostic value of endobronchial ultrasonography with a guide sheath for peripheral pulmonary lesions without x-ray fluoroscopy. *Chest* 2007;131: 1788–1793.
74. Yamada N, Yamakazi K, Kurimoto N, et al. Factors related to diagnostic yield of transbronchial biopsy using endobronchial ultrasonography with a guide sheath in small peripheral pulmonary lesions. *Chest* 2007;132:603–608.
75. Becker H, Herth F, Ernst A, et al. Bronchoscopic biopsy of peripheral lung lesions under electromagnetic guidance. A pilot study. *J Bronchol* 2005;12(1):9–13.
76. Hautmann H, Schneider A, Pinkau T, et al. Electromagnetic catheter navigation during bronchoscopy validation of a novel method by a conventional fluoroscopy. *Chest* 2005;128:382–387.
77. Schwarz Y, Greif J, Becker HD, et al. Real-time electromagnetic navigation bronchoscopy to peripheral lung lesions using overlaid CT images: the first human study. *Chest* 2006;129:988–994.
78. Gildea TR, Mazzone PJ, Karnak D, et al. Electromagnetic navigation diagnostic bronchoscopy: a prospective study. *Am J Respir Crit Care Med* 2006;174:982–989.
79. Wilson D, Bartlett R. Improved diagnostic yield of bronchoscopy in a community practice: combination of electromagnetic navigation system and rapid on-site evaluation. *J Bronchol* 2007;14:227–232.
80. Makris D, Scherpereel A, Leroy S, et al. Electromagnetic navigation diagnostic bronchoscopy for small peripheral lung lesions. *Eur Respir J* 2007;29:1187–1192.
81. Eberhardt R, Anantham D, Herth F, et al. Electromagnetic navigation diagnostic bronchoscopy in peripheral lung lesions. *Chest* 2007;131:1800–1805.
82. Eberhardt R, Anantham D, Ernst A, et al. Multimodality bronchoscopic diagnosis of peripheral lung lesions: a randomised controlled trial. *Am J Respir Crit Care Med* 2007;176:36–41.

CHAPTER 20

Simon D. Spivack
William Rom

Evolving Early Detection Modalities in Lung Cancer Screening

It would seem intuitively obvious that early detection efforts of a lethal disorder such as lung cancer would increase the chances for cure of that disease for individuals, and therefore, the population from which they derive, and thereby lead to a reduced death rate (reduced mortality) from that disease. This has proven to be the case for cervical and breast cancer screening.[1,2] However, to date, no molecular nor imaging modality of the lung, although suggestive, has yet been sufficiently evaluated to incontrovertibly confirm that it reduces mortality for early lung cancer detection.[3] Several studies of various lung imaging and other modalities are currently under way, are promising, and are described elsewhere in this textbook (see Chapters 15 to 17).

The lung is a visceral organ; therefore, access is necessarily limited. It is virtually impossible to directly examine all ramifications of the complex branching structures of the bronchial tree by external imaging, endobronchial fiberoptics, or other modalities. Therefore, certain aspects of a transforming epithelium must go unexamined, even by the most sophisticated sampling techniques. This inherent problem is reflected in imperfect sensitivity for all molecular lung cancer–screening modalities tested to date. Clearly, lung epithelial sampling approaches are evolving.

Also underappreciated is that any given screening modality will necessarily be imperfectly specific, in isolation, but two or more complementary stages in screening may, when coupled, offer vast improvements in predictive value of a positive test. That is, serial molecular monitoring for risk stratification could complement or even leverage imaging approaches to disease detection, by allowing enrichment of the disease prevalence ("risk") of the population destined for disease detection by more specific imaging approaches. Thus, in a typical population of otherwise unselected middle-aged smokers and ex-smokers, where lung cancer prevalence is about 2%, the positive predictive value (PPV) of a noncalcified nodule detected on spiral computed tomography (CT)—where typically specificities are ~90%—proves to be lung cancer in only about 18%.[4] However, if one uses a biomarker of risk to identify a higher-risk portion of the population, where prevalence for lung cancer is 20%, the PPV (probability that same CT-detected nodule represents lung cancer in this context), is much greater at ~70%.

Therefore, a staged approach to screening, first using a risk assessment tool, followed by a disease detection tool, implies that two different tiers or levels of performance can, when coupled, have synergistic effects on early detection efficacy. Here, the first tier of screening would identify less deterministic "risk factors," perhaps both demographic and molecular. Such nondeterministic but informative risk-assessment tools abound in the literature but are often underappreciated as such. Then, the second tier testing would entail much more stringent, and specific, conventional performance criteria for actual lung cancer detection markers or imaging features.[4]

Candidate noninvasive risk assessment tools for lung cancer screening might simply collect readily available clinical information in sophisticated risk prediction models.[5,6] Alternatively, as will be demonstrated, one can biologically sample the entire, or portions of, lung epithelium and include, for example, germline genetic polymorphisms in carcinogen metabolism or DNA repair genes (blood- or buccal cell–based); blood-based proteomic signatures; transcriptional signatures in a related airway specimen (e.g., brush-exfoliated buccal cells), sputum oncogene mutation, or tumor suppressor gene silencing (spontaneously exfoliating lung epithelial and inflammatory cells); or exhaled breath tests of volatile (alkanes or aldehydes) or nonvolatile compounds (DNA), derived from as yet undetermined airway origin (e.g., bronchial or alveolar lining fluids).

Conventional clinical disease detection tools might include anatomic-based CT scans, functional imaging such as positron emission tomography (PET) scans (see Chapter 27), various conventional and enhanced optical bronchoscopic techniques (see Chapters 19 and 28), or other localizing modalities, all discussed elsewhere in this text, followed by definitive tissue sampling where indicated, with attendant conventional or newer molecular assays applied. In this chapter, we will largely emphasize less invasive, molecular-oriented approaches to both risk assessment and disease detection that are inherently more easily applied to an asymptomatic population determined by clinical history to have some propensity to lung cancer.

AIRWAY IMAGING APPROACHES

Bronchoscopic Optical Techniques Although invasive, fiberoptic bronchoscopy has been considered in certain high-risk lung cancer screening contexts. Autofluorescence bronchoscopy (AFB), based on altered refractile properties of multilayered hyperplastic or dysplastic epithelium, has proven superior to conventional white-light bronchoscopy (WLB) in detecting moderate-to-severe dysplasia, and carcinoma in situ with 56% to 82% sensitivity (AFB), versus 9% to 58% sensitivity (WLB).[7,8] AFB is not universally available. Because there are several localized responses to detection of premalignancy and overt but confined bronchial malignancies (Nd:YAG laser therapy, photodynamic therapy [PDT], electrocautery, cryotherapy, and brachytherapy), some have advocated routine bronchoscopic screening of individuals determined as high risk by other means (e.g., high-grade sputum atypia, chronic obstructive pulmonary disease [COPD], asbestos exposure).[9,10] Specificity of AFB has been a question. Advancement of WLB techniques, including light-scattering technologies and videobronchoscopy, is imminent.[4,11–14] High-density radiographic CT image reconstruction has allowed for the development of *virtual bronchoscopy*, a technique that is completely noninvasive, although radiation dose is not trivial, and radiologist/computer evaluation strategies still evolving[15] (see Chapters 19 and 28).

LUNG TISSUE–BASED MOLECULAR ASSAYS

Of course, the gold standard for lung cancer detection is examination of lung tissue itself, either by conventional means (microscopy, immunohistochemistry, and the like), or by newer molecular means. Among the newer means, fluorescence in situ hybridization (FISH) for larger-region genomic deletions or duplications (see Chapter 49), microsatellite examinations (see Chapter 7), DNA methylation patterns (see Chapter 7), microarray messenger RNA (mRNA) expression signatures, candidate mRNA expression signatures, microRNA microarrays, candidate microRNA expression signatures, proteomic and antibody arrays, and metabolomic approaches are all in use in experimental and/or beta-testing for early clinical application. The National Cancer Institute (NCI) empowered, in the last decade, the Early Detection Research Network (EDRN) to create a consortium of tissue repositories and technology platforms for this purpose, and the technologies presented at the most recent 2008 meeting are truly astonishing. As this chapter emphasizes evolving early detection modalities, largely by molecular assays on noninvasively obtained tissues from individuals without symptoms, those molecular techniques requiring robust, large surgical level tissue specimens are covered elsewhere in this volume.

For noninvasively obtained tissues used in early detection studies on asymptomatic populations, such as exfoliated cells in sputum, or the circulating macromolecules of blood, polymerase chain reaction (PCR)-based assays of DNA and RNA are most often employed in the translational research setting. Their sensitivity is extraordinary, allowing analysis of these lung-surrogate tissues with greater ease. It must be acknowledged that although conferring great sensitivity, these nucleic acid end points may, even for cancer syndromes, often be considered more biologically proximate, or twice-removed end points, as opposed to direct measurement of the full-dimensional cancer biological phenotype (uncontrolled growth, invasion, metastasis), which is generally not feasible. Even other proximate markers (metabolites or proteins/enzymes generating those metabolites) that are the direct underpinnings of these cancer phenotypes are often beyond the level of sensitivity of current assays, although proteomic, and antibody microarray technologies are advancing rapidly as are informatic approaches to these multidimensional data sets.

DNA-based genome-wide search for aberrant copy number in tumors have revealed copy number aberrations using single nucleotide polymorphism (SNP) arrays or array comparative genomic hybridization (CGH) and reveal that many of the copy number alterations found to cluster in lung cancer involve unknown genes.[16]

DNA-based methylation markers in lung tissue, by example: cytosine-phosphodiester-guanine (CpG) methylation of gene promoter DNA is a major correlate of biologic pathway regulation and deregulation.[17–19] In many ways, progressive DNA methylation of tumor suppressor genes has been revealed over the last 10 to 15 years to be a strong correlate of lung carcinogenesis.

As a recent example of a comprehensive methylation biomarker search, a concerted genome-wide effort to assay in vitro genes likely to be methylated, and responsive to a methylation inhibitor, was checked for consistency with expression and methylation profiles in human lung. Those genes whose expression was most discriminatory for lung tumor from adjacent nontumor tissue (for lung, specifically) by methylation-specific PCR (MSP) sampling of one or a few (CpG) methylation sites in each gene locus, included *BNC1*, *MSX1*, *CCNA1*, *RASSF1A*, *p16*, *ALDH1A13*, *LOX*, and *CTSZ*. This is one of the first such comprehensive genome-wide searches for methylation-silenced genes in lung cancer[20] and has been followed up by others.[21]

In another study, a panel of candidate gene DNA methylation markers, using methylation-specific PCR sampling was constructed, and using the top four markers (*CDKN2A EX2*, *CDX2*, *HOXA1*, *OPCML*) could distinguish lung tumors from normal tissue with 94% sensitivity and 90% specificity.[22]

A workshop was convened in 2005 on the use of methylated DNA sequences as cancer biomarkers, in risk assessment and disease detection, enjoining the NCI's EDRN and the National Institute of Standards and Technology. The summary[23] has emphasized the importance of specimen choice and handling, bisulfite modification strategy, choice of assay based on scale, sensitivity and cost, tissue specificity, and other factors. These issues remain at play for current lung cancer screening biomarkers (see Chapter 7).

BLOOD-BASED MARKERS

Blood is an attractive surrogate specimen source because of its availability and the presumed pooling of metabolic processes in the circulation, as reflected, it is postulated, in that compartment.

DNA-Based Markers in Blood The quantity of DNA leaching into the blood itself has been proposed as a marker,[24] albeit controversially.[25,26] Attempts to detect DNA-based somatic markers in the blood have been myriad,[27] including oncogene mutations, somatic mutations, and other modifications, with mixed results. For the most proximate steps in tobacco carcinogenesis, the measurement of DNA adducts of known tobacco carcinogens in blood cells, several large European studies using ^{32}P postlabeling of adducts did not show consistent relation to smoking, nor risk.[28,29] A more recent large, pooled data analysis also suggests a weak association of bulky DNA adducts and lung cancer, perhaps apparent in current and recent smokers only.[30]

Aberrant DNA methylation in blood has been detected for the last decade, albeit its origin remains *unclear*, but these have been as disappointing as diagnostic tools.[31–33]

For risk assessment, blood-based genome-wide association and family linkage studies for germline variants associated with lung cancer have emerged, although in somewhat sparse number. A susceptibility locus on chromosome 6q23–25 was reported from a multi-institutional consortium examining high-risk family pedigrees, led by National Institute of Health (NIH) investigators[34] (see Chapter 4). The individual candidate genes in the region have not yet been confirmed with regard to association of their variants with lung cancer risk.

Individual variants in component enzymes in specific pathways have been explored in some detail in cross-sectional, case-control population-based studies, with particular attention paid to carcinogen metabolism,[35] DNA repair,[36–38] and inflammation.[39] In general, these data for individual variants have been inconsistent across populations but may have some incremental information when integrated into comprehensive risk assessment models that include demographic data. These are reviewed in greater detail in the cited references.

RNA-Based Markers in Blood There have been a small number of well-executed and suggestive studies of RNA expression in recovered circulating tumor cells[40–42] and/or peripheral blood lymphocytes.[43] Free circulating RNA studies are inherently challenging for quality template recovery, RNA-specific amplification, and detection of signal above background.

Proteomic-Based Markers in Blood A variety of proteomic-based approaches to obtaining patterns that distinguish cancer from noncancer tissue, premalignancy from normal tissue, and the corresponding signals reflected in the blood, have been approached[44] in a validation population, for example, a signature yielded a sensitivity of 58% and a specificity of 85.7%.[45] A more recent study combining proteomic-detected protein markers and proteins involved in known lung cancer pathways has suggested that a four-protein panel in blood may have significant diagnostic value.[46] None of the protein studies to date entail a temporal component.

Candidate Proteins in Blood Several academic and commercial ventures have proceeded from proteomics studies generating candidates to protein identification and construction of panels that distinguish lung cancer cases from appropriate controls with independent validation in separate populations.[45] Candidate proteins such as circulating serum carcinoembryonic antigen (CEA) and cytokeratin 19-fragment (CYFRA 21-1) values and lymphocyte antigen 6 complex locus K (LY6K) have demonstrated some signal in distinguishing lung cancer cases from controls, particularly in combination, although classification is not adequate for disease diagnosis, even in combination (sensitivity 65% to 70%).[47]

Autoantibodies with lung tumor–specific epitopes have been reported as showing some signal in lung cancer.[48] A recent report suggested that a panel of p53, c-myc, HER-2, NY-ESO-1, CAGE, MUC-1, and GBU4-5 autoantibodies detected by enzyme-linked immunosorbent assay (ELISA) in blood conferred a sensitivity of 76%, specificity of 92%.[49] On-chip synthesis of protein libraries that are used for detecting antitumor antibodies appear promising.

Metabolomics in Blood To our knowledge, the promise of metabolomics, using high-throughput generation of spectroscopic signatures representative of the metabolic states of a cell,[50–52] have not been applied to early detection of lung cancer. For candidate metabolites in blood, levels of S-adenosylmethionine have been reported as higher in lung cancer cases than in smoking controls.[53] Overall, there is a general paucity of investigations of lung cancer–related metabolites in blood.

Molecular Phenotypes in Blood Mutagen sensitivity and DNA repair capacity have been evaluated extensively in blood, particularly by several groups working at the MD Anderson Cancer Center in Houston, Texas. The identification of the phenotypes, measuring cytogenetic or more precisely ascertained DNA damage, presumably integrate a large number of genes and pathways into a cancer-relevant trait with impressive capacity to distinguish lung cancer cases versus controls in cross-sectional studies.[54,55,37] Performance in prospective studies in "integrative epidemiologic" investigations are pending.

AIRWAY-BASED MARKERS

Bronchoscopically Procured Airway Specimens for DNA and RNA and Protein Analyses It is clear that if directly procured, histologically dysmorphic airway specimens yield important clinical information, as discussed elsewhere in this volume. Newer molecular modalities have been applied to bronchial biopsy specimens and bronchoalveolar lavage (BAL). For example, computer-assisted fluorescence immunophenotyping and interphase cytogenetics as a tool for the investigation of neoplasms has been applied to BAL in the region of a nodule with provocative results.[56,57]

However, it also appears that field carcinogenesis patterns of transcriptome-wide gene expression can be obtained in the major airways, which reflect the likelihood that a radiographically detected peripheral lesion, far remote from the bronchoscope, is a malignancy.[58,59] Given that cigarette smoke creates a field of injury throughout the airway, Spira et al.[58,59] sought to determine if gene expression in histologically normal large-airway epithelial cells obtained at bronchoscopy from smokers with suspicion of lung cancer could be used as a lung cancer biomarker. Using gene-expression profiles from Affymetrix HG-U133A microarrays, an 80-gene biomarker that distinguished smokers with and without lung cancer was identified. When the biomarker was tested on an independent test set, an accuracy of 83% (80% sensitive, 84% specific) was obtained. The biomarker profile had 90% sensitivity for stage I cancer among all subjects. When cytopathology of lower airway cells obtained at bronchoscopy was combined with the biomarker, a 95% sensitivity and a 95% negative predictive value (NPV) were obtained. These findings indicate that gene expression in cytologically normal large-airway epithelial cells can serve as a lung cancer biomarker, potentially owing to a cancer-specific airway-wide response to cigarette smoke. This novel version of the field cancerization concept is now being tested in less invasively obtained airway specimens, such as exfoliated buccal and nasal epithelium. Justification for such an investigation comes from data that bronchial and nasal epithelium from nonsmokers were most similar in gene expression when compared with other epithelial and nonepithelial tissues and with several antioxidant, detoxification, and structural genes being highly expressed in both the bronchus and nose. Smoking had a similar effect on gene expression in nasal epithelium as in the bronchus.[60] The expression of several detoxification genes was commonly altered by smoking in all three respiratory epithelial tissues, suggesting a common airway-wide response to tobacco exposure (Fig. 20.1).

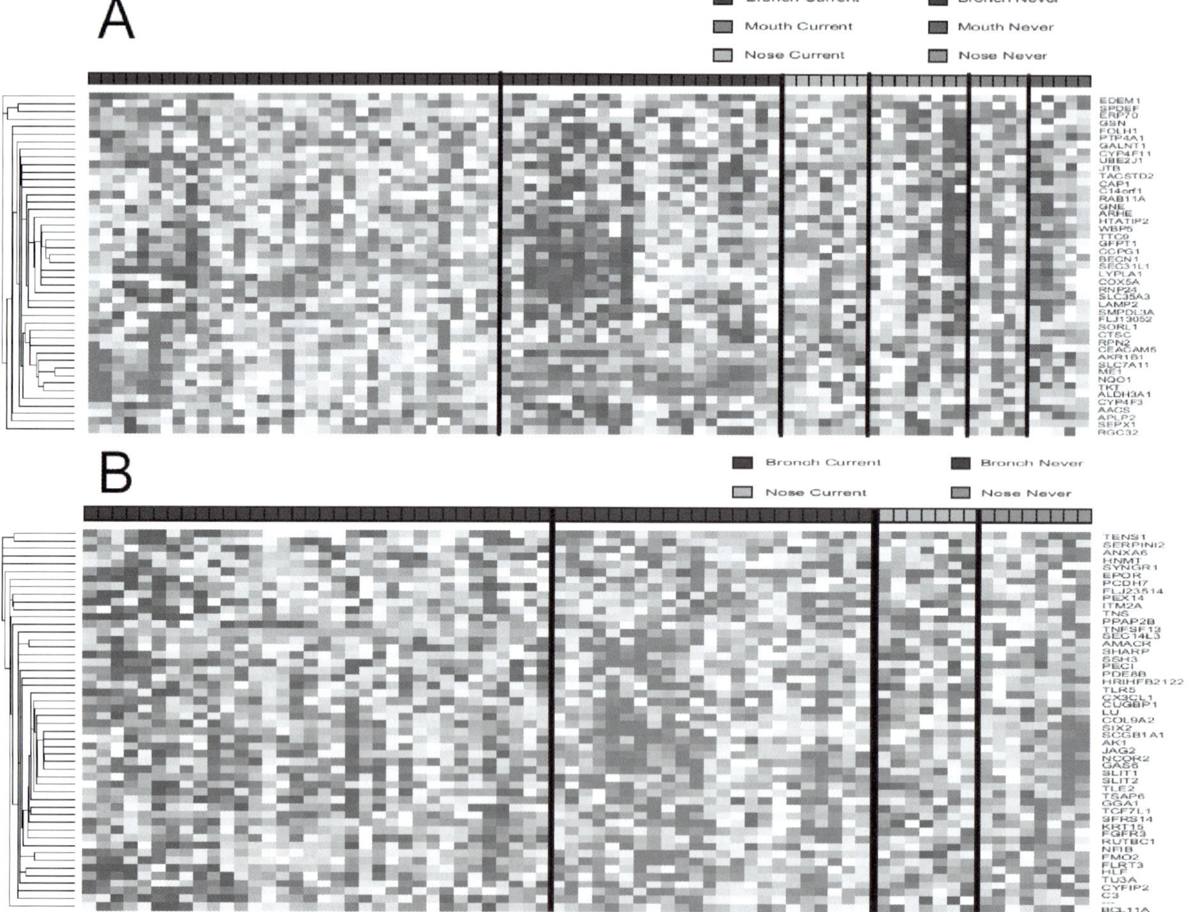

FIGURE 20.1 Hierarchical clustering of genes commonly perturbed by smoking across intrathoracic and extrathoracic airway epithelium. **A:** Supervised hierarchical clustering of the expression of 45 genes induced by smoking in the bronchial airway that are present in both the nasal and buccal "leading edge subsets" in samples from smokers and nonsmokers. These represent genes upregulated by smoking in bronchial, nasal, and buccal epithelium. **B:** Supervised hierarchical clustering of the expression of 50 genes repressed by smoking in the bronchial airway that are present in the nasal leading edge subset in samples from smokers and nonsmokers. High expression (*red*), average expression (*white*), low expression (*blue*). (See color plate.) (From Sridhar S, Schembri F, Zeskind J, et al. Smoking-induced gene expression changes in the bronchial airway are reflected in nasal and buccal epithelium. *BMC Genomics* 2008;9:259.)

Sputum-Based Cytology Although significant skepticism remains regarding the utility of standard sputum cytology as a lung cancer detection tool, and after the Mayo lung project and other NCI-sponsored studies yielded no overall mortality benefit, it has been long known that proximal and perhaps slower-growing lesions, such as that of squamous cell histopathology, could be detected in expectorated sputum with significant sensitivity (e.g., 30% to 50%). Additionally, automated, computerized image analysis can augment yield.[61]

Sputum for DNA-Based Markers Sputum-based detection has been studied extensively for somatic genetic and epigenetic alterations.

For *somatic genetic mutations*, credible studies have suggested a plethora of *k-ras* and *p53* mutations found in sputum that correlate, albeit imperfectly, with lung cancer prevalence, in the case-control context.[62,63] Of the more recent studies, one group has reported a correlation of FISH-detected HYAL2 and FHIT deletions in both tumor tissue and sputum in those with a smoking history in both lung cancer cases and smoking controls.[64] Another group examined three loci for loss of heterozygosity (LOH) and microsatellite instability (MSI) within the FHIT locus in sputum, with sensitivity of 55% and specificity of 82%.[65]

DNA Methylation by MSP in Sputa DNA methylation has been extensively studied in sputum for several presumed tumor suppressor gene promoters.[66] Among recent studies, Belinsky et al.[67] describe a case-control study nested within a high-risk cohort consisting of smokers with >30 pack-year smoking histories and spirometric airflow obstruction consistent with COPD. Results suggested qualitative sputum methylation increased with temporal proximity to the diagnosis, and with the number of genes methylated progressively conferring increased risk. Sensitivity and specificity of the 14-gene panel were both 64%. Methylation of three or more genes in sputum was associated with a 6.5-fold increased risk for lung cancer within 18 months. In stage III lung cancer, a methylation panel in sputum has been reported to reflect in the tumor itself, with 44% to 72% PPV and >70% NPV.[32] In most instances, sputum performed better than serum for the same gene panel (see Chapter 7).

A comprehensive study of quantitative MSP, using methylation-sensitive probes and primers, was carried out by Shivapurkar et al.[33] Eleven genes suggested to be silenced by methylation were examined in lung tumors, adjacent non-malignant lung tissues, and sputum. Of all genes, *3-OST-2*, *DCR-1*, and *RASSF1A* showed the highest levels in tumors and the lowest in adjacent nonmalignant tissues. Peripheral blood mononuclear cells (PBMCs) were uniformly nonmethylated at the probe sites. For sputum, when *3-OST-2*, *RASSF1A*, *mp16*, and *APC* were combined, significant discriminatory power in distinguishing cases from controls was apparent (ROC [receiver operating characteristic] − AUC [area under curve] = 0.8).

Sputum for RNA-Based Markers There are a few reports of RNA-based sputum studies in lung cancer detection that credibly identify the amplicon as RNA. Lacroix et al.[68] and Jheon et al.[69] reported an ability to amplify several transcripts (including preproGRP) from sputum, although in neither study there were no real-time controls employed to confirm the avoidance of contaminating DNA pseudogene amplification.

Sputum for Protein-Based Markers Claims of protein expression in sputum are more easily affirmed as credible than that for RNA, yet there have been relatively few to date. By example, the ribonucleoprotein has been suggested as a sputum-based biomarker by immunocytochemistry,[70] although there has been little follow-up data. A recent study correlating tumor and sputum telomerase activity found 68% sensitivity and 90% specificity, for concurrent lung cancer by sputum analyses, in a case-control context.[71]

Exhaled Breath for Volatile Small Compounds There is a considerable recent literature on the use of the gas phase of exhaled breath to identify individual volatile components or complex volatile mixtures that correlate with the presence of lung cancer. Study design has typically been case-control, such that predictive capacity for incident disease is largely unknown.

In a very carefully executed study, Wehinger et al.[72] collected tidal volume breathing mixed expiratory gas samples into 3-L pounds per cubic foot (pcf) bags, prior to any subject diagnostic or therapeutic interventions. They used a proton transfer reaction mass spectrometry (PTR-MS) approach to exhaled gas analysis, which avoids preconcentration steps otherwise required for gas chromatography-based techniques, but cannot distinguish compounds of the same mass. Among 17 predominantly early-stage lung cancer cases and 170 controls, mass-to-charge (m/z) = 31 or volative organic compound (VOC)-31 (tentatively protonated formaldehyde) and VOC-43 (tentatively a protonated fragment of isopropanol) were the most discriminatory; impressive twofold to threefold differences of cases versus smoker controls, with some overlap, were found. Overall test performance, in simulations, showed sensitivity for detecting lung cancer was 54%, accuracy was 96%, specificity was 99%, PPV (given 5% prevalence) was 90%, and NPV was 96%. ROC curves showed AUCs for those aged >50 years old of 0.82 and 0.95, respectively.

In some of the initial studies on volatile compounds in the gas phase that correlate to lung cancer, in a case-control context, Phillips et al.[73,74] reported significant correlations of gas chromatography–coupled mass spectrometry (GC-MS) patterns and the likelihood of having lung cancer. In one study, the approach yielded a training set sensitivity of 90% and specificity of 85% for lung cancer. In the test set, 83% sensitivity and 80% specificity was obtained.[74] Distinction from the exhaled volatile patterns of active or former cigarette smokers without apparent lung cancer was made.[74] Most recently, Phillips et al.[75] measured VOCs in 1-L alveolar breath from 193 subjects with primary lung cancer and 211 controls with a negative chest CT. Subjects were randomly assigned to a training set or to a prediction set in a 2:1 split. A fuzzy logic model of breath biomarkers of lung cancer was constructed in the training set and then tested in subjects in the prediction set by generating their typicality scores for lung cancer. Mean typicality scores employing a 16 VOC models were significantly higher in lung cancer patients than in the control group (p <0.0001 in all TNM stages). The model predicted primary lung cancer with 84.6% sensitivity, 80.0% specificity, and 0.88 AUC of the ROC curve. Predictive accuracy was similar in TNM stages I through IV, and was not affected by current or former tobacco smoking. The predictive model achieved near-maximal performance with six breath VOCs and was progressively degraded by random classifiers (Fig. 20.2). Predictions with fuzzy logic were consistently superior to multilinear analysis. If applied to a population with 2% prevalence of lung cancer, a screening breath test would have a NPV of 0.985 and a PPV of 0.163 (true-positive rate = 0.277, false-positive rate = 0.029).

Another group reported 71% sensitivity and 92% specificity for lung cancer detection in a case-control setting, using a commercialized sensor array "electronic nose."[76] In the sensor array method, the actual volatile components of the unique signal are not directly evaluated, although additional workup has revealed them to be predominantly volatile hydrocarbons. Corroborative later reports simplifying the sensor array have been reported,[77] although these patterns do not directly identify the responsible biomarker compounds. A recent uncorroborated study on training dogs, the ultimate biosensors, in study-blinded fashion, reports an extraordinary performance in distinguishing exhaled breath from those with lung cancer versus healthy controls (sensitivity and specificity both 99%).[78] A recent report that lung cancer cells in vitro evolve unique volatile metabolites in the gas phase above the culture dish lends some credence to the cancer specificity of the evolved exhaled gas detection approach.[79]

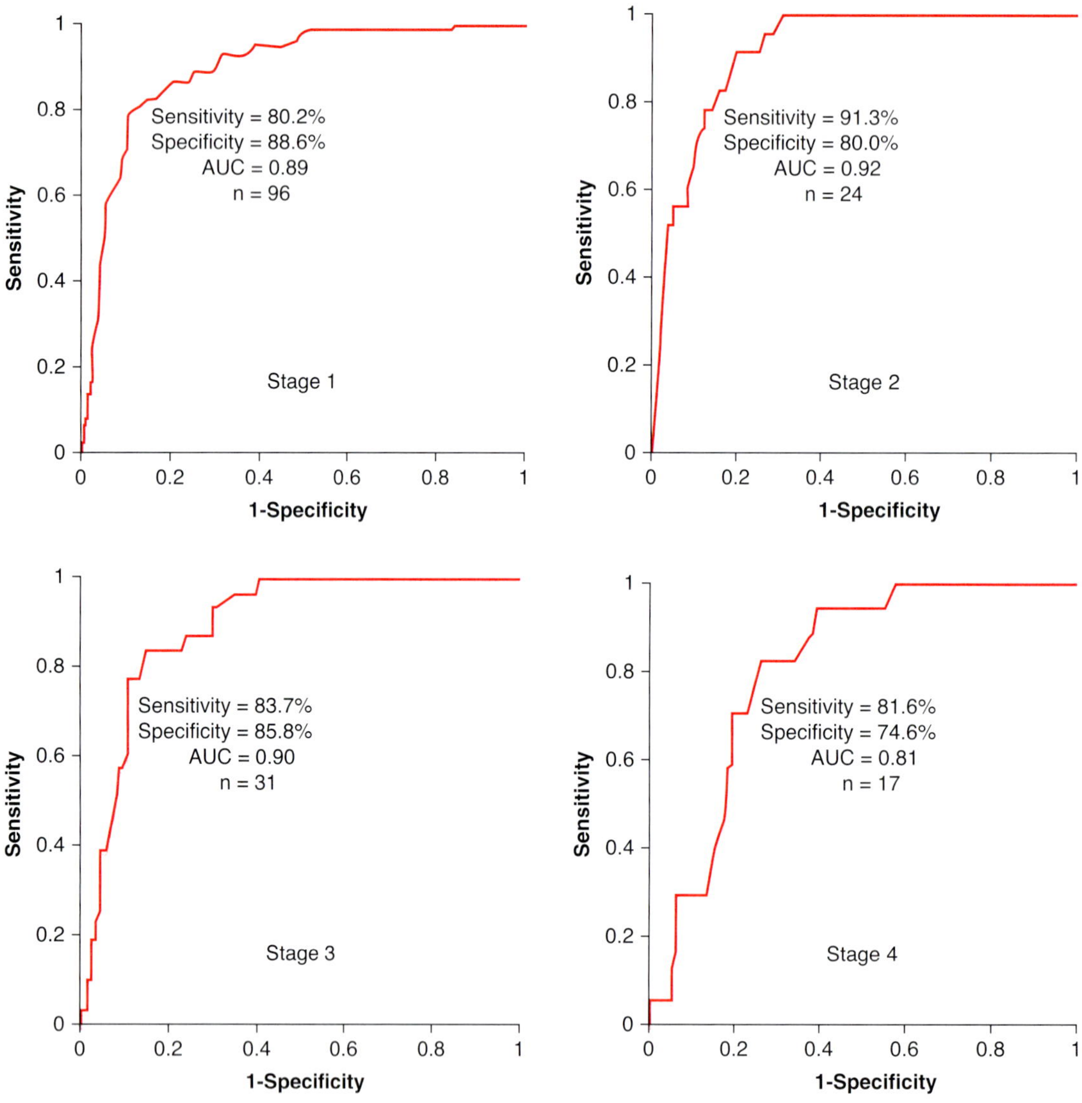

FIGURE 20.2 Measurement of VOCs from patients with various stages of lung cancer revealed accuracies of prediction that were similar across all stages. (From Phillips M, Altorki N, Austin JH, et al. Prediction of lung cancer using volatile biomarkers in breath. *Cancer Biomark* 2007;3:95–109.)

For molecules in the condensate (aqueous fraction) of exhaled breath, small molecules such as IL-2, tumor necrosis factor α (TNF-α), and leptin have been correlated to the presence of clinically apparent lung cancer cases versus controls.[80] Notable is that macromolecules directly reflective of carcinogenesis have also been detected in exhaled breath condensate. It is not intuitively obvious how large macromolecule markers of lung carcinogenesis, such as DNA and proteins, can be suspended in the breath, but there are multiple reports of this phenomenon from several laboratories, including our own. It is possible that a fraction of the components of bronchial lining fluid are suspended merely by entrainment by adjacent high-velocity airflow, or alternatively, alveolar lining fluid components are suspended by the agitation inherent in tidal volume inflation and deflation and/or the occasional opening snap of underinflated or atelectatic airspaces. Whatever the mechanism, several groups have reported the presence of DNA in exhaled breath, allowing DNA-based markers such as specific *p53* gene mutations,[81] microsatellite markers,[82,83] or DNA sequence annotated at high resolution for methylation.[84,85] In each case, a provocatively higher rate of carcinogenesis-related DNA aberrancy was detected in the lung cancer cases versus controls; the sensitivities and specificities are in the 80% range. Whether these case-control correlations will translate to meaningful predictive power for risk for lung cancer, in prospective studies, remains unevaluated.

SURROGATE AIRWAY EPITHELIA

Exfoliated Upper Airway Cells Brush-exfoliated buccal cells are transcriptionally active and potentially provide an easily procured window on gene–tobacco interaction that might be relevant to risk for tobacco-related malignancy. In one case-control study, expression of a candidate gene set of carcinogen metabolism pathway transcript in buccal epithelium was highly correlated with those in lung.[86] Genome-wide studies from other laboratories are underway for both buccal and nasal epithelia. Additionally, there have been intermittent reports of nasal epithelial access, in transcriptional and other studies, for gaining easier access to respiratory epithelium.

CONCLUSION

There is an impressive array of innovative approaches being developed for the early detection of lung cancer. Both optical and molecular-based methods are under study, in case-control discovery phase endeavors. Validation for a few of the most promising markers, be they somatic DNA mutation, DNA methylation, transcript assemblies, proteomic, or other markers, are underway, although prospective validation is clearly lacking. Rather than expect a single marker that is definitive and sensitive for both screening and diagnosis, it might be more practical to evolve a multistage approach employing population-wide risk assessment, followed by early disease detection approaches. The precise formulation of risk assessment approaches, and even disease detection tools, is in rapid flux. It is the high potential for public health impact of improvements in lung cancer diagnosis that has attracted a very considerable pool of innovations, strategies, and talent to focus on early detection approaches to this lethal disease.

REFERENCES

1. Koss LG. The Papanicolaou test for cervical cancer detection: a triumph and a tragedy. *JAMA* 1989;261:737–743.
2. Tabár L, Vitak B, Chen HH, et al. Beyond randomized controlled trials: organized mammographic screening substantially reduces breast carcinoma mortality. *Cancer* 2001;91:1724–1731.
3. Bach PB, Silvestri GA, Hanger M, et al. Screening for lung cancer. ACCP evidence-based clinical practice guidelines. (2nd edition). *Chest* 2007;132(3 Suppl);S69–S77.
4. Shaipanich T, McWilliams A, Lam S. Early detection and chemoprevention of lung cancer. *Respirology* 2006;11:366–372.
5. Bach PB, Kattan MW, Thornquist MD, et al. Variations in lung cancer risk among smokers. *J Natl Cancer Inst* 2003;95:470–478.
6. Spitz MR, Hong WK, Amos CI, et al. A risk model for prediction of lung cancer. *J Natl Cancer Inst* 2007;99:715–726.
7. Hirsch FR, Prindiville SA, Miller YA, et al. Fluorescence versus white-light bronchoscopy for detection of preneoplastic lesions: a randomized study. *J Natl Cancer Inst* 2001;93:1385–1391.
8. Haussinger K, Becker H, Stanzel F, et al. Autofluorescence bronchoscopy with white light bronchoscopy compared with white light bronchoscopy alone for the detection of precancerous lesions: a European randomized controlled multicentre trial. *Thorax* 2005;60(6):496–503.
9. Kennedy TC, McWilliams A, Edell E, et al. Bronchial intraepithelial neoplasia/early central airways lung cancer. ACCP evidence-based clinical practice guidelines (2nd edition). *Chest* 2007;132:S221–S233.
10. Loewen G, Natarajan N, Tan D, et al. Autofluorescence bronchoscopy for lung cancer surveillance based on risk assessment. *Thorax* 2007;62:335–340.
11. Chhajed PN, Shibuya K, Hoshino H, et al. A comparison of video and autofluorescence bronchoscopy in patients at high risk of lung cancer. *Eur Respir J* 2005;25:951–955.
12. Hanna N, Saltzman D, Mukai D, et al. Two-dimensional and 3-dimensional optical coherence tomographic imaging of the airway, lung, and pleura. *J Thorac Cardiovasc Surg* 2005;129:615–622.
13. Shulman L, Ost D. Advances in bronchoscopic diagnosis of lung cancer. *Curr Opin Pulm Med* 2007;13:271–277.
14. Kim YL, Turzhitsky VM, Liu Y, et al. Low-coherence enhanced backscattering: review of principles and applications for colon cancer screening. *J Biomed Opt* 2006;11:041125.
15. Horton KM, Horton MR, Fishman EK. Advanced visualization of airways with 64-MDCT: 3D mapping and virtual bronchoscopy. *AJR Am J Roentgenol* 2007;189:1387–1396.
16. Weir BA. Woo MS, Getz G, et al. Characterizing the cancer genome in lung adenocarcinoma. *Nature* 2007;450(7171):893–898.
17. Jones PA, Takai D. The role of DNA methylation in mammalian genetics. *Science* 2001;293:1068–1070.
18. Baylin SB, Schuebel KE. Genomic biology: the epigenomic era opens. *Nature* 2007;448:548–549.
19. Bird A. Perceptions of epigenetics. *Nature* 2007;447:396–398.
20. Shames DS, Girard L, Gao B, et al. A genome-wide screen for promoter methylation in lung cancer identifies novel methylation markers for multiple malignancies. *PLoS Med* 2006;3:E486.
21. Rauch TA, Zhong X, Wu X, et al. High-resolution mapping of DNA hypermethylation and hypomethylation in lung cancer. *Proc Natl Acad Sci U S A* 2008;105:252–257.
22. Tsou JA, Galler JS, Siegmund KD, et al. Identification of a panel of sensitive and specific DNA methylation markers for lung adenocarcinoma. *Mol Cancer* 2007;6:70.

23. Kagan J, Srivastava S, Barker PE, et al. Towards clinical application of methylated DNA sequences as cancer biomarkers: a joint NCI's EDRN and NIST workshop on standards, methods, assays, reagents, and tools. *Cancer Res* 2007;67:4545–4549.
24. Sozzi G, Conte D, Leon M, et al. Quantification of free circulating DNA as a diagnostic marker in lung cancer. *J Clin Oncol* 2003;21:3902–3908.
25. Herrera LJ, Raja S, Gooding WE, et al. Quantitative analysis of circulating plasma DNA as a tumor marker in thoracic malignancies. *Clin Chem* 2005;51:113–118.
26. Pathak AK, Bhutani M, Kumar S, et al. Circulating cell-free DNA in plasma/serum of lung cancer patients as a potential screening and prognostic tool. *Clin Chem* 2006;52:1833–1842.
27. Bremnes RM, Sirera R, Camps C. Circulating tumour-derived DNA and RNA markers in blood: a tool for early detection, diagnostics, and follow-up? *Lung Cancer* 2005;49:1–12.
28. Peluso M, Munnia A, Hoek G, et al. DNA adducts and lung cancer risk: a prospective study. *Cancer Res* 2005;65:8042–8048.
29. Godschalk RW, Van Schooten FJ, Bartsch H. A critical evaluation of DNA adducts as biological markers for human exposure to polycyclic aromatic compounds. *J Biochem Mol Biol* 2003;36:1–11.
30. Veglia F, Loft S, Matullo G, et al. DNA adducts and cancer risk in prospective studies: a pooled analysis and a meta-analysis. *Carcinogenesis* 2008;29(5):932–936.
31. Esteller M, Sanchez-Cespedes M, Rosell R, et al. Detection of aberrant promoter methylation of tumor suppressor genes in serum DNA from non-small cell lung cancer patients. *Cancer Res* 1999;59:67–80.
32. Belinsky SA, Grimes MJ, Casas E, et al. Predicting gene promoter methylation in non-small-cell lung cancer by evaluating sputum and serum. *Br J Cancer* 2007;96:1278–1283.
33. Shivapurkar N, Stastny V, Suzuki M, et al. Application of a methylation gene panel by quantitative PCR for lung cancers. *Cancer Lett* 2007;247:56–71.
34. Bailey-Wilson JE, Amos CI, Pinney SM, et al. A major lung cancer susceptibility locus maps to chromosome 6q23–25. *Am J Hum Genet* 2004;75:460–474.
35. Nair U, Bartsch H. Metabolic polymorphisms as susceptibility markers for lung and oral cavity cancer. *IARC Sci Publ* 2001;154:271–290.
36. Spitz MR, Wei Q, Dong Q, et al. Genetic susceptibility to lung cancer: the role of DNA damage and repair. *Cancer Epidemiol Biomarkers Prev* 2003;12:689–698.
37. Wu X, Lin J, Etzel CJ, et al. Interplay between mutagen sensitivity and epidemiological factors in modulating lung cancer risk. *Int J Cancer* 2007;120:2687–2695.
38. Hung RJ, Baragatti M, Thomas D, et al. Inherited predisposition of lung cancer: a hierarchical modeling approach to DNA repair and cell cycle control pathways. *Cancer Epidemiol Biomarkers Prev* 2007;16:2736–2744.
39. Engels EA, Wu X, Gu J, et al. Systematic evaluation of genetic variants in the inflammation pathway and risk of lung cancer. *Cancer Res* 2007;67:6520–6527.
40. Xi L, Nicatri DG, El-Hefnawy T, et al. Optimal markers for real-time quantitative reverse transcription PCR detection of circulating tumor cells from melanoma, breast, colon, esophageal, head and neck, and lung cancers. *Clin Chem* 2007;53:1206–1215.
41. Dom B, Timar J, Dobos J, et al. Identification and clinical significance of circulating endothelial progenitor cells in human non-small cell lung cancer. *Cancer Res* 2006;66:7341–7347.
42. Ge M-J, Shi D, Wu QC, et al. Observation of circulating tumour cells in patients with non-small cell lung cancer by real-time fluorescent quantitative reverse transcriptase-polymerase chain reaction in peroperative period. *J Cancer Res Clin Oncol* 2006;132:248–256.
43. Vogel U, Nexø BA, Tjønneland A, et al. ERCC1, XPD and RAI mRNA levels in lymphocytes are not associated with lung cancer risk in a prospective study of Danes. *Mutat Res* 2006;593:88–96.
44. Massion PP, Caprioli RM. Proteomic strategies for the characterization and the early detection of lung cancer. *J Thorac Oncol* 2006;1:1027–1039.
45. Yildiz PB, Shyr Y, Rahman JS, et al. Diagnostic accuracy of MALDI mass spectrometric analysis of unfractionated serum in lung cancer. *J Thorac Oncol* 2007;2:893–901.
46. Patz EF Jr, Campa MJ, Gottlin EB, et al. Panel of serum biomarkers for the diagnosis of lung cancer. *J Clin Oncol* 2007;25:5578–5583.
47. Ishikawa N, Takano A, Yasui W, et al. Cancer-testis antigen lymphocyte antigen 6 complex locus K is a serologic biomarker and a therapeutic target for lung and esophageal carcinomas. *Cancer Res* 2007;67:11601–11611.
48. Qiu J, Madoz-Gurpide J, Misek DE, et al. Development of natural protein microarrays for diagnosing cancer based on an antibody response to tumor antigens. *J Proteome Res* 2004;3:261–267.
49. Chapman CJ, Murray A, McElveen JE, et al. Autoantibodies in lung cancer—possibilities for early detection and subsequent cure. *Thorax* 2008;63:228–233.
50. Coen M, Holmes E, Lindon JC, et al. NMR-based metabolic profiling and metabonomic approaches to problems in molecular toxicology. *Chem Res Toxicol* 2008;21:9–27.
51. Nordstrom A, Want E, Northen T, et al. Multiple ionization mass spectrometry strategy used to reveal the complexity of metabolomics. *Anal Chem* 2008;80:421–429.
52. Chen H, Pan Z, Talaty N, et al. Combining desorption electrospray ionization mass spectrometry and nuclear magnetic resonance for differential metabolomics without sample preparation. *Rapid Commun Mass Spectrom* 2006;20:1577–1584.
53. Greenberg AK, Rimal B, Felner K, et al. S-adenosylmethionine as a biomarker for the early detection of lung cancer. *Chest* 2007;132:1247–1252.
54. Xing J, Spitz MR, Lu C, et al. Deficient G2-M and S checkpoints are associated with increased lung cancer risk: a case-control analysis. *Cancer Epidemiol Biomarkers Prev* 2007;16:1517–1522.
55. Wang W, Spitz MR, Yang H, et al. Genetic variants in cell cycle control pathway confer susceptibility to lung cancer. *Clin Cancer Res* 2007;13:5974–5981.
56. Chorostowska-Wynimko J, Szpechcinski A. The impact of genetic markers on the diagnosis of lung cancer: a current perspective. *J Thorac Oncol* 2007;2:1044–1051.
57. Ortiz-de-Solorzano C, Ucar-Vargas B, Pengo T, et al. Computer assisted detection of cancer cells in minimal samples of lung cancer. *Conf Proc IEEE Eng Med Biol Soc* 2007;2007:5517–5520.
58. Spira A, Beane J, Shah V, et al. Effects of cigarette smoke on the human airway epithelial cell transcriptome. *Proc Natl Acad Sci U S A* 2004;101:10143–10148.
59. Spira A, Beane JE, Shah V, et al. Airway epithelial gene expression in the diagnostic evaluation of smokers with suspect lung cancer. *Nat Med* 2007;13:361–366.
60. Sridhar S, Schembri F, Zeskind J, et al. Smoking-induced gene expression changes in the bronchial airway are reflected in nasal and buccal epithelium. *BMC Genomics* 2008;9:259.
61. Palcic B, Garner DM, Beveridge J, et al. Increase of sensitivity of sputum cytology using high-resolution image cytometry: field study results. *Cytometry* 2002;50:168–176.
62. Keohavong P, Gao WM, Zheng KC, et al. Detection of K-ras and p53 mutations in sputum samples of lung cancer patients using laser capture microdissection microscope and mutation analysis. *Anal Biochem* 2004;324:92–99.
63. Keohavong P, Lan Q, Gao WM, et al. Detection of p53 and K-ras mutations in sputum of individuals exposed to smoky coal emissions in Xuan Wei County, China. *Carcinogenesis* 2005;26:303–308.
64. Li R, Todd NW, Qiu Q, et al. Genetic deletions in sputum as diagnostic markers for early detection of stage I non-small cell lung cancer. *Clin Cancer Res* 2007;13:482–487.
65. Castagnaro A, Marangio E, Verduri A, et al. Microsatellite analysis of induced sputum DNA in patients with lung cancer, in heavy smokers, and in healthy subjects. *Exp Lung Res* 2007;33:289–301.
66. Belinsky SA. Gene promoter hypermethylation as a biomarker in lung cancer. *Nat Rev Cancer* 2004;4:707–717.

67. Belinsky SA, Liechty KC, Gentry FD, et al. Promoter hypermethylation of multiple genes in sputum precedes lung cancer incidence in a high-risk cohort. *Cancer Res* 2006;66:3338–3344.
68. Lacroix J, Becker HD, Woerner SM, et al. Sensitive detection of rare cancer cells in sputum and peripheral blood samples of patients with lung cancer by preproGRP-specific RT-PCR. *Int J Cancer* 2001; 92:1–8.
69. Jheon S, Hyun DS, Lee SC, et al. Lung cancer detection by a RT-nested PCR using MAGE A1—6 common primers. *Lung Cancer* 2004;43:29–37.
70. Sueoka E, Sueoka N, Goto Y, et al. Heterogeneous nuclear ribonucleoprotein B1 as early cancer biomarker for occult cancer of human lungs and bronchial dysplasia. *Cancer Res* 2001;61:1896–1902.
71. Pasrija T, Srinivasan R, Behera D, et al. Telomerase activity in sputum and telomerase and its components in biopsies of advanced lung cancer. *Eur J Cancer* 2007;43:1476–1482.
72. Wehinger A, Schmid A, Mechtcheriakov S, et al. Lung cancer detection by proton transfer reaction mass-spectrometric analysis of human breath gas. *Int J Mass Spectrometry* 2007;265:49–59.
73. Phillips M, Gleeson K, Hughes JM, et al. Volatile organic compounds in breath as markers of lung cancer: a cross-sectional study. *Lancet* 1999;353:1930–1933.
74. Phillips M, Cataneo RN, Cummin ARC, et al. Detection of lung cancer with volatile markers in the breath. *Chest* 2003;123: 2115–2123.
75. Phillips M, Altorki N, Austin JH, et al. Prediction of lung cancer using volatile biomarkers in breath. *Cancer Biomark* 2007;3(2):95–109.
76. Machado R, Laskowski D, Deffenderfer O, et al. Detection of lung cancer by sensor array analyses of exhaled breath. *Am J Respir Crit Care Med* 2005;171:1286–1291.
77. Mazzone PJ, Hammel J, Dweik R, et al. Diagnosis of lung cancer by the analysis of exhaled breath with a colorimetric sensor assay. *Thorax* 2007;62:565–568.
78. McCulloch M, Jezierski T, Broffman M, et al. Diagnostic accuracy of canine scent detection in early- and late-stage lung and breast cancers. *Integr Cancer Ther* 2006;5:30–39.
79. Chen X, Xu F, Wang Y, et al. A study of the volatile organic compounds exhaled by lung cancer cells in vitro for breath diagnosis. *Cancer* 2007;110:835–844.
80. Carpagnano GE, Spanevello A, Curci C, et al. IL-2, TNF-alpha, and leptin: local versus systemic concentrations in NSCLC patients. *Oncol Res* 2007;16:375–381.
81. Gessner C, Kuhn H, Toepfer K, et al. Detection of p53 mutations in exhaled breath condensate of non-small cell lung cancer patients. *Lung Cancer* 2004;43:215–222.
82. Carpagnano GE, Foschino-Barbaro MP, Mulé G, et al. 3p microsatellite alterations in exhaled breath condensate from patients with non-small cell lung cancer. *Am J Respir Crit Care Med* 2005;172:738–744.
83. Carpagnano GE, Foschino-Barbaro MP, et al. 3p microsatellite signature in exhaled breath condensate and tumor tissue of patients with lung cancer. *Am J Respir Crit Care Med* 2008;77:246–247.
84. Han W, Cauchi S, Herman JG, et al. Methylation mapping of DNA by tag-modified bisulfite genomic DNA sequencing. *Anal Biochem* 2006;355:50–61.
85. Han W, Wang T, Reilly AA, et al. Gene promoter methylation assayed in exhaled breath, with differences in smokers and lung cancer patients. *Respir Res* 2009;10:86.
86. Spivack SD, Hurteau GJ, Jain R, et al. Gene-environment interaction signatures by quantitative mRNA profiling in exfoliated buccal mucosal cells. *Cancer Res* 2004;64:6805–6813.

CHAPTER 21

Fadlo Khuri
Nico Van Zandwijk

Molecular Carcinogenesis and Chemoprevention of Lung Cancer

Lung cancer is by far the leading cause of cancer-related death, worldwide and in the United States.[1] Despite substantial progress in the treatment of lung cancer, which correlates with improvements in surgery, radiation oncology, and chemotherapy, 5-year survival has improved from 7% to only 16% over the last 2 decades. Although median survival in all stages of disease has improved somewhat, the low likelihood of obtaining a cure even with optimal modern therapy is largely because of the clinical presentation of this disease in its advanced stages The late diagnosis is almost certainly related to a covert carcinogenesis phase that often evolves over 10 to 20 years and requires multiple molecular genetic changes to facilitate the development of invasive lung cancer.[2,3] Thus, there exists a strong rationale for intervening in those stages of lung carcinogenesis that could result in arrest or delay of disease progression to the stage of frank cancer. Therefore, the strategies that are likely to be successful will likely optimally target both better biological understanding of lung cancer–mediated field carcinogenesis, and the development of reliable biomarkers that can accurately assess the likelihood of efficacy and toxicity across target populations. Ultimately, strategies involving screening and early detection, biomarker-based chemoprevention, smoking cessation, and better biological understanding of the phenomenon of lung carcinogenesis are all likely to be coupled with individualized risk stratification in the development of modern approaches to prevent this dreaded disease and reduce the societal burden of lung cancer.

LUNG CANCER EPIDEMIOLOGY

In most cases, lung cancer is strongly associated with direct consumption of tobacco products.[4] In fact, 87% of all lung cancers are detected in individuals who are active or former smokers, with an additional 6% to 7% composed of partners of smokers or their offspring (see Chapter 2). The second most common known cause of lung cancer is radon, which is associated with a significant increase in lung cancer risk, and with other risk factors including asbestos exposure. Nonetheless, despite the high degree of certainty that currently exists over the link between tobacco smoke and lung cancer, the understanding of these facts took several decades to clarify.

LUNG FIELD CARCINOGENESIS

The original description of *field carcinogenesis*, or *field cancerization* as it was originally called, dates back to Slaughter and coworkers,[5] who showed that multiple foci of epithelial hyperplasia, hyperkeratinization, atypia, dysplasia, and carcinoma in situ occurred in otherwise normal-appearing epithelium adjacent to cancers of the oral pharynx. This empiric evidence strongly suggested that carcinogen exposure has widespread effects throughout the entire carcinogen-damaged epithelial field. These diffuse histological changes suggested that the development of malignancy in the proximal upper aerodigestive tract is a result of the dose of carcinogen impacting exposed cell populations spread throughout this area. Auerbach and colleagues[6] observed and demonstrated the same pattern of heterogeneous, multifocal histological changes in the bronchial epithelium of smokers, many of whom have lung cancer. Thus, the concept of field cancerization or carcinogenesis was coined to describe the diffuse damage done by chronic exposure to carcinogens. Field carcinogenesis also forms the basis for the observation that individuals who survive a first cancer are often likely to develop a second malignancy in the region of the condemned epithelium.[7–9]

As these findings have been validated over the last several decades, increasing evidence has come to bear explaining the molecular genetic abnormalities that lead ultimately to the stepwise development of clonal invasion-competent cancer of the airway. Among the earliest findings in the aerodigestive tract of chronic smokers are loss of heterozygosity in chromosomes 3p, 9p, and 17p[2,10–14] (see Chapter 6). Clonal genetic abnormalities seen in normal histologic regions of the airway and not necessarily in areas that had detectable changes were further evidence that damage was scattered throughout the entire field (see Chapter 19). It also brought to bear the limitations of modern histologic techniques in detecting the extent of the damage induced by tobacco smoke in the airway. The importance of these losses of hererozygosity are crystallized in the fact that, for example, the short arm of chromosome 3, which is often the earliest loss and is demonstrated on occasion even in early hyperplasia,[10] results in the loss of a region rich in tumor suppressor genes. There is also evidence for losses of the short arms of chromosomes 9 and 17, resulting in loss of tumor suppressor genes in p16 and p53, both of which are important to the cell's ability to repair DNA damage done by the tobacco carcinogen. p53 in particular, acts as a transcription factor in the control of G1 arrest and apoptosis, or programmed cell death, thereby allowing the cell to repair existing DNA damage or make the determinant decision to push a cell into the apoptotic process once it is too far damaged for repair. p16, found on chromosome 9p, negatively controls cyclin-dependent kinases (CDK)–cyclin activity by overexpression of cyclin-D1. By inhibiting cyclin-D1/CDK, the damaged cell is also prevented from entering into mitosis and proliferating with damaged DNA (see also Chapter 14).

Increasing evidence shows that the loss of these and other tumor suppressor genes in lung cancer is augmented by the activation of several critical proto-oncogenes. For example, RAS, c-MYC, and the epidermal growth factor receptors (EGFRs), are all tumor-promoting genes that are activated progressively during lung carcinogenesis. K-ras mutations are particularly common in adenocarcinomas of the lung, with some studies showing 30% of lung adenocarcinomas in smokers containing K-ras mutations.[15] The EGFR is frequently amplified in non–small cell lung cancers (NSCLCs) and in fact in lung carcinogenesis[16] (see Chapter 49). Mutations have been detected in the EGFR tyrosine kinase binding domain conferring sensitivity to small molecule EGFR-tyrosine kinase inhibitors (EGFR-TKIs).[17,18] Interestingly, both K-ras mutations and EGFR mutations have been found in the airways of smokers and nonsmokers in regions distant from the primary tumor, suggesting that both play important roles in field carcinogenesis. Thus, modern molecular tools can help us better understand the process of field carcinogenesis and, as we will discuss, implement the development of targeted agents that can arrest or inhibit this otherwise inexorable progression.

Epigenetic Abnormalities in the Airway Loss of function of tumor suppressor genes and greater function of oncogenes through mutations or gene activations are not the only mechanisms by which carcinogenesis is augmented in lung cancer patients. A growing body of evidence suggests that gene silencing through epigenetic means can be crucial in lung carcinogenesis (see Chapter 7). For example, in NSCLC, some tumor suppressor genes such as RASSF1A, also located in the tumor suppressor gene–rich chromosome 3p, encodes a protein that heterodimerizes with Nore-1, an important RAS effector with pro-apoptotic effect.[19] Evidence from several groups suggests that in NSCLC, RASSF1A can be frequently inactivated by hypermethylation.[20,21] Another important gene that can be inactivated by epigenetic means is the retinoic acid receptor-β (RAR-β), which also maps to chromosome 3p. RAR-β is a nuclear retinoid receptor with vitamin A–dependent transcriptional activity.[22] RAR-β is a gene that is shown to be gradually lost in lung carcinogenesis,[23] and this can be regulated either by loss or by hypermethylation.[24,25] Interestingly, the maintenance of RAR-β in mature tumors is a factor for poor prognosis[26] and it is differentially regulated in current versus former smokers. For example, a recent retrospective study on methylation status and occurrence of second primary tumors (SPTs) in completely resected NSCLC patients revealed a strong association between RAR-β2 hypermethylation in the development of SPTs only in former smokers.[27] In current smokers, hypermethylation was associated with a protective effect, pointing to the critical value of context with regard to smoking status in understanding the biological effects of retinoid receptors in lung cancer.[27,28]

Lung Cancer Susceptibility and Risk Stratification Although there is little doubt that exposure to tobacco smoke is the major risk factor for the development of lung cancer, there is also progressive evidence that the risk of developing lung cancer, even among the heaviest smokers, varies widely according to genetic and perhaps even dietary factors. This is reinforced by the fact that 85% of heavy smokers will not develop lung cancer, implicating important differences in lung cancer susceptibility across the population in the likelihood of developing overt disease. However, there are significant competing risks for death of heavy smokers, including cardiovascular disease, chronic obstructive pulmonary disease, and other malignancies including those of the upper airway, bladder, cervix, kidney, and pancreas. Evidence exists, however, to show that every other smoker dies of a smoking-related cause.[29] Despite this, accumulating evidence suggests that genetic and epigenetic factors are critical in modulating individual susceptibility to lung cancer or other consequences of tobacco exposure.[30] The various carcinogens from cigarette smoke, benzpyrine and 4-(methylnitrosoamino)-1-(3-pyridil)-1 butanone (NNK) require metabolic activation before they can exert their full carcinogenic effects. Various activation pathways compete with detoxification pathways and the balance between the two is critical in modulating cancer risk. Cytochrome P450s serve as carcinogen-metabolizing enzymes, whereas glutathione transferases serve as detoxification enzymes. Both sets of these important genes are known to have significant polymorphisms correlating with variations in lung cancer risk (see Chapter 4).

Other important modulators of risk in lung cancer include diet and gender. Dietary factors play an important role as epigenetic modulators of lung cancer susceptibility. In several case-controlled studies, defective detoxification and defective repair of genetic damage have been shown to be associated with increased individual susceptibility to lung cancer.[31–34] However, certain food constituents appear to afford a significant degree of protection to individuals with limitations to their detoxification capacity.[35] This relationship between diet and lung cancer has been extensively explored and used as the basis

TABLE 21.1 Levels of Prevention in Lung and Aerodigestive Cancer

Level	Definition	Example
Primary	Diminish risk for normal healthy individuals	Smoking cessation or prevention; chemoprevention in asymptomatic smokers
Secondary	Decrease progression of preneoplasia	Reversal of preneoplasia or biomarkers of preneoplasia with chemoprevention
Tertiary	Decrease morbidity for patients treated or cured of an initial cancer	Chemoprevention of second primary tumor

for the development of novel approaches to the prevention of lung cancer. For example, large studies suggest that diets that have a high intake of fruits and vegetables are associated with a reduced risk of lung cancer.[36] Further evidence suggests that a Mediterranean diet is associated with a substantial reduction in several cancers, including lung cancer.[37]

Basis of Clinical Strategies in Lung Cancer Prevention As several dietary adjustments and micronutrients have been associated with lower risks of lung cancer, including vitamin E, selenium, isothiocyanates, and BMT-polyphenols, several large randomized trials have sought to delineate which compounds in complex human diets are most responsible for the protective effects seen.[36,38] Initially, the greatest degree of evidence existed around the potency of carotenoids and retinoids and the broad epidemiologic indications implicating them in reduction of cancer risk in general, and lung cancer risk in particular.[39,40] In fact, the original definition of chemoprevention coined by Michael Sporn as "attempts to reverse, suppress, and prevent carcinogenic progression to overt cancer"[41] is based on his and other's experimental work showing that vitamin A analogues are capable of reversing or preventing epithelial carcinogenesis in mouse models of cancer.

Consequently, the identification of populations at risk for development of this disease followed suit. For example, target populations in many of the early prevention studies included broad populations of individuals at risk because of their exposure to tobacco and/or asbestos. Others sought to develop strategies for uranium miners, also a population believed to be at enhanced risk for developing lung cancer. Thus, with several decades of broad epidemiologic and dietary investigation, augmented by important experimental systems showing several classes of compounds, especially the retinoids and carotenoids, were capable of reversing cell damage, a strong drive to develop this approach in human populations was born. The trials focused on broad patient populations, including those of individuals at even higher risk, in other words, individuals with known premalignancy of the airway, or those patients who had already developed a primary tobacco-related cancer, and thus were at the greatest risk for developing a second primary tumor.

Clinical Chemoprevention Trials Laudable as smoking cessation efforts have been, it is clear that lung cancers are developing in former smokers.[42,43] Thus, the design of lung cancer trials has taken the approach to develop strategies based on the different populations considered for each intervention. Risk categories were different across these populations, and thus the categories of chemoprevention were defined as primary, secondary, and tertiary prevention (Table 21.1). Primary prevention involved intervening in patient populations at increased risk but with no histological or clinical evidence of cancer. The end point here was reduction in incidence of lung cancer, and reduction in death from lung cancer. Secondary prevention involved attempts in individuals with evidence of lung premalignancy to prevent progression of that premalignancy or, ideally, to reverse it to an earlier stage of carcinogenesis. Finally, studies in the highest risk population were undertaken in those individuals who had already developed tobacco-related malignancy. Here, the goal was to prevent the development of SPTs. As expected, many of the early trials focused on using retinoids and carotenoids as the chemoprevention agents of choice, given that the weight of epidemiological and experimental evidence for these compounds was significantly greater than that for other classes of compounds.

Primary Chemoprevention Studies Several large randomized studies were undertaken in populations deemed to be at increased risk of lung cancer caused by exposure to tobacco, asbestos, or their occupation as uranium miners. Three major studies, the α-tocopherol/β-carotene (ATBC), β-carotene and retinol efficacy trial (CARET), and the U.S. Physician Study, were carried out using increasingly high doses of the carotenoid, β-carotene (Table 21.2). None of the three studies showed any reduction of lung cancer risk utilizing these compounds, and two of these studies, the ATBC and CARET studies, had surprising findings, both showing significant increases in lung cancer risk associated with supplementation with β-carotene. Both of these studies, which were 2 plus 2 factorial studies, also involved a second agent as an intervention. In these cases neither the second agent nor vitamin A itself was found to be associated with an increased risk of lung cancer, but neither were they protective against lung cancer incidence. Interestingly, both of these studies showed that the risk was increased only in populations

TABLE 21.2 Primary Randomized Chemoprevention Trials in Lung

	Intervention	End point	No. of Patients	Outcome
ATBC[39]	β-Carotene/ α-tocopherol	Lung cancer	29,133	Negative/harmful
CARET[46]	β-Carotene/ retinol	Lung cancer	18,314	Negative/harmful
Physician's Health Study[47]	β-Carotene	Lung cancer	22,071	Negative

that were heavy smokers, and particularly so in those individuals who had evidence of pulmonary asbestosis, as measured by manifestation of pleural plaques on chest radiograph.

The ATBC cancer prevention study was a randomized 2 by 2 factorial, double-blind, placebo-controlled, primary prevention study in which 29,133 Finnish male smokers received either α-tocopherol (50 mg/day alone), β-carotene (20 mg/day), both α-tocopherol and β-carotene, or a placebo. The participants, between 50 and 69 years of age, all of whom smoked at least five cigarettes per day, were enrolled on the study and received follow-up observation for 5 to 8 years. Although lung cancer incidence, the primary end point, was not modified by the addition of α-tocopherol alone, both groups who received β-carotene supplementation either alone or with α-tocopherol had an 18% increase in the incidence of lung cancer and a significant increase in lung cancer mortality. This study showed a stronger adverse effect from β-carotene in men who smoked more than 20 cigarettes per day, and was the first to raise the concern that pharmacologic doses of β-carotene could be harmful in active smokers. A recent update suggested that the excess risk for β-carotene recipients was no longer evident 4 to 6 years after any intervention and at that point, morbidity was largely caused by cardiovascular diseases.[39,44]

The CARET confirmed the results of the ATBC trial. This was also a randomized, double-blind, placebo-controlled trial testing the combination of 30 mg/day of β-carotene and 25,000 IU of retinyl palmitate in 18,314 men and women ages 50 to 69 years old who were considered at increased risk for lung cancer. The majority of participants had a smoking history of at least 20 pack-years, and were either current smokers or recent former smokers. Significant and even extensive occupational exposure to asbestos was noted in 4060 men on this trial.[45] The trial was stopped early by the Data Safety Monitoring Committee because of evidence of possible harm, consistent with the ATBC study. In fact, lung cancer incidence, the primary end point, increased 28% in the active intervention group, with an increase in overall mortality of 17% in this group.[46]

By contrast, the Physicians Health Study a randomized, double-blind, placebo-controlled trial studied 22,071 healthy male physicians, half of whom received 50 mg/day of β-carotene on alternate days and the other half received placebo. The use of supplemental β-carotene in this study comprising a majority of nonsmokers showed virtually no adverse or beneficial effects on cancer incidence or overall mortality rate during a 12-year follow-up.[47]

Subsequent subgroup analyses of the ATBC and the CARET studies have indicated that β-carotene had a harmful effect only in the high-risk heavy smokers, or those with previous exposure to asbestos.[48]

Reversal of Premalignancy or Secondary Prevention Although there has been much dispute over which are the optimal premalignant markers of lung cancer to follow, the success in developing chemoprevention agents in this arena has been extremely limited. To date, eight randomized trials have used various end points, including reversal of sputum atypia, reduction in DNA micronuclei, and reversal of dysplasia or hyperplasia (Table 21.3). Some of these trials have used retinoids, and have shown that in the absence of smoking cessation, retinoids are incapable of reversing premalignant lesions. Although some biomarker-driven studies utilizing novel pan-retinoids, such as 9-*cis*-retinoic acid, or atypical retinoids such as fenretinoid, have shown that these agents can modulate biomarkers such as RAR-β or human telomerase reverse transcriptase (hTERT) expression, respectively, there is little evidence to suggest that any of the compounds listed in Table 21.3 are capable of consistently reversing premalignant lesions. To date, one of the most positive studies has been one that utilized folate and vitamin B_{12}, which showed some improvement in bronchial epithelial metaplasia in smokers. Given the difficulty with validation of the end points, even these positive results must be viewed with caution. Larger trials using biologic end points are needed to confirm efficacy.[49]

Although several trials examining reversal of premalignancy in upper aerodigestive tumors with high doses of retinoids had shown significant initial efficacy, results have yet to be duplicated using retinoids in reversal of lung preneoplasia. Most importantly, findings from a trial by Lee et al.[50] indicated that retinoids could be effective in the presence of smoking cessation, but were highly ineffectual in active smokers. Recent studies employing novel retinoids have indicated that they may have significant promise. One such trial by Kurie et al.[51] reported the results of a randomized controlled trial in former smokers who received either 9-*cis*-retinoic acid or 13-*cis*-retinoic acid with α-tocopherol. The end point of this

TABLE 21.3 Secondary Randomized Chemoprevention Trials in Lung Cancer

	Intervention	End point	No. of Patients	Outcome
Lee et al.[50]	Isotretinoin	Metaplasia	86	Negative
Kurie et al.[88]	Fenretinide	Metaplasia	82	Negative
Arnold et al.[89]	Etretinate	Metaplasia	150	Negative
McLarty et al.[90]	β-Carotene/retinol	Sputum atypia	755	Negative
Heimburger et al.[91]	Vitamin B12/folic acid	Sputum atypia	73	Positive
Kurie et al.[51]	9-*cis*-retinoic acid	RAR-beta expression	226	Positive
Mao et al.[80]	Celecoxib	COX-2 expression and Ki-67	20	Positive
Kim et al.[81]	Celecoxib	COX-2 expression and Ki-67	204	Positive

trial was upregulation of RAR-β, the loss of which is gradually seen in pulmonary carcinogenesis. Of 177 evaluable patients, those treated with 9-*cis*-retinoic acid were found to have restoration of RAR-β expression ($p < 0.03$) and reduction of metaplasia ($p < 0.01$). There was no significant effect in the 13-*cis*-retinoic acid with α-tocopherol arm, encouraging this group of investigators to move forward with 9-*cis*-retinoic acid, a pan-retinoid agonist, targeting former smokers. Similar results were seen with fenretinide, an atypical retinoid that does not bind to any of the cognate X retinoid receptors, which was shown to downregulate hTERT, a critical component in human telomerase.[52] These promising data, albeit preliminary, suggest that continued investigation with novel retinoids may have substantial merit.

Second Primary Tumor Prevention Patients with tobacco-related cancers who have undergone successful treatment remain at a substantially elevated risk for developing subsequent tumors in the tobacco-damaged epithelium.[7,8,53–57] Although the treatment for the initial cancer can often be successful, these patients are at dramatically increased risk for developing and dying from a second primary tumor[58] (Table 21.4).The concept of SPTs initially described by Warren and Gates[59] explains the high likelihood of multiple oral and pharyngeal premalignancies, both synchronous and metachronous, disseminated throughout the condemned epithelium. Although modern molecular work by Sidransky et al.[60] has shown that the clonal origin of some of these SPTs can be indeterminate, some are a result of clonal evolution and the malignant clone can be found throughout the epithelium.[61,62] Clinical data continue to suggest that this remains a devastating long-term problem for patients definitively treated for primary tumor. The Warren and Gates criteria defined SPT as one that (a) is a new cancer of a different histological type, or (b) is a cancer, regardless of site, that occurs after more than 3 years, and (c) if it is also located in the head and neck region, the lesion is separated from the initial primary tumor by at least 2 cm of clinically normal epithelium, and (d) if found in the lung, and of squamous histologic subtype and developing within 3 years, it presents as a solitary mass with no evidence in the patient of local or regional disease, with changes consistent with dysplasia or carcinoma in situ within the surrounding bronchial epithelium. Using these criteria, the risk of local recurrence was shown by Vikram[58] to decline over time, whereas the risk of SPTs is constant for approximately the first decade following the initial head and neck cancer. Therefore, the lifetime risk of developing a SPT in the head and neck region is approximately 20%, with a similar incidence in the lung. Although estimates have varied between 3% to 7% per year, evidence remains incontrovertible that SPTs are the major cause of death after curative surgery in head and

TABLE 21.4 Lung and Aerodigestive Second Primary Tumor Prevention Studies

	Intervention	End point	No. of Patients	Outcome
Pastorino et al.[69]	Retinyl palmitate	SPT	307	Positive
EUROSCAN[71]	Retinyl palmitate /N-acetylcysteine	SPT	2592	Negative
Lippman et al.[72]	13-*cis*-retinoic acid	SPT	1166	Negative
Khuri et al.[68]	13-*cis*-retinoic acid	SPT	1190	Negative
Mayne et al.[73]	β-Carotene	SPT	264	Negative
Hong et al.[66]	Isotretinoin	SPT	103	Positive

neck cancer, and can be a major cause of death in early stage disease.[56–58,63–65]

Because of the high likelihood of both recurrence and SPTs in patients with advanced oral, oropharyngeal, or laryngeal squamous cell cancers, Hong et al.[66] launched a randomized, placebo-controlled study of 103 patients with stage I to IV head and neck squamous cell cancer, definitively treated with either previous surgery and/or radiation therapy. The patients were randomized to receive either high dose 13-*cis*-retinoic acid (100 mg/m^2/day) or placebo for 1 year after definitive local therapy. The dosage of 13-cRA was reduced to 50 mg/m^2/day after 13 of the first 44 patients experienced intolerable side effects. The primary end points were primary tumor recurrence and SPT development. In the two treatment arms, there was no difference in local recurrence or distant metastases. However, the patients treated with 13-cRA had a dramatically lower incidence of SPTs. Of the 103 patients followed for a median of 42 months, SPTs developed in 6% (3 of 49) of those in the 13-cRA arm, whereas 28% (14 of 51) of the patients on the placebo arm developed SPTs. Consistent with the findings of field carcinogenesis, the vast majority of the SPTs developed in the upper aerodigestive tract, esophagus, and lung, and 14 of 17 were found to be histologically of squamous cell type. Despite only 47% of the 13-cRA–treated patients completing the therapy as prescribed, the reduction in SPT development was still significant. Long-term follow-up has also revealed that the effects of 13-cRA decreased over time.[67]

A large scale follow-up to this trial using a much lower dose of 13-cRA was completed and presented a few years ago. In this trial, a randomized, double-blind, placebo-controlled study, launched in 1991, more than 1382 patients were registered and 1192 were randomized to either low dose 13-cRA at 30 mg/day versus placebo. These patients were definitively treated for stage I or II head and neck squamous cell cancer. With a median follow-up of 7 years, no effect was seen of the low dose retinoid on reducing the incidence of SPT in the lung or aerodigestive tract.[68]

Several other phase III trials have been launched in lung cancer in an attempt to prevent SPTs. The first of these was a trial by Pastorino et al.[69] that randomized over 300 patients with early stage lung cancer to retinyl palmitate or placebo. This study showed a significant reduction in the development of second primary lung cancers on the retinyl palmitate arm. A subsequent study by Bolla et al.[70] using a different synthetic retinoid, etretinate, failed to show a significant reduction in SPTs.

Two large phase III trials reported in the last decade include the EUROSCAN and the U.S. Intergroup NCI trial. EUROSCAN, a randomized adjuvant chemoprevention study of the European Organization for Research and Treatment of Cancer (EORTC), head and neck and lung groups studied the effects of vitamin A (retinyl palmitate) and N-acetylcysteine (NAC) in patients with early stage head and neck and lung cancer.[71] In this trial 2592 patients with cancers of the larynx, TIS-T3 and 0-N1, oral cavity, TIS-T2 and 0-N1, and NSCLC, T1-T2 and 0-N1, received retinyl palmitate, 300,000 IU per day in year 1, 150,000 IU/day in year 2, NAC 600 mg/day for 2 years, both drugs, or placebo. No significant differences were seen between the three active treatment arms and the placebo group in terms of recurrence rates, SPT development, or survival. More than 90% of the patient population was regular smokers, with 43 median pack-years of tobacco exposure.

The U.S. Intergroup NCI 91-0001 trial was a randomized, double-blind, placebo-controlled study utilizing the same low dose of 30 mg 13-cRA after complete resection of stage I NSCLC.[72] This trial completed accrual in 1997, having accrued 1486 participants. The study objectives were to evaluate the efficacy of low-dose daily 13-cRA for 3 years at 30 mg/day versus placebo in the prevention of SPTs. Patients were required to have complete resection of primary, stage I NSCLC (postoperative T1 or T2 and 0) and registered between 6 weeks to 3 years after completion of therapy. After a median follow-up of 3.5 years, no statistically significant differences were seen between the placebo and 13-cRA arms with respect to time to SPT development, recurrence rate, or mortality. Multivariate analyses showed that the rate of SPTs was not affected by any stratification factor, with recurrence rate affected only by treatment stage, and evidence for a treatment-by-smoking interaction (hazard ratio [HR] for treatment-by-current versus never-smoking status = 3.11, 95% confidence interval [CI], 1.00 to 9.71). Therefore, 13-cRA was not shown to affect overall survival rates or SPTs, recurrences, or mortality in stage I NSCLC. Subsequent subset analyses have indicated that 13-cRA was potentially harmful in current smokers and beneficial in never-smokers.

Finally, researchers at Yale University conducted a randomized, double-blind, placebo-controlled trial studying the effects of β-carotene at 50 mg/day in reducing local recurrence and SPTs in head and neck cancer.[73] Two hundred sixty-four patients with curatively treated early stage squamous cell carcinoma of the oral cavity, pharynx, or larynx were randomized to either 50 mg/day of β-carotene or placebo and were followed for 90 months for the development of SPTs and local recurrences. After a median follow-up of 51 months, no difference was seen between the two groups in time to failure, local recurrences or SPTs. Supplemental β-carotene had no effect on overall mortality, SPT rates, or rates of local recurrences.

FUTURE STRATEGIES IN LUNG CANCER PREVENTION

After more than 2 decades of unsuccessful interventions in NSCLC, evidence has now accumulated to suggest that approaches relying exclusively on the development of epidemiologic guidance for selection of compounds are unlikely to lead to effective interventions across broad and disparate populations. Although clues continue to emerge from the epidemiologic literature, including a study by Schabath et al.[74] showing that dietary phytoestrogens appear to significantly reduce lung cancer risk, few have suggested moving aggressive prevention approaches forward without further, well-designed, biomarker-driven trials.

Current targeted approaches focus on several pathways. To date, significant evidence exists to show that overexpression of the EGFR occurs throughout lung carcinogenesis,[16,75,76] and that mutations of the EGFR tyrosine kinase (EGFR-TK) binding domain can be seen diffusely across the normal-appearing airway in patients with resected adenocarcinomas who are nonsmokers and harbor an EGFR-TK binding domain mutation in their primary tumor. This discovery by Tang et al.[77] of a novel field effect in which EGFR-TK mutations are seen in apparently normal-appearing, nontobacco damaged airways suggests that despite the absence of an identifiable carcinogen leading to EGFR mutations, this represents a new and as yet etiologically unclear type of field effect. Several investigators have proposed novel chemoprevention approaches using the EGFR-TK inhibitors, erlotinib, and gefitinib, in high-risk patient populations. Given the fact that the incidence of EGFR-TK mutation-bearing adenocarcinoma of the lung is most frequently seen in Asian, female nonsmokers with lung cancer,[78,79] the identification of those individuals at greatest risk would likely lead to recognition of a target population, thereby enhancing the likelihood of a successful intervention with an EGFR-TKI.

Important data also implicate the progressive upregulation of cyclooxygenase-2 (COX-2) in lung carcinogenesis, and exciting preliminary trials targeting both suppression of COX-2 with selective COX-2 inhibitors by Mao et al.[80] and Kim et al.[81] have shown provocative results to date. Another approach taken by the University of Colorado group has sought to upregulate prostacycline, thereby downregulating prostaglandin E2 (PGE-2), potentially the critical downstream effector pathway for COX-2.[82] Another promising targeted approach is based on epidemiologic data. Govindarajan et al.[83] showed that thiazolidinediones (TZD), peroxisome proliferator-activated receptor (PPAR) stimulators, are able to induce cell cycle arrest. These investigators examined a large cohort study in 87,678 male veterans older than 40 years, and showed a 33% reduction of lung cancer risk among the 11,289 TZD users. Although the study failed to account for variations by smoking status, this represents a potentially exciting and useful chemopreventive approach. As reviewed by Nemenoff,[84,85] activation of PPARγ inhibits lung tumorigenesis as demonstrated by animal studies in which increased PPARγ may be chemopreventive against developing lung tumors. In established lung cancer, PPAR-γ activation inhibits proliferation, induces apoptosis, and promotes a less invasive phenotype by promoting epithelial differentiation, and perhaps blocking epithelial mesenchymal transition. PPAR-γ inhibition of chemokine production may also negatively impact tumor progression and metastasis. Although activation of PPAR-γ can occur by direct binding of pharmacological ligands to the molecule, emerging data indicate that PPAR-γ activation can occur through engagement of other signal transduction pathways, including Wnt signaling and prostaglandin production. Defining the molecular targets of TZDs mediating a specific response will be critical in the further development of second-generation PPAR-γ drugs. Cardiac events have been recorded with the use of TZDs, and the development of more selective PPAR-γ activators could potentially be therapeutically effective, without leading to adverse cardiac events.

Other methods have involved utilizing corticosteroids, both inhaled and oral, or inhaled retinoids, all of which have shown promise. Unfortunately, two randomized phase II studies in high-risk patients have failed to show a trend in favor of inhalational corticosteroids.[86,87]

While these and other data continue to be attractive, a surprising trial that sought to prevent SPT skin cancer in a selenium-poor population in Arizona resulted in the fortuitous finding of a dramatic reduction in lung cancer incidence (34% reduction).[38] The phase III Eastern Cooperative Oncology Group (ECOG) selenium trial, E5597, has accrued approximately 1300 of 1900 planned patients. This trial randomizes patients in a 2:1 ratio to receive selenium methionine at 200 μg/day versus placebo. Patients must have the identical criteria to the prior intergroup study, that is, a history of stage I to II NSCLC fully resected, patients being registered between 6 weeks and up to 3 years after surgery. Whether the selenium trial ultimately yields definitive answers, the recommendation must be to continue to build biomarker-driven, targeted, phase II approaches that appropriately pursue modulation of a critical biomarker, and confirm it prior to proceeding with aggressive, broad, studies in large patient populations. Once the appropriate biomarkers have been shown to be consistently modulated in selected populations, only then can we proceed with confidence to develop targeted agents that can meaningfully reduce the incidence of lung cancer in at-risk populations.

REFERENCES

1. Jemal A, Siegel R, Ward E, et al. Cancer statistics, 2008. *CA Cancer J Clin* 2008;58:71–96.
2. Mao L, Lee JS, Kurie JM, et al. Clonal genetic alterations in the lungs of current and former smokers. *J Natl Cancer Inst* 1997;89:857–862.
3. Bartsch H, Petruzzelli S, De Flora S, et al. Carcinogen metabolism in human lung tissues and the effect of tobacco smoking: results from a case—control multicenter study on lung cancer patients. *Environ Health Perspect* 1992;98:119–124.
4. Auerbach O, Forman JB, Gere JB, et al. Changes in the bronchial epithelium in relation to smoking and cancer of the lung; a report of progress. *N Engl J Med* 1957;256:97–104.
5. Slaughter DP, Southwick HW, Smejkal W. Field cancerization in oral stratified squamous epithelium; clinical implications of multicentric origin. *Cancer* 1953;6:963–968.
6. Auerbach O, Hammond EC, Garfinkel L. Changes in bronchial epithelium in relation to cigarette smoking, 1955–1960 vs. 1970–1977. *N Engl J Med* 1979;300:381–385.
7. Boice JD Jr, Fraumeni JF Jr. Second cancer following cancer of the respiratory system in Connecticut, 1935–1982. *Natl Cancer Inst Monogr* 1985;68:83–98.
8. de Vries N, Snow GB. Multiple primary tumours in laryngeal cancer. *J Laryngol Otol* 1986;100:915–918.
9. Vikram B, Strong EW, Shah JP, et al. Second malignant neoplasms in patients successfully treated with multimodality treatment for advanced head and neck cancer. *Head Neck Surg* 1984;6:734–737.
10. Hung J, Kishimoto Y, Sugio K, et al. Allele-specific chromosome 3p deletions occur at an early stage in the pathogenesis of lung carcinoma. *JAMA* 1995;273:1908.
11. Mao L. Tumor suppressor genes: does FHIT fit? *J Natl Cancer Inst* 1998; 90:412–414.

12. Wistuba, II, Lam S, Behrens C, et al. Molecular damage in the bronchial epithelium of current and former smokers. *J Natl Cancer Inst* 1997;89:1366–1373.
13. Kishimoto Y, Sugio K, Hung JY, et al. Allele-specific loss in chromosome 9p loci in preneoplastic lesions accompanying non-small-cell lung cancers. *J Natl Cancer Inst* 1995;87:1224–1229.
14. Kishimoto Y, Murakami Y, Shiraishi M, et al. Aberrations of the p53 tumor suppressor gene in human non-small cell carcinomas of the lung. *Cancer Res* 1992;52:4799–4804.
15. Westra WH, Slebos RJ, Offerhaus GJ, et al. K-ras oncogene activation in lung adenocarcinomas from former smokers. Evidence that K-ras mutations are an early and irreversible event in the development of adenocarcinoma of the lung. *Cancer* 1993;72:432–438.
16. Hirsch FR, Varella-Garcia M, Bunn PA Jr, et al. Epidermal growth factor receptor in non-small-cell lung carcinomas: correlation between gene copy number and protein expression and impact on prognosis. *J Clin Oncol* 2003;21:3798–3807.
17. Lynch TJ, Bell DW, Sordella R, et al. Activating mutations in the epidermal growth factor receptor underlying responsiveness of non-small-cell lung cancer to gefitinib. *N Engl J Med* 2004;350:2129–2139.
18. Paez JG, Jänne PA, Lee JC, et al. EGFR mutations in lung cancer: correlation with clinical response to gefitinib therapy. *Science* 2004;304:1497–1500.
19. Ortiz-Vega S, Khokhlatchev A, Nedwidek M, et al. The putative tumor suppressor RASSF1A homodimerizes and heterodimerizes with the Ras-GTP binding protein Nore1. *Oncogene* 2002;21:1381–1390.
20. Agathanggelou A, Honorio S, Macartney DP, et al. Methylation associated inactivation of RASSF1A from region 3p21.3 in lung, breast and ovarian tumours. *Oncogene* 2001;20:1509–1518.
21. Burbee DG, Forgacs E, Zöchbauer-Müller S, et al. Epigenetic inactivation of RASSF1A in lung and breast cancers and malignant phenotype suppression. *J Natl Cancer Inst* 2001;93:691–699.
22. Leid M, Kastner P, Chambon P. Multiplicity generates diversity in the retinoic acid signalling pathways. *Trends Biochem Sci* 1992;17: 427–433.
23. Xu XC, Sozzi G, Lee JS, et al. Suppression of retinoic acid receptor beta in non-small-cell lung cancer in vivo: implications for lung cancer development. *J Natl Cancer Inst* 1997;89:624–629.
24. Bérard J, Laboune F, Mukuna M, et al. Lung tumors in mice expressing an antisense RARbeta2 transgene. *FASEB J* 1996;10:1091–1097.
25. Toulouse A, Morin J, Dion PA, et al. RARbeta2 specificity in mediating RA inhibition of growth of lung cancer-derived cells. *Lung Cancer* 2000;28:127–137.
26. Khuri FR, Lotan R, Kemp BL, et al. Retinoic acid receptor-beta as a prognostic indicator in stage I non-small-cell lung cancer. *J Clin Oncol* 2000;18:2798–2804.
27. Kim JS, Lee H, Kim H, et al. Promoter methylation of retinoic acid receptor beta 2 and the development of second primary lung cancers in non-small-cell lung cancer. *J Clin Oncol* 2004;22:3443–3450.
28. Khuri FR, Lotan R. Retinoids in lung cancer: friend, foe, or fellow traveler? *J Clin Oncol* 2004;22:3435–3437.
29. Peto R, Lopez AD, Boreham J, et al. Mortality from tobacco in developed countries: indirect estimation from national vital statistics. *Lancet* 1992;339:1268–1278.
30. Xu H, Spitz MR, Amos CI, et al. Complex segregation analysis reveals a multigene model for lung cancer. *Hum Genet* 2005;116:121–127.
31. Denissenko MF, Pao A, Tang M, et al. Preferential formation of benzo[a]pyrene adducts at lung cancer mutational hotspots in P53. *Science* 1996;274:430–432.
32. Wei Q, Cheng L, Amos CI, et al. Repair of tobacco carcinogen-induced DNA adducts and lung cancer risk: a molecular epidemiologic study. *J Natl Cancer Inst* 2000;92:1764–1772.
33. Hecht SS. Tobacco smoke carcinogens and lung cancer. *J Natl Cancer Inst* 1999;91:1194–1210.
34. Spitz MR, Wu X, Wang Y, et al. Modulation of nucleotide excision repair capacity by XPD polymorphisms in lung cancer patients. *Cancer Res* 2001;61:1354–1357.
35. Spitz MR, Duphorne CM, Detry MA, et al. Dietary intake of isothiocyanates: evidence of a joint effect with glutathione S-transferase polymorphisms in lung cancer risk. *Cancer Epidemiol Biomarkers Prev* 2000;9:1017–1020.
36. Block G, Patterson B, Subar A. Fruit, vegetables, and cancer prevention: a review of the epidemiological evidence. *Nutr Cancer* 1992;18:1–29.
37. Fortes C, Forastiere F, Farchi S, et al. The protective effect of the Mediterranean diet on lung cancer. *Nutr Cancer* 2003;46(1):30–37.
38. Clark LC, Combs GF Jr, Turnbull BW, et al. Effects of selenium supplementation for cancer prevention in patients with carcinoma of the skin. A randomized controlled trial. Nutritional Prevention of Cancer Study Group. *JAMA* 1996;276:1957–1963.
39. The effect of vitamin E and beta carotene on the incidence of lung cancer and other cancers in male smokers. The Alpha-Tocopherol, Beta Carotene Cancer Prevention Study Group. *N Engl J Med* 1994;330:1029–1035.
40. Omenn GS. Chemoprevention of lung cancers: lessons from CARET, the beta-carotene and retinol efficacy trial, and prospects for the future. *Eur J Cancer Prev* 2007;16(3):184–191.
41. Sporn MB, Dunlop NM, Newton DL, et al. Prevention of chemical carcinogenesis by vitamin A and its synthetic analogs (retinoids). *Fed Proc* 1976;35:1332–1338.
42. Tong L, Spitz MR, Fueger JJ, et al. Lung carcinoma in former smokers. *Cancer* 1996;78:1004–1010.
43. Strauss G, DeCamp M, Dibiccaro E, et al. Lung cancer diagnosis is being made with increasing frequency in former cigarette smokers! *Proc Am Soc Clin Oncol* 1995;14:362.
44. Virtamo J, Pietinen P, Huttunen JK, et al. Incidence of cancer and mortality following alpha-tocopherol and beta-carotene supplementation: a postintervention follow-up. *JAMA* 2003;290:476–485.
45. Goodman M, Morgan RW, Ray R, et al. Cancer in asbestos-exposed occupational cohorts: a meta-analysis. *Cancer Causes Control* 1999;10: 453–465.
46. Omenn GS, Goodman GE, Thornquist MD, et al. Effects of a combination of beta carotene and vitamin A on lung cancer and cardiovascular disease. *N Engl J Med* 1996;334:1150–1155.
47. Hennekens CH, Buring JE, Manson JE, et al. Lack of effect of long-term supplementation with beta carotene on the incidence of malignant neoplasms and cardiovascular disease. *N Engl J Med* 1996;334: 1145–1149.
48. Cullen MR, Barnett MJ, Balmes JR, et al. Predictors of lung cancer among asbestos-exposed men in the {beta}-carotene and retinol efficacy trial. *Am J Epidemiol* 2005;161(3):260–270.
49. Slatore CG, Littman AJ, Au DH. Long-term use of supplemental multivitamins, vitamin C, vitamin E, and folate does not reduce the risk of lung cancer. *Am J Respir Crit Care Med* 2008;177:524–530.
50. Lee JS, Lippman SM, Benner SE, et al. Randomized placebo-controlled trial of isotretinoin in chemoprevention of bronchial squamous metaplasia. *J Clin Oncol* 1994;12:937–945.
51. Kurie JM, Lotan R, Lee JJ, et al. Treatment of former smokers with 9-cis-retinoic acid reverses loss of retinoic acid receptor-beta expression in the bronchial epithelium: results from a randomized placebo-controlled trial. *J Natl Cancer Inst* 2003;95:206–214.
52. Soria JC, Moon C, Wang L, et al. Effects of N-(4-hydroxyphenyl)retinamide on hTERT expression in the bronchial epithelium of cigarette smokers. *J Natl Cancer Inst* 2001;93:1257–1263.
53. Decker J, Goldstein JC. Risk factors in head and neck cancer. *N Engl J Med* 1982;306:1151–1155.
54. Wynder EL, Stellman SD. Impact of long-term filter cigarette usage on lung and larynx cancer risk: a case-control study. *J Natl Cancer Inst* 1979;62:471–477.
55. Gluckman JL, Crissman JD. Survival rates in 548 patients with multiple neoplasms of the upper aerodigestive tract. *Laryngoscope* 1983;93:71–74.
56. Yellin A, Hill LR, Benfield JR. Bronchogenic carcinoma associated with upper aerodigestive cancers. *J Thorac Cardiovasc Surg* 1986;91:674–683.
57. Vokes EE, Weichselbaum RR, Lippman SM, et al. Head and neck cancer. *N Engl J Med* 1993;328:184–194.

58. Vikram B. Changing patterns of failure in advanced head and neck cancer. *Arch Otolaryngol* 1984;110:564–565.
59. Warren S, Gates O. Multiple primary malignant tumors: a survey of the literature and statistical study. *Am J Cancer* 1932;16:1358–1403.
60. Califano J, Westra WH, Koch W, et al. Unknown primary head and neck squamous cell carcinoma: molecular identification of the site of origin. *J Natl Cancer Inst* 1999;91:599–604.
61. Califano J, Leong PL, Koch WM, et al. Second esophageal tumors in patients with head and neck squamous cell carcinoma: an assessment of clonal relationships. *Clin Cancer Res* 1999;5:1862–1867.
62. Scholes AG, Woolgar JA, Boyle MA, et al. Synchronous oral carcinomas: independent or common clonal origin? *Cancer Res* 1998;58: 2003–2006.
63. Lippman SM, Hong WK. Not yet standard: retinoids versus second primary tumors. *J Clin Oncol* 1993;11:1204–1207.
64. Lippman SM, Hong WK. Second malignant tumors in head and neck squamous cell carcinoma: the overshadowing threat for patients with early-stage disease. *Int J Radiat Oncol Biol Phys* 1989;17:691–694.
65. Larson JT, Adams GL, Fattah HA. Survival statistics for multiple primaries in head and neck cancer. *Otolaryngol Head Neck Surg* 1990; 103:14–24.
66. Hong WK, Lippman SM, Itri LM, et al. Prevention of second primary tumors with isotretinoin in squamous-cell carcinoma of the head and neck. *N Engl J Med* 1990;323:795–801.
67. Benner SE, Pajak TF, Lippman SM, et al. Prevention of second primary tumors with isotretinoin in patients with squamous cell carcinoma of the head and neck: long-term follow-up. *J Natl Cancer Inst* 1994; 86:140–141.
68. Khuri FR, Lee JJ, Lippman SM, et al. Randomized phase III trial of low-dose isotretinoin for prevention of second primary tumors in stage I and II head and neck cancer patients. *J Natl Cancer Inst* 2006;98:441–450.
69. Pastorino U, Infante M, Maioli M, et al. Adjuvant treatment of stage I lung cancer with high-dose vitamin A. *J Clin Oncol* 1993;11: 1216–1222.
70. Bolla M, Lefur R, Ton Van J, et al. Prevention of second primary tumours with etretinate in squamous cell carcinoma of the oral cavity and oropharynx. Results of a multicentric double-blind randomised study. *Eur J Cancer* 1994;30A:727–729.
71. van Zandwijk N, Dalesio O, Pastorino U, et al. EUROSCAN, a randomized trial of vitamin A and N-acetylcysteine in patients with head and neck cancer or lung cancer. For the European Organization for Research and Treatment of Cancer Head and Neck and Lung Cancer Cooperative Groups. *J Natl Cancer Inst* 2000;92:977–986.
72. Lippman SM, Lee JJ, Karp DD, et al. Randomized phase III intergroup trial of isotretinoin to prevent second primary tumors in stage I non-small-cell lung cancer. *J Natl Cancer Inst* 2001;93:605–618.
73. Mayne ST, Cartmel B, Baum M, et al. Randomized trial of supplemental beta-carotene to prevent second head and neck cancer. *Cancer Res* 2001;61:1457–1463.
74. Schabath MB, Hernandez LM, Wu X, et al. Dietary phytoestrogens and lung cancer risk. *JAMA* 2005;294:1493–1504.
75. Kurie JM, Shin HJ, Lee JS, et al. Increased epidermal growth factor receptor expression in metaplastic bronchial epithelium. *Clin Cancer Res* 1996;2:1787–1793.
76. Rusch V, Baselga J, Cordon-Cardo C, et al. Differential expression of the epidermal growth factor receptor and its ligands in primary non-small cell lung cancers and adjacent benign lung. *Cancer Res* 1993;53:2379–2385.
77. Tang X, Shigematsu H, Bekele BN, et al. EGFR tyrosine kinase domain mutations are detected in histologically normal respiratory epithelium in lung cancer patients. *Cancer Res* 2005;65:7568–7572.
78. Shepherd FA, Rodrigues Pereira J, Ciuleanu T, et al. Erlotinib in previously treated non-small-cell lung cancer. *N Engl J Med* 2005;353:123–132.
79. Thatcher N, Chang A, Parikh P, et al. Gefitinib plus best supportive care in previously treated patients with refractory advanced non-small-cell lung cancer: results from a randomised, placebo-controlled, multicentre study (Iressa Survival Evaluation in Lung Cancer). *Lancet* 2005;366:1527–1537.
80. Mao JT, Fishbein MC, Adams B, et al. Celecoxib decreases Ki-67 proliferative index in active smokers. *Clin Cancer Res* 2006;12:314–320.
81. Kim ES, Hong WK, Lee JJ, et al. A randomized double-blind study of the biological effects of celecoxib as a chemopreventive agent in current and former smokers. *J Clin Oncol* 2008;26S:1501.
82. Keith RL, Geraci MW. Prostacyclin in lung cancer. *J Thorac Oncol* 2006;1(6):503–505.
83. Govindarajan R, Ratnasinghe L, Simmons DL, et al. Thiazolidinediones and the risk of lung, prostate, and colon cancer in patients with diabetes. *J Clin Oncol* 2007;25:1476–1481.
84. Nemenoff RA, Weiser-Evans M, Winn RA. Activation and molecular targets of peroxisome proliferator-activated receptor-gamma ligands in lung cancer. *PPAR Res* 2008;2008:156875.
85. Nemenoff RA. Peroxisome proliferator-activated receptor-gamma in lung cancer: defining specific versus "off-target" effectors. *J Thorac Oncol* 2007;2(11):989–992.
86. Lam S, leRiche JC, McWilliams A, et al. A randomized phase IIb trial of pulmicort turbuhaler (budesonide) in people with dysplasia of the bronchial epithelium. *Clin Cancer Res* 2004;10(19):6502–6511.
87. van den Berg RM, van Tinteren H, van Zandwijk N, et al. The influence of fluticasone inhalation on markers of carcinogenesis in bronchial epithelium. *Am J Respir Crit Care Med* 2007;175(10):1061–1065.
88. Kurie JM, Lee JS, Khuri FR, et al. N-(4-hydroxyphenyl)retinamide in the chemoprevention of squamous metaplasia and dysplasia of the bronchial epithelium. *Clin Cancer Res* 2000;6:2973–2979.
89. Arnold AM, Browman GP, Levine MN, et al. The effect of the synthetic retinoid etretinate on sputum cytology: results from a randomised trial. *Br J Cancer* 1992;65:737–743.
90. McLarty JW, Holiday DB, Girard WM, et al. Beta-carotene, vitamin A, and lung cancer chemoprevention: results of an intermediate endpoint study. *Am J Clin Nutr* 1995;62:1431S–1438S.
91. Heimburger DC, Alexander CB, Birch R, et al. Improvement in bronchial squamous metaplasia in smokers treated with folate and vitamin B12. Report of a preliminary randomized, double-blind intervention trial. *JAMA* 1988;259:1525–1530.

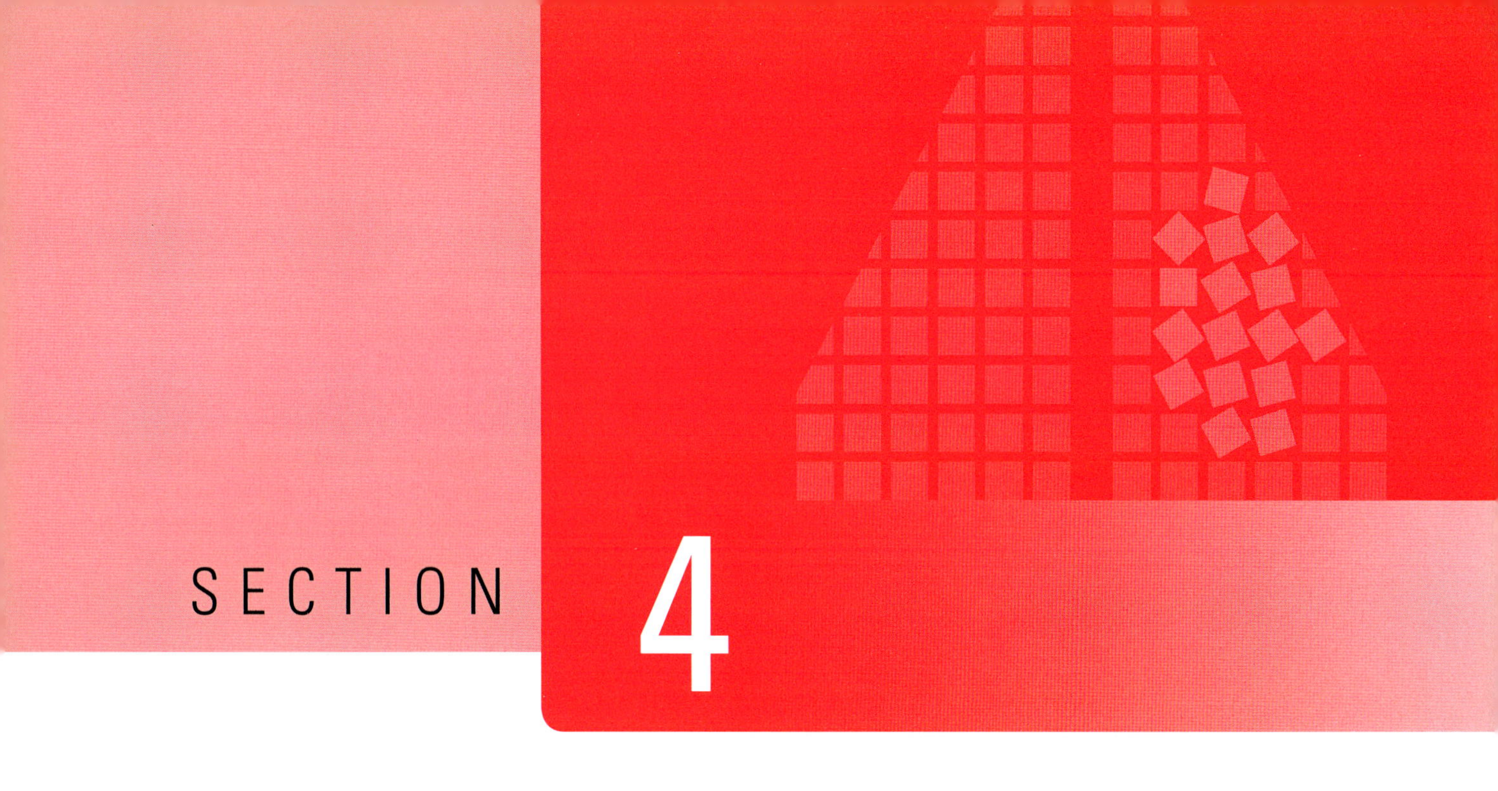

SECTION 4

Pathology

CHAPTER 22

Wilbur A. Franklin
Masayuki Noguchi
Adriana Gonzalez

Molecular and Cellular Pathology of Lung Cancer

Despite advances in imaging techniques and the molecular characterization of lung tumors described elsewhere in this volume, the histopathology of lung cancer remains the basis for diagnosis and treatment of the disease and is essential for the interpretation of imaging studies and molecular analyses. Histopathology has recently taken on added importance as it has been recognized that targeted agents affect specific lung tumor subtypes differently and that successful treatment may depend on histological distinctions that have been previously unrecognized or ignored. Historically, the classification of lung cancer rested on the expertise of individual pathologists but in 1967, an international panel was first assembled through the World Health Organization (WHO) to create a standard nomenclature for lung cancer. This classification with its periodic revisions has become the most widely used standard for diagnosis and treatment and is provided in Appendix A. The most recent edition of the WHO morphological classification was published in 2004 and is more comprehensive than previous editions' description of the classification, taking into account molecular data as well as morphology.[1] The purpose of this chapter is not so much to recapitulate the details of the WHO classification but rather to provide an understanding of the main categories of lung carcinoma, to highlight potential pitfalls in histopathological diagnosis of lung cancer, to summarize current information on molecular properties and cellular origin of individual lung tumor types, to relate pathology to biological behavior, and to provide review guidelines for reporting and pathological staging of lung cancer.

Nearly all lung cancers exhibit the morphological and molecular features of epithelial cells (described later) and are accordingly classified as carcinomas. The cells of origin of virtually all lung cancers reside in the epithelial lining of the airways. As more is learned about the origin of lung carcinoma, it is increasingly clear that the biology of lesions arising in the central airways is distinct from that of peripheral airway lesions. In addition, there are important distinctions between tumors from the two sites in histopathological appearances, molecular profiles, and diagnostic approaches. While the dichotomy between central and peripheral is not a sharp one, it is nevertheless useful to consider tumors of the central airways separately from peripheral tumors.

TUMORS PREDOMINANTLY OF THE CENTRAL BRONCHI

In this chapter, we use the term *central airway lesions* to refer to tumors and premalignant conditions predominantly arising proximal to the terminal bronchiolar and alveolar epithelium. Surprisingly, little information is available on the cells from which central airway carcinomas arise. It might be expected that since the high risk posed by tobacco exposure has been known for many years, the earliest changes in the airway lining cells would by now be well known and the subject of interventional trials. That this is not the case is because of the macroscopic invisibility of early carcinoma and its precursor lesions, to the inaccessibility of the lower airway epithelium to direct inspection and serial sampling and to the great extent of the lower airway epithelial surfaces. It has nevertheless been known for many years that, in the central airways, a distinct series of changes of variable severity may be seen in the airways of smokers. Typically these lesions, described in detail later in the chapter, have been regarded as precursors of squamous carcinoma but there is evidence that they may also represent precursors of other histological types of central airway carcinoma, including undifferentiated large and small cell lung carcinomas (SCLC).

Central Airway Precursor Lesions Lung carcinoma, like tumors in other organs, is thought to arise from a stepwise series of molecular and cellular alterations in precursor cells. The first studies to demonstrate significant histological changes in the lower airways of the human population were the autopsy analyses of Auerbach and colleagues[2] performed over 50 years ago. These studies consisted of serial cross sectioning of tracheobronchial tissue removed at autopsy from 1522 adult smokers and control nonsmoking patients without invasive carcinoma. Nearly 42,000 bronchial cross sections were evaluated and epithelial lesions consisting of *atypical cells* were found in 93% of sections from current smokers but in only 1.2% of sections from individuals who were never-smokers. Cellular abnormalities in smokers' lungs were often multifocal and were independent of age, sex, place of residence, and the presence of pneumonia. A significant number of individuals who were former smokers in this study also had cellular abnormalities, whereas they were rare in individuals who never smoked.[3]

Sputum Cytology and Risk Assessment Although these studies documented the prevalence of cellular lesions in the lower airways at a single time point in smokers who did not have carcinoma, prospective confirmation that these lesions represent precursor lesions for carcinoma has been problematic. A major difficulty is a lack of any creditable intervention strategy that can be offered to individuals who are found to have dysplasia. In other organs, preinvasive lesions can be excised and this has been a successful strategy in cervix and colon where screening has proven successful in reducing the incidence and mortality of invasive carcinoma.[4,5]

The most analogous studies in the lung are the lung cancer screening trials of the 1970s and 1980s. In these studies, the effectiveness of sputum cytology as a screening tool was evaluated in 21,000 subjects at Sloan-Kettering Medical Center and the Mayo Clinic. Spontaneous sputa were evaluated by conventional cytological criteria for the presence of carcinoma. Cytology proved to be an insensitive tool for detection of lung cancer. Only 41% of subjects were sputum positive among those who had carcinoma at an initial (*prevalence*) screen and 17% with carcinoma in subsequent (*incidence*) screenings. In the Mayo Clinic project, no effect on mortality could be demonstrated by chest radiograph or sputum cytology performed quarterly for 6 years. The only positive trend resulting from these interventions was a slightly improved median survival for screen-detected stage I carcinomas in comparison to those detected outside the screened group, a difference that was not statistically significant.[6]

The failure of sputum and radiograph screening to reduce mortality from lung cancer has largely been attributed to *overdiagnosis bias*.[7,8] Overdiagnosis bias refers to the detection of tumors through screening that, even if undetected, would not have affected mortality. It implies either that death may occur from other causes before any mortality effect from screened tumors can occur, or that the detected tumors were indolent and would not have affected survival. The lack of impact of screening on overall mortality has lead to the proposal that small screen-detected tumors are biologically distinct from advanced tumors that are responsible for the high mortality in lung cancer. Small screen-detected tumor are postulated to have lower growth rates and different epidemiological associations than those of advanced lethal tumors and, moreover, may not be precursors of advanced lesions,[9] as is widely believed. The morphological and biological features of screen-detected central airway tumors have been analyzed by Mayo pathologists.[10]

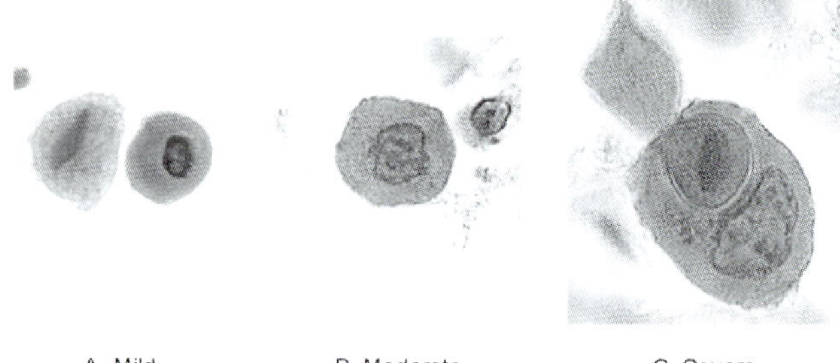

FIGURE 22.1 Dysplastic squamous cells in sputum. **A:** Mild dysplasia on the right consists of small rounded red cell with condensed nucleus and low N/C ratio. **B:** Moderately dysplastic orangophilic cell with large irregular nucleus and visible nucleolus. **C:** Carcinoma with large nucleus, high N/C ratio and visible nucleolus. Large cell appears to be ingesting smaller one. (See color plate.)

Only 86% of the screened tumors were unequivocally invasive with 14% regarded as preinvasive by one or more of the pathologists on the reviewing panel. Inclusion of preinvasive lesions in the outcome analysis may have contributed to overdiagnosis bias in the Mayo Lung Project and provides some biological basis for the outcome of the trial.

One crucial difference between the lung cancer screening trials and screening practices for colon and cervix is that the latter target preinvasive lesions rather than fully developed invasive carcinomas. A similar approach has not been fully explored in lung cancer. The significance of less than fully malignant cells in the sputum (Fig. 22.1) has recently been evaluated.[11,12] These studies have shown that cytologic atypia is a marker for increased lung cancer risk. The association of sputum atypia with lung cancer increases with the severity of the atypia, with short interval between sputum collection and with squamous tumor histology. Higher-grade cytological changes thus seem to arise from late events in the central airways. Whether sputum atypia can be a useful indicator for the presence of premalignant dysplasia in the central airways, whether the presence, grade, and extent of dysplasia predicts invasive carcinoma, and whether meaningful interruption or delay in neoplastic progression is possible when premalignant changes are identified are questions currently being investigated using new methods for visualizing and directly sampling bronchial mucosa for histological assessment.

HISTOLOGY OF SQUAMOUS DYSPLASIA

Because premalignant lesions and early carcinomas are not easily recognized by white-light bronchoscopy, the stimulus for evaluating the lower airways to identify lower airway neoplasia by this method has not been great. Only recently has it been possible to detect premalignant lesions using fluorescence bronchoscopy as described in this volume and elsewhere.[13,14]

This technical advance has engendered a need for a reproducible and less descriptive classification of bronchial premalignancy than that used in the earlier studies of Auerbach. The WHO pathology panel has recognized this need and has provided a suggested classification based largely on the earlier work of Saccomanno and illustrated in Figure 22.2. The classification is based on cellular changes that occur in the epithelium, which consist of a transformation of bilayered mucociliary epithelium to squamous epithelium that is associated with varying degrees of alteration in nuclear irregularity and mitotic activity. The classification includes seven categories including histologically normal epithelium, basal cell hyperplasia and squamous metaplasia, mild, moderate, and severe dysplasia, and carcinoma in situ (CIS). Independent studies have indicated that this classification is reproducible[15] and may be used in clinical trials targeting premalignant changes in the airways.

In addition to changes in the bronchial epithelium, changes in the stromal support tissues have also been described. Potentially, the most significant of these changes may be microscopic evidence neoangiogenesis that has been referred to as angiogenic squamous dysplasia (ASD).[16] ASD is characterized by the sprouting of capillaries into dysplastic squamous mucosa (Fig. 22.3). These lesions are frequently multifocal, may persist for several years at the same bronchial sites and are preferentially associated with squamous carcinoma.[17]

Although areas of squamous dysplasia are now more readily identified in the central airways, the risk posed by dysplastic lesions discovered at bronchoscopy has not been quantified. What is known is that CIS is associated with progression to invasive carcinoma in many cases[18] but not all and that CIS with aneuploidy in more likely to be associated in invasive carcinoma (discussed later).[19] One form of squamous CIS exhibits a horizontal pattern of spread that may extend a considerable distance along the airway mucosa without invasion or metastasis.[20] The prognosis in those few cases that have been reported has been excellent. The prognostic significance of lesser degrees of bronchoscopically detected dysplasia is not yet well defined but the association with invasive carcinoma is much weaker than with CIS.[19] It is likely that lesser degrees of dysplasia persist for many years before undergoing sufficient genetic alteration to progress to invasive tumor.

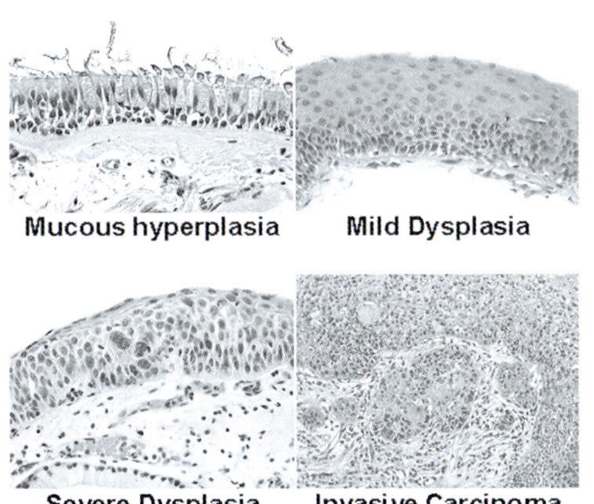

FIGURE 22.2 Chronological sequences of cellular and molecular changes that may occur during central airway carcinogenesis. Although this sequence is rarely observed in a single individual, these changes are well described in the high-risk population and the sequence provides a useful way to conceptualize multistep carcinogenesis in the lung. At the cellular level, the earliest smoking-related changes may consist of mucous gland hyperplasia (shown), basal cell hyperplasia, or squamous metaplasia, which are not recognizably premalignant changes. The earliest cellular abnormalities that suggest premalignancy are squamous dysplastic changes that may range from mild-to-severe carcinoma in situ. The appearance of stromal invasion marks progression to fully established malignancy. (See color plate.)

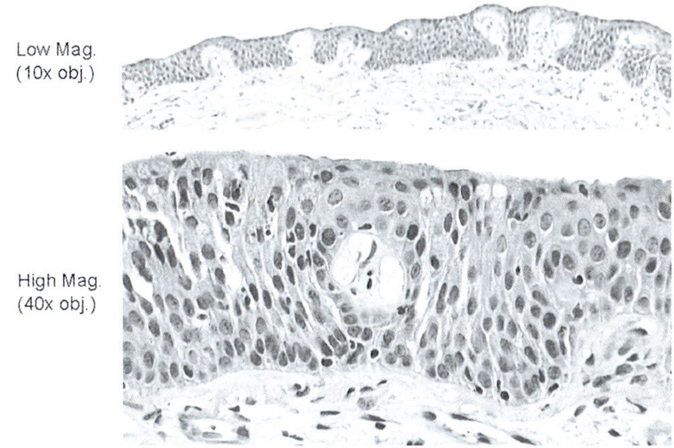

FIGURE 22.3 Premalignant changes in the bronchial epithelium. Mucociliary cells are converted to squamous cells and may elicit and angiogenic stromal response shown at low maginfication (**top**) and high magnification (**bottom**). Nuclear irregularity with clearly visible nucleoli is present in the cells surrounding the vascular loop in the lower frame. (See color plate.)

Finally, nonsquamous atypias of the respiratory mucosa have recently been reported.[21] In our experience, nonsquamous dysplasias of the central airways are less common and more difficult to recognize than squamous lesions. It will be important, however, to determine whether these lesions are significant predictors of nonsquamous carcinoma.

Immunohistochemical Changes in Bronchial Dysplasia

Premalignant squamous lesions in the lower airways are associated with a constellation of changes in protein expression that can be demonstrated by immunohistochemical methods, including overexpression of cytokeratin 5/6 (CK5/6),[22] epidermal growth factor receptor (EGFR),[23,24] human epidermal growth factor receptor 2 (HER-2)/*neu*,[24–26] and the cell cycle–associated protein Ki-67,[24,27,28] fatty acid synthase,[29] and MCM2.[24,30] Loss of FHIT,[31] p16,[32] E-cadherin,[33] and catenin[33] has also been demonstrated. Nuclear p53 accumulation has been described in dysplasia[32,34] but is usually focal and immunostained cells rarely have the robust signal present in tumors with homozygous mutation. Most of these immunohistochemical changes are first visible when normal mucociliary epithelium changes to squamous epithelium and do not visibly progress with the level of dysplasia. Exceptions to this rule are the biomarkers that are associated with cell proliferation. Generally, there is an increase in the level of expression of cell proliferation markers with increasing histological grade. Cyclin D1,[32,35,36] cyclin E,[37] PCNA,[38] Ki-67,[24,27,28] and MCM2[24,30] all increase with increasing grade of dysplasia, reflecting the increased proliferative capacity of more severely dysplastic cells. With the possible exception of proliferative immunohistochemical biomarkers, no single change in immunohistochemically demonstrable protein expression has to date added significantly to the information that can be gleaned from conventional histological examination.

Genetics of Preneoplasia Underlying the morphological and immunohistochemical changes that occur in the airways is a multistep sequence of molecular and chromosomal events illustrated in Figures 22.4 and 22.5. The initial event in lung carcinogenesis is the formation of DNA adducts, the physical complexes between DNA, and the reactive metabolites in tobacco smoke and industrial pollutants.[39–41] Among the most potent of the carcinogens are polycyclic aromatic hydrocarbons (PAH), aromatic amines, and metals. These compounds are largely metabolized to execrable products by cytochrome p450 and glutathione S transferase (GST). However, some small fraction of intermediates is highly reactive with DNA and forms bulky adducts with DNA in which the reactive metabolite is covalently bonded to specific DNA bases.[40]

DNA adducts activate complex DNA repair mechanisms, which are not completely effective in removing adducts from damaged DNA. Unrepaired DNA bases may be bypassed by DNA polymerase, creating mutations that are transmitted to daughter cells. Mutations formed in this way tend to favor GC→TA transversions. Many of the genetic changes that ultimately appear in lung carcinomas are thus thought to originate from misrepaired DNA adducts.

Among these changes are allelic losses, easily demonstrated by a simple molecular test based on the measurement of the length of polymorphic tandem repeat sequences that exist throughout the genome. In these tests, chromosomal loci that

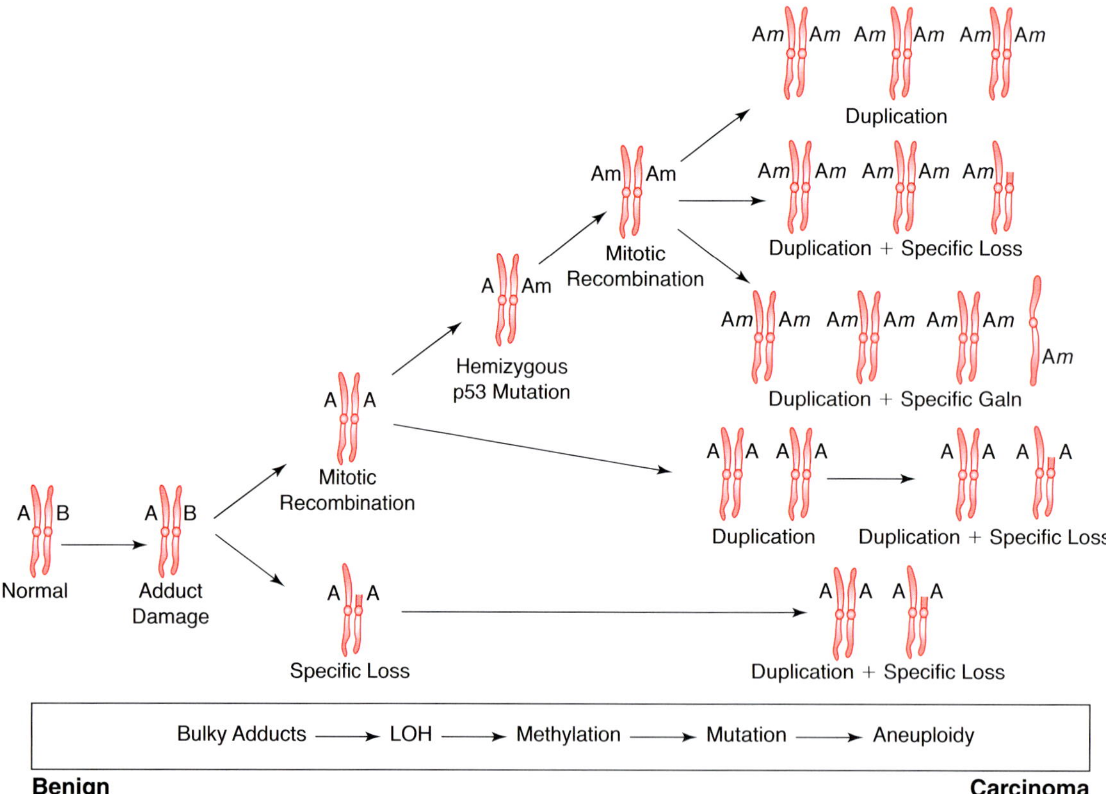

FIGURE 22.4 Lung carcinogenesis is thought to proceed through the accumulation of genetic and chromosomal abnormalities depicted in this diagram in approximate chronologic sequence. One of the earliest events is bulky DNA adduct formation as a result of exposure to carcinogens in tobacco smoke and which is not visible at the chromosomal level. Adducts may interfere with DNA repair and mitosis resulting in mitotic recombination or partial chromosomal loss. Recombination could explain the nearly ubiquitous occurrence of LOH that occurs early in lung carcinogenesis. Gene methylation, mutation, further mitotic recombination, and a high level of chromosomal rearrangement (chromosomal instability) may then occur resulting the high level of aneuploidy that is present in many lung carcinomas. *LOH*, loss of heterozygosity. (Reproduced from Franklin WA, Hirsch FR. Molecular and cell biology of lung carcinoma. In: Sculier JP, Fry WA, eds. *Malignant Tumors of the Lung*. New York: Springer-Verlag, 2003:3–17.)

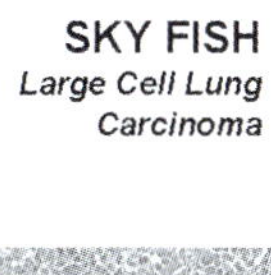

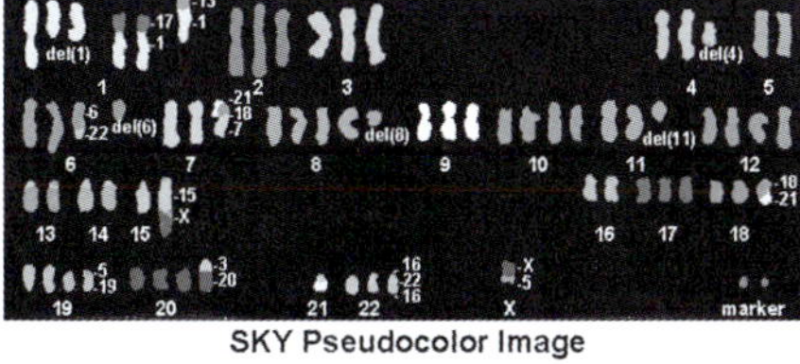

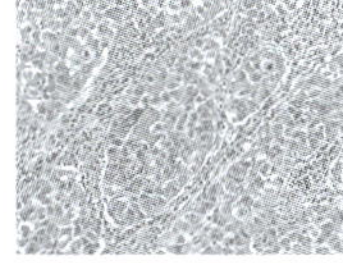

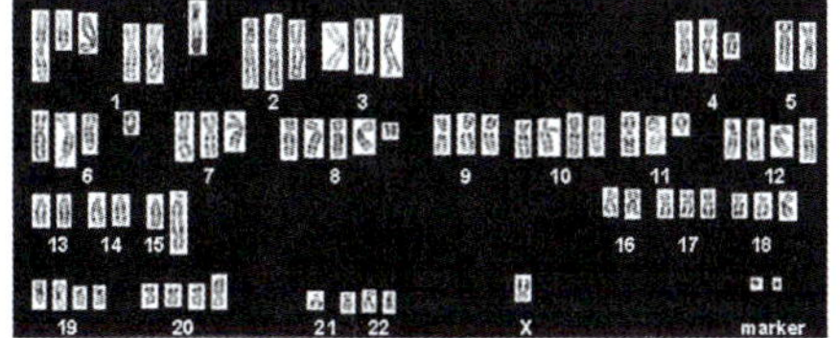

FIGURE 22.5 Chromosomal heterogeneity and instability. The high degree of chromosomal instability in lung carcinoma is reflected in numerous structural abnormalities that are visible through chromosomal imaging methods. Shown here is a spectral karyotype of a large cell undifferentiated carcinoma (H&E section). The SKY pseudocolor image of the karyotype provides a color code for each chromosome. In this figure, extra chromosomes 1, 2, 3, 4, 6, 7, 8, 9, 10, 11, 12, 18, 19, 20, and 22 are visible. A reciprocal translocation, several nonreciprocal translocations, deletions, and marker chromosomes are also present. *FISH*, fluorescence in situ hybridization; *H&E*, hematoxylin and eosin; *SKY*, spectral karyotyping. (See color plate.)

normally harbor two different polymorphic alleles are assessed for loss of one (loss of heterozygosity [LOH]) or both of these alleles. Loss of both alleles (homozygous deletion) results in silencing of the gene while loss of a single allele (heterozygous loss) causes loss of gene expression if the retained allele is mutated or inactivated by methylation. Loss of genes that are important in controlling cell growth, apoptosis, or error DNA replication can impart a malignant phenotype to lung cells and much effort has been expended in trying to identify candidate tumor suppressor genes in dysplastic epithelium and invasive tumors.[42]

Allelic losses at loci throughout the genome have been demonstrated in premalignant bronchial mucosa and detailed consideration of specific allelic losses is reviewed elsewhere.[43,44] Several conclusions may be drawn from LOH studies performed so far. First, many regions of allelic loss have been demonstrated in smoking damaged airways but few studies have demonstrated any effect of LOH on corresponding gene expression. Second, many loci demonstrate loss from the earliest exposure to tobacco smoke but allelic loss does not occur in individuals who have never smoked.[45] Finally, no specific loss appears to be crucial for progress to malignancy but rather it is the accumulation of multiple losses that is most tied to malignant progression.[46]

The molecular mechanism responsible for allelic loss is not fully known. It has been suggested that bulky adducts resulting from DNA oxidation could affect repair of double-stranded DNA breaks and result in the recombination of homologous recombination of DNA strands during the repair process. Fluorescence in situ hybridization (FISH) studies have indicated an increase rather than a decrease in gene copy number occurs at sites of allelic loss,[47] suggesting that tumor cells harbor multiple copies of the same allele and that gene dosage may in fact be increased. Allelic loss may result in functional loss of protein only when the retained allele is mutated or silenced by methylation.

A molecular property that distinguishes lung cancers and, to a lesser extent, premalignant lesions from normal bronchial cells is chromosomal instability, which is reflected as aneuploidy in tumor and premalignant cells. Aneuploidy is first detected in squamous dysplasia[48] and in one recent study, aneuploidy was found in cultured bronchial epithelial of 26% of high-risk smokers.[49] In invasive lung carcinomas, aneuploidy is nearly universal and involves multiple chromosomes.[50] Aneuploidy has been found in lung cancer by classical cytogenetics methods[51] but is more efficiently demonstrated by FISH. Numerical abnormalities have been demonstrated in every chromosome by FISH.[52–54]

New technologies such as spectral karyotyping (SKY) (Fig. 22.5) and comparative genomic hybridization indicate that not only are numerical chromosomal imbalances frequent but also structural chromosomal abnormalities such as translocations and amplifications are ubiquitous as well.[55] This high degree of chromosomal instability may explain the extreme molecular and cellular heterogeneity of lung cancers as well as their adaptability and resilience in the face of chemotherapeutic treatment.

Patients with squamous as well as large and SCLC frequently harbor dysplastic squamous lesions in the central airways although the precise frequency in which this occurs is not known. There is also increasing evidence of genomic and phenotypic plasticity in invasive carcinomas, and tumors of mixed histological type are a frequent finding in the lung suggesting that tumor cells of many histological types could arise from a common progenitor. Molecular evidence indicates that lung tumors recapitulate ontological development,[56,57] suggesting that central airway lesions of various histological types could represent arrested development at various stages in the same progenitor cells rather than origin from separate progenitor cell lineages.

Invasive Squamous Carcinoma of the Bronchus

Squamous carcinomas are in the most common of the central airway tumors and are highly associated with smoking.[58] Invasive squamous tumors are characterized by extension of malignant squamous cells beyond the basement membrane of the airway lining. Approximately 29% of lung cancers are of this histological type (Table 22.1).[59] The diagnosis of

TABLE 22.1 Frequencies of Histological Types

Histological Type (Subtype)	% Total
Squamous carcinoma	29%
SCLC	20%
LCLC	9%
LNEC	2%
Adenocarcinoma	32%
-(Bronchioloalveolar)	3%
Others	12%

squamous carcinoma and indeed of all non–small cell tumors has taken new importance with the recognition that new targeted agents may differentially affect non–small cell subtypes and it is therefore more important to recognize and report squamous lesions than in the past.

HISTOLOGY OF SQUAMOUS CARCINOMA

The histological features of squamous carcinoma are summarized and compared with other forms of lung cancer in Table 22.2. Invasion is recognized as angulated nests or individual tumor cells that have broken away from the surface epithelium and become embedded in the stromal tissues as shown in Figure 22.6. The invasive cells may form keratin pearls (KP) and intercellular bridges[60] and may develop irregular areas of central necrosis described as geographic necrosis. Nuclear features include irregular nuclei and coarse chromatin. The cytoplasm may show clearing, most clearly seen in clear cell variant of squamous cell carcinoma, which can resemble vacuolization as might be seen in adenocarcinomas. Squamous tumors also elicit a variable stromal response consisting of loose fibroblastic tissue with an inflammatory component that may include plasma cells, macrophages, and lymphocytes. In more poorly differentiated carcinomas, there is less keratinization and intercellular bridges may be difficult to identify. Here, the overall epithelioid architecture of the tumor cells is important for diagnosis. In these cases, there may be maturation of cells from a basilar zone to a central area where there is loss of the typical verticality of the epithelium.

Several variants of squamous cell carcinoma are described, which may mimic other tumors either clinically or histologically. A papillary variant of squamous cell carcinoma, for example, may present as an exophytic endobronchial mass and histologically show a prominent in situ pattern. While an

TABLE 22.2 Histological and Cytological Differences among Major Classes of Lung Cancer

Type (Subtype)	Nucleus	Cytoplasm	Defining Feature(s)
Squamous	Chromatin coarse, clumped Nucleoli often large and misshapen Mitoses frequent	Abundant Eosinophilic (red)	KP Intercellular bridges Epidermoid sheets Fibrotic stromal response
SCLC	Fine granularity (salt and pepper) Nucleoli inconspicuous Mitoses very frequent	Scant Basophilic	Small cell size (<21 mm) Nuclear configuration Nulear molding Cell clusters
LCLC	Chromatin coarse, clumped Nucleoli prominent Mitoses frequent	Abundant Basophilic/amphophilic	Lack of differentiated features Large cell size (>21 mm) Soid sheets and cell clusters
Carcinoid	Intermediate clumping Nucleoli inconspicous Mitotic rate <1/10 hpf	Intermediate abundance Granular Basophilic/amphophilic	Numerous neurosecretory granules Ribbonlike cords or solid sheets Spindle cell pattern Nuclear consistency Low mitotic rate
Atypical carcinoid	Intermediate clumping Nucleoli focally prominent Mitotic rate 1–10/10 hpf	Intermediate abundance Granular Basophilic/amphophilic	Neurosecretory granules Ribbonlike cords or solid sheets Intermediate mitotic rate Necrosis
LCNEC	Intermediated to fine granularity Nucleoli inconspicuous Mitotic rate >1/10 hpf	Abundant Basophilic/amphophilic	Lack of differentiated features Large size (>21 mm)
Adenocarcinoma	Intermediate clumping Prominent nucleoli Mitoses frequent	Abundant Basophilic/amphophilic	Mucin vacuoles (>10% of cells) Invasive glandlike nests and sheets Fibrotic stromal response
Bronchioloalveolar	Intermediate clumping Prominent nucleoli Mitoses usually infrequent	Abundant Basophilic/amphophilic	Lepidic along alveolar septae

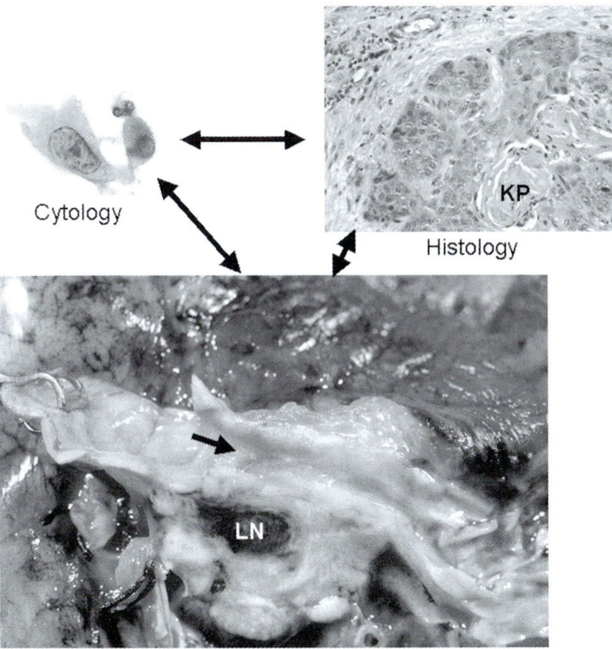

FIGURE 22.6 Various morphological appearances of squamous carcinoma. Cytological examination reveals bright orange, irregularly cells with conspicuous nucleolus. Histology of squamous cancers visible in both biopsy and resection specimens are characterized by irregular nests of cells, often with central KP. Early stage resected tumors are frequently ulcerated as indicated by the area of mucosal roughening and erythema (*arrow*). The ulcer overlies white invasive tumor tissue that surrounds a black anthrocotic LN. *KL*, keratin pearl; *LN*, lymph node. (See color plate.)

invasive component is usually present, a superficial biopsy may not be diagnostic of invasive tumor.

A small cell variant of squamous cell carcinoma may mimic neuroendocrine tumors including small cell carcinoma. Differences in nuclear pattern and mitotic activity are helpful in distinguishing these two tumors, as are neuroendocrine immunohistochemical stains. If sampled sufficiently, diagnostic squamous features (i.e., keratin, intercellular bridges) can be identified focally in basaloid squamous carcinomas.

Another consideration in the differential diagnosis is the distinction of squamous cell carcinoma from SCLC (discussed later). The nuclear architecture of squamous carcinoma uniquely contains large and atypical nucleoli that are not present in small cell carcinoma. There is also clumping of nuclear chromatin that permits distinction from the chromatin of SCLC.

Typically, squamous carcinomas spread directly through and replace tissue at the interface between normal lung and carcinoma. Squamous carcinomas can frequently be found spreading through the alveolar septae rather than along the surfaces of the alveolar walls as is typically observed in bronchioloalveolar carcinomas described later. However, a minority of tumors may also spread through the alveoli.

BRONCHIAL BIOPSIES AND THEIR PITFALLS

Endobronchial biopsy is the most commonly used procedure for obtaining a diagnosis in non–small cell carcinomas including squamous carcinoma and is described in detail elsewhere in this volume. In this procedure, a small fragment of bronchial mucosa is fixed in formalin and embedded in a block of paraffin wax for sectioning. Diagnostic tumor tissue my not be evenly distributed in the tissue and multiple sections of the block may be required to obtain a definitive histological result. Occasionally, squamous carcinomas may have an inaccessible endobronchial component and the easiest access to diagnostic material is through transbronchial biopsy. Here the same considerations of sampling artifact and representation of the tumor through all sections of the block are relevant.

Cytology Cytological specimens may be obtained through transbronchial or transthoracic fine-needle aspiration or through expectoration of sputum, either spontaneous or induced. Cytological specimens are fixed in alcohol-based fixatives and typically stained by the Papanicolaou method, which incorporates orange G dye that produces an intense waxy red-orange staining of squamous cell cytoplasm (Fig. 22.6).[61] Elongated single cells (*tadpole cells* or *fiber cells*) are frequent. Nuclei are large, irregular shaped, and irregularly condensed. Less differentiated tumors contain sheets of cells with high nuclear/cytoplasmic (N/C) ratios with fewer differentiated squamous cells. Although sheets of cells with well-defined cell borders can be suggestive of squamous cell carcinoma, intercellular bridges cannot be easily visualized in cytological specimens and therefore are not a reliable criterion. The appearance of the aspirate can vary with the technique used to sample the tumor. In squamous cell carcinoma, for example, a sputum specimen will more likely sample better differentiated superficial tumor cells, whereas techniques such as bronchial brushing or fine-needle aspiration will sample more cells from within a tumor mass that may show more of the tumor sheets and less differentiated cells.[61]

The overall sensitivity and specificity of cytological specimens in a recent literature review of 16 studies by the Duke University Center for Clinical Health Policy Research were 0.66 and 0.99, respectively.[62] The sensitivity of sputum specimens is highest for squamous cell carcinoma and small cell carcinoma (the centrally located tumors),[62,63] and is most specific for squamous cell carcinoma.[61] The diagnostic yield is better with larger tumors, which are centrally located, and in patients who present with bloody sputum.[63]

Differential Diagnosis A major differential diagnostic consideration in an endobronchial biopsy is the distinction between invasive squamous carcinoma and noninvasive squamous lesions in the respiratory mucosa. In some cases, in situ squamous carcinoma may exhibit considerable pleomorphism and may be difficult to distinguish from invasive carcinoma purely on the basis of the cytological appearances. An additional consideration is the extension of in situ tumor into the bronchial glands, which many mimic invasive carcinoma. Finally, the bronchial lining may respond to many different types of injury such as pneumonia, infarcts, and radiation or chemotherapy by converting from mucociliary epithelium to squamous epithelium that can mimic squamous cell carcinoma. It is therefore important that a history of these conditions accompany requests for pathological examination. In order to be completely confident of a diagnosis of invasive carcinoma, unequivocal invasion with nests of cells or single cell infiltrates eliciting a stromal response in the underlying mucosa is required.

The diagnosis of squamous carcinoma is usually made by conventional light microscopic examination of small biopsy or cytology specimens. Diagnosis can be difficult or misleading when small numbers of tumor cells are available for study and in approximately 30% of these small specimens, distinction of cell type cannot be made or the specimen is misdiagnosed. This can be a critical issue since agents such as the vascular endothelial growth factor (VEGF) blocker, bevacizimab,[64] may cause cavitation in squamous tumors that can be life threatening while pemetrexed may be less effective against squamous tumors than against adenocarcinoma.[65]

DIAGNOSTIC IMMUNOHISTOCHEMISTRY OF INVASIVE SQUAMOUS CARCINOMA

Immunohistochemical markers may be used for diagnosis, prognosis, or prediction of response to treatment with targeted agents. In this section, the focus is mainly on the diagnosis whereas in the next, molecular lesions that are important in squamous carcinogenesis are discussed. Immunohistochemical predictors of response to targeted therapy are discussed elsewhere in this volume.

Cytokeratin and Its Isotypes: Pan-CK, PCK5/6, CK7, and CK20 Immunohistochemical markers have been used in lung cancer largely to distinguish poorly differentiated metastatic tumors that may mimic the histological appearance of squamous carcinoma. Such tumors include large cell lymphoma, melanoma, germ cell malignancies, and sarcoma. The most helpful markers in this context are the cytokeratins (CKs). CK intermediate filaments are expressed in several different isotypic forms. Pan-CK antibodies recognize epitopes that are common to most of the CK isotypes. A pan-CK stain such as AE1/AE3 cocktail usually suffices to distinguish poorly differentiated squamous carcinomas from other poorly differentiated tumors. Occasionally, however, poorly differentiated tumors are pan-CK negative and these cases specific anti-CK isotypes such as CK5/6 may be positive and clarify the diagnosis.

A more complicated problem is the use of isotype-specific antikeratin antibodies to distinguish squamous carcinoma from other non–small cell lung carcinoma (NSCLC) types. With the emerging importance of squamous histology in predicting response to targeted agents, the question of whether immunohistochemical markers could be help to distinguish squamous from other non–small cell histologies has become more important. Several of the immunohistochemical markers useful for making this distinction are CKs (Table 22.3). The CKs form a large family of related proteins that associate to form mature filaments in

TABLE 22.3 Frequencies of Positive Diagnostic Immunohistochemistry Results by Histology

	Ki-67*	EGFR	CK5/6	CK-7	CK20	TTF-1	p63	CD56 (N-CAM)	CD57 (Leu7)	Neuron-Specific Enolase	Chromogranin A	CD-117 (c-KIT)	CEA	Ber-Ep4	MOC-31	CD-15	TAG72	Calretinin	Podoplanin (D2-40)	WT1
Sq Ca	++	+++	+++	+	−	+	+++	−	++	++	−	−	+++	+++	+++	+++	+++	+	+	−
BAC	+	+++	−	+++	−	++	++	+	++	++	−	−	+++	+++	+++	++	+++	+	−	−
AdCa	++	++	−	+++	−	++	++	+	++	++	−	−	+++	+++	+++	++	+++	+	−	−
LCLC	++	+++	−	+++	−	+++	++	+	++	++	−	−	+++	+++	+++	++	+++	+	−	−
LCNEC	++	+	−	+++	−	+++	++	+++	+++	+++	+	++	+++	+++	+++	++	+++	+	−	−
Carcinoid	+	−	−	+++	−	+++	+	+++	+++	+++	+++	−	+++	+++	+++	++	+++	+	−	−
SCLC	+++	−	−	+++	−	+++	++	+++	++	+++	++	+++	+++	+++	+++	++	+++	+	−	−
Meso	++	−	+	+++	−	−	+	−	−	−	−	−	−	−	−	−	−	+++	+++	+++
Met	++	++	++	++	++	−	++	+	++	+	+	−	+++	+++	+++	+++	+++	+	+	−

*Levels of expression as a function of the number of positive tumor cells for a specific marker.

−, <1%.

+, 1%–25%.

++, 25%–70%.

+++, >70.

epithelial cells and tumors.[66–68] Central airway squamous tumors express different CKs than tumors originating from peripheral airways. Squamous carcinomas express CK5/6 at a frequency of >80%,[69–71] but adenocarcinomas express this protein at a lesser frequency.[70–73] However, there is so much overlap in the expression of CK5/6 among the tumor types, staining for CK5/6 by itself is not a reliable marker for squamous carcinoma.[74]

A second CK protein that has been suggested as a useful diagnostic aid is CK7. In squamous carcinoma, CK7 is notable by its absence with three quarters of squamous carcinomas negative for this marker.[70,75–77] Here again, however, the number of positive cases found among squamous carcinoma is sufficient to limit the utility of the protein as a diagnostic discriminant of squamous carcinoma.

P63 P63 is a transcription factor and homologue of p53 that is important in epithelial cell differentiation. It is expressed by myoepithelial and reserve support cells and has been proposed as a possible marker of squamous phenotype. The marker is frequently expressed at high level in the nuclei of squamous carcinoma cells and overexpression is associated with *p63* gene amplification.[78] Several studies have shown that the marker has high sensitivity for squamous carcinoma with >95% of tumors immunoreactive with anti-p63 antibody.[69,79–81] However, specificity is variable, with several studies reporting that 0% to 30% of adenocarcinomas express *p63*.[79–82]

Antibodies against p63 or CK5/6 or both have been paired with anti–thyroid transcription factor-1 (TTF-1) (discussed later) in a single immunohistochemical panel to distinguish squamous carcinoma from adenocarcinoma. Sensitivities and specificities for the double antibody test are high (80% to 100%) but the numbers of cases reported is small.[82,83] Double antibody testing may ultimately prove useful for poorly differentiated tumors where little tissue is available but this test will require further validation in specific clinical contexts.

MOLECULAR PATHOLOGY OF SQUAMOUS CARCINOMA INCLUDING HIGH-THROUGHPUT GENE EXPRESSION ARRAYS

A variety of molecular abnormalities are present in squamous carcinoma that are not necessarily diagnostically useful but are part of the constellation of changes that accompany malignant transformation. Genetic changes in squamous tumors are numerous and can be grouped according to the molecular pathway they affect. Specific genetic lesions tend to group with specific histologies. To date, most mutations in squamous carcinoma are found to be associated with cell cycle genes and less frequently with tyrosine kinase pathway genes.[84,85] A list of the most common genetic abnormalities and their frequencies in specific tumor types is presented in Table 22.4 and discussed in the context of specific tumor types.

Cell Cycle Genes Genes of the cell cycle were the first to be evaluated in lung cancer and are the most commonly mutated genes in squamous carcinoma.

TP53 TP53 is a multifunctional transcription factor that plays a complex role in a variety of processes including cell cycle regulation, DNA repair, and apoptosis. Of particular interest is its role as a cell cycle checkpoint in which TP53 interacts with DNA repair and recombination enzymes.[86] This allows the cell to correct DNA damage during replication and the frequency of mutation and chromosomal rearrangement transmitted to daughter cells is thereby reduced. TP53 mutation interferes with DNA repair and may thus result in chromosomal instability, a major factor in malignant progression and resistance to chemotherapy. TP53 is the most commonly mutated gene in all lung carcinomas including squamous carcinoma.[87] TP53 mutation does not appear to be associated with outcome in squamous carcinoma although it is associated with reduced survival in adenocarcinoma.[88]

CDKN2A (p16) P16 protein inhibits cyclin-dependent kinase 4 (CDK4) and inactivation of this inhibitor removes a brake on cell proliferation, enhancing tumor growth. *P16* is one of the most frequently affected of the tumor suppressor genes and may be deleted[89,90] or methylated[91] in lung cancer. The gene is inactivated in approximately 60% squamous carcinoma.[92] Methylation of *p16* is an independent prognostic variable in NSCLC regardless of histological subtype.[93] By contrast, in SCLC *p16* is usually intact but the *RB1* gene, also affecting progression through the cell cycle, is almost universally inactivated (see succeeding discussion of SCLC). Immunohistochemical tests assessing cell cycle–related proteins have been of more limited prognostic value. In one recent

TABLE 22.4 Frequent Genetic Changes in Lung Cancer: Approximate Prevalence of Mutations by Histology*

Functional Pathway	Gene	Chromosome	Genetic Lesion	SCLC	Sq Ca	Adeno
Cell cycle /apoptosis	TP53	17p13.1	Point mutation	70%	60%	40%
	p16Ink4a	9p21	Deletion/methylation	<10%	60%	30%
	rb1	13q14.2	Mutation/inactivation	90%	<10%	<10%
TK signaling	K-*ras*	12p12.1	Point mutation	<1%	<5%	30%
	ErbB1 (EGFR)	7p12	Point mutation/in frame deletion	<5%	<1%	20%

*Adeno, adenocarcinoma; SCLC, small cell lung cancer; sq ca, squamous cell lung cancer; TK, tyrosine kinase.

study, no single cell cycle protein (including p16) was of prognostic importance[94,95] and only with combinations of markers could statistical significance be achieved.[95] Prediction of outcome in individual tumors based on immunohistochemical testing of cycle proteins is unlikely to be accurate or reliable and it appears that only direct assessment of *p16* gene methylation provides prognostic information.

Expression Microarrays other High-Throughput Technologies Until recently, biomarkers have been measured singly but oligonucleotide expression microarrays have permitted simultaneous evaluation of virtually all expressed genes in a single analysis. This technology has not yet found its way to broad clinical application but several important observations regarding lung tumors in general and squamous carcinoma in particular have been made utilizing this technology. First, microarray profiles strongly correlate with histology and clinical samples of squamous carcinoma can be distinguished from adenocarcinoma with a high degree of statistical certainty.[56,96,97] Second, microarray data is reproducible[98] and much of the variation in the reported literature can be attributed to differences in data interpretation that may be a complex exercise. Third, individual biomarkers are discoverable through application of microarrays and some of these markers may have clinical application. MAGE genes stand out in microarray experiments as some of the most highly overexpressed genes in central airway tumors including squamous carcinomas[99] providing a target for ongoing immunotherapy trials.[100,101] Fourth, it is possible to identify prognostically important subsets of genes[102] that may predict response chemotherapeutic intervention[103–105] or response to targeted agents.[106] Whether gene expression profiles can be used to prospectively select appropriate therapy for individual patients is an important and to date unanswered question.

Additional high-throughput technologies are currently under investigation including proteomics[107] and rapid large-scale gene sequencing that will permit identification of all mutations within individual tumors (see succeeding discussion of adenocarcinoma). These technologies potentially could reach a level accuracy that will compel their use in the clinical management of squamous and other non–small cell carcinomas. However, they require accessing larger amounts of tumor for clinical study and changes in the way tissue is processed. These requirements could transform surgical tissue acquisition and pathology practices but will need careful validation and cost/benefit analysis before transfer from bench to bedside.

LARGE CELL LUNG CARCINOMA

Large cell lung carcinoma (LCLC) is an undifferentiated malignancy without features of small cell carcinoma, squamous cell carcinoma, or adenocarcinoma.[60] Although the cell of origin of LCLC is not well defined, ultrastructural studies have revealed features of glandular or squamous differentiation that cannot be appreciated by light microscopy. LCLC thus represents an extremely poorly differentiated NSCLC without histological features that permit ready assignment to one of the more usual and better-differentiated forms of lung carcinoma. With loss of differentiating features comes extremely aggressive biological behavior. These tumors comprise approximately 9% of primary lung malignancies.[108]

Histology of Large Cell Lung Carcinoma LCLCs are composed of poorly differentiated large cells (>21 microns) with prominent nucleoli and abundant, clearly visible cytoplasm (Fig. 22.7). Cells and nuclei are usually separate and discrete and less prone to deformation than the cells of small cell carcinoma. Tumor cells are generally arranged in nests or sheets. Nuclei are large and N/C ratios may be high. Mitoses are numerous and areas of necrosis are common.

The category of LCLC is heterogeneous and several variants of this tumor type have been described based on histology and immunohistochemical properties. These include clear cell carcinoma, large cell carcinoma with rhabdoid phenotype (rhabdoid carcinoma), and lymphoepithelioma-like carcinoma as well as two variants discussed elsewhere in this chapter, basaloid carcinoma and large cell neuroendocrine carcinoma (LCNEC). Clear cell carcinoma and rhabdoid carcinoma are terms that convey the essential cytological appearances of these neoplasms. The rhabdoid type has a particularly poor prognosis.[109–112]

The lymphoepithelioma-like variant resembles the lymphoepithelial carcinoma seen in the nasopharynx (undifferentiated epithelial cells with an intermixed prominent lymphoid infiltrate); this rare variant that affects young, Asian, nonsmokers[113,114] is associated with Epstein-Barr virus (EBV). These tumors are Bcl-2 positive by immunohistochemistry (IHC) and express EBER-1 by in situ hybridization,[114] suggesting viral etiology. Surgery is the treatment for early stage tumors, while multimodality treatment is used in advanced cases. Although quick to metastasize, this variant shows a favorable response to chemotherapy.[114–118]

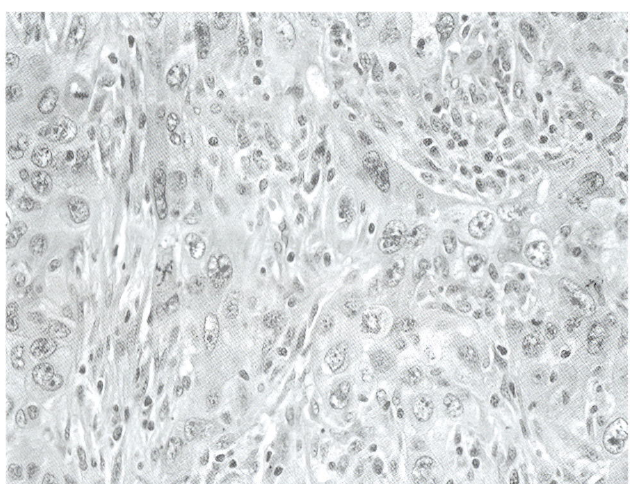

FIGURE 22.7 Large cell undifferentiated lung carcinoma exhibits no differentiating features and is composed of large cells with coarsely clumped nuclei and prominent nucleoli. Mitoses are abundant. (See color plate.)

Cytology

Because the diagnosis of large cell carcinoma is made after the exclusion of squamous, glandular, or small cell components, it is often classified as a *non–small cell carcinoma* on small tissue specimens such as transbronchial biopsies and cytological specimens. Cytological smears show an undifferentiated carcinoma without squamous, glandular, or small cell features. Smears are usually cellular and composed of both single cells and syncytial aggregates. Cells are large with high N/C ratios, large nuclei with prominent or multiple nucleoli in a background of necrosis.

Immunohistochemistry of Large Cell Lung Carcinoma

The immunohistochemical staining properties of LCLC are listed in Table 22.3. In general, they are similar to other forms of NSCLC with the exception of a higher level of expression of proliferation markers, reflecting the rapid growth of these tumors.

UNCOMMON BUT SIGNIFICANT VARIANTS OF NON–SMALL CELL LUNG CARCINOMA

Several histological variants of NSCLC are significant because of their distinct morphology and prognosis. The most prominent among these variants are basaloid carcinoma and pleomorphic carcinoma.

Basaloid Carcinoma

This variant histology may be found admixed with other forms of non–small cell carcinoma or as the sole cell type in a subgroup of lung carcinomas. Basaloid histological features include lobular growth of relatively small cells with dense nuclei, inconspicuous nucleoli, scant cytoplasm, a high mitotic rate, and peripheral palisading.[119] Misinterpretation of these tumors as SCLC has been described in fine-needle aspirations.[120,121] Small cell variant of squamous carcinoma is also distinguished from undifferentiated small cell carcinoma by nuclear features including prominent nucleoli and a coarse clumping of the chromatin. In doubtful cases, immunohistochemical stains for neuroendocrine markers may be applied (see succeeding discussion).

The reported frequency is about 6% of all lung cancers.[119] The reported prognostic significance of basaloid histology has been inconsistent with one study finding reduced actuarial 5-year survival for basaloid tumors in comparison to poorly differentiated squamous tumors[122] but a second similar-sized study finding similar survival for the two tumor types.[123] Since these tumors are rare, additional studies, perhaps through a multicenter registry, will be necessary to better characterize their behavior.

Carcinomas with Pleomorphic, Sarcomatoid, or Sarcomatous Elements

These carcinomas have been recognized under various names for many years including spindle cell carcinoma, giant cell carcinoma, pleomorphic carcinoma, and carcinosarcoma. This category consists of tumors that are composed exclusively of sarcoma or pleomorphic tumor cells or of tumors that contain a component of sarcomatoid or pleomorphic cells along with tumor of a more usual histological type. In the most recent WHO classification,[1] these tumors are grouped in a single diagnostic category. These tumors are uncommon and usually reported as single cases but two larger series have also been published.[124,125] The median survival in these series is 10 months.

Sarcomatoid tumor histology is characterized by the presence of spindle areas that resemble sarcoma.[124,125] The sarcomatous element in this variant type may contain muscle, bone, or cartilage as well as undifferentiated spindle cells.[124,125] There also may be mixtures of epithelial tumor and sarcomatous components, referred to as carcinosarcoma. The giant cell variant of the category consists of highly pleomorphic cells that form multinucleated giant cells, usually accompanied by a heavy inflammatory infiltrate. In most cases, these tumors have biomarker profiles similar to those of other lung tumors, expressing CK7 and TTF-1.[125] However, in approximately 25%, either one or the other or both of these biomarkers is (are) absent and these negative tumors tend to be those with the most sarcomatous histological appearance.

The biological significance of this category of tumor has been emphasized by the recent description of the stromal molecular and cellular properties in tumors that are otherwise considered epithelial. This pattern of differentiation has been referred to as *epithelial mesenchymal transition* (EMT). Properties associated with EMT include change in cell culture characteristics from the sheetlike pattern of epithelial cells to a more single cell infiltrative stromal pattern of growth.[126] This morphological change is accompanied by increased expression of vimentin intermediate filament and the transcription factor ZEB1 and by reduced expression of the adhesion molecule E-cadherin, the transcription factor SNAIL, and EGFR.[127] Such molecular changes are most evident in tumors that exhibit elements of sarcomatoid differentiation but poorly differentiated tumors without sarcomatous elements may also lose expression of E-cadherin. Loss of E-cadherin imparts a poor prognosis independent of stage[128] and resistance to EGFR blockade.[77,106,127,129–131] It seems likely that the loss of E-cadherin represents part of a continuum of dedifferentiation that at its most extreme is reflected in the pleomorphic tumor category. This category will require unique therapeutic consideration, especially as targeted drugs become increasingly available for tumors with specific molecular phenotypes.

SMALL CELL LUNG CARCINOMA

The separate and unique histological features of SCLC were first recognized in 1926 by Bernard who introduced the tumor as *oat cell sarcoma*.[132] This subcategory took on greater importance when it was shown that the response to chemotherapy in these tumors differed substantially from the response of other tumor types with the SCLC being particularly sensitive to mitotic inhibitors.[133] It is for this reason that the main dichotomy of clinical relevance in lung cancer pathological diagnosis remains the distinction between SCLC and all other forms of lung carcinoma (NSCLC).

Histology of Small Cell Lung Carcinoma SCLC is an invasive carcinoma composed of small (<21 microns or <3 lymphocyte diameters) cells with scanty cytoplasm (Fig. 22.8). Histologically, these tumors are distinguished by their finely granular nuclei (*salt and pepper* chromatin), by their small and relatively inconspicuous nucleoli, and by the tendency for the nuclei to become easily deformed by contact with other cells and other structures (*nuclear molding*). These tumors are highly proliferative and rarely is the mitotic rate less than 10 mitoses per 10 high-power fields (hpf) so that virtually every hpf contains one or more mitoses. The neoplastic cells in this tumor type are fragile, and crush artifact is common particularly in small biopsy samples. Lymphocytes and other inflammatory cells can also undergo crush artifact and it is therefore of some importance that definitive diagnosis be based on examination of well-preserved cells where nuclei are clearly visible. A unique feature of SCLC is the *Azzopardi effect* consisting of an accumulation of chromatin in the vascular walls supplying the tumor. In a great majority of cases, the diagnosis of SCLC is obvious by histological examination alone. However, in some cases, immunohistochemical studies can serve to buttress the diagnosis and provide confirmation of diagnosis.

Within the category of SCLC, there is considerable variation in cell size and cellular configuration. For several years, subsets of SCLC were included in the SCLC category. The 1967 WHO classification included *oat cell* carcinoma and an intermediate cell variant that differed from classical oat cell carcinoma in cell size and amount of cytoplasm. These categories proved to be of no prognostic significance and the two categories were combined in the latest classification into a single small cell category. This tumor type comprises 15% to 20% of all lung cancers but its frequency may be decreasing.[59,134] Typically, small cell carcinomas present as an endophytic lesion in a central bronchus with mediastinal lymph node (LN) metastases.

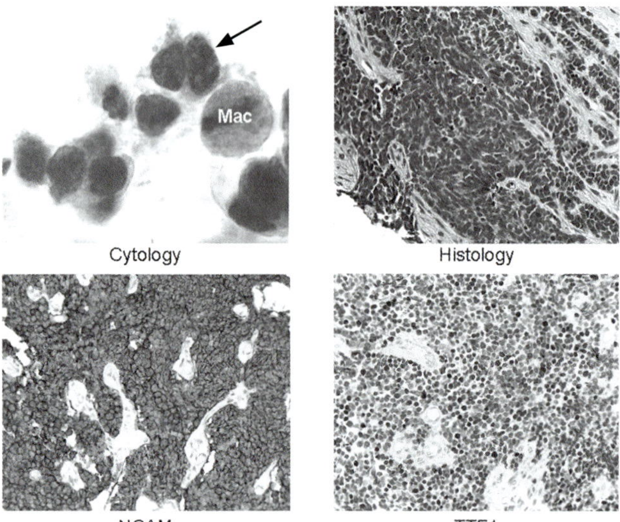

FIGURE 22.8 SCLC as found on cytology, histology, and IHC. On the upper left are clusters of small cells with scant cytoplasm, nuclear molding (*arrow*), and finely granular nuclei with inconspicuous nucleoli. Macrophage (*Mac*) provides size comparison. The frame on the upper right shows the histology of SCLC with closely packed cells with scanting cytoplasm with streaming nuclei. NCAM and TTF-1 stains are strongly positive along plasma membranes and in the nuclei. *Mac*, macrophage; *NCAM*, neural cell adhesion molecule; *TTF-1*, thyroid transcription factor-1. (See color plate.)

Cytology Success in identifying SCLC by cytological examination is partially dependent on the type of specimen available for examination. SCLC may be readily identified bronchial washings and brushings where the cells are well preserved and in these cases, cytology may be crucial in arriving at a definitive diagnosis. However, SCLC has been infrequently identified in screening trials[135,136] in part because SCLC is not well preserved in expectorated sputum and also perhaps because the disaggregation process may damage the fragile cell of SCLC. The cytological features of SCLC correspond to what is seen in well-preserved tissue sections. Single cells or small clusters of cells less than 21 microns in diameter have a high N/C ratio with only a thin sometimes barely visible rim of cytoplasm around and enlarged nucleus (Fig. 22.8). Nuclear fragmentation is often present in association with better-preserved cells. The nucleus again has finely granular (salt and pepper) chromatin and small, inconspicuous nuclei. In small clusters of cells, nuclei are often molded against one another. Nuclear features are crucial and excellent preservation of cells is required for diagnosis. Cells that may resemble SCLC are basilar cells of the respiratory mucosa that usually are smaller and more uniform that the cells of SCLC. Lymphocytes may also cause confusion but usually only in poorly preserved specimens.

Diagnostic Immunohistochemisty of Small Cell Lung Carcinoma Immunohistochemical stains can be used to verify the neuroendocrine nature of the tumor or help distinguish SCLC from other NSCLC (Fig. 22.8). SCLC almost always expresses CK but the amount of this intermediate filament may be quite small, particularly in less than that optimally preserved specimens. CK expression serves to distinguish SCLC from other small blue cell tumors such as lymphoma, which occasionally can mimic SCLC. SCLC, like adenocarcinomas of the lung (see succeeding discussion), is usually positive for the primitive lung differentiation gene TTF-1 with several studies documenting expression rate in at least 85% of these tumors.[71,137–144] In specific contexts, TTF-1 may be useful in distinguishing SCLC from small cell tumors of other sites. For example, while this marker is expressed in a large percentage of SCLC, histologically similar Merkel cell tumor of dermal origin and small cell carcinoma of ovary are virtually always negative for this marker.[140–142,144–146] Small cell cervical and colon carcinomas are occasionally positive (10% to 15%[140,146,147]) but up to 50% of transitional carcinomas of bladder[140,147–149] and over 70% of esophageal small cell tumors are reported positive.[150] Reported results for small cell prostate carcinomas have been variable with some studies indicating high frequency of expression[147] and other low frequency of expression.[140,151] The utility of TTF-1 in distinguishing site of origin of unknown primary is therefore highly context dependent.

A distinguishing feature of SCLC is its expression of neuroendocrine markers including neuron specific enolase, synaptophysin, neural cell adhesion molecule (NCAM) (CD56), and Leu-7 (CD57).[152–154] Approximately 50% of SCLCs also express chromogranin A in sufficient quantity to be detectable in conventional immunohistochemical tests so that in doubtful cases a negative chromogranin is uninformative. The quantity of chromogranin in SCLC is usually less than that present in carcinoid, so that in cases with strongly positive chromogranin stains carcinoid tumor should be excluded. A salient feature of SCLC is its high growth fraction; as determined by Ki-67 labeling procedures, the growth fraction usually exceeds 50%. Ki-67 may be helpful in distinguishing SCLC from other neuroendocrine tumors of the lung. A negative differentiating marker is EGFR, which is expressed in NSCLC but not in SCLC.[154] Finally, it has been reported that c-kit receptor (CD117) is nearly always expressed by high-grade neuroendocrine carcinomas including SCLC and LCNEC,[155–158] an observation that has been fully exploited neither diagnostically nor therapeutically. The expression of CD117 is apparently not associated with mutation of the c-kit receptor gene[159] and no relationship to survival or response to chemotherapy has been shown to date.[160]

The application of immunohistochemical staining procedures to lung tumors has revealed considerable overlap in staining properties. It is known for example that about 20% of adenocarcinomas are focally positive for NCAM, a molecule that otherwise is almost universally expressed by SCLC. This suggests a degree of phenotypic plasticity in lung tumors that is confirmed in gene profiling studies (see discussion that follows).

Molecular Pathology in Small Cell Lung Carcinoma

The unique histological and immunohistochemical features of this tumor are a reflection of underlying genetic changes that are increasingly better defined. SCLC was among the first of the lung tumor types in which genetic changes were defined. These changes included structural chromosomal abnormalities (deletion [3p(14–23)[161]] and the mutations described and listed in Table 22.4. The pathways most frequently affected by mutation involve cell regulation and tyrosine kinase signaling genes including KRAS[84,162] and EGFR[84,163] are rarely mutated. In the succeeding discussion, genetic lesions are grouped by pathway as in the previous discussion of squamous carcinoma.

Cell Cycle Genes A number of the mutations and chromosomal rearrangements that affect cell cycle genes are present in SCLC.

RB1/CDKN2A (p16) *RB1* was first identified as a tumor suppressor gene in retinoblastoma. Knudson's "two-hit" model of carcinogenesis, whereby a dominant tumor suppressor gene is inactivated by two mutational events eliciting tumor formation, was formulated in 1971 to explain retinoblastoma tumorigenesis.[164] Fifteen years later, the retinoblastoma gene, *RB1*, was cloned[165] and the relevance of *RB1* to lung cancer was demonstrated.

RB1 encodes a phosphoprotein that binds to the transcription factor E2F. Phosphorylation of RB1 releases E2F and transition from the G1 to S phase of the mitotic cycle occurs. *RB1* is therefore an important cell cycle regulator and tumor suppressor gene. Loss of *RB1* results in an increase in cell proliferation and more rapid tumor growth.

Structural changes in the *RB1* gene in SCLC lines and tumors have been reported and complete absence of RB1 protein has been reported to affect all SCLC.[166–168] The mechanism of *RB1* inactivation in human tumors is still not completely understood. Although RB protein is absent in SCLC, DNA sequencing has identified mutations in only a minority of tumors and these consist primarily of deletions resulting in frame shifts or stop codons.[169]

The mutational pattern evident in cell cycle genes in SCLC is distinct from that in NSCLC with the latter frequently affected by loss of p16 with and overexpression of cyclin D1 rather than the near universal loss of *RB1*[168] observed in SCLC.

TP53 TP53 is more frequently mutated in SCLC than in the other non–small cell forms of lung cancer. Loss of TP53 function with associated loss of cell cycle checkpoint function and impairment of apoptotic pathways undoubtedly contributes to the aggressive growth and hypermutability that are features of this tumor.

Gene Expression Profiles In virtually all the nucleotide microarray analyses, small cell tumors emerge as a separate phenotypic category with numerous gene expression difference with the non–small cell tumors.[170] Available microarray data for SCLC has considerably expanded the number of potential biomarkers that may be useful in the differential diagnosis and detection of SCLC. Moreover, these studies have indicated that many of the genes expressed in SCLC are also found during lung differentiation (see succeeding discussions).

To date, however, the molecular features of SCLC have not been sufficiently definitive nor have they added sufficient independent information to histological diagnosis to justify the general application of diagnostic molecular testing in this tumor. The diagnosis of this neoplasm therefore continues to rest on histological examination supplemented by immunohistochemical studies in difficult cases.

MIXED SMALL CELL AND NON–SMALL CELL CARCINOMA

It is of interest that a large proportion of small cell carcinomas contain a component of non–small cell tumor. These tumors include large cell carcinoma, adenocarcinoma, and squamous carcinoma. In a recent review of 100 small cell carcinomas,

Nicholson et al.[171] found 72 pure small cell carcinomas and 28 combined small cell carcinomas. Sixteen cases were combined with large cell carcinoma, nine with adenocarcinoma, and three with squamous cell carcinoma.

BRONCHIAL CARCINOID, ATYPICAL CARCINOID AND LARGE CELL NEUROENDOCRINE CARCINOMA

The term *carcinoid* was originally coined in 1907 to describe a subset of gastrointestinal epithelial tumors that were less aggressive than the conventional gastrointestinal carcinoma and were therefore designated carcinoid tumors rather than *carcinoma*.[172] It was subsequently demonstrated that similar tumors existed in the lower respiratory tract.[173] Currently, these tumors together with SCLC and LCNEC are regarded as *neuroendocrine* and are considered part of a continuum. Carcinoid tumor is the lowest grade and least aggressive of this group and SCLC is the highest grade and most aggressive.[174,175] This category also includes atypical carcinoid, which characteristically has an elevated mitotic rate in comparison to typical carcinoid and behaves more aggressively with a metastatic rate of approximately 50%. Finally, LCNEC is an aggressive, high-grade tumor that was first described in 1991[175] as an undifferentiated tumor that is intermediate in morphological features and prognosis between atypical carcinoid and SCLC.

Typical Carcinoid Tumor

Typical carcinoid tumors may arise in the either central or peripheral airways. They usually have strikingly different macroscopic features in the two locations. The central airway tumors are relatively large (mean diameter 3 cm)[176] and grow as endobronchial masses that may obstruct the large bronchi (Fig. 22.9). The secretory products of these tumors also may induce swelling of adjacent tissues that augments the obstruction caused by the tumor itself. These tumors may extend into the bronchial wall but such infiltration does not necessarily imply aggressive growth and is not a criterion for atypical carcinoid. The sectioned surface of carcinoid tumor is usually gray and homogeneous. The histological features that distinguish carcinoid tumors from NSCLC are relative uniformity of the tumors cells, abundant grayish granular cytoplasm, lack of tumor cell necrosis, and round to oval nuclei with finely granular (salt and pepper) nuclear chromatin and inconspicuous nucleoli. Carcinoid cells form small clusters without true gland formation in a pattern that is variously described as organoid or insular. Cells and nuclei are frequently oriented perpendicularly to the basement membrane, forming palisading or rosettelike patterns. To distinguish slow-growing typical carcinoids from more aggressive tumors, the diagnosis is limited to those tumors with <2 mitoses per 2 mm^2 (<10 hpf) and no necrosis. [60]

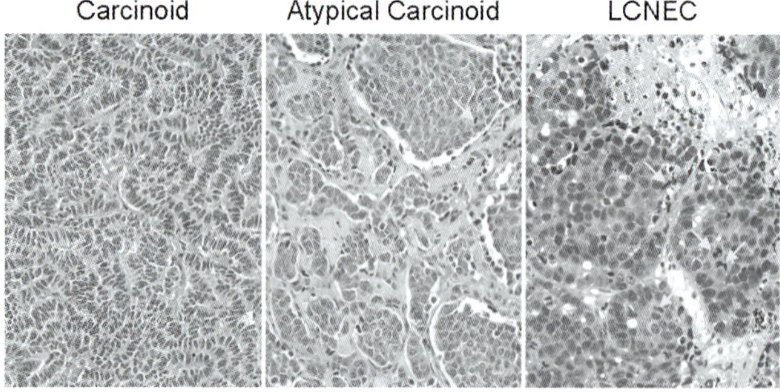

FIGURE 22.9 Histological comparison of various forms of neuroendocrine tumor of the lung. On the left is a classical carcinoid tumor with a ribbonlike pattern of growth. The central image shows more sheetlike tumor growth with occasional mitotic figures (see text). This tumor type also is defined by the presence of focal areas of necrosis. The figure on the right shows the high level of mitotic activity (*arrows*) and areas of necrosis that characterize LCNEC. *LCNEC*, large cell neuroendocrine carcinoma. (See color plate.)

Carcinoid tumors may also grow in the peripheral lung. Minute (<5 mm) peripheral carcinoid tumors, referred to as *tumorlets*,[177] are frequent incidental findings in lungs resected for other lung diseases and are benign. Larger carcinoid tumors may also occur in the peripheral lung. The uniform cellular appearances of the central airway tumors are recapitulated in the peripheral tumors with the exception that tumor cells are found in the bronchioles and in some cases, the tumors have a spindled appearance (spindle cell carcinoid tumor[178]).

Symptomatic carcinoid tumors represent 1% to 2% of all lung carcinomas and survival at both 5 and 10 years is 87%.[174,179]

Atypical Carcinoid

A mitotic rate of 2 to 10 per 2 mm^2 and foci of necrosis are the features that separate atypical from typical carcinoid (Fig. 22.9) as first defined by Arrigoni et al.[180]

In contrast to the low mortality of typical carcinoid, atypical carcinoid tumors have a survival rate of 50% to 60% at 5 years and 35% at 10 years, a mortality effect that remains significant in multivariate analysis.[174,181] Patients with atypical carcinoid are reported to have higher tobacco smoke exposure than the general population or patients with typical carcinoid.[182] A smoking association is supported by an increase in the prevalence of smoking-associated genetic changes including LOH and p53 mutation in atypical carcinoid in comparison to typical carcinoid.[183]

Large Cell Neuroendocrine Carcinoma

In the LCNEC, necrosis is also frequently present and mitotic rate exceeds 10 mitoses per 2 mm^2 areas. Cells often retain a neuroendocrine appearance with organoid nesting, trabeculae, rosettelike structures, and peripheral palisading[175] (Fig. 22.9). Nuclei may exhibit the fine granularity seen in SCLC but there are often more conspicuous nucleoli. Immunostains for neuroendocrine markers may or may not be positive and are not necessary for diagnosis when neuroendocrine differentiation is evident. Conversely, the diagnosis of LCNEC in an undifferentiated large tumor may be based purely on immunohistochemical staining results (Table 22.3). LCNEC is distinguished from SCLC on the basis of the aforementioned features as well as cell size >21 microns (3 lymphocyte diameters).

The incidence of LCNEC carcinoma is approximately 3% of all primary pulmonary malignancies[184,185] and is strongly associated with smoking history.[186] It is generally thought that LCNEC carries a worse prognosis than other non–small cell carcinomas.[179,187] Five-year survival for this tumor from several studies varies from 15%[179] to 27%,[174,186] and 10-year survival is reported at 9%.[174,187] Another study of 87 cases of LCNEC reported significantly worse survival for stage I patients[185] but overall 5-year survival was not significantly different from an overall 5-year survival of or the NSCLC at 57%. Although currently treated as NSCLC, the prognosis for LCNEC approaches that of small cell carcinoma, and treatment options may change in the future.[188,189]

Cytology of Carcinoid Tumor and Large Cell Neuroendocrine Carcinoma

Although most carcinoid tumors are centrally located, their cytologic features are better seen on fine-needle aspiration specimens than in sputum. Smears show small uniform cells with central to eccentric round nuclei with smooth nuclear outlines. There is no molding as seen with high-grade neuroendocrine carcinomas. A minority of carcinoid tumors can have spindle-shaped cells. Cytologically, atypical carcinoids show more pleomorphism, atypia, higher N/C ratios, more irregular membranes, and coarser chromatin than typical carcinoids. Cells are arranged as single cells and syncytial aggregates, and necrosis may be present[190]; however, these features are only suggestive and tissue is required for a definitive diagnosis.

Suggested cytological criteria for LCNEC include flattened three-dimensional groups of cells with peripheral palisading, moderate to large cells, some molding and crush artifact, prominent nucleoli, mitoses, necrosis, and positive neuroendocrine markers.[191,192] Distinction between SCLC and NSCLC may be difficult on cytological examination[193] unless enough material is available for a cell block to evaluate architectural features and immunohistochemical biomarker expression.

Immunohistochemisty of Carcinoid Tumor and Large Cell Neuroendocrine Carcinoma

As mentioned previously, expression of immunohistochemical markers is currently one of the two defining criteria of neuroendocrine tumors. Table 22.3 lists antibodies that distinguish among neuroendocrine tumor types. Antibodies that are most generally useful in the evaluation of neuroendocrine tumors include NCAM, synaptophysin, and chromogranin.[194–201] LCNEC frequently expresses one or more neuroendocrine markers.[153,202] However, staining tends to be more focal and weaker than that observed with SCLC or carcinoid tumor (Table 22.3). In a small subset of LCNEC, immunostains for these markers are negative and diagnosis is made on the basis of histology alone.

Electron microscopy has, in the past, been useful in characterizing neuroendocrine tumors but has largely been replaced by less expensive and often more informative immunohistochemical tests.

Cell of Origin: Small Cell Lung Carcinoma and the Neuroendocrine Tumor Hypothesis

Since the original description of SCLC, the cell of origin has been the subject of much speculation. In the 1960s, the hypothesis was advanced that these tumors were derived from Kulchitsky (K) cells that are scattered along the airway surfaces.[203] K cells were considered to be a part of a dispersed neuroendocrine system.[204] These cells were thought to be derived from neural crest and thus separately derived from the rest of the lung. However, the neuroendocrine cells were later shown to be derived locally.[205] Although K cells populate the bronchial epithelium at a density of approximately one cell per millimeter, these cells are infrequently observed in premalignant conditions. Moreover, SCLC arises in a milieu similar to that of non–small cell central airway lesions including widespread squamous metaplasia and dysplasia. This, together with the frequent combination of small cell and non–small cell elements in lung carcinomas, suggests that the small cell tumors may have the same progenitor cells of origin as NSCLC.

The hypothesis that tumors with neuroendocrine properties should be grouped into a single category is not universally accepted[206] for several reasons. First, a large proportion of lung carcinomas have mixed nonneuroendocrine and neuroendocrine properties. This is particularly evident in molecular profiling studies where otherwise unremarkable adenocarcinomas have been shown to express clusters of genes that are thought to reflect neuroendocrine differentiation.[96,97,207] Adenocarcinomas having this gene expression profile have a worse prognosis than other adenocarcinomas. Second, many of the markers that are regarded as neuroendocrine markers are expressed in a variety of cells in addition to neuroendocrine cells.[206] Third, neuroendocrine markers including NCAM are expressed during embryonic development of the lung.[208] For example,[209] gastrin-releasing peptide signaling has been to shown to determine airway branching in the embryonic mouse lung.[210] Expression of neuroendocrine biomarkers in LCNEC could be regarded as evidence of dedifferentiation to a more primitive developmental stage rather than neuroendocrine differentiation.

At the present time then, expression of neuroendocrine biomarkers may be regarded as an interesting but not yet fully understood property of lung carcinomas that may be prognostically important within specific histological categories. Moreover, expression of neuroendocrine-associated genes may provide therapeutic targets but does not necessarily indicate ontological relationships among tumors. The biological rationale for grouping diverse lung tumors into a single neuroendocrine diagnostic category is problematic and this grouping has not yet been unequivocally proven to be clinically relevant. It may yet prove to be more useful to annotate conventional histological categories with biomarker expression data rather than retain the neuroendocrine designation to refer to such a divergent group of tumors.

DIFFUSE IDIOPATHIC PULMONARY NEUROENDOCRINE CELL HYPERPLASIA: A POSSIBLE CARCINOID PRECURSOR

Neuroendocrine cells may also proliferate in the bronchiolar walls without forming tumors, a condition referred to as diffuse idiopathic pulmonary neuroendocrine cell hyperplasia (DIPNECH).[211] Histologically, multifocal, patchy collections of neuroendocrine cells may involve the full circumference of the bronchiolar walls and form tumorlets or small carcinoid tumors. The proliferative cells in this condition are considered to be benign but because the disorder gives rise to carcinoid tumors, it is considered a premalignant condition. To date, more aggressive forms of lung carcinoma, including SCLC, have not been associated with DIPNECH. The condition may cause an obliterative bronchiolitis that is often a presenting symptom. It has also been described in association with hypoxic childhood pulmonary emphysema, tachypnea of infancy, and adult dyspnea.[212–214] There is currently no effective treatment.

Peripheral Airway Lesions: Adenocarcinoma and Its Precursors In this chapter, we use the term *peripheral airway lesions* to refer to tumors and premalignant conditions predominantly arising from airway epithelium distal to the terminal bronchiolar and alveolar epithelium. Most but not all adenocarcinomas of the lung arise in the peripheral airways and are divided into invasive adenocarcinoma, which is distinguished by a fibrous stromal response around individual tumor cell nests, bronchioloalveolar carcinoma, which grows exclusively along the alveolar surfaces and does not invade stromal tissues, and the putative adenocarcinoma precursor lesion atypical adenomatous hyperplasia (AAH).

The incidence of adenocarcinoma is rising.[108] This cell type now represents over 30% of primary lung malignancies. Although adenocarcinoma is associated with smoking, the association is weaker than for squamous cell carcinoma or small cell carcinoma and a large subset of adenocarcinomas occur in never-smokers. This histological type is the most common type seen in women and in nonsmokers.[215]

Emerging evidence suggests and indicates that peripheral adenocarcinomas may arise from different progenitor lesions than squamous carcinoma as discussed later. During the past 2 decades, the existence of stepwise sequential morphological changes corresponding to the progression from atypia to carcinoma has been described in the peripheral lung. The prognostic significance of histology in small early lesions is increasingly better understood. Moreover, the increasing sensitivity of imaging technology during the past several years has allowed for the detection of smaller lesions in previously inaccessible peripheral airways. All this has created a pressing need for accurate classification of the peripheral airway lesions.

ATYPICAL ADENOMATOUS HYPERPLASIA AND THE ORIGIN OF PERIPHERAL LUNG ADENOCARCINOMA

AAH (also referred to as *atypical alveolar hyperplasia* or *bronchial adenoma*) is a small (<5 mm) proliferation of alveolar cells that was originally described in lungs resected for invasive adenocarcinoma.[216] Since its original description, a high frequency of AAH in patients with adenocarcinoma has been documented in many studies. AAH has been found in 14% to 57% of lungs with adenocarcinoma[217–223] and in 3% to 30% with squamous carcinoma.[218,220–223] It has also been found at autopsy in 2.8% of elderly Japanese population without carcinoma.[224] The frequent occurrence of AAH in association with adenocarcinoma and bronchioloalveolar carcinoma (BAC)[223] suggests that AAH may be a precursor of adenocarcinoma and BAC, and AAH has been defined as a preinvasive lesion of adenocarcinoma in the current WHO classification.[1] This hypothesis is supported by the similarity in molecular profiles between AAH and BAC.

Histopathology of Atypical Adenomatous Hyperplasia AAH can be recognized by careful examination of freshly resected lung, but is usually invisible to the naked eye and is detected only incidentally on microscopic examination. In hematoxylin and eosin (H&E)–stained sections, AAH (Fig. 22.10) is observed as well-circumscribed cluster of alveoli lined by a single uniform layer of well-formed type II pnuemocytes or Clara type (*hobnail*) cells without scarring or significant inflammation in the area. Involved alveoli are frequently clustered around a terminal bronchiole. The cells of AAH are sparsely concentrated along the alveoli and have dense nuclei with inconspicuous nucleoli.

AAH may be difficult to histologically discriminate from BAC. Histological evidence of malignancy includes

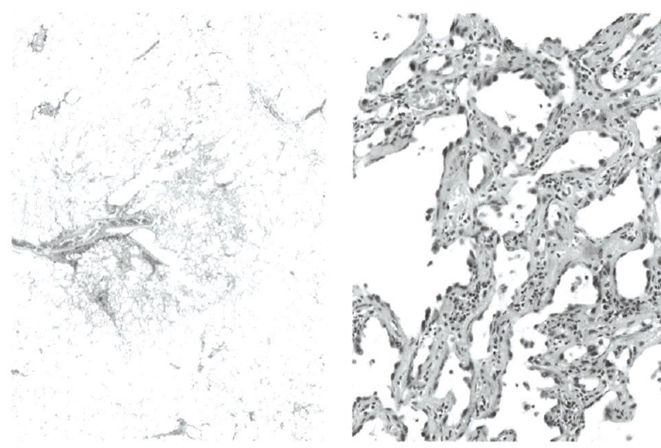

FIGURE 22.10 Atypical adenomatous hyperplasia. On the left is a low magnification view showing the small overall size of the lesion. At higher magnification (*right*), a single layer of cuboidal cells covers the alveolar septae with minimal associated inflammation. (See color plate.)

cellular crowding, nuclear chromatin granularity and prominence of nucleoli, increase in cell height, and stratification of cells.[225] Lesions containing larger, more crowded cells with cytological atypia may be impossible to distinguish from BAC and some observers have suggested that lesions smaller than 5 mm be classified as AAH, while larger lesions be classified as BAC.

Molecular Correlates of Atypical Adenomatous Hyperplasia

Immunohistochemistry It has been difficult to characterize AAH immunohistochemically because it is usually detected incidentally after surgery as a very small lesion. However, several studies have reported an immunohistochemical relationship between AAH and BAC. AAH expresses high levels of several markers that are also upregulated in lung carcinomas including survivin,[227] Mre11 (telomere maintenance),[228] telomerase, Dicer (microRNA-related protein),[229] and matrix metalloproteinases.[230] Overexpression is consistent with a likely pathogenetic relationship among AAH (preinvasion lesion), BAC (in situ adenocarcinoma), and invasive adenocarcinoma.

Genetic Changes That AAH represents a true neoplasm is also supported by morphometric and molecular studies. AAH has proven to be aneuploid by morphometric analysis[231–234] and flow cytometry,[235] is monoclonal, and may harbor the same genetic changes listed for adenocarcinoma in Table 22.4 including mutations of *KRAS*[236,237] and *EGFR*.[237] AAH also has demonstrated LOH at chromosomal sites of putative tumor suppressor genes including 3p,[238,239] 9p,[238,239] 9q,[240,241] 16p,[241] 17p,[239] 17q,[240] and chromosomal imbalance by comparative genomic hybridization.[242] One study[239] has shown that increasing frequency of LOH and *TP53* mutation correlates with increasing histological grade from AAH to invasive carcinoma, suggesting an increasing frequency of genetic abnormalities with progression from premalignant to invasive disease.

Natural History of Atypical Adenomatous Hyperplasia The evidence that AAH is a precursor lesion for peripheral adenocarcinoma is also supported by the coexistence AAH with non–small cell carcinoma, but because the lesion is rarely identified in patients without tumor, longitudinal studies have not been possible. Combined molecular and available epidemiological data support a stepwise sequence of changes in the peripheral airways similar to the adenomatous polyp/invasive carcinoma sequence that has been well described in the colon.[218] The lesion following AHH in sequential peripheral lung carcinogenesis is BAC.

Bronchioloalveolar Carcinoma BAC was described many years before AAH. Recently, there has been renewed interest in this tumor type for several reasons. First, BAC is unique among lung tumors in its capacity to spread through the airways without tissue destruction. Metastasis through the airways may result in nodular growths anywhere in the airways. Direct extension of tumor along the alveolar septae can result in a pneumonic pattern of growth that has a pneumonia-like appearance on imaging studies, the pneumonic form of BAC.[243] Second, the pathological definition of BAC has changed during the past 10 years and continues to evolve. Third, although 70% of BAC occurs in smokers, it is one of the few lung cancers in which a substantial minority of the affected population is nonsmoking.[244] Fourth, molecular mechanisms that drive tumor cells of this type have been dramatically elucidated through genetic analyses.[245,246] Finally, it is a tumor that is most frequently detected by new high-resolution computed tomography (CT) imaging methods.[247] The extension of tumor cells along the alveolar septae with retained aeration or low-density mucous production may provide BAC with a unique ground-glass appearance in CT imaging studies,[248–250] the so-called *ground glass opacity* (GGO). The small peripheral GGO is often a presenting feature of BAC. Its incidence has been increasing with the use of CT screening for lung cancer. An account of the development of the concept of BAC is provided in the succeeding discussion.

Histology of Bronchioloalveolar Carcinoma: A Changing Concept The notion that tumors may develop in the peripheral lung from alveolar epithelium is an old one that was first advanced in 1876.[251] The premise was in doubt for another three quarters century since it was not until 1953 that electron microscopic studies demonstrated a thin pneumocyte layer continuously lining the alveolar septae and abutting the bronchiolar epithelium.[252] During the intervening years, there was much speculation about the nature of the subset of well-differentiated peripheral lung cancers that grew by extending along the alveolar septae, that were frequently multicentric and that preserved the underlying architecture of the lung.[253] In the early 20th century, South African sheep suffering an endemic infectious disease (jaagsiekte) were found to have nonmetastasizing epithelial proliferations in the lungs,[254] microscopically similar to human alveolar tumors.[255] The term *adenomatosis* was proposed to refer to this disease. Jaagsiekte eventually proved to have a viral etiology and but to date, no causative viral agent has yet been confirmed in morphologically similar human tumors.[256] The term *adenomatous* was applied to human tumors as well but was not wholly satisfactory since sheep rarely developed metastases but that were frequent in the analogous human tumors.

By 1960, it had become clear that peripheral lung tumors that spread along the alveolar surfaces could resemble bronchiolar or alveolar epithelium. The term *bronchiolo-alveolar* carcinoma was introduced by Liebow[257] and quickly accepted to describe "…well-differentiated adenocarcinomas primary in the periphery of the lung beyond a grossly recognizable bronchus, with a tendency to spread chiefly within the confines of the lung by aerogenous and lymphatic routes…"

This definition persisted without change until 1980 when Shimosato et al.[258] recognized that peripheral adenocarcinomas <3.0 cm without fibrosis have a significantly longer mean survival than those with a central scar. Noguchi et al.[259] later confirmed that the 5-year survival of patients with pure BAC with no fibroblastic foci is 100%, with no cancer-related death. Fibroblastic foci were presumed to indicate host response to invasion by tumor cells and the presence of fibroblastic foci reduced 5-year survival to 75%. This fibrosis of invasion was distinguished from *collapse* of alveolar walls with accumulation of residual elastic fibers and basement membrane into consolidated nodules.[259] The importance of fibrosis to predict outcome in early stage alveolar tumors has been supported by more recent studies from Japan that indicate fibrosis <5 to 10 mm in maximum diameter is a favorable prognostic indicator.[260,261] The WHO/International Association for the Study of Lung Cancer (IASLC) panel lung tumor recognized these observations in the most recent classification published in 2004.[1] By current definition, BAC is an in situ lesion that may spread through the alveolar spaces but exhibits no evidence of stromal invasion and does not metastasize to distant sites through the blood or lymphatics. To accommodate those numerous tumors with both BAC and invasive carcinoma components, the category of *adenocarcinoma, mixed subtype*, sometimes referred to as *adenocarcinoma*, mixed subtype with BAC features.

To determine whether or not fibroblastic foci are present in a peripheral nodule and whether vascular, lymphatic, or pleural invasion are present, it is necessary to carefully examine the entire tumor. Elastic staining is useful for distinguishing alveolar collapse from tumor invasion. If the lesion is small (<1 cm) the entire tumor should be embedded for microscopic examination. This is not possible when diagnosis is based on needle biopsy or aspiration.

BAC may be mucinous or nonmucinous (Fig. 22.11). Mucinous tumors are composed of mucus-producing goblet cells with large cytoplasmic mucous vacuoles that may compress and deform nuclei. These cells are often evenly distributed in single layers along alveoli. Nuclei are low grade but may be difficult to visualize well. Surrounding alveoli often contain pools of mucus. Nonmucinous cells may differentiate along the lines of Clara-type cells, type 2 pneumocytes, or a mixture of both. In the nonmucinous Clara-type tumor, cells are columnar and eosinophilic, with apical cytoplasmic extensions (*snout*) projecting above the level of adjacent epithelium. The less frequent tumors composed of nonmucinous, type II pneumocyte-like cells contain cuboidal or low columnar cells that may have foamy, vacuolated cytoplasm. Nuclei are located centrally in nonmucinous tumors, nuclear grade is usually low, and mitoses infrequent in both cell types. Rare mixtures of mucinous and nonmucinous types may coexist in the same tumor.[262]

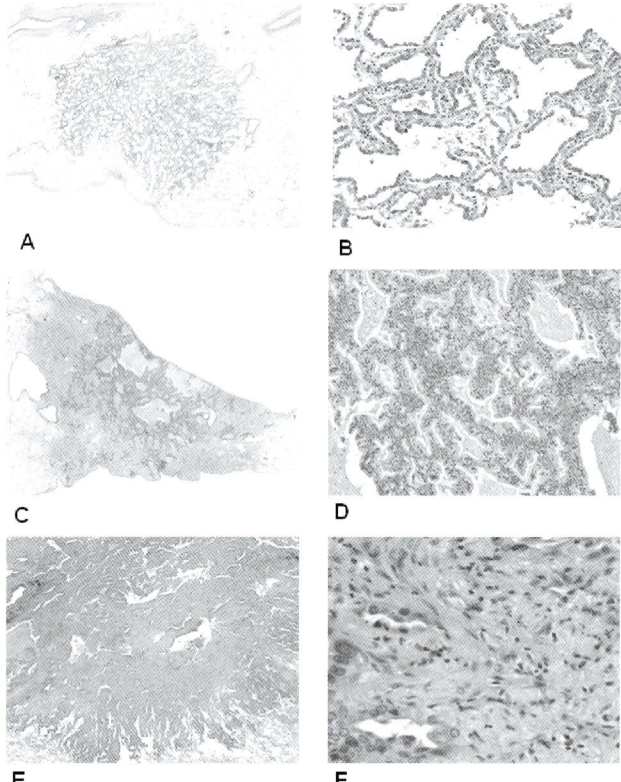

FIGURE 22.11 Histology of various forms of BAC, BAC mixed with invasive carcinoma, and pure invasive carcinoma. **A:** Small nonmucinous BAC at low magnification without evidence of stromal invasion. **B:** High magnification of **A** shows lepidic spread of well-differentiated malignant pneumocytes along alveolar septae. **C:** Pink acellular mucus fills the alveoli of this mucinous BAC photographed at low magnification. **D:** At higher magnification of **C**, mucous vacuoles are present in apex of columnar cells lining alveoli. **E:** In this invasive adenocarcinoma, there is fibrosis at the center of a tumor that exhibits extension of tumor cells. **F:** High magnification of this tumor (**E**) reveals a sclerotic response to tumor cells with pink fibers aligned parallel to the elongated fibroblastic nuclei. (See color plate.)

Cytology of Bronchioloalveolar Carcinoma

Fine-needle aspiration may be readily used to evaluate peripheral lung nodules and cytological specimens from these aspirates can be diagnostic of carcinoma. However, accurate distinction of BAC from invasive carcinoma is not possible without the view of lung architecture afforded by tissue sections. Athough BAC has been reported to have characteristic cytological features,[263–265] these features do not directly reflect the presence or absence of stromal invasion and cannot be reliably used to make this important distinction.

Generally, the aspirate of BAC[266] is cellular with minimal inflammatory infiltrate and contains two-dimensional monolayer sheets of uniform cells.[263,264] In contrast, cytological features such as three-dimensional balls, papillary clusters, marked nuclear atypia, and background necrosis are characteristic of invasive adenocarcinoma, but not BAC, and it is important not to overlook these invasive signs. Nuclei are pale staining and round with nuclear grooves in cells from nonmucinous tumors. In mucinous tumors, extracellular mucin is visible.[267] These cytological features may also be evident in advanced and invasive adenocarcinomas and in part responsible for the 35% overall accuracy of FNA for specific diagnosis of adenocarcinoma.[268] It is currently recommended that a specific diagnosis of BAC not be made on a cytology specimen.[226]

Immunohistochemisty of Bronchioloalveolar Carcinoma BAC is a relatively slow-growing tumor and difficult to culture in immunohistochemical studies support this biological behavior in vivo. Growth fraction estimated by Ki-67 labeling is reported to be 11% in pure BAC and increases to 35% in invasive adenocarcinoma.[269,270] These tumors often have proliferative margins but nonproliferating central zones. Otherwise, the immunohistochemical and other molecular features of BAC are similar to invasive carcinoma and are discussed later.

INVASIVE ADENOCARCINOMA

Invasive adenocarcinoma, in contrast to BAC, destroys the alveolar septae rather than using them as a framework for spread and metastasizes through the lymphatics to LNs rather than through the airways. Invasive adenocarcinoma is now the most common form of lung carcinoma.[271] Metastatic rates for even small (stage I to II) peripheral adenocarcinomas overall is 17% and is higher (31%) in more poorly differentiated carcinomas.[272] Distant metastases are also common even in stage I tumors particularly those that are high grade.[273] The invasive adenocarcinoma category is quite heterogeneous in its both morphological and molecular features, as discussed later.

Histology of Adenocarcinoma Invasive adenocarcinoma (Fig. 22.11) is distinguished from pure BAC by extension of nests of glandlike cells frequently containing mucus vacuoles into a proliferative, fibroblastic stroma with destruction of bronchi and alveolar walls. Tissue invasion permits cells to gain access to the lymphatic and vascular channels of the lung so that spread of invasive adenocarcinoma is typically by LN or hematogenous metastasis, in contrast to BAC with its exclusively intrapulmonary spread.

The scarring (desmoplasia) that occurs in invasive tumors is chemically and morphologically distinct from that occuring in response to infection or ischemia.[274–276] Rather than representing a preexisting focus from which tumor arises, as implied in the now-outmoded term *scar carcinoma*, scarring is thought to be stimulated directly by tumor. Scarring of invasive adenocarcinoma is also distinct from collapse of the stromal framework that occurs in BAC.[232]

The histological features that distinguish adenocarcinoma from other invasive carcinomas are glandular differentiation and mucin production. The glandular elements and mucin vacuoles of adenocarcinoma may be arranged in many different patterns and these various arrangements are the basis of the division of adenocarcinoma into several different subgroups. The most common pattern is the acinar pattern in which tumor cells form glandlike or tubular structures. More uncommon are the papillary, solid, and signet ring patterns of growth. Detailed discussion of the many different variants is contained in several excellent reviews and atlases.[1,60,271,277] The papillary and micropapillary subtypes are composed of tufts of cells projecting into alveolar spaces with central vascular cores in the papillary variant and without vascular cores in the micropapillary variant. The significance of papillary and micropapillary patterns is their poor prognosis[278,279] and their relatively high EGFR mutation rate (approximately 35%).[280]

Demonstration of mucus vacuoles in mucicarmine or alcian blue stains may be crucial for the diagnosis of this tumor type. However, small amounts of mucin are also produced by other types of NSCLC and for this reason, the presence of mucin in 10% or more of tumor cells has been set as a threshold for the diagnosis of adenocarcinoma.[60]

Current grading of adenocarcinoma is based on the resemblance of tumor to normal lung tissue. Recent studies have suggested that tumor grade,[272] nuclear grade,[281] necrosis,[281] lymphatic invasion,[281,282] and the presence of >25% papillary growth component[282] have may be indicators of aggressive behavior. Even so, the predictive accuracy of these features is not sufficient to allow extrapolation to individual cases. Eight percent of small, well-differentiated adenocarcinoma is reported to have metastases at the time of surgery. The presence of an intratumoral fibrotic response may prove to be a valuable grading marker but is difficult to quantify in cross sections and impossible to evaluate in needle biopsies.

Cytology of Adenocarcinoma The cytological appearances of adenocarcinoma are complicated by the heterogeneity of this group of tumors. Diagnosis is based on overall architecture and individual cellular details (Fig. 22.12). Cytological specimens may show groups of cells with glandular, papillary, or bronchioloalveolar patterns but as noted previously, diagnosis of specific subtypes of adenocarcinoma is not possible by cytological examination alone. Cell aggregates may form monolayer sheets, three-dimensional cell balls, papillary structures, or flat groups with a central lumen. Cytoplasm may

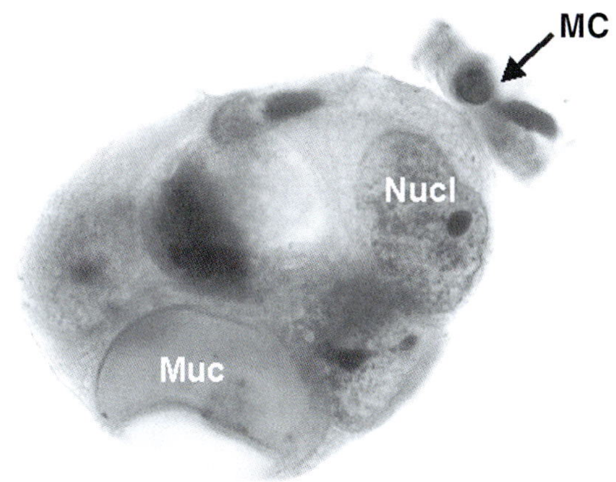

FIGURE 22.12 Cytology of adenocarcinoma showing Papanicolaou-stained cluster of adenocarcinoma cells. These are large cells with high N/C ratio and prominent nucleoli (dark circular structure in nucleus [Nucl]). Under the microscope, the cell cluster has a three-dimensional structure and a mucus vacuole (Muc) is present at one margin of the cluster. *MC* indicates smaller mucociliary cell. (See color plate.)

be vacuolization or may be granular and is usually translucent. Nuclei are eccentrically placed and have prominent nucleoli that may be misshapen rather that perfectly rounded. Micropapillary adenocarcinomas, a variant with poor prognosis and EGFR association reported by Miyoshi et al.[279] as mentioned previously, are recognizable in cytology preparation by their micropapillary structures. These are composed of tumor cell aggregates without central fibrovascular tufts. Adenocarcinomas are only infrequently detected in sputum and because the majority of adenocarcinomas are more peripheral tumors. Transthoracic FNA is most likely to yield a diagnosis especially in peripheral nodules >2.0 cm with a sensitivity and specificity of 0.9 and 0.97, respectively.[62]

Diagnostic Immunohistochemistry of Adenocarcinoma A major practical question facing the pathologist on discovery of adenocarcinoma in the lung is the organ site of origin since many adenocarcinomas found in the lung are metastatic. The detailed immunophenotypic characterization of lung adenocarcinoma has done much to address this question. Perhaps the most useful protein biomarker in this regard is TTF-1 (Fig. 22.13). This protein is one of the master regulatory genes for lung development. It is a transcription factor that regulates the expression of surfactant, Clara cell proteins, and several others that are important in lung development.[283,284] TTF-1 is first expressed in the laryngotracheal diverticulum, then, for the next few weeks, in the bronchial epithelium. Expression then shifts to the alveolar epithelium where it is found in the adult.[285] In lung cancers, this protein is expressed by many types of primary lung tumors including adenocarcinoma, SCLC, LCLC, and carcinoid but usually not by squamous carcinoma (Table 22.3). The *TTF1* gene has recently been shown to reside in a region of amplification.[286,287] Gene amplification is associated with overexpression of the protein, but overexpression may occur in the absence of amplification.[288]

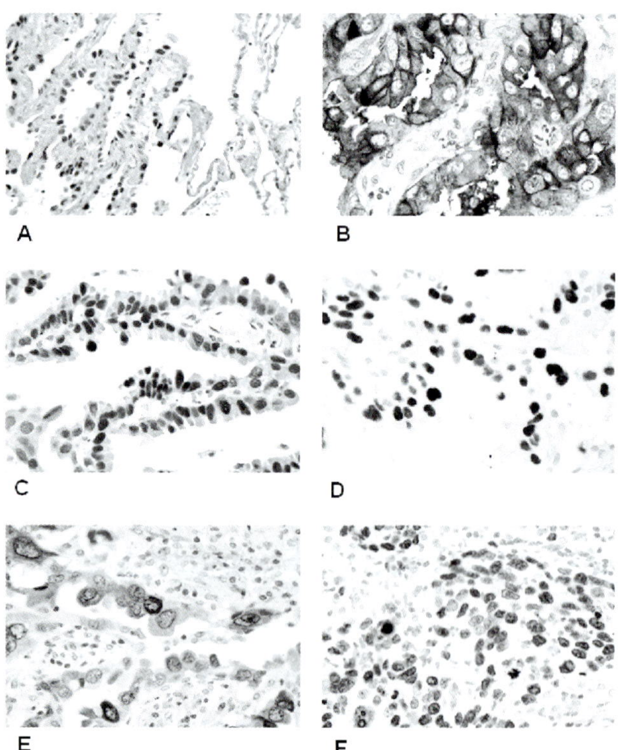

FIGURE 22.13 Immunohistochemical staining patterns for several biomarkers reported to be of diagnostic and prognostic significance in adenocarcinoma (see text). **A:** TTF-1, nuclear staining; **B:** CEA, cytoplasmic staining; **C:** p27, nuclear staining; **D:** p53; strong nuclear staining (mutant pattern); **E:** COX-2, cytoplasmic staining; **F:** MIB-1 (Ki67); nuclear staining. (See color plate.)

A second marker set that addresses the question of tumor site of origin are the CKs. Well-differentiated lung adenocarcinoma has a CK profile that is distinct from squamous carcinoma and from metastasic adenocarcinomas arising below the diaphragm. Most pulmonary adenocarcinomas are CK5/6−/CK7+/p63−/CK20−, while squamous tumors are usually CK 5/6+/CK7−/p63/CK20−. Other primaries such as breast, ovary, pancreas, and endometrium may also be CK7+/CK20−.[289,290] Carcinomas of colon are usually CK7−/CK20+[291,292] and may, in addition, produce the gastrointestinal marker, caudal-related homeobox 2 (CDX2).[290,293,294] A CK7/CK20/CDX immunohistochemical panel may thus be useful in the distinction of pulmonary adenocarcinoma from tumors of the gastrointestinal tract metastatic to the lung.[295]

Other proteins that could reflect peripheral airway origin are the surfactant proteins including surfactant protein A (SPA) and surfactant protein C (SPC), which are expressed in more than half of adenocarcinomas.[296–299] The utility of these markers is limited by relatively low sensitivity[70,300–302] of the immunohistochemical assay and by expression of many of the surfactant proteins by nonpulmonary tumors.[303] TTF-1 and the CKs are generally the more specific and useful of the discriminators of pulmonary adenocarcinoma.

Molecular Pathology of Adenocarcinoma The rapid expansion of technologies available to examine adenocarcinomas during the past 2 decades has led to the deciphering of complex molecular pathology that drives growth and metastases of these tumors. The molecular abnormalities of adenocarcinoma are not only of intrinsic biological interest but also provide targets for therapeutic intervention and can be used to predict response to new targeted agents. Molecular pathology is probably better defined for adenocarcinoma than for other tumor types because of its high frequency, surgical accessibility, and heterogeneity and because of the early success in identifying clinically important molecular pathways in this tumor type.

Gene Mutations in Adenocarcinoma

KRAS Among the first of the molecular changes of clinical significance identified in pulmonary adenocarcinoma was point mutation in the *KRAS* gene. This gene encodes a membrane-associated protein that is a key link in the tyrosine kinase signaling cascade in cancer cells. Mutation in this gene results in a constitutively active protein that enhances cell proliferation and induces malignant transformation.[304,305] In 1988, Rodenhuis et al.[306] reported that *KRAS* mutation was present in 9 of 35 clinical samples of adenocarcinoma and subsequently *KRAS* mutation prevalence has ranged from approximately 10% to 40%.[307–315] The frequency of *KRAS* mutation increases with disease stage,[316] ranging from 12.5% of single nodules to 40% of tumors with satellite nodules to 60% of cases of intrathoracic spread of tumor. Initially, *KRAS* mutation was reported as negative prognostic marker[307] but the prognostic significance of mutation was not initially confirmed. A recent analysis of available prognostic data concludes that *KRAS* is a weakly negative prognostic indicator.[317] There is a strong association between smoking and *KRAS* mutation in adenocarcinoma.[318–320]

TP53 Point mutation in the *TP53* gene is also common in lung adenocarcinomas, occurring in 35% of these tumors and has been associated with poor outcome.[321,322] Mutation is uncommon in pure BAC but is found in 11% of adenocarcinomas of mixed invasive/BAC subtype and in 48% of tumors that are purely invasive,[323] suggesting a role for *TP53* in progression to aggressive forms of invasive peripheral lung cancer. *TP53* mutation occurs in association with *KRAS* in a small proportion (<5%) of adenocarcinomas and appears to occur independently.[320,324]

EGFR EGFR-blocking agents are now available that are most effective in *EGFR* mutant tumors and for this reason, the most clinically relevant of the mutations reported to date in lung cancer are point mutations and deletions of the EGFR gene. Reported independently by two Boston groups in 2004,[245,246] point mutations were found in exons 18 and 21 and deletions in exon 19, the coding region for the tyrosine kinase domain of EGFR. The mutations increase sensitivity of tumor cells to small molecule EGFR blockers, erlotinib (Tarceva) and gefitinib (Iressa). In a large series of tumors from Japan, Taiwan, Australia, and United States, EGFR mutation is closely correlated with gender (female), nonsmoker status, and Asian ethnicity.[84] Not all EGFR mutations are equally predictive of survival or response to EGFR blockers and mean survival in treated tumors with exon 19 deletion is longer than survival in treated tumors with point mutation.[325,326] Finally, resistance to EGFR blockade may be acquired during treatment and has been attributed to mutation in *EGFR* exon 20 (T790M) in half of the cases[327,328] and acquired amplification of the *c-met* gene in another 20%.[329,330] C-met amplification is present in <5% of untreated tumors.[330]

As indicated previously, adenocarcinoma is a histologically heterogeneous tumor with many different patterns of growth. The correlation between histological subtype and *EGFR* mutational status is not completely resolved. Initially, it was reported that mutations occurred predominantly in BAC.[246] Subsequent studies using strict noninvasive WHO criteria have had conflicting results with some studies finding few if any tumors with pure or predominant BAC to be mutant,[84,280] while others find the frequency of *EGFR* mutation in pure nonmucinous BAC higher than in invasive adenocarcinoma[331] or mucinous BAC.[332] Recently, it has also been reported that adenocarcinomas with predominantly papillary or micropapillary morphology are more likely to be *EGFR* mutant[280] than nonpapillary tumors. In view of these complexities, it seems likely that direct mutational analysis of adenocarcinoma will continue to be required for accurate assessment of biological behavior and prediction of treatment outcome regardless of histological subtype.

Several studies have reported that there is a mutually exclusive relationship between EGFR mutation and Ki-RAS mutation and cases harboring both mutations are unusual.[84] While EGFR mutation is associated in nonmucinous tumors in nonsmokers, Ki-RAS mutation is often present in mucinous tumors and in smokers, suggesting different carcinogens may affect neoplastic development in tumors harboring the separate mutations.

STK11 (LKB1) *STK11 (LKB1)* encodes a serine-theonine kinase that coordinates a variety of cellular processes including cell polarity, regulation of proliferation, and control of protein synthesis.[333] STK11 is mutated in the germline DNA of patients with Peutz-Jeghers syndrome,[334,335] an hereditary condition that includes melanocytic macules of the lips, multiple gastrointestinal hamartomatous polyps, and an increased risk for various neoplasms, including gastrointestinal cancer and is thus considered a tumor suppressor gene. Approximately 30% of lung adenocarcinomas harbor an inactivating mutation of STK1,[336–338] but mutation is rare in other lung tumor types. Mutations consist of nonsense point mutations and frame shifts all of which predict a truncated protein with an incomplete catalytic domain.[336] Mutational inactivation of SKT11 is frequently associated with mutation of *KRAS*,[337] suggesting synergy between the tumor SKT11 tumor suppressor gene and the *KRAS* oncogene. The full clinical relevance of mutated SKT11 is to be determined and it is not yet clear whether mutation can be a prognostic marker or predictor of response to targeted agents.

***EML4-ALK* Fusion Gene** A new oncogene has recently been discovered that is the result of a small inversion in chromosome 2p.[339] The inversion results in the fusion in opposite orientations of a gene called echinoderm microtubule-associated protein-like 4 (*EML4*) and anaplastic lymphoma kinase (*ALK*), a gene that is also a fusion partner in large cell lymphomas. The new gene was discovered in a complementary DNA (cDNA) expression library created from a patient with NSCLC and was shown to transform T3T fibroblasts. The gene has been detected in 4% of a large series of adenocarcinomas from Japan[340] but not in other tumor types. Emerging data indicates that the mutation is also present in Western tumors at approximately the same frequency and tumors harboring the mutation have a consistent invasive adenocarcinomatous morphology. It seems that oncogenes resulting from rearrangements of tumor

DNA are likely to be frequent and could present therapeutic targets in the future.

High-Throughput Mutational Analysis Finally, the mutations described previously were discovered separately over many years. Recent technical advances have made it possible to rapidly sequence the genome of separate tumors to provide a complete mutational profile of all expressed genes.[338] Recently, this technological approach has been employed to evaluate 188 adenocarcinomas for the presence of mutations in 623 genes with known or potential relationships to cancer. Over 1000 mutations were identified in 163 of the tumors. Mutations were found in 26 genes at a significant frequency. The four most commonly mutated genes unsurprisingly were *p53*, *KRAS*, *STK11*, and *EGFR*. Most of the remaining mutations were point mutations and were present in less than 10% of tumors. Notably, most tumors had more than one mutation and the number of mutations per tumor was significantly higher in smokers (maximum 49) than in nonsmokers (maximum 5) consistent with a higher degree of genetic instability in tumors of smokers. This project identified several new potential targets for therapeutic intervention that will take considerably more time to fully assess than it took to identify them. The relatively low frequency of the mutations suggests that in the future, sequencing of a large number of genes will be required to identify therapeutic targets and that sequencing of single genes may be replaced by high-throughput global sequencing of individual tumor genomes.

Molecular Changes Detectable by In Situ Methods: Immunohistochemistry and Fluorescence In Situ Hybridization IHC and FISH have been used to assess levels molecules that may be therapeutically useful or elucidate the biology of adenocarcinoma. IHC was applied in adenocarcinoma to demonstrate that the expression of the tyrosine kinase receptor, EGFR, is less frequent and more heterogeneous in adenocarcinoma than in squamous carcinoma.[25] EGFR is strongly expressed in nonmucinous BAC (Fig. 22.14) and early anecdotal reports of dramatic responses of tumors with nonmucinous BAC morphology suggested that expression levels of EGFR might predict response to EGFR blockade. However, large subsequent IHC studies have had mixed outcomes with some studies indicating no relationship between EGFR level[341,342] and effectiveness of anti-EGFR treatment but others suggesting improved response in EGFR *positive* non–small cell tumors regardless of histology type.[343,344] Whatever the explanation for this discrepancy, it seems unlikely that EGFR protein level by itself will be a reliable predictive marker but may provide added insight into the biology of adenocarcinoma and, in the proper context, could be of clinical use.

A mechanism for the overexpression of EGFR was elucidated when it was observed and subsequently confirmed that high EGFR gene copy number is associated with overexpression of EGFR protein[345,346] in NSCLC including adenocarcinoma.

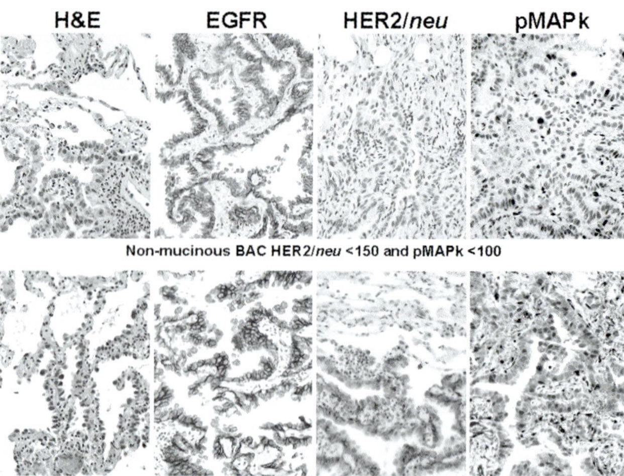

FIGURE 22.14 Immunohistochemical stains of two morphologically similar BAC. Both tumors strongly express EGFR but on the upper tumor sufficient levels of HER-2/*neu* to be visible in immunostains. Activation of intracellular signaling through the mitogen-activated protein (MAP) kinase pathway as reflected in phosphorylated MAPK (pMAPk) immunostaining levels is strongest in the lower tumor. *BAC*, bronchioloalveolar carcinoma; *EGFR*, epidermal growth factor receptor; *H&E*, hematoxylin and eosin; *pMAPk*, phosphorylated MAPK. (See color plate.)

However, EGFR protein overexpression may occur in the absence of high gene copy number and protein level does not therefore predict gene copy number. As reviewed elsewhere in this volume, high EGFR gene copy number has been found to independently predict outcome in patients treated by EGFR blockade.[343,344,347,348]

Many markers have been reported to be related to prognosis in adenocarcinoma including carcinoembryonic antigen (CEA),[349] p53,[331] p27,[350] cyclooxygenase-2 (COX-2),[351] and MIB-1 index (Ki67 labeling) (Fig. 22.13).[352] However, only two markers are significantly correlated with the prognosis of early stage adenocarcinomas including BAC and their clinical impact has been minor to date.

High-Throughput Gene Expression Arrays Heterogeneity in lung cancer histomorphology is now increasingly evident but the first studies to highlight the extent of this striking heterogeneity were molecular. Gene expression array analyses have demonstrated that adenocarcinomas can be divided into several groups, at least one of which has prognostic importance.[96,97,207,353–355] This prognostically important group expresses markers that have been previously associated with neuroendocrine differentiation and has a significantly worse prognosis than other forms of pulmonary adenocarcinoma.

Histogenesis of Central Airway Adenocarcinoma Many aspects of the histogenesis of invasive adenocarcinoma have been discussed under BAC. However, it should be pointed out here that a minority of adenocarcinomas is thought to arise from the bronchial gland or mucosal epithelium. These are endobronchial or central airway lesions that grow as plaques or polyploid lesions frequently with preservation of the overlying epithelium.[356] Histologically, these tumors have acinar or cribriform patterns, such as salivary glandtype adenocarcinoma and occur about 10 years earlier than adenocarcinomas of the peripheral airways.[107] Tumor cells are mostly positive for lactoferrin. The frequency of central adenocarcinoma type is not entirely clear since, in many cases, growth to large size and destruction of tissue around the sites of origin of invasive carcinoma may result in underestimation of the true frequency of this tumor type. These tumors have not been well characterized as to cell of origin and it is possible that they arise from the same central respiratory mucosa as squamous carcinoma and large cell carcinoma.

MESOTHELIOMA

Mesothelioma is a malignant tumor of cells lining the pleural cavity. It is a tumor that results from exposure to asbestos fibers, but other causative factors may be involved in its genesis including exposure to SV-40 virus and radiation. Most patients with mesothelioma present between the ages of 50 and 70 with chest pain and dyspnea and less often with weight loss, cough, or fever.[357] Eighty to ninety-five percent of patients have pleural effusion. The tumor may begin with multiple small lesions on the parietal pleura that later coalesce and encase the lung. Findings associated with a better prognosis include epithelial histology, younger age, absence of pain and weight loss, and good performance status.[358] Median survival in mesothelioma is less than 1 year.[359,360] The poor survival is due to uncontrolled growth of neoplastic mesothelial cells with spread of tumor over pleural surfaces and nodal metastases but distant metastases are infrequent. Death is usually due to respiratory failure and treatment is aimed at local control.

Asbestos and Mesothelioma

Although interstitial lung disease caused by asbestos was recognized at the turn of the 20th century,[361] the carcinogenic properties of asbestos were not appreciated and it was another 60 years before an association between mesothelioma was established.[362]

Since that time, the risk posed by the various types of asbestos has been quantified.[357,363] Asbestos is a group of silicate minerals that form fibers with somewhat variable properties. There are two forms of asbestos, serpentine and amphibole. These two forms are further subdivided. The only form of serpentine asbestos is chrysotile fiber, which is long, curly, and pliable and is more easily broken down and removed from the lungs.[364] It is considered less hazardous than amphibole fibers. Amphibole asbestos is divided into several types including amosite, crocidolite, and anthophyllite, which form short, straight, and stiff fibers that are favored in commercial and industrial processes for their chemical and physical stability. Several forms of nonindustrial asbestos are also found in soils including tremolite, actinolite, and zeolite. Asbestos fibers in lungs of patients with mesothelioma are over 95% amphibole[365] and amphibole exposure is much more likely to result in mesothelioma than chrysotile exposure.[363]

Asbestos exposure may result in several pleural changes that precede mesothelioma including pleural effusion and pleural plaque. Pleural effusion has a peak incidence in the 2nd decade after exposure and pleural plaque progressively increases in frequency from 10 to 50 years after exposure.[366] By contrast, the prevalence of mesothelioma begins to increase approximately 25 years after exposure and continues to increase indefinitely thereafter.[366,367] However, a direct relationship between the benign pleural lesions associated with asbestos exposure and the future occurrence of mesothelioma has not been established.[357]

The prevalence of mesothelioma has increased in parallel with increasing use of asbestos[367] and its occurrence is associated with cumulative exposure.[363] The incidence may be five times higher in heavily exposed workers[368] than in those with low to moderate exposure.[369] However, not all cases are associated with heavy asbestos exposure and the roll of radiation and SV-40 exposure in these patients is currently under study (see succeeding discussion).

Histology of Mesothelioma

Mesothelioma is frequently difficult to diagnose, in part, because it is histologically heterogeneous and, in part, because in well, differentiated cases, it may resemble reactive pleural conditions or adenocarcinoma of lung (Fig. 22.15). Four subtypes of mesothelioma are recognized in the most recent WHO classification,[60] the epithelial, sarcomatoid, desmoplastic, and biphasic. Epithelial mesothelioma shows a pattern of tumor cell growth that resembles that of reactive mesothelium but includes formation

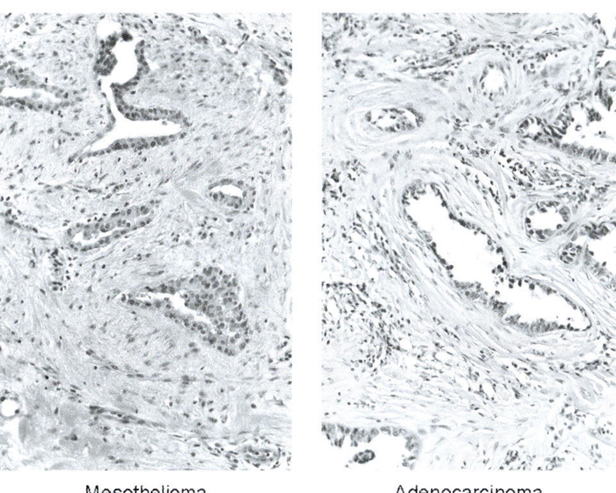

FIGURE 22.15 Histological sections showing similarity between epithelial type mesothelioma and adenocarcinoma. (See color plate.)

of tubules, acini, papillae, or sheets. These tumors invade normal adjacent tissues including fat and skeletal muscle. Fifty percent of mesotheliomas are of this type.[359] Sarcomatoid mesothelioma is composed of malignant spindle cells that resemble sarcoma but may express CKs demonstrable in immunohistochemical tests. This type represents about 16% of mesotheliomas and carries a worse prognosis than the epithelial type.[370] Desmoplastic mesothelioma is defined as a bland-appearing sarcomatoid mesothelioma in which more than 50% of the tumor consists of hypocellular, dense collagenous stroma containing slitlike spaces.[371] Due to its bland appearance, this histological subtype may be a diagnostic challenge for the pathologist and may be misinterpreted as a reactive fibrosing process. The last histological subtype is biphasic mesothelioma, which contains both epithelial and sarcomatoid components and accounts for the remaining 34%.

Cytology of Mesothelioma Cytological specimens are cellular and composed of cells that resemble benign mesothelial cells, but show more atypia, nuclear enlargement, and large cell clusters. Cells show a range of atypia within the same specimen rather than two obvious populations of cells (normal mesothelial cells and malignant cells), as would be seen with involvement by carcinoma. Giant cells and signet ring forms can be seen. The differential diagnosis includes primary or metastatic carcinoma. Thus, a cell block preparation on which immunohistochemical stains can be performed is essential. In some cases, electron microscopy can be applied to cytologic specimens.[372]

Immunohistochemistry of Mesothelioma Mesothelioma may resemble lung carcinoma, especially adenocarcinoma. While in some cases, the clinical, radiographic, and histologic features point to the correct diagnosis, in many cases, mesothelioma cannot be distinguished from carcinoma on purely morphological grounds. The most common diagnostic problem in this regard is distinguishing mesothelioma from epithelial tumors, particularly adenocarcinoma. Several studies testing large numbers of cases with panels of antibodies against candidate markers to distinguish mesothelioma from carcinoma have been reported. In a study by Ordonez,[373] 19 candidate immunohistochemical biomarkers were evaluated on a set of 110 lung tumors including 60 mesotheliomas and 50 adenocarcinomas. Antibodies that proved most sensitive in identifying mesothelioma were those against calretinin (100% sensitivity, 92% specificity), CK5/6 (100% sensitivity, 98% specificity), and WT1 (93% sensitivity, 100% specificity). Antibodies most accurate for identifying adenocarcinoma were TTF-1 (74% sensitivity, 100% specificity), TAG72 (88% sensitivity, 100% specificity), CEA (88% sensitivity, 100% specificity), and CD15 (72% sensitivity, 100% specificity). Another candidate marker recently added to this list is podoplanin, which is recognized by monoclonal antibody D2-40.[374] This marker has nearly 90% sensitivity for epithelioid mesothelioma[375–377] but has low sensitivity for sarcomatoid mesothelioma and cross-reacts with metastatic 65% of serous carcinomas[375] and approximately 15% of squamous carcinomas.[378]

Thus, a substantial list of antibodies is now available with reasonable sensitivity and specificity for distinguishing mesothelioma from other tumors in tissue sections (Table 22.3). It is likely that no single panel will distinguish all mesotheliomas and a small number of poorly differentiated tumors will not be identifiable through IHC. Optimal panels for distinguishing mesothelioma from adenocarcinoma have been suggested[379–381] and most include a limited number of antibodies. Which antibodies are employed in these panels will ultimately depend not only on sensitivity and specificity but also on clinical context and local resources available for addressing this problem as well.

Electron microscopy can also be helpful in the diagnosis of mesothelioma. By electron microscopy, tumor cells have microvilli, which are longer and thinner than those seen in adenocarcinomas, and the length/diameter ratio can be used to favor one tumor versus the other. Of note, electron microscopy is less useful in poorly differentiated epithelial tumors and in sarcomatous tumors.[382]

High-Throughput Gene Expression Arrays Several studies utilizing gene expression microarray technology to evaluate mesothelioma have been published in the past few years.[383,384–387] A substantial gene expression database is available for mining the high-density data that is the product of these studies. The objectives of these studies have been to detect genes that are overexpressed and underexpressed in mesothelioma in comparison to normal tissue, to identify prognostic markers, and to define subsets of genes that predict response to treatment. These studies have constructed gene classifiers that are reported to predict outcome with an accuracy in the range of 68% to 88%.[384,386,387] However, there is little overlap in the genes incorporated into the various classifiers and when compared to clinical predictors such as stage, histology, and *p16* deletion status, no independent or additive predictive value is found.[387] At the present time, therefore, expression microarrays can be regarded as a valuable source of biological data that is not completely explored and does not yet have an established clinical role.

Molecular Correlates The mutations, gene copy number abnormalities, and patterns of protein expression that drive carcinogenesis in epithelial lung tumors are largely absent from mesothelioma. The underlying molecular lesions responsible for uncontrolled tumor cell growth in mesothelioma are not well understood. It is known that asbestos may induce phosphorylation of EGFR[388] stimulating tumor cell growth and spread but *EGFR* mutations commonly present in adenocarcinoma have not been found in mesothelioma.[389] Genes that are overexpressed and may represent activation of growth signal transduction include *hepatocyte growth factor (HGF)*[390] and *notch*,[391] but mutations and structural alterations affecting these genes have not been explored to date. In fact, genomic alterations in mesothelioma are numerous[392] but consistent abnormalities affecting specific genes are not defined.

It has been proposed that reactive oxygen and nitrogen species produced in response to asbestos fibers directly induce DNA damage in mesothelial cells, causing adduct formation and ultimately mutation of important tumor suppressor genes inducing NF2, p15, and p16. In addition, SV-40 sequences have been identified in mesothelioma.[393] SV-40 large T antigen is able to bind RB and p53 protein. Binding of these proteins may result in tumor cell proliferation and chromosomal instability. The role of SV-40 in mesothelioma, however, has yet to be confirmed and clinical consequences of this possible association are not established.

PATHOLOGICAL STAGING OF LUNG CANCER

Pathological staging remains a definitive means of quantifying extent of disease. Staging considerations differ for non–small cell carcinoma and small cell carcinoma and are discussed separately.

Staging of Non–Small Cell Carcinoma Revised staging definitions for NSCLC have recently been compiled by the IASLC and are summarized in Table 22.5. This revision is the result of an international effort involving 46 data sources from 19 countries that began in 1996.[394–398] Data from 67,725 NSCLC patients with 5-year follow-up and complete staging information were analyzed to arrive at the final revision. Changes made in the staging system include refinement of the T-stage criteria, revision of the classification of intrapulmonary multifocal tumor, and stratification of the M category as follows:

1. Analysis of T1 tumors indicated separation of Kaplan-Meier survival curves for tumors less than 2 cm (median survival 103 months) versus tumors between 2 and 3 cm (median survival 124 months). To accommodate this difference, the T stages 1a and 1b were introduced.
2. Analysis of outcome data prompted the reclassification of tumors with separate nodules in the same lobe from the T4 to T3, those with nodules in separate ipsilateral lobes as T4 and those with nodules in the contralateral lung as M1.
3. M1 disease was subdivided into an M1a category that consists of intrathoracic metastases to the contralateral lung or to either pleura and an M1b category that includes distant metastasis.

Details of the changes that are incorporated into the new staging scheme are provided elsewhere.[394–398]

An important component of staging is the assessment of pleural invasion. Assessment of pleural invasion is not always straightforward since tumors may abut the visceral pleura without invading it. Recent studies have indicated that elastic stains may be helpful and in some cases definitive in assessing whether true invasion of the pleura has occurred.[399–403]

If staging is based on pathologic evaluation of lung tissue and LNs, there is generally a migration from lower- to higher-stage disease (Table 22.6). Clinical staging tends to underestimate the extent of disease. It is important to note that the presence of enlarged LNs on CT scanning is not a reliable indicator of metastatic disease within those LNs. The specificity of this finding is only 70%. If enlarged size is taken as equivalent to metastatic disease, significant numbers of patients will be denied surgical therapy who might otherwise benefit. Mediastinoscopy can aid in the staging of these patients.

Staging of Small Cell Carcinoma SCLC is clinically staged as either limited or extensive disease. Limited stage generally refers to those tumors that are confined to the chest including supraclavicular LNs but without pleural effusion. Extensive stage refers to tumors that have metastasized beyond the chest and is equivalent to stage IV in the NSCLC staging system. Combination of chemotherapy and radiation is curative in approximately 10% of limited stage SCLC patients but is rarely curative in extensive stage disease. Limited stage SCLC therefore is initially treated with concurrent chemotherapy and radiation to the site of the primary lesion. This regimen results in more cures but may not be well tolerated. Patients with extensive-stage SCLC are initially treated with chemotherapy alone and radiation therapy is reserved for either resistant or symptomatic disease. It is therefore important for proper choice of treatment that SCLC be properly staged both clinically and pathologically.

MICROMETASTATIC DISEASE

Despite apparently complete surgical resection, patients without detectable metastases have a 40% rate of relapse within 24 months. Furthermore, this group has an overall 5-year survival rate of roughly 60%. These numbers indicate that NSCLC disseminates early in its progression and causes significant mortality. Conventional histological sections may not be sufficiently sensitive to detect small numbers of tumor cells in regional LNs or distant tissue, such as bone marrow. By most accounts, a micrometastasis is defined as less than 0.2 cm in size, although many studies include much smaller cell clusters and even single tumor cells as micrometastasis. Several studies have suggested that micrometastatic disease may be efficiently detected by IHC. NSCLC tumor cells have been detected in up to 45%[404] of histologically negative LNs and 60% of histologically negative bone marrows.[405] Antibodies used tumor cell

TABLE 22.5 Pathologic Tumor-Node-Metastasis Staging for Lung Cancer with Proposed Changes (*Italics*)

Descriptor			Definition
Tumor (T)	T0		No tumor
	TX		Positive sputum or bronchial cytology, no apparent tumor
	TIS		Carcinoma in situ
	T1		≤3 cm in greatest dimension, surrounded by lung or visceral pleura, without bronchoscopic evidence of invasion more proximal than lobar bronchus (i.e., not in the main bronchus)
		T1a	*Tumor ≤2 cm diameter; no visceral pleural or lobar bronchial involvement*
		T1b	*Tumor ≤3 cm diameter; no visceral pleural or lobar bronchial involvement*
	T2		Tumor >3 cm but ≤7 cm or involve main bronchus ≥2 cm distal to carina or visceral pleura; or with hilar obstructive pneumonitis or atelectasis
		T2a	*T2a Tumor >3 cm but ≤5 cm in greatest dimension*
		T2b	*>5 cm but ≤7 cm in greatest dimension*
	T3		>7 cm or invades chest wall (including superior sulcus tumors), diaphragm, phrenic nerve, mediastinal pleura, parietal pericardium; or tumor in main bronchus <2 cm distal to the carina but without involvement of carina; or associated atelectasis or obstructive pneumonitis of entire lung; *or separate tumor nodule(s) in the same lobe*
	T4		Invades mediastinum, heart, great vessels, trachea, recurrent laryngeal nerve, esophagus, carina, or vertebrae; or *separate tumor nodule(s) in different ipsilateral lobe*
Nodes (N)	NX		Not assessed
	N0		No LN involvement
	N1		Ipsilateral peribronchial, hilar, or intrapulmonary node(s)
	N2		Ipsilateral mediastinal or subcarinal node(s)
	N3		Contralateral mediastinal or hilar nodes; any supraclavicular or scalene nodes
Metastasis (M)	MX		Not assessed
	M0		No distant metastasis
	M1		Distant metastasis
		M1a	*Separate nodule(s) in a contralateral lobe; pleural nodules or malignant pleural (or pericardial) effusion*
		M1b	*Distant metastasis*
Grade (G)	GX		Not assessed
	G1		Well differentiated
	G2		Moderately differentiated
	G3		Poorly differentiated
	G4		Undifferentiated
Lymphatic Invasion	LX		Not assessed
	L0		Lymphatic invasion absent
	L1		Lymphatic invasion present
Vascular Invasion	VX		Not assessed
	V0		Vascular invasion absent
	V1		Vascular invasion present

detection have included BerEP4, AE1/AE3, p53,[404,406] and CK2.[405,406] Patients with IHC detectable NSCLC in LNs and bone marrow show an increased risk for both relapse and shortened survival times.[404,407] However, whether IHC improves tumor cell detection sensitivity significantly beyond careful LN sectioning and thorough H&E evaluation is still debated.[408] Micrometastases do not have a specific designation in the current or revised staging systems. Whether patients diagnosed with micrometastatic disease could benefit from postoperative adjuvant chemotherapy and/or immunotherapy therapy is yet to be determined.

Reverse transcriptase-polymerase chain reaction (RT-PCR) has also been evaluated as a method of detecting micrometastases and has been shown to be more sensitive than routine H&E.[409] However, both false-positive and false-negative results may occur. Correlation with histology to verify malignant

TABLE 22.6 Outcomes by Clinical Stage in Comparison to Pathology Stage

Stage	Definition	5-Year Survival Clinical Stage	5-Year Survival Pathology Stage
IA	T1 N0 M0	61%	67%
IB	T2 N0 M0	38%	57%
IIA	T1 N1 M0	34%	55%
IIB	T2 N1 M0	24%	39%
	T3 N0 M0		
IIIA	T1 N2 M0	13%	23%
	T2 N2 M0		
	T3 N1 M0		
	T3 N2 M0		
IIIB	T1–3 N3 M0	<5%	
	T4 Any N M0		
IV	Any T, Any N, M1	~1%	

cytology, and use of more than one marker may be helpful.[409,410] In one study by Xi et al.,[411] 39 benign LNs and 38 tumor LNs were evaluated by screening for a panel of six markers by RT-PCR, resulting in a combination of three markers (SFTPB, TACSTD1, PVA), which provided the best classification of benign and malignant LNs. Such panels may increase the accuracy of this method.[411]

Micrometastatic tumor has been evaluated intraoperatively using intratumoral injections of color markers or radioactive isotope (technetium-99m) to detect grossly inapparent tumor in thoracic LNs (sentinel nodes). To date, results of these procedures have been promising[412–416] but controlled trials have not been reported, and clinical benefit has not been demonstrated. It is also not yet clear how positron emission tomography (PET) and PET/CT imaging, which improve the sensitivity of radiological staging procedures,[417–419] will affect the need to perform sentinel node sampling.

MOLECULAR STAGING

Increasing understanding of the biology of specific tumor types and the availability of targeted therapies have prompted detailed molecular assessment of tumors and other biospecimens not only for diagnostic purposes but also to assess treatment strategies as well. Genomic analysis by gene expression array is already being used in the treatment of breast cancer, for example, and similar methods are being developed to assess recurrence or predict response to therapy of lung cancer patients. Potti et al.,[105] for example, studied 89 early stage NSCLC by Affymetrix microarray, using a lung metagene model to analyze numerous gene expression profiles that predict recurrence. The gene expression data predicted recurrence better than clinical data.[105] More recently, Taguchi et al.[107] in a multi-institutional proteomic study discovered eight distinct mass/charge ratios that identified patients likely to respond to tyrosine kinase inhibitors (TKIs). The features were not predictive of response to standard chemotherapy. This is a promising study in that it was able to show reproducible results between institutions and suggests that it may not be necessary to directly sample tumor to predict response to targeted agents. Continued progress in this area of investigation could potentially alter the approach to treatment selection in lung carcinoma.

THE PATHOLOGY REPORT

Despite the importance of the pathological diagnosis in lung cancer until recently, the surgical pathology report was not standardized and was left to the discretion of individual pathologists. The increasing standardization of diagnoses and requirements for specific information by clinicians, clinical trial administrators, billing personnel, and statistical/epidemiological workers has resulted in development of guidelines for the reporting of pathological diagnoses by several organizations.[420,421] A summary of the information that can be reasonably expected to appear on an adequate pathology report is listed in Table 22.7.

TABLE 22.7 Checklist for Lung Cancer Pathology Report

1 Patient and specimen identifiers (forms, labels)
2 Type procedure performed to generate specimen
3 Fixation, processing (formalin, frozen, etc.)
4 Part of lung removed (bronchial site, lobe, lung)
5 Tumor size (preferably three dimensions)
6 Bronchus of origin
7 Distance from closest pleural margin
8 Pleural puckering
9 Distance from closest bronchial margin
10 Histological type (WHO classification)
11 Histological grade
12 Special procedures (immunohistochemistry, electron microscopy, etc.)
13 Other lesions in lung (2nd tumor, pneumonia, emphysema, clots, etc.)
14 LNs location
15 LNs positive
16 LNs negative
17 Invasion of other intrathoracic structures
18 Submitted metastasis
19 Pathology stage (pTNM, stage grouping)

Appendix A. World Health Organization Classification of Lung Cancer

Tumor Type	Code*
MALIGNANT EPITHELIAL TUMORS	
Squamous cell carcinoma	8070/3
Variants:	
Papillary	8052/3
Clear cell	8084/3
Small cell	8073/3
Basaloid	8083/3
Small cell carcinoma	8041/3
Variant:	
Combined small cell carcinoma	8045/3
Adenocarcinoma	8140/3
Adenocarcinoma, mixed subtype	8255/3
Acinar adenocarcinoma	8550/3
Papillary adenocarcinoma	8260/3
Bronchioloalveolar carcinoma	8250/3
Nonmucinous	8252/3
Mucinous	8253/3
Mixed nonmucinous and mucinous or indeterminate	8254/3
Solid adenocarcinoma with mucin production	8230/3
Variants:	
Fetal adenocarcinoma	8333/3
Mucinous ("colloid") carcinoma	8480/3
Mucinous cystadenocarcinoma	8470/3
Signet ring adenocarcinoma	8490/3
Clear cell adenocarcinoma	8310/3
Large cell carcinoma	8012/3
Variants:	
Large cell neuroendocrine carcinoma	8013/3
Combined large cell neuroendocrine carcinoma	8013/3
Basaloid carcinoma	8123/3
Lymphoepithelioma-like carcinoma	8082/3
Clear cell carcinoma	8310/3
Large cell carcinoma with rhabdoid phenotype	8014/3
Adenosquamous carcinoma	8560/3
Sarcomatoid carcinoma	8033/3
Pleomorphic carcinoma	8022/3
Spindle cell carcinoma	8032/3
Giant cell carcinoma	8031/3
Carcinosarcoma	8980/3
Pulmonary blastoma	8972/3
Carcinoid Tumor	8240/3
Typical carcinoid	8240/3
Atypical carcinoid	8249/3
Salivary Gland Tumors	
Mucoepidermoid carcinoma	8430/3
Adenoid cystic carcinoma	8200/3
Epithelial-myoepithelial carcinoma	8562/3
PREINVASIVE LESIONS	
Squamous carcinoma in situ	8070/2
Atypical adenomatous hyperplasia	
Diffuse idiopathic pulmonary neuroendocrine cell Hyperplasia	
MESENCHYMAL TUMORS	
Epithelioid hemangioendothelioma	9133/1
/Angiosarcoma	9120/3
Pleuropulmonary blastoma	11012
Chondroma	9220/0
Congenital peribronchial myofibroblastic tumor	8827/1
Diffuse pulmonary lymphangiomatosis	
Inflammatory myofibroblastic tumor	8825/1
Lymphangioleiomyomatosis	9174/1
Synovial sarcoma	9040/3
Monophasic	9041/3
Biphasic	9043/3
Pulmonary artery sarcoma	8800/3
Pulmonary vein sarcoma	8800/3
BENIGN EPITHELIAL TUMORS	
Papillomas	
Squamous cell papilloma	8052/0
Exophytic	8052/0
Inverted	8053/0
Glandular papillomas	8260/0
Mixed squamous cell and glandular papilloma	8560/0
Adenomas	
Alveolar adenoma	8251/0
Papillary adenoma	8260/0
Adenomas of the salivary gland type	
Mucous gland adenoma	8140/0
Pleomorphic adenoma	8940/0
Others	
Mucinous cystadenoma	8470/0

Appendix A. World Health Organization Classification of Lung Cancer *(continued)*

Tumor Type	Code*	Tumor Type	Code*
LYMPHOPROLIFERATIVE TUMORS		Clear cell tumor	8005/0
Marginal zone B-cell lymphoma of the mucosa-associated lymphoid tissue (MALT) type	9699/3	Germ cell tumors	
		Teratoma, mature	9080/0
Diffuse large B-cell lymphoma	9680/3	immature	9080/3
Lymphomatoid granulomatosis	9766/1	Other germ cell tumors	
Langerhans cell histiocytosis	9751/1	Intrapulmonary thymoma	8580/1
		Melanoma	8720/3
MISCELLANEOUS TUMORS			
Hamartoma		**METASTATIC TUMORS**	
Sclerosing hemangioma	8832/0	**UNCLASSIFIED TUMORS**	

*Morphology code of the International Classification of Diseases for Oncology (ICD-O) and the Systematized Nomenclature of Medicine (SNOMED).

REFERENCES

1. Travis WD, Muller-Hermelink, HK, Harris CC, et al. Pathology and genetics of tumours of the lung, pleura, thymus and heart. *World Health Organization Classification of Tumours: Pathology and Genetics.* Lyon: IARC Press. WHO Blue Books, 2004.
2. Auerbach O, Stout AP, Hammond EC, et al. Changes in bronchial epithelium in relation to sex, age, residence, smoking and pneumonia. *N Engl J Med* 1962;267(3):111–119.
3. Auerbach O, Stout AP, Hammond EC, et al. Bronchial epithelium in former smokers. *N Engl J Med* 1962;267(3):119–125.
4. Mitchell MF, Tortolero-Luna G, Wright T, et al. Cervical human papillomavirus infection and intraepithelial neoplasia: a review. *J Natl Cancer Inst Monogr* 1996;(21):17–25.
5. Bond JH. Colorectal cancer update. Prevention, screening, treatment, and surveillance for high-risk groups. *Med Clin North Am* 2000;84:1163–1182.
6. Marcus PM, Bergstralh EJ, Fagerstrom RM, et al. Lung cancer mortality in the Mayo Lung Project: impact of extended follow-up. *J Natl Cancer Inst* 2000;92:1308–1316.
7. Parkin DM, Moss SM. Lung cancer screening: improved survival but no reduction in deaths—the role of "overdiagnosis." *Cancer* 2000;89: 2369–2376.
8. Marcus PM. Lung cancer screening: an update. *J Clin Oncol* 2001;19: S83–S86.
9. Bach PB. Is our natural-history model of lung cancer wrong? *Lancet Oncol* 2008;9:693–697.
10. Colby TV, Tazelaar HD, Travis WD, et al. Pathologic review of the Mayo Lung Project. Is there a case for misdiagnosis or overdiagnosis of lung carcinoma in the screened group? *Cancer* 2002;95:2361–2365.
11. Prindiville SA, Byers T, Hirsch FR, et al. Sputum cytological atypia as a predictor of incident lung cancer in a cohort of heavy smokers with airflow obstruction. *Cancer Epidemiol Biomarkers Prev* 2003;12:987–993.
12. Byers T, Wolf HJ, Franklin WA, et al. Sputum cytologic atypia predicts incident lung cancer: defining latency and histologic specificity. *Cancer Epidemiol Biomarkers Prev* 2008;17:158–162.
13. Hirsch FR, Prindiville SA, Miller YE, et al. Fluorescence versus white-light bronchoscopy for detection of preneoplastic lesions: a randomized study. *J Natl Cancer Inst* 2001;93:1385–1391.
14. Kennedy TC, McWilliams A, Edell E, et al. Bronchial intraepithelial neoplasia/early central airways lung cancer: ACCP evidence-based clinical practice guidelines (2nd edition). *Chest* 2007;132(3 Suppl): S221–S233.
15. Nicholson AG, Perry LJ, Cury PM, et al. Reproducibility of the WHO/IASLC grading system for pre-invasive squamous lesions of the bronchus: a study of inter-observer and intra-observer variation. *Histopathology* 2001;38:202–208.
16. Keith RL, Miller YE, Gemmill RM, et al. Angiogenic squamous dysplasia in bronchi of individuals at high risk for lung cancer. *Clin Cancer Res* 2000;6:1616–1625.
17. Keith RL, Miller YE, Kennedy TC, et al. Angiogenic squamous dysplasia (ASD): a biomarker highly associated with squamous cell lung carcinoma. *Lung Cancer* 2003;41(Suppl 2):S161.
18. Venmans BJ, van Boxem TJ, Smit EF, et al. Outcome of bronchial carcinoma in situ. *Chest* 2000;117:1572–1576.
19. Jonsson S, Varella-Garcia M, Miller YE, et al. Chromosomal aneusomy in bronchial high-grade lesions is associated with invasive lung cancer. *Am J Respir Crit Care Med* 2008;177:342–347.
20. Nagamoto N, Saito Y, Sato M, et al. Clinicopathological analysis of 19 cases of isolated carcinoma in situ of the bronchus. *Am J Surg Pathol* 1993;17:1234–1243.
21. Wang GF, Lai MD, Yang RR, et al. Histological types and significance of bronchial epithelial dysplasia. *Mod Pathol* 2006;19:429–437.
22. Wiest JS, Franklin WA, Drabkin H, et al. Genetic markers for early detection of lung cancer and outcome measures for response to chemoprevention. *J Cell Biochem Suppl* 1997;28–29:64–73.
23. Rusch V, Klimstra D, Linkov I, et al. Aberrant expression of p53 or the epidermal growth factor receptor is frequent in early bronchial neoplasia and coexpression precedes squamous cell carcinoma development. *Cancer Res* 1995;55:1365–1372.
24. Merrick DT, Kittelson J, Winterhalder R, et al. Analysis of c-ErbB1/epidermal growth factor receptor and c-ErbB2/HER-2 expression in bronchial dysplasia: evaluation of potential targets for chemoprevention of lung cancer. *Clin Cancer Res* 2006;12:2281–2288.
25. Franklin WA, Veve R, Hirsch FR, et al. Epidermal growth factor receptor family in lung cancer and premalignancy. *Semin Oncol* 2002;29:3–14.
26. Hirsch FR, Scagliotti GV, Langer CJ, et al. Epidermal growth factor family of receptors in preneoplasia and lung cancer: perspectives for targeted therapies. *Lung Cancer* 2003;41(Suppl 1):S29–S42.
27. Meert AP, Feoli F, Martin B, et al. Ki67 expression in bronchial preneoplastic lesions and carcinoma in situ defined according to the new 1999 WHO/IASLC criteria: a preliminary study. *Histopathology* 2004;44:47–53.
28. Hittelman WN, Liu DD, Kurie JM, et al. Proliferative changes in the bronchial epithelium of former smokers treated with retinoids. *J Natl Cancer Inst* 2007;99:1603–1612.

29. Orita H, Coulter J, Tully E, et al. Inhibiting fatty acid synthase for chemoprevention of chemically induced lung tumors. *Clin Cancer Res* 2008;14:2458–2464.
30. Tan DF, Huberman JA, Hyland A, et al. MCM2—a promising marker for premalignant lesions of the lung: a cohort study. *BMC Cancer* 2001;1:6.
31. Sozzi G, Pastorino U, Moiraghi L, et al. Loss of FHIT function in lung cancer and preinvasive bronchial lesions. *Cancer Res* 1998;58:5032–5037.
32. Brambilla E, Gazzeri S, Moro D, et al. Alterations of Rb pathway (Rb-p16INK4-cyclin D1) in preinvasive bronchial lesions. *Clin Cancer Res* 1999;5:243–250.
33. Kato Y, Hirano T, Yoshida K, et al. Frequent loss of E-cadherin and/or catenins in intrabronchial lesions during carcinogenesis of the bronchial epithelium. *Lung Cancer* 2005;48:323–230.
34. Boers JE, ten Velde GP, Thunnissen FB. P53 in squamous metaplasia: a marker for risk of respiratory tract carcinoma. *Am J Respir Crit Care Med* 1996;153:411–416.
35. Ratschiller D, Heighway J, Gugger M, et al. Cyclin D1 overexpression in bronchial epithelia of patients with lung cancer is associated with smoking and predicts survival. *J Clin Oncol* 2003;21:2085–2093.
36. Jeanmart M, Lantuejoul S, Fievet F, et al. Value of immunohistochemical markers in preinvasive bronchial lesions in risk assessment of lung cancer. *Clin Cancer Res* 2003;9:2195–2203.
37. Jeanmart M, Lantejoul S, Fievet F, et al. Value of immunohistochemical markers in preinvasive bronchial lesions in risk assessment of lung cancer. *Clin Cancer Res* 2003;9:2195–2203.
38. Pendleton N, Dixon GR, Burnett HE, et al. Expression of proliferating cell nuclear antigen (PCNA) in dysplasia of the bronchial epithelium. *J Pathol* 1993;170:169–172.
39. Hecht SS. Cigarette smoking and lung cancer: chemical mechanisms and approaches to prevention. *Lancet Oncol* 2002;3:461–469.
40. Pfeifer GP, Denissenko MF, Olivier M, et al. Tobacco smoke carcinogens, DNA damage and p53 mutations in smoking-associated cancers. *Oncogene* 2002;21:7435–7451.
41. Wiencke JK. DNA adduct burden and tobacco carcinogenesis. *Oncogene* 2002;21:7376–7391.
42. Zochbauer-Muller S, Gazdar AF, Minna JD. Molecular pathogenesis of lung cancer. *Annu Rev Physiol* 2002;64:681–708.
43. Girard L, Zochbauer-Muller S, Virmani AK, et al. Genome-wide allelotyping of lung cancer identifies new regions of allelic loss, differences between small cell lung cancer and non-small cell lung cancer, and loci clustering. *Cancer Res* 2000;60:4894–4906.
44. Franklin WA, Hirsch FR. Molecular and cell biology of lung carcinoma. In: Sculier JP, Fry WA, eds. *Malignant Tumors of the Lung*. 1st Ed. New York: Springer, 2003:3–27.
45. Wistuba II, Behrens C, Virmani AK, et al. High resolution chromosome 3p allelotyping of human lung cancer and preneoplastic/preinvasive bronchial epithelium reveals multiple, discontinuous sites of 3p allele loss and three regions of frequent breakpoints. *Cancer Res* 2000;60:1949–1960.
46. Wistuba II, Behrens C, Milchgrub S, et al. Sequential molecular abnormalities are involved in the multistage development of squamous cell lung carcinoma. *Oncogene* 1999;18:643–650.
47. Varella-Garcia M, Gemmill RM, Rabenhorst SH, et al. Chromosomal duplication accompanies allelic loss in non-small cell lung carcinoma. *Cancer Res* 1998;58:4701–4707.
48. Smith AL, Hung J, Walker L, et al. Extensive areas of aneuploidy are present in the respiratory epithelium of lung cancer patients. *Br J Cancer* 1996;73:203–209.
49. Romeo MS, Sokolova IA, Morrison LE, et al. Chromosomal abnormalities in non-small cell lung carcinomas and in bronchial epithelia of high-risk smokers detected by multi-target interphase fluorescence in situ hybridization. *J Mol Diagn* 2003;5:103–112.
50. Taguchi T, Zhou JY, Feder M, et al. Detection of aneuploidy in interphase nuclei from non-small cell lung carcinomas by fluorescence in situ hybridization using chromosome-specific repetitive DNA probes. *Cancer Genet Cytogenet* 1996;89:120–125.
51. Balsara BR, Testa JR. Chromosomal imbalances in human lung cancer. *Oncogene* 2002;21:6877–6883.
52. Testa JR, Siegfried JM. Chromosome abnormalities in human non-small cell lung cancer. *Cancer Res* 1992;52(9 Suppl):S2702–S2706.
53. Schenk T, Ackermann J, Brunner C, et al. Detection of chromosomal aneuploidy by interphase fluorescence in situ hybridization in bronchoscopically gained cells from lung cancer patients. *Chest* 1997;111:1691–1696.
54. Haruki N, Harano T, Masuda A, et al. Persistent increase in chromosome instability in lung cancer: possible indirect involvement of p53 inactivation. *Am J Pathol* 2001;159:1345–1352.
55. Luk C, Tsao MS, Bayani J, et al. Molecular cytogenetic analysis of non-small cell lung carcinoma by spectral karyotyping and comparative genomic hybridization. *Cancer Genet Cytogenet* 2001;125:87–99.
56. Borczuk AC, Gorenstein L, Walter KL, et al. Non-small-cell lung cancer molecular signatures recapitulate lung developmental pathways. *Am J Pathol* 2003;163:1949–1960.
57. Watkins DN, Berman DM, Burkholder SG, et al. Hedgehog signalling within airway epithelial progenitors and in small-cell lung cancer. *Nature* 2003;422:313–317.
58. Khuder SA. Effect of cigarette smoking on major histological types of lung cancer: a meta-analysis. *Lung Cancer* 2001;31:139–148.
59. Wahbah M, Boroumand N, Castro C, et al. Changing trends in the distribution of the histologic types of lung cancer: a review of 4,439 cases. *Ann Diagn Pathol* 2007;11:89–96.
60. Travis WD, Colby TV, Corrin B, et al. Histological typing of tumours of lung and pleura. In: Sobin LH. *World Health Organization International Classification of Tumours*. Berlin, Heidelberg, New York: Springer-Verlag.
61. DeMay RM. *The Art and Science of Cytopathology*. Chicago: ASCP Press, 1996:209.
62. Rivera MP, Detterbeck F, Mehta AC. Diagnosis of lung cancer: the guidelines. *Chest* 2003;123(1 Suppl):S129–S136.
63. Risse EK, van't Hof MA, Vooijs GP. Relationship between patient characteristics and the sputum cytologic diagnosis of lung cancer. *Acta Cytol* 1987;31:159–165.
64. Sandler A, Gray R, Perry MC, et al. Paclitaxel-carboplatin alone or with bevacizumab for non-small-cell lung cancer. *N Engl J Med* 2006;355:2542–2550.
65. Scagliotti GV, Parikh P, von Pawel J, et al. Phase III study comparing cisplatin plus gemcitabine with cisplatin plus pemetrexed in chemotherapy-naive patients with advanced-stage non-small-cell lung cancer. *J Clin Oncol* 2008;26:3543–3551.
66. Moll R, Franke WW, Schiller DL, et al. The catalog of human cytokeratins: patterns of expression in normal epithelia, tumors and cultured cells. *Cell* 1982;31:11–24.
67. Fuchs E, Cleveland DW. A structural scaffolding of intermediate filaments in health and disease. *Science* 1998;279:514–519.
68. Chu PG, Weiss LM. Keratin expression in human tissues and neoplasms. *Histopathology* 2002;40:403–439.
69. Ordonez NG. The diagnostic utility of immunohistochemistry in distinguishing between epithelioid mesotheliomas and squamous carcinomas of the lung: a comparative study. *Mod Pathol* 2006;19:417–428.
70. Camilo R, Capelozzi VL, Siqueira SA, et al. Expression of p63, keratin 5/6, keratin 7, and surfactant-A in non-small cell lung carcinomas. *Hum Pathol* 2006;37:542–546.
71. Kargi A, Gurel D, Tuna B. The diagnostic value of TTF-1, CK 5/6, and p63 immunostaining in classification of lung carcinomas. *Appl Immunohistochem Mol Morphol* 2007;15:415–420.
72. Ordonez NG. Value of cytokeratin 5/6 immunostaining in distinguishing epithelial mesothelioma of the pleura from lung adenocarcinoma. *Am J Surg Pathol* 1998;22:1215–1221.
73. Chu PG, Weiss LM. Expression of cytokeratin 5/6 in epithelial neoplasms: an immunohistochemical study of 509 cases. *Mod Pathol* 2002;15:6–10.
74. Au NH, Cheang M, Huntsman DG, et al. Evaluation of immunohistochemical markers in non-small cell lung cancer by unsupervised hierarchical clustering analysis: a tissue microarray study of 284 cases and 18 markers. *J Pathol* 2004;204:101–109.

75. Lyda MH, Weiss LM. Immunoreactivity for epithelial and neuroendocrine antibodies are useful in the differential diagnosis of lung carcinomas. *Hum Pathol* 2000;31:980–987.
76. Chu P, Wu E, Weiss LM. Cytokeratin 7 and cytokeratin 20 expression in epithelial neoplasms: a survey of 435 cases. *Mod Pathol* 2000;13:962–972.
77. Jerome Marson V, Mazieres J, Groussard O, et al. Expression of TTF-1 and cytokeratins in primary and secondary epithelial lung tumours: correlation with histological type and grade. *Histopathology* 2004;45:125–134.
78. Massion PP, Taflan PM, Jamshedur Rahman SM, et al. Significance of p63 amplification and overexpression in lung cancer development and prognosis. *Cancer Res* 2003;63:7113–7121.
79. Wang BY, Gil J, Kaufman D, et al. P63 in pulmonary epithelium, pulmonary squamous neoplasms, and other pulmonary tumors. *Hum Pathol* 2002;33:921–926.
80. Au NH, Gown AM, Cheang M, et al. L. P63 expression in lung carcinoma: a tissue microarray study of 408 cases. *Appl Immunohistochem Mol Morphol* 2004;12:240–247.
81. Pelosi G, Pasini F, Olsen Stenholm C, et al. p63 immunoreactivity in lung cancer: yet another player in the development of squamous cell carcinomas? *J Pathol* 2002;198:100–109.
82. Downey P, Cummins R, Moran M, et al. If it's not CK5/6 positive, TTF-1 negative it's not a squamous cell carcinoma of lung. *APMIS* 2008;116:526–529.
83. Kalhor N, Zander DS, Liu J. TTF-1 and p63 for distinguishing pulmonary small-cell carcinoma from poorly differentiated squamous cell carcinoma in previously pap-stained cytologic material. *Mod Pathol* 2006;19:1117–1123.
84. Shigematsu H, Lin L, Takahashi T, et al. Clinical and biological features associated with epidermal growth factor receptor gene mutations in lung cancers. *J Natl Cancer Inst* 2005;97:339–346.
85. Tsao AS, Tang XM, Sabloff B, et al. Clinicopathologic characteristics of the EGFR gene mutation in non-small cell lung cancer. *J Thorac Oncol* 2006;1:231–239.
86. Sengupta S, Harris CC. p53: traffic cop at the crossroads of DNA repair and recombination. *Nat Rev Mol Cell Biol* 2005;6:44–55.
87. Greenblatt MS, Bennett WP, Hollstein M, et al. Mutations in the p53 tumor suppressor gene: clues to cancer etiology and molecular pathogenesis. *Cancer Res* 1994;54:4855–4878.
88. Mitsudomi T, Hamajima N, Ogawa M, et al. Prognostic significance of p53 alterations in patients with non-small cell lung cancer: a meta-analysis. *Clin Cancer Res* 2000;6:4055–4063.
89. Cairns P, Polascik TJ, Eby Y, et al. Frequency of homozygous deletion at p16/CDKN2 in primary human tumours. *Nat Genet* 1995;11:210–212.
90. Kamb A, Gruis NA, Weaver-Feldhaus J, et al. A cell cycle regulator potentially involved in genesis of many tumor types. *Science* 1994;264:436–140.
91. Belinsky SA, Nikula KJ, Palmisano WA, et al. Aberrant methylation of p16(INK4a) is an early event in lung cancer and a potential biomarker for early diagnosis. *Proc Natl Acad Sci U S A* 1998;95:11891–11896.
92. Toyooka S, Toyooka KO, Maruyama R, et al. DNA methylation profiles of lung tumors. *Mol Cancer Ther* 2001;1:61–67.
93. Brock MV, Hooker CM, Ota-Machida E, et al. DNA methylation markers and early recurrence in stage I lung cancer. *N Engl J Med* 2008;358:1118–1128.
94. Geradts J, Fong KM, Zimmerman PV, et al. Correlation of abnormal RB, p16ink4a, and p53 expression with 3p loss of heterozygosity, other genetic abnormalities, and clinical features in 103 primary non-small cell lung cancers. *Clin Cancer Res* 1999;5:791–800.
95. Burke L, Flieder DB, Guinee DG, et al. Prognostic implications of molecular and immunohistochemical profiles of the Rb and p53 cell cycle regulatory pathways in primary non-small cell lung carcinoma. *Clin Cancer Res* 2005;11:232–241.
96. Bhattacharjee A, Richards WG, Staunton J, et al. Classification of human lung carcinomas by mRNA expression profiling reveals distinct adenocarcinoma subclasses. *Proc Natl Acad Sci U S A* 2001;98:13790–13795.
97. Garber ME, Troyanskaya OG, Schluens K, et al. Diversity of gene expression in adenocarcinoma of the lung. *Proc Natl Acad Sci U S A* 2001;98:13784–13789.
98. Barash Y, Dehan E, Krupsky M, et al. Comparative analysis of algorithms for signal quantitation from oligonucleotide microarrays. *Bioinformatics* 2004;20:839–846.
99. Sugita M, Geraci M, Gao B, et al. Combined use of oligonucleotide and tissue microarrays identifies cancer/testis antigens as biomarkers in lung carcinoma. *Cancer Res* 2002;62:3971–3979.
100. Atanackovic D, Altorki NK, Cao Y, et al. Booster vaccination of cancer patients with MAGE-A3 protein reveals long-term immunological memory or tolerance depending on priming. *Proc Natl Acad Sci U S A* 2008;105:1650–1655.
101. Vansteenkiste JF, Zielinski M, Dahabreh IJ, et al. Association of gene expression signature and clinical efficacy of MAGE-A3 antigen-specific cancer immunotherapeutic (ASCI) as adjuvant therapy in resected stage IB/II non-small cell lung cancer (NSCLC). *J Clin Oncol* 2008;26:7501.
102. Raponi M, Zhang Y, Yu J, et al. Gene expression signatures for predicting prognosis of squamous cell and adenocarcinomas of the lung. *Cancer Res* 2006;66:7466–7472.
103. Riedel RF, Porrello A, Pontzer E, et al. A genomic approach to identify molecular pathways associated with chemotherapy resistance. *Mol Cancer Ther* 2008;7:3141–3149.
104. Minna JD, Girard L, Xie Y. Tumor mRNA expression profiles predict responses to chemotherapy. *J Clin Oncol* 2007;25:4329–4336.
105. Potti A, Mukherjee S, Petersen R, et al. A genomic strategy to refine prognosis in early-stage non-small-cell lung cancer. *N Engl J Med* 2006;355:570–580.
106. Coldren CD, Helfrich BA, Witta SE, et al. Baseline gene expression predicts sensitivity to gefitinib in non-small cell lung cancer cell lines. *Mol Cancer Res* 2006;4:521–528.
107. Taguchi F, Solomon B, Gregorc V, et al. Mass spectrometry to classify non-small-cell lung cancer patients for clinical outcome after treatment with epidermal growth factor receptor tyrosine kinase inhibitors: a multicohort cross-institutional study. *J Natl Cancer Inst* 2007;99:838–846.
108. Travis WD, Travis LB, Devesa SS. Lung cancer. *Cancer* 1995;75:191–202.
109. Tamboli P, Toprani TH, Amin MB, et al. Carcinoma of lung with rhabdoid features. *Hum Pathol* 2004;35:8–13.
110. Chetty R, Bhana B, Batitang S, et al. Lung carcinomas composed of rhabdoid cells. *Eur J Surg Oncol* 1997;23:432–434.
111. Shimazaki H, Aida S, Sato M, et al. Lung carcinoma with rhabdoid cells: a clinicopathological study and survival analysis of 14 cases. *Histopathology* 2001;38:425–434.
112. Hiroshima K, Shibuya K, Shimamura F, et al. Pulmonary large cell carcinoma with rhabdoid phenotype. *Ultrastruct Pathol* 2003;27:55–59.
113. Ho JC, Wong MP, Lam WK. Lymphoepithelioma-like carcinoma of the lung. *Respirology* 2006;11:539–545.
114. Ho JC, Lam WK, Wong MP, et al. Lymphoepithelioma-like carcinoma of the lung: experience with ten cases. *Int J Tuberc Lung Dis* 2004;8:890–895.
115. Chow LT, Chow WH, Tsui WM, et al. Fine-needle aspiration cytologic diagnosis of lymphoepithelioma-like carcinoma of the lung. Report of two cases with immunohistochemical study. *Am J Clin Pathol* 1995;103:35–40.
116. Chan AT, Teo PM, Lam KC, et al. Multimodality treatment of primary lymphoepithelioma-like carcinoma of the lung. *Cancer* 1998;83:925–929.
117. Hekelaar N, van Uffelen R, van Vliet AC, et al. Primary lymphoepithelioma-like carcinoma within an intralobular pulmonary sequestration. *Eur Respir J* 2000;16:1025–1027.
118. Han AJ, Xiong M, Gu YY, et al. Lymphoepithelioma-like carcinoma of the lung with a better prognosis. A clinicopathologic study of 32 cases. *Am J Clin Pathol* 2001;115:841–850.
119. Brambilla E, Moro D, Veale D, et al. Basal cell (basaloid) carcinoma of the lung: a new morphologic and phenotypic entity with separate prognostic significance. *Hum Pathol* 1992;23:993–1003.

120. Dugan JM. Cytologic diagnosis of basal cell (basaloid) carcinoma of the lung. A report of two cases. *Acta Cytol* 1995;39:539–542.
121. Vesoulis, Z. Metastatic laryngeal basaloid squamous cell carcinoma simulating primary small cell carcinoma of the lung on fine needle aspiration lung biopsy. A case report. *Acta Cytol* 1998;42:783–787.
122. Moro D, Brichon PY, Brambilla E, et al. Basaloid bronchial carcinoma. A histologic group with a poor prognosis. *Cancer* 1994;73: 2734–2739.
123. Kim DJ, Kim KD, Shin DH, et al. Basaloid carcinoma of the lung: a really dismal histologic variant? *Ann Thorac Surg* 2003;76:1833–1837.
124. Fishback NF, Travis WD, Moran CA, et al. Pleomorphic (spindle/giant cell) carcinoma of the lung. A clinicopathologic correlation of 78 cases. *Cancer* 1994;73:2936–2945.
125. Rossi G, Cavazza A, Sturm N, et al. Pulmonary carcinomas with pleomorphic, sarcomatoid, or sarcomatous elements: a clinicopathologic and immunohistochemical study of 75 cases. *Am J Surg Pathol* 2003;27:311–324.
126. Lee JM, Dedhar S, Kalluri R, et al. The epithelial-mesenchymal transition: new insights in signaling, development, and disease. *J Cell Biol* 2006;172:973–981.
127. Witta SE, Gemmill RM, Hirsch FR, et al. Restoring E-cadherin expression increases sensitivity to epidermal growth factor receptor inhibitors in lung cancer cell lines. *Cancer Res* 2006;66:944–950.
128. Bremnes RM, Veve R, Gabrielson E, et al. High-throughput tissue microarray analysis used to evaluate biology and prognostic significance of the e-cadherin pathway in non-small-cell lung cancer. *J Clin Oncol* 2002;20:2417–2428.
129. Rho JK, Choi YJ, Lee JK, et al. Epithelial to mesenchymal transition derived from repeated exposure to gefitinib determines the sensitivity to EGFR inhibitors in A549, a non-small cell lung cancer cell line. *Lung Cancer* 2009;63(2):219–226.
130. Yauch RL, Januario T, Eberhard DA, et al. Epithelial versus mesenchymal phenotype determines in vitro sensitivity and predicts clinical activity of erlotinib in lung cancer patients. *Clin Cancer Res* 2005;11: 8686–8698.
131. Deeb G, Wang J, Ramnath N, et al. Altered E-cadherin and epidermal growth factor receptor expressions are associated with patient survival in lung cancer: a study utilizing high-density tissue microarray and immunohistochemistry. *Mod Pathol* 2004;17:430–439.
132. Barnard WG. The nature of "oat-celled sarcoma" of the mediastinum. *J Pathol* 1926;29:241–244.
133. Sandler AB. Chemotherapy for small cell lung cancer. *Semin Oncol* 2003;30:9–25.
134. Wingo PA, Ries LA, Giovino GA, et al. Annual report to the nation on the status of cancer, 1973–1996, with a special section on lung cancer and tobacco smoking. *J Natl Cancer Inst* 1999;91:675–690.
135. Frost JK, Ball WC Jr, Levin ML, et al. Early lung cancer detection: results of the initial (prevalence) radiologic and cytologic screening in the Johns Hopkins study. *Am Rev Respir Dis* 1984;130:549–554.
136. Flehinger BJ, Melamed MR, Zaman MB, et al. Early lung cancer detection: results of the initial (prevalence) radiologic and cytologic screening in the Memorial Sloan-Kettering study. *Am Rev Respir Dis* 1984;130:555–560.
137. Fabbro D, Di Loreto C, Stamerra O, et al. TTF-1 gene expression in human lung tumours. *Eur J Cancer* 1996;32A:512–517.
138. Di Loreto C, Di Lauro V, Puglisi F, et al. Immunocytochemical expression of tissue specific transcription factor-1 in lung carcinoma. *J Clin Pathol* 1997;50:30–32.
139. Folpe AL, Gown AM, Lamps LW, et al. Thyroid transcription factor-1: immunohistochemical evaluation in pulmonary neuroendocrine tumors. *Mod Pathol* 1999;12:5–8.
140. Ordonez NG. Value of thyroid transcription factor-1 immunostaining in distinguishing small cell lung carcinomas from other small cell carcinomas. *Am J Surg Pathol* 2000;24:1217–1223.
141. Byrd-Gloster AL, Khoor A, Glass LF, et al. Differential expression of thyroid transcription factor 1 in small cell lung carcinoma and Merkel cell tumor. *Hum Pathol* 2000;31:58–62.
142. Leech SN, Kolar AJ, Barrett PD, et al. Merkel cell carcinoma can be distinguished from metastatic small cell carcinoma using antibodies to cytokeratin 20 and thyroid transcription factor 1. *J Clin Pathol* 2001;54:727–729.
143. Sturm N, Rossi G, Lantuejoul S, et al. Expression of thyroid transcription factor-1 in the spectrum of neuroendocrine cell lung proliferations with special interest in carcinoids. *Hum Pathol* 2002;33:175–182.
144. Bobos M, Hytiroglou P, Kostopoulos I, et al. Immunohistochemical distinction between merkel cell carcinoma and small cell carcinoma of the lung. *Am J Dermatopathol* 2006;28:99–104.
145. Llombart B, Monteagudo C, Lopez-Guerrero JA, et al. Clinicopathological and immunohistochemical analysis of 20 cases of Merkel cell carcinoma in search of prognostic markers. *Histopathology* 2005;46: 622–634.
146. Carlson JW, Nucci MR, Brodsky J, et al. Biomarker-assisted diagnosis of ovarian, cervical and pulmonary small cell carcinomas: the role of TTF-1, WT-1 and HPV analysis. *Histopathology* 2007;51: 305–312.
147. Agoff SN, Lamps LW, Philip AT, et al. Thyroid transcription factor-1 is expressed in extrapulmonary small cell carcinomas but not in other extrapulmonary neuroendocrine tumors. *Mod Pathol* 2000;13: 238–242.
148. Alijo Serrano F, Sanchez-Mora N, Angel Arranz J, et al. Large cell and small cell neuroendocrine bladder carcinoma: immunohistochemical and outcome study in a single institution. *Am J Clin Pathol* 2007;128:733–739.
149. Jones TD, Kernek KM, Yang XJ, et al. Thyroid transcription factor 1 expression in small cell carcinoma of the urinary bladder: an immunohistochemical profile of 44 cases. *Hum Pathol* 2005;36:718–723.
150. Yun JP, Zhang MF, Hou JH, et al. Primary small cell carcinoma of the esophagus: clinicopathological and immunohistochemical features of 21 cases. *BMC Cancer* 2007;7:38.
151. Yao JL, Madeb R, Bourne P, et al. Small cell carcinoma of the prostate: an immunohistochemical study. *Am J Surg Pathol* 2006;30:705–712.
152. Kaufmann O, Georgi T, Dietel M. Utility of 123C3 monoclonal antibody against CD56 (NCAM) for the diagnosis of small cell carcinomas on paraffin sections. *Hum Pathol* 1997;28:1373–1378.
153. Lantuejoul S, Moro D, Michalides RJ, et al. Neural cell adhesion molecules (NCAM) and NCAM-PSA expression in neuroendocrine lung tumors. *Am J Surg Pathol* 1998;22:1267–1276.
154. Franklin WA. Diagnosis of lung cancer: pathology of invasive and preinvasive neoplasia. *Chest* 2000;117(4 Suppl 1):80S-89S.
155. Rossi G, Cavazza A, Marchioni A, et al. Kit expression in small cell carcinomas of the lung: effects of chemotherapy. *Mod Pathol* 2003;16:1041–1047.
156. Boldrini L, Ursino S, Gisfredi S, et al. Expression and mutational status of c-kit in small-cell lung cancer: prognostic relevance. *Clin Cancer Res* 2004;10:4101–4108.
157. Rohr UP, Rehfeld N, Pflugfelder L, et al. Expression of the tyrosine kinase c-kit is an independent prognostic factor in patients with small cell lung cancer. *Int J Cancer* 2004;111:259–263.
158. Lonardo F, Pass HI, Lucas DR. Immunohistochemistry frequently detects c-Kit expression in pulmonary small cell carcinoma and may help select clinical subsets for a novel form of chemotherapy. *Appl Immunohistochem Mol Morphol* 2003;11:51–55.
159. Mojica WD, Saxena R, Starostik P, et al. CD117+ small cell lung cancer lacks the asp 816→val point mutation in exon 17. *Histopathology* 2005;47:517–522.
160. Lopez-Martin A, Ballestin C, Garcia-Carbonero R, et al. Prognostic value of KIT expression in small cell lung cancer. *Lung Cancer* 2007; 56:405–413.
161. Whang-Peng J, Kao-Shan CS, Lee EC, et al. Specific chromosome defect associated with human small-cell lung cancer; deletion 3p(14–23). *Science* 1982;215:181–182.
162. Wistuba II, Gazdar AF, Minna JD. Molecular genetics of small cell lung carcinoma. *Semin Oncol* 2001;28:3–13.
163. Tatematsu A, Shimizu J, Murakami Y, et al. Epidermal growth factor receptor mutations in small cell lung cancer. *Clin Cancer Res* 2008;14:6092–6096.

164. Knudson AG Jr. Mutation and cancer: statistical study of retinoblastoma. *Proc Natl Acad Sci U S A* 1971;68:820–823.
165. Friend SH, Bernards R, Rogelj S, et al. A human DNA segment with properties of the gene that predisposes to retinoblastoma and osteosarcoma. *Nature* 1986;323:643–646.
166. Harbour JW, Lai SL, Whang-Peng J, et al. Abnormalities in structure and expression of the human retinoblastoma gene in SCLC. *Science* 1988;241:353–357.
167. Yokota J, Akiyama T, Fung YK, et al. Altered expression of the retinoblastoma (RB) gene in small-cell carcinoma of the lung. *Oncogene* 1988;3:471–475.
168. Schauer IE, Siriwardana S, Langan TA, et al. Cyclin D1 overexpression vs. retinoblastoma inactivation: implications for growth control evasion in non-small cell and small cell lung cancer. *Proc Natl Acad Sci U S A* 1994;91:7827–7831.
169. Gouyer V, Gazzeri S, Bolon I, et al. Mechanism of retinoblastoma gene inactivation in the spectrum of neuroendocrine lung tumors. *Am J Respir Cell Mol Biol* 1998;18:188–196.
170. Meyerson M, Franklin WA, Kelley MJ. Molecular classification and molecular genetics of human lung cancers. *Semin Oncol* 2004; 31:4–19.
171. Nicholson SA, Beasley MB, Brambilla E, et al. Small cell lung carcinoma (SCLC): a clinicopathologic study of 100 cases with surgical specimens. *Am J Surg Pathol* 2002;26:1184–1197.
172. Oberndorfer S. Tumoren des Dunndarms. *Frankf Z Pathol* 1907; 1:426.
173. Hamperl H. Uber gutartige Bronchialtumoren (Cylindrome und Carcinoide). *Virchows Arch* 1937;300:46–88.
174. Travis WD, Rush W, Flieder DB, et al. Survival analysis of 200 pulmonary neuroendocrine tumors with clarification of criteria for atypical carcinoid and its separation from typical carcinoid. *Am J Surg Pathol* 1998;22:934–944.
175. Travis WD, Linnoila RI, Tsokos MG, et al. Neuroendocrine tumors of the lung with proposed criteria for large-cell neuroendocrine carcinoma. An ultrastructural, immunohistochemical, and flow cytometric study of 35 cases. *Am J Surg Pathol* 1991;15:529–553.
176. McCaughan BC, Martini N, Bains MS. Bronchial carcinoids. Review of 124 cases. *J Thorac Cardiovasc Surg* 1985;89:8–17.
177. Churg A, Warnock ML. Pulmonary tumorlet. A form of peripheral carcinoid. *Cancer* 1976;37:1469–1477.
178. Ranchod M, Levine, GD. Spindle-cell carcinoid tumors of the lung: a clinicopathologic study of 35 cases. *Am J Surg Pathol* 1980;4: 315–331.
179. Skuladottir H, Hirsch FR, Hansen HH, et al. Pulmonary neuroendocrine tumors: incidence and prognosis of histological subtypes. A population-based study in Denmark. *Lung Cancer* 2002;37:127–35.
180. Arrigoni MG, Woolner LB, Bernatz PE. Atypical carcinoid tumors of the lung. *J Thorac Cardiovasc Surg* 1972;64:413–421.
181. Beasley MB, Thunnissen FB, Brambilla E, et al. Pulmonary atypical carcinoid: predictors of survival in 106 cases. *Hum Pathol* 2000;31: 1255–1265.
182. Fink G, Krelbaum T, Yellin A, et al. Pulmonary carcinoid: presentation, diagnosis, and outcome in 142 cases in Israel and review of 640 cases from the literature. *Chest* 2001;119:1647–1651.
183. Onuki N, Wistuba II, Travis WD, et al. Genetic changes in the spectrum of neuroendocrine lung tumors. *Cancer* 1999;85:600–607.
184. Jiang SX, Kameya T, Shoji M, et al. Large cell neuroendocrine carcinoma of the lung: a histologic and immunohistochemical study of 22 cases. *Am J Surg Pathol* 1998;22:526–537.
185. Takei H, Asamura H, Maeshima A, et al. Large cell neuroendocrine carcinoma of the lung: a clinicopathologic study of eighty-seven cases. *J Thorac Cardiovasc Surg* 2002;124:285–292.
186. Flieder DB. Neuroendocrine tumors of the lung: recent developments in histopathology. *Curr Opin Pulm Med* 2002;8:275–280.
187. Mazieres J, Daste G, Molinier L, et al. Large cell neuroendocrine carcinoma of the lung: pathological study and clinical outcome of 18 resected cases. *Lung Cancer* 2002;37:287–292.
188. Iyoda A, Hiroshima K, Toyozaki T, et al. Clinical characterization of pulmonary large cell neuroendocrine carcinoma and large cell carcinoma with neuroendocrine morphology. *Cancer* 2001;91: 1992–2000.
189. Hage R, Seldenrijk K, de Bruin P, et al. Pulmonary large-cell neuroendocrine carcinoma (LCNEC). *Eur J Cardiothorac Surg* 2003;23: 457–460.
190. Frierson HF Jr, Covell JL, Mills SE. Fine needle aspiration cytology of atypical carcinoid of the lung. *Acta Cytol* 1987;31:471–475.
191. Wiatrowska BA, Krol J, Zakowski MF. Large-cell neuroendocrine carcinoma of the lung: proposed criteria for cytologic diagnosis. *Diagn Cytopathol* 2001;24:58–64.
192. Kakinuma H, Mikami T, Iwabuchi K, et al. Diagnostic findings of bronchial brush cytology for pulmonary large cell neuroendocrine carcinomas: comparison with poorly differentiated adenocarcinomas, squamous cell carcinomas, and small cell carcinomas. *Cancer* 2003;99: 247–254.
193. Yang YJ, Steele CT, Ou XL, et al. Diagnosis of high-grade pulmonary neuroendocrine carcinoma by fine-needle aspiration biopsy: nonsmall-cell or small-cell type? *Diagn Cytopathol* 2001;25:292–300.
194. Loy TS, Darkow GV, Quesenberry JT. Immunostaining in the diagnosis of pulmonary neuroendocrine carcinomas. An immunohistochemical study with ultrastructural correlations. *Am J Surg Pathol* 1995;19:173–82.
195. Gosney JR, Gosney MA, Lye M, et al. Reliability of commercially available immunocytochemical markers for identification of neuroendocrine differentiation in bronchoscopic biopsies of bronchial carcinoma. *Thorax* 1995;50:116–120.
196. Graziano SL, Tatum AH, Newman NB, et al. The prognostic significance of neuroendocrine markers and carcinoembryonic antigen in patients with resected stage I and II non-small cell lung cancer. *Cancer Res* 1994;54:2908–2913.
197. Abbona G, Papotti M, Viberti L, et al. Chromogranin A gene expression in non-small cell lung carcinomas. *J Pathol* 1998;186: 151–156.
198. Al-Khafaji B, Noffsinger AE, Miller MA, et al. Immunohistologic analysis of gastrointestinal and pulmonary carcinoid tumors. *Hum Pathol* 1998;29:992–999.
199. Pujol JL, Simony J, Demoly P, et al. Neural cell adhesion molecule and prognosis of surgically resected lung cancer. *Am Rev Respir Dis* 1993;148:1071–1075.
200. Brambilla E, Veale D, Moro D, et al. Neuroendocrine phenotype in lung cancers. Comparison of immunohistochemistry with biochemical determination of enolase isoenzymes. *Am J Clin Pathol* 1992; 98:88–97.
201. Totsch M, Muller LC, Hittmair A, et al. Immunohistochemical demonstration of chromogranins A and B in neuroendocrine tumors of the lung. *Hum Pathol* 1992;23:312–316.
202. Hiroshima K, Iyoda A, Shida T, et al. Distinction of pulmonary large cell neuroendocrine carcinoma from small cell lung carcinoma: a morphological, immunohistochemical, and molecular analysis. *Mod Pathol* 2006;19:1358–1368.
203. Bensch KG, Gordon GB, Miller LR. Electron microscopic and biochemical studies on the bronchial carcinoid tumor. *Cancer* 1965;18: 592–602.
204. Pearse AG. The cytochemistry and ultrastructure of polypeptide hormone-producing cells of the APUD series and the embryologic, physiologic and pathologic implications of the concept. *J Histochem Cytochem* 1969;17:303–313.
205. Fontaine J, Le Douarin NM. Analysis of endoderm formation in the avian blastoderm by the use of quail-chick chimaeras. The problem of the neurectodermal origin of the cells of the APUD series. *J Embryol Exp Morphol* 1977;41:209–222.
206. Yesner R. Heterogeneity of so-called neuroendocrine lung tumors. *Exp Mol Pathol* 2001;70:179–182.
207. Beer DG, Kardia SL, Huang CC, et al. Gene-expression profiles predict survival of patients with lung adenocarcinoma. *Nat Med* 2002;8: 816–824.

208. Bobrow LG, Happerfield L, Patel K. The expression of small cell lung cancer related antigens in foetal lung and kidney. *Br J Cancer Suppl* 1991;14:56–58.
209. Wuenschell CW, Sunday ME, Singh G, et al. Embryonic mouse lung epithelial progenitor cells co-express immunohistochemical markers of diverse mature cell lineages. *J Histochem Cytochem* 1996;44:113–123.
210. King KA, Torday JS, Sunday ME. Bombesin and [Leu8]phyllolitorin promote fetal mouse lung branching morphogenesis via a receptor-mediated mechanism. *Proc Natl Acad Sci U S A* 1995;92:4357–4361.
211. Aguayo SM, Miller YE, Waldron JA Jr, et al. Brief report: idiopathic diffuse hyperplasia of pulmonary neuroendocrine cells and airways disease. *N Engl J Med* 1992;327:1285–1288.
212. Miller RR, Muller NL. Neuroendocrine cell hyperplasia and obliterative bronchiolitis in patients with peripheral carcinoid tumors. *Am J Surg Pathol* 1995;19:653–658.
213. Alshehri M, Cutz E, Banzhoff A, et al. Hyperplasia of pulmonary neuroendocrine cells in a case of childhood pulmonary emphysema. *Chest* 1997;112:553–556.
214. Resl M, Kral B, Simek J. Carcinoid tumorlets and pulmonary hypoxia [in Czech]. *Cesk Patol* 1995;31:84–86.
215. Charloux A, Quoix E, Wolkove N, et al. The increasing incidence of lung adenocarcinoma: reality or artefact? A review of the epidemiology of lung adenocarcinoma. *Int J Epidemiol* 1997;26:14–23.
216. Shimosato Y, Kodama T, Kameya T. Morphogenesis of peripheral type adenocarcinoma of the lung. In: Shimosato Y, Melamed MR, Nettesheim P, eds. *Morphogenesis of Lung Cancer*, vol. 1. Boca Raton, Florida: CRC Press, 1982:65–69.
217. Kodama T, Nishiyama H, Nishiwaki Y, et al. Histopathological study of adenocarcinoma and hyperplastic epithelial lesions of the lung. *Jpn J Lung Cancer (Haigan)* 1988;28:325–333.
218. Miller RR. Bronchioloalveolar cell adenomas. *Am J Surg Pathol* 1990;14:904–912.
219. Nakanishi K. Alveolar epithelial hyperplasia and adenocarcinoma of the lung. *Arch Pathol Lab Med* 1990;114:363–368.
220. Weng SY, Tsuchiya E, Kasuga T, et al. Incidence of atypical bronchioloalveolar cell hyperplasia of the lung: relation to histological subtypes of lung cancer. *Virchows Arch A Pathol Anat Histopathol* 1992;420:463–471.
221. Chapman AD, Kerr KM. The association between atypical adenomatous hyperplasia and primary lung cancer. *Br J Cancer* 2000;83:632–636.
222. Nakahara R, Yokose T, Nagai K, et al. Atypical adenomatous hyperplasia of the lung: a clinicopathological study of 118 cases including cases with multiple atypical adenomatous hyperplasia. *Thorax* 2001;56: 302–305.
223. Koga T, Hashimoto S, Sugio K, et al. Lung adenocarcinoma with bronchioloalveolar carcinoma component is frequently associated with foci of high-grade atypical adenomatous hyperplasia. *Am J Clin Pathol* 117:464–470.
224. Yokose T, Ito Y, Ochiai A. High prevalence of atypical adenomatous hyperplasia of the lung in autopsy specimens from elderly patients with malignant neoplasms. *Lung Cancer* 2000;29:125–130.
225. Minami Y, Matsuno Y, Iijima T, et al. Prognostication of small-sized primary pulmonary adenocarcinomas by histopathological and karyometric analysis. *Lung Cancer* 2005;48:339–348.
226. Flieder DB. Screen-detected adenocarcinoma of the lung. Practical points for surgical pathologists. *Am J Clin Pathol* 2003;119(Suppl):S39–S57.
227. Akyurek N, Memis L, Ekinci O, et al. Survivin expression in preinvasive lesions and non-small cell lung carcinoma. *Virchows Arch* 2006;449:164–170.
228. Nakanishi K, Kumaki F, Hiroi S, et al. Mre11 expression in atypical adenomatous hyperplasia and adenocarcinoma of the lung. *Arch Pathol Lab Med* 2006;130:1330–1334.
229. Chiosea S, Jelezcova E, Chandran U, et al. Overexpression of Dicer in precursor lesions of lung adenocarcinoma. *Cancer Res* 2007;67: 2345–3250.
230. Kerr KM, MacKenzie SJ, Ramasami S, et al. Expression of Fhit, cell adhesion molecules and matrix metalloproteinases in atypical adenomatous hyperplasia and pulmonary adenocarcinoma. *J Pathol* 2004;203:638–644.
231. Kodama T, Biyajima S, Watanabe S, et al. Morphometric study of adenocarcinomas and hyperplastic epithelial lesions in the peripheral lung. *Am J Clin Pathol* 1986;85:146–151.
232. Mori M, Chiba R, Takahashi T. Atypical adenomatous hyperplasi of the lung and its differentiation from adenocarcinoma. Characterization of atypical cells by morphometry and multivariate cluster analysis. *Cancer* 1993;72:2331–2340.
233. Kitamura H, Kameda Y, Nakamura N, et al. Atypical adenomatous hyperplasia and bronchoalveolar lung carcinoma. Analysis by morphometry and the expressions of p53 and carcinoembryonic antigen. *Am J Surg Pathol* 1996;20:553–562.
234. Kitamura H, Kameda Y, Ito T, et al. Atypical adenomatous hyperplasia of the lung. Implications for the pathogenesis of peripheral lung adenocarcinoma. *Am J Clin Pathol* 1999;111:610–622.
235. Nakayama H, Noguchi M, Tsuchiya R, et al. Clonal growth of atypical adenomatous hyperplasia of the lung: cytofluorometric analysis of nuclear DNA content. *Mod Pathol* 1990;3:314–320.
236. Westra WH, Baas IO, Hruban RH, et al. K-ras oncogene activation in atypical alveolar hyperplasias of the human lung. *Cancer Res* 1996;56:2224–2228.
237. Yoshida Y, Shibata T, Kokubu A, et al. Mutations of the epidermal growth factor receptor gene in atypical adenomatous hyperplasia and bronchioloalveolar carcinoma of the lung. *Lung Cancer* 2005;50:1–8.
238. Kohno H, Hiroshima K, Toyozaki T, et al. p53 mutation and allelic loss of chromosome 3p, 9p of preneoplastic lesions in patients with nonsmall cell lung carcinoma. *Cancer* 1999;85:341–347.
239. Yamasaki M, Takeshima Y, Fujii S, et al. Correlation between genetic alterations and histopathological subtypes in bronchiolo-alveolar carcinoma and atypical adenomatous hyperplasia of the lung. *Pathol Int* 2000;50:778–785.
240. Anami Y, Matsuno Y, Yamada T, et al. A case of double primary adenocarcinoma of the lung with multiple atypical adenomatous hyperplasia. *Pathol Int* 1998;48:634–640.
241. Takamochi K, Ogura T, Suzuki K, et al. Loss of heterozygosity on chromosomes 9q and 16p in atypical adenomatous hyperplasia concomitant with adenocarcinoma of the lung. *Am J Pathol* 2001;159:1941–1948.
242. Ullmann R, Bongiovanni M, Halbwedl I, et al. Is high-grade adenomatous hyperplasia an early bronchioloalveolar adenocarcinoma? *J Pathol* 2003;201:371–376.
243. Akata S, Fukushima A, Kakizaki D, et al. CT scanning of bronchioloalveolar carcinoma: specific appearances. *Lung Cancer* 1995;12: 221–230.
244. Rolen KA, Fulton JP, Tamura DJ, et al. Bronchoalveolar carcinoma is linked to cigarette smoking: a case-control study from Rhode Island. *Proc Am Soc Clin Oncol* 2003;22:674.
245. Paez JG, Janne PA, Lee JC, et al. EGFR mutations in lung cancer: correlation with clinical response to gefitinib therapy. *Science* 2004;304:1497–1500.
246. Lynch TJ, Bell DW, Sordella R, et al. Activating mutations in the epidermal growth factor receptor underlying responsiveness of non-small-cell lung cancer to gefitinib. *N Engl J Med* 2004;350: 2129–2139.
247. Swensen SJ, Jett JR, Sloan JA, et al. Screening for lung cancer with low-dose spiral computed tomography. *Am J Respir Crit Care Med* 2002;165:508–513.
248. Wislez M, Massiani MA, Milleron B, et al. Clinical characteristics of pneumonic-type adenocarcinoma of the lung. *Chest* 2003;123: 1868–1877.
249. Kakinuma R, Ohmatsu H, Kaneko M, et al. Progression of focal pure ground-glass opacity detected by low-dose helical computed tomography screening for lung cancer. *J Comput Assist Tomogr* 2004;28: 17–23.
250. Gaeta M, Caruso R, Barone M, et al. Ground-glass attenuation in nodular bronchioloalveolar carcinoma: CT patterns and prognostic value. *J Comput Assist Tomogr* 1998;22:215–219.
251. Malassez L. Examen histologique d'un cas de cancer encephaloide du poumon (epithelioma). *Arch Physiol Norm Pathol* 1876;3:353.

252. Low FN. The pulmonary alveolar epithelium of laboratory mammals and man. *Anat Rec* 1953;117:241–263.
253. Delarue NC, Graham EA. Alveolar cell carcinoma of the lung (pulmonary adenomatosis, Jagziekte?) a multicentric tumor of epithelial origin. *J Thorac Surg* 1949;18:237–251.
254. Cowdry EV. Studies on the etiology of Jagziekte: origin of the epithelial proliferations and subsequent changes. *J Exp Med* 1925;42:335.
255. Bonne C. Morphological resembalance of pulmonary adenomatosis (jaagseikte in she and certain cases of cancer of the lung in man). *Am J Cancer* 1939;35:491–501.
256. Yousem SA, Finkelstein SD, Swalsky PA, et al. Absence of jaagsiekte sheep retrovirus DNA and RNA in bronchioloalveolar and conventional human pulmonary adenocarcinoma by PCR and RT-PCR analysis. *Hum Pathol* 2001;32:1039–1042.
257. Liebow AA. Bronchiolo-alveolar carcinoma. *Adv Intern Med* 1960;10: 329–358.
258. Shimosato Y, Suzuki A, Hashimoto T, et al. Prognostic implications of fibrotic focus (scar) in small peripheral lung cancers. *Am J Surg Pathol* 1980;4:365–373.
259. Noguchi M, Morikawa A, Kawasaki M, et al. Small adenocarcinoma of the lung. Histologic characteristics and prognosis. *Cancer* 1995;75:2844–2852.
260. Suzuki K, Yokose T, Yoshida J, et al. Prognostic significance of the size of central fibrosis in peripheral adenocarcinoma of the lung. *Ann Thorac Surg* 2000;69:893–897.
261. Maeshima AM, Niki T, Maeshima A, et al. Modified scar grade: a prognostic indicator in small peripheral lung adenocarcinoma. *Cancer* 2002;95:2546–2554.
262. Clayton F. Bronchioloalveolar carcinomas. Cell types, patterns of growth, and prognostic correlates. *Cancer* 1986;57:1555–1564.
263. Tao LC, Weisbrod GL, Pearson FG, et al. Cytologic diagnosis of bronchioloalveolar carcinoma by fine-needle aspiration biopsy. *Cancer* 1986;57:1565–1570.
264. Auger M, Katz RL, Johnston DA. Differentiating cytological features of bronchioloalveolar carcinoma from adenocarcinoma of the lung in fine-needle aspirations: a statistical analysis of 27 cases. *Diagn Cytopathol* 1997;16:253–257.
265. Morishita Y, Fukasawa M, Takeuchi M, et al. Small-sized adenocarcinoma of the lung. Cytologic characteristics and clinical behavior. *Cancer* 2001;93:124–131.
266. Elson CE, Moore SP, Johnston WW. Morphologic and immunocytochemical studies of bronchioloalveolar carcinoma at Duke University Medical Center, 1968–1986. *Anal Quant Cytol Histol* 1989;11: 261–274.
267. MacDonald LL, Yazdi HM. Fine-needle aspiration biopsy of bronchioloalveolar carcinoma. *Cancer* 2001;93:29–34.
268. Edwards SL, Roberts C, McKean ME, et al. Preoperative histological classification of primary lung cancer: accuracy of diagnosis and use of the non-small cell category. *J Clin Pathol* 2000;53:537–540.
269. Kitamura H, Kameda Y, Nakamura N, et al. Proliferative potential and p53 overexpression in precursor and early stage lesions of bronchioloalveolar lung carcinoma. *Am J Pathol* 1995;146:876–887.
270. Terasaki H, Niki T, Matsuno Y, et al. Lung adenocarcinoma with mixed bronchioloalveolar and invasive components: clinicopathological features, subclassification by extent of invasive foci, and immunohistochemical characterization. *Am J Surg Pathol* 2003;27: 937–951.
271. Colby TV, Koss MN, Travis WD. Tumors of the lower respiratory tract. In: Rosai J, ed. *Atlas of Tumor Pathology.* Washington, DC: Armed Forces Institute of Pathology, 1995:65–90.
272. Takizawa T, Terashima M, Koike T, et al. Lymph node metastasis in small peripheral adenocarcinoma of the lung. *J Thorac Cardiovasc Surg* 1998;116:276–280.
273. Stenbygaard LE, Sorensen JB, Olsen JE. Metastatic pattern in adenocarcinoma of the lung. An autopsy study from a cohort of 137 consecutive patients with complete resection. *J Thorac Cardiovasc Surg* 1995;110: 1130–1135.
274. Madri JA, Carter D. Scar cancers of the lung: origin and significance. *Hum Pathol* 1984;15:625–631.
275. el-Torkey M, Giltman LI, Dabbous M. Collagens in scar carcinoma of the lung. *Am J Pathol* 1985;121:322–326.
276. Barsky SH, Huang SJ, Bhuta S. The extracellular matrix of pulmonary scar carcinomas is suggestive of a desmoplastic origin. *Am J Pathol* 1986;124:412–419.
277. Franklin WA. The pathology and pathogenesis of peripheral lung adenocarcinoma. *Lung Cancer*, 3rd Ed. Oxford: Blackwell Publishing, 2008:121–143.
278. Silver SA, Askin FB. True papillary carcinoma of the lung: a distinct clinicopathologic entity. *Am J Surg Pathol* 1997;21:43–51.
279. Miyoshi T, Satoh Y, Okumura S, et al. Early-stage lung adenocarcinomas with a micropapillary pattern, a distinct pathologic marker for a significantly poor prognosis. *Am J Surg Pathol* 2003;27:101–109.
280. Motoi N, Szoke J, Riely GJ, et al. Lung adenocarcinoma: modification of the 2004 WHO mixed subtype to include the major histologic subtype suggests correlations between papillary and micropapillary adenocarcinoma subtypes, EGFR mutations and gene expression analysis. *Am J Surg Pathol* 2008;32:810–827.
281. Goldstein NS, Mani A, Chmielewski G, et al. Prognostic factors in T1 NO MO adenocarcinomas and bronchioloalveolar carcinomas of the lung. *Am J Clin Pathol* 1999;112:391–402.
282. Yokose T, Suzuki K, Nagai K, et al. Favorable and unfavorable morphological prognostic factors in peripheral adenocarcinoma of the lung 3 cm or less in diameter. *Lung Cancer* 2000;29:179–188.
283. Warburton D, Zhao J, Berberich MA, et al. Molecular embryology of the lung: then, now, and in the future. *Am J Physiol* 1999;276: L697–L704.
284. Mendelson CR. Role of transcription factors in fetal lung development and surfactant protein gene expression. *Annu Rev Physiol* 2000;62: 875–915.
285. Yatabe Y, Mitsudomi T, Takahashi T. TTF-1 expression in pulmonary adenocarcinomas. *Am J Surg Pathol* 2002;26:767–773.
286. Kendall J, Liu Q, Bakleh A, et al. Oncogenic cooperation and coamplification of developmental transcription factor genes in lung cancer. *Proc Natl Acad Sci U S A* 2007;104:16663–16668.
287. Weir BA, Woo MS, Getz G, et al. Characterizing the cancer genome in lung adenocarcinoma. *Nature* 2007;450:893–898.
288. Perner S, Wagner P, Soltermann A, et al. TTF1 expression in non-small cell lung carcinoma: association with TTF1 gene amplification and improved survival. *J Pathol* 2009;217:65–72.
289. Tot T. The value of cytokeratins 20 and 7 in discriminating metastatic adenocarcinomas from pleural mesotheliomas. *Cancer* 2001;92: 2727–2732.
290. Mazziotta RM, Borczuk AC, Powell CA, et al. CDX2 immunostaining as a gastrointestinal marker: expression in lung carcinomas is a potential pitfall. *Appl Immunohistochem Mol Morphol* 2005;13:55–60.
291. Tan J, Sidhu G, Greco MA, et al. Villin, cytokeratin 7, and cytokeratin 20 expression in pulmonary adenocarcinoma with ultrastructural evidence of microvilli with rootlets. *Hum Pathol* 1998;29:390–396.
292. Rubin BP, Skarin AT, Pisick E, et al. Use of cytokeratins 7 and 20 in determining the origin of metastatic carcinoma of unknown primary, with special emphasis on lung cancer. *Eur J Cancer Prev* 2001;10:77–82.
293. Saad RS, Cho P, Silverman JF, et al. Usefulness of Cdx2 in separating mucinous bronchioloalveolar adenocarcinoma of the lung from metastatic mucinous colorectal adenocarcinoma. *Am J Clin Pathol* 2004;122:421–427.
294. Rossi G, Marchioni A, Romagnani E, et al. Primary lung cancer presenting with gastrointestinal tract involvement: clinicopathologic and immunohistochemical features in a series of 18 consecutive cases. *J Thorac Oncol* 2007;2:115–120.
295. Kummar S, Fogarasi M, Canova A, et al. Cytokeratin 7 and 20 staining for the diagnosis of lung and colorectal adenocarcinoma. *Br J Cancer* 2002;86:1884–1887.
296. Linnoila RI, Mulshine JL, Steinberg SM, et al. Expression of surfactant-associated protein in non-small-cell lung cancer: a discriminant between biologic subsets. *Monogr Natl Cancer Inst* 1992;(13):61–66.

297. Bejarano PA, Baughman RP, Biddinger PW, et al. Surfactant proteins and thyroid transcription factor-1 in pulmonary and breast carcinomas. *Mod Pathol* 1996;9:445–452.
298. Khoor A, Whitsett JA, Stahlman MT, et al. Utility of surfactant protein B precursor and thyroid transcription factor 1 in differentiating adenocarcinoma of the lung from malignant mesothelioma. *Hum Pathol* 1999;30:695–700.
299. Takezawa C, Takahashi H, Fujishima T, et al. Assessment of differentiation in adenocarcinoma cells from pleural effusion by peripheral airway cell markers and their diagnostic values. *Lung Cancer* 2002;38:273–281.
300. Kaufmann O, Dietel M. Thyroid transcription factor-1 is the superior immunohistochemical marker for pulmonary adenocarcinomas and large cell carcinomas compared to surfactant proteins A and B. *Histopathology* 2000;36:8–16.
301. Uzaslan E, Stuempel T, Ebsen M, et al. Surfactant protein A detection in primary pulmonary adenocarcinoma without bronchioloalveolar pattern. *Respiration* 2005;72:249–253.
302. Inamura K, Satoh Y, Okumura S, et al. Pulmonary adenocarcinomas with enteric differentiation: histologic and immunohistochemical characteristics compared with metastatic colorectal cancers and usual pulmonary adenocarcinomas. *Am J Surg Pathol* 2005;29:660–665.
303. Braidotti P, Cigala C, Graziani D, et al. Surfactant protein A expression in human normal and neoplastic breast epithelium. *Am J Clin Pathol* 2001;116:721–728.
304. McCoy MS, Toole JJ, Cunningham JM, et al. Characterization of a human colon/lung carcinoma oncogene. *Nature* 1983;302:79–81.
305. McCoy MS, Bargmann CI, Weinberg RA. Human colon carcinoma Ki-ras2 oncogene and its corresponding proto-oncogene. *Mol Cell Biol* 1984;4:1577–1582.
306. Rodenhuis S, Slebos RJ, Boot AJ, et al. Incidence and possible clinical significance of K-ras oncogene activation in adenocarcinoma of the human lung. *Cancer Res* 1988;48:5738–5741.
307. Slebos RJ, Kibbelaar RE, Dalesio O, et al. K-ras oncogene activation as a prognostic marker in adenocarcinoma of the lung. *N Engl J Med* 1990;323:561–565.
308. Mitsudomi T, Steinberg SM, Oie HK, et al. Ras gene mutations in non-small cell lung cancers are associated with shortened survival irrespective of treatment intent. *Cancer Res* 1991;51:4999–5002.
309. Rosell R, Li S, Skacel Z, et al. Prognostic impact of mutated K-ras gene in surgically resected non-small cell lung cancer patients. *Oncogene* 1993;8:2407–2412.
310. Keohavong P, DeMichele MA, Melacrinos AC, et al. Detection of K-ras mutations in lung carcinomas: relationship to prognosis. *Clin Cancer Res* 1996;2:411–418.
311. Cooper CA, Carby FA, Bubb VJ, et al. The pattern of K-ras mutation in pulmonary adenocarcinoma defines a new pathway of tumour development in the human lung. *J Pathol* 1997;181:401–404.
312. Cho JY, Kim JH, Lee YH, et al. Correlation between K-ras gene mutation and prognosis of patients with nonsmall cell lung carcinoma. *Cancer* 1997;79:462–467.
313. Siegfried JM, Gillespie AT, Mera R, et al. Prognostic value of specific KRAS mutations in lung adenocarcinomas. *Cancer Epidemiol Biomarkers Prev* 1997;6:841–847.
314. Nemunaitis J, Klemow S, Tong A, et al. Prognostic value of K-ras mutations, ras oncoprotein, and c-erb B-2 oncoprotein expression in adenocarcinoma of the lung. *Am J Clin Oncol* 1998;21:155–160.
315. Nelson HH, Christiani DC, Mark EJ, et al. Implications and prognostic value of K-ras mutation for early-stage lung cancer in women. *J Natl Cancer Inst* 1991;91:2032–2038.
316. Holst VA, Finkelstein S, Yousem SA. Bronchioloalveolar adenocarcinoma of lung: monoclonal origin for multifocal disease. *Am J Surg Pathol* 1998;22:1343–1350.
317. Aviel-Ronen S, Blackhall FH, Shepherd FA, et al. K-ras mutations in non-small-cell lung carcinoma: a review. *Clin Lung Cancer* 2006;8:30–38.
318. Slebos RJ, Hruban RH, Dalesio O, et al. Relationship between K-ras oncogene activation and smoking in adenocarcinoma of the human lung. *J Natl Cancer Inst* 1991;83:1024–1027.
319. Ahrendt S A, Decker PA, Alawi EA, et al. Cigarette smoking is strongly associated with mutation of the K-ras gene in patients with primary adenocarcinoma of the lung. *Cancer* 2001;92:1525–1530.
320. Le Calvez F, Mukeria A, Hunt JD, et al. TP53 and KRAS mutation load and types in lung cancers in relation to tobacco smoke: distinct patterns in never, former, and current smokers. *Cancer Res* 2005;65:5076–5083.
321. Kwiatkowski DJ, Harpole DH Jr, Godleski J, et al. Molecular pathologic substaging in 244 stage I non-small-cell lung cancer patients: clinical implications. *J Clin Oncol* 1998;16:2468–2477.
322. Mitsudomi T, Hamajima N, Ogawa M, et al. Prognostic significance of p53 alterations in patients with non-small cell lung cancer: a meta-analysis. *Clin Cancer Res* 2000;6:4055–4063.
323. Koga T, Hashimoto S, Sugio K, et al. Clinicopathological and molecular evidence indicating the independence of bronchioloalveolar components from other subtypes of human peripheral lung adenocarcinoma. *Clin Cancer Res* 2001;7:1730–1738.
324. Fukuyama Y, Mitsudomi T, Sugio K, et al. K-ras and p53 mutations are an independent unfavourable prognostic indicator in patients with non-small-cell lung cancer. *Br J Cancer* 1997;75:1125–1130.
325. Jackman DM, Yeap BY, Sequist LV, et al. Exon 19 deletion mutations of epidermal growth factor receptor are associated with prolonged survival in non-small cell lung cancer patients treated with gefitinib or erlotinib. *Clin Cancer Res* 2006;12:3908–3914.
326. van Zandwijk N, Mathy A, Boerrigter L, et al. EGFR and KRAS mutations as criteria for treatment with tyrosine kinase inhibitors: retro- and prospective observations in non-small-cell lung cancer. *Ann Oncol* 2007;18:99–103.
327. Kosaka T, Yatabe Y, Endoh H, et al. Analysis of epidermal growth factor receptor gene mutation in patients with non-small cell lung cancer and acquired resistance to gefitinib. *Clin Cancer Res* 2006;12:5764–5769.
328. Balak MN, Gong Y, Riely GJ, et al. Novel D761Y and common secondary T790M mutations in epidermal growth factor receptor-mutant lung adenocarcinomas with acquired resistance to kinase inhibitors. *Clin Cancer Res* 2006;12:6494–6501.
329. Engelman JA, Zejnullahu K, Mitsudomi T, et al. MET amplification leads to gefitinib resistance in lung cancer by activating ERBB3 signaling. *Science* 2007;316:1039–1043.
330. Bean J, Brennan C, Shih JY, et al. MET amplification occurs with or without T790M mutations in EGFR mutant lung tumors with acquired resistance to gefitinib or erlotinib. *Proc Natl Acad Sci U S A* 2007;104:20932–20937.
331. Matsumoto S, Iwakawa R, Kohno T, et al. Frequent EGFR mutations in noninvasive bronchioloalveolar carcinoma. *Int J Cancer* 2006;118:2498–2504.
332. Yatabe Y, Kosaka T, Takahashi T, et al. EGFR mutation is specific for terminal respiratory unit type adenocarcinoma. *Am J Surg Pathol* 2005;29:633–639.
333. Spicer J, Ashworth A. LKB1 kinase: master and commander of metabolism and polarity. *Curr Biol* 2004;14:R383-R385.
334. Jenne DE, Reimann H, Nezu J, et al. Peutz-Jeghers syndrome is caused by mutations in a novel serine threonine kinase. *Nat Genet* 1998;18:38–43.
335. Hemminki A, Markie D, Tomlinson I, et al. A serine/threonine kinase gene defective in Peutz-Jeghers syndrome. *Nature* 1998;391:184–187.
336. Sanchez-Cespedes M, Parrella P, Esteller M, et al. Inactivation of LKB1/STK11 is a common event in adenocarcinomas of the lung. *Cancer Res* 2002;62:3659–3662.
337. Matsumoto S, Iwakawa R, Takahashi K, et al. Prevalence and specificity of LKB1 genetic alterations in lung cancers. *Oncogene* 2007;26:5911–5198.
338. Ding L, Getz G, Wheeler DA, et al. Somatic mutations affect key pathways in lung adenocarcinoma. *Nature* 2008;455:1069–1075.
339. Soda M, Choi YL, Enomoto M, et al. Identification of the transforming EML4-ALK fusion gene in non-small-cell lung cancer. *Nature* 2007;448:561–566.

340. Takeuchi K, Choi YL, Soda M, et al. Multiplex reverse transcription-PCR screening for EML4-ALK fusion transcripts. *Clin Cancer Res* 2008;14:6618–6624.
341. Gandara DR, West H, Chansky K, et al. Bronchioloalveolar carcinoma: a model for investigating the biology of epidermal growth factor receptor inhibition. *Clin Cancer Res* 2004;10:4205S–4209S.
342. Miller VA, Riely GJ, Zakowski MF, et al. Molecular characteristics of bronchioloalveolar carcinoma and adenocarcinoma, bronchioloalveolar carcinoma subtype, predict response to erlotinib. *J Clin Oncol* 2008;26:1472–1478.
343. Tsao MS, Sakurada A, Cutz JC, et al. Erlotinib in lung cancer—molecular and clinical predictors of outcome. *N Engl J Med* 2005;353: 133–144.
344. Hirsch FR, Varella-Garcia M, Cappuzzo F, et al. Combination of EGFR gene copy number and protein expression predicts outcome for advanced non-small-cell lung cancer patients treated with gefitinib. *Ann Oncol* 2007;18:752–760.
345. Hirsch FR, Varella-Garcia M, Bunn PA Jr, et al. Epidermal growth factor receptor in non-small-cell lung carcinomas: correlation between gene copy number and protein expression and impact on prognosis. *J Clin Oncol* 2003;21:3798–3807.
346. Li AR, Chitale D, Riely GJ, et al. EGFR mutations in lung adenocarcinomas: clinical testing experience and relationship to EGFR gene copy number and immunohistochemical expression. *J Mol Diagn* 2008;10:242–248.
347. Cappuzzo F, Hirsch FR, Rossi E, et al. Epidermal growth factor receptor gene and protein and gefitinib sensitivity in non-small-cell lung cancer. *J Natl Cancer Inst* 2005;97:643–655.
348. Zhu CQ, da Cunha Santos G, Ding K, et al. Role of KRAS and EGFR as biomarkers of response to erlotinib in National Cancer Institute of Canada Clinical Trials Group Study BR.21. *J Clin Oncol* 2008;26:4268–4275.
349. Kitamura H, Kameda Y, Nakamura N, et al. Atypical adenomatous hyperplasia and bronchoalveolar lung carcinoma. Analysis by morphometry and the expressions of p53 and carcinoembryonic antigen. *Am J Surg Pathol* 1996;20:553–562.
350. Yatabe Y, Masuda A, Koshikawa T, et al. p27KIP1 in human lung cancers: differential changes in small cell and non-small cell carcinomas. *Cancer Res* 1998;58:1042–1047.
351. Niki T, Kohno T, Iba S, et al. Frequent co-localization of Cox-2 and laminin-5 gamma2 chain at the invasive front of early-stage lung adenocarcinomas. *Am J Pathol* 2002;160:1129–1141.
352. Puglisi F, Aprile G, Bruckbauer M, et al. Combined analysis of MIB-1 and thyroid transcription factor-1 predicts survival in non-small cell lung carcinomas. *Cancer Lett* 2001;162:97–103.
353. Golub TR, Slonim DK, Tamayo P, et al. Molecular classification of cancer: class discovery and class prediction by gene expression monitoring. *Science* 1999;286:531–537.
354. Fujiwara T, Tanaka N, Kanazawa S, et al. Multicenter phase I study of repeated intratumoral delivery of adenoviral p53 in patients with advanced non-small-cell lung cancer. *J Clin Oncol* 2006;24: 1689–1699.
355. Garnis C, Lockwood WW, Vucic E, et al. High resolution analysis of non-small cell lung cancer cell lines by whole genome tiling path array CGH. *Int J Cancer* 2006;118:1556–1564.
356. Kodama T, Shimosato Y, Koide T, et al. Endobronchial polypoid adenocarcinoma of the lung. Histological and ultrastructural studies of five cases. *Am J Surg Pathol* 1984;8:845–854.
357. Cugell DW, Kamp DW. Asbestos and the pleura: a review. *Chest* 2004;125:1103–1117.
358. Baas P. Predictive and prognostic factors in malignant pleural mesothelioma. *Curr Opin Oncol* 2003;15:127–130.
359. Hillerdal, G. Malignant mesothelioma 1982: review of 4710 published cases. *Br J Dis Chest* 1983;77:321–343.
360. Yates DH, Corrin B, Stidolph PN, et al. Malignant mesothelioma in south east England: clinicopathological experience of 272 cases. *Thorax* 1997;52:507–512.
361. Murray M. Departmental Committee for Compensation of Industrial Disease. HMSO. 7. London, UK.
362. Wagner JC, Sleggs CA, Marchand P. Diffuse pleural mesothelioma and asbestos exposure in the North Western Cape Province. *Br J Ind Med* 1960;17:260–271.
363. McDonald JC, McDonald AD. The epidemiology of mesothelioma in historical context. *Eur Respir J* 1996;9:1932–1942.
364. Roggli VL, Sanders LL. Asbestos content of lung tissue and carcinoma of the lung: a clinicopathologic correlation and mineral fiber analysis of 234 cases. *Ann Occup Hyg* 2000;44:109–117.
365. Roggli VL, Pratt PC, Brody AR. Asbestos fiber type in malignant mesothelioma: an analytical scanning electron microscopic study of 94 cases. *Am J Ind Med* 1993;23:605–614.
366. Epler GR, McLoud TC, Gaensler EA. Prevalence and incidence of benign asbestos pleural effusion in a working population. *JAMA* 1982;247:617–622.
367. Price B. Analysis of current trends in United States mesothelioma incidence. *Am J Epidemiol* 1997;145:211–218.
368. Kielkowski D, Nelson G, Rees D. Risk of mesothelioma from exposure to crocidolite asbestos: a 1995 update of a South African mortality study. *Occup Environ Med* 2000;57:563–567.
369. Berry G, Newhouse ML, Wagner JC. Mortality from all cancers of asbestos factory workers in east London 1933–80. *Occup Environ Med* 2000;57:782–785.
370. Boutin C, Schlesser M, Frenay C, et al. Malignant pleural mesothelioma. *Eur Respir J* 1998;12:972–981.
371. Cantin R, Al-Jabi M, McCaughey WT. Desmoplastic diffuse mesothelioma. *Am J Surg Pathol* 1982;6:215–222.
372. Kobzik L, Antman KH, Warhol MJ. The distinction of mesothelioma from adenocarcinoma in malignant effusions by electron microscopy. *Acta Cytol* 1985;29:219–225.
373. Ordonez NG. The immunohistochemical diagnosis of mesothelioma: a comparative study of epithelioid mesothelioma and lung adenocarcinoma. *Am J Surg Pathol* 2003;27:1031–1051.
374. Schacht V, Dadras SS, Johnson LA, et al. Up-regulation of the lymphatic marker podoplanin, a mucin-type transmembrane glycoprotein, in human squamous cell carcinomas and germ cell tumors. *Am J Pathol* 2005;166:913–921.
375. Chu AY, Litzky LA, Pasha TL, et al. Utility of D2-40, a novel mesothelial marker, in the diagnosis of malignant mesothelioma. *Mod Pathol* 2005;18:105–110.
376. Kimura N, Kimura I. Podoplanin as a marker for mesothelioma. *Pathol Int* 2005;55:83–86.
377. Ordonez NG. D2-40 and podoplanin are highly specific and sensitive immunohistochemical markers of epithelioid malignant mesothelioma. *Hum Pathol* 2005;36:372–380.
378. Ordonez NG. The diagnostic utility of immunohistochemistry in distinguishing between epithelioid mesotheliomas and squamous carcinomas of the lung: a comparative study. *Mod Pathol* 2006;19:417–428.
379. Ordonez NG. What are the current best immunohistochemical markers for the diagnosis of epithelioid mesothelioma? A review and update. *Hum Pathol* 2007;38:1–16.
380. Mimura T, Ito A, Sakuma T, et al. Novel marker D2-40, combined with calretinin, CEA, and TTF-1: an optimal set of immunodiagnostic markers for pleural mesothelioma. *Cancer* 2007;109:933–938.
381. Marchevsky AM, Wick MR. Evidence-based guidelines for the utilization of immunostains in diagnostic pathology: pulmonary adenocarcinoma versus mesothelioma. *Appl Immunohistochem Mol Morphol* 2007;15:140–144.
382. Hirano H, Maeda H, Sawabata N, et al. Desmoplastic malignant mesothelioma: two cases and a literature review. *Med Electron Microsc* 2003;36:173–178.
383. Singhal S, Wiewrodt R, Malden LD, et al. Gene expression profiling of malignant mesothelioma. *Clin Cancer Res* 2003;9:3080–3097.
384. Pass HI, Liu Z, Wali A, et al. Gene expression profiles predict survival and progression of pleural mesothelioma. *Clin Cancer Res* 2004;10:849–859.

385. Gordon GJ, Rockwell GN, Jensen RV, et al. Identification of novel candidate oncogenes and tumor suppressors in malignant pleural mesothelioma using large-scale transcriptional profiling. *Am J Pathol* 2005;166:1827–1840.
386. Holloway AJ, Diyagama DS, Opeskin K, et al. A molecular diagnostic test for distinguishing lung adenocarcinoma from malignant mesothelioma using cells collected from pleural effusions. *Clin Cancer Res* 2006;12:5129–5135.
387. Lopez-Rios F, Chuai S, Flores R, et al. Global gene expression profiling of pleural mesotheliomas: overexpression of aurora kinases and P16/CDKN2A deletion as prognostic factors and critical evaluation of microarray-based prognostic prediction. *Cancer Res* 2006;66: 2970–2979.
388. Mossman BT, Gruenert DC. SV40, growth factors, and mesothelioma: another piece of the puzzle. *Am J Respir Cell Mol Biol* 2002;26: 167–170.
389. Cortese JF, Gowda AL, Wali A, et al. Common EGFR mutations conferring sensitivity to gefitinib in lung adenocarcinoma are not prevalent in human malignant mesothelioma. *Int J Cancer* 2006;118: 521–522.
390. Ramos-Nino ME, Blumen SR, Sabo-Attwood T, et al. HGF mediates cell proliferation of human mesothelioma cells through a PI3K/MEK5/Fra-1 pathway. *Am J Respir Cell Mol Biol* 2008;38: 209–217.
391. Graziani I, Eliasz S, De Marco MA, et al. Opposite effects of Notch-1 and Notch-2 on mesothelioma cell survival under hypoxia are exerted through the Akt pathway. *Cancer Res* 2008;68:9678–9685.
392. Ivanov SV, Miller J, Lucito R, et al. Genomic events associated with progression of pleural malignant mesothelioma. *Int J Cancer* 2009;124:589–599.
393. Gazdar AF, Butel JS, Carbone M. SV40 and human tumours: myth, association or causality? *Nat Rev Cancer* 2002;2:957–964.
394. Goldstraw P, Crowley J, Chansky K, et al. The IASLC Lung Cancer Staging Project: proposals for the revision of the TNM stage groupings in the forthcoming (seventh) edition of the TNM Classification of malignant tumours. *J Thorac Oncol* 2007;2:706–714.
395. Groome PA, Bolejack V, Crowley JJ, et al. The IASLC Lung Cancer Staging Project: validation of the proposals for revision of the T, N, and M descriptors and consequent stage groupings in the forthcoming (seventh) edition of the TNM classification of malignant tumours. *J Thorac Oncol* 2007;2:694–705.
396. Postmus PE, Brambilla E, Chansky K, et al. The IASLC Lung Cancer Staging Project: proposals for revision of the M descriptors in the forthcoming (seventh) edition of the TNM classification of lung cancer. *J Thorac Oncol* 2007;2:686–693.
397. Rusch VW, Crowley J, Giroux DJ, et al. The IASLC Lung Cancer Staging Project: proposals for the revision of the N descriptors in the forthcoming seventh edition of the TNM classification for lung cancer. *J Thorac Oncol* 2007;2:603–612.
398. Rami-Porta R, Ball D, Crowley J, et al. The IASLC Lung Cancer Staging Project: proposals for the revision of the T descriptors in the forthcoming (seventh) edition of the TNM classification for lung cancer. *J Thorac Oncol* 2007;2:593–602.
399. Mulligan CR, Meram AD, Proctor CD, et al. Lung cancer staging: a case for a new T definition. *Ann Thorac Surg* 2006;82:220–226.
400. Butnor KJ, Cooper K. Visceral pleural invasion in lung cancer: recognizing histologic parameters that impact staging and prognosis. *Adv Anat Pathol* 2005;12:1–6.
401. Flieder DB. Commonly encountered difficulties in pathologic staging of lung cancer. *Arch Pathol Lab Med* 2007;131:1016–1026.
402. Shimizu K, Yoshida J, Nagai K, et al. Visceral pleural invasion classification in non-small cell lung cancer: a proposal on the basis of outcome assessment. *J Thorac Cardiovasc Surg* 2004;127:1574–1578.
403. Taube JM, Askin FB, Brock MV, et al. Impact of elastic staining on the staging of peripheral lung cancers. *Am J Surg Pathol* 2007;31:953–956.
404. Gu CD, Osaki T, Oyama T, et al. Detection of micrometastatic tumor cells in pN0 lymph nodes of patients with completely resected non-small cell lung cancer: impact on recurrence and survival. *Ann Surg* 2002;235:133–139.
405. Passlick, B. Micrometastases in non-small cell lung cancer (NSCLC). *Lung Cancer* 2001;34(Suppl 3):S25–S29.
406. Osaki T, Oyama T, Gu CD, et al. Prognostic impact of micrometastatic tumor cells in the lymph nodes and bone marrow of patients with completely resected stage I non-small-cell lung cancer. *J Clin Oncol* 2002;20:2930–2936.
407. Kubuschok B, Passlick B, Izbicki JR, et al. Disseminated tumor cells in lymph nodes as a determinant for survival in surgically resected non-small-cell lung cancer. *J Clin Oncol* 1999;17:19–24.
408. Junker K. Histopathologic evaluation of mediastinal lymph nodes in lung cancer. *Lung Cancer* 2004;45(Suppl 2):S79–S83.
409. Maeda J, Inoue M, Okumura M, et al. Detection of occult tumor cells in lymph nodes from non-small cell lung cancer patients using reverse transcription-polymerase chain reaction for carcinoembryonic antigen mRNA with the evaluation of its sensitivity. *Lung Cancer* 2006;52:235–240.
410. Wang XT, Sienel W, Eggeling S, et al. Detection of disseminated tumor cells in mediastinoscopic lymph node biopsies and lymphadenectomy specimens of patients with NSCLC by quantitative RT-PCR. *Eur J Cardiothorac Surg* 2005;28:26–32.
411. Xi L, Coello MC, Litle VR, et al. A combination of molecular markers accurately detects lymph node metastasis in non-small cell lung cancer patients. *Clin Cancer Res* 2006;12:2484–2491.
412. Little AG. Sentinel node biopsy for staging lung cancer. *Surg Clin North Am* 2002;82:561–571, vii.
413. Liptay, MJ, Masters GA, Winchester DJ, et al. Intraoperative radioisotope sentinel lymph node mapping in non-small cell lung cancer. *Ann Thorac Surg* 2000;70:384–389; discussion 389–390.
414. Minamiya Y, Ogawa J. The current status of sentinel lymph node mapping in non-small cell lung cancer. *Ann Thorac Cardiovasc Surg* 2005;11:67–72.
415. Minamiya Y, Ito M, Katayose Y, et al. Intraoperative sentinel lymph node mapping using a new sterilizable magnetometer in patients with nonsmall cell lung cancer. *Ann Thorac Surg* 2006;81:327–330.
416. Schirren J, Bergmann T, Beqiri S, et al. Lymphatic spread in resectable lung cancer: can we trust in a sentinel lymph node? *Thorac Cardiovasc Surg* 2006;54:373–380.
417. Pieterman RM, van Putten JW, Meuzelaar JJ, et al. Preoperative staging of non-small-cell lung cancer with positron-emission tomography. *N Engl J Med* 2000;343:254–261.
418. Lardinois D, Weder W, Hany TF, et al. Staging of non-small-cell lung cancer with integrated positron-emission tomography and computed tomography. *N Engl J Med* 2003;348:2500–2507.
419. Ung YC, Maziak DE, Vanderveen JA, et al. 18Fluorodeoxyglucose positron emission tomography in the diagnosis and staging of lung cancer: a systematic review. *J Natl Cancer Inst* 2007;99:1753–1767.
420. Gephardt GN, Baker PB. Lung carcinoma surgical pathology report adequacy: a College of American Pathologists Q-Probes study of over 8300 cases from 464 institutions. *Arch Pathol Lab Med* 1996;120:922–927.
421. Association of Directors of Anatomic and Surgical Pathology. Recommendations for the reporting of resected primary lung carcinomas. *Am J Clin Pathol* 1995;104:371–374.

SECTION 5

Presentation, Diagnosis, and Staging

CHAPTER 23

Antoinette J. Wozniak
Shirish M. Gadgeel

Clinical Presentation of Non–Small Cell Carcinoma of the Lung

Lung cancer is a major cause of cancer-related mortality worldwide and is expected to remain a major health problem for the foreseeable future.[1] Although lung cancer remains predominantly a disease of men, the number of women diagnosed with the disease has risen dramatically over the last 2 decades. The median age at presentation in the United States is around 67 years old. However, about 10% of the cases occur in patients younger than the age of 50.[2]

The clinical manifestations of lung cancer are varied. Patients are usually asymptomatic in early stages of the disease. This is related to the sparse pain fiber innervation of the lungs and the significant respiratory reserve that both lungs provide. The lack of symptoms is particularly true for lung cancers that originate in the periphery of the lungs. Approximately 5% to 10 % of lung cancer patients are asymptomatic at presentation.[3,4] These cancers are often detected during evaluation for an unrelated medical problem or on a chest radiograph performed for preoperative evaluation. Screening to identify a greater proportion of lung cancer patients has been the focus of much effort over the last 3 decades, and this may lead to an increase in the percentage of lung cancer patients who are asymptomatic at diagnosis. In recent years, promising results have been reported with the use of high-resolution computed tomography (CT) scans. The applicability of CT scans or other methods as screening tools for lung cancer remains to be determined.

Most lung cancer patients who are symptomatic have advanced disease. In a series of more than 600 patients, 27% presented with symptoms related to the primary tumor.[5] Most of the patients had either symptoms related to metastatic disease (32%) or nonspecific constitutional symptoms such as anorexia, fatigue, and weight loss (Table 23.1). Outcomes of patients appeared to be better when they were asymptomatic at presentation, whereas patients who presented with symptoms related to metastatic disease fared the worst. Furthermore, patients with absence of symptoms and abnormalities on standard laboratory tests were very unlikely to have scan evidence of metastatic disease.[6,7]

A delay in reporting of new symptoms or change of existing symptoms by lung cancer patients has been observed. In a series from the United Kingdom, the median time between onset of symptoms and patients seeking medical attention was 12 months.[8] A further delay often occurs since primary care physicians may not consider lung cancer in the differential diagnosis.[9] Various reasons account for the delay in considering lung cancer as a diagnosis by physicians, including the nonspecific nature of lung cancer symptoms and the fact that common lung cancer symptoms are more often attributable to benign etiologies. The impact of this observed delay on patient prognosis is unclear.

MANIFESTATIONS OF LOCAL DISEASE

Cough Cough is the most common symptom reported at presentation by lung cancer patients. Cough is present at diagnosis in 50% or more of patients and eventually develops in nearly all patients who are not cured.[10,11] Cough in lung cancer may be related to many factors, including a central tumor, obstructive pneumonia, multiple parenchymal metastases, lymph node involvement, and pleural effusion. Even though cough is the most common symptom of lung cancer, it accounts as the only cause in about 2% of patients with chronic cough.[12]

Many lung cancer patients have underlying chronic obstructive pulmonary disease (COPD) and therefore may suffer from a chronic cough. Some smokers and former smokers also have a chronic cough referred to as *smoker's cough*. Hence, the patient or the patient's physician may ignore a gradual change in such a cough. A persistent change in the cough or acute exacerbation of COPD that fails to respond to therapy should prompt performance of a chest radiograph or even a CT scan. This evaluation is particularly important if the cough is not associated with fever or symptoms of upper respiratory tract infection or persists for longer than a week. Some of these patients are treated with multiple courses of antibiotics under the

TABLE 23.1 Symptoms at Diagnosis of Non–Small Cell Lung Cancer[3,53,87–89]

Symptoms	Present at Diagnosis (%)
Cough	45–75
Dyspnea	40–60
Weight loss	20–70
Chest pain	30–45
Hemoptysis	25–35
Bone pain	6–25
Fatigue	0–20
Dysphagia	0–2
Wheezing and stridor	0–2
None	2–5

presumption of bronchitis or pneumonia, thereby delaying the diagnosis of lung cancer.

Treatment of cough is most successful if the underlying etiology can be addressed. Thus, tumor-specific therapy is most successful in relieving lung cancer–related cough. In patients with airway involvement by the tumor, patients may also benefit from the addition of beta$_2$-agonists such as albuterol.

Many lung cancer patients continue to suffer from a persistent, distressing cough despite appropriate tumor-specific therapy. It is important to evaluate and treat other potential causes of cough such as postnasal drip, gastroesophageal reflux, and bronchospasm. Opiates have been used with some success for their antitussive properties.[9] There is no evidence that one preparation of opiates is better than the other. Other antitussives such as guaifenesin, dextromethorphan, benzonatate, and levodropropizine may be tried, but they have had variable success in treating cancer-related cough.[13–16]

Inhaled lidocaine has been used to suppress cough.[13,17–19] A starting dose of 5 mL of 2% lidocaine solution, via a nebulizer, every 4 to 6 hours may be used. The dose may be increased if required. Generally, dosages greater than 15 mL of 2% lidocaine solution are avoided to decrease the risk of seizures, from systemic absorption of lidocaine through the airways. Patients should be warned about the potential for aspiration resulting from oropharyngeal anesthesia. Corticosteroids can also be helpful in treating cough, particularly when the cough is related to underlying bronchitis, radiation-induced lung damage, or lymphangitic metastases. In addition, inhaled sodium cromoglycate may help cough of lung cancer through the inhibition of afferent unmyelinated C-fiber activation. C-fibers are involved in cancer-related cough, probably from the release of bradykinin by cancer cells and from the stimulation of the C-fibers by the cancer.[20]

Hemoptysis Hemoptysis in lung cancer varies in severity but commonly consists of blood-streaked sputum. The most common description by the patient is that of coughing up blood-tinged sputum for several days in succession. Again, these patients are presumed to have bronchitis and are treated with antibiotics. The index of suspicion is raised if the symptom persists or recurs particularly in a patient who has a smoking history. It is prudent to initiate a workup immediately in a patient younger than 40 years with a smoking history who presents with hemoptysis. Although chest radiographs are usually abnormal in these patients, some may have a normal study. In these patients, further diagnostic studies such as sputum cytology, bronchoscopy,[21] and CT scans should be considered. Detailed history of hemoptysis is essential because presence of hemoptysis is a contraindication for the use of bevacizumab. In the clinical trial, Eastern Cooperative Oncology Group phase III trial (ECOG 4599) that evaluated the role of bevacizumab, presence of half a teaspoon of hemoptysis per episode was an exclusion criteria.[22]

The management of hemoptysis in lung cancer patients depends on the severity. Blood-streaked sputum does not require any specific therapy other than the therapy for lung cancer. More severe hemoptysis requires use of antitussives and advising the patient to sleep with the affected lung in the dependent position. In patients with advanced lung cancer, chest radiotherapy is the preferred treatment for moderate hemoptysis. In patients who have received prior radiotherapy, management of hemoptysis can be challenging.[23]

In certain cases, emergent thoracotomy with resection of the affected area could be considered. However, technical difficulties or the general condition of the patient may preclude such an approach. Endobronchial brachytherapy is another alternative for control of hemoptysis in patients who have received prior external beam radiotherapy. Selective embolization of bronchial arteries feeding the hemorrhagic area can also be considered in settings where such expertise exists.[24,25]

Massive hemoptysis, which is fairly uncommon in lung cancer patients, is immediately fatal in many cases. The initial management of these patients is securing the airway with intubation or emergent tracheostomy to allow efficient suctioning of the blood that floods the alveoli, leading to respiratory failure. Bronchoscopy can be performed for both diagnostic and therapeutic purposes. Bronchoscopic instillation of cold saline solution or vasoconstrictive agents and bronchial balloon tamponade are some of the therapeutic interventions that could be implemented.[26] Further management of hemorrhage should proceed based on the clinical condition of the patient. Management of hemoptysis in lung cancer patients requires sound clinical judgment. Many patients with this problem have a poor prognosis, and any interventions chosen for the hemoptysis must be consistent with the patient's prognosis.

Chest Pain Chest pain or discomfort is a common symptom that may occur even in early stage lung cancer, without frank evidence of invasion of the pleura, chest wall, or mediastinum. The origin of such discomfort is unclear because the lung parenchyma is not supplied with pain fibers. Patients may develop retrosternal pain from hilar and mediastinal adenopathy or at times from pericardial involvement. Pain from pleural involvement or rib metastasis is usually more localized and severe than the nonspecific chest pain associated with lung cancer. Appropriate analgesics, including narcotics, should be used along with definitive antitumor therapy.

It is not unusual for patients with chest pain to undergo evaluation for coronary artery disease, including cardiac catheterization. Given the prevalence of coronary artery disease among smokers, it is not surprising that such patients have been discovered to have lung cancer from a chest radiograph performed prior to or after coronary artery bypass surgery.

Dyspnea Dyspnea is a fairly common symptom in patients with lung cancer. Most lung cancer patients have dyspnea during the course of their disease.[27] Dyspnea could be from various causes, including the tumor itself or the underlying chronic lung disease, and/or could be multifactorial (Table 23.2). Patients could also experience dyspnea from the complications of radiation therapy administered with or without chemotherapy. Incidence of dyspnea is often higher when pain and anxiety are high.[28]

Management of dyspnea requires proper identification and treatment of the underlying etiology, with recognition that the tumor is not always the primary cause of the dyspnea. Symptomatic management of dyspnea includes judicious use of oxygen, opioids, and sedatives. Use of oxygen is clearly beneficial in the treatment of hypoxic patients with dyspnea.[29,30] The role of oxygen, in treating dyspnea in patients who are not hypoxic, is unclear. There are studies that suggest that oxygen may be helpful in patients with nonhypoxic dyspnea,[31,32] and based on this limited data, it is appropriate to offer a trial of oxygen in all cancer patients with dyspnea.

Opioids have been used to relieve dyspnea for many years. There is a concern about the potential of inducing respiratory failure with opioid use, particularly in patients with preexisting respiratory impairment.[33] However, studies in cancer patients suggest that opioids do not compromise respiratory function when titrated correctly.[34,35] Respiratory depression is more a function of rate of change of the dose of opioids and the history of previous exposure to opioids.[36] Opioids administered through both parenteral and oral routes appear to be beneficial in relieving dyspnea.[37] Nebulized morphine was also assessed but was found to be no better than nebulized saline, when the data of randomized trials were analyzed.[37] Sedatives and tranquilizers have also been used to relieve dyspnea. Evidence supports the use of promethazine or chlorpromazine alone or in combination with morphine for the treatment of dyspnea, but the evidence for the use of benzodiazepines is lacking.[38–41] Systemic steroids should be considered in patients with acute exacerbation of COPD and in patients with treatment-related lung toxicity.

Dyspnea is an extremely distressing symptom for the patient and the family. Relief of dyspnea to the maximum extent possible should be a primary goal of the treating physician. Education regarding complimentary methods such as breathing and relaxation techniques has been shown to be helpful for patients dealing with dyspnea.[42] It is also important to educate the patient and the family about measures that can be taken to relieve dyspnea such as anticipatory administration of opioids, taking frequent rests during physical activities, and sitting near an open window or in front of a fan.

TABLE 23.2 Causes of Dyspnea in Lung Cancer

Causes of Dyspnea
Loss of alveolar space due to extensive tumor
Atelectasis/obstruction
Lymphangitic spread
Pleural effusion
Pericardial effusion
Pneumonia
Hemoptysis with aspiration
Bronchospasm
Chronic obstructive pulmonary disease
Cardiac failure
Pulmonary embolism

Wheezing Localized wheezing may be the presenting symptom in patients with disease in the major airways, particularly in the mainstem bronchi. This symptom should be distinguished from the generalized wheezing of bronchospasm. The patient is often able to tell from where the wheezing is emanating. This type of localized wheezing is often associated with cough.

Lesions that are primarily endobronchial, but are too proximal for resection, often require special management techniques. Newer techniques have improved the ability to control such cancers and thus the symptoms from these lesions. High-dose brachytherapy, either alone or in combination with external beam radiation, can be highly effective in palliating such lesions.[43] Photodynamic therapy techniques have improved recently with the development of better photosensitizing agents and can be effectively employed in this setting.[44] Laser therapy can also be useful for this problem, particularly when other treatments have failed.[45] Stents made of different materials have been used, following tumor debridement to relieve airway obstruction, primarily when the obstruction is in central airways.[46,47]

Pneumonia Pneumonia can be a common presentation of lung cancer. Patients may not have the classical symptoms of pneumonia such as high fever, pleuritic chest pain, cough, and dyspnea but may have more generalized symptoms such as fatigue. A chest x-ray performed for evaluation may reveal lobar consolidation or atelectasis. These patients may not necessarily have pneumonia but are treated for pneumonia based on chest x-ray findings and despite lack of resolution are continued on different antibiotics. It is essential that follow-up x-rays are performed for evaluating resolution of the original findings.

MANIFESTATIONS OF LOCALLY ADVANCED DISEASE

Hoarseness Hoarseness in lung cancer patients is almost always caused by the involvement of the left recurrent laryngeal nerve resulting in left vocal cord paralysis. Because the left recurrent laryngeal nerve passes under the arch of the aorta, it is susceptible to involvement by primary tumors or lymphadenopathy in the aortopulmonary window. It is not unusual for patients with hoarseness to have had laryngoscopy and CT scans of the neck performed and then told that they have vocal cord paralysis, without any chest evaluation. New-onset hoarseness caused by involvement of the left recurrent laryngeal nerve is usually indicative of surgically unresectable lung cancer. Hoarseness may also be observed after surgery for lung cancer, because the recurrent laryngeal nerve may have to be sacrificed for complete resection of the tumor.

Vocal cord paralysis leads to voice change, in addition to hoarseness, and could also cause aspiration, dyspnea, and/or dysphagia. Hoarseness may improve with treatment of lung cancer, but more often it is persistent because of inadequate control of the primary tumor or irreversible damage to the nerve. Management of vocal cord paralysis includes Teflon or Gore-Tex injection of the vocal cord or phonosurgery.[48,49] These procedures can improve the vocal quality, as well as improve other symptoms such as dysphagia and aspiration. Some patients may require feeding tubes to prevent aspiration pneumonia.

Phrenic Nerve Paralysis The phrenic nerve courses along the pericardium bilaterally and is subject to injury caused by invasion from the primary tumor or bulky adenopathy. The left phrenic nerve is more commonly affected than the right, probably because of the relatively greater proximity of the left phrenic nerve to lymph nodes of the aortopulmonary window. Damage to the left phrenic nerve results in paralysis of the left hemidiaphragm, with consequent volume loss in the left hemithorax. Because the left hemidiaphragm is normally lower than the right, this condition has a rather characteristic x-ray appearance. The proximity of the left recurrent laryngeal nerve to the phrenic nerve in the aortopulmonary window occasionally results in coexisting hoarseness and left diaphragmatic paralysis. Phrenic nerve paralysis is always indicative of locally advanced disease. This condition is generally not reversible.

Dysphagia Dysphagia can result from esophageal obstruction by bulky mediastinal adenopathy. Although bulky adenopathy is a relatively common occurrence, this symptom is surprisingly uncommon. Another potential cause of dysphagia is recurrent laryngeal nerve damage that can lead to dysfunction of the pharyngeal swallowing mechanism. This problem may be associated with aspiration as well (see preceding discussion under "Hoarseness"). Treatment of the mediastinal adenopathy with radiotherapy (with or without concurrent chemotherapy) may improve dysphagia caused by this mechanism. However, radiation-induced esophagitis could lead to acute odynophagia and dysphagia with a few patients developing chronic dysphagia from esophageal strictures. Selected patients may require nutritional support until effective swallowing is reestablished.

Stridor Stridor results from compromise of the lumen of the trachea. It can be caused by invasion of the trachea by tumor, or less commonly, bilateral vocal cord paralysis. An aggressive approach to management of stridor is necessary, because this problem is life threatening and extremely distressing. Prompt initiation of treatment, including radiotherapy or brachytherapy, with or without chemotherapy, is essential. For lesions located high in the trachea, or stridor caused by vocal cord paralysis, a tracheostomy may permit placement of a rigid canula beyond the obstruction. Considerations could be given to treatments, such as photodynamic therapy or laser therapy, to improve the airways prior to proceeding with more definitive therapy. Because flow is related to diameter in an exponential fashion, a small increase in diameter can result in a dramatic improvement in symptoms. This increase can sometimes be accomplished via laser fulguration.[50,51]

Symptoms can be eased by the use of a helium–oxygen mixture (70:30), in place of room air or oxygen alone. Helium has a much lower viscosity than nitrogen, thus reducing obstruction to flow.[52] Patients whose disease progresses despite therapy may require significant doses of morphine for control of symptoms.

Superior Vena Cava Syndrome Superior vena cava (SVC) syndrome is a relatively common complication of lung cancer.[53,54] It is generally a consequence of obstruction of the SVC by right paratracheal adenopathy or central extension of primary tumor in the right upper lobe. The syndrome is characterized by facial swelling, flushing, cough, and neck and chest wall vein distention. The extent and severity of symptoms greatly depends on how rapidly the obstruction progresses and on the speed and extent of the development of collateral circulation. Rapidly developing obstruction is most dangerous because it can result in central nervous system symptoms, including coma and death. Much more commonly, the onset is insidious, with swelling of the face, upper extremities, and breasts, causing the patient to seek medical attention.

In the undiagnosed patient, the principal differential diagnosis is between lung cancer and lymphoma. Approximately 80% of patients with SVC syndrome in the United States have an underlying diagnosis of lung cancer, divided approximately equally between small cell and non–small cell histologies. Once considered an emergency, current practice is to obtain a tissue diagnosis expeditiously prior to the initiation of appropriate therapy.[55] Bronchoscopy, mediastinoscopy, or mediastinotomy usually yield a diagnosis with little risk to the patient. Radiotherapy remains the preferred treatment for non–small cell lung cancer (NSCLC) and in selected situations, concurrent chemotherapy may be appropriate. Percutaneous stenting of the SVC is being increasingly used as the first treatment modality.[56,57] Stents are also considered in patients who have not responded to other treatment modalities. In uncommon circumstances, surgery could be considered for bypass or replacement of the SVC.

Pleural Effusion Approximately 15% of lung cancer patients present with pleural effusion. Although most of these effusions are ultimately determined to be malignant, about one half are initially cytologically negative. Diagnostic thoracentesis should be performed to determine the origin of the effusion, with an adequate amount of fluid sent for cytology. The differential diagnosis for causes of effusion can include atelectasis, pneumonia, lymphatic obstruction from enlarged lymph nodes, and congestive heart failure, among others. It is important to identify malignant effusion if possible. Proper classification of an effusion can both prevent the application of ineffective local measures (i.e., surgery or radiotherapy) as well as ensure that resectable patients are not denied the benefits of surgery.

The management of malignant pleural effusion varies greatly, depending on the clinical situation. Patients with good performance status and reasonable life expectancy can benefit from aggressive interventions such as video-assisted thoracoscopy and talc insufflation. Traditional thoracostomy tube placement can also be beneficial to patients who are in good physical condition.[58,59] Patients with more advanced stages of disease are better served by placement of a flexible small-bore catheter, which does not require hospitalization. It is also important to understand that patients with trapped lung caused by parenchymal or pleural disease will not benefit from pleural fluid drainage.

Pleural effusions may resolve with effective chemotherapy, especially in patients with small cell lung cancer (SCLC). In NSCLC patients who are not symptomatic from the effusion and do not have a large effusion, chemotherapy may be tried as the initial management, but most patients in this category eventually require more aggressive local measures.

Pericardial Effusion Pericardial effusion develops in 5% to 10% of lung cancer patients. At autopsy, cardiac involvement occurs in approximately 15% of cases.[60,61] Pericardial effusion typically occurs in the setting of locally advanced disease. Patients usually have dyspnea and orthopnea as the initial symptoms. The other symptoms and signs associated with pericardial effusion are anxiety, substernal chest tightness, jugular venous distension, and hepatomegaly.

Pericardial effusion causing cardiac tamponade is missed in up to one third of patients. The symptoms can be only dyspnea and anxiety and are often attributed to progression of parenchymal lung disease. The finding of dyspnea without concurrent hypoxia in an anxious, dyspneic patient with locally advanced lung cancer should prompt an investigation for pericardial disease.

Management of pericardial disease is dependent on whether the patient has cardiac tamponade. Patients with tamponade require immediate intervention with the preferred treatment being pericardiotomy (pericardial window) via a subxiphoid approach.[62] Patients with very short expected survival or patients who do not have tamponade could be treated with pericardiocentesis. If appropriate expertise is available, placement of a small bore pericardial catheter can be effective. Such a catheter could be used to instill a sclerosing agent, which may help achieve long-term control of the effusion in many patients.[63]

Pericardial effusion can be a late complication of chest radiation therapy (with or without chemotherapy) when significant portions of the pericardium are included in the radiation field.[64] Therefore, occurrence of pericardial effusion in a patient who has received chest radiation should not be assumed to be tumor recurrence.

Pancoast Syndrome Pancoast syndrome is the occurrence of shoulder and upper chest wall pain caused by the presence of a tumor in the apex of the lung with invasion of adjacent structures. It could be accompanied by Horner syndrome, brachial plexopathy, and reflex sympathetic dystrophy. The chest pain is caused by direct invasion of the chest wall, the first and second ribs, and in some cases, the transverse processes and bodies of the upper thoracic vertebrae. Some of these patients develop spinal cord compression. Horner syndrome results from the involvement of the superior cervical ganglion, and consists of ipsilateral ptosis, meiosis, enophthalmos, and anhydrosis. When the upper sympathetic chain is also destroyed, autonomic innervation to the ipsilateral limb is lost, leading to reflex sympathetic dystrophy. This is characterized by pain and swelling, resulting from loss of vascular tone regulation. Involvement of the brachial plexus results in radiating pain to the arm and forearm.

The typical patient has symptoms for long periods and is often evaluated for local shoulder problems without attention to the chest. Treatment of patients with pancoast tumors is based on the stage of the disease. Patients with no mediastinal involvement are treated with preoperative chemotherapy and radiation followed by surgery.[65,66] Patients who have mediastinal involvement are treated usually with radiation and chemotherapy. Pain control can be problematic in these patients requiring large doses of long-acting narcotics. In patients who do not undergo surgery, radiation can achieve pain control. However, the pain control in many of these patients is transient, requiring further interventions such as placement of an epidural or intradural catheter.

Lymphangitic Spread Lymphangitic spread of the tumor through the lung parenchyma is an ominous development. This spread is characterized by progressive dyspnea, cough, and hypoxia associated with an expanding infiltrate. Fever may be observed with these developments.

Lymphangitic spread often presents a diagnostic dilemma. The nonspecific nature of the infiltrate often results in diagnostic uncertainty. The differential diagnosis typically includes infection and radiation pneumonitis. High-resolution

CT scanning might reveal characteristic changes associated with lymphangitic spread.[67] Bronchoscopy with bronchoalveolar lavage can also be useful in establishing a diagnosis. In many cases, empiric use of antibiotics and high-dose steroids may be preferable in many patients. High-dose steroids may be transiently beneficial in relieving dyspnea caused by lymphangitic spread.

MANIFESTATIONS OF EXTRATHORACIC SPREAD

Brain Metastases Lung cancer is the most common cause of brain metastases.[68] There are some data to suggest that with improved disease control in locally advanced disease increased incidence of brain metastases is being observed.[69,70] The manifestations of brain metastases are variable and depend on the location of the lesion and the amount of associated edema and/or hemorrhage. Patients may present with headache, nausea/emesis, focal weakness, seizures, confusion, ataxia, or visual disturbances. Leptomeningeal carcinomatosis may present as cranial nerve palsies. Patients with persistent headaches without any structural abnormalities on brain imaging should undergo spinal fluid evaluation for leptomeningeal carcinomatosis. A positive cytology is found on an initial lumbar puncture in 50% to 70% of the patients. In patients with clinical signs and symptoms suggestive of leptomeningeal metastases, repeat lumbar puncture is required if the first cytology evaluation is negative.

Magnetic resonance imaging (MRI) is clearly the gold standard for identifying brain metastases and is more sensitive than CT scanning.[71,72] MRI is particularly useful when resection of solitary brain metastases is being contemplated because an MRI scan with gadolinium contrast may reveal other smaller lesions missed on CT scans. MRI could also be useful in the diagnosis of leptomeningeal involvement.

Initial management of brain metastases consists of corticosteroids given intravenously or orally, based on the patient's condition.[73] Patients with seizures should be treated with antiseizure medications. However, prophylactic use of antiseizure medications is not essential and carries with it a high potential for adverse effects.[74] Subsequent management of brain metastases depends on size, number, location of the lesions as well as the status of the extracranial disease, and the general condition of the patient.[75]

Leptomeningeal carcinomatosis is a particularly difficult challenge in lung cancer patients. It is poorly responsive to therapy and generally occurs in the setting of progressive systemic disease. In selected patients, intrathecal chemotherapy can be beneficial, but in many patients, supportive care alone is optimal.[76]

Bone Metastases Lung cancer can metastasize to almost any bone, although the axial skeleton and proximal long bones are most commonly involved. Bone pain is present in up to 25% of all lung cancer patients at presentation. In lung cancer, positron emission tomography (PET) scans have similar sensitivity to isotope bone scans although less specificity.[77] Therefore, patients with PET scans that do not show any abnormality in bones, and have no signs or symptoms suggestive of metastases, do not need an additional bone scan. In patients with bone metastases, radiograph evaluation of weight-bearing bones may be important to detect the risk of and prevent pathologic fractures. Most symptomatic bone metastases in lung cancer patients are treated with radiation therapy. In selected patients with weight-bearing bony metastases, surgical options could be considered.[78,79]

Patients with bone metastases may require significant pain medications. Pain related to bone metastases may respond well to nonsteroidal anti-inflammatory drugs (NSAIDs) and should be considered in addition to narcotic analgesics. Recent data suggests that the new generation nitrogen-containing bisphosphonate, zoledronic acid, has clinical benefits in solid tumor patients with bone metastases, including lung cancer patients. In a randomized study that included NSCLC patients, zoledronic acid significantly decreased the incidence of skeletal-related events and increased the time to the first skeletal-related event.[80] There are also data to suggest that the addition of bisphosphonates to radiation therapy for bone metastases was beneficial.[81]

Liver, Adrenal Glands, and Intra-abdominal Lymph Node Metastases Liver involvement is fairly common in patients with lung cancer. Liver metastases most commonly cause fatigue, weight loss, epigastric discomfort, and nausea/emesis. Patients may have upper quadrant pain from large metastases. Liver function tests could be normal, and liver dysfunction occurs only in the presence of numerous metastases. Presence of liver metastases carries a poor prognosis.

Adrenal and intra-abdominal lymph node metastases are usually detected on CT scans performed to evaluate lung cancer. In most cases, these lesions are asymptomatic. Large adrenal metastases may cause pain. Adrenal insufficiency is usually not observed but should be considered in patients who present with appropriate clinical symptoms and laboratory abnormalities, with bilateral adrenal metastases. There have been reports of surgical resection of solitary adrenal metastases, particularly metachronous lesions.[82,83] However, many of these reports have demonstrated limited benefits from such a strategy.

Other Metastatic Sites Since lung cancer is a common tumor, metastases are occasionally seen at a variety of other sites. These include skin, soft tissue, pancreas, bowel, ovary, and thyroid. Management of these other metastatic sites is primarily symptomatic.

Constitutional Symptoms Several constitutional symptoms affect lung cancer patients. These symptoms include depression, fatigue, anxiety, and insomnia. Depression is fairly common in lung cancer patients.[84,85] Impaired functional status was the most important risk factor for presence of depression.[85] Inadequate recognition of depression has been observed among cancer patients. Presence of depression and anxiety can worsen other symptoms such as pain and fatigue. Appropriate interventions, including use of drug therapy, have shown benefits in cancer patients.[86]

Fatigue is a frequent symptom in lung cancer patients and is commonly a result of multiple factors including anemia, dyspnea, cachexia, and therapy-related side effects. Identification of the factors contributing to fatigue in a particular patient is important for the management of the symptom. Similarly, multiple different factors cause and contribute to insomnia. Appropriate assessment of these symptoms and management of the causes can reduce the symptom burden of the patient, particularly in patients with advanced cancer.

PARANEOPLASTIC SYNDROMES

Carcinomas of the lung most often present with symptoms related to the locoregional effects of the primary tumor or to the manifestation of extrathoracic spread. However, patients can also present with paraneoplastic syndromes, which are remote effects of the primary tumor that can result in organ dysfunction.[90] The development of paraneoplastic syndromes is not necessarily related to the extent of disease and can precede the clinical diagnosis of cancer. They can also occur later in the course of the disease or herald a cancer recurrence. The mechanistic etiology of these syndromes is not entirely understood but, in some instances, may be related to a humoral substance produced by the tumor or to an immunologic response to the cancer.[91] Several different paraneoplastic syndromes are clinically apparent in 10% to 20% of patients with bronchogenic carcinoma. These syndromes occur with more frequency in patients with SCLC. Table 23.3 lists the common and not-so-common paraneoplastic syndromes associated with thoracic malignancies.[92] This discussion will be devoted to those syndromes that occur in NSCLC patients.

Cachexia Cancer cachexia syndrome is characterized by anorexia, weight loss, and weakness, resulting in impaired immune status, tissue wasting, and decline in performance status.[93] Cancer-associated anorexia and cachexia entails weight loss of more than 5% of baseline weight during the previous 2 to 6 months.

The syndrome of cancer cachexia occurs commonly in lung cancer patients but usually in the case of advanced disease. The origin of cancer cachexia is not totally understood but is probably multifactorial. Several cytokines, tumor factors, and hormones have been implicated, including tumor necrosis factor α (TNF-α), interleukins (IL), proteoglycan, insulin, corticotropin, epinephrine, human growth factor, and insulin-like growth factor.[94,95] The cancer patient may also have a maladaptive metabolism, resulting in a poor utilization of nutrients, in addition to decreased caloric intake.[96] The abnormalities associated with cachexia include alterations in carbohydrate, lipid, and protein metabolism.[97] Anorexia can also be potentiated by pain, gastrointestinal involvement by tumor, development of food aversions, and the systemic effect of cancer treatment.[98] Cachexia in lung cancer patients has been associated with reduction in performance status, quality of life, and poorer prognosis.

The cachexia syndrome is not easily managed. A careful assessment of the patient's symptoms, clinical condition, and the disease status is required to properly address the issues of anorexia and cachexia. It is important to detect and treat reversible causes such as dry mouth, stomatitis, severe constipation, pain, depression, and others. Simply increasing nutritional support even by central or parenteral means is not clinically efficacious.[99] Several pharmacologic agents have been utilized to improve anorexia in cancer patients.[100] The most commonly used agent is megestrol acetate. In a trial by Loprinzi et al.,[101] a positive dose–response effect on appetite resulted with increasing doses of megestrol acetate (no benefit beyond 800 mg/day), and a trend toward nonfluid weight gain was apparent. Steroids have limited benefit; tetrahydrocannabinol derivatives may be useful in improving appetite and symptoms of nausea. The treatment of cancer-related cachexia is a fertile area of research. Some novel approaches have included the use of ghrelin, melanocortin antagonists, and anticytokine strategies.[102] A better understanding of the mechanism of cancer-related anorexia/cachexia will clearly be needed before more advances can be made.

Endocrinologic Syndromes

Hypercalcemia Hypercalcemia is a fairly common metabolic problem associated with malignancies.[103] Several pathologic mechanisms have been proposed, including osteolytic bone metastases or humoral and cytokine factors such as parathyroid hormone–related protein (PTHrP), transforming growth factor-α, IL-1, TNF, prostaglandins, and lymphotoxin.[104,105] Bender and Hansen[106] reviewed 200 consecutive cases of bronchogenic lung cancer and found a 12.5% incidence of hypercalcemia. Hypercalcemia associated with carcinoma of the lung can occur with bone metastases but often occurs in the absence of osseous involvement. Squamous cell carcinoma is the most common histology associated this paraneoplastic presentation, generally in advanced-stage disease.[107] Hypercalcemia rarely occurs in small cell carcinoma even though other paraneoplastic syndromes are common in this malignancy.[108] Benign conditions may be responsible for hypercalcemia in cancer patients. An example of this relationship would be coexistence of primary hyperparathyroidism with the malignancy.[109]

Calcium is controlled by the interaction of parathyroid hormone (PTH), 1,25-dihydroxyvitamin D, and calcitonin in the bone, kidney, and gastrointestinal tract. PTH stimulates bone resorption, renal calcium reabsorption in the distal renal tubules, and production of vitamin D by the kidney. Patients with cancer-related hypercalcemia can have increased PTH activity in their blood.[110] Immunoreactive PTH levels are usually low or normal; however, a PTHrP can be detected in the serum.[111] This protein product is homologous with PTH at the amino terminus, which is the portion that binds to the

TABLE 23.3 Paraneoplastic Syndromes Associated with Lung Cancer

Endocrinologic	Hematologic/Coagulopathies
Hypercalcemia (PTHrP)	Anemia
Hyponatremia (SIADH)	Autoimmune hemolytic anemia
Cushing syndrome (ACTH)	Leukocytosis
Gynecomastia (β-hCG)	Eosinophilia
Galactorrhea (prolactin)	Monocytosis
Hypoglycemia (insulin-like substance)	Thrombocytosis
Acromegaly (growth hormone)*	Idiopathic thrombocytopenic purpura
Calcitonin†	Thrombophlebitis
Thyroid stimulating hormone†	Trousseau syndrome
	Nonbacterial thrombotic endocarditis
Neurologic	Disseminated intravascular coagulation
Necrotizing myelopathy	
Intestinal pseudo-obstruction	**Renal/Metabolic**
Lambert-eaton myasthenic syndrome	Lactic acidosis
Retinopathy	Hyperuricemia/hypouricemia
Peripheral neuropathy (motor and/or sensory)	Hypertension (renin)
Cerebellar degeneration	Nephrotic syndrome
Limbic encephalitis	Membranous nephropathy
Encephalomyelitis	
Stiff-man syndrome	**Systemic**
Opsoclonus/myoclonus	Fever
	Anorexia/cachexia
Musculoskeletal/Collagen Vascular	
Clubbing	
Hypertrophic pulmonary osteoarthropathy	
Vasculitis	
Dermatomyositis	
Polymyositis	
Myopathy	
Systemic lupus erythematosus	
Mucocutaneous	
See Table 23.4	

*Associated with carcinoid tumors.

†No significant clinical syndrome.

PTH receptor.[112] The gene responsible for PTHrP expression is located on the short arm of chromosome 12. PTHrP acts as a hormone that stimulates bone resorption and renal phosphate wasting, resulting in hypercalcemia and hypophosphatemia. It has been suggested that lung cancer patients with hypercalcemia and elevated PTHrP levels may have a higher likelihood of bone metastases and a shorter survival.[113]

Clinical symptoms associated with hypercalcemia can be variable depending on the level of serum calcium and rapidity with which the level was achieved. Early manifestations can include nausea and vomiting, fatigue, lethargy, anorexia, muscle weakness, constipation, pruritus, polyuria, and polydipsia. The symptoms may not be recognized because they can be related to the existing malignancy, treatment toxicities (i.e., chemotherapy, narcotics), and other comorbid conditions. If untreated, patients can become severely dehydrated, subsequently developing renal insufficiency. Glomerular filtration is decreased, and a reversible defect in the kidney can result in loss of urine-concentrating ability.[114] Neurologic manifestations can also be significantly worsened, resulting in confusion, obtundation, psychosis, seizures, and coma. Further effects on the gastrointestinal tract can lead to obstipation and ileus. Electrocardiographic changes can occur with a prolonged PR interval, shortened QT interval, and a wide T wave. This can result in bradycardia and atrial or ventricular arrhythmias. Poor performance status, advanced age, and preexisting renal and hepatic dysfunction can add to the effects of hypercalcemia.

Patients who have serum calcium levels higher than 13 mg/dL or who exhibit symptoms related to hypercalcemia usually require treatment. Goals of treatment should include hydration, inhibition of bone resorption and/or promotion of calcium excretion, and treatment of the underlying malignancy.[115]

Because hypercalcemic patients are often dehydrated, rehydration has become the mainstay of treatment. Vigorous hydration with isotonic saline (200 to 400 mL/hr) can be used for several hours to restore intravascular volume and glomerular filtration to promote calcium excretion.[116] Care must be taken in the patient with cardiovascular compromise or renal insufficiency to avoid volume overload. In cases of renal failure, dialysis may have to be employed. Diuretics should be used judiciously once rehydration is achieved. Thiazide diuretics should be avoided because they can increase calcium resorption in the distal tubule. Furosemide is the diuretic of choice and can promote calcium excretion by interfering with calcium reabsorption in the ascending limb of Henle's loop. Diuretics should be primarily used to balance fluid intake and output. The use of saline hydration and forced diuresis for treatment of hypercalcemia is no longer recommended. Along with hydration, a pharmaceutical agent that helps decrease bone resorption should be employed.

The bisphosphonates are the safest and most effective agents used for the treatment of hypercalcemia. These compounds are structural analogues of pyrophosphate and by binding to hydroxyapatite are potent inhibitors of bone crystal dissolution and osteoclast reabsorption. Pamidronate and zoledronate are the drugs most commonly used for the treatment of hypercalcemia. In a randomized trial, zoledronate (4 and 8 mg) proved to be statistically superior to pamidronate (90 mg) in that it yielded a more rapid and sustained decrease in serum calcium.[117] The recommended dose of zoledronic acid is 4 mg by a 15-minute infusion. The drugs have an acceptable safety profile but should be administered with caution in patients with renal insufficiency.

Gallium nitrate is a potent inhibitor of bone resorption via inhibition of an ATPase-dependent pump in the osteoclast.[118] Gallium nitrate is usually administered at a dose of 100 to 200 mg/m^2/day by continuous infusion for up to 5 days, making it somewhat inconvenient. Urine output has to be maintained during administration and nephrotoxic drugs should be avoided because of a potential for renal toxicity. Calcitonin (4 to 8 IU/kg intramuscularly or subcutaneously every 12 hours) exerts its hypocalcemic effect by inhibiting bone resorption and promoting calcium excretion.[119] The main advantage is that it has a rapid onset of action and can be used in patients even if they have renal insufficiency. The main disadvantage of the drug is that the hypocalcemic effect is weak and transient. Plicamycin (Mithramycin) is an antineoplastic agent that is toxic to osteoclasts.[120] Its use is currently limited secondary to lack of availability and potential adverse side effects. Corticosteroids are useful agents in patients whose diseases are often treated with these drugs (i.e., hematologic malignancies, breast cancer). Steroids are not particularly useful in lung cancer–related hypercalcemia.

Ultimately, successful treatment of the malignancy controls hypercalcemia. This goal is particularly difficult in the case of advanced lung cancer. No effective oral agents are available for maintenance of a desired serum calcium level. Patients who have continued problems with symptomatic hypercalcemia may require intermittent treatment with a bisphosphonate, which can easily be given as an outpatient infusion.

Other Endocrinologic Paraneoplastic Syndromes The syndrome of inappropriate antidiuretic hormone (SIADH) is most commonly associated with SCLC. Other cancers including NSCLC, prostate, adrenal cortex, esophageal, pancreas, colon, head and neck, thymoma, mesothelioma, bladder, carcinoid tumors, and hematologic malignancies have been associated with SIADH.[121] Nonmalignant conditions, such as an intracranial process (i.e., trauma, cerebral vascular accident, infection), pulmonary infection, or drug-related toxicity, can also be associated with SIADH. Chemotherapeutic agents (vincristine, cisplatin, cyclophosphamide), narcotics, chlorpropamide, thiazides, clofibrate, and carbamazepines have all been implicated.[122] Other causes for hyponatremia in the lung cancer patient include cardiac, liver and renal disease, adrenal insufficiency, hypothyroidism, and gastrointestinal and renal losses that are not SIADH related.

Most normal tumor tissues produce a precursor adrenocorticotropin hormone (ACTH) molecule, whereas carcinomas can produce this same precursor in much larger quantities. Some neoplasms convert the precursor ACTH to biologically active ACTH, resulting in clinically apparent Cushing syndrome.[123] The most common malignancy associated with ectopic Cushing syndrome is SCLC. Lung cancers other than SCLC tend to produce precursor ACTH that does not result in Cushing syndrome.[124] Other neoplasms associated with ectopic ACTH production include carcinoid tumors, thymic cancer, islet cell tumors, pheochromocytoma, neuroblastoma, medullary carcinoma of the thyroid, and various malignancies.[125]

Lung cancers, particularly SCLCs, can produce other hormone substances, but this process does not always result in a clinically significant paraneoplastic syndrome. Gonadotropin secretion can occur from bronchogenic carcinomas.[126] Production of the β-subunit of human chorionic gonadotropin (hCG) can result in the male patient presenting with gynecomastia. Other causes of β-hCG elevation, such as germ cell tumors, should be ruled out in this situation. Galactorrhea as a result of increased prolactin level has been reported.[127] Thyroid-stimulating hormone can be produced by tumors but rarely results in clinical hyperthyroidism. Acromegaly has been attributed to the release of a growth hormone–releasing factor by a bronchial carcinoid.[128] Hypoglycemia is rarely associated with non–islet cell malignancies. Mesothelioma is the most common neoplasm associated with hypoglycemia. The suspected cause is the tumor secretion of a nonsuppressible insulin-like substance.[129]

Neurologic Syndromes Neurologic paraneoplastic syndromes are relatively rare and can involve any portion of the nervous system.[130] Effects can be relatively focal or involve multiple levels of the nervous system. These syndromes may often develop before the actual diagnosis of the cancer. SCLC is the most common histologic type associated with neurologic paraneoplastic syndromes.

Musculoskeletal Paraneoplastic Syndromes Hypertrophic pulmonary osteoarthropathy (HPO) has long been associated with carcinoma of the lung. It is characterized by digital clubbing, painful arthralgias, and periostosis of the tubular bones.[131] Digital clubbing involves paronychial soft tissue expansion with loss of the angle between the base of the nail bed and cuticle and can involve both fingers and toes. Clubbing can present as an isolated finding. In one series, clubbing was present in 29% of the patients and was more common in women.[132] HPO is seen in less than 5% of patients with NSCLC.[133] Adenocarcinoma and squamous cell carcinoma are the most common histologies, with SCLC accounting for a small number of cases.[134] The origin of HPO is not really known. It has been suggested that a humoral mechanism, specifically growth hormone, may be involved.[135] An overexpression of vascular endothelial growth factor has recently been implicated in the pathogenesis of HPO and clubbing.[136] Diagnosis is made with radiographs of the long bones, which show periosteal elevation. A radioisotope bone scan can be very sensitive in detecting HPO before it is evident on radiographs. Treatment of the malignancy does not usually alleviate symptoms because patients often have advanced NSCLC. NSAIDs can be useful in treating the painful arthralgias.

Dermatomyositis and polymyositis are inflammatory conditions characterized by muscle weakness and tenderness, and skin changes, in the case of dermatomyositis. Breast and lung cancers are the most common associated malignancies. Most cases are idiopathic in nature and unrelated to cancer. Some controversy exists as to whether there is an actual increase in cancer risk in patients who have either disorder.[137,138] The course of these conditions may not parallel the course of the malignancy. Immunosuppressives, particularly steroids, have been used for treatment.

Mucocutaneous Manifestations Many cutaneous syndromes are associated with cancer. Many of these skin lesions are uncommon, and the association with malignancy is stronger. Some of the cutaneous findings are common and may be associated with benign conditions. It is beyond the scope of this review to describe all of these mucocutaneous manifestations. Table 23.4 shows a compilation of the syndromes associated with lung cancer.[122,139,140]

TABLE 23.4 Mucocutaneous Syndromes

Associated with Lung Cancer
Pigmented/Keratoses
Acanthosis nigricans
Tripe palms
Generalized melanosis (ACTH production)
Bazex disease
Acquired tylosis
Erythema
Erythroderma
Erythema annulare centrifugum
Erythema gyratum repens
Erythema multiforme
Miscellaneous
Dermatomyositis
Pachydermoperiostosis
Hypertrichosis lanuginosa
Pruritus/urticaria
Scleroderma
Exfoliative dermatitis
Sweet syndrome
Leser-Trélat sign

Hematologic Syndromes and Vascular Manifestations Anemia is a common problem in cancer patients, with many possible causes such as bleeding, nutritional deficiencies, and bone marrow involvement by the malignancy. Anemias with no apparent cause can be termed *paraneoplastic*. Red blood cells are usually normochromic or slightly hypochromic, ferritin levels and iron stores are normal or increased, and erythropoietin levels and reticulocyte counts are inappropriately low. The anemia may be related to several cytokines that blunt erythropoietin response.[141] Rarely autoimmune hemolytic anemia, red cell aplasia, and microangiopathic hemolytic anemia have been associated with lung cancers.[142,143]

Leukocytosis is observed in some patients and may be related to the effects of IL-1 or granulocyte-stimulating factor.[144] Leukopenia is rare. Both eosinophilia and monocytosis can occur infrequently. Thrombocytosis is a fairly common occurrence and may be related to cytokine release of IL-6 or thrombopoetin.[145,146] An idiopathic thrombocytopenia purpura-like syndrome can rarely be seen in lung cancer.[147]

Trousseau syndrome is one of the earliest paraneoplastic syndromes described. It represents an association between thrombosis and malignancy. It is seen in several malignancies, including gastrointestinal, lung, breast, ovarian, and prostate cancers.[148] Deep vein thrombosis of the lower extremities and pulmonary embolism are the most common presentations, although unusual location of thromboses can occur. The origin is probably multifactorial and can include release of procoagulant materials (particularly from mucin), release of cytokines that have procoagulant activity, platelet hyperactivity, and the release of tissue factors via abnormal tumor vasculature.[149] Therapy with heparin or warfarin may not provide satisfactory treatment.

Nonbacterial thrombotic endocarditis is associated with sterile verrucous fibrin platelet lesions in the left-sided heart valves. It is most commonly associated with adenocarcinoma of the lung.[150] This syndrome can cause tumor embolisms to the brain and other organs. Anticoagulants are usually not useful.

REFERENCES

1. Jemal A, Siegel R, Ward E, et al. Cancer statistics 2008. *CA Cancer J Clin* 2008;58:71–96.
2. Jemal A, Murray T, Samuels A, et al. Cancer statistics, 2003. *CA Cancer J Clin* 2003;53:5–26.
3. Chute CG, Greenberg ER, Baron J, et al. Presenting conditions of 1539 population-based lung cancer patients by cell type and stage in New Hampshire and Vermont. *Cancer* 1985;56:2107–2111.
4. Buccheri G, Ferrigno D. Lung cancer: clinical presentation and specialist referral time. *Eur Respir J* 2004;24:898–904.
5. Carbone PP, Frost JK, Feinstein AR, et al. Lung cancer: perspectives and prospects. *Ann Intern Med* 1970;73:1003–1024.
6. Hooper RG, Tenholder MF, Underwood GH, et al. Computed tomographic scanning of the brain in the initial staging of bronchogenic carcinoma. *Chest* 1984;85:774–776.
7. Silvestri GA, Lenz JE, Harper SN, et al. The relationship of clinical findings to CT scan evidence of adrenal gland metastases in the staging of bronchogenic carcinoma. *Chest* 1992;102:1748–1751.
8. Corner J, Hopkinson J, Fitzsimmons D, et al. Is late diagnosis of lung cancer inevitable? Interview study of patient's recollections of symptoms before diagnosis. *Thorax* 2005;60:314–319.
9. Hamilton W, Sharp D. Diagnosis of lung cancer in primary care: a structured review. *Fam Pract* 2004;21:605–611.
10. Patel AM, Peters SG. Clinical manifestations of lung cancer. *Mayo Clin Proc* 1993;68:273–277.
11. Muers MF, Round CE. Palliation of symptoms in non-small cell lung cancer: a study by the Yorkshire Regional Cancer Organisation Thoracic Group. *Thorax* 1993;48:339–343.
12. Pratter MR, Bartter T, Akers S, et al. An algorithmic approach to chronic cough. *Ann Intern Med* 1993;119,977–983.
13. Fuller RW, Jackson DM. Physiology and treatment of cough. *Thorax* 1990;45:425–430.
14. Hagen NA. An approach to cough in cancer patients. *J Pain Symptom Manage* 1991;6:257–262.
15. Irwin RS, Curley FJ, Bennett FM. Appropriate use of antitussives and protussives: a practical review. *Drugs* 1993;46:80–91.
16. Homsi J, Walsh D, Nelson KA. Important drugs for cough in advanced cancer. *Support Care Cancer* 2001;9,565–574.
17. Cowcher K, Hank GW. Long-term management of respiratory symptoms in advanced cancer. *J Pain Symptom Manage* 1990;5: 320–330.
18. Howard P, Cayton RM, Brennan SR, et al. Lidocaine aerosol and persistent cough. *Br J Dis Chest* 1977;71:19–24.
19. Sanders RV, Kirkpatrick MB. Prolonged suppression of cough after inhalation of lidocaine in a patient with sarcoid. *JAMA* 1984;252:2456–2457.
20. Moroni M, Porta C, Gualtieri G, et al. Inhaled sodium cromoglycate to treat cough in advanced lung cancer patients. *Br J Cancer* 1996;74,309–311.
21. Poe RH, Israel RH, Marin MA, et al. Utility of fiberoptic bronchoscopy in patients with hemoptysis and a nonlocalizing chest roentgenogram. *Chest* 1988;93:70–75.
22. Sandler A, Gray R, Perry MC, et al. Paclitaxel-carboplatin alone or with bevacizumab for non-small cell lung cancer. *N Engl J Med* 2007;356:318.
23. Hoegter D. Radiotherapy for palliation of symptoms in incurable cancer. *Curr Probl Cancer* 1997;21:129–183.
24. Cremaschi P, Nascimbene C, Vitulo P, et al. Therapeutic embolization of bronchial artery: a successful treatment in 209 cases of relapse hemoptysis. *Angiology* 1993;44:295–299.
25. Hayakawa K, Tanaka F, Torizuka T, et al. Bronchial artery embolization for hemoptysis: immediate and long term results. *Cardiovasc Intervent Radiol* 1992;15:154–158.
26. Valipour A, Kreuzer A, Koller H, et al. Bronchoscopy-guided topical hemostatic tamponade therapy for the management of life-threatening hemoptysis. *Chest* 2005;127,2113–2118.
27. Muers MF, Round CE. Palliation of symptoms in non-small cell lung cancer: a study by the Yorkshire Regional Cancer Organisation Thoracic Group. *Thorax* 1993;48,339–343.
28. Smith EL, Hann DM, Ahles TA, et al. Dyspnea, anxiety, body consciousness, and quality of life in patients with lung cancer. *J Pain Symptom Manage* 2001;21:323–329.
29. Bruera E, de Stoutz, Velasco-Leiva A, et al. The effects of oxygen on the intensity of dyspnea in hypoxemic terminal cancer patients. *Lancet* 1993;342:13–14.
30. Bruera E, Schoeller T, MacEachern T. Symptomatic benefit of supplemental oxygen in hypoxemic patients with terminal cancer: the use of the N of 1 randomized controlled trial. *J Pain Symptom Manage* 1992;7:365–368.
31. Woodcock AA, Gross ER, Geddes DM. Oxygen relieves breathlessness in "pink puffers." *Lancet* 1981;6:907–909.
32. Booth S, Kelly M, Cox NP, et al. Does oxygen help dyspnea in patients with cancer? *Am J Respir Crit Care Med* 1996;153:1515–1518.
33. Wilson RH, Hoseth W, Dempsey ME. Respiratory acidosis: I. Effects of decreasing respiratory minute volume in patients with severe chronic pulmonary emphysema, with specific reference to oxygen, morphine and barbiturates. *Am J Med* 1954;17:464–470.
34. Bruera E, MacMillan K, Pither J, et al. Effects of morphine on the dyspnea of terminal cancer patients. *J Pain Symptom Manage* 1990;5: 341–344.
35. Mazzocato C, Buclin T, Rapin CH. The effects of morphine on dyspnea and ventilatory function in elderly patients with advanced cancer: a randomized double-blind controlled trial. *Ann Oncol* 1999;10:1511–1514.
36. Dudgeon DJ. Managing dyspnea and cough. *Hematol Oncol Clin N Am* 2002;16:557–577.
37. Jennings AL, Davies A, Higgins JPT, et al. Opioids for the palliation of breathlessness in terminal illness (Cochrane Review). In: *The Cochrane Library*. 4th issue. Oxford: Update software, 2001.
38. O'Neill PA, Morton PB, Stark RD. Chlorpromazine- a specific effect on breathlessness? *Br J Clin Pharmacol* 1985;19:793–797.
39. Woodcock AA, Gross ER, Geddes DM. Drug treatment of breathlessness: contrasting effects of diazepam and promethazine in pink puffers. *BMJ* 1981;283:343–346.
40. Light RW, Stansbury DW, Webster JS. Effects of 30 mg of morphine alone or with promethazine or prochlorperazine on the exercise capacity of patients with COPD. *Chest* 1996;109:975–981.
41. Sen D, Jones G, Leggat PO. The response of the breathless patient treated with diazepam. *Br J Clin Pract* 1983;37:232–233.
42. Corner J, Plant H, A'Hern R, et al. Non-pharmacological intervention for breathlessness in lung cancer. *Palliat Med* 1996;10:299–305.
43. Gejerman G, Mullokandov EA, Bagiella E, et al. Endobronchial brachytherapy and external beam radiotherapy in patients with endobronchial obstruction and extrabronchial extension. *Brachytherapy* 2002;1:204–210.
44. Moghissi K, Dixon K, Stringer M, et al. The place of bronchoscopic photodynamic therapy in advanced unresectable lung cancer: experience of 100 cases. *Eur J Cardiothorac Surg* 1999;15:1–6.

45. Lui JS, Amemiya R, Chung FM, et al. The present status of bronchoscopic Nd:YAG laser. *J Clin Laser Med Surg* 1991;9:63–70.
46. Dutau H, Toutblanc B, Lamb C, et al. Use of the Dumon Y-stent in the management of malignant disease involving the carina: a retrospective review of 86 patients. *Chest* 2004;126:951–988.
47. Miyazawa T, Yamakido M, Ikeda S, et al. Implantation of ultraflex nitinol stents in malignant tracheobronchial stenoses. *Chest* 2000;118: 959–965.
48. Kraus DH, Ali MK, Ginsberg RJ, et al. Vocal cord medialization for unilateral paralysis associated with intrathoracic malignancies. *J Thorac Cardiovasc Surg* 1996;111:334–339.
49. Abraham MT, Bains MS, Downey RJ, et al. Type I thyroplasty for acute unilateral vocal cord paralysis following intrathoracic surgery. *Ann Oto Rhinol Laryngol* 2002;111:667–671.
50. Torre M, Amari D, Barbieri B, et al. Emergency laser vaporization and helium oxygen administered for acute malignant tracheobronchial obstruction. *Am J Emerg Med* 1989;7:294–296.
51. Chen K, Baron J, Wenker OC. Malignant airway obstruction: recognition and management. *J Emerg Med* 1998;16:83–92.
52. Curtis JL, Mahlmeister M, Fink JB, et al. Helium-Oxygen gas therapy. Use and availability for the emergency treatment of inoperable airway obstruction. *Chest* 1986;90;455–457.
53. Hyde L, Hyde CI. Clinical manifestations of lung cancer. *Chest* 1974;65:299–306.
54. Yellin A, Rosen A, Reichert N, et al. Superior vena cava syndrome. *Am Rev Respir Dis* 1990;141:1114–1118.
55. Schraufnagel D, Hill R, Leech J, et al. Superior vena caval obstruction. Is it a medical emergency? *Am J Med* 1981;70:1169–174.
56. Tanigawa N, Sawada S, Mishima K, et al. Clinical outcome of stenting in superior vena cava syndrome associated with malignant tumors: comparison with conventional treatment. *Acta Radiol* 1998;39: 669–674.
57. Nicholson AA, Ettles DF, Arnold A, et al. Treatment of malignant superior vena cava obstruction: metal stents or radiation therapy. *J Vasc Interv Radiol* 1997;8:781–788.
58. Light RW. Malignant pleural effusion. In: *Pleural Diseases*. Philadelphia: Williams & Wilkins, 1990:94.
59. Kvale PA, Simoff M, Prakash UB. Palliative Care. *Chest* 2003;123: S284–S311.
60. Mukai K, Shinkai T, Tominaga K, et al. The incidence of secondary tumors of the heart and pericardium. *Jpn J Clin Oncol* 1988;18: 195–201.
61. Onuiigbo WI. The spread of lung cancer to the heart, pericardium and great vessels. *Jpn Heart J* 1974;15:234–238.
62. Park JS, Rentsehler R, Wilbur D. Surgical management of pericardial effusion in patients with malignancies. Comparison of subxiphoid window versus pericardiectomy. *Cancer* 1991;67:76–80.
63. Bellon RJ, Wright WH, Unger EC. CT-guided pericardial drainage catheter placement with subsequent pericardial sclerosis. *J Comput Assist Tomogr* 1995;19:672–673.
64. Caret RW, Sawicka JM, Choi NC. Cytologically negative pericardial effusion complicating combined modality therapy for localized small-cell carcinoma of the lung. *J Clin Oncol* 1987;5:818–824.
65. Rusch VW, Giroux DJ, Kraut MJ, et al. Induction chemoradiation and surgical resection for superior sulcus non-small cell lung carcinomas: long term results of Southwest Oncology Group trial 9416 (Intergroup Trial 0160). *J Clin Oncol* 2007;25:313–318.
66. Kunitoh H, Kato H, Tsuboi M, et al. A phase II trial of pre-operative chemoradiotherapy followed by surgical resection in pancoast tumors: Initial report of Japan Clinical Oncology Group trial (JCOG 9806). *Proc Am Soc Clin Oncol* 2003;22:634. Abstract 2549.
67. Munk PL, Müller NL, Miller RR, et al. Pulmonary lymphangitic carcinomatosis: CT and pathologic findings. *Radiology* 1988;166: 705–709.
68. Merchut MP. Brain metastases from undiagnosed systemic neoplasms. *Arch Intern Med* 1989;149:1076–1080.
69. Ceresoli GL, Reni M, Chiesa G, et al. Brain metastases in locally advanced nonsmall cell lung carcinoma after multimodality treatment: risk factor analysis. *Cancer* 2002;95:605–612.
70. Gandara DR, Chansky K, Albain KS, et al. Long-term survival with concurrent chemoradiation therapy followed by consolidation docetaxel in stage IIIB non-small-cell lung cancer: a phase II Southwest Oncology Group Study (S9504). *Clin Lung Cancer* 2006;8: 116–121.
71. Sze G, Milano E, Johnson C, et al. Detection of brain metastases: comparison of contrast-enhanced MR with unenhanced MR and contrast CT. *Am J Neuroradiol* 1990;11:785–791.
72. Davis PC, Hudgins PA, Peterman SB, et al. Diagnosis of cerebral metastases: double dose delayed CT vs contrast-enhanced MR imaging. *Am J Neuroradiol* 1991;12:293–300.
73. Coia LR, Aaronson N, Linggood R, et al. A report of the consensus workshop panel on the treatment of brain metastases. *Int J Radiat Oncol Biol Phys* 1992;23:223–227.
74. Cohen N, Strauss G, Lew R, et al. Should prophylactic anticonvulsants be administered to patients with newly diagnosed cerebral metastases? A retrospective analysis. *J Clin Oncol* 1988;6:1621–1624.
75. Kelly K, Bunn PA Jr. Is it time to reevaluate our approach to the treatment of brain metastases in patients with non-small cell lung cancer. *Lung Cancer* 1998;20:85–91.
76. Kesari S, Batchelor TT. Leptomeningeal metastases. *Neurol Clin* 2003;21:25–66.
77. Fogelman I, Cook G, Israel O, et al. Positron emission tomography and bone metastases. *Semin Nucl Med* 2005;35:135–142.
78. Haentjens P, Casteleyn PP, Opdecam P. Evaluation of impending fractures and indications for prophylactic fixation of metastases in long bones: review of literature. *Acta Orthop Belg* 1993;59 (suppl 1):6–11.
79. Broos P, Reynders P, Van Den Bogert W, et al. Surgical treatment of metastatic fracture of the femur improvement of quality of life. *Acta Orthop Belg* 1993;59(Suppl 1):52–56.
80. Rosen LS, Gordon D, Tchekmedyian NS, et al. Long-term efficacy and safety of zoledronic acid in the treatment of skeletal metastases in patients with nonsmall cell lung carcinoma and other solid tumors: a randomized, Phase III, double-blind, placebo-controlled trial. *Cancer* 2004;100:2613–2621.
81. Bloomfield DJ. Should bisphosphonates be part of the standard therapy of patients with multiple myeloma or bone metastases from other cancers? An evidence-based review. *J Clin Oncol* 1998;16: 1218–1225.
82. Porte H, Siat J, Guibert B, et al. Resection of adrenal metastases from non-small cell lung cancer: A multiinstitutional study. *Ann Thorac Surg* 2001;71:981–985.
83. Pham DT, Dean DA, Detterbeck FC. Adrenalectomy as the new treatment paradigm for solitary adrenal metastasis from lung cancer. Paper presented at: Thirty-Seventh Annual Meeting of the Society of Thoracic Surgeons; January 30, 2001, New Orleans, LA.
84. Néron S, Correa JA, Dajczman E, et al. Screening for depressive symptoms in patients with unresectable lung cancer. *Support Care Cancer* 2007;15:1207–1212.
85. Hopwood P, Stephens RJ. Depression in patients with lung cancer: prevalence and risk factors derived from quality-of-life data. *J Clin Oncol* 2000;18:893–903.
86. Patrick DL, Ferketich SL, Frame PS, et al. National Institutes of Health State-of-the-Science Conference Statement: symptom management in cancer: pain, depression, and fatigue, July 15–17, 2002. *J Natl Cancer Inst Monogr* 2004;32:9–16.
87. Anderson HA, Prakash UBS. Diagnosis of symptomatic lung cancer. *Semin Respir Med* 1982;3:165–175.
88. Grippi MA. Clinical aspects of lung cancer. *Semin Roentgenol* 1990;25:12–24.
89. Cromartie RS III, Parker EF, May JE, et al. Carcinoma of the lung. *Ann Thorac Surg* 1980;30:30–35.

90. Hall TC, ed. Paraneoplastic syndromes. *Ann NY Acad Sci* 1974; 230:1–577.
91. Spiro SG, Gould MK, Colice GL. Initial evaluation of the patient with lung cancer: symptoms, signs, laboratory tests, and paraneoplastic syndromes: ACCP evidenced-based clinical practice guidelines (2nd edition). *Chest* 2007;132:S149–S160.
92. Gerber RB, Mazzone P, Arroliga AC. Paraneoplastic syndromes associated with bronchogenic carcinoma. *Clin Chest Med* 2002;23: 257–264.
93. Puccio M, Nathanson L. The cancer cachexia syndrome. *Semin Oncol* 1997;24:277–287.
94. Langstein HN, Norton JA. Mechanisms of cancer cachexia. *Hematol Oncol Clin North Am* 1991;5:103–123.
95. Todorov P, Cariuk P, McDevitt T, et al. Characterization of cancer cachectic factor. *Nature* 1996;379:739–742.
96. Tisdale MJ. Cancer cachexia: metabolic alterations and clinical manifestations. *Nutrition* 1997;13:1–7.
97. Bosaeus I. Nutritional support in multimodal therapy for cancer cachexia. *Support Care Cancer* 2008;16:447–451.
98. Nelson KA, Walsh D, Sheehan FA. The cancer anorexia-cachexia syndrome. *J Clin Oncol* 1994;12:213–225.
99. Body JJ. The syndrome of anorexia-cachexia. *Curr Opin Oncol* 1999;11:255–260.
100. Ottery FD, Walsh D, Strawford A. Pharmacologic management of anorexia/cachexia. *Semin Oncol* 1998;25(Suppl 6):35–44.
101. Loprinzi CL, Michalak JC, Schaid DJ, et al. Phase III evaluation of four doses of megestrol acetate as therapy for patients with cancer, anorexia and/or cachexia. *J Clin Oncol* 1993;11:762–767.
102. Argilés JM, López-Soriano FJ, Busquets S. Novel approaches to the treatment of cachexia. *Drug Discov Today* 2008;13:73–78.
103. Stewart AF. Hypercalcemia associated with cancer. *N Engl J Med* 2005;352:373–379.
104. Mundy GR. Hypercalcemic factors other than parathyroid hormone-related protein. *Endocrinol Metab Clin North Am* 1989;18: 795–806.
105. Mundy GR, Martin TJ. The hypercalcemia of malignancy: pathogenesis and management. *Metabolism* 1982;31:1247–1277.
106. Bender RA, Hansen H. Hypercalcemia in bronchogenic carcinoma. *Ann Intern Med* 1974;80:325.
107. Coggeshall J, Merrill W, Hande K, et al. Implications of hypercalcemia with respect to diagnosis and treatment of lung cancer. *Am J Med* 1986;80:325–328.
108. Hayward ML Jr, Howell DA, O'Donnell JF, et al. Hypercalcemia complicating small-cell lung cancer. *Cancer* 1981;48:1643–1646.
109. Farr HW, Fahey TJ Jr, Nash AG, et al. Primary hyperparathyroidism and cancer. *Am J Surg* 1973;126:539–543.
110. Goltzman D, Stewart AF, Broadus AE. Malignancy associated hypercalcemia: evaluation with a cytochemical bioassay for parathyroid hormone. *J Clin Endocrinol Metab* 1981;53:899–904.
111. Rankin W, Grill V, Martin TJ. Parathyroid hormone-related protein and hypercalcemia. *Cancer* 1997;80:1564–1571.
112. Suva LJ, Winslow GA, Wettenhall RE, et al. A parathyroid-related protein implicated in malignant hypercalcemia: cloning and expression. *Science* 1987;237:893–896.
113. Hiraki A, Ueoka H, Bessho A, et al. Parathyroid hormone-related protein measured at the time of first visit is an indicator of bone metastases and survival in lung carcinoma patients with hypercalcemia. *Cancer* 2002;95:1706–1713.
114. Bajorunas DR. Clinical manifestations of cancer-related hypercalcemia. *Semin Oncol* 1990;17:16–25.
115. Bilezikian JP. Management of acute hypercalcemia. *N Engl J Med* 1992;326:1196–1203.
116. Ritch PS. Treatment of cancer-related hypercalcemia. *Semin Oncol* 1990;17:26–33.
117. Major P, Lortholary A, Hon J, et al. Zoledronic acid is superior to pamidronate in the treatment of hypercalcemia of malignancy: a pooled analysis of two randomized, controlled clinical trials. *J Clin Oncol* 2001;19:558–567.
118. Blair HC, Teitelbaum SL, Tan HL, et al. Reversible inhibition of osteoclastic activity by bone-bound gallium (III). *J Cell Biochem* 1992;48:401–410.
119. Warrell RP Jr. Oncologic emergencies: metabolic emergencies. In: DeVita VT Jr, Hellman S, Rosenberg SA, eds. *Cancer: Principles and Practice of Oncology*. 6th ed. Philadelphia: Lippincott Williams & Wilkins, 2001;2633–2643.
120. Kiang DT, Loken MK, Kennedy BJ. Mechanism of the hypocalcemic effect of mithramycin. *J Clin Endocrinol Metab* 1979;48:341–344.
121. Glover DJ, Glick JH. Metabolic oncologic emergencies. *CA Cancer J Clin* 1987;37:302–320.
122. Arnold SM, Lowy AM, Patchell R, et al. Paraneoplastic syndromes. In: DeVita VT Jr, Hellman S, Rosenberg SA, eds. *Cancer: Principles and Practice of Oncology.* 6th ed. Philadelphia: JB Lippincott, 2001;2511.
123. Odell WD. Endocrine/metabolic syndromes of cancer. *Semin Oncol* 1997;214:299–317.
124. Yalow RS, Eastridge CE, Higgins G Jr, et al. Plasma and tumor ACTH in carcinoma of the lung. *Cancer* 1979;44:1789–1792.
125. Liddle GW, Island DP, Ney RL, et al. Nonpituitary neoplasms and Cushing's syndrome. Ectopic "adrenocorticotropin: produced by nonpituitary neoplasms as a cause of Cushing's syndrome. *Arch Intern Med* 1963;11:471–475.
126. Faiman C, Colwell JA, Ryan RJ, et al. Gonadotropin secretion from a bronchogenic carcinoma. *N Eng J Med* 1967;277:1395–1399.
127. Blackman MR, Rosen SW, Weintraub BD. Ectopic hormones. *Adv Intern Med* 1978;23:85–113.
128. Scheithauer BW, Block B, Carpenter PC, et al. Ectopic secretion of a growth hormone-releasing factor: report of a case of acromegaly with bronchial carcinoid tumor. *Am J Med* 1984;76:605–616.
129. Gordon P, Hendricks CM, Kahn CR, et al. Hypoglycemia associated with non-islet cell tumor and insulin-like growth factors. *N Engl J Med* 1981;305:1452–1455.
130. Darnell RB, Posner JB. Paraneoplastic syndromes involving the nervous system. *N Engl J Med* 2003;349:1543–1554.
131. Martinez-Lavín M, Matucci-Cerinic M, Jajic J, et al. Hypertrophic osteoarthropathy: consensus on its definition, classification, assessment and diagnostic criteria. *J Rheumatol* 1993;20:1386–1387.
132. Sridhar KS, Lobo CF, Altman RD. Digital clubbing and lung cancer. *Chest* 1998;114:1535–1537.
133. Prakash U. Hypertrophic pulmonary osteoarthropathy and clubbing. In: Sackner MA, ed. *Weekly Updates: Pulmonary Medicine*; lesson 30. Princeton NJ: Biomedia, 1978:2–7.
134. Stenseth JH, Clagett OT, Woolner LB. Hypertrophic pulmonary osteoarthropathy. *Dis Chest* 1967;52:62–68.
135. Ennis GC, Cameron DP, Burger HG. On the etiology of hypertrophic pulmonary osteoarthropathy in bronchogenic carcinoma: lack of relationship to elevated growth hormone levels. *Aus NZ J Med* 1973;3:157–161.
136. Olán F, Portela M, Navarro C, et al. Circulating vascular endothelial growth factor concentrations in a case of pulmonary hypertrophic osteoarthropathy. *J Rheumatol* 2004;31:614–616.
137. Sigurgeirsson B, Lindelöf B, Edhag O, et al. Risk of cancer in patients with dermatomyositis or polymyositis: a population-based study. *N Eng J Med* 1992;326:363–367.
138. Lakhampal S, Bunch TW, Ilstrup DM, et al. Polymyositis-dermatomyositis and malignant lesions: does an association exist. *Mayo Clin Proc* 1986;61: 645–653.
139. Cohen PR, Kurzrock R. Mucocutaneous paraneoplastic syndromes. *Semin Oncol* 1997;24:334–359.
140. Pipkin CA, Lio PA. Cutaneous manifestations of internal malignancies: an overview. *Dermatol Clin* 2008;26:1–15.
141. Spivak JL. Cancer-related anemia: its causes and characteristics. *Semin Oncol* 1994;21(Suppl 3):3–8.
142. Spira MA, Lynch EC. Autoimmune hemolytic anemia and carcinoma: an unusual association. *Am J Med* 1979;67:753–758.

143. Antman KH, Skarin AT, Mayer RJ, et al. Microangiopathic hemolytic anemia and cancer: a review. *Medicine (Baltimore)* 1979;58:377–384.
144. Shimasaki AK, Hirata T, Kawamura T, et al. The level of granulocyte colony-stimulating factor in cancer patients with leukocytosis. *Internal Med* 1992;31:861–365.
145. Gastl G, Plante M, Finstead CL, et al. High IL-6 levels in ascitic fluid correlate with reactive thrombocytosis with epithelial ovarian cancer. *Br J Hematol* 1993;83:433–441.
146. Estrov Z, Talpaz M, Maligit G, et al. Elevated plasma thrombopoetin activity in patients with cancer related thrombocytosis. *Am J Med* 1995;98;551–558.
147. Doan C, Bouroncie BA, Wiseman BK. Idiopathic and secondary thrombocytopenic purpura: clinical study and evaluation of 381 cases over a period of 28 years. *Ann Intern Med* 1960;53:861.
148. Sack GH Jr, Levin J, Bell WR. Trousseau's syndrome and other manifestations of chronic disseminate coagulopathy in patients with neoplasms. *Medicine (Baltimore)* 1977;56:1–37.
149. Green KB, Silverstein RL. Hypercoagubility in cancer. *Hematol Oncol Clin North Am* 1996;10:499–530.
150. Gonzáles Quintela A, Candela M, Vidal C, et al. Non-bacterial thrombotic endocarditis in cancer patients. *Acta Cardiol* 1991;46: 1–9.

CHAPTER 24

Gregory A. Masters

Clinical Presentation of Small Cell Lung Cancer

The clinical presentation of small cell lung cancer (SCLC), including signs and symptoms of the disease, is important in the understanding of this disease to help make a proper diagnosis and ultimately decide on the best therapy. Various clinical factors can help predict outcome in patients with SCLC, including tumor-related factors and host-related factors. This chapter will discuss the clinical presentation of SCLC and paraneoplastic syndromes associated with this disease.

INITIAL PRESENTATION: SYMPTOMS AND SIGNS

Nearly all patients with SCLC present with symptomatic disease, and less than 10% of lung cancer patients will be diagnosed prior to clinical presentation of symptoms.[1] More effective screening, including use of chest x-rays, and more recently, low-dose spiral computed tomography (CT) scanning, as well as more sensitive molecular or genomic techniques may allow for improvement in the ability to diagnose this disease at an earlier stage,[2] but SCLC will likely be the more difficult histologic subtype to find early because of its proclivity for early dissemination. Lung cancer also tends to affect the elderly population, and nearly half of all patients presenting with SCLC will be older than the age of 60 years.[3]

A thorough understanding of the symptoms associated with SCLC can help in the appropriate diagnostic workup and, ultimately, in more effective control of these symptoms in these patients. Clinical reports have identified the most common symptoms at the time of presentation.[4] Table 24.1[5] delineates the frequency of these various signs and symptoms.[6] These can be classified as localized symptoms from the primary tumor, regional spread of disease, and distant effects from metastatic disease, as well as general symptoms, which may be attributed to a paraneoplastic effect. Presenting symptoms can also help predict prognosis in this disease.[7] It has been shown that early presentation of lung cancer is often associated with a specific pattern of symptoms.[8] Limited versus extensive disease stage, the fewer sites of metastatic involvement, good performance status, and absence of weight loss are all consistently found to correlate with survival in this disease.[9]

General Systemic Symptoms Most patients with lung cancer, and particularly SCLC, present with symptoms from their disease. Generalized systemic symptoms can include fatigue, anorexia, weight loss, and depression. These symptoms occur to a greater degree than would be expected for the extent of tumor spread.

Attempts have been made to investigate the etiology for the anorexia/cachexia syndrome associated with malignant disease, including lung cancer. This syndrome has been described as the most common cause of death in cancer patients.[10] Cachexia comes from Greek meaning "bad condition" and causes significant morbidity in lung cancer patients. No definite etiology has been determined, but loss of appetite and weight loss are commonly attributed to circulating cytokines.[11] Up to 40% of patients may experience anorexia and cachexia,[12] often requiring interventions to improve appetite and weight gain.

Fatigue is another presenting symptom commonly associated with lung cancer.[13] Commonly found at presentation, fatigue can be exacerbated by antineoplastic therapy including surgery, radiation, chemotherapy, and biologics. Evaluation for contributing secondary causes of fatigue, including anemia, endocrine dysfunction, and depression can identify readily treatable and reversible causes. Treatment of the primary tumor may be the most effective way to manage this symptom.

Depression can be another symptom in lung cancer patients.[14] With such a poor prognosis, reactive depression is a common initial reaction to a lung cancer diagnosis. Other factors may be involved in the development of depression in patients with lung cancer. Recent clinical trials have demonstrated that quality of life can be severely impacted by a diagnosis of lung cancer. Contributing to the depression are the specific symptoms from the disease as well as the psychosocial adjustment necessary with this diagnosis and its associated

TABLE 24.1 Signs and Symptoms of Small Cell Lung Cancer at Presentation

Symptom/Sign	Frequency (%)
Chest pain	20–49
Anorexia	18–33
Superior vena cava syndrome	10–15
Cough	8–75
Hemoptysis	6–35
Bone pain	6–25
Dyspnea	3–60
Hoarseness	2–18
Weight loss	0–68
Weakness	0–42
Clubbing	0–20
Fever	0–20
Dysphagia	0–2
Wheezing/stridor	0–2

treatments.[15] Further refinement of quality of life analysis in lung cancer patients is being attempted by several groups.[16]

Paraneoplastic symptoms associated with SCLC will be discussed later in this chapter. These symptoms are characterized by a systemic manifestation of disease not explained by local tumor effects.

Local Symptoms SCLC frequently presents as a large central tumor, often with symptoms of bronchial obstruction. Therefore, many patients present with local symptoms at the time of diagnosis of lung cancer.[17] Most commonly observed are chest pain, cough, and shortness of breath.[18] Cough occurs in lung cancer patients when the tumor irritates bronchial nerve fibers or leads to increased sputum production or atelectasis. Obstruction of the airway may lead to postobstructive atelectasis and/or pneumonia. These symptoms are present in at least 50% of patients at the time of diagnosis and develop in many of the remaining patients.[19] Chest x-ray can identify sites of disease and evidence for postobstructive changes. A CT scan and possibly fiberoptic bronchoscopy are necessary to identify the exact location of the tumor and to help determine appropriate ways to manage respiratory symptoms.

Central tumors can erode into blood vessels, and cough can be associated with bleeding. Hemoptysis has been noted to occur in up to 35% of patients presenting with lung cancer.[20] Hemoptysis does not necessarily imply more advanced disease but can be associated with cavitation or local extension into blood vessels. In fact, hemoptysis does not in and of itself imply malignancy.[21] Hemoptysis at times can be mild or can lead to fatal hemorrhage in lung cancer patients. Therefore, management of hemoptysis depends on the severity and specific etiology of the process. Various techniques from surgical resection, to external beam radiation, to bronchoscopic techniques including laser treatment, brachytherapy, cryotherapy, or photodynamic therapy can control symptoms effectively.[22]

Chest pain is another common symptom in SCLC, occurring in up to 49% of patients who present with primary lung cancer.[23] Pain is generally not caused by a primary tumor in the lung parenchyma, but it can be associated with chest wall involvement or local extension of disease affecting adjacent nerve fibers. Chest pain can also be attributed to unrelated causes, such as cardiac disease, esophageal disease, or vascular disease such as aortic dissection. Thus, careful evaluation of lung cancer patients with chest pain is crucial. Alternatively, lung cancer can be diagnosed serendipitously in patients presenting with acute chest pain of unrelated etiology when the chest radiograph or CT identifies a pulmonary nodule or mass.

Dyspnea or shortness of breath is also common in patients with SCLC.[24] Primary tumors are unlikely to directly result in true hypoxia. However, more advanced disease, such as obstructing tumors, lymphangitic cancer spread, or central lesions that produce significant sputum can be a cause of dyspnea in these patients. Evaluation of the differential diagnosis of shortness of breath is important to determine the underlying etiology, even in patients with malignancy. Patients may have underlying pulmonary pathology resulting from chronic obstructive pulmonary disease (COPD), and acute events such as pulmonary embolism, congestive heart failure, pneumonia, pneumothorax, and cardiac ischemia are also possibilities. In addition, regional extension and pleural effusion with compression of the remaining lung can lead to shortness of breath in this population. A thorough workup for other causes of dyspnea is necessary in lung cancer patients with worsening shortness of breath.

Lung cancer patients also present with wheezing, which can be wrongly attributed to reactive airway disease such as asthma or COPD. Obstructing pulmonary lesions can lead to wheezing in SCLC patients and should be thoroughly evaluated. Primary treatment techniques such as radiation and chemotherapy may be useful in controlling this symptom, as can standard medical therapy such as bronchodilators or corticosteroids.

Involvement of the heart or pericardium can result in tachyarrhythmias. These can present with palpitations or lightheadedness. Unexplained tachycardia in lung cancer patients should be evaluated with an electrocardiogram and/or echocardiogram whenever pericardial involvement is suspected. Pericardial metastasis or effusion may be the offending etiology, and urgent attention may benefit this population.

Locally advanced SCLC can produce esophageal compression from the primary tumor or mediastinal lymphadenopathy. Patients may have dysphagia or odynophagia, and should be evaluated endoscopically or with upper gastrointestinal imaging to evaluate the etiology of the dysphagia. Local radiation provides appropriate palliation but occasionally stenting can be helpful.[25] Particularly in SCLC, chemotherapy may provide adequate tumor shrinkage for symptom relief.

Multimodality management of SCLC patients with significant pulmonary symptoms including a thoracic surgeon, pulmonologist, primary care physician, radiation oncologist, radiologist, and medical oncologist leads to the most effective management of these local symptoms from lung cancer.

Regional Metastasis SCLC is notorious for its regional symptoms from locally advanced disease. Growth to adjacent structures near the lung as well as involvement of regional lymph nodes lead to these symptoms in patients with locally advanced disease. Patients with right-sided tumors can develop superior vena cava (SVC) obstruction as a result of the primary cancer or involvement of lymph nodes in the right paratracheal area. This can lead to the clinical manifestation, SVC syndrome. This is typically characterized by swelling of the arms, neck, face, and head. This syndrome can also be associated with shortness of breath, cyanosis, headaches, nausea, blurred vision, and more serious neurological sequelae.[26] This syndrome can also be associated with distention or dilatation of the neck and chest wall veins because of collateral blood flow. SVC syndrome can appear indolently, delaying diagnosis because of the slow changes that occur. More rapidly growing tumors or thrombosis associated with SVC syndrome can lead to a more acute presentation with rapidly developing symptoms.

In SCLC, SVC syndrome occurs in 10% to 15% of patients, more commonly than in non–small cell carcinoma.[27] A careful differential diagnosis is important in patients with SVC syndrome. Other malignancies including breast cancer and lymphoma, as well as other mediastinal tumors and occasionally benign disease such as tuberculosis or other infections can cause SVC syndrome and need to be considered in the differential diagnosis.

For patients presenting with SCLC and SVC syndrome, chemotherapy is generally the standard treatment approach, and radiotherapy is used only when chemotherapy has failed or there is a need for more rapid tumor cell kill. More aggressive interventions may become necessary, including vascular stenting of the SVC, therapeutic anticoagulation, or corticosteroids to decrease vascular inflammation and obstruction and alleviate clinical symptoms. Invasive procedures may be more hazardous because of the extensive collateral vascularity commonly observed with this syndrome.

Hoarseness is another regional symptom associated with SCLC. This is most commonly attributed to mediastinal lymph node involvement and compression of the left recurrent laryngeal nerve. This is nearly always associated with pathologic involvement of the levels 4 and 5 left-sided mediastinal lymph nodes. Evaluation with laryngoscopy can help confirm the diagnosis of vocal cord paralysis. CT scanning of the neck and chest with intravenous contrast can help document involved nodes in this region. Occasionally, local treatment may be necessary to improve symptoms resulting from vocal cord paralysis from recurrent nerve involvement.[28] Hoarseness may improve with treatment of the underlying cancer, but this symptom is commonly irreversible because of permanent nerve injury or progressive cancer in this region.

Stridor can also develop because of tracheal compression with involvement of the upper airways or bilateral recurrent laryngeal nerve involvement. This may be a result of local tumor involvement or extrinsic compression from lymphadenopathy. This can be a life-threatening emergency in patients with malignancies of the lung and/or head and neck and requires urgent airway management, usually tracheostomy. Laryngoscopic therapy can be useful in controlling upper airway tumors, but more aggressive intervention is often required, including radiation, chemotherapy, or rarely in SCLC, surgical therapy.[29]

Patients with SCLC can present with malignant effusions in the pleural or pericardial space. These effusions are most commonly directly related to tumor involvement, either with direct invasion of the pleura or with hematologic spread to the pleura, but can also be a result of lymphatic obstruction from adenopathy or the primary tumor. Effusions can also be caused by late effects of prior therapy including surgery or radiation. Prompt management of pericardial effusions can prevent life-threatening consequences, including cardiac tamponade. Pericardial effusions, which become clinically symptomatic resulting from pressure on the ventricles, may require surgical intervention with a pericardial window or pericardial stripping, or can be managed less invasively with percutaneous catheter drainage.[30]

Malignant pleural effusions occur in up to 20% of patients with lung cancer[31] and may be the initial presenting sign of malignant disease.[32] Lung cancer is the most common cause of malignant pleural effusion.[33] The incidence of malignant effusions in SCLC is comparable to that of non–small cell lung cancers (NSCLC) in general but less than for the adenocarcinoma histologic subtype. Some authors have argued that patients with small cell with an isolated malignant effusion as the only site of metastatic disease may have a comparable outcome to patients with limited stage disease and should therefore be treated as such.[34] Nonetheless, this strategy has not gained widespread acceptance. Initial evaluation should be with diagnostic and therapeutic thoracentesis. Exudative effusions should be assumed to be malignant, unless a satisfactory benign etiology can be assigned.[35] These effusions may require chest tube drainage and pleurodesis for optimal management, although SCLC patients may be appropriately treated with chemotherapy alone. Less invasive options are becoming available in the management of malignant pleural effusions, such as smaller catheters and home drainage.

Horner syndrome can be observed in lung cancer patients with apical lung carcinoma in the superior sulcus because of involvement of the sympathetic chain of nerves. This syndrome, more commonly associated with NSCLC, is often associated with Pancoast syndrome. SCLC more commonly is a central mass with bulky mediastinal lymphadenopathy, and therefore is not commonly involving the lung apex.[36] Horner syndrome is characterized by ptosis, myosis, and anhydrosis of the affected side most commonly from apical lung tumors. Pancoast syndrome is characterized by Horner syndrome plus the additional local–regional effects of involvement of the brachial plexus, chest wall, ribs, and thoracic spine.[37] Again, chemotherapy often provides rapid symptomatic relief from this syndrome in SCLC, and the cancer is managed according to clinical stage.

Systemic Metastasis SCLC can spread at a rapid rate, and early diagnosis before regional or metastatic spread is rare. Nearly two thirds of patients with small cell present with systemic disease at the time of initial diagnosis. Involved sites affected by metastatic disease can cause significant symptoms. The most commonly involved sites with metastatic lung cancer include the brain, contralateral lung, liver, adrenals, and bones.[38] Other less common sites can also be affected, including visceral organs, skin and subcutaneous tissues, kidneys, pancreas, and spinal cord and meninges. Specific symptoms related to each of these sites of disease can appear at the time of initial diagnosis or may develop as the disease progresses. Symptomatic patients should be further evaluated with the appropriate diagnostic test (CT, magnetic resonance imaging [MRI], or radionuclide scan) to exclude additional sites of disease. Asymptomatic patients, however, may not need full evaluation for metastatic disease in the absence of clinical findings.[39]

Optimal evaluation of patients with SCLC for evidence of metastasis generally includes a CT scan of the chest to include adrenals and liver, and consideration of brain imaging with CT or MRI, bone scanning, and possibly bone marrow biopsy. This procedure became part of standard staging of SCLC because of the frequent involvement of bone marrow by metastatic disease. More recent evidence suggests that having marrow involvement as the sole site of metastasis occurs in less than 5% of patients and may not have the prognostic significance previously thought.[40] In fact, these patients were found to have no difference in overall survival compared with patients with extensive disease without marrow involvement. Newer imaging techniques including positron emission tomography (PET) are still being evaluated in SCLC, but may play a role in defining disease stage in some patients.[41]

Brain metastasis is common in SCLC, occurring in 50% of patients in one autopsy series.[42] Symptomatic patients presenting with brain metastasis from SCLC may develop headaches, nausea, fatigue, weakness, seizures, visual change, or ataxia. These symptoms can often be the presenting symptoms of the cancer and are generally controlled with treatment. Patients may also harbor metastatic disease to the brain in the absence of symptoms. Some have debated the roll of screening asymptomatic patients with brain scanning. One study found that 63% of SCLC patients with any neurologic symptoms had brain metastases on CT scan, whereas only 18% of patients with no neurologic symptoms had evidence for brain metastasis.[43] The more sensitive technique of MRI scanning may have picked up additional patients with small volume metastases, but the clinical implications of this are unclear, especially given the chemosensitivity of this tumor.

Options for treatment of brain metastasis include surgery, radiation, chemotherapy, or some combination. More recent data suggests that some patients with SCLC may have control of central nervous system (CNS) disease with chemotherapy alone.[44] Leptomeningeal metastasis carries a particularly grave prognosis[45] and may produce the similar neurological symptoms, changes in mental status, or the signs of meningeal irritation including stiff neck and photophobia.

Bony metastasis is another common site of metastasis and can lead to significant problems with pain. Aggressive management of symptomatic bone metastasis is necessary in this disease. Patients who present with bony pain should be evaluated with whole body bone scanning, and specific sites of involvement can be further evaluated with plain x-rays and CT or MRI scanning. Sites of symptomatic metastasis should be considered for palliative radiotherapy. Weight-bearing regions in the hip, epidural spinal cord compression, or proximal humerus lesions should also be considered for surgical evaluation and possible prophylactic fixation. However, the role of aggressive local therapy for metastatic disease must be weighed carefully with the need for systemic therapy in this aggressive neoplasm. Data has emerged suggesting that bisphosphonates may be effective in reducing bony complications and discomfort caused by metastatic tumor to bone.[46] Definitive clinical trials are not yet available in SCLC patients.

Patients presenting with metastatic SCLC to the adrenal gland are generally those with systemic manifestations of their disease.[47] It is relatively uncommon for patients with adrenal metastasis to develop clinical hypoadrenalism, but bilateral metastases can produce adrenal insufficiency.[48]

Patients with liver metastasis may present with abdominal pain, asymptomatic hepatomegaly, or jaundice. Evaluation with ultrasound, CT scan, or MRI is often useful in evaluating for metastases to the liver. Generally, chemotherapy is the treatment of choice, but in unique cases, radiation, surgery, or other local treatment modalities such as chemoembolization, cryotherapy or radiofrequency ablation may play a role.[49]

THE ROLE OF CLINICAL EXAMINATION DURING DISEASE EVALUATION

As in all cancer patients, the clinical examination is a crucial component of the initial evaluation of patients presenting with SCLC. A thorough patient history is important to evaluate for local, regional, and systemic symptoms of cancer as listed in the previous sections. The clinical examination may reveal additional abnormal findings in these patients who most often present with advanced disease at the time of diagnosis. The initial approach to the physical examination in SCLC patients includes a general assessment of the patient and his or her overall well-being and performance status. Most patients with SCLC do present with physical symptoms, which often lead to a change in a patient's general appearance. The general examination may reveal cachexia associated with weight loss, and may also reveal changes in skin tone or color characteristic of the anemia often present in patients with advanced disease (or the plethora seen in patients with emphysema). Vital signs are another important element of the examination because patients may have developed abnormal heart rates or rhythms based on systemic illness or involvement of the cardiopulmonary system. Specifically, resting tachycardia is common in patients with underlying hypoxia. Patients may also exhibit postural hypotension related to poor oral intake leading to dehydration. Fever can be associated with postobstructive pneumonia, and tachypnea is a typical finding because many patients have pulmonary compromise from their cancer or underlying pulmonary disease.

The physical examination of the head and neck region in patients with SCLC can help detect spread to this region and associated abnormalities. Subcutaneous metastasis can occur in the scalp, and these can be demonstrated on physical examination by observation and palpation. In addition, cervical or supraclavicular, or even occipital lymphadenopathy can be associated with locally advanced or metastatic SCLC. SVC syndrome may reveal neck vein distension or facial or periorbital swelling in this region as well. Cranial nerve abnormalities can be associated with CNS disease, meningeal carcinomatosis, or sympathetic nerve involvement with the occasional small cell cancer affecting the superior sulcus producing Horner syndrome.

The pulmonary examination is crucial in evaluating patients with lung cancer. Local consolidation from mass effect or atelectasis can occur and often shows other specific findings such as pneumonia leading to crackles, rhonchi, wheezing, or dullness to percussion. SCLC can also produce pleural effusions demonstrated by dullness to percussion and decreased breath sounds. Pleural involvement may lead to a pleural friction rub. Most patients with SCLC have a history of heavy tobacco exposure and may therefore demonstrate changes associated with COPD such as wheezing and decreased air movement.

Cardiac examination in SCLC patients may reveal tachyarrhythmias such as sinus tachycardia or atrial fibrillation if pericardial disease (or pulmonary hypertension) is present. The cardiac examination may reveal a friction rub consistent with pericarditis or a pericardial effusion. Pulmonary artery hypertension can also accompany lung cancer, and a right ventricular heave may be identified on physical examination.

Examination of the bones including spine may reveal areas of tenderness consistent with bony metastatic disease. Less often observed in small cell histology is digital clubbing or hypertrophic pulmonary osteoarthropathy (HPOA), with tenderness of the bones of the lower extremities, more characteristic of non–small cell carcinoma.

Careful examination of all lymph node stations is important in patients with SCLC because of the proclivity of this disease to metastasize to lymph nodes. The palpable regions most commonly involved are the cervical and supraclavicular lymph node chains. Enlarged axillary lymph nodes may also be detected. Inguinal lymph nodes are less commonly involved, but when present, they indicate disseminated stage IV disease.

The abdominal examination may demonstrate liver, adrenal, or intraperitoneal metastases. Small cell carcinoma can also spread to the periportal or pancreatic region. Examination may show hepatomegaly or abdominal fullness consistent with abdominal metastasis. Ascites can develop in patients with metastatic SCLC related to intra-abdominal tumor or liver disease and produce abdominal distension.

The extremity examination in patients with NSCLC can show digital clubbing, but this occurs less commonly in small cell histology. Other abnormalities in the extremity examination can include wasting of the muscles, fingernail changes, or cyanosis in these patients.

Skin examination may show changes in patients with SCLC, including pallor associated with anemia, skin rashes that may be paraneoplastic in nature, or jaundice associated with liver dysfunction (or occasionally hemolysis). Small cell carcinoma can also spread to the skin or subcutaneous tissues, producing symptomatic or asymptomatic nodules.

The neurologic examination requires particularly careful attention in SCLC patients. Various manifestations can include dementia, changes in mental status, weakness (focal or diffuse), loss of sensation, cerebellar findings such as ataxia, loss of coordination and gait disturbances, and cranial nerve abnormalities. These findings need to be viewed in the context of the overall clinical situation to make an appropriate diagnosis and direct further evaluation and treatment. A careful neurologic examination helps to evaluate for CNS involvement from metastatic tumor or paraneoplastic neurologic effects. Neurologic consultation is often helpful as are imaging studies such as CT or MRI scans, and electromyogram (EMG)/nerve conduction velocity (NCV) studies in localizing the lesion and narrowing down the differential diagnosis of neurologic abnormalities. Serum and cerebrospinal fluid antibodies may be helpful in suspected paraneoplastic syndromes.

PARANEOPLASTIC SYNDROMES

Paraneoplastic syndromes are associated with malignancy, but are not directly related to the primary tumor, regional spread, or distant metastasis. Paraneoplastic syndromes are particularly common in SCLC patients, occurring in up to 50% of patients with SCLC, but in only about 10% of patients with NSCLC.[50] Paraneoplastic syndromes may precede the diagnosis of malignancy, or at any time during the course of the disease, but worsening of these symptoms generally signals disease progression. The extent of symptoms from paraneoplastic syndromes may be unrelated to the size of the primary tumor or bulk of metastatic disease, and may, in fact, be the dominant cause for a patient to seek medical attention.[51] These syndromes are clinically important because of the disabling effect on patients. Clinical improvement may result from treating the underlying malignancy, leading to improvement in quality of life. Paraneoplastic syndromes can be useful markers of tumor activity and may also carry prognostic value (Table 24.2).

TABLE 24.2 The Paraneoplastic Syndromes Associated with Small Cell Lung Cancer

Category	Syndrome	Predominant Cell Type
General	Cachexia/anorexia	Any
	Depression	Any
Endocrinologic	Hypercalcemia	Squamous cell
	Cushing syndrome	Small cell
	SIADH	Small cell
Neurologic	LEMS	Small cell
	Cerebellar degeneration	Small cell
	Peripheral neuropathy	Small cell
	Myotonia	Small cell
	Retinopathy	Small cell
	Optic neuropathies	Small cell
Hematologic	Anemia	Any
	Thrombocytosis	Any
	Thrombosis	Any
Musculoskeletal	Digital clubbing	Adenocarcinoma
	HPOA	Adenocarcinoma
	Polymyositis	Any
Dermatologic	Dermatomyositis	Any
	Acquired tylosis	Small cell
	Trip palms	Small cell
	Erythema gyratum repens	Small cell
Renal	Nephrotic syndrome	Any
	Glomerulonephritis	Any

General Patients with SCLC can present with a wasting syndrome characterized by anorexia, cachexia, weight loss, weakness, and fatigue that is unresponsive to increased caloric intake. The etiology of such paraneoplastic cachexia is not known but is likely multifactorial, involving cytokines and hormonal factors.[52] The increased metabolic needs of an increasing tumor burden, and failure to efficiently incorporate nutrients may explain the difficulty in gaining or even maintaining weight despite adequate caloric intake. Patients appear to have a syndrome of maladaptive metabolism that results in decreased nutrient intake, increased hepatic gluconeogenesis, failure to efficiently use glucose, and increased proteolysis and lipolysis. Neuropeptides produced in the hypothalamus stimulate appetite in a normal individual[53]; whether qualitative or quantitative abnormalities of these peptides play a role in the anorexia of cancer is not clear. Other mediators may be involved in the pathophysiology of the wasting syndrome including cytokines such as tumor necrosis factor α (TNF-α), hormones (insulin, corticotropin, epinephrine, growth hormone), and other tumor-related factors.[54] Retrospective studies have consistently found that patients experiencing weight loss have an inferior survival compared with those who have maintained their weight.[55]

Endocrine Paraneoplastic endocrine syndromes commonly associated with SCLC are caused by the production of protein hormones or precursors to these hormones. Two potential mechanisms may explain the production of these hormones. One hypothesis states that cancers producing ectopic endocrine syndromes are derived from amine precursor uptake and deamination (APUD) cells.[56,57] Another more recent hypothesis states that these hormones are not produced ectopically, but rather represent an increased expression of a normal cell function.[58] The most common endocrine syndromes associated with SCLC are Cushing syndrome and syndrome of inappropriate secretion of antidiuretic hormone (SIADH). Other paraneoplastic abnormalities can include hyperglycemia, hypoglycemia, hypercalcemia, and gynecomastia.

Ectopic adrenocorticotropic hormone (ACTH) can produce Cushing syndrome. This syndrome is seen in up to half of the patients with lung cancer[59] and is most commonly associated with SCLC. Studies have shown that normal tissues can produce small amounts of the precursor pro-ACTH.[34] Carcinomas seem to produce a greater amount. SCLC cells can convert pro-ACTH to the biologically active ACTH, and therefore produce the clinical syndrome of weakness, muscle wasting, drowsiness, confusion, edema, hypokalemic alkalosis, and hyperglycemia. However, severe symptoms develop in less than 5% of patients with SCLC.[60] These patients may have a worse prognosis than SCLC patients who do not demonstrate ectopic ACTH production. One study found a response rate of only 46% to chemotherapy in these patients, with a median survival of only 3.6 months.[61]

Paraneoplastic Cushing syndrome can be differentiated from pituitary-dependent Cushing disease by five factors: (a) both the serum and urine cortisol levels are markedly elevated in cancer-related Cushing syndrome, but only moderately increased in Cushing disease; (b) serum ACTH levels are markedly higher in cancer-related Cushing syndrome compared with Cushing disease; (c) hypokalemia is more commonly seen in cancer-related Cushing syndrome; (d) the elevated levels of ACTH and cortisol are generally not suppressed by high doses of dexamethasone in cancer-related Cushing syndrome in contrast to Cushing disease; (e) corticotropin-releasing hormone (CRH) increases ACTH and cortisol secretion in Cushing disease but not in cancer-related Cushing syndrome.[62] Effective therapy of the underlying disease in SCLC can often improve the paraneoplastic Cushing syndrome.

Lung cancer is the most common malignancy associated with SIADH, and SIADH can be seen in 40% of patients with small cell carcinoma.[63] This syndrome produces hyponatremia, hypervolemia, increased loss of renal sodium, and inappropriately high urine osmolality. This clinical syndrome was first described in cancer patients by Vorherr et al.[64] in 1968. Increased levels of antidiuretic hormone (ADH) were found in these patients. Despite the laboratory abnormality, not all of these patients have symptoms attributed to SIADH. In order to develop symptoms, increased water intake is also needed.[65,66] Symptomatic patients can present with confusion, somnolence, and may lead to seizures. SIADH does not seem to lead to a worse prognosis in these patients, and often resolves with effective treatment of the cancer,[67] but tends to recur with tumor recurrence or progression.

Neurologic Paraneoplastic syndromes of the nervous system are rare, affecting less than 1% of cancer patients.[68] These syndromes can be caused by a systemic autoimmune reaction to an "onconeural" antigen shared by both the cancer and the nervous system.[69] Specific autoantibodies have been identified in some patients with paraneoplastic syndromes of the nervous system, and these can be associated with specific tumors. Treatment of neurologic paraneoplastic syndromes consists of (a) treatment of the underlying cancer, which has been shown to diminish the neurologic impairment in some cases,[70] and (b) suppression of the antibody with steroids, cyclophosphamide, plasma exchange, and intravenous immune globulin (IVIG). Such immunosuppression may also lead to significant clinical improvement.[71]

Lambert-Eaton myasthenic syndrome (LEMS) can affect up to 3% of patients with SCLC.[72] LEMS provides strong support for the autoimmune basis for neurologic paraneoplastic syndromes. Patients develop immunoglobulin G (IgG) antibodies against voltage-gated calcium channels (VGCC) in the presynaptic neurons. Decreased calcium entry leads to decreased acetylcholine release, leading to a pure motor neuropathy characterized by muscular weakness. Patients present with muscle weakness preferentially affecting the lower limbs and proximal muscles. Commonly associated is autonomic dysfunction such as dry mouth, impotence, constipation, and blurred vision. On physical examination, deep tendon reflexes in lower extremities are diminished or absent, and patients have increased strength after repeated contraction of the involved muscles, differentiating LEMS from typical myasthenia. Treatment of the underlying tumor usually results in improvement of LEMS, and plasma exchange or IVIG may also improve the clinical symptoms.[73] One case-control report suggested that these patients affected by LEMS may actually have a better survival outcome than SCLC patients who are not affected.[74] The authors hypothesized that these patients with LEMS may have a slower rate of tumor growth in part related to tumor macrophage infiltration.

Paraneoplastic cerebellar degeneration (PCD) may have an indolent or a more sudden onset, often evolves rapidly, and can lead to ataxia, dysarthria, and dysphagia. Symptoms may be purely cerebellar, or they can also be associated with other neurologic manifestations. The disease course for this effect may be independent of that of the underlying tumor. This syndrome has been shown to result from autoantibodies against the Purkinje cells of the cerebellum.[75] In half the patients of PCD associated with SCLC, circulating anti-Hu antibodies are found.[76] Limbic encephalitis is a paraneoplastic effect consisting of memory failure, seizures, and agitation.[77] Most of these patients also have detectable anti-Hu antibodies in both the serum and cerebrospinal fluid.

Peripheral neuropathies in SCLC patients may indicate a paraneoplastic syndrome. Four types of paraneoplastic peripheral neuropathies can occur: pure motor, pure sensory, sensorimotor, and autonomic.[75] SCLC is most strongly associated with peripheral sensory neuropathy, a rapidly developing severe disorder in which patients lose sensory modalities in all four extremities. Symptoms usually start proximally and progress distally. Neurologic symptoms usually precede the diagnosis of cancer, and anti-Hu antibodies are often present in high titers.[78] Autonomic neuropathy can also develop in patients with the anti-Hu antibody. These patients can have the entire autonomic nervous system affected or may present with isolated dysfunction, involving the sympathetic or the parasympathetic nervous system. These patients may develop gastroparesis and intestinal pseudo-obstruction resulting from dysfunction of autonomic innervation to the gastrointestinal tract as well.

SCLC can be associated with myotonia. In neuromyotonia, spontaneous and continuous muscle fiber activity causes stiffness and cramping. The muscle activity continues during sleep, general anesthesia, and peripheral nerve block, but can be inhibited by blocking the neuromuscular junction. This condition is differentiated from the stiff-man syndrome in which muscle activity goes into quiescence during sleep and general anesthesia.[79] In stiff-man syndrome, the axial lower extremity muscles are affected most, causing such severe spasms that bone deformities and fractures have been reported.

Cancer-associated retinopathy (CAR) is a rare complication of SCLC. Patients present with night blindness, photosensitivity, and impaired color vision. Symptoms often develop prior to the detection of cancer, and the disease usually progresses to painless visual loss. Visual field testing reveals peripheral and ring scotomata and loss of visual acuity. The electroretinogram is abnormal and establishes the diagnosis. This paraneoplastic phenomenon is thought to be caused by autoimmune destruction of photoreceptors with preservation of the rest of the optic pathway. Steroids, plasmapheresis, or intravenous IgG (IVIgG) can reduce antibody titer and stabilize vision in some cases, but progressive total loss of vision is more the rule.[80] Paraneoplastic optic neuropathies can also occur in SCLC.[81] These are characterized by visual loss, as well as other neurologic changes, and may respond to immunosuppressive therapy.

Hematologic Cancer-related anemia is generally characterized by a normochromic to slightly hypochromic morphology and a low serum iron, but with increased bone marrow iron stores and ferritin. Other causes of anemia must be ruled out such as nutritional deficiencies, bleeding, concurrent inflammatory disorders or other causes of chronic disease, and bone marrow suppression from treatment such as chemotherapy or radiation. Treatment of the underlying malignancy may occasionally reverse the anemia, but more commonly, transfusion or recombinant erythropoietin may be required because of suppressed erythropoietin levels. Paraneoplastic anemia may be related to cytokines such as the tumor necrosis factor and interleukin-1.[82]

Thrombocytosis can be observed as a paraneoplastic effect in SCLC patients. Up to 35% of patients with platelet counts greater than 400,000/μL will have an underlying malignancy, and thrombocytosis is present in 40% of patients with lung cancer.[83] Interleukin-6 (IL-6) has been shown to stimulate production of platelets in vivo and in vitro, and patients with cancer have been observed to possess elevated serum levels of IL-6.[84] Thrombopoietin simulates megakaryocyte proliferation and may play a role in platelet overproduction; however, the definitive cause of thrombocytosis in cancer patients has not yet been determined.

There is no clear link between thrombocytosis and the elevated risk of venous thrombosis, or Trousseau syndrome, in patients with cancer.[85] As many as 17% of patients with recurrent venous thromboembolism have an underlying malignancy.[86] Clotting may be caused by the release of procoagulants or cytokines from tumor cells, inappropriately initiating the coagulation cascade and activating platelet aggregation.[87] Patients who develop deep venous thrombosis and do not have a contraindication to systemic anticoagulation should receive intravenous heparin or low–molecular weight heparin, and anticoagulation should be continued for a minimum of 6 months.[88] Patients with a documented deep venous thrombosis or pulmonary embolism with a contraindication to anticoagulation should be considered for placement of an inferior venous cava filter.

Musculoskeletal Digital clubbing and HPOA can be associated with many types of lung disease. With bronchogenic carcinoma, this association is strongest with adenocarcinoma histology and least common with small cell cancer. The mechanism for these paraneoplastic disorders is unknown, but may involve neurogenic, hormonal, and vascular mechanisms. Circulating vasodilators have been postulated as one underlying mechanism of this condition.[89] In a study of 111 patients with lung cancer, clubbing was present in 29%.[90] Clubbing is more commonly observed in women than men (40% vs. 19%). About 10% to 20% of patients also have HPOA. HPOA is characterized by digital clubbing as well as pain, swelling, and tenderness of distal extremities with or without joint effusions, and periosteal new bone formation along the shafts of long bones. Lower extremity involvement predominates. In patients who present with HPOA, malignancy and NSCLC in particular are found in 90% of patients.[91]

Polymyositis, an inflammatory myopathy, can represent a paraneoplastic effect in SCLC patients. Characterized by muscle pain, weakness, and inflammation, this condition may predate the diagnosis of malignancy by up to 5 to 10 years.[92] In one retrospective study of polymyositis, the relative risk of cancer in patients diagnosed with this condition was 1.8, and 14% of these patients ultimately died of cancer. It remains a rare condition, however, and may be difficult to recognize and diagnose in lung cancer patients with a host of other ailments.

Dermatologic Many dermatologic manifestations can be associated with malignancy. Most commonly associated with lung cancer are dermatomyositis, acquired tylosis, tripe palms, and erythema gyratum repens.[93] Dermatomyositis is identified by a bluish purple "heliotrope" rash on the upper eyelids, a flat rash on the face and trunk, and erythema and scaling of the knuckles that often precede muscle weakness.[94] Acquired tylosis presents with keratoderma in palmar and plantar areas. Tripe palms are thickened palms with the fingers acquiring a velvety texture. This condition can occur independently or can be found in association with acanthosis nigricans. More than 90% of patients with tripe palms have an underlying or associated malignancy.[95] Erythema gyratum repens is a reactive erythema presenting with lesions that produce a "wood-grain" appearance of the affected skin, especially on the trunk and proximal extremities. Pruritus can become debilitating. An associated malignancy is usually present with erythema gyratum repens, with lung cancer observed most frequently.

Renal An association has been made between the development of nephrotic syndrome and glomerulonephritis and malignancy.[96] This paraneoplastic effect is rare, however, occurring in less than 1% of lung cancer patients. Nonetheless, smokers who develop an otherwise idiopathic renal disorder should be evaluated for an underlying malignancy.

CONCLUSION

In summary, the clinical presentation of patients with SCLC, including paraneoplastic syndromes often begins with new or changing symptoms of pulmonary origin, but may be characterized by a host of regional or systemic complaints. The vast majority of this population will present with significant symptoms at the time of initial diagnosis, and generally, they have abnormal findings on the physical examination. This stresses the importance of the basic technique of a thorough medical history and physical examination in the population of SCLC patients. A careful and detailed discussion with patients will assist in the proper diagnosis and staging of such patients. This can also help guide further evaluation and management decisions to determine the appropriate interventions to maximize treatment efficacy and improve quality of life, and ultimately prevent future complications from this disease.

The clinician must be particularly aware of the diverse signs and symptoms of patients presenting with SCLC, including those related to the local tumor, regional spread of disease to the surrounding structures, distant spread of cancer, and general symptoms or paraneoplastic syndromes that affect these patients. It is crucial to establish the baseline condition of these patients to differentiate new or progressive symptoms related to the cancer itself versus toxicities arising from diagnostic or therapeutic interventions and therapy.

The careful clinical evaluation of lung cancer patients can help determine an individual patient's stage of disease as well as help address the need for interventions to maximize symptom control, provide effective curative treatment when possible, and individualize palliative measures for the maximum improvement of overall quality of life and survival. Measuring symptom control and quality of life may also ultimately lead to better monitoring and evaluation of the effectiveness of our treatments.

REFERENCES

1. Soni MK, Cella DF, Masters GA, et al. The validity and clinical utility of symptom monitoring in advanced lung cancer: a literature review. *Clin Lung Cancer* 2002;4:1–2.
2. Henschke CI, McCauley DI, Yankelevitz DF, et al. Early lung cancer action project: overall design and findings from baseline screening. *Lancet* 1999;354:99–105.
3. Mountain C. Clinical biology of small cell carcinoma: relationship to surgical therapy. *Semin Oncol* 1978;5:272–279.
4. Feinstein MB, Stover D. Clinical features of lung cancer. In: Ginsburg RJ, ed. *The American Cancer Society Atlas of Clinical Oncology.* Hamilton, Canada: BC Decker, Inc., 2002:43–56.
5. Beckles MA, Spiro SG, Colice GL, et al. Initial evaluation of the patient with lung cancer. *Chest* 2003;123:S97–S104.
6. Chute CG, Greenberg ER, Baron J, et al. Presenting conditions of 1539 population based lung cancer patients by cell type and stage in New Hampshire and Vermont. *Cancer* 1985;56:2107–2111.
7. Abrams J, Doyle LA, Aisner J. Staging, prognostic factors, and special considerations in small cell lung cancer. *Semin Oncol* 1988;15:261–277.
8. Buccheri G, Ferrigno D. Symptomatic pattern, alarm symptoms and diagnostic delay in a cohort of 1277 consecutive lung cancer patients. *Lung Cancer* 2003;41:S196 (abst P-411).
9. Osterlind K, Ihde DC, Ettinger DS, et al. Staging and prognostic factors in small cell carcinoma of the lung. *Cancer Treat Rep* 1983;67:3–9.
10. Warren S. The immediate causes of death in cancer. *Am J Med Sci* 1932;184:610–615.
11. Nathanson L, Puccio M. The cancer cachexia syndrome. *Semin Oncol* 1997;24:277–287.
12. Nelson KA, Walsh D, Sheehan FA. The cancer anorexia-cachexia syndrome. *J Clin Oncol* 1994;12:213–225.
13. Okuyama T, Tanaka K, Akechi G, et al. Fatigue in ambulatory patients with advanced lung cancer: prevalence, correlated factors, and screening. *J Pain Symptom Manage* 2001;22:554–564.
14. Stommel M, Given BA, Given CW. Depression and functional status as predictors of death among cancer patients. *Cancer* 2002;94:2719–2727.
15. Naughton MJ, Herndon JE, Shumaker SA, et al. The health-related quality of life and survival of small-cell lung cancer patients: results of a companion study to CALGB 9033. *Qual Life Res* 2002;11:235–248.
16. Chang CH, Cella D, Masters GA, et al. Real-time clinical application of quality of life assessment in advanced lung cancer. *Clin Lung Cancer* 2002;4:104–109.
17. Grippi MA. Clinical aspects of lung cancer. *Semin Roentgen* 1990;25:12–24.
18. Filderman AE, Shaw C, Matthay RA. Lung cancer. Part 1: etiology, pathology, natural history, manifestions, and diagnostic techniques. *Invest Radiol* 1986;21:80–90.
19. Patel AM, Peters SG. Clinical manifestations of lung cancer. *Mayo Clin Proc* 1993;68:273–277.
20. Hirshberg B, Biran I, Glazer, M, et al. Hemoptysis: etiology evaluations and outcome in a tertiary referral hospital. *Chest* 1997;112:440–444.
21. O'Neil KM, Lazarus AA. Hemoptysis: indications for bronchoscopy. *Arch Intern Med* 1991;151:171–174.
22. Poe RH, Israel RH, Marin MA, et al. Utility of fiberoptic bronchoscopy in patients with hemoptysis and a non-localizing chest roentgenogram. *Chest* 1988;93:70–75.
23. Hyde L, Hyde CI. Clinical manifestations of lung cancer. *Chest* 1974;65:299–306.
24. Farber SM, Mandel W, Spain DM. *Diagnosis and Treatment of Tumors of the Chest.* New York: Grune and Stratton, 1960.
25. Christie NA, Buenaventura PO, Fernando HC, et al. Results of expandable metal stents for malignant esophageal obstruction in 100 patients: short-term and long-term follow-up. *Ann Thorac Surg* 2001;71:1797–801.
26. Fincher RE. Superior vena cava syndrome: Experience in a teaching hospital. *South Med J* 1987;80:1243–1245.
27. Urban T, Lebeau B, Chastang C, et al. Superior vena cava syndrome in small cell lung cancer. *Arch Intern Med* 1993;153:384–387.
28. Kraus DH, Ali MK, Ginsberg RJ, et al. Vocal cord medialization for unilateral paralysis associated with intrathoracic malignancies. *J Thorac Cardiovasc Surg* 1996;111:334–339.
29. Torre M, Amari D, Barbieri B, et al. Emergency laser vaporization and helium oxygen administered for acute malignant tracheobronchial obstruction. *Am J Emerg Med* 1989;7:294–296.
30. Park JS, Rentschler R, Wilbur D. Surgical management of pericardial effusion in patients with malignancies. Comparison of subxiphoid window versus pericardiectomy. *Cancer* 1991;67:76–80.
31. Lynch TJ. Management of malignant pleural effusions. *Chest* 1993;103(Suppl 4):S385–S389.
32. Chernow B, Sahn SA. Carcinomatous involvement of the pleura. *Am J Med* 1977;63:695–702.
33. Johnston WW. The malignant pleural effusion. *Cancer* 1985;56:905–909.
34. Livingston RB, McCracken JD, Trauth CJ, et al. Isolated pleural effusion in small cell lung carcinoma: Favorable prognosis. *Chest* 1982;81:208–211.
35. Light RW. Pleural effusion. *N Engl J Med* 2002;346:1971–1977.

36. Johnson DH, Hainsworth JD, Greco FA. Pancoast's syndrome and small cell lung cancer. *Chest* 1982;82:602–606.
37. Paulson D. Carcinomas in the superior pulmonary sulcus. *J Thorac Cardiovasc Surg* 1975;70:1095–1094.
38. Luketich JD, Ginsberg RJ. Diagnosis and staging of lung cancer. In: Johnson BE, Johnson DH, eds. *Lung Cancer.* New York: Wiley-Liss, Inc., 1995:161–173.
39. Silvestri GA, Littenberg B, Colice GL. The clinical evaluation for detecting metastatic lung caner: a meta-analysis. *Am J Respir Crit Care Med* 1995;152:225–230.
40. Tritz DB, Doll DC, Ringenberg S, et al. Bone marrow involvement in small cell lung cancer. *Cancer* 1989;63:763–766.
41. Kut V, Spies W, Spies S, et al. FDG-positron emission tomography in the staging and monitoring of small cell lung cancer. *Lung Cancer* 2003;41:S200 (abstr. P-429).
42. Pederson AG. Diagnosis of CNS metastases from SCLC. In: Hansen HH, ed. *Lung Cancer: Basic and Clinical Aspects.* Boston: Martinus Nijhoff, 1986:153–182.
43. Hooper RG, Tenholder MF, Underwood GH, et al. Computed tomographic scanning of the brain in initial staging of bronchogenic carcinoma. *Chest* 1984;85:774–776.
44. Postmus PE. Brain Metastases from small cell lung cancer: chemotherapy, radiotherapy, or both? *Semin Radiat Oncol* 1995;5:69–73.
45. Grossman SA, Krabak MJ. Leptomeningeal carcinomatosis. *Cancer Treat Rev* 1999;25:103–119.
46. Rosen L, Gordon D, Tchekmedyian V, et al. Zoledronic acid (Zol) significantly reduces skeletal-related events (SREs) in patients with bone metastases from solid tumors. *Proc Am Soc Clin Oncol* 2002;21: No.1179 (abstr).
47. Silvestri GA, Lenz JE, Harper SN, et al. The relationship of clinical findings to CT scan evidence of adrenal gland metastases in the staging of bronchogenic carcinoma. *Chest* 1992;102:1748–1751.
48. Potti A, Schell DA. Unusual presentations of thoracic tumors: case 1. Acute adrenal insufficiency due to metastatic lung cancer. *J Clin Oncol* 2001;19:3780–3782.
49. Bhattacharya R, Rao S, Kowdley KV. Liver involvement in patients with solid tumors of nonhepatic origin. *Clin Liver Dis* 2002;6: 1033–1043.
50. Richardson GE, Johnson BE. Paraneoplastic syndromes in lung cancer. *Curr Opin Oncol* 1992;4:323–333.
51. Greenberg E, Divertie MB, Woolner LB. A review of unusual systemic manifestations associated with cancer. *Am J Med* 1964;36:106–120.
52. Heber D, Tchekmedyian NS. Mechanism of cancer cachexia. *Contemp Oncol* 1995;6–10.
53. Wilding JD. Neuropeptides and appetite control. *Diabet Med* 2002;19:619–627.
54. Lanstein HN, Norton JA. Mechanism of cancer cachexia. *Hematol Oncol Clin North Am* 1991;5:103–123.
55. DeWys WD, Begg C, Lavin PT, et al. Prognostic effect of weight loss prior to chemotherapy in cancer patients. *Am J Med* 1980;69: 491–497.
56. Pearse AG. Common cytochemical and ultrastructural characteristics of cells producing polypeptide hormones and their relevance to thyroid and ultimobronchial C cells and calcitonin. *Proc R Soc Lond B Biol Sci* 1968;170:71–80.
57. Yellin A, Benfield JR. The pulmonary Kulchitsky cell (neuroendocrine) cancers: from carcinoid to small cell carcinomas. *Curr Probl Cancer* 1985;9:1–38.
58. Odell WD. Endocrine/metabolic syndromes of cancer. *Semin Oncol* 1997;24:299–317.
59. Mendelsohn G, Baylin SB. Ectopic hormone production—biological and clinical implications. *Prog Clin Biol Res* 1984;142:291–316.
60. Hansen M, Bork E. Peptide hormones in patients with lung cancer. *Recent Results Cancer Res* 1985;99:180–186.
61. Shepherd FA, Laskey J, Evans WK, et al. Cushing's syndrome associated with ectopic corticotropin production and small cell lung cancer. *J Clin Oncol* 1992;10:21–27.
62. Nieman LK, Chrousos GP, Oldfield EH, et al. Diagnosis and management of ACTH-dependent Cushing's syndrome: comparison and the features in ectopic and pituitary ACTH production. *Clin Endocrinol* 1986;24:699–713.
63. Gilby ED, Rees LH, Bondy PK. *Ectopic Hormones as Markers of Response to Therapy in Cancer. Advances in Tumour Prevention, Detection and Characterization,* Vol. 3. Proceedings of the 6th International Symposium on Biological Characterization of Human Tumours. New York: Elsevier, 1976:132.
64. Vorherr H, Massry SG, Utiger RD, et al. Anti-diuretic principle in malignant tumor extracts from patients with inappropriate ADH syndrome. *J Clin Endocrinol Metab* 1968;28:162–168.
65. Odell WD, Wolfesen A, Yoshimoto Y, et al. Ectopic peptide synthesis: a universal concomitant of neoplasia. *Trans Assoc Am Physicians* 1977; 90:204–227.
66. North WG, LaRochelle FT Jr, Melton J, et al. Human neurophysins (HNPs) as potential tumor markers for small-cell carcinomas (SCC). *Clin Res* 1978;26:536A (abstr).
67. List AF, Hainsworth JD, Davis BW, et al. The syndrome of inappropriate secretion of antidiuretic hormone (SIADH) in small cell lung cancer. *J Clin Oncol* 1986;4:1191–1198.
68. van Oosterhort AG, van de Pol M, ten Velde GP, et al. Neurologic disorders in 203 consecutive patients with small cell lung cancer. *Cancer* 1996;77:1434–1441.
69. Dalmau JO, Posner JB. Paraneoplastic syndromes affecting the nervous system. *Semin Oncol* 1997;24:318–328.
70. Grisold W, Drlicek M, Liszka-Setinek U, et al. Anti-tumour therapy in paraneoplastic neurologic disease. *Clin Neurol Neurosurg* 1995;97: 112–116.
71. Graus F, Delattre J. Immune modulation of paraneoplastic disorders. *Clin Neurol Neurosurg* 1995;97:112–116.
72. Erlington GM, Murray NM, Spiro SG, et al. Neurological paraneoplastic disorders in patients with small cell lung cancer: a prospective survey of 150 patients. *J Neurol Neurosurg Psychiatr* 1991;54:764–767.
73. Latov N, Chaudhry V, Koski CL, et al. Use of intravenous gamma globulins in neuroimmunologic diseases. *J Allergy Clin Immunol* 2001;108(4 Suppl):S126–S132.
74. Maddison P, Newsom-Davis J, Mills KR, et al. Favourable prognosis in Lambert-Eaton myasthenic syndrome and small cell lung carcinoma. *Lancet* 1999;353:117–118.
75. Lieberman FS, Schold SC. Distant effects of cancer on the nervous system. *Oncology* 2002;16:1539–1548.
76. Mason WP, Graus F, Valideoriola F, et al. Paraneoplastic cerebellar degeneration (PCD) in small-cell lung cancer: impact of anti-Hu antibody (HuAb) on clinical presentation and survival. *Neurology* 1996;46: A127–A128 (abstr).
77. Gultekin SH, Rosenfeld MR, Voltz R, et al. Paraneoplastic limbic encephalitis: neurological symptoms, immunological findings, and tumour association in 50 patients. *Brain* 2000;123:1481–1494.
78. Dalmau J, Grau F, Rosenblum MK, et al. Anti-Hu-associate paraneoplastic encephalomyelitis/sensory neuropathy. A clinical study of 71 patients. *Medicine* 1992;71:59–72.
79. Meinck HM, Thompson PD. Stiff man syndrome and related conditions. *Mov Disord* 1992;110:853–866.
80. Keltner JL, Thirkill CE, Tyler NK, et al. Management and monitoring of cancer associated retinopathy. *Arch Ophthalmol* 1992;110:48–53.
81. Luiz JE, Lee AG, Keltner JL, et al. Paraneoplastic optic neuropathy and autoantibody production in small cell carcinoma of the lung. *J Neuroophthalmol* 1998;18:178–181.
82. Spivak JL. Cancer-related anemia: its causes and characteristics. *Semin Oncol* 1994;21(Suppl 3):3–8.
83. Richard MS. Metastatic cancer of unknown primary site. In: Fauci AS, Braunwald E, Isselbacher KJ, et al., eds. *Harrison's Principles of Internal Medicine.* 14th ed. New York: McGraw-Hill, 1998:614–622.
84. Gastl G, Plante M, Finstead CI, et al. High IL-6 levels in ascetic fluid correlate with reactive thrombocytosis with epithelial ovarian cancer. *Br J Hematol* 1993;83:433–441.

85. Estrov Z, Talpaz M, Maligit G, et al. Elevated plasma thrombopoietin activity in patients with cancer related thrombocytosis. *Am J Med* 1995;98:551–558.
86. Prandoni P, Lensing AW, Butler HR, et al. Deep-vein thrombosis and the incidence of subsequent symptomatic cancer. *N Engl J Med* 1992;327:1128–1133.
87. Green KB, Silverstein RL. Hypercoagulability in cancer. *Hematol Oncol Clin North Am* 1996;10:506–507.
88. Schulman S, Lindmarker P. Incidence of cancer after prophylaxis with warfarin against recurrent venous thromboembolism. *N Engl J Med* 2000;342:1953–1958.
89. Schneerson JM. Digital clubbing and hypertrophic osteoarthropathy: The underlying mechanisms. *Br J Dis Chest* 1981;75:113–131.
90. Sridhar KS, Lobo CF, Altman RD. Digital clubbing and lung cancer. *Chest* 1998;114:1535–1537.
91. Segal AM, Mackenzie AH. Hypertrophic osteoarthropathy: a 10 year retrospective analysis. *Semin Arthrit Rheum* 1982;12:220–232.
92. Sigurgeirsson B, Lindelof B, Edhag O, et al. Risk of cancer in patients with dermatomyositis and polymyositis: A population based study. *N Engl J Med* 1992;326:363–367.
93. Cohen PR, Razelle R. Mucocutaneous paraneoplastic syndromes. *Semin Oncol* 1997;41:334–359.
94. Dalakas MC. Polymyositis, dermatomyositis, and inclusion body myositis. In: Braunwald E, Fauci A, Kasper DL, et al., eds. *Principles of Internal Medicine,* 15th ed. New York: McGraw-Hill, 2001: 2524–2529.
95. Cohen PR, Grossman ME, Almeida L, et al. Tripe palms and malignancy. *J Clin Oncol* 1989;7:669–678.
96. Lee JC, Yamauchi H, Hopper J. The association of cancer and the nephritic syndrome. *Ann Int Med* 1966;64:41–51.

CHAPTER 25

Silvia Novello
Julie R. Brahmer
Laura P. Stabile
Jill M. Siegfried

Gender-Related Differences in Lung Cancer

For several decades, lung cancer has been mainly viewed as a malignant disease affecting men; however, over the past 30 years, as a consequence of the dramatic increase in tobacco consumption in women, there has been an exponential increase in the incidence of the disease among women.[1] Starting from 1990 to 1995, in many parts of the western world, the incidence of lung cancer in men has progressively declined as a consequence of antitobacco campaigns. If the worldwide sharp increase in women continues, the incidence of this malignancy is projected to be identical for women and men over the next decade.[2] Overall, lung cancer causes the death of more women than the other three most common female cancers (breast, colorectal, and ovarian cancer) combined.

Sex differences in terms of susceptibility to carcinogens and natural history of the disease have been observed. When compared with men, women are more likely to develop adenocarcinoma and small cell carcinoma than squamous cell carcinoma, are more likely to be younger (<50 years old) at the time of diagnosis, are less likely to have a positive smoking history, and have a better survival at any stage (Table 25.1).[3–6]

EPIDEMIOLOGY

Internationally, lung cancer is the most often diagnosed cancer and is the leading cause of cancer-related deaths in men and women.[7] In the United States, prostate cancer has the highest incidence in men, and in women, breast cancer has the highest incidence.[8]

Tobacco smoking became popular among women at the end of World War II, and the number of lung cancer cases and deaths in women started to increase around the 1960s and 1970s. The prevalence of smoking is extremely epidemic especially in high school girls: the percentage of American high school girls who smoke rose from 17.9% in 1991 to 27.7% in 2001.[9]

United States Data In the United States, the lung cancer incidence and mortality are different between men and women. The incidence rate is higher in men than in women regardless of age.[3] In 2006, among new lung cancer cases, it has been estimated that 92,700 men (53% of the lung cancer cases) were diagnosed with lung cancer and 90,330 died of their disease. For women, 81,770 (47% of lung cancer cases) were diagnosed with lung cancer and 72,130 died of their disease.[8] Lung cancer is the leading cause of cancer-related death in both sexes. Although the lung cancer incidence and mortality have been decreasing, since the early 1990s, in men, the incidence and mortality from lung cancer in women has been rising until just recently.[10,11] The incidence in women peaked in 1991 at 33.1 per 100,000 person-years and has leveled off at 30.2 to 32.3 per 100,000 person-years between 1992 and 1999.[3]

Several other epidemiologic differences exist between the sexes. Utilizing the National Surveillance, Epidemiology, and End Results (SEER) database from 1975 to 1999, Fu et al.[3] found that the median age at the time of diagnosis was 66 years for both men and women. However, more women were diagnosed at an age younger than 50 compared to men (8.6% vs. 6.9%, respectively; $p = 0.0001$). Overall incidence rates in both men and women younger than 50 years old have decreased. In those patients older than 50 years, the incidence of lung cancer decreased by 13.5% in men but increased by 37.3% in women from 1975 to 1987 and from 1988 to 1999. Lung cancer rates in women older than the age of 50 continue to rise.[4–6,12,13] Among 228,572 patients with lung cancer registered in the SEER database, and diagnosed from 1975 to 1999, 35.8% were women. Women accounted for 40.9% of patients who were younger than 50 years of age.

The proportional occurrence of histologic subtypes also differed significantly between men and women ($p < 0.0001$): in women, adenocarcinoma (44.7%) was the most common histologic subtypes, followed by small cell carcinoma (22.6%) and squamous cell carcinoma (21.4%).[3] The incidence rate of adenocarcinoma increased in both men and women from 1975 to 1987, with an

TABLE 25.1 Sex Differences at Diagnosis in Different Studies

First Author	Fu[3]	Radzikowska[4]	de Perrot[5]	Minami[6]
No. of patients	228.572	16.791	1.046	1.242
Men	64.2%	86.1%	80%	72.9%
Women	35.8%	13.9%	20%	27.1%
Histology				
Adenocarcinoma				
Men	33.2%	9.6%	26%	48.3%
Women	44.7%	21.6%	54%	86.0%
Small cell				
Men	18.4%	19.9%	—	—
Women	22.6%	26.6%	—	—
Squamous				
Men	36.3%	55.2%	65%	45.4%
Women	21.4%	32.5%	31%	9.5%
Other				
Men	12.1%	15.3%	—	6.3%
Women	11.3%	19.3%	—	4.5%
Age at diagnosis				
Men	66	62	61	64
Women	66	60	62	62
Smoking habits				
Men	NR	97.6%	98%	91.4%
Women	NR	81.2%	73%	12.8%

NR, no record.

increase seen in women of 40.5% versus 9.3% in men. In the same period, incidence rates for squamous cell and small cell carcinoma decreased in men, while increasing in women (Fig. 25.1). In the previously mentioned group of patients registered in SEER, the sex-related survival difference was greatest in patients with local disease and declined as the extent of disease increased.[3]

European Data Data from European cancer registries are slightly different than the U.S. statistics. In Europe, lung cancer accounts for 10% of cancer deaths in women compared to 28% in the United States.[14] Lung cancer is not the most common cause of cancer-related deaths in women.[15] Lung cancer ranks third behind breast and colon cancer in European women

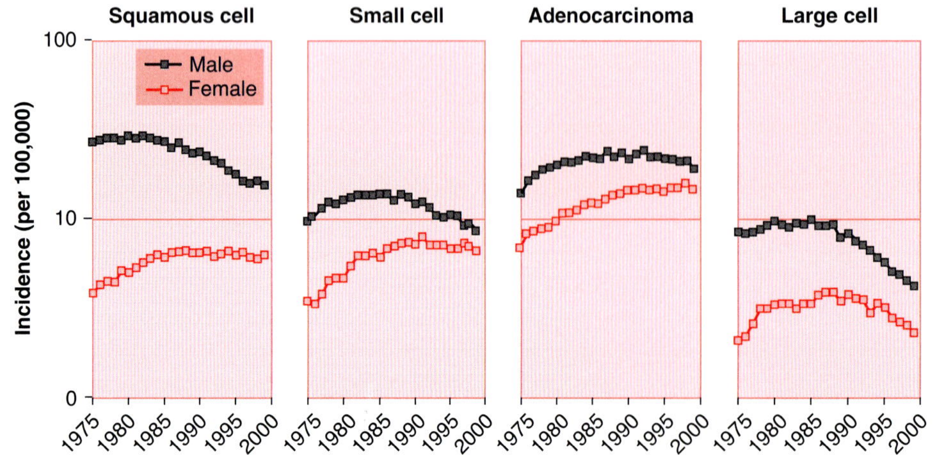

FIGURE 25.1 Age-adjusted, gender-specific incidence rates of histologic subtypes of lung cancer, from 1975 to 1999. (From Fu JB, Kau TY, Severson RK, et al. Lung cancer in women: analysis of the national Surveillance, Epidemiology, and End Results database. *Chest* 2005;127:768–777.)

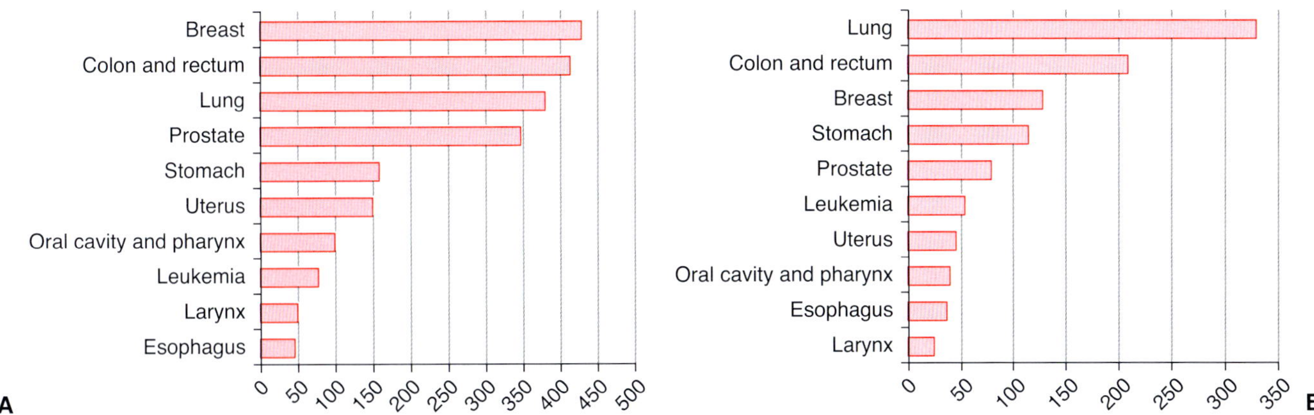

FIGURE 25.2 Estimated incidence of cancer **(A)** and estimated mortality from cancer **(B)** in Europe in 2006. (Data from Ferlay J, Autier P, Boniol M, et al. Estimates of the cancer incidence and mortality in Europe in 2006. *Ann Oncol* 2007 Mar;18[3]:581–592.)

(Fig. 25.2). Of course these data vary from country to country; the lung cancer–related deaths have increased in the United Kingdom and northern European countries, where lung cancer is now the leading cause of cancer-related deaths in women. The risk of lung cancer for women is highest in Denmark and Iceland. Data published from a Polish community-based cancer registry revealed that the age at diagnosis was younger for women compared to men (60.02 vs. 62.18 years, respectively; $p < 0.001$).[4] Squamous cell cancer was the most common type of lung cancer in both sexes in Poland. Similarly to U.S. data, more women were diagnosed at an age younger than 50 years compared to men (23% vs. 12%, respectively). Also, women were more frequently nonsmokers (18.8%) than men (2.4%).

Asian Data In Asia, the lung cancer mortality rates for women are lower than in the United States and Europe. However, the lung cancer mortality rates are increasing across several Asian countries including China, South Korea, and Japan.[16–18] Adenocarcinoma tends to be the most common histology in women in Asia, and this proportion continues to increase over time.[19–24] Although tobacco smoke is the most common cause of lung cancer in women throughout the rest of the world, the cause of lung cancer in the Asian woman is more complex. The proportion of female lung cancer patients who are never-smokers is 61% to 83%.[25,26] In fact, only Filipino and Japanese women have a smoking rate higher than 10%.[27] In comparison, the smoking prevalence is 22% in U.S. women.[27] Environmental tobacco smoke and indoor pollutants, including cooking oil fumes and burning coal, have been implicated in increasing risks of lung cancer in nonsmoking Asian women.[28–39]

SUSCEPTIBILITY

Never-Smokers The risk of lung cancer is 2.5 times more common in female lifetime nonsmokers compared to male nonsmokers.[40] Several studies have shown an association of increased risk of lung cancer, particularly adenocarcinoma, in never-smoking women with smoking husbands.[41] Reasons for this are unclear; however, hormonal factors may play a role.[42,43]

Thun et al.[44] investigated lung cancer death rates in lifelong nonsmokers. The age-standardized lung cancer death rate was 17.1 for men and 14.7 for women per 100,000 person-years. A small increase in death rate was seen between the periods of 1959 to 1972 and 1982 to 2000 in white and African American women, but not for men. The increase in death rate was only significant in women aged 70 to 84 years ($p < 0.001$).

Smokers Epidemiologic studies demonstrate mixed results regarding female smokers and their susceptibility to develop lung cancer. Some studies note an increased risk of developing lung cancer in women compared to men (Fig. 25.3). Other

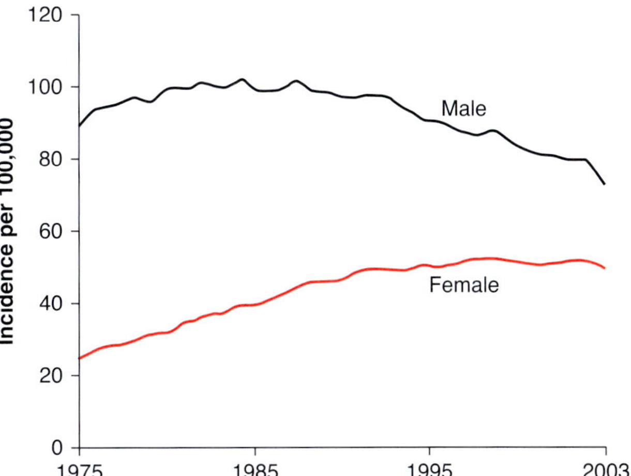

FIGURE 25.3 Age-adjusted incidence rates for men and women, 1975 to 2004. The decline in the incidence of lung cancer in men has not been seen in the female population. (From SEER program, Fast Stats: Lung and Bronchus Cancer, 9 registries, Age-adjusted incidence rates, 1975–2004. Available at: http://seer.cancer.gov/faststats/sites.php?site = Lung%20and%20Bronchus%20Cancer&stat = Incidence.Accessed September 10, 2009.)

trials found similar risks between the sexes when controlling for smoking exposure.[45–48] One trial concluded that smoking women had a 1.5-fold higher relative risk (RR) of lung cancer compared to men.[49] Another study noted an odds ratio (OR) for developing lung cancer in a 40–pack-year smoker compared to a never-smoker of 27.9 in women versus 9.6 in men.[50] In 2004, Henschke and Miettinen[51] reported an increased risk of lung cancer of 2.7 (prevalence OR with 95% interval estimate of 1.6 to 4.7) in women versus men, controlled for age and smoking history, in a regression analysis done among smokers undergoing screening by computed tomography (CT) in the Early Lung Cancer Action Project.

GENETIC/FAMILIAL FACTORS

Polymorphisms of genes that encode for enzymes, important in the breakdown of tobacco-derived carcinogens, may play a role in the development of lung cancer in female smokers and never-smokers. N-acetyltransferase (NAT2) activity can modify risk as well as cytochrome P450 (CYP) CYP1A2 activity (see Chapter 4). In Chinese female nonsmokers, low NAT2 activity and fast CYP1A2 activity had an adjusted OR of 6.9 compared to high NAT2 activity and slow CYP1A2 activity, making them at higher risk of developing lung cancer. Also, CYP1A1 is associated with an increased risk of lung cancer in female nonsmokers (OR = 3.97; 95% confidence interval [CI], 1.85 to 7.28).[52] CYP1A1 is important in converting tobacco carcinogens into DNA-binding metabolites important in DNA adduct formation. Glutathione S-transferase M1 (GSTM1) and T1 (GSTT1) are important for detoxification of carcinogens. GSTM1 null genotype is associated with an increased risk of lung cancer in some series but not in others.[52–55] One study conducted among Japanese women demonstrated an association between GSTM1 null genotype and the increased risk of lung cancer particularly in lifetime nonsmoking women with the null genotype and the increased risk of lung cancer in never-smoker women with the null genotype and significant environmental tobacco smoke exposure (OR = 2.27; 95% CI, 1.13 to 2.7) compared with women without the null genotype and no significant environmental tobacco smoke (ETS) exposure.[56] Similar to GSTM1, the null genotype of GSTT1 has shown an increased risk for the development of lung cancer in never-smokers.[57]

Nitadori et al.[58] evaluated the association of lung cancer incidence and family history in the Japanese population. The study found that women had higher risks of lung cancer if a first-degree relative was diagnosed with lung cancer with a hazard ratio (HR) of 2.65 compared to similar men with an HR of 1.69. Other case-control studies found similar findings.[59]

VIRAL FACTORS

Human papillomavirus (HPV) may play a role in the development of lung cancer. In lung cancer, one study reported that female lung cancer patients who were never-smokers and older than 60 years of age had a higher prevalence of infection with HPV-16 and HPV-18.[60,61] However, other studies have not demonstrated this same result in similar populations.[62]

DIET, RADON, OCCUPATIONAL EXPOSURES, AND PREEXISTING LUNG DISEASE

Sex differences have not been well studied regarding the risk of developing lung cancer related to occupational exposures independent of smoking (asbestosis, radiation, and other chemicals), diet, and radon. In one study of never-smoking women, researchers found that women exposed to asbestos (OR = 3.5; 95% CI, 1.2 to 10) and pesticides (OR = 2.4; 95% CI, 1.1 to 5.6) had an increased risk for developing lung cancer.[63] Dry-cleaning workers were also found to have an elevated risk (OR = 1.8; 95% CI, 1.1 to 3.0). Exposure to radiation in the workplace or for treatment of other malignancies has been linked to the development of lung cancer. A recent study reported that breast cancer radiotherapy increased the risk of developing lung cancer particularly in smokers. Adjusted OR for smokers who received postmastectomy radiation was 18.9 (95% CI, 7.9 to 45.4). Nonsmokers in this study, who received postmastectomy radiation, did not have an increased risk for the development of lung cancer.[64]

Exposure to high levels of radon is also associated with an increased risk for developing lung cancer particularly in smokers or those with exposure to secondhand smoke.[65] Bonner et al.[66] studied women pooled from several case-control studies that measured exposure to secondhand smoke and radon. The researchers also looked at the GSTM1 status of the person and found that in individuals exposed to residential radon who had GSTM1 null genotype, the risk of lung cancer was threefold higher than GSTM1 carriers (OR = 3.41; 95% CI, 1.10 to 10.61) even when adjusting for age, smoking status, and secondhand smoke exposure. In case-control and cohort studies, high dietary intake of fruits and vegetables decrease the risk of developing lung cancer.[67] Of the fruits and vegetables studied, tomatoes and cruciferous have been associated with decreased risk for lung cancer.[68–70]

Other potential risk factors for lung cancer include preexisting lung diseases such as asthma and chronic obstructive pulmonary diseases. Several case-control studies demonstrate an increased risk for developing lung cancer in both men and women affected of these lung diseases.[71] Even when controlling for active and passive tobacco exposure, some studies show an increased risk for lung cancer.[72] Wu et al.[73] studied nonsmoking women with previous lung disease and demonstrated an increased risk for lung cancer (adjusted OR = 1.56; 95% CI, 1.2 to 2.0).

STEROID HORMONES IN LUNG CANCER

Classical steroid hormone pathways have been successfully targeted in the treatment of breast and prostate cancer, where hormone-dependent growth has been well established. Steroid hormone receptors are known to be expressed in tissues outside the reproductive tract and to have biological effects in nonreproductive tumors. Some effects mediated by steroid receptors appear to be independent of steroid ligands and result from activation of steroid receptors by phosphorylation pathways. Steroid hormone receptors could thus have biological activity via steroid-induced signaling or steroid-independent signaling. Because estrogen receptor (ER) signaling pathways that induce proliferation have been repeatedly found in non–small cell lung cancer (NSCLC), the ER is a promising target for lung cancer therapy. The progesterone receptor (PR) may play a role in lung cancer biology as well.

ESTROGEN RECEPTORS IN LUNG CANCER

Studies of sex differences in lung cancer risk and disease presentation suggest that estrogens may be involved in the aetiology of this disease.[74] For example, female patients are more likely to present with adenocarcinoma of the lung and to be never-smokers compared to male patients.[75] As detailed previously, data have recently emerged that the rate of diagnosis of lung cancer in never-smoking women is higher than in never-smoking men.[76] ERs, members of the nuclear steroid receptor superfamily, mediate cellular response to estrogen. Two forms of the ER have been identified, ERα and ERβ, which are encoded by separate genes and display different tissue distributions. These proteins function either as ligand-activated transcription factors or can be activated by phosphorylation independent of ligand (Fig. 25.4).[77]

There have been inconsistent results reported concerning the presence of ERs in lung tumors. With the identification of antibodies that distinguish between ERα and ERβ and more standard immunohistochemical procedures, it is now clear that ERβ is expressed and functional in most human NSCLC cell lines and is present in primary specimens of human NSCLCs from both men and women.[78–82] There is less consensus on the expression of ERα in the lung. ERα was mainly found in the cytoplasm and membrane in immunohistochemical studies and was found to be comprised of mostly alternatively spliced variants based on immunoblot and RNA analysis.[78] This non-nuclear ERα pool may be comprised of a variant isoform that lacks the amino-terminus, because it is differentially detected

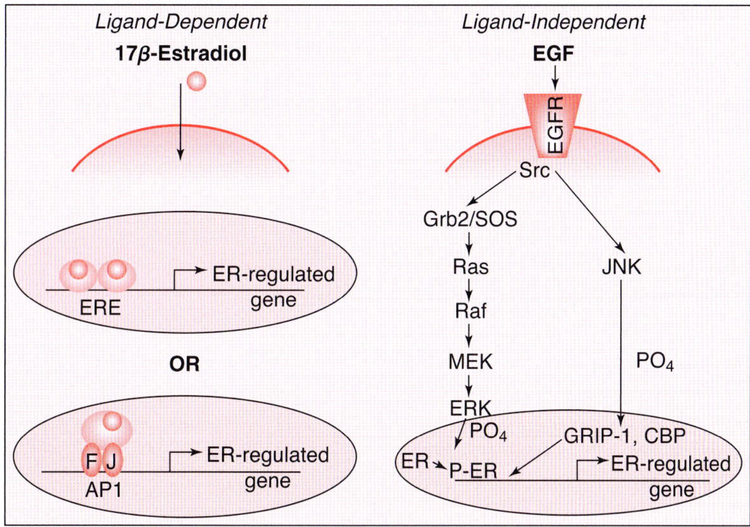

FIGURE 25.4 Classic nuclear estrogenic effects in the lung. Nuclear estrogen receptors can be activated in a ligand-dependent manner by 17-β-estradiol binding to nuclear ERs at either estrogen responsive elements (ERE) or AP1 sites utilizing the fos (F) and jun (J) transcription factors in the promoters of estrogen-regulated genes. Alternatively, nuclear ERs can be activated in a ligand-independent manner such as through growth factor–mediated estrogen receptor phosphorylation. Epidermal growth factor receptor activation is an example of such a pathway. *AP1*, activator protein 1; *CBP*, calcium binding protein; *EGF*, epidermal growth factor; *EGFR*, epidermal growth factor receptor; *ER*, estrogen receptor; *ERE*, estrogen responsive elements; *ERK*, extracellular regulated MAP kinase; *ER-regulated gene*, estrogen receptor–regulated gene; *F*, fos; *Grb2/SOS*, growth factor receptor bound protein 2/son of sevenless; *GRIP-1*, glutamate receptor interacting protein 1; *J*, jun; *JNK*, c-jun N-terminal kinase; *MEK*, MAP kinase-ERK kinase; *P-ER*, phosphorylated estrogen receptor; *PO_4*, phosphate; *Raf*, cellular homolog of viral raf gene (v-raf); *Ras*, rat sarcoma; *Src*, Rous sarcoma oncogene.

by antibodies that recognize the ERα amino- and carboxy-terminal.[79] ERβ, on the other hand, was found mainly localized to the nucleus with some cytoplasmic staining also observed and to be comprised of mainly full-length protein in addition to some variants.[78] ER-mediated RNA transcription and proliferation in lung tumor cell lines support the hypothesis that at least some forms of ER are functional.[78]

Several reports relating ER status to NSCLC patient survival have been completed. Nuclear localization of ERβ was observed in 45.8% to 69% of lung cancer cases[79–82] and found to be a favorable prognostic indicator in all studies. In some cases, the prognostic significance was only observed in male patients. Nuclear ERα expression is either never detected or rarely detected in NSCLC patient tumors.[79–83] Prognostic significance of ERα was shown to have either no effect on survival or to correlate with poor prognosis.[79,80] Kawai et al.[79] reported that the presence of cytoplasmic ERα and the absence of ERβ is associated with worse prognosis among NSCLC patients. Patients at higher risk at histopathologic stage I were those with no ERβ expression.[79] These results are opposite of what has been demonstrated for ER status and prognosis of breast cancer patients.[84,85] Whether or not this relationship is observed in other patient populations is not known at the present time, and the specificity of some ERβ antibodies has been disputed. Clearly, both nuclear and cytoplasmic ERs are important, and each component should be assessed separately and together, when examining patient tissue specimens for clinical evaluation.

Several studies have shown that women with advanced NSCLC live longer than men.[4,86,87] A population study examining lung cancer presentation and survival in premenopausal versus postmenopausal women revealed that the premenopausal women presented with more advanced disease including poorly differentiated tumors with less favorable histologies.[88] However, in this study, there was not a significant survival difference between premenopausal and postmenopausal women. In a more recent study, women older than the age of 60 had a statistically significant survival advantage over both men and younger women; the difference compared to younger women is potentially caused by higher levels of circulating estrogens in the younger population.[89] Men did not show a survival difference by age.

Hormone replacement therapy (HRT) has also been examined in relation to lung cancer risk and survival and has yielded conflicting results. Ganti et al.[90] have reported that in almost 500 female lung cancer patients examined, a significant association between both a lower median age at lung cancer diagnosis and a shorter median survival time in women who used HRT around the time of diagnosis versus those who did not. This effect was more pronounced in smoking women versus nonsmokers, suggesting an interaction between estrogens and tobacco carcinogens. However, other reports suggest that HRT use prior to diagnosis could actually protect women from developing lung cancer, especially if they smoked.[91] An inverse relationship was also observed between HRT use and NSCLC risk in postmenopausal women with ER-positive lung tumors, but not ER-negative lung tumors.[92] This may suggest that there are different effects on the balance between induction of cell differentiation and cell proliferation by estrogen in normal lung epithelium compared to malignant epithelium. Because lung tumors are also known to produce aromatase (see discussion that follows), it is possible that exogenous hormone use reduced local estrogen production by inhibiting aromatase expression. Exact HRT used, duration of use and timing of use, is critical information needed to elucidate the exact role of HRT on lung cancer risk and survival of lung cancer patients in future studies.

Although epidemiologic studies evaluating the effects of estrogen on lung cancer risk have yielded varying results, preclinical evidence clearly shows that estrogen acts to induce cell proliferation of NSCLC cells in vitro and in vivo and can modulate expression of genes in NSCLC cell lines that are important for inducing cell proliferation.[78,83,93] Genomic estrogen signaling has been demonstrated to occur mainly through ERβ in NSCLC cells.[94] Furthermore, fulvestrant, an ER antagonist with no agonist effects, inhibits cell proliferation in vitro and lung tumor xenograft growth in severe combined immunodeficient mice by ~40%.[78] Thus, preclinical evidence strongly suggests that targeting the estrogen signaling pathway may have therapeutic value to treat or prevent lung cancer.

There are currently three available strategies to target the estrogen signaling pathway in cancer cells: (a) antagonists of ER function through drugs such as tamoxifen and raloxifene; (b) downregulation of ER function through agents such as fulvestrant; and (c) reduction of estrogen levels through aromatase inhibitors, such as the reversible nonsteroidal agents letrozole and anastrozole and the irreversible steroidal inactivator exemestane.[95,96] Tamoxifen and raloxifene have partial agonist effects in certain tissues, such as endometrium. Tamoxifen has been shown to increase lung tumor xenograft growth and is not an appropriate choice of therapy for NSCLC.[94] Additionally, results from the Tamoxifen Breast Cancer Prevention trial as part of the National Surgical Adjuvant Breast and Bowel Project did not show any decreased risk of lung cancer.[97] Seventeen tumors of the lung, trachea, and bronchus were reported among the placebo group and 20 in the women who had received tamoxifen therapy. Although not statistically significant, these results suggest that tamoxifen could have some agonistic effects in the lung.

Aromatase in Lung Cancer Lung cancer cells can also produce their own estrogen.[98] The aromatase enzyme, a member of the CYP family, catalyzes the conversion of the androgens androstenedione and testosterone to estrone and estradiol, respectively, and is expressed in the lung.[99,100] Aromatase protein was expressed in lung tumor cell lines and tumor tissue and was demonstrated to be functional.[98] Additionally, a large decrease in growth of lung tumor xenografts treated with anastrozole was observed.[98] Aromatase inhibitor therapy in lung cancer is further supported by Coombes et al.,[101] who reported a decreased incidence of primary lung cancer in breast. Preclinical work suggests that aromatase inhibitors are also potential inhibitors for lung cancer therapy. Cancer patients treated with exemestane after 2 to 3 years of tamoxifen therapy (4 cases) compared with continued tamoxifen treatment (12 cases).

Mah et al.[102] have recently identified aromatase as an early stage predictive biomarker of lung cancer survival. In this regard, in women older than the age of 65, lower levels of aromatase in tumor tissue predicted a greater chance of survival compared to women with higher aromatase expression levels. Furthermore, the prognostic value of aromatase expression was greatest in early stage lung cancer patients (stages I and II). In this population of patients where circulating estrogen levels are low because of decreased production by the ovaries, tumor cells could compensate for this loss by producing estrogen through aromatase. These results strongly suggest the use of aromatase inhibitors, already approved for breast cancer treatment, to treat or possibly prevent lung cancer in women whose lung cancers have high levels of aromatase and may give clinicians a new tool to predict survival at an early stage of disease where more treatment options are available.

Nongenomic Estrogen Signaling and Interactions with the Epidermal Growth Factor Receptor Signaling Pathway In addition to the nuclear mechanisms of ER action such as increased cell proliferation and gene transcription, estrogens can also rapidly activate signaling in seconds to minutes. These rapid signaling effects are often referred to as nongenomic effects and are thought to occur via ERs located in the membrane (Fig. 25.5). In human breast cancer cells, this membrane receptor was identified as a G-protein–coupled receptor called GPR30.[103,104] In NSCLC cells, extranuclear ERs have been identified in plasma membrane fractions and have been shown to promote rapid stimulation of signaling pathways.[105] These effects can be inhibited by the addition of fulvestrant. Current work is focusing on the role of GPR30 in NSCLC.

Nongenomic ER signaling acts in concert with growth factor signaling pathways, such as the epidermal growth factor receptor (EGFR/HER-1). EGFR is a member of the tyrosine kinase receptor family that also includes HER-2, HER-3, and HER-4.[106] These receptors have been implicated in proliferation, cell motility, angiogenesis, cell survival, and differentiation.[107] Clinically, overexpression of EGFR correlates with poor prognosis in NSCLC patients.[79,108] Furthermore, combined overexpression of EGFR and ERα correlates was demonstrated to be an independent indicator of poorer prognosis in lung cancer, consistent with cross talk between these two pathways.[79]

An interaction between the ER and EGFR has been demonstrated in lung cancer cells.[94,109] In this regard, estrogen can rapidly activate the EGFR in lung cancer cell lines (ligand-dependent signaling) and the combination of fulvestrant and gefitinib, an EGFR tyrosine kinase inhibitor (TKI), in NSCLC can maximally inhibit cell proliferation, induce apoptosis and affect downstream signaling pathways both in vitro and in vivo.[94] The more clinically relevant EGFR TKI, erlotinib, also gave superior antitumor activity in NSCLC tumor xenograft experiments when used in combination with fulvestrant compared to single-agent therapy.[109] Furthermore, membrane ERs were found to be colocalized with EGFR in lung tumors.[105] Ligand-independent nongenomic signaling can also occur. In this regard, EGFR could directly phosphorylate ER at specific serine residues.[110] These residues were found to be phosphorylated in 87.5% of ER-positive lung tumors examined.[109]

A reciprocal control mechanism was also observed between ER and EGFR in lung cancer cells. In this respect, EGFR protein expression was downregulated in response to estrogen and upregulated in response to fulvestrant in vitro, suggesting that the EGFR pathway is activated when estrogen is depleted.[94] Conversely, ERβ protein expression was downregulated in response to EGF and upregulated in response to gefitinib providing a rationale to target these two pathways simultaneously.[94]

Targeting the EGFR through small molecule TKIs is of limited use in the absence of an EGFR mutation, which only occurs in a minority of patients. Interestingly, the patients who respond to EGFR TKIs are mainly women and never-smokers.[111] Recently, a phase I clinical trial using drugs that target these two signaling pathways was performed to assess the

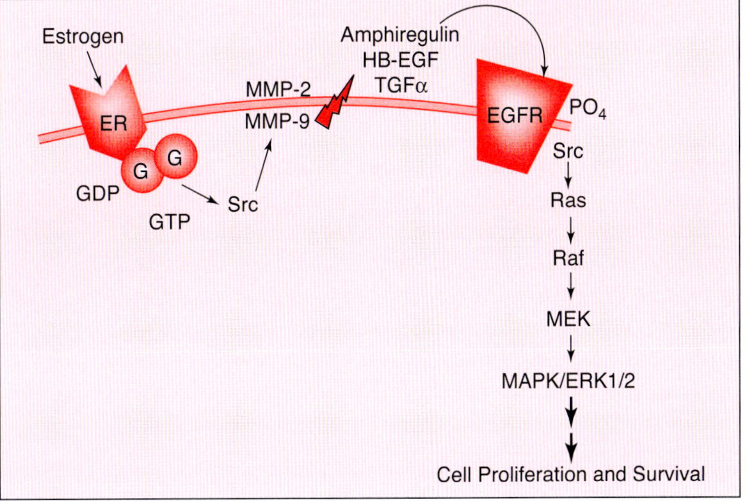

FIGURE 25.5 Non-nuclear mechanism of estrogen action in the lung through rapid activation of EGFR in the cell membrane. Estrogen can bind to the ER and activate G-proteins, which can activate Src and cause matrix metalloproteinases (MMPs) to cleave EGFR ligands (amphiregulin, HB-EGF, TGF-α) to allow them to bind to EGFR. The ERK downstream signaling pathway is then activated, which ultimately leads to cell proliferation and survival. *EGFR*, epidermal growth factor receptor; *ER*, estrogen receptor; *G*, G protein subunits; *GDP*, guanosine diphosphate; *GTP*, guanosine triphosphate; *HB-EGF*, heparin-binding epidermal growth factor; *MAPK/ERK1/2*, mitogen-activated kinase-like protein/elk-related tyrosine kinase; *MEK*, MAP kinse-ERK kinase; *MMP-2*, matrix metallopeptidase 2; *MMP-9*, matrix metallopeptidase 9; PO_4, phosphate; *Raf*, cellular homolog of viral raf gene (v-raf); *Ras*, rat sarcoma; *Src*, Rous sarcoma oncogene; *TGF-α*, transforming growth factor alpha.

toxicity of combined treatment of gefitinib with fulvestrant in 22 postmenopausal women.[112] Targeting both pathways was found to be safe and have antitumor activity in women with stage IIIB/IV NSCLC. Additionally, immunohistochemical staining of nuclear ERβ was correlated with improved patient survival. Phase II trials examining the combination of erlotinib with fulvestrant are also underway. Targeting the estrogen signaling pathway via both nuclear and extranuclear receptors in conjunction with the EGFR signaling pathway should have increased beneficial antitumor effects in NSCLC as has been observed in breast cancer cells.[113] Combination therapy may increase the duration of response in patients whose tumors harbor an EGFR mutation as well as an improved response in patients whose tumors do not contain an EGFR mutation.

Progesterone Receptors in Lung Cancer

Progesterone mediates cell differentiation through the PR. Presence of PR in breast cancer is, in general, an indication of a more differentiated tumor that is responsive to antiestrogen therapy, and PR is a known estrogen-responsive gene. There are several reports of expression of PR by primary NSCLC, although there is a great deal of variability in the reported frequency of expression.[114,115] One report found no PR in NSCLC.[116] A recent report used a monoclonal antibody that recognizes both the A and B forms of PR and found positive PR expression in 46% of cases, with a preponderance of positive PR expression in tumors from women.[117] Enzymes capable of synthesizing progesterone were also detected in many NSCLC, and a positive correlation was observed between intratumoral levels of progesterone and the presence of three enzymes that participate in progesterone synthesis. Exposure of NSCLCs to progesterone led to growth inhibition of tumor xenografts and concomitant induction of apoptosis, in agreement with clinical data, suggesting that the presence of PR was correlated with longer overall survival in NSCLC patients.

Progesterone derivatives have been useful in the treatment of both endometrial cancer and breast cancer.[118,119] Agents such as medroxyprogesterone acetate, which can be given orally, have a potential role in the treatment of lung cancer, perhaps in combination with agents that suppress either the ER pathway or act on growth factor pathways such as EGFR, mesenchymal–epithelial transition factor (c-Met), or other TKIs. Long-term progesterone treatment might even be feasible for chemoprevention of lung cancer.

Implications for Lung Cancer Therapy

Research on estrogen in lung cancer is likely to benefit both men and women. Because lung tumors from both men and women express ERs and aromatase and cell lines derived from both sexes respond to estrogens, antiestrogens, and aromatase inhibitors, these types of therapeutic treatments may be beneficial for both populations, not solely women. However, data are strongest for aromatase and estrogen levels playing an important role in survival of female lung cancer patients. Further understanding of the role of estrogen, estrogen synthesis and ERs in lung cancer will provide rationale for future targeting of this pathway for therapy earlier in the course of disease and possibly for lung cancer prevention. Additional understanding of the role of non-nuclear versus nuclear ERs as well as PRs in lung cancer and which drugs affect which receptors will be important for designing new effective treatments.

Sex as a Prognostic Factor in Early Stage Lung Cancer

Several authors have reported a more favorable prognosis of lung cancer in women than in men and this regardless of a longer life expectancy or the influence of other prognostic factors (Fig. 25.6). In a large population-based analysis conducted in patients with local disease, more women underwent surgery than men (64% vs. 56%; $p < 0.001$), and men were more frequently treated with radiotherapy (23% vs. 18%; $p < 0.001$). A similar trend, although to a lesser extent, was also reported for patients with locoregional extent of the disease.[4] In a Polish cancer registry information, about 20,561 patients diagnosed from 1995 to 1998 were collected and women had an RR of death of 1 compared to 1.21 ($p = 0.001$) for men at univariate analysis.[4] In a French cohort of 208 patients, when the data were adjusted for stage, women lived significantly longer in each stage of the disease.[13] Similarly, in a retrospective review of 7553 patients treated for NSCLC between 1974 and 1998, the overall median survival was 12.4 months for women and 10.3 months for men ($p < 0.001$) and the survival advantage was uniformly detected across all stages ($p < 0.001$).[120] In all the previously mentioned studies, the lack of information about smoking status and cause-specific mortality does not allow any definitive conclusion about the prognostic influence of sex.

In a prospective cohort of 4618 patients diagnosed with NSCLC, sex was found at the multivariate analysis to be an independent prognostic factor after adjusting for age at diagnosis, tumor histology and grade, stage, pack-years smoked, and treatment received (resection, radiation, or chemotherapy). Stage of the disease, at diagnosis and treatment received, did not differ between men and women. The estimated 1- and 5-year survival

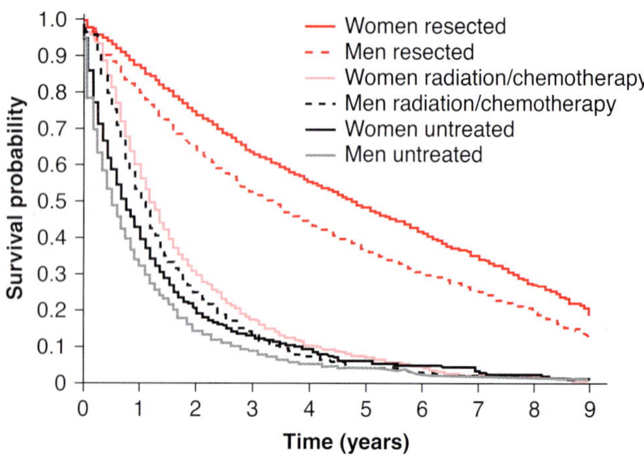

FIGURE 25.6 Lung cancer–specific survival curves by sex and type of treatment. Women had a statistically significant survival benefit compared with men regardless of the type of treatment received.

time in men was 51% (95% CI, 49%, 53%) and 15% (95% CI, 12%, 17%), respectively, whereas in women, the 1- and 5-year survival time was 60% (95% CI, 58%, 62%) and 19% (95% CI, 16%, 22%). Men were at a significantly increased risk of mortality compared to women, following a diagnosis of NSCLC (adjusted RR = 1.20; 95% CI, 1.11, 1.30), particularly for patients with stage III/IV disease or adenocarcinoma.[2]

These data have been confirmed in other prospective studies. Cerfolio et al.[121] analyzed a cohort of 1085 patients and detected an overall age-adjusted and stage-adjusted 5-year survival rate favoring women (60% vs. 50%; $p < 0.001$). Women had better stage-specific 5-year survival rates (stage I disease, 69% vs. 64%, [$p = 0.034$]; stage II disease, 60% vs. 50%, [$p = 0.042$]; and stage III disease, 46% vs. 37%, respectively [$p = 0.024$]). Women who received neoadjuvant chemotherapy were more likely to achieve a complete or partial response compared to men ($p = 0.025$).

In a single institution study in completely resected NSCLC, it was found that pathological stage, female sex, and squamous cell type were independent predictors of survival. According to stage, women had a significant survival advantage at pathological stage I ($p = 0.01$) and a moderately better survival at stage II and stage III disease ($p = 0.3$)[122] (Table 25.2). A similar survival trend according to stage with a more pronounced survival difference in stage I and II was also confirmed in two other studies,[5,123] and the impact of sex on survival independent from smoking status was also reported in a large Japanese cohort, which studied 12,703 cases of resected NSCLC.[124]

Survival advantage by female sex is also maintained among elderly patient population. In a population-based analysis from the SEER database, 18,967 elderly patients (<65 years old) with stage I and II NSCLC, diagnosed between 1991 and 1999, were considered. Patients were grouped into three categories according to the treatment received: surgery, radiation or chemotherapy, and untreated cases. Survival data were controlled for competing risks, including lung cancer–specific survival, overall survival adjusting for comorbidities, and relative survival. Women in all treatment groups had better lung cancer–specific, overall, and relative survival than men ($p < .0001$), and this benefit was retained with multivariate analysis. Sensitivity analyses demonstrated that these survival differences were not related to a different smoking behavior. Sex differences were also observed among untreated patients, and this may suggest that lung cancer in women has a different natural history.[125] An ongoing South Western Oncology Group (SWOG) trial is investigating molecular epidemiology of NSCLC in smoking and never-smoking men and women, evaluating the influence of hormonal and reproductive factors in 720 stage I to III lung cancer patients.

The epidemiological findings from population-based studies indicate that more women are diagnosed at earlier stages. A higher adherence rate among women in ongoing early detection studies raises the issue of whether or not the survival advantage by sex may be attributable only to a more frequent medical consultation and radiological assessment rather than related to differences in genetic predisposition and natural history of the neoplastic disease.

As previously described, the ELCAP screening project gave insights into women and lung cancer.[51] In the International Early Lung Cancer Action Program (I-ELCAP), 14,435 asymptomatic volunteers with no previous history of cancer and fit to undergo thoracic surgery (6296 women), at least 40 years of age, and past or current cigarette smokers underwent baseline CT screening for lung cancer. Lung cancer was diagnosed in 111 of 6296 women and 93 of 8139 men: in terms of prevalence, the women-to-men OR was 1.6 ($p = .001$). Women diagnosed with lung cancer were at a comparable age to men (67 vs. 68 years) but had a significantly reduced tobacco exposure (47 vs. 64 pack-years, respectively). Additionally, women were more frequently diagnosed in clinical stage I disease (89% vs. 80%), but the resection rate in stage I was only slightly higher than men (90% vs. 88%). The proportion of adenocarcinoma subtype among women and men was 73% versus 59%, respectively.[126]

From this study, the hypothesis that women may be more susceptible to tobacco carcinogens appears biologically plausible: if lung cancer risk for women who smoke is indeed higher than the risk for men of the same age who smoke, this suggests that antismoking efforts directed toward girls and women need to be even more serious than those directed toward boys and men. For the same reason, in consideration that early detection programs are conducted among smokers, female sex calls for screening at lower levels of tobacco exposure than the corresponding indication threshold in men.

Overall, the evidence suggests that women with lung cancer survive longer than men and that this difference is more pronounced in very early stages. Cancer stage at diagnosis, cell type, or treatment do not appear to be entirely explanatory of this difference, and it is not clear whether this survival difference is because lung cancer in women tends to be more commonly curable or less malignant.

TABLE 25.2 Five-Year Survival in Women and Men with Early Stage Non–Small Cell Lung Cancer, in Different Studies

First Author	Ouellette[13]	Cerfolio[121]	Alexiou[122]
No. of subjects	208	1085	833
Women (%)	104 (50%)	414 (38%)	252 (30%)
5-year survival			
Stage I	47.2%	69%	56%
II	63.1%	60%	41%
III	14.5%	46%	21%
Men (%)	104 (50%)	671 (62%)	581 (70%)
5-year survival			
Stage I	32.7%	64%	42%
II	51.5%	50%	32%
III	6.1%	37%	16%

PROGNOSTIC/PREDICTIVE ROLE OF SEX IN ADVANCED DISEASE

Insights from Therapeutic Trials: Chemotherapy

Although the potential prognostic influence of sex may be established in surgical series alone or in those patients treated with supportive care alone, in advanced disease, sex may be either prognostic or predictive of a higher effectiveness of chemotherapy. In fact, a prognostic factor mainly reflects the natural history of the disease (i.e., survival after surgery), whereas the predictive factor more precisely reflects the impact of a therapeutic intervention (i.e., predicts response and/or survival from chemotherapy or a biologic agent). For instance, HER-2 positive status in breast cancer is associated with poor prognosis, but this status carries on a positive predictive value for benefit from trastuzumab.

Theoretically, as consequence of the prognostic significance, a hypothetical clinical trial of a new therapy that includes lower stage patients, only PS 0-1, and a high percentage of women will yield favorable results based on these selection factors alone and this independently from the efficacy of therapy.

A large retrospective study reviewed 13 SWOG trials in which 2531 women were enrolled in the period of time between 1974 and 1987. A survival advantage for women was reported. The median survival time was 5.7 and 4.8 months for women and men, respectively and 1-year survival rates were 19% versus 14% (p <0.01). This benefit, however, was not maintained with a multivariate analysis.[127] Similarly, a nonsignificant difference in survival by sex was reported in the setting of multimodality therapy for locally advanced disease (median survival of 21 months for women vs. 12 months for men)[128] (Table 25.3).

The European Lung Cancer Working Party (ELCWP) retrospectively analyzed 1052 patients treated between 1980 and 1991, for locally advanced or metastatic NSCLC. The statistical analysis included 23 pretreatment variables: female sex was one of eight variables significantly associated with improved survival with an RR of death of 0.7 (p = 0.03) at the multivariate analysis.[129] Survival advantage according to gender was also reported by O'Connell et al.[130] in a single institution study, in 378 patients with advanced stage NSCLC treated with chemotherapy. Female sex was one of four predictors of improved survival at the multivariate analysis (median survival time for women was 12.4 months vs. 8.8 months for men, p = 0.001).

Most of the published randomized trials cannot be pooled because of survival differences between the arms, but in the Eastern Cooperative Oncology Group (ECOG) 1594 study, this evaluation was possible, considering the lack of survival difference among the four arms.[131] In this study, 1207 patients were enrolled (1157 were eligible) with stage IIIB and IV NSCLC and randomized to four different chemotherapy treatment arms.[132] The median survival for all 1207 patients was 8 months, and all the other efficacy outcomes were comparable among four arms in the study. Consequently, it was possible to make a pooled analysis of this trial and to investigate the role of sex in survival. Men were more likely to have weight loss (65% for men vs. 58% for women, p = 0.02) and be slightly older (mean age 61.9 vs. 60.5 years for women, p = 0.02). Women were more likely to have adenocarcinoma histology (63% of women vs. 53% of men, p = 0.003). There was no difference in RR by sex (19% in both cohorts, p = 0.15). Median progression-free survival (PFS) and median survival times (MST) were different by sex: median PFS for women was 3.8 versus 3.5 months for men (p = 0.022) and MST 9.2 months for women and 7.3 months for men, respectively (p = 0.004). Survival was also better at 1, 2, and 3 years being for women, 38%, 14%, and 7%, respectively, versus 31%, 11%, and 5%, respectively, for men. This survival difference remained statistically significant after adjusting for performance status, weight

TABLE 25.3 Survival Data in Men and Women with Advanced Non–Small Cell Lung Cancer

First Author	Therapies	No. of Patients	Sex (M/F)	Median Survival Time (months)		p Value	1-Year Survival	
				Men	Women		Men	Women
Albain[127]	Different phase II/III trials platinum and nonplatinum-based therapy.	2531	1949/582	4.8	5.7	<0.01	14%	19%
O'Connell[130]	CDDP/vinca alkaloids	378	265/113	8.8	12.4	0.001	NR	
Schiller[132]	CDDP/paclitaxel CDDP/GMC CDDP/docetaxel CBDCA/paclitaxel	1207	760/447	7.3	9.2	0.004	31%	38%

NR, not reported.

loss >10%, presence of brain metastases and stage (IIIB vs. IV). No difference in survival was found by chemotherapy regimen for both sex cohorts. In terms of toxicity, women tended to have more nausea, vomiting, alopecia, neurosensory deficits, and neuropsychiatric deficits.

Sex-related differences in survival were not identified in a recent study by the North Central Cancer Treatment Group (NCCTG). Nine trials (six phase II and three phase III, five of them platinum-based), conducted from 1985 to 2001, were retrospectively considered. In the multivariate analysis, sex was not an independent prognostic factor for improved overall survival and time to progression. Similar to the previously mentioned study, a difference in toxicity was observed: both grade ≥3 hematologic and nonhematologic toxicities were higher in women than in men with OR of 1.60 ($p = 0.0007$) and 1.71 ($p < 0.001$), respectively.[133]

The TAX 326 trial was a multinational, phase III study of docetaxel plus carboplatin (DCb) or docetaxel plus cisplatin (DC) versus the reference regimen of vinorelbine plus cisplatin (VC). Baseline characteristics were well balanced across treatment groups. Approximately two thirds of the patients in each treatment group had stage IV disease. In the pairwise comparison of DC versus VC, the overall survival times were 11.3 versus 10.1 months, respectively ($p = 0.044$). The 1- and 2-year survival rates were 46% versus 41% and 21% versus 14% for DC versus VC, respectively. The overall response rates were 31.6% for DC and 24.5% for VC ($p = 0.029$). MST and overall response rates were similar in the pairwise comparison of DC versus VC, and within each arm of the study, it has been reported a trend favoring a survival advantage for women.[134,135] Similar to ECOG 1594, sex differences in toxicity were also noted: women were more likely than men to develop grade ≥3 nausea and vomiting and neurotoxicity across all three treatment arms, whereas the other hematological and nonhematological toxicity was similar for both groups.

One potential explanation for this better survival outcome in women is differences in DNA-repair capacities between the sexes, making women more responsive to platinum-based chemotherapies. DNA repair machinery should be, on average, more defective in women, making them more susceptible to respiratory carcinogens but also more sensitive to DNA-interfering agents.

NSCLC is considered a neoplastic disease relatively resistant to chemotherapy, and this resistance has been associated with elevated nucleotide excision repair (NER) in tumor tissue.

In a case-control study, 375 patients with newly diagnosed NSCLC were accrued, and NER activity was estimated by the DNA repair capacity (DRC) measured in the patient's peripheral blood lymphocytes by the host cell reactivation assay. For every unit of increase in DRC, a progressive increase in the RR of death was observed. Of those 86 patients treated with chemotherapy, patients in the top quartile of the DRC distribution were at twice the RR of death as those in the lowest quartile (RR = 2.72; 95% CI, 1.24 to 5.95; $p = 0.01$), whereas effective DRC was not a risk factor for death in patients who were not treated with chemotherapy. In univariate analysis of the relationship between DRC and clinical and demographic variables, DRC was significantly higher in men than in women (8.37% ± 2.92% vs. 7.13% ± 2.37%, respectively; $p < 0.001$) but was not related stage of disease, histology, differentiation of the tumor, or self-reported weight loss.[136]

Some interesting data regarding differential activity by sex are emerging for paclitaxel poliglumex, a drug that combines paclitaxel with poly-L-glutamic acid, a biodegradable polymer that is broken down to the active form by cathepsin B, which is modulated by estrogens. In two phase III studies, paclitaxel poliglumex did not show any advantage over standard chemotherapy. However, in a subgroup of 198 women from these two studies, it was found that it produced a better survival in younger premenopausal women, especially those with higher circulating levels of estrogens.[137] On the basis of these results, a phase III study comparing paclitaxel poliglumex plus carboplatin versus paclitaxel plus carboplatin was designed, recruiting only female patients with advanced lung cancer patients, who are premenopausal or taking estrogen replacement therapy. Further studies evaluating estrogen levels and outcomes in lung cancer patients are needed to understand the mechanism and significance of these findings. It is possible that estrogens not only influence tumor proliferation, but also alter chemotherapy efficacy and/or carcinogen metabolism to affect patient survival.

Insights from Therapeutic Trials: Targeted Therapies

Data reported from several phase II and III clinical trials evaluating the role of EGFR TKI, erlotinib, and gefitinib, in the setting of second and third line, NSCLC claim for a higher responsiveness to these agents in women. In the Iressa Dose Evaluation in Advanced Lung Cancer (IDEAL) 1 and 2 studies, gefitinib was tested in patients with advanced NSCLC previously treated with one or two lines of chemotherapy, and female sex was associated with improved outcomes.[138,139] In the IDEAL 2 study, 50% of women had symptom improvements compared to 31% in men and, additionally, 82% of partial responses occurred in women (Table 25.4).

In a randomized double-blind, placebo-controlled phase III trial in second- and third-line advanced NSCLC,[140] patients treated with daily erlotinib had a response rate of 8.9% with a median survival of 6.7 months, resulting in a 42% improvement in median survival compared to patients receiving placebo that had a median survival of 4.7 months. One-year survival rate was 31% in the erlotinib arm and 21% in the placebo arm. Response rate was statistically superior in women (14.4% vs. 6.0% in men) but in the multivariate analysis, sex did not predict increased response to erlotinib. In another large randomized study, a statistically significant higher response rate was observed for gefitinib-treated women compared to men (14.7% vs. 5.1%, respectively). This study included 1692 patients and failed to demonstrate a survival improvement with gefitinib over placebo in either overall population (5.6 vs. 5.1 months) or in adenocarcinomas (6.3 vs. 5.4 months).

TABLE 25.4 Gender Differences in NSCLC Patients Treated with EGFR Inhibitors

First Author	Therapies	No. of Patients	Sex (M/F)	Response Rate (RR)	Gender Differences
Fukuoka[138]	Gefitinib 250 mg	104	78/26	18.4%	OR F:M 2.6 ($p = 0.017$)
	Gefitinib 500 mg	106	70/36	19.0%	
Kris[139]	Gefitinib 250 mg	102	60/42	12%	RR male 2% – female 10%
	Gefitinib 500 mg	114	63/51	10%	RR male 2% – female 8%
Shepherd[140]	Erlotinib	488	315/173	8.9%	Overall RR male 6.0%
	Placebo	243	160/83	<1%	Overall RR female 14.4%

In a large phase II study, 138 patients with a diagnosis of bronchoalveolar carcinoma were treated with gefitinib as first- or second-line treatment. An exploratory subset analysis found gefitinib more active in women, and a statistically significant difference in survival was observed in the previously untreated women versus men ($p = 0.04$).[141]

The improved survival observed in women treated with these EGFR TKIs may be related to differences in frequency of mutations in tyrosine kinase domain of the EGFR (20% in women vs. 9% in men),[142] an increased percentage of high EGFR copy number by fluorescence in situ hybridization (FISH) or a higher EGFR expression by immunohistochemistry.

In the ECOG 4599 study, the benefit on survival of adding bevacizumab to the doublet of carboplatin/paclitaxel was consistently reported in all subgroups of patients (measurable vs. nonmeasurable disease, prior radiation therapy versus no prior radiation therapy, prior weight loss of less than 5% vs. 5% or more, stage IIIB with pleural effusion vs. stage IV), but not in women and in the elderly patient population. Among men, the median overall survival was 8.7 months in the standard arm and 11.7 months in the experimental arm, whereas in women, 13.1 and 13.3 months, respectively. This unexpected increased survivorship of women may be attributable to imbalances between the two groups related to known or unknown baseline prognostic factors, to the use of second- and third-line therapies may be related to statistical chance or a true sex-based difference[143] (Table 25.5).

TABLE 25.5 Bevacizumab in Advanced NSCLC: Efficacy by Gender[143]

Parameter	Men		Women	
	PC (n = 230)	PCB (n = 191)	PC (n = 162)	PCB (n = 190)
OS, mo	8.7	11.7*	13.1	13.3
PFS, mo	4.3	6.3*	5.3	6.2*
RR, %	16	29*	14	41*

*Statistically significant.

OS, overall survival; PC, paclitaxel carboplatin; PCB, paclitaxel carboplatin bevacizumab; PFS, progression-free survival; RR, response rate.

Insights from Therapeutic Trials: Small Cell Lung Cancer Less extensive information about sex-related differences in survival have been documented in small cell lung cancer: the analysis of four consecutive prospective trials showed a better overall survival favoring women.[144] A total of 2580 patients from 10 SWOG trials with limited (LD) and extensive disease (ED) were analyzed for prognostic factors. Only in LD, female sex ($p = <0.0001$) was a significant favorable independent predictor of survival.[145]

CONCLUSION

Although lung cancer death rates in recent years have reached a plateau, the number of women who will die from lung cancer remains alarmingly high. A better understating of the genetic, metabolic, and hormonal factors that affect the way women react to carcinogens and lung cancer represents a research priority. This information could affect the way patients who smoke are screened and evaluated, as well as the way smoking cessation and lung cancer prevention programs are directed.

Evidence suggests that the development of lung cancer is different in women compared with men. Female smokers are more likely than men to develop adenocarcinoma of the lung. Women who have never smoked are more likely to develop lung cancer than men who have never smoked. Women with lung cancer also live longer than men with lung cancer, regardless of therapy and stage. These differences are most likely caused by hormonal, genetic, and metabolic differences between the sexes.

The response variations seen with the EGFR inhibitors and antiangiogenesis drugs are intriguing but insufficient to allow the sex of the patient to guide the choice of therapy. All large trials in lung cancer should stratify patients according to gender, and as we enter the era of more personalized medicine, gender will clearly be a critical factor in therapeutic choice in the future.

REFERENCES

1. Jemal A, Murray T, Samuels A, et al. Cancer statistics, 2003. *CA Cancer J Clin* 2003;53:5–26.
2. Visbal AL, Williams BA, Nichols FC III, et al. Gender differences in non-small-cell lung cancer survival: an analysis of 4,618 patients diagnosed between 1997 and 2002. *Ann Thorac Surg* 2004;78:209–215.

3. Fu JB, Kau TY, Severson RK, et al. Lung cancer in women: analysis of the national Surveillance, Epidemiology, and End Results database. *Chest* 2005;127:768–777.
4. Radzikowska E, Glaz P, Roszkowski K. Lung cancer in women: age, smoking, histology, performance status, stage, initial treatment, and survival. Population-based study of 20 561 cases. *Ann Oncol* 2002;13: 1087–1093.
5. de Perrot M, Licker M, Bouchardy C, et al. Sex differences in presentation, management, and prognosis of patients with non-small cell lung carcinoma. *J Thorac Cardiovasc Surg* 2000;119:21–26.
6. Minami H, Yoshimura M, Miyamoto Y, et al. Lung cancer in women: sex-associated differences in survival of patients undergoing resection for lung cancer. *Chest* 2000;118:1603–1609.
7. World Health Organization, International Agency for Research on Cancer. *World cancer report*. Lyon, France: IARC Press, 2003.
8. Jemal A, Siegel R, Ward E, et al. Cancer statistics, 2006. *CA Cancer J Clin* 2006;56:106–130.
9. French SA, Perry CL, Leon GR, et al. Weight concerns, dieting behavior, and smoking initiation among adolescents: a prospective study. *Am J Public Health* 1994;84:1818–1820.
10. Jemal A, Siegel R, Ward E, et al. Cancer statistics, 2009. *CA Cancer J Clin* 2009;59(4):225–249. Epub 2009 May 27.
11. Ries LAG, Eisner MP, Kosary CL, et al., eds. *Cancer statistics review*, 1975–2002. Bethesda, MD: National Cancer Institute, 2005.
12. Ferguson MK, Skosey C, Hoffman PC, et al. Sex-associated differences in presentation and survival in patients with lung cancer. *J Clin Oncol* 1990;8:1402–1407.
13. Ouellette D, Desbiens G, Emond C, et al. Lung cancer in women compared with men: stage, treatment, and survival. *Ann Thorac Surg* 1998;66:1140–1143; discussion 1143–1144.
14. Boyle P, Ferlay J. Cancer incidence and mortality in Europe, 2004. *Ann Oncol* 2005;16:481–488.
15. Ferlay J, Autier P, Boniol M, et al. Estimates of the cancer incidence and mortality in Europe in 2006. *Ann Oncol* 2007 Mar;18(3):581–592.
16. Jee SH, Kim IS, Suh I, et al. Projected mortality from lung cancer in South Korea, 1980–2004. *Int J Epidemiol* 1998 Jun;27(3):365–369.
17. Yang L, Parkin DM, Li LD, et al. Estimation and projection of the national profile of cancer mortality in China: 1991–2005. *Br J Cancer* 2004;90: 2157–2166.
18. Chen K, Wang PP, Sun B, et al. Twenty-year secular changes in sex specific lung cancer incidence rates in an urban Chinese population. *Lung Cancer* 2006 Jan;51(1):13–19.
19. Devesa SS, Shaw GL, Blot WJ. Changing patterns of lung cancer incidence by histological type. *Cancer Epidemiol Biomarkers Prev* 1991 Nov-Dec;1(1):29–34.
20. Perng DW, Perng RP, Kuo BI, et al. The variation of cell type distribution in lung cancer: a study of 10,910 cases at a medical center in Taiwan between 1970 and 1993. *Jpn J Clin Oncol* 1996 Aug;26(4): 229–233.
21. Seow A, Duffy SW, Ng TP, et al. Lung cancer among Chinese females in Singapore 1968–1992: time trends, dialect group differences, and implications for aetiology. *Int J Epidemiol* 1998 Apr;27(2):167–172.
22. Lam KY, Fu KH, Wong MP, et al. Significant changes in the distribution of histologic types of lung cancer in Hong Kong. *Pathology* 1993 Apr;25(2):103–105.
23. Yoshimi I, Ohshima A, Ajiki W, et al. A comparison of trends in the incidence rate of lung cancer by histological type in the Osaka Cancer Registry, Japan and in the Surveillance, Epidemiology, and End Results Program, USA. *Jpn J Clin Oncol* 2003 Feb;33(2):98–104.
24. Au JS, Mang OW, Foo W, et al. Time trends of lung cancer incidence by histologic types and smoking prevalence in Hong Kong 1983–2000. *Lung Cancer* 2004 Aug;45(2):143–152.
25. Jindal SK, Malik SK, Dhand R, et al. Bronchogenic carcinoma in Northern India. *Thorax* 1982 May;37(5):343–347.
26. Badar F, Meerza F, Khokhar RA, et al. Characteristics of lung cancer patients–the Shaukat Khanum Memorial experience. *Asian Pac J Cancer Prev* 2006 Apr-Jun;7(2):245–248.
27. Stratton K, Shetty P, Wallace R, et al. *Clearing the smoke: assessing the science base for tobacco harm reduction*. Washington DC: National Academy Press, 2001.
28. Yu IT, Chiu YL, Au JS, et al. Dose-response relationship between cooking fumes exposures and lung cancer among Chinese nonsmoking women. *Cancer Res* 2006 May 1;66(9):4961–4967.
29. Gao YT, Blot WJ, Zheng W, et al. Lung cancer among Chinese women. *Int J Cancer* 1987 Nov 15;40(5):604–609.
30. Wang TJ, Zhou BS, Shi JP. Lung cancer in nonsmoking Chinese women: a case-control study. *Lung Cancer* 1996 Mar;(14 Suppl 1): S93–S98.
31. Wu-Williams AH, Dai XD, Blot W, et al. Lung cancer among women in north-east China. *Br J Cancer* 1990 Dec;62(6):982–987.
32. Ko YC, Cheng LS, Lee CH, et al. Chinese food cooking and lung cancer in women nonsmokers. *Am J Epidemiol* 2000 Jan 15;151(2):140–147.
33. Metayer C, Wang Z, Kleinerman RA. Cooking oil fumes and risk of lung cancer in women in rural Gansu, China. *Lung Cancer* 2002 Feb;35(2):111–117.
34. Kleinerman RA, Wang Z, Lubin J, et al. Lung cancer and indoor air pollution in rural China. *Ann Epidemiol* 2000 Oct 1;10(7):469.
35. Zhong L, Goldberg MS, Gao YT, et al. Lung cancer and indoor air pollution arising from Chinese-style cooking among nonsmoking women living in Shanghai, China. *Epidemiology* 1999 Sep;10(5):488–494.
36. Seow A, Poh WT, Teh M, et al. Fumes from meat cooking and lung cancer risk in Chinese women. *Cancer Epidemiol Biomarkers Prev* 2000 Nov;9(11):1215–1221.
37. Zhao Y, Wang S, Aunan K, et al. Air pollution and lung cancer risks in China–a meta-analysis. *Sci Total Environ* 2006 Aug 1;366(2–3):500–513. Epub 2006 Jan 10.
38. Mumford JL, He XZ, Chapman RS, et al. Lung cancer and indoor air pollution in Xuan Wei, China. *Science* 1987 Jan 9;235(4785):217–220.
39. Zhou BS, Wang TJ, Guan P, et al. Indoor air pollution and pulmonary adenocarcinoma among females: a case-control study in Shenyang, China. *Oncol Rep* 2000 Nov-Dec;7(6):1253–1259.
40. Parkin DM, Bray F, Ferlay J, et al. Global cancer statistics, 2002. *CA Cancer J Clin* 2005 Mar-Apr;55(2):74–108.
41. Kurahashi N, Inoue M, Liu Y, et al. Passive smoking and lung cancer in Japanese non-smoking women: a prospective study. *Int J Cancer* 2008 Feb 1;122(3):653–657.
42. Siegfried JM. Women and lung cancer: does oestrogen play a role? *Lancet Oncol* 2001 Aug;2(8):506–513.
43. Taioli E, Wynder EL. Re: Endocrine factors and adenocarcinoma of the lung in women. *J Natl Cancer Inst* 1994 Jun 1;86(11):869–870.
44. Thun MJ, Henley SJ, Burns D, et al. Lung cancer death rates in lifelong nonsmokers. *J Natl Cancer Inst* 2006 May 17;98(10):691–699.
45. Agudo A, Ahrens W, Benhamou E, et al. Lung cancer and cigarette smoking in women: a multicenter case-control study in Europe. *Int J Cancer* 2000 Dec 1;88(5):820–827.
46. Kreuzer M, Boffetta P, Whitley E, et al. Gender differences in lung cancer risk by smoking: a multicentre case-control study in Germany and Italy. *Br J Cancer* 2000 Jan;82(1):227–233.
47. Koyi H, Hillerdal G, Brandén E. A prospective study of a total material of lung cancer from a county in Sweden 1997–1999: gender, symptoms, type, stage, and smoking habits. *Lung Cancer* 2002 Apr;36(1):9–14.
48. Patel JD. Lung cancer in women. *Clin Oncol* 2005 May 10;23(14):3212–3218. Review.
49. Zang EA, Wynder EL. Differences in lung cancer risk between men and women: examination of the evidence. *J Natl Cancer Inst* 1996;88: 183–192.
50. Risch HA, Howe GR, Jain M, et al. Are female smokers at higher risk for lung cancer than male smokers? A case control analysis by histologic type. *Am J Epidemiol* 1993;138:281–293.
51. Henschke CI, Miettinen OS. Women susceptibility to tobacco carcinogens. *Lung Cancer* 2004;43:1–5.
52. Yang XR, Wacholder S, Xu Z, et al. CYP1A1 and GSTM1 polymorphisms in relation to lung cancer risk in Chinese women. *Cancer Lett* 2004 Oct 28;214(2):197–204.

53. Hung RJ, Boffetta P, Brockmöller J, et al. CYP1A1 and GSTM1 genetic polymorphisms and lung cancer risk in Caucasian non-smokers: a pooled analysis. *Carcinogenesis* 2003 May;24(5):875–882.
54. Raimondi S, Boffetta P, Anttila S, et al. Metabolic gene polymorphisms and lung cancer risk in non-smokers. An update of the GSEC study. *Mutat Res* 2005 Dec 30;592(1–2):45–57. Epub 2005 Jul 11.
55. Bennett WP, Alavanja MC, Blomeke B, et al. Environmental tobacco smoke, genetic susceptibility, and risk of lung cancer in never-smoking women. *J Natl Cancer Inst* 1999 Dec 1;91(23):2009–2014.
56. Kiyohara C, Wakai K, Mikami H. Risk modification by CYP1A1 and GSTM1 polymorphisms in the association of environmental tobacco smoke and lung cancer: a case-control study in Japanese nonsmoking women. *Int J Cancer* 2003 Oct 20;107(1):139–144.
57. Chan-Yeung M, Tan-Un KC, Ip MS, et al. Lung cancer susceptibility and polymorphisms of glutathione-S-transferase genes in Hong Kong. *Lung Cancer* 2004 Aug;45(2):155–160.
58. Nitadori J, Inoue M, Iwasaki M, et al. Association between lung cancer incidence and family history of lung cancer: data from a large-scale population-based cohort study, the JPHC study. *Chest* 2006 Oct;130(4):968–975.
59. Schwartz AG, Yang P, Swanson GM. Familial risk of lung cancer among nonsmokers and their relatives. *Am J Epidemiol* 1996 Sep 15;144(6):554–562.
60. zur Hausen H. Papillomaviruses causing cancer: evasion from host-cell control in early events in carcinogenesis. *J Natl Cancer Inst* 2000 May 3;92(9):690–698. Review.
61. Cheng YW, Chiou HL, Sheu GT, et al. The association of human papillomavirus 16/18 infection with lung cancer among nonsmoking Taiwanese women. *Cancer Res* 2001 Apr 1;61(7):2799–2803.
62. Fei Y, Yang Y, Hsieh WC, et al. Different human papillomavirus 16/18 infection in Chinese non-small cell lung cancer patients living in Wuhan, China. *Jpn J Clin Oncol* 2006;36:274–279.
63. Brownson RC, Alavanja MC, Chang JC. Occupational risk factors for lung cancer among nonsmoking women: a case-control study in Missouri (United States). *Cancer Causes Control* 1993 Sep;4(5):449–454.
64. Kaufman EL, Jacobson JS, Hershman DL, et al. Effect of breast cancer radiotherapy and cigarette smoking on risk of second primary lung cancer. *J Clin Oncol* 2008 Jan 20;26(3):392–398.
65. International Agency for Research on Cancer (IARC). IARC monographs on the evaluation of carcinogenic risks to humans. Man-made mineral fibres and radon. Lyon, France: IARC, 1988.
66. Bonner MR, Bennett WP, Xiong W, et al. Radon, secondhand smoke, glutathione-S-transferase M1, and lung cancer among women. *Int J Cancer* 2006 Sep 15;119(6):1462–1467.
67. Alberg AJ, Samet JM. Epidemiology of lung cancer. In: Sadler MJ, Caballero B, Strain JJ, eds. Encyclopedia of human nutrition. London, UK: Academic Press, 2005:272–284.
68. Bond GG, Thompson FE, Cook RR. Dietary vitamin A and lung cancer: results of a case-control study among chemical workers. *Nutr Cancer* 1987;9(2–3):109–121.
69. Brennan P, Fortes C, Butler J, et al. A multicenter case-control study of diet and lung cancer among non-smokers. *Cancer Causes Control* 2000 Jan;11(1):49–58.
70. Hu J, Mao Y, Dryer D, et al, and the Canadian Cancer Registries Epidemio logy Research Group. Risk factors for lung cancer among Canadian women who have never smoked. *Cancer Detect Prev* 2002;26(2):129–138.
71. Brownson RC, Alavanja MC. Previous lung disease and lung cancer risk among women (United States). *Cancer Causes Control* 2000 Oct;11(9):853–858.
72. Mayne ST, Buenconsejo J, Janerich DT. Previous lung disease and risk of lung cancer among men and women nonsmokers. *Am J Epidemiol* 1999 Jan 1;149(1):13–20.
73. Wu AH, Fontham ET, Reynolds P, et al. Previous lung disease and risk of lung cancer among lifetime nonsmoking women in the United States. *Am J Epidemiol* 1995 Jun 1;141(11):1023–1032.
74. Patel JD, Bach PB, Kris MG. Lung cancer in US women: a contemporary epidemic. *JAMA* 2004;29:1763–1768.
75. Zang EA, Wynder EL. Differences in lung cancer risk between men and women: Examination of the evidence. *J Natl Cancer Inst* 1996;88: 183–192.
76. Wakelee HA, Chang ET, Gomez SL, et al. Lung cancer incidence in never smokers. *J Clin Oncol* 2007;25:472–478.
77. Levin ER. Bidirectional signaling between the estrogen receptor and the epidermal growth factor receptor. *Mol Endocrinol* 2003;17:309–317.
78. Stabile LP, Davis AL, Gubish CT, et al. Human non-small cell lung tumors and cells derived from normal lung express both estrogen receptor alpha and beta and show biological responses to estrogen. *Cancer Res* 2002;62:2141–2150.
79. Kawai H, Ishii A, Washiya K, et al. Combined overexpression of EGFR and estrogen receptor alpha correlates with a poor outcome in lung cancer. *Anticancer Res* 2005;25:4693–4698.
80. Wu CT, Chang YL, Shih JY, et al. The significance of estrogen receptor beta in 301 surgically treated non-small cell lung cancers. *J Thorac Cardiovasc Surg* 2005;130:979–986.
81. Schwartz AG, Prysak GM, Murphy V, et al. Nuclear estrogen receptor beta in lung cancer: expression and survival differences by sex. *Clin Cancer Res* 2005;11:7280–7287.
82. Skov BG, Fischer BM, Pappot H. Oestrogen receptor b over expression in males with non-small cell lung cancer is associated with better survival. *Lung Cancer* 2008;59:88–94.
83. Hershberger PA, Vasquez AC, Kanterewicz B, et al. Regulation of endogenous gene expression in human non-small cell lung cancer cells by estrogen receptor ligands. *Cancer Res* 2005;65:1598–1605.
84. Osborne CK, Yochmowitz MG, Knight WA III, et al. The value of estrogen and progesterone receptors in the treatment of breast cancer. *Cancer* 1980;46:2884–2888.
85. Thorpe SM, Rose C, Rasmussen BB, et al. Prognostic value of steroid hormone receptors: multivariate analysis of systemically untreated patients with node negative primary breast cancer. *Cancer Res* 1987;47:6126–6133.
86. O'Connell JP, Kris MG, Gralla RJ, et al. Frequency and prognostic importance of pretreatment clinical characteristics in patients with advanced non-small-cell lung cancer treated with combination chemotherapy. *J Clin Oncol* 1986;4:1604–1614.
87. Albain KS, Crowley JJ, LeBlanc M, et al. Survival determinants in extensive-stage non-small-cell lung cancer: the Southwest Oncology Group experience. *J Clin Oncol* 1991;9:1618–1626.
88. Moore KA, Mery CM, Jaklitsch MT, et al. Menopausal effects on presentation, treatment, and survival of women with non-small cell lung cancer. *Ann Thorac Surg* 2003;766:1789–1795.
89. Wakelee HA, Dahlberg SE, Schiller JH, et al. Menopausal status of women may affect survival in advanced NSCLC: Analysis of recent Eastern Cooperate Oncology Group (ECOG) studies using age of 60 years or older as a surrogate marker: P1-052. *J Thorac Oncol* 2007; 2:S570.
90. Ganti AK, Sahmoun AE, Panwalkar AW, et al. Hormone replacement therapy is associated with decreased survival in women with lung cancer. *J Clin Oncol* 2006;24:59–63.
91. Schabath MB, Wu X, Vassilopoulou-Sellin R, et al. Hormone replacement therapy and lung cancer risk: a case-control analysis. *Clin Cancer Res* 2004;10:113–123.
92. Schwartz AG, Wenzlaff AS, Prysak GM, et al. Reproductive factors, hormone use, estrogen receptor expression, and risk of non-small cell lung cancer in women. *J Clin Oncol* 2007;25:5785–5792.
93. Sun S, Schiller JH, Gazdar AF. Lung cancer in never smokers–a different disease. *Nat Rev Cancer* 2007;7:778–790.
94. Stabile LP, Lyker JS, Gubish CT, et al. Combined targeting of the estrogen receptor and the epidermal growth factor receptor in non-small cell lung cancer shows enhanced antiproliferative effects. *Cancer Res* 2005;65:1459–1470.
95. Hamilton A, Piccart M. The third-generation non-steroidal aromatase inhibitors: a review of their clinical benefits in the second-line hormonal treatment of advanced breast cancer. *Ann Oncol* 1999;10: 377–384.

96. Giudici D, Ornati G, Briatico G, et al. 6-Methylenandrosta-1,4-diene-3,17-dione (FCE 24304): a new irreversible aromatase inhibitor. *J Steroid Biochem* 1988;30:391–394.
97. Fisher B, Costantino JP, Wickerham DL, et al. Tamoxifen for prevention of breast cancer: report of the National Surgical Adjuvant Breast and Bowel Project P-1 Study. *J Natl Cancer Inst* 1998;90:1371–1388.
98. Weinberg OK, Marquez-Garban DC, Fishbein MC, et al. Aromatase inhibitors in human lung cancer therapy. *Cancer Res* 2005;65:11287–11291.
99. Martel C, Melner MH, Gagné D, et al. Widespread tissue distribution of steroid sulfatase, 3 beta-hydroxysteroid dehydrogenase/delta 5-delta 4 isomerase (3 beta-HSD), 17 beta-HSD 5 alpha-reductase and aromatase activities in the rhesus monkey. *Mol Cell Endocrinol* 1994;104:103–111.
100. Price T, Aitken J, Simpson ER. Relative expression of aromatase cytochrome P450 in human fetal tissues as determined by competitive polymerase chain reaction amplification. *J Clin Endocrinol Metab* 1992;74:879–883.
101. Coombes RC, Hall E, Gibson LJ, et al., and the Intergroup Exemestane Study. A randomized trial of exemestane after two to three years of tamoxifen therapy in postmenopausal women with primary breast cancer. *N Engl J Med* 2004;35011:1081–1092.
102. Mah V, Seligson DB, Li A, et al. Aromatase expression predicts survival in women with early-stage non small cell lung carcinoma. *Cancer Res* 2007;67:10484–10490.
103. Thomas P, Pang Y, Filardo EJ, et al. Identity of an estrogen membrane receptor coupled to a G protein in human breast cancer cells. *Endocrinology* 2005;146:624–632.
104. Revankar CM, Cimino DF, Sklar LA, et al. A transmembrane intracellular estrogen receptor mediates rapid cell signaling. *Science* 2005;307:1625–1630.
105. Pietras RJ, Márquez-Garbán DC. Membrane-associated estrogen receptor signaling pathways in human cancers. *Clin Cancer Res* 2007;13:4672–4676.
106. Rajkumar T, Gullick WJ. The type I growth factor receptors in human breast cancer. *Breast Cancer Res Treat* 1994;29:3–9.
107. Yarden Y, Sliwkowski MX. Untangling the ErbB signalling network. *Nat Rev Mol Cell Biol* 2001;2:127–137.
108. Selvaggi G, Novello S, Torri V, et al. Epidermal growth factor receptor overexpression correlates with a poor prognosis in completely resected non-small-cell lung cancer. *Ann Oncol* 2004;151:28–32.
109. Márquez-Garbán DC, Chen HW, Fishbein MC, et al. Estrogen receptor signaling pathways in human non-small cell lung cancer. *Steroids* 2007;72:135–143.
110. Kato S, Endoh H, Masuhiro Y, et al. Activation of the estrogen receptor through phosphorylation by mitogen-activated protein kinase. *Science* 1995;270:1491–1494.
111. Yang SH, Mechanic LE, Yang P, et al. Mutations in the tyrosine kinase domain of the epidermal growth factor receptor in non-small cell lung cancer. *Clin Cancer Res* 2005;11:2106–2110.
112. Traynor AM, Schiller JH, Stabile LP, et al. Combination treatment with gefitinib and fulvestrant for post-menopausal women with advanced non-small cell lung cancer. *ASCO Annual Meeting Proceedings*. Orlando, FL; 2005. abstract 7224.
113. Okubo S, Kurebayashi J, Otsuki T, et al. Additive antitumour effect of the epidermal growth factor receptor tyrosine kinase inhibitor gefitinib (Iressa, ZD1839) and the antioestrogen fulvestrant (Faslodex, ICI 182,780) in breast cancer cells. *Br J Cancer* 2004;901:236–244.
114. Su JM, Hsu HK, Chang H, et al. Expression of estrogen and progesterone receptors in non-small-cell lung cancer: immunohistochemical study. *Anticancer Res* 1996;16:3803–3806.
115. Kaiser U, Hofmann J, Schilli M, et al. Steroid-hormone receptors in cell lines and tumor biopsies of human lung cancer. *Int J Cancer* 1996;67:357–364.
116. Di Nunno L, Larsson LG, Rinehart JJ, et al. Estrogen and progesterone receptors in non-small cell lung cancer in 248 consecutive patients who underwent surgical resection. *Arch Pathol Lab Med* 2000;124: 1467–1470.
117. Ishibashi H, Suzuki T, Suzuki S, et al. Progesterone receptor in non-small cell lung cancer–a potent prognostic factor and possible target for endocrine therapy. *Cancer Res* 2005;65:6450–6458.
118. Sutton G. Hormonal aspects of endometrial cancer. *Curr Opin Obstet Gynecol* 1990;2:69–73.
119. Kelley RM, Baker WH. Progestational agents in the treatment of carcinoma of the endometrium. *N Engl J Med* 1961;264:216–222.
120. Moore R, Doherty D, Chamberlain R, et al. Sex differences in survival in non-small cell lung cancer patients 1974–1998. *Acta Oncol* 2004;43:57–64.
121. Cerfolio RJ, Bryant AS, Scott E, et al. Women with pathologic stage I, II, and III non-small cell lung cancer have better survival than men. *Chest* 2006;130:1796–1802.
122. Alexiou C, Onyeaka CVP, Beggs D, et al. Do women live longer following lung resection for carcinoma? *Eur J Cardiothorac Surg* 2002;21:319–325.
123. Båtevik R, Grong K, Segadal L, et al. The female gender has a positive effect on survival independent of background life expectancy following surgical resection of primary non-small cell lung cancer: a study of absolute and relative survival over 15 years. *Lung Cancer* 2005;47:173–181.
124. Hajime M, Shimao F, Hikotaro K, et al. Gender differences and smoking affect the prognosis of patients with non-small cell lung cancer. JTO 2007, P3-247.
125. Wisnivesky JP, Halm EA. Sex differences in lung cancer survival: do tumors behave differently in elderly women? *J Clin Oncol* 2007;25 (13):1705–1712.
126. International Early Lung Cancer Action Program Investigators. Women's susceptibility to tobacco carcinogens and survival after diagnosis of lung cancer. *JAMA* 2006;296:180–184.
127. Albain KS, Crowley JJ, LeBlanc M, et al. Survival determinants in extensive-stage non-small cell lung cancer: the Southwest Oncology Group Experience. *Am J Clin Oncol* 1991;9:1618–1626.
128. Albain KS, Rusch VW, Crowley JJ, et al. Concurrent cisplatin/etoposide plus chest radiotherapy followed by surgery for stages IIIA (N2) and IIIB non-small cell lung cancer: mature results of Southwest Oncology Group phase II study 8805. *J Clin Oncol* 1995;13:1880–1992.
129. Paesmans M, Sculier JP, Libert P, et al. Prognostic factors for survival in advanced non-small cell lung cancer: univariate and multivariate analyses including recursive partitioning and amalgamation algorithms in 1,052 patients. *J Clin Oncol* 1995;13:1221–1230.
130. O'Connell JP, Kris MG, Gralla RJ, et al. Frequency and prognostic importance of pretreatment clinical characteristics in patients with advanced non-small-cell lung cancer treated with combination chemotherapy. *J Clin Oncol* 1986;4:1604–1614.
131. Wakelee HA, Wang W, Shiller JH, et al. Survival differences by sex for patients with advanced non-small-cell lung cancer on Eastern Cooperative Oncology Group trial 1594. *J Thorac Oncol* 2007;1(5):441–446.
132. Schiller JH, Harrington D, Belani CP, et al. Comparison of four chemotherapy regimens for advanced non-small-cell lung cancer. *N Engl J Med* 2002;346:92–98.
133. Mandrekar S, Schild SE, Hillman SL, et al. A pooled analysis of 11 NCCTG advanced stage non-small cell lung cancer (NSCLC) trials reveal the importance of baseline blood counts on clinical outcomes. *J Clin Oncol* 2003;21:3016–3024.
134. Fossella F, Pereira JR, von Pawel J, et al. Randomized, multinational, phase III study of docetaxel plus platinum combinations versus vinorelbine plus cisplatin for advanced non-small-cell lung cancer: the TAX 326 study group. *J Clin Oncol* 2003;21:3016–3024.
135. Belani CP, von Pawel J, Pluzanska A, et al. Phase III study of docetaxel-cisplatin (DC) or docetaxel-carboplatin (D-Cb) versus vinorelbine-cisplatin (VC) as first line treatment in advanced non-small cell lung cancer (NSCLC): analyses by gender. *Lung Cancer* 2006;49:S235–S236.
136. Bosken CH, Wei Q, Amos CI, et al. An analysis of DNA repair as a determinant of survival in patients with non-small-cell lung cancer. *J Natl Cancer Inst* 2002;94:1091–1099.

137. Ross H, Bonomi P, Langer C, et al. Effect of gender on outcome in two randomized phase III trials of paclitaxel poliglumex (PPX) in chemonaive pts with advanced NSCLC and poor performance status (PS2). *Proc Am Soc Clin Oncol* 2006;24:373. Abstract 7039.
138. Fukuoka M, Yano S, Giaccone G, et al. Multi-institutional randomized phase II trial of gefitinnib for previously treated patients with advanced non-small-cell lung cancer. *J Clin Oncol* 2003;21:2237–2246.
139. Kris MG, Natale RB, Herbst RS, et al. Efficacy of gefitinib, an inhibitor of the epidermal growth factor receptor tyrosine kinase, in symptomatic patients with non-small cell lung cancer. A randomized trial. *JAMA* 2003;290:2149–2158.
140. Shepherd FA, Rodrigues Pereira J, Ciuleanu T, et al. Erlotinib in previously treated non-small-cell lung cancer. *N Engl J Med* 2005;353:123–132.
141. West H, Franklin WA, Gumerlock PH, et al. Gefitinib (ZD1839) therapy for advanced bronchioloalveolar lung cancer (BAC): Southwest Oncology Group (SWOG) study S0126. *Proc Am Soc Clin Oncol* 2004;22:145. Abstract 7014.
142. Paez JG, Jänne PA, Lee JC, et al. EGFR mutations in lung cancer: correlation with clinical response to gefitinib therapy. *Science* 2004;304: 1497–1500.
143. Sandler A, Gray R, Perry MC, et al. Paclitaxel-Carboplatin alone or with bevacizumab for non-small-cell lung cancer. *N Engl J Med* 2006 Dec 14;24:2542–2550.
144. Johnson BE, Steinberg SM, Phelps R, et al. Female patients with small cell lung cancer liver longer than male patients. *Am J Med* 1988;85:194–196.
145. Albain KS, Crowley JJ, LeBlanc M, et al. Determinants of improved outcome in small-cell lung cancer: an analysis of the 2,580-patient Southwest Oncology Group database. *J Clin Oncol* 1990;8: 1563–1574.

CHAPTER 26

Leslie E. Quint
Naama R. Bogot
Sheila C. Rankin

Conventional Imaging of Non–Small Cell Lung Cancer

Bronchogenic carcinoma is generally first imaged, and often first detected, by chest radiography. Chest radiography is the preferred initial imaging modality because of its availability, low cost, low-radiation dose, and high sensitivity.[1] Computed tomography (CT) and occasionally magnetic resonance (MR) imaging of the chest and upper abdomen are used to stage a known or suspected lung cancer.

MORPHOLOGIC APPEARANCES OF LUNG CANCER

Lung cancer morphology depends, to a certain extent, on cell type. Although prediction of cell type from morphology is far from 100% accurate, the following generalizations are often correct[2]:

1. Adenocarcinoma usually presents as a solitary pulmonary nodule (SPN), and most malignant SPNs are adenocarcinomas (Fig. 26.1). Squamous cell is also a common SPN (Fig. 26.2), whereas SPN is the typical manifestation of alveolar cell carcinoma.
2. Large central masses frequently represent squamous cell carcinoma or small cell carcinoma; small cell cancers especially involve mediastinal and hilar lymph nodes, sometimes without a recognizable parenchymal lesion, whereas squamous cell cancer is generally centered at or adjacent to the hilum (Fig. 26.3).
3. A large peripheral mass most commonly represents large cell carcinoma or squamous cell carcinoma; adenocarcinoma occasionally manifests this way. Large cell carcinoma is usually a large peripheral mass, but a large central mass is its next most common manifestation.
4. Multiple nodules generally occur with bronchioloalveolar cell carcinoma (BAC) (Fig. 26.4); adenocarcinoma also occasionally manifests this way.[3] With BAC, multiple nodules are a late manifestation, usually reflecting aerogenous, or less commonly hematogenous, dissemination.
5. Airspace disease is another late manifestation of BAC. It may be focal, lobar, or more diffuse (Fig. 26.5).
6. BAC as well as other types of adenocarcinoma may present as ground glass attenuation nodules, semisolid attenuation, containing solid and ground glass components, or irregular solid nodules.[4,5]

MISSED LUNG CANCER

Experience teaches that larger lesions are more easily diagnosed than smaller lesions, and peripheral lesions are more readily detected than central lesions. Radiologic diagnosis is facilitated by the presence of typical radiographic features; uncommon manifestations of lung cancer, such as spontaneous regression, may prove misleading.[6,7] In one study of 27 missed lung cancers, the single most frequently identified cause of missed diagnoses was failure of the radiologist to compare the current chest radiographs with previous chest radiographs.[8] Other important factors were upper lobe location of the lesion (81%) and female gender of the patient (67%). A follow-up study from the same institution[9] featured 40 missed non–small cell lung cancers (NSCLC) over an 8-year period. In this series, gender did not play a role, but 72% of missed lesions were again in the upper lobes, and 22% were obscured by a clavicle.

Application of computerized automated lung nodule detection methods (computer-aided diagnosis [CAD]) to digital chest radiographs may improve the detection rate of lung cancers. One preliminary study using a commercial, computerized detection system on radiographs with T1 lesions showed a detectability rate of 74% (37/50) using CAD.[10] However, the CAD system showed a false-positive rate of 2.3 per case in 50 normal chest radiographs. The mean area under the receiver operating characteristic (ROC) curve for all observers increased significantly from 0.896 without CAD to 0.923 with CAD in the lung cancer cases. The primary reason for the improvement in performance was caused by a decrease in the number

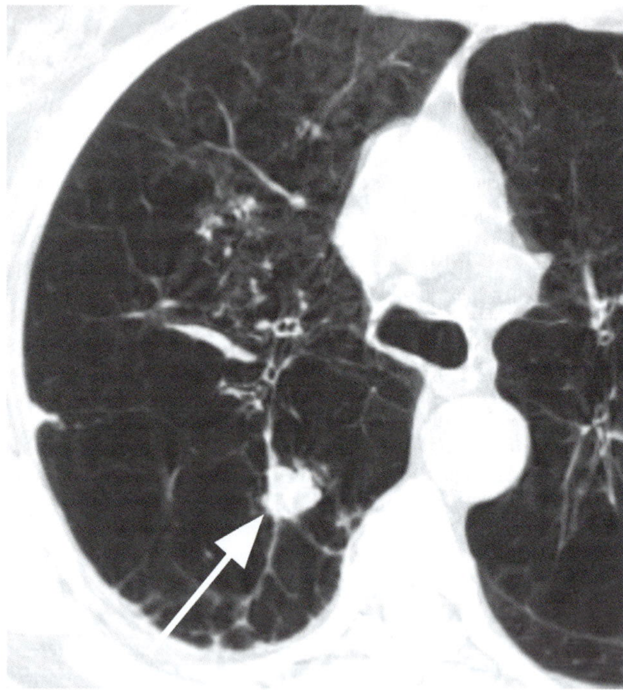

FIGURE 26.1 T1 adenocarcinoma (*arrow*) surrounded by emphysematous lung.

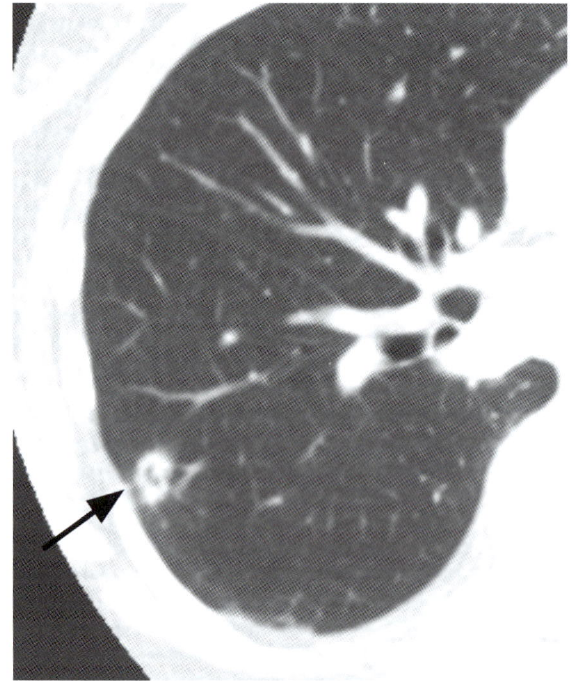

FIGURE 26.2 Small, cavitary squamous cell cancer with soft tissue stranding, extending to the pleural surface (*arrow*). Histopathological examination of the resected specimen revealed tumor invasion of the visceral pleura.

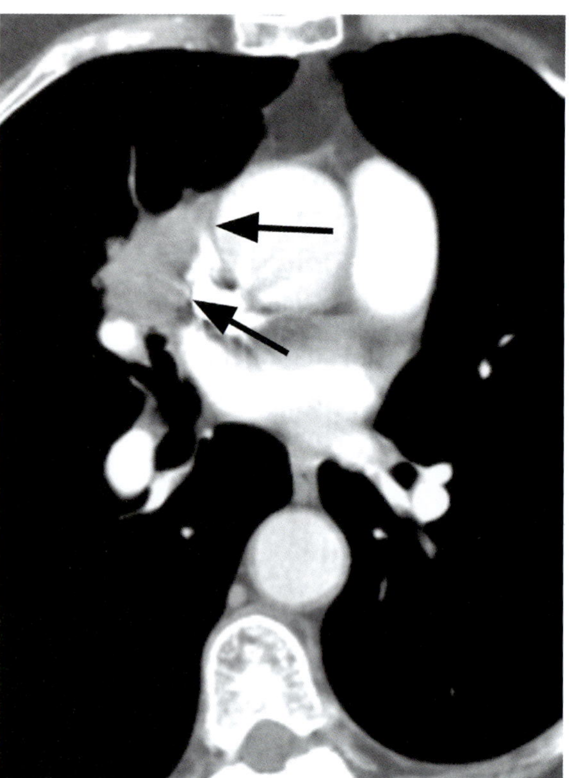

FIGURE 26.3 Middle lobe squamous cell cancer showing broad contact with the mediastinal vascular structures (*arrow*); CT findings are equivocal for mediastinal invasion. The tumor was resected via right upper and middle lobectomies; histological examination showed tumor extending to, but not through, the pericardium.

of false negatives and a concomitant increase in the number of true positives.[10]

The novel technique of single-exposure, dual-energy digital chest radiography appears promising for the detection of pulmonary nodules and lung cancers. In a preliminary study assessing the detectability of lung nodules in 77 patients with lung cancer and 77 normal subjects, the combination of standard radiography and single-exposure, dual-energy digital radiography improved nodule detection compared to standard radiography alone.[11]

Some authors have analyzed the detectability of lung cancers based on size and extent of ground-glass opacity at thin-section CT.[12] They reviewed 75 peripheral NSCLC (26 localized BACs and 49 other cell types). The chest radiographs were mixed with 60 normals and blindly reviewed. Sensitivity for detection was 58.5% for BACs and 78.6% for the other cell types. Lesions <15 mm in size and those with ≥70% ground-glass opacity proved to be statistically significantly more difficult to detect. A similar result was obtained in a study analyzing lung cancers missed at low-dose helical CT screening.[13] In this study, 32 of 83 lung cancers found by annual low-dose CT screening had initially been missed. Nodules missed because of detection errors more frequently were ground glass (91%), and also, more frequently were judged to be "subtle" (91%).

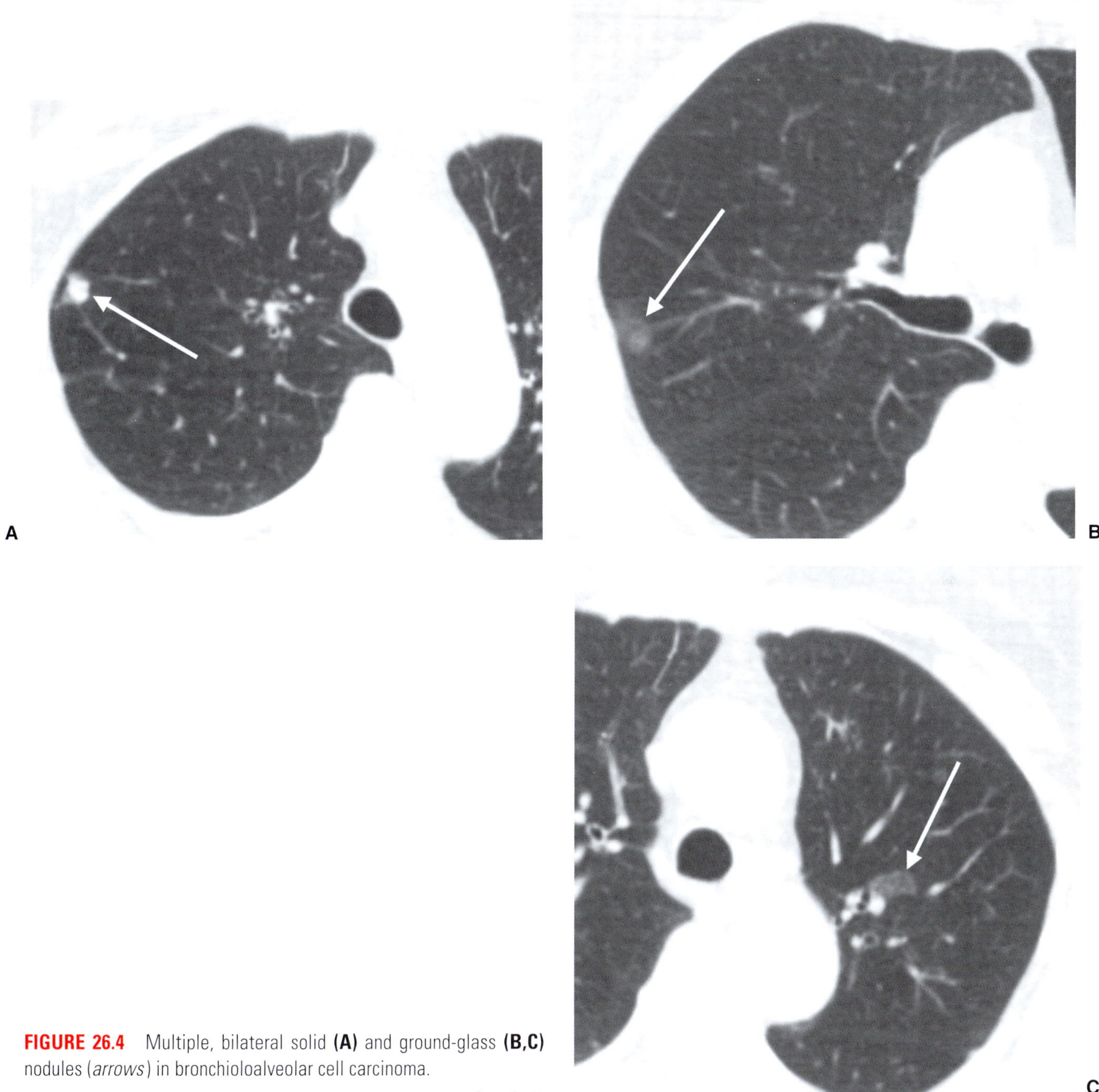

FIGURE 26.4 Multiple, bilateral solid **(A)** and ground-glass **(B,C)** nodules (*arrows*) in bronchioloalveolar cell carcinoma.

Application of a computerized automated lung nodule detection method to proven lung cancers missed at low-dose CT screening may improve the detection rate significantly.[14] In a series of 38 missed lung cancers, such a method allowed identification of 32 (84%) of the missed lesions.

Similar to its use in chest radiography, CAD is an emerging tool for automatic detection of pulmonary nodules on CT; it may be used as a second reader, drawing the attention of the radiologist to possible abnormalities in order to increase the detection rate of small pulmonary nodules. High-resolution data (thin sections obtained during a single breath hold) acquired with multidetector CT (MDCT) has led to improvements in the sensitivity of various CAD systems and a decrease the false-positive rate. There are diverse methods of CAD, each based on different detection algorithms.[15] One recent study compared two CAD systems in 25 patients with 116 nodules, evaluated by three radiologists with varying levels of expertise[16]; this study showed that sensitivity for pulmonary nodule detection increased with the use of CAD. For example, in nodules smaller than 5 mm, sensitivity increased from 55% to 71% to 68% to 74%. There was no significant difference in the performance of the two CAD systems.

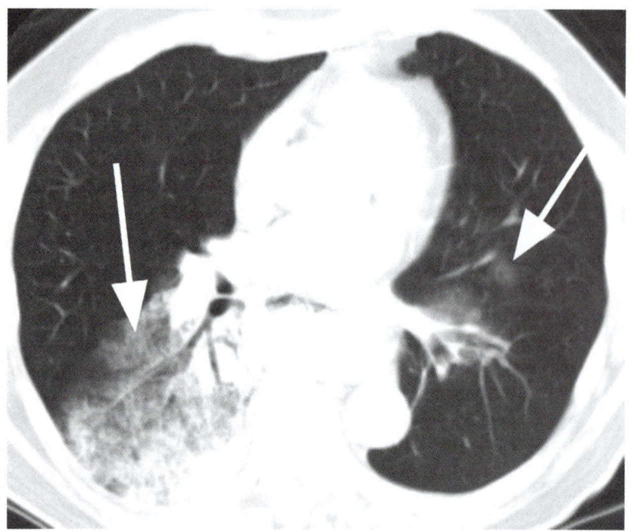

FIGURE 26.5 Bronchioloalveolar cell carcinoma manifesting as bilateral air space disease (*arrows*).

Other CT evaluation methods have also been shown to decrease perception error and improve detection of pulmonary nodules. These dedicated computer applications involve alternative two- (2D) and three-dimensional (3D) displays of CT data.[17,18] For example, on maximum intensity projection (MIP) images, pulmonary nodules tend to stand out against background structures, such as lung and tubular vessels (Fig. 26.6); several studies have demonstrated the superiority of MIP over standard axial images. In one study, five readers evaluated examinations of 25 patients with 122 nodules (3 to 9 mm in diameter). Readings were performed with and without MIP.[17] MIP enhanced the detection of peripheral nodules for the junior readers, and of central nodules for both the junior and senior readers. Volume rendering (VR) in 3D techniques display the entire volume data, assigning relative opacity values to each voxel (ranging from 0% to 100%). In a study comparing MIP and VR computer applications among three readers, VR was superior to MIP in the detection of pulmonary nodules smaller than 11 mm and was associated with a statistically significant shorter reading time.[18]

Is missed lung cancer automatically evidence of malpractice? In the Mayo Clinic lung cancer screening article

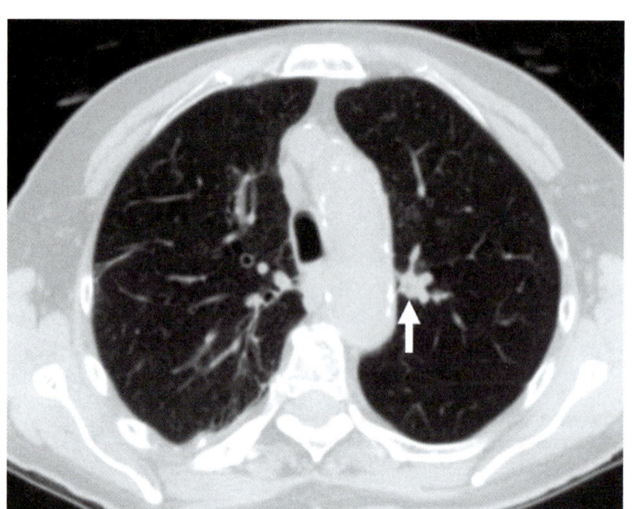

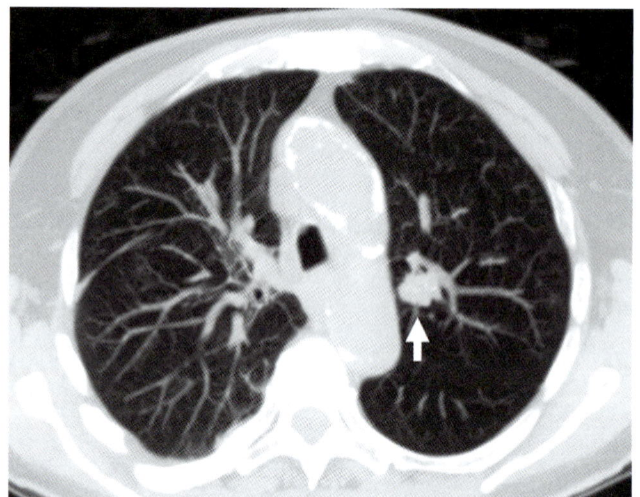

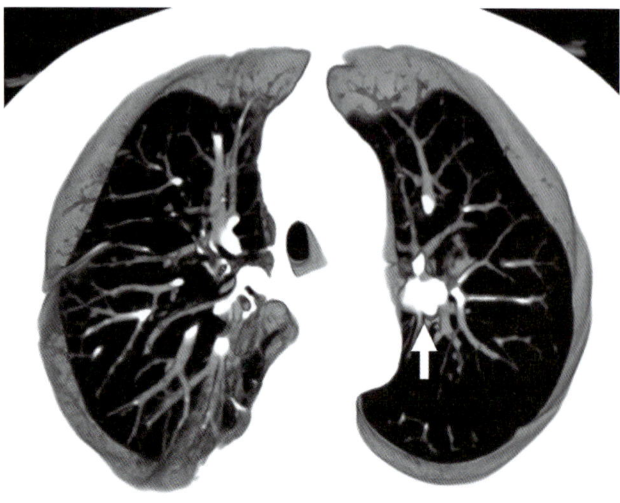

FIGURE 26.6 Small central lung cancer (*arrow*) is more obvious on MIP **(B)** and VR **(C)** images compared to axial CT image **(A)**.

previously cited,[19] each radiographic study was reviewed by two (and often three), trained and interested observers (chest radiologists or chest physicians) specifically to answer the question: "Is there lung cancer?" Amazingly, 45 of 50 peripheral carcinomas that they diagnosed were visible in retrospect, with 18 visible for more than 1 year and four for more than 2 years; one was visible in retrospect for 53 months. Furthermore, 12 of 16 perihilar carcinomas and 13 of 20 carcinomas presenting as hilar or paratracheal lymph node enlargement were visible in retrospect, although not generally for as long as the peripheral carcinomas. The authors concluded that ". . . failure to detect a small pulmonary nodule on a single examination should not constitute negligence or be the basis for malpractice litigation." In an elegant letter to the editor, Hendrix[20] pointed out the need for an analogy to explain to members of a lay audience (the jury) how a well-qualified, careful radiologist could miss the lesion that they now easily see on a radiograph. He likens the radiologist's analysis of the image to the search for Waldo in the series of *Where's Waldo?* books. As Dr. Hendrix pointed out, everyone understands how hard it can be to locate Waldo in a given illustration. However, once he has been found, Waldo is amazingly obvious when the same illustration is reviewed. As Dr. Hendrix added, it is even harder to look for lung cancer (or any other radiographic finding) because, although Waldo is definitely present on every page of a *Where's Waldo* book, a radiograph may be normal. Even with these potentially helpful legal strategies, defending missed lung cancer is generally an unpleasant experience.[21]

SOLITARY PULMONARY NODULE

The SPN is a common presentation of lung cancer. However, most SPNs are benign. Summarizing five large series of resected SPNs seen on chest radiographs,[22–26] Siegelman et al.[27] noted that 53.9% were granulomas, 28.3% were bronchogenic carcinomas or other primary malignancies, 6.6% were hamartomas, and 3.5% were metastases. An even higher percentage of all radiographically detected SPNs are presumably benign, because nodules that appear calcified on chest radiographs are rarely resected.

The challenge in evaluating SPNs is to avoid invasive procedures in patients who have benign nodules without allowing potentially curable bronchogenic carcinomas the time to progress to more advanced or even unresectable disease. This is an area of active, ongoing research; however, the many approaches that have been tried attest to the lack of complete success for most modalities to date. A proper SPN evaluation acknowledges the following key points:

1. Imaging at a single point in time relies heavily on morphologic characteristics in distinguishing benign from malignant SPNs.
2. Calcification is the single best morphologic indicator of benignancy.
3. Behavior (i.e., lack of growth) is *far* better than any morphologic criterion at predicting benignancy.
4. Any predictor of benignancy must err on the side of intervention—it is better to resect a benign SPN unnecessarily than erroneously to call a malignant SPN benign.

With these key points in mind and realizing the significant expense (and in some cases radiation dose) of radiologic tests, it is always best to start the evaluation of the SPN by seeking old radiographs for comparison. This saves money, radiation, and often time, and provides the possibility for proving that a lesion is benign, no matter what its morphology is. A lesion that is stable for 2 years or more is considered to be benign, although the exception occurs for ground glass nodules at CT, which may represent very indolent adenocarcinomas. The flip side is that almost no matter what the morphology is, a growing lesion has declared itself to be one that should be resected. The lack of vigor with which old films are pursued is generally disappointing; if the patient were a close relative, we would all try a lot harder to spare him or her unnecessary tests that involve (potentially fatal) injection of intravenous contrast. And consider this—how many adults 40 years of age or older have never had a prior chest radiograph? In the United States, the number must be vanishingly small.

Whereas the concept of stability appears, on the surface, to be fairly straightforward, in practice it can be quite difficult to determine if a nodule has grown, particularly if it is small (e.g., less than 1 cm in diameter). This is true for both conventional radiography and for CT. For instance, a nodule that has increased from 10 to 11 mm in diameter may show no apparent, significant change in size at radiography or on axial CT scans; however, this represents a volume increase of 33%. To maximize the ability to detect such changes in size, it is important to optimize both CT imaging parameters, as well as postprocessing techniques. Particularly for small nodules, the best results may be obtained using thin section (1 to 2.5 mm), overlapping CT sections with 3D volumetric reconstructions (Fig. 26.7).[28,29] In addition, all follow-up scans should be performed using the same techniques. Volumetric measurements may be affected by many factors, including section thickness and spacing, x-ray dose, motion artifact, respiratory or cardiac phase, nodule location, and intraobserver/extraobserver variability; therefore, in general, volume differences less than about 25% should be regarded with skepticism.[28,30–36]

Sometimes, the clinical decision is made to prospectively follow an SPN with imaging, to demonstrate stability; this raises questions about appropriate scanning intervals. One study based on phantom exams and in vivo nodules, using automatic segmentation for lesion boundary definition, found that CT follow-up at 30 days could detect interval growth for all malignant lesions larger than 1 cm, and for lesions as small as 5 mm with a doubling time faster than 150 days.[37] Even for 5-mm lesions with slower doubling times, a second follow-up CT 30 days later rendered growth detectable in all cases. In a subsequent study of 13 patients, all five malignant nodules had doubling times less than 177 days, and all eight benign nodules had doubling times greater than 395 days.[38] However, other authors have found that a significant proportion of

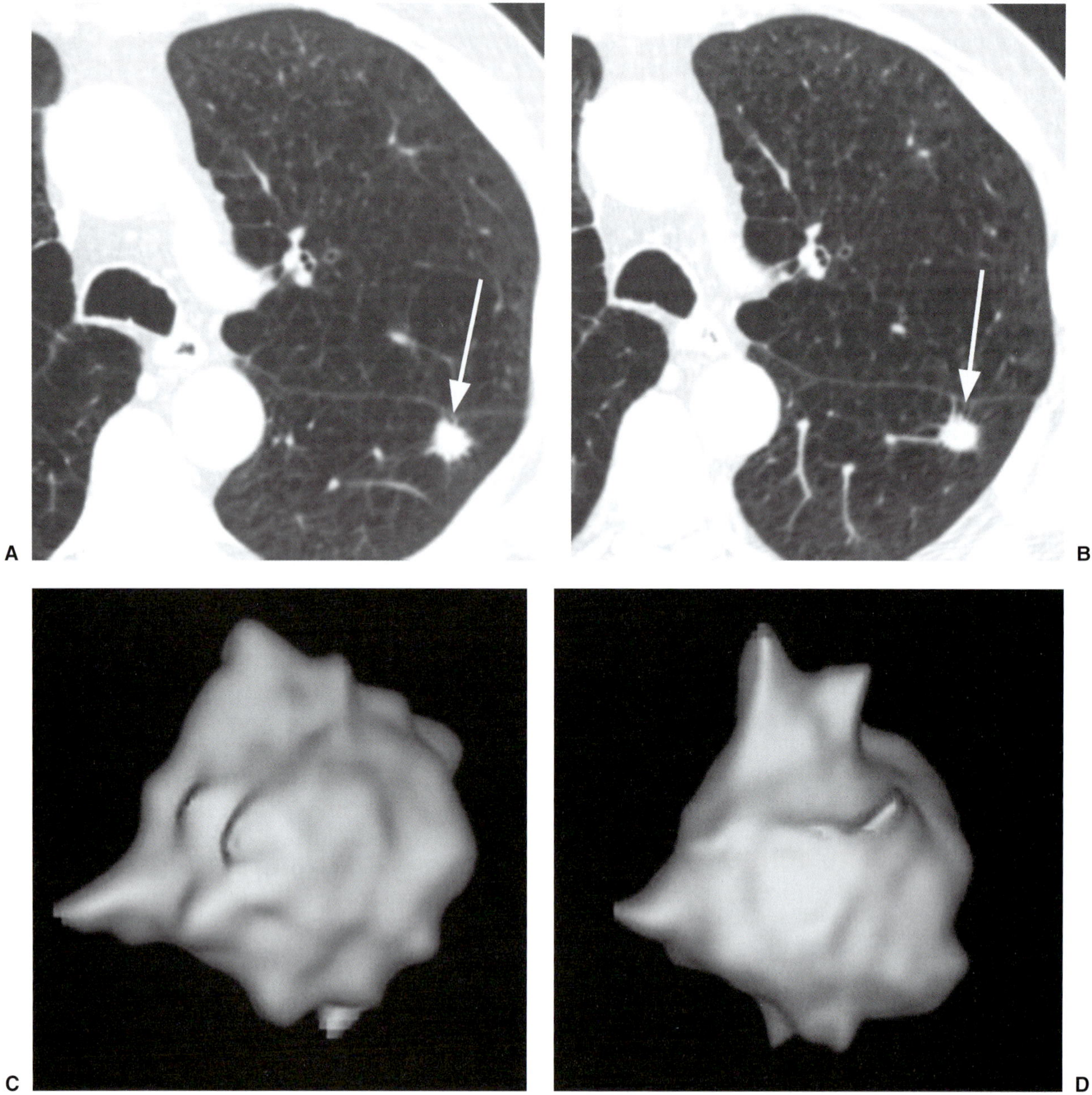

FIGURE 26.7 Small, spiculated left lower lobe tumor (*arrow*) on initial axial CT **(A)** shows minimal change in area by visual assessment on 6-month follow-up scan **(B)**. Corresponding 3D-volume reconstructions **(C,D)** show asymmetric growth and approximately 49% interval increase in volume (from 1.23 cm^3 to 1.83 cm^3).

malignant tumors have much longer doubling times (>465 days), and therefore short-term follow-up may not be helpful in many patients.[5,29,39,40]

For a small indeterminate SPN seen at CT, follow-up guidelines have been published by the Fleischner Society[41] (Table 26.1), as well as others,[42] regarding the suggested time intervals for repeat CT scanning, taking into account nodule size and whether the patient is clinically at low or high risk for developing lung cancer. These guidelines suggest follow-up out to 2 years, unless the nodule is nonsolid (ground glass) or partly solid; it is probably prudent to follow these nodules out to at least 3 years, because they could represent indolent adenocarcinomas, including BACs.

If a nodule is stable over a substantial period of time (e.g., 2 to 3 years), then it is almost certainly benign. However, it is well-known that not all growing nodules are malignant; various types of benign nodules may increase in size over time, including hamartomas, granulomas, and various other infectious or inflammatory lesions. In general, benign nodules tend to grow either extremely fast or extremely slowly, compared to

TABLE 26.1 Fleischner Society Recommendations for Follow-up and Management of an Incidental, Newly Detected, Indeterminate Nodule in Persons Older Than or Equal To Age 35 Years[41]

Nodule Size (mm)[a]	Low-Risk Patients[b]	High-Risk Patients[c]
≤4	No follow-up needed (<1% chance of malignancy)	Follow-up CT at 12 mo; if unchanged, no further follow-up[d]
>4–6	Follow-up CT at 12 mo; if unchanged, no further follow-up[d]	Initial follow-up CT at 6–12 mo then at 18–24 months if no change[d]
>6–8	Initial follow-up CT at 6–12 mo, then at 18–24 mo if no change	Initial follow-up CT at 3–6 mo then at 9–12 and 24 mo if no change[d]
>8	Follow-up CT at ~3, 9, and 24 mo, dynamic contrast CT, PET, +/or biopsy	Same as for low-risk patient

[a]Average of length and width.

[b]Minimal or absent history of smoking and of other known risk factors.

[c]History of smoking or of other known risk factors.

[d]Nonsolid (ground-glass) or partly solid nodules may require longer follow-up to exclude indolent adenocarcinoma.

malignancies. Therefore, it has been postulated that growth rates of nodules may be helpful in distinguishing benign from malignant nodules. However, a recent study addressing this issue, using data based on serial, thin section CT scans, found extensive overlap among the growth rates of benign and malignant, clinically suspicious, pathologically proven lung nodules.[29]

When comparison studies are not available to establish stability, assessment of morphologic features is the next step in an SPN evaluation. Various morphologic features are suggestive of malignancy, including spiculation; ill-defined, lobulated, or irregular margins, with distortion of adjacent vessels; heterogeneity; central cavity with thick, irregular walls; and air bronchograms (Figs. 26.1 and 26.7). In addition, a ground-glass nodular opacity on CT, particularly with a new solid component (Fig. 26.8), adjacent pleural thickening or retraction (Fig. 26.2), and large lesion size are features associated with malignancy. On the other hand, benign features include calcification, smooth, well-defined margins; concave, linear, branching or polygonal shape; subpleural location; homogeneous and solid opacity; and a cavity with thin, smooth walls. Unfortunately, there is great overlap in these features between benign and malignant lesions.

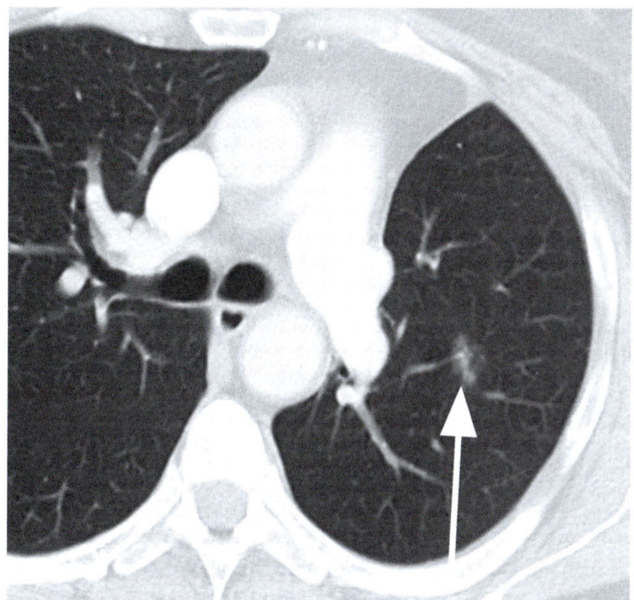

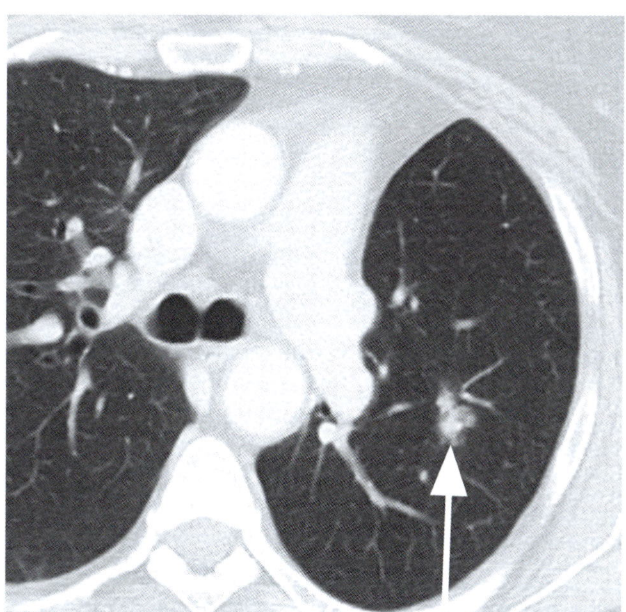

FIGURE 26.8 Small left upper lobe adenocarcinoma manifesting as a ground-glass nodule on the initial CT (*arrow*) **(A)**; follow-up CT 22 months later shows a new solid component (*arrow*) **(B)**.

Helical CT was used in one study to evaluate the surface morphology of lesions, with particular attention to vascular involvement; 29 patients with noncalcified SPNs less than 3 cm in size were examined.[43] Eighteen SPNs were malignant (nine bronchogenic carcinoma, nine metastatic) and eleven were benign (six granulomas, two hamartomas, one mixed granuloma, one arteriovenous malformation, one inflammatory infiltrate). Venous involvement was present in all 18 malignant SPNs, but also in 4 of 11 benign SPNs. Arterial involvement was seen in all nine bronchogenic carcinomas, in five of nine metastatic lesions, and in 2 of 11 benign SPNs. Thus vascular involvement does not distinguish between benign and malignant SPNs.

Of all the morphologic features that can be examined, it appears that demonstration of calcification is the best way to attempt to establish a benign etiology. Unfortunately, analysis of lung nodule calcification on chest radiographs is inaccurate. In a review of 35 nodules seen on posteroanterior (PA) and lateral chest radiographs and thin-section CT, radiologists were asked to predict lesion calcification at radiography with one of six levels of confidence.[44] Among the nodules thought to be "definitely calcified," 7% were not actually calcified. The authors suggested that nodules without documentation of long-term stability may warrant a low threshold for CT correlation. In fact, the demonstration of calcification on chest radiographs has been made more difficult by current widely used techniques that employ high kilovolt (peak). For that reason, chest fluoroscopy with low kilovolt (peak) spot films would be a good next step in looking for calcification. Unfortunately, few centers still perform chest fluoroscopy. Computed chest radiography with selective windowing may be an alternative possibility.[45] In addition, dual energy subtraction radiography is occasionally performed to improve confidence in the detection or exclusion of nodule calcification.[46]

At CT, assessment for calcification is currently performed by visual assessment of thin section images, making sure that the section thickness is less than one half the nodule diameter, to avoid partial volume effects. In addition, such scans should be performed using helical technique, during a single breath hold, in order to avoid scan plane misregistration and motion artifact. It should, however, be remembered that not all calcifications seen at CT indicate benignancy. Benign forms of calcification include diffuse, near complete, laminated or central nidus patterns, and these lesions usually represent old granulomas. Hamartomas may contain coarse, scattered "popcornlike" calcification, either with or without foci of fat. (Depiction of fat within a nodule is essentially diagnostic for a pulmonary hamartoma, regardless of the presence or absence of calcification, and, like calcification, is best detected using thin sections.)[47] On the other hand, malignant forms of calcification include amorphous, stippled, or eccentric patterns (Fig. 26.9). Approximately 10% of lung cancers[48] and up to 30% of carcinoids[49] contain calcification. Malignancies may calcify if dystrophic calcification is formed by the tumor cells, if the neoplasm arises in a preexisting, calcified scar, or if the tumor engulfs a nearby granuloma.

If morphologic features are indeterminate for benignancy, various diagnostic procedures may be attempted. One technique is the assessment of contrast enhancement. Preliminary studies with follow-up of noncalcified SPNs have reported that all or nearly all malignant SPNs enhance by at least 20 Hounsfield units (HU) within 2 to 4 minutes after contrast injection; few benign SPNs enhance to that degree.[50–52] Based on these promising preliminary results, a multicenter study[53] evaluated 356 SPNs that were ≥5 mm, solid, relatively spherical, homogeneous, and without calcification or fat on noncontrast images. Contrast-enhanced, single- or dual-detector helical CT images were obtained at 1, 2, 3, and 4 minutes after onset of injection (3-mm collimation, 420 mgI/kg, 300 mgI/mL administered at 2 mL/sec). Using a threshold increase in attenuation of 15 HU resulted in 98% sensitivity, 58% specificity, and 77% accuracy in diagnosing malignancy. Prevalence of malignancy in this patient group was 48% (171 of 356 nodules). A later study using a four-slice multidetector scanner and a slightly faster contrast injection rate found nearly identical results and also noted that peak attenuation of the nodules correlated with microvessel density.[54] Although uncommon, false-negative exams may occur occasionally in mucin-producing or necrotic tumors. Because of the latter pitfall, it is recommended that the technique not be used in large (>2 cm), potentially necrotic lesions. Given its overall high sensitivity, it is somewhat surprising that this technique has not become a standard tool in the workup of SPNs. However, another study demonstrated overlap in enhancement of malignant lesions and benign, active inflammatory lesions,[55] which may explain the low specificity and the current minor role of this technique.

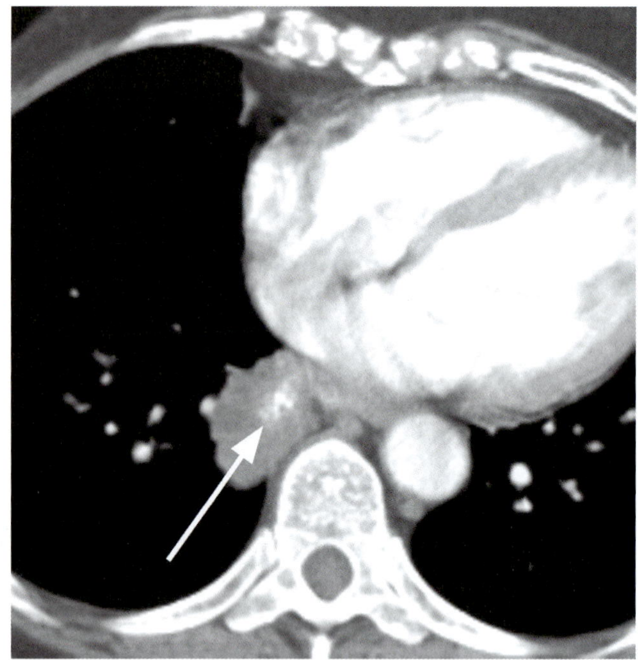

FIGURE 26.9 Right lower lobe carcinoma with amorphous calcifications (*arrow*).

Some preliminary work has been published on the use of combined contrast wash-in and wash-out, as an attempt to increase the specificity of contrast enhancement techniques. One study examined 107 nodules (49 malignant, 58 benign) using multidetector helical CT images obtained out to 15 minutes after the onset of contrast injection.[56] Using an increase in attenuation (wash-in threshold) of ≥25 HU resulted in 100% sensitivity, 48% specificity, and 72% accuracy in diagnosing malignancy; however, the addition of a wash-out threshold of 5 to 31 HU led to greatly improved results, showing 94% sensitivity, 90% specificity, and 92% accuracy. False-positive cases were seen in pneumonias and false negatives in adenocarcinomas. Only 57% of malignancies reached peak enhancement within 2 minutes; 92% reached peak within 5 minutes and 98% within 9 minutes. These data suggest that images should be obtained out to at least 9 minutes after administration of the contrast bolus. These results are quite promising; however, a larger, follow-up study by the same group found somewhat less sanguine findings (89% sensitivity, 79% specificity, and 84% accuracy) and suggested that the combination of wash-in plus evaluation of morphologic features gives equivalent results to wash-in plus wash-out.[57]

The degree of lung nodule contrast enhancement has been used not only for diagnostic purposes, but also for regional staging. A recent report has suggested that peak enhancement of a lung nodule ≥110 HU or net enhancement ≥60 HU is indicative of the presence of mediastinal nodal metastases, showing sensitivity, specificity, and accuracy figures of 65%, 89%, and 83%, respectively; these figures were similar to the results of ^{18}F-fluorodeoxyglucose–positron emission tomography (FDG–PET) scanning, performed in the same group of patients.[58]

Magnetic resonance imaging (MRI) is infrequently used for the detection and characterization of pulmonary nodules. The use of 2D half-Fourier single-shot turbo spin echo (HASTE) sequences allows the detection of pulmonary nodules greater than 5 mm in diameter. In a study using this sequence with MDCT as the gold standard, the sensitivity of MRI was 92% for lesions greater than 3 mm and 98% for nodules greater than 5 mm.[59] However, characterization using MRI is more difficult, partly because calcification is hard to identify on MRI. In an early study of 28 patients with SPNs, it was suggested that signal intensity measurements of nodules on dynamic contrast-enhanced MR studies may provide information about the nature of the nodules[60]; in addition, other investigations have suggested that dynamic contrast enhanced MRI, including relative enhancement and rate of enhancement, may be helpful in differentiating benign from malignant nodules.[61] In a study by Schaefer et al.,[62] time–intensity curves showing contrast enhancement profiles were 100% sensitive and 75% specific for malignancy. The absence of enhancement and thin, peripheral rim enhancement are features suggesting a benign lesion.[61–64]

In many centers, nodules that are suspicious for malignancy at CT are percutaneously biopsied using fluoroscopic or CT guidance; this is a relatively safe procedure and high accuracies have been reported, with positive predictive values (PPV) of at least 99%. The key number, however, is the negative predictive value (NPV): How reliable is a negative result? Can a nodule with a negative biopsy be safely watched, or should it be resected regardless of the biopsy result? Reported NPVs for fine-needle aspiration biopsy (FNAB) of lung nodules range from 59% to 82%.[65–68] There is little data regarding the NPV of core needle biopsies in this setting, and the available results are also somewhat conflicting, ranging from 67% to 92%.[68–71] The NPVs for core biopsies showing nonspecific benign tissue or insufficient tissue for diagnosis were 76% and 50%, respectively, according to one recent study; on the other hand, the NPV for a biopsy revealing a specific, benign diagnosis, such as hamartoma or fungus, approached 100%.[69] Published studies have suggested that the use of core needle biopsy technique increases the frequency of obtaining a specific benign diagnosis, compared to FNAB[72,73]; the proportion of specific benign diagnoses compared to all benign diagnoses ranged from 21% to 83% in recent investigations.[68–71] Given these results, surgeons at many institutions believe that a percutaneous biopsy of an SPN is not indicated: except for the uncommon instance when a specific benign diagnosis is established, they will resect the nodule regardless of the biopsy results. (An exception might occur in the patient with a history of previous extrathoracic primary neoplasm.) At other institutions, where percutaneous biopsy is routinely performed for SPNs, it is advocated that a nonspecific negative biopsy be followed by a repeat biopsy. If the repeat biopsy is also negative for malignancy, then close follow-up is advised.

The various approaches to the SPN described previously have largely been overshadowed by the growing acceptance of PET scanning. PET has the obvious advantage of evaluating the metabolic behavior of the nodule rather than its morphology, and it is of great value in differentiating benign and malignant SPNs. PET is covered in Chapter 27.

Whereas in the general population, the major issue with regard to an SPN is distinguishing the benign nodule from the malignant nodule, the issue is slightly different in the patient with a current or previous extrapulmonary primary cancer. In this type of patient, it can be important to distinguish between a solitary metastasis and a new bronchogenic carcinoma. The relative likelihood that a new SPN seen on a chest radiograph is a solitary metastasis versus a new lung cancer depends on the histology of the previous primary tumor. In some instances, the odds favor a new lung primary, such as for head and neck carcinoma (15.8:1), bladder carcinoma (8.3:1), and cervical carcinoma (6:1).[74] In fact, with some primaries, all malignant SPNs in one series were lung cancers (prostate, 26 patients; stomach, 7 patients; esophagus, 4 patients; pancreas, 3 patients). In other cases, a solitary metastasis is favored, such as in patients with soft tissue sarcoma (17.5:1), osteosarcoma (6.7:1), melanoma (4.1:1), and testicular carcinoma (2:1)[74] With most primaries the answer is in between, but slightly favoring lung cancer; examples include breast carcinoma (1.7:1), colon carcinoma (1.4:1), renal cell carcinoma (1.2:1), and endometrial carcinoma (1.1:1).[74]

Because CT is more sensitive at detecting lung nodules, the CT demonstration of a SPN more reliably indicates that there is really only one nodule. A recent study used CT to readdress the issue of a patient with a previous extrathoracic primary neoplasm and a new SPN.[75] In this study, breast cancer was grouped with cancers of bladder, cervix, biliary tree, esophagus, ovary, prostate, and stomach, and the overall result was that 26 SPNs were lung cancers, and 8 were solitary metastases (3.3:1). For head and neck cancer, the ratio of lung cancers to solitary metastases was 8.3:1. For patients with carcinoma of the salivary glands, adrenal glands, colon, kidney, thyroid, thymus, or uterus the corresponding ratio was 0.8:1, whereas patients with melanoma, sarcoma, or testicular carcinoma had many more solitary metastases than new lung primaries (3.8:1).[75]

STAGING OF LUNG CANCER

Initial tumor staging in patients with NSCLC is important in order to identify those patients with locoregional disease who are likely to benefit from surgical resection or other potentially curative therapies, such as definitive radiation therapy or radiofrequency ablation. Staging may be performed using a combination of modalities, although the workhorses are CT and FDG–PET scanning[76]; other techniques, such as MRI, ultrasonography, bone radiography, bone scintigraphy, and endoscopic ultrasound are usually reserved for specific problem solving and/or to enable tissue biopsy. The TNM staging system of the American Joint Committee on Cancer (AJCC) and the International Union Against Cancer (Union Internationale Contre le Cancer [UICC]) is the most widely accepted and used classification system for preoperative and postoperative staging,[77–80] although this will be replaced by the new International Association for the Study of Lung Cancer (IASLC) staging system in 2009 (see Chapter 30). In the most current version of TNM staging classification (published in 2002),[77,81] T1 tumors are small (≤3 cm in diameter), are surrounded by lung or visceral pleura, and are without bronchoscopic evidence of invasion more proximal than the lobar bronchus. T2 tumors show one or more of the following features: larger than 3 cm; involvement of a mainstem bronchus 2 cm or more distal to the carina; invasion of visceral pleura; and atelectasis extending to the hilum, without involvement of the entire lung. T3 tumors show invasion of the chest wall, diaphragm, pericardium, mediastinal pleura, or mainstem bronchus (less than 2 cm distal to the carina), or have postobstructive atelectasis or pneumonia of an entire lung. T4 cancers invade the mediastinum, heart, great vessels, trachea, esophagus, or vertebral body, have an associated malignant pleural effusion, or have satellite nodule(s) within the ipsilateral primary-tumor lobe of the lung. Metastatic spread to lymph nodes is classified as N1 for peribronchial or ipsilateral hilar nodes and for intrapulmonary nodes involved by direct extension of the primary tumor. Metastatic disease to ipsilateral mediastinal or subcarinal nodes falls into the N2 category and into the N3 category for involvement of contralateral mediastinal or hilar nodes, and ipsilateral or contralateral scalene or supraclavicular lymph nodes. The M0 category comprises patients with no distant metastases; presence of distant metastases confers M1 status.

In the current TNM system, stage I tumors have no lymph node metastases. Stage II tumors either have no lymph node metastases or spread is confined to hilar lymph nodes. Stage IIIA includes tumors with spread to ipsilateral mediastinal or subcarinal nodes, whereas stage IIIB includes tumors with involvement of contralateral mediastinal or hilar nodes, or ipsilateral or contralateral scalene or supraclavicular lymph nodes. Tumors with distant metastases are classified as stage IV.[77]

In the summer of 2007, the IASLC published a series of articles outlining recommendations for amendments to the TNM staging system based on data from more than 100,000 patients in its Lung Cancer Staging Project.[82–86] These amendments will likely be reflected in the next official version of the TNM classification system, due to be published in 2009. These changes include the following: the T1 and T2 categories are broken down by tumor diameter (T1a: ≤2 cm; T1b: >2 to 3 cm; T2a: >3 to 5 cm, T2b: >5 to 7 cm). Furthermore, T3 includes tumors >7 cm in diameter. If a patient has a satellite nodule (or nodules) in the same lobe of the lung as the primary tumor, this falls into the T3 category; if the satellite nodule is in a different, ipsilateral lobe, this represents T4 disease; and if it is in a contralateral lobe, this presents M1a disease. There are no changes in the N classification. The M category has been divided into M1a and M1b. M1a includes patients with distant metastatic disease confined to the lung and pleura, for example, malignant pleural nodules, malignant pleural or pericardial effusion, or separate tumor nodule(s) in a contralateral lobe. The M1b category includes distant metastases outside of the lung and pleura. The stage groupings have also shifted somewhat to better align the classifications with prognosis and treatment.[82]

COMPUTED TOMOGRAPHY

Evaluation of the Primary Tumor

Pleural Invasion A pleural effusion in a patient with lung cancer may be malignant, caused by pleural metastases, or it may be benign, particularly in a patient with postobstructive pneumonia. The CT hallmark for a malignant effusion is soft tissue nodularity along the pleural surfaces, accompanying the effusion, although this finding is not always present (Fig. 26.10). It has been reported that pleural nodularity and/or fissural thickening are indicative of pleural metastases, even in the absence of pleural effusion.[87] Pleural tumor dissemination is currently classified as T4 disease and is generally considered unresectable.

Chest Wall Invasion CT has shown somewhat disparate results in assessing for chest wall invasion by tumor, with sensitivity ranging from 38% to 87% and specificity from 40% to 90%.[88–94] Signs of invasion may include bone destruction, tumor mass extending into the chest wall, pleural thickening, loss of the extrapleural fat plane, obtuse angle between mass and chest wall, and greater than 3 cm of contact between mass and chest wall (Figs. 26.2 and 26.11 to 26.14). In a series of 112 patients with cancers adjacent to the pleural surface, Ratto et al.[91] found that CT was 83% sensitive and 80% specific for

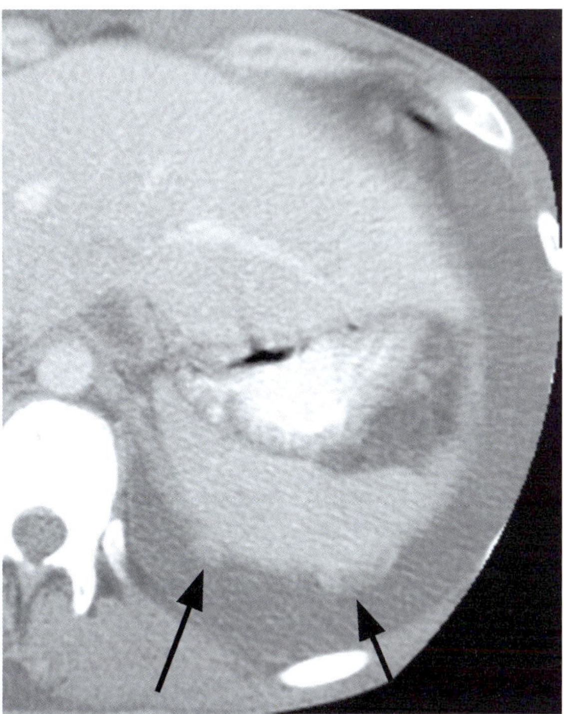

FIGURE 26.10 Malignant pleural effusion from adenocarcinoma of the lung. Note pleural tumor nodules (*arrows*).

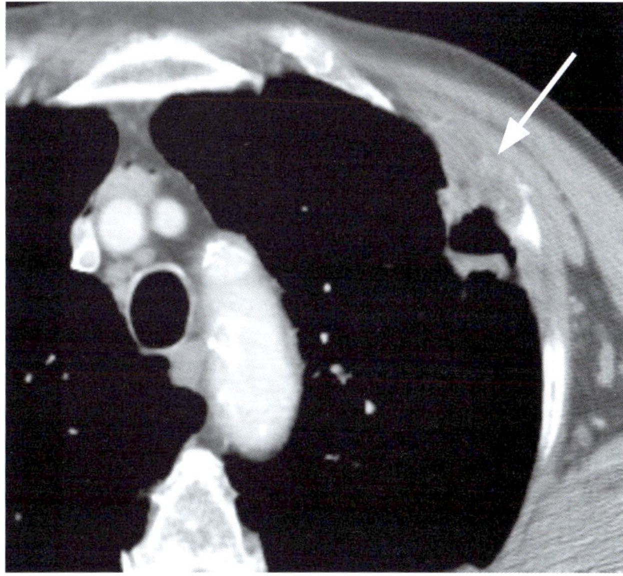

FIGURE 26.11 Cavitary non–small cell lung cancer with chest wall invasion. Note abnormal soft tissue in chest wall with accompanying rib destruction (*arrow*).

chest wall invasion using a cutoff of 0.9 for the ratio between the length of tumor–pleura contact and tumor diameter. They also found that obliteration of the extrapleural fat plane was 85% sensitive and 87% specific for invasion. However, they noted that the extrapleural fat plane was not always visible, particularly when the tumor contacted the ribs; on the other hand, this plane was usually visible when the tumor contacted the pleural surface in between the ribs. Length of tumor–pleura contact, angle between the tumor and the pleura, presence of soft tissue mass involving the chest wall, and rib destruction were less accurate indicators of chest wall invasion in this series. Pennes et al.[90] noted that in their series of 33 patients with peripheral pulmonary malignancies, 5 patients showed encroachment on or increased density of the extrapleural fat; however, only 3 of these 5 had chest wall or pleural invasion at surgery. In the other two patients, lymphoid aggregates were present in the extrapleural fat, suggesting that nonspecific

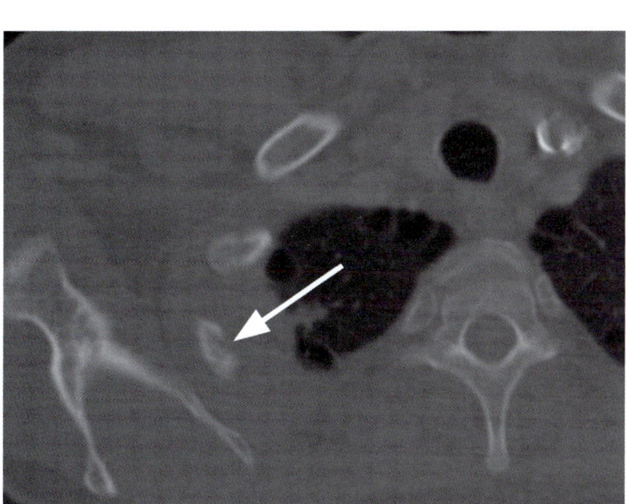

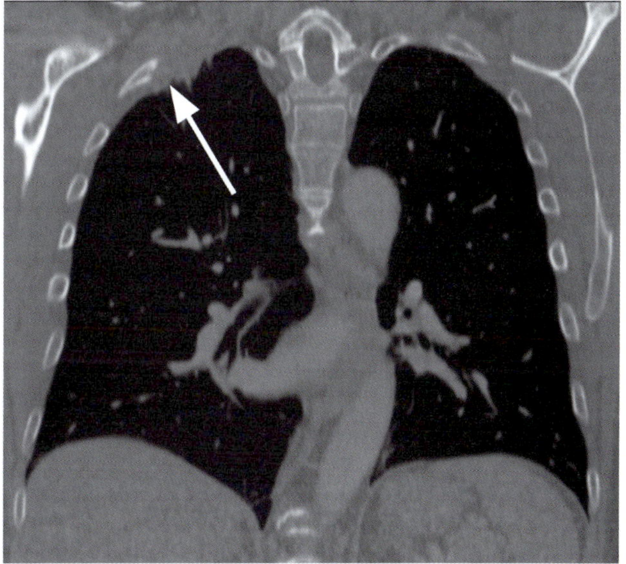

FIGURE 26.12 Peripheral right upper lobe adenocarcinoma showing rib invasion (*arrow*) on axial **(A)** and coronal **(B)** CT images.

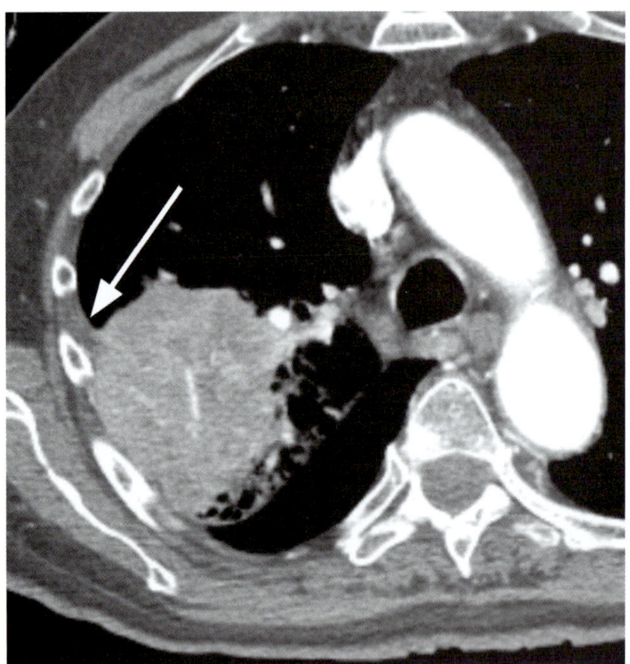

FIGURE 26.13 Right upper lobe adenocarcinoma. CT shows broad contact between the tumor and the chest wall, with mild soft tissue infiltration into the adjacent extrapleural fat (*arrow*). These findings are indeterminate for chest wall invasion.

inflammatory processes involving the pleura may extend into the adjacent extrapleural soft tissues. Pleural thickening was a very sensitive (100%) indicator of chest wall invasion in this study, although very poor specificity (44%) led to poor accuracy (58%). In the 20 patients with peripheral lung malignancies studied by Pearlberg et al.,[94] definite bone destruction at CT showed 100% PPV (11 of 11). Soft tissue extension around ribs into fat or muscle of the chest wall had a PPV of 33% (three of nine). In each of these six false-positive cases, fibrous, inflammatory, and/or hemorrhagic changes were shown in the adjacent pleural or extrapleural tissues, but no tumor extension was seen.

Some investigators have employed artificial (i.e., induced) pneumothorax in order to increase the accuracy of CT in diagnosing chest wall and mediastinal pleural invasion. For example, Watanabe et al.[95] found 100% sensitivity, 80% specificity and 88% accuracy for CT using this technique in 12 patients. In one patient with no separation between the tumor and the mediastinal pleura, only adhesions were found at surgery, with no mediastinal tumor invasion. In a different study of 43 patients with equivocal chest wall invasion on routine CT, artificial pneumothorax yielded 100% accuracy for diagnosing chest wall invasion and 76% accuracy for mediastinal invasion.[96] These authors noted difficulty when the tumor was near the root of the pulmonary arteries and veins, because it was occasionally hard to introduce air into this region of the pleural space.

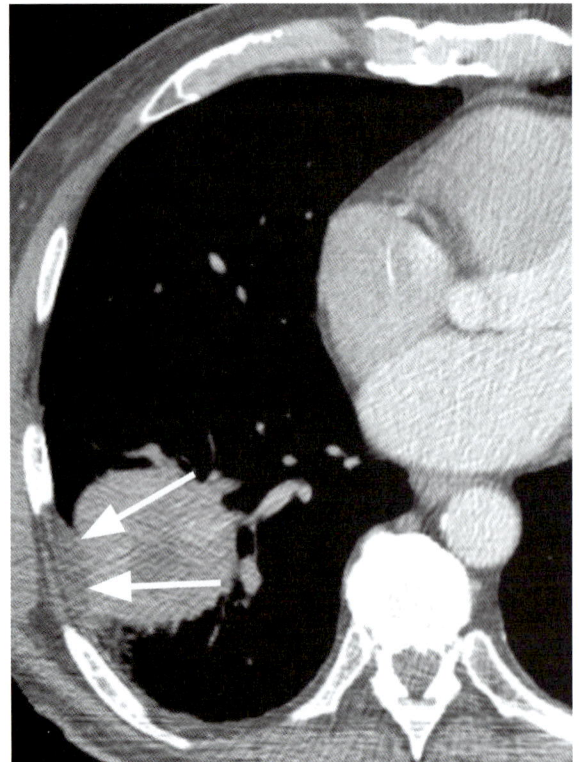

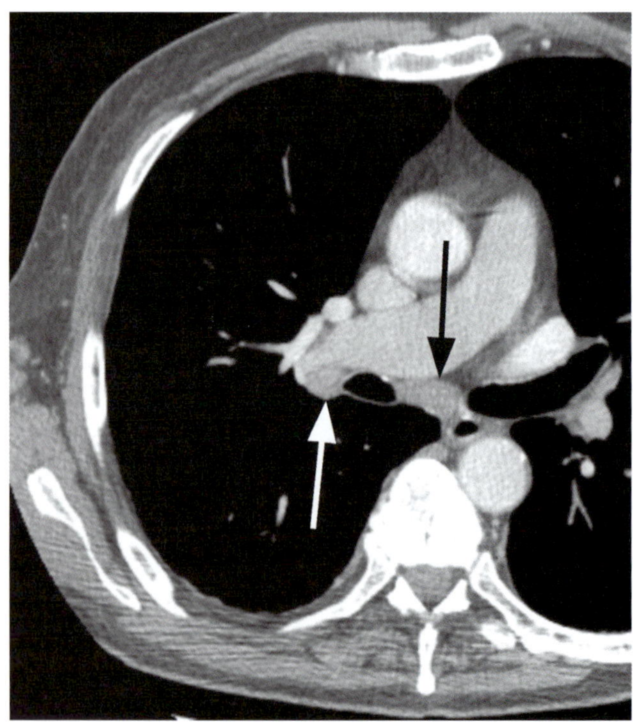

FIGURE 26.14 Right lower lobe adenocarcinoma showing broad contact with pleura and adjacent pleural thickening **(A)** (*arrows*); CT findings are indeterminate for pleural and chest wall invasion. Mildly enlarged right hilar (*white arrow*) and subcarinal (*black arrow*) lymph nodes are seen at CT **(B)**. At surgery, there was a benign pleural plaque adjacent to the tumor, without pleural tumor invasion. Tumor involved hilar lymph nodes (N1), without mediastinal nodal involvement.

Other techniques for diagnosing chest wall invasion rely on the absence of relative movement between the chest wall and the adjacent tumor during respiration. Investigators have used inspiratory or expiratory CT, ultrasonography, and cine MR during deep breathing to evaluate this feature, with moderately successful results.[97–99]

In summary, these studies suggest that the best and the only reliable criterion for diagnosing chest wall invasion with routine CT is definite bone destruction, with or without tumor mass extending into the chest wall. Thin sections are often helpful in making this assessment. It should be noted that chest wall invasion does not preclude surgical resection, because the surgeon can perform en bloc resection and chest wall reconstruction (see Chapter 34). However, this procedure is associated with increased operative morbidity and mortality. In addition, patients with known mediastinal nodal metastases and chest wall invasion are felt to have a very poor prognosis (7% reported 5-year survival following surgical resection), and surgery is usually not advocated in these patients.[100,101] Superior sulcus tumors invading extrapleurally are usually treated with radiation therapy followed by surgical resection.

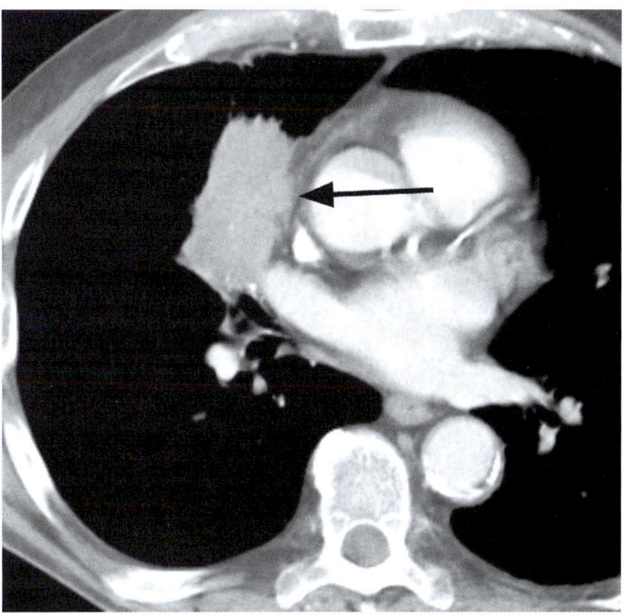

FIGURE 26.15 Minimal mediastinal fat invasion (*arrow*) by middle lobe neoplasm, proven at surgery and successfully resected using a middle lobe sleeve lobectomy.

Mediastinal Invasion Although invasion of the mediastinum falls into the T4 category in the TNM staging classification, minimal invasion of fat only (without invasion of vascular or other structures) is generally considered resectable by many surgeons. Therefore, it is not usually necessary to preoperatively diagnose minimal mediastinal fat invasion (Fig. 26.15); on the other hand, gross invasion is considered to be unresectable (Fig. 26.16). In addition, a reliable diagnosis of invasion of mediastinal vessels, trachea, esophagus, and/or vertebral body would usually preclude surgical resection. Several studies have investigated the usefulness of CT in detecting mediastinal invasion and in predicting resectability

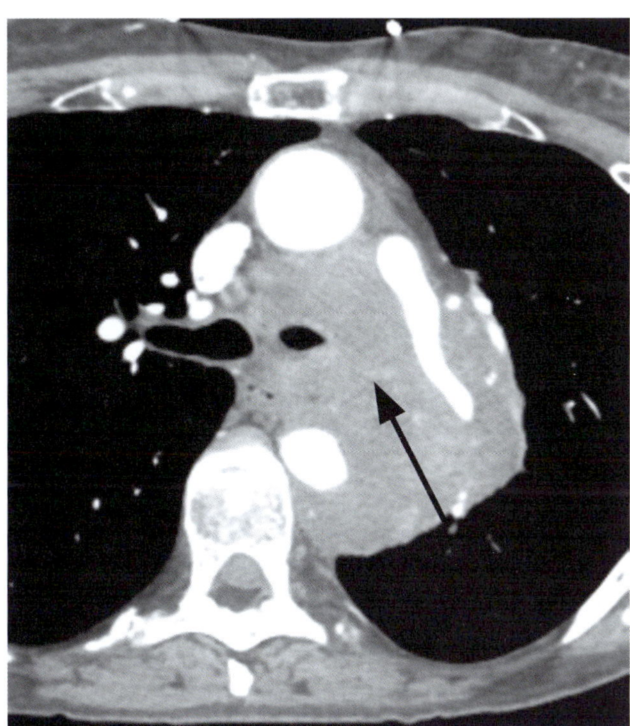

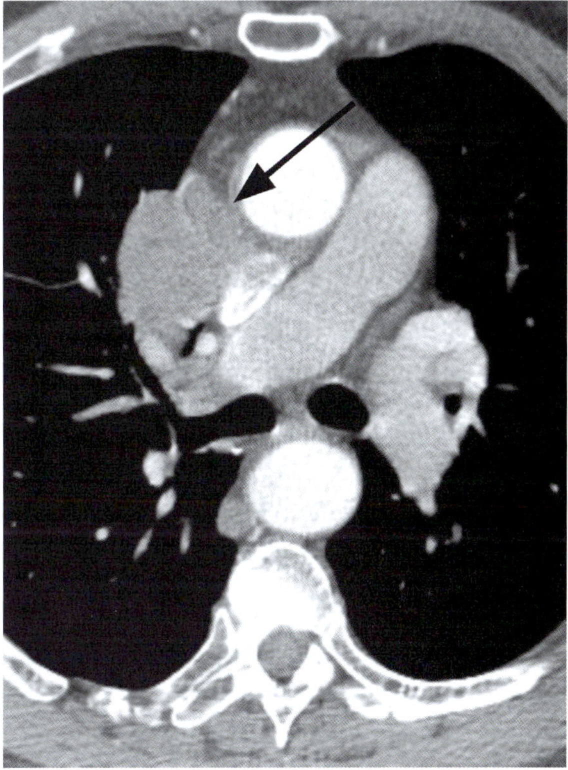

FIGURE 26.16 Two different patients **(A, B)** showing gross, unresectable invasion of mediastinal fat (*arrow*).

of the primary tumor.[88,92,102–109] Accuracy for distinguishing between T0 to T2 and T3 to T4 tumors has been reported to be 56% to 89%.[106–109] However, this information is not particularly helpful, because the clinically important distinction is between resectable (T3) and unresectable (T4) cancers.

In one retrospective study of 80 patients with an indeterminate CT for mediastinal invasion (i.e., mass contiguous with the mediastinum but without definite infiltration into the mediastinal fat or extension around the central vessels or mainstem bronchi), the authors were able to identify a large group of masses that were likely to be technically resectable using one or more of the following criteria: contact of 3 cm or less with mediastinum, less than 90 degrees of contact with aorta, and mediastinal fat between the mass and mediastinal structure.[102] A total of 36 out of 37 masses in this category were resectable; 28 of 36 masses had no mediastinal invasion, and 8 of 36 had focal limited invasion. However, more than 3-cm contact with mediastinum, more than 90 degrees of contact with aorta, obliteration of the fat plane between the mass and mediastinal structures, presence of mass effect on adjacent mediastinal structures, and pleural or pericardial thickening were not reliable signs of either invasion or unresectability. Kameda et al.[104] studied 52 patients with lung cancer, including 21 with central tumors. CT was 100% sensitive although not specific (60% to 67%) in evaluating for superior vena cava or right pulmonary artery invasion. For the left pulmonary artery and the left atrium or pulmonary vein, CT had high specificity (94% to 100%) but poor sensitivity (56% to 62%). In a CT study of 108 patients, Izbicki et al.[105] reported one false-positive case for aortic invasion and multiple false-negative cases for invasion of an atrium, pulmonary artery, superior vena cava, or mediastinal bronchus. Choe et al.[110] found that obliteration of the superior pulmonary vein at CT was consistent with intrapericardial extension of tumor through the pulmonary vein in 10 of 10 patients. On the other hand, only four of nine patients with obliteration of the inferior pulmonary vein at CT showed intrapericardial tumor extension at surgery.

In summary, CT diagnosis of mediastinal fat or mediastinal structure invasion is generally unreliable (Figs. 26.3, 26.17, and 26.18), and a patient should not be denied of surgery based on unproven CT findings. Gross mediastinal fat invasion may be proved via mediastinoscopy or transtracheal Wang needle biopsy, if the location is accessible using these techniques. Findings suggestive of central tracheobronchial invasion at CT are usually further evaluated using bronchoscopy. CT and bronchoscopy are complementary procedures: bronchoscopy is superior to CT in evaluating the mucosal surface of the airway, whereas CT is superior in visualizing tumor spread extraluminally and occasionally within the wall of the bronchus. Transesophageal echocardiography (TEE) may aid in evaluating for direct aortic invasion by tumor.[111] Occasionally, secondary signs are helpful in diagnosing mediastinal invasion;

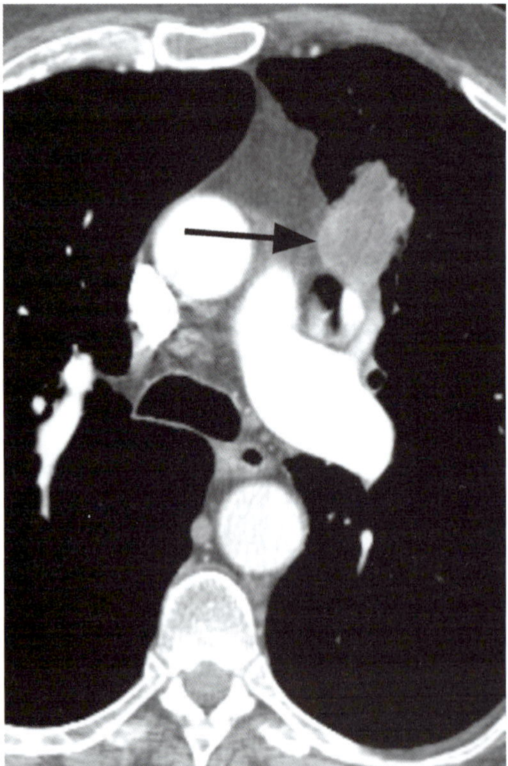

FIGURE 26.17 Squamous cell cancer of the left upper lobe. Broad, convex margin between the tumor and the mediastinum (*arrow*) is suggestive of mediastinal invasion; the tumor was surgically resected, and there was no mediastinal or pleural invasion.

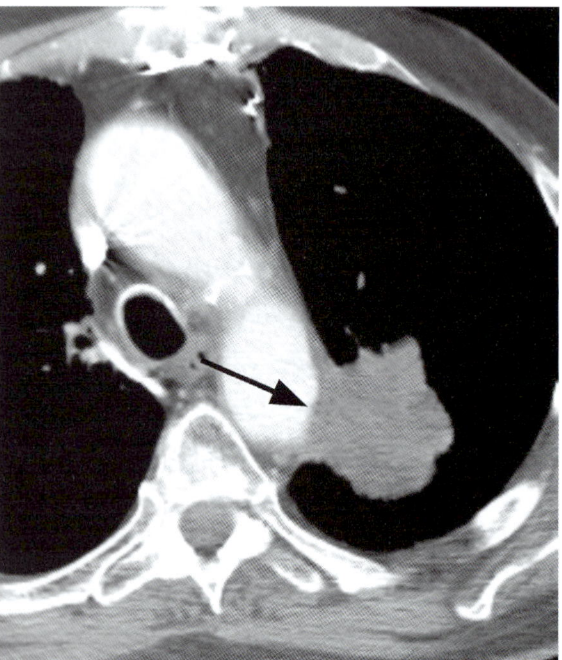

FIGURE 26.18 Obliteration of fat plane between left upper lobe tumor and aorta (*arrow*); CT findings are equivocal for aortic invasion. The tumor was unresectable because of aortic invasion at surgical exploration.

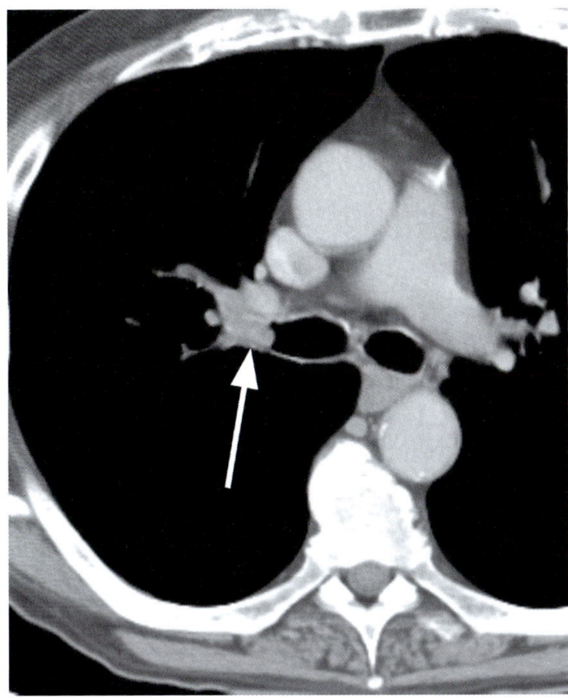

FIGURE 26.19 Squamous cell cancer (*arrow*) obstructing the right upper lobe bronchus, with minimal extension into the right mainstem bronchus. The tumor was resected using a right upper sleeve lobectomy.

for example, deviation of the left vocal cord and hoarseness in a patient with a left lung cancer is suggestive of mediastinal tumor invasion involving the recurrent laryngeal nerve.

Prediction of Need for Lobectomy versus Pneumonectomy Tumor invasion of central pulmonary arteries and veins, as well as tumor extension across the major fissure (anywhere on the left; above the minor fissure on the right), are findings that would generally require pneumonectomy for resection rather than lobectomy. In many cases, tumor involvement of a mainstem bronchus also necessitates pneumonectomy, although some of these tumors may be resected with lobectomy using a sleeve resection and bronchoplasty (Fig. 26.19). The assessment of the need for lobectomy versus pneumonectomy is important in the patient with poor pulmonary function who cannot tolerate a pneumonectomy. Quint et al.[112] found CT to be inaccurate in making this assessment, although thin sections (1.5 to 3.0 mm) helped in evaluating for tumor spread across a fissure. The recent use of multidetector helical scanning modes enables acquisition of large numbers of thin sections during a single breath hold. These capabilities facilitate optimal evaluation of the central airways and other central structures, particularly by using sagittal, coronal, and off-axis planar reformatted images, as well as 3D reconstructions. Some surgeons find that 3D displays of CT data are helpful in preoperative surgical planning,[113] and 3D reconstructions may improve accuracy in evaluating for central pulmonary vascular invasion.[114]

Differentiation between Tumor and Adjacent Atelectasis/Pneumonia Another use for CT in evaluating local extension of the primary tumor is in distinguishing central tumor from adjacent collapsed lung. After an intravenous bolus of urographic contrast material, the atelectatic lung may enhance much more than the adjacent tumor, thus giving a more accurate assessment of tumor size.[115] However, in many cases, it remains difficult to distinguish tumor from adjacent postobstructive atelectasis or pneumonia.

CT Evaluation of Hilar and Mediastinal Lymph Nodes

Significance Metastatic disease to hilar lymph nodes (N1 disease) adversely affects patient prognosis, although it does not generally affect resectability. Usually, involved hilar nodes can be easily removed from the hilar vessels at surgery. Thus, although preoperative detection of tumor spread to hilar nodes is useful, it is generally not crucial in directing surgical treatment planning. Moreover, the presence or absence of hilar node metastases is an unreliable indicator of mediastinal node metastases.[116,117]

In the past, the presence of mediastinal node metastases has been considered a contraindication to thoracotomy, and preoperative detection of mediastinal spread of disease has generally precluded surgical resection. However, some investigators have found reasonable 3- and 5-year survival rates for patients with positive ipsilateral mediastinal nodes, and many surgeons now feel that certain groups of patients with limited N2 disease may be surgical candidates.[118–120] Naruke et al.[121] found significantly increased 5-year survival in patients with N2 disease (14%) as compared to patients with N3 disease (0%) following pulmonary resection in 1479 patients with no distant metastatic disease. It has been suggested that resection may be worthwhile in patients with ipsilateral mediastinal nodal disease as long as the nodes are not in the high paratracheal region, are not numerous or bulky, and can be completely resected.[122,123] Some groups have advocated surgical resection in conjunction with postoperative radiation therapy in patients with mediastinal metastases.[116,124,125] Other investigators have suggested that patients with N2 (or even N3) disease may benefit from chemotherapy or combined chemotherapy and radiation, either alone or prior to surgical resection.[126–132] However, most clinicians believe that metastatic disease to contralateral hilar or mediastinal lymph nodes or metastases to any scalene or supraclavicular lymph nodes (N3 disease) precludes surgery. It has been observed that metastases to mediastinal lymph nodes indicates aggressive tumor biology, suggesting the presence of distant metastases and implying poor survival.[126]

CT Criteria for Detection of Lymph Node Metastases Given the importance of preoperative nodal staging for treatment planning, a noninvasive imaging modality such as CT is of great potential value for assessment of mediastinal nodes, both ipsilateral and contralateral to the primary lung tumor. Mediastinal lymph nodes are generally identified on axial CT images as nonenhancing, oval, soft tissue density structures surrounded by mediastinal fat. Nodal size may be estimated by measuring the short and long-axis diameters of a node as seen on the axial images. Glazer et al.[133] stated that the short-axis diameter is a more accurate predictor of nodal size than the long-axis diameter, because long-axis measurements are more dependent on the spatial orientation of the node. The long-axis diameter is accurate on transverse CT images only when the longest axis of the ovoid, 3D lymph node is oriented in the plane of section that is, the transverse plane. If the lymph node is vertically oriented, the long-axis diameter on CT has no relation to the true long-axis measurement of the lymph node. Short-axis diameters are also affected by nodal orientation, although to a lesser extent. In a CT or autopsy correlation study, Quint et al.[134] found that the short-axis diameter of the nodes at CT was the best predictor of actual nodal volume.

CT criteria for lymph node malignancy theoretically include morphological features such as nodal density and margination, as well as nodal size. In practice, however, most of these features are not helpful, and increased nodal size is the only useful criterion for malignancy. One exception to this rule is the occasional finding of central nodal low density, suggesting necrosis; this is a good indicator for malignant nodal disease. Occasionally, the central low density will show the attenuation of fat, and this finding is reliable for benignancy. In addition, another study suggested that rounding of the contour of a hilar lymph node, where it meets the lung margin, is indicative of metastatic disease.[135]

Several groups have investigated the normal size limits for mediastinal lymph nodes, studying normal patients and those with lung cancer. Genereux and Howie[136] studied CT scans of normal patients and compared their findings with dissection of 12 cadaver mediastina. The largest mediastinal nodes at CT were in the precarinal or subcarinal and aortopulmonary regions, and at autopsy, the largest nodes were in the pretracheal and precarinal or subcarinal regions. These authors measured long-axis lymph node diameters at CT and found that 95% were less than 11 mm. In another CT study by Schnyder and Gamsu,[137] the mean diameter of normal lymph nodes in the pretracheal, retrocaval space was 5.5 mm plus or minus 2.8 SD (short vs. long axis not specified), with 91% (116 of 127) being less than or equal to 1 cm. A CT or autopsy study in five cadavers by Quint et al.[134] showed excellent correlation for the number of nodes in right-sided mediastinal regions, with poorer correlation in left-sided regions. Mean short-axis nodal diameters at CT ranged from 3.2 to 7.3 mm, depending on exact nodal location. Kiyono et al.[138] dissected 40 cadaver mediastina from patients without chest malignancy or infection, and recorded the number, size (short and long axes in the transverse plane), and American Thoracic Society (ATS) location of each lymph node identified. Based on their findings, these authors proposed standards for maximum short-axis diameters as follows: 12 mm for ATS region 7 (subcarinal), 10 mm for ATS regions 4 (right lower paratracheal) and 10R (right tracheobronchial angle), and 8 mm for other regions. They found that maximum long-axis diameters showed a wider variation.

Glazer et al.[133] examined normal mediastinal lymph nodes on CT scans from 56 normal patients and tabulated the number and size of lymph nodes in each anatomical region as specified by the ATS lymph node mapping scheme. In this study, 1 cm was the optimal upper limit of normal for the short axis of a mediastinal node at CT, with slight variations according to specific location (range 7 to 11 mm). The largest nodes were in the subcarinal and right tracheobronchial regions, whereas the smallest nodes were in the upper paratracheal and left peribronchial regions. A prior CT study by the same group involving patients with NSCLC similarly found 1 cm as the optimal size threshold for diagnosing metastatic disease in mediastinal nodes.[139] Platt et al.[140] confirmed 11 mm as the upper limit of normal size at CT for subcarinal lymph nodes in 46 patients with NSCLC.

To address the issue of lymph node size versus presence/absence of metastases, Medina Gallardo et al.[141] conducted a pathological study of lymph nodes resected from 67 patients with NSCLC. The authors correlated lymph node size (as measured on the fresh, resected nodes in the pathology department) with presence or absence of tumor at histological examination. Using a size threshold of 10 mm (short vs. long axis not specified), 73 of 167 (44%) patients had enlarged mediastinal nodes and 58 of 167 (35%) had enlarged hilar nodes. There are 18 out of 73 (25%) and 12 out of 58 (21%) patients who had neoplastic involvement of enlarged mediastinal and hilar nodes at pathological examination, respectively (25% mediastinal nodal PPV). The PPV for enlarged mediastinal lymph nodes in squamous cell carcinoma was 23% and in adenocarcinoma was 18%. These low values were reflective of the large number of false-positive cases caused by enlarged, benign lymph nodes.

These results highlight one pitfall in using a nodal size threshold to distinguish benign from malignant lymph nodes at CT. Benign nodes may be enlarged because of reactive hyperplasia, anthracosis, inflammation, or infection (Fig. 26.20). Conversely, malignant nodes may be normal in size if they contain only microscopic metastases. Daly et al.[142] reported that enlarged, benign nodes were a particular problem for central tumors with postobstructive pneumonia. Gross et al.[143] addressed the issue of microscopic metastases to normal-sized nodes in a study of 39 patients with bronchogenic carcinoma. Five of thirty-nine (13%) patients had metastases limited to normal-sized nodes as measured at surgery and pathology; however, two of these five patients showed enlarged nodes at CT owing to inaccurate CT depiction of nodal size in the subcarinal region. In one patient, multiple normal-sized subcarinal nodes containing metastatic tumor were visualized only as a single large mass at CT. In the second patient, a 10 × 9 mm subcarinal node containing metastatic tumor measured 12 × 11 mm at CT, and was therefore identified as abnormal. Thus metastatic disease to normal-sized mediastinal lymph nodes was missed at CT in only 3 of 39 (8%) patients, and the authors concluded that metastatic disease to normal-sized mediastinal lymph nodes was not a major problem in CT staging of lung cancer. Similarly, Daly et al.[142] reported that

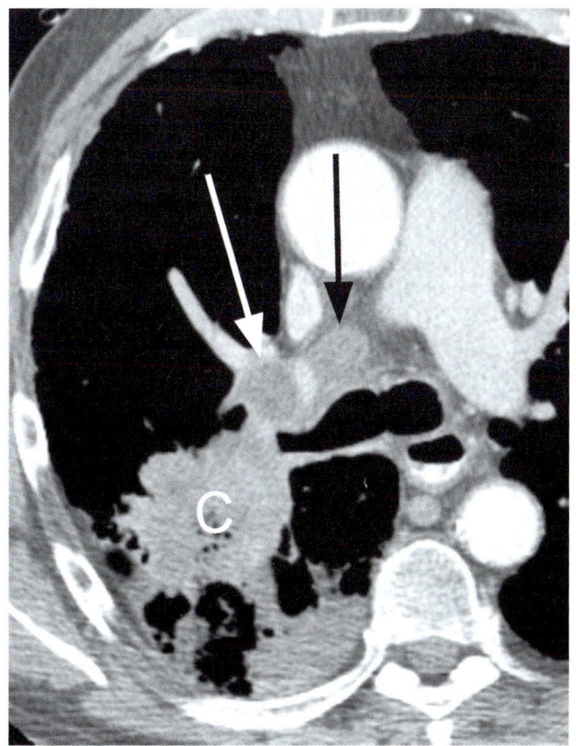

FIGURE 26.20 Squamous cell cancer (*C*) that obstructs the right upper lobe bronchus, with postobstructive pneumonia. Enlarged right hilar (*white arrow*) and tracheobronchial angle (*black arrow*) lymph nodes could be neoplastic or reactive in nature.

of 146 patients studied, only two of eight CT false-negative cases were attributable to microscopic metastases. On the other hand, 10 of 25 (40%) patients with mediastinal metastases in one study[122] and 7 of 11 (64%) patients in another study[144] had no enlarged nodes. There is no obvious explanation for these discrepant results.

Regardless of the actual frequency of microscopic lymph node metastases, it has been suggested that microscopic disease may have a better prognosis than metastases to enlarged nodes, and thus it may not be as crucial to detect microscopic spread of tumor preoperatively.[119,145,146] For instance, Pearson et al.[123] reported that the survival rate in patients whose N2 status was established at mediastinoscopy was significantly worse than in those with a negative mediastinoscopy, in whom the N2 status was established at subsequent thoracotomy. Similarly, Cybulsky et al.[147] found that patients with false-negative CT studies for mediastinal nodal metastases did better than those with true-positive CT studies (5-year survival following resection was 13.5% vs. 6.6%, respectively). These differences may relate to the distinction between normal-sized nodes with microscopic metastases versus enlarged metastatic lymph nodes, because enlarged nodes are more likely to be detected by mediastinoscopy and called abnormal at CT. Moreover, in a study of 115 patients who had undergone resection for NSCLC, Ishida et al.[148] found increased survival for patients with microscopic nodal metastases compared to those with moderate or gross nodal metastases. These findings are supported by one small CT series which suggested that metastases to enlarged mediastinal nodes were more likely to have extracapsular spread of tumor than microscopic metastases to normal-sized nodes.[143] Because extracapsular spread is thought to be a poor prognostic indicator,[149,150] microscopic metastases to normal-sized nodes may have a less dire prognosis than enlarged malignant nodes.

In summary, although different size threshold values for normal mediastinal lymph nodes have been suggested, the current consensus is that this figure should generally be approximately 1 cm in short-axis diameter.[133,134,136,137,139,146,151–155] Some authors have preferred to use nodal size criteria that vary with the precise mediastinal nodal location, based on the studies described previously.[156,157]

Evaluation of Hilar Lymph Node Metastases (N1 Disease) Conventional radiography and tomography have been used extensively in the past to evaluate patients with bronchogenic carcinoma. In one study of 47 lung cancer patients, the reported sensitivity of conventional radiography for hilar disease was 53%, with specificity of 84% and accuracy of 71%[154] (Fig. 26.21). In a subsequent study of 84 patients with suspected intrathoracic neoplasm, sensitivity and accuracy were 64% and specificity was 65%.[158] Conventional tomography has been only slightly better, although it has been replaced by CT at the current time.

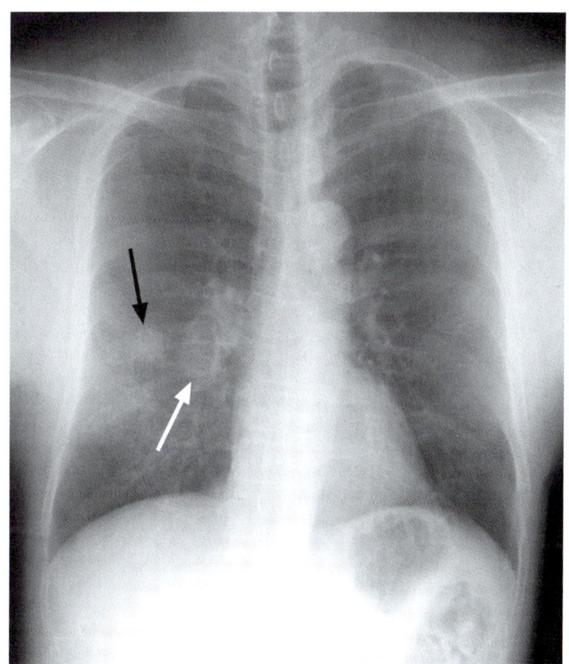

FIGURE 26.21 Frontal chest radiograph shows a small nodule in the right mid lung (*black arrow*) and enlarged lymph nodes in the right hilum (*white arrow*) consistent with T1N1 disease.

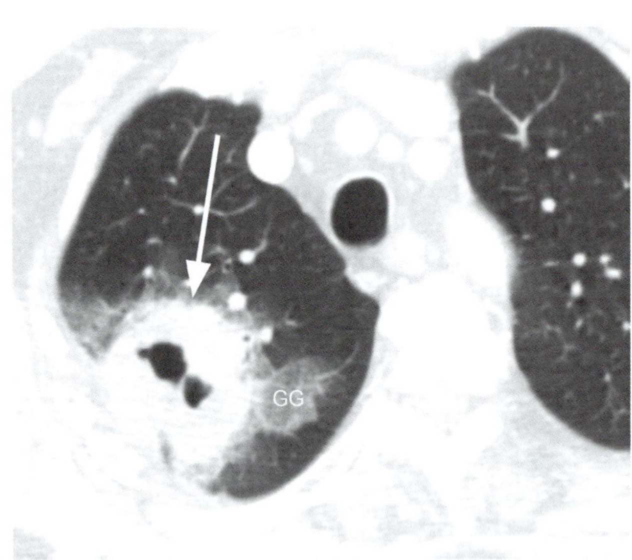

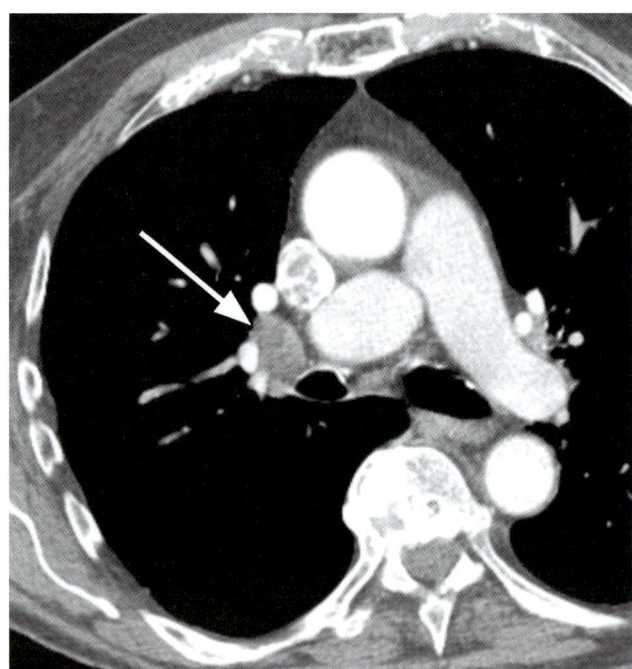

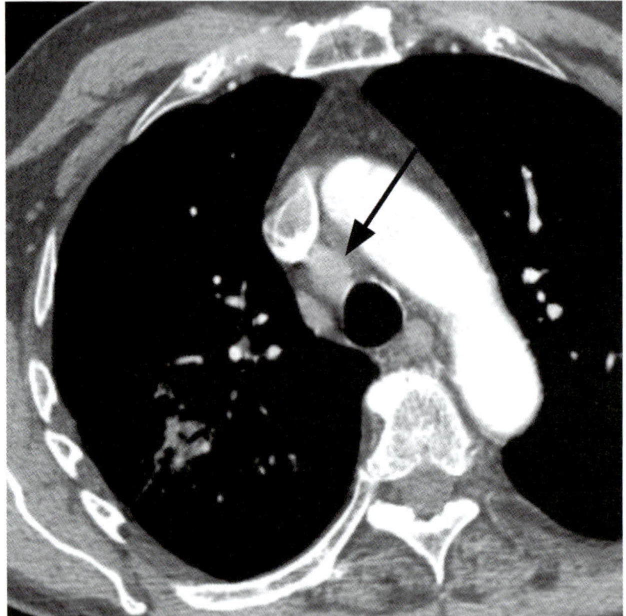

FIGURE 26.22 Cavitary right upper lobe non–small cell lung cancer **(A)** (*arrow*); adjacent ground-glass (*GG*) opacity may represent local lymphangiectic spread of neoplasm. CT shows enlarged right hilar **(B)** and right paratracheal **(C)** lymph nodes (*arrows*); subsequent FDG–PET scan was consistent with nodal involvement by tumor only in the right paratracheal region.

The accuracy of CT in detecting hilar lymph node metastases is unclear (Figs. 26.14, 26.20, and 26.22). Three lung cancer studies reported low sensitivity (45% to 63%) and PPV (38% to 68%) and moderately high NPV (79% to 85%).[105,159,160] Two of these studies showed high specificity (92% to 93%), whereas the other reported only 58% specificity. Accuracies ranged from 59% to 82%.

Evaluation of Mediastinal Lymph Node Metastases (N2/N3 Disease) The accuracy of conventional radiography in diagnosing mediastinal lymph node metastases has generally been quite low because of poor sensitivity (6% to 81%).[107,142,153,154,161–164] Disparate results have been reported regarding the accuracy of CT in this setting (Figs. 26.14 and 26.22 to 26.25; Table 26.2). Many studies have found fairly high sensitivity for CT (>85%)[93,108,139,152,154,156,161,165–167] and high NPV (>85%; Table 26.2).[156,157,160,166–170] Others have found high specificity (>85%).[105,142,155–157,162,166,167,169–174] On the other hand, some of the more recent studies have shown low accuracy, resulting from both poor sensitivity and poor specificity.[88,106,159,175–177] Low sensitivity in some studies was attributed to the high frequency of microscopic metastases within normal-sized nodes.[105] Low specificity arose from the frequent occurrence of enlarged, hyperplastic nodes, particularly in patients with postobstructive pneumonitis.[159] Dales et al.[178] performed a metaanalysis of CT accuracy in staging

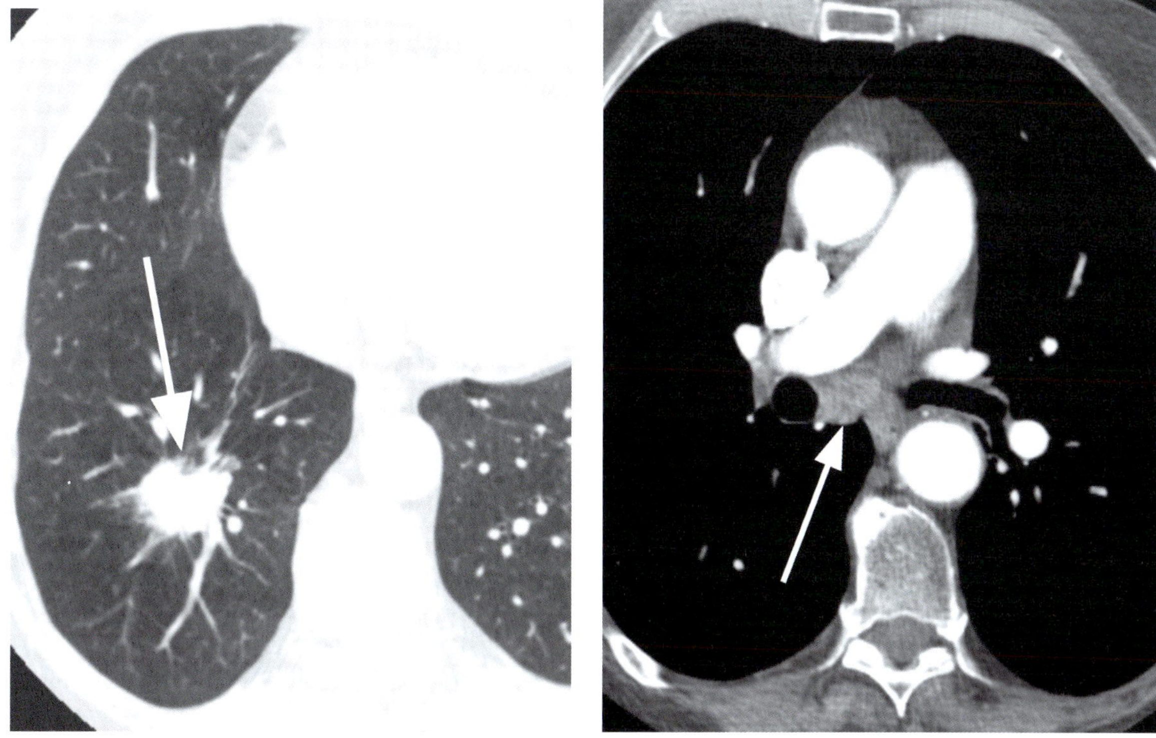

FIGURE 26.23 Right lower lobe non–small cell lung cancer **(A)** (*arrow*). Metastatic disease in subcarinal lymph nodes **(B)** (*arrow*), proven via transtracheal Wang needle biopsy.

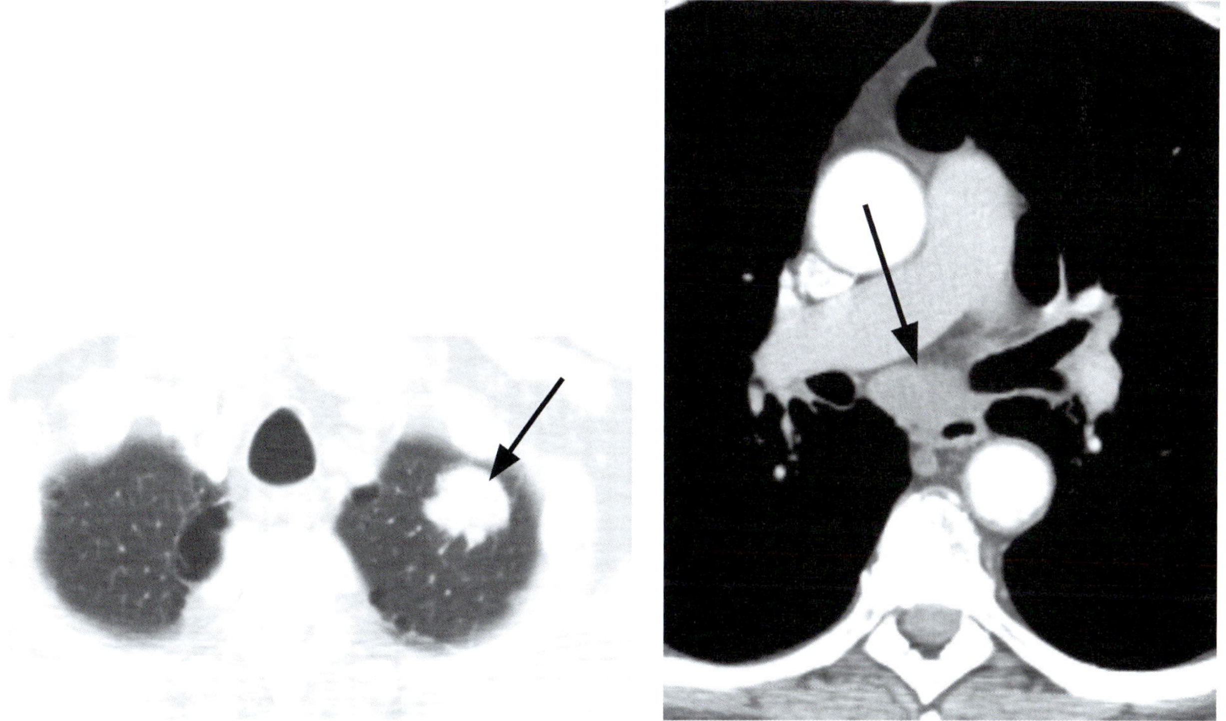

FIGURE 26.24 Right upper lobe non–small cell lung cancer **(A)** (*arrow*). Enlarged subcarinal lymph **(B)** (*arrow*) showed no tumor upon transtracheal Wang needle biopsy; tumor involvement was proven via subsequent transesophageal endoscopic ultrasound (EUS)-guided biopsy.

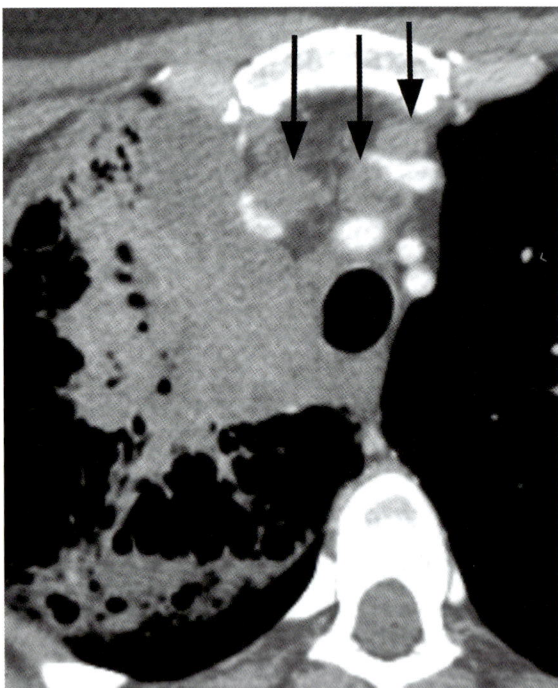

FIGURE 26.25 Right upper lobe squamous cell cancer with enlarged ipsilateral and contralateral mediastinal lymph nodes (*arrows*). Uptake in these nodes on a subsequent FDG–PET scan was consistent with metastatic disease (N3 disease).

mediastinal lymph nodes in NSCLC using data from studies published between 1980 and 1988. Pooled data revealed accuracy, sensitivity, and specificity figures that were approximately 80% each. They found no significant differences between the results from studies performed using fourth-generation versus third-/second-generation CT scanners. Moreover, there is no data to suggest that the helical or spiral scanners (either single or multidetector) improve CT accuracy in this setting.

Results within some of the individual studies quoted previously varied according to the size and morphologic criteria used for diagnosing metastatic disease to mediastinal lymph nodes. For example, Seely et al.[169] found that sensitivity increased and specificity decreased if long-axis diameter measurements were used instead of short-axis measurements or if adjacent nodal stations were considered together instead of considering each nodal station alone. Buy et al.[156] found maximal sensitivity when individual size thresholds were used for each individual nodal station, rather than using a uniform 10-mm size cutoff. In contrast, the data of Ikezoe et al.[157] showed slightly better sensitivity, albeit significantly worse specificity and accuracy, using a uniform 10-mm threshold rather than two separate criteria (13 mm for nodes in the subcarinal, precarinal, and tracheobronchial regions and 10 mm for nodes in other regions). Specificity in the study of Buy et al.[156] was maximized when the criterion for nodal abnormality was defined as follows: the short axis of the largest mediastinal node in the lymphatic drainage territory of the cancer was greater than or equal to 10 mm and the difference between this node and the largest node in the other territories was greater than 5 mm. According to the investigation of Ratto et al.,[167] specificity increased dramatically if nodes 10 to 15 mm in short-axis diameter were considered indeterminate and excluded from analysis. However, 36% (44 of 123) of patients fell into this category, limiting the usefulness of this criterion. These authors also found increased specificity if the criterion for abnormal nodes was modified to include nodes 10 to 20 mm in short axis diameter with central necrosis and/or a discontinuous capsule.

In some studies, CT accuracy also appeared to depend on the precise anatomic location within the mediastinum being analyzed. In the study of McLoud et al.,[159] sensitivity of CT using a single size criterion (10-mm short-axis diameter) varied for individual nodal stations, ranging from 17% to 83%. Highest sensitivity was found in ATS regions 4R and 5, and lowest in 7, 4L, 10R, 10L. Specificity ranged from 72% to 94%, being highest in 10L and lowest in 10R. Platt et al.[151] compared staging of right and left lung tumors. Although prior reports have shown that CT is more accurate in evaluating right-sided mediastinal lymph nodes,[134,179] Platt et al.[151] found no statistically significant difference in staging accuracy between left and right lung cancers. This is probably a result of involvement of subcarinal and contralateral mediastinal lymph nodes, which are present more often in left lung cancers as compared to right-sided lesions.[180]

There were also some reported differences when the data were broken down according to cell type of the tumor. Ikezoe et al.[157] found that sensitivity for cases of adenocarcinoma (61%) was lower than that for squamous cell carcinoma (86%), but specificity for these two groups was almost the same (93% to 94%). There was an increased number of false-negative cases for adenocarcinomas, as compared to squamous cell carcinomas in both this study and two others[105,147]; the authors postulated that this probably indicated a higher frequency of microscopic metastases in adenocarcinomas. On the other hand, Ratto et al.[167] reported no difference in staging accuracy between squamous cell carcinoma and adenocarcinoma.

When calculated on a nodal station-by-station basis, results in some studies varied according to whether or not adjacent nodal stations were included in the analysis. For instance, inclusion of adjacent nodal stations led to an increase in sensitivity and a decrease in specificity in one investigation.[169] However, it is important to note that the clinical usefulness of a staging modality does not depend on accurate detection of disease in any individual node or nodal group, but rather on accurate detection of mediastinal nodal malignancy in the individual patient, either ipsilateral or contralateral to the neoplasm. Moreover, several authors have reported increased sensitivity in mediastinal lymph node evaluation when calculated on a patient-by-patient basis rather than on a nodal station-by-station basis.[143,159,169]

There are many possible reasons for the different reported CT accuracies among studies in detecting mediastinal metastases. Differences in patient populations and prevalence of mediastinal nodal disease would affect CT accuracy. Some investigations included all patients with known or suspected

TABLE 26.2 CT Staging of Mediastinal Lymph Node Metastases in Patients with Known or Suspected Lung Cancer

Authors	No. of Patients	Patient Selection Criteria	Upper Limit Normal Lymph Node Size at CT (mm)	Basis	Prevalence (%)	Sensitivity (%)	Specificity (%)	Accuracy (%)	PPV (%)	NPV (%)
Lewis et al.[160]	418	Known lung cancer	10	Per patient	29	84	84	84	69	93
Ikezoe et al.[157]	208	Known lung cancer; only adenocarcinoma and squamous cell carcinoma included	13 SAD for subcarinal, precarinal and tracheobronchial regions; 10 SAD other regions	Per patient	31	69	94	86	83	91
Webb et al.[106]	155	Known or suspected non–small cell lung cancer	NS	Per patient	21	52	69	65	31	84
Cybulsky et al.[147]	124	Proven N2 disease	<10 LAD	Per patient	NS	51	NS	NS	NS	NS
Izbicki et al.[105]	108	Known lung cancer	10 SAD	Per station	19*	24*	93*	80*	44*	84*
				Per patient	26*	NS	NS	58*	NS	NS
McLoud et al.[159]	143	Known or suspected lung cancer	10 SAD	Per station	15	44	85	79	34	89
				Per patient	31	64	62	63	44	79
Daly et al.[168]	681	Known lung cancer	<10–15†	Per patient	NS	NS	NS	NS	NS	93
Seeley et al.[169]	104	Known lung cancer; only T1 lesions	10 LAD	Per station	8	55	86	83	25	96
			10 SAD	Per station	8	41	93	89	35	95
			10 LAD	Per station including adjacent stations	8	77	73	71	14	98
			10 SAD	Per station including adjacent stations	8	59	91	88	36	96
			10 LAD	Per patient	21	77	73	74	44	92
			10 SAD	Per patient	21	59	91	85	65	89
Gdeedo et al.[88]	74	Known non–small cell lung cancer; negative mediastinoscopy	10 SAD	Per patient	9.5	43	57	55	9	90
Kernstine et al.[176]	64	Known lung cancer	10 SAD	Per side of mediastinum	16	65	79	76	37	92
Kamiyoshihara et al.[174]	546	Known lung cancer	10 SAD	Per patient	20	33	90	79	46	84

*Excludes ATS region 10.

†<15 mm (1979–1986); <10 mm (1987–1991).

LAD, long-axis diameter; NPV, negative predictive value; NS, not specified; SAD, short-axis diameter.

lung cancer, and some included only those with biopsy proven cancer. Others focused on clinical T1N0M0 cancers, that is, small lesions surrounded by lung parenchyma, with no conventional radiographic signs of mediastinal disease. Seely et al.[169] found higher specificity in their study of T1 cancers as compared to historical controls for all cancers. They postulated that this was partly caused by lack of obstructive pneumonitis with resultant enlarged, hyperplastic nodes.

In addition, there were substantial variations in scanning techniques. Some studies used older CT scanners (second generation) with long scan times (18 to 20 seconds), resulting in image blur from biologic motion; studies done on third- and fourth-generation scanners did not have this problem. CT examinations were performed using different section thicknesses, section spacing, and methods of administration of intravenous urographic contrast material. Gaps between slices[172,173,181] and motion artifact from long scan times[153,171–173] probably contributed to insensitive detection of enlarged lymph nodes. There were no uniform criteria for interpreting the scans, and definitions of nodal enlargement ranged from "any visible node" to 2-cm diameter, with or without morphological nodal changes. Some investigators interpreted their results on a patient-by-patient basis, some on a nodal station-by-station basis, and some on a nodal station-by-station basis including adjacent nodal stations. It can be quite difficult at CT and surgery to precisely determine the boundaries between one nodal station and an adjacent one, and some studies, including the large study of McLoud et al.[159] made no allowances for this pitfall. Many studies appeared to lack precise radiologic/surgical/pathologic correlation, and different methods of proof were employed. This is important because certain mediastinal node groups are accessible only at thoracotomy and would be missed at mediastinoscopy. Moreover, it is plausible that those studies employing thorough mediastinal lymph node dissection rather than nodal palpation and biopsy would show decreased CT sensitivity because of the inability to detect microscopic metastases within normal sized lymph nodes. However, Daly et al.[142] were unable to substantiate this premise. They divided their patients into two surgical groups: in group I (51 cases) mediastinal nodes were removed only if palpably abnormal, if CT showed enlarged nodes, or if hilar nodes were grossly tumorous. In group II (97 cases), the mediastinum was explored in every patient and all nodes were resected. There was no statistically significant difference in CT sensitivity between these two groups (88% and 75%, respectively).

CT Evaluation of Distant Metastases

Several autopsy series have demonstrated an overall prevalence of distant metastases in patients with end-stage lung cancer as high as 93%. Key sites involved include liver (33% to 40%), adrenal (18% to 38%), brain (15% to 43%), bone (19% to 33%), kidney (16% to 23%), and abdominal lymph nodes (29%).[182–184] Autopsy studies performed in the immediate postoperative period as well as one report of abdominal exploratory surgery prior to thoracotomy for bronchogenic carcinoma have shown lower prevalences of metastatic spread to individual organs (liver 7% to 14%, adrenal 1% to 9%, brain 4%, bone 1% to 5%, kidney 0% to 4%, abdominal lymph nodes 5% to 8%). Nonetheless, the overall prevalence of occult metastatic disease was fairly high (18% to 36%) in these pre-CT-era studies.[185–188] One of these studies found that extrathoracic metastases were more common among men with adenocarcinoma than among those with squamous cell carcinoma.[185] A more recent autopsy report also found a moderately high frequency (19% of 103 = 18%) of distant metastases in patients dying in the perioperative period after lung cancer resection.[186]

Out of 95 patients with newly diagnosed NSCLC and N0 disease at CT, one report demonstrated CT evidence of extrathoracic tumor spread in 24 of 95 (25%) patients. These included metastases to brain (10), bone (8), liver (6), adrenal (6), and soft tissue (2) (some patients had involvement at more than one site).[189] An additional, prospective study of 146 patients with potentially resectable NSCLC (clinical T3 or less and N2 or less)[190] revealed distant metastatic disease in 30 of 146 (30%) patients. These metastases were detected by chest or abdominal CT, brain CT, abdominal ultrasonography, and/or bone scan, and presumably each finding was proved. The lesions were distributed as follows: 13% bone, 13% brain, 12.3% liver, 7.5% adrenal, 1.4% kidney, and 1.4% subdiaphragmatic nodules. (In 17 patients the metastases were "multiorganic.") The authors indicated that patients with nonsquamous cell carcinomas (adenocarcinoma or large cell carcinoma) were at significantly greater risk for metastases outside the thorax than those with squamous cell cancer (p = less than 0.5). No relationship was detected between the TN stage and the existence of metastases in adenocarcinoma and large cell adenocarcinoma. There was, however, an association between advanced N stage (IIIa) and presence of extrathoracic metastases for squamous cell cancers. None of the stage I intrathoracic squamous cell cancers had metastases. Many patients with metastases to brain, bone, liver, and adrenal were asymptomatic. Thus these authors advocated the routine performance of preoperative upper abdominal CT and/or ultrasonography in all patients except those with asymptomatic stage I squamous cell cancers. Brain CTs were suggested for all patients with adenocarcinoma and large cell carcinoma, as well as for those with squamous cell cancer and neurologic symptoms. Bone scanning was suggested only in those patients with clinical and laboratory indications of possible bone involvement by metastatic disease.

A study by Quint et al.[191] found 21% overall prevalence of distant metastases in 348 patients with newly diagnosed NSCLC. In 56% of patients with distant metastases, the lesions were detected using chest or abdominal CT. Brain, bone, liver, and adrenal glands were the most common sites of disease, in decreasing order (Fig. 26.26). Brain metastases often occurred as an isolated finding. On the other hand, isolated liver metastases were uncommon, and therefore the incremental yield of abdominal CT over chest CT was quite small. Thus these authors concluded that abdominal CT does not appear to be an effective method of screening for metastases if chest CT has been performed. A recent report that examined clinical predictors of metastatic disease to the brain from NSCLC found that

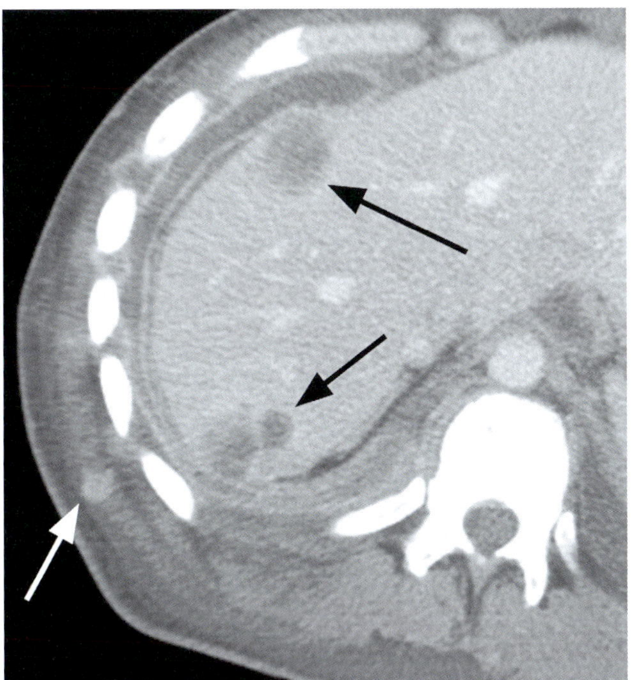

FIGURE 26.26 Liver metastases (*black arrows*) and body wall metastasis (*white arrow*) in a patient with metastatic adenocarcinoma of the lung. Also note right pleural thickening and effusion caused by metastatic disease.

the probability of brain metastases correlated with size of the primary tumor, cell type, and intrathoracic lymph node stage, but not with gender, patient age, or central versus peripheral location of the tumor; adenocarcinomas and undifferentiated cell types were more commonly associated with tumor spread to the brain compared to squamous cell carcinoma.[192]

Despite the high prevalence of adrenal metastases from bronchogenic carcinoma, approximately two thirds of adrenal masses in patients with NSCLC actually represent adenomas, rather than metastases.[193] Adrenal adenomas are found in about 3% to 9% of autopsies on adults,[194,195] and approximately 1% of patients undergoing abdominal CT have benign incidental adrenal masses larger than 1 cm.[196] In a study of 546 patients with lung cancer, 22 of 546 (4%) patients had one or more adrenal masses on preoperative CT.[197] Seventeen of twenty-two had proof of adrenal status via either biopsy or follow-up. A total of 5 of these 17 were malignant (29%) and 12 of 17 were benign (71%). These authors reported that adenomas were well defined and low in attenuation and showed a smooth, high attenuation rim and involvement of only part of gland. Features of metastases included a low attenuation, large (larger than 5 cm) mass without a rim and irregular, mixed attenuation.[197] Unfortunately, there is significant overlap in the appearance of adrenal metastases and benign adenomas on routine, contrast-enhanced CT. Therefore detection of an adrenal mass on such a study requires further workup. Unenhanced CT densitometry can be used to distinguish between lipid-rich adenomas and nonadenomatous masses. Using a cutoff of 10 HU, an accuracy of more than 90% can be achieved for the diagnosis of a lipid-rich adenoma.[198,199] In addition, considerable work has recently been done using dedicated adrenal CT with a combination of noncontrast, postcontrast and delayed enhanced images in evaluating wash-out characteristics in adrenal masses.[200–203] Using these techniques, it is usually possible definitively to diagnose benign adrenal cortical adenomas without biopsy. If these imaging studies suggest the presence of a metastasis, biopsy proof is generally required before altering therapy.

Usefulness of CT in Clinical T1N0M0 Patients

There has been controversy over the usefulness of CT in the preoperative evaluation of patients with radiographic T1N0M0 cancers. Reports in the surgical and radiologic literature give varying figures for the prevalence of proven mediastinal lymph node or distant metastases in this set of patients, ranging from 3% to 33%.[139,204–211] The lower prevalences may be underestimations, reflecting incomplete mediastinal nodal sampling and/or lack of good-quality preoperative upper abdominal CT scanning. Because distant metastases remain a contraindication to thoracotomy, and known mediastinal metastases will alter treatment at many institutions, CT is potentially useful by detecting such occult disease. In the series of Parker et al.[206] CT evidence for unresectable spread of disease was obtained in 12 of 36 patients with radiographic T1N0M0 disease, including metastases to the liver (four patients), the adrenal (one patient), an axillary lymph node (one patient), and mediastinal lymph nodes (eight patients). Conces et al.[211] reported CT signs of inoperability in 7 of 26 radiographic T1N0M0 cases with surgical correlation (27%). Metastatic disease was confirmed in four of these seven cases, including mediastinal metastases in three (3 of 26, 12% prevalence) and one contralateral lung malignancy. Of 31 radiographic T1N0M0 patients reported by Heavey et al.,[210] eight (26%) had proven spread of disease, including six patients with malignant mediastinal lymph nodes (19% prevalence), one with an adrenal metastasis, and one patient with a metastasis to the contralateral lung. CT detected 5 of these 8 cases, thus preventing thoracotomy in 5 of 31 (16%) patients. As noted by Heavey et al.,[210] preventing thoracotomy in only 16% of patients resulted in significant overall cost savings, even when the cost of CT scans and prethoracotomy biopsies is taken into account. Thus these studies suggest that CT is highly useful in the preoperative workup of such patients.

On the other hand, another study of radiographic T1N0M0 tumors by Pearlberg et al.[209] found only 2 of 23 (8.7%) patients with proven mediastinal metastases; however, these patients did not undergo total mediastinal nodal sampling, and thus the true prevalence may have been somewhat higher. CT findings averted thoracotomy in only one patient, due to mediastinal adenopathy subsequently proven at mediastinotomy to contain metastatic disease. Becker et al.,[207] in a prospective investigation of 38 patients with presumed lung cancer (radiographic T1N0M0), found proven mediastinal nodal metastases in only one patient. Eleven of thirty-eight lesions turned out to be benign. Thus, preliminary data indicate that CT may be helpful and cost-effective in the preoperative assessment of patients with radiographic T1N0M0 lesions when the diagnosis of lung cancer has been proven.

Predicting Resectability with CT Prediction of resectability depends on accurate detection of T4, N3, and/or M1 tumors. One prospective study of 96 patients with lung cancer and preoperative CT found a 12% prevalence of unresectability.[212] CT criteria for unresectability included encasement of the proximal pulmonary arteries or carina, or gross mediastinal involvement by tumor, or widespread lymphadenopathy or distant metastases. Using these criteria, CT was 96% accurate and showed 97% PPV and 50% NPV for resectability. Another, more recent study found that CT erred in predicting resectability in 12 of 50 patients (24%).[213] In three patients, a malignant pleural effusion was missed at CT, and in nine patients, operable patients were deemed inoperable at CT due to incorrect diagnosis of malignant pleural effusion (three patients) or direct mediastinal tumor invasion (six patients). Therefore the usefulness of CT in this setting is uncertain.

Current Usefulness of Pretreatment CT It is important for the radiologist to know what treatment options are available at his or her particular institution and what features of the tumor or its spread would affect treatment decisions. At most institutions, proven T4, N3, or M1 disease is considered unresectable. Patients with N2 disease may be treated with preoperative chemotherapy and radiation therapy. CT findings are used to help define the extent of the primary nodule or mass, look for calcifications that might indicate benignancy, determine its relationships with nearby structures, assess for resectability, and suggest the type of surgery required for resection. If enlarged mediastinal lymph nodes are detected, CT may be used to direct preoperative lymph node sampling via transbronchoscopic Wang needle biopsy, TEE, EBUS, mediastinoscopy, mediastinotomy, or video-assisted thoracoscopic surgery (VATS). Nodes accessible to transbronchoscopic Wang needle biopsy include the paratracheal, tracheobronchial, and subcarinal groups. Transbronchial Wang needle biopsy may be facilitated by ultrasound guidance. Nodes accessible to mediastinoscopy include pretracheal, anterior subcarinal, and anterior tracheobronchial groups. Lymph nodes in the aortopulmonary window are not accessible using these techniques, and tissue sampling requires other approaches such as VATS or anterior thoracotomy. As an alternative to surgical staging procedures, some groups advocate the use of CT-guided hilar and mediastinal lymph node biopsies,[214–216] although this is not common practice unless the nodal masses are large.

In summary, at many institutions, preoperative chest CT, including the adrenal glands, is routinely performed on all patients suspected of having NSCLC. Dedicated abdominal CT is not generally necessary, given the low frequency of isolated liver metastases. Intravenous contrast material is usually administered to help distinguish vessels from lymph nodes and to aid in evaluation of primary tumor extent. However, some investigators believe that intravenous contrast is unnecessary, because the added information obtained from the use of contrast material rarely changes tumor stage and does not substantially influence management decisions.[217]

Many CT studies have reported high NPVs in detecting metastatic disease to mediastinal lymph nodes. In addition, Daly et al.[168] reported that overall projected 2- and 5-year survival rates for 37 CT false-negative patients in their series were 40% and 28%, respectively. Given this information, many investigators believe that a negative CT obviates the need for mediastinoscopy, and these patients should go directly to thoracotomy.[146,160,168] An exception may be made for patients with T3 tumors or central adenocarcinomas, due to the high incidence of positive mediastinal lymph nodes and low NPV of CT in this setting.[168] In addition, patients with suspected chest wall invasion, including Pancoast tumors, should probably have mediastinoscopy regardless of CT findings, because mediastinal nodal metastases and chest wall invasion portend a poor prognosis, and these patients are not usually felt to be surgical candidates.[100,101] In a dissenting opinion, Pearson et al.[218] recommended mediastinoscopy for all T2 and T3 tumors and for T1 adenocarcinomas and large cell carcinomas, even in the setting of a negative CT. A more recent study by Kernstine et al.[176] took this a step further, concluding that CT was not sensitive or specific enough to change their current recommendation to perform surgical evaluation for mediastinal lymph node staging in all patients. On the other hand, it is generally agreed that all patients with abnormal mediastinal lymph nodes at CT need lymph node biopsy (or futher imaging with FDG–PET); therapy should not be planned based on unproven, positive CT findings. Mediastinal and hilar lymph node stations, as delineated by the ATS, have been mapped using axial CT scans in a recently published atlas[219]; reference to such standard locations is essential in directing accurate lymph node sampling.

CT Imaging in Evaluating Response to Therapy
Published reports have shown mixed results regarding the usefulness of CT in evaluating for tumor response to therapy. A study of 21 patients who were treated with neoadjuvant concurrent chemoradiotherapy followed by surgery found that CT findings in the primary tumor and mediastinal lymph nodes were not helpful in evaluating tumor response.[220] A more recent study of 57 patients receiving chemotherapy for NSCLC reported that early restaging CT scans (within 1 month after treatment) identified six patients with tumor progression, thereby allowing a change to more appropriate therapy.[221] However, one neoadjuvant chemotherapy study noted that CT findings underestimated the frequency of pathologic complete response.[222] Moreover, another small study concluded that the therapeutic effect on tumors is generally underestimated using CT size criteria after chemotherapy and/or radiation therapy; these authors suggested that CT criteria for response should include change in shape (from round to oval or irregular) and disappearance of contrast enhancement.[223] Other studies have suggested that serial CT scans obtained early during radiation therapy may accurately predict final tumor volume; however, the clinical significance of tumor volume reduction is uncertain, because it does not necessarily indicate histologic tumor clearance.[224,225] The bottom line seems to be that posttherapeutic increase in tumor size at CT indicates lack of tumor response. Decrease in tumor size is consistent with tumor response, but does not necessarily either indicate or exclude complete pathologic response.

MAGNETIC RESONANCE IMAGING

Magnetic resonance imaging is used infrequently in the staging of lung carcinoma. The development of MDCT (up to 64 detector rows) now allows the rapid acquisition of volumetric data sets that may be reformatted in any plane, giving multiplanar capabilities similar to MRI. The current major advantages of MRI over CT include its superior contrast resolution and ability to image vascular structures without the use of intravascular contrast material. However, MRI is susceptible to motion artifacts, has poorer spatial resolution than CT, calcification is difficult to image, and the relatively low signal from the air containing lung parenchyma limits the evaluation of parenchymal abnormalities. Given these limitations, the role of MRI in the detection and staging of bronchogenic carcinoma has been limited, and MRI tends to be used only to answer very specific questions that CT has been unable to resolve.[226–233]

Evaluation of the Primary Tumor

Chest Wall Invasion MRI maybe slightly superior to CT for the staging of local tumor extent into the adjacent chest wall, because of its superior contrast resolution[234,235] (Figs. 26.27 and 26.28). Chest wall invasion is best depicted as disruption of the normal high signal intensity extrapleural fat by moderate-intensity soft tissue on spin-echo (SE) T1-weighted images or as abnormal high-signal intensity tissue on T2-weighted images. The use of surface coils may provide high-resolution images depicting these findings. However, unfortunately, inflammatory and malignant tissues may have similar appearances on MRI, making it difficult to distinguish between these two entities.[235–238] Like CT, in the absence of a pleural effusion, MRI cannot differentiate the visceral from the parietal pleura. In most studies that have compared the two modalities, the accuracy rates for assessing chest wall invasion have been similar.

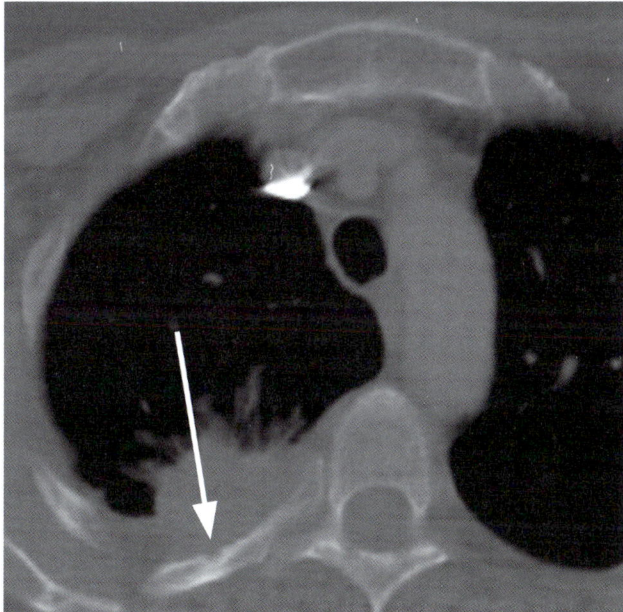

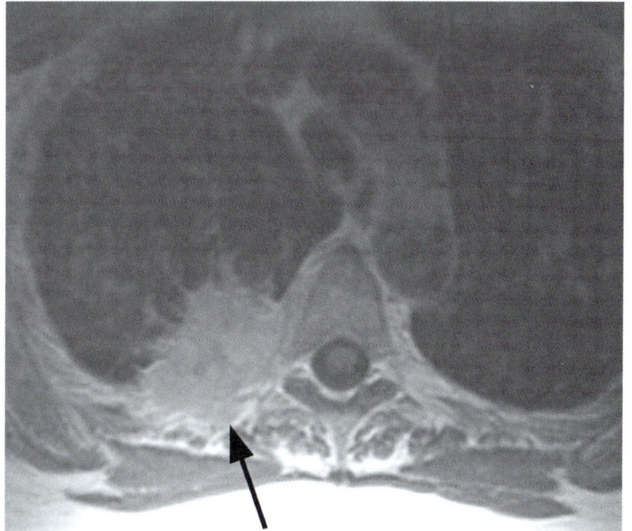

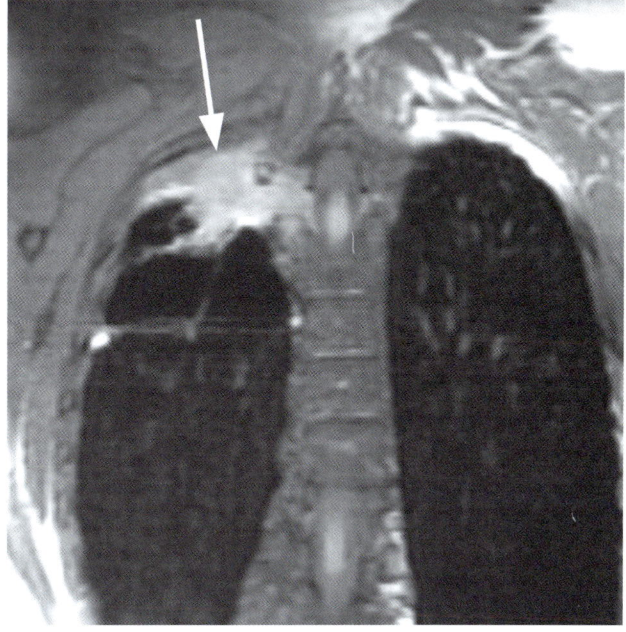

FIGURE 26.27 Right upper lobe adenocarcinoma with chest wall invasion. Note rib erosion (*arrow*) at CT **(A)** and abnormal soft tissue in the chest wall (*arrow*) on axial **(B)** and coronal **(C)** MR.

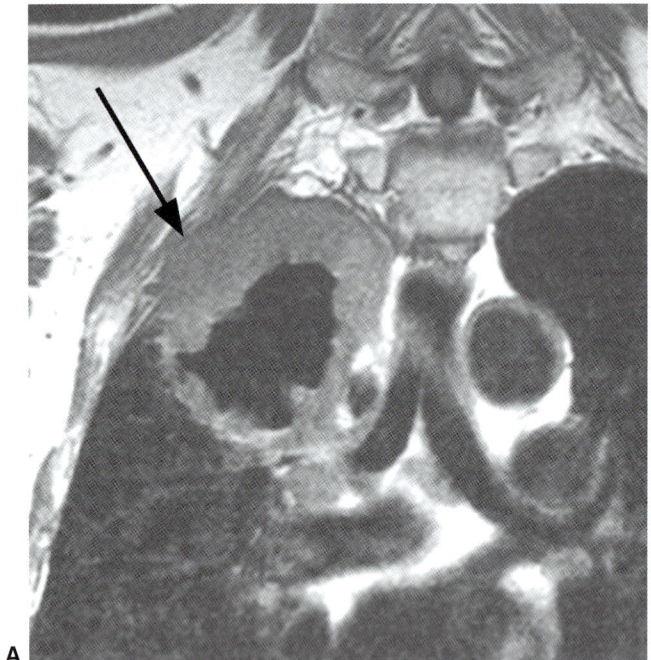

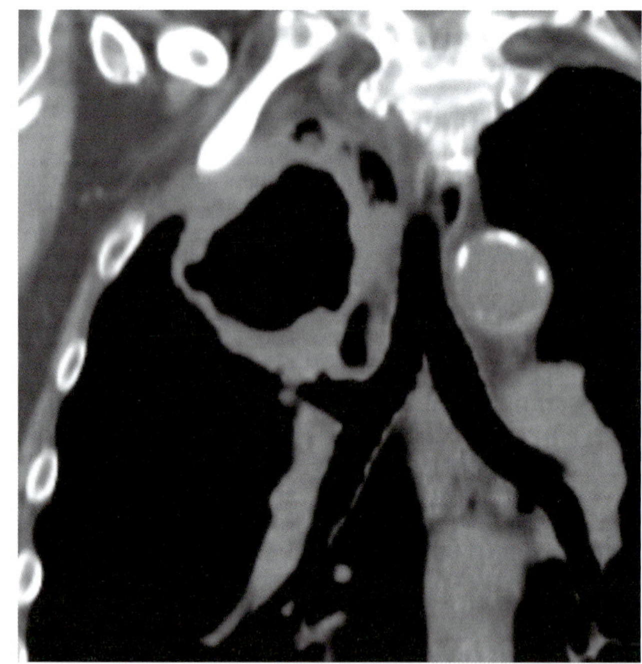

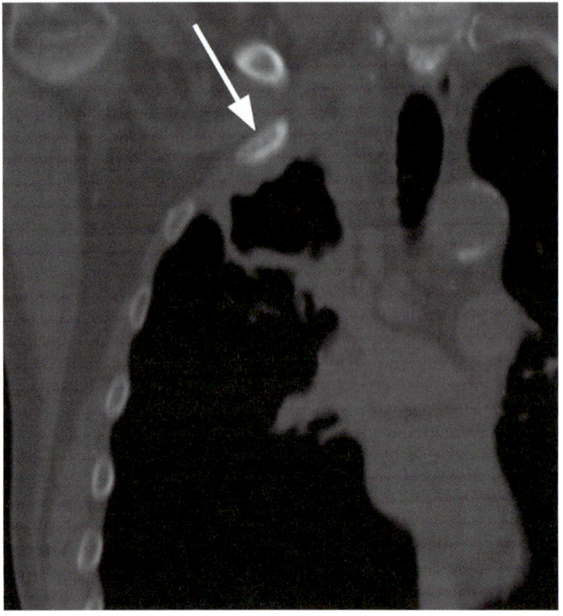

FIGURE 26.28 Cavitary right upper lobe poorly differentiated non–small cell carcinoma. Soft tissue invading into the chest wall (*arrow*) on MR **(A)** is difficult to appreciate on a coronal CT reconstruction **(B)**. However, another coronal CT section **(C)** shows rib sclerosis (*arrow*), consistent with tumor involvement.

The overall reported sensitivity for chest wall invasion by MRI is 63% to 90%, with a specificity of 84% to 86%.[106,239,240] Haggar et al.[241] demonstrated that SE MRI had a NPV of 100% for chest wall invasion. More importantly, in nine cases in which CT was equivocal, MRI accurately resolved the issue. Therefore, MRI may be helpful in cases with equivocal CT findings.[242] There have, however, been no studies comparing MDCT and MRI.

Superior Sulcus Tumors MRI is still the modality of choice in evaluating superior sulcus tumors.[243–246] Coronal and sagittal MR images facilitate evaluation for brachial plexus and mediastinal vascular involvement; although contrast enhanced MDCT is good for delineating the vascular anatomy, it will not always identify the brachial plexus (Fig. 26.29).[106,235,242–244,247] In addition, vertebral body invasion, involvement of the neural foramina and marrow infiltration can be readily determined on MRI.[244] Accuracy rates of 94% have been reported with MRI, as compared to 63% with CT, in assessing the true extent of superior sulcus tumors.[234,243,244]

Mediastinal Invasion MRI has the same limitations as CT in differentiating a tumor that abuts the mediastinal structures from one invading the mediastinum.[108,248] Both CT and MRI

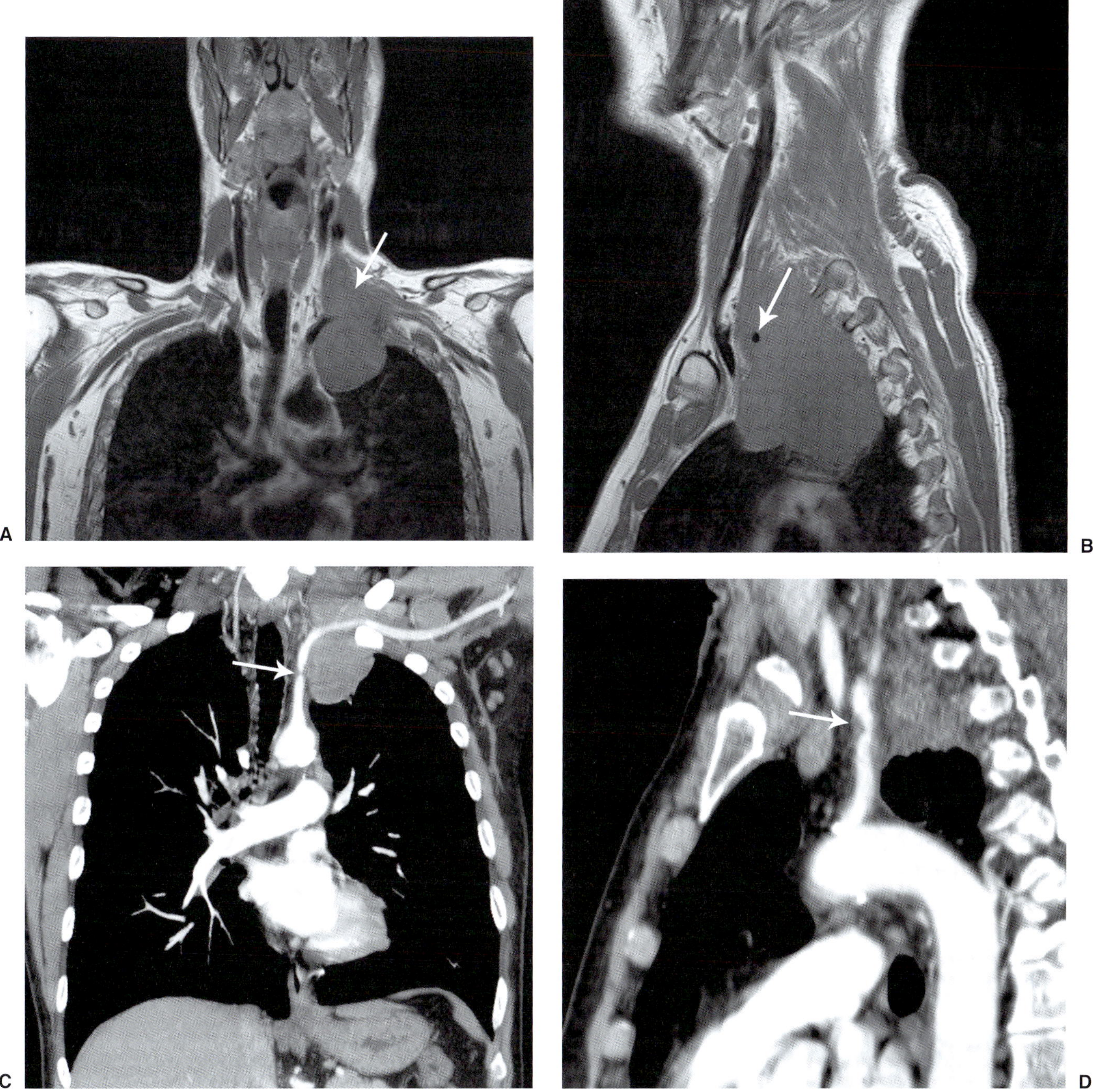

FIGURE 26.29 Superior sulcus tumor. Coronal T1-weighted MRI **(A)** shows involvement of the lower roots of the brachial plexus (*arrow*), and sagittal T1-weighted MRI **(B)** shows encasement of the subclavian artery (*arrow*). Coronal **(C)** and sagittal **(D)** CT reformats reveal the vascular invasion (*arrow*), but not the brachial plexus involvement.

depict mediastinal invasion by lung carcinoma with equal accuracy ranging between 56% to 89% for CT and 50% to 93% for MR.[102,106–108,230,242,249] The Radiology Diagnostic Oncology Group (RDOG) Trials, showed slight superiority for MRI in diagnosing mediastinal invasion in a small group of patients as compared to CT, with areas under the ROC for MRI being 0.924 (SE 0.034) versus 0.832 (SE 0.041) for CT.[106]

Involvement of the cardiac chambers, although rare, and the pericardium can be easily evaluated with MRI. If the normal 2 to 3 mm thick curvilinear low–signal-intensity rim representing the pericardium is disrupted, then tumor extension to the pericardium is to be suspected, although this alone is not a contraindication to tumor resection.[250,251] Using cine MR to identify the sliding motion between the mass and adjacent structures, cardiovascular invasion can be assessed, showing a reported accuracy of 94%.[252]

MRI Evaluation of Hilar and Mediastinal Lymph Nodes

Although nodal size is a nonspecific criterion, it is routinely used to help distinguish normal from tumor-containing lymph nodes; generally a size threshold of 1 cm is used.[253] CT and MR are fairly accurate in detecting enlarged lymph nodes in the hilar and mediastinal regions. However, the cause for nodal enlargement maybe reactive hyperplasia or metastases, and these cannot be easily differentiated using either modality.[159] One limitation of MRI for assessing nodal staging is its poor spatial resolution; small adjacent nodes that are discrete on CT may appear as one large, indistinct mass at MRI, leading to an erroneous diagnosis of nodal enlargement.[254] In addition, MRI is poor for detecting calcification, and thus enlarged benign nodes containing calcification may be misclassified as being malignant. CT and MRI have accuracies of 62% to 68% and 68% to 74%, respectively, for detecting metastatic disease to hilar lymph nodes and neither modality will identify micrometatastases within normal size lymph nodes.[106,107,251,254–258] Lymph node morphology and signal characteristics on MR have not been useful in predicting the presence or absence of metastatic disease.[106,108,239,253,256,259]

MRI performed after intravenous infusion of ultra small iron-oxide particles that are taken up by the reticuloendothelial system has been used to distinguish between nontumorous lymph nodes and tumor-containing lymph nodes.[260,261] This technique has been shown to be of value in distinguishing between normal and tumor-containing lymph nodes in small series of patients with head and neck and pelvic malignancies,[262–264] but the results in the chest have been disappointing, with a reported specificity of only 37%.[265] The developments of PET/CT and endobronchial ultrasound combined with fine needle cytology hold more promise.[266]

MRI Evaluation of Distant Metastases

Whole-body MRI, using fast breath-hold T2W sequences with a rolling table top, has been suggested as a screening method for metastatic disease and would appear to be as good as conventional imaging for the detection of cerebral, hepatic and bone metastases.[267] With regard to adrenal masses, like CT, MRI is able to identify lipid-rich adenomas. On lipid-sensitive out-of-phase images, lipid-rich adrenal adenomas show signal loss and appear dark in comparison to a reference organ such as the spleen,[268] whereas most adrenal metastases do not show this change on the out-of-phase images. This technique has an accuracy rate of >90% in the diagnosis of a lipid-rich adenoma.[269–271] Thus either CT or MR can be used to diagnose adrenal lipid-rich adenomas and distinguish them from metastases. However, contrast enhanced CT with delayed imaging can distinguish both lipid-rich and lipid-poor adenomas from nonadenomas,[201,272] and this is an advantage that CT currently has over MR.

The incidence of brain metastases in patients with NSCLC is approximately 12% to 28% over the entire course of the disease. Imaging is usually undertaken when the patient becomes symptomatic, although early screening of asymptomatic patients has been suggested in an attempt to instigate early treatment and improve survival. In a study by Kim et al.,[273] using a modified MR technique, the incidence of asymptomatic brain metastases at the time of initial staging was 21%, with upstaging in 16% of patients who were initially considered suitable for surgery. These authors therefore suggested that a limited MRI, which was both sensitive and cost-effective, should be offered during initial staging for all patients.

REFERENCES

1. Heelan R. Lung cancer imaging: primary diagnosis, staging, and local recurrence. *Semin Oncol* 1991;18:87–98.
2. McCarthy M, Ros P, Sobin L. Scientific exhibit-carcinoma of the lung: updated imaging-pathologic correlations. *Radial Soc N Am* 1985: 17–22.
3. Zwirewich CV, Miller RR, Müller NL. Multicentric adenocarcinoma of the lung: CT-pathologic correlation. *Radiology* 1990;176:185–190.
4. Lindell RM, Hartman TE, Swensen SJ, et al. Five-year lung cancer screening experience: CT appearance, growth rate, location, and histologic features of 61 lung cancers. *Radiology* 2007;242:555–562.
5. Hasegawa M, Sone S, Takashima S, et al. Growth rate of small lung cancers detected on mass CT screening. *Br J Radiol* 2000;73:1252–1259.
6. Felson B, Wiot JF. Some less familiar roentgen manifestations of carcinoma of the lung. *Semin Roentgenol* 1977;12:187–206.
7. Woodring JH. Unusual radiographic manifestations of lung cancer. *Radiol Clin North Am* 1990;28:599–618.
8. Austin JH, Romney BM, Goldsmith LS. Missed bronchogenic carcinoma: radiographic findings in 27 patients with a potentially resectable lesion evident in retrospect. *Radiology* 1992;182:115–122.
9. Shah PK, Austin JH, White CS, et al. Missed non-small cell lung cancer: radiographic findings of potentially resectable lesions evident only in retrospect. *Radiology* 2003;226:235–241.
10. Sakai S, Soeda H, Takahashi N, et al. Computer-aided nodule detection on digital chest radiography: validation test on consecutive T1 cases of resectable lung cancer. *J Digit Imaging* 2006;19:376–382.
11. Ide K, Mogami H, Murakami T, et al. Detection of lung cancer using single-exposure dual-energy subtraction chest radiography. *Radiat Med* 2007;25:195–201.
12. Tsubamoto M, Kuriyama K, Kido S, et al. Detection of lung cancer on chest radiographs: analysis on the basis of size and extent of ground-glass opacity at thin-section CT. *Radiology* 2002;224:139–144.
13. Li F, Sone S, Abe H, et al. Lung cancers missed at low-dose helical CT screening in a general population: comparison of clinical, histopathologic, and imaging findings. *Radiology* 2002;225:673–683.
14. Armato SG III, Li F, Giger ML, et al. Lung cancer: performance of automated lung nodule detection applied to cancers missed in a CT screening program. *Radiology* 2002;225:685–692.
15. Wiemker R, Rogalla P, Blaffert T, et al. Aspects of computer-aided detection (CAD) and volumetry of pulmonary nodules using multislice CT. *Br J Radiol* 2005;78 Spec No 1:S46–S56.
16. Das M, Mühlenbruch G, Mahnken AH, et al. Small pulmonary nodules: effect of two computer-aided detection systems on radiologist performance. *Radiology* 2006;241:564–571.
17. Gruden JF, Ouanounou S, Tigges S, et al. Incremental benefit of maximum-intensity-projection images on observer detection of small pulmonary nodules revealed by multidetector CT. *AJR Am J Roentgenol* 2002;179:149–157.
18. Peloschek P, Sailer J, Weber M, et al. Pulmonary nodules: sensitivity of maximum intensity projection versus that of volume rendering of 3D multidetector CT data. *Radiology* 2007;243:561–569.

19. Muhm J, Miller WE, Fontana RS, et al. Lung cancer detected during a screening program using four-month chest radiographs. *Radiology* 1983;148:609–615.
20. Hendrix RW. In defense of a missed lesion. *Radiology* 1995;195: 578–579.
21. Berlin L. Failure to diagnose lung cancer: anatomy of a malpractice trial. *AJR Am J Roentgenol* 2003;180:37–45.
22. Good CA, Hood RT Jr, McDonald JR. Significance of a solitary mass in the lung. *Am J Roentgenol Radium Ther Nucl Med* 1953;70: 543–554.
23. Davis EW, Katz S, Peabody JW Jr. The solitary pulmonary nodule; a ten-year study based on 215 cases. *J Thorac Surg* 1956;32:728–770.
24. Walske B. The solitary pulmonary nodule. *Dis Chest* 1956;49: 302–304.
25. Taylor RR, Rivkin LN, Salyer JM. The solitary pulmonary nodule; a review of 236 consecutive cases, 1944 to 1956. *Ann Surg* 1958;147:197–202.
26. Steele JD. The solitary pulmonary nodule. Report of a cooperative study of resected asymptomatic solitary pulmonary nodules in males. *J Thorac Cardiovasc Surg* 1963;46:21–39.
27. Siegelman SS, Zerhouni EA, Leo FP, et al. CT of the solitary pulmonary nodule. *AJR Am J Roentgenol* 1980;135:1–13.
28. Petrou M, Quint LE, Nan B, et al. Pulmonary nodule volumetric measurement variability as a function of CT slice thickness and nodule morphology. *AJR Am J Roentgenol* 2007;188:306–312.
29. Quint LE, Cheng J, Schipper M, et al. Lung lesion doubling times: values and variability based on method of volume determination. *Clin Radiol* 2008;63:41–48.
30. Winer-Muram HT, Jennings SG, Meyer CA, et al. Effect of varying CT section width on volumetric measurement of lung tumors and application of compensatory equations. *Radiology* 2003;229:184–194.
31. Boll DT, Gilkeson RC, Fleiter TR, et al. Volumetric assessment of pulmonary nodules with ECG-gated MDCT. *AJR Am J Roentgenol* 2004;183:1217–1223.
32. Zhao B, Schwartz LH, Moskowitz CS, et al. Pulmonary metastases: effect of CT section thickness on measurement—initial experience. *Radiology* 2005;234:934–939.
33. Goo JM, Tongdee T, Tongdee R, et al. Volumetric measurement of synthetic lung nodules with multi-detector row CT: effect of various image reconstruction parameters and segmentation thresholds on measurement accuracy. *Radiology* 2005;235:850–856.
34. Wormanns D, Kohl G, Klotz E, et al. Volumetric measurements of pulmonary nodules at multi-row detector CT: in vivo reproducibility. *Eur Radiol* 2004;14:86–92.
35. Kostis WJ, Yankelevitz DF, Reeves AP, et al. Small pulmonary nodules: reproducibility of three-dimensional volumetric measurement and estimation of time to follow-up CT. *Radiology* 2004;231:446–452.
36. Revel MP, Lefort C, Bissery A, et al. Pulmonary nodules: preliminary experience with three-dimensional evaluation. *Radiology* 2004;231:459–466.
37. Yankelevitz DF, Gupta R, Zhao B, et al. Small pulmonary nodules: evaluation with repeat CT—preliminary experience. *Radiology* 1999; 212:561–566.
38. Yankelevitz DF, Reeves AP, Kostis WJ, et al. Small pulmonary nodules: volumetrically determined growth rates based on CT evaluation. *Radiology* 2000;217:251–256.
39. Winer-Muram HT, Jennings SG, Tarver RD, et al. Volumetric growth rate of stage I lung cancer prior to treatment: serial CT scanning. *Radiology* 2002;223:798–805.
40. Revel MP, Merlin A, Peyrard S, et al. Software volumetric evaluation of doubling times for differentiating benign versus malignant pulmonary nodules. *AJR Am J Roentgenol* 2006;187:135–142.
41. MacMahon H, Austin JH, Gamsu G, et al. Guidelines for management of small pulmonary nodules detected on CT scans: a statement from the Fleischner Society. *Radiology* 2005;237:395–400.
42. Winer-Muram HT. The solitary pulmonary nodule. *Radiology* 2006; 239:34–49.
43. Strunk H, Schweden F, Schild H, et al. Spiral CT with 3D surface reconstruction in assessing solitary pulmonary foci. *Rofo* 1993;158:26–30.
44. Berger WG, Erly WK, Krupinski EA, et al. The solitary pulmonary nodule on chest radiography: can we really tell if the nodule is calcified? *AJR Am J Roentgenol* 2001;176:201–204.
45. Sherrier RH, Chiles C, Johnson GA, et al. Differentiation of benign from malignant pulmonary nodules with digitized chest radiographs. *Radiology* 1987;162:645–649.
46. Gilkeson RC, Sachs PB. Dual energy subtraction digital radiography: technical considerations, clinical applications, and imaging pitfalls. *J Thorac Imaging* 2006; 21:303–313.
47. Siegelman SS, Khouri NF, Scott WW Jr, et al. Pulmonary hamartoma: CT findings. *Radiology* 1986;160:313–317.
48. Grewal RG, Austin JH. CT demonstration of calcification in carcinoma of the lung. *J Comput Assist Tomogr* 1994;18:867–871.
49. Chong S, Lee KS, Chung MJ, et al. Neuroendocrine tumors of the lung: clinical, pathologic, and imaging findings. *Radiographics* 2006;26: 41–57; discussion 57–48.
50. Swensen S, Brown LR, Colby TV, et al. Pulmonary nodules: CT evaluation of enhancement with iodinated contrast material. *Radiology* 1995;194:393–398.
51. Yamashita K, Matsunobe S, Tsuda T, et al. Solitary pulmonary nodules: preliminary study of evaluation with incremental dynamic CT. *Radiology* 1995;194:399–405.
52. Swensen SJ, Brown LR, Colby TV, et al. Lung nodule enhancement at CT: prospective findings. *Radiology* 1996;201:447–455.
53. Swensen SJ, Viggiano RW, Midthun DE, et al. Lung nodule enhancement at CT: multicenter study. *Radiology* 2000;214:73–80.
54. Yi CA, Lee KS, Kim EA, et al. Solitary pulmonary nodules: dynamic enhanced multi-detector row CT study and comparison with vascular endothelial growth factor and microvessel density. *Radiology* 2004; 233:191–199.
55. Zhang M, Kono M. Solitary pulmonary nodules: evaluation of blood flow patterns with dynamic CT. *Radiology* 1997;205:471–478.
56. Jeong YJ, Lee KS, Jeong SY, et al. Solitary pulmonary nodule: characterization with combined wash-in and washout features at dynamic multi-detector row CT. *Radiology* 2005;237:675–683.
57. Lee KS, Yi CA, Jeong SY, et al. Solid or partly solid solitary pulmonary nodules: their characterization using contrast wash-in and morphologic features at helical CT. *Chest* 2007;131:1516–1525.
58. Yi CA, Lee KS, Kim BT, et al. Efficacy of helical dynamic CT versus integrated PET/CT for detection of mediastinal nodal metastasis in non-small cell lung cancer. *AJR Am J Roentgenol* 2007;188:318–325.
59. Schroeder T, Ruehm SG, Debatin JF, et al. Detection of Pulmonary Nodules Using a 2D HASTE MR Sequence: Comparison with MDCT. *Am J Roentgenol* 2005;185:979–984.
60. Gückel C, Schnabel K, Deimling M, et al. Solitary pulmonary nodules: MR evaluation of enhancement patterns with contrast-enhanced dynamic snapshot gradient-echo imaging. *Radiology* 1996;200:681–686.
61. Ohno Y, Hatabu H, Takenaka D, et al. Solitary pulmonary nodules: potential role of dynamic MR imaging in management initial experience. *Radiology* 2002;224:503–511.
62. Schaefer JF, Schneider V, Vollmar J, et al. Solitary pulmonary nodules: Association between signal characteristics in dynamic contrast enhanced MRI and tumor angiogenesis. *Lung Cancer* 2006;53:39–49.
63. Kono M, Adachi S, Kusumoto M, et al. Clinical utility of Gd-DTPA-enhanced magnetic resonance imaging in lung cancer. *J Thorac Imaging* 1993;8:18–26.
64. Sakai F, Sone S, Maruyama A, et al. Thin-rim enhancement in Gd-DTPA-enhanced magnetic resonance images of tuberculoma: a new finding of potential differential diagnostic importance. *J Thorac Imaging* 1992;7:64–69.
65. Ohno Y, Hatabu H, Takenaka D, et al. CT-guided transthoracic needle aspiration biopsy of small (< or = 20 mm) solitary pulmonary nodules. *AJR Am J Roentgenol* 2003;180:1665–1669.
66. Romano M, Griffo S, Gentile M, et al. CT guided percutaneous fine needle biopsy of small lung lesions in outpatients. Safety and efficacy of the procedure compared to inpatients. *Radiol Med* 2004;108: 275–282.

67. Savage C, Walser EM, Schnadig V, et al. Transthoracic image-guided biopsy of lung nodules: when is benign really benign? *J Vasc Interv Radiol* 2004;15:161–164.
68. Yamagami T, Iida S, Kato T, et al. Usefulness of new automated cutting needle for tissue-core biopsy of lung nodules under CT fluoroscopic guidance. *Chest* 2003;124:147–154.
69. Quint LE, Kretschmer M, Chang A, et al. CT-guided thoracic core biopsies: value of a negative result. *Cancer Imaging* 2006;6:163–167.
70. Montaudon M, Latrabe V, Pariente A, et al. Factors influencing accuracy of CT-guided percutaneous biopsies of pulmonary lesions. *Eur Radiol* 2004;14:1234–1240.
71. Satoh S, Ohdama S, Matsubara O, et al. CT-guided automated cutting needle biopsy by a combined method for accurate specific diagnosis of focal lung lesions. *Radiat Med* 2005;23:30–36.
72. Klein J, Salomon G, Stewart E. Transthoracic needle biopsy with a coaxially placed 20-gauge automated cutting needle: results in 122 patients. *Radiology* 1996;198:715–720.
73. Hayashi N, Sakai T, Kitagawa M, et al. CT-guided biopsy of pulmonary nodules less than 3 cm: usefulness of the spring-operated core biopsy needle and frozen-section pathologic diagnosis. *AJR Am J Roentgenol* 1998;170:329–331.
74. Cahan WG, Shah JP, Castro EB. Benign solitary lung lesions in patients with cancer. *Ann Surg* 1978;187:241–244.
75. Quint LE, Park CH, Iannettoni MD. Solitary pulmonary nodules in patients with extrapulmonary neoplasms. *Radiology* 2000;217:257–261.
76. Quint LE. Staging non-small cell lung cancer. *Cancer Imaging* 2007; 7:148–159.
77. AJCC Cancer Staging Handbook. New York: Springer-Verlag, 2002.
78. Mountain CF. Staging classification of lung cancer. A critical evaluation. *Clin Chest Med* 2002;23:103–121.
79. Mountain CF. Revisions in the International System for Staging Lung Cancer. *Chest* 1997;111:1710–1717.
80. Mountain CF, Dresler CM. Regional lymph node classification for lung cancer staging. *Chest* 1997;111:1718–1723.
81. Sobin L, Wittekind C, eds. *TNM Classification of Malignant Tumours*, 6th ed. New York: Wiley-Liss, 2002.
82. Goldstraw P, Crowley J, Chansky K, et al. The IASLC Lung Cancer Staging Project: proposals for the revision of the TNM stage groupings in the forthcoming (seventh) edition of the TNM Classification of malignant tumours. *J Thorac Oncol* 2007;2:706–714.
83. Groome PA, Bolejack V, Crowley JJ, et al. The IASLC Lung Cancer Staging Project: validation of the proposals for revision of the T, N, and M descriptors and consequent stage groupings in the forthcoming (seventh) edition of the TNM classification of malignant tumours. *J Thorac Oncol* 2007;2:694–705.
84. Postmus PE, Brambilla E, Chansky K, et al. The IASLC Lung Cancer Staging Project: proposals for revision of the M descriptors in the forthcoming (seventh) edition of the TNM classification of lung cancer. *J Thorac Oncol* 2007;2:686–693.
85. Rami-Porta R, Ball D, Crowley J, et al. The IASLC Lung Cancer Staging Project: proposals for the revision of the T descriptors in the forthcoming (seventh) edition of the TNM classification for lung cancer. *J Thorac Oncol* 2007;2:593–602.
86. Rusch VW, Crowley J, Giroux DJ, et al. The IASLC Lung Cancer Staging Project: proposals for the revision of the N descriptors in the forthcoming seventh edition of the TNM classification for lung cancer. *J Thorac Oncol* 2007;2:603–612.
87. Murayama S, Murakami J, Yoshimitsu K, et al. CT diagnosis of pleural dissemination without pleural effusion in primary lung cancer. *Radiat Med* 1996;14:117–119.
88. Gdeedo A, Van Schil P, Corthouts B, et al. Comparison of imaging TNM [(i)TNM] and pathological TNM [(p)TNM] in staging of bronchogenic carcinoma. *European Journal of Cardio-Thoracic Surgery* 1997; 12:224–227.
89. Glazer HS, Duncan-Meyer J, Aronberg DJ. Pleural and chest wall invasion in bronchogenic carcinoma: CT evaluation. *Radiology* 1985;157: 191–194.
90. Pennes DR, Glazer GM, Wimbish KJ, et al. Chest wall invasion by lung cancer: limitations of CT evaluation. *AJR Am J Roentgenol* 1985; 144:507–511.
91. Ratto GB, Piacenza G, Frola C, et al. Chest wall involvement by lung cancer: computed tomographic detection and results of operation. *Ann Thorac Surg* 1991;51:182–188.
92. Venuta F, Rendina E, Ciriaco P, et al. Computed tomography for preoperative assessment of T3 and T4 bronchogenic carcinoma. *Eur J Cardiothorac Surg* 1992;6:238–241.
93. Rendina EA, Bognolo DA, Mineo TC, et al. Computed tomography for the evaluation of intrathoracic invasion by lung cancer. *J Thorac Cardiovasc Surg* 1987;94:57–63.
94. Pearlberg JL, Sandler MA, Beute GH, et al. Limitations of CT in evaluation of neoplasms involving chest wall. *J Comput Assist Tomogr* 1987;11:290–293.
95. Watanabe A, Shimokata K, Saka H, et al. Chest CT combined with artificial pneumothorax: value in determining origin and extent of tumor. *AJR Am J Roentgenol* 1991;156:707–710.
96. Yokoi K, Mori K, Miyazawa N, et al. Tumor invasion of the chest wall and mediastinum in lung cancer: evaluation with pneumothorax CT. *Radiology* 1991;181:147–152.
97. Yokozaki M, Nawano S, Nagai K, et al. Cine magnetic resonance imaging, computed tomography and ultrasonography in the evaluation of chest wall invasion of lung cancer. *Hiroshima J Med Sci* 1997;46:61–66.
98. Murata K, Takahashi M, Mori M, et al. Chest wall and mediastinal invasion by lung cancer: evaluation with multisection expiratory dynamic CT. *Radiology* 1994;191:251–255.
99. Suzuki N, Saito T, Kitamura S. Tumor invasion of chest wall in lung cancer: diagnosis with US. *Radiology* 1993;187:39–42.
100. Piehler JM, Pairolero PC, Weiland LH, et al. Bronchogenic carcinoma with chest wall invasion: factors affecting survival following en bloc resection. *Ann Thoracic Surg* 1982;34:684–691.
101. Paone JF, Spees EK, Newton CG, et al. An appraisal of en bloc resection of peripheral bronchogenic carcinoma involving the thoracic wall. *Chest* 1982;81:203–207.
102. Glazer HS, Kaiser LR, Anderson DJ. Indeterminate mediastinal invasion in brochogenic carcinoma: CT evaluation. *Radiology* 1989;173:37–42.
103. Würsten H, Vock P. Mediastinal infiltration of lung carcinoma (T4NO-1): the positive predictive value of computed tomography. *Thorac Cardiovasc Surg* 1987;35:355–360.
104. Kameda K, Adachi S, Kono M. Detection of T-factor in lung cancer using magnetic resonance imaging and computed tomography. *J Thorac Imag* 1988;3:73–80.
105. Izbicki JR, Thetter O, Karg O, et al. Accuracy of computed tomographic scan and surgical assessment for staging of bronchial carcinoma. A prospective study. *J Thorac Cardiovasc Surg* 1992;104:413–420.
106. Webb WR, Gatsonis C, Zerhouni EA, et al. CT and MR imaging in staging non-small cell bronchogenic carcinma: report of the radiologic diagnostic oncology group. *Radiology* 1991;178:705–713.
107. Martini N, Heelan R, Westcott J, et al. Comparative merits of conventional, computed tomographic, and magnetic resonance imaging in assessing mediastinal involvement in surgically confirmed lung carcinoma. *J Thorac Cardiovasc Surg* 1985;90:639–648.
108. Musset D, Grenier P, Carette MF. Primary lung cancer staging: prospective comparative study of MR imaging with CT. *Radiology* 1986;160: 607–611.
109. Laurent F, Drouillard J, Dorcier F, et al. Bronchogenic carcinoma staging: CT versus MR imaging. Assessment with surgery. *Eur J Cardiothorac Surg* 1988;2:31–36.
110. Choe DH, Lee JH, Lee BH, et al. Obliteration of the pulmonary vein in lung cancer: significance in assessing local extent with CT. *J Comput Assist Tomogr* 1998;22:587–591.
111. Schröder C, Schönhofer B, Vogel B. Transesophageal echographic determination of aortic invasion by lung cancer. *Chest* 2005;127:438–442.
112. Quint LE, Glazer GM, Orringer MB. Central lung masses: prediction with CT of need for pneumonectomy versus lobectomy. *Radiology* 1987;165:735–738.

113. Hu Y, Malthaner RA. The feasibility of three-dimensional displays of the thorax for preoperative planning in the surgical treatment of lung cancer. *Eur J Cardiothorac Surg* 2007;31:506–511.
114. Quint LE, McShan DL, Glazer GM, et al. Three dimensional CT of central lung tumors. *Clin Imaging* 1990;14:323–329.
115. Tobler J, Levitt RG, Glazer HS, et al. Differentiation of proximal bronchogenic carcinoma from post-obstructive lobar collapse by magnetic resonance imaging: comparison with computed tomography. *Invest Radiol* 1987;22:538–543.
116. Kirsh MM, Kahn DR, Gago O, et al. Treatment of bronchogenic carcinoma with mediastinal metastases. *Ann Thorac Surg* 1971;12:11–21.
117. Martini N, Flehinger BJ, Zaman MB, et al. Results of resection in non-oat cell carcinoma of the lung with mediastinal lymph node metastases. *Ann Surg* 1983;198:386–397.
118. Naruke T, Suemasu K, Ishikawa S. Lymph node mapping and curability at various levels of metastasis in resected lung cancer. *J Thorac Cardiovasc Surg* 1978;76:832–839.
119. Watanabe Y, Shimizu J, Oda M, et al. Aggressive surgical intervention in N2 non-small cell cancer of the lung. *Ann Thorac Surg* 1991;41: 253–261.
120. Mountain CF. Expanded possibilities for surgical treatment of lung cancer. *Chest* 1990;97:1045–1051.
121. Naruke T, Goya T, Tsuchiya R, et al. Prognosis and survival in resected lung carcinoma based on the new international staging system. *J Thorac Cardiovasc Surg* 1988;96:440–447.
122. McKenna RJ Jr, Libshitz HI, Mountain CE, et al. Roentgenographic evaluation of mediastinal nodes for preoperative assessment in lung cancer. *Chest* 1985;88:206–210.
123. Pearson FG, DeLarue NC, Ilves R, et al. Significance of positive superior mediastinal nodes identified at mediastinoscopy in patients with resectable cancer of the lung. *J Thorac Cardiovasc Surg* 1982;83:1–11.
124. Martini N, Flehinger B. The role of surgery in N2 lung cancer. *Surg Clin North Am* 1987;67:1037–1049.
125. Patterson GA, Piazza D, Pearson FG, et al. Significance of metastatic disease in subaortic lymph nodes. *Ann Thorac Surg* 1987;43:155–159.
126. Patel V, Shrager JB. Which patients with stage III non-small cell lung cancer should undergo surgical resection? *Oncologist* 2005;10:335–344.
127. Taylor SG IV, Trybula M, Bonomi PD, et al. Simultaneous cisplatin fluorouracil infusion and radiation followed by surgical resection in regionally localized stage III, non-small cell lung cancer. *Ann Thorac Surg* 1987;43:87–91.
128. Faber L, Kittle C, Warren W. Preoperative chemotherapy and irradiation for stage III non-small cell lung cancer. *Ann Thorac Surg* 1989;47:669–677.
129. Skarin A, Jochelson M, Sheldon T. Neoadjuvant chemotherapy in marginally resectable stage III M0 non-small cell lung cancer: long-term follow-up in 41 patients. *J Surg Oncon* 1989;40:266–274.
130. Sugarbaker D, Herndon J, Kohman L, et al. Results of Cancer and Leukemia Group B protocol 8935: a multi-institutional phase II trimodality trial of stage HIA (N2) non-small cell lung cancer. *J Thorac Cardiovasc Surg* 1995;109:473–485.
131. Roth JA, Fossella F, Komaki R, et al. A randomized trial comparing perioperative chemotherapy and surgery with surgery done in resectable stage IIIA non-small cell lung cancer. *J Natl Cancer Inst* 1994;86: 673–680.
132. Rosell R, Gómez-Codina J, Camps C, et al. A randomized trial comparing chemotherapy plus surgery with surgery alone in patients with non-small cell lung cancer. *N Engl J Med* 1994;330:153–158.
133. Glazer GM, Gross BH, Quint LE, et al. Normal mediastinal lymph nodes: number and size according to American thoracic society mapping. *AJR Am J Roentgenol* 1985;144:261–265.
134. Quint LE, Glazer GM, Orringer MB, et al. Mediastinal lymph node detection and sizing at CT and autopsy. *AJR Am J Roentgenol* 1986;147:469–472.
135. Shimoyama K, Murata K, Takahashi M, et al. Pulmonary hilar lymph node metastases from lung cancer: evaluation based on morphology at thin-section, incremental dynamic CT. *Radiology* 1997;203:187–195.
136. Genereux GP, Howie JL. Normal mediastinal lymph node size and number: CT and anatomic study. *AJR Am J Roentgenol* 1984;142:1095–1100.
137. Schnyder PA, Gamsu G. CT of the pretracheal retrocaval space. *AJR Am J Roentgenol* 1981;136:303–308.
138. Kiyono K, Sone S, Sakai F, et al. The number and size of normal mediastinal lymph nodes: a postmortem study. *AJR Am J Roentgenol* 1988;150:771–776.
139. Glazer GM, Orringer MB, Gross BH, et al. The mediastinum in non-small cell lung cancer: CT-surgical correlation. *AJR Am J Roentgenol* 1984;142:1101–1105.
140. Platt JF, Glazer GM, Orringer MB, et al. Radiologic evaluation of the subcarinal lymph nodes: a comparative study. *AJR Am J Roentgenol* 1988;151:279–282.
141. Medina Gallardo JF, Borderas Naranjo F, Torres Cansino M, et al. Validity of enlarged mediastinal nodes as markers of involvement by non-small cell lung cancer. *Am Rev Respir Dis* 1992;146:1210–1212.
142. Daly BJ Jr, Faling LJ, Pugatch RD, et al. Computed tomography. An effective technique for mediastinal staging in lung cancer. *J Thorac Cardiovasc Surg* 1984;88:486–494.
143. Gross BH, Glazer GM, Orringer MB, et al. Bronchogenic carcinoma metastatic to normal-sized lymph nodes: frequency and significance. *Radiology* 1988;166:71–74.
144. Arita T, Matsumoto T, Kuramitsu T, et al. Is it possible to differentiate malignant mediastinal nodes from benign nodes by size? Reevaluation by CT, transesophageal echocardiography, and nodal specimen. *Chest* 1996;110:1004–1008.
145. Pretreatment evaluation of non-small-cell lung cancer. The American Thoracic Society and The European Respiratory Society. *Am J Respir Crit Care Med* 1997;156:320–332.
146. Faling LJ, Pugatch RD, Jung-Legg Y, et al. Computed tomographic scanning of the mediastinum in the staging of bronchogenic carcinoma. *Am Rev Respir Dis* 1981;124:690–695.
147. Cybulsky IJ, Lanza LA, Ryan MB, et al. Prognostic significance of computed tomography in resected N2 lung cancer. *Ann Thorac Surg* 1992;54:533–537.
148. Ishida T, Tateishi M, Kaneko S, et al. Surgical treatment of patients with nonsmall-cell lung cancer and mediastinal lymph node involvement. *J Surg Oncol* 1990;43:161–166.
149. Bergh NP, Schersten T. Bronchogenic carcinoma: a follow-up study of a surgically treated series with special reference to the prognostic significance of lymph node metastases. *Acta Chir Scand* 1965;347:1–42.
150. Fisher ER, Gregorio RM, Redmond C, et al. Pathologic findings from the National Surgical Adjuvant Breast Project (protocol no. 4). III. The significance of extranodal extension of axillary metastases. *Am J Clin Pathol* 1976;65:439–444.
151. Platt JF, Glazer GM, Gross BH, et al. CT evaluation of mediastinal lymph nodes in lung cancer: influence of the lobar site of the primary neoplasm. *AJR Am J Roentgenol* 1987;149:683–686.
152. Baron R, Levitt RG, Sagel SS, et al. Computed tomography in the preoperative evaluation of bronchogenic carcinoma. *Radiology* 1982;145: 727–732.
153. Moak GCD, Cockerill EM, Farber MO, et al. Computed tomography vs standard radiology in the evaluation of mediastinal adenopathy. *Chest* 1982;82:69–75.
154. Osborne DR, Korobkin M, Ravin CE, et al. Comparison of plain radiography, conventional tomography, and computed tomography in detecting intrathoracic lymph node metastases from lung carcinoma. *Radiology* 1982;142:157–161.
155. Rea HH, Shevland JE, House AJ. Accuracy of computed tomographic scanning in assessment of the mediastinum in bronchial carcinoma. *J Thorac Cardiovasc Surg* 1981;81:825–829.
156. Buy JN, Ghossain MA, Poirson F, et al. Computed tomography of mediastinal lymph nodes in nonsmall cell lung cancer. *J Comput Assist Tomogr* 1988;12:545–552.
157. Ikezoe J, Kadowaki K, Morimoto S, et al. Mediastinal lymph node metastases from nonsmall cell bronchogenic carcinoma: reevaluation with CT. *J Comput Assist Tomogr* 1990;14:340–344.

158. Glazer GM, Francis IR, Shirazi KK, et al. Evaluation of the pulmonary hilum: comparison of conventional radiography, 55° posterior oblique tomography, and dynamic computed tomography. *J Comput Assist Tomogr* 1983;7:983–989.
159. McLoud TC, Bourgouin PM, Greenberg RW, et al. Bronchogenic carcinoma: analysis of staging in the mediastinum with CT by correlative lymph node mapping and sampling. *Radiology* 1992;182:319–323.
160. Lewis JW Jr, Pearlberg JL, Beute GH, et al. Can computed tomography of the chest stage lung cancer? yes and no. *Ann Thorac Surg* 1990;49:591–596.
161. Lewis JW Jr, Madrazo BL, Gross SC, et al. The value of radiographic and computed tomography in the staging of lung carcinoma. *Ann Thorac Surg* 1982;34:553–558.
162. Patterson GA, Ginsberg RJ, Poon PY, et al. A prospective evaluation of magnetic resonance imaging, computed tomography, and mdiastinoscopy in the preoperative assessment of mediastinal node status in bronchogenic carcinoma. *J Thorac Cardiovasc Surg* 1987;94:679–684.
163. Müller NL, Webb WR, Gamsu G. Paratracheal lymphadenopathy: Radiologic findings and correlation with CT. *Radiology* 1985;156: 761–765.
164. Thermann M, Poser H, Müller-Hermelink KH, et al. Evaluation of tomography and mediastinoscopy for the detection of mediastinal lymph node metastases. *Ann Thorac Surg* 1984;37:443–447.
165. Hirleman MT, Yiu-Chiu VS, Chiu LC, et al. The resectability of primary lung carcinoma: a diagnostic staging review. *J Comput Tomogr* 1980;4:146–163.
166. Lähde S, Hyrynkangas K, Merikanto J, et al. Computed tomography and mediastinoscopy in the assessment of resectability of lung cancer. *Acta Radiol* 1989;30:169–173.
167. Ratto GB, Frola C, Cantoni S, et al. Improving clinical efficacy of computed tomographic scan in the preoperative assessment of patients with non-small cell lung cancer. *J Thorac Cardiovasc Surg* 1990;99: 416–425.
168. Daly BD, Mueller JD, Faling LJ, et al. N2 lung cancer: outcome in patients with false-negative computed tomographic scans of the chest. *J Thorac Cardiovasc Surg* 1993;105:904–910; discussion 910–911.
169. Seely JM, Mayo JR, Miller RR, et al. T1 lung cancer: prevalence of mediastinal nodal metastases and diagnostic accuracy of CT. *Radiology* 1993;186:129–132.
170. Daly BD Jr, Faling LJ, Bite G, et al. Mediastinal lymph node evaluation by computed tomography in lung cancer. *J Thorac Cardiovasc Surg* 1987;94:664–672.
171. Underwood GH Jr, Hooper RG, Alelbaum SP, et al. Computed tomographic scanning of the thorax in the staging of bronchogenic carcinoma. *N Engl J Med* 1979;300:777–778.
172. Modini C, Passariello R, Iascone C, et al. TNM staging in lung cancer: role of computed tomography. *J Thorac Cardiovasc Surg* 1982;84:569–574.
173. Goldstraw P, Kurzer M, Edwards D. Preoperative staging of lung cancer: role of computed tomography. *Thorax* 1983;38:10–15.
174. Kamiyoshihara M, Kawashima O, Ishikawa S, et al. Mediastinal lymph node evaluation by computed tomographic scan in lung cancer. *J Cardiovasc Surg (Torino)* 2001;42:119–124.
175. Suzuki K, Nagai K, Yoshida J, et al. Clinical predictors of N2 disease in the setting of a negative computed tomographic scan in patients with lung cancer. *J Thorac Cardiovasc Surg* 1999;117:593–598.
176. Kernstine KH, Stanford W, Mullan BF, et al. PET, CT, and MRI with Combidex for mediastinal staging in non-small cell lung carcinoma. *Ann Thorac Surg* 1999;68:1022–1028.
177. Gupta NC, Graeber GM, Rogers JS II, et al. Comparative efficacy of positron emission tomography with FDG and computed tomographic scanning in preoperative staging of non-small cell lung cancer. *Ann Surg* 1999;229:286–291.
178. Dales RE, Stark RM, Raman S. Computed tomography to stage lung cancer. *Am Rev Respir Dis* 1990;144:1096–1101.
179. Ferguson MK, MacMahon H, Little AG, et al. Regional accuracy of computed tomography of the mediastinum in staging of lung cancer. *J Thorac Cardiovasc Surg* 1986;91:498–504.
180. Nohl HC. An investigation into the lymphatic and vascular spread of carcinoma of the bronchus. *Thorax* 1956;11:172–185.
181. Nakata H, Ishimaru H, Nakayama C, et al. Computed tomography for preoperative evaluations of lung cancer. *J Comp Tomogr* 1986;10:147–151.
182. Abrams HL, Spiro R, Goldstein N. Metastases in carcinoma. Analysis of 1000 autopsied cases. *Cancer* 1950;3:74–85.
183. Anderson EE. Nonfunctioning tumors of the adrenal gland. *Urol Clin North Am* 1977;4:263–271.
184. Matthews MJ. Problems in morphology and behavior of bronchopulmonary malignant disease. In: Israel L, Chahinian P, eds. *Lung cancer: natural history, prognosis and therapy*. New York: Academic Press, 1976; 23–62.
185. Weiss W, Gillick JS. The metastatic spread of bronchogenic carcinoma in relation to the interval between resection and death. *Chest* 1977;71:725–729.
186. Smith RA. Evaluation of long-term results of surgery for bronchial carcinoma. *J Thorac Cardiovasc Surg* 1981;82:325–333.
187. Bell JW. Abdominal exploration in one-hundred lung carcinoma suspects prior to thoracotomy. *Ann Surg* 1968;167:199–203.
188. Matthews MJ, Kanhouwa S, Pickren J, et al. Frequency of residual and metastatic tumor in patients undergoing curative surgical resection for lung cancer. *Cancer Chemother Rep 3* 1973;4:63–67.
189. Salvatierra A, Baamonde C, Llamas JM, et al. Extrathoracic staging of bronchogenic carcinoma. *Chest* 1990;97:1053–1058.
190. Sider L, Horejs D. Frequency of extrathoracic metastases from bronchogenic carcinoma in patients with normal-sized hilar and mediastinal lymph nodes on CT. *AJR Am J Roentgenol* 1988;151:893–895.
191. Quint LE, Tummala S, Brisson LJ, et al. Distribution of distant metastases from newly diagnosed non-small cell lung cancer. *Ann Thorac Surg* 1996;62:246–250.
192. Mujoomdar A, Austin JH, Malhotra R, et al. Clinical predictors of metastatic disease to the brain from non-small cell lung carcinoma: primary tumor size, cell type, and lymph node metastases. *Radiology* 2007;242:882–888.
193. Oliver TW Jr, Bernardino ME, Miller JI, et al. Isolated adrenal masses in nonsmall-cell bronchogenic carcinoma. *Radiology* 1984;153:217–218.
194. Commons RR, Callaway CP. Adenomas of the adrenal cortex. *Arch Med Interna* 1948;81:37–41.
195. Hedeland H, Ostberg G, Hökfelt B. On the prevalence of adrenocortical adenomas in an autopsy material in relation to hypertension and diabetes. *Acta Med Scand* 1968;184:211–214.
196. Glazer HS, Weyman PJ, Sagel SS, et al. Nonfunctioning adrenal masses: incidental discovery on computed tomography. *AJR Am J Roentgenol* 1982;139:81–85.
197. Gillams A, Roberts CM, Shaw P, et al. The value of CT scanning and percutaneous fine needle aspiration of adrenal masses in biopsy-proven lung cancer. *Clin Radiol* 1992;46:18–22.
198. Lee MJ, Hahn PF, Papanicolaou N, et al. Benign and malignant adrenal masses: CT distinction with attenuation coefficients, size and observer analysis. *Radiology* 1991;179:415–418.
199. Korobkin M, Brodeur FJ, Yutzy GG, et al. Differentiation of adrenal adenomas from nonadenomas using CT attenuation values. *AJR Am J Roentgenol* 1996;166:531–536.
200. Blake MA, Kalra MK, Sweeney AT, et al. Distinguishing benign from malignant adrenal masses: Multi-detector row CT protocol with 10-minute delay. *Radiology* 2006;238:578–585.
201. Caoili EM, Korobkin M, Francis IR, et al. Adrenal masses: characterization with combined unenhanced and delayed enhanced CT. *Radiology* 2002;222:629–633.
202. Korobkin M. CT characterization of adrenal masses: the time has come. *Radiology* 2000;217:629–632.
203. Jhaveri KS, Wong F, Ghai S, et al. Comparison of CT Histogram Analysis and Chemical Shift MRI in the Characterization of Indeterminate Adrenal Nodules. *AJR Am J Roentgenol* 2006;187: 1303–1308.
204. Whitcomb ME, Barham E, Goldman AL, et al. Indications for mediastinoscopy in bronchogenic carcinoma. *Am Rev Respir Dis* 1976; 113:189–195.

205. Duncan KA, Gomersall LN, Weir J. Computed tomography of the chest in T1N0M0 non-small cell bronchial carcinoma. *Br J Radiol* 1993;66:20–22.
206. Parker LA, Mauro MA, Delany DJ, et al. Evaluation of T1N0M0 lung cancer with CT. *J Comput Assist Tomogr* 1991;15:943–947.
207. Becker GL, Whitlock WL, Schaefer PS, et al. The impact of thoracic computed tomography in clinically staged T1, N0, M0 chest lesions. *Arch Intern Med* 1990;150:557–559.
208. Baker ME, Spritzer C, Blinder R, et al. Benign adrenal lesions mimicking malignancy on MR imaging: report of two cases. *Radiology* 1987;163:669–671.
209. Pearlberg JL, Sandler MA, Beute GH, et al. T1N0M0 bronchgenic carcinoma: assessment by CT. *Radiology* 1985;157:187–190.
210. Heavey LR, Glazer GM, Gross BH, et al. The role of CT in staging radiographic T1N0M0 lung cancer. *AJR Am J Roentgenol* 1986;146:285–290.
211. Conces DJ Jr, Klink JF, Tarver RD, et al. T1N0M0 lung cancer: evaluation with CT. *Radiology* 1989;170:643–646.
212. Lähde S, Päivänsalo M, Rainio P. CT for predicting the resectability of lung cancer. A prospective study. *Acta Radiol* 1991;32:449–454.
213. Roberts JR, Blum MG, Arildsen R, et al. Prospective comparison of radiologic, thoracoscopic, and pathologic staging in patients with early non-small cell lung cancer. *Ann Thorac Surg* 1999;68:1154–1158.
214. Akamatsu H, Terashima M, Koike T, et al. Staging of primary lung cancer by computed tomography-guided percutaneous needle cytology of mediastinal lymph nodes. *Ann Thorac Surg* 1996;62:352–355.
215. Westcott JL. Percutaneous needle aspiration of hilar and mediastinal masses. *Radiology* 1981;141:323–329.
216. Williams RA, Haaga JR, Karagiannis E. CT guided paravertebral biopsy of the mediastinum. *J Comput Assist Tomogr* 1984;8:575–578.
217. Patz EF Jr, Erasmus JJ, McAdams HP, et al. Lung cancer staging and management: comparison of contrast-enhanced and nonenhanced helical CT of the thorax. *Radiology* 1999;212:56–60.
218. Pearson F. Staging of the mediastinum. Role of mediastinoscopy and computed tomography *Chest* 1993;103:S346–S348.
219. Chapet O, Kong FM, Quint LE, et al. CT-based definition of thoracic lymph node stations: an atlas from the University of Michigan. *Int J Radiat Oncol Biol Phys* 2005;63:170–178.
220. Lee KS, Shim YM, Han J, et al. Primary tumors and mediastinal lymph nodes after neoadjuvant concurrent chemoradiotherapy of lung cancer: serial CT findings with pathologic correlation. *J Comput Assist Tomogr* 2000;24:35–40.
221. Bruzzi JF, Truong M, Zinner R, et al. Short-term restaging of patients with non-small cell lung cancer receiving chemotherapy. *J Thorac Oncol* 2006;1:425–429.
222. Milleron B, Westeel V, Quoix E, et al. Complete response following preoperative chemotherapy for resectable non-small cell lung cancer: accuracy of clinical assessment using the French trial database. *Chest* 2005;128:1442–1447.
223. Seto M, Kuriyama K, Kasugai T, et al. Comparison of computed tomography and pathologic examination for evaluation of response of primary lung cancer to neoadjuvant therapy. *J Thorac Imaging* 1999;14:69–73.
224. Siker ML, Tomé WA, Mehta MP. Tumor volume changes on serial imaging with megavoltage CT for non-small-cell lung cancer during intensity-modulated radiotherapy: how reliable, consistent, and meaningful is the effect? *Int J Radiat Oncol Biol Phys* 2006;66:135–141.
225. Seibert RM, Ramsey CR, Hines JW, et al. A model for predicting lung cancer response to therapy. *Int J Radiat Oncol Biol Phys* 2007;67:601–609.
226. Laurent F, Montaudon M, Corneloup O. CT and MRI of Lung Cancer. *Respiration* 2006;73:133–142.
227. Patz EF Jr. Imaging bronchogenic carcinoma. *Chest* 2000;117: S90–S95.
228. Templeton PA, Caskey CI, Zerhouni EA. Current uses of CT and MR imaging in the staging of lung cancer. *Radiol Clin North Am* 1990; 28:631–646.
229. Lau CL, Harpole DH Jr, Patz E. Staging techniques for lung cancer. *Chest Surg Clin N Am* 2000;10:781–801.
230. Haramati LB, White CS. MR imaging of lung cancer. *Magn Reson Imaging Clin N Am* 2000;8:43–57, viii.
231. Haberkorn U, Schoenberg SO. Imaging of lung cancer with CT, MRT and PET. *Lung Cancer* 2001;34:S13–S23.
232. MacDonald SL, Hansell DM. Staging of non-small cell lung cancer: imaging of intrathoracic disease. *Eur J Radiol* 2003;45:18–30.
233. Toloza EM, Harpole L, McCrory DC. Noninvasive staging of non-small cell lung cancer: a review of the current evidence. *Chest* 2003;123: S137–S146.
234. Rapoport S, Blair DN, McCarthy SM, et al. Brachial plexus: correlation of MR imaging with CT and pathologic findings. *Radiology* 1988;167:161–165.
235. Webb WR, Sostman HD. MR imaging of thoracic disease: clinical uses. *Radiology* 1992;182:621–630.
236. Gefter WB. Magnetic resonance imaging in the evaluation of lung cancer. *Semin Roentgenol* 1990;25:73–84.
237. White CS, Templeton PA, Belani CP. Imaging in lung cancer. *Semin Oncol* 1993;20:142–152.
238. White CS, Templeton PA. Radiologic manifestations of bronchogenic cancer. *Clin Chest Med* 1993;14:55–67.
239. Padovani B, Mouroux J, Seksik L, et al. Chest wall invasion by bronchogenic carcinoma: evaluation with MR imaging. *Radiology* 1993;187:33–38.
240. Quint LE, Francis IR, Wahl RL, et al. Preoperative staging of non-small-cell carcinoma of the lung: imaging methods. *AJR Am J Roentgenol* 1995;164:1349–1359.
241. Haggar AM, Pearlberg JL, Froelich JW. Chest-wall invasion by carcinoma of the lung: detection by MR imaging. *AJR Am J Roentgenol* 1987;148:1075–1078.
242. Klein JS, Webb WR. The radiologic staging of lung cancer. *J Thorac Imaging* 1991;7:29–47.
243. Heelan RT, Demas BE, Caravelli JF, et al. Superior sulcus tumors: CT and MR imaging. *Radiology* 1989;170:637–641.
244. McLoud TC, Filion RB, Edelman RR, et al. MR imaging of superior sulcus carcinoma. *J Comput Assist Tomogr* 1989;1989:233–239.
245. Takasugi JE, Rapoport S, Shaw C. Superior sulcus tumors: the role of imaging. *J Thorac Imaging* 1989;4:41–48.
246. Freundlich IM, Chasen MH, Varma DG. Magnetic resonance imaging of pulmonary apical tumors. *J Thoracic Imaging* 1996;11: 210–222.
247. Castagno AA, Shuman WP. MR imaging in clinically suspected brachial plexus tumor. *AJR Am J Roentgenol* 1987;149:1219–1222.
248. Mayr B, Lenhard M, Fink U, et al. Preoperative evaluation of bronchogenic carcinoma: value of MR in T- and N-staging. *Eur J Radiol* 1992;14:245–251.
249. McLoud TC. CT of bronchogenic carcinoma: indeterminate mediastinal invasion. *Radiology* 1989;173:15–16.
250. Barakos JA, Brown JJ, Higgins CB. MR imaging of secondary cardiac and paracardiac lesions. *AJR Am J Roentgenol* 1989; 153: 47–50.
251. Amparo EG, Higgins CB, Farmer D, et al. Gated MRI of cardiac and paracardiac masses: initial experience. *AJR Am J Roentgenol* 1984;143:1151–1156.
252. Seo JS, Kim YJ, Choi BW, et al. Usefulness of magnetic resonance imaging for evaluation of cardiovascular invasion: evaluation of sliding motion between thoracic mass and adjacent structures on cine MR images. *J Magn Reson Imaging* 2005;22:234–241.
253. Glazer GM, Orringer MB, Chenevert TL, et al. Mediastinal lymph nodes: relaxation time/pathologic correlation and implications in staging of lung cancer with MR imaging. *Radiology* 1988;168: 429–431.
254. Webb WR, Jensen BG, Sollitto R, et al. Bronchogenic carcinoma: staging with MR compared with staging with CT and surgery. *Radiology* 1985;156:117–124.
255. Heelan RT, Martini N, Westcott JW, et al. Carcinomatous involvement of the hilum and mediastinum: computed tomographic and magnetic resonance evaluation. *Radiology* 1985;156:111–115.

256. Grenier P, Dubray B, Carette M, et al. Preoperative thoracic staging of lung cancer: CT and MR evaluation. *Diagn Interv Radiol* 1989;1: 23–28.
257. Bonomo L, Ciccotosto C, Guidotti A, et al. Lung cancer staging: the role of computed tomography and magnetic resonance imaging. *Eur J Radiol* 1996;23:35–45.
258. Boiselle PM. MR imaging of thoracic lymph nodes. A comparison of computed tomography and positron emission tomography. *Magn Reson Imaging Clin N Am.* 2000;8:33–41.
259. Dooms GC, Hricak H, Moseley ME, et al. Characterization of lymphadenopathy by magnetic resonance relaxation times: preliminary results. *Radiology* 1985;155:691–697.
260. Anzai Y, Blackwell KE, Hirschowitz SL, et al. Initial clinical experience with dextran-coated superparamagnetic iron oxide for detection of lymph node metastases in patients with head and neck cancer. *Radiology* 1994;192:709–715.
261. Harisinghani MG, Saini S, Hahn PF, et al. MR imaging of lymph nodes in patients with primary abdominal and pelvic malignancies using ultra small superparamagnetic iron oxide (Combidex). *Acad Radiol* 1998;5(suppl 1):S167–S169.
262. Harisinghani MG, Barentsz J, Hahn PF, et al. Noninvasive detection of clinically occult lymph-node metastases in prostate cancer. *N Engl J Med* 2003;348:2491–2499.
263. Anzai Y, Piccoli CW, Outwater EK, et al. Evaluation of neck and body metastases to nodes with ferumoxtran 10-enhanced MR imaging: phase III safety and efficacy study. *Radiology* 2003;228:777–788.
264. Rockall AG, Sohaib SA, Harisinghani MG, et al. Diagnostic performance of nanoparticle-enhanced magnetic resonance imaging in the diagnosis of lymph node metastases in patients with endometrial and cervical cancer. *J Clin Oncol* 2005;23(12):2813–2821,
265. Pannu HK, Wang KP, Borman TL, et al. MR imaging of mediastinal lymph nodes: evaluation using a superparamagnetic contrast agent. *J Magn Reson Imaging* 2000;12:899–904.
266. Herth FJ, Rabe KF, Gasparini S, et al. Transbronchial and transoesophageal (ultrasound-guided) needle aspirations for the analysis of mediastinal lesions. *Eur Respir J* 2006;28:1264–1275.
267. Lauenstein TC, Goehde SC, Herborn CU, et al. Whole-body MR Imaging: evaluation of patients for metastases. *Radiology* 2004;233: 139–148.
268. Mitchell DG, Crovello M, Matteucci T, et al. Benign adrenocortical masses: diagnosis with chemical shift MR imaging. *Radiology* 1992; 185:345–351.
269. McNicholas MM, Lee MJ, Mayo-Smith WW, et al. An imaging algorithm for the differential diagnosis of adrenal adenomas and metastases. *AJR Am J Roentgenol* 1995;165:1453–1459.
270. Outwater EK, Siegelman ES, Radecki PD, et al. Distinction between benign and malignant adrenal masses: value of T1-weighted chemical-shift MR imaging. *AJR Am J Roentgenol* 1995;65:579–583.
271. Heinz-Peer G, Hönigschnabl S, Schneider B, et al. Characterization of adrenal masses using MR imaging with histopathologic correlation. *AJR Am J Roentgenol* 1999;173:15–22.
272. Caoili EM, Korobkin M, Francis IR, et al. Delayed enhanced CT of lipid-poor adrenal adenomas. *AJR Am J Roentgenol* 2000;175:1411–1415.
273. Kim SY, Kim JS, Park HS, et al. Screening of brain metastasis with limited magnetic resonance imaging (MRI): clinical implications of using limited brain MRI during initial staging for non-small cell lung cancer patients. *J Korean Med Sci* 2005;20:121–126.

CHAPTER 27

Johan Vansteenkiste
Christophe Dooms
Sigrid Stroobants

Positron Emission Tomography in Lung Cancer

BASIC PRINCIPLES AND TECHNICAL ASPECTS

Positron emission tomography (PET) is the most selective and sensitive (picomolar to nanomolar range) imaging technique for measuring molecular pathways and interactions in vivo. Positron-emitting isotopes are radioactive variants of elements naturally occurring in organic molecules and can be incorporated without changing the chemical and biological characteristics of the labeled molecule. They decay by emission of a positron, which is the subatomic, positively charged, antiparticle of the negatively charged electron. The positron will annihilate with an electron and create two 511-keV photons, emitted in opposite directions. The detection of numerous of these annihilations by the detector rings of the PET camera generates high-resolution pictures (5 to 10 mm) indicating the sites of tracer accumulation in the body.

The most frequently used tracer in PET oncology is the glucose analogue ^{18}F-fluorodeoxyglucose (FDG). Its use is based on the increased glycolysis of cancer cells compared with normal tissues. This increased glycolysis is linked to an increase in glucose membrane transporters and upregulation of the principal enzymes that control the glycolytic pathway.[1] FDG uptake is, however, not specific for cancer cells, and increased FDG uptake is also seen in some inflammatory conditions, the most common cause of false-positive FDG–PET findings.[2] The ability to perform whole-body imaging within one examination makes PET an ideal technique for cancer staging. In clinical oncology, the FDG uptake is often quantified as the standardized uptake value (SUV; i.e., the ratio of the activity in tissue per unit volume to the injected dose per patient body weight). In vitro studies demonstrated that the amount of FDG uptake in tumor tissue is mainly related to the number of viable cancer cells[3] and their proliferation capacity.[4] Therefore, SUV changes on FDG-PET can be used to evaluate treatment efficacy, because tumor cell kill results in a proportional reduction of the FDG signal.[5] Furthermore, the correlation between FDG uptake and proliferation capacity allows in vivo evaluation of tumor aggressiveness.

Interpretation of PET scans is hampered by the lack of anatomical detail, which makes it sometimes difficult to correctly localize hot spots or differentiate tumor tissue from benign structures with physiologically high FDG uptake (e.g., muscle, brown fat, gut). Therefore, PET always has to be interpreted in conjunction with anatomical images such as computed tomography (CT). Attempts to align or coregister CT and PET data sets acquired on separate machines with fusion software are generally only successful in the brain, whereas in the remainder of the body differences in patient setup present a challenge to the software approaches. Recently, integrated PET/CT systems were introduced, which enable acquisition of PET and CT data in the same session without changing the patients' position. Since the installation of the first clinical PET/CT in 2001, the technology has gained widespread use and all new PET scanners installed today are integrated PET/CT machines. Another advantage of PET/CT is the possibility to use the CT component for attenuation correction of the PET images and reduce the scan time substantially (~50%), but specific artifacts can sometimes be a problem.[6] An example are the errors in localization of lesions caused by breathing and the difference in scan time to acquire a PET (minutes) and CT image (seconds). This can result in incorrect anatomical localization of lesions near the diaphragm on the attenuation-corrected images (Fig. 27.1). High-density objects (dental fillings, chemotherapy ports, barium contrast) can lead to an overestimation of tracer uptake, thereby producing false-positive PET findings. Therefore, non–attenuation-corrected PET images, which do not manifest these errors, should always be reviewed in parallel to recognize these artifacts.

Although FDG has made the way for PET in clinical oncology, several other radiopharmaceuticals can be used to study

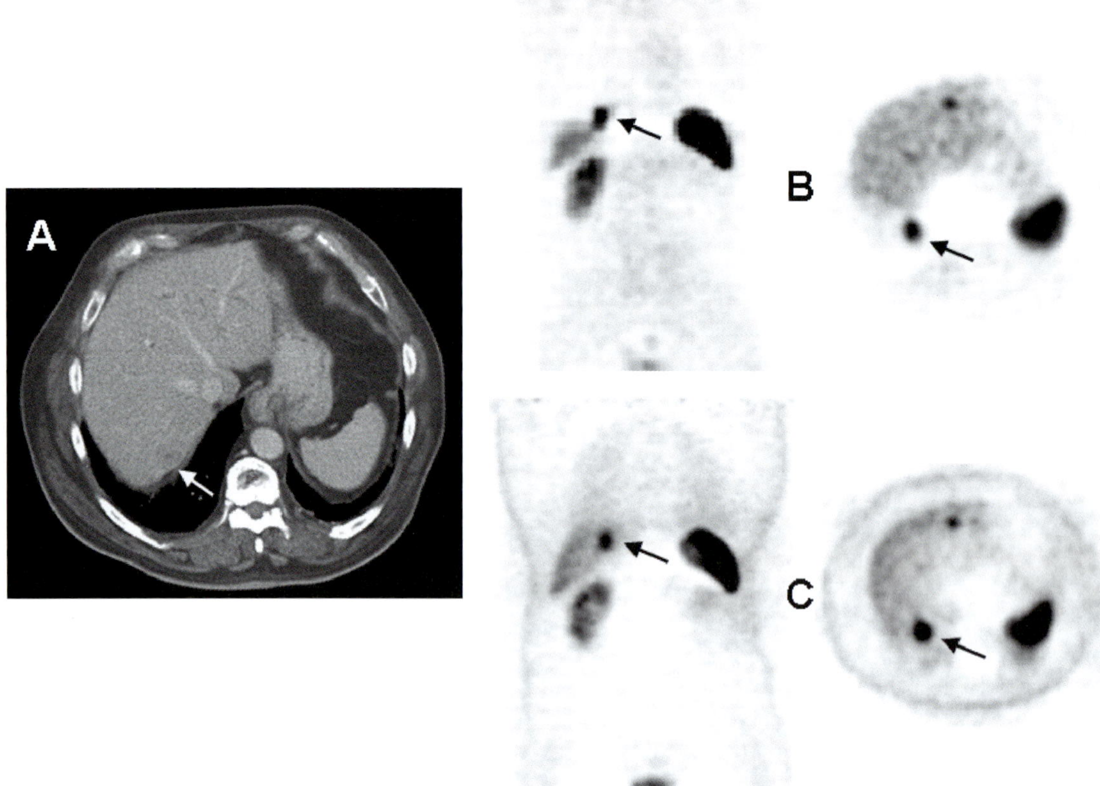

FIGURE 27.1 Ga-68 DOTATOC scan of patient with a typical carcinoid of the left lung (not shown). Existing liver metastasis were rather difficult to discern on the portal phase of CT **(A)**, but Ga-68 DOTATOC PET proved to be a valuable adjunct to establish the liver lesion **(B,C)**. Misalignment of PET and CT caused by breathing introduced attenuation artifacts and caused erroneous projection of the liver metastasis in the base of the right lung on attenuation-corrected (AC) PET images **(B)**. Therefore, non-AC images (which do not harbor these artifacts) should always be reviewed **(C)**.

processes such as blood flow ($H_2{}^{15}O$), hypoxia (^{18}F-MISO), DNA synthesis (^{18}F-fluorothymidine [FLT]), and somatostatin receptor expression (Ga-68 DOTATOC). Certainly, with the rapid development of molecular-targeted treatments, noninvasive assessment of metabolic processes will become increasingly important to assess efficacy of these drugs. However, in the succeeding text, PET always refers to FDG-PET, unless otherwise specified. It summarizes the standard indications, other applications, and innovative use of this imaging technique (Table 27.1).

Interpretation of PET Images

If the aim of the PET study is just to stage the patient, visual analysis of non–attenuation-corrected images (i.e., hot spots higher than background activity being regarded positive for tumor) is probably just as good as SUV images, as has been pointed out by different prospective studies, both for the discrimination of nodules as well as for the evaluation of mediastinal involvement.[7]

There is a low degree of physiologic uptake of FDG in thoracic structures, including the lung, the heart, the aorta and large arteries, esophagus, thymus, trachea, thoracic muscles, bone marrow, and joints and soft tissues. This low background tracer activity builds the image contour. The high degree of FDG uptake in the brain and the excretory system impedes sensitive detection in these organs.

False-negative results may be lesion or technique dependent (Table 27.2). A critical mass of metabolically active malignant cells is required for PET detection.[8] Interpretation should be careful in tumors with decreased FDG uptake such as very well-differentiated adenocarcinoma, bronchioloalveolar carcinoma, or carcinoid tumors. FDG-avid lesions smaller than 5 mm may be false negative because of the limitations in spatial resolution of the PET scanner and partial volume effects in small lesions. In the lower lung fields, the detection limit may even go up to 10 mm as a result of additional respiratory motion. Factors inherent to the technique are paravenous FDG injection or high-baseline glucose serum levels. Blood glucose levels should be checked, and it is advised to proceed only if the glucose level is within a normal range prior to tracer injection. Although diabetic patients were often excluded

TABLE 27.1 Applications of FDG–PET Scan in Lung Cancer

Diagnosis of Pulmonary Nodules and Masses
Differentiation of malignant vs. benign nodules
Reduce the need of unwanted invasive procedures
Aid in decision algorithms
False positives
Inflammatory respiratory disorders
False negatives
Small tumors (<8–10 mm)
Tumors with low glucose metabolism
Mediastinal LN staging
High negative predictive value for LN metastasis
Reduce the number of invasive tests, without loss of accuracy
Better guidance of invasive procedures
False positives
Inflammatory LNs
False negatives
Low FDG uptake in primary tumor
LNs obscured by centrally located tumors or hilar nodes
Extrathoracic Staging
Complement to conventional imaging
Detection of unexpected metastasis
Characterization of equivocal lesions
False positives
Inflammatory lesions
Second primary tumor
False negatives
Low FDG uptake in primary tumor
Small metastatic deposits
Other Applications
Prognosis (independent from TNM stage)
Early response evaluation during chemotherapy
Reassessment after induction treatment
Planning of radiotherapy
Diagnosis of recurrence after radical therapy
Selective use in lung cancer screening
Innovative Indications
Use of tracers other than FDG
Improvements in PET/CT cameras
Response evaluation in molecular therapy

TABLE 27.2 Caveats in the Interpretation of PET in Lung Cancer Patients

Causes of False-Negative Findings
Lesion dependent
Small tumors (<8–10 mm)
Ground-glass opacity neoplasms (BAC)
Carcinoid tumors
Technique dependent
Hyperglycemia
Paravenous FDG injection
Excessive time between injection and scanning
Causes of False-Positive Findings
Infectious/Inflammatory lesions
(Postobstructive) pneumonia/abscess
Mycobacterial or fungal infection
Granulomatous disorders (sarcoidosis, Wegener)
Chronic nonspecific lymphadenitis
(Rheumatoid) arthritis
Occupational exposure (anthracosilicosis)
Bronchiectasis
Organizing pneumonia
Reflux esophagitis
Iatrogenic causes
Invasive procedure (puncture, biopsy)
Talc pleurodesis
Radiation esophagitis and pneumonitis
Bone marrow expansion postchemotherapy
Colony-stimulating factors
Thymic hyperplasia postchemotherapy
Benign mass lesions
Salivary gland adenoma (Whartin)
Thyroid adenoma
Adrenal adenoma
Colorectal dysplastic polyps
Focal physiological FDG uptake
Gastrointestinal tract
Muscle activity
Brown fat
Unilateral vocal cord activity
Atherosclerotic plaques

BAC, bronchioloalveolar cell carcinoma.

in prospective studies, FDG uptake is probably not significantly influenced in these patients if the blood glucose levels are reasonably controlled.

False-positive findings are a result of the fact that FDG uptake is not tumor specific, and can be found in all active tissues with high glucose metabolism, in particular inflammation (Table 27.2). Therefore, clinically relevant FDG-positive findings, especially if isolated and decisive for patient management, require confirmation. The differentiation between metastasis, a benign or inflammatory lesion, or even an unrelated second malignancy should be made by other tests or tissue diagnosis. The major causes of false-positive results in lung patients are infectious, inflammatory and granulomatous disorders, and iatrogenic procedures, such as thoracocentesis, placement of a chest tube, percutaneous needle biopsy, mediastinoscopy, and talc pleurodesis.

Diagnosis of Pulmonary Nodules and Masses

Peripheral solitary pulmonary nodules (SPNs) represent a diagnostic challenge, especially if they are noncalcified. With the increased interest in the use of low-dose spiral CT for early lung cancer detection, the number of coincidental SPNs will only increase.

Multiple studies—often using a threshold maximum SUV (SUV_{max}) of >2.5 for the diagnosis of malignancy—have proven the accuracy of PET in the differentiation of malignant from benign lesions (Fig. 27.2). In a metaanalysis, based on series with nearly all nodules larger than 1 cm, an overall sensitivity, specificity, positive and negative predictive value of 96%, 78%, 91%, and 92% was reported.[9]

False-negative findings may occur if a critical mass of metabolic active cells for detection on PET is not in place; therefore, exclusion of malignancy is more hazardous in small lesions.[10] In that respect, the use of the SUV_{max} threshold of >2.5 should better be abandoned, because quite some lesions with SUV_{max} ≤2.5 are malignant.[11] A large prospective series (n = 585) looked at the accuracy of integrated PET/CT scan in SPNs ≤2.5 cm.[12] If the SUV_{max} was between 0 and 2.5, there was a 24% chance of malignancy; if between 2.6 and 4.0, it was 80%; and if >4, it was 96%. Likewise, the accuracy of PET is also challenged in small nodules detected in lung cancer screening studies.[13] Nonetheless, selective use of PET was reported to be useful in some series,[14–16] but with more limitations than in the daily practice population presenting with SPNs.

False-negative images are also common in tumors with low metabolic activity, bronchioloalveolar cell carcinomas in particular,[17,18] because they have significantly lower expression of the glucose transporter Glut-1 compared with other non–small cell lung cancer (NSCLC) subtypes.[19] Carcinoid tumors also have a low FDG uptake,[20,21] but the presence of somatostatin receptors in these neuroendocrine tumors allows PET imaging with radiolabeled somatostatine analogues, such as Ga-68-DOTATOC[22] (Fig. 27.1).

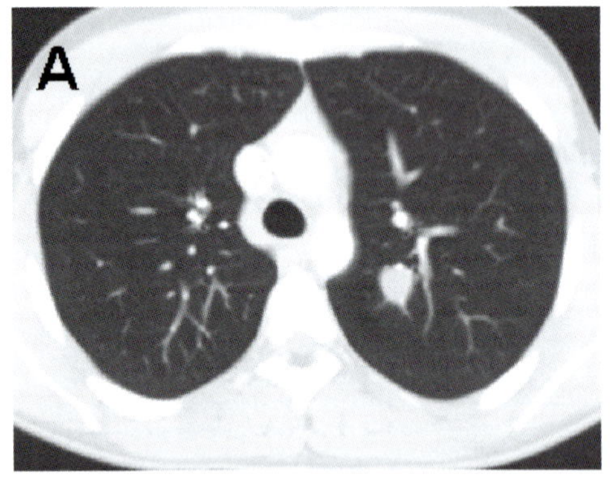

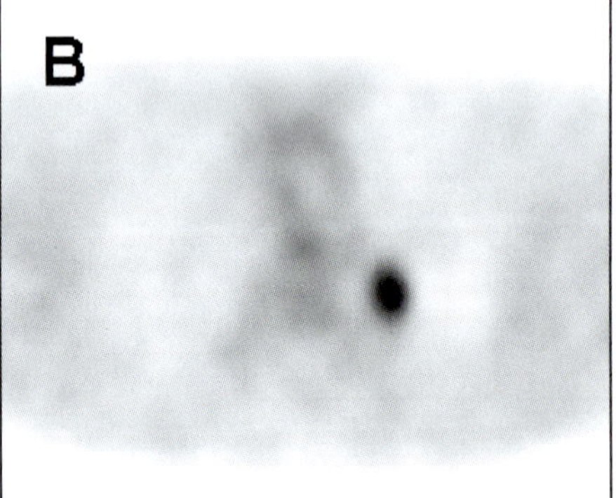

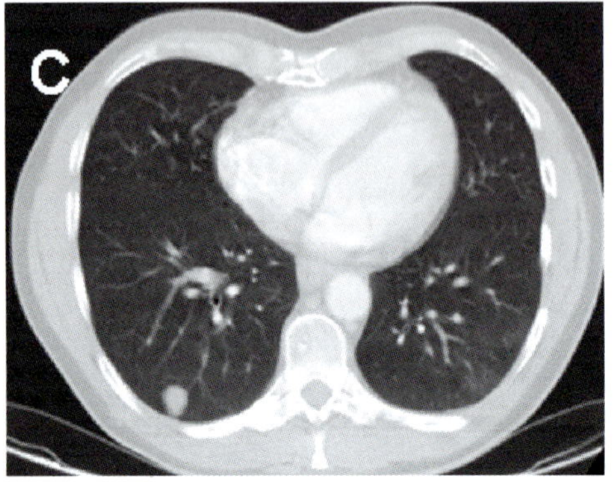

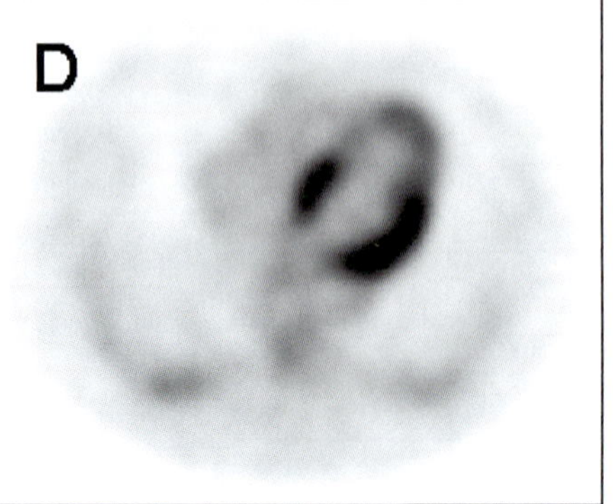

FIGURE 27.2 Solitary pulmonary nodule in the left upper lobe **(A)**, with clear FDG uptake on PET **(B)**. Surgery revealed pT1N0 adenocarcinoma. Solitary nodule in the right upper lobe **(C)**, no uptake higher than lung background on PET **(D)**. No change during follow-up, probably hamartoma.

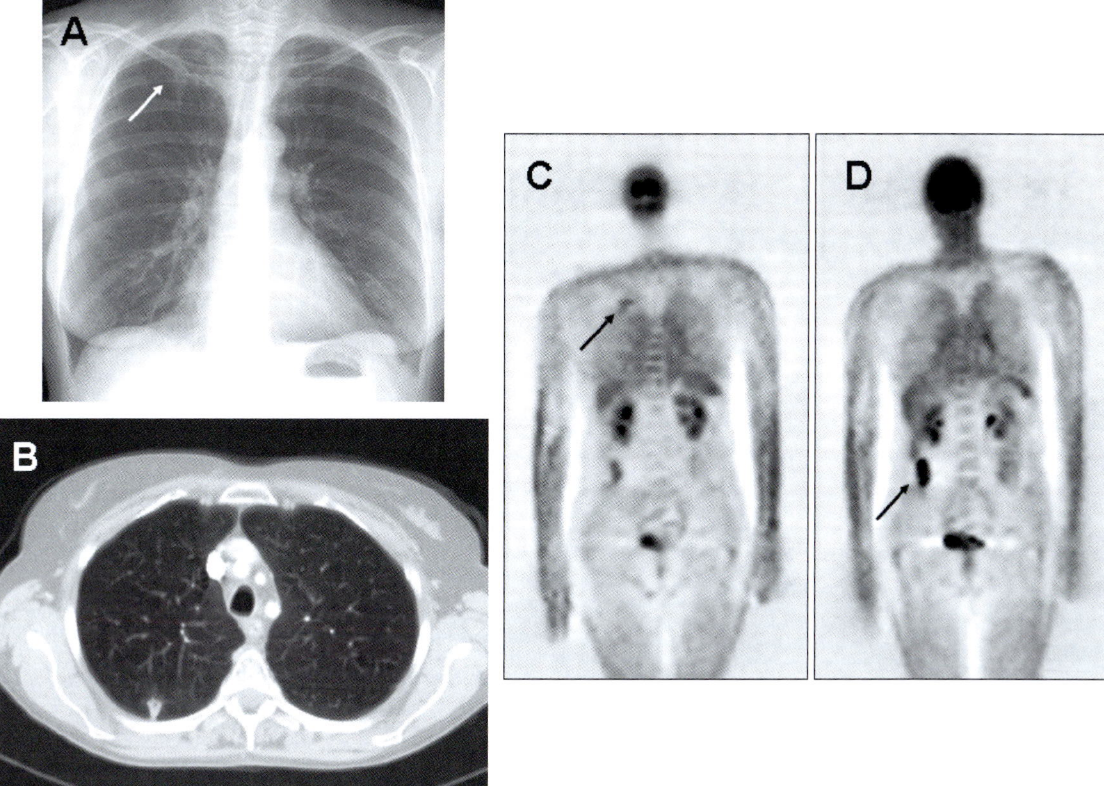

FIGURE 27.3 A 54-year-old woman in follow-up after radical radiotherapy for right vocal cord squamous cell carcinoma. Detection of a nodule in the right upper lobe on chest radiograph **(A)**, confirmed at CT scan **(B)**. PET showed some FDG avidity in the lesion **(C)**, and in addition, a prominent FDG-positive lesion in the right hemicolon **(D)**. Further studies pointed at postradiotherapy inflammation in the right lung and adenocarcinoma of the ascending colon.

False positives occur because of trapping of FDG in activated granulocytes and/or macrophages in several inflammatory conditions[23–25] (Fig. 27.3), and this leads to a variable specificity (50% to 100%) in different series, according to the prevalence of certain inflammatory or infectious diseases, such as tuberculosis or histoplasmosis. A nice pictorial overview of false-positive findings is given in Shim et al.[26] In special situations, specificity can be improved by looking at the FDG uptake kinetics using dual-time–point imaging at 1 and 2 hours (FDG continued uptake in malignant versus rapid uptake followed by washout in benign lesions).[27]

Lung Cancer Staging CT, with its excellent anatomic detail, remains the method of choice to assess the *T-factor*, that is, the extent of the primary tumor in relation to lung fissures, mediastinal structures, pleura, or chest wall. PET on its own has little to add to the accuracy of CT because of its lower spatial resolution.[28] For the *N-factor*, one of the main limitations of CT—using only a size criterion—is its low accuracy in differentiating benign from malignant lymph nodes (LNs).[29,30] Since about a decade, PET imaging—with its metabolic information—was proven to be superior,[31,32] a finding confirmed in different meta-analyses based on a multitude of prospective studies.[33–35] PET on its own is more accurate, but is still not perfect in defining the N-status. Lack of anatomical detail is one important reason, for example, PET images often do not allow to distinguish hilar from mediastinal LNs (Fig. 27.4), or to exclude LNs in patients with a large centrally located tumor. Many well-designed prospective studies also demonstrated a gain in accuracy in the *M-factor*, mainly because PET is able to detect additional metastatic lesions in 5% to 25% of the patients.[36–45] There is a substantial variation in the proportion of patients with additional lesions, because authors differ in the definitions of "unexpected" lesions; in most series, an equivocal lesion on conventional imaging, found to be metastatic on PET, was not regarded as unexpected, although this was the case in some series.[37,40] If PET helps to characterize equivocal lesions, this is usually for adrenal lesions, contralateral lung nodules, or bone scintigraphy abnormalities.[36–38,40]

Nowadays, the best combination of morphologic and metabolic information is obtained by integrated PET/CT

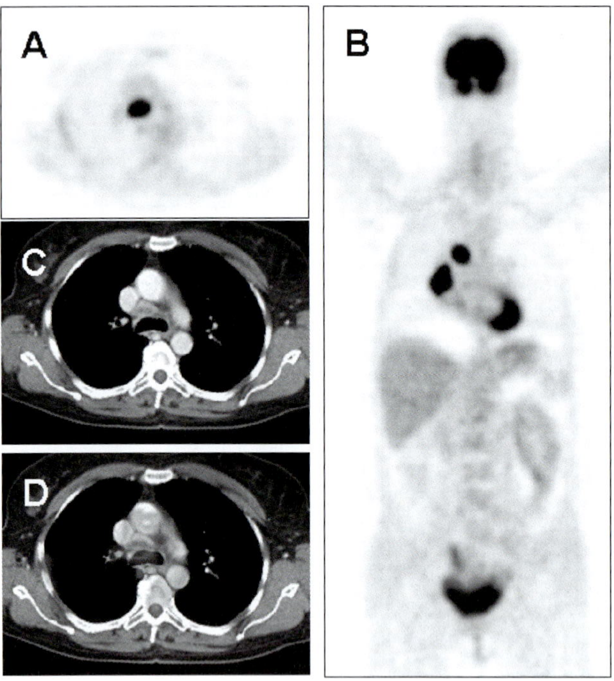

FIGURE 27.4 Transaxial **(A)** and coronal **(B)** PET images with a right lung tumor and accompanying adenopathy, either in the right hilar or mediastinal station. On CT, there is a suspect LN **(C)**, on integrated PET/CT, right paratracheal adenopathy is confirmed **(D)**. (See color plate.)

scanners. Comparative results for the *T-factor* are listed in Table 27.3. Comparisons are often made with PET alone or with PET images in visual correlation with CT images. Although the first comparison may be of scientific interest, it is of little clinical relevance. Papers in the late 1990s already pointed out that interpretation of PET images in visual correlation with CT images was the minimum standard.[31,46] Three studies reported better results with PET/CT in comparison with PET alone.[47–49] This superiority can be assigned to the CT component of this examination because of poor performance of PET alone in measuring tumor size or assessing potential infiltration of adjacent structures. The integrated images allow more precise evaluation of chest wall and mediastinal infiltration in some patients, and better differentiation between tumor and accompanying inflammation or atelectasis in others. In the Zurich group report, there was a benefit in comparison with side-by-side reading of PET and CT images as well, which was not in the place in the Leuven experience.[50] Results for the *N-factor* display a similar picture (Table 27.4), with PET/CT superior to PET alone. Accurate anatomic correlation allows exact location of involved nodes, and thus better distinction between N1, N2, and N3. Furthermore, the role of PET/CT in identifying supraclavicular N3 nodes and in the distinction between FDG-avid brown fat and a metastatic LN is indisputable[47–49] (Fig. 27.5). Here again, in the study of the Zurich group, PET/CT was superior to visual comparison, but the accuracy of the latter in this study was unexpectedly low at 59%.[47] In the Leuven experience, there was little difference between integrated and visually compared imaging,[50] confirming a similar previous experience with software fusion.[51] Finally, for the *M-factor*, only a few results are available. In a large retrospective study, there was a significant superiority of PET/CT versus PET alone or CT alone, but not versus side-to-side correlation.[28]

There are far less data on the use of PET or PET/CT in small cell lung cancer (SCLC), probably because it is far less frequent, and because the disease is often disseminated at the time of diagnosis.[52] The most relevant question is the distinction between limited disease (LD) and extensive disease (ED).

One prospective study examined how often PET detects ED SCLC in patients considered to have LD based on conventional staging.[53] PET correctly upstaged 2 of 24 patients (8%) to ED. PET also correctly depicted all tumor sites in the primary mass and nodal stations. PET impacted on the radiotherapy planning because of detection of unsuspected locoregional

TABLE 27.3 Comparative Data on PET/CT regarding T-Stage

Study	Year	N	Imaging	Accuracy (%)	*p* Value
Lardinois et al.[47]	2003	50	PET	40	0.013
			PET and CT	65	
			PET/CT	88	
Cerfolio et al.[48]	2004	129	PET	47	0.001
			PET/CT	64	
Halpern et al.[49]	2005	36	PET	67	0.01
			PET/CT	97	
De Wever et al.[50]	2007	50	PET and CT	72	NS
			PET/CT	86	

NS, non significant; PET/CT, integrated PET and CT scan; PET and CT, side-to-side comparison of PET and CT images.

TABLE 27.4 Comparative Data on PET/CT regarding N-Stage

Study	Year	N	Imaging	Accuracy (%)	p Value
Lardinois et al.[47]	2003	50	PET	49	0.021
			PET and CT	59	
			PET/CT	81	
Cerfolio et al.[48]	2004	129	PET	56	0.008
			PET/CT	78	
Halpern et al.[49]	2005	36	PET	69	NS
			PET/CT	78	
De Wever et al.[50]	2007	50	PET and CT	80	NS
			PET/CT	84	

NS, non significant; PET/CT, integrated PET and CT scan; PET and CT, side-to-side comparison of PET and CT images.

LN metastasis in 6 of 24 patients. In the largest study to date, a total of 91 SCLC patients underwent conventional staging (including cranial magnetic resonance imaging [MRI] or CT) and PET.[54] In 14 patients, PET caused a stage migration, correctly upstaging 10 patients (11%) to ED and downstaging three patients to LD. PET was significantly superior to CT in the detection of extrathoracic metastases except for the brain. In a recent prospective study with 29 patients, a correct overall change in stage in 10% of the patients was noted with PET/CT, in comparison with staging by means of CT, bone scintigraphy and bone marrow analysis.[55] Interestingly, these authors reported similar results in staging of bone metastases and bone marrow invasion with PET/CT in comparison with bone scintigraphy and bone marrow biopsy. Despite the fact that there is less evidence in SCLC compared with NSCLC, it seems fair to say that about 10% of patients with LD will have their staging upgraded to ED when PET is used, because lesions that may escape standard clinical examination and conventional imaging are detected on whole-body PET/CT imaging (Fig. 27.6).

Prognostic Value Apart from the TNM stage at diagnosis, the classical prognostic factor for NSCLC patient groups, metabolic imaging using the FDG uptake expressed as SUV_{max} was reported to have prognostic value for the individual patient as well. Several retrospective studies—mostly in operable NSCLC patients—demonstrated that survival was significantly better in patients with a tumor of lower metabolic activity (i.e., below the study-specific cutoff value or below the median value),[56–65] and this was confirmed in a recent literature-based metaanalysis.[66] Recently, one retrospective[67] and one prospective study[68] argued that tumor FDG uptake did not provide additional prognostic information apart from

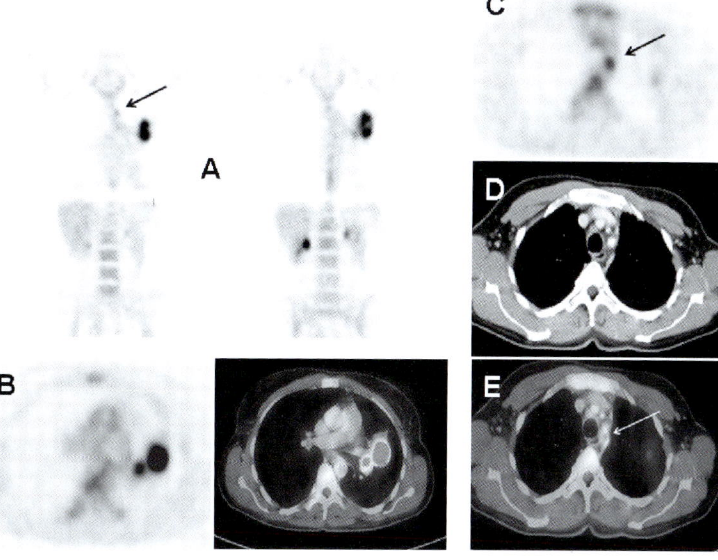

FIGURE 27.5 PET/CT in a patient with squamous cell carcinoma of the left upper lobe. FDG uptake is present in the primary tumor and an adjacent hilar LN **(A,B)**. PET also shows a focal hot spot suspected for N2 disease in level 2L (**A,C** *arrow*). PET/CT fusion images project the hot spot in brown fat tissue **(D,E)**. At thoracotomy with LN, dissection confirmed the absence of mediastinal involvement (pT2N1). (See color plate.)

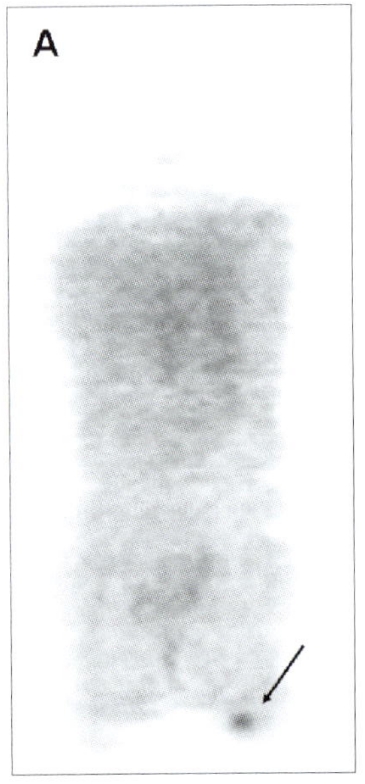

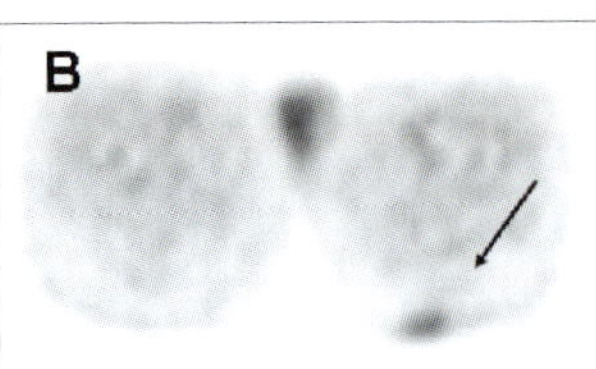

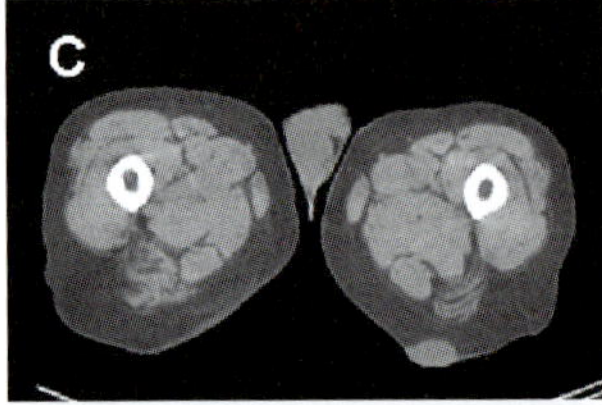

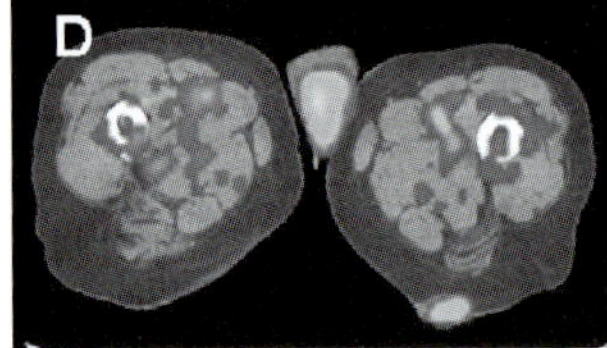

FIGURE 27.6 Patient with limited disease SCLC on conventional staging, with unexpected lesion in the left thigh on PET **(A,B)**, and on accompanying CT and PET/CT images **(C,D)**. Biopsy confirmed subcutaneous SCLC metastasis. (See color plate.)

pathologic TNM stage in multivariate analysis. Further studies and individual patient-based metaanalysis are needed to clarify the prognostic role of PET, taking into account methodological issues such as the intercenter reproducibility of the PET acquisition protocol and SUV measurement (such as max or mean). A survival analysis using a stage-specific median SUV_{max} cutoff significantly correlated with long-term overall survival for stage IB, stage II, and stage IIIA (median SUV_{max} of 10, 13, and 14, respectively).[63] Whether PET could be of help in deciding on adjuvant chemotherapy for early stage resected NSCLC is a challenging question that deserves further research.

Evaluation of Therapy Quantitative changes in tumor metabolism on PET during or after completion of chemo(radio)therapy have been studied in different settings.[69,70]

Two small prospective studies reported on the use of PET to predict clinical outcome of chemotherapy at an early stage of treatment in patients with advanced NSCLC. In one series, a predefined decrease in SUV_{max} of >20% after one cycle of cisplatin-based chemotherapy significantly correlated with prognosis.[71] In the other, a reduction of SUV_{max} by >30% also significantly correlated with survival.[72] The broader application of PET response to clinical practice—as is the case for serial CT in the Response Evaluation Criteria in Solid Tumors (RECIST) system—is hampered by technical and methodological differences between different PET cameras and centers. Although serial FDG-PET on one single camera is valid for treatment monitoring, much more work is still needed to align acquisition and interpretation of SUV data across centers.

More data are available on the use of PET in surgical combined modality treatment for stage III NSCLC.[73–82] Factors associated with good prognosis after induction treatment and surgical resection for stage IIIA-N2 are complete resection, downstaging of mediastinal LNs, and the degree of pathologic response in the primary tumor. These factors are poorly predicted by CT, and classically only available after resection. More than a decade ago, a prospective pilot study reported that the combination of LN downstaging on PET and an SUV_{max} decrease of >50% in the primary tumor after neoadjuvant chemotherapy for stage IIIA-N2 NSCLC significantly predicted a better outcome.[83] Since then, many studies have addressed the value of PET and PET/CT in assessment of LN downstaging, estimation of pathologic response, and relation of these findings with survival outcome.

Results for mediastinal LN restaging are listed in Table 27.5. Again, these studies differ in methodological aspects, such as type of induction (chemotherapy or chemoradiotherapy), timing of imaging (interval 3 to 4 weeks, straight after, or at a variable

TABLE 27.5 Results of PET and Integrated PET/CT in Mediastinal Lymph Node Restaging after Induction Treatment for Locally Advanced NSCLC

Study	Year	N	Stage	CTRT	Imaging	Sensitivity	Specificity
Vansteenkiste et al.[73]	2001	31	IIIA-N2	0%	PET and CT	71%	88%
Akhurst et al.[74]	2002	56	I–III	29%	PET and CT	67%	61%
Ryu et al.[75]	2002	26	III	100%	PET and CT	58%	93%
Cerfolio et al.[76]	2003	34	IB–IIIA	21%	PET and CT	50%	99%
Hellwig et al.[77]	2004	37	III	70%	PET and CT	50%	88%
Port et al.[78]	2004	25	I–IIIA	0%	PET and CT	20%	71%
Hoekstra et al.[79]	2005	25	IIIA-N2	0%	PET and CT	50%	71%
Cerfolio et al.[80]	2006	93	IIIA-N2	100%	PET/CT	62%	88%
Pottgen et al.[81]	2006	37	IIIA/B	100%	PET/CT	73%	89%
De Leyn et al.[82]	2006	30	IIIA-N2	0%	PET/CT	77%	92%

CTRT, % patients with chemoradiotherapy; PET/CT, integrated PET and CT scan; PET and CT, side-to-side comparison of PET and CT images.

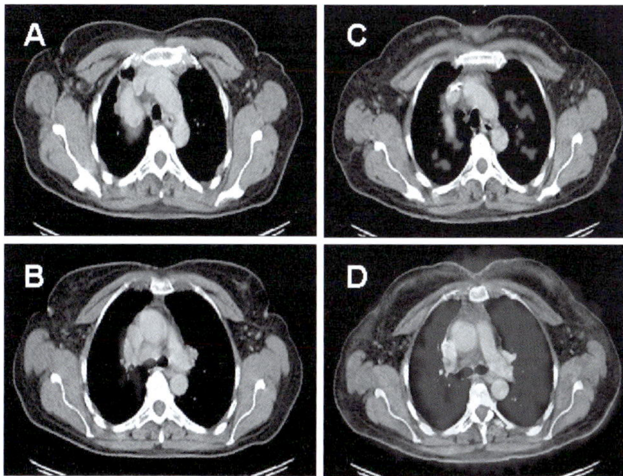

FIGURE 27.7 Right upper lobe large cell carcinoma **(A)** with right hilar and paratracheal adenopathy **(B)**, both clearly FDG avid on PET/CT fusion images. After induction chemotherapy, a major decrease in the metabolic activity of the primary tumor **(C)** and absence of FDG uptake in the mediastinum **(D)** is noted. Patient underwent complete resection, pT1N0. (See color plate.)

interval 4 to 10 weeks after neoadjuvant therapy, respectively), and interpretation of imaging (visual correlation with CT or integrated PET/CT). Nonetheless, it is clear that the sensitivity and specificity are lower than for baseline LN staging, but better if studies with PET/CT are considered.

A unique feature of repeat PET after induction is that it assesses not only mediastinal nodes but response in the primary tumor as well (Fig. 27.7). The earliest studies reported a sensitivity of 81% to 97% and a specificity of 64% to 67% to predict a pathological complete response on PET after neoadjuvant therapy.[74–77] Other studies used the percentage change in the SUV_{max} on PET before and after neoadjuvant therapy, and described a strong but imperfect correlation between this decrease and the residual amount of viable tumor in the resection specimen.[77,80,81]

Several recent studies also confirmed the relevance of changes on PET for survival outcome. In one study, a cutoff value of 60% decrease in SUV_{max} after induction chemotherapy was a significant predictor of 5-year survival (60% vs. 15%; $p = 0.0007$).[84] The picture was less clear for repeat PET after neoadjuvant chemoradiotherapy ($p = 0.02$), mainly because the chemoradiotherapy caused no further decrease in SUV_{max}, and because the repeat PET was performed too early (days) after the last dose of radiation therapy. The optimal interval for scanning after induction was recently suggested to be 4 weeks after the last radiotherapy dose.[85] One study even found that the residual glucose metabolic rate after one single cycle of induction chemotherapy provided a statistically significant prediction of outcome.[79]

In a recent paper, a prognostic stratification model, based on the combination of pathologic response in mediastinal nodes and primary tumor response on serial PET was presented, in an attempt to refine the decision regarding which patients are candidate for surgery after induction therapy for stage IIIA-N2 NSCLC.[86]

Planning of Radiotherapy Although most of the PET studies on locoregional extension of NSCLC were performed in a preoperative setting—in order to have histological verification of the findings—the use of this technique is of equivalent importance in patients scheduled for radiotherapy. Accurate noninvasive PET staging of the tumor and nodes not only influences the treatment intention (i.e., curative or palliative),[87] but also the volumes to be treated, and therefore may reduce the chances of geographic miss[88] or decrease the risk of toxicity to be expected. Classical radiotherapy planning uses CT to describe the tumor and nodes and to draw the gross tumor volume (GTV). The main limitations are the poor demarcation of some tumors on CT, especially in the presence of atelectasis, and poor accuracy of CT in distinguishing benign and malignant LNs.

A simulation study based on 105 NSCLC patients with surgery verified PET findings looked at the impact on GTV when adding PET information to CT.[89] For 73 of these patients, with positive nodes on CT and/or on PET, the completeness of tumor coverage by the CT-GTV and PET-GTV was calculated, using the available surgical pathology data as gold standard. Tumor coverage improved from 75% with CT to 89% with PET ($p = 0.0005$). In one study, the PET-GTV was actually used for planning radiation fields, and only 1 of 44 patients developed an isolated nodal recurrence.[90]

PET, and especially integrated PET/CT, also alters the GTV by a better discrimination between tumor and peritumoral atelectasis or necrosis (Fig. 27.8),[91,92] thereby reducing the interobserver variability in tumor delineation.[93]

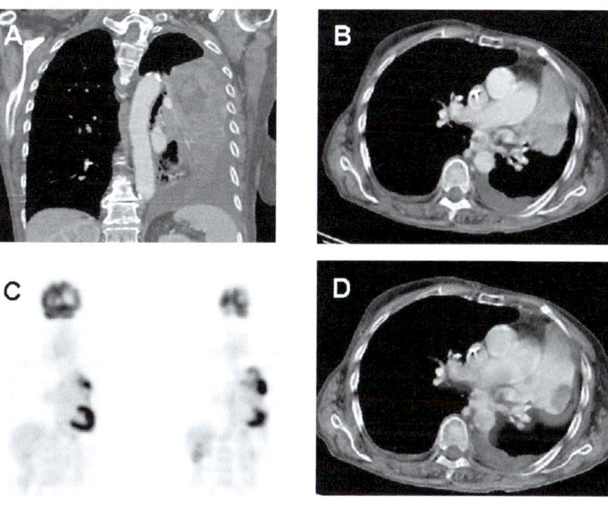

FIGURE 27.8 Patient with a squamous cell carcinoma in the left hilum (cT3N3) with atelectasis of the left upper lobe resulting in a shift of heart and mediastinum **(A,B)**. For a better discrimination of atelectasis and tumor, PET/CT was performed to optimize radiation treatment planning **(C, D)**. (See color plate.)

A major remaining issue for improvement is the optimal tumor contouring by PET, depending on the size of the tumor and the tumor-to-background ratio,[94,95] and on respiratory motion as PET images—acquired over several minutes during free breathing—result in enlargement of the metabolic lesion in the axis of the respiratory movement. For the latter, respiratory gating techniques should be implemented.[96] Finally, future prospective comparative studies should ascertain that use of PET/CT in radiation treatment planning will actually result in reduced toxicity, better local control, and increased survival.

Follow-up after Therapy How to follow patients after a radical primary treatment is a matter of debate, as re-treatment after radical surgery, radiotherapy or combined modality treatment may be rewarding in selected cases. Three prospective studies correlated a repeat PET scan performed "late" after primary treatment at >6 months, at median 8 months, and at 19 months, respectively, to a long-term clinical follow-up of median 19, 34, and 30 months, respectively.[97–99] A significantly better long-term outcome was found for patients with a negative compared with positive late repeat PET scan. In patients with confirmed relapse, the long-term survival rate was significantly better for patients with a cutoff for FDG uptake below the median SUV_{max}.[99]

After radical surgery or radiotherapy, it can be difficult to differentiate therapy-induced fibrosis from tumor on conventional imaging. In this situation, PET was able to correctly confirm or exclude disease relapse in an indeterminate lesion on CT scan with a sensitivity of 97% to 100%, a specificity of 62% to 100%, and an accuracy of 78% to 98%.[98,100]

Impact on Clinical Practice and Recommendations

A large number of different types of accuracy studies—summarized in metaanalyses—have confirmed that assessment of an SPN, mediastinal staging, and detection of extrathoracic metastases are improved by PET in combination with CT compared with CT alone.[9,33] How should this improved test performance be implemented in patient management?

In the evaluation of SPNs, PET should be seen in conjunction with the pretest probability of malignancy, judged according to clinical experience either based on factors such as review of previous radiographs, age, smoking habits, size, and aspect of the lesions on radiological documents or based on a validated calculator model.[101] PET will be most contributive in SPNs with intermediate (5% to 60%) probability of malignancy.[102] For lesions of at least 8 to 10 mm in diameter, the negative predictive value of PET is high. If such a lesion does not show any FDG uptake higher than the surrounding lung parenchyma (thus not using an SUV threshold for interpretation), follow-up with serial CT scans—repeated at months 3, 6, 12, and 24 months—is an acceptable strategy.[10] False negatives can occur in lesions smaller than 1 cm and in ground-glass opacities.

If the SPN is FDG avid, histological exploration by transthoracic needle biopsy, endobronchial ultrasound-guided bronchoscopy, or thoracoscopic wedge excision is recommended, unless there is evidence for a specific benign etiology such as tuberculosis, sarcoidosis, etc.

Patients with NSCLC, considered for treatment with curative intent, benefit from PET scanning for mediastinal and extrathoracic staging.

Patients with a clinical stage I tumor and negative mediastinal PET findings can proceed to direct surgical resection, on the condition that the primary tumor is not centrally located and that there is no major hilar LN involvement (which may obscure mediastinal LN disease on PET), and that the primary tumor is sufficiently FDG avid (thereby avoiding false-negative LN findings).[103] Patients with mediastinal LN enlargement on CT preferably have invasive confirmation of the LN status (by either esophageal or endobronchial ultrasound aspiration or mediastinoscopy, depending on local expertise),[104] as their pretest probability of LN metastases is higher.[105]

Patients with extensive or bulky mediastinal LN infiltration, do not really need PET to assess LNs, but PET is nonetheless useful because it will quite often detect distant metastatic findings undetected at conventional imaging, with a major impact on treatment intent.[44]

Because PET detects additional metastatic lesions and characterizes lesions left equivocal on CT, its use in clinical studies resulted in stage shift from the one determined by conventional imaging in 27% to as high as 62% of the patients with NSCLC and a change in patient management in 25% to even 52% of the patients.[37,39,43,106–108] Multiple intense abnormal foci in different organs usually point at disseminated disease (Fig. 27.9). However, patients should not be excluded from potentially radical treatment based on isolated abnormal finding on PET suggestive for distant metastasis. In these instances, additional confirmation by other imaging procedures or by tissue confirmation should be sought, to rule out a false-positive finding (Fig. 27.10), or a second primary tumor not affecting the stage of the lung cancer[109] (Fig. 27.3).

This clinical trial experience was confirmed in questionnaires and surveys in broader clinical practice.[110–112]

The additive value of PET was also investigated through comparing implementation of PET added to conventional staging compared with the conventional process alone in randomized controlled trials. One trial randomly allocated 188 clinical stage I to III NSCLC patients to either conventional workup

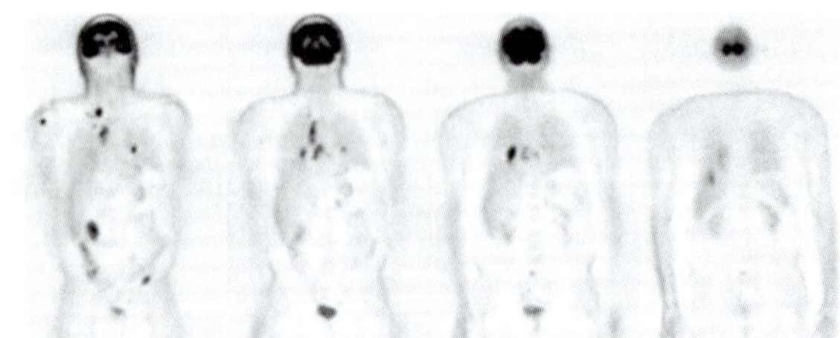

FIGURE 27.9 Patient with a large cell carcinoma of the right lower lobe with N3 mediastinal LN spread and multifocal metastatic disease (bone, contralateral lung, abdominal LNs, and bilateral adrenal metastases).

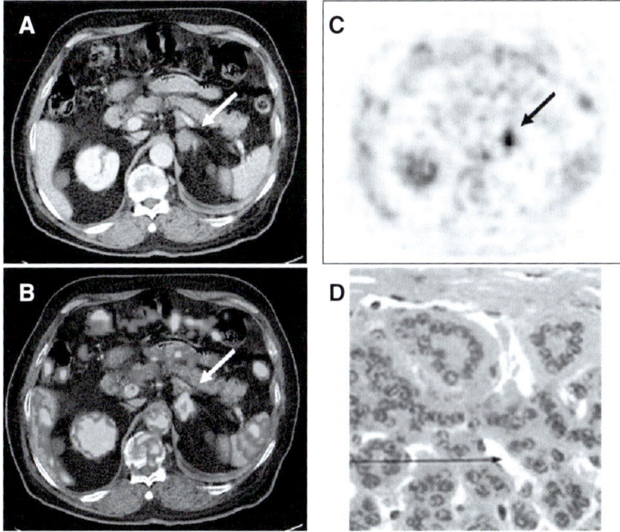

FIGURE 27.10 Patient with left upper lobe adenocarcinoma (not shown) and abnormal left adrenal gland on CT **(A)**, PET **(C)**, and fusion image **(B)**. Needle aspiration biopsy revealed normal cortical adrenal tissue **(D)**. No change in the adrenal gland during follow-up postlobectomy. (See color plate.)

or conventional workup plus PET.[113] A clear reduction in the number of futile surgical procedures in the latter arm was found: five patients needed a PET to prevent one futile surgery. A similar trial in clinical stage I to II patients revealed no difference between a PET-guided or conventional strategy.[114] As with therapeutic interventions, multiple trials should be performed to provide a valid estimation of the effect.

Another prospective randomized study compared staging with upfront PET (i.e., directly after first presentation) versus routine clinical staging in 465 patients.[115] In this study, patients with FDG avid, noncentrally located tumors without signs of mediastinal or distant spread on PET proceeded directly to surgical resection, without conventional staging tests. Quality of staging was measured by comparison of the clinical stage with the final stage, and was similarly good in both arms. Noninvasive tests to reach a clinical TNM were similar in both arms, but invasive tests (i.e., mainly mediastinoscopy) were significantly less needed in the upfront PET group.

Future Technical Developments FDG-PET allows excellent discrimination between normal tissues and tissues with enhanced glucose metabolism, but false-positive uptake of FDG in inflammatory tissues is one of the major limitations of this tracer. Therefore, tracers with an equally high sensitivity but a better specificity are in the focus of ongoing research, but none have shown a clear improvement over FDG at this time in clinical lung cancer imaging. Results with ^{11}C-methionine, a marker of protein metabolism,[116,117] and ^{11}C-choline, a component of phospholipids in the cell membrane,[118] were disappointing. The most exciting new tracer is the thymidine analogue FLT, a marker of cell proliferation.[119] Although FLT itself is not incorporated in DNA, FLT uptake is cycle dependent because trapping occurs only after phosphorylation by cytosolic thymidine kinase-1 activity, an enzyme only functional in the S phase of the cell cycle. In the differentiation of SPNs, FLT proved to be more specific than FDG, although false-positive uptake is also described in acute infections.[120–122] Because the absolute uptake of FLT uptake is usually lower than FDG, especially in slowly proliferating tumors, the sensitivity of FLT-PET is reduced. In one study, the sensitivity on a lesion-by-lesion analysis was only 58%, compared with 79% for FDG-PET.[121] Therefore, FLT-PET will never replace but rather be complementary to FDG-PET in special situations of SPNs. Furthermore, a whole new field using PET is molecular imaging in order to study cellular functions such as receptors, transport proteins, or intracellular enzymes. These results are eagerly awaited, as targeted agents are the emerging new treatments for lung cancer, and targeting these expensive drugs by proper selection of patients by predictive markers is a key question.

With the advent of integrated PET and multislice spiral CT, the hardware for lung cancer imaging has actually come to a high technical standard. Future expectations are a further decrease of the spatial resolution of PET cameras to as low as 2 mm, which will probably be the limit of this technique, as the emitted photons are emitted with some scatter and with a slight deviation from the 180-degree angle of the detectors.

Another feature that could improve the quality of the images, especially in respiratory medicine, is respiratory gating of PET acquisition. Because of respiratory motion, the volume of a lung lesion is smeared out and thus overestimated, whereas the FDG intensity is underestimated, especially in the lower lung fields. Synchronization of the acquisition of the PET emission images with respiratory motion may overcome this problem.

REFERENCES

1. Pauwels EK, McCready VR, Stoot JH, et al. The mechanism of accumulation of tumour-localising radiopharmaceuticals. *Eur J Nucl Med* 1998;25:277–305.
2. Shreve PD, Anzai Y, Wahl RL. Pitfalls in oncologic diagnosis with FDG PET imaging: physiologic and benign variants. *Radiographics* 1999;19:61–77.
3. Higashi K, Clavo AC, Wahl RL. Does FDG uptake measure proliferative activity of human cancer cells? In vitro comparison with DNA flow cytometry and titrated thymidine uptake. *J Nucl Med* 1993;34:414–419.
4. Minn H, Joensuu H, Ahonen A, et al. Fluorodeoxyglucose imaging: a method to assess the proliferative activity of human cancer in vivo. Comparison with DNA flow cytometry in head and neck tumors. *Cancer* 1988;61:1776–1781.
5. Spaepen K, Stroobants S, Dupont P, et al. [(18)F]FDG PET monitoring of tumour response to chemotherapy: does [(18)F]FDG uptake correlate with the viable tumour cell fraction? *Eur J Nucl Med Mol Imaging* 2003;30:682–688.
6. Mawlawi O, Pan T, Macapinlac HA. PET/CT imaging techniques, considerations, and artifacts. *J Thorac Imaging* 2006;21:99–110.
7. Vansteenkiste JF. PET scan: current recommendations and innovation. *J Thorac Oncol* 2006;1:71–73.

8. Fischer BM, Olsen MW, Ley CD, et al. How few cancer cells can be detected by positron emission tomography? A frequent question addressed by an in vitro study. *Eur J Nucl Med Mol Imaging* 2006;33:697–702.
9. Gould MK, Maclean CC, Kuschner WG, et al. Accuracy of positron emission tomography for diagnosis of pulmonary nodules and mass lesions: a meta-analysis. *JAMA* 2001;285:914–924.
10. Vansteenkiste JF. Nodules, CT-scans and PET-scans: a good partnership [editorial]. *Lung Cancer* 2004;45:29–30.
11. Vansteenkiste J, Dooms C. Postiron emission tomography in non-small cell lung cancer. *Curr Opin Oncol* 2007;19:78–83.
12. Bryant AS, Cerfolio RJ. The maximum standardized uptake values on integrated FDG-PET/CT is useful in differentiating benign from malignant pulmonary nodules. *Ann Thorac Surg* 2006;82:1016–1020.
13. Dooms C, Vansteenkiste J. Postiron emission tomography in non-small cell lung cancer. *Curr Opin Pulm Med* 2007;13:256–260.
14. Pastorino U, Bellomi M, Landoni C, et al. Early lung-cancer detection with spiral CT and positron emission tomography in heavy smokers: 2-year results. *Lancet* 2003;362:593–597.
15. Lindell RM, Hartman TE, Swensen SJ, et al. Lung cancer screening experience: a retrospective review of PET in 22 non-small cell lung carcinomas detected on screening chest CT in a high-risk population. *AJR Am J Roentgenol* 2005;185:126–131.
16. Bastarrika G, Garcia-Velloso MJ, Lozano MD, et al. Early lung cancer detection using spiral computed tomography and positron emission tomography. *Am J Respir Crit Care Med* 2005;171:1378–1383.
17. Nomori H, Watanabe K, Ohtsuka M, et al. Evaluation of F-18 fluorodeoxyglucose (FDG) PET scanning for pulmonary nodules less than 3 cm in diameter, with special reference to the CT images. *Lung Cancer* 2004;43:19–27.
18. Heyneman LE, Patz EF. PET imaging in patients with bronchioloalveolar cell carcinoma. *Lung Cancer* 2002;38:261–266.
19. Higashi K, Ueda Y, Yagishita M, et al. FDG PET measurement of the proliferative potential of non-small cell lung cancer. *J Nucl Med* 2000;41:85–92.
20. Erasmus JJ, McAdams HP, Patz EF, et al. Evaluation of primary pulmonary carcinoid tumors using FDG PET. *AJR Am J Roentgenol* 1998;170:1369–1373.
21. Belhocine T, Foidart J, Rigo P, et al. Fluorodeoxyglucose positron emission tomography and somatostatin receptor scintigraphy for diagnosing and staging carcinoid tumours: correlations with the pathological indexes p53 and Ki-67. *Nucl Med Commun* 2002;23:727–734.
22. Buchmann I, Henze M, Engelbrecht S, et al. Comparison of 68Ga-DOTATOC PET and 111In-DTPAOC (Octreoscan) SPECT in patients with neuroendocrine tumours. *Eur J Nucl Med Mol Imaging* 2007;34:1617–1626.
23. Bakheet SM, Saleem M, Powe J, et al. F-18 fluorodeoxyglucose chest uptake in lung inflammation and infection. *Clin Nucl Med* 2000;25:273–278.
24. Goo JM, Im JG, Do KH, et al. Pulmonary tuberculoma evaluated by means of FDG PET: findings in 10 cases. *Radiology* 2000;216:117–121.
25. Nishiyama Y, Yamamoto Y, Fukunaga K, et al. Comparative evaluation of 18F-FDG PET and 67Ga scintigraphy in patients with sarcoidosis. *J Nucl Med* 2006;47:1571–1576.
26. Shim SS, Lee KS, Kim BT, et al. Focal parenchymal lung lesions showing a potential of false-positive and false-negative interpretations on integrated PET/CT. *AJR Am J Roentgenol* 2006;186:639–648.
27. Matthies A, Hickeson M, Cuchiara A, et al. Dual time point 18F-FDG PET for the evaluation of pulmonary nodules. *J Nucl Med* 2002;43:871–875.
28. Antoch G, Stattaus J, Nemat AT, et al. Non-small cell lung cancer: dual-modality PET/CT in preoperative staging. *Radiology* 2003;229:526–533.
29. Schrevens L, Lorent N, Dooms C, et al. The role of PET-scan in diagnosis, staging and management of non-small cell lung cancer. *Oncologist* 2004;9:633–643.
30. Vansteenkiste JF, Stroobants SG. Positron emission tomography in the management of non-small lung cancer. *Hematol Oncol Clin North Am* 2004;18:269–288.
31. Vansteenkiste JF, Stroobants SG, De Leyn PR, et al. Mediastinal lymph node staging with FDG-PET scan in patients with potentially operable non-small cell lung cancer: a prospective analysis of 50 cases. *Chest* 1997;112:1480–1486.
32. Vansteenkiste JF, Stroobants SG, De Leyn PR, et al. Lymph node staging in non-small cell lung cancer with FDG-PET scan: a prospective study on 690 lymph node stations from 68 patients. *J Clin Oncol* 1998;16:2142–2149.
33. Fischer BM, Mortensen J, Hojgaard L. Positron emission tomography in the diagnosis and staging of lung cancer: a systematic, quantitative review. *Lancet Oncol* 2001;2:659–666.
34. Toloza EM, Harpole L, McCrory DC. Noninvasive staging of non-small cell lung cancer: a review of the current evidence. *Chest* 2003;123(Suppl 1):137S–146S.
35. Gould MK, Kuschner WG, Rydzak CE, et al. Test performance of positron emission tomography and computed tomography for mediastinal staging in patients with non-small cell lung cancer: a meta-analysis. *Ann Intern Med* 2003;139:879–892.
36. Stroobants S, Dhoore I, Dooms C, et al. Additional value of whole-body fluorodeoxyglucose positron emission tomography in the detection of distant metastases of non-small cell lung cancer. *Clin Lung Cancer* 2003;4:242–247.
37. Bury T, Dowlati A, Paulus P, et al. Whole-body 18FDG positron emission tomography in the staging of non-small cell lung cancer. *Eur Respir J* 1997;10:2529–2534.
38. Marom EM, McAdams HP, Erasmus JJ, et al. Staging non-small cell lung cancer with whole-body PET. *Radiology* 1999;212:803–809.
39. Pieterman RM, Van Putten JW, Meuzelaar JJ, et al. Preoperative staging of non-small cell lung cancer with positron emission tomography. *N Engl J Med* 2000;343:254–261.
40. Valk PE, Pounds TR, Hopkins DM, et al. Staging non-small cell lung cancer by whole-body positron emission tomographic imaging. *Ann Thorac Surg* 1995;60:1573–1581.
41. Weder W, Schmid RA, Bruchhaus H, et al. Detection of extrathoracic metastases by positron emission tomography in lung cancer. *Ann Thorac Surg* 1998;66:886–892.
42. Vesselle H, Pugsley JM, Vallieres E, et al. The impact of fluorodeoxyglucose F18 positron emission tomography on the surgical staging of non-small cell lung cancer. *J Thorac Cardiovasc Surg* 2002;124:511–519.
43. Saunders CA, Dussek JE, O'Doherty MJ, et al. Evaluation of fluorine-18-fluorodeoxyglucose whole body positron emission tomography imaging in the staging of lung cancer. *Ann Thorac Surg* 1999;67: 790–797.
44. Mac Manus MP, Hicks RJ, Matthews JP, et al. High rate of detection of unsuspected distant metastases by PET in apparent stage III non-small cell lung cancer: implications for radical radiation therapy. *Int J Radiat Oncol Biol Phys* 2001;50:287–293.
45. Eschmann SM, Friedel G, Paulsen F, et al. FDG PET for staging of advanced non-small cell lung cancer prior to neoadjuvant radio-chemotherapy. *Eur J Nucl Med Mol Imaging* 2002;29:804–808.
46. Weng E, Tran L, Rege S, et al. Accuracy and clinical impact of mediastinal lymph node staging with FDG-PET imaging in potentially resectable lung cancer. *Am J Clin Oncol* 2000;23:47–52.
47. Lardinois D, Weder W, Hany TF, et al. Staging of non-small cell lung cancer with integrated positron-emission tomography and computed tomography. *N Engl J Med* 2003;348:2500–2507.
48. Cerfolio RJ, Ojha B, Bryant AS, et al. The accuracy of integrated PET-CT compared with dedicated PET alone for the staging of patients with non-small cell lung cancer. *Ann Thorac Surg* 2004;78:1017–1023.
49. Halpern BS, Schiepers C, Weber WA, et al. Presurgical staging of non-small cell lung cancer: positron emission tomography, integrated positron emission tomography/CT, and software image fusion. *Chest* 2005;128:2289–2297.
50. De Wever W, Ceyssens S, Mortelmans L, et al. Additional value of PET-CT in the staging of lung cancer: comparison with CT alone, PET alone and visual correlation of PET and CT. *Eur Radiol* 2007; 17:23–32.

51. Vansteenkiste JF, Stroobants SG, Dupont PJ, et al. FDG-PET scan in potentially operable non-small cell lung cancer: do anatometabolic PET-CT fusion images improve the localisation of regional lymph node metastases? *Eur J Nucl Med* 1998;25:1495–1501.
52. Wynants J, Stroobants S, Dooms C, et al. Staging of lung cancer. *Radiol Clin North Am* 2007;45:609–625.
53. Bradley JD, Dehdashti F, Mintun MA, et al. Positron emission tomography in limited-stage small cell lung cancer: a prospective study. *J Clin Oncol* 2004;22:3248–3254.
54. Brink I, Schumacher T, Mix M, et al. Impact of 18F-FDG-PET on the primary staging of small cell lung cancer. *Eur J Nucl Med Mol Imaging* 2005;31:1614–1620.
55. Fischer BM, Mortensen J, Langer SW, et al. A prospective study of PET/CT in initial staging of small cell lung cancer: comparison with CT, bone scintigraphy and bone marrow analysis. *Ann Oncol* 2007;18:338–345.
56. Ahuja V, Coleman RE, Herndon J, et al. The prognostic significance of fluorodeoxyglucose positron emission tomography imaging for patients with nonsmall cell lung carcinoma. *Cancer* 1998;83:918–924.
57. Vansteenkiste JF, Stroobants SG, De Leyn PR, et al. Prognostic importance of the Standardized Uptake Value on FDG-PET-scan in non-small cell lung cancer: an analysis of 125 cases. *J Clin Oncol* 1999;17:3201–3206.
58. Higashi K, Ueda Y, Arisaka Y, et al. 18F-FDG uptake as a biologic prognostic factor for recurrence in patients with surgically resected non-small cell lung cancer. *J Nucl Med* 2002;43:39–45.
59. Dhital K, Saunders CA, Seed PT, et al. [(18)F]Fluorodeoxyglucose positron emission tomography and its prognostic value in lung cancer. *Eur J Cardiothorac Surg* 2000;18:425–428.
60. Jeong HJ, Min JJ, Park JM, et al. Determination of the prognostic value of [(18)F]fluorodeoxyglucose uptake by using positron emission tomography in patients with non-small cell lung cancer. *Nucl Med Commun* 2002;23:865–870.
61. Sasaki R, Komaki R, Macapinlac H, et al. 18F-fluorodeoxyglucose uptake by positron emission tomography predicts outcome of non-small cell lung cancer. *J Clin Oncol* 2005;23:1136–1143.
62. Downey RJ, Akhurst T, Gonen M, et al. Preoperative F-18 fluorodeoxyglucose-positron emission tomography maximal standardized uptake value predicts survival after lung cancer resection. *J Clin Oncol* 2004;22:3255–3260.
63. Cerfolio RJ, Bryant AS, Ohja B, et al. The maximum standardized uptake values on positron emission tomography of a non-small cell lung cancer predict stage, recurrence, and survival. *J Thorac Cardiovasc Surg* 2005;130:151–159.
64. Borst GR, Belderbos JS, Boellaard R, et al. Standardised FDG uptake: a prognostic factor for inoperable non- small cell lung cancer. *Eur J Cancer* 2005;41:1533–1541.
65. Ohtsuka T, Nomori H, Watanabe K, et al. Prognostic significance of [18F]fluorodeoxyglucose uptake on positron emission tomography in patients with pathologic stage I lung adenocarcinoma. *Cancer* 2006; 107:2468–2473.
66. Berghmans T, Dusart M, Paesmans M, et al. Primary tumor standardized uptake value (SUV_{max}) measured on fluorodeoxyglucose positron emission tomography (FDG-PET) is of prognostic value for survival in non-small cell lung cancer (NSCLC): a systematic review and meta-analysis (MA) by the European Lung Cancer Working Party for the IASLC Lung Cancer Staging Project. *J Thorac Oncol* 2008;3:6–12.
67. Downey RJ, Akhurst T, Gonen M, et al. Fluorine-18 fluorodeoxyglucose positron emission tomographic maximal standardized uptake value predicts survival independent of clinical but not pathologic TNM staging of resected non-small cell lung cancer. *J Thorac Cardiovasc Surg* 2007;133:1419–1427.
68. Vesselle H, Freeman JD, Wiens L, et al. Fluorodeoxyglucose uptake of primary non-small cell lung cancer at positron emission tomography: new contrary data on prognostic role. *Clin Cancer Res* 2007;1;13: 3255–3263.
69. Detterbeck FC, Vansteenkiste JF, Morris DE, et al. Seeking a home for a PET, part 3: emerging applications of positron emission tomography (PET) imaging in the management of patients with lung cancer. *Chest* 2004;126:1656–1666.
70. Vansteenkiste J, Fischer BM, Dooms C, et al. Positron-emission tomography in prognostic and therapeutic assessment of lung cancer: systematic review. *Lancet Oncol* 2004;5:531–540.
71. Weber WA, Petersen V, Schmidt B, et al. Positron emission tomography in non-small cell lung cancer: prediction of response to chemotherapy by quantitative assessment of glucose use. *J Clin Oncol* 2003; 21:2651–2657.
72. De Geus-Oei LF, Van der Heijden HF, Visser EP, et al. Chemotherapy response evaluation with 18F-FDG PET in patients with non-small cell lung cancer. *J Nucl Med* 2007;.48:1592–1598.
73. Vansteenkiste J, Stroobants S, Hoekstra C, et al. 18fluoro-2-deoxyglucose positron emission tomography (PET) in the assessment of induction chemotherapy (IC) in stage IIIA-N2 NSCLC: a multi-center prospective study. *Proc ASCO* 2001;20:313A (abstract).
74. Akhurst T, Downey RJ, Ginsberg MS, et al. An initial experience with FDG-PET in the imaging of residual disease after induction therapy for lung cancer. *Ann Thorac Surg* 2002;73:259–266.
75. Ryu JS, Choi NC, Fischman AJ, et al. FDG-PET in staging and restaging non-small cell lung cancer after neoadjuvant chemoradiotherapy: correlation with histopathology. *Lung Cancer* 2002;35:179–187.
76. Cerfolio RJ, Ojha B, Mukherjee S, et al. Positron emission tomography scanning with 2-fluoro-2-deoxy-d- glucose as a predictor of response of neoadjuvant treatment for non-small cell carcinoma. *J Thorac Cardiovasc Surg* 2003;125:938–944.
77. Hellwig D, Graeter TP, Ukena D, et al. Value of F-18-fluorodeoxyglucose positron emission tomography after induction therapy of locally advanced bronchogenic carcinoma. *J Thorac Cardiovasc Surg* 2004;128:892–899.
78. Port JL, Kent MS, Korst RJ, et al. Positron emission tomography scanning poorly predicts response to preoperative chemotherapy in non-small cell lung cancer. *Ann Thorac Surg* 2004;77:254–259.
79. Hoekstra CJ, Stroobants SG, Smit EF, et al. Prognostic relevance of response evaluation using [18F]-2-fluoro-2-deoxy-D-glucose positron emission tomography in patients with locally advanced non-small cell lung cancer. *J Clin Oncol* 2005;23:8362–8370.
80. Cerfolio RJ, Bryant AS, Ojha B. Restaging patients with N2 (stage IIIa) non-small cell lung cancer after neoadjuvant chemoradiotherapy: a prospective study. *J Thorac Cardiovasc Surg* 2006;131: 1229–1235.
81. Pottgen C, Levegrun S, Theegarten D, et al. Value of 18F-fluoro-2-deoxy-D-glucose-positron emission tomography/computed tomography in non-small cell lung cancer for prediction of pathologic response and times to relapse after neoadjuvant chemoradiotherapy. *Clin Cancer Res* 2006;12:97–106.
82. De Leyn P, Stroobants S, De Wever W, et al. Prospective comparative study of integrated positron emission tomography-computed tomography compared with remediastinoscopy in the assessment of residual mediastinal lymph node disease after induction chemotherapy for mediastinoscopy proven stage IIIA-N2 non-small cell lung cancer: a Leuven Lung Cancer Group study. *J Clin Oncol* 2006;24: 3333–3339.
83. Vansteenkiste JF, Stroobants SG, De Leyn PR, et al. Potential use of FDG-PET scan after induction chemotherapy in surgically staged IIIA-N2 non-small cell lung cancer: a prospective pilot study. *Ann Oncol* 1998;9:1193–1198.
84. Eschmann SM, Friedel G, Paulsen F, et al. Repeat (18)F-FDG PET for monitoring neoadjuvant chemotherapy in patients with stage III non-small cell lung cancer. *Lung Cancer* 2007;55:165–171.
85. Cerfolio RJ, Bryant AS. When is it best to repeat a 2-fluoro-2-deoxy-D-glucose positron emission tomography/computed tomography scan on patients with non-small cell lung cancer who have received neoadjuvant chemoradiotherapy? *Ann Thorac Surg* 2007;84: 1092–1097.

86. Dooms C, Verbeken E, Stroobants S, et al. Prognostic stratification of stage IIIA-N2 non-small cell lung cancer after induction chemotherapy: a model based on the combination of morphometric-pathologic response in mediastinal nodes and primary tumor response on serial 18-fluoro-2-deoxy-glucose positron emission tomography. *J Clin Oncol* 2008;26:1128–1134.
87. Mah K, Caldwell CB, Ung YC, et al. The impact of 18 FDG-PET on target and critical organs in CT-based treatment planning of patients with poorly defined non-small cell lung carcinoma: a prospective study. *Int J Radiat Oncol Biol Phys* 2002;52:339–350.
88. Erdi YE, Rosenzweig K, Erdi AK, et al. Radiotherapy treatment planning for patients with non-small cell lung cancer using positron emission tomography (PET). *Radiother Oncol* 2002;62:51–60.
89. Vanuytsel LJ, Vansteenkiste JF, Stroobants SG, et al. The impact of (18)F-fluoro-2-deoxy-D-glucose positron emission tomography (FDG-PET) lymph node staging on the radiation treatment volumes in patients with non-small cell lung cancer. *Radiother Oncol* 2000;55: 317–324.
90. De Ruysscher D, Wanders S, Van Haren E, et al. Selective mediastinal node irradiation based on FDG-PET scan data in patients with non-small cell lung cancer: A prospective clinical study. *Int J Radiat Oncol Biol Phys* 2005;62:988–994.
91. Nestle U, Walter K, Schmidt S, et al. 18F-deoxyglucose positron emission tomography (FDG-PET) for the planning of radiotherapy in lung cancer: high impact in patients with atelectasis. *Int J Radiat Oncol Biol Phys* 1999;44:593–597.
92. Bradley J, Thorstad WL, Mutic S, et al. Impact of FDG-PET on radiation therapy volume delineation in non-small cell lung cancer. *Int J Radiat Oncol Biol Phys* 2004;59:78–86.
93. Steenbakkers RJ, Duppen JC, Fitton I, et al. Reduction of observer variation using matched CT-PET for lung cancer delineation: a three-dimensional analysis. *Int J Radiat Oncol Biol Phys* 2005;64:435–448.
94. Nestle U, Kremp S, Schaefer-Schuler A, et al. Comparison of different methods for delineation of 18F-FDG PET positive tissue for target volume definition in radiotherapy of patients with non-small cell lung cancer. *J Nucl Med* 2005;46:1342–1348.
95. Yaremko B, Riauka T, Robinson D, et al. Threshold modification for tumour imaging in non-small cell lung cancer using positron emission tomography. *Nucl Med Commun* 2005;26:433–440.
96. Boucher L, Rodrigue S, Lecomte R, et al. Respiratory gating for 3-dimensional PET of the thorax: feasibility and initial results. *J Nucl Med* 2004;45:214–219.
97. Patz EF, Connolly J, Herndon J. Prognostic value of thoracic FDG PET imaging after treatment for non-small cell lung cancer. *AJR Am J Roentgenol* 2000;174:769–774.
98. Hicks RJ, Kalff V, Mac Manus MP, et al. The utility of (18)F-FDG PET for suspected recurrent non-small cell lung cancer after potentially curative therapy: impact on management and prognostic stratification. *J Nucl Med* 2001;42:1605–1613.
99. Hellwig D, Groschel A, Graeter TP, et al. Diagnostic performance and prognostic impact of FDG-PET in suspected recurrence of surgically treated non-small cell lung cancer. *Eur J Nucl Med Mol Imaging* 2006;33:13–21.
100. Bury T, Corhay JL, Duysinx B, et al. Value of FDG-PET in detecting residual or recurrent non-small cell lung cancer. *Eur Respir J* 1999;14: 1376–1380.
101. Swensen SJ, Silverstein MD, Ilstrup DM, et al. The probability of malignancy in solitary pulmonary nodules. Application to small radiologically indeterminate nodules. *Arch Int Med* 1997;157:849–855.
102. Gould MK, Fletcher J, Iannettoni MD, et al. Evaluation of patients with pulmonary nodules: when is it lung cancer?: ACCP evidence-based clinical practice guidelines (2nd edition). *Chest* 2007;132(3 Suppl): 108S–130S.
103. Vansteenkiste JF. FDG-PET for lymph node staging in NSCLC: a major step forward, but beware of the pitfalls [editorial]. *Lung Cancer* 2005;47:151–153.
104. Detterbeck FC, Jantz M, Wallace M, et al. American College of Chest Physicians (ACCP). Invasive mediastinal staging of lung cancer: ACCP evidence-based clinical practice guidelines (2nd edition). *Chest* 2007;132(3 Suppl):202S–220S.
105. De Langen AJ, Raijmakers P, Riphagen I, et al. The size of mediastinal lymph nodes and its relation with metastatic involvement: a meta-analysis. *Eur J Cardiothorac Surg* 2006;29:26–29.
106. Hicks RJ, Kalff V, Mac Manus MP, et al. 18F-FDG PET provides high-impact and powerful prognostic stratification in staging newly diagnosed non-small cell lung cancer. *J Nucl Med* 2001;42:1596–1604.
107. Tucker R, Coel M, Ko J, et al. Impact of fluorine-18 fluorodeoxyglucose positron emission tomography on patient management: first year's experience in a clinical center. *J Clin Oncol* 2001;19:2504–2508.
108. Hoekstra CJ, Stroobants SG, Hoekstra OS, et al. The value of [18F]fluoro-2-deoxy-D-glucose positron emission tomography in the selection of patients with stage IIIA-N2 non-small cell lung cancer for combined modality treatment. *Lung Cancer* 2003;39:151–157.
109. Lardinois D, Weder W, Roudas M, et al. Etiology of solitary extrapulmonary positron emission tomography and computed tomography findings in patients with lung cancer. *J Clin Oncol* 2005;23: 6846–6853.
110. Seltzer MA, Yap CS, Silverman DH, et al. The impact of PET on the management of lung cancer: the referring physician's perspective. *J Nucl Med* 2002;43:752–762.
111. Herder GJ, Van Tinteren H, Comans EF, et al. Prospective use of serial questionnaires to evaluate the therapeutic efficacy of 18F-fluorodeoxyglucose (FDG) positron emission tomography (PET) in suspected lung cancer. *Thorax* 2003;58:47–51.
112. McCain TW, Dunagan DP, Chin R, et al. The usefulness of positron emission tomography in evaluating patients for pulmonary malignancies. *Chest* 2000;118:1610–1615.
113. Van Tinteren H, Hoekstra OS, Smit EF, et al. Effectiveness of positron emission tomography in the preoperative assessment of patients with suspected non-small cell lung cancer: the PLUS multicentre randomised trial. *Lancet* 2002;359:1388–1393.
114. Viney RC, Boyer MJ, King MT, et al. Randomized controlled trial of the role of positron emission tomography in the management of stage I and II non-small cell lung cancer. *J Clin Oncol* 2004;22:2357–2362.
115. Herder GJ, Kramer H, Hoekstra OS, et al. Traditional versus up-front [18F] fluorodeoxyglucose positron emission tomography staging of non-small cell lung cancer: a Dutch cooperative randomized study. *J Clin Oncol* 2006;24:1800–1806.
116. Nettelbladt OS, Sundin AE, Valind SO, et al. Combined fluorine-18-FDG and carbon-11-methionine PET for diagnosis of tumors in lung and mediastinum. *J Nucl Med* 1998;39:640–647.
117. Sasaki M, Kuwabara Y, Yoshida T, et al. Comparison of MET-PET and FDG-PET for differentiation between benign lesions and malignant tumors of the lung. *Ann Nucl Med* 2001;15:425–431.
118. Pieterman RM, Que TH, Elsinga PH, et al. Comparison of (11)C-choline and (18)F-FDG PET in primary diagnosis and staging of patients with thoracic cancer. *J Nucl Med* 2002;43:167–172.
119. Vesselle H, Grierson J, Muzi M, et al. In vivo validation of 3′deoxy-3′-[(18)F]fluorothymidine (18F-FLT) as a proliferation imaging tracer in humans: correlation of 18F-FLT uptake by positron emission tomography with Ki-67 immunohistochemistry and flow cytometry in human lung tumors. *Clin Cancer Res* 2002;8:3315–3323.
120. Buck AK, Schirrmeister H, Hetzel M, et al. 3-deoxy-3-[(18)F] fluorothymidine-positron emission tomography for noninvasive assessment of proliferation in pulmonary nodules. *Cancer Res* 2002;62:3331–3334.
121. Yap CS, Czernin J, Fishbein MC, et al. Evaluation of thoracic tumors with 18F-fluorothymidine and 18F- fluorodeoxyglucose positron emission tomography. *Chest* 2006;129:393–401.
122. Tian J, Yang X, Yu L, et al. A multicenter clinical trial on the diagnostic value of dual-tracer PET/CT in pulmonary lesions using 3′-deoxy-3′-18F-fluorothymidine and 18F-FDG. *J Nucl Med* 2008;49:186–194.

CHAPTER 28

Thomas G. Sutedja
Thomas Santo
Michael Zervos
Felix J.F. Herth

Bronchoscopy in the Diagnosis and Evaluation of Lung Cancer

Rigid optics to examine the central airways were designed by Gustav Killian in Heidelberg more than a century ago and were revolutionized with the creation of the fiberoptic bronchoscope by Shigeto Ikeda.[1] Recent and continuing advancements in catheter-based tissue imaging and therapeutics have significantly increased the role of bronchoscopy in the management of lung cancer patients because of its minimal invasive nature.[2–6] Bronchoscopy provides us with less morbid and tailored strategies for each individual at risk with regard to extended diagnostics and therapeutics by the application of many techniques currently available.[3–7] Thus, bronchoscopic activities also encompass early detection, staging, and treatment for at-risk individuals with various pulmonary pathologies, and its role for the management of lung cancer has become an integral part in the thoracic oncology discipline as well.[3,4,7]

From the perspectives of interventional pulmonology, target lesions are either centrally located inside or adjacent to the major airways or located in the lung parenchyma beyond the segmental bronchi, in which current fiberoptic bronchoscopes with an average diameter of ≈6 mm have limited access. However, the standard use of fluoroscopy and current advancement of computerized digital four-dimensional (4D) imaging computed tomography (CT), magnetic resonance imaging (MRI), ultrasound, and tissue spectral analysis can be further exploited to refine bronchoscopic applications in studying dynamic disease processes in pulmonary parenchyma beyond our direct vision and toward visualization of subcellular processes.[8–12]

The aim of this chapter is to describe current and future perspectives of various bronchoscopic techniques that are used in the management of lung cancer. Recent advancements in nodal staging and therapeutic strategy for early detected lesion will be more extensively discussed.

THE CONCEPT OF BRONCHOSCOPIC DIAGNOSIS, STAGING, AND TREATMENT

For most patients with clinically overt lung cancer based on current World Health Organization (WHO) histology classification, the squamous and small cell types are primarily located in the central airways, whereas adeno and large cell neuroendocrine types are mostly located in the lung parenchyma distal to the segmental bronchi. As the majority of patients are still diagnosed at advanced stage, central bulky tumor and nodal disease involvement adjacent to the central airways can be (re-)staged by acquiring specimens for tissue diagnosis with relative ease.[3,6]

Bronchoscopic sampling of specimens for histological evaluation in the central airways can be performed under direct vision, and the use of coagulative techniques (e.g., lasers, electrocautery, and argon plasma) and cryotherapy can better control bleeding that may occur.[3] Extended use of various debulking techniques for obtaining immediate relief in patients with imminent suffocation will not be dealt here (see Chapter 61).

Adjacent to the central airways are the mediastinal lymph nodes (MLN) (Fig. 28.1), which can be staged using transbronchial (and transesophageal) needle aspiration as alternatives for conventional staging (e.g., mediastinoscopy and video-assisted thoracoscopic surgery [VATS]).[6,13,14] These aspiration techniques are a major improvement for reducing morbidity in those with advanced cancers, with improved accuracy and safety caused by the advent of esophageal and endobronchial ultrasound (EUS and EBUS), allowing real-time puncturing of the nodes.[13,14] It is important to know that mediastinal nodes move during respiration, such that in dealing with especially small unforeseen ^{18}F-fluorodeoxyglucose positron emission tomography (FDG-PET)-positive nodes, one cannot presume the locations to be static during aspiration.[15,16] It is therefore quite obvious that with expertise and real-time puncturing of the nodes, diagnosis can be obtained in >90% accuracy.[13,14] These endoscopic alternatives are straightforward and least morbid in staging procedures, despite the great potential of noninvasive imaging techniques such as PET/CT. Tissue will remain the issue for still a considerable period of time as FDG-PET avidity is showing metabolic function not exclusively for malignancies alone.[17,18]

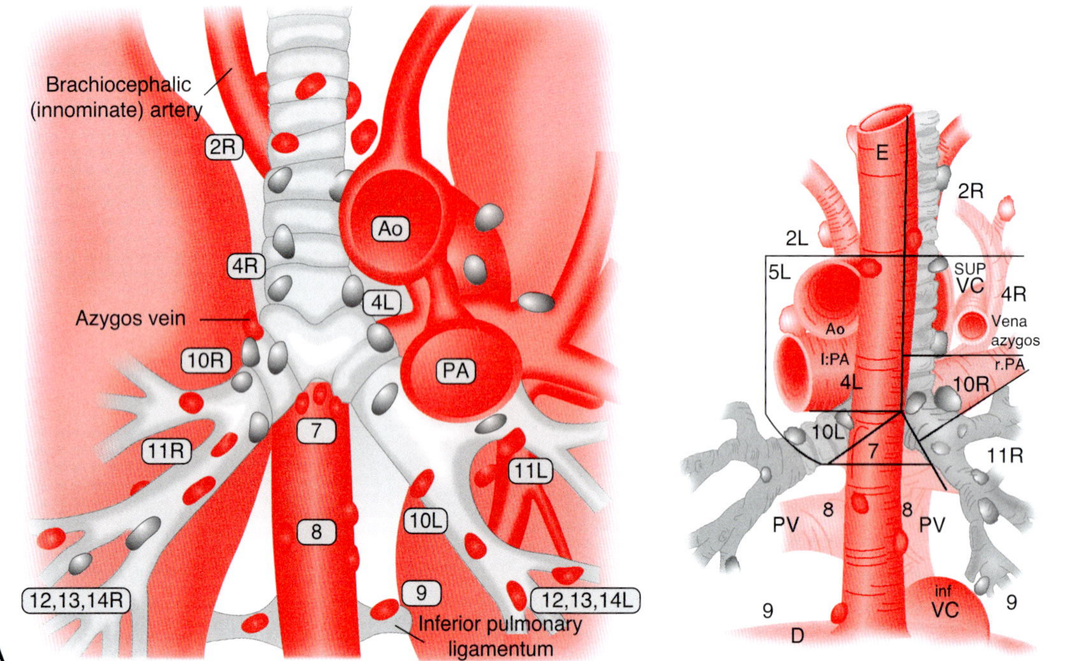

FIGURE 28.1 Lymph nodes map for transbronchoscopic (left, anterior view) and transesophageal (right, posterior view) endoscopic punctures. *Ao*, aorta; *inf VC*, inferior vena cava; *l:PA*, left pulmonary artery; *PA*, pulmonary artery; *PV*, pulmonary vein; *r:PA*, right pulmonary artery; *SUP VC*, superior vena cava. (**A:** from Krasnik M, Vilmann P, Herth F. EUS-FNA and EBUS-TBNA: the pulmonologist's and surgeon's perspective. *Endoscopy* 2006:38:S105–S109; **B:** from Herth FJF, Rabe KF, Gasparini S, et al. Transbronchial and transoesophageal [ultrasound-guided] needle aspirations for the analysis of mediastinal lesions. *Eur Resp J* 2006;28:1264–1275.)

Currently, for lesions in the lung parenchyma, tissue sampling under fluoroscopy, CT, or ultrasound guided may prevent the need for more invasive surgical diagnostics.[12,19,20] However, 30% of pulmonary parenchymal lesions do not have proximity to the smaller airways. Therefore, transthoracic approaches may still be required with the inherent risk for causing a pneumothorax—a potential complication often overrated as an interventional specialist should anticipate any procedure-related complication.

The issue of huge numbers of submillimeter parenchymal lesions detected in current CT screening programs cannot be easily addressed with either fluoroscopic or endobronchial techniques. Targeting all these lesions will be a colossal task. The entire strategy regarding CT screening requires thorough understanding of all screening controversies (see Chapter 16).[21–25]

4D navigational techniques based on CT data seem promising. Nevertheless, the requirement for tissue biopsy should be put in the proper perspective of the CT screening controversies.[25–28] The issues of potential overdiagnosis, relatively high number of only bronchioloalveolar cell carcinoma (BAC) lesions found, the lack of any proof that stage shift has been accomplished, together with potential difficulty for proper histological classification if only based on tiny pieces of tissue specimens collected, are among the few aspects to consider.[22,25,26,29,30] The poor negative predictive value (NPV) of CT-detected subcentimeter lesions in lung cancer screening study may encourage bronchoscopists to accomplish tissue diagnosis to exclude malignancy, but is practically unrealistic because of the sheer numbers of these lesions that are found, of which most will be nonmalignant.[22–25] Consideration of theoretical and practical issues should prevent tunnel vision for interventional pulmonologist in dealing with CT screen–detected nodules.[25]

When there is a strong suspicion for lung malignancy, PET/CT may soon be expected to become the standard initial staging procedure.[26–28] Improved spatial resolution of current PET/CT machines can greatly assist the bronchoscopist for optimal selection of techniques, for example, in using ultrathin bronchoscope, steerable catheters (e.g., virtual bronchoscopic navigation).[19,20,31–33] This may ease targeting lesions beyond bronchoscopic reach, thus distal to the segmental bronchi deep in the lung parenchyma, also for first-station nodal disease.

The epidemiological shift of lung cancer cell type to ≈40% adenocarcinoma makes it mandatory for bronchoscopists to be proficient in understanding the potential and limitations of 4D noninvasive spatial data for targeting these lesions.[26,27] Small parenchymal lesions are difficult moving targets because of respiratory cycles and may require adjuncts such as using real-time ultrasound sensor probes.[12,15,16,20] Great promise about the possibility of 4D navigational assistance may improve our ability herein, similar to recent achievements in stereotactic body radiation therapy (see Chapter 43).[34]

For central airway lesions within bronchoscopic reach, minute early preneoplastic lesions at the clonal level located in the bronchial mucosa of the central airways are difficult to detect.[8] Preneoplastic lesions are aberrant clonal cell groups of several hundred cells with an average thickness of five cells only. The role of autofluorescence bronchoscopy (AF) herein has been established.[4] Tumor infiltration beyond the bronchial wall can be visualized accurately using thin cuts high-resolution CT (HRCT),[5] EBUS,[35] with optical coherence tomography (OCT) as a promising tool (see Chapter 19).[36]

Standard bronchoscopic biopsies may prove sufficient to obtain a diagnosis, and by using tiny biopsy forceps, repeat biopsies can be obtained. Autofluorescence-guided[37,38] sampling can improve accuracy of detection and staging of early squamous cell type lesions, and these can be completely eradicated using intraluminal treatment. Moreover, bronchoscopic approaches are clearly a cost-effective alternative method.[4,5,8,39–41]

Expert opinion as well as international and national guidelines are available on bronchoscopy and interventional pulmonology.[3,4] Optimizing cytological and histological yields requires support from a panel of experienced pathologists based on current WHO classification.[29,30]

Recent Issues in Mediastinal Nodal Staging The variable yield (Table 28.1) in puncturing CT-enlarged lymph nodes is understandable, because there is no real-time guidance during bronchoscopic session while these are moving targets if transbronchial needle aspiration (TBNA) is performed under conscious sedation in spontaneously breathing and coughing patient.[13–16]

Currently, many patients with advanced stage cancers have bulky multilevel MLN involvement. Patients' population in each particular medical practice should be put in the proper perspective about the likelihood for obtaining good yields.[42,43] Also, the proper time window for TBNA restaging after induction chemotherapy should be a point for consideration.[44,45] With the advent of ultrasound and 4D PET/CT virtual bronchoscopy previously mentioned, needle aspiration can be executed in real time with utmost accuracy, with excellent yield.[13,14,28]

TABLE 28.1 Factors Influencing Diagnostic Yield of Needle Aspiration of Lymph Nodes Adjacent to the Central Airways

Presence of lymph node enlargement on computed tomography scan
Type of needle employed
Site of the tumor and lymph node
Lymph node size
Number of aspirates performed
Availability of rapid on-site cytopathologic examination
Ability and experience of the operators
Nature of the lesion (malignancy, type of malignancy)

(From Herth FJ, Rabe KF, Gasparini S, et al. Transbronchial and transoesophageal [ultrasound-guided] needle aspirations for the analysis of mediastinal lesions. *Eur Respir J* 2006;28:1264–1275.)

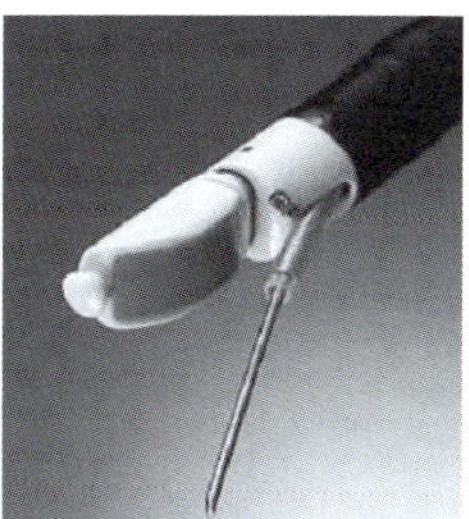

FIGURE 28.2 EBUS bronchoscope with needle extruded. (Photo courtesy of Felix Herth.)

A major recent advancement in MLN staging is the incorporation of (curvi-)linear ultrasound transducer video/bronchoscope with color flow Doppler that visualized target lymph node and adjacent vessels, allowing accurate needle aspiration with great safety. Endobronchial ultrasound–guided transbronchial needle aspiration (EBUS-TBNA) allows for direct sampling of mediastinal and hilar lymph nodes in real time. The procedure is performed using an ultrasound biopsy bronchoscope, with a 7.5 MHz convex linear array ultrasonic transducer located at the distal tip, encased by a water inflatable balloon. There is also a separate working channel through which the biopsy needle is extended, allowing for real-time biopsy (convex probe EBUS [CP-EBUS], XBF-UC260 F-OL8, Olympus; Figs. 28.2 and 28.3). Once a lymph node is visualized, the balloon is inflated to maintain adequate contact with the bronchial wall and to better visualize the lymph node. The bronchoscope is also supported by Doppler function for the identification of blood vessels. The Doppler is used prior to needle insertion to ensure that a suspected lymph node is not, in fact, a blood vessel. Once the physician is confident that the structure in question is a lymph

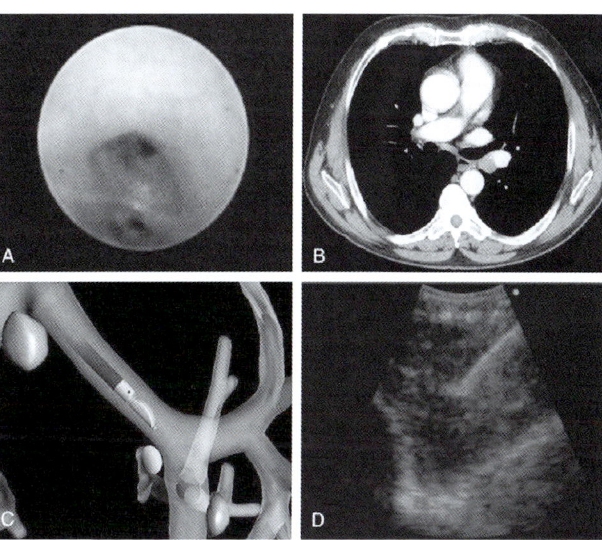

FIGURE 28.3 **A:** Intraluminal view of the carina left upper and lower lobe. **B:** CT image of node station 10 L. **C:** Position of the bronchoscope. **D:** EBUS image of the puncture procedure, the needle is visible. (Photo courtesy of Felix Herth.) (See color plate.)

node, the 22-gauge needle is passed through the bronchial wall and into the lymph node once the outer sheath has been positioned and brought in contact with the airway. The balloon is deflated prior to deployment of the needle to prevent balloon rupture. The needle is passed back and forth through the lymph node once a vacuum syringe has been connected to the needle in order to aspirate lymphatic tissue either in the form of cells or actual tissue cores.

EBUS-TBNA is a promising alternative to mediastinoscopy for the staging of MLN in patients who present with mediastinal lymphadenopathy on CT scan. Compared with mediastinoscopy, EBUS-TBNA is less invasive, can be performed under conscious sedation (as opposed to general anesthesia), and does not require overnight hospitalization (less costly). More importantly, EBUS-TBNA allows access to posterior subcarinal,[7] hilar,[10] and intrapulmonary (≥11) lymph nodes, which are inaccessible by mediastinoscopy. Also, unlike mediastinoscopy, EBUS-TBNA can be performed multiple times on the same patient without deleterious effect, all while preserving the integrity of the mediastinum. This is an important fact if future mediastinal restaging is anticipated, as is often the case with stage IIIA-N2 disease following induction chemotherapy. A recent study by Herth et al.[46] investigated the ability of EBUS-TBNA to accurately restage the mediastinum following induction chemotherapy in patients with stage IIIA-N2 non–small cell lung cancer (NSCLC). Between February 2003 and March 2006, 124 patients who had completed induction chemotherapy, underwent EBUS-TBNA, followed by thoracotomy with resection and systematic lymph node dissection with curative intent. The sensitivity, specificity, positive predictive value (PPV), NPV, and diagnostic accuracy of EBUS-TBNA were 76%, 100%, 100%, 20%, and 77%, respectively. These results compare favorably with those observed in studies that have performed remediastinoscopy[47–50] or EUS-TNA[51,52] in the mediastinal restaging of similar cohorts.

In the largest study published to date on EBUS-TBNA sampling of MLN, Herth et al.[53] biopsied 572 enlarged (>1 cm on CT) lymph nodes from 502 patients, between June 2002 and September 2004. The average lymph node size as measured during EBUS examination was 1.6 cm. (range 0.8 to 3.2). EBUS-TBNA established a diagnosis in 535 of the 572 lymph nodes biopsied, providing a diagnostic yield of 93.5%. On a per patient basis, a diagnosis was obtained in 470 of 502 patients, establishing a diagnostic yield of 93%. Overall, EBUS-TBNA had a sensitivity, specificity, accuracy, PPV, and NPV of 94%, 100%, 94%, 100%, and 11%, respectively. Given the low NPV, which reflects a high number of false negatives, the authors have suggested that a negative EBUS-TBNA be followed by a more definitive diagnostic procedure, presumably, a mediastinoscopy.

Current guidelines for the noninvasive staging of NSCLC recommend that a PET scan be administered to any patient with clinical stage IA to IIIB disease that is being treated with curative intent.[54]

Moreover, it is recommended that any abnormal (positive standardized uptake value [SUV]) lymph nodes on FDG-PET should be further evaluated via tissue sampling. The question then becomes, "What procedure should be performed to obtain tissue samples from PET-positive lymph nodes?" A recent study evaluated the use of real-time EBUS-TBNA for the sampling of PET-positive lymph nodes in 106 patients with proven (29 patients) or suspected (77 patients) lung cancer.[55]

All procedures were done under conscious sedation, and patients were managed on an outpatient basis. Based on the 90 assessable patients, the sensitivity, specificity, PPV, NPV, and accuracy of EBUS-TBNA for PET-positive lymph node staging were 93%, 100%, 100%, 91%, and 97%. Furthermore, surgical intervention was avoided by the use of EBUS-TBNA in 56% (59 of 106) of the patients. In experienced hands, these findings suggest that EBUS-TBNA should be considered as the initial method of sampling in patients with suspected/proven lung cancer and PET-positive lymph nodes. However, subsequent surgical sampling should be performed following a negative EBUS-TBNA, based on a 10% false-negative EBUS-TBNA rate. Lastly, at the time of procedure, EBUS-TBNA also allows the sampling of any PET-normal MLN that are visualized. This provides a simple means to rule out occult N2/N3 disease. EBUS-TBNA found lymph node metastasis in PET-negative nodes in 4 of 58 positive patients, upstaging these patients from suspected N1 and N2 based on PET, to N2 and N3, respectively.

Data exist, which demonstrate that a significant percentage of NSCLC patients with clinical stage I disease do, in fact, harbor lymph node metastases. Anywhere between 15% to 37% of patients with negative lymph nodes on CT scan are found to have nodal involvement upon surgical staging,[56] depending on what data is referenced.[57–60] This is a reflection of the low sensitivity and accuracy of CT scan in staging the mediastinum in lung cancer patients. This percentage drops to 9% to 11% in patients with solely T1 lesions.[61,62]

Even at this lower estimation, MLN staging prior to surgical intervention in clinical stage I NSCLC patients is justified. Between January 2003 and March 2005, Herth et al.[63] evaluated EBUS-TBNA as a means of sampling lymph nodes in NSCLC patients with CT scans showing no enlarged lymph nodes (no node >1 cm) in the mediastinum. In 100 patients, 119 lymph nodes between 5 to 10 mm were sampled, with a mean diameter of 8.1 mm. EBUS-TBNA correctly identified 19 out of 21 lymph node–positive patients and all 79 lymph node–negative patients. Of the 19 positive cases identified by EBUS-TBNA, 3 had N3 disease, 13 had N2 disease, and 3 had N1 disease. Sensitivity, specificity, and NPV of EBUS-TBNA were 92.3%, 100%, and 96.3%, respectively. These findings suggest that EBUS-TBNA can be used as an accurate way to preoperatively stage the mediastinum in NSCLC patients with normal-appearing lymph nodes, a procedure, which in the past was only reserved for mediastinoscopy.

Because of the fact that PET scan is now being incorporated into the standard workup on lung cancer patients, EBUS-TBNA has also been evaluated as a means of staging the mediastinum in NSCLC patients with a CT *and* PET-normal mediastinum.[64]

From January 2004 to May 2007, EBUS-TBNA was used to sample 156 lymph nodes (5 to 10 mm in size) in 97 NSCLC patients. Mean diameter of punctured lymph nodes was 7.9 mm. The sensitivity, specificity, and NPV of EBUS-TBNA in detecting malignancy were 89%, 100%, and 98.9%, respectively. This demonstrates that EBUS-TBNA is an accurate means of staging the mediastinum in NSCLC patients with no evidence of mediastinal involvement on CT and PET scans.

In light of the promising data that have been published on the use of EBUS-TBNA for MLN staging in NSCLC patients, direct comparison with mediastinoscopy (the gold standard) is necessary to establish the appropriate clinical approach to mediastinal staging in patients with NSCLC. Thus far, a study by Ernst et al.[65] is the only one to draw such a comparison. Included in the study were 66 patients with suspected NSCLC and mediastinal adenopathy (≥1 cm) on CT scan that was confined to lymph node stations 2, 4, or 7. Biopsies from 120 lymph nodes (mean size 15 mm, range 10 to 21) in these 66 patients were obtained by both EBUS-TBNA and mediastinoscopy. In a per lymph node analysis, EBUS-TBNA had a higher overall diagnostic yield (91%) than mediastinoscopy (78%). Specifically, EBUS-TBNA had a statistically significant ($p < 0.05$) higher diagnostic yield than mediastinoscopy in subcarinal (98% vs. 78%) and malignant (86% vs. 66%) lymph nodes. There was also a trend toward obtaining a definite histologic diagnosis with EBUS-TBNA (59%) compared with mediastinoscopy (47%), but this did not reach statistical significance. Overall, the sensitivity, specificity, and NPV of EBUS-TBNA were 87%, 100%, and 78%, respectively. The sensitivity, specificity, and NPV of mediastinoscopy were 68%, 100%, and 59%, respectively.

Complementary use of transesophageal MLN sampling further improves staging of aortic window, paraesophageal LN stations and adrenals, still more cumbersome to be tackled using alternative surgical approaches.[13,17] Current screening efforts may increasingly confront clinicians with subcentimeter's lesions in the lung parenchyma, and the potential role for EBUS for obtaining diagnosis have been pusblihsed.[12,20]

For daily practice, the use of bronchial needle aspiration by bronchoscopists is frequently underutilized, resulting from lack of awareness of its potential for accurate and safely sampling nodal stations based on the proximity of many important nodal stations to the central airways. Experts' opinion herein and recent American College of Chest Physicians (ACCP) guidelines have addressed this issue in details.[6,13,66] It is obvious that scalene, aortic, paraesophageal nodes, left adrenal, require EUS and other measures.[17]

Recent Issues on Bronchoscopic Treatment of Early Lung Cancer

Accurate staging of early central airway cancer is extremely important for the selection of appropriate treatment.[4,5] Although surgery is still the preferred option, many patients harboring early squamous cancer in the central airways have smoking-related comorbidities that place them at high surgical risk, with 20% to 30% multifocal cancers in the event of field cancerization, justifying less morbid early interventional approach.[38–40]

The need for maximal lung preservation strategy has propelled the interest for applying various local treatment alternatives by bronchoscopy, which is a further implementation of its potentials for quick recanalisation in central airway tumor obstruction (see Chapter 61).

Criteria of early central airway cancers suitable for local, thus bronchoscopic treatment are radiographically (currently HRCT) occult without lymph node or distant metastasis, mainly squamous cell cancer–type measuring <1 cm^2 in longitudinal axis with visible distal margin confined within the cartilaginous layer of the tracheobronchial tree.[4,5,7,21] It is clear from the point of intraluminal tumor growth that tumor dimensions are the most important determinant for cure, as pathological studies have shown repeatedly the strong correlation between tumor volume in intraluminal growing squamous cell cancer and its nodal status.[4,38,67,68] Hence, excellent local control can be achieved by using local therapy (e.g., bronchoscopic treatment in carefully selected cases), such as has been shown in photodynamic series previously reported. Recent ACCP guidelines have addressed this issue.[4]

The combined use of autofluorescence bronchoscopy, high-resolution CT, FDG-PET, and EBUS can now better select true early stage squamous cancer, which correlated well with excellent cure rate in smaller =1 cm^2 flat-type lesions as reported previously in the photodynamic therapy studies.[4,5,35,39]

Whether OCT (Fig. 28.4) and confocal microendoscopy will provide significant clinical benefit in early intervention remains to be seen.[10,36] OCT detects backscattered light instead of sound waves, and because light is 200,000 times faster than sound, low coherence interferometry is required to integrate reflectance properties of tissue scanned for obtaining high-resolution cross-sectional microscopic images of the bronchial wall, with potential in vivo microdynamic imaging without the necessity for biopsy for studying carcinogenesis.[36]

OCT and confocal microendoscopy may facilitate our understanding of dynamic processes in the continuous damage and repair processes of clonal cells over time. Very early carcinogenesis at the clonal level cannot be properly studied, because biopsy in itself may completely eradicate these minute

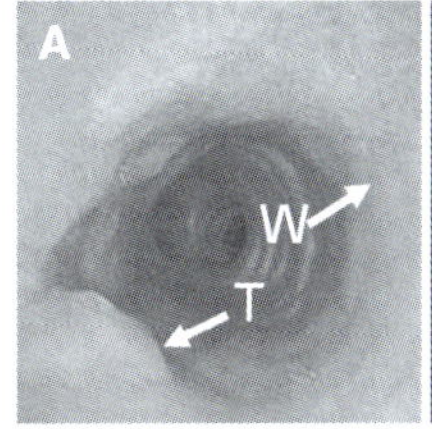

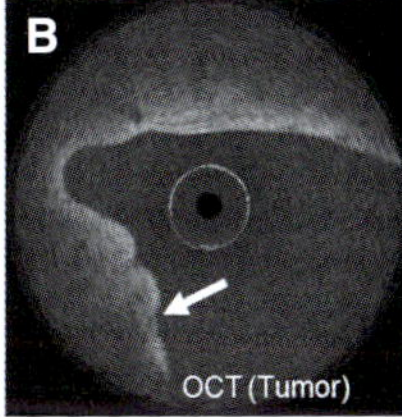

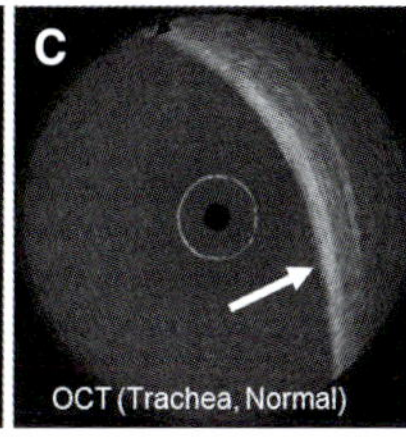

FIGURE 28.4 Optical coherence tomography (OCT) of an intraluminal squamous cell cancer in the tracheal wall. **A:** Bronchoscopic image showing nodular tumor (*T*) and normal tracheal wall (*W*). **B:** OCT showing tumor (*T*) infiltrating beyond the cartilage. **C:** Normal OCT. (From Tsuboi M, Hayashi A, Ikeda N, et al. Optical coherence tomography in the diagnosis of bronchial lesions. *Lung Cancer* 2005;49:387–394; courtesy of N. Ikeda, Mita Hospital, Japan.) (See color plate.)

lesions at the initial bronchoscopic study. The relatively high "spontaneous" regression rate for lower-grade dysplasias after bronchoscopic biopsy hampers further study on molecular carcinogenesis,[41] further emphasizing the need for novel optical biopsy techniques.[2,10,36]

CONCLUSION

The relative inaccessibility of thoracic organs has pushed bronchoscopic techniques to the limit. With the refinements of various catheter techniques and advancements of 4D real-time digital imaging, further exploration is aimed to optimize the use of minimally invasive techniques in thoracic medicine. Activities currently encompass the complete array of diagnostic staging and treatment intervention in patients and individuals at highest risk to develop preneoplastic lesions in their asymptomatic phase. Resolution has allowed us to study tissue at the clonal and subcellular level.

As such, practical exploitation of minimally invasive endoscopy for extended diagnostics in central airway tumor and for accurate staging of MLN suit sell in our common practice, because the majority of patients still have advanced disease.

Early minimally invasive intervention provides great opportunity for true stage shift by significantly reducing morbidity and mortality of early intervention, because quality of life in both patients with advanced cancer and cohort of asymptomatic individuals in lung cancer screening protocols is important.

REFERENCES

1. Ikeda S, Yanai N, Ishikawa S. Flexible bronchofiberscope. *Keio J Med* 1968;17(1):1–16.
2. Sutedja G. New techniques for early detection of lung cancer. *Eur Resp J Suppl* 2003;39:57s–66s.
3. Bolliger CT, Mathur PN, Beamis JF, et al. ERS/ATS statement on interventional pulmonology. European Respiratory Society/American Thoracic Society. *Eur Respir J* 2002;19:356–373.
4. Downie G, Yung R, Gazdar A, et al. Evidence-based clinical practice guidelines central airways lung cancer: ACCP (2nd Edition). *Chest* 2007;132;221–233.
5. Sutedja G, Codrington H, Risse EK, et al. Autofluorescence bronchoscopy improves staging of radiographically occult lung cancer and has an impact on therapeutic strategy. *Chest* 2001;120:1327–1332.
6. Krasnik M, Vilmann P, Herth F. EUS-FNA and EBUS-TBNA; the pulmonologist's and surgeon's perspective. *Endoscopy* 2006:38:S105–S109.
7. Bolliger CT, Sutedja TG, Strausz J, et al. Therapeutic bronchoscopy with immediate effect: laser, electrocautery, argon plasma coagulation and stents. *Eur Respir J* 2006;27:1258–1271.
8. Lam S, Hung J, LeRiche J, et al. Detection of dysplasia and carcinoma in situ with a lung imaging fluorescence endoscope device. *J Thorac Cardiovasc Surg* 1993;105:1035–1040.
9. Huang Z, McWilliams A, Lui H, et al. Near-infrared raman spectroscopy for optical diagnosis of lung cancer. *Int J Cancer* 2003;107:1047–1052.
10. Thiberville L, Moreno-Swirc S, Vercauteren T, et al. In vivo imaging of the bronchial wall microstructure using fibered confocal fluorescence microscopy. *Am J Respir Crit Care Med* 2007;175(1):22–31.
11. Schnall M, Rosen M. Primer on imaging technologies for cancer. *J Clin Oncol* 2006;24:3225–3233.
12. Eberhardt R, Anantham D, Ernst A, et al. Multimodality bronchoscopic diagnosis of peripheral lung lesions: a randomized controlled trial. *Am J Respir Crit Care Med* 2007;176(1):36–41.
13. Herth FJ, Rabe KF, Gasparini S, et al. Transbronchial and transoesophageal (ultrasound-guided) needle aspirations for the analysis of mediastinal lesions. *Eur Respir J* 2006;28:1264–1275.
14. Yasufuku K, Nakajima T, Motoori K, et al. Comparison of endobronchial ultrasound, positron emission tomography, and CT for lymph node staging of lung cancer. *Chest* 2006;130;710–718.
15. Goerres GW, Kamel E, Heidelberg TN, et al. PET-CT image co-registration in the thorax: influence of respiration. *Eur J Nucl Med Mol Imaging* 2002;29:351–360.
16. Piet AH, Lagerwaard FJ, Kunst PW, et al. Can mediastinal nodal mobility explain the low yield rates for transbronchial needle aspiration without real-time imaging? *Chest 2007*;131:1783–1787.
17. Cerfolio RJ, Ayesha S. Bryant AS, et al. Routine mediastinoscopy and esophageal ultrasound fine-needle aspiration in patients with non-small cell lung cancer who are clinically N2 negative. A prospective study. *Chest* 2006;130:1791–1795.
18. Dooms C, Vansteenkiste J. Positron emission tomography in nonsmall-cell lung cancer. *Curr Opin Pulm Med* 2007;13:256–260.
19. Shinagawa N, Yamazaki K, Onodera Y, et al. CT-guided transbronchial biopsy using an ultrathin bronchoscope with virtual bronchoscopic navigation. *Chest* 2004;125:1138–1143.
20. Herth FJ, Eberhardt R, Becker HD, et al. Endobronchial ultrasound-guided transbronchial lung biopsy in fluoroscopically invisible solitary pulmonary nodules: a prospective trial. *Chest* 2006;129(1):147–150.
21. Pasic A, Postmus PE, Sutedja G. What is early lung cancer? A review of the literature. *Lung Cancer* 2004;45:267–277.
22. Black WC. Randomized clinical trials for cancer screening: rationale and design considerations for imaging tests. *J Clin Oncol* 2006;24:3252–3260.
23. Black C, de Verteuil R, Walker S, et al. Population screening for lung cancer using computed tomography, is there evidence of clinical effectiveness? A systematic review of the literature. *Thorax* 2007; 62:131–138.
24. MacMahon H, Austin JH, Gamsu G, et al. Guidelines for management of small pulmonary nodules detected on CT scans: a statement from the Fleischner Society. *Radiology* 2005;237:395–400.
25. Lee P, Sutedja G. Lung cancer screening: has there been any progress? Computed tomography and autofluroescence bronchoscopy. *Curr Opin Pulm Med* 2007;13:243–248.
26. Schöder H, Gönen M. Screening for cancer with PET and PET/CT: potential and limitations. *J Nucl Med* 2007;48(Suppl 1):4S–18S.
27. Truong MT, Pan T, Erasmus JJ. Pitfalls in integrated CT-PET of the thorax: implications in oncologic imaging. *J Thorac Imaging* 2006;21:111–122.
28. Seemann MD, Schaefer JF, Englmeier KH. Virtual positron emission tomography/computed tomography-bronchoscopy: possibilities, advantages and limitations of clinical application. *Eur Radiol* 2007;17:709–715.
29. Flieder DB, Vazquez M, Carter D, et al. Pathologic findings of lung tumors diagnosed on baseline CT screening. *Am J Surg Pathol* 2006;30:606–613.
30. Thunnissen FB, Kerr KM, Brambilla E, et al. EU-USA pathology panel for uniform diagnosis in randomised controlled trials for HRCT screening in lung cancer. *Eur Respir J* 2006;28:1186–1189.
31. Quon A, Napel S, Beaulieu CF, et al. Flying through and "flying around" a PET/CT scan: pilot study and development of 3D integrated 18F-FDG PET/CT for virtual bronchoscopy and colonoscopy. *J Nucl Med* 2006;47:1081–1087.
32. Makris D, Scherpereel A, Leroy S, et al. Electromagnetic navigation diagnostic bronchoscopy for small peripheral lung lesions. *Eur Respir J* 2007;29:1187–1192.
33. McAdams HP, Goodman PC, Kussin P. Virtual bronchoscopy for directing transbronchial needle aspiration of hilar and mediastinal lymph nodes: a pilot study. *AJR Am J Roentgenol* 1998;170:1361–1364.
34. Cover KS, Lagerwaard FJ, Senan S. Color intensity projections: a rapid approach for evaluating four-dimensional CT scans in treatment planning. *Int J Oncol Rad Biol Phys* 2006;64:954–961.

35. Miyazu Y, Miyazawa T, Kurimoto N, et al. Endobronchial ultrasonography in the assessment of centrally located early-stage lung cancer before photodynamic therapy. *Am J Respir Crit Care Med* 2002;165:832–837.
36. Tsuboi M, Hayashi A, Ikeda N, et al. Optical coherence tomography in the diagnosis of bronchial lesions. *Lung Cancer* 2005;49:387–394.
37. Pasic A, Vonk Noordegraaf A, Risse EK, et al. Multiple suspicious lesions detected by autofluorescence bronchoscopy predict malignant development in the bronchial mucosa in high risk patients. *Lung Cancer* 2003;41:295–301.
38. Nakamura H, Kawasaki N, Hagiwara M, et.al. Early hilar lung cancer risk for multiple lung cancers and clinical outcome. *Lung Cancer* 2001;33:51–55.
39. Pasic A, Brokx HA, Vonk NA, et al. Cost-effectiveness of early intervention: comparison between intraluminal bronchoscopic treatment and surgical resection for T1N0 lung cancer patients. *Respiration* 2004;71:391–396.
40. van Boxem TJ, Westerga J, Venmans BJ, et al. Photodynamic therapy, Nd-YAG laser and electrocautery for treating early-stage intraluminal cancer. Which to choose? *Lung Cancer* 2001;31:31–36.
41. Breuer RH, Pasic A, Smit EF, et al. The natural course of preneoplastic lesions in bronchial epithelium. *Clin Cancer Res* 2005;11:537–543.
42. Holty JE, Kuschner WG, Gould MK. Accuracy of transbronchial needle aspiration for mediastinal staging of non-small cell lung cancer: a meta-analysis. *Thorax* 2005;60:949–55.
43. Diacon AH, Schuurmans MM, Theron J, et al. Transbronchial needle aspirates: How many passes per target site? *Eur Resp J* 2007;29:112–116.
44. Cerfolio RJ, Bryant AS, Buddhiwardhan O. Restaging patients with N2 (stage IIIA) non-small cell lung cancer after neoadjuvant chemoradiotherapy: A prospective study. *J Thorac Cardiovasc Surg* 2007;131;1229–1235.
45. Kunst PW, Lee P, Paul MA, et al. Restaging of mediastinal nodes with transbronchial needle aspiration after induction chemoradiation for locally advanced non-small cell lung cancer. *J Thorac Oncol* 2007;2:912–915.
46. Herth F, Annema JT, Eberhardt R, et al. Endobronchial ultrasound with transbronchial needle aspiration for restaging the mediastinum in lung cancer. *J Clin Oncol* 2008;26(20):3346–3350.
47. Stamatis G, Fechner S, Hillejan L, et al. Repeat mediastinoscopy as a restaging procedure. *Pneumologie* 2005;59(12):862–866.
48. De Leyn P, Stroobants S, De Wever W, et al. Prospective comparative study of integrated positron emission tomography: computed tomography scan compared with remediastinoscopy in the assessment of residual mediastinal lymph node disease after induction chemotherapy for mediastinoscopy-proven stage IIIA-N2 non–small-cell lung cancer: a Leuven Lung Cancer Group study. *J Clin Oncol* 2006;24(21):3333–3339.
49. Van Schil P, Stamatis G. Sensitivity of remediastinoscopy: influence of adhesions, multilevel N2 involvement, or surgical technique? *J Clin Oncol* 2006;24(33):5338.
50. Van Schil PE, De Waele M. A second mediastinoscopy: how to decide and how to do it? *Eur J Cardiothorac Surg* 2008;33:703–706.
51. Annema JT, Veseliç M, Versteegh MI, et al. Mediastinal restaging: EUS-FNA offers a new perspective. *Lung Cancer* 2003;42:311–318.
52. Varadarajulu S, Eloubeidi M. Can endoscopic ultrasonography-guided fine-needle aspiration predict response to chemoradiation in non–small-cell lung cancer? A pilot study. *Respiration* 2006;73:213–220.
53. Herth F, Eberhardt R, Vilmann P, et al. Real-time endobronchial ultrasound guided transbronchial needle aspiration for sampling mediastinal lymph nodes. *Thorax* 2006;61:795–798.
54. Silvestri GA, Gould MK, Gould MK, et al. Noninvasive staging of non-small cell lung cancer: ACCP evidence-based clinical practice guidelines (2nd edition). *Chest* 2007;132:178–201.
55. Bauwens O, Dusart M, Pierard P, et al. Endobronchial ultrasound and value of PET for prediction of pathological results of mediastinal hot spots in lung cancer patients. *Lung Cancer* 2008;61(3):356–361.
56. Herth F, Ernst A, Eberhardt R, et al. Endobronchial ultrasound-guided transbronchial needle aspiration of lymph nodes in the radiologically normal mediastinum. *Eur Respir J* 2006;28:910–914.
57. LeBlanc JK, Devereaux BM, Imperiale TF, et al. Endoscopic ultrasound in non-small cell lung cancer and negative mediastinum on computed tomography. *Am J Respir Crit Care Med* 2005;171:177–182.
58. Hoffmann H. Invasive staging of lung cancer by mediastinoscopy and video-assisted thoracoscopy. *Lung Cancer* 2001;34:3–5.
59. Luke WP, Pearson FG, Todd TR, et al. Prospective evaluation of mediastinoscopy for assessment of carcinoma of the lung. *J Thorac Cardiovasc Surg* 1986;91:53–56.
60. Coughlin M, Deslauriers J, Beaulieu M, et al. Role of mediastinoscopy in pretreatment staging of patients with primary lung cancer. *Ann Thorac Surg* 1985;40:556–560.
61. Tahara RW, Lackner RP, Graver LM. Is there a role for routine mediastinoscopy in patients with peripheral T1 lung cancers? *Am J Surg* 2000;180(6):488–491.
62. De Leyn P, Vansteenkiste J, Cuypers P, et al. Role of cervical mediastinoscopy in staging of non-small cell lung cancer without enlarged mediastinal lymph nodes on CT scan. *Eur J Cardiothorac Surg* 1997;12(5):706–712.
63. Herth F, Ernst A, Eberhardt R, et al. Endobronchial ultrasound-guided transbronchial needle aspiration of lymph nodes in the radiologically normal mediastinum. *Eur Respir J* 2006;28:910–914.
64. Herth F, Eberhardt R, Krasnik M, et al. Endobronchial ultrasound-guided transbronchial needle aspiration of lymph nodes in the radiologically and positron emission tomography-normal mediastinum in patients with lung cancer. *Chest* 2008;133:887–889.
65. Ernst A, Anantham D, Eberhardt R, *et al.* Diagnosis of mediastinal adenopathy: real-time endobronchial ultrasound-guided needle aspiration versus mediastinoscopy. *J Thorac Oncol* 2008;3(6):577–582.
66. Rivera P, Mehta A. Initial diagnosis of lung cancer. Evidence-based clinical practice guidelines central airways lung cancer: ACCP (2nd edition). *Chest* 2007;132:131S–148S.
67. Woolner LB, Fontana RS, Cortese DA, et al. Roentgenographically occult lung cancer: pathologic findings and frequency of multicentricity during a 10-year period. *Mayo Clin Proc* 1984;59:453–466.
68. Konaka C, Hirano T, Kato H, et al. Comparison of endoscopic features of early-stage squamous cell lung cancer and histological findings. *Br J Cancer* 1999;80:1435–1439.

CHAPTER 29

Frank C. Detterbeck

Surgical Evaluation of the Mediastinum

At first glance, surgical mediastinal staging may appear to be a mundane and lackluster topic, extensively reviewed with little new information to be added. However, beneath this surface lie many nuances and issues that often lead to confusion, misinterpretation of data, and erroneous conclusions. Furthermore, there are many new developments, both with respect to surgical techniques and in regard to alternative approaches to mediastinal evaluation. Because mediastinal staging remains a key factor in selecting a treatment approach for patients with lung cancer, an understanding of the issues and developments is crucial to achieve optimal clinical outcomes.

Definition of the role of surgical mediastinal staging is complex and depends on many characteristics of the patients being considered. In fact, lack of attention to details of the patients involved is probably the major factor leading to inappropriate application of results from one population to a different cohort. The patients may have undergone minimal imaging (chest x-ray [CXR] or computed tomography [CT]) or more sophisticated imaging (positron emission tomography [PET] or PET/CT). Whether the patient has undergone a careful clinical evaluation for signs and symptoms of distant metastases is often glossed over, and patients may (e.g., those with symptoms of metastases or asymptomatic clinical stage III [cIII]) or may not (e.g., asymptomatic cI) have an indication for extrathoracic imaging for metastases. It is important to note whether the patients have normal-sized or enlarged mediastinal nodes. Finally, results of a procedure done as a staging test are very different from a procedure done merely to make a diagnosis (often including many patients that do not have lung cancer). A lack of awareness of these issues often leads to inappropriate application of the results of a study to a different type of patient.

Even when the focus is limited only to surgical mediastinal staging, there are issues regarding the extent and quality of the procedure. Newer techniques of surgical mediastinal staging can provide a much more accurate assessment, but the biggest issue is simply whether traditional mediastinoscopy is performed according to accepted standards. It is clear that there are frequent breaches in quality that are likely to have serious consequences for patients,[1] although this has not been studied in detail. Furthermore, there are differences in pathologists' assessment of nodes, and newer techniques can provide more sensitive assessments (i.e., immunohistochemistry of micrometastases). Having said this, the prognostic value of such pathologic investigations is questionable at present.[2–4]

Many alternative techniques have been developed to allow less invasive, "nonsurgical" mediastinal tissue staging. These are discussed in more detail in Chapter 31, but how these techniques can be integrated is discussed here. It is important not to view the various techniques of tissue staging as competitive. To a large extent, the techniques have been used in different patient populations (i.e., anatomic location of particular enlarged or normal-sized nodes), making a simple comparison of test performance characteristics inappropriate. How the different procedures best complement one another depends on patient characteristics, the primary question to be addressed (i.e., to rule in cancer or to rule out cancer), and the level of proficiency available with a particular approach.

Finally, the role of surgical mediastinal staging is a matter of judgment. No test can be expected to yield perfect results, so it becomes a question of how much uncertainty one is willing to accept. This threshold is influenced by the risk and morbidity of the procedures involved. Although mediastinoscopy is done as an outpatient procedure in most centers and is associated with low morbidity (2%) and mortality (0.08%), it is somewhat invasive.[5] It is proposed that in general, invasive staging is justified if there is a >10% chance of error in the mediastinal stage from imaging alone, and noninvasive testing (i.e., PET) for a >5% chance of error. Performing a test for a low prevalence of disease runs the risk of either a test-related complication or an erroneous result without a high chance of benefiting from the test.

SCOPE

This chapter focuses on surgical methods of mediastinal staging, namely, mediastinoscopy and variation of this technique (videomediastinoscopy, video-assisted mediastinal lymphadenectomy [VAMLA], and transcervical extended mediastinal lymphadenectomy [TEMLA]). The chapter also includes a discussion of thoracoscopic approaches as well as the Chamberlain procedure (anterior mediastinotomy). The focus is on primary staging of patients with non–small cell lung cancer (NSCLC). Restaging of the mediastinum after induction therapy is not covered thoroughly. In addition, mediastinal procedures done only to make a diagnosis (i.e., lymphoma, thymoma) are not discussed.

DEFINITIONS

It is important to clearly define the major terms used to avoid confusion. *Pathologic staging*, according to the American Joint Committee on Cancer (AJCC), refers to the stage after surgical *resection* and complete pathologic evaluation of the specimen and any other tissues submitted. Clinical stage is the stage as determined by any and all information that is available prior to resection. Thus, clinical stage can involve imaging (radiographic staging) or biopsies such as transbronchial needle aspiration (TBNA) or a mediastinoscopy (tissue staging). Although mediastinoscopy is considered a surgical procedure and involves a pathology report, it is still part of clinical staging.

Various parameters can be used to assess the reliability of a test, including sensitivity, specificity, and false-negative (FN) and false-positive (FP) rates (typically expressed as a percentage). The latter two measures are sometimes expressed in a less intuitive manner as the converse, known as the negative predictive value (NPV = 1 − FN rate) or positive predictive value (PPV = 1 − FP rate). Sensitivity and specificity are derived from patient populations in whom the true disease status is already known, who either all have or do not have the condition in question. These parameters provide data about how often the test will be positive or negative for these respective populations. Thus, these measures provide information about the *test*, because the disease status has already been determined in the patients. In theory, these measures can be used to compare different tests, but *only if* the patient populations in which the tests are used are the same. Unfortunately, particularly with regard to invasive staging tests, the patients selected for different tests are not the same, limiting the value of the measures of sensitivity and specificity.

The FN and FP rates of a test are of much greater practical use to the clinician, who must interpret the reliability of a test result (positive or negative) in an individual patient. The clinician does not know the true disease status of the patient; he/she only knows that the patient has a negative or a positive test result. Interpretation of a test result for an individual patient requires knowledge of the FN or FP rate. It is important to point out that the FN or FP rate of the test *cannot* be estimated from the sensitivity or specificity, because each of these is derived from different formulas. This is a common misconception that frequently creates confusion and inappropriate interpretation of test results. The only exception to this fact is in the case of "perfect" test performance: a sensitivity of 100% does, in fact, imply an FN rate of 0, and a specificity of 100% implies an FP rate of 0.

In general, patients with lung cancer can be separated into four groups (Fig. 29.1) with respect to intrathoracic radiographic characteristics of the primary tumor and the mediastinal nodes.[5,6] Briefly, the groups are patients with extensive mediastinal infiltration (radiographic group A), those with enlargement of discrete mediastinal nodes (radiographic group B), patients with normal mediastinal nodes by CT but a central tumor or suspected N1 disease (radiographic group C), and those with normal nodes, mediastinal nodes, and a peripheral cI tumor (radiographic group D).

A widely accepted definition of normal-sized mediastinal lymph nodes is a short-axis diameter of ≤1 cm on a transverse CT image.[6] Discrete nodal enlargement implies that discrete nodes are seen on the CT scan and are defined well enough to be able to measure their size (and are >1 cm). Mediastinal infiltration is present when there is abnormal tissue in the mediastinum that does not have the appearance and shape of distinct lymph nodes, but instead has an irregular, amorphous shape.[6] In this case, it is difficult to distinguish discrete nodes and impossible to come up with a measurement of the size of nodes. This occurs when multiple nodes are matted together to the point where the boundary between them is obscured and can be assumed to involve extensive extranodal spread of tumor. It may progress to the point where mediastinal vessels and other structures are partially or completely encircled. Finally, the distinction between a central versus a peripheral tumor has also not been codified, but most authors consider any tumor in the outer two thirds of the hemithorax to be peripheral.[6]

TECHNIQUE AND OUTCOMES OF STANDARD MEDIASTINOSCOPY

Mediastinoscopy has been the mainstay of invasive mediastinal staging for the past 40 years. The procedure is performed in the operating room, usually under general anesthesia. It is currently done as an outpatient in most U.S. centers.[7–9] Mediastinoscopy involves an incision just above the suprasternal notch, insertion of a mediastinoscope alongside the trachea, and biopsy of mediastinal nodes. Rates of morbidity and mortality as a result of this procedure are low (2% and 0.08%).[10] Right and left high and low paratracheal nodes (stations 2R, 2L, 4R, 4L), pretracheal nodes (stations 1, 3), and anterior subcarinal nodes (station 7) are accessible via this approach. Node groups that cannot be biopsied with this technique

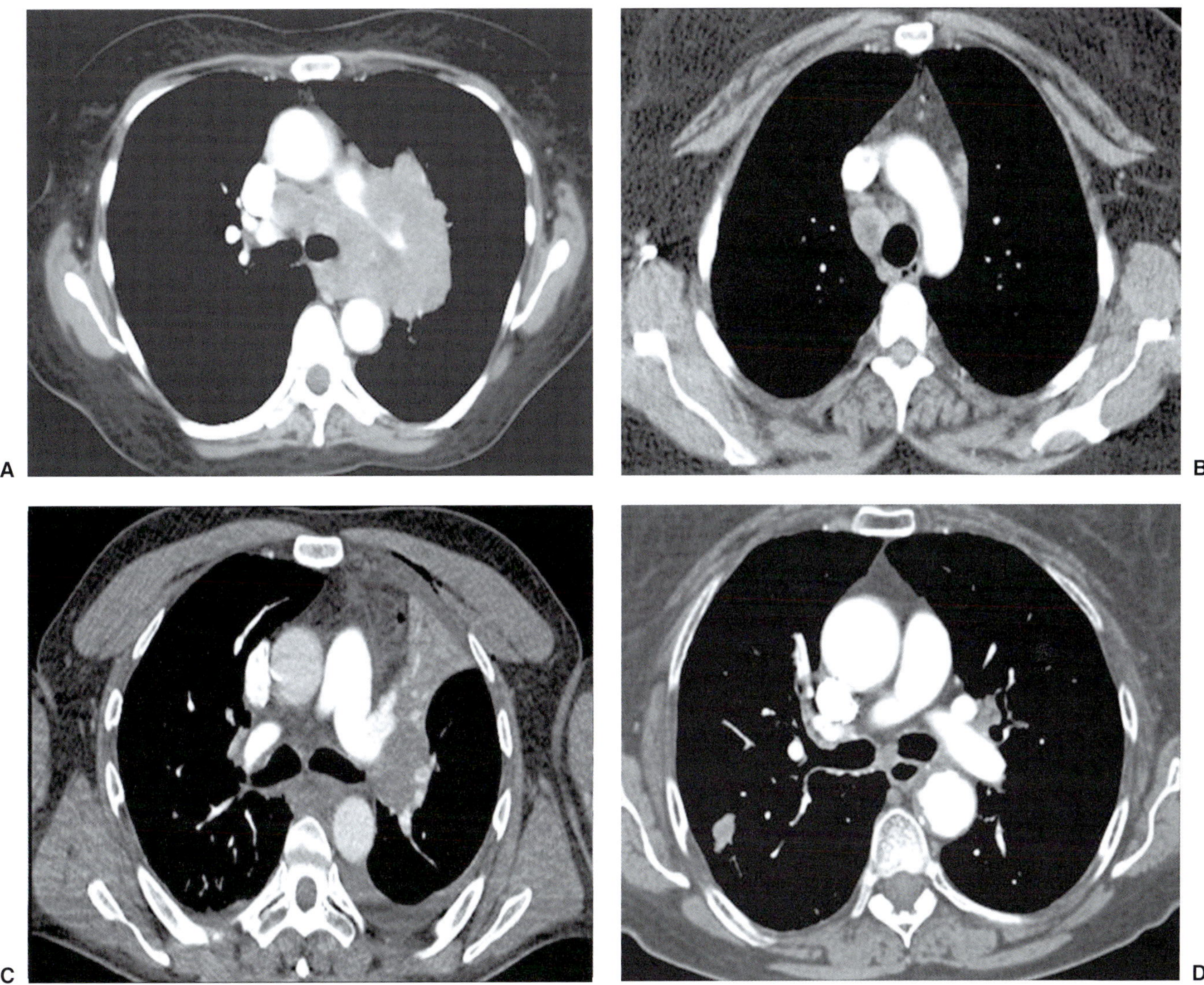

FIGURE 29.1 Radiographic categories of mediastinal appearance in patients with lung cancer. **A:** Mediastinal infiltration by tumor. **B:** Enlarged discrete N2, N3 nodes. **C:** A central tumor or a tumor with enlarged N1 nodes, but a normal mediastinum. **D:** A peripheral small tumor (lower left corner of image) with normal-sized lymph nodes. (From Silvestri G, Gould MK, Margolis ML, et al. Noninvasive staging of non-small cell lung cancer: ACCP evidenced-based clinical practice guidelines (2nd edition). *Chest* 2007;132:178S–201S.)

include posterior subcarinal (station 7), inferior mediastinal (stations 8, 9), aortopulmonary window (APW) (station 5), and anterior mediastinal (station 6) nodes.

The average sensitivity of mediastinoscopy to detect mediastinal node involvement from cancer is approximately 80%, and the average FN rate is approximately 10% to 15% (Table 29.1), as has been compiled in several systematic reviews.[5,11] Several authors have shown that approximately half (42% to 57%) of the FN cases were caused by nodes that were not accessible by the mediastinoscope.[12–17] The specificity and the FP rates of mediastinoscopy are reported to be 100% and 0, respectively. Strictly speaking, these values cannot really be assessed because patients with a positive biopsy were not subjected to any further procedures (e.g., thoracotomy) to confirm the results. The results of mediastinoscopy are fairly consistent among studies.[5]

Quality of Surgical Staging The results cited in the preceding paragraph outline the experience in dedicated thoracic centers with a specific interest in thoracic surgery. However, there are indications that what is practiced more broadly is not the same.[1,18] In the United States, many patients with lung cancer undergo resection either by general surgeons or cardiothoracic surgeons whose primary scope of practice is cardiac surgery. A fair amount of data suggests that both short- and long-term outcomes of patients with lung cancer are affected by the quality of care as well as the extent of specialization in thoracic surgery.[19–21]

TABLE 29.1 Performance Characteristics of Mediastinoscopy

Author	Year	N	Patient Type	Proc. Type	Sens	Spec	FP	FN	Prev
Hammoud et al.[16]	1999	1369	cI–III	Med	85	100	0	8	36
Coughlin et al.[12]	1985	1259	cI–III	Med	92	100	0	3	29
Luke et al.[71]	1986	1000	cI–III	Med	85	100	0	9	39
De Leyn et al.[72]	1996	500	cI–III	Med	76	100	0	13	39
Brion et al.[73]	1985	153	cI–III	Med	67	100	0	15	35
Jolly et al.[74]	1991	136	cI–III	Med	92	100	0	9	54
Ratto et al.[75]	1990	123	cI–III	Med	88	100	0	6	33
Ebner et al.[76]	1999	116	cI–III	Med	81	100	0	18	50
Gdeedo et al.[14]	1997	100	cI–III	Med	78	100	0	9	32
Deneffe et al.[77]	1983	124	cI–III	Med	68	100	0	12	31
Aaby et al.[78]	1995	57	cI–III	Med	84	100	0	11	44
Page et al.[79]	1987	345	cII–III[a]	Med	73	100	0	20	48
Dillemans et al.[80]	1994	331	cII,III[a]	Med	72	100	0	16	41
Riordan et al.[81]	1991	74	cII–III	Med	81	100	0	16	50
Choi et al.[82]	2003	291	cI	Med	44	100	0	9	15
Gürses et al.[83]	2002	67	cI	Med	40	100	0	7	15
Subtotal		**5922**	**cI–III**	**Med**	**79**	**100**	**0**	**13**	**47**
Lardinois et al.[17]	2003	181	cI–III	VMS	87	100	0	8	34
Venissac et al.[27]	2003	154	cIII	VMS	97	100	0	6	71
Kimura et al.[28]	2003	125	cII,III	VMS	85	100	0	8	36
Subtotal		**460**	**cII,III**	**VMS**	**90**	**100**	**0**	**7**	**47**
Witte et al.[29]	2006	130	cI–III	VAMLA	94	100	0	1	-
Leschber et al.[30]	2003	18	—	VAMLA	100	100	0	(0)	4
Zieliński[32]	2007	256	cI–III	TEMLA	94	100	0	3	31
Subtotal		**404**	**cI–III**	**TCMLA**	**96**	**100**	**0**	**1**	**18**

[a]Excluded peripheral cI. Included central cII and cIII.

Feas, feasibility; FN, false-negative rate; FP, false-positive rate; Med, mediastinoscopy; Prev, prevalence; Proc., procedure; Sens, sensitivity; Spec, specificity; TCMLA, transcervical mediastinal lymphadenectomy (either TEMLA or VAMLA); TEMLA, transcervical extended mediastinal lymphadenectomy; VAMLA, video-assisted mediastinal lymphadenectomy; VMS, videomediastinoscopy.

With regard to mediastinal staging, it seems obvious that the FN rate depends on the diligence with which nodes are dissected and sampled at mediastinoscopy. Ideally, five nodal stations (stations 2R, 4R, 7, 4L, 2L) should routinely be examined, with at least one node sampled from each station unless none are present after *actual dissection* in the region of a particular node station. The difference between this and what is actually done is underscored in a report by Little et al.[1] Analysis of national data in the United States on 11,688 surgically treated patients disclosed that only about half of the patients underwent either PET or mediastinoscopy to define the status of mediastinal nodes. Even more striking was the fact that in more than half of the mediastinoscopies performed, *not even a single mediastinal node was biopsied*. Finally, in almost half of the patients, no mediastinal nodes were biopsied at the time of thoracotomy.

The survival of patients with intraoperatively discovered "surprise N2" disease discovered at the time of resection varies dramatically according to the extent of preoperative staging that was undertaken.[22] Extrapolation of this data suggests that the differences between good- and poor-quality preoperative staging overshadow any differences that might be realized by integration of newer alternative techniques (esophageal ultrasound-guided needle aspiration [EUS-NA], endobronchial ultrasound-guided needle aspiration [EBUS-NA]). It is probably more important to have expertise in at least one technique of invasive mediastinal staging by a dedicated individual than to quibble about the relative value of one technique versus another. PET alone is clearly not adequate to stage the mediastinum, even in centers with a dedicated interest and expertise in PET for lung cancer.[6,23–25]

The recommendation that five nodal stations (stations 2R, 4R, 7, 4L, 2L) should routinely be examined at mediastinoscopy has been endorsed by the American College of Chest Physicians (ACCP),[5] the American Thoracic Society (ATS), and the European Society of Thoracic Surgeons (ESTS).[26] The ESTS recommends, but does not mandate, that sampling of stations 2R and 2L be done.

NEWER SURGICAL STAGING TECHNIQUES

Videomediastinoscopy The traditional mediastinoscope consists in principle of a tube with a light. This has been modified to include an optical system that provides a much more detailed view and allows a much more extensive dissection of nodes and other structures. Qualitatively, videomediastinoscopy allows actual dissection of nodal stations and removal of entire nodes. In addition, the fascial plane separating the anterior pretracheal space and the subcarinal space can be opened. Dissection directly adjacent to the carina and bronchi allows the subcarinal nodes to be mobilized, providing access to the posterior subcarinal nodes that are thought to be relatively inaccessible via traditional mediastinoscopy. Data from several series confirms an advantage over traditional mediastinoscopy for staging of the mediastinum: the average reported sensitivity is 90%, FN rate 7% (compared with approximately 80% and 13% for traditional mediastinoscopy).[17,27,28]

Video-Assisted Mediastinal Lymphadenectomy The videomediastinoscope has allowed development of techniques to completely remove all mediastinal nodes, which has been called VAMLA. The feasibility of carrying out a complete dissection is reported to be 86% (because of calcified or scarred nodes).[29] Only a few studies of this technique have been published.[29–31] Procedure-related complications have been uncommon (6%) and include recurrent nerve paralysis (five patients), bleeding from the azygous vein (two patients), and infection (one patient).[29,30] At the time of thoracotomy, 19% of patients had residual mediastinal nodes (primarily involving those VAMLA procedures that were deemed not completely feasible).[29] Some mediastinal stations appear to be quite completely dissected (stations 2R, 4R, 4L, and 7), whereas residual nodes were fairly common in others (stations 1, 2L, 3, 5).[30,31] Thus, this procedure results in a partial mediastinal lymphadenectomy, albeit a rather complete lymphadenectomy of the most important nodal stations. Parameters of sensitivity, specificity, and FN and FP rates are reported as 88, 100, 2, and 0, respectively, in a series of 130 patients that included incomplete VAMLA procedures (prevalence of N2, N3 disease of 13%), and 94%, 100, 1, and 0, respectively among only complete VAMLA cases.[29]

Transcervical Mediastinal Lymphadenectomy The technique of TEMLA has been developed by Dr. Zielinski in Zakopane, Poland.[32–34] This involves a collar incision that is wider than for a traditional mediastinoscopy, followed by dissection of the right and left carotid and the innominate arteries and the right and left innominate veins. This mobilization of the vessels allows them to be moved aside and provides excellent exposure to the entire mediastinum. Both of the recurrent nerves are visualized and carefully protected. A complete mediastinal node dissection can be performed, including nodes above the innominate vein (level 1), bilateral paratracheal (2, 4), subcarinal and periesophageal (7, 8), as well as the para-aortic nodes (5, 6). Complications in an experience of 256 cI to III patients were seen in 11% (including transient recurrent nerve palsy in 2.3%, pleural effusion in 4%, pneumothorax in 0.4%).[32] A mean of 39 nodes per patient were removed. At thoracotomy, residual benign nodes were found in 9% and missed malignant nodes in 4%, occurring exclusively early in their experience. The sensitivity of TEMLA for the detection of mediastinal node involvement is 94%, with a specificity of 100%, FN rate of 3%, and FP rate of 0.[32] It is not known at this point whether a small deposit found by such an extensive staging investigation carries the same poor prognosis as a deposit detected by routine mediastinoscopy.

Thoracoscopy Thoracoscopy (video-assisted thoracoscopic surgery [VATS]) for mediastinal staging has been reported in a limited number of studies.[5,35–40] Overall, a sensitivity of 75% and an FN rate of 7% have been reported.[5] However, the sensitivity varies widely (from 37% to 100%) without any obvious explanation. The low results stem primarily from the only prospective multicenter study.[36] Thus, in general, the results of VATS for staging appear to be not as good as that of other techniques, although the degree to which this has been defined is limited. This is coupled with the fact that VATS is associated with more discomfort than all of the other mediastinal staging procedures. VATS for staging is probably best reserved for specific situations, such as in patients with a cervical tracheostomy, or assessment of nodes in stations 5, 6, or 9 if other techniques cannot be used or are not available.

Nonsurgical Invasive Techniques Several newer techniques of invasive staging that are nonsurgical are available, including esophageal ultrasound (EUS) and endobronchial ultrasound (EBUS) coupled with needle aspiration. A full discussion of these is beyond the scope of this chapter, but one cannot discus surgical staging in a vacuum. Details of EBUS are discussed in Chapter 28. A summary of the performance characteristics of these newer tests, taken from a systematic review,[5] is provided in Table 29.2. It must be emphasized that a direct comparison between different techniques is inappropriate because of differences in the patient population, both in terms of the radiographic groups as well as the location of suspicious lymph nodes.

Like mediastinoscopy, these needle techniques generally do not require hospitalization, but in contrast to mediastinoscopy they are generally performed only with sedation (not general anesthesia).[5] Thus, these procedures have an advantage of being less invasive and complex. Unfortunately, the needle-based techniques carry an FN rate of approximately 20% to 25%. The sensitivity of a traditional (non–image guided) TBNA is lower (around 75%) than traditional mediastinoscopy, even though this has been done almost exclusively in patients with markedly enlarged nodes.[5] The sensitivity of EUS (also primarily in enlarged nodes) is similar to traditional mediastinoscopy.[5] On the other hand, EBUS appears to have a higher sensitivity (around 90%) and has been used in both enlarged and normal-sized nodes.[5]

TABLE 29.2 Average Performance Characteristics of Mediastinal Staging Tests[a]

	Patient Groups[b]		%				
Test	**Majority**	**Minor**	**Prev**	**Sens**	**Spec**	**FP**	**FN**
Mediastinoscopy (traditional)	B,C	D	47	79	100	0	13
Videomediastinoscopy	B,C	D	47	90	100	0	7
Mediastinal lymphadenectomy[c]	C,D	—	18	96	100	0	1
Thoracoscopy of mediastinum	B	C	44	75	100	0	7
Transbronchial needle aspiration	A,B	—	75	78	99	1	28
Endobronchial ultrasound[d]	B	A,C	68	90	100	0	20
Esophageal ultrasound[d]	B	A,C	61	84	100	1	19

[a]Results are not directly comparable because the patient populations differ.

[b]Groups as defined in Figure 29.1.

[c]Via transcervical approach.

[d]With needle aspiration.

FN, false-negative rate; FP, false-positive rate; prev, prevalence; sens, sensitivity; spec, specificity.

Data taken from Table 29.1 and Tables in Systematic Review conducted by the American College of Chest Physicians.[5] Transthoracic needle biopsy omitted because it is generally used to establish a diagnosis in patients with mediastinal infiltrative tumors, rather than as a staging test.

The major limitation of needle-based techniques is the FN rate (about 20% to 25%, likely even higher in normal-sized nodes). In general, a negative EUS, EBUS, or TBNA should be followed by a mediastinoscopy.[5] Thus, these techniques are less useful in patients with normal-sized mediastinal nodes. This is both because in general, the sensitivity of the needle techniques is lower in patients with normal-sized nodes (as is also in mediastinoscopy) and a negative result is more likely, but is relatively unreliable (because of the high FN rate).

The various surgical and nonsurgical invasive staging techniques should be viewed as complimentary.[41] Furthermore, all of the techniques depend on the skill of the operator. The results published from the best centers with a dedicated interest in a particular technique cannot often be duplicated more broadly. The presence of a dedicated interest and expertise with a particular test may be a key factor in determining the best way to integrate the various staging techniques in a particular institution. Ideally, the performance characteristics of staging tests at a particular institution should be collected and assessed to have a sound basis for making these decisions.

WHEN IS TISSUE STAGING NOT NEEDED?

Tissue confirmation of the mediastinal stage is not needed in patients with SCLC, stage IV NSCLC, or malignant pleural effusion.[5] In these patients, the status of the mediastinum is irrelevant to defining the appropriate treatment. In patients with extensive mediastinal infiltration (radiographic group A, Fig. 29.1), the radiographic stage is widely accepted as accurate without tissue confirmation.[5] It must be acknowledged that this is based on general clinical experience, because there is no published data to prove this. These recommendations are summarized in Table 29.3.

Tissue confirmation of the mediastinal stage is unnecessary in patients with cI tumors based on a chest CT and a clinical evaluation (i.e., history and physical examination) (radiographic group D, Fig. 29.1).[5] This is based on extensive data that N2 node involvement (as assessed at thoracotomy) is found in <10% of such patients.[5] The chance of making the diagnosis of N2 involvement by preoperative invasive staging is lower, because the sensitivity of these tests is not perfect. A PET scan to evaluate the mediastinum also appears not to be needed in patients with cI tumors.[6,23,42,43] This is because the chance of finding a PET-positive N2 nodal metastasis is <5%.[23,43] In fact, there is a higher chance of being misled by PET (FP mediastinal uptake or FP distant site of uptake) than the chance of correctly identifying disease spread in patients with cI tumors.[23,43]

WHEN IS TISSUE STAGING NECESSARY?

Tissue staging of the mediastinum is clearly needed if there is PET activity in mediastinal nodes (unless there is extensive mediastinal infiltration). This is because the FP rate of PET in the mediastinum is approximately 15% to 20%,[5,25] although the largest and most recent metaanalysis found an average FP rate of 27% (on a per patient basis, excluding studies with a prevalence of <10%).[6] These recommendations are summarized in Table 29.3.

Tissue staging is particularly important with increasing wide variability in the quality of PET scans. Furthermore, the accuracy of the scan interpretation is increasingly an issue with the movement to bring PET scanners out into smaller

TABLE 29.3 Algorithm for Confirmation of Mediastinal Stage

Clinical Scenario[a] (H & P; Chest CT)	Recom. Imaging[b] (& Result)[c]	Justification for Bx. Confirmation[c]	Recommended Invasive Mediastinal Staging Procedure	Justification for Choice of Procedure
Peripheral cI (D)[d]	None	<10% FN of CT	None	—
cII, central cI (C)[d]	PET (neg)	20% FN of CT & PET	Med	Low FN; neg result anticipated
	PET (pos)	20% FP of PET	1. Med	Low FN, more definitive
	" "	"	2. EUS/EBUS; if neg → Med	Less invasive; high FN
cIII, discrete N2,3 (B)[d]	PET (neg)	20% FN of PET	1. Med	Low FN, more definitive
	" "	"	2. EUS/EBUS/TBNA; if neg → Med	Less invasive; high FN
	PET (pos)	15% FP of PET	1. EUS/EBUS/TBNA; if neg → Med	Less invasive; pos result anticipated
	" "	"	2. Med	Low FN, more definitive
cIII, infiltration (A)[d]	None[e]	Low FP of CT	None	—
cIV	None[e]	Will not affect Tmt	None	—

[a]Applies to patients with a clinical diagnosis of NSCLC.

[b]Recommendation based on ACCP Guidelines.[5,6]

[c]Pertains to status of the mediastinal nodes.

[d]Radiographic group as defined in Figure 29.1.

[e]PET needed for evaluation of distant metastases.

1.,2., Reasonable alternative approaches, choice of EUS/EBUS/TBNA depends on size, location of nodes and availability of expertise; Bx., biopsy; cI, clinical stage I; cII, clinical stage II; cIII, clinical stage III; cIV, clinical stage IV; CT, computed tomography scan; EBUS, endobronchial ultrasound (and needle aspiration); EUS, esophageal ultrasound (and needle aspiration); FN, false-negative rate; FP, false-positive rate; H & P, history and physical examination; Med, mediastinoscopy; neg, negative; NSCLC, non–small cell lung cancer; PET, positron emission tomography; pos, positive; TBNA, transbronchial needle aspiration; Tmt, treatment.

communities (especially mobile scanners), which hampers communication between the reader of the PET scan and a physician experienced in treating lung cancer. There are data that the interpretation of a CT scan is much more accurate when it is done with input from the treating clinician,[44] and there are multiple reasons that would suggest that this is even more true with PET imaging. Important aspects in this regard include a mechanism for meaningful interaction between a dedicated PET radiologist and a clinician with experience in lung cancer (enabling collective judgment) as well as a mechanism for feedback of final results to the radiologist.[45,46] Little formal study of these issues has been done, but they suggest that one should be cautious about simply accepting PET interpretation without tissue confirmation, especially when the PET is done in a smaller center.

Tissue staging of the mediastinum is also needed in the face of a negative PET in the mediastinum in patients with discrete mediastinal node involvement (radiographic group B) and in patients with central tumors or N1 node enlargement (radiographic group C, Fig. 29.1).[5] The basis for this statement is the finding of an FN rate of PET of approximately 25% in these situations.[5,25,47–49] CT alone is also notoriously inaccurate in these patient cohorts (an FP rate of 40% with discrete mediastinal node involvement and an FN rate of 25% in patients with central tumors of N1 node enlargement).[11] Therefore, tissue staging is necessary in such patients whether or not a PET is performed.

It is worth noting that accurate mediastinal staging is important whenever treatment with curative intent is being planned, not only when the treatment involves surgery. The principles of accurate staging are specific to the disease and not to the modality used. Thus, the same data and, therefore, the same rules about the need for tissue staging of the mediastinum apply if the curative treatment being considered is chemoradiation alone, radiofrequency ablation, or stereotactic radiosurgery.

LEFT UPPER LOBE TUMORS AND AORTOPULMONARY WINDOW NODES

Cancers in the left upper lobe (LUL) have a predilection for involvement of the nodes in the APW (station 5). These nodes are classified as mediastinal nodes and represent the most important group of N2 nodes that are not accessible by standard cervical mediastinoscopy. It has been suggested that nodes in this region should not be viewed as mediastinal nodes and that resection of patients should be performed regardless of APW node involvement, making assessment of these nodes superfluous.[50] This was based on a selected subgroup of 23 completely resected patients who had APW node involvement as the only site of N2 disease. However, analysis of all of the data in this regard shows that survival of patients with only APW node involvement is not substantially different than that of patients with involvement of only a single N2 node station in another location.[22,51] Therefore, the issue is more a matter of whether patients with involvement of a single mediastinal node station should undergo surgical resection and not whether APW nodes should be classified as N2 nodes.

The classic way of invasively assessing this area is a Chamberlain procedure (also known as an anterior mediastinotomy), which involves an incision in the second or third intercostal space just to the left of the sternum. Traditionally, an overnight hospital stay was necessary, but in many institutions, this is no longer found to be necessary, especially as surgeons have used visualization between the ribs more frequently as opposed to removal of a costal cartilage. The reliability of this procedure has not been extensively documented, despite its common use. The sensitivity of a Chamberlain procedure in addition to a standard cervical mediastinoscopy in patients with LUL tumors is approximately 87%, and the FN rate is approximately 10%.[5] These patients are primarily from radiographic group B, with probably a few from group C. Two additional studies regarding this procedure have not really addressed the reliability of the procedure for staging of NSCLC. In one study, no actual biopsies were performed in most patients, and the procedure was used to assess resectability (resectable patients included those with bulky APW nodal involvement in this series).[52] The other study used anterior mediastinotomy primarily for diagnosis (not staging), and included pulmonary biopsies and evaluation of patients with mediastinal masses.[53] In fact, only a few patients included in this study had lung cancer.

Extended cervical mediastinoscopy offers an alternative way of invasive assessment of APW nodes, but is used in only a few institutions.[5] With this procedure, a mediastinoscope is inserted through the suprasternal notch and directed lateral to the aortic arch.[54] In 100 consecutive patients with LUL cancers, standard mediastinoscopy and extended mediastinoscopy were found to have a sensitivity of 69% and an FN rate of 11% for detection of N2, N3 disease (prevalence, 29%).[54] Similar results (sensitivity, 81%; FN rate, 9%) were reported in another series of 93 such patients, all of whom had enlarged APW nodes.[55] These patients are primarily from radiographic group B, with probably a few from group C. In approximately 550 patients undergoing extended cervical mediastinoscopy, two major complications (one stroke and one aortic injury) have been reported.[54–58]

Thoracoscopy has been used to assess APW lymph nodes.[5,35] The only study specifically addressing this techniques found complete accuracy in 39 patients.[35] However, the study is limited because it involved only three patients without station 5 or 6 node involvement. EUS-NA also provides an alternative method of sampling APW nodes (see previous discussion). Only one study has specifically addressed EUS-NA for stations 5 and 6, but the data reported do not allow calculation of sensitivity, specificity, and FN or FP rates. However, a high FN rate is suggested.[35]

In conclusion, it appears that the sensitivity of either a Chamberlain or VATS assessment of the APW is high, whereas the results for extended cervical mediastinoscopy, and perhaps also EUS-NA, are somewhat lower. The FN rate appears to be low for all procedures with the exception of EUS-NA. However, these conclusions are somewhat speculative because the amount of data available is limited.

INTEGRATION OF INVASIVE STAGING TECHNIQUES

The various techniques of tissue staging should be viewed as complementary and not as competitive procedures.[41] There are many reasons for this. First of all, one cannot compare the performance characteristics (sensitivity, specificity, and FN and FP rates) of two tests unless they are being applied to the same patient population.[5] It is quite clear that in most published studies, the patient populations included are *not* the same. They differ relative to whether lymph nodes were enlarged or normal sized, which node stations were most suspicious, and whether the issue at hand was simply to establish a diagnosis or to establish a tissue stage. Furthermore, in assessing the results of a particular technique, it is important to recognize that the performance characteristics will be different in patients with enlarged or normal-sized mediastinal nodes. One should not use data from patients with enlarged nodes to estimate the value of a test for a patient with normal-sized nodes. Therefore, patient characteristics are important determinants in selection of the best method of tissue staging.

The results of staging procedures are also strongly affected by the expertise of the physicians performing the test. It is likely that the difference between the same procedure performed by an expert with a dedicated interest and someone who performs the procedure only occasionally is far greater than differences between different tests. Therefore, appropriate integration of staging procedures is dependent on the local experience. This must be evaluated critically, ideally in a multidisciplinary manner and based on actual local data.

A suggested algorithm (Table 29.3) is to perform mediastinoscopy as the generally preferred tissue staging method in patients with normal-sized mediastinal nodes (e.g., in patients with a central tumor or N1 node enlargement who have a 20% to 25% incidence of N2 involvement). This is because the primary issue is to rule out node involvement, and needle-based techniques carry a high FN rate, especially in normal-sized nodes. Because a negative needle biopsy (EUS-NA, EBUS-NA, or TBNA) should be followed by a mediastinoscopy, most patients would undergo both tests if a needle technique is used as the first step. On the other hand, a needle-based approach may be a good first step in patients with enlarged nodes, because it may spare many patients the need for mediastinoscopy; however, a negative needle test in patients with enlarged nodes should generally still be followed by a mediastinoscopy. Of course, these recommendations are affected by the locations of the nodes that are most in question as well as the local expertise, as previously discussed.

INTRAOPERATIVE SURGICAL STAGING

Resection of a lung cancer includes a thorough assessment of hilar and mediastinal lymph nodes, and anything less than this constitutes a substandard operation.[59,60] It is important to recognize the differences between a selective node sampling (limited sampling directed by "judgment"), a systematic sampling (at least one representative node from each ipsilateral mediastinal station), a complete mediastinal lymph node dissection (LND, removal of all ipsilateral nodal tissue), and a lobe-specific node dissection (removal of all nodal tissue in the mediastinal node stations most commonly affected for that lobe). Either a systematic sampling or a complete node dissection should be done, although a lobe-specific systematic node dissection may be appropriate in some circumstances.[60]

Several randomized and controlled studies have demonstrated that systematic sampling or node dissection provides more accurate staging information than a selective-node sampling.[61–63] Stage classification is the same after systematic mediastinal node sampling versus a formal lymph node dissection.[61,64–66] There is no increase in morbidity or mortality after LND.[65] Because adjuvant therapy is recommended for patients with nodal involvement, an operation that omits a thorough nodal assessment must be condemned as being of unacceptable quality. This is true whether the procedure is performed via thoracotomy or thoracoscopy, and applies to sublobar resection as well.

Whether there is a therapeutic benefit to a complete lymph node dissection is controversial.[63,67–69] Two randomized studies have found no differences in recurrence rates or survival in patients undergoing LND versus systematic lymph node sampling (in 115 patients with ≤2-cm pathologic stage I [pI] NSCLC and 182 cI to IIIa patients).[68,69] Another randomized study found a benefit to LND as compared with selective sampling, although this was potentially confounded by better staging after LND.[63] Finally, two retrospective studies have found conflicting results.[67,70] The long-term survival results of the completed American College of Surgeons Oncology Group randomized trial of mediastinal node dissection (ACOSOG Z0030) are not yet available.[65]

CONCLUSION

Surgical evaluation of the mediastinum has evolved, and newer techniques such as videomediastinoscopy or transcervical mediastinal lymphadenectomy are safe and more accurate than traditional mediastinoscopy. At the same time, nonsurgical, needle-based techniques such as EUS-NA and EBUS-NA have been developed. The sensitivity of these techniques is fairly similar, but the needle-based techniques have a higher FN rate that limits their utility, especially in patients with normal-sized mediastinal nodes.

The quality of surgical staging preoperatively is a major issue, and it appears that the difference between high- and poor-quality staging is likely to be much larger than differences between various surgical and nonsurgical techniques. Invasive mediastinal staging remains important in many patients with lung cancer. Careful attention to mediastinal staging is crucial and, ideally, should be addressed in a multidisciplinary fashion.

REFERENCES

1. Little AG, Rusch VW, Bonner JA, et al. Patterns of surgical care of lung cancer patients. *Ann Thorac Surg* 2005;80:2051–2056.
2. Osaki T, Oyama T, Gu CD, et al. Prognostic impact of micrometastatic tumor cells in the lymph nodes and bone marrow of patients with completely resected stage I non-small-cell lung cancer. *J Clin Oncol* 2002;20:2930–2936.
3. Wu J, Ohta Y, Minato H, et al. Nodal occult metastasis in patients with peripheral lung adenocarcinoma of 2.0 cm or less in diameter. *Ann Thorac Surg* 2001;71:1772–1777.
4. Maddaus M, Wang X, Vollmer R, et al. CALGB 9761: a prospective analysis of IHC and PCR based detection of occult metastatic disease in stage I NSCLC. *ASCO Annual Meeting Proceedings Part I, 2006. J Clin Oncol* 2006;24:7030.
5. Detterbeck F, Jantz M, Wallace M, et al. Invasive mediastinal staging of lung cancer: an ACCP evidence-based clinical practice guideline (2nd edition). *Chest* 2007;132:202S–220S.
6. Silvestri G, Gould MK, Margolis ML, et al. Non-invasive staging of non-small cell lung cancer: ACCP evidenced-based clinical practice guidelines (2nd edition). *Chest* 2007;132:178S–201S.
7. Cybulsky IJ, Bennett WF. Mediastinoscopy as a routine outpatient procedure. *Ann Thorac Surg* 1994;58:176–178.
8. Vallières E, Pagé A, Verdant A. Ambulatory mediastinoscopy and anterior mediastinotomy. *Ann Thorac Surg* 1991;52:1122–1126.
9. Selby JH Jr, Leach CL, Heath BJ, et al. Local anesthesia for mediastinoscopy: experience with 450 consecutive cases. *Am Surg* 1978;44:679–682.
10. Kiser AC, Detterbeck FC. General aspects of surgical treatment. In: Detterbeck FC, Rivera MP, Socinski MA, et al., eds. *Diagnosis and Treatment of Lung Cancer: An Evidence-Based Guide for the Practicing Clinician*. Philadelphia, PA: WB Saunders, 2001:133–147.
11. Detterbeck FC, Jones DR, Parker LA Jr. Intrathoracic staging. In: Detterbeck FC, Rivera MP, Socinski MA, et al., eds. *Diagnosis and Treatment of Lung Cancer: An Evidence-Based Guide for the Practicing Clinician*. Philadelphia: WB Saunders, 2001:73–93.
12. Coughlin M, Deslauriers J, Beaulieu M, et al. Role of mediastinoscopy in pretreatment staging of patients with primary lung cancer. *Ann Thorac Surg* 1985;40:556–560.
13. Staples CA, Müller NL, Miller RR, et al. Mediastinal nodes in bronchogenic carcinoma: comparison between CT and mediastinoscopy. *Radiology* 1988;167:367–372.
14. Gdeedo A, Van Schil P, Corthouts B, et al. Prospective evaluation of computed tomography and mediastinoscopy in mediastinal lymph node staging. *Eur Respir J* 1997;10:1547–1551.
15. Van den Bosch JM, Gelissen HJ, Wagenaar SS. Exploratory thoracotomy in bronchial carcinoma. *J Thorac Cardiovasc Surg* 1983;85:733–737.
16. Hammoud ZT, Anderson RC, Meyers BF, et al. The current role of mediastinoscopy in the evaluation of thoracic disease. *J Thorac Cardiovasc Surg* 1999;118:894–899.
17. Lardinois D, Schallberger A, Betticher D, et al. Postinduction video-mediastinoscopy is as accurate and safe as video-mediastinoscopy in patients without pretreatment for potentially operable non-small cell lung cancer. *Ann Thorac Surg* 2003;75:1102–1106.
18. Smulders SA, Smeenk FW, Janssen-Heijnen ML, et al. Surgical mediastinal staging in daily practice. *Lung Cancer* 2005;47:243–251.
19. Bach PB, Cramer LD, Schrag D, et al. The influence of hospital volume on survival after resection for lung cancer. *N Engl J Med* 2001;345:181–188.

20. Silvestri GA, Handy J, Lackland D, et al. Specialists achieve better outcomes than generalists for lung cancer surgery. *Chest* 1998;114:675–680.
21. Hillner BE, Smith TJ, Desch CE. Hospital and physician volume or specialization and outcomes in cancer treatment: importance in quality of cancer care. *J Clin Oncol* 2000;18:2327–2340.
22. Detterbeck F. What to do with "surprise" N2: intraoperative management of patients with non-small cell lung cancer. *J Thorac Oncol* 2008;3:289–302.
23. Detterbeck F, Falen S, Rivera M, et al. Seeking a home for a PET, part 2: defining the appropriate place for positron emission tomography imaging in the staging of patients with suspected lung cancer. *Chest* 2004;125:2300–2308.
24. Gonzalez–Stawinski GV, Lemaire A, Merchant F, et al. A comparative analysis of positron emission tomography and mediastinoscopy in staging non-small cell lung cancer. *J Thorac Cardiovasc Surg* 2003;126:1900–1905.
25. Gould MK, Kuschner WG, Rydzak CE, et al. Test performance of positron emission tomography and computed tomography for mediastinal staging in patients with non-small-cell lung cancer: a meta-analysis. *Ann Intern Med* 2003;139:879–892.
26. De Leyn P, Lardinois D, Van Schil P, et al. ESTS guidelines for preoperative lymph node staging for non-small cell lung cancer. *Eur J Cardiothorac Surg* 2007;32:1–8.
27. Venissac N, Alifano M, Mouroux J. Video-assisted mediastinoscopy: experience from 240 consecutive cases. *Ann Thorac Surg* 2003;76:208–212.
28. Kimura H, Iwai N, Ando S, et al. A prospective study of indications for mediastinoscopy in lung cancer with CT findings, tumor size, and tumor markers. *Ann Thorac Surg* 2003;75:1734–1739.
29. Witte B, Wolf M, Huertgen M, et al. Video-assisted mediastinoscopic surgery: clinical feasibility and accuracy of mediastinal lymph node staging. *Ann Thorac Surg* 2006;82:1821–1827.
30. Leschber G, Holinka G, Linder A. Video-assisted mediastinoscopic lymphadenectomy (VAMLA):a method for systematic mediastinal lymph node dissection. *Eur J Cardiothorac Surg* 2003;24:192–195.
31. Hurtgen M, Friedel G, Toomes H, et al. Radical video-assisted mediastinoscopic lymphadenectomy (VAMLA):technique and first results. *Eur J Cardiothorac Surg* 2002;21:348–351.
32. Zieliński M. Transcervical extended mediastinal lymphadenectomy: results of staging in two hundred fifty-six patients with non-small cell lung cancer. *J Thorac Oncol* 2007;2:370–372.
33. Kuzdzal J, Zielinski M, Papla B, et al. Transcervical extended mediastinal lymphadenectomy—the new operative technique and early results in lung cancer staging. *Eur J Cardiothorac Surg* 2005;27:384–390.
34. Kuzdzal J, Zielinski M, Papla B, et al. The transcervical extended mediastinal lymphadenectomy versus cervical mediastinoscopy in non-small cell lung cancer staging. *Eur J Cardiothorac Surg* 2007;31:88–94.
35. Cerfolio RJ, Bryant AS, Eloubeidi MA. Accessing the aortopulmonary window (#5) and the para-aortic (#6) lymph nodes in patients with non-small cell lung cancer. *Ann Thorac Surg* 2007;84:940–945.
36. Sebastian–Quetglas F, Molins L, et al. Clinical value of video-assisted thoracoscopy for preoperative staging of non-small cell lung cancer: a prospective study of 105 patients. *Lung Cancer* 2003;42:297–301.
37. Eggeling S, Martin T, Bottger J, et al. Invasive staging of non-small cell lung cancer: a prospective study. *Eur J Cardiothorac Surg* 2002;22:679–684.
38. Landreneau RJ, Hazelrigg SR, Mack MJ, et al. Thoracoscopic mediastinal lymph node sampling: useful for mediastinal lymph node stations inaccessible by cervical mediastinoscopy. *J Thorac Cardiovasc Surg* 1993;106:554–558.
39. Massone PP, Lequaglie C, Magnani B, et al. The real impact and usefulness of video-assisted thoracoscopic surgery in the diagnosis and therapy of clinical lymphadenopathies of the mediastinum. *Ann Surg Oncol* 2003;10:1197–1202.
40. Roberts JR, Blum MG, Arildsen R, et al. Prospective comparison of radiologic, thoracoscopic, and pathologic staging in patients with early non-small cell lung cancer. *Ann Thorac Surg* 1999;68:1154–1158.
41. Detterbeck F. Integration of mediastinal staging techniques for lung cancer. *Semin Thorac Cardiovasc Surg* 2007;19:217–224.
42. Boyer M, Viney R, Fulham M, et al. A randomised trial of conventional staging with or without positron emission tomography (PET) in patients with stage 1 or 2 non-small cell lung cancer (NSCLC). *ASCO Proc* 2001;20:309a.
43. Farrell MA, McAdams HP, Herndon JE, et al. Non-small cell lung cancer: FDG PET for nodal staging in patients with stage I disease. *Radiology* 2000;215:886–890.
44. Leslie A, Jones AJ, Goddard PR. The influence of clinical information on the reporting of CT by radiologists. *Br J Radiol* 2000;73:1052–1055.
45. Smulders S, Gundy C, van Lingen A, et al. Observer variation of 2-deoxy-2-[F-18]fluoro-d-glucose-positron emission tomography in mediastinal staging of non-small cell lung cancer as a function of experience, and its potential clinical impact. *Mol Imaging Biol* 2007;9: 318–322.
46. Brehmer B. In one word: not from experience. *Acta Psychologica* 1980;45:223–241.
47. Serra M, Cirera L, Rami-Porta R, et al. Routine positron emission tomography (PET) and selective mediastinoscopy is as good as routine mediastinoscopy to rule out N2 disease in non-small cell lung cancer (NSCLC). *J Clin Oncol* 2006;24(No. 18S Part I of II):S371.
48. Cerfolio RJ, Bryant AS, Ojha B, et al. Improving the inaccuracies of clinical staging of patients with NSCLC: a prospective trial. *Ann Thorac Surg* 2005;80:1207–1214.
49. Dietlein M, Weber K, Gandjour A, et al. Cost-effectiveness of FDG-PET for the management of potentially operable non-small cell lung cancer; priority for a PET-based strategy after nodal-negative CT results. *Eur J Nucl Med* 2000;27:1598–1609.
50. Patterson GA, Piazza D, Pearson FG, et al. Significance of metastatic disease in subaortic lymph nodes. *Ann Thorac Surg* 1987;43:155–159.
51. Detterbeck FC, Jones DR. Surgical treatment of stage IIIa (N2) non-small cell lung cancer. In: Detterbeck FC, Rivera MP, Socinski MA, et al., eds. *Diagnosis and Treatment of Lung Cancer: An Evidence-Based Guide for the Practicing Clinician.* Philadelphia: WB Saunders, 2001:244–256.
52. Jiao J, Magistrelli P, Goldstraw P. The value of cervical mediastinoscopy combined with anterior mediastinotomy in the peroperative evaluation of bronchogenic carcinoma of the left upper lobe. *Eur J Cardiothorac Surg* 1997;11:450–454.
53. Best LA, Munichor M, Ben-Shakhar M, et al. The contribution of anterior mediastinotomy in the diagnosis and evaluation of diseases of the mediastinum and lung. *Ann Thorac Surg* 1987;43:78–81.
54. Ginsberg RJ, Rice TW, Goldberg M, et al. Extended cervical mediastinoscopy: a single staging procedure for bronchogenic carcinoma of the left upper lobe. *J Thorac Cardiovasc Surg* 1987;94:673–678.
55. Freixinet Gilart J, Gámez-Garcia P, Rodríguez de Castro F, et al. Extended cervical mediastinoscopy in the staging of bronchogenic carcinoma. *Ann Thorac Surg* 2000;70:1641–1643.
56. Urschel JD, Vretenar DF, Dickout WJ, et al. Cerebrovascular accident complicating extended cervical mediastinoscopy. *Ann Thorac Surg* 1994;57:740–741.
57. Lopez L, Varela A, Freixinet J, et al. Extended cervical mediastinoscopy: prospective study of fifty cases. *Ann Thorac Surg* 1994;57:555–558.
58. Ginsberg RJ. In discussion of: Lopez L, Varela A, Freixinet J, et al. Extended cervical mediastinoscopy: prospective study of fifty cases. *Ann Thorac Surg* 1994;57:557–558.
59. Scott W, Howington J, Feigenberg S, et al. Treatment of non-small cell lung cancer - stage I & II: ACCP evidence-based clinical practice guideline (2nd ed). *Chest* 2007;132:234S–242S
60. Lardinois D, De Leyn P, Van Schil P, et al. ESTS guidelines for intraoperative lymph node staging in non-small cell lung cancer. *Eur J Cardiothorac Surg* 2006;30:787–792.
61. Bollen EC, van Duin CJ, Theunissen PH, et al. Mediastinal lymph node dissection in resected lung cancer: morbidity and accuracy of staging. *Ann Thorac Surg* 1993;55:961–966.

62. Gaer JA, Goldstraw P. Intraoperative assessment of nodal staging at thoracotomy for carcinoma of the bronchus. *Eur J Cardiothorac Surg* 1990;4:207–210.
63. Wu Y, Huang ZF, Wang SY, et al. A randomized trial of systematic nodal dissection in resectable non-small cell lung cancer. *Lung Cancer* 2002;36:1–6.
64. Izbicki JR, Passlick B, Karg O, et al. Impact on radical systematic mediastinal lymphadenectomy on tumor staging in lung cancer. *Ann Thorac Surg* 1995;59:209–214.
65. Allen MS, Darling GE, Pechet TT, et al. Morbidity and mortality of major pulmonary resections in patients with early-stage lung cancer: initial results of the randomized, prospective ACOSOG Z0030 Trial. *Ann Thorac Surg* 2006;81:1013–1020.
66. Magnanelli G, Scanagatta P, Benato C, et al. Is sampling really effective in staging non-small cell lung cancer? A prospective study. *Chir Ital* 2006;58:19–22.
67. Keller SM, Adak S, Wagner H, et al. Mediastinal lymph node dissection improves survival in patients with stages II and IIIa non-small cell lung cancer; from the Eastern Cooperative Oncology Group. *Ann Thorac Surg* 2000;70:358–365.
68. Sugi K, Nawata K, Fujita N, et al. Systematic lymph node dissection for clinically diagnosed peripheral non-small-cell lung cancer less than 2 cm in diameter. World J Surg 1998;22:290–294.
69. Izbicki JR, Thetter O, Habekost M, et al. Radical systematic mediastinal lymphadenectomy in non-small cell lung cancer: a randomized controlled trial. *Br J Surg* 1994;81:229–235.
70. Funatsu T, Matsubara Y, Ikeda S, et al. Preoperative mediastinoscopic assessment of N factors and the need for mediastinal lymph node dissection in T1 lung cancer. *J Thorac Cardiovasc Surg* 1994;108:321–328.
71. Luke WP, Pearson FG, Todd TR, et al. Prospective evaluation of mediastinoscopy for assessment of carcinoma of the lung. *J Thorac Cardiovasc Surg* 1986;91:53–56.
72. De Leyn P, Schoonooghe P, Deneffe G, et al. Surgery for non-small cell lung cancer with unsuspected metastasis to ipsilateral mediastinal or subcarinal nodes (N2 disease). *Eur J Cardiothorac Surg* 1996;10:649–655.
73. Brion JP, Depauw L, Kuhn G, et al. Role of computed tomography and mediastinoscopy in preoperative staging of lung carcinoma. *J Computer Assist Tomogr* 1985;9:480–484.
74. Jolly PC, Hutchinson CH, Detterbeck F, et al. Routine computed tomographic scans, selective mediastinoscopy, and other factors in evaluation of lung cancer. *J Thorac Cardiovasc Surg* 1991;102:266–271.
75. Ratto GB, Frola C, Cantoni S, et al. Improving clinical efficacy of computed tomographic scan in the preoperative assessment of patients with non-small cell lung cancer. *J Thorac Cardiovasc Surg* 1990; 99:416–425.
76. Ebner H, Marra A, Butturini E, et al. Clinical value of cervical mediastinoscopy in the staging of bronchial carcinoma. *Ann Ital Chir* 1999;70:873–879.
77. Deneffe G, Lacquet L, Gyselen A. Cervical mediastinoscopy and anterior mediastinotomy in patients with lung cancer and radiologically normal mediastinum. *Eur J Respir Dis* 1983;64:613–619.
78. Aaby C, Kristensen S, Nielsen SM. Mediastinal staging of non-small-cell lung cancer: computed tomography and cervical mediastinoscopy. *ORL J Otorhinolaryngol Relat Spec* 1995;57:279–285.
79. Page A, Nakhle G, Mercier C, et al. Surgical treatment of bronchogenic carcinoma: the importance of staging in evaluating late survival. *Ca J Surg* 1987;30:96–99.
80. Dillemans B, Deneffe G, Verschakelen J, et al. Value of computed tomography and mediastinoscopy in preoperative evaluation of mediastinal nodes in non-small cell lung cancer: a study of 569 patients. *Eur J Cardiothorac Surg* 1994;8:37–42.
81. Riordan D, Buckley D, Aherne T. Mediastinoscopy as a predictor of resectability in patients with bronchogenic carcinoma. *Ir J Med Sci* 1997;160:291–292.
82. Choi YS, Shim YM, Kim J, et al. Mediastinoscopy in patients with clinical stage I non-small cell lung cancer. *Ann Thorac Surg* 2003;75:364–366.
83. Gürses A, Turna A, Bedirhan M, et al. The value of mediastinoscopy in preoperative evaluation of mediastinal involvement in non-small-cell lung cancer patients with clinical NO disease. *Thorac Cardiovasc Surg* 2002;50:174–177.

CHAPTER 30

Peter Goldstraw

The International Staging System for Lung Cancer

Over the last 40 years, the International Staging System (ISS) has become an essential tool for all those involved in the care of patients suffering from cancer or undertaking research in this field. Increasingly, patients are becoming empowered by understanding this system and are making use of this knowledge in their search for information in the literature, on the Internet, and in discussions with their medical advisors. At the heart of the ISS lies an international shorthand that utilizes the TNM-based system to describe the anatomical extent of the disease: the T category describing the size and extent of the primary tumor, the N category describing the extent of involvement of regional lymph nodes, and the M category describing the presence or absence of distant metastatic spread. Each category is defined by ascending numerical descriptors that indicate increasingly advanced disease. All possible combinations of the T, N, and M categories are then used to create TNM subsets. TNM subsets with similar prognoses are then combined into stage groupings. The term *stage*, without further classification, relates to the pretreatment, clinical stage or cTNM. This is derived using the evidence available from clinical history and examination, blood tests, imaging, endoscopic examination, biopsy material, surgical examination, and any other test considered necessary prior to making a decision as to the appropriate treatment in any individual. If this decision leads to surgical treatment, then additional information becomes available at surgery and by pathological examination allowing a more accurate assessment of disease extent, the pathological, postsurgical stage or pTNM. This does not replace the cTNM, which should remain as a record in the patient's notes. If the patient undergoes preoperative, "induction" therapy, usually with chemotherapy and/or radiotherapy, then a reassessment is made after this treatment, prior to a final decision on surgical treatment. The evidence available from this process is used to create the ycTNM, and after surgical treatment in these circumstances, the postsurgical pathological extent of disease is described as ypTNM. At various points in the patient's journey, events may allow or demand a reassessment of disease extent. An rTNM may be established if relapse occurs after a disease-free interval. An aTNM may be formulated if the disease is first discovered at an autopsy. In each case, previous assessments of TNM are retained in the patient records.

The TNM classification is administered by two nongovernmental bodies: the American Joint Committee on Cancer (AJCC) and the Union Internationale Contre le Cancer (UICC) now referred to by the anglicized form of its title, the International Union Against Cancer. Each produces its own publication on cancer staging, denoted as a *Cancer Staging Manual* by the AJCC and the *TNM Classification of Malignant Tumours* by the UICC. In addition, there are several other publications from each organization, such as supplements, atlases, pocket guides, and textbooks on additional prognostic factors. Periodic revisions of *TNM Classification of Malignant Tumours* are undertaken, now on a 7-year cycle. Close collaboration between these organizations in recent years has ensured that for all cancer sites, the definitions of TNM are identical. The 7th edition of both publications was published in 2009.

The anatomical extent of disease, as described by TNM, is not the only prognostic indicator. Many other such indices have been identified.[1] They may be classified as "tumor-related" factors, which include TNM but also other features such as histologic type and grade, "host-related" factors such as gender, age, weight loss, and performance status, and "treatment-related" factors such as the adequacy of resection margins, radiotherapy dose, and chemotherapy response. These can be further categorized as those that are considered "essential," those that provide supplementary guidance by giving "additional" information, and those that are as yet unproven but are "new and promising." These, for lung cancer, are depicted in Tables 30.1 to 30.3.[2] In recent years, advances in molecular biology have taught us much

TABLE 30.1 Prognostic Factors in Surgically Resected NSCLC*

Prognostic Factors	Tumor Related	Host Related	Environment Related
Essential	T category N category Extracapsular nodal extension Superior sulcus location Intrapulmonary metastasis	Weight loss Performance status	Resection margins Adequacy of mediastinal dissection
Additional	Histologic type Grade Vessel invasion Tumor size	Gender Age	Radiotherapy dose Adjuvant radiation
New and promising	Molecular/biologic markers	Quality of life Marital status	

*From Gospodarowicz MK, O'Sullivan B, Sobin LH, eds. Lung cancer. In: *Prognostic Factors in Cancer.* 3rd Ed. New York: Wiley-Liss, 2006:chapter 19. Reproduced with kind permission by the UICC.

about the process of carcinogenesis, the genetic basis for predisposition in certain tumor types, the mechanisms by which cancers progress and metastasize, and the reasons for varying responses to treatment and, in some cancers, have provided additional prognostic information. In lung cancer, as yet, there is no consensus as to which molecular markers are of prognostic importance.[3] The anatomical extent of disease, as described by TNM stage, remains the most useful prognostic tool.[4]

The aims of TNM may be summarized as the following:

- To aid the clinician in the planning of treatment
- To give some indication of prognosis
- To assist in evaluation of the results of treatment
- To facilitate the exchange of information between treatment center
- To contribute to the continuing investigation of human cancer

TABLE 30.2 Prognostic Factors in Advanced (Locally Advanced or Metastatic) NSCLC*

Prognostic Factors	Tumor Related	Host Related	Environment Related
Essential	Stage SVCO Solitary brain Solitary adrenal metastasis Number of sites	Weight loss Performance status	Chemoradiotherapy Chemotherapy
Additional	Number of metastatic sites Pleural effusion Liver metastases Hemoglobin LDH Albumin	Gender Symptom burden	
New and promising	Molecular/biologic markers	Quality of life Marital status Anxiety/depression	

*From Gospodarowicz MK, O'Sullivan B, Sobin LH, eds. Lung cancer. In: *Prognostic Factors in Cancer.* 3rd Ed. New York: Wiley-Liss, 2006:chapter 19. Reproduced with kind permission by the UICC.

LDH, lactate dehydrogenase; SVCO, superior vena cava obstruction.

TABLE 30.3 Prognostic Factors in SCLC*

Prognostic Factors	Tumor Related	Host Related	Environment Related
Essential	Stage	Performance Status Age Comorbidity	Chemotherapy Thoracic radiotherapy Prophylactic cranial RT
Additional	LDH Alkaline phosphatase Cushing syndrome M0—Mediastinal involvement M1—Number of sites —Bone or brain involvement —WBC, platelet count	—	—
New and promising	Molecular/biologic markers		

*From Gospodarowicz MK, O'Sullivan B, Sobin LH, eds. Lung cancer. In: *Prognostic Factors in Cancer.* 3rd Ed. New York: Wiley-Liss, 2006:chapter 19. Reproduced with kind permission by the UICC.

LDH, lactate dehydrogenase; RT, radiotherapy; WBC, white blood cell.

THE HISTORY OF TNM IN LUNG CANCER[5]

The TNM system for the classification of malignant tumors was developed by Pierre Denoix, a surgeon at the Institute Gustave Roussy in Paris, and published in a series of articles between 1943 and 1952.[6] The following year, 1953, this system was adopted by the recently formed UICC Committee on Tumour Nomenclature and Statistics under the auspices of the League of Nations. The UICC process at this time developed proposals by consensus between experts in the field. These proposals were disseminated in a series of 23 brochures or fascicles published between 1960 and 1967, which covered the TNM classification of cancers in 23 sites, lung being included in the brochure published in 1966. Subsequently, the recommendations were brought together in the 1st edition of the UICC *TNM Classification of Malignant Tumours* published in 1968 in a compact *Livre de Poche* format.[7] The proposals were for "trial" from 1967 to 1971. At that time, there was insufficient information on lung cancer to merit a section of its own, and it was listed under "other sites." The T descriptors included T0 for cases in which there was no evidence of the primary tumor, T1 for tumors confined to a segment or segmental bronchus, T2 where there was lobar involvement, T3 if there was involvement of more than one lobe, and T4 for tumors extending beyond the lung. The N descriptors were NX, N0, or N1, this last category being applied if *intrathoracic* nodes were involved. Intrathoracic nodes were described as *hilar* or *peripheral* with no mention of nodes in the mediastinum. The M1 descriptor was subdivided into M1a in which there was a pleural effusion with malignant cells present, M1b cases with palpable cervical nodes, and M1c for cases in which other distant sites were involved. Stage groupings were not proposed at that time.

The AJCC, formed in 1959 as the American Joint Committee (AJC) for Cancer Staging and End Results Reporting, developed a separate and distinctive process in which "Task Forces" were set up to gather data, which were used to inform its proposals. There was clearly a possibility that these two organizations would make different, and possibly conflicting, recommendations to the cancer community. Therefore, at a series of meetings between the UICC and the AJC, a rapprochement was reached, which ensured that these two organizations would not produce further recommendations without consultation between themselves and other National TNM Committees and International nongovernmental professional organizations.

In 1973, the Task Force on Lung Cancer of the AJC accepted proposals from Dr. Mountain, Dr. Carr, and Dr. Anderson for "A Clinical Staging System for Lung Cancer."[8] This was based on data from 2155 cases of lung cancer, of which 1712 were cases of non–small cell lung cancer (NSCLC), diagnosed at least 4 years before analysis. The majority of the T, N, and M descriptors in use today were introduced at that time, including the impact on T category of such features as the 3-cm cutoff between T1 and T2 tumors, the bronchoscopic extent of disease, the extent of atelectasis/consolidation of the lung parenchyma, and the invasion of chest wall, diaphragm, or mediastinum. The T categories 0 to 3 were retained but T4 was dropped, N categories 0 to 1 were retained but N2 was added to address the issue of mediastinal node involvement, and M categories 0 to 1 were retained. Pleural effusions were removed from the M1 category and became a T3 descriptor.

The resultant TNM subsets were grouped into stages I to III. Four of the possible eighteen TNM subsets had too few cases for analysis and seven others contained less than 100 cases. Survival curves showed distinct differences between prognosis in overall T, N, and M categories and the three-stage groupings to 5 years and beyond. A table showed the differing survival at 12 and 18 months for those TNM subsets for which data was available. No assessment of statistical significance was presented, and there was no validation of the individual descriptors. These proposals were incorporated in the 2nd edition of the UICC *TNM Classification of Malignant Tumours* published in 1975[9] and the 1st edition of the *Manual for Staging of Cancer* published by the AJC in 1977.[10]

The 3rd edition of the UICC manual, published in 1978[11] and revised in 1982, further divided stage I into Ia and Ib (note that at that time, stage subgroups were lowercase) and established stage IV for cases with M1 disease. The "x" descriptor, erratically applied to some categories in earlier editions, was, for the first time, introduced as an option in all three categories of T, N, and M.

The American committee, now the AJCC, did not make these changes in its 2nd edition, which was published in 1983.[12]

By 1986, Dr. Mountain had assembled a new database containing 3753 cases of lung cancer with a minimum follow-up of 2 years. The proposals from this source were accepted by the AJCC, and subsequently by the UICC and cancer committees in Germany and Japan, creating "A new International Staging System for Lung Cancer."[13] The recommendations were published in the 4th edition of the UICC *TNM Classification of Malignant Tumours* in 1987[14] and in the 3rd edition of the American manual in 1988.[15] Changes proposed in this edition include the addition of "visceral pleural invasion" as a T2 descriptor, the designation of superficial tumors limited to the bronchial wall as T1 irrespective of location, a recommendation that the occasional pleural effusion that was cytologically negative could be ignored in defining the T category, the reemergence of the T4 category, and the creation of an N3 category. The existing T3 descriptors were split between T3 and the new T4 category on the basis that the former would retain those descriptors that indicated that such tumors were "candidates for complete resection," whereas the latter would be "inoperable." The previous descriptor of mediastinal invasion was split into its component parts, with invasion of the mediastinal pleura or pericardium remaining T3, whereas invasion of the great vessels, heart, trachea, esophagus, carina, and vertebral bodies became T4 descriptors, along with the presence of a pleural effusion. The situation was confused by additional definitions of T3 and T4 given in the text. Those tumors with "limited, circumscribed extrapulmonary extension" were to be retained within the T3 category, whereas those with "extensive extrapulmonary extension" became T4. These conflicting definitions resulted in a lack of clarity as to whether tumors invading such structures as the pericardium remained T3 if there was extensive invasion and were considered inoperable or became T4, or if invasion limited to a circumscribed area of the esophagus and resected completely at surgery should be considered to be T3 or T4. Metastases to the ipsilateral mediastinal nodes and subcarinal nodes remained within the N2 category, and the new N3 category was added to accommodate metastases to the contralateral mediastinal nodes, contralateral hilum or ipsilateral, and contralateral supraclavicular or scalene lymph nodes. Additional changes in that edition include the moving of T1N1M0 cases from stage I to stage II and the division of stage III into IIIA (containing T3 and N2 cases) and IIIB (containing T4 and N3 cases). Once again, a table showed the differing survival prospects for TNM subsets, and a graph showed statistically significant survival differences between stage groupings. No validation was presented for the individual descriptors or to substantiate the movement of some into T3 and others T4.

The AJCC made no changes in the classification for lung cancer in its 4th edition published in 1992.[16]

At the time of the next revision in 1997, the database of Dr. Mountain has increased to include 5319 cases, all but 66 being NSCLC, 4351 cases treated at the MD Anderson Cancer Center between 1975 and 1988, and 968 cases referred there from the National Cancer Institute Cooperative Lung Cancer Study Group for confirmation of stage and histology.[17] Tables showed statistically significant differences in survival as far as 5 years between clinical/evaluative cTNM categories and pathological/postsurgical pTNM categories T1N0M0 and T2N0M0 and these were divided into a new stage IA and stage IB, respectively. Similarly, T1N1M0 cases were placed in a new stage IIA, and T2N1M0 and T3N0M0 cases became stage IIB. The remaining TNM categories in stages IIIA, IIIB, and IV remained unchanged although statistically significant differences were found between some TNM categories. An additional paragraph determined that "the presence of *satellite* tumor(s), not lymph nodes, within the primary-tumor lobe of the lung should be classified as T4. Intrapulmonary ispilateral [sic] *metastasis* in a distant, that is, nonprimary lobe(s) of the lung, should be classified M1."[17] No data was presented to support these suggestions and the wording used to describe such additional pulmonary nodules was loaded to underline the apparent logic of considering some to be "satellite" lesions and, therefore, a T descriptor, whereas those in other lobes were a "metastasis" and, therefore, an M descriptor.

These recommendations were accepted by the AJCC and the UICC-TNM Prognostic Factors Project Committee and appeared in the 5th edition of their publications in 1997.[18,19]

There were no changes in the lung cancer classification in the 6th edition of *TNM Classification of Malignant Tumours* published in 2002.[20,21]

THE NEED FOR CHANGE

Undoubtedly, the lung cancer community owes an enormous debt of gratitude to the pioneers of TNM, especially to Dr. Clifton Mountain. However, over the last decade, there has grown a feeling among lung cancer clinicians and scientists that changes were needed to the process for revision of the *TNM Classification for Lung Cancer*. The Mountain database, which had been the major source of data to inform revisions of the TNM system up to and including the 6th edition had, by 1996, enlarged to include 5319 cases. Thus, it was a relatively small database, accumulated over 20 years, during which period many advances had been made in the techniques available for pretreatment staging, most noticeably the routine application of computed tomography (CT) scanning. The great majority of cases in this database had been referred for surgical treatment and had been recruited from a single center. There were understandable concerns as to whether the recommendations emanating from such a database were historically valid, globally relevant, and appropriate for evaluating treatment by nonsurgical or combined modality care. Oncologists treating small cell lung cancer (SCLC) had abandoned TNM for all, except those very limited cases in which surgery was considered and instead were using a simpler classification based on the single distinction between "limited" or "extensive" disease.[22] Even when used in a surgical setting and for NSLC, the lack of validation in previous editions of the *TNM Classification of Malignant Tumours* had led to many of the descriptors being increasingly challenged. Data had been published supporting size cutoffs other than the 3-cm limit separating T1 and T2 tumors, ranging from less than 1 cm to more than 9 cm. "Irresectable" T4 tumors had been resected with good results in selected cases. The descriptors applied to cases in which there were additional tumor nodules in the lobe of the primary and other ipsilateral lobes were generally regarded as harsh. Oncologists had long treated cases with pleural effusion, the "wet" IIIB cases, with the therapeutic strategies used for patients with metastatic, stage IV disease. Clearly, if the TNM classification was to retain its central role in the day-to-day care of patients with lung cancer in an evidence-based era, its recommendations had to be intensively validated and the process for change had to be modernized to make the staging system fit for purpose. These concerns crystallized at an International Association for the Study of Lung Cancer (IASLC) workshop on "Intrathoracic Staging" held at the Brompton Hospital in London in October 1996.[23] One of the published recommendations of this meeting was "the establishment by the IASLC of a staging committee."

THE IASLC STAGING PROJECT[24]

At the 8th World Conference on Lung Cancer in Dublin in 1997, the board of the IASLC considered a submission from the late Dr. RJ Ginsberg and Dr. P Goldstraw to create an international staging committee. The board agreed that the IASLC, as the only global organization dedicated to the study of lung cancer, representing all clinical and research aspects of lung cancer care, had a responsibility to become involved in the revision process and to develop a new database to inform future revisions. At its next meeting in December 1998, the board agreed to provide pump-priming funds for such a project. Meetings were held in London in 1999 and 2000, during which the composition of the committee was developed to ensure speciality and geographical representation and the involvement of stakeholders such as the UICC, the AJCC, and the joint Japanese societies involved in the study of lung cancer. At the next World Conference in 2000, collaboration was established with colleagues from Cancer Research and Biostatistics (CRAB), a not-for-profit medical statistics and data management organization based in Seattle with extensive experience with multicenter data collection and analysis. At that meeting, sufficient funds were guaranteed from the pharmaceutical industry to allow a major meeting in London in 2001, to which database proprietors were invited to present an outline of the data they held. Over the 2-day workshop, data on 80,000 cases were presented from 20 databases across the globe. In was decided to estimate the budget based on the assumption that 30,000 suitable cases could be recruited and that the length of the project would be the 5-year cycle used by the UICC and AJCC at that time. Cases would be solicited from databases worldwide, treated by all modalities of care, between 1990 and 2000, a period during which there had been relative stability in staging methods. This would ensure a 5-year follow-up by the time of analysis. In collaboration with CRAB, the data fields and data dictionary were finalized. Later that year, full funding was obtained by the IASLC via a partnership agreement with the pharmaceutical industry.

Meetings continued to be held on an annual basis utilizing the world conferences, now held biennially, wherever possible.

The UICC was well aware of the need to update the revision process and, around this time, established a "TNM Process Subcommittee. Criteria were established for instituting changes to the TNM classification and for the evaluation of proposals for such changes."[25] A system for continuous monitoring of the proposals in the literature, a "literature watch," was set up. For each cancer type, a "TNM expert panel" was established to review the sifted literature and help in the evaluation of proposals for change. In May 2003, the UICC and AJCC extended the revision cycle to 7 years, which resulted in publication of the 7th edition of the *TNM Classification of Malignant Tumours* being deferred until 2009. The internal review processes within these organizations required that the IASLC submitted its proposals to the UICC in January 2007 and the AJCC in June 2008.

Data collection was discontinued in April 2005, by which time, over 100,000 cases had been submitted to the data center at CRAB. After an initial sift, which excluded cases with insufficient data on stage, treatment, or follow-up, cases outside the designated study period and cases in which the cell type was unsuited or unknown 81,015 were available for analysis, 67,725 cases of NSCLC, and 13,290 cases of SCLC. The proposals for the 7th edition of *TNM Classification of Malignant Tumours* were formulated on the NSCLC cases alone. The geographical distribution of the data sources in this cell type is illustrated in Figure 30.1 and the spread of treatment modalities is shown in Figure 30.2. This enormous task was divided among subcommittees, each charged with collaborating with CRAB to analyze the data and develop proposals for given aspects of the study. These covered the T, N, and M descriptors, the relevance of TNM in SCLC and in carcinoid tumors, the development of an internationally agreed nodal chart, and a thorough review of the value of additional prognostic factors

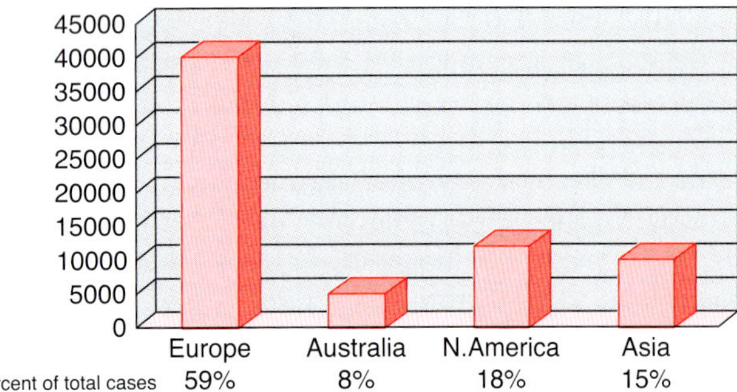

FIGURE 30.1 The geographical spread, by continent, for the 67,725 cases of NSCLC that informed the IASLC recommendations for the 7th edition of *TNM Classification of Malignant Tumours*.

and biological markers. As validation had been an issue with previous revisions, a separate subcommittee was created to undertake a comprehensive validation process and to ensure that revisions were compatible with the methodology of the UICC and AJCC. This committee was closely involved with the work of the other groups as their proposals evolved.

a) Validation and methodology subcommittee[26]

All exploratory analyses were examined for their relevance in the clinical/evaluative, cTNM population and the postsurgical/pathological pTNM population. There was cTNM data on 53,640 cases, pTNM on 33,933 cases, and both c and p TNM in 20,006 cases. The recommendations of the T descriptors subcommittee were assessed in M0 cases with all combinations of N category and completeness of resection, R, category. Internal validation of the recommendations was checked for consistency across all geographical areas and between differing types of data source. Where the volume of data permitted, in the T descriptors and the TNM stage grouping analysis, the recommendations were created using a "training set" of a randomly selected subgroup comprising two thirds of all cases and then validated against the other one third of cases in the "validation set." External validation was mainly established by studying the appropriateness of all recommendations against the Surveillance, Epidemiology, and End Results (SEER) database for 1998 to 2000. Consistency with suggestions raised in the literature was undertaken in collaboration with the UICC Literature Watch program.

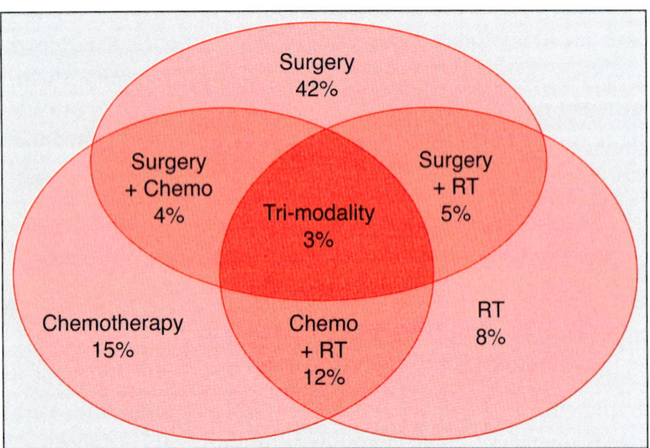

FIGURE 30.2 The treatment modalities utilized in the 67,725 cases of NSCLC that informed the IASLC recommendations for the 7th edition of *TNM Classification of Malignant Tumours*. RT, radiotherapy.

b) T descriptors subcommittee[27]

There was a paucity of data on many T descriptors. However, data on tumor size was well represented within the database. A running log-rank analysis of size as a continuous variable in T1 tumors revealed a significant cut point at 2 cm. When tested in the validation subset, there was a statistically significant difference in survival between T1 tumors up to 2 cm in size compared with those more than 2 cm but not more than 3 cm.

Recommendation: T1 tumors should be subclassified as T1a for tumors up to 2 cm in size and T1b tumors for those that are more than 2 cm in size but not greater than 3 cm in size.

A similar analysis of size in larger tumors showed two additional cut points, one at 5 cm and another at 7.3 cm. For clinical utility, the latter was taken as 7 cm. Using these cut points, three additional size groupings were identified in the training set; those patients whose tumors were larger than 3 cm but not more than 5 cm in size, those with tumors more than 5 cm in size but not more than 7 cm in size, and those whose tumors were more than 7 cm in size. When the survival of these groups was assessed in the validation subset, there were distinctly different survival curves for each group. Furthermore, survival of those with the largest tumors, larger than 7 cm in size, was similar to cases classified as T3 by other criteria.

Recommendation: T2 tumors should be subclassified into T2a tumors, more than 3 cm in size but not more than 5 cm, and T2b tumors, more than 5 cm but not more than 7 cm in size. Tumors more than 7 cm in size should be reclassified as T3 tumors.

When the survival of cases classified by the 6th edition of *TNM Classification of Malignant Tumours* as T4 on the basis of additional tumor nodules in the lobe of the primary was compared with that of cases classified as T3 or T4 by other criteria, the survival of the former was found to be different to that of T4 tumors but similar to that of T3 tumors.

Recommendation: Reclassify T4 tumors by additional nodules in the lobe of the primary tumor as T3.

Similarly, the survival of cases with additional tumor nodules in ipsilateral lobes other than that of the primary tumor, classified as M1 in the 6th edition of *TNM Classification of Malignant Tumours*, compared with T4 and M1 cases by other criteria, was in line with T4 cases and much better than other M1 cases.

Recommendation: Reclassify M1 tumors by additional nodules in other ipsilateral lobes (other than the lobe of the primary tumor) as T4.

Cases classified by the 6th edition of *TNM Classification of Malignant Tumours* as T4 by the presence of a malignant pleural effusion had a survival that was much worse than T4 tumors and similar to that of M1 cases.

Recommendation: Reclassify tumors by malignant pleural or pericardial effusion as M1 disease.

c) N descriptors subcommittee[28]

This subcommittee studied the prognostic significance of the nodal categories in the 6th edition and found that the current N0 to N3 descriptors defined distinct prognostic groups for both clinical and pathologic staging. They undertook exploratory analyses on the prognostic impact of individual nodal stations in the hilum and mediastinum, and combinations and permutations of cell type, lobe of the primary, patterns of nodal involvement in N1 and N2 locations, and the impact of "skip" metastases to the mediastinal nodes without hilar node disease. Although these analyses showed some interesting results, the groups were small and compromised geographically and by treatment modality. They concluded that further prospective studies were necessary before taking these suggestions forward. Such studies would be facilitated by an agreed set of international definitions for nodal stations, and a new "IASLC" international nodal chart, which, for the first time, could reconcile the differences between the Japanese nodal chart and the Mountain/Dressler chart. The concept of "nodal zones" was suggested, amalgamating nodal stations into larger units within the anatomical region. It was hoped that this would ensure that nodal mapping was relevant to oncologists and radiologists used to dealing with bulky disease that often transgressed the boundaries of adjacent nodal stations.

Recommendation: The existing categories of N0 to N3 should be retained for the 7th edition. An IASLC nodal chart was created, incorporating the concept of nodal zones.[29]

d) M descriptors subcommittee[30]

An analysis of those cases suggested for reclassification as M1 caused by malignant pleural effusion showed a similar survival to those classified as M1 in the 6th edition because of additional tumor nodules in the contralateral lung. These two groups had a better survival than that of cases classified in the 6th edition as M1 by the presence of distant metastases, by a small but significant difference.

Recommendation: Reclassify M1 because of additional tumor nodules in the contralateral lung as M1a. Reclassify T4 tumors caused by malignant pleural or pericardial effusions as M1a. Reclassify M1 caused by distant metastatic disease as M1b.

e) Changes to the TNM stage groupings in the 7th edition[31]

This aspect of the project raised issues that affected the way that the recommendations derived from the T, N, and M descriptor subcommittees were presented in the final documents. Where analysis suggested that new descriptors were necessary to accommodate patients whose prognosis differed from the other cases within any particular T or M category, two alternative strategies were considered: (a) Retain that descriptor in the existing category, identified by alphabetical subsets. For example, additional pulmonary nodules in the lobe of the primary, considered to be T4 in the 6th edition, would remain T4 but identified as T4a, whereas additional pulmonary nodules in other ipsilateral lobes, designated as M1 in the 6th edition, would become M1a. (b) Allow descriptors to move between categories, to a category containing other descriptors with a similar prognosis, for example, additional pulmonary nodules in the lobe of the primary would move from T4 to T3, and additional pulmonary nodules in other ipsilateral lobes would move from M1 to T4. The first strategy had the advantage of allowing, to a large extent, retrograde compatibility with existing databases. Unfortunately, this strategy generated a large number of descriptors (approximately 20) and an impractically large number of TNM subsets (>180). For this reason, backward compatibility was compromised and strategy *b* was preferred for its clinical utility. The recommendations were therefore formatted as previously described. These changes to T and M descriptors were then incorporated into the resultant TNM subsets. A small number of candidate stage grouping schemes were developed initially, based on a "training" set, using a recursive partitioning and amalgamation (RPA) algorithm.[32] This generated a tree-based model for the survival data using log-rank test statistics for recursive partitioning and, for selection of the important groupings, bootstrap resampling to correct for the adaptive nature of the splitting algorithm. An ordered list of groupings from the terminal nodes of the "survival tree" was created, and with this as a guide, several proposed stage groupings were created by combining adjacent groups. Selection of a final stage grouping proposal from among the candidate schemes was based on its statistical properties in the training set and its relevance to clinical practice, and was arrived at by consensus.

The survival of cases within our database stratified by the 6th edition of *TNM Classification of Malignant Tumours* and by the IASLC proposals for the 7th edition are shown for cases staged clinically in Figure 30.3 and for pathologically staged cases in Figure 30.4. The proposed system better delineated the early stage cases, where problems with overlap between IB and IIA have been noted with the 6th edition of *TNM Classification of Malignant Tumours*.[33] Improvement was also seen in the distinction between clinical IIA and IIB, as well as the proportion of cases assigned to stage IIA, another weakness of the 6th edition of *TNM Classification of Malignant Tumours*. For both the clinical and pathological stage models, there was an increase in the value for R^2, an estimate of the percent variance explained (PVE) by the model.[34] The proposals for the 7th edition made use of well-justified changes to T and M, and served to identify subsets of patients with tumors of different sizes with differing prognoses. Both the proposed new system and the 6th edition of *TNM Classification of Malignant Tumours* showed a reversal on pathological staging from the expected survival for advanced stage disease (IIIB and IV). This result, although anomalous, could be explained by the selective nature of advanced cases undergoing surgery, many of which were taken to surgery on the assessment that their disease was limited only to be discovered to have advanced disease at thoracotomy.

Recommendation: The new descriptors and the recommended stage groupings, now enacted in the 7th edition, are shown in Tables 30.4 and 30.5.

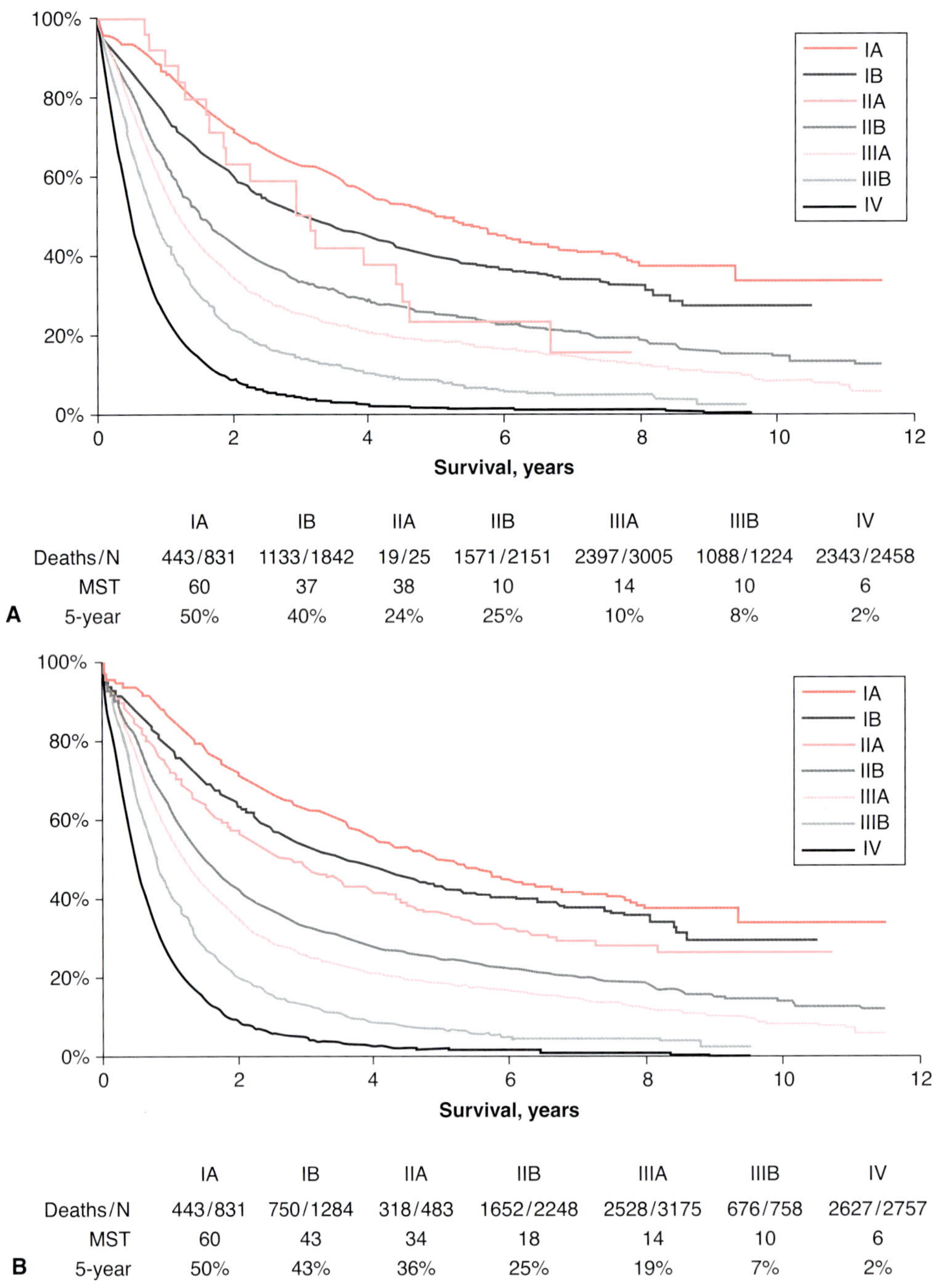

A

	IA	IB	IIA	IIB	IIIA	IIIB	IV
Deaths/N	443/831	1133/1842	19/25	1571/2151	2397/3005	1088/1224	2343/2458
MST	60	37	38	10	14	10	6
5-year	50%	40%	24%	25%	10%	8%	2%

B

	IA	IB	IIA	IIB	IIIA	IIIB	IV
Deaths/N	443/831	750/1284	318/483	1652/2248	2528/3175	676/758	2627/2757
MST	60	43	34	18	14	10	6
5-year	50%	43%	36%	25%	19%	7%	2%

FIGURE 30.3 Survival of pretreatment, clinical staged cases by **(A)** 6th edition of *TNM Classification of Malignant Tumours* and **(B)** 7th edition of *TNM Classification of Malignant Tumours*. *MST*, median survival time.

f) SCLC subcommittee[35,36]

There were 13,290 cases of SCLC in the IASLC database, of which details on clinical TNM stage were available in 8088. Survival was found to be reliably related to both T and N categories. Differences were more pronounced in patients without mediastinal or supraclavicular nodal involvement. Stage grouping, using the 6th edition of *TNM Classification of Malignant Tumours*, also differentiated survival except between IA and IB. Patients with pleural effusion regardless of the cytology were found to have an intermediate prognosis between those with limited and extensive disease. The IASLC proposals for the 7th edition of the TNM classification were found to be applicable to this series of SCLC and to the SEER database.

Recommendation: TNM staging is recommended in the staging of SCLC, and stratification by stage I to III should be incorporated in clinical trials of early stage disease. Further studies are needed to clarify the impact of pleural effusion and the extent of N3 disease.

g) Carcinoid tumors subcommittee[37]

Previously, carcinoid tumors had been excluded from the TNM classification, although TNM was frequently used in the literature to describe the anatomical extent of disease in surgical and pathology reviews of carcinoid tumors. Data on carcinoid tumors were not specifically requested for our database, but nevertheless, we received details on 520 cases. The SEER data for the corresponding period (1990 to 2002) also contained TNM data on 1998 cases of carcinoid tumors. Unfortunately, the distinction between "typical" and "atypical" tumors was infrequently and unreliably recorded. Our analysis of these cases found that the TNM classification, by the 6th edition and using our proposals for the 7th edition of *TNM Classification of Malignant Tumours*, was a useful predictor of survival and a strong predictor when assessing N and M descriptors. The analysis of T descriptors was confounded by the lack of clarity on several aspects of the pathology reports such as

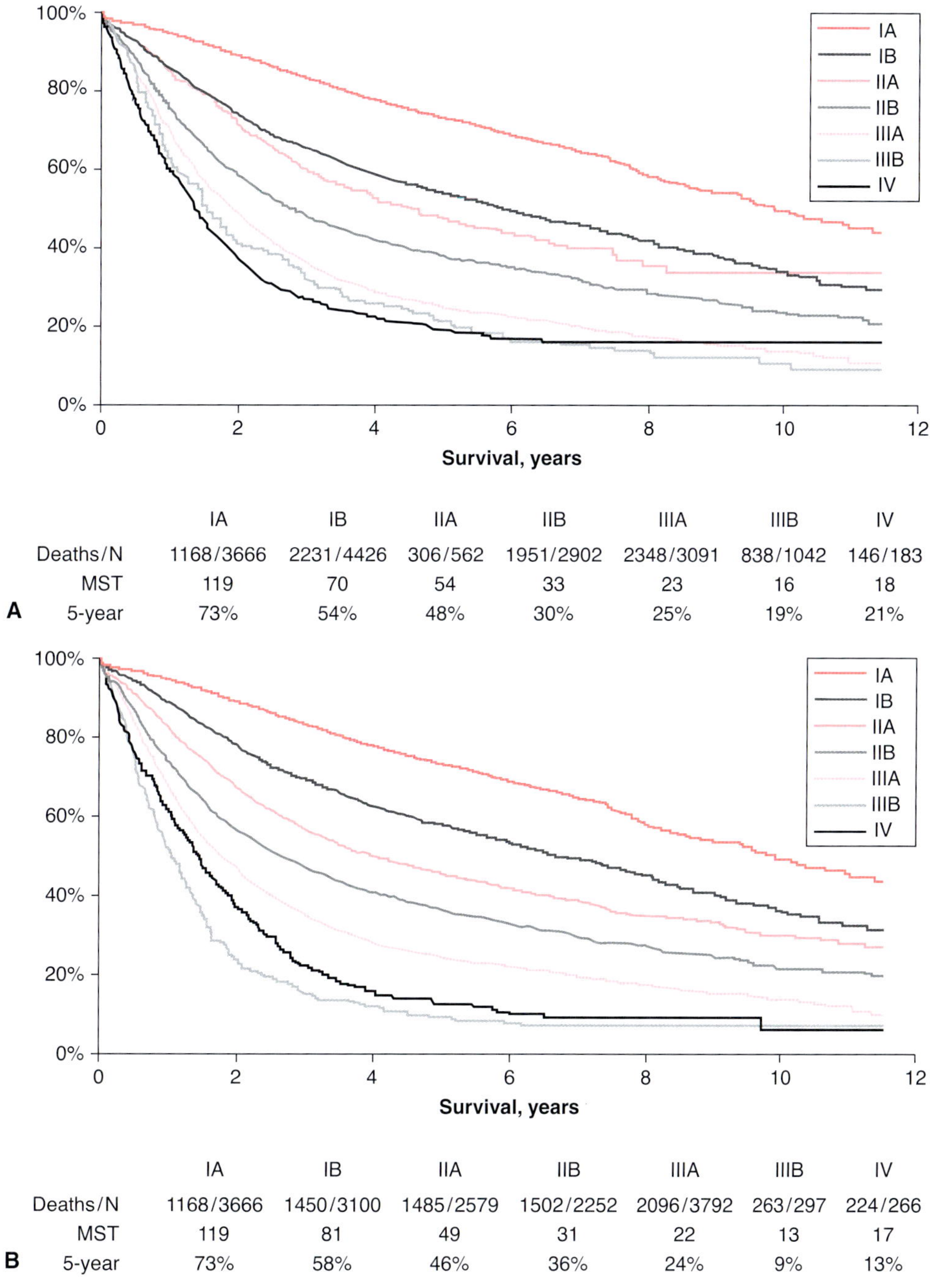

A

	IA	IB	IIA	IIB	IIIA	IIIB	IV
Deaths/N	1168/3666	2231/4426	306/562	1951/2902	2348/3091	838/1042	146/183
MST	119	70	54	33	23	16	18
5-year	73%	54%	48%	30%	25%	19%	21%

B

	IA	IB	IIA	IIB	IIIA	IIIB	IV
Deaths/N	1168/3666	1450/3100	1485/2579	1502/2252	2096/3792	263/297	224/266
MST	119	81	49	31	22	13	17
5-year	73%	58%	46%	36%	24%	9%	13%

FIGURE 30.4 Survival of postsurgical, pathological staged cases by **(A)** 6th edition of *TNM Classification of Malignant Tumours* and **(B)** 7th edition of *TNM Classification of Malignant Tumours. MST*, median survival time.

TABLE 30.4 The T, N, and M Descriptors in the 7th Edition of *TNM Classification of Malignant Tumours**

T: Primary Tumor

TX Primary tumor cannot be assessed, *or* tumor proven by the presence of malignant cells in sputum or bronchial washings but not visualized by imaging or bronchoscopy

T0 No evidence of primary tumor

Tis Carcinoma in situ

T1 Tumor 3 cm or less in greatest dimension, surrounded by lung or visceral pleura, without bronchoscopic evidence of invasion more proximal than the lobar bronchus (i.e., not in the main bronchus)[1]

T1a Tumor 2 cm or less in greatest dimension

T1b Tumor more than 2 cm but not more than 3 cm in greatest dimension

T2 Tumor more than 3 cm but not more than 7 cm;

or tumor with *any* of the following features*:

- Involves main bronchus, 2 cm or more distal to the carina
- Invades visceral pleura
- Associated with atelectasis or obstructive pneumonitis that extends to the hilar region but does not involve the entire lung

T2a Tumor more than 3 cm but not more than 5 cm in greatest dimension

T2b Tumor more than 5 cm but not more than 7 cm in greatest dimension

*T2 tumors with these features are classified T2a if 5 cm or less

T3 Tumors more than 7 cm or one that directly invades any of the following: chest wall (including superior sulcus tumors), diaphragm, phrenic nerve, mediastinal pleura, parietal pericardium; *or* tumor in the main bronchus less than 2 cm distal to the carina[1] but without involvement of the carina; *or* associated atelectasis or obstructive pneumonitis of the entire lung or separate tumor nodule(s) in the same lobe

T4 Tumor of any size that invades any of the following: mediastinum, heart, great vessels, trachea, recurrent laryngeal nerve, esophagus, vertebral body, carina; separate tumor nodule(s) in a different ipsilateral lobe

N: Regional Lymph Nodes

NX Regional lymph nodes cannot be assessed

N0 No regional lymph node metastasis

N1 Metastasis in ipsilateral peribronchial and/or ipsilateral hilar lymph nodes and intrapulmonary nodes, including involvement by direct extension

N2 Metastasis in ipsilateral mediastinal and/or subcarinal lymph node(s)

N3 Metastasis in contralateral mediastinal, contralateral hilar, ipsilateral or contralateral scalene, or supraclavicular lymph node(s)

M: Distant Metastasis

MX Distant metastasis cannot be assessed

M0 No distant metastasis

M1 Distant metastasis

M1a Separate tumor nodule(s) in a contralateral lobe; tumor with pleural nodules or malignant pleural (or pericardial) effusion[2]

M1b Distant metastasis

Notes: 1. The uncommon superficial spreading tumor of any size with its invasive component limited to the bronchial wall, which may extend proximal to the main bronchus, is also classified as T1a.

2. Most pleural (and pericardial) effusions with lung cancer are due to tumor. In a few patients, however, multiple cytopathological examinations of pleural (pericardial) fluid are negative for tumor, and the fluid is nonbloody and is not an exudate. Where these elements and clinical judgment dictate that the effusion is not related to the tumor, the effusion should be excluded as a staging element and the patient should be classified as T1, T2, T3, or T4.

*From UICC. *TNM Classification of Malignant Tumours*. 7th Ed. New York: Wiley-Liss, 2009. Reproduced with kind permission by the UICC.

size, atelectasis, the presence of multiple nodules, pleural invasion, and bronchoscopic extent.

Recommendation: Carcinoid tumors will be included under the 7th edition. A registry of such tumors will form part of the next phase of the IASLC Staging Project.

h) Visceral pleural invasion subcommittee[38]

Visceral pleural invasion was identified as a T2 descriptor in the 4th edition of *TNM Classification of Malignant Tumours* published in 1987.[14] It has persisted into the 6th edition of *TNM Classification of Malignant Tumours* and will remain so according

TABLE 30.5 The TNM Stage Groupings in the 7th Edition of *TNM Classification of Malignant Tumours**

Occult carcinoma	TX	N0	M0
Stage 0	Tis	N0	M0
Stage IA	T1a,b	N0	M0
Stage IB	T2a	N0	M0
Stage IIA	T1a,b	N1	M0
	T2a	N1	M0
	T2b	N0	M0
Stage IIB	T2b	N1	M0
	T3	N0	M0
Stage IIIA	T1, T2	N2	M0
	T3	N1, N2	M0
	T4	N0, N1	M0
Stage IIIB	T4	N2	M0
	Any T	N3	M0
Stage IV	Any T	Any N	M1a,b

*From UICC. *TNM Classification of Malignant Tumours*. 7th Ed. New York: Wiley-Liss, 2009. Reproduced by kind permission of the UICC.

to our recommendations for the 7th edition. However, pathologists have struggled to arrive at an internationally agreed definition of such invasion. The UICC states in the *TNM Supplement: A Commentary on Uniform Use*[39] that "invasion of visceral pleura (T2) includes not only perforation of the mesothelium but also invasion of the lamina propria serosae" although the Japan Lung Cancer Society only considers that "p2," defined as "tumor that is exposed on the pleural surface but does not invade adjacent anatomic structures" is by itself a T2 descriptor.[40] The IASLC Staging Project has undertaken a literature review of this subject and has proposed a standardized definition.

Recommendation: Invasion of the visceral pleura should be defined as "invasion beyond the elastic layer including invasion to the visceral pleural surface." The use of elastic stains is recommended when this feature is not clear on routine histology.

i) Additional prognostic factors subcommittee[3]

There is a growing debate as to how additional prognostic factors should be integrated with the TNM classification. As suggested earlier, some of these will have prognostic importance and others are predictive of response to treatment. Ultimately, the UICC and AJCC must decide whether such factors are incorporated within TNM or, as seems more probable, are added to TNM in a composite prognostic model. The IASLC database contained limited information of patient-related factors such as age, gender, and performance status; tumor-related factors such as cell type and degree of differentiation; and laboratory variables such as serum albumen, hemoglobin, white blood cell count, and sodium. An analysis of the value and interaction of these variables with TNM stage in clinically and pathologically staged cases on NSCLC was undertaken and the results were published.[3,4]

We did not collect data on positron emission tomography (PET) studies but a metaanalysis, based on a literature review, was undertaken by the European Lung Cancer Study Party in collaboration with the IASLC Staging Project. This showed the prognostic significance of the PET maximum standardized uptake value (SUV_{max}) in the primary tumor at diagnosis[41] to be an independent prognostic factor in lung cancer.

THE 7TH EDITION OF TNM IN LUNG TUMORS

The recommendations from the IASLC Staging Project were submitted to the UICC and AJCC on time, underwent internal review, and were accepted without change as the 7th edition of *TNM in Lung and Pleural Tumours*. Because of the central role of the IASLC Staging Project in the creation of the 7th edition and delays in the publishing schedules of the UICC and the AJCC, the IASLC was accorded the privilege of being the first to publish this new classification, at the 13th World Conference on Lung Cancer in August 2009.[42,43] The 7th editions of this classification were subsequently published later in 2009 by the UICC and AJCC.[44,45] The T, N, and M descriptors are listed in Table 30.4 and the resultant stage groupings in Table 30.5.

Additional Changes in the 7th Edition of *TNM Classification of Malignant Tumours* The additional proposals, suggested by analyses within the IASLC Staging Project, have all been incorporated into the 7th edition of *TNM Classification of Malignant Tumours*, along with clarification on other aspects of the classification. These include the following:

1. The "IASLC" nodal chart and the accompanying table of definitions has been accepted as the recommended means of describing the regional lymph node involvement for lung cancers. It is also recommended that at least six lymph nodes/stations be removed/sampled and confirmed on histology to be free of disease to confer pN0 status. Three of these nodes/stations should be mediastinal, including the subcarinal nodes (#7) and three from N1 nodes/stations.
2. There is greater emphasis on the use of the TNM classification in SCLC.
3. Bronchopulmonary carcinoid tumors are, for the first time, covered by the TNM classification.
4. The definition of visceral pleural invasion is included within the TNM classification.
5. In cases in which there is more than one tumor in the lung(s), the distinction between metastases and multiple synchronous primary tumors has traditionally been based on the Martini and Melamed[46] paper. In the 7th edition, these definitions are retained but supplemented by a new emphasis on the role of the pathologist, utilizing where necessary special studies such as immunohistochemistry and molecular markers. In this distinction, lung differs from other organ sites as additional tumor nodules that are microscopic or otherwise only discovered on pathological examination are also covered in the classification.

6. In the application of the "V" classification, lung also differs from other organ sites as, in lung, invasion of arterioles is not uncommon. The V classification in lung therefore covers vascular invasion, whether venous or arteriolar.

Proposals for Testing The *TNM Classification of Malignant Tumours* allows for the formulation of "proposals for testing." This section is largely aspirational allowing additional classifications to be trialed for some years. Often, these have been suggested by inquiries to the UICC TNM Helpdesk or in published studies scrutinized by their systematic annual literature search. For some, there is already supportive data, but for all, additional data and validation are required before considering their inclusion into future revisions. In the 7th edition, these proposals include the following:

1. Where the pN0 category has been based on less than the recommended number of lymph nodes (six lymph nodes/stations, three mediastinal, including the subcarinal nodes [#7], and three N1) or where the highest node removed contains metastases, it is proposed that the resection be categorized as an "**Uncertain Resection**," and designated "**R0(un)**."[47]
2. The concept of nodal zones has been suggested as a simpler, more utilitarian system for clinical staging where surgical exploration of lymph nodes has not been performed.[28] An exploratory analysis suggested that nodal extent could be grouped into three categories with differing prognoses: (a) involvement of a single N1 zone, designated as N1a, (b) involvement of more than one N1 zone, designated as N1b, or a single N2 zone, designated N2a, and (c) involvement of more than one N2 zone, designated as N2b. It is suggested that radiologists, clinicians, and oncologists use the classification prospectively, where more detailed data on nodal stations is not available, to assess the utility of such a classification for future revision.
3. A recent metaanalysis[48] has confirmed that pleural lavage cytology (PLC), undertaken immediately on thoracotomy and shown to be positive for cancer cells, has an adverse and independent prognostic impact following complete resection. Such patients may be candidates for adjuvant chemotherapy. Surgeons and pathologists are encouraged to undertake this simple addition to intraoperative staging and collect data on PLC+ve and PLC–ve cases. Where the resection fulfils all of the requirements for classification as a "Complete Resection," R0 but PLC has been performed and is positive the resection should be classified as "**R1(cy+)**."
4. A standardized definition of visceral pleural invasion (VPI) has been incorporated into the 7th edition of *TNM Classification of Malignant Tumours*.[38] A subclassification has been proposed using a "PL" category be used to describe the pathological extent of pleural invasion:
   PL0 tumor within the subpleural lung parenchyma or invades superficially into the pleural connective tissue beneath the elastic layer
   PL1 tumor invades beyond the elastic layer
   PL2 tumor invades to the pleural surface
   PL3 tumor invades into any component of the parietal pleura
5. There are suggestions that the depth of chest wall invasion may influence prognosis following resection of lung cancer. A subclassification has been proposed, based on the histopathologic findings of the resection specimen, dividing such pT3 tumors into pT3a if invasion is limited to the parietal pleura (PL 3), pT3b if invasion involves the endothoracic fascia, and pT3c if invasion involves the rib or soft tissue.
6. Imaging evidence of lymphangitis carcinomatosa is usually a contraindication to surgical treatment. The "L" category, which is used to assess pathological evidence of "lymphatic invasion," is therefore not applicable. The radiological extent of lymphangitis is thought to be of prognostic importance. An exploratory analysis of this feature is proposed using a "cLy" category in which cLy0 indicates that radiological evidence of lymphangitis is absent, cLy1 indicates lymphangitis is present and confined to the area around the primary tumor, cLy2 indicated lymphangitis at a distance from the primary tumor but confined to the lobe of the primary, cLy3 indicates lymphangitis in other ipsilateral lobes, and cLy4 indicates lymphangitis affecting the contralateral lung.
7. All cases in which there is metastatic spread to distant organs are classified as M1b disease. However, there are clear differences in prognosis based on tumor burden and the critical nature of some organ sites. Such differences will influence the choice of treatment and the intent of treatment by all modalities of care. Selected patients with isolated metastases to a single organ may benefit from surgical treatment. Data on M1b cases should record the number of metastases and the number of metastatic sites as far as is practicable. It should prove feasible in all cases to record if metastases are single or multiple.
8. The categories assigned to cases in which there are additional tumor nodules of similar histological appearance in the lung(s) has been reclassified in the 7th edition of *TNM Classification of Malignant Tumours*. We cannot determine that this is valid for cases in which multiple deposits are encountered and prospective data collection is necessary to fully validate this reclassification. It is recommended that the number of nodules in the lobe of the primary, other ipsilateral lobes and the contralateral lung, and the diameter of the largest deposit in each location be documented as far as is practicable.
9. Bronchopulmonary carcinoid tumors are included within the 7th edition of *TNM Classification of Malignant Tumours*. However, further data are needed to assess the prognostic impact of certain features in carcinoid tumors; typical versus atypical features, T size cut points, the prognostic impact of multiple deposits, and whether these are associated with the syndrome of diffuse idiopathic pulmonary neuroendocrine cell hyperplasia (DIPNECH). In addition, in carcinoid tumors, long-term survival can be expected even when associated with multiple tumor nodules or nodal disease. It is therefore important to collect data on disease-specific survival

10. PET scanning using ^{18}F-fluorodeoxyglucose (FDG) is now widely utilized and has had an impact of the accuracy of clinical staging and referrals for surgical treatment. In addition, a metaanalysis has shown that PET features, such as the maximum value of the SUV_{max} in the primary tumor prior to treatment is an independent prognostic factor.[41] Where PET scans are performed, it is suggested that data is collected on features such as SUV_{max} in the primary and any nodal and/or metastatic sites.

We encourage clinicians, radiologist, nuclear medicine specialists, and pathologists to collect data on these aspects of lung cancer staging for subsequent analysis.

Clinical Implications of the 7th Edition

Intensive validation formed a central feature of the IASLC Staging Project resulting in robust changes for the 7th edition of *TNM Classification of Malignant Tumours*. However, it is recognized that some of these changes will create problems for colleagues in this field. The necessity to sacrifice backward compatibility with existing databases in the search for a staging system, which is manageable in clinical practice, has already been mentioned. It is also recognized that moving some descriptors within stage categories and recommending the proposed changes to the stage groupings will cut across established treatment algorithms. The moving of the larger, node-negative T2 tumors (T2b cases more than 5 cm in greatest dimension) and tumors more than 7 cm in greatest dimension (which would become T3) from stage IB into stage IIA and stage IIB, respectively, will clearly raise the question as to whether such cases should have adjuvant chemotherapy after complete resection. Although there is still doubt as to the value of adjuvant chemotherapy after complete resection for node-negative cases in stage IB,[49,50] at least two large trials have shown a benefit for node-positive cases in stages II and IIIA.[51,52] The question as to whether these larger, node-negative tumors benefit from adjuvant therapy after complete resection will only be resolved by large, prospective randomized trials. The reassignment of cases with additional nodules in an ipsilateral, nonprimary bearing lobe into a T4 descriptor rather than an M1 descriptor and the relocation of T4 N0 M0 and T4 N1 M0 cases into stage IIIA will also lead to questions as to the appropriate treatment algorithm. One limitation of our database was that it does not allow us to be certain whether this reassignment is appropriate for cases with multiple additional tumor nodules or for all T4 cases. Multimodality treatment models, some including surgery, will no doubt evolve, informed by appropriate trials. In other situations, the changes included in the 7th edition of the *TNM Classification of Malignant Tumours* better reflect current practice as with the move of cases with malignant pleural effusions into an M category from a T category. Within the IASLC database, there was a clear difference in prognosis between patients with metastases to the contralateral lung or associated with a pleural effusion and those with metastases at distant sites outside the thorax. In general, the latter have the worst prognosis and have been historically considered as stage IV, and candidates for primarily systemic treatment. It therefore seems relevant to subclassify, within an expanded stage IV, those cases with spread within the thorax as M1a and those with metastases to distant sites as M1b.

The Future for TNM

The 7th edition was based on the IASLC international database, the largest databases ever accumulated for this purpose. The number of cases recruited was 15 to 20 times larger than that which informed any previous revision. Data were donated by 46 sources in over 19 countries. The IASLC is grateful for the support offered by colleagues around the world, which has ensured the success of the staging project. Although the treatment of these cases included surgery in 53% of the patients, there were 30% in which chemotherapy was used and 29% in which radiotherapy was utilized. The data were collected from cases treated over a relatively short period during which the techniques used in clinical staging were reasonably standardized worldwide. The recommendations have been, for the first time, intensively validated. Internal validation has ensured that the recommendations are supported by data from all geographical areas and across all types of database. External validation has been established against the SEER database.

There are, however, limitations to this project. The volume of data and the international nature of the data sources has made data audit extremely difficult and, as a result, only limited checks for consistency have been possible. There are glaring deficiencies in the global distribution of the data with no data at all being included from Africa, South America, or the Indian subcontinent. Other vast countries such as Russia, China, and Indonesia are not represented or only poorly represented. Although less surgically dominated than previous databases, the spread of treatment modalities does not reflect the practice in most institutions. The period under study predates the widespread and routine use of PET scanning, which has had an enormous impact on clinical staging algorithms. In any retrospective database, one has to collect the data that were considered important by each source and this reflects the use for which the data were collected. Although we have an enormous amount of data on some descriptors, such as tumor dimension, we have too little on many to prove or disprove the validity of some descriptors.

It is hoped that our colleagues in clinical practice will recognize that the changes suggested by this project are driven by the data available to us from a database of over 68,000 cases. Even with the acknowledged limitations of the database, its breadth has allowed the application of evidence-based standards in terms of statistical power, reliability, and scientific validity that were not possible in previous revisions. Inevitably, existing treatment algorithms will be challenged but it is hoped that by the rigorous analysis of large volumes of data, the utility of the TNM classification for lung cancer will be strengthened. The IASLC Staging Project is now entering its next phase. This will see the scope of the project expand to include neuroendocrine tumors, including carcinoid tumors, mesothelioma, and possibly other thoracic malignancies. A prospective data set has been established and web-based data collection has been trialed.[53] We hope that these features will ensure further, carefully validated proposals concerning thoracic malignancies for the 8th edition of the *TNM Classification of Malignant Tumours* and beyond. Any institution that wishes to contribute can receive additional information by sending an email to information@crab.org with the phrase "IASLC Staging Project" in the subject line. The success of the next cycle of revision, as in this cycle, totally depends on the support we receive from the global lung cancer community.

CONCLUSION

The *TNM Classification of Malignant Tumours* has stood the test of time and remains the most powerful prognostic tool in lung cancer.[4] The IASLC Staging Project created robust proposals for the 7th edition and the resultant 7th edition of *TNM Classification of Malignant Tumours*, which more accurately correlates the anatomical extent of disease and prognosis. In the future, the challenge will be to integrate TNM with other prognostic factors as they are identified and validated.

REFERENCES

1. Gospodarowicz MK, O'Sullivan B, Sobin LH. *Prognostic Factors in Cancer*. 3rd Ed. New Jersey: Wiley-Liss, 2006.
2. Brundage MD, Mackillop WJ. Lung cancer. In: Gospodarowicz MK, O'Sullivan B, Sobin LH, eds. *Prognostic Factors in Cancer*. 3rd Ed. New Jersey: Wiley-Liss, 2006:159–163.
3. Sculier JP, Chansky K, Crowley JJ, et al. The impact of additional prognostic factors on survival and their relationship with the anatomical extent of disease as expressed by the 6th Edition of the TNM Classification of Malignant Tumours and the proposals for the 7th Edition. *J Thorac Oncol* 2008;3:457–466.
4. Chansky K, Sculier JP, Crowley JJ, et al. The International Association for the Study of Lung Cancer Staging Project: prognostic factors and pathological TNM stage in surgically managed non-small cell lung cancer. *J Thorac Oncol* 2009;4:792–801.
5. Goldstraw P. History of TNM in Lung Cancer. In: Goldstraw P, ed. *IASLC Staging Manual in Thoracic Oncology*. 1st Ed. Florida: EditorialRx, 2009:16–29.
6. Denoix PF. The TNM Staging System. *Bull Inst Nat Hyg (Paris)* 1952; 7:743.
7. UICC. *TNM Classification of Malignant Tumours*. 1st Ed. Geneva: UICC, 1968.
8. Mountain CF, Carr DT, Anderson WA. A system for the clinical staging of lung cancer. *Am J Roentogenol Rad Ther Nucl Med* 1974;120: 130–138.
9. UICC. *TNM Classification of Malignant Tumours*. 2nd Ed. Geneva: UICC, 1975.
10. American Joint Committee on Cancer Staging and End Results Reporting. *AJC Cancer Staging Manual*. 1st Ed. Philadelphia: Lippincott-Raven, 1977.
11. UICC. *TNM Classification of Malignant Tumours*. 3rd Ed. Geneva: UICC, 1978.
12. American Joint Committee on Cancer. Manual for Staging of Cancer. In: Beahrs OH, Myers MH, eds. 2nd Ed. Philadelphia: JB Lippincott, 1978.
13. Mountain CF. A new international staging system for lung cancer. *Chest* 1986;89S:S225–S232.
14. Hermanek P, Sobin LH, UICC. *TNM Classification of Malignant Tumours*. 4th Ed. Berlin: Springer Verlag, 1987.
15. American Joint Committee on Cancer. Manual for Staging of Cancer. In: Beahrs OH, Henson DE, Hutter RVP, et al., eds. 3rd Ed. Philadelphia: JB Lippincott, 1988.
16. American Joint Committee on Cancer. Manual for Staging of Cancer. In: Beahrs OH, Henson DE, Hutter RVP, et al., eds. 4th Ed. Philadelphia: JB Lippincott, 1992.
17. Mountain CF. Revisions in the International System for Staging Lung Cancer. *Chest* 1997;111:1710–1717.
18. UICC International Union Against Cancer. TNM Classification of Malignant Tumours. In: Sobin LH, Wittekind C, eds. 5th Ed. New York: Wiley-Liss, 1997.
19. American Joint Committee on Cancer. AJCC Cancer Staging Manual. In: Fleming ID, Cooper JS, Henson DE, et al., eds. 5th Ed. Philadelphia: Lipincott Raven, 1997.
20. UICC International Union Against Cancer. *TNM Classification of Malignant Tumours*. 6th Ed. New York: Wiley-Liss, 2002.
21. American Joint Committee on Cancer. *AJCC Cancer Staging Manual*. 6th Ed. New York: Springer, 2002.
22. Micke P, Faldum A, Metz T, et al. Staging small cell lung cancer: Veterans Administration Lung Study Group versus International Association for the Study of Lung Cancer—what limits limited disease? *Lung Cancer* 2002;37:271–276.
23. Goldstraw P. Report on the International workshop on intrathoracic staging. London, October 1996. *Lung Cancer* 1997;18:107–111.
24. Goldstraw P, Crowley JJ, Chansky K, et al. The IASLC International Staging Project on Lung Cancer. *J Thorac Oncol* 2006;1:281–286.
25. Gospodarowicz MK, Miller D, Groome PA, et al. The process for continuous improvement of the TNM classification. *Cancer* 2004;100:1–5.
26. Groome PA, Bolejack V, Crowley JJ, et al. The IASLC Lung Cancer Staging Project: Validation of the proposals for revision of the T, N, and M descriptors and consequent stage groupings in the forthcoming (seventh) TNM classification for lung cancer. *J Thorac Oncol* 2007;2:694–705.
27. Rami-Porta R, Ball D, Crowley J, et al. The IASLC Lung Cancer Staging Project: Proposals for the revision of the T descriptors in the forthcoming (seventh) edition of the TNM classification for lung cancer. *J Thorac Oncol* 2007;2:593–602.
28. Rusch VR, Crowley JJ, Giroux DJ, et al. The IASLC Lung Cancer Staging Project: proposals for revision of the N descriptors in the forthcoming (seventh) edition of the TNM classification for lung cancer. *J Thorac Oncol* 2007;2:603–612.
29. Rusch VW, Asamura H, Watanabe H, et al. The IASLC lung cancer staging project: a proposal for a new international node map in the forthcoming seventh edition of the TNM classification for lung cancer. *J Thorac Oncol* 2009;4:568–577.
30. Postmus PE, Brambilla E, Chansky K, et al. The IASLC Lung Cancer Staging Project: proposals for revision of the M descriptors in the forthcoming (seventh) edition of the TNM classification for lung cancer. *J Thorac Oncol* 2007;2:686–693.
31. Goldstraw P, Crowley JJ, Chansky K, et al. The IASLC Lung Cancer Staging Project: proposals for revision of the stage groupings in the forthcoming (seventh) edition of the TNM classification for lung cancer. *J Thorac Oncol* 2007;2:706–714.
32. Crowley JJ, LeBlanc M, Jacobson J, et al. Some exploratory tools for survival analysis. In: Lin DY, Fleming TR, eds. *Proceedings of the First Seattle Symposium in Biostatistics: Survival analysis*. 1st Ed. New York: Springer, 1997:199–229.
33. Asamura H, Goya T, Koshlishi Y, et al. How should the TNM staging system for lung cancer be revised? A simulation based on the Japanese Lung Cancer Registry populations. *J Thorac Cardiovasc Surg* 2006;132:316–319.
34. O'Quigley J, Xu R. Explained variation in proportional hazards regression. In: Crowley J, Ankerst D, eds. *Handbook of Statistics in Clinical Oncology*. 2nd Ed. New York: Chapman and Hall/CRC Press, 2006:347–363.
35. Shepherd FA, Crowley J, Van Houtte P, et al. The IASLC Lung Cancer Staging Project: proposals regarding the clinical staging of small-cell

lung cancer in the forthcoming (seventh) edition of the TNM classification for lung cancer. *J Thorac Oncol* 2007;2:1067–1077.

36. Vallieres E, Shepherd FA, Crowley J, et al. The IASLC Lung Cancer Staging Project: proposals regarding the relevance of TNM in the pathological staging of small-cell lung cancer in the forthcoming (seventh) edition of the TNM classification for lung cancer. *J Thorac Oncol* 2009; 4:1049–1059.
37. Travis WD, Giroux DJ, Chansky K, et al. The IASLC Lung Cancer Staging Project: proposals for the inclusion of carcinoid tumours in the forthcoming (seventh) edition of the TNM classification for lung cancer. *J Thorac Oncol* 2008;3:1213–1223.
38. Travis WD, Brambilla E, Rami-Porta R, et al. Visceral pleural invasion: Pathologic criteria and use of elastic stains: proposals for the 7th edition of the TNM classification for lung cancer. *J Thorac Oncol* 2008;3:1384–1390.
39. Wittekind C, Greene FL, Henson DE, et al. *TNM Supplement: A Commentary on Uniform Use*. 3rd Ed. New Jersey: Wiley-Liss, 2003.
40. Shimizu K, Yoshida J, Nagai K, et al. Visceral pleural invasion classification in non-small cell lung cancer: a proposal on the basis of outcome assessment. *J Thorac Cardiovasc Surg* 2004;127:1574–1578.
41. Berghmans T, Dusart M, Paesmans M, et al. Primary tumour standardized uptake value (SUVmax) measured on florodeoxyglucose emission tomography (PDG-PET) is of prognostic value for survival in non-small cell lung cancer (NSCLC): a systematic review and meta-analysis (MA) by the European Lung Cancer Working Party for the IASLC Lung Cancer Staging Project. *J Thorac Oncol* 2008;3:6–12.
42. Goldstraw P. *IASLC Staging Handbook in Thoracic Oncology.* 1st Ed. Florida, USA: EditorialRx Press, 2009.
43. Goldstraw P. *IASLC Staging Manual in Thoracic Oncology.* 1st Ed. Florida, USA: EditorialRx Press, 2009.
44. Sobin LH, Wittekind C. *TNM Classification of Malignant Tumours.* 7th Ed. New York: Wiley Liss, 2009.
45. *AJCC Cancer Staging Handbook.* 7th Ed. New York, Springer, 2009.
46. Martini N, Melamed MR. Multiple primary lung cancers. *J Thorac Cardiovasc Surg* 1975;70:606–612.
47. Rami-Porta R, Wittekind C, Goldstraw P. Complete resection in lung cancer surgery:proposed definition. *Lung Cancer* 2005;49:25–33.
48. Lim E, Clough R, Goldstraw P, et al. Impact of positive pleural lavage cytology on survival in patients undergoing lung cancer resection for non-small cell lung cancer: an International multicentre meta-analysis. *J Thorac Cardiovasc Surg* In press 2009.
49. Strauss GM, Herndon JE, Maddaus MA, et al. Adjuvant chemotherapy in stage IB non-small cell lung cancer (NSCLC): update of Cancer And Leukemia Group B (CALGB) protocol 9633. *J Clin Oncol* 2006; 24[Abstract 7007], 18s.
50. Pignon JP, Tribodet H, Scagliotti GV, et al. Lung Adjuvant Cisplatin Evaluation (LACE): a pooled analysis of five randomized clinical trials including 4,584 patients. *J Clin Oncol* 2006;24[Abstract 7008], 18s.
51. Winton T, Livingston R, Johnson D, et al. Vinorelbine plus Cisplatin vs Observation in resected non-small-cell lung cancer. *N Engl J Med* 2005;352:2589–2597.
52. Douillard JY, Rosell R, Delena M, et al. Adjuvant vinorelbine plus cisplatin versus observation in patients with completely resected stage IB-IIIA non-small-cell lung cancer (Adjuvant Navelbine International Trialists Association [ANITA]): a randomised controlled trial. *Lancet Oncol* 2006;7:719–727.
53. Giroux DJ, Rami-Porta R, Chansky K, et al. The IASLC Lung Cancer Staging Project: data elements for the prospective project. *J Thorac Oncol* 2009;4:679–683.

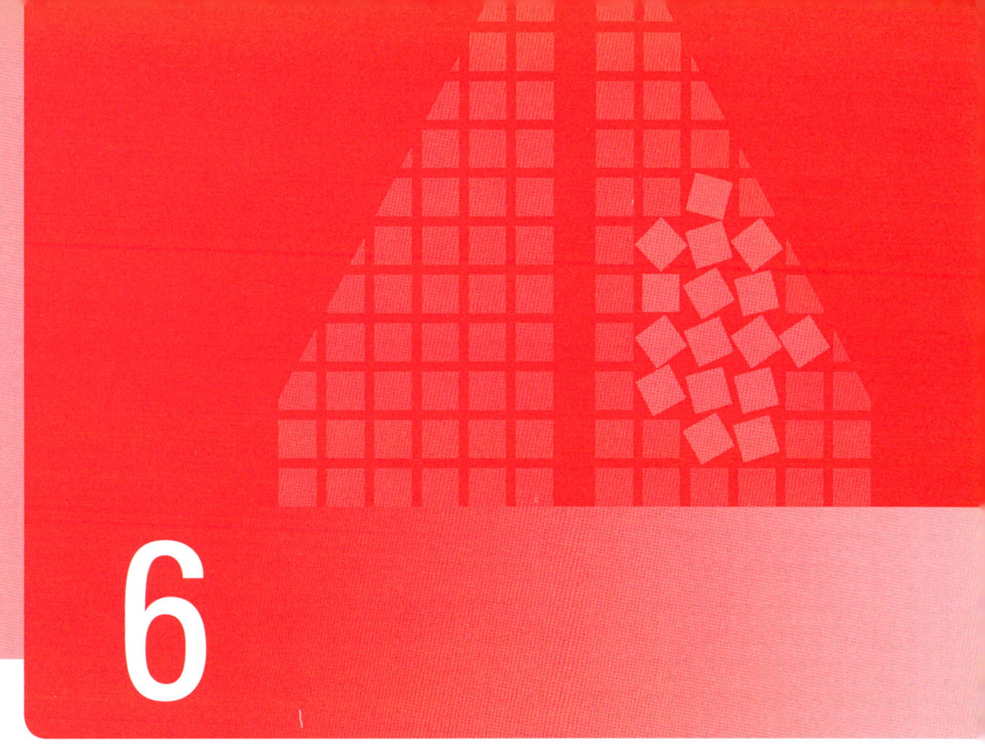

SECTION 6

Surgical Management of Lung Cancer

CHAPTER 31

Robert J. McKenna, Jr.

Minimally Invasive Techniques for the Management of Lung Cancer

The hope for video-assisted thoracic surgery (VATS) treatment of lung cancer is that it would reduce morbidity, mortality, and hospital stay and allow quicker return to regular activities for patients after procedures that formerly required major incisions. However, since the first VATS lobectomy (VL) with anatomic hilar dissection was performed in 1992, some have questioned the safety and benefits reported for a VATS approach.[1–3] Although there is no large, randomized prospective study from around the world, the experience is now sufficiently large enough to compare VATS with open thoracotomy for pulmonary resection. Large series of VATS lobectomies show impressive results. More and more, thoracic surgeons offer their patients minimally invasive pulmonary resections. This chapter will provide the current data regarding minimally invasive procedures for the management of lung cancer.

QUESTIONS ABOUT VATS LOBECTOMY

The following are the current questions about VATS for lobectomy:

- What is the definition of a VATS lobectomy?
- How is it done?
- Is it safe?
- Is it an adequate cancer operation?
- Are there advantages over a thoracotomy?

DEFINITION

There are some controversies about the exact definition of a VL, and these issues include rib spreading, instrumentation, and anatomic dissection. However, most agree that a VL should include an anatomic dissection of pulmonary vessels, a nodal sampling or dissection, an incision ≤10 cm long, and, most importantly, no rib spreading. Visualization should be on a monitor, not through the incision. A retractor to hold open the soft tissue may be helpful to prevent expansion of the lung during intrapleural suctioning. The use of standard, open instruments or disposable, minimally invasive instruments does not matter and should not be part of the definition. Simultaneous ligation of the hilar structures[1] should be discouraged. A "hybrid" operation that involves rib spreading through a small incision has only recently been addressed in the literature, and surely is used by many surgeons as a compromise between complete VATS and open thoracotomy. There are few reports comparing these techniques[4] and patients undergoing lobectomy and lymph node dissection with a complete VATS had less blood loss, faster recovery, shorter hospitalization, and longer operating times than did patients undergoing the lobectomy with the open approaches. At a mean follow-up of 38.8 months, Kaplan-Meier probabilities of survival at 5 years were complete VATS, 96.7%; hybrid VATS, 95.2%; and open techniques, 97.2%. There was no significant difference in the rate of recurrence among the three different procedures. It was concluded that VATS lobectomy is an acceptable cancer operation for patients with peripheral non–small cell lung cancer less than or equal to 2 cm in diameter (clinical stage IA) with the same long-term survivals as open surgery.

GENERAL APPROACH FOR A VATS LOBECTOMY

Philosophically, a lobectomy should be the same operation, whether it is performed through a thoracotomy or by VATS. The arteries, veins, and bronchi should all be individually ligated and a lymph node dissection or sampling should be performed.[5]

With current technology, most lobectomies can be performed by VATS. In 2005, although 94% of the 239 lobectomies performed by our group were VATS, only 18% of lobectomies in the 2005 Society of Thoracic Surgeons General Thoracic Surgery Database were performed by VATS (personal communication). The adoption for VATS lobectomy was slow after the first VATS lobectomy in 1992, but the momentum is currently growing rapidly, because patients demand the procedure and thoracic surgeons gain an understanding of the techniques to perform the procedure.

TABLE 31.1 Indications and Contraindications for VATS Lobectomy

Indications
Clinical stage I lung cancer
Tumor size <6 cm
Physiologic operability
Possible Contraindications
Nodal disease (benign or malignant)
Pancoast tumors
Chest wall or mediastinal invasion (T3 or T4 tumor)
Need for sleeve lobectomy
Neoadjuvant chemotherapy
Neoadjuvant radiation therapy
Contraindications
Nodal disease densely adherent to vessels
Chest wall or mediastinal invasion (T3 or T4 tumor)
Neoadjuvant chemotherapy and radiation therapy

INDICATIONS AND CONTRAINDICATIONS

The indications for a lobectomy (Table 31.1) are similar whether the procedure is performed by VATS or via a thoracotomy. For VATS, the ideal case is a T1N0 peripheral tumor; however, we have removed an 8-cm tumor through a 5-cm incision by cutting one rib. Centrally located tumors that require a bronchial sleeve resection are generally performed via a thoracotomy, although VATS sleeve resections have been performed with good results.[6] VATS may expand the indications to include patients with marginal performance status and who are not candidates for a thoracotomy.

The contraindication and possible contraindications to a VATS lobectomy are also shown in Table 31.1. Safe dissection around the vessels and in the mediastinum after neoadjuvant chemotherapy and/or radiation is challenging and may require a thoracotomy. Reports do show that VATS lobectomies after neoadjuvant chemotherapy, and sometimes after chemotherapy and radiation treatment, can be performed safely.[7]

TECHNIQUE FOR VATS LOBECTOMY

Procedure Typical placement of incisions for a VATS lobectomy is seen in Figure 31.1. The utility incision is 4 to 6 cm, and the ribs are not spread. The fissure, bronchus, and pulmonary vessels larger than 5 mm are individually transected with the endoscopic stapler. Smaller vessels may be tied or clipped. The completeness of the fissure is not a factor in determining the feasibility of performing a VATS lobectomy, because the vessels are stapled anteriorly and then the fissure is completed. Vessels are dissected anteriorly, not through the

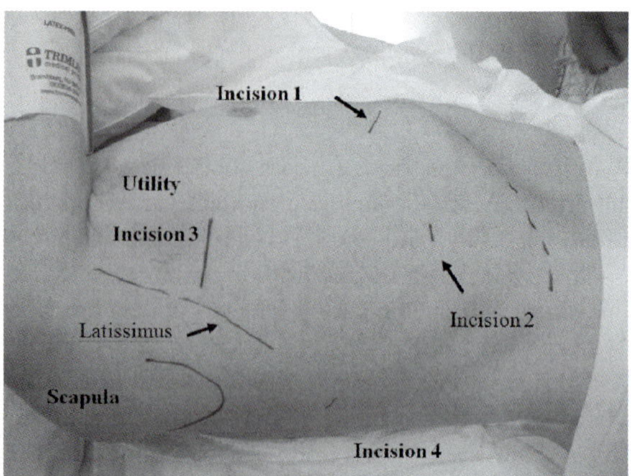

FIGURE 31.1 The incisions for our approach to video-assisted thoracic surgical lobectomy include the following: (*1*) incision 1 in the auscultatory triangle for an assistant's instrument, (*2*) an incision 2 for the trocar and the thoracoscope, (*3*) the utility thoracotomy incision 3, and (*4*) incision 4 in the midclavicular line for the stapler.

fissure; the fissure is usually completed after the vessels and bronchus are transected. To minimize the risk of contaminating the incision with the tumor, the lung specimen is placed in a bag for removal through the utility incision.

Lymph Node Dissection Mediastinal node sampling or complete lymph node dissection should be part of all lobectomies for cancer; and they can properly be performed by VATS. In a prospective study, after one surgeon performed a VATS nodal dissection, another thoracic surgeon then performed a thoracotomy to remove any additional lymphatic tissue that could be found.[8] For the right-sided procedures, the mean numbers of lymph nodes resected by VATS was 40.3 (weight = 10 g), and mean number of additional nodes found at thoracotomy was 1.2 (weight = 0.2 g). Therefore, a good node dissection can be performed by VATS.

IS A VATS LOBECTOMY SAFE?

Table 31.2 shows the result of several large series. The morbidity and mortality are low in these series, and the length of stay is short. These statistics are comparable or better than those for lobectomy by thoracotomy. The mortality, morbidity, and length of stay for the VATS approach are comparable or better than the results with current series utilizing a thoracotomy.[9] A small randomized study showed fewer complications for the VATS approach (18% vs. 50%).[10]

Conversion to Thoracotomy Conversion from VATS to thoracotomy is not a failure for a VATS lobectomy. Conversion to thoracotomy was necessary in 0% to 19.5% of patients in large series of VATS lobectomy referenced in this chapter. This was most often required for oncologic reasons, such as a centrally located tumor requiring vascular control,

TABLE 31.2 Results after VATS Lobectomy for Several Large Series

Reference	No. of Patients	Mortality	Morbidity	Length of Stay*
McKenna Jr. et al.[1]	1100	0.8	15%	4.8/4
Onaitis et al.[24]	500	1%	15%	/3
Yim et al.[25]	214	0.5%	22%	6.8/NR
Kaseda et al.[27]	204	0.8%	2.3%	NR
Swanson et al.[9]	180	0.6%	21%	NR/4
Roviaro[28]	171	0.6%	8.7%	NR
Walker et al.[3]	159	1.8%	NR	NR/6
Iwasaki[29]	140	0%	NR	NR

*mean/median days
NR, not reported.

a sleeve resection, or an unsuspected T3 tumor, attached to the chest wall, diaphragm, or superior vena cava, prompted the conversion. Abnormal hilar nodes with granulomatous or metastatic disease adherent to the superior pulmonary vein may be better evaluated and more safely resected with thoracotomy. Approximately 30% of the conversions to thoracotomy are for nononcologic reasons, such as pleural symphysis.

Intraoperative Hemorrhage Although bleeding during a VATS procedure can be dangerous because access is limited, this occurs rarely when an experienced surgeon performs VATS resections. The scrub nurse should always keep a sponge stick available to immediately apply pressure for controlling hemorrhage in the event that bleeding occurs. After the bleeding is controlled, the surgeon can then deal with the bleeding by VATS or thoracotomy. Significant bleeding occurs in <1% of cases and can usually be managed with low risk.[11]

Tumor Seeding of the Incision Although tumor recurrence in a VATS incision with a poor prognosis, the incidence appears to be very low (<0.5%). The risk of tumor seeding in an incision can be minimized with the use of proper bags to protect the incisions during removal of specimens.

Immunologic Effect of VATS versus Thoracotomy
There appears to be less impact after a VATS procedure than after a thoracotomy. VATS is associated with a reduced stress response, reduced postoperative C-reactive protein, reduced IL-6 levels, and better cellular immune function.[12–14] However, the clinical significance of this is unclear.

ADEQUACY OF VATS AS A CANCER OPERATION

The ultimate measure of any cancer treatment is long-term disease-free survival. Although, in general, the 5-year survival for stage I lung cancer after resection is about 60%, the 5-year survival after a VATS lobectomy for stage I lung cancer has been reported to be 72% to 94%. This may be related to patient selection, rather than any true benefit from the VATS approach.

BENEFITS OF VATS OVER THORACOTOMY FOR LOBECTOMY

Nonrandomized studies suggest that there are benefits for VATS compared with a thoracotomy for lobectomy (Table 31.3). Patients generally appear to have less pain after a VATS than after a lobectomy by thoracotomy ($p < 0.02$).[15–17] VATS patients averaged less morphine, less breakthrough narcotic, less sleep disturbance, and a better pain analogue score than the thoracotomy patients. The incidence of postthoracotomy pain syndrome after VATS lobectomy (2.2%) is lower than expected after thoracotomy.[1] The VATS patients also experienced less pain and greater shoulder strength in the first 6 months postoperatively, but there was no difference after 1 year.

In single-institution series, other benefits to VATS appear to be the following: reduced blood loss and need for transfusion,[18] atrial fibrillation,[1] incidence of pneumonia.[19] VATS appears to be easier for elderly patients and allows surgeons to offer a lobectomy to older patients than can tolerate a thoracotomy.[20]

Cost analysis favors a VATS approach, with fewer lab charges, anesthesia charges, less disposable charges, and fewer hospital charges.[21]

TABLE 31.3 Studies Showing Benefits of VATS

Benefit	Author
Fewer complications	Hoksch et al.[10]
Less pain	Walker et al.,[3] Li et al.[22]
Better shoulder ROM	Li et al.[22]
Better PFT	Nakata et al.[26]
Better quality of life, earlier recovery	Sugiura et al.,[23] Demmy and Curtis[18]
Less pneumonia	Whitson et al.[19]
Easier for octogenarians	McVay et al.,[20] Demmy and Curtis[18]
Less cost	Nakajima et al.[21]
Receive more adjuvant chemotherapy	Peterson et al.[2]
Less impact on immunotherapy	Walker et al.,[3] Ng et al.[14]

PFT, pulmonary function test; ROM, range of motion.

There are also benefits after discharge from the hospital. These include reduced need for pain medicine,[22] an earlier recovery,[18] reduced need for skilled nursing unit,[18] and better quality of life.[23] Acutely, pulmonary function[23] and shoulder strength and range of motion[16,22] are better after VATS than after thoracotomy; although at 1 year, the results are the same.

Furthermore, VATS benefits patients who need postoperative adjuvant chemotherapy. Adjuvant treatment for other cancers show that the benefit from adjuvant treatment only occurs if patients receive a high percentage of their chemotherapy, so presumably that is also important for lung cancer patients. More patients receive at least 75% of their planned chemotherapy after VATS lobectomy than after a thoracotomy (61% vs. 40%).[2]

CONCLUSION

The experience and techniques for minimally invasive thoracic procedures have progressed. With VATS, thoracic surgeons can perform the same major lung resections with the same long-term survival as with thoracotomy; whereas VATS appears to offer patients lower complication rates and earlier recovery.

REFERENCES

1. McKenna RJ Jr, Houck W, Fuller CB. Video-assisted thoracic surgery lobectomy: experience with 1,100 cases. *Ann Thorac Surg* 2006; 81:421–426.
2. Peterson RP, Pham D, Burfeind WR, et al. Thoracoscopic lobectomy facilitates the delivery of chemotherapy after resection for lung cancer. *Ann Thorac Surg* 2007;83:1245–1249.
3. Walker WS, Codispoti M. Soon SY, et al. Long-term outcomes following VATS lobectomy for non-small cell bronchogenic carcinoma. *Eur J Cardio Thorac Surg* 2003;23(3):397–402.
4. Okada M, Sakamoto T, Yuki T, et al. Hybrid surgical approach of video-assisted minithoracotomy for lung cancer: significance of direct visualization on quality of surgery. *Chest* 2005;128(4):2696–2701.
5. McKenna RJ Jr. VATS lobectomy with mediastinal lymph node sampling or dissection. *Chest Surg Clin N Am* 1995;4:223.
6. Mahtabifard A, Fuller CB, McKenna RJ Jr. Video-assisted thoracic surgery sleeve lobectomy: a case series. *Ann Thorac Surg* 2008;85(2): S729–S732.
7. Petersen RP, Pham D, Burfeind WR, et al. Thoracoscopic lobectomy facilitates the delivery of chemotherapy after resection for lung cancer. *Ann Thorac Surg* 2007;83(4):1245–1249; discussion 1250.
8. Sagawa M, Sato M, Sakurada A, et al. A prospective trial of systematic nodal dissection for lung cancer by video-assisted thoracic surgery: can it be perfect? *Ann Thorac Surg* 2002;73:900–904.
9. Swanson SJ, Herndon JE 2nd, D'Amico TA, et al. Video-assisted thoracic surgery lobectomy: report of CALGB 39802—a prospective, multi-institution feasibility study. *J Clin Oncol* 2007;25(31):4993 -4997.
10. Hoksch B, Ablassmaier B, Walter M, et al. Complication rate after thoracoscopic and conventional lobectomy. *Zentralblatt fur Chirurgie* 2003;128(2):106–110.
11. Mackinlay TA. VATS lobectomy: an international survey. Presented at the IVth International Symposium on Thoracoscopy and Video-Assisted Thoracic Surgery. Sao-Paulo, Brazil, May, 1997.
12. Yim AP, Wan S, Lee TW, et al. VATS lobectomy reduces cytokine responses compared with conventional surgery. *Ann Thorac Surg* 2000; 70(1):243–247.
13. Walker WS, Leaver HA. Immunologic and stress responses following video-assisted thoracic surgery and open pulmonary lobectomy in early stage lung cancer. *Thorac Surg Clin* 2007;17(2):241–249, ix.
14. Ng CS H, Song W, Connie H, et al. Video-assisted thoracic surgery lobectomy for lung cancer is associated with less immunochemokine disturbances than thoracotomy. *Eur J Cardio Thorac Surg* 2007;31(1):83–87.
15. Walker WS, Pugh GC, Craig SR, et al. Continued experience with thoracoscopic major pulmonary resection. *Int Surg* 1996;81:255–258.
16. Landreneau RJ, Mack MJ, Hazelrigg SR, et al. Prevalence of chronic pain after pulmonary resection by thoracotomy or video-assisted thoracic surgery. *J Thorac Cardiovasc Surg* 1994;107:1079–1085.
17. Giudicelli R, Thomas P, Lonjon T, et al. Video-assisted minithoracotomy versus muscle-sparing thoracotomy for performing lobectomy. *Ann Thorac Surg* 1994;58:712–717.
18. Demmy TL, Curtis JJ. Minimally invasive lobectomy directed toward frail and high-risk patients: a case-control study. *Ann Thorac Surg* 1999;68(1):194–200.
19. Whitson BA, Andrade RS, Boettcher A, et al. Video-assisted thoracoscopic surgery is more favorable than thoracotomy for resection of clinical stage I non-small cell lung cancer. *Ann Thorac Surg* 2007; 83:1965–1970.
20. McVay C, Houck W, Fuller CB, et al. VATS lobectomy on octogenarians. *Amer Surg* 2005;71(9):791–793.
21. Nakajima J, Takamoto S, Kohno T, et al. Costs of videothoracoscopic surgery versus open resection for patients with of lung carcinoma. *Cancer* 2000;89(11 Suppl):2497–2501.
22. Li WW, Lee RL, Lee TW, et al. The impact of thoracic surgical access on early shoulder function: video-assisted thoracic surgery versus posterolateral thoracotomy. *Eur J Card Thorac Surg* 2003;23(3):390–396.
23. Sugiura H, Morikawa T, Kaji M, et al. Long-term benefits for the quality of life after video-assisted thoracoscopic lobectomy in patients with lung cancer. *Surg Lap Endo* 1999;9(6):403–410.
24. Onaitis MW, Petersen RP, Balderson SS, et al. Thoracoscopic lobectomy is a safe and versatile procedure: experience with 500 consecutive patients. *Ann Surg* 2006;244(3):420–425.
25. Yim APC, Izzat MB, Liu HP, et al. Thoracoscopic major lung resections: an Asian perspective. *Semin Thorac Cardiovasc Surg* 1998;10:326–331.
26. Nakata M, Saeki H, Yokoyama N, et al. Pulmonary function after lobectomy: video-assisted thoracic surgery versus thoracotomy. *Ann Thorac Surg* 2000;70:938–941.
27. Kaseda S, Aoki T, Hangai N. Video-assisted thoracic surgery (VATS) lobectomy: the Japanese experience. *Semin Thorac Cardiovasc Surg* 1998;10:300–304.
28. Roviaro G, Varoli F, Vergani C, et al. Video-assisted thoracoscopic surgery (VATS) major pulmonary resections: the Italian experience. *Semin Thorac Cardiovasc Surg* 1998;10:313–320.
29. Iwasaki A, Shirakusa T, Shiraishi T, et al. Results of video-assisted thoracic surgery for stage I/II non-small cell lung cancer. *Eur J Cardiothorac Surg* 2004;26(1):158–164.

CHAPTER 32

Paul C. Lee
Nasser K. Altorki

Extent of Resection for Stage I Lung Cancer

HISTORICAL BACKGROUND

The surgical management of lung cancer has undergone tremendous evolution since the first case series of pulmonary resection for lung cancer was reported by Oschner and DeBakey in 1939.[1] Since that time, the extent of surgical resection for lung cancer has been a point of heated debate among thoracic surgeons. In the early 20th century, most surgeons considered pneumonectomy the treatment of choice for lung cancer despite its associated high operative mortality.[1] Later, noncomparative retrospective case series showed that lobar resection can result in equivalent survival to that achieved by pneumonectomy with lower morbidity and mortality.[2] Anatomic segmentectomy was first described by Churchill and Belsey[3] in 1939 for resection of bronchiectasis and tuberculosis. Anatomic segmentectomy for resection of lung cancer was performed by some thoracic surgeons.[4–7] However, the relative complexity of the operation and the perceived higher risk of local recurrence dampened the enthusiasm of most surgeons.[8] In 1995, the Lung Cancer Study Group (LCSG) reported a randomized trial of 247 patients with clinical T1N0 (cT1N0) peripheral non–small cell lung cancer (NSCLC) who were randomly assigned to either limited resection (anatomical segmentectomy or wedge resection) or lobectomy.[9] Absence of nodal metastases to the draining segmental, lobar, hilar, and mediastinal lymph nodes was confirmed by frozen section examination prior to randomization. The study showed that locoregional recurrence was significantly higher in patients treated by sublobar resections. Locoregional recurrence rates per person-year were 0.022 following lobectomy, 0.044 following segmental resection, and 0.086 after wedge resection. Although patients treated by lobectomy had a higher 5-year survival compared with those treated by limited resection, the difference in survival did not achieve statistical significance (73% vs. 56%, $p = 0.06$).[9] This trial established lobectomy as the surgical standard of care for early stage disease. Limited resection (segmentectomy or wedge) has since been largely reserved for patients with compromised cardiopulmonary function who could not tolerate a lobectomy.

Recently, there has been renewed enthusiasm for the use of limited resection as a result of increased detection of smaller tumors by more widespread use of computed tomography (CT). Evidence derived mostly from retrospective case series and a few prospective studies suggested that sublobar resection was feasible and possibly associated with 5-year survival comparable to that attained by lobectomy in patients with stage I peripheral NSCLC measuring 2 cm or less in size. Ongoing prospective randomized clinical trials are currently underway to determine the relative merits of sublobar resection compared with lobectomy in this subset of patients. In this chapter, we will review the results reported after limited resection done either as a compromise procedure in patients with suboptimal cardiopulmonary reserve or intentionally in patients considered suitable candidates for lobar resection. We will also discuss some of the factors one needs to consider in selecting patients for limited resection including tumor size, location, intralobar satellites, cell type, nodal metastases, and surgical margins. Methods such as brachytherapy to extend the effective surgical margin will also be discussed.

LIMITED RESECTION AS A COMPROMISE PROCEDURE

Several studies have examined the outcome of limited resection as a compromise procedure in patients with limited cardiopulmonary reserve. For example, Landreneau et al.[10] analyzed the results of 219 consecutive patients with pathologic T1N0 NSCLC who underwent wedge resection or lobectomy. The wedge resection group of patients was significantly older and had reduced pulmonary function. At 5 years, overall survival (OS) was 58% following treatment by open wedge resection, 65% for patients treated by video-assisted wedge resection, and 70% for those treated by lobectomy. The difference in survival between the lobectomy group and the entire wedge resection group approached but did not attain statistical significance ($p = 0.56$). The difference in survival at 5 years was a result of a significantly greater frequency of non–cancer-related deaths among patients treated by open wedge resection (38% vs. 18% for the lobectomy group; $p = 0.014$). Furthermore, there was no significant difference in the local/systemic recurrence rates between patients treated by wedge resection and those treated by lobectomy. The authors concluded that wedge resection was a viable surgical option for patients with stage I NSCLC who have impaired cardiopulmonary function.

Keenan et al.[11] retrospectively reviewed patients with stage I NSCLC who had either lobectomy (n = 147) or anatomical segmentectomy (n = 54). The segmentectomy group of patients had a significantly greater degree of preoperative pulmonary impairment compared with the lobectomy group. The authors reported no statistically significant difference in overall and disease-free survival (DFS) between the two groups of patients. The 4-year OS was 67% for lobectomy and 62% for segmentectomy ($p = 0.86$). The authors also compared pulmonary function between the two groups 1 year postoperatively. Patients treated by segmentectomy had preservation of forced vital capacity, forced expiratory volume in 1 second, and maximum voluntary ventilation postoperatively. In contrast, patients treated by lobectomy experienced a significant decline in all pulmonary function parameters.

In 2006, El-Sherif et al.[12] reported the results of sublobar resection for stage I NSCLC in 207 patients with cardiopulmonary impairment and compared them with the results following lobectomy in 577 patients with similar stage disease. For stage IA patients, both sublobar resection and lobectomy resulted in identical DFS of 65% at 7 years ($p = 0.308$). For stage IB patients, there was a significantly worse DFS after sublobar resection compared with lobectomy, 50% versus 58% ($p = 0.009$). The authors concluded that sublobar resection seemed appropriate for stage IA patients.

INTENTIONAL LIMITED RESECTION

Most, if not all, of the evidence supporting the use of limited resection in early stage NSCLC is derived from case series reported by Japanese surgeons (Table 32.1). For example, Kodama et al.[13] reported a case-control series of 46 patients with cT1N0 NSCLC treated by intentional limited resection with curative intent. All patients had peripheral tumors less than 2 cm in size, and all were treated by segmentectomy with regional lymph node dissection. The comparator or control group comprised 77 patients with stage I treated by lobectomy. The segmentectomy group had a 5-year survival of 93%, which was similar to survival in the control group. Locoregional recurrence was 2.2% in the segmentectomy group and 1.3% in the lobectomy group.

Similarly, Okada et al.[14] reviewed their prospective experience with 70 patients who had T1N0 NSCLC 2 cm or less treated by intentional limited resection. The authors performed what they termed an *extended segmentectomy*, which is essentially a segmental resection where parenchymal division extends slightly beyond the anatomical segmental boundary. In this study, segmentectomy was performed only after frozen section examination of the segmental, hilar, and mediastinal nodes confirmed the absence of metastatic disease. Patients with nodal disease were treated by lobar resection. Five-year survival of pathologic T1N0 patients was 87.1% in the extended segmentectomy group compared with 87.7% in the lobectomy group ($p = 0.8$). There were no local recurrences after limited resection. The local recurrence rate

TABLE 32.1 Studies of Intentional Limited Resection for Stage I NSCLC

Study	n	Type of Resection	Tumor Sizes	Recurrence (%)	5-Yr Survival (%)
Kodama et al.[13]	46	Segmentectomy with frozen nodal analysis	Avg 16.7 mm	Local 2.2 Distant 4.3	93 88
	77	Lobectomy with nodal dissection	Avg 22.9 mm	Local 1.3 Distant 5.2	
Okada et al.[14]	70	Extended segmentectomy with frozen nodal analysis	≤2 cm T1N0 NSCLC	Local 0 Distant 1.4	87.1 87.7
	139	Lobectomy		N/A	
Yoshikawa et al.[15]	55	Extended segmentectomy with frozen nodal analysis	Peripheral <2 cm T1N0 NSCLC	Local 1.8 Distant 5.5	81.8
Koike et al.[16]	74	Segmentectomy (60) and wedge (14) with frozen nodal analysis	Peripheral ≤2 cm T1N0 NSCLC	Local 2.7 Distant 4.1	89.1 90.1
	159	Lobectomy		Local 1.3 Distant 4.4	
Watanabe et al.[17]	34	Extended segmentectomy (20) and wedge (14) with frozen nodal analysis	Peripheral ≤2 cm T1N0 NSCLC	Local 0 Distant 2.9	93 84
	57	Lobectomy		N/A	

Avg, average; N/A, not applicable.

for the lobectomy group was not reported in that study. The authors concluded that extended segmentectomy is an acceptable alternative to lobectomy for T1N0 NSCLC 2 cm or less.

Yoshikawa et al.[15] published their multi-institutional prospective Japanese trial of limited resection for peripheral NSCLC less than 2 cm. A total of 55 patients were enrolled. Intraoperatively, an extended segmentectomy with frozen section of hilar and mediastinal lymph node was performed. The authors reported a 5-year OS of 81.8% and lung cancer–specific survival of 91.8%.

Koike et al.[16] reported their results of intentional limited resection for peripheral T1N0 NSCLC 2 cm or less. The limited resection group consisted of 60 segmentectomies and 14 wedge resections, which was compared with 159 patients treated by lobectomy. Intraoperative frozen analysis of hilar and mediastinal lymph nodes was performed, and a standard lobectomy was done when lymph node metastasis were detected. The 3- and 5-year OS was 94.0% and 89.1% in the limited resection group compared with 97.0% and 90.1% in the lobectomy group. Tumor recurrence was noted in five patients after limited resection and in nine patients after lobectomy. Both the OS and the local recurrence rate were not significantly different between the two groups.

Watanabe et al.[17] reported their results of intentional limited resection for T1N0 peripheral NSCLC 2 cm or less in size. Limited resection was done in 34 patients, wedge resection in 14 patients, and extended segmentectomy in 20 patients. Again, intraoperative examination of hilar and mediastinal lymph nodes showed no evidence of nodal metastases. Impressively, the 5-year survival after extended segmentectomy was 93% with no local recurrences. This compared favorably with 5-year survival after lobectomy patients, which was 84%.

Collectively, these studies suggest equivalence between anatomical segmentectomy (the data are less robust for wedge resection) and lobectomy in a select group of patients with peripheral small (≤2 cm) NSCLC who are meticulously staged to rule out the presence of segmental, hilar, and mediastinal nodal metastases. Nonetheless, the data are largely derived from retrospective or prospective noncomparative studies that are inherently limited by unavoidable selection biases. Furthermore, one cannot reasonably exclude the possibility of a significant impact of ethnicity on biological tumor characteristics and survival.

CONSIDERATIONS IN LIMITED RESECTION

Tumor Size Tumor size is a critical factor in determining the feasibility and safety of limited resection. It is well established that tumor size is an important prognostic factor for survival in NSCLC.[18–23] The current staging system recognizes a difference in survival between tumors >3 cm and those ≤3 cm. This is supported by several retrospective studies that showed a survival advantage for T1 tumors compared with T2.[24–28] Even within T1 tumors, several retrospective studies have shown that survival is better with smaller tumor size. Gajra et al.[29] reported their experience with 246 patients surgically resected for stage IA NSCLC. Patients with tumors ≤1.5 cm had a significantly improved DFS and OS compared with those patients with tumors 1.6 to 3.0 cm. Tumor size was an independent prognostic factor for survival in their multivariate analysis. Similarly, Port et al.[18] reviewed 244 patients with resected stage IA NSCLC. The 5-year OS for patients with tumors ≤2 cm was 77.2% compared with 60.3% in patients with tumor >2 cm in size, again supporting the relationship between tumor size and survival. For subcentimeter stage IA tumors, Lee et al.[19] reported 5- and 10-year OS of 94% and 75%, respectively, with the disease-specific survival was 100% at both time points without any recurrences. Other investigators have also reported excellent survival following resection of subcentimeter tumors.[30,31] The aforementioned studies along with many others have led to the new proposed staging system, which divides T1 tumors into T1a and T2b at the 2-cm cutoff.[32–36] Given the preceding evidence of tumor sizes, sublobar resection may be more appropriate for the T1a tumors ≤2 cm in size.

Tumor Location Tumors for which wedge resections are planned *must* be peripherally located at or close to the costal or diaphragmatic pleural surface. Tumors considered for limited resection by a segmentectomy must be confined within the anatomical segmental boundaries without crossing intersegmental planes. Although segmentectomy may be performed for central tumors, the bulk of the evidence supporting segmentectomy with curative intent is accumulated from series with peripheral tumors located within the outer third of the lung. The traditional TNM classification does not consider tumor location as a prognostic factor. However, some studies suggested that central tumors are more likely to harbor lymph node metastases and have a poorer prognosis. For example, Ketchedjian et al.[37] reported that central T1 tumors had a 50% incidence of lymph node involvement.[37] Similarly, Lee et al.[38] reported that for centrally located tumors, the incidence of occult N2 disease was 21.6% and was as high as 26.7% for tumor greater than 2 cm in size. In that same study, the incidence of occult N2 disease was 2.9% for peripherally located tumors. The high prevalence of nodal metastasis in central tumors suggests that these tumors may be best treated by a lobar rather than a sublobar resection.

Intralobar Satellite Tumors One of the theoretical criticisms of a limited resection is the risk of intralobar satellite lesions that were not recognized by preoperative radiographic studies or intraoperative palpation. The incidence of intralobar satellite lesions in small peripheral tumors is actually quite small in published series. Koike et al.[21] have examined 496 patients with cT1N0 peripheral NSCLC, and found that the incidence of intrapulmonary satellite lesions was only 1% to 2%. In a study by Lee et al.[19] of 84 patients with resected subcentimeter NSCLC, 5 patients (6%) had intralobar satellite lesions in the resected specimen that were unrecognized in preoperative CT or positron emission tomography (PET) scanning. Even though the incidence of intralobar satellites may be low, great care must be taken at the time of a sublobar resection to carefully palpate the entire lobe. Clearly, if suspicious lesions are found, a lobectomy rather than a limited resection may be more appropriate once the malignant nature of the satellite is histologically confirmed. Current evidence from our group and others suggests that patients with resected T4 NSCLC have a reasonable survival, with the 5-year OS as high as 58% for properly selected T4N0 patients.[39–41]

Cell Type The traditional TNM classification does not consider cell type as a prognostic factor. Several studies have suggested that there is a difference in the incidence of lymph node metastases between squamous cell carcinoma and adenocarcinoma. Asamura et al.[42] have shown that in squamous cell carcinoma ≤2 cm, lymph node involvements are rare. They examined 337 patients with peripheral resected NSCLC in regard to lymph node involvement. The authors have found that lymph node involvement was very rare among squamous cell carcinoma of 2 cm or less in diameter, and concluded that the rarity of lymphatic spread might justify not performing a lymphadenectomy in this subset of patients. Lee et al.[38] made similar observations in a study of occult mediastinal metastases in clinical stage I NSCLC. In that report, all 16 patients with occult N2 disease had adenocarcinoma as the primary tumor cell type. None of the 34 patients with squamous cell carcinomas harbored any occult N2 metastases. Although this was not statistically significant ($p = 0.082$), the trend certainly suggests that adenocarcinoma cell type as compared with squamous cell carcinoma is a relative risk factor for occult N2 metastases. Suzuki et al.[42a] have investigated predictors of lymph node and intrapulmonary metastases in clinical stage IA NSCLC. Multivariate analyses showed that the grade of tumor differentiation was a significant predictor of regional lymph node metastases.

The only possible relevance of these findings to limited resection is the extent of lymphadenectomy that may be required in the event a sublobar resection is performed for a peripheral squamous cell cancer. Until the results of prospective randomized trials offer further insight into this subject, the standard of care during a sublobar resection, regardless of the histology of the cancer, remains a complete hilar and mediastinal nodal examination to confirm N0 status.

Nodal Metastases The prevalence of mediastinal metastases increases with tumor size. Asamura et al.[42] have found that among patients with resected peripheral NSCLC, the prevalence of lymph node metastases increased from 19.5% in tumor 2 cm or smaller to 32.5% in tumors 2 to 3 cm in diameter. Even for subcentimeter tumors, it appears that a subset of tumors may have aggressive biologic behavior. In a report by Lee et al.[19] on 83 patients with NSCLC 1 cm or less, six patients (7.2%) had nodal metastases, with N1 nodal metastases in four patients and N2 metastases in two patients. The survival in this non-IA group was significantly diminished compared with node-negative patients with deaths associated exclusively with tumor recurrence.

Additionally, occult nodal micrometastasis may occur in NSCLC patients who have histologically negative nodes. Wu et al.[43] studied a total of 103 N0 patients with peripheral lung adenocarcinomas 2 cm or less. A total of 1438 regional lymph nodes were examined for occult micrometastasis by immunohistochemically staining for cytokeratins. Micrometastases were detected in 49 lymph nodes (3.4%) of 21 patients (20.4%). The 5-year survival of patients with micrometastasis was significantly lower (61.9%) compared with those patients free of micrometastases (86.3%). Similarly, Ohta et al.[33] reported that nodal micrometastases were found in 20% of patients with adenocarcinoma 1.1 to 2.0 cm in size, and in 4 of 11 patients with tumor 1 cm or less in size. Interestingly, nodal micrometastases were not found in patients with squamous cell carcinoma of 2 cm or less.

When lymphatic vessel invasion was examined, Ichinose et al.[25] have found a direct correlation between tumor size and incidence of lymphatic vessels invasion in completely resected pathologic stage I peripheral NSCLC. The incidence of lymphatic invasion was 25% for tumors size 1 cm or less, 40% for those 1.1 to 2.0 cm in size, 49% for tumors 2.1 to 3.0 cm in size, and up to 57% for tumor size greater than 3.1 cm. In light of these findings, whenever a limited resection is entertained for a curative resection for NSCLC, it is imperative that a thorough intraoperative examination of hilar and mediastinal lymph nodes be performed. If nodal metastases were found, a lobectomy should be performed.

Surgical Margins The greatest concern after limited resection is a possible increase in the rate of local recurrence. Studies examining the minimal margin necessary in limited resection are sparse. Generally, the margin is considered adequate if it is equal to or greater than the maximal tumor diameter as measured in the deflated lung.[44–46] Adequacy of the resection margin should, whenever possible, be confirmed by frozen section examination. Despite a negative surgical margin, local relapse is not uncommon. New techniques have been recently described to further examine the surgical lung margin and confirm complete tumor resection. Higashiyama et al.[47] developed a novel intraoperative lavage technique to assess surgical margin status at the time of limited resection. Both wide wedge resections and segmentectomies were done. Wide wedge resection was defined by the authors as a macroscopically assessed margin that was greater than the maximal tumor diameter. The margins of the resected specimen were lavaged and the fluid was centrifuged. An on-site cytologist then examined the sediment after proper fixation. In a total of 112 resections, they observed that 11 lesions (10%) had cytological evidence of tumor at the margin. This was significantly higher for patients with more advanced stage, those in whom a compromise limited resection was performed and those with large tumor size. In four cases with positive cytology at the margins, a wider resection by lobectomy or segmentectomy was done in three patients and laser ablation in one patient who later developed recurrence at the surgical margin. Interestingly, all four patients were originally treated by wedge resections. During follow-up, local recurrence at the surgical margin occurred in four patients, all of whom were treated by a wedge resection because of impaired cardiopulmonary function. Remarkably, there were no local recurrences at the surgical margins among lesions with negative cytology at the margin. The main limitation of this technique is the risk of tumor cell contamination from the visceral pleural surface. The success of this technique also depends very much on the expertise and availability of an on-site cytologist.

Sawabata et al.[48] reported a different test of surgical margins using another cytologic technique (run-across method) in which a glass slide is run across the stapled site. They examined 15 NSCLC excised by limited resection. The rate of positive cytology was 47% compared with the rate of positive histology of 20%. Of the seven patients with positive cytology margins, four patients had margin relapse, with no margin relapse in the negative cytology group ($p = 0.03$). The authors concluded that despite a negative histology margin, a positive cytology margin could lead to margin relapse. In contrast to the lavage technique described by Higashiyama et al.,[47] Sawabata reported a much higher sensitivity rate of 47%, possibly because of a direct extraction of cells or tissues from the surgical margin by the glass slides.

The presence of occult tumor cells at the time of limited resection might very well account for an increase in local relapse rate especially following wedge resection. The incidence of occult tumors at the surgical margins appears to increase with larger tumor size and advanced stage. This is an important consideration during a limited resection for NSCLC, and may account for the increase in local recurrence in earlier studies of limited resection such as the trial conducted by the LCSG. In general, when performing a limited resection (especially wedge resection), one should attempt to achieve a wide resection margin equivalent at least to the longest diameter of the tumor.

In addition to achieving a wide resection margin, techniques have been described to effectively increase the local resection margin. Yoshikawa et al.[15] published their results of extended segmentectomy as an alternative method of resection for small <2-cm peripheral tumors. The essential point of the technique is to divide the lung beyond the tumorous segment. After the segmental bronchus is isolated, the tumorous segment is inflated and the affiliated segmental bronchus is tied. The rest of the surrounding segments are left deflated. Using stapling or electrocautery, the resection line is placed on the adjacent collapsed segment so that the margin is beyond the affected segment. A hilar and mediastinal lymph nodes dissection is done concomitantly.

BRACHYTHERAPY

Because of the concerns regarding higher local recurrences following sublobar resection, adjuvant radiotherapy has been used in an attempt to sterilize any residual microscopic tumor cells adjacent to the primary tumor. Miller and Hatcher Jr.[49] has reported a small group of sublobar resection patients in whom postoperative focal radiotherapy significantly decreased local recurrence. However, difficulties in three-dimensional radiation planning of resection site as well as the risk of radiation-induced lung injury in patients who often have compromised pulmonary function has dampened the enthusiasm for adjuvant external beam radiotherapy.

Other investigators have used intraoperative brachytherapy with ^{125}Iodine (^{125}I) as a means to achieve further local control in cases where the resection margins were close or positive. The theoretical advantage of this approach is that surgeons can place the brachytherapy seeds directly at the margins of concern without delay. D'Amato et al.[50] described their experience of intraoperative brachytherapy following thoracoscopic wedge of stage I lung cancer with clear surgical margins. ^{125}I pellets were embedded along a polyglycolate suture at 1-cm interval, with the sutures sewn onto a polyglocolate hernia mesh template. The mesh template was then sutured onto the stapled line. The technique was calculated to deliver very high intensity radiation of 10,000 cGy to a 1-cm depth, thereby extending resection margin by another centimeter. Various studies have demonstrated that risk of local recurrence can be diminished with this technique.[51,52] Fernando et al.[52] conducted a retrospective multicenter study of 291 patients with surgical resected T1N0 disease, where 124 patients had sublobar resection and 167 patients had lobar resection. Brachytherapy with ^{125}I seeds were used in conjunction with sublobar resection in 60 patients. Brachytherapy decreased the local recurrence rate significantly to 3.3%, compared with 17.7% in the sublobar resection group without brachytherapy. Interestingly, for tumors smaller than 2 cm, there was no difference in survival between the sublobar and lobar resection groups. However, for larger tumors 2 to 3 cm in size, the median survival was significantly better in the lobar resection group, 70 versus 44.7 months ($p = 0.003$). More recently, Birdas et al.[53] have extended the use of ^{125}I brachytherapy to larger T2 tumors chosen for sublobar resection. They compared the results of 41 patients treated by sublobar resection and ^{125}I brachytherapy with 126 lobectomy patients, and found similar local recurrence rates of 4.8% and 3.2%, respectively. There was no difference in DFS and OS between the two groups. Although these preliminary results regarding the use of ^{125}I brachytherapy as an adjunctive therapy for sublobar resection are promising, they should be validated in a prospective randomized manner prior to adoption as the standard of care. Currently, an American College of Surgeons Oncology Group prospective randomized trial (Z04042) of sublobar resection (segmentectomy or wedge) with and without intraoperative ^{125}I brachytherapy in stage IA NSCLC is underway.

CURRENT CLINICAL TRIALS

Cancer and Leukemia Group B (CALGB) has recently activated a phase III randomized trial (CALGB 140503) of lobectomy versus sublobar resection for ≤2-cm peripheral node-negative NSCLC. Eligibility criteria consist of peripheral lung nodule ≤2 cm on preoperative CT scan, with the

TABLE 32.2 Comparison of CALGB 140503 and JCOG0802 Trials

	CALGB 140503	JCOG0802
Design	Randomized phase III	Randomized phase III
Preregistration eligibility criteria	Peripheral ≤2-cm NSCLC	Peripheral ≤2-cm NSCLC part-solid to solid on chest CT
Intraoperative randomization criteria	N0 status confirmed by frozen exam: right (level 4,7,10), left (level 5–7,10)	Free of noncurative factor (i.e., malignant pleural effusion and dissemination) Frozen exam of lymph nodes not required
Exclusion criteria	Pure ground-glass lesions Carcinoid tumor	Carcinoid tumors
Control arm	Lobectomy	Lobectomy
Study arm	Segmentectomy or wedge resection	Segmentectomy
Primary end point	Disease-free survival	Overall survival
Secondary end points	Overall survival, local and systemic recurrence rates, pulmonary function at 6 months	Pulmonary function at 3 months and 1 year, disease-free survival, local recurrence rate, adverse events, hospitalization, chest drainage amount, operative time, bleeding amount, number of autostaplers
Target number/entry period/follow-up	1297 cases, 908 eligible cases after randomization/5 years/3.25 years	1100 cases/3 years/5 years
Postoperative follow-up	CT chest at 6 months, 1 year then yearly for 4 years	CT chest every 6 months

center of the tumor located in the outer third of the lung field. Patients are randomized intraoperatively into lobectomy versus sublobar resection (segmentectomy or wedge). Confirmation of N0 status by frozen section of mediastinal and major hilar nodal stations is required prior to randomization. The primary end point of the trial is DFS. Secondary end points include OS, rate of locoregional and systemic recurrence, and pulmonary function as measured by pulmonary expiratory flow rate 6 months after the surgery. The target accrual is 908 randomized patients over 5 years with 3 years of follow-up. The trial is supported by most American cooperative groups as well as National Cancer Institute of Canada (NCI-Canada).

Concurrently, a multi-institutional trial is in the planning phase by the Japan Clinical Oncology Group (JCOG0802). The trial will randomize patients with ≤2-cm peripheral NSCLC to lobectomy or segmentectomy. Target accrual is 1100 cases over 3 years with 5 years of follow-up. Table 32.2 highlights the similarities and differences between the CALGB 140503 and the JCOG0802 trials.

CONCLUSION

Since the report of the LCSG, lobectomy has been regarded by most thoracic surgeons as the gold standard for resection of early stage NSCLC. Limited resection has been largely reserved for those patients with compromised cardiopulmonary status. However, recent evidence supports the use of intentional limited resection (segmentectomy or wedge) for small peripheral stage I NSCLC 2 cm or less in size. Careful intraoperative analysis of hilar and mediastinal lymph node must be performed to exclude occult lymph node metastases and ensure accurate staging in determining the need of adjuvant chemotherapy. Future results from the randomized phase III limited resection trials CALGB 140503 and JCOG0802 for peripheral ≤2-cm NSCLC will hopefully elucidate the role of sublobar resection as a viable alternative to lobectomy.

REFERENCES

1. Oschner A, DeBakey M. Primary pulmonary malignancy: treatment by total pneumonectomy. Analysis of 79 collected cases and presentation of 7 personal cases. *Surg Gynecol Obstret* 1939;68:435–441.
2. Churchill ED, Sweet RH, Souter L, et al. The surgical management of carcinoma of the lung; a study of cases treated at the Massachusetts General Hospital from 1930 to 1950. *J Thorac Cardiovasc Surg* 1950; 20:349–365.
3. Churchill ED, Belsey R. Segmental pneumonectomy in bronchiectasis: the lingula segment of the left upper lobe. *Ann Surg* 1939;109:481–499.
4. Churchill ED, Sweet RH, Souter L, et al. Further studies in the surgical management of carcinoma of the lung; a further study of the cases treated at the Massachusetts General Hospital from 1950 to 1957. *J Thorac Surg* 1958;36:301–308.
5. Bonfils-Roberts EA, Clagett OT. Contemporary indication for pulmonary segmental resections. *J Thorac Cardiovasc Surg* 1972;63:433–438.
6. Jensik RJ, Faber LP, Milloy FJ, et al. Segmental resection for a lung cancer. A fifteen year experience. *J Thorac Cardiovasc Surg* 1973;66:563–572.
7. Read RC, Yoder G, Schaeffer RC. Survival after conservative resection for T1N0M0 non-small cell lung cancer. *Ann Thorac Surg* 1990;49:391–400.
8. Warren WH, Faber LP. Segmentectomy versus lobectomy in patients with stage I pulmonary carcinoma. Five-year survival and patterns of intrathoracic recurrence. *J Thorac Cardiovasc Surg* 1994;107:1087–1093.
9. Ginsberg RJ, Rubinstein LV. Randomized trial of lobectomy versus limited resection for T1 N0 non–small cell lung cancer. Lung Cancer Study Group. *Ann Thorac Surg* 1995;60:615–622.

10. Landreneau RJ, Sugarbaker DJ, Mack MJ, et al. Wedge resection versus lobectomy for stage I (T1 N0 M0) non–small cell lung cancer. *J Thorac Cardiovasc Surg* 1997;113:691–700.
11. Keenan RJ, Landreneau RJ, Maley RH Jr, et al. Segmental resection spares pulmonary function in patients with stage I lung cancer. *Ann Thorac Surg* 2004;78:228–233.
12. El-Sherif A, Gooding WE, Santos R, et al. Outcomes of sublobar resection versus lobectomy for stage I non-small cell lung cancer: a 13-year analysis *Ann Thorac Surg* 2006;82:408–416.
13. Kodama K, Doi O, Higashiyama M, et al. Intentional limited resection for selected patients with T1 N0 M0 non-small-cell lung cancer. a single-institution study. *J Thorac Cardiovasc Surg* 1997;114:347–353.
14. Okada M, Yoshikawa K, Hatta T, et al. Is segmentectomy with lymph node assessment an alternative to lobectomy for non–small cell lung cancer of 2 cm or smaller? *Ann Thorac Surg* 2001;71:956–960.
15. Yoshikawa K, Tsubota N, Kodama K, et al. Prospective study of extended segmentectomy for small lung tumors: the final report. *Ann Thorac Surg* 2002;73:1055–1058.
16. Koike T, Yamato Y, Yoshiya K, et al. Intentional limited pulmonary resection for peripheral T1N0M0 small-sized lung cancer. *J Thorac Cardiovasc Surg* 2003;125:924–928.
17. Watanabe T, Okada A, Imakiire T, et al. Intentional limited resection for small peripheral lung cancer based on intraoperative pathologic exploration. *Jpn J Thorac Cardiovasc Surg* 2005;53:29–35.
18. Port JL, Kent MS, Korst RJ, et al. Tumor size predicts survival within stage IA non-small cell lung cancer. *Chest* 2003;124:1828–1833.
19. Lee PC, Korst RJ, Port JL, et al. Long-term survival and recurrence in patients with resected non-small cell lung cancer 1 cm or less in size. *J Thorac Cardiovasc Surg* 2006;132(6):1382–1389.
20. Birim O, Kappetein AP, Takkenberg JJ, et al. Survival after pathological stage IA nonsmall cell lung cancer: tumor size matters. *Ann Thorac Surg* 2005;79:1137–1141.
21. Koike T, Terashima M, Takizawa T, et al. Clinical analysis of small-sized peripheral lung cancer. *J Thorac Cardiovasc Surg* 1998;115:1015–1020.
22. Okada M, Nishio W, Sakamoto T, et al. Effect of tumor size on prognosis in patients with non–small cell lung cancer: the role of segmentectomy as a type of lesser resection. *J Thorac Cardiovasc Surg* 2005;129:87–93.
23. Nesbitt JC, Putnam JB Jr, Walsh GL, et al. Survival in early-stage non-small cell lung cancer. *Ann Thorac Surg* 1995;60:466–472.
24. Suzuki K, Nagai K, Yoshida J, et al. Conventional clinicopathologic prognostic factors in surgically resected nonsmall cell lung carcinoma. A comparison of prognostic factors for each pathologic TNM stage based on multivariate analyses. *Cancer* 1999;86:1976–1984.
25. Ichinose Y, Yano T, Asoh H, et al. Prognostic factors obtained by a pathologic examination in completely resected non-small cell lung cancer. An analysis of each pathologic stage. *J Thorac Cardiovasc Surg* 1995;110:601–605.
26. Suzuki K, Nagai K, Yoshida J, et al. Prognostic factors in clinical stage I non-small cell lung cancer. *Ann Thorac Surg* 1999;67:927–932.
27. Padilla J, Peñalver J, Calvo V, et al. Model of mortality risk in stage I non-small cell bronchogenic carcinoma [in Spanish]. *Arch Bronconeumol* 2001;37:287–291.
28. Rena O, Oliaro A, Cavallo A, et al. Stage I non-small cell lung carcinoma: really an early stage? *Eur J Cardiothorac Surg* 2002;21:514–519.
29. Gajra A, Newman N, Gamble GP, et al. Impact of tumor size on survival in stage IA non-small cell lung cancer: a case for subdividing stage IA disease. *Lung Cancer* 2003;42:51–57.
30. Martini N, Bains MS, Burt ME, et al. Incidence of local recurrence and second primary tumors in resected stage I lung cancer. *J Thorac Cardiovasc Surg* 1995;109:120–129.
31. Miller DL, Rowland CM, Deschamps C, et al. Surgical treatment of non-small cell lung cancer 1 cm or less in diameter. *Ann Thorac Surg* 2002;73:1545–1551.
32. Wisnivesky JP, Yankelevitz D, Henschke CI. The effect of tumor size on curability of stage I non-small cell lung cancers. *Chest* 2004;126,761–765.
33. Ohta Y, Oda M, Wu J, et al. Can tumor size be a guide for limited surgical resection in patients with peripheral non-small cell lung cancer? Assessment from the point of view of nodal micrometastasis. *J Thorac Cardiovasc Surg* 2001;122:900–906.
34. Flieder DB, Port JP, Korst RJ, et al. Tumor size is a determinant of stage distribution in T1 non–small cell lung cancer. *Chest* 2005;128: 2304–2308.
35. Okada M, Sakamoto T, Nishio W, et al. Characteristics and prognosis of patients after resection of nonsmall cell lung carcinoma measuring 2 cm or less in greatest dimension. *Cancer* 2003;98:535–541.
36. López-Encuentra A, Duque-Medina JL, Rami-Porta R, et al. Staging in lung cancer: is 3 cm a prognostic threshold in pathologic stage I non-small cell lung cancer? A multicenter study of 1,020 patients. *Chest* 2002;121:1515–1520.
37. Ketchedjian A, Daly BD, Fernando HC, et al. Location as an important predictor of lymph node involvement for pulmonary adenocarcinoma. *J Thorac Cardiovasc Surg* 2006;132:544–548.
38. Lee PC, Port JL, Korst RJ, et al. Risk factors for occult mediastinal metastases in clinical stage I non-small cell lung cancer. *Ann Thorac Surg* 2007;84:177–181.
39. Port JL, Korst RJ, Lee PC, et al. Surgical resection for multifocal (T4) non-small cell lung cancer: is the T4 designation valid? *Ann Thorac Surg* 2007;83:397–401.
40. Bryant AS, Pereira SJ, Miller DL, et al. Satellite pulmonary nodule in the same lobe (T4N0) should not be staged as IIIB non-small cell lung cancer. *Ann Thorac Surg* 2006;82:1808–1814.
41. Battafarano RJ, Meyers BF, Guthrie TJ, et al. Surgical resection of multifocal non-small cell lung cancer is associated with prolonged survival. *Ann Thorac Surg* 2002;74:988–983.
42. Asamura H, Nakayama H, Kondo H, et al. Lymph node involvement, recurrence, and prognosis in resected small, peripheral, non–small cell lung carcinomas. are these carcinomas candidates for video-assisted lobectomy? *J Thorac Cardiovasc Surg* 1996;111:1125–1134.
42a. Suzuki K, Nagai K, Yoshida J, et al. Predictors of lymph node and intrapulmonary metastasis in clinical stage IA non-small cell lung carcinoma. *Ann Thorac Surg* 2001;72(2):352–356.
43. Wu J, Ohta Y, Minato H, et al. Nodal occult metastasis in patients with peripheral lung adenocarcinoma of 2.0 cm or less in diameter. *Ann Thorac Surg* 2001;71:1772–1777; discussion 1777–1778.
44. Kodama K, Doi O, Yasuda T, et al. Radical laser segmentectomy for T1 N0 lung cancer. *Ann Thorac Surg* 1992;54:1193–1195.
45. Kodama K, Doi O, Higashiyama M, et al. Intentional limited resection for selected patients with T1 N0 M0 non-small-cell lung cancer: a single-institution study. *J Thorac Cardiovasc Surg* 1997;114: 347–353.
46. Kodama K, Higashiyama M, Yokouchi H, et al. Natural history of pure ground-glass opacity after long-term follow-up of more than two years. *Ann Thorac Surg* 2002;73:386–393.
47. Higashiyama M, Kodama K, Takami K, et al. Intraoperative lavage cytologic analysis of surgical margins in patients undergoing limited surgery for lung cancer. *J Thorac Cardiovasc Surg* 2003;125:101–107.
48. Sawabata N, Ohta M, Nagakawa K. Optimal distance of malignant negative margin excision of non-small cell lung cancer: a multicenter prospective study. *Ann Thorac Surg* 2004;77:415–420.
49. Miller JI, Hatcher CR Jr. Limited resection of bronchogenic carcinoma in the patient with marked impairment of pulmonary function. *Ann Thorac Surg* 1987;44:340–343.
50. d'Amato TA, Galloway M, Szyldowski G, et al. Intraoperative brachytherapy following thoracoscopic wedge resection of stage I lung cancer. *Chest* 1998;114(4):1112–1115.
51. Santos R, Colonias A, Parda D, et al. Comparison between sublobar resection and 125 iodine bracytherapy after sublobar resection in high-risk patients with stage I non-small-cell lung cancer. *Surgery* 2003;124:691–697.
52. Fernando HC, Santos RS, Benfield JR, et al. Lobar and sublobar resection with and without brachytherapy for small stage 1A NSCLC. *J Thorac Cardiovasc Surg* 2005;129:261–267.
53. Birdas TJ, Koehler RP, Colonias A, et al. Sublobar resection with brachytherapy versus lobectomy for stage Ib non-small cell lung cancer. *Ann Thorac Surg* 2006;81(2):434–438.

CHAPTER 33

Hisao Asamura

Management of Ground-Glass Opacity Lesions

Recently, smaller and fainter nodules are being found on computed tomography (CT) imaging.[1,2] This is partly a result of the markedly improved quality of CT images and the increased likelihood of CT examinations in screening programs. On CT images, all noncalcified nodules should be carefully checked because of the possibility of lung cancer. A nodule might manifest as a focal nonlinear opacity regardless of its characteristics (i.e., solid or subsolid, parenchymal or endobronchial). The term *ground-glass opacity* (GGO) is used to describe noncalcified, subsolid nodules. The pathobiological nature, natural history, and proper management of GGOs have become of greater concern in the thoracic community.

According to recent studies on the relationship between appearance on CT and the histopathology of GGOs, a considerable portion of these lesions, although not all, correspond to preinvasive, noninvasive, or early forms of neoplastic growth, especially those of adenocarcinoma lineage.[3–11] The clinicopathological entity of these tumors has been established only recently, and has never been the subject of clinical studies. Interestingly, some of these tumors show obvious progression to more advanced, invasive tumors, and some show a constant shape for more than 10 years. The rate of growth, if any, is generally slow. A diagnostic workup for these tumors has not yet been developed. Therefore, these tumors are outside the scope of the standard management of lung cancer. Surgical intervention is difficult with regard to the indication and proper mode of surgical resection. The present surgical management of lung cancer, in which at least lobectomy is performed in conjunction with systematic lymph node dissection/sampling, cannot be applied to these GGOs.[12] A standard care for these lesions is currently being established. Clear-cut indications and the rationale for limited resection have not been demonstrated. Some of the treatment strategies for GGO lesions will require future clinical trials.

DEFINITION OF GROUND-GLASS OPACITY

The term GGO is currently being used more often to describe the CT appearance of a focal, noncalcified lesion with a slight/moderate increase in CT density. Routine CT images with 1-cm thick slices are not suitable for the diagnosis of GGO, and usually the GGO is characterized on high-resolution CT scan images with a slice thickness of 1 to 3 mm. The CT appearance of GGO is characterized as a "focal, transparent" lesion. GGO refers to a localized or focal lesion regardless of multicentricity, and the diffuse ground-glass appearance seen for interstitial pneumonitis should be excluded from this category. GGO lesions are well characterized by a slight/mild increase in CT density, which does not obscure preexisting lung structures such as blood vessels and bronchi. This appearance refers to CT transparency (Fig. 33.1). When the shape of the pulmonary vessels in the nodules is not recognized in the nodule, the lesion is no longer considered GGO, and instead is called a "solid" lesion. GGO lesions, therefore, can be either homogeneous or heterogeneous.

GGO lesions are classified according to the absence or presence of a solid part. If GGO lesions are homogeneous and do not contain a solid part, they are called *nonsolid GGO* or *pure GGO* (Fig. 33.2). If GGO lesions contain a solid, cystic, or linear part inside the nodule, they are called nonsolid GGO or complex GGO (Fig. 33.3). The solid part is more likely to be located in the center of the nodule and surrounded by the GGO part, which shows a so-called fried egg appearance. The solid part might be scant or prominent, with various proportions of solid to GGO parts. In the classic solid tumor, the GGO part no longer exists within the nodule (Fig. 33.4). The relationships between the subtype of CT appearance and histopathologic findings are discussed later.

HISTOPATHOLOGIC FEATURES OF GROUND-GLASS OPACITY LESIONS

With regard to histopathology (see Chapter 22), GGO lesions are either neoplastic or inflammatory. A focal inflammation of the lung parenchyma sometimes presents with a GGO on

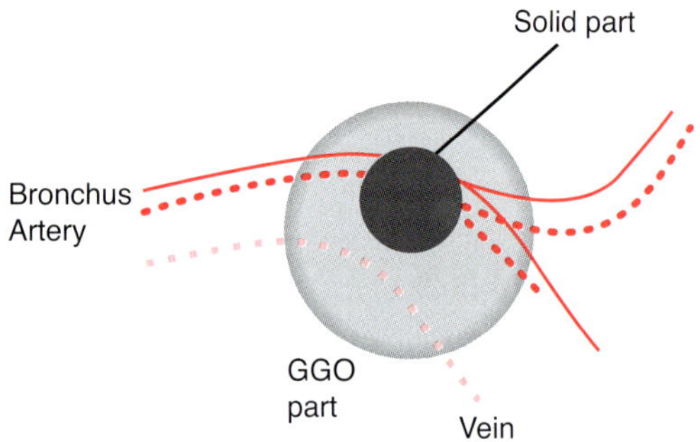

FIGURE 33.1 Schematic drawing of CT appearance of ground-glass opacity (GGO). In the GGO lesion, preexisting anatomical structures such as bronchus and blood vessels are apparent.

the CT image, and pathologically this pattern is described as *organizing pneumonia*. These changes are more likely to be temporary. In contrast, persistent GGOs are more likely to be neoplastic. According to the World Health Organization (WHO) histological classification of lung and pleural tumors, GGO lesions are associated with three pathological entities.[5] Atypical adenomatous hyperplasia (AAH) is described as a preinvasive lesion, in which slightly atypical tumor cells line the involved alveoli and respiratory bronchioles. Nonmucinous bronchioloalveolar carcinoma (BAC) is an adenocarcinoma with Clara cells and/or type II pneumocytes growing along alveolar walls, and without stromal invasion. The important feature of BAC is "noninvasive" growth of the tumor, and therefore, this lesion could be considered in situ carcinoma. The third category is adenocarcinoma with mixed subtypes, which shows a mixture of histologic subtypes as well as obvious invasive growth.

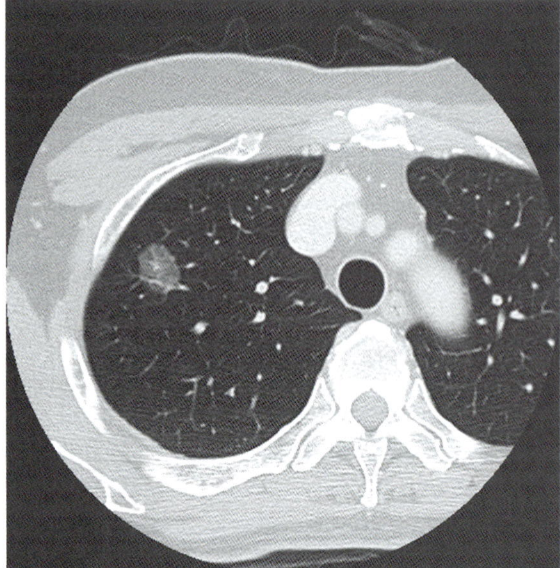

FIGURE 33.2 CT appearance of nonsolid GGO. There is no solid or linear part in the lesion.

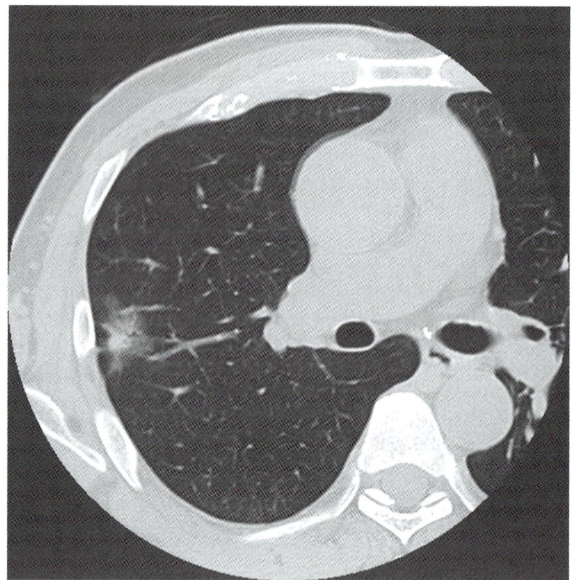

FIGURE 33.3 CT appearance of part-solid GGO. There is a region of increased density in the center of the lesion.

The relationship between CT appearance and histology has been studied.[6–8] Most nonsolid GGOs are AAH or BAC. Invasive growth is rarely seen in the pathology of nonsolid GGO. On the other hand, most part-solid GGOs are BAC and adenocarcinoma with mixed subtypes. A solid lesion usually exhibits invasive growth and is diagnosed as adenocarcinoma with mixed

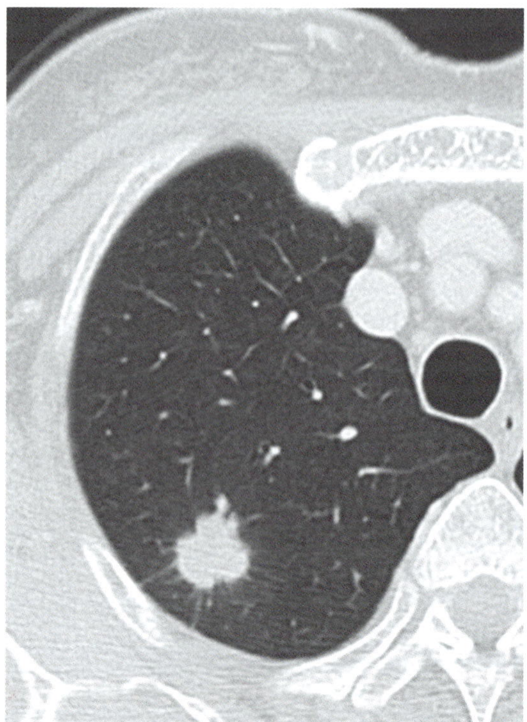

FIGURE 33.4 CT appearance of a solid lesion. The CT density of the whole area is increased, and intrinsic structures are no longer obvious.

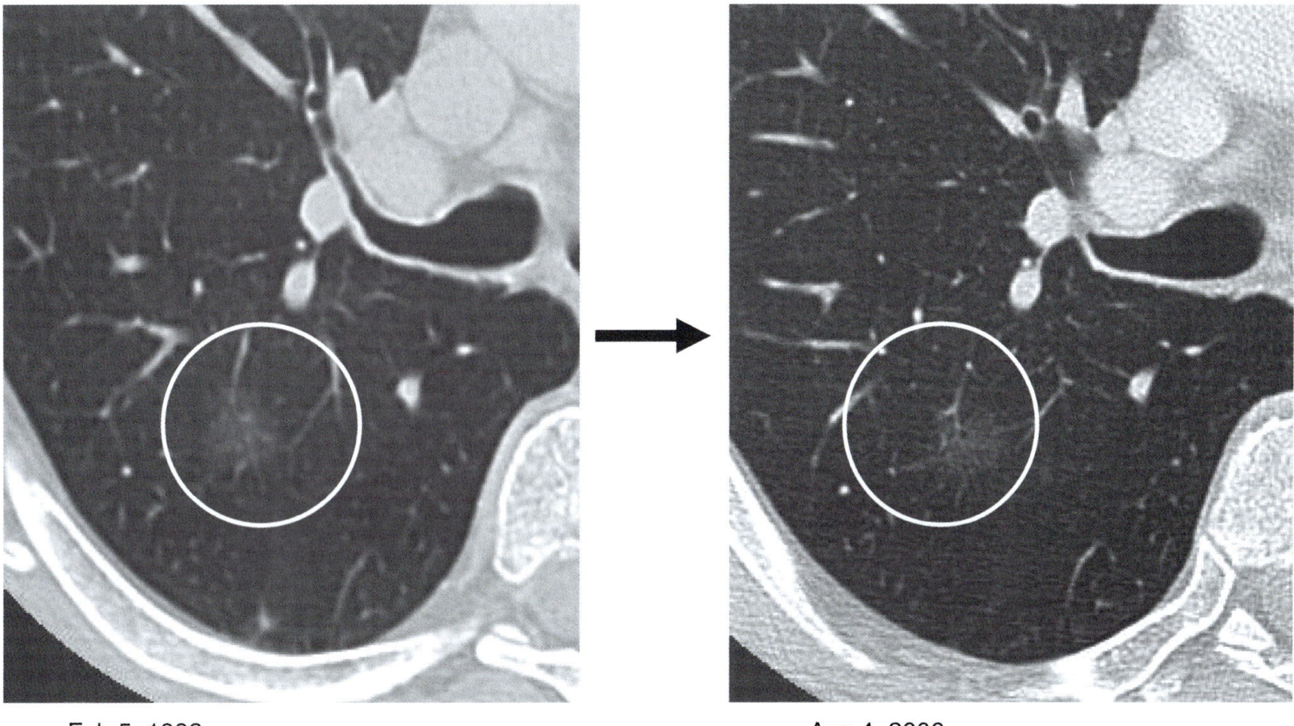

FIGURE 33.5 Indolent GGO (nonsolid GGO). The appearance of GGO remained unchanged for 8 years.

subtypes. Although the image findings on high-resolution CT cannot precisely reveal the pathology with special reference to invasive growth of the tumor, the value of high-resolution CT should be addressed.

The pathobiological background of GGO–BAC tumors has been studied by several investigators.[9,10] GGO–BAC tumors are more likely to arise in nonsmoking women in their 50s and 60s. They also tend to be multicentric, both synchronously and heterochronously. Interestingly, among nonsolid GGOs, some are followed up for more than 10 years without any intervention, and there has been no overt growth (Fig. 33.5). In contrast, some show overt growth with consolidation (Fig. 33.6). These observations indicate that GGOs do not always grow or they only grow slowly, and as a result, they are indolent for considerably long periods. These observations have also shown that GGOs with a smaller size or with a scarce solid component tend to be stable in size, and GGOs in patients with a history of lung cancer tend to grow faster. Other factors that may affect the growth of GGO tumors need to be defined in future studies. In case series from many institutions, noninvasive BAC has been shown to have a superb prognosis, which supports the notion that BAC is carcinoma in situ. According to the degree of invasive growth of adenocarcinoma, the prognosis is determined in a step-ladder fashion.[11]

INTERVENTION FOR GGO–BAC TUMORS

The intervention strategy for GGO lesions has been established only very recently, and future clinical trials to validate the suggested approaches are still needed. Several factors are related to the management strategy: the size of lesions, image characteristics (nonsolid vs. part solid), and a history of previous lung cancer. The indolent nature of small-sized, nonsolid GGOs needs to be stressed. For these tumors, immediate surgical intervention should be avoided. Furthermore, the physical condition of the patient, such as age and coexisting medical conditions, must also be taken into consideration. When we consider surgical intervention, the location of the lesion (outer vs. inner) is also an important issue from a technical point of view. For tumors that are located deep within the lung parenchyma, sublobar resection is generally amenable because of the lack of sufficient surgical margin.

The intraoperative localization of a GGO can be challenging, even if the procedure is performed via an open rather than videothoracoscopic method. GGOs tend to be soft lesions that are painfully difficult to feel, and palpating these lesions are like feeling a sponge within a sponge. If they are located at the very periphery of the lung, one can see a faint change in the color of the visceral pleura, which is greyer than usual and circumscribed. Usually, however, for pure GGOs or those with a minimal solid component, it is best to employ methods for the marking of the lesion using interventional radiologic techniques using methylene blue or isotopic localization. Although all of the methods are effective in locating the target lesion, their limitations are obvious. The needle-wire technique is associated with several complications, such as lung hemorrhage, pleuritic pain, and pneumothorax.[13] A hookwire dislodgement rate of 7.5% has been reported.[14] A failure rate

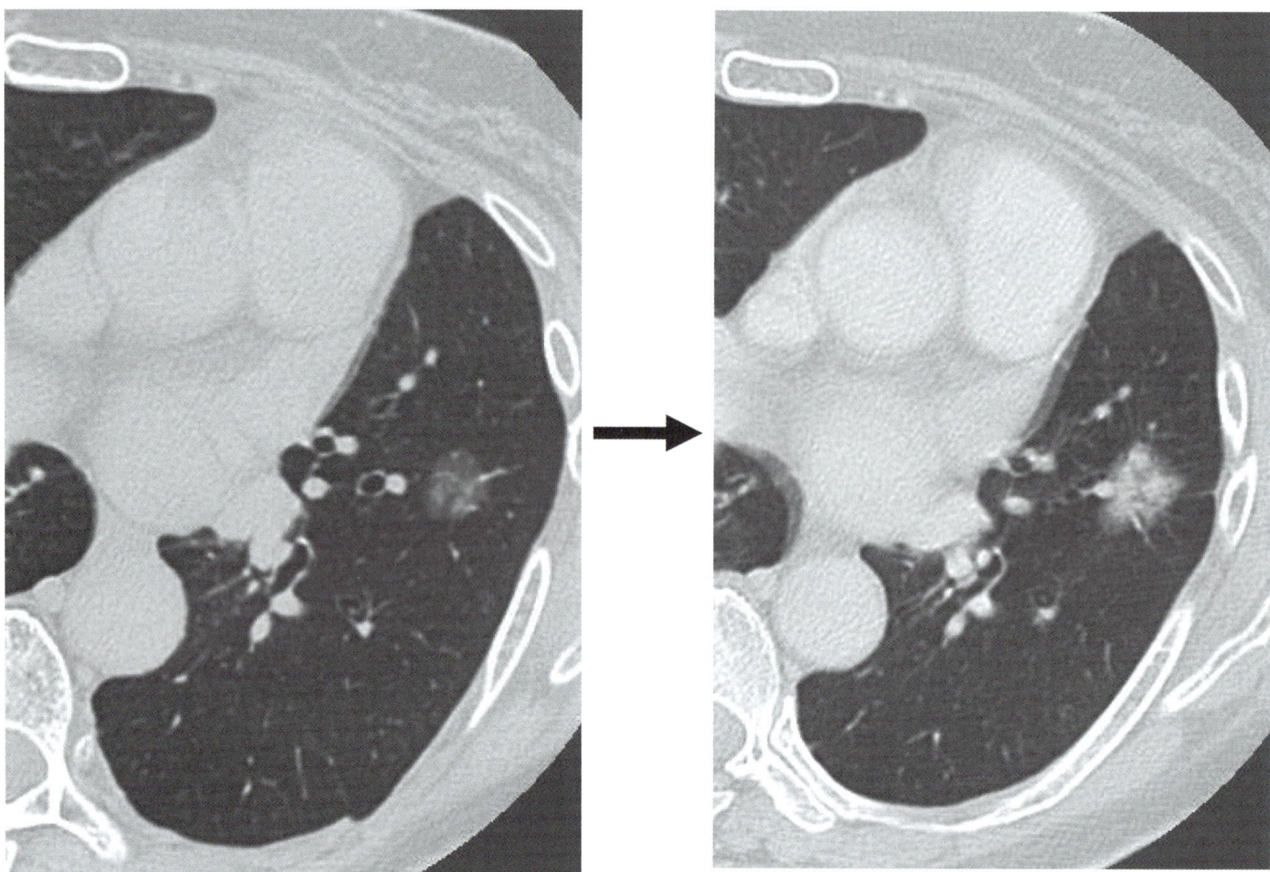

FIGURE 33.6 Obvious growth of GGO in a 54-year-old woman (part-solid GGO).

of approximately 13% for preoperative methylene blue injection under the CT fluoroscopic guidance has been reported because of either an excess of liquid injection or an error in nodule localization. Moreover, the dye frequently dissipates over a large area by the time the surgical procedure is done, making its localization features inadequate.[15] The localization of pulmonary nodules by radio-guided technique[16] also has drawbacks including fast diffusion of contrast medium in the pulmonary parenchyma surrounding the nodule. Moreover, special radiation protection precautions in the operating room or in handling the surgical specimens are required. Injection of coils[17] or agar[18] under CT guidance into the lesion will also assist the surgeon in palpating the lesion intraoperatively.

Nonsolid Ground-Glass Opacities Less than 15 mm in Diameter These small lesions without any solid part in the nodule (nonsolid GGO) are watched carefully with repeated high-resolution CT. The appropriate interval between repeated CTs has not been clearly demonstrated but may range from 3 to 6 months. If overt growth or a newly developing solid component is seen, surgical intervention should be considered.

Part-Solid Ground-Glass Opacities Less than 15 mm in Diameter The solid component in part-solid GGOs represents a fibrotic scar and/or collapse of the lung in which the proliferation of collagen fibers and active fibroblast is generally seen, and these findings reflect invasive growth. Therefore, tumors in this category should be resected. Careful observation should be indicated only for patients with poor physical condition, which would compromise surgical resection. However, if we consider their minimally invasive nature and small size, sublobar resection should be a reasonable option. For these tumors, segmentectomy should be preferable to wedge resection. The location of the tumor should be carefully evaluated. When the tumor is located in the outer two thirds of the lung parenchyma, segmental resection should be acceptable. When the tumor is located in the inner third of the lung, segmentectomy may not be able to ensure a safe surgical margin. Thus, lobectomy, instead of segmentectomy, must be chosen. Furthermore, the lymph nodes at the hilum and, preferably, mediastinum should also be evaluated during surgery. If any of the nodes is positive, the surgery should be converted to traditional lobectomy.

Nonsolid Ground-Glass Opacities Larger than 15 mm in Diameter As with smaller nonsolid GGOs, these lesions should not be resected immediately. However, larger GGOs are more likely to grow faster even if they do not contain a solid part. Therefore, if the lesion stays the same in size (i.e., does not decrease in size as an inflammatory lesion would) after an appropriate follow-up period of 3 to 6 months, these GGOs should be resected. Similarly, resection should be performed with a sublobar resection, such as segmentectomy, rather than lobectomy. The location of the lesion is also considered when choosing the surgical mode.

Part-Solid Ground-Glass Opacities Larger than 15 mm in Diameter Part-solid GGOs of this size are more likely to be invasive adenocarcinomas. When the solid part exceeds 50% of the whole area of the lesion, invasive features become more common. Therefore, the standard of care for such a lesion would, at present, be a lobectomy. The hilar/mediastinal lymph nodes should also be evaluated during surgery.

Lobectomy versus Segmentectomy in the Surgical Management of Small-Sized Lung Cancer Including Ground-Glass Opacity Whether limited resection such as segmentectomy or wedge resection can replace lobectomy or not in the surgical management of smaller (less than 2 cm) lung cancer including both GGO and solid appearance is a great concern. The definitive answer to this crucial question is only given by the controlled randomized, phase III trial (see Chapter 32). Although more than 1000 patients need to be enrolled in such studies for enough statistical power, the results might revise the standard surgical care for tumors without nodal involvement. Such studies are already open in North America or will be launched very soon in Japan.

REFERENCES

1. Henschke CI, McCauley DI, Yankelvitz DF, et al. Early lung cancer action project: overall design and findings from baseline screening. *Lancet* 1999;354:99–105.
2. Sone S, Takashima S, Li F, et al. Mass screening for lung cancer with mobile spiral computed tomography scanner. *Lancet* 1998;351:1242–1245.
3. Yankelevitz DF, Henschke CI. Small solitary pulmonary nodules. *Radiol Clin North Am* 2000;38:471–478.
4. Adler B, Padley S, Miller RR, et al. High-resolution CT of bronchioloalveolar carcinoma. *AJR Am J Roentgenol* 1992;159:275-277.
5. Travis WD, Colby TV, Corrin B, et al. *Histological Typing of Lung and Pleural Tumors. World Health Organization International Histological Classification of Tumors*. Berlin: Springer, 1999.
6. Aoki T, Tomoda Y, Watanabe H, et al. Peripheral lung adenocarcinoma: correlation of thin-section CT findings with histologic prognostic factors and survival. *Radiology* 2001;220:803–809.
7. Kodama K, Higashiyama M, Yokouchi H, et al. Prognostic value of ground-glass opacity found in small lung adenocarcinoma on high-resolution CT scanning. *Lung Cancer* 2001;33:17–25.
8. Takamochi K, Nagai K, Yoshida J, et al. Pathologic N0 status in pulmonary adenocarcinoma is predictable by combining serum carcinoembryonic antigen level and computed tomographic findings. *J Thorac Cardiovasc Surg* 2001;122:325–330.
9. Asamura H, Suzuki K, Matsuno Y, et al. A clinicopathological study of resected subcentimeter lung cancers: a favorable prognosis for ground-glass opacity (GGO) lesions. *Ann Thorac Surg* 2003;76:1016–1022.
10. Suzuki K, Asamura H, Kusumoto M, et al. “Early” peripheral lung cancer: prognostic significance of ground glass opacity on thin-section computed tomographic scan. *Ann Thorac Surg* 2002;74:1635–1639.
11. Sakurai H, Maeshima A, Watanabe S, et al. Grade of stromal invasion in small adenocarcinoma of the lung: histopathological minimal invasion and prognosis. *Am J Surg Pathol* 2004;28:198–206.
12. Lung Cancer Study Group, Ginsberg RJ, Rubinstein LV. Randomized trial of lobectomy versus limited resection for T1N0 non-small cell lung cancer. *Ann Thorac Surg* 1995;60:615–623.
13. Carcoforo P, Sortini D, Pozza E, et al. Necessity of needle wire localization during video assisted thoracic surgery for patients with solitary pulmonary nodule. *Eur J Cardiothorac Surg* 2004;26:233–234.
14. Gonfiotti A, Davini F, Vaggelli L, et al. Thoracoscopic localization techniques for patients with solitary pulmonary nodule: hookwire versus radio-guided surgery. *Eur J Cardiothorac Surg* 2007;32:843–847.
15. Lenglinger FX, Schwarz CD, Artmann W. Localization of pulmonary nodules before thoracoscopic surgery: value of percutaneous staining with methylene blue. *AJR Am J Roentgenol* 1994;163:297–300.
16. Grogan EL, Jones DR, Kozower BD, et al. Identification of small lung nodules: technique of radiotracer-guided thoracoscopic biopsy. *Ann Thorac Surg* 2008;85:S772–S777.
17. Powell TI, Jangra D, Clifton JC, et al. Peripheral lung nodules: fluoroscopically guided video-assisted thoracoscopic resection after computed tomography-guided localization using platinum microcoils. *Ann Surg* 2004;240:481–488.
18. Tsuchida M, Yamato Y, Aoki T, et al. CT-guided agar marking for localization of nonpalpable peripheral pulmonary lesions. *Chest* 1999;116:139–143.

CHAPTER 34

Matthew Steliga
Ashish Patel
Ara Vaporciyan

Management of Stage II Non–Small Cell Lung Cancer and Pancoast Tumors

STAGE II TUMORS

Lung cancer remains the single most deadly cancer in the United States with an incidence of 170,000 per year and a 5-year overall mortality of 84%. This poor prognosis is secondary to the fact that most patients are diagnosed at higher stage (III and IV) on presentation.[1,2] The best chance for cure is provided by surgical resection of early stage (stage I and II) non–small cell lung cancer (NSCLC). This chapter focuses on surgical management of stage II NSCLC. The treatment, and even the definition, of stage II lung cancer have undergone significant changes over the last decade. Data examining the role of chemotherapy have expanded treatment options for patients with stage II NSCLC through adjuvant and neoadjuvant regimens. Although surgical therapy still remains the mainstay of therapy, a complete understanding of the role of multimodality therapy is crucial in the management of stage II NSCLC.

This chapter will first review the definition of stage II NSCLC along with the proposed modifications to the staging system. The presentation, diagnosis, and staging of stage II lung cancers will be reviewed followed by a discussion of the surgical treatment. Pancoast tumors without nodal involvement, a distinct subgroup of stage II NSCLC, will be discussed separately secondary to their unique presentation and treatment approach.

TNM CLASSIFICATION

The TNM classification for lung cancer, developed by Dr. Clifford Mountain in 1972, has been revised once in 1997. More recently, an international effort organized through the International Association for the Study of Lung Cancer (IASLC) has led to a further revision outlined in greater detail earlier in this book.

Stage II NSCLC is currently defined as tumors confined to the lung or obstructing a bronchus >2 cm distal from the carina (T1 to T2) with involvement of nodes within the ipsilateral visceral pleura (N1). Stage II also includes tumors adherent to surrounding structures such as chest wall, mediastinal pleura, diaphragm, or pericardium (T3) without nodal involvement (N0).[1,3] Stage II, therefore, includes T1N1, T2N1, and T3N0 tumors.

The new proposed system for stage II NSCLC will include T1a, T1b, and T2a lesions with N1 disease or T2b or T3 lesions without nodal involvement (N0). T1a are tumors <2 cm, T1b are tumors 2 to 3 cm in size, T2a lesions are 3 to 5 cm in size, and T2b lesions are tumors 5 to 7 cm in size. The term T3 will not only refer to tumors causing postobstructive lung collapse and/or tumors invading the surrounding structures, but will also involve intraparenchymal lesions greater than 7 cm in size or tumors with satellite nodules in the same lobe of the lung (prior T4). N1 definition will remain as nodes within the ipsilateral visceral pleura (stations 10 to 14.)[1–3] Thus, large tumors (>7 cm) with negative nodes, previously stage I, will now be considered stage II. Tumors with satellite nodules, which were previously considered T4N0 and therefore stage IIIB, will now be considered T3N0 stage IIB.

These changes to the stage groupings and the T descriptors will clearly have an impact on which patients are now considered resectable. In a recent validation, Kassis et al.[3] studied the impact of the new staging system on 1154 pathologically staged patients. Stage assignments changed in a total of 202 patients (17.5%) using the new proposed system, (79 patients [6.3%] upstaged and 129 [11.2%] downstaged). However, it is important to note that no patient was upstaged into a nonsurgical stage (i.e., stage IIIB or IV). Downstaging from a traditionally nonsurgical stage to a surgical stage occurred in 59 patients previously staged IIIB and in 2 patients who had been staged IV. What remains to be determined, however, is what the impact of this redistribution of patients will be on recent adjuvant chemotherapy data. The recent studies demonstrating adjuvant chemotherapies' effectiveness was performed on stage I to IIIA patients staged using the prior systems. Whether this new system alters those results is yet to be seen.

EVALUATION AND STAGING

Clinical Presentation Risk factors for lung cancer include age, history of smoking, and history of lung cancer. Of the 170,000 new patients with lung cancer diagnosed each year in the United States, 90% are older than age 45, and 85% have a history of smoking.[1] When present, clinical symptoms of lung cancer include cough, weight loss, dyspnea, hemoptysis, chest pain, and hoarseness in decreasing order.[1,2,4] There is limited data regarding symptoms at presentation of a clinical stage II lung cancer. Therefore, we reviewed our prospective database at the MD Anderson Cancer Center, and found 280 clinical stage II patients over the last 7 years. Symptoms were reported in 69.6% of patients at presentation. The most common symptom for the entire group was cough. For those with T3N0 caused by chest wall invasion, chest wall pain was a very common symptom. The remaining patients presented with an incidental finding of a lung lesion on chest radiograph or a computed tomography (CT) scan.

Imaging Earlier chapters have addressed imaging in lung cancer (see Chapters 26 and 27), but some specific aspects of imaging related to stage II lung cancer are discussed here.

Chest radiograph has traditionally been the modality of choice for screening and evaluating lung cancer. The advantages of chest radiographs include widespread availability, low-radiation dose, and low cost. The disadvantages include low sensitivity and specificity, especially for small tumors. The role of chest radiographs in stage II lung cancer is confined to excluding more advanced stage through identification of a pleural effusion or an extrathoracic bony metastasis.

During the past 20 years, development of the CT technology has made CT scans of the chest a standard of care in the evaluation of lung cancer. Patients with suspected lung cancer should receive CT scan of the chest with inclusion of the liver and adrenals. The latest versions of high-resolution CT scanners provide 1.2-mm thick slice capabilities, and this resolution improves almost yearly. These scans carry a sensitivity of 98%, a specificity of 58%, and an accuracy of 77% in the diagnosis of lung cancer.[1] Specifically with regard to stage II lung cancer, CT scans can assess both the nodal and tumor status of a lesion. The T status including size, ipsilateral/ipsilobar satellite lesions (now considered T3 based on the IASLC staging recommendations), involvement of central lobar structures, and proximity to the carina are easily assessed by CT imaging. However, for the latter two, bronchoscopy remains the gold standard to confirm the lobar involvement and the distance from the carina to the tumor. Pleural and chest wall involvement, distinguishing characteristics of T2 and T3 tumors, respectively, are also addressed by CT scanning. CT scans have an 80% sensitivity and specificity at predicting chest wall involvement using established criteria such as obliteration of the extrapleural fat plane, length of tumor–pleura contact, high ratio of contact length to tumor diameter, and obviously, rib destruction. However, when these criteria are absent and the patient has no symptoms consistent with chest wall involvement (constant or episodic pleuritic chest pain), surgery remains the gold standard approach for elucidating chest wall involvement. If the presence of chest wall involvement is a significant factor to determine respectability (e.g., a patient with marginal performance status and limited cardiopulmonary reserve), a thoracoscopy may be necessary to establish chest wall involvement.

Hilar nodal involvement (N1 disease), a hallmark of most stage II patients, is also assessed by CT scanning although its accuracy is limited. In the absence of significant N1 nodal enlargement, many stage II lung cancers will be difficult to distinguish from stage I lung cancer based on CT alone. Several studies have evaluated CT criteria for predicting lymph node involvement. These studies have focused on the predictive ability of CT for N2 disease (mediastinal nodal involvement) and have a pooled positive predictive value of 0.56.[4] Extrapolating from this data, one can estimate that a solitary peripheral lung cancer can carry 26% to 44% risk of lymph node involvement (hilar or mediastinal), despite a negative CT scan for nodal enlargement.[1] Data specifically assessing the diagnosis of N1 (hilar) disease is limited, because preoperative determination of N1 disease has limited clinical relevance. Currently, both stage I and II patients are offered surgical resection, and it is only the preoperative identification of N2 (mediastinal) disease that alters treatment. For this reason, most investigators have not addressed the diagnosis of N1 disease specifically. However, if appropriate application of lung sparing techniques, such as stereotactic radiotherapy, radiofrequency ablation, and cryoknife are to be made, then accurate information on the presence or absence of N1 disease will be mandatory to prevent early recurrence within the hilum.

Positron emission tomography (PET) and PET/CT scans have been the latest addition in the armamentarium for the evaluation and staging of lung cancer. PET scans are excellent at discerning metastatic disease; however, their poor spatial resolution makes evaluation of nodal disease less than optimal. Similarly, this poor spatial resolution limits PET's contribution to the evaluation of the T status. PET/CT has greatly improved the spatial resolution of the PET scan and thus improved the nodal evaluation of the test, although T status is still best evaluated by CT scanning. Where PET/CT scanning excels is in its negative predictive value. A negative CT and PET scan of the mediastinum has a high sensitivity. A recent study by Cerfolio et al.[5] addressed this issue, where 129 consecutive patients with NSCLC underwent PET and integrated PET/CT. Patients then underwent mediastinal node biopsy, and if negative, went on to pulmonary resection. Their study reported a negative predictive value of 99% for N2 nodal disease. Their positive predictive value was only 49%; however, the positive predictive value is hampered by endemic chronic inflammatory conditions (i.e., histoplasmosis) and acute inflammatory processes (i.e., postobstructive pneumonia secondary to a central lobar tumor). For this reason, PET or PET/CT positive N1 or N2 lymph nodes that are accessible should be biopsied to confirm their involvement, especially when the node is normal or only slightly enlarged on CT imaging.

Bronchoscopy Bronchoscopy, as indicated previously, has a prominent role in stage II disease. As mentioned earlier, it remains the gold standard for evaluation of lobar involvement and proximity to the carina. The treating surgeon should perform the bronchoscopy or be present when it is performed. This is especially true of central lobar T2 lesions that may require a sleeve resection. In this case, accurate assessment of the airway anatomy by the operating surgeon is required to assist with surgical planning.

Mediastinoscopy Evaluation of the mediastinum in stage II lung cancer is paramount. Although imaging has provided significant advances in noninvasive staging, there still remains a significant role for direct biopsy. Mediastinoscopy and its ability to assess mediastinal nodes are discussed in detail in Chapter 29. It remains a vital component in the evaluation of stage II disease. The obvious benefits of assessing ipsilateral and contralateral mediastinal nodes are well established. Many stage II tumors already involve hilar nodes and microscopic nodal involvement in the mediastinum can easily escape detection by imaging. However, an additional benefit of mediastinoscopy is its ability to assess the degree of mediastinal involvement. Mediastinal invasion by central tumors abutting the trachea or the proximal pulmonary artery can be difficult to assess by radiographic imaging. Mediastinoscopy is perfectly suited to evaluate this aspect of a tumor distinguishing a T4 tumor from a T3 or lesser tumor. However, mediastinoscopy, performed in this setting, can lead to scarring and distortion of normal-tissue planes. Although this degree of scarring is limited, it can increase the difficulty of subsequent planned complex resections such as a sleeve resection. If a sleeve resection or central dissection is anticipated, then the mediastinoscopy should be performed concurrently or within 2 to 3 days of the resection.

Endobronchial Ultrasound and Esophageal Ultrasound Similar to mediastinoscopy, endobronchial ultrasound (EBUS) allows sampling of mediastinal nodes for pathologic evaluation. Unlike mediastinoscopy, EBUS is less invasive and allows some hilar (level 10) nodes to be assessed. Esophageal ultrasound (EUS) coupled with transesophageal fine-needle aspiration (FNA) has the capability of reaching paraesophageal and inferior pulmonary ligament nodes (levels 8 and 9) as well as some of the nodes reached by EBUS (levels 7 and less frequently level 4). When combined, these two complimentary procedures have the capability of sampling seven nodal stations[2,4,6–10] versus only four stations with mediastinoscopy.[2,4,6,11] Discussed in Chapter 29, EBUS is quickly becoming a powerful tool in the evaluation of patients with lung cancer. Its high specificity has been consistently reported, but its sensitivity, especially compared with mediastinoscopy, is still debated. The high resolution of some EBUS and EUS probes can even supplant the evaluation of mediastinal invasion performed by mediastinoscopy.

The complete evaluation of mediastinal nodal involvement and assessment of mediastinal invasion has a clear impact on the subsequent treatment of a lung cancer. Until recently, the preoperative identification of hilar nodal involvement had fewer treatment-related consequences. When the treatment of stage I or II lung cancers were confined to lobectomy or conventional radiation, the preoperative determination of N1 nodal disease was of prognostic value only. However, the use of lobectomy as the sole treatment of subcentimeter node negative peripheral tumors is no longer the sole modality offered. Lung sparing techniques including stereotactic radiotherapy, percutaneous treatments such as radiofrequency ablation, or techniques such as wedge resections or segmentectomies (see also Chapters 32, 37, and 43), may be appropriate options. In these cases, preoperative identification of N1 involvement will play a significant role in treatment decisions. Similarly, the use of neoadjuvant chemotherapy, although currently not extensively utilized for early stage lung cancer, may be an option in the future. Again, pretreatment identification of N1 disease may be paramount in making these treatment-related decisions. The role of EBUS and EUS will undoubtedly increase in the evaluation and confirmation of stage II lung cancer.

All patients with stage II NSCLC without signs of metastatic disease should be evaluated for surgery. Exercise testing and preoperative evaluation of the patient with lung cancer is applicable to patients with stage II disease. Considerations that are specific for stage II disease stem from the frequently central location of some of these tumors. The involvement of a lobar bronchus by either the primary tumor (T2) or a hilar lymph node (N1) is encountered in stage II disease. These tumors can be approached by a sleeve resection rather than a pneumonectomy, and this should be considered when calculating the postoperative pulmonary reserve. In addition, the distal collapse caused by large >7-cm tumors (T3) or the lobar obstruction requires a split perfusion scan to be performed when calculating the postoperative pulmonary reserve. Additional considerations applicable to Pancoast tumors are discussed later in this chapter.

SURGICAL TREATMENT

Surgical Approach Possible approaches include an open thoracotomy or a minimally invasive approach. The open thoracotomy remains the dominant approach for stage II disease, and it can include various methods. These include the posterolateral thoracotomy with division of the latissimus muscle and ± the serratus muscle. Muscle-sparing techniques are also quite common and include a posterior, anterior, or axillary approach. In rare cases a sternotomy, a hemiclamshell incision can also be utilized. These incisions are useful for centrally placed tumors that abut the anterior mediastinum.

The minimally invasive approaches have included several approaches that are nothing more than an open thoracotomy with an additional port for the thoracoscope to a completely thoracoscopic procedure. The definition most widely accepted for minimally invasive pulmonary resection was outlined in the feasibility trial of video-assisted thoracic surgery (VATS) lobectomy (Cancer and Leukemia Group B [CALGB] 39802).[12] The study mandated no rib spreading; a maximum length of

8 cm of the access incision for removal of the lobectomy specimen; individual dissection of the vein, arteries, and airway for the lobe in question; and standard node sampling or dissection (identical to an open thoracotomy). All specimens were placed in an impermeable bag and removed through the access incision. Although other approaches and techniques that have been reported included minimal rib spreading and hilar ligation, the authors agree with the intergroup investigators in maintaining a rigorous adherence to the principles utilized in an open thoracotomy.

The use of a VATS lobectomy in stage II disease may be limited by the tumor size. To effectively remove a tumor without rib spreading, most authors feel that the primary must be less than 5 to 6 cm in greatest diameter. Of course, flat tumors larger than 6 cm can be removed if the specimen is appropriately oriented in the impermeable bag. Additional concerns about a VATS approach in stage II disease center on the dissection of enlarged hilar nodes. Although lymph node dissection via a VATS approach has been shown to be very effective,[13] the intergroup investigators did comment on factors that required conversion to an open procedure. In 25% of the case (4 of 12), conversion was secondary to the difficulty dissecting lymph nodes from the vascular structures. Although this is not an absolute contraindication for a VATS approach, the surgeon should consider the size of the hilar nodes, the presence of calcifications or scarring from prior induction therapy, and the technical experience with a VATS approach.

Open Thoracotomy Although there are several types of open thoracotomy, the most commonly employed versions include a posterolateral thoracotomy, a posterior muscle-sparing thoracotomy, and perhaps an axillary thoracotomy. All are performed with the patient in a lateral decubitus position. Attention to the method of pain control should also be given with the most common approach being a thoracic epidural. Local delivery of analgesics with a self-contained pump and catheter positioned in the extrapleural space are also gaining acceptance.

Although each has slight advantages and disadvantages when compared with one another, they are all appropriate for resection of most stage II lung cancers. The posterolateral thoracotomy is the most commonly employed incision and is the gold standard with regard to hemithoracic exposure. Its primary drawback remains the pain associated with this large incision and the division of the latissimus dorsi muscle, which has implications in postoperative function and the muscle's availability as a rotational flap. The posterior muscle–sparing thoracotomy uses the posterior two thirds of the posterolateral thoracotomy incision and mobilizes the latissimus dorsi and serratus anterior muscle anteriorly. Although the incision is slightly smaller, almost all procedures performed via a posterolateral thoracotomy can be safely approached through this incision. Exceptions, although not absolute, include complex sleeve resections and chest wall resections. The preservation of the latissimus dorsi muscle (and perhaps the speed of closure) is its primary advantage. The axillary thoracotomy utilizes either a vertical incision in the low axilla aligned with the anterior border of the latissimus dorsi muscle or a transverse incision centered on the anterior border of the latissimus dorsi muscle. The fibers of the serratus anterior muscle are separated exposing the third or fourth intercostal space through which the thorax is entered. The entry through the lateral aspect of the chest wall, where the ribs are most mobile, allows for distraction of the ribs with the least force being applied to the costovertebral junction. The main disadvantage is the limited exposure of lower lobe lesions.

For stage II tumors, each of these approaches can be used at the discretion and comfort of the surgeon. Patients with significant hilar disease or central lesions requiring sleeve resections may be best approached through a larger posterolateral thoracotomy. The limitations of an axillary thoracotomy make this approach the least utilized incision.

Video-Assisted Thoracic Surgery In the past, the definition of a VATS resection has been variable in the literature. The range of definitions has included everything from a limited posterior muscle–sparing thoracotomy with thoracoscopic visualization, to a completely thoracoscopic approach without any rib spreading. Most thoracic surgeons today will agree that a true VATS resection should include absolutely no rib spreading, although the conduct of the resection should duplicate an open resection. The technical considerations for this approach have been discussed in detail previously in this text.

Although the effectiveness of this technique for early stage malignancies seems apparent, there are some concerns when applying the technique to stage II malignancies. Enlarged hilar N1 nodes, especially where there is concern of arterial or bronchial invasion, can magnify the technical complexity of a VATS resection. Although reports of VATS sleeve resections and pneumonectomies exist, these require advanced skills and will be adopted more slowly. A more practical limitation of the VATS technique in stage II malignancies is the size of the tumor that can be physically removed. Tumors larger than 5 to 6 cm cannot be removed through the utility thoracotomy without rib spreading. Correspondingly, these large tumors may limit visualization of and accessibility to the hilar structures increasing the technical complexity of the resection. Finally, the utility of combining a chest wall resection with VATS lobectomy may be questionable. Reports of chest wall resections accomplished by VATS do exist. However, the main advantage of a VATS resection, which is of rapid recovery of function, may be lost when coupled with a chest wall resection.

Extent of Resection Although some debate exists regarding the extent of resection for stage I tumors, the options are less contentious for stage II disease. The frequent involvement of hilar lymph nodes in stage II disease mandates a resection that encompasses the nodal basin of the tumor. Although the new staging system includes some tumors that are without nodal involvement (T2bN0 and T3N0), the large size of these tumors (greater than 5 cm) and their aggressive features (chest wall invasion and interlobar satellite lesions) would make lung-sparing techniques difficult or less advantageous. For these reasons, there is relatively uniform agreement that an anatomical lobectomy with complete hilar nodal dissection should be performed.

For the same reasons mentioned previously, most surgeons would also advocate a systematic mediastinal nodal dissection rather than a nodal sampling. However, definitive data demonstrating an advantage from complete nodal dissection on survival has yet to be established. The ACOSOG Z0030 trial randomizing clinical stage I patients to systematic node dissection versus node sampling have not yet reported long-term results. The early results exhibited no difference in morbidity associated with the performance of a systematic node dissection.[14] Mediastinal nodal involvement was identified in 3.8% of clinical stage I patients. Considering the higher likelihood of occult N2 disease in clinical stage II patients and the lack of evidence for increased morbidity associated with complete lymph node dissection, we would endorse complete lymph node dissection in all stage II patients.

Pneumonectomy Pneumonectomy, or the complete removal of an entire lung, entails the division of the ipsilateral main pulmonary artery, both pulmonary veins and the mainstem bronchus. Ipsilateral hilar nodes are removed en bloc with the lung, and the mediastinal lymph nodes are removed as part of a systematic nodal sampling or dissection. A conventional pneumonectomy implies division of the vessels within the thoracic cavity. An intrapericardial pneumonectomy entails entry into the pericardium for division of any of the pulmonary vessels.

The definition of stage II disease includes several features that can require a pneumonectomy for complete resection. The most common is hilar nodal disease with concomitant invasion of the mainstem bronchus or the proximal pulmonary artery. This is especially true when the primary tumor resides in the lower lobes and the nodal disease involves the upper lobe bronchi or vasculature. Other reasons are large tumors (>7-cm tumors now classified as T3) that cross the fissure and involve the upper and lower lobes or tumors that obstruct the mainstem bronchus not amenable to a sleeve resection.

Bilobectomy As the name implies, a bilobectomy is the removal of two lobes and can only be performed on the right lung. The indication for such a procedure is a large tumor that extends across the fissure to involve a substantial portion of an adjacent lobe. Additionally, hilar nodal disease that invades the central bronchi of two lobes can also necessitate bilobectomy. The later indication is not uncommonly seen in stage II disease.

Lobectomy The definition of a lobectomy is, as expected, the removal of the entire lobe of a lung. The vascular and bronchial branches are individually identified and ligated along with the resection of any hilar lymph nodes surrounding these branches. Intraparenchymal lymph nodes associated with the lobe are removed en bloc with the specimen. Similar to a pneumonectomy, the mediastinal lymph nodes are removed as part of a systematic nodal sampling or dissection.

Lobectomy is the most common procedure for stage II lung cancer. The frequent central location of the tumor or the associated hilar nodal disease necessitates resection of the entire lobe. Even if the hilar nodal disease can be resected without sacrificing the lobar structures, most thoracic surgeons would not advocate a wedge or segmental resection of the primary tumor. A lobectomy should be performed to remove the entire nodal draining basin.

Wedges or Segmental Resection These techniques resect a portion of lung surrounding the lesion or a segment of the lung. Segments are anatomically distinct with 10 named segments in the right lung and 8 in the left lung. These segments have a discrete arterial, venous, and bronchial anatomy, and a true segmentectomy would involve their isolation and division similar to a lobectomy.

As discussed earlier, these lung-sparing techniques are not frequently an option in stage II disease. The need to resect the hilar lymph nodes and their parenchymal nodal basin usually necessitates a lobectomy at the least. However, in some cases, such as a chest wall lesion without nodal disease (T3N0), one of these lung-sparing techniques can be used especially in patients with marginal pulmonary function.

Sleeve Resections Sleeve resection, also referred to as bronchoplastic procedures, are techniques that preserve normal lung tissue when the lesions are small but located at or near the main bronchi. The technique involves resection of a portion of the main bronchus followed by an end-to-end anastomosis to preserve the lung tissue distal to the resection. Examples are shown in Figure 34.1.[15] In stage II disease, common indications for sleeve resection are involved hilar nodes that invades the origin of the lobar bronchus or small central tumors within 2 cm of the carina without lymph node involvement (T3N0). Although these tumors can also be resected with a pneumonectomy, there is clear data that the morbidity and mortality following a sleeve resection is less than a pneumonectomy. The added oncologic benefit of a pneumonectomy has not been clearly demonstrated.

Chest Wall Resections Isolated chest wall involvement outside of the superior sulcus is also encountered in lung cancer. In the current staging system, a chest wall lesion without lymph node involvement is considered stage II disease, in the proposed changes to the staging system a T3 tumor with hilar nodal disease (N1) will also be considered stage II. Both of these tumors could be offered surgical resection. The goal of resection is an en bloc anatomical resection. Most investigators have identified completeness of resection as a prognostic factor in long-term survival.[16–18] The depth of invasion seems to be less predictive of survival.

There are areas of controversy that exist regarding the treatment of lung cancer invading the chest wall. The first is the use of an extrapleural dissection for tumors limited to parietal pleural involvement. Several publications have decried the use of this technique reporting worse outcomes.[19,20] Although the series from Memorial Sloan Kettering[21] failed to demonstrate a difference, the authors stated that patients with any suspicion of parietal pleural involvement were addressed with

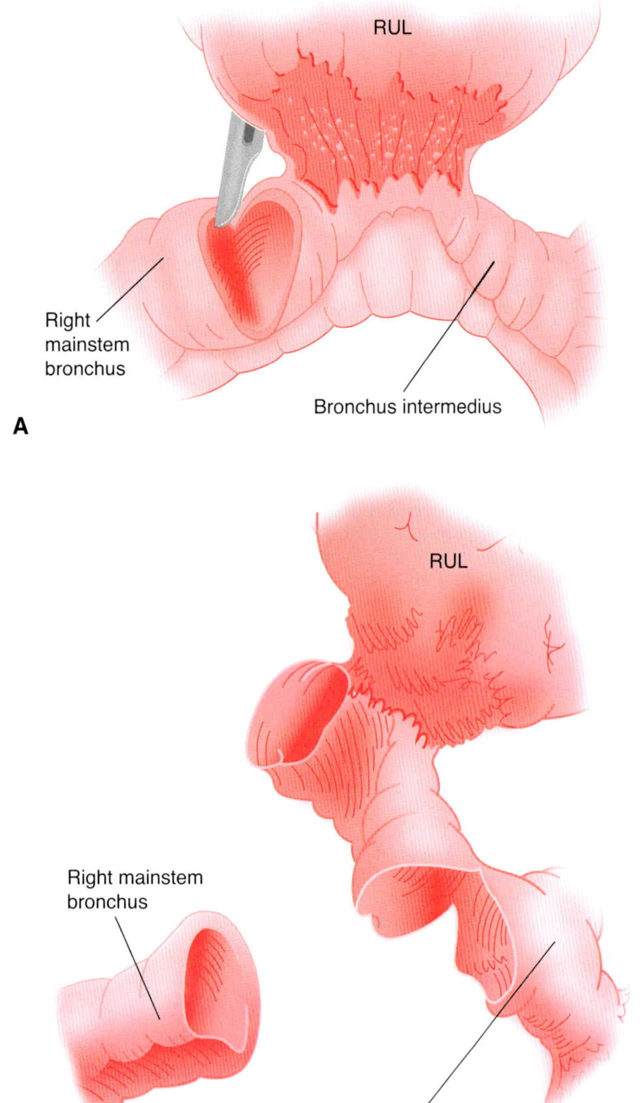

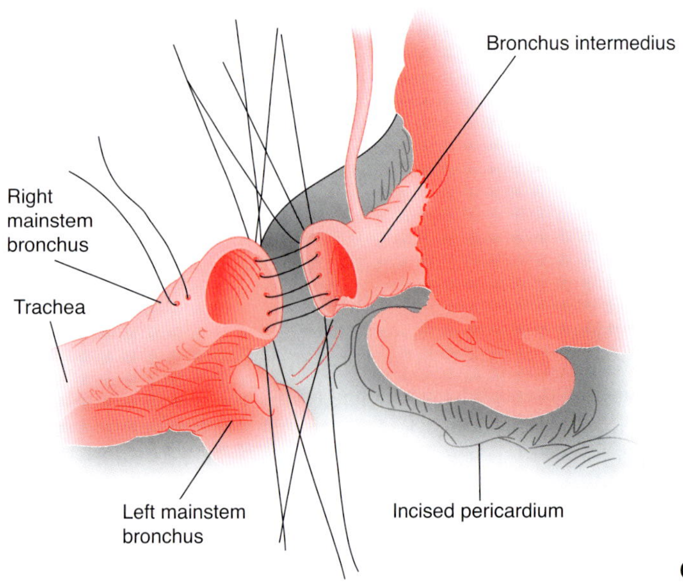

FIGURE 34.1 Sleeve resection involves resection of a segment of the airway with anastomosis of the more distal bronchus to the more proximal bronchus, allowing noninvolved distal lung parenchyma to be spared from resection. Shown here is a right upper lobe (RUL) tumor involving the proximal aspect of the right upper lobe bronchus. **A:** The right mainstem bronchus is divided proximal to the origin of the right upper lobe bronchus and the tumor. **B:** The bronchus intermedius is now divided distal to the right upper lobe bronchus allowing the tumor and the right upper lobe to be removed. **C:** The bronchial anastomosis is constructed. (From Nesbitt JC, Wind GG. Thoracic Surgical Oncology: Exposures and Techniques. Philadelphia, PA: Lippincott Williams and Wilkins, 2003:58–60.)

a chest wall resection. Extrapleural resection was reserved only for those with filmy inflammatory adhesions to the chest.

A second area of controversy surrounds the impact of nodal disease. Most series have shown a significant decrease in survival with increasing nodal involvement.[22–25] Evidence of N2 disease should be aggressively sought during evaluation of these patients. Identification of N2 or N1 disease may prompt the use of induction chemotherapy followed by resection for patients with a favorable response. However, data regarding the advantage of this approach, outside Pancoast tumors, do not exist.

Other controversies center on the use of radiation therapy after a complete resection and the extent of the pulmonary resection. Neither of these issues has been addressed with a randomized study, and an attempt at addressing the former question by the North American Lung Cancer Study group during the 1980s was closed for poor accrual. Our approach has been to not offer adjuvant radiation therapy for completely resected chest wall lesions. Positive margins are offered radiation therapy if the area of positivity is clearly delineated. Wedge or segmental resections are avoided with a preference for a lobectomy unless comorbidities or pulmonary function dictates a lesser resection.

Mediastinal Lymph Node Dissection Mediastinal lymph node dissection in the right chest includes dissecting and removing all visible nodes at level 2R, 4R, 7, and 9R position. Left chest mediastinal lymph node dissection involves removing all nodes at level 5, 6, 7, and 9L position. Levels 10 to 14 nodes of the corresponding lobe should have been removed with the specimen. Care should be taken to avoid injury to the right phrenic and right recurrent laryngeal nerves during dissection of levels 2R and 4R and the left phrenic and left recurrent nerve during dissection of levels 5 and 6.

The preference of a complete dissection in stage II disease was discussed earlier. Data comparing a complete node dissection versus a systematic nodal sampling has been evaluated in a randomized setting, but these studies have had mixed results with regard to long-term oncologic benefit.[26,27] These trials were limited by small numbers of patients, but a recent trial sponsored by the American College of Surgeons Oncology Group is hoped to address this issue definitively. Early results demonstrate no additional morbidity, but long-term survival data are still pending.[28]

Adjuvant Therapy The role of adjuvant chemotherapy in the treatment of NSCLC is discussed in Chapter 45. For many decades, adjuvant chemotherapy, radiotherapy, or a combination was not offered for completely resected stage II lung cancer. Recent results generated from large multi-institutional and multinational trails have begun to identify early stage patients who do benefit from adjuvant chemotherapy. Stage II disease, specifically, has been identified in many of these studies as a favorable stage to receive therapy.

Follow-up Stage II NSCLC patients should be followed postoperatively for two reasons. First, long-term survival is only 30% to 40% even with the best available treatment. Majority of patients (90%) present with metastatic disease, whereas a few (10%) develop local recurrence. Those who develop local recurrence can be treated with additional radiation therapy for symptomatic control. Those who develop systemic disease can be helped with palliative treatment. Secondly, lung cancer is a risk factor for a second cancer. Thirty percent of patients with lung cancer develop a new malignancy. Patients with history of lung cancer also have 1% to 4% per year risk of developing a new primary lung cancer.[1] Thus, patients followed aggressively may benefit from detection of early new primary lung cancers.

The recommendations for follow-up include at least 6 months with the specialist providing care and then a systematic follow-up every 6 to 12 months. The focus should be on detecting metastatic disease within the first 2 years and then detecting any new malignancies subsequently.

PANCOAST TUMORS

In 1932, Henry Pancoast,[29] a radiologist from Philadelphia, addressed the American Medical Association describing for the first time what he termed a *superior pulmonary sulcus tumor* that was associated with Horner syndrome, rib destruction, and atrophy of the hand muscles. Although Hare[30] had first described this tumor in 1838, it was Pancoast's classic clinical presentation of pain of the eighth cervical or the first and second thoracic trunk distribution that has become known as Pancoast syndrome.

A Pancoast tumor is defined as a tumor arising in or near the apex of the lung, at or above the level of the second rib, with involvement of extrathoracic structures of the apical chest wall. The tumor originates peripherally and extends over the apex of the lung to involve the apical chest wall. This involvement can be seen by clinical and radiological evidence and can include the parietal pleura, lymphatics, endothoracic fascia, intercostal nerves, ribs, vertebral bodies, lower roots of the brachial plexus, the sympathetic chain (stellate ganglion), and subclavian vessels. The clinical triad of shoulder or arm pain, atrophy of the hand muscles, and Horner syndrome is the sine qua non of a Pancoast tumor. Lack of rib involvement accompanied by these symptoms is frequently included in the definition of a Pancoast tumor.[31]

An apical lung tumor with invasion of similar structures but without the symptom triad that defines a Pancoast tumor has been developed as a broader group termed a *superior sulcus tumor*. The anatomic definition of the superior sulcus of the chest has been debated with various definitions offered. Most seem to agree that the sulcus is the costovertebral gutter, and the superior sulcus is the uppermost extent of this.[32] These tumors may have some of the symptoms seen in a Pancoast tumor but are defined as an apical tumor with extension into the chest wall (the upper two or three ribs), the vertebral body, or the subclavian vessels.[31,33] Because the treatment of superior sulcus tumors and their narrower subgroup of Pancoast tumors are similar, most studies have evaluated all superior pulmonary sulcus tumors.

EVALUATION AND STAGING

Clinical Presentation and Diagnosis The incidence of superior sulcus tumors is uncommon, and it is estimated that only 5% of NSCLC will present in this manner. By definition, a Pancoast tumor includes shoulder or arm pain or paresthesias, Horner syndrome, and atrophy of the intrinsic muscles of the arm. However, as described previously, not all superior pulmonary sulcus tumors will present with a complete Pancoast syndrome. Therefore, patients with risk factors for lung cancer who present with any combination of these symptoms should be evaluated for an apical tumor. Although the history and physical exam can be suggestive, the diagnosis is commonly made after radiographic examination.

The chest radiograph is regrettably very uninformative in many cases with only a small homogenous apical cap or pleural thickening visible (see Fig. 34.2). With advanced tumors, chest radiographs can visualize bony destruction of ribs and vertebral bodies. Unfortunately, the low sensitivity of chest radiographs can lead to a delay in diagnosis. A high level of clinical suspicion on the part of the treating physician is necessary for diagnosis of these lesions. This is especially true for early and hence more treatable tumors.

CT scans are highly accurate at detecting apical abnormalities. An apical mass apparent on a CT scan in a patient with symptoms of a Pancoast tumor can be diagnostic but nonmalignant, and metastasis presenting with similar findings have been

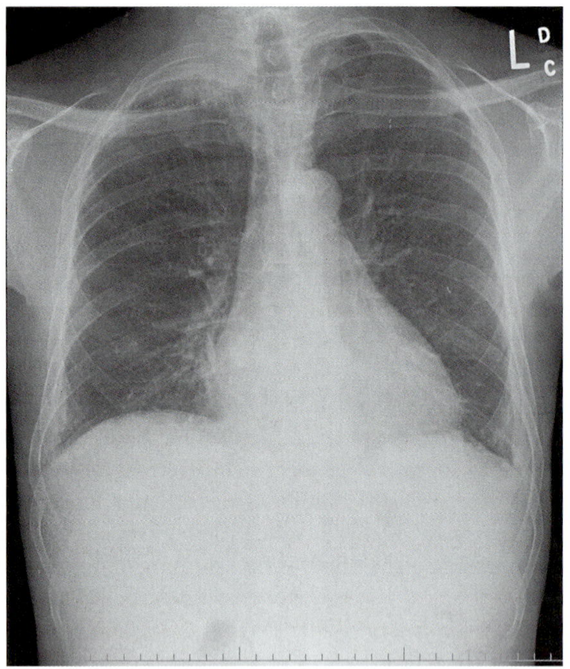

FIGURE 34.2 Posteroanterior (PA) chest radiograph of a patient with a right-sided Pancoast tumor with the apical cap on the right. This tumor invaded the subclavian artery and vein, as well as the T1 nerve root. This patient had classic symptoms consistent with Pancoast syndrome.

reported.[34–36] Therefore, the diagnosis should be confirmed by a biopsy. Transthoracic biopsies can be obtained without significant complications. The biopsy can also assist in staging. In patients without symptoms or radiographic evidence of chest wall invasion a transthoracic biopsy complicated by a small pneumothorax can differentiate an apical tumor without chest wall invasion from a true superior pulmonary sulcus tumor.

Staging Pancoast tumors are lung malignancies, and therefore, staged with the same TNM classification system. Because of the involvement of the chest wall, all Pancoast tumors are by definition at least stage IIB. If the proposed changes to the staging system take effect, there will be some shifting of stages IIIA and IIIB Pancoast tumors into the stage IIB category. These changes are primarily a result of changes in the TNM groupings (Table 34.1).

T Descriptors Inherent in the definition of a Pancoast tumor is chest wall involvement. Identification of any extension into nearby structures is paramount to establishing the T status of the tumor and, more importantly, determining its resectability. Although the new definitions of the T descriptors proposed by the IASLC may alter the staging of Pancoast tumors, most of these changes occur in the T1 and T2 descriptors. Their effect on Pancoast staging is negligible. The majority of the changes will express themselves as a shift of previously stage IIIA and IIIB tumors into earlier stages. Although these changes were established based on considerable data, there is some concern that applying these definitions to a Pancoast tumor will not yield similar results. Pancoast tumors with extension into the vertebral body (T4 extension) and any nodal disease have historically done very poorly.[37]

Although CT imaging is adequate for the initial evaluation of these tumors, determination of resectability requires greater resolution. Magnetic resonance imaging (MRI) has been the modality of choice for this anatomic region. Sagittal imaging allows better visualization of the brachial plexus and the subclavian vessels but additionally, evaluation for invasion of the vertebral body and the neural foramina is improved with MRI.[38,39] An MRI can help characterize C8 and T1 roots. Although the T1 nerve root can be sacrificed distal to its contribution to the brachial plexus with little impact on arm and hand function, preservation of the C8 nerve root is required for adequate hand function. Establishing their involvement is a key to the determination of resectability. In a study comparing CT with MRI, Heelan et al.[39] found CT scan to have a sensitivity of 60%, a specificity of 65%, and an accuracy of 63% in determining resectability. MRI was 88% sensitive, 100% specific, and 94% accurate. Thus, most centers today will obtain a CT and an MRI to best assess the local extension of the tumor (see Fig. 34.3). Improvements in CT resolution continue and CT coronal and sagittal reconstructions combined with refinements in CT imaging may eventually supersede MRI's role in the evaluation of these tumors.

TABLE 34.1 Proposed Stage Grouping Changes that Would Effect Pancoast Tumor Staging by the IASLC Staging System

Existing UICC Stage				Proposed IASLC Stage
Stage	T	N	M	
IIIB	T4 (same lobe nodule)	N0	M0	IIB
IIIB	T4 (same lobe nodule)	N1–N2	M0	IIIA
IIIB	T4 (extension)	N0–N1	M0	IIIA
IV	Any T	N0–N1	M1 (ipsilateral lung)	IIIA
IV	Any T	N2–N3	M1 (ipsilateral lung)	IIIB

IASLC, International Association for the Study of Lung Cancer; UICC, Union Internationale Contre le Cancer.

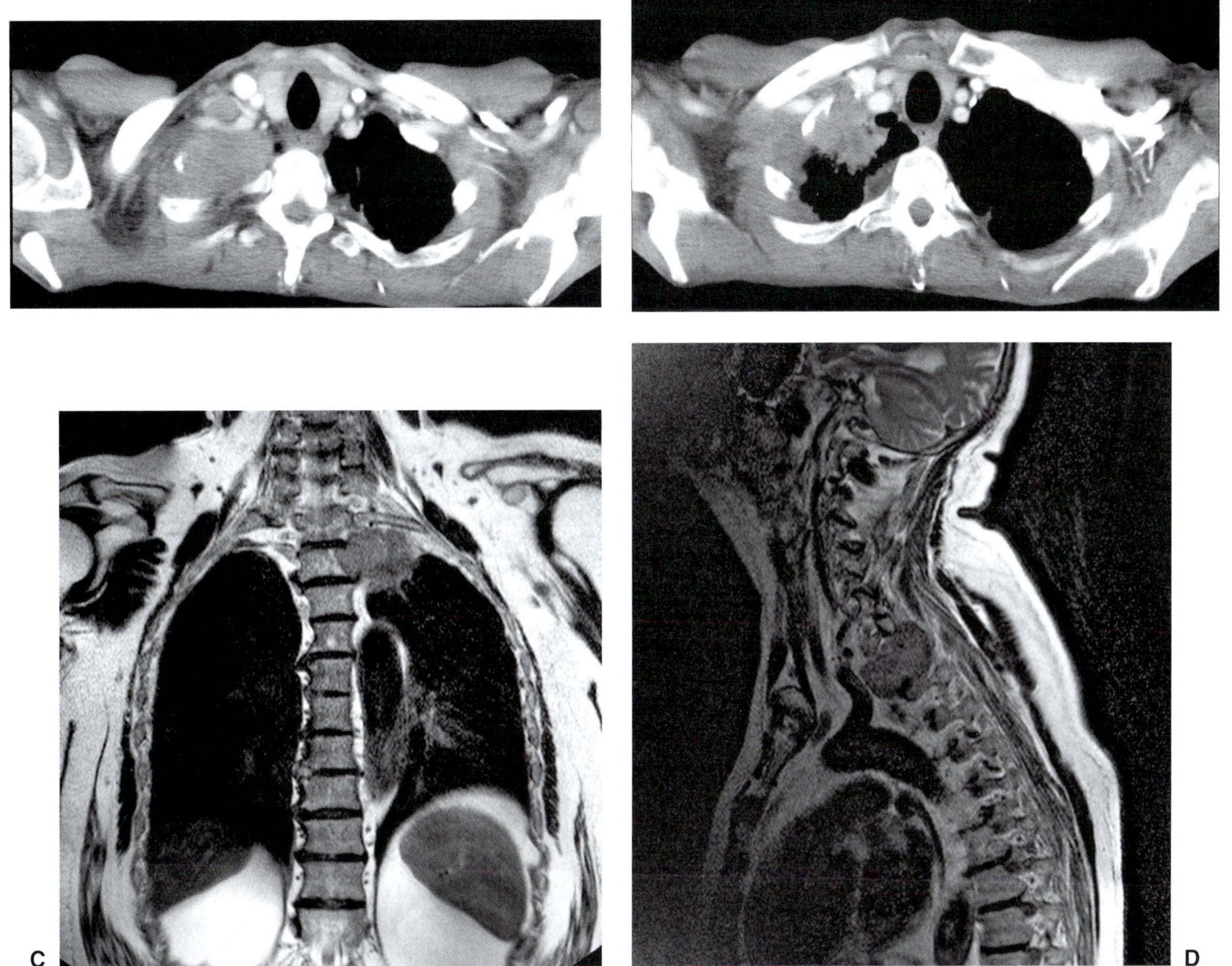

FIGURE 34.3 Pancoast tumor with direct extension to apical chest wall, abutting brachial plexus and involving subclavian vessels. **A,B:** The CT scans clearly show the abutment of the tumor and the subclavian vessels. MRI allows greater resolution of this region, however, and the multiplanar reconstructions are useful for preoperative assessment and evaluation of vascular structures as well as involvement of the brachial plexus. **C,D:** MRI images of a different patient whose tumor can be seen involving the T2 vertebral body on the coronal images. The sagittal image **(D)** demonstrates a clear plane between the tumor and the left subclavian artery.

N Descriptors Pancoast tumors with positive mediastinal nodes (N2 or N3) have a uniformly poor prognosis. Mediastinoscopy is required in all clinical trials and should be strongly considered when evaluating patients for surgery. The use of endoscopic bronchial ultrasound can also be considered in centers with sufficient experience in its use. An added advantage of EBUS is its ability to biopsy some hilar nodes, allowing tissue confirmation of N1 disease. In patients with suspicious scalene nodes, an ultrasound-guided FNA or a scalene node dissection is also strongly recommended.

M Descriptors PET/CT scanning is a powerful tool to assess for metastatic disease and should be performed during the evaluation of these patients. Any suspicious lesions should be confirmed with a biopsy of the region before finalizing the patient's stage. The brain and long bones, areas poorly visualized by conventional PET/CT should also be evaluated with a CT or MRI of the brain and a bone scan. Although the new IASLC staging system has downstaged ipsilateral lung lesions as T4 rather than M1, most would continue to approach Pancoast tumors and an ipsilateral lung lesion with trepidation.

Histology The origin of Pancoast tumor was uncertain in the early years. Pancoast believed these tumors originated from a brachial pouch, and it was not until 1932 that the pulmonary origin of these tumors was identified. Despite its peripheral position in the lung, many of these tumors were squamous cell histology; however, recent series have demonstrated an increase in the number of adenocarcinomas. The most recent published series from France reported nearly identical rates of each of these histologies and a large number of large cell histology as well. Only 3% to 5% of total Pancoast tumors are small cell carcinomas. Other rare etiologies include adenoid cystic carcinoma, hemangiopericytoma, and localized mesothelioma. Rarely, Pancoast syndrome has been reported in patients without pulmonary etiologies because of apical chest involvement by hematologic malignancies and infectious agents such as tuberculosis.[40]

MULTIMODALITY TREATMENT

There is no definitive or agreed-upon treatment strategy for Pancoast tumors. The treatment regimens have varied from radiotherapy, chemoradiotherapy, induction radiotherapy followed by surgical resection, induction chemotherapy with or without radiotherapy followed by resection, and surgical resection followed by adjuvant chemoradiotherapy.

Historically speaking, Pancoast tumors were considered universally fatal until the 1950s because of technical limitations of resection and lack of effective multimodality therapy. Chardack and MacCallum[41] reported the first successful resection of a Pancoast tumor in 1953. An en bloc lobectomy and chest wall resection was employed followed by adjuvant radiation therapy (65 Gy over 54 days). The patient died almost 6 years later and a postmortem revealed no evidence of malignancy.[42] In 1961, Shaw and colleagues [42a] treated their first in a series of 18 patients with superior sulcus tumors employing preoperative radiation therapy (30 to 35 Gy over 2 weeks) followed by en bloc surgery 4 to 6 weeks later. Although retrospective and a small series, the data demonstrated that high resectability with minimal morbidity could be achieved. The reported survival rate was also greater than expected leading to wide spread acceptance of this treatment approach. For the next 30 years, numerous investigators confirmed Shaw's findings and few alterations were made.[43]

This began to change approximately 2 decades ago as researchers around the globe began not only to expand the definition of resectability but also to address the systemic nature of the disease through multimodality therapy. The definition of resectability was initially confined to chest wall lesions with limited involvement of the spine (i.e., the transverse process). Improvements in surgical techniques and a multidisciplinary approach to surgical resection allowed resection of tumors involving the vascular structures of the thoracic inlet and the vertebral bodies. Dartevelle et al.[44] anterior transcervical approach was one such advance. This approach allowed safe access to the subclavian vessels and demonstrated that their resection could achieve comparable survival rates. Rapid acceptance of the anterior approach followed throughout the world. A similar extension of the definition of resectability occurred with the multidisciplinary approach to vertebral involvement. Advances in spine stabilization developed by neurosurgeons and orthopedic surgeons were applied to Pancoast tumors with surprisingly effective rates of local control.[45]

The addition of systemic therapy to the treatment regimen of Pancoast tumors was the next appropriate step considering the survival advantages seen with induction chemotherapy for stage IIIA NSCLC. The Southwest Oncology Group (SWOG 9416, INT 0160) was a phase II trial that addressed this in a prospective multi-institutional fashion. The induction regimen was similar to previous trials in stage IIIA disease and was known to be well tolerated and effective.[46] The initial results were reported in 2001[31] and updated in 2003.[47] Over 4 years, 111 patients were eligible for this trial with surgery performed by 26 surgeons throughout five cooperative groups. Seven patients did not complete their induction therapy as planned with three deaths (2.7%). A total of 87 patients were eventually registered for the surgical arm of the trial although four were not resected at the discretion of the individual investigators. The final number taken to surgery, 83, represented 75% of the 111 enrolled patients.

The next major development was the North American Southwest Oncology Group trial (9416) of induction chemoradiotherapy followed by resection, which has now become the most widely used approach for Pancoast tumors with survival ranging as high as 53%. One hundred ten patients with T3N0 to T4N0 disease received induction chemoradiotherapy with etoposide and cisplatin and 45 Gy radiation. Patients with resectable disease postinduction underwent thoracotomy. The 5-year survival was 41% for all patients and 53% for complete resection.

The morbidity of the induction regimen was well tolerated with only 18 patients suffering a reduction in their performance status. At restaging, there were 0%, 36%, and 41% complete, partial, and stable responses, respectively. Resection was performed with various anatomic resection, the most common being lobectomy and en bloc chest wall (67.5%). Interestingly, 12 patients (14%) had lung resection without chest wall resection. Although this may represent effective induction therapy, another consideration must be that these patients were clinically overstaged and were not true pathologic T3 tumors at the time of their registration. The morbidity and mortality of surgery was not substantially different from other series with two deaths (2.4%) and 10 pneumonias (12%), and a median hospital stay of 7 days.

The pathologic response was encouraging with 65% of patients demonstrating a complete pathologic response or only minimal microscopic disease. The individual frequencies of these two groups were evenly distributed between the two groups. Also apparent was the striking inaccuracy of the preoperative radiographic assessment of the response.

The overall survival in this initial report with a median follow up of 21 months was 55% at 2 years. In the group who enjoyed a complete pathologic response, the 2-year survival was 70% (Fig. 34.4).[48] At the time of the initial report, there was no statistically significant prognostic factor evident, the

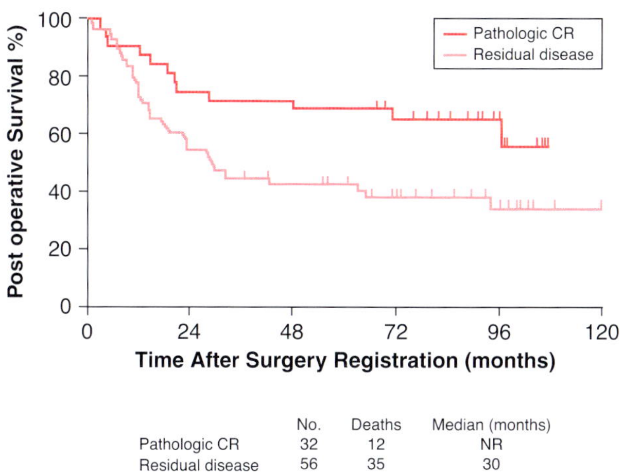

	No.	Deaths	Median (months)
Pathologic CR	32	12	NR
Residual disease	56	35	30

$P = .02$

FIGURE 34.4 Results of the SWOG trial 9416 comparing patients with pathologic complete response and patients with residual disease at final pathology. *CR*, complete response; *NR*, no record. (From Rusch VW, Giroux DJ, Kraut MJ, et al. Induction chemoradiation and surgical resection for superior sulcus non-small-cell lung carcinomas: long-term results of Southwest Oncology Group trial 9416 [Intergroup trial 0160]. *J Clin Oncol* 2007;25:313–318.)

updated results in 2003 demonstrated that the pathological response, but not tumor stage, predicted the overall survival. Updated survival data demonstrated 5-year survivals of 41% overall and 53% in the complete pathologic response group.

Since its publication, two additional small studies have supported the findings of this trial.[49] Clearly, their results demonstrate the feasibility of induction chemoradiotherapy for this challenging group of patients. These data will also serve as a benchmark for future studies. It is clear that multimodality must play an integral part in the treatment of these tumors. Although the overall survival has been enhanced and the size of the patient population offered treatment with curative intent, expanded surgery remains the basis of any meaningful approach to Pancoast tumors.

SURGICAL TREATMENT

Surgical Approach

Posterior Approach This approach was utilized in the initial reports of successful resection of Pancoast tumors and has remained the mainstay in exposing most Pancoast tumors. The patient is positioned in a lateral decubitus position with careful attention to expose the base of the cervical spine and support the head. A posterolateral thoracotomy incision is performed and based on the position of the tumor, a safe interspace is chosen to enter the thorax. Exploration is performed to confirm resectability. The incision is then extended posteriorly and superiorly between the medial border of the scapula and the spine up to the seventh cervical vertebra (Fig. 34.5). After division of the trapezius and rhomboid muscles, the scapula can be elevated away from the chest wall allowing visualization up to the first rib. Retraction can be achieved with one arm of the rib spreader, an internal mammary retractor, or a customizable frame mechanical retractor such as the Thompson retractor (Fig. 34.6).

The scalene muscles can now be divided exposing the upper border of the first rib and the subclavian vessels. Involvement of these vessels can be assessed as well as the superior extent of

FIGURE 34.5 The posterior approach to Pancoast tumors is an extension of the standard posterolateral thoracotomy incision with division of the latissimus, trapezius, and rhomboid muscles, permitting access to the apex of the chest. The planned incision begins the base of the neck posteriorly, extends between the scapula and the spine, and curves beneath the scapula to extend across the lateral chest wall similar to a standard posterolateral thoracotomy. (From Nesbitt JC, Wind GG. Thoracic Surgical Oncology: Exposures and Techniques. Philadelphia, PA: Lippincott Williams and Wilkins, 2003:164.)

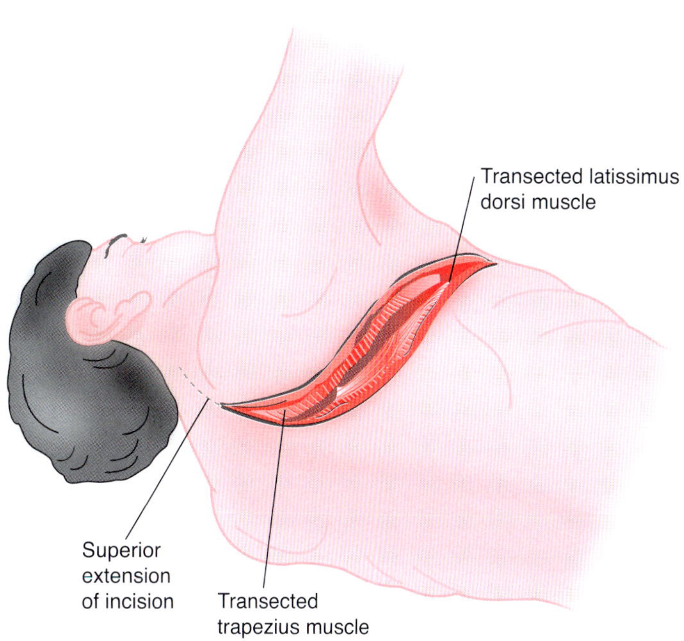

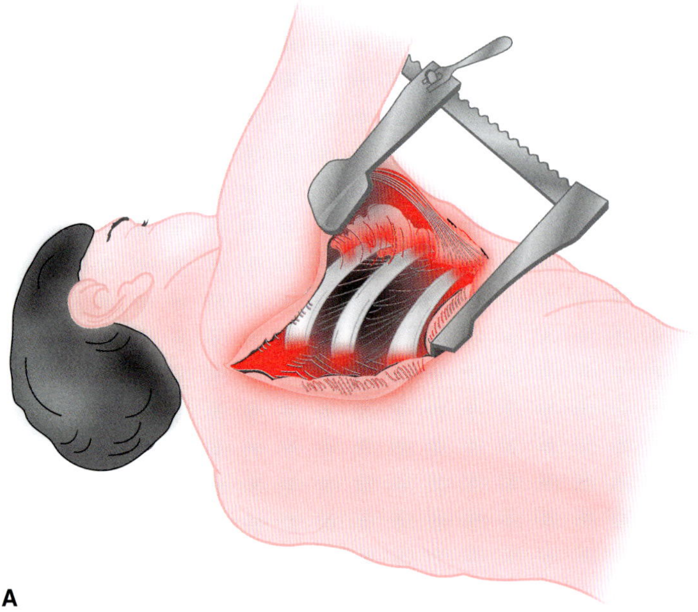

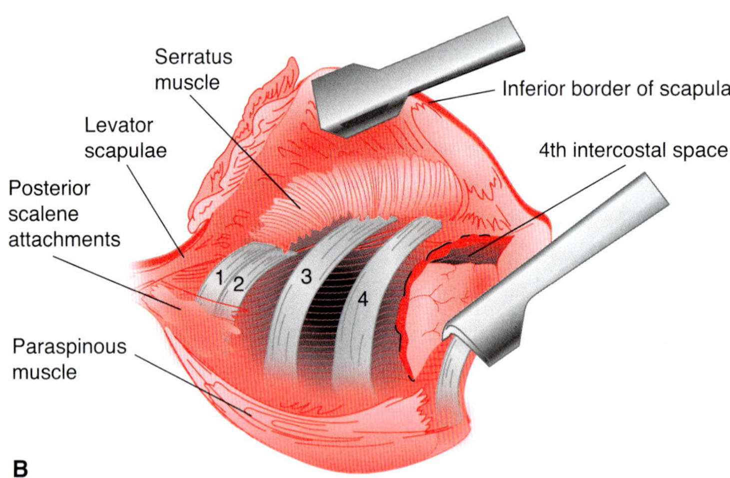

FIGURE 34.6 A self-retaining retractor is used to elevate the scapula during the posterior approach. This permits the division of the scalene muscles and resection of the first rib. **A:** The use of a standard rib retractor, although a mammary retractor or a self-retaining retractor could be used. **B:** View of the apex of the chest with the scapula elevated. (From Nesbitt JC, Wind GG. Thoracic Surgical Oncology: Exposures and Techniques. Philadelphia, PA: Lippincott Williams and Wilkins, 2003:164–165.)

the tumor. If the lesion appears resectable, then the chest wall resection can begin with the anterior division of the ribs. It is sometimes useful to resect a small portion (<1 cm) of each rib to allow easier manipulation of the chest wall segment during the subsequent disarticulation of the ribs from the spine. Every effort is made to achieve a 4-cm margin at the anterior division of the ribs.

The posterior disarticulation of the chest wall is begun at the inferior most rib and then progresses superiorly. Each rib has two synovial plane joints: the medial costovertebral joint that articulates the vertebral column with the heads of the ribs and the more lateral costotransverse joint. Between these two facets lies the neural foramen. A surgeon operating in this area should become very familiar with the bony anatomy and the position of the neural vascular structures. If there is any concern over vertebral involvement or unfamiliarity with operating in this region, a spine surgeon should be engaged to assist with this portion of the dissection.

The transverse processes should be exposed posteriorly by elevating the erector spinae muscle. If involved, these can then be divided at their base with either an osteotome or rongeurs with care not to injure the nerve roots. More commonly, the transverse process can be preserved, and the dissection begins with anterior and medial distraction of the chest wall segment. The costotransverse ligaments are then carefully divided with cautery or sharp dissection. If accomplished correctly, the costotransverse joint is exposed and disarticulated. (Fig. 34.7) This joint has a superior (larger) and inferior (smaller) facet resulting from its intervertebral location and both facets will need to be exposed. If compression of the chest wall segment is insufficient to achieve disarticulation (common during the dissection of the initial lowest rib), disarticulation can be assisted with a Cobb retractor placed in the joint and used to apply forceful anterior retraction. Medial force or leveraging with these instruments should be avoided because the instrument may slip into the neural foramen.

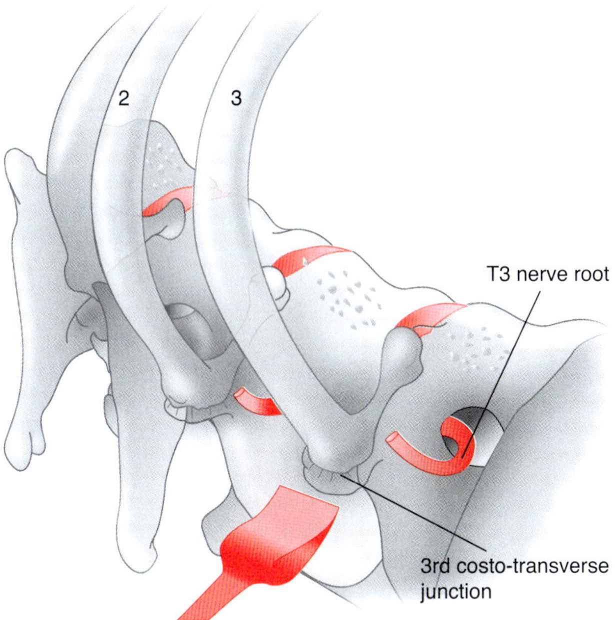

FIGURE 34.7 Tumors abutting or invading the proximal rib near the vertebral body may require disarticulation of the costovertebral junction. (From Nesbitt JC, Wind GG. Thoracic Surgical Oncology: Exposures and Techniques. Philadelphia, PA: Lippincott Williams and Wilkins, 2003:171.)

With the more lateral costotransverse joint disarticulated, the nerve root must now be identified and ligated. The neural foramen, an oval opening located at the base of the transverse process, can be exposed by continuing the division of the costotransverse ligaments, the levator costorum muscles, and distracting the chest wall segment. As the chest wall segment begins to loosen, care should be taken to not distract the segment aggressively and risk avulsing the nerve root before they can be identified, ligated, and divided. Ligation can be accomplished with surgical clips or a silk ligature and is advocated, because the dura may be incompletely fused with the nerve root resulting in a postoperative cerebrospinal fluid leak. After division of the nerve root, the vascular structures can also be identified and ligated with clips, ties, or even bipolar cautery and attention can be turned to the costovertebral joint.

This medial joint can be disarticulated by continuing to apply anterior and medial compression on the chest wall. Use of a Cobb retractor can also be employed although involvement of the rib with tumor can sometimes weaken the bone leading to fracture. If this occurs, the remaining fragments of the rib will need to be removed. Sometimes, if the tumor is situated laterally, the costovertebral joint can be approached intrapleurally. This helps define the location of mediastinal vascular structures and define the medial extent of the dissection.

Although these techniques are useful, they must be used with caution at the level of the first rib. Two aspects of the first rib require greater attention to the dissection. The first is the close approximation of the C8 nerve root to the superior border of the first rib head. If the costotransverse joint of the first rib is aggressively distracted, inadvertent avulsion of this root can occur with resulting hand weakness. Even more attention must be paid when approaching the more medial costovertebral joint. One technique is to grasp the first rib with a Kocher forceps and apply purely lateral retraction during dissection of the joint.

The second aspect of the first rib is that the T1 nerve root, after leaving the foramen, provides a branch to the brachial plexus that joins the C8 nerve root. If the tumor is positioned lateral to this branch, the T1 nerve can be divided distal to this branch preserving this sensory nerve contribution to the arm. In addition, the costovertebral joint can be left undisturbed lessening the risk of injury to the C8 root.

There are a few additional structures that need to be recognized and, in some cases preserved, during the medial–superior mobilization of the chest wall. A structure that can be sacrificed if involved is the superior stellate ganglion of the sympathetic chain. Frequently, these patients already have a Horner syndrome, but infrequently the Horner is new, and appropriate patient education will need to be provided. Other structures that rarely can be involved are the vertebral arteries and, on the left side, the esophagus and the thoracic duct. The proximity to the vertebral artery and esophagus should be established by preoperative imaging, but the thoracic duct may be encountered intraoperatively. In tumors that approach these structures, even greater care should be taken when completing the medial portion of the dissection after division of the costovertebral joint.

Anterior Approach Superior sulcus tumors include the classic Pancoast tumors that invade posteriorly leading to the classic Pancoast syndrome but can also invade anteriorly toward the subclavian vessels. The posterior approach, although sufficient to assess vessel involvement, does not provide adequate distal control of the artery or vein to allow resection. The anterior approach popularized by Dartevelle et al.[44] has become the ideal approach for these presentations of superior sulcus tumors. Alterations to this approach have allowed even greater exposure of posterior elements and the hilum of the lung allowing access to more posteriorly placed tumors and performance of greater lung resections.

The patient is positioned supine with the neck rotated toward the contralateral side and extended. The actual incision has varied with modifications both in the position of the incision and the method of exposing the subclavian vessels. Dartevelle utilized a transclavicular approach with the incision following the anterior border of the sternocleidomastoid muscle then extending laterally along the clavicle. Masaoka et al.[50] utilized a median sternotomy with extension into the fourth intercostal space and an incision along the superior border of the clavicle (similar to a hemiclamshell incision). Grunenwald and Spaggiari[51] addressed the limitations of a clavicular resection by developing a transmanubrial approach with sparing of the clavicle and the sternoclavicular joint. (Fig. 34.8)

The transclavicular approach proceeds with elevation of the pectoralis major as a myocutaneous flap, allowing exposure of the chest wall. The scalene nodes are completely dissected, and

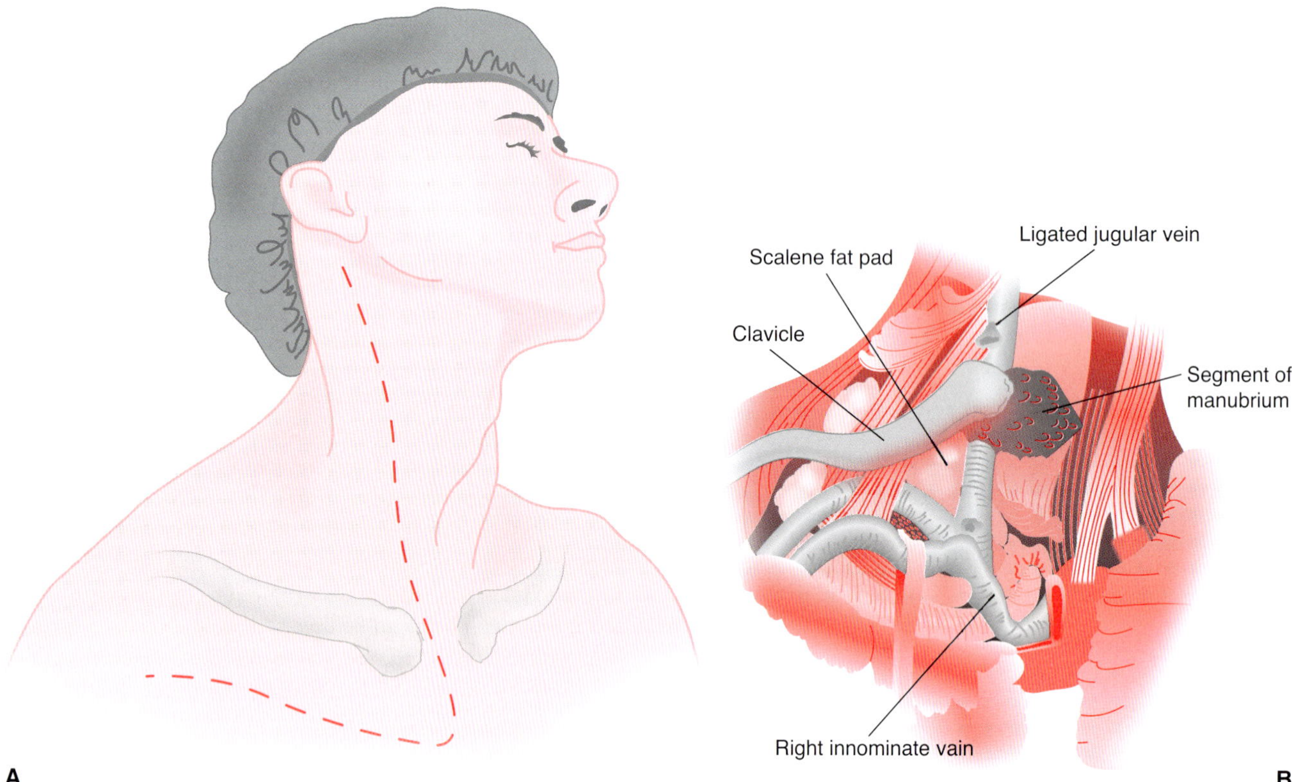

FIGURE 34.8 **A:** The anterior approach involves an incision along the sternocleidomastoid, extending inferiorly across the manubrium then turning laterally below the clavicle across the superior anterior chest wall. **B:** This permits safe access to vascular structures. (From Nesbitt JC, Wind GG. Thoracic Surgical Oncology: Exposures and Techniques. Philadelphia, PA: Lippincott Williams and Wilkins, 2003:182,184.)

the chest is entered through a safe intercostal space below the tumor. If deemed resectable, the clavicular head of the sternocleidomastoid muscle is divided and the medial third of the clavicle resected. The subclavian vein can be dissected free or, if involved, resected. On the left side, care should be taken to preserve or ligate the thoracic duct, if involved. The anterior scalene is now exposed, and the phrenic nerve should be sought and mobilized medially. Division of the anterior scalene muscle above the level of the tumor will expose the subclavian artery and the brachial plexus. If the artery can be preserved, it is carefully dissected, and every attempt is made to preserve the vertebral artery if possible. If preoperative imaging suggested involvement of the vertebral artery, then a cranial ultrasound or MR cerebral angiogram should be performed to confirm an intact circle of Willis, which would allow safe division of this vessel. If the subclavian artery cannot be dissected free, the excellent proximal and distal exposure of the artery allows resection if so indicated. The final dissection addresses the brachial plexus and allows complete release of the superior aspect of the tumor.

Attention is now turned to the chest wall resection. The first rib can be disarticulated from the manubrium followed by division of any additional ribs as indicated. With increasing experience, the posterior attachments of the ribs can also be approached and disarticulated using posterior and medial compression of the chest wall segment to distract the costotransverse and costovertebral joints. Although this exposure is sufficient for limited posterior extension, tumors that involve anterior structures as well as the vertebral body should be mobilized anteriorly then approached with a posterior approach to achieve an en bloc resection. Finally, the resulting chest wall defect is usually sufficient to perform a lobectomy and an adequate lymph node dissection.

The transmanubrial approach preserves the sternoclavicular joint by creating an L-shaped incision in the manubrium. The first rib is disarticulated from the manubrium and with gradual elevation of the manubrial–clavicular segment, the internal mammary vessels are identified and ligated. The remainder of the anterior dissection then proceeds in a manner similar to that described by Dartevelle. Grunenwald then proceeded to perform a posterolateral thoracotomy for the remainder of the dissection, whereas others have used an anterolateral thoracotomy.[52] The combination of a pure anterior transcervical approach, or a modified anterior approach with various other methods to gain access to the chest (sternotomy, posterolateral, or anterolateral thoracotomy) can be confusing. Each approach has subtle advantages and disadvantages and the reader is recommended a recent concise review by Macchiarini.[15]

Extent of Resection and Reconstruction

Anatomic versus Limited Resection Early series sometimes utilized a limited aggressive wedge resection when performing the pulmonary resection of a Pancoast tumor. This was logical because early series had such high rates of local recurrence in the thoracic inlet (around 40% in most series) that the advantage of a lobectomy versus a limited resection would not be apparent. However, later larger series began to identify an advantage associated with lobectomy rather than limited resections.[53] Currently, most investigators agree that a lobectomy should be offered if the patient is an appropriate candidate physiologically.

The role of a pneumonectomy in the resection of a Pancoast tumor, although rare, is not unheard of. In the SWOG trial, 3.6% of patients required a pneumonectomy, whereas the French trial, reported by Martinod et al.,[10] performed a pneumonectomy in 5% of patients. Although both series reported acceptable morbidity and mortality rates, the ubiquitous application of these data to all patients must be done cautiously. If the work by the SWOG investigators is correct and induction chemoradiotherapy becomes the standard approach to these tumors, then further data on the risks of induction chemoradiotherapy coupled with a pneumonectomy will be needed. Cause for this concern is evident in reports of significant increase in mortality following induction therapy and a right pneumonectomy.[54]

Chest Wall Reconstruction Chest wall reconstruction after a Pancoast resection is rarely performed, because most of the resection is subsequently covered by the scapula. The scapula provides adequate structural rigidity, allowing adequate ventilation to continue. However, if the chest wall resection extends to or below the fourth rib, postoperative trapping of the scapula inside the chest can occur. This occurs when the arm is elevated, drawing the scapula superiorly. As the arm is brought down, the tip of the scapula can herniate into the chest restricting the patient's ability to lower his/her arm. Two solutions are available. At the time of resection, a limited chest wall reconstruction can be performed using nonabsorbable material. The lower ribs should be covered and the material secured to the inferior rib, so that the scapula can ride over the material and not herniate into the chest. Alternatively, the lower 3 cm of the scapula can be exposed with a periosteal elevator and then resected using a sternal or oscillating saw. Either method is appropriate at the time of the tumor resection, although the latter is ideal when this complication is first identified postoperatively.

Vertebrectomy Originally, vertebral involvement was thought to be a contraindication to resection in these difficult patients because of poor long-term survival. Advances in spine technology combined with multispecialty approaches have led investigators to look at the feasibility of vertebral body resection in conjunction with superior sulcus tumor resection. Gandhi et al.[55] found a 2-year survival of 54% in patients with a superior sulcus tumor and vertebral body resection. The survival was 80% for negative margins and 0% for patients with positive margins. A recent update confirmed the earlier findings and also demonstrated the very poor results in these patients with any nodal disease. A more complete discussion of vertebral involvement and the techniques of resection is found in Chapter 35.

Subclavian Vessel Involvement Subclavian vessel involvement, once considered unresectable, is now addressed through an anterior approach popularized by Dartevelle. The vein can be resected without reconstruction, because there is frequently extensive collateralization already in place to provide adequate drainage of the arm. Arterial resection requires reconstruction. Although a direct reconstruction from the two divided ends of the vessel using a ringed polytetrafluoroethylene (PTFE) material is the most common method of reconstruction, a reversed venous graft can also be used. An alternative method for reconstruction to consider is a carotid–subclavian bypass. This method is especially useful for extensive tumors that cannot be completely mobilized from the anterior approach. These tumors will need to remain in place after completion of the anterior dissection until they can be released posteriorly. Rather than performing a direct end-to-end reconstruction, which will take a circuitous route around the tumor, a carotid subclavian bypass can be constructed very close to its final length with the tumor still in place or with limited proximal subclavian artery exposure.

The impact of subclavian arterial resection on long-term survival appears to be negligible in these highly selected patients. Dartevelle et al.[44] reported 12 patients in 1993 who underwent subclavian artery resection and reconstruction with 5-year 30% survival. Martinod et al. have reported 25 patients with subclavian artery involvement with 40% 5-year survival.[10]

Postoperative Morbidity and Mortality The most current data on the morbidity and mortality of Pancoast resection comes from the data obtained in the SWOG trial. Although this trial did use induction chemoradiation therapy, the modern nature of the series gives the best reflection of the current status in the United States. The surgical mortality rate in that series was very low at 2.4%. There was an additional three treatment-related deaths for a final mortality rate of 4.5%. Earlier series have reported similar rates of mortality and are summarized in Table 34.2. The morbidity in all the series was similar to what was seen in the SWOG trial. The dominant complications were pulmonary with pneumonia rates around 12%.

Local recurrences also varied considerably between series ranging from 9% in the recently updated SWOG data[47] to as high as 72% in a series of 124 patients treated with surgery and brachytherapy.[56] Although this variation is very multifactorial, including tumor-specific and treatment-related factors, more modern series appear to be able to achieve local recurrence rates below 30%.

TABLE 34.2 Mortality and Local Recurrence Rates Reported in Major Series on Pancoast Tumor Resections

Preoperative Treatment	N	Mortality	Local Recurrence
Chemo/XRT[48]	110	4.5%	9%
Chemo, XRT or Chemo/XRT[53]	225	4%	40%
XRT or Chemo/XRT[49]	35	NR	30%
Chemo, XRT, Chemo/XRT or Surgery alone[10]	139	7.2%	35%

Chemo, chemotherapy; NR, not reported; XRT, x-ray therapy.

FUTURE ADVANCES

There are several areas where future advances can be directed in the treatment of these malignancies. One area is common to both stage II disease, and the subset of Pancoast tumors is the integration of targeted therapies either preoperatively or as adjuvant therapy.

Many of the trials of adjuvant chemotherapy have demonstrated the challenges of administering postoperative platinum-based systemic therapy.[57] Induction therapy is better tolerated, but even in the SWOG trial it was clear that, when combined with radiotherapy, platinum-based therapy administration is still challenging.[31] The use of targeted therapies initiated preoperatively or postoperatively may have a role in this disease. Certainly, minimally invasive approaches may improve patient's tolerance of adjuvant therapy, but in the case of Pancoast tumors, there is little that can be done presently to reduce the physiologic stress of surgery. Agents targeting angiogenesis (e.g., bevacizumab) or epithelial growth factor receptor antagonists (e.g., erlotinib) are just a few examples of these agents. As improvements develop in genetic and proteomic analysis of lung cancers, even more intelligent choices on chemotherapeutics can be applied to these malignancies limiting the toxicities that already accompany the treatment of these advanced malignancies. To this end, the SWOG has initiated a trial (0220) to examine the effect of a less toxic regimen, docetaxel, in an adjuvant setting for Pancoast tumors.

Novel radiotherapy techniques are becoming available as well. It is clear that a multidisciplinary approach to Pancoast tumors is necessary to achieve the lowest local recurrence rates. The development of proton radiation techniques with their decreased collateral radiation damage may have a significant effect in these tumors. Additionally, the high rate of brain metastases seen in these patients may lead to prophylactic cranial irradiation in high-risk patients after resection.

CONCLUSION

Stage II NSCLC and their subset of Pancoast tumors, although considered surgically resectable, still suffer from relatively poor survival statistics. Overall, this group, when clinically staged, has a survival at 5 years of less than 30% to 40%. Although disappointing, this also provides the greatest opportunity for significant improvement. As we have shown, the local therapy for stage II lesions and even the technically challenging Pancoast patients have improved considerably. The majority of failures in these patients are a result of systemic failures. As investigators now concentrate their efforts on improving cytotoxic and biologic therapies, we have an opportunity to diminish these failures and greatly impact on their overall outcome.

REFERENCES

1. American Lung Association Web site. http://www.lungusa.org/. Accessed October 2, 2009.
2. Chute CG, Greenberg ER, Baron J, et al. Presenting conditions of 1539 population-based lung cancer patients by cell type and stage in New Hampshire and Vermont. *Cancer* 1985;56:2107–2112.
3. Kassis ES, Vaporciyan AA, Swisher SG. et al. Application of the revised lung cancer staging system (IASLC Staging Project) to a cancer center population. *J Thorac Cardiovasc Surg* 2009;138(2):412–418.
4. Le Roux BT. Bronchial carcinoma. *Thorax* 1968;23:136–143.
5. Cerfolio RJ, Ojha B, Bryant AS, et al. The accuracy of integrated PET-CT compared with dedicated PET alone for the staging of patients with nonsmall cell lung cancer. *Ann Thorac Surg* 2004;78:1017–1023.
6. Hyde L, Hye CI. Clnical manifestations of lung cancer. *Chest* 1974; 65:299.
7. Toloza EM, Harpole L, McCrory DC. Noninvasive staging of non-small cell lung cancer: a review of the current evidence. *Chest* 2003; 123:137S–146S.
8. Rusch VW. Surgery for stage III non-small cell lung cancer. *Cancer Control* 1994;1:455–466.
9. Rice DC, Kim HW, Sabichi A, et al. The risk of second primary tumors after resection of stage 1 non-small cell lung cancer. *Ann Thorac Surg* 2003;76:1001–1008.
10. Martinod E, D'Audiffret A, Thomas P, et al. Management of superior sulcus tumors: experience with 139 cases treated by surgical resection. *Ann Thorac Surg* 2002;73:1534–1539.
11. Toloza EM, Harpole L, McCrory DC. Noninvasive staging of non-small cell lung cancer: a review of the current evidence. *Chest* 2003;123: 137S–146S.
12. Swanson SJ, Herndon JE, D'Amico TA, et al. Video-assisted thoracic surgery lobectomy: report of CALGB 39802—a prospective, multi-institution feasibility study. *J Clin Oncol* 2007;25:4993–4997.
13. Sagawa M, Sato M, Sakurada A, et al.–a prospective trial of systematic nodal dissection for lung cancer by video-assisted thoracic surgery: can it be perfect? *Ann Thorac Surg* 2002;73:900–904.

14. Allen MS, Darling GE, Pechet TTV, et al. Morbidity and mortality of major pulmonary resections in patients with early-stage lung cancer: Initial results of the randomized, prospective ACOSOG Z0030 trial. *Ann Thorac Surg* 2006;81:1013–1019.
15. Macchiarini P. Resection of superior sulcus carcinomas (anterior approach). *Thorac Surg Clin* 2004;14:229–240.
16. Voltolini L, Rapicetta C, Luzzi L, et al. Lung cancer with chest wall involvement: predictive factors of long-term survival after surgical resection. *Lung Cancer* 2006;52:359–364.
17. Matsuoka H, Nishio W, Okada M, et al. Resection of chest wall invasion in patients with non-small cell lung cancer. *Eur J Cardio Thorac Surg* 2004;26:1200–1204.
18. Downey RJ, Martini N, Rusch VW, et al. Extent of chest wall invasion and survival in patients with lung cancer. *Ann Thorac Surg* 1999;68:188–193.
19. Piehler JM, Pairoler PC, Weiland LH, et al. Bronchogenic carcinoma with chest wall invasion: factors affecting survival following en bloc resection. *Ann Thorac Surg* 1982;34:684–691.
20. McCaughan BC, Martini N, Bains MS, et al. Chest wall invasion in carcinoma of the lung. *J Thorac Cardiovasc Surg* 1985;89:836–841.
21. Downey RJ, Martini N, Rusch VW, et al. Extent of chest wall invasion and survival in patients with lung cancer. *Ann Thorac Surg* 1999; 68:188–193.
22. Voltolini L, Rapicetta C, Luzzi L, et al. Lung cancer with chest wall involvement: predictive factors of long-term survival after surgical resection. *Lung Cancer* 2006;52:359–364.
23. Matsuoka H, Nishio W, Okada M, et al. Resection of chest wall invasion in patients with non-small cell lung cancer. *Eur J Cardio Thorac Surg* 2004;26:1200–1204.
24. Downey RJ, Martini N, Rusch VW, et al. Extent of chest wall invasion and survival in patients with lung cancer. *Ann Thorac Surg* 1999; 68:188–193.
25. Burkhart HM, Allen MS, Nichols FC III, et al. Results of en bloc resection for bronchogenic carcinoma with chest wall invasion. *J Thorac Cardiovasc Surg* 2002;123:670–675.
26. Izbicki JR, Thetter O, Habekost M, et al. Radical systematic mediastinal lymphadenectomy in non-small cell lung cancer: a randomized controlled trial. *Br J Surg* 1994;81:229–235.
27. Wu YL, Huang ZF, Wang SY, et al. A randomized trial of systematic nodal dissection in resectable non-small cell lung cancer. *Lung Cancer* 2002;36:1–6.
28. Allen MS, Darling GE, Pechet TTV, et al. Morbidity and mortality of major pulmonary resections in patients with early-stage lung cancer: initial results of the randomized, prospective ACOSOG Z0030 trial. *Ann Thorac Surg* 2006;81:1013–1019.
29. Pancoast HK. Superior pulmonary sulcus tumor. *JAMA* 1932;99:16–17.
30. Hare ES. Tumors involving certain nerves. *Med Gaz* 1838;1:16–18.
31. Rusch VW, Giroux DJ, Kraut MJ, et al. Induction chemoradiation and surgical resection for non-small cell lung carcinomas of the superior sulcus: initial results of Southwest Oncology Group trial 9416 (Intergroup trial 0160). *J Thorac Cardiovas Surg* 2001;121:472–483.
32. Teixeira JP. Concerning the Pancoast tumor: what is the superior pulmonary sulcus? *Ann Thorac Surg* 1983;35:577–578.
33. Attar S, Krasna MJ, Sonett JR, et al. Superior sulcus (pancoast) tumor: experience with 105 patients. *Ann Thorac Surg* 1998;66:193–198.
34. Comet R, Monteagudo M, Herranz S, et al. Pancoast's syndrome secondary to lung infection with cutaneous fistulisation caused by Staphylococcus aureus. *J Clin Patholo* 2006;59:997–998.
35. Hung JJ, Lin SC, Hsu WH. Pancoast syndrome caused by metastasis to the superior mediastinum of hepatocellular carcinoma. *J Thorac Cardiovasc Surg* 2007;55:463–465.
36. Beshay M, Roth T, Stein RM, et al. Tuberculosis presenting as Pancoast tumor. *Ann Thorac Surg* 2003;76:1733–1735.
37. Bolton WD, Rice DC, Goodyear, A et al. Superior sulcus tumors with vertebral body involvement. *J Thorac Cardiovasc Surg* 2009;137(6): 1379–1387.
38. Freundlich IM, Chasen MH, Varma DG. Magnetic resonance imaging of pulmonary apical tumors. *J Thorac Imaging* 1996;11:210–222.
39. Heelan RT, Demas BE, Caravelli JF, et al. Superior sulcus tumors: CT and MR imaging. *Radiology* 1989;170:637–641.
40. Beshay M, Roth T, Stein RM, et al. Tuberculosis presenting as Pancoast tumor. *Ann Thorac Surg* 2003;76:1733–1735.
41. Chardack WM, MacCallum JD. Pancoast syndrome due to bronchogenic carcinoma: successful surgical removal and postoperative irradiation: a case report. *J Thorac Surg* 1953;25:402–412.
42. Chardack W, MacCallum J. Pancoast tumor: 5-year survival without recurrence or metastases following radical resection and postoperative irradiation. *J Thorac Cardiovasc Surg* 1956;31:535–542.
42a. Shaw RR, Paulson DL, Kee JL. Treatment of the Superior Sulcus Tumor by Irradiation Followed by Resection. *Ann Surg* 1961;154:29–40.
43. Attar S, Miller JE, Satterfield J, et al. Pancoast's tumor: irradiation or surgery? *Ann Thorac Surg* 1979;28:578–586.
44. Dartevelle PG, Chapelier AR, Macchiarini P, et al. Anterior transcervical-thoracic approach for radical resection of lung tumors invading the thoracic inlet. *J Thorac Cardiovas Surg* 1993;105: 1025–1034.
45. Mazel C, Grunenwald D, Laudrin P, et al. Radical excision in the management of thoracic and cervicothoracic tumors involving the spine: results in a series of 36 cases. *Spine* 2003;28:782–792.
46. Albain KS, Rusch VW, Crowley JJ, et al. Concurrent cisplatin/etoposide plus chest radiotherapy followed by surgery for stages IIIA (N2) and IIIB non-small-cell lung cancer: mature results of Southwest Oncology Group phase II study 8805. *J Clin Oncol* 1995;13:1880–1892.
47. Rusch VW, Giroux D, Kraut MJ. Induction chemoradiotherapy and surgical resetion for non-small cell lung carcinomas of the superior sulcus: prediction and impact of pathologic complete response. *Lung Cancer* 2003;41:S78.
48. Rusch VW, Giroux DJ, Kraut MJ, et al. Induction chemoradiation and surgical resection for superior sulcus non-small-cell lung carcinomas: long-term results of Southwest Oncology Group trial 9416 (Intergroup trial 0160). *J Clin Oncol* 2007;25:313–318.
49. Wright CD, Menard MT, Wain JC, et al. Induction chemoradiation compared with induction radiation for lung cancer involving the superior sulcus. *Ann Thorac Surg* 2002;73:1541–1544.
50. Masaoka A, Ito Y, Yasumitsu T. Anterior approach for tumor of the superior sulcus. *J Thorac Cardiovasc Surg* 1979;78:413–415.
51. Grunenwald D, Spaggiari L. Transmanubrial osteomuscular sparing approach for apical chest tumors. *Ann Thorac Surg* 1997;63: 563–566.
52. Spaggiari L, Pastorino U. Transmanubrial approach with antero-lateral thoracotomy for apical chest tumor. *Ann Thorac Surg* 1999;68:590–593.
53. Rusch VW, Parekh KR, Leon L, et al. Factors determining outcome after surgical resection of T3 and T4 lung cancers of the superior sulcus. *J Thorac Cardiovas Surg* 2000;119:1147–1153.
54. Martin J, Ginsberg RJ, Abolhoda A, et al. Morbidity and mortality after neoadjuvant therapy for lung cancer: the risks of right pneumonectomy. *Ann Thorac Surg* 2001;72:1149–1154.
55. Gandhi S, Walsh GL, Komaki R, et al. A multidisciplinary surgical approach to superior sulcus tumors with vertebral invasion. *Ann Thorac Surg* 1999;68:1778–1785.
56. Ginsberg RJ, Martini N, Zaman M, et al. Influence of surgical resection and brachytherapy in the management of superior sulcus tumor. *Ann Thorac Surg* 1994;57:1440–1445.
57. Betticher DC. Adjuvant and neoadjuvant chemotherapy in NSCLC: a paradigm shift. *Lung Cancer* 2005;50:S9–S16.

CHAPTER 35

Linda W. Martin
Garrett L. Walsh

Vertebral Body Resection

Non–small cell lung cancer (NSCLC) that extends to the vertebrae is classified in the TNM system as T4 disease. The T4 description is historically used for locally advanced tumors involving a structure that is considered "unresectable" for cure. Incomplete resection offers no survival advantage, and until recently, surgical techniques provided few options for removing and reconstructing the vertebral body. Nonsurgical therapy for T4 tumors leads to dismal survival rates (5% to 10% 5-year survival for superior sulcus tumors treated without surgery[1,2]), which has prompted thoracic surgeons to attempt resection of supposedly unresectable structures in the last 2 decades. Complete resection of T4N0 NSCLC invading the vertebrae can achieve 5-year survival of approximately 45% to 50% in some series.[1,3–5]

Lung cancer with spinal involvement usually occurs in the upper thoracic spine, most frequently seen as a superior sulcus tumor (see Chapter 34). Approximately 2% to 3% of all NSCLC presents as a superior sulcus, or *Pancoast* tumor. Pancoast syndrome is defined as the triad of (a) shoulder and arm pain, (b) wasting of the hand muscles, and (c) ipsilateral Horner syndrome (ptosis, miosis, and anhidrosis caused by invasion of the stellate ganglion); not every case of superior sulcus tumors will present with the Pancoast syndrome, but it is more commonly seen with vertebral invasion because of the posterior location of the tumor within the thoracic inlet. The remainder of this chapter will refer to the entity of superior sulcus tumor with vertebral invasion unless otherwise specified.

Collaborative efforts between thoracic and spine surgeons for spinal resection for metastatic disease has greatly increased knowledge and surgical skills that can be applied to this small subset of patients with T4 Pancoast tumors who may now be considered for cure. Furthermore, improved outcomes with multidisciplinary treatment approaches for superior sulcus tumors has engendered optimism for achieving complete resection and even cure for these difficult tumors. Not surprisingly, careful patient selection, meticulous attention to detail both in the clinic and the operating room, and diligent postoperative care are necessary elements for success with vertebral resection for Pancoast tumors.

PATIENT SELECTION

As always, a complete history and physical exam should be performed. The usual imaging and cardiopulmonary evaluation are required (Table 35.1). Tissue diagnosis is important to obtain preoperatively; there are reports of lymphoma, metastatic tumors, or mycobacterial infections masquerading as superior sulcus NSCLC.[6] Percutaneous image-guided biopsy is usually very high yield with these peripherally located tumors, whereas bronchoscopy is rarely helpful for obtaining tissue.

For a multimodality treatment strategy that includes major pulmonary resection with concomitant rib and vertebral resection, patients need to be in optimal condition. Performance status must be satisfactory, and patients must have adequate cardiac, pulmonary, and renal function. Pulmonary complications are the most frequent source of postoperative morbidity; thus, patients with marginal respiratory status preoperatively are unlikely to have a good result. Smoking cessation is also critical to minimize perioperative respiratory events.

Other important factors in patient selection include a thorough assessment of any neurologic deficits. Brachial plexus involvement above the lower trunk of the plexus is likely to lead to significant limb dysfunction with resection, so most surgeons consider this a contraindication to resection. Lower extremity weakness may indicate direct extension of tumor into the spinal cord, or perhaps unstable bony elements of the vertebrae because of tumor destruction. Spinal cord impingement typically causes pain, followed by weakness, and less frequently sensory deficits and bowel or bladder dysfunction.[7,8] Although spinal canal involvement portends a worse prognosis, it is not strictly a contraindication. It is important to query the patient about subtle symptoms, and involve a spine surgeon early on in case impending neurologic damage may ensue. In some instances, these patients may be well palliated by undergoing resection to prevent or limit lower extremity neurologic deficits, even when an R0 resection is not possible.

Neurosurgical or orthopedic spine consultation should be obtained whenever there is suspicion of vertebral involvement.

TABLE 35.1 Preoperative Assessment

History and physical exam
Chest radiograph
Chest CT including liver and adrenals
FDG–PET/CT scan whole body
Brain MRI or enhanced CT
MRI chest/thoracic inlet/upper thoracic spine
Percutaneous needle aspirate to confirm NSCLC
Invasive mediastinal staging prior to resection*
Pulmonary function testing
Cardiac assessment
Spine surgeon consultation
Electromyography in select cases

*Mediastinoscopy, thoracoscopy, or transbronchial needle aspiration to confirm absence of N2 or contralateral N3 disease, may be performed after induction therapy.

FDG, ^{18}F-fluorodeoxyglucose; MRI, magnetic resonance imaging; NSCLC, non–small cell lung carcinoma; PET/CT, positron emission tomography and computed tomography scan.

In some cases, electromyography or nerve conduction studies may be helpful to delineate the extent and reversibility of neurologic dysfunction. Magnetic resonance imaging (MRI) of the chest and spine with contrast usually accurately demonstrates the extent of vertebral body involvement, nerve impingement, vascular invasion, and juxtaposition of the tumor with the thecal sac. Vertebral artery and anterior spinal artery invasion can also be determined with MR angiography, or in some cases, computed tomography (CT) arteriography can be helpful. Brain MRI is highly recommended given the frequency of brain metastases in this population (7% at presentation, up to 25% within 10 months of diagnosis).[9] For the same reason, fused imaging with positron emission tomography (PET) and CT is also critical to evaluate for metastatic disease.

Brachial plexus involvement should be evaluated clinically and by MRI and CT imaging. It is useful to review the sensory and motor findings expected with invasion of the brachial plexus and lower nerve roots to assist in the preoperative assessment; in addition, these potential neurologic changes should be discussed with patients before resection and possible nerve ligation. The C8 and T1 nerve roots make up the lower trunk of the plexus as it crosses the first rib. The T1 dermatome extends across the upper chest onto the anteromedial aspect of the forearm. The C8 dermatome follows the ulnar nerve distribution along the medial aspect of the arm and the fourth and fifth digits. C7 innervates sensation for the index and middle fingers, C6 for the thumb. A C7 nerve motor function abnormality is manifested by weakness of forearm extension (triceps). C8 motor nerve impingement leads to weakness of finger flexors and wasting of interosseous muscles of the hand.[10] T1 weakness leads to inability to abduct the little finger. If the clinical exam is equivocal, MRI of the brachial plexus as well as nerve conduction studies can be helpful.

Most agree that division of T1 is acceptable with minimal hand and arm morbidity, whereas the ligation of C8 will be associated with hand deformity that is excessive. Uniformly, C7 ligation is not acceptable. The rationale is that it makes little sense to perform an aggressive surgical resection to preserve a functionless upper extremity that is a source of severe pain or is completely insensate. Although it sounds extreme, sometimes forequarter amputation may provide better palliation than preservation of a useless limb.[11] Having an experienced neurosurgeon perform plexus neurolysis may allow for resection with nerve preservation in cases of significant brachial plexus displacement or invasion.

Many authors have recognized poor outcomes with N2 or N3 metastases particularly in the setting of T4 primary tumor.[12–14] Thus, invasive mediastinal staging is a necessary step in the preoperative workup, and if mediastinal nodal disease is identified, radical resection should not be offered. The possibility of downstaging these nodes to N0 or N1 with induction chemoradiation with a reasonable long-term result is a subject of debate. N3 status on the basis of ipsilateral supraclavicular nodal metastases (rather than contralateral mediastinal N3) is considered local spread by some authors, analogous to N1 disease with a typical lung primary[15,16] and not a contraindication to resection, whereas others exclude any N2 or N3 disease from surgical consideration.[5] Recent series have reinforced the importance of nodal disease as it pertains to curative resection, as outcomes have been uniformly poor with N1, N2, or N3 diseases.[4]

To summarize, contraindications to resection (Table 35.2) include involvement of the anterior spinal artery,[17,18] brachial plexus compromise at or above C7, poor cardiopulmonary reserve, distant metastases, N3 disease, and persistent N2 disease after preoperative therapy. Relative contraindications are involvement of more than three vertebral bodies, N2 disease prior to induction therapy, and invasion of the C8 nerve root.

TABLE 35.2 Contraindications to Resection of Lung Cancer with Vertebral Invasion

Absolute
Inadequate cardiopulmonary reserve
Metastatic disease
Brachial plexus invasion at or above C7 level
Invasion of the anterior spinal artery
N3 disease: contralateral mediastinal or ipsilateral supraclavicular lymph node metastases
Persistent N2 disease after induction therapy
Relative
Presence of N2 disease at diagnosis
Functionless upper extremity
Spinal cord invasion
Invasion of C8 nerve root

THERAPEUTIC APPROACH

For most stage IIIB NSCLC, chemoradiation alone is offered, either concurrently or sequentially, depending on performance status.[19] However, local control rates are only about 17% at 1 year,[20] and distant failure more than 50% at 2 years,[21] prompting interest in trimodality therapy. Several series of locally advanced T4, N0 or N1, NSCLC cases with adjacent structure invasion have been treated aggressively with resection alone, resulting in 5-year survival rates in the 20% to 35% range.[21] Distant failure is still a problem even after complete resection. Clearly, multidisciplinary care is necessary; questions remain about which chemotherapeutic agents are best, optimal dose of radiation, and the order in which chemotherapy, radiation, and surgery are used. Regardless of these questions, the lessons learned from this aggressive treatment for locally advanced lung cancers are that not all T4 designations are created equal, and most structures deemed unresectable in the last iteration of the lung cancer staging system have indeed been successfully resected with reasonable oncologic and functional outcomes. Surgery alone is almost never going to be adequate treatment, and it must be combined with other therapy. These lessons have been learned over the last 4 to 5 decades for superior sulcus tumors with or without vertebral body invasion.

Since 1961, the standard treatment for superior sulcus tumors has been radiation followed by surgery. This is based on the Shaw et al.[22] publication where 30 Gy radiation was given followed by successful resection for a subset of patients who had previously been offered no treatment. The treatment scheme and radiation dose delivered was empiric, and not challenged for many years. Rates of complete resection (around 50%) and overall 5-year survival (average 30%)[22,23] remained suboptimal, prompting the introduction of concurrent chemoradiation prior to surgery. The recently published phase II Intergroup 0160 study[5] of 110 patients resulted in a 76% rate of complete resection, partial or complete pathologic response in 56%, and overall 5-year survival of 44% after induction with cisplatin, etoposide, and 45 Gy radiation to the primary tumor bed, resection, then consolidation chemotherapy. A total of 32 of the 110 patients had T4 disease based on vertebral or subclavian vessel involvement; outcomes for these patients were surprisingly equivalent to T3 patients. Another phase II trial involving 76 patients conducted by the Japan Clinical Oncology Group (9806) using mitomycin, vindesine, and 45 Gy radiation as induction therapy yielded a 68% complete resection rate and 5-year survival of 56%.[15] Many consider induction chemotherapy with 45 Gy external beam radiation followed by surgery to be the new standard of care. Questions remain as to the optimal dose of radiation. Kwong et al.[24] used high-dose radiation in conjunction with induction chemotherapy in 36 patients, 15 of which had either N2 or N3 disease pretreatment or solitary brain metastases. Pathologic complete response occurred in 40.5%. Median survival was 2.6 years, and perioperative complications were similar to lower-dose radiation schemes. These excellent results will need to be repeated in a multicenter setting before becoming accepted practice.

Some institutions favor reserving chemotherapy and radiation for the adjuvant setting.[16] The rationale is to allow for treatment of the anticipated positive microscopic margin, to allow for an uninterrupted course of radiotherapy postoperatively, and to preserve tissue planes without the added adhesions and treatment effect of neoadjuvant radiation. Finally, immediate resection offers perhaps better, more rapid palliation of what is often debilitating pain from chest wall and brachial plexus invasion.[4] The argument for this strategy is that outcomes and patterns of failure are no different for preoperative versus postoperative therapy. In a French series, 67 patients were treated without induction therapy; 53 of 61 patients who survived the operative period had postoperative treatment, most commonly, concurrent chemoradiotherapy. After complete resection, 5-year survival was 44.9% (0% with incomplete resection).[25] It is unlikely that the two main strategies outlined previously will ever be compared head to head in a randomized trial; surgeon and institutional preference will likely drive the therapeutic plan.

TECHNIQUES OF RESECTION

There are several particular considerations for the operative planning of these complex cases. Beginning with anesthesia monitoring and positioning, standard practice includes use of a double lumen endotracheal tube, preoperative antibiotics, and deep vein thrombosis prophylaxis. A central line is not mandatory but highly recommended for reliable intravenous access, and to monitor central venous pressure during and after surgery. It is best placed in the contralateral neck, as it may be in the way of the dissection that frequently goes up to the neck or requires anterior exposure. Similarly, the arterial line should be placed in the contralateral extremity in case subclavian artery resection is necessary on the surgical side. An esophageal bougie may be helpful for large tumors to help identify the course of the esophagus during the dissection; with a large, invasive tumor, it can be easy to inadvertently enter the esophagus when working close to the vertebral bodies.[26] This has been a source of postoperative complications in some centers and a bougie, in our experience, has helped to avoid this problem. Patients are positioned in the lateral decubitus position; we favor use of a beanbag for stabilization. Cervical tongs are very helpful to enhance access to the upper thoracic spine, and they help with the critical step of attaining perfect horizontal alignment of the spine to allow for proper spinal hardware placement. Evoked potential monitoring of spinal cord function intraoperatively is recommended.

There are two main schools of thought on resectional technique for vertebrectomy. The technique championed by Grunenwald et al.[27] involves an en bloc total vertebrectomy, whereas the MD Anderson Cancer Center (MDACC) approach involves intralesional resection. There are several advantages and disadvantages to each choice, which will be discussed later.

The MD Anderson Cancer Center Technique In most superior sulcus tumors invading the spine, the tumor is centered posteriorly within the thoracic inlet; satisfactory exposure is achieved through a posterolateral thoracotomy with extension to the upper chest parallel to the spine. A second vertical incision is made directly over the spinous processes when extensive vertebral body involvement is present and posterior stabilization will be required. More recently, posterior stabilization has been accomplished first, then the patient returns to the operating room 2 or 3 days later for the anterior approach and tumor resection. It is also a critical step to carefully plan the intersection of the two incisions so that it is perpendicular (Fig. 35.1). Otherwise, if the angles between the incisions are acute, there is an island of skin that is at high risk of necrosis directly overlying spinal hardware—a set up for disaster. When the tumor extends more anteriorly, medially, or extensively involves the brachial plexus, an anterior L-shaped incision along the sternocleidomastoid and clavicle is added.

The chest is entered one interspace below the tumor. The involved ribs are divided several centimeters anterior to the tumor. For smaller tumors, dissection is greatly facilitated by dividing the lung between the tumor and the hilum with a linear cutting stapler; a completion lobectomy is performed with hilar dissection and individual vessel ligation in the standard fashion after the chest wall has been removed (Fig. 35.2A). In some cases, only a wedge resection is performed when pulmonary function is limited; several series have shown no difference in long-term results with wedge resection compared with lobectomy in this circumstance.[4,28] The portion of the lung attached to the chest wall is removed en bloc with the specimen after complete mobilization of the bony elements (Fig. 35.2B).

If necessary, a laminectomy for the involved vertebral levels is performed. The involved ribs are then disarticulated at the costotransverse and costovertebral ligaments unless the tumor transgresses these joints, in which case en bloc resection may be done with an osteotome through the vertebral body. The anterior spinal ligament and parietal pleura are mobilized off the vertebral bodies toward the lung and the entire specimen, short of the vertebral bodies, are removed. With better exposure, the vertebral bodies can now be carefully assessed for extent of involvement. If only the foramen or pedicle is invaded, these bony elements can be removed with the high-speed drill, preserving the vertebral body. When the cancellous bone of the vertebral body is invaded, at least a partial corpectomy is carried out with an intralesional resection technique using a high-speed drill. Once the lateral and posterior elements are removed, the dural sac is well exposed and any intracanal component of tumor can be safely removed. Nerve roots are directly ligated as they exit the dural sac (Fig. 35.3).

Spinal reconstruction techniques have evolved with the experience of over 2000 resections for metastatic lesions to the spine at MDACC. Initially, anterior stabilization was accomplished

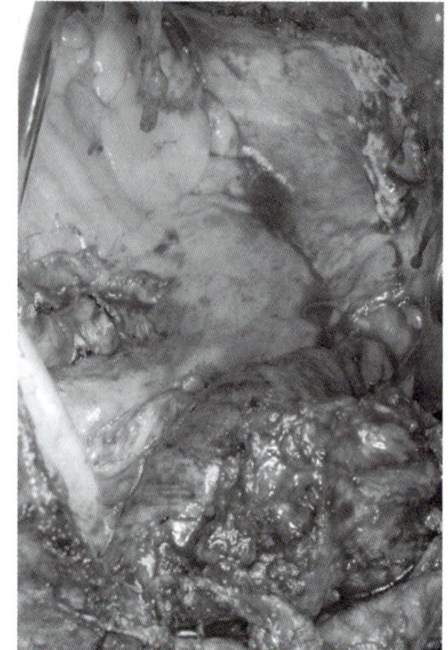
A

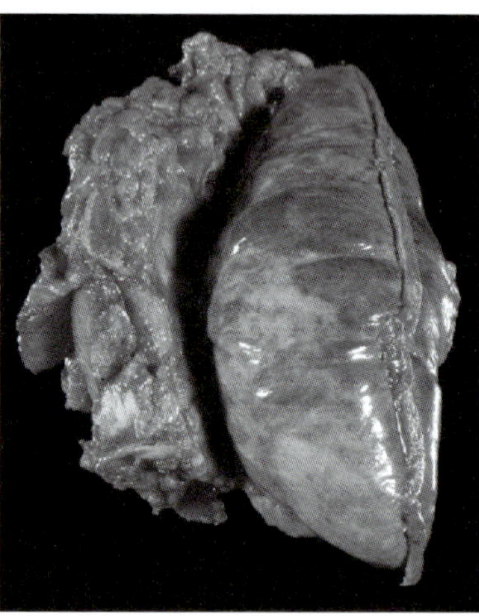
B

FIGURE 35.2 **A:** View through a left posterolateral thoracotomy for resection of a left upper lobe tumor invading the T1 and T2 vertebral bodies. Ligated hilar vessels are visible on the left side of the photograph. The lung tumor is still attached to the chest wall (right side of photograph); a linear staple line marks where the lobe was bisected to allow for en bloc chest wall resection after the proximal lobe is removed. **B:** Specimen from resection. Peripheral portion of lung is removed en bloc with chest wall and vertebral bodies.

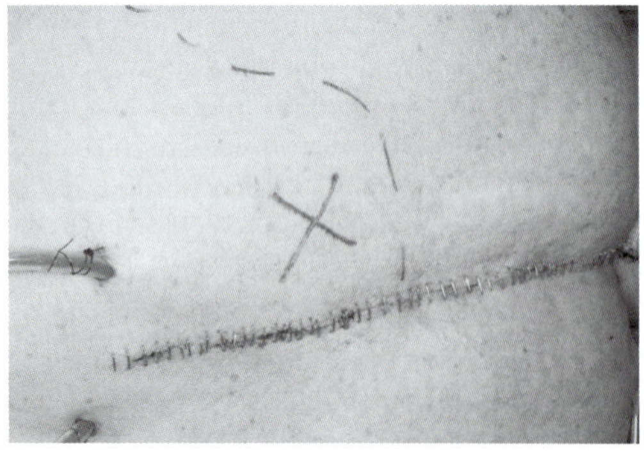

FIGURE 35.1 Mapping of thoracotomy incision for a posterior approach to a combination lung and vertebral resection. The patient had laminectomy and posterior instrumentation 2 days previously. The patient's head is to the right; drains exit caudal to the stapled incision. Note the perpendicular intersection of the thoracotomy incision with the posterior midline incision.

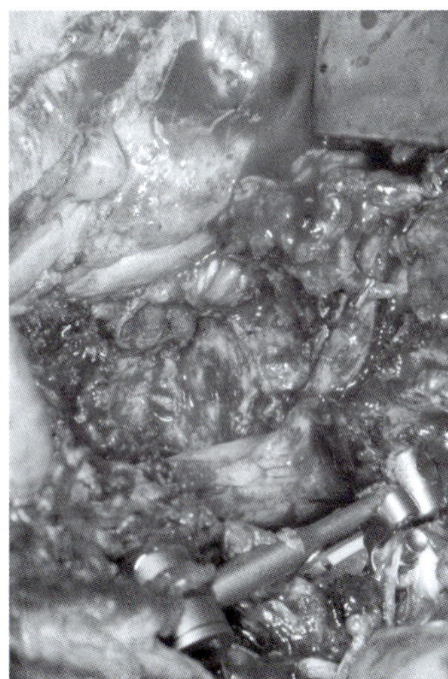

FIGURE 35.3 Operative view of chest wall and left pleural cavity after resection. The top of the photograph is anterior; the bottom is posterior chest wall. The dural sac with intact nerve root is nicely exposed; in this case, nerve root ligation was not necessary. Posterior hardware is already in place from laminectomy 2 days prior. The vertebral body defect (T1 and T2) is anterior to the dural sac.

with methyl methacrylate injected through a 32 French chest tube strut as described by Errico, Cooper, and Miller,[29,30] with additional anterior plate fixation and posterior instrumentation. More recently, expandable titanium cages have been used that will lock into the adjacent vertebral body end plates (Fig. 35.4A,B), and can facilitate fusion when packed with bone chips. Drilling adjacent vertebral bodies is avoided. When needed, the posterior elements are stabilized with wires, screws, rods, hooks, and cervical lateral mass plates (Fig. 35.4C). Care should be taken to preserve paraspinous muscles and soft tissues to cover the hardware. In addition, avoidance of a dural tear is optimal but should one occur, efforts should be made to recognize it intraoperatively, as it can be repaired with monofilament suture and buttressed with a tissue flap such as intercostal muscle.

In most cases, chest wall reconstruction is not required as the scapula covers the area of resection. If the tip of the scapula is close to the chest wall edge, there is a risk of scapular entrapment that presents similarly to shoulder dislocation. To avoid this, the chest wall can be reconstructed with taut, 2-mm thick polytetrafluoroethylene, or the tip of the scapula may be resected. Two chest tubes should be placed intrapleurally in the standard fashion. Soft tissue closure is performed in layers, again taking great care to provide adequate coverage for spinal hardware. Most patients are extubated in the operating room, and early ambulation commences as soon as possible postoperatively. Radiographic confirmation of hardware alignment is usually done prior to discharge (Fig. 35.5).

European Approach Vertebral resection for direct extension from Pancoast tumor was first described by Grunenwald et al.[27] in 1996. The technique was initially described as a three-step procedure—first an anterior cervical incision, then a standard thoracotomy to divide the ribs, wedge resection of the lung leaving the tumor-bearing portion attached to the chest wall, followed by a posterior midline incision for the vertebrectomy. Currently, a transmanubrial approach is used followed by a posterior midline incision, with the patient positioned prone with a head holder.

A 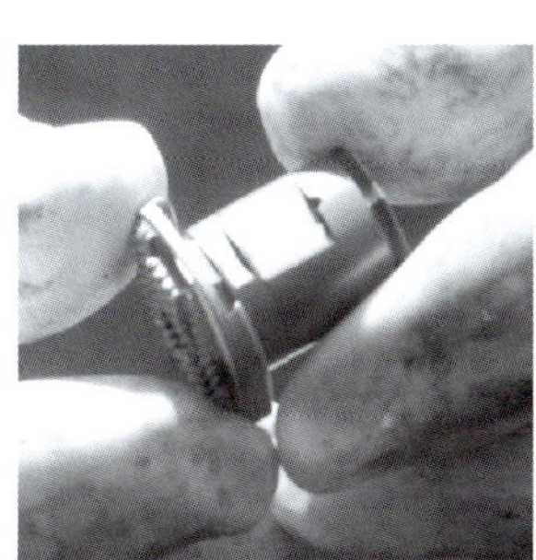 B 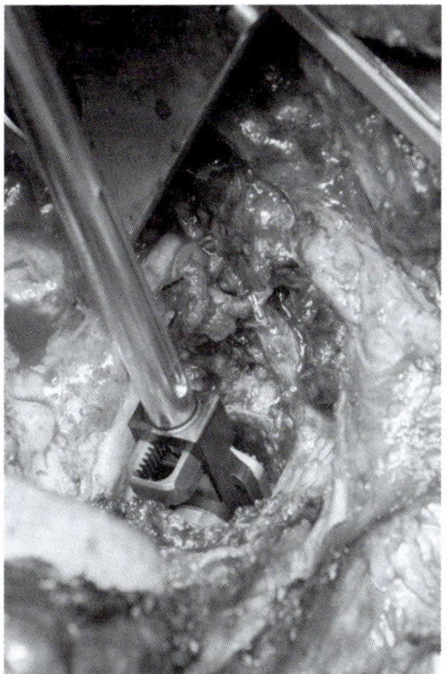 C 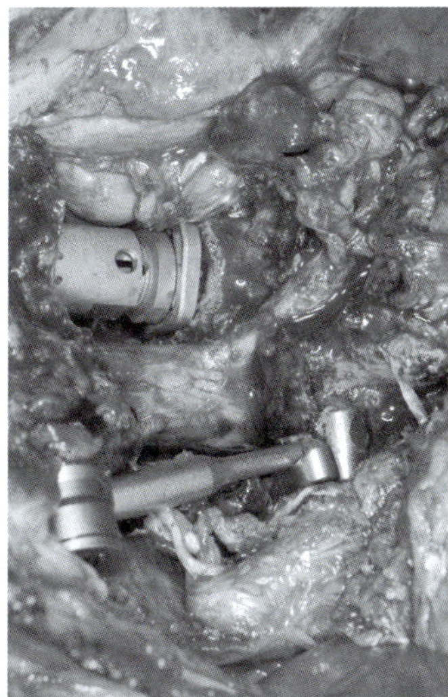

FIGURE 35.4 **A:** Titanium cage (Synthes, West Chester, PA) used for anterior spinal stabilization. **B:** Insertion of titanium cage into vertebral body defect. Great care must be taken to properly align the device. **C:** Completed spinal reconstruction. The inflated lung is present at the top of the photograph. The titanium cage is replacing the resected vertebral body, and posterior instrumentation is affixed to transverse processes of the vertebral bodies above and below the area of resection. Note the proximity of the lung to the dural sac, which illustrates how a pulmonary parenchymal air leak might communicate with an opening in the dural sac, leading to postoperative pneumocephalus.

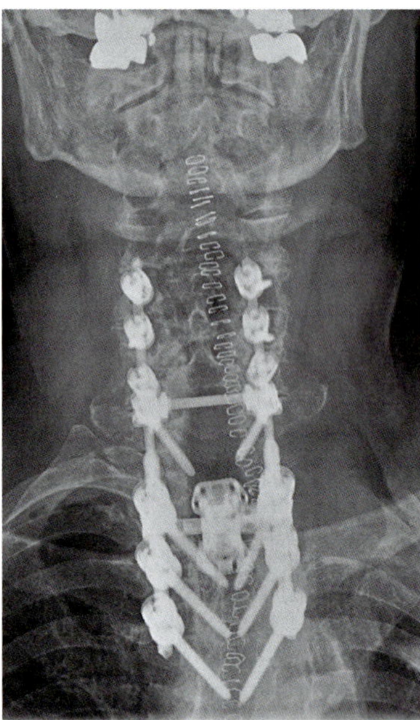

FIGURE 35.5 Postoperative radiograph confirming proper hardware position.

A laminectomy is performed one level above and below the tumor; facets and pedicles are removed bilaterally including a portion of contralateral rib, just beyond the costotransverse juncture. The posterior longitudinal ligament is divided, then the vertebral body is rotated into the chest toward the tumor and subsequently removed en bloc with the lung and chest wall.[18,31]

Reconstruction is performed with a clavicular or fibular bone graft for anterior fusion, and posterior fixation with transpedicular screws. For further stability, patients are required to wear a plastic jacket for 6 months until bone engraftment occurs. When only the foramina or costovertebral junction is invaded, a partial vertebrectomy can be performed using an osteotome in an oblique pathway, after contralateral transpedicular screws have been placed to maintain spinal stability.[18,31] This concept of partial vertebrectomy has also been embraced by other groups when less than 30% of the vertebral body is involved.[32,33]

The advantages of the MD Anderson technique are relative ease of exposure through one incision, and decreased morbidity and complexity using intralesional resection rather than en bloc vertebrectomy. The need for a plastic vest in the European series for 6 months is far from ideal, not only for patient comfort, but also the mechanical failure rate is notably higher than when anterior and posterior internal fixation is used. Although the MDACC approach does not strictly follow principles of "no touch" en bloc cancer surgery, local and distant failure rates are quite similar.

POSTOPERATIVE COMPLICATIONS

Patients undergoing resection of Pancoast tumors with vertebral involvement are subject to all the usual risks seen with any lung resection. It is noteworthy that even with these more complex operations, the most common postoperative event is respiratory in nature[25]—pneumonia, reintubation, or atelectasis requiring bronchoscopy occur in about 20% to 40%[4,25,31] of patients. The usual risk of respiratory complications following any lung resection is compounded by the added chest wall resection, disruption of accessory muscles, and risk of phrenic nerve injury with thoracic inlet dissection. The best way to avoid these problems is to carefully select good-risk patients preoperatively. Neoadjuvant radiation may increase the risk of pulmonary complications especially when pneumonectomy is required. Smoking cessation for at least 2 weeks, and preferably 4 weeks preoperatively is mandatory for active smokers. Aggressive pulmonary toilet and early mobilization are always helpful as well. When a corset is required (European approach) or if a cerebrospinal fluid (CSF) leak occurs mandating bed rest and lumber drainage, the propensity for respiratory complications is increased in this already high-risk population. Other complications, such as atrial fibrillation, stroke, myocardial infection, pulmonary embolism, and prolonged air leak occur at similar frequency to any lung resection. Bleeding risk seems to be slightly higher because of extensive chest wall resection, but most series have not reported significant numbers of reoperations for bleeding. Intraoperative blood loss tends to be much higher than expected for a standard lobectomy, with several authors reporting average blood loss in the range of 2 L or more.[31,32]

There are unique concerns related to this complex operation including hardware infection, neurologic complications, CSF leak, pneumocephalus, and esophageal injury (Table 35.3). Providing adequate, well-vascularized soft tissue coverage for hardware, as outlined previously, will avoid hardware infection in most cases. Prevention of esophageal injury and prolonged air leak, both of which will eventually lead to empyema, are obviously beneficial also. Neurologic complications caused by spinal instability have not occurred in the MD Anderson series[4] where anterior and posterior fixation are used, but were reported in 3 of 36 cases with an additional two long-term mechanical problems with spinal hardware in the French series.[31]

CSF leak usually results from inadequate ligation of nerve roots, or sometimes from dural tear. Intraoperative recognition allows for repair with fine monofilament suture buttressed with an intercostal muscle flap, but when it occurs in the

TABLE 35.3 Unique Postoperative Complications of Concomitant Lung and Vertebral Resection

Cerebrospinal fluid leak
Hardware infection or skin breakdown
Sensory or motor deficits
Pneumocephalus
Esophageal injury
Chylothorax
Spinal instability
Meningitis

postoperative period, it can manifest in one of two ways: CSF coming out of the chest drains or wound, or pneumocephalus caused by pulmonary air leak entry into the subarachnoid space (see Fig. 35.4C). When chest tube output is thin and profuse, a few drops of fluid can be placed on filter paper to check for the "double-ring sign"—an inner ring of blood with an outer ring of clear fluid. More definitively, it can be sent for beta-2 transferrin or beta-trace protein to confirm the presence of CSF. There is almost always a CSF collection locally when a leak occurs, and this can be demonstrated by MRI if suspected postoperatively. Lumbar drain placement and bed rest will usually heal the leak. Subarachnoid pleural fistula may be demonstrated by the development of altered mental status or seizure, frequently presumed to be because of brain metastases, but brain imaging will show air within the ventricles. This phenomenon seems to happen several months postoperatively[16,31] for unclear reasons. The mechanism is communication between pulmonary parenchyma and the subarachnoid space. Treatment is reoperation to close the dural leak and patch it with vascularized autogenous tissue. Esophageal injury is briefly mentioned earlier and can often be avoided by using a bougie intraoperatively to facilitate identification of the esophagus in the thoracic inlet and upper chest.

CONCLUSION

Surgical treatment for Pancoast tumors has been increasingly aggressive over the last few decades, and what was previously considered inoperable can now be successfully resected with good oncologic and functional results. Vertebral body resection and reconstruction with lung resection is a complex procedure, but can be accomplished in experienced centers. When combined with chemotherapy and radiation, T4 superior sulcus tumors have similar outcomes to T3 tumors and long-term survival up to 50% has been documented. Careful pretreatment evaluation with extensive imaging allows for optimal patient selection. Neurosurgical or orthopedic spine specialist collaboration is a must. There are several unique complications, such as hardware infection or failure, CSF leak, or subarachnoid–pleural fistula that require increased vigilance and awareness if they are to be properly managed. Ongoing areas of controversy include the sequence and dose of trimodality care, technique of vertebral resection (intralesional vs. en bloc), and whether or not patients with N2 or N3 disease should be offered curative resection. Overall, successful resection of superior sulcus tumors with vertebral body invasion represents a significant advancement in the treatment of a subset of lung cancer that previously was considered uniformly fatal.

REFERENCES

1. Komaki R, Roth JA, Walsh GL, et al. Outcome predictors for 143 patients with superior sulcus tumors treated by multidisciplinary approach at the University of Texas M. D. Anderson Cancer Center. *Int J Radiat Oncol Biol Phys* 2000;48:347–354.
2. Mountain CF. Revisions in the International System for Staging Lung Cancer. *Chest* 1997;111:1710–1717.
3. Bilsky MH, Vitaz TW, Boland PJ, et al. Surgical treatment of superior sulcus tumors with spinal and brachial plexus involvement. *J Neurosurg* 2002;97:301–309.
4. Bolton WD, Rice DC, Goodyear A, et al. Superior sulcus tumors with vertebral body involvement: a multimodality approach. *J Thorac Cardiovasc Surg* 2009;137(6):1379–1387.
5. Rusch VW, Giroux DJ, Kraut MJ et al. Induction chemoradiation and surgical resection for superior sulcus non-small-cell lung carcinomas: long-term results of Southwest Oncology Group Trial 9416 (Intergroup Trial 0160). *J Clin Oncol* 2007;25:313–318.
6. Arcasoy SM, Bajwa MK, Jett JR. Non-Hodgkin's lymphoma presenting as Pancoast's syndrome. *Respir Med* 1997;91:571–573.
7. Arcasoy SM, Jett JR. Superior pulmonary sulcus tumors and Pancoast's syndrome. *N Engl J Med* 1997;337:1370–1376.
8. Helweg-Larsen S, Sørensen PS. Symptoms and signs in metastatic spinal cord compression: a study of progression from first symptom until diagnosis in 153 patients. *Eur J Cancer* 1994;30A:396–398.
9. Shah H, Anker C, Bogart J, et al. Brain: the common site of relapse in patients with pancoast or superior sulcus tumors. *J Thorac Oncol* 2006;1:1020–1022.
10. Bilsky MH, Vitaz TW, Boland PJ, et al. Surgical treatment of superior sulcus tumors with spinal and brachial plexus involvement. *J Neurosurg* 2002;97(3 Suppl):301–309.
11. Wittig JC, Bickels J, Kollender Y, et al. Palliative forequarter amputation for metastatic carcinoma to the shoulder girdle region: indications, preoperative evaluation, surgical technique, and results. *J Surg Oncol* 2001;77:105–113.
12. Detterbeck FC. Pancoast (superior sulcus) tumors. *Ann Thorac Surg* 1997;63:1810–1818.
13. Vallières E, Karmy-Jones R, Mulligan MS, et al. Pancoast tumors. *Curr Probl Surg* 2001;38:293–376.
14. Ginsberg RJ, Martini N, Zaman M, et al. Influence of surgical resection and brachytherapy in the management of superior sulcus tumor. *Ann Thorac Surg* 1994;57:1440–1445.
15. Kunitoh H, Kato H, Tsuboi M, et al. Phase II trial of preoperative chemoradiotherapy followed by surgical resection in patients with superior sulcus non-small-cell lung cancers: report of Japan Clinical Oncology Group trial 9806. *J Clin Oncol* 2008;26:644–649.
16. Martin LW, Walsh GL. Vertebral body resection. *Thorac Surg Clin* 2004;14:241–254.
17. Fadel E, Missenard G, Chapelier A, et al. En bloc resection of non-small cell lung cancer invading the thoracic inlet and intervertebral foramina. *J Thorac Cardiovasc Surg* 2002;123:676–685.
18. Grunenwald DH, Mazel C, Girard P, et al. Radical en bloc resection for lung cancer invading the spine. *J Thorac Cardiovasc Surg* 2002;123:271–279.
19. Jett JR, Scott WJ, Rivera MP, et al. Guidelines on treatment of stage IIIB non-small cell lung cancer. *Chest* 2003;123(1 Suppl):221S–225S.
20. Arriagada R, Le CT, Quoix E, et al. ASTRO (American Society for Therapeutic Radiology and Oncology) plenary: effect of chemotherapy on locally advanced non-small cell lung carcinoma: a randomized study of 353 patients. GETCB (Groupe d'Etude et Traitement des Cancers Bronchiques), FNCLCC (Féderation Nationale des Centres de Lutte contre le Cancer) and the CEBI trialists. *Int J Radiat Oncol Biol Phys* 1991;20:1183–1190.
21. Grunenwald DH. Surgery for advanced stage lung cancer. *Semin Surg Oncol* 2000;18:137–142.
22. Shaw RR, Paulson DL, Kee JL. Treatment of superior sulcus tumor by irradiation followed by resection. *Ann Surg* 1961;154:29–40.
23. Martinod E, D'Audiffret A, Thomas P, et al. Management of superior sulcus tumors: experience with 139 cases treated by surgical resection. *Ann Thorac Surg* 2002;73:1534–1539.
24. Kwong KF, Edelman MJ, Suntharalingam M, et al. High-dose radiotherapy in trimodality treatment of Pancoast tumors results in high pathologic complete response rates and excellent long-term survival. *J Thorac Cardiovasc Surg* 2005;129:1250–1257.

25. Alifano M, D'Aiuto M, Magdeleinat P, et al. Surgical treatment of superior sulcus tumors: results and prognostic factors. *Chest* 2003;124:996–1003.
26. York JE, Walsh GL, Lang FF, et al. Combined chest wall resection with vertebrectomy and spinal reconstruction for the treatment of Pancoast tumors. *J Neurosurg* 1999;91:74–80.
27. Grunenwald D, Mazel C, Girard P, et al. Total vertebrectomy for en bloc resection of lung cancer invading the spine. *Ann Thorac Surg* 1996;61:723–725.
28. Gandhi S, Walsh GL, Komaki R, et al. A multidisciplinary surgical approach to superior sulcus tumors with vertebral invasion. *Ann Thorac Surg* 1999;68:1778–1784.
29. Errico TJ, Cooper PR. A new method of thoracic and lumbar body replacement for spinal tumors: technical note. *Neurosurgery* 1993;32:678–680.
30. Miller DJ, Lang FF, Walsh GL,et al. Coaxial double-lumen methylmethacrylate reconstruction in the anterior cervical and upper thoracic spine after tumor resection. *J Neurosurg* 2000;92:181–190.
31. Mazel C, Grunenwald D, Laudrin P, et al. Radical excision in the management of thoracic and cervicothoracic tumors involving the spine: results in a series of 36 cases. *Spine* 2003;28:782–792.
32. Koizumi K, Haraguchi S, Hirata T, et al. Surgical treatment of lung cancer with vertebral invasion. *Ann Thorac Cardiovasc Surg* 2004;10:229–234.
33. Yokomise H, Gotoh M, Okamoto T, et al. En bloc partial vertebrectomy for lung cancer invading the spine after induction chemoradiotherapy. *Eur J Cardiothorac Surg* 2007;31:788–790.

CHAPTER 36

Yvonne M. Carter
Dan J. Raz
David M. Jablons

Surgical Management of Second Primary and Metastatic Lung Cancer

More than half of the approximately 160,000 patients diagnosed with lung cancer annually in the United States have metastatic disease at the time of presentation.[1] In the past, a selected few patients with metastases to other lung segments or the brain have been treated surgically; otherwise, there has not been a defined role for surgery in the treatment of advanced lung cancer. Recently, however, there have been increasing reports of surgical management of adrenal, liver, bone, and pleural metastases from primary lung cancer. Surgical resection is also indicated for a heterogeneous group of patients with multiple primary lung cancers (MPLCs). This chapter presents a guideline for addressing these special considerations in lung cancer.

MULTIPLE PRIMARY LUNG CANCERS

Patients with a history of current or previously treated lung cancer are at high risk for additional primary lung cancers because of a high prevalence of tobacco exposure. Although Bilroth and von Winiwarter[2] first described MPLCs over 100 years ago, it is Beyreuther who is credited with directing attention to this subgroup of cancer patients with his 1924 report of two primary lung cancers in a tuberculosis patient. A review of the English literature from 1983 to 2002 identified MPLCs occurring in only 2.7% of more than 36,000 patients (Table 36.1). The true incidence of MPLCs has been difficult to estimate because diagnostic criteria have not been agreed upon and the staging system for lung cancer has changed multiple times in the last decade. Despite their rarity, the incidence and reports of such lesions seem to be increasing (Table 36.2). Martini and Melamed[3] described diagnostic criteria for MPLC (Table 36.3).

EVALUATION AND MANAGEMENT OF SYNCHRONOUS PULMONARY TUMORS

Synchronous Primary Carcinomas of Lung Originally defined by Bilroth and von Winiwarter[2] to (a) have different histologic characteristics, (b) originate from different locations, and (c) produce individual metastases, synchronous primary lung cancers are now frequently distinguished by different histologic patterns and locations—the same or different lobes. Controversy remains among investigators about the involvement of mediastinal lymph nodes as a factor in the classification of synchronous primary lung carcinomas. Many would, however, agree with Antakli et al.,[4] who have suggested that tumors of the same histologic subtype only be categorized as synchronous in the absence of mediastinal nodal disease (Tables 36.4 and 36.5).

Primary Lung Carcinoma with Intrapulmonary Metastasis These tumors are similar in histology, but differ in anatomic location. Satellite nodules are metastatic lesions that occur within the same lobe as the index tumor. The American Joint Commission on Cancer (AJCC) has long defined satellite nodules as T4 (stage IIIb) disease, and ipsilateral intrapulmonary metastases as M1 disease (stage IV). However, in the absence of nodal involvement, several centers have reported that with lobar resection, patients with satellite nodules have 5-year survival of close to 60% comparable to patients with Ib or IIa disease.[5,6] Meanwhile, Deslauriers et al.[7] reported only a 22% 5-year survival among the 84 patients with satellite nodules. Zell et al.[8] analyzed Surveillance, Epidemiology, and End Results (SEER) data and reported improved survival outcomes among patients with ipsilateral pulmonary metastases compared with other stage IV patients. The recent International Association for the Study of Lung Cancer (IASLC) proposed staging system downgrades satellite nodules to T3 disease and ipsilateral intrapulmonary metastases to T4 disease (see Chapter 30).[9] This change is supported by validation studies carried out using population-based data.[8,10] The role of chemotherapy either in a neoadjuvant or adjuvant setting for these patients has not been carefully studied. It is the bias of the authors of this chapter to treat patients with presumed or questionable T4 satellites with up-front chemotherapy, resection, and adjuvant therapy based on intraoperative findings.

There are little data to support surgical resection of intrapulmonary metastases from lung cancer, although some patients

TABLE 36.1 Incidence of Multiple Primary Lung Cancers

Author	Lung Cancer Patients	Frequency of MPLCs
Bewtra[91]	12,685	382 (1.7%)
Mathisen et al.[31]	341	26 (7.6%)
Wu et al.[36]	3815	30 (0.8%)
Verhagen et al.[23]	1004	32 (3.2%)
Deschamps et al.[27]	9611	117 (1.2%)
Okunaka et al.[22]	1180	24 (2.0%)
Antakli et al.[4]	1572	65 (4.1%)
Yoshino[92]	509	42 (8.3%)
Adebonojo et al.[37]	1325	68 (5.1%)
van Rens[93]	3086	127 (4.1%)
Aziz et al.[38]	892	51 (5.7%)
Total	36,020	964 (2.7%)

MPLCs, multiple primary lung cancers.

anecdotally are cured after complete resection. Patients with multifocal bronchioloalveolar carcinoma (BAC) are exceptions to the poor prognosis of multifocal lung cancer. Patients with multifocal BAC who undergo complete resection can achieve 5-year survivals of upward of 60%.[11,12] These patients have a high rate of intrapulmonary recurrence. Epidermal growth factor tyrosine kinase inhibitors (EGFR TKIs) have been a useful adjuvant treatment in such patients, although the optimal time course of treatment has not been well studied. Lung transplantation has been used at selected centers in patients with unresectable multifocal BAC, who have no evidence of nodal or distant metastases with promising long-term results. The largest reported series (29 patients) reported a 5-year survival of 51%, although there was tumor recurrence in 13 patients (45%).[13]

TABLE 36.2 Incidence of Synchronous and Metachronous Lung Cancer in Patients with Multiple Primary Tumors

Author	Patients	Synchronous	Metachronous
Razzuk[26]	34	5 (15%)	29 (85%)
Abbey-Smith et al.[32]	55	10 (18%)	45 (72%)
Mathisen et al.[31]	90	10 (11%)	80 (89%)
Wu et al.[36]	30	10 (33%)	20 (67%)
Deschamps et al.[27]	80	36 (45%)	44 (55%)
Rosengart et al.[25]	111	33 (30%)	78 (70%)
Antakli et al.[4]	65	26 (40%)	39 (60%)
Adebonojo et al.[37]	52	15 (29%)	37 (71%)
Aziz et al.[38]	51	41 (80%)	10 (20%)
Total	568	186 (33%)	382 (67%)

TABLE 36.3 Criteria for the Diagnosis of Multiple Primary Lung Cancers

A. Metachronous tumors
- I. Different histology
- II. Same histology, if:
  - a. free interval between cancers at least 2 years, or
  - b. origin from carcinoma in situ, or
  - c. second cancer in different lobe or lung, and
    - i. no carcinoma in lymphatics common to both
    - ii. no extrapulmonary metastases at time of diagnosis

B. Synchronous tumors
- I. Tumors physically distinct and separate
- II. Histologic type:
  - a. different
  - b. same, but different segment, lobe, or lung, if:
    - i. origin from carcinoma in situ
    - ii. no carcinoma in lymphatics common to both
    - iii. no extrapulmonary metastasis at time of diagnosis

From Martini N, Melamed MR. Multiple primary lung cancers. *J Thorac Cardiovasc Surg* 1975;20:606–612, with permission.

One Primary Carcinoma and One Benign Lesion

A significant proportion of the second pulmonary nodules discovered preoperatively by Kunitoh et al.[14] were found to be benign. Pathologic diagnoses included infarction, granuloma, fibrosis, and hamartoma. A thorough metastatic evaluation is indicated in patients with a known lung carcinoma and a second indeterminate parenchymal mass. Positron emission tomography (PET) and fusion computed tomography (CT)/PET scanning are useful both for staging and to estimate the probability that a lesion is benign or malignant. Once there is no proof of metastatic disease, one could either observe the second lesion or opt to obtain a tissue sample for a histologic diagnosis. In the case of an ipsilateral nodule, the assessment can be performed at the time of thoracotomy. For contralateral

TABLE 36.4 Modified Criteria for Multiple Primary Lung Cancers

A. Different histologic condition

B. Same histologic condition with two or more of the following:
1. anatomically distinct
2. associated premalignant lesion
3. no systemic metastases
4. no mediastinal spread
5. different DNA ploidy

From Antakli T, Schaefer RF, Rutherford JE, et al. Second primary lung cancer. *Ann Thorac Surg* 1995;59:863–866, with permission.

TABLE 36.5 Incidence of Synchronous Primary Lung Cancer

Author	Lung Cancer Patients	Synchronous Tumors
Mathisen et al.[31]	2041	10 (0.48%)
Ferguson et al.[95]	2100	28 (1.33%)
Wu et al.[36]	3815	10 (0.26%)
Deschamps et al.[27]	9611	44 (0.46%)
Antakli et al.[4]	1572	26 (1.65%)
Pommier[94]	3034	27 (0.8%)
Yoshino[92]	509	42 (8.3%)
Adebonojo et al.[37]	1309	15 (1.1%)
Okada[96]	889	89 (10%)
Total	24,880	291 (1.2%)

lesions, CT-guided fine-needle aspiration biopsy (FNAB), video-assisted thoracoscopic surgery (VATS) wedge resection, or Wang biopsy as well as mediastinoscopy at the time of surgery may be required.

Evaluation Specific questions must be addressed in the evaluation of two distinct lung cancers.

1. Does the lesion(s) represent an extrathoracic primary carcinoma with pulmonary metastases?
2. Are mediastinal lymph nodes involved?
3. In the case of a primary lung cancer, is there evidence of distant metastatic disease?
4. What is the histologic diagnosis of the nodule(s)?

The accuracy of a cytologic diagnosis from an FNAB ranges from 60% to 80%.[15–17] Treatment of two lung nodules should be based on a histologic diagnosis from either a core needle or a wedge biopsy. Disseminated neoplastic disease should be assessed with CT, PET, and brain magnetic resonance imaging (MRI).

Bronchoscopy allows for evaluation of the bronchial lumen, assessing for tumor involvement, communication with the esophagus, and obstruction. McElvaney et al.[18] discovered synchronous endobronchial foci of adenocarcinoma in nearly 20% of surgical patients evaluated with bronchoscopy before surgical resection—only two of which were identified preoperatively. These data support the universal requirement for bronchoscopic examination prior to proceeding with any planned surgical resection.

Mediastinoscopy has been established as an important component in the evaluation of patients with lung cancer. The use of endoscopic ultrasound (EUS) and endobronchial ultrasound (EBUS) to perform fine-needle aspiration (FNA) of mediastinal lymph nodes for staging have been increasing. EUS and EBUS offer less invasive staging of the mediastinum, but are operator dependent and result in far less tissue for analysis. Tournoy et al.[19] recently reported similar diagnostic yields for EUS and mediastinoscopy, whereas Wallace et al.[20] reported excellent yields when combining both EUS and EBUS. We currently employ EUS and EBUS in patients who have previously undergone mediastinoscopy, or who have other contraindications to mediastinoscopy or general anesthesia.

Treatment Surgical resection is indicated when there are two primary lung carcinomas without evidence of mediastinal lymph nodes or distant metastases—clinical stage I or II.[21] Those patients with N1 disease (stage II) should be offered surgery and referred for adjuvant chemotherapy. The clinical stage of the tumors should be used to determine which lesion should be pursued initially.[22–26] Other factors to consider before surgical resection of the second tumor are pathologic stage of the first tumor, extent of the second tumor, extent of resection required for the second tumor, and the patient's pulmonary reserve. Also, possible benefit of systemic therapy prior to either initial resection or second resection should be considered.

In such cases where a second cancer is discovered intraoperatively in a different lobe, N2 disease should be ruled out and pulmonary function should be reviewed. In all cases, a mediastinal and hilar lymph node dissection should be performed initially with intraoperative frozen section analysis for accurate pathologic staging. Presence of N1 disease and certainly N2 would preclude pneumonectomy. Regardless of the surgical procedure chosen, the goal should always be complete resection of the tumors, as this has an evident impact on survival. If the patient has adequate respiratory reserve and no evidence of N2 disease, an anatomical resection should be pursued. If pulmonary function is insufficient, wedge resection should be considered. On the other hand, there are proponents of nonsurgical treatment in patients found to have positive hilar or mediastinal lymph nodes intraoperatively, based on a median survival of 11 months compared to 26 months in those with negative lymph nodes.[24,27] Patients who do not undergo surgical resection are referred for definitive chemoradiation. In addition, ablative procedures such as radiofrequency ablation and CyberKnife should be considered.

Prognosis Stage for stage comparison, survival after resection of synchronous primary lung cancers is worse than for a solitary bronchogenic neoplasm.[28] These data have led some to believe that synchronous lesions should be classified as stage IV disease.[29] The lower survival rates may be explained by an overall greater probability of recurrent disease given two independent cancers, more aggressive biologic behavior, an inherent increased risk of developing a neoplastic process.[25,27] The fact that the second lesion is usually treated with wedge or segmental resection—procedures associated with increased incidence of locoregional recurrence and lower survival—may also explain these poor survival results.[30] Compared to other treatment methods (i.e., radiation therapy, ablative procedures, chemotherapy), surgery has still been shown to significantly prolong survival.

Metachronous Tumors The minimum duration of time, between treatment of a first primary tumor and the appearance second primary tumor, that defines metachronous tumor is considered to be 2 years.[3,23,27,30–35] Multiple series have cited a median of 48 months or longer between the treatment of the first lung tumor and the presentation of a second,[23,31,32,36] whereas others report shorter time periods, between 24 and 48 months.[27,33,34] Most recently, Aziz et al. reported an average tumor-free interval of 46 ± 14 months in patients with metachronous lesions; however, the 3-, 5-, and 10-year survival rates of 39%, 15%, and 2%, respectively, were no different than those in studies with a median interval of 24 months.[37,38] Additionally, there is no consistent evidence relating the tumor-free interval to either the type of surgical resection or histologic cell type of the tumors.

The incidence of metachronous second primary lung cancers is estimated to be 0.5% overall, including 2.5% of the surgical patients and 10% to 32% of long-term survivors. The risk of developing a metachronous primary lung cancer after curative resection of an initial early stage NSCLC is 0.65% to 5% annually (Table 36.6).[26,27,35,39–40] Pairolero et al.[29] reviewed 346 surgically treated stage I patients from the Mayo Clinic and discovered a metachronous second lung primary in 10% of their NSCLC patients. A more aggressive approach to surveillance and the increasing sensitivity of surveillance modalities (i.e., CT, PET, PET/CT) may contribute to what appears to be an increased incidence of these tumors. As far as location, there appears to be a prevalence for metachronous lesions to develop on the same side as the initial primary lung cancer. Feld et al.[41] reported the metachronous second primary lung cancers in 390 stage I and II NSCLC patients to occur twice as often on the ipsilateral side compared to the contralateral side; 26% and 13%, respectively.

Evaluation The majority of patients (80%) are asymptomatic, with lesions revealed on surveillance chest roengenograph.[8,23,25,26,31] This statistic supports the need for close follow-up and surveillance of all patients with lung cancer. Smoking cessation should be encouraged, as there is certainly an increased risk of developing a second primary lung cancer in patients who continue to smoke after treatment of the index tumor.[14] Evaluation of the second tumor should mimic the initial workup and should certainly include close assessment for locoregional and distant metastatic disease.

TABLE 36.6 Incidence of Metachronous Lung Cancer in Resected Lung Cancer Patients

Author	Resected Lung Cancer Patients	Metachronous Lesions
Abbey-Smith et al.[32]	1400	45 (3.2%)
Wu et al.[36]	3815	20 (0.5%)
Verhagen et al.[23]	1004	25 (1.5%)
Adebonojo et al.[37]	1309	37 (2.8%)
van Rens[93]	3086	127 (4.1%)
Aziz et al.[38]	892	41 (4.6%)
Doddoli[97]	1900	38 (2%)
Total	13,406	333 (2.5%)

Treatment Most of these lesions—approximately 75%—are stage I, and it is estimated that 65% are amenable to surgical resection.[42] Complete resection is indicated to treat these lesions, of which two thirds of the patients will require extended surgical resection. The surgical decision must be based on the site of neoplasm, previous surgical procedures, and the extent of disease.

Residual/Contralateral Lung

The gold standard for an early stage NSCLC is lobectomy, based on Lung Cancer Study Group (LCSG) data and on the Memorial Sloan Kettering data, demonstrating a significantly higher rate of recurrence and decreased 5-year survival with limited resection.[43] Despite this, there were very few patients with cancers smaller than 2 cm in the LCSG trial, and clinical trials comparing wedge resection to lobectomy in patients with very small tumors are currently underway. Limited surgical resection should only be considered in patients with inadequate pulmonary reserve or in patients who are high operative risk, in which case either a segmentectomy or wedge resection with lymph node sampling is appropriate. In those patients who experience a metachronous pulmonary cancer after limited resection, a completion lobectomy should be considered. When a metachronous tumor is ipsilateral, and in a different lobe than the index tumor, a completion pneumonectomy may be considered but usually lobectomy of the index tumor and generous wedge resection of the synchronous lesion is also reasonable.[44,45] Emerging experience with high energy, focal radiotherapy (CyberKnife radiation, etc.) may provide comparable local control to surgery in small (less than 3 cm) lesions in patients with limited pulmonary reserve or postpneumonectomy.

Endobronchial Lesions

Recurrences can be limited to the mucosa/submucosa of the bronchial stump, sparing the peribronchial lymphatics. This small subset of patients experiences a better prognosis than those with lymphatic involvement. Although these endobronchial recurrences can be addressed with local treatment (i.e., photodynamic therapy, brachytherapy), surgery does play a role in selected patients. Either a sleeve lobectomy or completion pneumonectomy should be considered worthwhile given the potentially curative intent. Compared to an initial pneumonectomy, there is a higher morbidity and mortality rate (MR = 0% to 15%). The postoperative mortality rate and 5-year survival (25%) are the same whether the completion pneumonectomy is performed for a local recurrence or second primary lung cancer. Increasing evidence supports the use of sleeve resections wherever possible over pneumonectomy. Long-term survival and disease-free recurrence are comparable, and sleeve resection preserves parenchyma and lung function.

Nodal Recurrence Metastatic disease involving the lymph nodes can occur in the mediastinal, hilar, or intraparenchymal nodes. Rarely is metastatic disease limited to the intraparenchymal or hilar nodes; however, these patients are potentially curable with surgery. In the absence of mediastinal lymph node involvement, one should consider a surgical resection using a similar treatment approach as that used for the index tumor. A positive mediastinoscopy revealing mediastinal (N2) lymph node involvement should preclude thoracotomy in most cases. Select patients may benefit from induction chemotherapy and subsequent restaging. Those with sterilization of their N2 disease (verified by repeat mediastinoscopy, etc.) can do well, long term, with resection (see Chapter 55).

Pleura/Chest Wall Involvement of the pleura or chest wall with malignancy is usually indicative of a diffuse process involving the entire pleural space. There are, however, some rare true solitary recurrences involving either the pleura or chest wall. These lesions should be approached with complete surgical resection (i.e., chest wall resection), with the curative intent. The majority of these cases are better treated with local external beam radiation therapy.

Prognosis The best chance for cure and long-term survival for all of these patients is surgical resection. Undoubtedly, the morbidity and mortality rates are higher with re-resection; up to 39%[35] and 4.5% to 9.3%,[27,31,34] respectively. Overall, the 5-year survival in patients treated surgically is 20% to 30%, and 20% at 10 years.[10,25,46,47] Multiple studies cite improved 5-year survival (36%) with complete resection of the metachronous lesion. Complete surgical resection increases survival to 36%.[10,25,27,37,48,49]

BRAIN METASTASIS

The brain is the most common site of metastasis for bronchogenic carcinoma,[50] and is found in approximately 25% of patients with stage IV NSCLC[51] (see also Chapter 63). The discovery of brain metastases is usually a manifestation of widely disseminated disease. Occasionally, however, the brain is the only site of distant disease as Arbit and Wronski[52] reported to be the case in 18.9% of their patients. Unfortunately, it is estimated that 40% of patients with NSCLC will develop brain metastases during the course of their disease.[53–57]

A correlation has been found between the treatment of brain metastases and median survival. Patients not receiving directed therapy can expect a less than 3-month median survival.[58,59] In addition to symptomatic relief gained with treatment, patients experience prolonged survival of up to 6 months when treated with whole-brain radiotherapy (WBRT).[51,60,61] Arbit and Wronski[52] demonstrated improved median survival to 9.4 months by using stereotactic radiosurgery to treat brain metastases. The availability of steroids and modern advances in neurologic imaging (i.e., MRI) with gadolinium, neurosurgical technique, and postoperative care has led to an increase in surgery in the treatment of these patients.[62–64] In addition to prolonged survival, the associated operative mortality is reported to be approximately 5% on average.[51]

Evaluation Upon discovering a brain lesion in a patient with a history of NSCLC, efforts should be directed at determining if it represents metastasis. Patients considered to be candidates for surgical resection should undergo extensive metastatic evaluation to assess for other sites of distant disease, as only 3% of patients with NSCLC develop an isolated and single operable brain metastasis. The use of highly sensitive brain MRI with contrast has significantly increased the rate at which occult, small asymptomatic brain lesions are identified. Nearly 10% to 15% of patients with advanced stage cancer (IIIb or IV) harbor occult brain metastasis. As imaging modalities continue to improve, a greater focus on the treatment of prevalent brain metastases will be required.

Symptomatic brain lesions are common, nearly half of all patients with brain metastasis experience, at the minimum, headaches.[65] Neurologic signs such as focal weakness or hemiparesis are almost as common, occurring in roughly 40% of patients. Other symptoms, such as dysphasia, seizures, and visual changes occur less frequently.[54,55,65] Interestingly, Pladdet et al.[65] found patients with metastatic adenocarcinoma tended, on the whole, to be less symptomatic than other non–small cell histologic types. Thus, we recommend that these patients be considered for further evaluation (i.e., brain MRI) if one has sufficient suspicion even in the absence of symptoms. Most patients with bulky hilar tumors (greater than T3) or suspicious or proven N2 (stage IIIa) disease should undergo brain MRI. CT scanning is much less sensitive.

CT and MRI scans are the primary radiologic studies used to evaluate brain lesions. CT scanning is occasionally better for smaller lesions as well as assessing the effect of steroid therapy, whereas MRI is better to evaluate the brainstem.[65,66] Considering that the majority of patients with brain metastases have up to three lesions at presentation, less than 50% can be offered surgical resection for local control. Unfortunately, only 30% to 50% of these patients are surgical candidates.[50,52,56,65,67–71] The presence of any of the criteria listed in Table 36.7 render a patient inoperable for brain metastasis.

TABLE 36.7 Criteria for Inoperable Brain Metastases

Surgically inaccessible location
Detection of other distant sites of metastatic non–small cell lung cancer
Poor medical condition
Anticipated life expectancy is less than 3 months

From Patchell RA, Cirrineione C, Thales HT, et al. Single brain metastases: surgery plus radiation or radiation alone. *Neurology* 1988;36:447–453.

A thorough search for other sites of recurrent NSCLC should be conducted prior to deciding if a patient is a candidate for curative treatment. Given the short survival of patients with brain metastases, aggressive treatment with surgical resection or radiosurgery should be considered as a palliative attempt to increase survival. In those patients with a solitary focus of metastasis, however, these approaches may offer potential chance of cure.

Treatment Treatment of brain metastases involves chemotherapy, external beam radiation (EBRT), brachytherapy, surgery, stereotactic radiosurgery, or a combination thereof. Selection of appropriate treatment modality is based on the patient's symptoms, medical condition, extent of cerebral disease, and the presence of extracranial disease. Unfortunately, there are no randomized trials comparing surgical resection and radiosurgery. A comparison of palliative treatment approaches, however, has yielded similar survival, disease control, morbidity, and mortality rates between the two modalities.[50,72] Chemotherapy should be considered as an adjunct to surgery or radiotherapy in the management of brain metastases after they have been controlled. Surgical resection and radiosurgery are considered to be comparable at this time, and the decision of which modality to use is individualized (Table 36.8), based on the characteristics of the metastatic bronchogenic lesions.

Prognosis The data reported by Detterbeck et al.[42] suggest better outcome for patients who are younger, of female gender, have metachronous lesions or supratentorial lesions, and tumors under 3 cm in diameter. These relative considerations, however, should not exclude other patients from complete resection. Regardless of whether the goal is cure or palliation, patients universally report an improvement in their symptoms with treatment,[69,73,74] and surgery combined with WBRT has been demonstrated to result in a survival benefit over WBRT alone. In fact, Magilligan Jr. et al.[70] experienced an average 2.3-year survival in their patients with a solitary brain metastasis treated with surgical resection. Average 5-year survival in completely resected patients has been reported to be approximately 20%,[50,70] with patients experiencing a only 2% operative mortality. Such survival data combined with low operative mortality support a more aggressive approach to such patients.

TABLE 36.8 Surgical Decision Making for Brain Metastases

	Surgery	Radiosurgery
Solitary with edema		✓
Large size	✓	
Superficial	✓	
Immediate symptom relief	✓	
Associated hemorrhage	✓	
Deep but diameter <3 cm	✓	
Medical contraindications for surgery		✓
Recurrent tumor	✓	

From Patchell RA, Cirrinicione C, Thaler HT, et al. Single brain metastases: surgery plus radiation or radiation alone. *Neurology* 1986;36:447–453.

ADRENAL METASTASIS

Although enlarged adrenal glands have been demonstrated in an appreciable proportion (4.1% to 15%)[2,75–77] of patients with operable bronchogenic carcinoma, only half of these lesions are proven to be metastatic lung cancer.[2,75] The majority of patients with adrenal metastases are asymptomatic, because more than 90% of the gland must be replaced before dysfunction is clinically evident. The solitary adrenal metastasis is extremely rare, occurring in 1.6% to 3.5% of patients.[78]

Evaluation CT is the primary modality used to evaluate the adrenal glands, and it is common practice to extend chest imaging to the level of the adrenals in patients with lung cancer. The rate of "incidentalomas" is 21%, with two thirds being benign adenomas. The sensitivity of CT scan is reported to be only 40% for adrenal metastasis[79]; however, Silverman et al.[28] cited a 96% accuracy when CT scanning is combined with FNAB. Percutaneous fine-needle biopsies may be nondiagnostic, and we consider a history of recent lung cancer and corroborating PET scan as sufficient for diagnosis of metastasis. We do not recommend routine needle biopsy of suspected adrenal metastases, unless biopsy findings will alter the treatment plan. If fine-needle biopsy is to be performed, the diagnosis of pheochromocytoma should be excluded first by measuring urine metanephrines.

According to Shea and Lillington,[80] MRI appears to be comparable to CT by detecting adrenal abnormalities in 10% to 20% of patients with lung cancer, with one third of the abnormalities representing metastatic lung cancer. Schwartz et al.[81] actually found the powerful technique of chemical shift MRI to be valuable in evaluating adrenal masses in patients with lung cancer. Its ability to detect fat within an adrenal mass with better specificity than CT scan yields a 96% sensitivity and 100% specificity for adenomas obviates the need for percutaneous biopsy in over one half of the patients.

PET or PET/CT has become a routine part of lung cancer staging. The sensitivity and specificity for adrenal metastasis were 100% and 80%, respectively, in 33 patients with bronchogenic carcinomas and adrenal masses.[82]

Treatment Neither laterality, histologic type, nor timing of the adrenal mass has been determined as prognostic factors in patients with lung cancer. Only nodal disease and the resectability of the primary lung tumor are important.[83–85] The literature suggests potential long-term survival benefit after adrenalectomy for metastatic NSCLC, with small series and isolated case reports. The treatment of isolated adrenal metastasis is surgical resection, preferably with a laparoscopic approach. Expedient resection of isolated adrenal mass as a laparoscopic approach may not be possible because of large tumor size or regional invasion of tumor. Most surgeons would initially address the lung tumor; however, there have been reports of combined resection with improved survival.[83,85]

Prognosis A recent systematic review by Tanvetyanon et al.[86] showed a 5-year survival of 25% for patients with surgically resected isolated adrenal metastases. Metachronous metastases have a somewhat better median survival compared with synchronous metastases that are surgically resected, but long-term survival is similar among the two groups. Long-term survival is rare without surgical resection.

OTHER METASTASIS

Surgery has sporadically been suggested to have a role in the management of metastatic bronchogenic carcinoma to other sites,[2,83,87] but it is mostly performed at the adrenal gland. Excluding the brain and adrenal gland, surgery should be considered for palliation in the management of metastatic NSCLC. Most skeletal metastatic lesions involve the axial skeleton, and only 5% of patients have an isolated bony lesion.[88] These patients are treated with palliative radiation therapy with the goal of restoring function.

Small bowel metastases have been described as an epiphenomenon of NSCLC, consisting of yet unidentified biologic characteristics that portend a higher metastatic potential of the bronchogenic carcinoma. Stenbygaard and Sørenson[89] reported a 4.6% incidence of small bowel involvement in 218 autopsy cases, with concurrent metastatic lesions in additional sites in all patients with small bowel metastases. Further investigation of small bowel involvement may lead to suggestions for neoadjuvant or adjunctive chemotherapy that may have an impact on long-term survival of patients with NSCLC.

Unfortunately, surgical extirpation has been reported in only a small group of advanced-stage patients, but has not been found to have a significant impact on cure or survival. Hasse[87] investigated the benefit of pleurectomy in five patients, and noted only one patient to be disease free postoperatively. Certainly, the presence of pleural metastases or malignant pleural effusion suggests surgery for palliation only.[90]

REFERENCES

1. LoCicero J III, Ponn RB, Daly BDT. Surgical treatment of non-small cell lung cancer. In: Shields TW, LoCicero J III, Ponn RB, eds. *General Thoracic Surgery*. Philadelphia: Lippincott Williams & Wilkins, 2000:1311.
2. Bilroth T, von Winiwarter A. *General Surgical Pathology and Therapeutics*. 10th Ed. [Translated from German ed.] New York: Appleton-Century-Crofts, 1983.
3. Martini N, Melamed MR. Multiple primary lung cancers. *J Thorac Cardiovasc Surg* 1975;70:606–612.
4. Antakli T, Schaefer RF, Rutherford JE, et al. Second primary lung cancer. *Ann Thorac Surg* 1995;59:863–866.
5. Rao J, Sayeed RA, Tomaszek S, et al. Prognostic factors in resected satellite-nodule T4 non-small cell lung cancer. *Ann Thorac Surg* 2007;84:934–938.
6. Bryant AS, Pereira SJ, Miller DL, et al. Satellite pulmonary nodule in the same lobe (T4N0) should not be staged as IIIB non-small cell lung cancer. *Ann Thorac Surg* 2006;82:1808–1813.
7. Deslauriers J, Brisson J, Cartier R, et al. Carcinoma of the lung. Evaluation of satellite nodules as a factor influencing prognosis after resection. *J Thorac Cardiovasc Surg* 1989;97(4):504–512.
8. Zell JA, Ou SH, Ziogas A, et al. Survival improvements for advanced stage nonbronchioloalveolar carcinoma-type nonsmall cell lung cancer cases with ipsilateral intrapulmonary nodules. *Cancer* 2008;112:136–143.
9. Mountain CF. Revisions in the international system for staging lung cancer. *Chest* 1997;111:1710–1717.
10. Ou SH, Zell JA. Validation study of the proposed IASLC staging revisions of the T4 and M non-small cell lung cancer descriptors using data from 23,583 patients in the California Cancer Registry. *J Thorac Oncol* 2008;3:216–227.
11. Roberts PF, Straznicka M, Lara PN, et al. Resection of multifocal non-small cell lung cancer when the bronchioloalveolar subtype is involved. *J Thorac Cardiovasc Surg* 2003;126:1597–1602.
12. Raz DJ, He B, Rosell R, et al. Bronchioloalveolar carcinoma: a review. *Clin Lung Cancer* 2006;7:313–322.
13. de Perrot M, Chernenko S, Waddell TK, et al. Role of lung transplantation in the treatment of bronchogenic carcinomas for patients with end-stage pulmonary disease. *J Clin Oncol* 2004;22:4351–4356.
14. Kunitoh H, Eguchi K, Yamada K, et al. Intrapulmonary sublesions detected before surgery in patients with lung cancer. *Cancer* 1992;70:1876–1879.
15. Jolly PC, Hutchinson CH, Detterbeck F, et al. Routine computed tomographic scans, selective mediastinoscopy, and other factors in evaluation of lung cancer. *Thorac Cardiovasc Surg* 1991;102:266–270.
16. Truong LD, Underwood RD, Greenberg SD, et al. Diagnosis and typing of lung carcinomas by cytopathologic methods: a review of 108 cases. *Acta Cytol* 1985;29:379–384.
17. Cataluña JJ, Perpiñá M, Greses JV, et al. Cell type accuracy of bronchial biopsy specimens in primary lung cancer. *Chest* 1996;109:1199–1203.
18. McElvaney G, Miller RR, Muller NL, et al. Multicentricity of adenocarcinoma of the lung. *Chest* 1989;95:151–154.
19. Tournoy KG, De Ryck F, Vanwalleghem LR, et al. Endoscopic ultrasound reduces surgical mediastinal staging in lung cancer: a randomized trial. *Am J Respir Crit Care Med* 2008;177:531–535.
20. Wallace MB, Pascual JM, Raimondo M, et al. Minimally invasive endoscopic staging of suspected lung cancer. *JAMA* 2008;299:540–546.
21. Ferguson MK, DeMeester TR, DesLauriers J, et al. Diagnosis and management of synchronous lung cancers. *J Thorac Cardiovasc Surg* 1985;89:378–385.
22. Okunaka T, Kato H, Konaka C, et al. Photodynamic therapy for multiple primary bronchogenic carcinoma. *Cancer* 1991;68:253–258.
23. Verhagen AF, van de Wal HJ, Cox AL, et al. Surgical treatment of multiple primary lung cancers. *J Thorac Cardiovasc Surg* 1989;37:107–111.
24. Klingman RR, DeMeester TR. Surgical approach to non-small cell lung cancer stage I and II. *Hematol Oncol Clin North Am* 1990;4:1079–1091. Review.
25. Rosengart TK, Martini N, Ghosn P, et al. Multiple primary lung carcinoma: prognosis and treatment. *Ann Thorac Surg* 1991;52:773–778.
26. Razzuk MA, Pockey M, Urschel HC Jr, et al. Dual primary bronchogenic carcinoma. *Ann Thorac Surg* 1974;17:425–433.
27. Deschamps C, Pairlero PC, Trastek VF, et al. Multiple primary lung cancers. Results of surgical treatment. *J Thorac Cardiovasc Surg* 1990;99:769–777.
28. Silverman SG, Mueller PR, Pinkney LP, et al. Predictive value of image-guided adrenal biopsy: analysis of results of 101 biopsies. *Radiology* 1993;187:715–718.

29. Pairolero PC, Williams DE, Bergstrahl EJ, et al. Postsurgical stage I bronchogenic carcinoma: morbid implications of recurrent disease. *Ann Thorac Surg* 1984;38:331–338.
30. Darteville P, Khlife J. Surgical approach to local recurrence and the second primary lesion. In: Delarue NC, Eschapasse H, eds. International Trends in General Thoracic Surgery. Philadelphia: WB Saunders, 1985:156.
31. Mathisen DJ, Jensik RJ, Faber LP, et al. Survival following resection for second and third primary lung cancers. *J Thorac Cardiovasc Surg* 1984;88:502–510.
32. Abbey-Smith R, Nigam BK, Thompson JM. Second primary lung carcinoma. *Thorax* 1976;17:425.
33. Salerno TA, Munro DD, Blundell PE, et al. Second primary bronchogenic carcinoma: life-table analysis of surgical treatment. *Ann Thorac Surg* 1979;27:3–6.
34. Rohwedder JJ, Weatherbee L. Multiple primary bronchogenic carcinoma with a review of the literature. *Am Rev Resp Dis* 1974;109: 435–445.
35. Shields TW. Multiple primary bronchial carcinomas. *Ann Thorac Surg* 1979;27:1–2.
36. Wu SC, Lin ZQ, Xu CW, et al. Multiple primary lung cancers. *Chest* 1987;92:892–896.
37. Adebonojo SA, Moritz DM, Danby CA. The results of modern surgical therapy for multiple primary lung cancers. *Chest* 1997;112:693–701.
38. Aziz TM, Saad RA, Glasser J, et al. The management of second primary lung cancers. A single centre experience in 15 years. *Eur J Cardiothorac Surg* 2002;21:527–533.
39. Bower SL, Choplin RH, Muss HB. Multiple primary bronchogenic carcinomas of the lung. *AJR Am J Roentgenol* 1983;140:253–258.
40. Spaggiaria L, Grunewal D, Girard P, et al. Cancer resection on the residual lung after pneumonectomy for bronchogenic carcinoma. *Ann Thorac Surg* 1996;62:1598–1602.
41. Feld R, Rubinstein LV, Weisenberger TH. Sites of recurrence in resected stage I non-small cell lung cancer: a guide for future studies. *J Clin Oncol* 1984;2:1352–1358.
42. Detterbeck FC, Jones DR, Funkhouser WK Jr. Satellite nodules and multiple primary cancers. In: Detterbeck FC, Rivera MP, Socinski MA, et al, eds. *Diagnosis and Treatment of Lung Cancer: an Evidence-Based Guide for the Practicing Clinician*. Philadelphia: WB Saunders, 2001:437.
43. Martini N, Bains MS, Burt ME, et al. Incidence of local recurrence and second primary tumors in resected stage I lung cancer. *J Thorac Cardiovasc Surg* 1995;109:120–129.
44. Spaggiari L, Grunewald D, Girard P, et al. Cancer resection on the residual lung after pneumonectomy for bronchogenic carcinoma. *Ann Thorac Surg* 1996;62:1598–1602.
45. Vaaler AK, Hosannah HO, Wagner RB. Pneumonectomy after contralateral lobectomy: is it reasonable? *Ann Thorac Surg* 1995;59:178–182.
46. Payne CR, Hadfield JW, Stovin PG, et al. Diagnostic accuracy of cytology and biopsy in primary bronchial carcinoma. *J Clin Pathol* 1981;34:773–778.
47. Verhagen AF, Tavilla G, van de Wal HJ, et al. Multiple primary lung cancers. *Thorac Cardiovasc Surg* 1994;42:40–44.
48. Van Bodegom PC, Wagenaar SS, Corrin B, et al. Second primary lung cancer: importance of long term follow up. *Thorax* 1989;44:788–793.
49. Ribet M, Dambron P. Multiple primary lung cancers. *Eur J Cardiothorac Surg* 1995;9:231–236.
50. Merchut MP. Brain metastases from undiagnosed systemic neoplasms. *Arch Int Med* 1989;149:1076–1080.
51. Detterbeck FC, Jones DR, Molina PL. Extrathoracic staging. In: Detterbeck FC, Rivera MP, Socinski MA, et al., eds. *Diagnosis and Treatment of Lung Cancer: An Evidence-Based Guide for the Practicing Clinician*. Philadelphia: WB Saunders, 2001:94.
52. Arbit E, Wronski M. Clinical decision making in brain metastases. *Neurosurg Clin North Am* 1996;7:447–457.
53. Mandell L, Hilaris B, Sullivan M, et al. The treatment of single brain metastasis from non-oat cell lung carcinoma. *Cancer* 1986;58:641–649.
54. Sundaresan N, Galicich JH, Beattie EJ Jr. Surgical treatment of brain metastases from lung cancer. *J Neurosurg* 1983;58:666–671.
55. Torre M, Quaini E, Chiesa G, et al. Synchronous brain metastasis from lung cancer: result of surgical treatment in combined resection. *J Thorac Cardiovasc Surg* 1988;95:994–997.
56. Rizzi A, Tondini M, Rocco G, et al. Lung cancer with a single brain metastasis: therapeutic options. *Tumori* 1990;76:579–581.
57. Cox JD, Yesner RA. Adenocarcinoma of the lung: recent results from VA lung group. *Am Rev Resp Dis* 1979;120:1025–1029.
58. Richards P, McKissock W. Intracranial metastases. *Br Med J* 1963;1:15–18.
59. Stoier M. Metastatic tumors of the brain. *Acta Neurol Scand* 1965;41:262–278.
60. Galicich JH, French LA, Melby JC. Use of dexamethasone in treatment of cerebral edema associated with brain tumors. *Lancet* 1961;1:46–53.
61. Posner JB, Shapiro WR. Brain tumor: current status of treatment and its complications. *Arch Neurol* 1975;32:781–784.
62. Winston KR, Walsh JW, Fischer EG. Results of operative treatment of intracranial metastatic tumors. *Cancer* 1980;45:2639–2645.
63. Galicich JH, Sundaresan N, Thaler HT. Surgical treatment of single brain metastasis: evaluation of results by computerized tomography scanning. *J Neurosurg* 1980;53:63–67.
64. Sundaresan N, Galicich JH. Surgical treatment of brain metastases: clinical and computerized tomography evaluation of the results of treatment. *Cancer* 1985;55:1382–1388.
65. Pladdet I, Boven E, Nauta J, et al. Palliative care for brain metastasis of solid tumor types. *Neth J Med* 1989;34:10–21.
66. Tarver RD, Richmond BD, Klatte EC. Cerebral metastases from lung carcinoma: neurological and CT correlation. *Radiology* 1984;153:689–692.
67. Galuzzi S, Payne PM. Bronchial carcinoma: a statistical study of 741 necropsies with special reference to the distribution of blood born metastases. *Br J Cancer* 1955;9:511–527.
68. Vieth RG, Odom GL. Intracranial metastases and their neurosurgical treatment. *J Neurosurg* 1965;23:375–383.
69. Magilligan DJ Jr, Rogers JS, Knighton RS, et al. Pulmonary neoplasm with solitary cerebral metastasis: results of combined excision. *J Thorac Cardiovasc Surg* 1976;76:690–698.
70. Magilligan DJ Jr, Duvernoy C, Malik G, et al. Surgical approach to lung cancer with solitary cerebral metastasis: twenty-five years experience. *Ann Thorac Surg* 1986;42:360–364.
71. Deviri E, Schachner A, Halevy A, et al. Carcinoma of lung with a solitary cerebral metastasis: surgical management and review of the literature. *Cancer* 1983;52:1507–1509. Review.
72. Bindal AK, Bindal RK, Hess KR, et al. Surgery versus radiosurgery in the treatment of brain metastases. *J Neurosurg* 1996;84:748–754.
73. Patchell RA, Cirrinicione C, Thaler HT, et al. Single brain metastases: surgery plus radiation or radiation alone. *Neurology* 1986;36:447–453.
74. Burt M, Wronski M, Arbit E, et al. Resection of brain metastases from non-small cell lung carcinoma: results of treatment. *Thorac Cardiovasc Surg* 1992;103:399–410.
75. Oliver TW Jr, Bernardino ME, Miller JI, et al. Isolated adrenal masses in non small-cell bronchogenic carcinoma. *Radiology* 1984;153:217–218.
76. Dunnick NR, Ihde DC, Johnston-Early A. Abdominal CT in the evaluation of small cell carcinoma of the lung. *AJR Am J Roentgenol* 1979;133:1085–1088.
77. Cromartie RS III, Parker EF, May JE, et al. Carcinoma of the lung: a clinical review. *Ann Thorac Surg* 1980;30:30–35.
78. Porte H, Siat J, Guibert B, et al. Resection of adrenal metastases from non-small cell lung cancer: a multi-institutional study. *Ann Thorac Surg* 2001;71:981–985.
79. Allard P, Yankaskas BC, Fletcher RH, et al. Sensitivity and specificity of computed tomography for the detection of adrenal metastatic lesions among 91 autopsied lung cancer patients. *Cancer* 1990;66:457–462.
80. Shea J, Lillington GA. Preoperative staging of lung cancer. *West J Med* 1994;161:508–509.
81. Schwartz LH, Ginsberg MS, Burt ME, et al. MRI as an alternative to CT-guided biopsy of adrenal masses in patients with lung cancer. *Ann Thorac Surg* 1998;65:193–197.

82. Erasmus JJ, Patz EF Jr, McAdams HP, et al. Evaluation of adrenal masses in patients with bronchogenic carcinoma using 18F-fluorodeoxyglucose positron emission tomography. *AJR Am J Roentgenol* 1997;168:1357–1360.
83. Warren S, Gates O. Multiple primary malignant tumors: a survey of the literature and a statistical study. *Am J Cancer* 1932;16:1358.
84. Raviv G, Klein E, Yellin A, et al. Surgical treatment of solitary adrenal metastases from lung cancer. *J Surg Oncol* 1990;43:123–124.
85. Reyes L, Parvez Z, Nemoto T, et al. Adrenalectomy for adrenal metastasis from lung carcinoma. *J Surg Oncol* 1990;44:32–34.
86. Tanvetyanon T, Robinson LA, Schell MJ, et al. Outcomes of adrenalectomy for isolated synchronous versus metachronous adrenal metastases in non-small-cell lung cancer: a systematic review and pooled analysis. *J Clin Oncol* 2008;26:1142–1147.
87. Hasse J. Surgery in bronchial carcinoma with metastasis. *Lung* 1990; 168(Suppl):1145–1152.
88. Krishnamuthy GT, Tubis M, Hiss J, et al. Distribution pattern of metastatic bone disease. A need for total body skeletal image. *JAMA* 1977;237(23):2504–2506.
89. Stenbygaard LE, Sørensen JB. Small bowel metastases in non-small cell lung cancer. *Lung Cancer* 1999;26:95–101.
90. Lynch TJ Jr. Management of malignant pleural effusions. *Chest* 1996; 103:S385–S389.
91. Bewtra C. Multiple primary bronchogenic carcinomas with a review of the literature. *J Surg Oncol* 1984;25:207–213.
92. Yoshino I, Nakanishi R, Osaki T, et al. Postoperative prognosis in patients with non-small cell lung cancer with synchronous ipsilateral intrapulmonary metastasis. *Ann Thorac Surg* 1997;64(3):809–813.
93. van Rens MT, Zanen P, de la Rivière AB, et al. Survival after resection of metachronous non-small cell lung cancer in 127 patients. *Ann Thorac Surg* 2001;71(1):309–313.
94. Pommier RF, Vetto JT, Lee JT, et al. Synchronous non-small cell lung cancers. *Am J Surg* 1996;171(5):521–524.
95. Ferguson MK, DeMeester TR, DesLauriers J, et al. Diagnosis and management of synchronous lung cancers. *J Thorac Cardiovasc Surg* 1985;89(3):378–385.
96. Okada M, Tsubota N, Yoshimura M, et al. Evaluation of TMN classification for lung carcinoma with ipsilateral intrapulmonary metastasis. *Ann Thorac Surg* 1999;68(2):326–330.
97. Doddoli C, Thomas P, Ghez O, et al. Surgical management of metachronous bronchial carcinoma. *Eur J Cardiothorac Surg* 2001;19(6): 899–903.

CHAPTER 37

Shawn Haji-Momenian
Ricardo S. Santos
Hiran C. Fernando
Damian E. Dupuy

Percutaneous Therapeutic Technologies for Medically Inoperable Lung Cancer

Lung cancer is the number one cause of cancer death in the United States, accounting annually for approximately 160,000 deaths per year.[1] If diagnosed at an early stage, surgical resection of non–small cell lung cancer (NSCLC) offers the best opportunity for local control and survival. However, it is estimated that more than 15% of all patients and 30% of those aged 75 years or older diagnosed with stage I or II NSCLC will be considered medically inoperable.[2] The majority of these patients are not surgical candidates because of their poor cardiopulmonary function.

For many years since the first pulmonary resections described by Churchill et al.[3] in the early 20th century, pneumonectomy and, subsequently, lobectomy were considered the standard operations for lung cancer. Sublobar resection for stage I NSCLC then emerged as an attractive option, but was subsequently demonstrated to be associated with a threefold increase in local recurrence in the randomized trial conducted by the Lung Cancer Study Group[4] during the late 1980s and early 1990s (see Chapters 32 and 33).

Since the publication of that study, most surgeons consider sublobar resections (such as a wedge or segmentectomy) a compromise operation that should be reserved for patients who are felt to be at increased risk for lobectomy, but can still tolerate a smaller pulmonary resection.[5,6] With the increasing identification of smaller cancers, particularly with implementation of computed tomography (CT) screening programs, this approach is being challenged, particularly for small stage I cancers. Further discussion of sublobar resection for small-diameter cancers is found in Chapters 32 and 33.

One approach that has been described to minimize local recurrence when sublobar resection is performed is the use of adjuvant intraoperative brachytherapy.[7] Initial results have been encouraging, with a multicenter trial of this technique currently underway. For patients that are considered too high risk for any resection, the standard therapy has been external beam radiation. An alternative to radiotherapy (XRT) is percutaneous image-guided tumor ablation, which has been used for various solid tumors, including liver, kidney, breast, bone, adrenal, and is now proving to be an important tool in the treatment of primary and secondary lung neoplasms. Radiofrequency ablation (RFA) is the current ablative method of choice, although other techniques including microwave ablation (MWA) and cryoablation are also available. In this chapter, we review these alternative therapies that can be used for the high-risk patient with NSCLC.

SUBLOBAR RESECTION AND BRACHYTHERAPY

Higher local recurrence remains the primary problem of sublobar resection for NSCLC. In an effort to improve local control, postoperative external beam XRT following sublobar resection can be used. Miller and Hatcher[8] used this approach on a small group of patients who were treated with sublobar resection followed by "postage stamp" external beam radiation. The authors reported a significant decrease in local recurrence compared with an earlier group of patients they had managed with sublobar resection alone.

Unfortunately, this approach is not easy to apply to most of the high-risk patients with NSCLC where sublobar resection is selected. Many of these elderly patients are unwilling to travel for several radiation treatments. Additionally, radiation treatment planning is challenging, because it can be difficult to target small areas around the staple line, particularly if this is in a region of lung that moves with respiration. Radiation pneumonitis is also a potentially life-threatening problem, particularly for patients with impaired pulmonary function, who are the typical candidates referred for these compromise therapies.

An alternative option is the intraoperative placement of ^{125}Iodine (^{125}I) brachytherapy seeds along the staple line after sublobar resection.[7,9] This brachytherapy technique utilizes a commercially available vicryl suture that contains 10 ^{125}I pellets incorporated at 1-cm intervals along the length of the suture (Oncura, Arlington Heights, IL). In the first report describing this technique, these vicryl sutures were placed on a vicryl mesh. Usually 40 to 60 ^{125}I pellets with four to five lines of suture material are used with each brachytherapy implant. The total delivered radiation dose to the local tissues (staple line) is usually around 10,000 cGY at a 1-cm distance from the staple line. In essence, this technique effectively extended the margin of resection by another centimeter. The advantage of using intraoperative brachytherapy compared with external beam radiation therapy is that this is a one-time treatment, with 100% patient compliance. There is no burden placed on the patient to return for several radiation therapies after recovering from their operation. Additionally, the radiation is delivered directly at the staple line with minimal injury to surrounding lung parenchyma.

An alternative technique to that described previously is to place the ^{125}I sutures directly adjacent to the staple line without the use of mesh. This technique of "paired" ^{125}I suture lines was described by Lee et al.[10] The authors reported the use of brachytherapy "paired-suture line" technique in 33 high-risk patients, primarily after wedge resection. The local recurrence rate was 6.1%, which was similar to the 6.4% reported after lobectomy in the Lung Cancer Study Group study.

A larger study from Pittsburgh utilizing the mesh technique compared the results of sublobar resection with adjuvant ^{125}I brachytherapy in 101 patients with a historical control group of 102 patients who underwent sublobar resection alone; both groups had poor cardiopulmonary function.[9] A significant reduction in local recurrence was noticed with the use of brachytherapy (18% vs. 2%). There was no evidence of radiation fibrosis or implant migration among patients receiving ^{125}I brachytherapy (Fig. 37.1). Another multicenter study of stage IA patients undergoing lobar and sublobar resection was also reported.[11] Included in the study cohort were 124 patients who underwent sublobar resection. Brachytherapy was used in 60 of 124 patients. A decrease in local recurrence from 17.2% to 3.3% was demonstrated in the patients treated with adjuvant brachytherapy. More recently, Birdas et al.[12] analyzed the local recurrence, disease-free survival, and overall survival for patients with stage IB cancer who underwent lobectomy (n = 126) versus sublobar resection with brachytherapy (n = 41). Local recurrence was similar between the groups (3% to 5%), with no statistical difference in survival or disease-free interval.

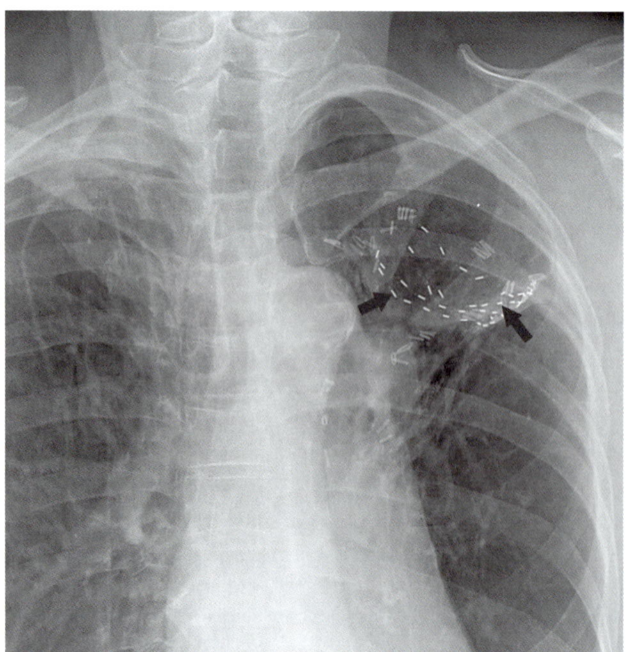

FIGURE 37.1 Chest radiograph demonstrating the ^{125}Iodine implant following sublobar resection.

One concern with the technique of brachytherapy is the radiation risk posed to the staff caring for the patient, as well as to the patient's family. Smith et al.[13] have addressed this risk in a prospective study of 22 patients who underwent ^{125}I vicryl mesh implantations. Diodes to measure radiation exposure were placed on the back of each hand of the primary radiation oncologist and primary surgeon during the creation and implantation of the mesh. A control reading was obtained by placing diodes on the posterior shoulder of the patient. The authors concluded that there is very little radiation exposure: 1 and 2 mrem/h for the radiation oncologist and surgeon, respectively. Median dose to the control diode on the patient was 5.4 mrem/h. Although the ALARA (as low as reasonably achievable) principle should still be followed, this is a safe method of lung cancer treatment for healthcare professionals. As a precaution beyond state and national radiation guidelines, general recommendations postoperatively for the patients include avoiding close contact with small children or pregnant women for the first 3 months following surgery.

The results of these single-center studies of sublobar resection and brachytherapy have been encouraging. A phase III study of this technique in stage IA NSCLC patients who are at high risk for lobectomy is currently underway by the American College of Surgeons Oncology Group (Z4032). This study will better define the role of adjuvant brachytherapy when sublobar resection is selected for NSCLC.

PERCUTANEOUS IMAGE-GUIDED ABLATION FOR NSCLC

Mechanism Percutaneous image-guided ablation is performed using various thermal energy sources, including radiofrequency (RF), microwave (MW), high-intensity focused ultrasound, laser, and cryoablation to kill tumor cells. These techniques are being applied with increasing frequency for several cancers. The most commonly used ablative modality for NSCLC has been RFA, although some centers are using MWA and cryoablation.

Heat-based ablative methods are effective means of depositing energy into a discrete focus via percutaneously placed electrodes. The volume of heat ablation is dependent on the temperature distribution within the tissue, which often has heterogeneous composition and perfusion. The heat distribution in a target lesion was described by Pennes' "bioheat" equation[14] in 1948. This equation can be simplified to a first approximation as "necrosis = energy deposited × local tissue interactions − heat loss."[15]

Cellular homeostasis can be achieved with mild temperature elevation of approximately 40°C. Hyperthermic states (42°C to 45°C) cause cellular susceptibility to chemotherapy and radiation therapy.[16,17] Cellular death does not occur at these elevated temperatures, however, and continued cellular proliferation has been observed even after prolonged exposure to these temperatures. Long-term exposure to temperatures above 46°C can cause irreversible cellular damage. Increasing the temperature by a few degrees to 50°C to 52°C markedly shortens the time necessary to induce cytotoxicity (down to 4 to 6 minutes).

Between 60°C and 100°C, there is near instantaneous induction of protein coagulation that results in irreversible damage to critical cytosolic and mitochondrial proteins and nucleic acid–histone complexes. Cells experiencing this degree of thermal damage immediately die and undergo coagulative necrosis over the course of several days. *Coagulative necrosis* denotes irreversible thermal damage and cellular death regardless of the ultimate microscopic findings, which may not meet histologic criteria for coagulation necrosis. Temperatures greater than 105°C to 115°C result in tissue boiling, vaporization, and carbonization.[18] These processes limit optimal ablation as a result of the insulating effects of the produced gas, which decreases the amount of energy deposited, and reduces thermal conduction into the lesion. The goal of ablative therapies is to achieve stable temperatures ranging between 60°C and 100°C throughout the entire volume of the lesion.

Technique

Radiofrequency Ablation RFA is currently the most robust technique for the treatment of solid malignancies. RFA has become the ablative method of choice because of its relatively low cost, its capability of creating large regions of coagulative necrosis in a controlled fashion, and its relatively low toxicity. RFA applies to all electromagnetic energy sources with frequencies less than 30 MHz, although most clinically available devices function in the 375- to 500-kHz range. The technique for thermal ablation utilizing RFA was first described in animal lung tumor models in 1995,[19] and reported in human lungs in 2000.[20]

Percutaneous RFA deposits energy into the local tissue environment by converting RF waves into heat via ionic vibrations, elevating cellular temperatures, and causing necrosis. RF electrodes are available in various lengths and have an insulated shaft and an uninsulated conductive "active tip" that emits the RF current (Fig. 37.2). When possible, the electrode is positioned along the long axis of the lesion, and advanced into deepest margin of the lesion for the first treatment. The more proximal margins of the tumor can then be treated by retracting the electrode and administering an additional treatment. Larger tumors can be treated by repositioning the electrode into a new portion of the tumor 1.5 to 2 cm away from the initial longitudinal axis of the previous treatment.

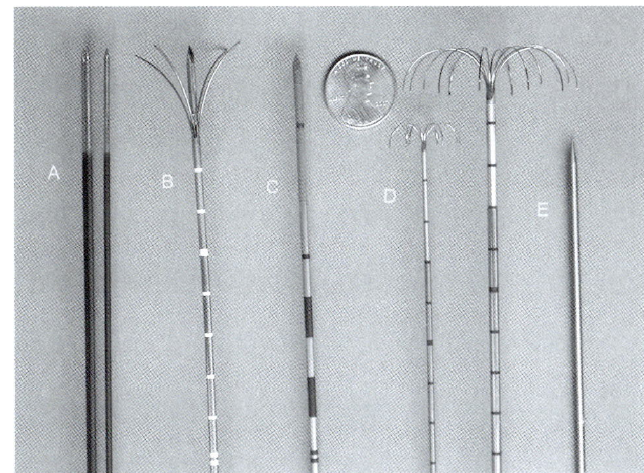

FIGURE 37.2 Commercially available radiofrequency, microwave, and cryoablation probes. (*A*) Valleylab Cool-tip Cluster RF electrode. (*B*) RITA Talon infusion RF electrode. (*C*) Valleylab Vivawave MW antenna. (*D*) Boston Scientific small and large Levine RF electrode. (*E*) Endocare PERC-24 cryoapplicator.

The RF electrode is coupled to the RF generator and grounded by means of a grounding pad applied to the opposite side of the chest wall or the thigh. The generator produces a voltage between the two electrodes, establishing lines of electrical field that oscillate with the alternating current. This oscillating electrical field causes ionic vibrations in proportion to the field intensity. Tissue heating occurs by frictional or resistive energy loss caused by ionic motion from the current.[21] Tissue heating more than temperatures of 60°C for varying amounts of time leads to coagulation necrosis and, ultimately, cell death.[22]

The volume of ablation is based on the energy balance between heat conduction of the local RF energy and the heat convection from the circulating blood and extracellular fluid. In the lung, RF energy is efficiently deposited because the surrounding air acts as an insulator (concentrating the energy within the lesion), and the high pulmonary vascular flow acts as a "heat sink" that dissipates heat from normal parenchyma. Although this will have a protective effect on the surrounding normal parenchyma and pulmonary vasculature, this peripheral heat sink will also limit the therapeutic ablation margins surrounding the lesion, which is important to prevent local recurrence.

Currently in the United States, there are three commercially available RFA systems. Two of the systems (Radiotherapeutics, Boston Scientific, Watertown, MA and RITA Medical Systems Inc., Mountain View, CA) utilize a deployable array RF electrode that consists of 4 to 16 small wires (tines) deployed through a 14- to 17-gauge needle. Because the tines curve backward toward the handle, the Boston Scientific device (Leveen electrode) is initially deployed at the deep aspect of the tumor. In contrast, the RITA electrode tines course forward and lateral so the probe is deployed on the near surface of the tumor. The Leveen electrode measures only impedance, and treatment time depends on repeated rises in impedance during active heating to achieve adequate thermocoagulation. With the RITA system electrodes, temperature readings are obtained throughout the ablation cycle through multiple peripheral thermocouples. The third RF system (Radionics CC-1, Valleylab, Boulder, CO) utilizes a single or triple "cluster" (three single electrodes spaced 5 mm apart) perfused electrode; the tip is positioned at the deepest aspect of the tumor. The single or cluster RF electrode contains a thermocouple embedded in its tip, used to measure intratumoral temperature. A switching controller can be used with the Valleylab system, allowing for the placement of up to three separate single electrodes spaced 2 to 2.5 cm apart, increasing the duty cycle of the generator and allowing for the creation of a greater volume of tissue thermocoagulation compared with three separate ablations with a single electrode.

The effective local control and safety profile of percutaneous RFA has been firmly established in the treatment of numerous solid malignancies, including those in liver, bone, lung, breast, kidney, and adrenals. As of this writing, there have been no head-to-head comparisons of safety and efficacy between these devices in the lung.

Microwave Ablation Like RFA, MWA utilizes electromagnetic waves to produce tissue heating effects. Unlike RFA, however, the microwave energy spectrum lies in a much higher frequency range, extending from 300 MHz to 300 GHz; microwave probes available for clinical use generally operate in the 900- to 2450-MHz range.[23] Microwave tissue heating occurs as a result of the induction of kinetic energy in surrounding water molecules. Because of their electron configuration, water molecules are highly polar and function as small electrical dipoles with the negative charges preferentially localized around the oxygen nucleus. The rapidly alternating electric field of the microwave probe causes water molecules to rapidly spin in an attempt to align with electromagnetic charges of opposite polarity. These spinning water molecules interact with neighboring tissues, transferring a portion of their kinetic energy. Because temperature is merely a proxy measurement of molecular kinetic energy, this energy transfer results in local tissue hyperthermia. Currently, in the United States, there is one commercially available microwave system (VivawWave, Valleylab, Boulder, CO) that utilizes a 915-MHz generator and straight antennae with active tips of 3.7 cm (Fig. 37.2). Cooling of the antennae shaft with infused room temperature saline reduces conductive heating of the nonactive portion of the applicator, thus preventing damage to the skin and tissues proximal to the active tip.

Cryoablation Cryoablation, with the local application of liquid nitrogen directly or within sealed metal cryoprobes, has been used to treat tumors in the operating room setting for more than 3 decades. With the development of the argon-based cryoablation systems, which are now widely available, cryotherapy applicator diameters have decreased significantly, making the percutaneous utilization of this technique to other sites of disease more feasible than ever before.[24]

Cryoablation involves the insertion of one or more hollow needles (cryoprobes) directly into a tumor, under image guidance. The probes are filled with pressurized argon gas and cooled to temperatures as low as −140°C via the Joule-Thomson effect (in which the expansion of compressed gas through a small gap causes a temperature drop). The extreme cold at the tip of the probe creates an expanding ice ball that freezes the surrounding tissue as it progresses. At temperatures of below −40°C, cryogenic destruction of living tissue occurs via several mechanisms, including protein denaturation, osmotic shifts in intracellular and extracellular water, membrane destabilization, cell rupture, and tissue ischemia. Currently, there are two commercially available percutaneous argon-based cryoablation devices available (CryoHit, Galil Medical, Plymouth Meeting, PA and Cryocare, Endocare Inc., Irvine, CA; Fig. 37.2). These systems allow the placement of between 1 and 15 individual 1.5- to 2.4-mm diameter cryoprobes. Typically, a freeze-thaw-freeze cycle in a single probe position is used to achieve local tumor necrosis. Ice ball visualization under CT or MR imaging allows for direct comparison of kill zone with respect to tumor margins, and allows for accounting of a cytotoxic ice margin of 3 to 5 mm within the most peripheral aspect of the ice ball.

Clinical Results of Thermal Ablative Therapies

The current standard therapy for patients considered high risk for surgical resection is external beam XRT. A previous study[25] of 71 node-negative patients who received at least 60 Gy showed 3- and 5-year survival rates of 19% and 12%, respectively. In another report of 60 patients treated with XRT for stage I/II cancers, local progression occurred in 53% of patients, with a median progression-free survival of 18.5 months and overall median survival of 20 months.[26] A metaanalysis[27] evaluating the efficacy of radical XRT alone for stage I/II medically inoperable NSCLC patients found an overall 5-year survival rate of 0% to 42%, with local failure rates ranging from 6% to 70%. These studies demonstrate marginal efficacy of XRT in eradicating pulmonary tumors and argue for the development of minimally invasive therapies such as RFA to treat these high-risk NSCLC patients.

Radiofrequency Ablation RFA has been used in the treatment of lung tumors for several years. In 2000, Dupuy et al.[28] published the first report of the use of RFA for the treatment of lung malignancies. As previously mentioned, many factors affect the efficacy of complete tumor ablation, including tumor histology, size, and location. Studies have demonstrated that complete tumor ablation is more likely in lesions less than 3 to 5 cm. The majority of these studies are retrospective reviews of institutional experience.

In a series of 27 patients with NSCLC and 4 patients with lung metastases by Lee et al.,[29] complete tumor necrosis (as confirmed by a mean follow-up imaging of 12.5 months) was demonstrated in all 6 patients with lesions less than 3 cm, but only 23% complete ablation (in 6 of 26 patients) in lesions greater than 3 cm. There was at least 50% tumor necrosis among the 20 lesions (62%) with incomplete necrosis. They also noted at least a 5-mm well-demarcated nonenhancing zone of ground-glass opacity surrounding the ablated lesion in 8 of the 12 cases of complete necrosis. None of these patients demonstrated any local tumor recurrence on follow-up imaging (mean 22.2 months).

Akeboshi et al.[30] similarly demonstrated higher rates of complete tumor necrosis in a series of 54 ablated lung neoplasms. There was a 69% rate of complete tumor necrosis in 36 lesions less than 3 cm, and 39% complete necrosis in 18 tumors larger than 3 cm; tumor type did not influence the rate of necrosis. Yasui et al.[31] achieved a 91% rate of complete tumor necrosis among 99 neoplasms with a mean diameter of 1.9 cm (based on stable CT size and follow-up biopsy of one third of the lesions). All of the studies mentioned used the Valleylab RFA system, and most used a single electrode rather than a cluster probe. The expandable RFA electrodes such as the Boston Scientific or RITA probes theoretically allow a larger diameter of ablation.

In another study,[32] using the Boston Scientific system, 33 tumors were ablated in 18 patients. Results were superior in patients with tumors 5 cm or less. Response (as defined by a composite score comprising of tumor mass, tumor quality, and, when indicated, [positron emission tomography] PET) was seen in 66% of the patients with tumors 5 cm or less compared with only 33% in those patients with tumors >5 cm. Additionally, 33% of the patients with small tumors were not alive at follow-up, compared with 66% in those patients with larger tumors. This experience demonstrates that that recurrence rates are directly related to completeness of tumor necrosis, which not surprisingly is dependent on tumor diameter.

Another series of 18 NSCLC patients with RFA has also been previously reported.[33] The median tumor diameter was 2.8 cm. Nine patients had stage I cancers. Fifteen (83.3%) of the patients were alive at a median follow-up of 14 months. For the stage I cancers, the mean progression–free interval in this study was 17.6 months. The median progression–free interval was not reached, with only three (33%) of these patients demonstrating local progression. More recently, these results have been updated in a group of 19 stage I NSCLC patients,[34] who had a median forced expiratory volume (FEV) 1% of 29%, making them high-risk surgical candidates. During follow-up, local progression occurred in eight (42%) patients, with a median time to progression of 27 months. There were no procedure-related mortalities, and six deaths occurred during follow-up. The probability of survival at 1 year was estimated to be 95%.

A large multicenter study known as the RAPTURE (Radiofrequency Ablation of Pulmonary Tumors Response Evaluation) trial[35] included 106 patients. In this study, there were 33 NSCLC patients. The 2-year overall survival was 48%. However, most of these high-risk patients died from noncancer-related causes, as indicated by their cancer-specific survival, which was much higher at 92%.

The long-term outcomes in a cohort of 153 patients were also recently reported.[36] This study included 75 stage I NSCLC patients. Median survival for the NSCLC group was 29 months. Overall survival at 1, 2, 3, 4, and 5 years was 78%, 57%, 36%, 27%, and 27%, respectively. Local tumor progression was reported for all tumors rather than by tumor type. The key finding was that there were differences in local control between tumors 3 cm or less in size compared with tumors larger than 3 cm. In patients with smaller tumors, median time to progression was 45 months, and 1-, 2-, 3-, 4-, and 5-year progression-free rates were 83%, 64%, 57%, 47%, and 47%, respectively. In the patients with larger tumors, median time to progression was 12 months and the progression-free rates at 1, 2, 3, 4, and 5 years were 45%, 25%, 25%, 25%, and 25%, respectively. It should be noted that all ablations were performed using the single-electrode or cluster-tip Valleylab probes, which may not as effective for tumors larger than 3 cm. However, this study supports the earlier argument that therapeutic outcomes will be better with smaller cancers.

Microwave Ablation To date, there have been two reports regarding MWA[37,38] of pulmonary tumors. The largest study is by Wolf et al., using a 914-MHz VivaWave microwave system in 50 patients who underwent 66 percutaneous MWAs for 82 intraparenchymal pulmonary masses without chest wall involvement. Patients were followed for a mean period of 10 ± 6.8 months, and during this time, 22% of patients (11 of 50) were found to have recurrent disease distant from the ablation site. Progressive disease within the treated lobe, but not at the ablation site, was found in 9 of 11 patients, and new metastatic foci in untreated lobes or organs were found in 2 of 11 patients as evidenced by enhancement on routine contrast-enhanced CT or ^{18}F-fluorodeoxyglucose (FDG) avidity on PET scan. This resulted in a 1-year local control rate of 67% ± 10% with a mean of 16.2 ± 1.3 months to first recurrence distant from the ablation site. Presence of residual enhancing tumor was more commonly found in follow-up of treated tumors greater than 3 cm. Thus, index tumor size greater than 3 cm was predictive of residual disease in these patients (p = 0.01). The Kaplan-Meier median time to death for all patients (n = 50) resulting from any cause, including the pulmonary malignancy being treated, was 19 ±1 months. The 1-, 2-, and 3-year actuarial survival rates were 65% ± 7%, 55% ± 9%, and 45% ± 11%, respectively. Analysis of cancer-specific mortality yielded a median time to death of 22 ± 1 months, and 1-, 2-, and 3-year survival rates of 83% ± 6%, 73% ± 9%, and 61% ± 13%, respectively.

Wolf et al. also discussed the radiographic evolution of an ablated tumor, noting that the ablated index tumor changed in appearance, demonstrating the effects of thermally induced coagulation necrosis. A hazy, "ground-glass" opacification was most commonly observed within and extending from the zone of ablation penetrated by well-defined antennae tracts. At 1-, 3-, and 6-month intervals, ablated tumors (zones of ablation) were measured, and mean maximum postablation diameters were compared with index dimensions. Preliminary data revealed an initial increase in size ($t[158] = 2.4$ cm; $p = 0.02$), with a mean increase in maximum diameter of 0.65 ± 0.27 cm, caused by thermal changes in adjacent lung tissue, followed by a persistent reduction in diameter consistent with consolidation. Cavitary changes were identified in 35 of 82 (43%) treated tumors (26 of 50 patients, 52%), and had a statistically significant relation to cancer-specific mortality ($p = 0.02$). No intraprocedural deaths occurred; pneumothoraces occurred in 39% of the ablations, 69% of which did not require chest tube placement. Of the 26 pneumothoraces, 8 required chest tube placement. Two patients experienced intraprocedural skin burns, one of which required surgical debridement and plastic surgery reconstruction.

Cryoablation To date, there is only one report of percutaneous lung cryoablation. Wang et al.[39] reported the technique, feasibility, and safety profile of the procedure for thoracic malignancy in 187 patients (89% of patients had advanced cancer and had failed conventional therapy). Complete ice ball coverage for peripheral lesions less than 4 cm was 100%, with 80% success rate for complete ice ball coverage in lesions greater than 4 cm. Tumor size and location were highly predictive of tumor ice coverage even when controlled for tumor stage and type. By 6 months, 86% of the CT scans available were stable or smaller than the original tumor. A short follow-up period precluded any accurate survival estimates, but palliative benefits of cryoablation were noted in terms of the Karnofsky Performance Status scale and general health status (e.g., increased dietary intake and weight gain).

Combination Ablation and Radiotherapy As discussed earlier, local tissue factors and vital adjacent structures can limit the volume of coagulation necrosis, leaving incomplete tumor margins with potential for residual disease. This provides ample argument for the combining thermal therapy with other treatments, including chemotherapy, chemoembolization, and XRT. Multimodality insult to tumor cells can only serve to increase the potential for cell death. Synergy between chemotherapeutic agents and hyperthermic temperatures (42°C to 45°C) has already been established.[40,41] Combining RFA with additional therapies is one of the many topics of ablation currently under research, intended to mirror the current literature supporting the multidisciplinary approach that includes surgery, chemotherapy, and XRT. Preliminary results are already suggesting that combination therapy of RFA and XRT has improved local control and survival rates as compared with XRT alone, without any additional major side effects.[42,43] The combination of RFA and radiation is intriguing. The center of a tumor tends to be more hypoxic and, therefore, more resistant to radiation. RFA is more effective in the central dense portion of a tumor that conducts heat easily, but has gradually decreasing potential for coagulation necrosis as the radius from the electrode tip increases, which creates a potential for incomplete tumor margin ablation. Radiation can complement RFA in treating tumor margins, particularly if the there is a good inflammatory response with resultant neovascularity post-RFA.

Dupuy et al.[44] published the first series of 24 RFA stage I NSCLC tumors (mean size of 3.4 cm) that were subsequently treated with XRT (average of 66 Gy), demonstrating survival rates of 50% and 39% at 2 and 5 years, respectively. Grieco et al. reported a series of 41 patients who underwent RFA and MWA of inoperable stage I/II NSCLC tumors coupled with external beam XRT or brachytherapy. Local tumor recurrence was 11.8% for tumors less than 3 cm (after an average of 45.6 months), and 33.3% in tumors larger than 3 cm (occurring after an average of 34.0 months). There was no difference between the XRT and brachytherapy groups.

Imaging Features Post-RFA An understanding of the radiographic evolution of ablated tumors is important to accurately assess the efficacy of this therapy and to differentiate normal post-RFA changes from incomplete tumor necrosis and local recurrence. Given the multiple factors that create a potential for incomplete tumor ablation, long-term follow-up surveillance imaging is mandated. The goal of surveillance is to detect recurrent malignant disease at its earliest stages, and offer re-treatment with RFA or other types of therapy. Blood-pool contrast agents are typically used to differentiate between nonenhancing coagulated tissue and enhancing viable incompletely treated residual tumor. Nonionic iodinated contrast enhanced CT and gadolinium-chelate contrast enhanced MRI are being used. The choice of modality depends on the target organ of interest, user experience, and clinical factors including contrast allergies and renal function.

Immediate post-RFA CT imaging demonstrates vaporization and wrinkling surrounding the margins of the lesion. The ablated lesion is typically surrounded by concentric rings of varying densities, referred to as a "cockade phenomenon,"[45] which is thought to represent the thermal gradient between the tumor and the surrounding parenchyma. This has also been described as a rim of ground-glass parenchymal opacity surrounding the lesion, which typically resolves within 1 to 3 months. Lee et al.[46] noted at least a 5-mm well-demarcated nonenhancing zone of ground-glass opacity surrounding ablated lesion in 8 of the 12 cases of complete necrosis. None of these patients demonstrated any local tumor recurrence on follow-up imaging (mean of 22.2 months), suggesting better treatment of tumor margins. Similar findings were noted in rabbit animal models and were found to correlate with coagulation necrosis on histology.[47]

Tumor size is variable within the first 6 months following RFA. Short-term follow-up imaging within the first 3 months has shown that lesions may increase in size. Bojarski et al.[48] report of a series of 32 RF-ablated pulmonary neoplasms: 64% of lesions increased in size, 32% remained unchanged, and 4% decreased in size at 1-month post-RFA. It is believed that the peripheral rim of ground-glass opacity contributes to the apparent increase in the size of treated tumors in the short term. Tumors that demonstrate continued growth beyond 6 months are highly suspicious for residual malignant disease, however. Cavitation was also noted within the first 3 months post-RFA in 31% of lesions in this series by Bojarski et al., typically occurring in larger lesions (with a mean of 3.8 cm in diameter). The majority of these cavitations decreased or completely collapsed on long-term follow-up (Fig. 37.3). Subcentimeter bubble-like lucencies are also noted in treated neoplasms, and also resolve within the first year. Pleural changes are occasionally noted within the first 3 months, consisting primarily of pleural thickening (usually in the area of pleura traversed by the electrode). Reactive pleural effusions are relatively uncommon after RFA.

The use of nodule CT densitometry for solitary pulmonary nodule has received considerable attention[49] for ablation surveillance. This involves measuring the enhancement of the lesion after the administration of intravenous contrast, and is based on the hypervascular nature of most malignancies. Suh et al.[50] demonstrated that RFA-treated malignancies have marked diminution of mean contrast enhancement at 1- to 2-month follow-up. Only one lesion demonstrated enhancement greater than baseline on initial follow-up, and this patient went on to develop a malignant effusion and expired during the course of the study. These lesions demonstrated mildly increased enhancement at 3-month follow-up, which remained below the pretreatment baseline levels. The marked decrease of mean contrast enhancement at follow-up is secondary to local vascular damage caused by RFA. The mild delayed increase in contrast enhancement is likely a result of local angiogenesis in the setting of granulation tissue formation. Peripheral nodular enhancement that increases in size on follow-up imaging would, therefore, be most suggestive of residual malignant disease.

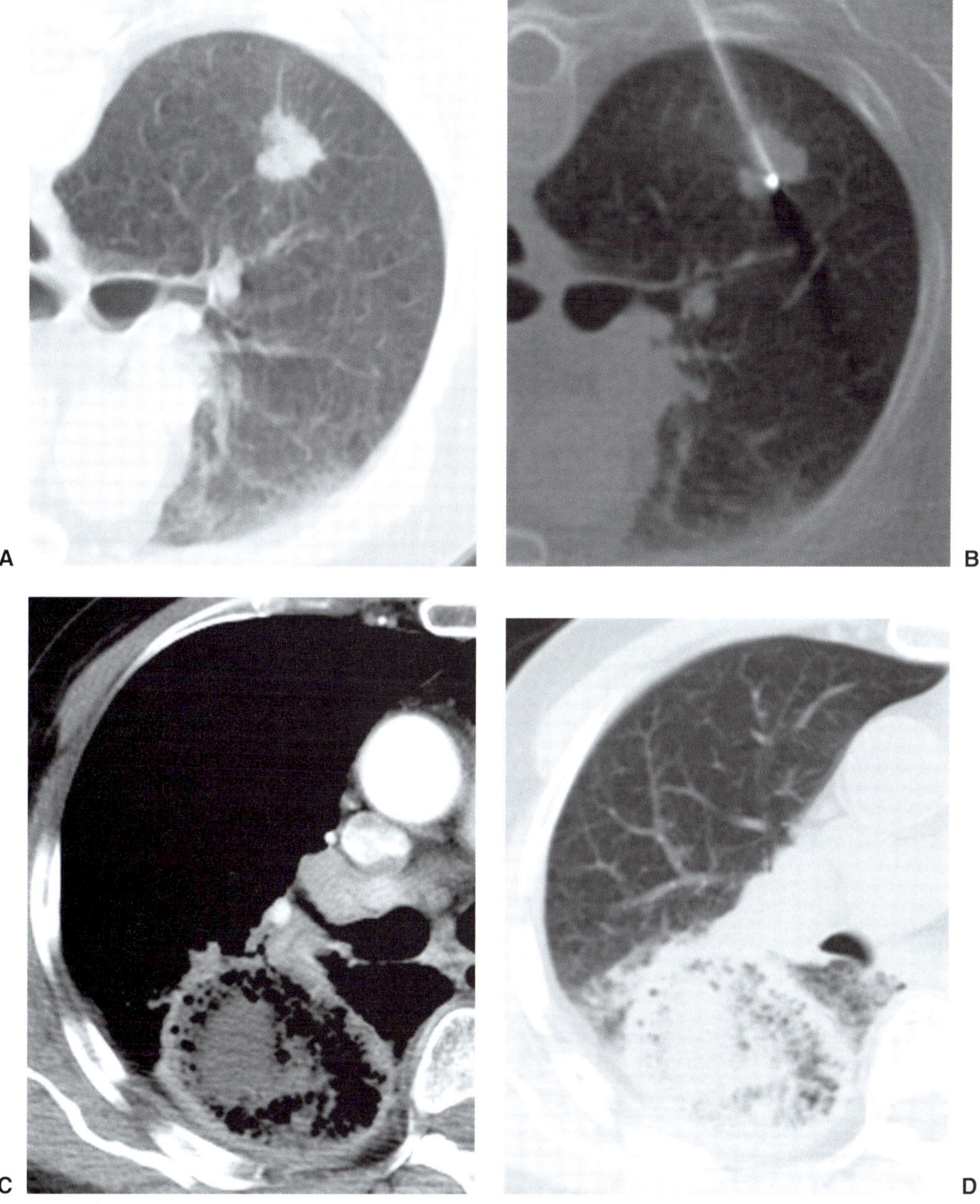

FIGURE 37.3 **A:** Initial study showing a stage IA squamous cell carcinoma. **B:** Radiofrequency ablation of the lesion. **C,D:** Two-week follow-up imaging shows a large cavitary mass with reactive rim enhancement and bubble-like lucencies, containing nonenhancing central necrotic debris. *(continues)*

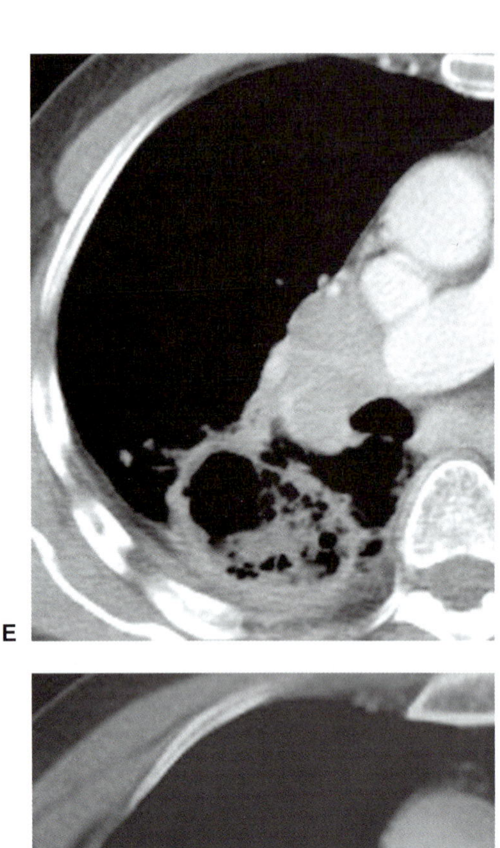
E

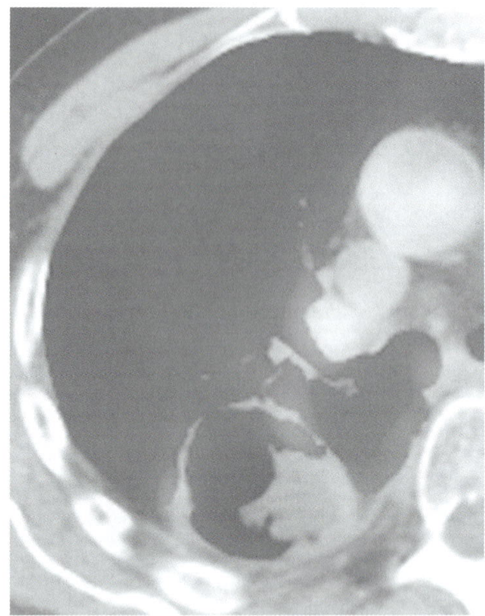
F

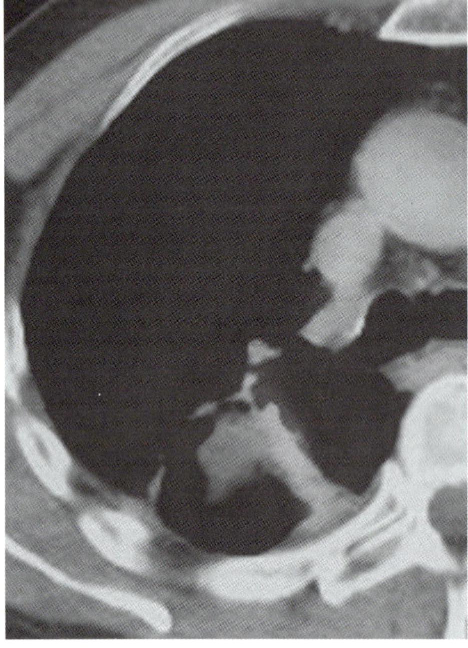
G

FIGURE 37.3 *(continued)* **E:** One-month follow-up demonstrates slight involution of the cavitating ablation site. Reactive lymphadenopathy is also noted. **F:** Three-month follow-up PET demonstrates mild FDG activity surrounding the ablation cavity, consistent with inflammatory scar tissue, with no FDG activity within the central necrotic debris. FDG avid right hilar reactive lymph node persists. **G:** Six-month follow-up PET shows mild peripheral FDG activity, without evidence of tumor recurrence. There is also resolution of the reactive lymphadenopathy.

Functional imaging with FDG-PET also holds great potential. Akeboshi et al. have shown that preablation high FDG uptake in malignant lesions on PET is eliminated on post-RFA scans. Other studies have demonstrated that complete disappearance of FDG activity within a malignant pulmonary lesion after any treatment (surgery, XRT, or chemotherapy) is a good prognostic indicator,[51,52] and this principle is similarly applied to RFA. Limitations of PET imaging include its low resolution and the prominent FDG avidity of the inflammatory reaction surrounding an ablated lesion on short-term follow-up imaging, which has a uniform circumferential appearance. Residual or recurrent malignant disease typically appears as increased asymmetric focus of FDG uptake, often at the periphery of the lesion.

Lesion size and enhancement pattern may therefore be used to evaluate ablated lesions for recurrent or residual malignant disease. Figure 37.4 illustrates this multimodality approach to follow-up imaging of tumor ablation and recurrence. CT densitometry and FDG–PET imaging will likely become the preferred methods of surveillance for ablated pulmonary lesions.

Complications after Lung Ablation Patients undergo screening for bleeding diathesis, and anticoagulants and antiplatelet drugs are discontinued prior to ablation. When using conscious sedation, many patients experience mild-to-moderate pain during the procedure, which is controlled with intravenous fentanyl. Mild fevers can occur up to 1 week following the therapy. Productive cough producing brown sputum may last 1 to 2 weeks in a minority of patients after ablation. Postprocedural pleurisy or small pleural effusions have also occurred in patients with pleural-based or peripheral lesions, although symptoms have rarely warranted thoracocentesis. Although there is a case report of massive pulmonary hemorrhage in a patient on clopidogrel,[53] significant pulmonary hemorrhage and hemoptysis are extremely rare complications.

Pneumothoraces occur in approximately 20% to 35% of patients after RFA[31,46,54] with approximately 6% to 16% requiring placement of a chest catheter.[45] This higher rate of pneumothorax and chest tube placement, as compared with pulmonary needle biopsy rate, is likely attributed to the larger

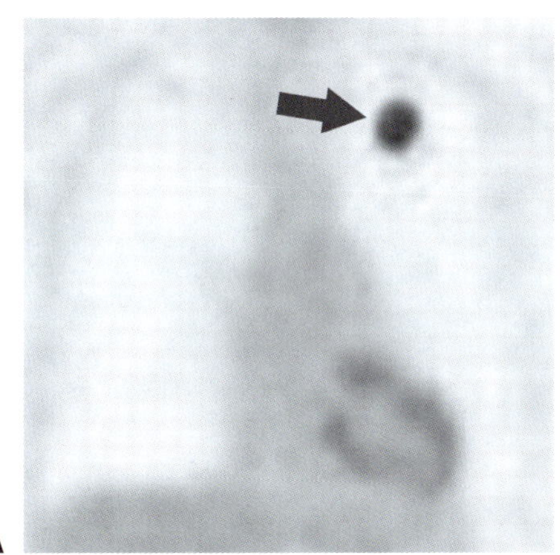

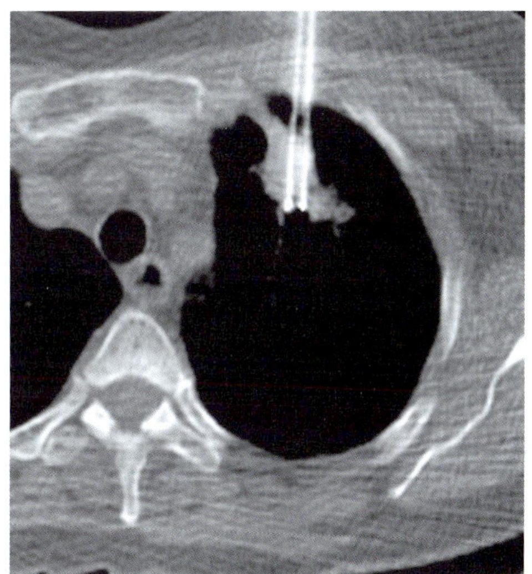

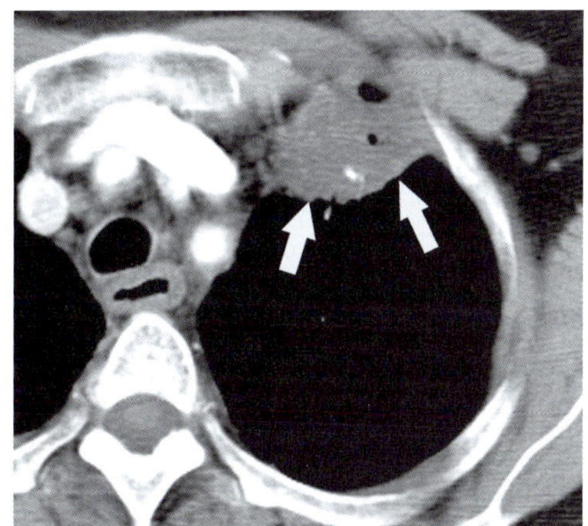

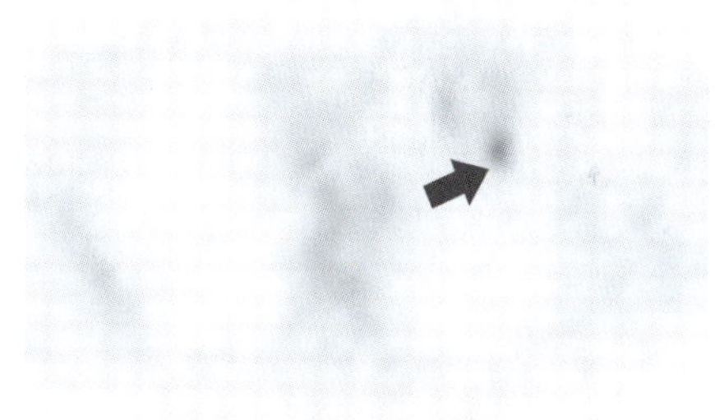

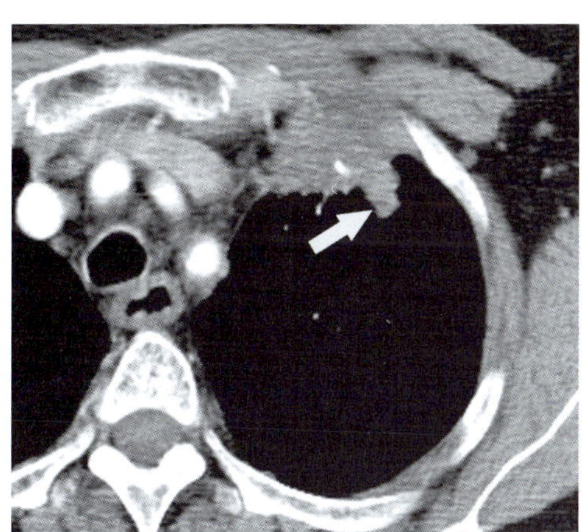

FIGURE 37.4 **A:** Initial PET showing a stage IB NSCLC. **B:** Radiofrequency ablation of the lesion. **C:** One-week postcontrast image shows thermal scar without any enhancement within the lesion, consistent with tumor necrosis. The punctuate high attenuation density in the periphery of the lesion was present on noncontrast images and is consistent with calcification. **D,E:** Six-month follow-up PET shows mild peripheral FDG activity surrounding the lesion, typical of surrounding inflammatory changes. There is a more focal focus of intense uptake at the periphery of the lesion (*arrow*), suspicious for residual tumor. This is also supported by CT imaging, which shows a similar enhancing soft tissue density along the ablation margin (*arrow*). *(continues)*

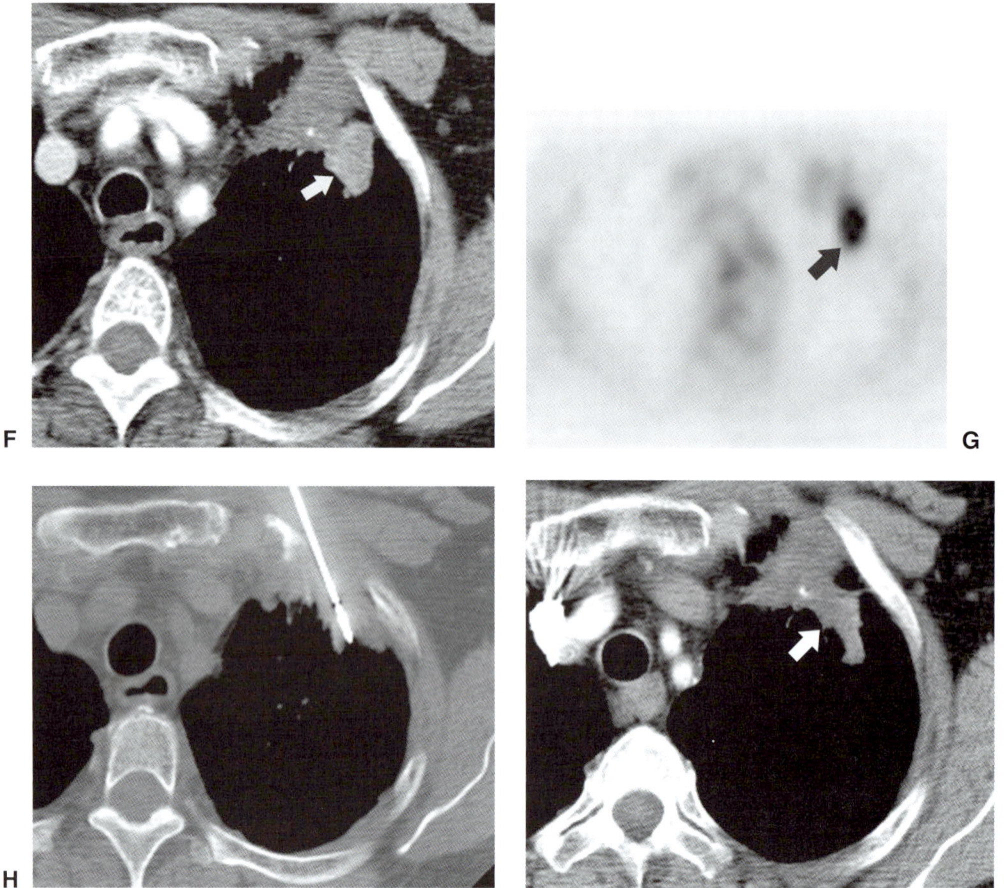

FIGURE 37.4 *(continued)* **F,G:** Ten-month follow-up PET demonstrates more intense focal FDG uptake along the tumor margin (*arrow*), which correlates with a growing enhancing soft tissue mass (*arrow*), consistent with tumor recurrence. **H:** Patient undergoing microwave ablation of recurrent malignant disease at the tumor margin. **I:** Follow-up imaging demonstrating lack of enhancement along ablated lesion (*arrow*).

electrode size (often a 14- to 17-gauge electrode as compared with a 20-gauge needle biopsy), and a selection bias toward patients with severe emphysema who are nonsurgical candidates. Preventative measures include planning the electrode access route to avoid bullae and interlobular fissures when possible. Most chest tubes are typically removed within 24 hours, and patients may be followed in the outpatient setting with the addition of a Heimlich valve.

Pulmonary complications include pneumonia, exacerbation of existing chronic obstructive pulmonary disease, abscess, and bronchopleural fistula. Pulmonary abscess and bronchopleural fistulae are felt to be more common following ablation of larger tumors; however, as seen in Table 37.1, the incidence of these specific complications is extremely low.

One unique risk of RFA within the lung is systemic embolization, including potential risk for stroke. Experience with liver ablation had previously demonstrated the generation of microbubbles that are thought to occur from vapor formation from blood and intracellular and extracellular water. This raises the possibility of microbubbles flowing into the pulmonary veins, and resulting in cerebral microemboli. Yamamoto et al.[55] prospectively monitored 17 patients who underwent RFA of lung tumors with carotid sonography, noting echogenic microbubbles ascending the carotid arteries of three patients (who all had larger tumor diameters ranging from 2.5 to 6.5 cm). None of their patients demonstrated any evidence of acute infarct on MRI imaging that was performed within 24 hours. Microbubbles are used as a sonographic contrast agent, and the incidence of acute infarction is very low with the 35.5-μm microbubbles commonly used for this technique. Microbubbles generated by RFA are reported to be 3 to 8 μm, and are therefore of unlikely clinical significance. Jin et al.[56] have reported a case of an acute cerebral infarction following the ablation of a 4-cm atypical carcinoid tumor that resulted in left hemifacial palsy and grade 3 left upper and lower extremity weakness that improved following course of anticoagulation.

There is no definitive evidence of RFA interfering with pacemaker devices. Hayes et al.[57] reported no adverse events with pacemaker function in the ablation of liver tumors. Tong et al.[58]

TABLE 37.1 Types and Frequency of Lung Ablation–Related Complications

Type	Frequency
Pneumothorax requiring chest tube or aspiration	0%–54% (most <20%)
Pneumonia	0%–22%
COPD exacerbation	0%–6%
ARDS	0%–3%
Pulmonary abscess	0%–6%
Hemoptysis	0%–12%
Hemothorax	0%–2%
Pleural effusion requiring drainage	0%–4%
Parenchymal hemorrhage	0%–1%
Death	4 case reports[36,61]
Bronchopleural fistula	1 case report
Acute renal failure	1 case report
Vocal cord paralysis	1 case report
Atrial fibrillation	1 case report
Pulmonary embolus	1 case report
Third-degree skin burn	1 case report
Stroke	1 case report
Tumor tract seeding	1 case report

Adapted from Rose SC, Thistlethwaite PA, Sewell PE, et al. Lung cancer and radiofrequency ablation. *J Vasc Interv Radiol* 2006;17:927–951.

ARDS, acute respiratory distress syndrome; COPD, chronic obstructive pulmonary disease.

report of a single case of irregular pacing rhythm in the ablation of an adrenal lesion, with resumption of normal paced rhythm posttreatment, with no evidence of malfunction or damage on interrogation.

Finally, skin burns associated with improper ground pad placement can occur, but this is rare if the pads are placed appropriately. Rare cases of pulmonary emboli and periprocedural atrial fibrillation are likely secondary to associated comorbid conditions in this patient population, including advanced age and debilitation and tumor-related coagulopathy. A single case of tumor tract seeding has also been reported.[59]

Equally important, RFA does not appear to affect the overall pulmonary function. In a series of 97 ablated lesions by de Baère et al.,[60] 47 patients in the 60-patient study underwent spirometry between 3 and 5 weeks after RFA. There was no significant change in their forced expiratory volume in 1 second (FEV_1) or their vital capacity as compared to pretreatment spirometry.

CONCLUSION

Sublobar resection in combination with adjuvant brachytherapy appears to be a reasonable option for the patient considered high risk for lobectomy. Preliminary results are encouraging, and a current randomized trial will better define the role of this approach. Thermal ablation is an alternative for patients who are high risk for any resection or those patients with tumors in anatomic locations that preclude a sublobar resection. Thermal ablation is more successful with smaller tumors and results may be improved if used in combination with radiation therapy. MWA may also be preferable to RFA, although studies to confirm this are still needed.

REFERENCES

1. American Cancer Society. *Cancer Facts and Figures 1999.* Atlanta: American Cancer Society, 1999.
2. Bach PB, Cramer LD, Warren JL, et al. Racial differences in the treatment of early stage non-small cell lung cancer. *N Eng J Med* 1999;341:1198–205.
3. Churchill ED, Sweet RH, Sutter L, et al. The surgical management of carcinoma of the lung: a study of cases treated at the Massachusetts General Hospital from 1930–50. *J Thorac Cardiovasc Surg* 1950;20:349–365.
4. Ginsberg RJ, Rubenstein LV. Lung Cancer Study Group: randomized trial of lobectomy versus limited resection for T1N0 non-small cell lung cancer. *Ann Thorac Surg* 1995;60:615–623.
5. Warren WH, Faber LP. Segmentectomy versus lobectomy in patients with stage I pulmonary carcinoma. *J Thorac Cardiovasc Surg* 1994;107:1087–1094.
6. Landreneau RJ, Sugarbaker DJ, Mack MJ, et al. Wedge resection versus lobectomy for stage I (T1N0M0) non-small cell lung cancer. *J Thorac Cardiovasc Surg* 1997;113(4):691–700.
7. D'Amato TA, Galloway M, Szydlowski G, et al. Intraoperative brachytherapy following thoracoscopic wedge resection of stage I lung cancer. *Chest* 1998;114(4):1112–1115.
8. Miller JI, Hatcher CR. Limited resection of bronchogenic carcinoma in the patient with marked impairment of pulmonary function. *Ann Thorac Surg* 1987;44:340–343.
9. Santos R, Colonias A, Parda D, et al. Comparison between sublobar resection and 125Iodine brachytherapy after sublobar resection in high-risk patients with stage I non-small-cell lung cancer. *Surgery* 2003;134:691–697.
10. Lee W, Daly BD, DiPetrillo TA, et al. Limited resection for non-small cell lung cancer: observed local control with implantation of I-125 brachytherapy seeds. *Ann Thorac Surg* 2003;75(1):237–242.
11. Fernando HC, Santos, RS, Benfield JR, et al. Lobar and sublobar resection with and without brachytherapy for small stage IA NSCLC. *J Thorac Cardiovasc Surg* 2005;129(2):261–267.
12. Birdas J, Koehler P, Colonias A, et al. Sublobar resection with brachytherapy versus lobectomy in stage IB NSCLC. Presented, Society of Thoracic Surgeons, January 2005.
13. Smith RP, Schuchert M, Komanduri K, et al. Dosimetric evaluation of radiation exposure during I-125 vicryl mesh implants: implications for ACOSOG z4032. *Ann Surg Oncol* 2007;14(12):3610–3613.
14. Pennes HH. Analysis of tissue and arterial blood temperatures in the resting human forearm. *J Appl Physiol* 1948;1:93–122.
15. Goldberg SN, Gazelle GS, Mueller PR. Thermal ablation therapy for focal malignancy: a unified approach to underlying principles, techniques, and diagnostic imaging guidance. *AJR Am J Roentgenol* 2000;174:323–331.
16. Seegenschmiedt MH, Brady LW, Sauer R. Interstitial thermoradiotherapy: review on technical and clinical aspects. *AJR Am J Clin Oncol* 1990;13:352–363.
17. Trembley BS, Ryan TP, Strohbehn JW. Interstitial hyperthermia: physics, biology and clinical aspects. In: Urano M, Douple E, eds. *Physics of Microwave Hyperthermia in Hyperthermia and Oncology.* Vol 3. Utrecht, The Netherlands: Verlag Springer, 1992:11–98.

18. Kruskal JB, Goldberg SN, Huertas JC, et al. In vivo identification of cellular events that may be used to potentiate the effects of radiofrequency (RF) ablation of liver tissue. *Radiology* 2000;217(suppl):26.
19. Goldberg SN, Gazelle GS, Compton CC, et al. Radiofrequency tissue ablation in the rabbit lung: efficacy and complications. *Acad Radiol* 1995;2(9):776–784.
20. Dupuy DE, Zagoria RJ, Akerley W, et al. Percutaneous radiofrequency ablation of malignancies in the lung. *AJR Am J Roentgenol* 2000;174:57–59.
21. Organ LW. Electrophysiologic principles of radiofrequency lesion making. *Appl Neurophysiol* 1976;39:69–76.
22. Goldberg SN, Dupuy DE. Image-guided radiofrequency tumor ablation: challenges and opportunities—part I. *J Vasc Interv Radiol* 2001;12:1021–1032.
23. Beland M, Mueller PR, Gervais DA. Thermal ablation in interventional oncology. *Semin Roentgenol* 2007;42(3):175–90.
24. Gage AA. History of cryosurgery. *Semin Surg Oncol* 1998;14(2):99–109.
25. Kupelian PA, Komaki R, Allen P. Prognostic factors in the treatment of node-negative non-small cell lung carcinoma with radiotherapy alone. *Int J Radiat Oncol Biol Phys* 1996;36:607–613.
26. Zierhut D, Bettscheider C, Shubert K, et al. Radiation therapy of stage I and II non-small cell lung cancer. *Lung Cancer* 2001;34:S39–S43.
27. Rowell NP, William CJ. Radical radiotherapy for stage I/II non-small cell lung cancer in patients not sufficiently fit for or declining surgery (medically inoperable): a systemic review. *Thorax* 2001;56:628–638.
28. Dupuy DE, Zagoria RJ, Akerly W, et al. Percutaneous radiofrequency ablation of malignancies in the lung. *AJR Am J Roentgenol* 2000;174:57–59.
29. Lee JM, Jin GY, Goldberg SN, et al. Percutaneous radiofrequency ablation for inoperable non-small cell lung cancer and metastases: preliminary report. *Radiology* 2004;230(1):125–134. Epub 2003 Nov 26.
30. Akeboshi M, Yamakado K, Nakatsuka A, et al. Percutaneous radiofrequency ablation of lung neoplasms: initial therapeutic response. *J Vasc Int Rad* 2004;15:463–470.
31. Yasui K, Kanazawa S, Sano Y, et al. Thoracic tumors treated with CT-guided radiofrequency ablation: initial experience. *Radiology* 2004;231:850–857.
32. Herrera LJ, Fernando HC, Perry Y, et al. Radiofrequency ablation of pulmonary malignant tumors in nonsurgical candidates. *J Thorac Cardiovasc Surg* 2003;125(4):929–937.
33. Fernando HC, De Hoyos A, Landreneau RJ, et al. Radiofrequency ablation for the treatment of non-small cell lung cancer in marginal surgical candidates. *J Thorac Cardiovasc Surg* 2005;129(3):639–644.
34. Pennathur A, Luketich JD, Abbas G, et al. Radiofrequency ablation for the treatment of stage I non-small cell lung cancer in high-risk patients. *J Thorac Cardiovasc Surg* 2007;134(4):857–864.
35. Lencioni R, Crocetti DW, Glen DL, et al. Radiofrequency ablation of pulmonary tumors response evaluation (RAPTURE) trial. Proceedings Society of Interventional Radiology, *30th Annual Meeting*. New Orleans, LA, 2005.
36. Simon CJ, Dupuy DE, DiPetrillo TA, et al. Pulmonary radiofrequency ablation: long-term safety and efficacy in 153 patients. *Radiology* 2007;243(1):268–275.
37. Feng W, Liu W, Li C, et al. Percutaneous microwave coagulation therapy for lung cancer. *Zhonghua Zhong Liu Za Zhi* 2002;24(4): 388–390.
38. Wolf F, DiPetrillo T, Machan, J et al. Microwave ablation of lung malignancies: effectiveness, CT findings and safety in 50 patients. *Radiology* 2008;247(3):871–879.
39. Wang H, Littrup PJ, Duan Y, et al. Thoracic masses treated with percutaneous cryotherapy: initial experience with more than 200 procedures. *Radiology* 2005;235:289–298.
40. Seegenschmiedt MH, Brady LW, Sauer R. Interstitial thermoradiotherapy: review on technical and clinical aspects. *Am J Clin Oncol* 1990;13:352–363.
41. Trembley BS, Ryan TP, Strohbehn JW. Interstitial hyperthermia: physics, biology and clinical aspects. In: Urano M, Douple E, eds. *Physics of Microwave Hyperthermia in Hyperthermia and Oncology*. Vol 3. Utrecht, The Netherlands: Verlag Springer, 1992:11–98.
42. Dupuy D, DiPetrillo T, Gandhi S, et al. Radiofrequency ablation followed by conventional radiotherapy for medically inoperable stage I non-small cell lung cancer. *Chest* 2006;129:738–745.
43. Grieco CA, Simon CJ, Mayo-Smith WW, et al. Percutaneous image-guided thermal ablation and radiation therapy: outcomes of combined treatment for 41 patients with inoperable stage I/II non–small-cell lung cancer. *J Vasc Interv Radiol* 2006;17:1117–1124.
44. Dupuy DE, Dipetrill T, Gandhi S, et al. Radiofrequency ablation followed by conventional radiotherapy for medically inoperable stage I non-small cell lung cancer. *Chest* 2006;129:738–745.
45. Cosmo G, Vittorio M, Giuseppe C, et al. Radiofrequency ablation of 40 lung neoplasms: preliminary results. *AJR Am J Roentgenol* 2004;183:361–368.
46. Lee JM, Jin GY, Goldberg SN, et al. Percutaneous radiofrequency ablation for inoperable non-small cell lung cancer and metastases: preliminary report. *Radiology* 2004;230:125–134.
47. Goldberg SN, Gazelle GS, Compton CC, et al. Radiofrequency tissue ablation in the rabbit lung: efficacy and complications. *Acad Radiol* 1995;2:776–784.
48. Bojarski JD, Dupuy DE, Mayo-Smith W. CT imaging findings of pulmonary neoplasms after treatment with radiofrequency ablation: results in 32 tumors. *AJR Am J Roentgenol* 2005;185:466–471.
49. Swensen SJ, Viggiano RW, Midthun DE, et al. Lung nodule enhancement at CT: a multicenter study. *Radiology* 2000;214:73–80.
50. Suh RD, Wallace AB, Sheehan RE, et al. Unresectable pulmonary malignancies: CT-guided percutaneous radiofrequency ablation—preliminary results. *Radiology* 2003;229:821–829.
51. Patz EF Jr, Connolly J, Herndon J. Prognostic value of thoracic FDG PET imaging after treatment for non-small cell lung cancer. *AJR Am J Roentgenol* 2000;174(3):769–774.
52. Akhurst T, Downey RJ, Ginsberg MS, et al. An initial experience with FDG-PET in the imaging of residual disease after induction chemotherapy for lung cancer. *Ann Thorac Surg* 2002;73:259–264.
53. Vaughn C, Mychaskiw G II, Sewell P, et al. Massive hemorrhage during radiofrequency ablation of a pulmonary neoplasm. *Anesth Analg* 2002;94(5):1149–1151.
54. Steinke K, King J, Glenn D, et al. Percutaneous radiofrequency ablation of lung tumors with expandable needle electrodes: tips from preliminary experience. *AJR Am J Roentgenol* 2004;183:605–611.
55. Yamamoto A, Matsuoka T, Toyoshima M, et al. Assessment of cerebral microembolism during percutaneous radiofrequency ablation of lung tumors using diffusion weighted imaging. *AJR Am J Roentgenol* 2004;183:1785–1789.
56. Jin GY, Lee JM, Lee YC, et al. Acute cerebral infarction after radiofrequency ablation of an atypical carcinoid pulmonary tumor. *AJR Am J Roentgenol* 2004;182(4):990–992.
57. Hayes DL, Charboneau JW, Lewis BD, et al. Radiofrequency treatment of hepatic neoplasms in patients with permanent pacemakers. *Mayo Clin Proc* 2001;76:950–952.
58. Tong NY, Hsieh JR, Ling, et al. Extracardiac radiofrequency ablation interferes with pacemaker unction but does not damage the device. *Anesthesiology* 2004;100:1041.
59. Yamakado K, Akeboshi M, Nakatsuka A, et al. Tumor seeding following lung radiofrequency ablation: a care report. *Cardiovasc Intervent Radiol* 2005;28:530–532.
60. De Baère T, Palussière J, Aupérin A, et al. Midterm local efficacy and survival after radiofrequency ablation of lung tumors with minimum follow-up of 1 year: prospective evaluation. *Radiology* 2006;240:587–596.
61. Steinke K, Sewell PE, Dupuy D, et al. Pulmonary radiofrequency ablation—an international study survey. *Anticancer Res* 2004;24(1):339–343.

CHAPTER 38

Theolyn Price
Francis Nichols

Surgical Management of Small Cell Lung Cancer

Small cell lung cancer (SCLC) is a virulent, rapidly growing, early metastasizing, invasive cancer. SCLC represents approximately 15% of all lung cancers and up to 25% of lung cancer deaths each year in the United States.[1] At diagnosis, approximately 90% of patients will have regional or distant spread. Although the incidence of SCLC in the United States is decreasing, there have been only modest improvements in survival noted over the past 30 years.[2]

Although several decades ago, surgery for SCLC was the treatment of choice, this was abandoned following the 1973 report of the British Medical Research Council, which randomized patients with limited disease SCLC to either surgery or radiotherapy alone.[3–5] It was concluded from this study that radiotherapy was preferable to surgery. Subsequently, it has been shown that SCLC can exhibit an initial dramatic response rate to chemotherapy and radiation therapy.[2] Numerous clinical trials have reported response rates of 80% to 90%. Nevertheless, despite this initial response to therapy, most patients ultimately die from this disease. For patients with limited-stage disease, the most frequent site of chemoradiotherapy treatment failure is localized recurrence.[6,7] It is this sobering fact that has led many to reconsider surgery as part of the treatment armamentarium of SCLC. This chapter will review four clinical circumstances in which surgery may be beneficial in the treatment of SCLC: (a) SCLC presenting as a solitary pulmonary nodule (SPN) and diagnosed at the time of surgery, (b) mixed histology (i.e., SCLC and non-SCLC combined) lung cancers, (c) salvage therapy for local failure of chemoradiotherapy, and (d) planned multimodality therapy consisting of induction chemotherapy followed by surgery for limited-stage SCLC.

HISTORICAL BACKGROUND

Mountain[8] reported the MD Anderson Hospital and Tumor Institute's surgical experience for 368 patients with pathologically proven SCLC and found only one patient surviving greater than 5 years as compared to 15% to 25% 5-year survival for non–small cell lung cancer (NSCLC). Mountain[8] did not identify any prognostic factors positively influencing survival and concluded that SCLC was a nonsurgical disease warranting systemic treatment.

To try and determine if it was ever appropriate to utilize surgery as primary treatment for SCLC, a prospective randomized trial was undertaken by the Medical Research Council of Great Britain.[3–5] In this study, 144 patients were diagnosed with SCLC by bronchoscopy, and then randomized with 71 having surgical resection and 73 radiotherapy (>30 Gy over 20 to 40 days). Median survival for the surgical patients was 199 days compared to 300 days for the radiotherapy patients. At 5 years, one and three patients were alive in the surgical and radiotherapy arms, respectively ($p = 0.04$), and at 10 years, only the three radiotherapy patients remained. This study discredited surgery for SCLC for years to come. Retrospectively, the British Medical Research Council study has been criticized in several areas: (a) initial staging was crude compared with today's preoperative staging modalities, and many of the patients likely would have been deemed inoperable, (b) only patients with central tumors were included since all required bronchoscopy for diagnosis, peripheral tumors, which might have received the most benefit were excluded, (c) only 48% of the surgical patients had complete surgical resection, all of which entailed pneumonectomy, and (d) no intraoperative staging was performed.[9–12] Subsequently, the addition of preoperative radiotherapy was examined; however, no survival advantage was achieved.[13–15] Considering these facts, some surgeons still believed in the role for surgery in select patients with SCLC; therefore, further investigations were continued. Table 38.1 outlines the results of surgery alone for SCLC.

It became evident to the 1960s and 1970s investigators that most patients with SCLC were dying from systemic metastatic disease, and that effective systemic treatment was needed. Bergsagel et al.[25] showed an improved overall survival with the addition of low-dose cyclophosphamide to radiation therapy. Similarly, the British Medical Research Council Lung Cancer Working Party[26] showed improved disease-free survival with multiagent chemotherapy and radiation. Concurrently, other investigators were applying the same adjuvant chemotherapy

TABLE 38.1 Survival of Patients with Small Cell Lung Cancer Treated with Surgery Alone

Author	Number of Patients	Percent 5-Year Survival by Stage			
		I	II	III	Overall
Mountain[8,a]	368	—	—	—	Only 1 patient
Shah et al.[16,a]	28	57.1%	0%	55.5%	43.5%
Sørensen et al.[17,a]	77	12%	13%	0%	8%
Shore and Paneth[18,a]	40	—	—	—	25%
Lennox et al.[19,a]	275	—	—	—	Lobectomy: 18% Pneumonectomy: 7%
Prasad et al.[20,b]	56	35%	23%	—	—
Inoue et al.[21,c]	9	22%	22%	—	—
Coolen et al.[22,c]	19	11%	—	—	—
Lucchi et al.[23,c]	20	0%	0%	0%	—
Wada et al.[24,c]	6	0%	0%	0%	—
British MRC[3,4,5,a]	71	—	—	—	Only 1 patient

[a]Reports include surgery alone.

[b]Report includes surgery alone for stages I and II, with surgery followed by adjuvant chemotherapy for stage III.

[c]Reports on patients treated with multiple modalities with the data for surgery-alone patients shown.

MRC, Medical Research Council.

principles to surgical SCLC patients. The Veterans Administration Surgical Adjuvant Group (VASOG) in the United States showed no survival benefit in 417 lung cancer patients (both SCLC and NSCLC) treated by either surgery alone, surgery plus single-agent chemotherapy, or surgery plus multiagent chemotherapy.[27] When considering those patients specifically diagnosed with SCLC, 4 out of 18 total patients were alive at 3 years, none being in the surgery alone arm. This was the first study demonstrating a possible increased survival for patients with SCLC who underwent adjuvant chemotherapy following complete surgical resection.[27]

In 1982, Shields et al.[28] evaluated four of the VASOG adjuvant chemotherapy trials, which resulted in the reawakening of surgical interest in the treatment of limited disease SCLC. This study analyzed 148 patients diagnosed with SCLC who had undergone potentially curative resection. There were 16 operative deaths, and in the remaining 132 patients, the overall 5-year survival was 23%. Although in this study, there was no benefit shown with adjuvant chemotherapy, the importance of the TNM (tumor, node, metastasis) staging SCLC was demonstrated. SCLC patients with T1N0M0 tumors had a 60% 5-year survival, T1N1M0 31%, T2N0M0 28%, T2N1M0 9%, and any T3 or N2 3.6%.[28] (Fig. 38.1) SCLC may occasionally present as an SPN. In 1975, Higgins et al.[29] reported on a VASOG trial involving 1134 patients with asymptomatic SPN. The 392 patients underwent resection for lung cancer, and 15 (4%) were found to have SCLC. The 1-, 5-, and 10-year survivals were 64%, 36%, and 18%, respectively.[29] In a retrospective review of 40 patients who underwent potentially curative resection for SCLC between 1959 and 1972, overall 5-year survival was 25%, and long-term survival was 40% in patients without

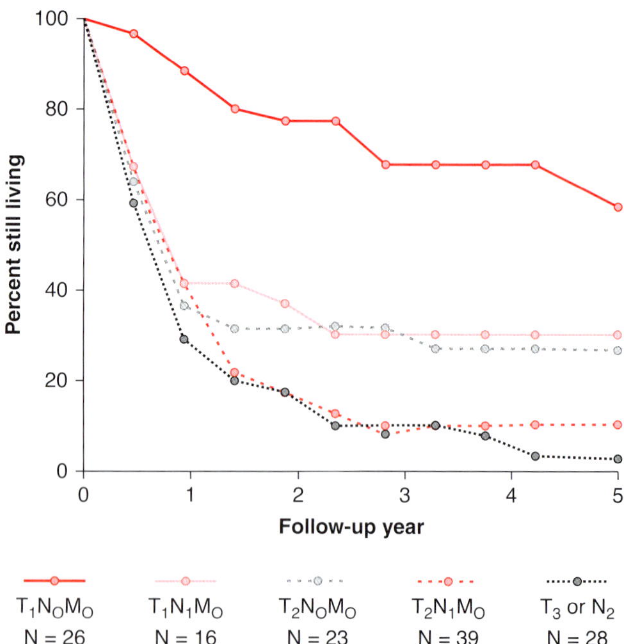

FIGURE 38.1 Survival, computed by the life-table method, from postoperative day 30 (early trials) or from randomization (recent trials) by TNM classification for patients with undifferentiated small cell carcinoma who had undergone a "curative" resection in the VASOG lung trials. (From Shields TW, Higgins GA, Matthews MG, et al. Surgical resection in the management of small cell carcinoma of the lung. *J Thorac Cardiovasc Surg* 1982;84:481–488, with permission.)

metastatically involved lymph nodes.[18] Similarly, Angeletti et al.[30] suggested that survival was statistically influenced by the N stage rather than T stage. Their results demonstrated that patients with T1, T2, and T3 SCLC tumors, without evidence of lymph node involvement, might benefit from surgical resection and adjuvant chemotherapy. SCLC typically presents as a central mass. Lennox et al.[19] observed that patients with more proximal tumors requiring pneumonectomy had worse survival than patients requiring lobectomy. The 2- and 5-year survival rates for patients undergoing lobectomy were 32% and 18%, respectively, compared with 14% and 7% for patients having pneumonectomy.[19]

Although some authors may consider the combination of chemoradiotherapy to be the standard of care for limited disease SCLC,[31] from this historical review, it is suggested that various subpopulations of patients with SCLC might benefit from surgery. Whether surgery can offer any substantial advantage over radiotherapy in terms of local control is still an unanswered question. However, we concede that if surgery is to have any meaningful role in the treatment of SCLC, it must be in the context of a combined modality treatment regimen, which includes systemic chemotherapy and possibly radiotherapy.

SURGICAL INDICATIONS IN THE MANAGEMENT OF SMALL CELL LUNG CANCER

Solitary Pulmonary Nodule The SCLC that presents as an SPN is often diagnosed at the time of therapeutic resection. This represents a small percentage of patients that carry the diagnosis of SCLC ranging from 4% to 12%.[29,32,33] These patients usually have solitary peripheral nodules on chest radiograph and computerized tomography (CT). Bronchoscopy tends to be nondiagnostic, and the definitive diagnosis often is not made until the time of surgical resection. Some investigators have hypothesized that SCLC presenting as an SPN has an inherently different biology and, in turn, natural history than the more typical SCLC.[32,34]

The VASOG trial reported by Higgins et al.[29] is one of the earliest studies confirming an improved outcome (5-year survival 36%) for patients with resected SCLC presenting as an SPN. Several series of peripheral SCLC treated by surgery alone have been previously discussed and show survivals similar to resected NSCLC (Table 38.1). A 5-year survival of approximately 50% can be seen with pathologic stage I SCLC patients treated with surgery and adjuvant chemotherapy.[27] Randomized trials have not been carried out in this subset of patients with resected peripheral SCLC, and it is therefore impossible to know if this more favorable outcome is caused by the surgical resection, the adjuvant chemotherapy that many receive, or the natural history of this subset of SCLC. The accuracy of the pathologic diagnosis must always come to mind in any of the older series of resected peripheral SCLC. Some of these SCLCs may, in fact, be atypical carcinoids or other well-differentiated neuroendocrine carcinomas.[35] Some surgeons have questioned the necessity for adjuvant chemotherapy following resection of peripheral SCLC.[16] Many clinical series of surgery and chemotherapy have shown improved survival when compared to historical groups of patients treated by surgery alone (Table 38.2).

TABLE 38.2 Survival According to Pathologic Stage for Patients Treated with Adjuvant Chemotherapy after Surgery for Small Cell Lung Cancer

		Percent 5-Year Survival			
Author	**Number of Patients**	**Stage I**	**Stage II**	**Stage III**	**Overall**
Shields et al.[27,28]	132	51%	20%	3%	28%
Hayata[37]	72	26%	17%	0%	11%
Meyer et al.[37,38]	30	>50%	50%	0	—
Osterlind et al.[39]	36	22%	—	—	25% (3 yrs)
Maassen et al.[40]	124	34%	21%	11%	20% (3 yrs)
Shepherd et al.[41]	63	48%	24%	24%	31%
Ulsperger et al.[42]	146	50%	31%	23%	37 (4 yrs)
Macchiarini et al.[43]	42	52%	—	13%	36%
Ichinose et al.[44]	37	68%	18%	16%	27%
Davis et al.[45]	32	50%	35%	21%	36%
Wada et al.[24]	17	37% (stages I and 2)	33%	32%	—
Lucchi et al.[23]	92	47%	15%	14%	32%
Cataldo[46]	60	46%	36%	15%	—
Angeletti et al.[30]	34	—	—	—	26%[a]
Friess et al.[47]	15	—	—	—	45% (2 yrs)

[a]All survivors were T1, T2, or T3 with N0 disease. No patients with N1 or N2 disease survived.

Chandra et al.[36] from the Mayo Clinic recently reviewed 77 patients who, from January 1985 to July 2002, underwent thoracotomy for SCLC. Many of the SCLC were solitary nodules or masses. The median tumor diameter was 4 cm (range: 1 to 10 cm) Surgical procedures included wedge resection in 30 patients (6 with concomitant talc pleurodesis), lobectomy in 28, segmentectomy in 4, bilobectomy in 3, pneumonectomy in 2, and thoracotomy with biopsy of the hilar mass in 10. Mediastinal lymphadenectomy was performed in 50 patients, mediastinal lymph node sampling in 19, and no mediastinal lymph nodes were biopsied in 8. Patients were classified using the TNM staging system according to the criteria established by the American Joint Committee for Cancer and End Results Reporting for NSCLC. Postsurgical stage was IA in 7 patients, IB in 11, IIA in 8, IIB in 7, IIIA in 30, IIIB in 10, and IV in 4. Five patients had combined chemoradiotherapy prior to thoracotomy. Adjuvant therapy included chemotherapy in 20 patients, radiation therapy in 3, and both in 40. Figure 38.2 shows the 5-year survival for these patients according to stage. Five-year survival for patients with stage I disease was 36%, stage II 40%, stage III 17%, and stage IV 0% ($p = 0.06$). Five-year survival for patients with stages I and II combined was 38% compared with 16% for patients with stages III and IV combined. After multivariable analysis, surgical stage I/II versus III/IV was the only significant predictor identified.

In patients whose performance status is acceptable for surgical resection, we do not routinely perform transthoracic needle aspirations (TTNA) of peripheral lung nodules. In patients who, for some reason, have had a TTNA and a diagnosis of SCLC is obtained, consideration for surgical resection is still given. This is because the cytologic diagnosis may be in error as mentioned previously. Additionally, some SCLC are mixed tumors with NSCLC being present as well.[48,49] Surgical resection clarifies the pathology and eliminates the NSCLC portion of the tumor.

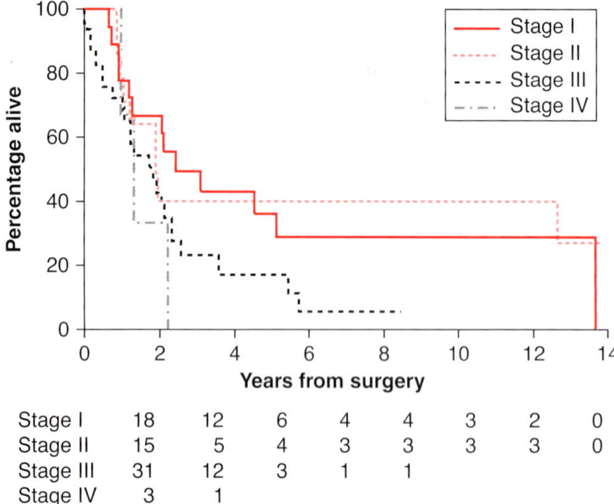

FIGURE 38.2 Survival of patients following resection of SCLC. Probability of survival (death from any cause) in patients who underwent resection of SCLC. Zero time on the abscissa represents the date of lung resection. Patients who had surgical biopsy only are excluded. Numbers under the graph represent the number of patients at risk. (From Chandra V, Allen MS, Nichols FC III, et al. The role of pulmonary resection in small cell lung cancer. *Mayo Clin Proc* 2006;81:619–624, with permission.)

Preoperative staging for patients with peripheral SCLC is more thorough than that for NSCLC. Noninvasive staging includes a CT scan of the chest and abdomen, whole body positron emission tomography (PET), and head magnetic resonance imaging (MRI). Depending on the results of the noninvasive staging, invasive preoperative staging may include endoscopic bronchoscopic ultrasound (EBUS), esophageal endoscopic ultrasound (EUS) both with fine-needle aspirations as appropriate, and finally mediastinoscopy. The intraoperative management of peripheral SCLC is similar to that of NSCLC. Complete resection of the tumor most commonly includes lobectomy and mediastinal lymphadenectomy. For those patients where the diagnosis of SCLC is made at the time of surgical resection, missing parts of the noninvasive metastatic workup are completed postoperatively. This allows for accurate cancer staging and appropriate adjuvant therapy.

Mixed Histology Tumors Approximately 5% to 10% of patients diagnosed with SCLC will have "mixed tumors," meaning other pathologies such as adenocarcinoma or squamous cell carcinoma can be found within the pathologic specimen.[48,49] The University of Toronto Lung Oncology Group reported a mixed histology in 17.7% of surgical patients with adjuvant chemotherapy and in 7.5% of surgical patients with neoadjuvant chemotherapy.[49] There appears to be a higher percentage of surgical patients with mixed histology. This, in part, is thought to be a result of the more peripheral location of most mixed SCLC.[48] Other factors may also contribute to the increased incidence of mixed histology in resected SCLC including: (a) the surgical cases have more pathologic tissue available for analysis increasing the likelihood of finding other histopathology, and (b) the NSCLC component is much less sensitive to chemoradiation therapy and is often the major histology found in residual tumors undergoing resection.[50] This latter fact should be remembered when limited disease SCLC fails to respond as expected to chemotherapy. In such a situation, repeat biopsy should be considered, and if NSCLC is identified and there is no evidence for metastatic disease, then the operative criteria for NSCLC should be followed. Based on these facts, it is reasonable to consider surgical resection for patients with mixed SCLC, as the standard chemoradiation therapy will manage the small cell component, and surgery will eliminate the non–small cell component potentially curing this small subset of patients.[2,10]

Salvage Surgery for Initial Treatment Failure or Relapse When treatment in limited disease SCLC is unsuccessful with either persistence of disease or localized recurrence, second-line chemoradiotherapy is usually ineffective.[50] This sparked interest in the concept of salvage surgery. Shepherd et al.[51]

reported on 28 patients who underwent salvage surgery after neoadjuvant chemotherapy ± radiation therapy. The patients considered had either relapse following complete remission, no response to neoadjuvant therapy, a partial response followed by local progression while on chemotherapy, or a residual tumor mass >3 cm.[51] Histopathology revealed SCLC alone in 18 patients, mixed in 4, and NSCLC alone in 6. Postsurgical stage was stage I in 4 patients, stage II in 10, and stage III in 14. Overall 5-year survival was 25%, and all patients with pathologic stage I were still alive at the time of publication.[51] Yamada et al.[52] reported on salvage surgery following chemotherapy for SCLC in 9 patients. Four patients experienced long-term disease-free survival ranging from 3 to 11 years. Three of the long-term survivors had stage I tumors. Although the outcome data is limited, surgical resection in carefully selected patients with persistent or recurrent localized SCLC offers the best chance for local control and may improve long-term survival in a group of patients whose prognosis is otherwise dismal.

In long-term survivors of successfully treated SCLC, there is an increased frequency of second primary tumors, most commonly NSCLC. This was demonstrated by Heyne et al.[53] at the MD Anderson Cancer Center when they reviewed 47 patients with more than 2-year survival following successful treatment of SCLC and identified 14 patients with second malignancies. The risk of developing these secondary cancers increases with time from 2% at 2 to 4 years, 12.6% to 14.4% after 10 years, to a 70% actuarial cumulative risk after 15 years.[53–55] The University of Toronto reported on eight patients who developed apparent relapse after long-term survival from successful treatment of SCLC. Two patients had NSCLC and achieved successful long-term survival after surgical treatment of their second malignancy.[49,56] Any patient who develops a second lung lesion, after long-term survival following successful SCLC treatment, should not be assumed to have recurrent SCLC. Many times, the histopathology is NSCLC, which can potentially be cured with surgical resection. Needless to say, the patients with these new lung lesions should be evaluated in the same manner as any other patient with a newly diagnosed pulmonary lesion. In these cases, we would consider biopsy of the new lesion if possible. Pending the pathology, clinical stage, and performance status of the patient, surgery may be warranted with the potential of long-term cure.[10,56]

Prospective Trials of Induction Chemotherapy Followed by Surgical Resection As some of the promising results from adjuvant chemotherapy for SCLC were reported, an interest in neoadjuvant chemotherapy was begun. Several institutions developed phase II prospective trials to further evaluate the benefit. The results of 15 such studies can be found summarized in Table 38.3.

TABLE 38.3 Prospective Phase II Trials of Induction Chemotherapy Followed by Surgery for Limited Small Cell Lung Cancer

Author	N	Clinical Stage			Drug Regimen	ORR(%)/ Path CR(%)	No. Surgery: Thoracotomy/CSR	5-Year Survival
		I	II	III				
Prager et al.[57]	39	2	12	25	CAVE × 2–4	88/5	1/8 (21%)	—
Williams et al.[58]	38	—	—	—	CAE × 3	82/11	25/21 (55%)	38%
Johnson et al.[59]	24	3	7	14	CAV × 6 ±EP	100/37	23/15 (62%)	—
Baker et al. [60]	37	—	—	—	CAE × 2	54/5	20/20 (54%)	58% (2 yrs)
Shepherd et al.[61]	72	21	16	35	CAV × 6 ±EP	80/4	38/33 (36%)	36%
Benfield et al.[62]	8	—	5	3	CAEV × 2	88/0	8/8 (100%)	—
Zatopek et al.[63]	25	10	1	24	COPE × 3	96/20	14/10 (40%)	—
Hara et al.[64]	17	4	6	7	Various	82/?	17/17 (100%)	33%
Eberhardt et al.[65]	46	6	2	38	EP	94/24	32/23 (50%)	46%
Fujimori et al.[66]	22	11	4	7	CAV	96/25	21/21 (96%)	64% (3 yrs)
Rea et al.[67]	53	—	—	—	Various	—/—	38/37 (70%)	20%
Gridelli et al.[68]	33	0	1	32	Car, Ep, E	90/9	5/4 (12%)	9% (4 yrs)
Wada et al.[24]	17				Various	?/13	—	31%
Lewinski et al.[69]	75	6[a]	12[a]	17[a]	EP × 3	75/16	46/35 (4%7)	29%
Müller et al.[70]	27	—	—	27	Various	—	48/45 (94%)[b]	36%

[a]Stage reported only for surgical patients.

[b]Includes patients who had surgery before chemotherapy.

From Darling GE, Shepherd FA. Surgical management of small cell lung cancer. In: Pass HI, Carbone DP, Johnson DH, Minna JD, Turrisi AT, eds. Lung Cancer Principles and Practice. 3rd Ed. Philadelphia: Lippincott Williams & Wilkins, 2005;475–490, with permission.

A, doxorubicin; C, cyclophosphamide; Car, carboplatin; CR, complete response; CSR, complete surgical resection; E, etoposide; Ep, epirubicin; O, vincristine; ORR, overall response rate; P, cisplatin; V, vincristine.

Each of the studies administered multiple courses of combination chemotherapy. Approximately 60% of patients were rendered resectable after neoadjuvant therapy with more than 80% of those being completely resected.[71] Although there is mention of a more difficult surgical dissection after neoadjuvant therapy, the overall morbidity/mortality did not appear to be significantly increased or different from that seen in patients without neoadjuvant therapy. The complete pathologic response rate ranged from 4% to 37%, with an average of about 10%, not dissimilar to the results found in patients with NSCLC treated with surgery and neoadjuvant chemotherapy. Patients with no viable tumor identified within the surgical specimen had the best survival with some patients cured.[71] The importance of pathologic TNM staging was verified, with stage I tumors having a 5-year survival of approximately 70% when complete resection was performed. The results were not as good for stages II and III, but all series report at least few patients with N2 disease that achieved long-term survival and appeared cured by the multimodality therapy.[71]

The objective of these trials was to look at the combination of induction chemotherapy followed by surgical resection in terms of long-term survival and cure by reducing the rate of local recurrence. The local failure rate of most studies ranged from 10% to 20% in patients with complete resection (Table 38.4). Of the patients who responded to chemotherapy and proceeded to surgery, approximately 15% had unresectable tumors. If the unresectable patients are combined with those patients who locally relapsed, the local failure rate is approximately 25% of the surgical patients.

In 2007, Veronesi et al.[72] reported a single-center prospective trial to evaluate the utility of surgical resection after neoadjuvant chemotherapy (cisplatin/carboplatin and etoposide ± ifosfamide) in patients with limited disease SCLC. Data from 1998 to 2004 on 23 consecutive patients was accumulated. Nineteen patients underwent curative surgery. Four patients had a complete pathologic response, with 7 being stage I, 7 stage II, and 5 stage III. Overall 3-year survival was 25%, but in the 11 with pathologic stage 0 or I, it was 90% at 2 years versus 20% in those with pathologic stage II or III. Local recurrence rate was 17%, and the brain was the most common site of distant metastases occurring in 39% of the patients. They concluded that patients with limited clinical disease (N0), or those pathologically downstaged to pN0 following neoadjuvant therapy would benefit from surgery with the result being good local control. They also recommend prophylactic brain irradiation for all responders, because this was the most common site of distant metastatic recurrence.

Although these phase II trials would suggest a benefit to including surgery with neoadjuvant chemotherapy for limited small cell carcinoma, there has still been question as to whether patient selection was the reason for the outcomes seen in these trials. The Toronto Group has emphasized the importance of selection bias.[73] A significant survival advantage was found for patients who had no clinical involvement of mediastinal lymph nodes.

Randomized Trials To further determine the role of surgery combined with chemoradiotherapy in the treatment of SCLC, Lad et al.,[74] as part of the Lung Cancer Study Group, organized a prospective randomized trial of induction chemotherapy and surgery in 1983. The patients received five courses of induction chemotherapy, which included cyclophosphamide, doxorubicin, vincristine, and etoposide in the early phase, and cyclophosphamide, doxorubicin, and vincristine in the later phase. Afterward, patients were evaluated for response to chemotherapy. Induction therapy had to be received by all patients, the tumor had to be

TABLE 38.4 Pattern of Relapse for Patients with Small Cell Lung Cancer Treated with Induction Chemotherapy followed by Surgery[a]

Author	Thoracotomy/ Complete Resection	Number of Patients with Relapse		
		Local Only	Distant Only	Both
Prager et al.[57]	11/8	—	4	—
Williams et al.[58]	25/21	3	6	—
Johnson et al.[59]	23/15	3	7	3
Shepherd et al.[61]	38/33	3	20	—
Benfield et al.[62]	8/8	—	6	0
Zatopek et al.[63]	14/10	—	5	—
Hara et al.[64]	17/17	3	7	—
Yamada et al.[52]	20/18	3	7	—
Müller et al.[70]	48/45	4	15	—
Lewinski et al.[69]	46/35	3	16	2
Total	**250/210**	**22**	**93**	**5**

[a]Excluding patients who did not have complete surgical resection at time of thoracotomy.

From Darling GE, Shepherd FA. Surgical management of small cell lung cancer. In: Pass HI, Carbone DP, Johnson DH, Minna JD, Turrisi AT, eds. *Lung Cancer Principles and Practice.* 3rd Ed. Philadelphia: Lippincott Williams & Wilkins, 2005;475–490, with permission.

judged resectable, and there had to be no evidence of spread of disease. They were then randomized to receive surgery followed by thoracic radiation and prophylactic cranial radiation versus the same without surgery. There were 340 patients entered into the trial with a 68% clinical response rate, 28% complete, and 37% partial. Sixty-eight patients were randomized to surgery, 76 patients to no surgery, 6 patients refused surgery, and 8 had off-protocol surgery, totalling 70 patients that underwent surgery. Fifty-four patients (77%) were thought to have complete resection with an 18% complete pathologic response. The median survival for all patients was 14 months, with a 15.4-month median survival for the surgical arm and 18.6 for the no surgery arm. The 2-year survival rate was only 20%, with a local failure rate of approximately 38% in both arms.

Several groups are currently in the process of randomized trials to further define the specific role of surgery in limited disease SCLC. Eberhardt and Korfee,[75,76] of the Essen Thoracic Oncology Group, have a randomized phase II trial where patients will receive neoadjuvant chemotherapy with etoposide and cisplatin for three cycles, followed by twice-daily radiation (45 Gy) with concurrent chemotherapy, followed by randomization. The first arm will be definitive surgery and the second arm will be small-volume chemoradiation boost (20/26 Gy daily). The primary end point will be a comparison of locoregional relapse-free survival in 4 years.[75] Fukuoka and Tada, of the West Japan Lung Cancer Group, are performing a prospective randomized trial to evaluate trimodality therapy in patients with mainly stage IIIA disease.[75,76] One arm includes neoadjuvant chemotherapy with etoposide and cisplatin for three cycles, followed by twice-daily radiation (45 Gy) with concurrent chemotherapy, followed by surgery. The second arm includes one cycle of chemotherapy, followed by two cycles of hyperfractionated accelerated twice-daily radiation therapy (45 Gy), followed by two more cycles of chemotherapy. Thomas and Passlick are part of a German multicenter randomized trial, where patients are randomized to five cycles of chemotherapy with paclitaxel, etoposide, and carboplatin, followed by surgery with or without once-daily radiation therapy (50 Gy) versus the same neoadjuvant chemotherapy, followed by once daily-radiation therapy (50 Gy) only.[75,76] Hopefully, these trials will yield insight into improved treatment options for limited disease SCLC.

CONCLUSION

It is clear that surgery plays a less definitive role in the treatment of SCLC than in NSCLC. Moreover, the exact role of surgery in treating SCLC remains elusive because of the paucity of up-to-date information. For the patient where SCLC is diagnosed intraoperatively at the time of SPN or presumed NSCLC resection, surgical staging followed by appropriate surgical resection is the preferred treatment. This should be followed postoperatively by noninvasive staging, which might not have been preoperatively obtained and adjuvant chemotherapy.

Based on several historical series, clinical T1 and T2 SCLC without evidence of lymph node involvement (N0) can be considered for surgical resection. Careful patient selection is of paramount importance. When making decisions about the best treatment for SCLC, it must be remembered that a substantial percentage of patients have a higher pathologic stage than clinical stage. Therefore, prior to any surgery, an extensive mediastinal and distant metastatic disease evaluation, both noninvasive and, if necessary, invasive, should be performed. There is unanimous emphasis on the importance of TNM staging which has been shown to correlate with long-term survival and possible cure.

With regard to stage II disease, it is not possible to make generalized recommendations regarding surgery, and treatment decisions must be individualized. If surgery is part of the treatment approach, it is likely best offered as adjuvant therapy to patients with a demonstrated response to chemotherapy.

The poor prognosis for stage III SCLC clearly does not justify surgical therapy outside of the setting of a prospective randomized trial. For stage IV SCLC, surgery is reserved for palliation of symptoms such as treatment of symptomatic pleural effusion or central airway obstruction.

The final group of SCLC patients that might benefit from surgical resection is those patients with mixed histopathology. For such patients, the treatment might be up-front resection for early stage disease, followed by adjuvant chemotherapy or neoadjuvant chemotherapy to control the small cell component followed by surgery for the NSCLC remnant. For patients who experience an unexpectedly poor chemotherapeutic response or develop a localized relapse, repeat biopsy should be performed, and if NSCLC is found, surgical resection should be considered therapy.

REFERENCES

1. Sher T, Dy GK, Adjei AA. Small cell lung cancer. *Mayo Clin Proc* 2008;83:355–367.
2. Govindan R, Page N, Morgensztern D, et al. Changing epidemiology of small-cell lung cancer in the United States over the last 30 years: analysis of the surveillance, epidemiologic, and end results database. *J Clin Oncol* 2006;24:4539–4544.
3. Working-party on the evaluation of different methods of therapy in carcinoma of the bronchus. Comparative trial of surgery and radiotherapy for the primary treatment of small-celled or oat-celled carcinoma of the bronchus. *Lancet* 1966;2:979–986.
4. Miller AB, Fox W, Tall R. Five-year follow-up of the Medical Research Council comparative trial of surgery and radiotherapy for the primary treatment of small-celled or oat-celled carcinoma of the bronchus. *Lancet* 1969;2:501–505.
5. Fox W, Scadding JG. Medical Research Council comparative trial of surgery and radiotherapy for primary treatment of small-celled or oat-celled carcinoma of the bronchus. Ten-year follow-up. *Lancet* 1973;2:63–65.
6. Elliott JA, Osterlind K, Hirsch FR, et al. Metastatic patterns in small-cell lung cancer: correlation of autopsy findings with clinical parameters in 537 patients. *J Clin Oncol* 1987;5:246–254.
7. Passlick B. Can surgery improve local control in small cell lung cancer? *Lung Cancer* 2001;33(Suppl 1):S147–S151.
8. Mountain CF. Clinical biology of small cell carcinoma: relationship to surgical therapy. *Semin Oncol* 1978;5:272–279.
9. Szczesny TJ, Szczesna A, Shepherd FA, et al. Surgical treatment of small cell lung cancer. *Semin Oncol* 2003;30(1):47–56.

10. Dusmet M, Goldstraw P. Surgery for small cell lung cancer. *Hematol Oncol Clin North Am* 2004;18:323–341.
11. Deslauriers J. Surgery for small cell lung cancer. *Lung Cancer* 1997; 17(Suppl 1):S91–S98.
12. Leo F, Pastorino U. Surgery in small-cell lung carcinoma. Where is the rationale? *Semin Surg Oncol* 2003;21:176–181.
13. Bates M, Levison V, Hurt R, et al. Treatment of oat-cell carcinoma of the bronchus by preoperative radiotherapy and surgery. *Lancet* 1975; 1:1134–1135.
14. Levison V. Pre-operative radiotherapy and surgery in the treatment of oat-cell carcinoma of the bronchus. *Clin Radiol* 1980;31:345–348.
15. Sherman DM, Neptune W, Weichselbaum R, et al. An aggressive approach to marginally resectable lung cancer. *Cancer* 1978;41:2040–2045.
16. Shah S, Thompson J, Goldstraw P. Results of operation without adjuvant therapy in the treatment of small cell lung cancer. *Ann Thorac Surg* 1992;54:498–501.
17. Sørensen HR, Lund C, Alstrup P. Survival in small cell lung carcinoma after surgery. *Thorax* 1986;41:479–482.
18. Shore DF, Paneth M. Survival after resection of small cell carcinoma of the bronchus. *Thorax* 1987;35:819–822.
19. Lennox SC, Flavell G, Pollock DJ, et al. Results of resection for oat-cell carcinoma of the lung. *Lancet* 1968;2:925–927.
20. Prasad US, Naylor AR, Walker WS, et al. Long term survival after pulmonary resection for small cell carcinoma of the lung. *Thorax* 1989;44:784–787.
21. Inoue M, Miyoshi S, Yasumitsu T, et al. Surgical results for small cell lung cancer based on the new TNM staging system. Thoracic Surgery Study Group of Osaka Universuty, Osaka, Japan. *Ann Thorac Surg* 2000; 70:1615–1619.
22. Coolen L, Van den Eeckhout A, Deneffe G, et al. Surgical treatment of small cell lung cancer. *Eur J Cardiothorac Surg* 1995;9:59–64.
23. Lucchi M, Mussi A, Chella A, et al. Surgery in the management of small cell lung cancer. *Eur J Cardiothorac Surg* 1997;12:689–693.
24. Wada H, Yokomise H, Tanaka F, et al. Surgical treatment of small cell lung carcinoma of the lung: advantage of preoperative chemotherapy. *Lung Cancer* 1995;13:45–56.
25. Bergsagel DE, Jenkin RD, Pringle JF, et al. Lung cancer: clinical trial of radiotherapy alone versus radiotherapy plus cyclophosphamide. *Cancer* 1972;30:621–627.
26. Medical Research Council Lung Working Party. Radiotherapy alone or with chemotherapy in the treatment of small-cell carcinoma of the lung. *Br J Cancer* 1979;40:1–10.
27. Shields TW, Humphrey EW, Eastridge CE, et al. Adjuvant cancer chemotherapy after resection of carcinoma of the lung. *Cancer* 1977; 40:2057–2062.
28. Shields TW, Higgins GA Jr, Matthews MJ, et al. Surgical resection in the management of small cell carcinoma of the lung. *J Thorac Cardiovasc Surg* 1982;84:481–488.
29. Higgins GA, Shields TW, Keehn RJ. The solitary pulmonary nodule. Ten-year follow-up of Veteran's Administration-Armed Forces Cooperative study. *Arch Surg* 1975;110:570–575.
30. Angeletti CA, Macchiarini P, Mussi A, et al. Influence of T and N stages on long-term survival in resectable small cell lung cancer. *Eur J Surg Oncol* 1989;15:337–340.
31. Simon GR, Wagner H. Small cell lung cancer. *Chest* 2003;123(1 Suppl): S259–S271.
32. Quoix E, Fraser R, Wolkove N, et al. Small cell lung cancer presenting as solitary pulmonary nodule. *Cancer* 1990;66:577–582.
33. Muhm JR, Miller WE, Fontana RS, et al. Lung cancer detected during a screening program using four months chest radiographs. *Radiology* 1983;148:609–615.
34. Kreisman H, Wolkove N, Quoix E. Small cell lung cancer presenting as a solitary pulmonary nodule. *Chest* 1992;101:225–231.
35. Warren WH, Faber LP, Gould VE. Neuroendocrine neoplasms of the lung: a clincopathologic update. *J Thorac Cardivasc Surg* 1989;98:321–332.
36. Chandra V, Allen MS, Nichols FC III, et al. The role of pulmonary resection in small cell lung cancer. *Mayo Clin Proc* 2006;81:619–624.
37. Meyer JA, Gullo JJ, Ikins PM, et al. Adverse prognostic effect of N2 disease in treated small-cell carcinoma of the lung. *J Thorac Cardiovasc Surg* 1984;88:495–501.
38. Meyer JA, Comis RL, Ginsberg SJ, et al. The prospect of disease control by surgery with chemotherapy in stage I and stage II small cell carcinoma of the lung. *Ann Thorac Surg* 1983;36:37–41.
39. Osterlind K, Hansen M, Hansen HH, et al. Influence of surgical resection prior to chemotherapy on the long-term results in small-cell lung cancer. A study of 150 operable patients. *Eur J Cancer Clin Oncol* 1986;22:589–593.
40. Maassen W, Greschuchna D. Small-cell carcinoma of the lung—to operate or not? Surgical experience and results. *J Thorac Cardiovasc Surg* 1986;34:71–76.
41. Shepherd FA, Evans WK, Feld R, et al. Adjuvant chemotherapy following surgical resection for small-cell carcinoma of the lung. *J Clin Oncol* 1988;6:832–838.
42. Ulsperger E, Karrer K, Denck H. Multimodality treatment for small-cell bronchial carcinoma. Preliminary results of a prospective, multicenter trial. The ISC-Lung Cancer Study Group. *Eur J Cardiothorac Surg* 1991;5:306–309; discussion 310.
43. Macchiarini P, Hardin M, Basolo F, et al. Surgery plus adjuvant chemotherapy for T1–3N0M0 small-cell lung cancer. *Am J Clin Oncol* 1991; 14:218–224.
44. Ichinose Y, Hara N, Ohta M, et al. Comparison between resected and irradiated small cell lung cancer in patients in stages I through IIIa. *Ann Thorac Surg* 1992;53(1):95–100.
45. Davis S, Crino L, Tonato M, et al. A prospective analysis of chemotherapy following surgical resection of clinical stage I–II small-cell lung cancer. *Am J Clin Oncol* 1993;16:93–95.
46. Cataldo I. Long-term survival for resectable small cell lung cancer. *Lung Cancer* 2000;29(Suppl 1):130(abst 428).
47. Friess GG, McCracken JD, Troxell ML, et al. Effect of initial resection of small-cell carcinoma of the lung: a review of Southwest Oncology Group Study 7628. *J Clin Oncol* 1985;3(7):964–968.
48. Magnum MD, Greco FA, Hainsworth JD, et al. Combination small-cell and non-small-cell lung cancer. *J Clin Oncol* 1989;7:607–612.
49. Shepard FA, Ginsberg RJ, Feld R, et al. Surgical treatment for limited small-cell lung cancer. *J Thorac Cardiovasc Surg* 1991;101:385–393.
50. Anraku M, Waddell TK. Surgery for small-cell lung cancer. *Semin Thorac Cardiovasc Surg* 2006;18:211–216.
51. Shepherd FA, Ginsberg R, Patterson GA, et al. Is there ever a role for salvage operations in limited small cell lung cancer? *J Thorac Cardiovasc Surg* 1991;101:196–200.
52. Yamada K, Saijo N, Kojima A, et al. A retrospective analysis of patients receiving surgery after chemotherapy for small cell lung cancer. *Jpn J Clin Oncol* 1991;21:39–45.
53. Heyne KH, Lippman SM, Lee JJ, et al. The incidence of second primary tumors in long-term survivors of small cell lung cancer. *J Clin Oncol* 1992;10:1519–1524.
54. Govindan R, Ihde DC. Practical issues in the management of the patient with small cell lung cancer. *Chest Surg Clin N Am* 1997;7(1):167–181.
55. Richardson GE, Tucker MA, Venzon DJ, et al. Smoking cessation after successful treatment of small cell lung cancer is associated with fewer smoking-related second primary cancers. *Ann Int Med* 1993;119: 383–390.
56. Shepherd FA. The role of surgery in SCLC. In: Movsas B, Langer CJ, Goldberg M, eds. *Controversies in Lung Cancer A Multidisciplinary Approach*. New York: Marcel Dekker, Inc, 2001:125–148.
57. Prager RL, Foster JM, Hainsworth JD, et al. The feasibility of adjuvant surgery in limited-stage small cell carcinoma: a prospective evaluation. *Ann Thorac Surg* 1984;38:622–626.
58. Williams CJ, McMillan I, Lea R, et al. Surgery after initial chemotherapy for localized small cell carcinoma of the lung. *J Clin Oncol* 1987;5:1579–1588.
59. Johnson DH, Einhorn LH, Mandelbaum I, et al. Postchemotherapy resection of residual tumor in limited stage small cell lung cancer. *Chest* 1987;92:241–246.

60. Baker RR, Ettinger DS, Ruckdeschel JD, et al. The role of surgery in the management of selected patients with small-cell carcinoma of the lung. *J Clin Oncol* 1987;5:697–702.
61. Shepherd FA, Ginsberg RJ, Patterson GA, et al. A prospective study of adjuvant surgical resection after chemotherapy for limited small cell cancer. A University of Toronto Lung Oncology Group trial. *J Thorac Cardiovasc Surg* 1989;97:177–186.
62. Benfield GF, Matthews HR, Watson DC, et al. Chemotherapy plus adjuvant surgery for local small cell lung cancer. *Eur J Surg Oncol* 1989; 15:341–344.
63. Zatopek NK, Holoye PY, Ellerbroek NA, et al. Resectability of small-cell lung cancer following induction chemotherapy in patients with limited disease (stage II–IIIb). *Am J Clin Oncol* 1991;14:427–432.
64. Hara N, Ichinose Y, Kuda T, et al. Long-term survivors in resected and nonresected small cell lung cancer. *Oncology* 1991;48:441–447.
65. Eberhardt W, Wilke H, Stamatis G, et al. Preliminary results of a stage oriented multimodality treatment including surgery for selected subgroups of limited disease small cell lung cancer. *Lung Cancer* 1997; 18(Suppl 1):61.
66. Fujimori K, Yokoyam A, Kurita Y, et al. A pilot phase II study of surgical treatment after induction chemotherapy for respectable stage I to stage IIIA small cell lung cancer. *Chest* 1997;111:1089–1093.
67. Rea F, Callagaro D, Favaretto A, et al. Long-term results of surgery and chemotherapy in small cell lung cancer. *Eur J Cardiothorac Surg* 1998;14:398–402.
68. Gridelli C, D'aprile M, Curcio C, et al. Carboplatin plus epirubicin plus VP-16 concurrent "split-course" radiotherapy and adjuvant surgery for limited small cell lung cancer. *Lung Cancer* 1994;11: 83–91.
69. Lewinski T, Zulawski M, Turski C, et al. Small cell lung cancer stage I-IIIA: a cytoreductive chemotherapy followed by resection with continuation of chemotherapy. *Eur J Cardiothorac Surg* 2001;20:391–398.
70. Müller LC, Salzer GM, Huber H, et al. Multimodal therapy of small cell lung cancer in NM stages I–IIIa. *Ann Thorac Surg* 1992;54: 493–497.
71. Darling GE, Shepherd FA. Surgical management of small cell lung cancer. In Pass HI, Carbone DP, Johnson DH, Minna JD, Turrisi AT, eds. *Lung Cancer Principles and Practice.* 3rd Ed. Philadelphia: Lippincott Williams & Wilkins, 2005:475–490.
72. Veronesi G, Scanagatta P, Leo F, et al. Adjuvant surgery after carboplatin and VP16 in resectable small cell lung cancer. *J Thorac Oncol* 2007;2(2):131–134.
73. Shepherd FA, Ginsberg RJ, Haddad R, et al. Importance in clinical staging in limited small-cell lung cancer: a valuable system to separate prognostic subgroups. *J Clin Oncol* 1993;8:1592–1597.
74. Lad T, Piantadosi S, Thomas P, et al. A prospective randomized trial to determine the benefit of surgical resection of residual disease following response of small cell lung cancer to combination chemotherapy. *Chest* 1994;7(Suppl 6):3205–3235.
75. Eberhardt W, Korfee S. New approaches for small-cell lung cancer: local treatments. *Cancer Control* 2003;10(4):289–296.
76. Koletsis EN, Prokakis C, Karanikolas M, et al. Current role of surgery in small cell lung carcinoma. *J Cardiothorac Surg* 2009;4:30.

CHAPTER 39

Traves D. Crabtree
Chadrick E. Denlinger

Complications of Surgery for Lung Cancer

BACKGROUND

Surgery remains the primary therapy for patient with early stage non–small cell lung cancer. Nonsurgical modalities of local therapy such as focused stereotactic radiation and radiofrequency ablation have been used recently, particularly in patients thought to be of high operative risk. In an era of multimodality therapy, with the availability of several emerging treatment options for local therapy, it is imperative that we understand the potential complications of surgery for lung cancer as well as treatment strategies for these complications to select the best treatment options for individual patients.

The risks for pulmonary resection depend primarily on the preoperative status of the patient with regard to factors such as comorbidities, overall functional status, and preoperative pulmonary function. Complications of pulmonary resection that are well described and will be discussed in this chapter include pneumonia, respiratory failure, empyema, bronchopleural fistulae, prolonged air leaks, chylothorax, postpneumonectomy pulmonary edema, postpneumonectomy syndrome, and death.

OPERATIVE RISKS ASSESSMENT

Several contemporary studies have demonstrated improved outcomes in patients undergoing pulmonary resection for malignancies compared to resections performed in an earlier era. Recent improvements in patient survival and reduction in complications have been attributed to better patient selection for surgery as well as improved postoperative care, although these perceptions are not well supported by objective data.

Recently, the American College of Surgeons Oncology Group (ACOSOG) Z0030 trial randomized patients with non–small cell lung cancer undergoing an anatomic resection for clinical T1 to T2, N0 to N1 tumors to mediastinal lymph node sampling or mediastinal lymph node dissection.[1] This study included 1023 patients from 63 different institutions and 102 different surgeons. There were 42 pneumonectomies, 42 bilobectomies, 766 lobectomies, 70 segmentectomies, and 101 patients with a combination of resections. The overall mortality rate in this patient group was 1.4%, and the overall morbidity rate was 38%. The most frequent morbidities were atrial arrhythmias (14%) followed by chest tube drainage >7 days (11%), air leak >7 days (8%), respiratory (7%), hemorrhage (3%), chylothorax (1%), and recurrent laryngeal nerve injury (1%). Table 39.1 outlines the incidence of significant complications occurring in both historical and contemporary series of lung cancer resections for comparison. The ACOSOG Z0030 multi-institutional study provides a contemporary benchmark of morbidity and mortality for patients undergoing major pulmonary resections for stage I and II lung cancers when performed by surgeons specializing in thoracic surgery.

In published series of major pulmonary resections for lung cancer, the reported mortality rates have ranged from 1.3% to 5.5% (Table 39.2).[2–8] Wada et al.[8] reported a series of 7099 thoracic procedures with significant differences in mortality noted depending on the extent of lung resection. The mortality rates were 3.2% for pneumonectomy, 1.2% for lobectomy, and 0.8% for sublobar resections. There were also significantly more deaths in patients with increasing age where the mortality rates were 0.4% for patients younger than 60 years, 1.3% for patients aged 60 to 69, 2.0% for patients 70 to 79, and 2.2% for patients 80 years or older. In the Z030 trial, there were no trends toward increased mortality or complications with larger pulmonary resections although the trial was not designed to examine differences in resection strategy.[1] Romano and Mark[5] reported a direct correlation between the extent of pulmonary resection and mortality. In this retrospective study, the mortality rates were 3.8% for wedge resections, 3.7% for segmentectomy, 4.2% for lobectomy, and 11.6% for pneumonectomy. Factors that significantly correlated with patient mortality were patients older than 60 years, extent of resection, male gender, chronic lung or heart disease, diabetes, and volume of pulmonary cases performed at each participating institution. The finding that mortality rates are higher when cases are performed by general surgeons rather than surgeons

TABLE 39.1 Incidence of Postoperative Complications following Lung Cancer Resection

Author	Year	N	Air Leak >7 Days	Chest Drain >7 Days	Chylothorax	Hemorrhage	Recurrent Nerve Injury	Arrhythmia	Respiratory	Pulmonary Embolus	Bronchopleural Fistula	Empyema	New O2 Requirement	Pneumonia	Wound Infection
Licker[102]	2006	1222	5.0%	—	—	—	—	—	16.3%	—	1.5%	5.0%	—	4.0%	—
Allen et al.[1]	2006	1023	8.0%	11%	1.0%	3.0%	1.0%	14.0%	7.0%	—	0.5%	1.1%	—	2.5%	—
Ventura[103]*	2006	379	7.0%	—	1.0%	1.0%	2.0%	21.0%	—	—	—	1.0%	7.0%	4.0%	—
Harpole Jr. et al.[9]	1999	3516	—	—	—	2.9%	—	—	—	0.8%	—	—	—	11.3%	2.6%
Deslauriers et al.[2]	1994	783	—	—	—	—	—	4.7%	7.5%	5.4%	5.1%	5.0%	—	6.4%	—

*All patients ≥80 years old.

specializing in thoracic surgery has been suggested in other studies but remains controversial.[6,7]

RISK STRATIFICATION

Clinical stage of disease plays an important role in identifying the high-risk surgical patient for two reasons. The first is the perceived likelihood of achieving the goal of cure of cancer. Patients with early stage disease have improved survival over patients with advanced stage disease. As a rule, only patients with stage I to IIIA disease are even considered for surgical therapy. Within this group, patients with stage I disease have improved survival over those with stage IIIA disease. The surgical team may favor a more aggressive approach in a patient with earlier stage disease because of an increased likelihood of cure. The second reason clinical stage is important is because of the extent of resection needed to obtain tumor free margins. Tumors requiring chest wall resection, sleeve resection, vascular reconstruction, and pneumonectomy have higher rates of complications. At times, the risk of complications is high enough to avoid recommending surgery to less surgically fit candidates with more advanced tumors.

Although a basic understanding of the expected morbidity and mortality rates is important for discussions with patients before and after major lung resections, further risk stratification based on patient comorbidities and the extent of the planned operation are also necessary. Strand et al.[7] reviewed the Norwegian experience of patients undergoing pulmonary resections between 1993 and 2005. During this period, there

TABLE 39.2 Operative Mortality following Lung Cancer Resection

			Mortality %				
Author	Date	N	Overall	Pneumonectomy	Bilobectomy	Lobectomy	Sublobar
Strand et al.[7]	2007	4395	4.4%	8.6% (92/1071)	7.3% (28/383)	2.5% (67/2663)	2.2% (6/278)
Licker et al.[102]	2006	1222	2.9%	—	—	—	—
Allen et al.[1]	2006	1023	1.4%	0 (0/42)	5% (2/42)	1% (10/766)	3% (2/70)
Ventura et al.[103]*	2006	379	6.3%	8.0% (2/25)	14.3% (1/7)	5.0% (12/240)	8.4% (9/107)
Harpole et al.[9]	1999	3516	5.2%	11.5% (119/2949)	—	4.0% (65/567)	0.8% (7/904)
Silvestri et al.[6]	1998	1583	5.2%	16.8% (28/167)	—	4.2% (59/1416)	—
Wada et al.[8]	1998	7099	1.3%	3.2% (19/586)	—	1.2% (67/5609)	0.8% (7/904)
Deslauriers et al.[2]	1994	783	3.8%	—	—	—	—
Ginsberg et al.[4]	1983	2220	3.8%	6.2% (44/569)	—	2.9% (35/1058)	1.4% (2/143)
Nagasaki et al.[104]	1982	759	2.1%	5.5% (4/72)	—	1.6% (9/570)	2.6% (3/117)
Weiss et al.[105]	1974	547	12.4%	17% (36/212)	—	10.0% (15/149)	0 (0/3)

*All patients ≥80 years old.

were 4395 procedures with an overall mortality rate of 4.4%. Multivariate analysis identified several procedure-related factors associated with an increased risk of mortality including male gender (odds ratio [OR] = 1.76), age 70 to 79 or ≥80 (OR = 3.38 and 9.94 compared to patients ≤50), right-sided tumors (OR = 1.73), and bilobectomy or pneumonectomy (OR = 3.06 and 4.54, respectively). In this study, neither the extent of local–regional advancement nor tumor size had any impact on 30-day mortality. The presence of metastatic disease was the only tumor-related factor that had a negative impact on survival. The largest observational study evaluating the impact of patient's age found a direct correlation between the patient's age and mortality with the most significant increased risk occurring after the age of 70.[7] The 30-day mortality OR for patients aged 70 to 79 and 80 to 89 were 4.91 and 19.71, respectively, when compared to patients ≤50 years. Most studies have shown that advanced age is a predictor of morbidity and mortality after pulmonary resection,[7–10] although studies in carefully selected patients older than 80 years of age undergoing pulmonary resection have shown similar morbidity and mortality rates to younger patient cohorts.[11]

In addition to factors associated with the extent of resection required, scoring systems exist to further stratify patients according to medical comorbidities.[3] Algorithms for identifying higher risk patients include the Cardiopulmonary Risk Index (CPRI),[12] the Physiological and Operative Severity Score for Enumeration of Mortality and Morbidity (POSSUM),[13] and the EVAD scoring system. The EVAD scoring system is primarily based on the patient's forced expiratory volume in 1 second (FEV_1), age, and diffusing capacity of lung for carbon monoxide (DLCO).[3] In a comparison of these three systems in a cohort of 400 patients, POSSUM scores that were retrospectively calculated did not correlate with either fatal or nonfatal complications of surgery.[3] The CPRI scoring system did not correlate with patient mortality but did correlate with nonfatal complications when analyzed together. More specifically, the CPRI calculations correlated significantly with pulmonary and cardiopulmonary complications but did not correlate with cardiovascular, infectious, or other complications. The EVAD scoring system showed trends toward prediction of mortality and did correlate significantly with all types of morbidity evaluated with the exception of infectious complications. Unfortunately, the statistical predictive power of this scoring system is, at this point, not sufficient for application to individual patients and has not been further evaluated in other institutions. In addition, scoring systems specifically developed for lung resection, such as the Predictive Respiratory Quotient (PRQ)[14] and the Predicted Postoperative Product (PPP),[15] have not gained widespread use. Although the surgical team may not rely completely on a particular scoring system to determine the surgical fitness of a patient, many of the factors that make up these scoring systems along with surgical judgment are used to make the ultimate decision. Some of these factors may include clinical stage of disease, patient age, spirometry, and presence of comorbidities.

PREOPERATIVE SPIROMETRY

An important component of risk assessment is to determine whether there is sufficient pulmonary reserve to sustain the patient postoperatively. Pulmonary function testing is used to assess airflow, lung volume, lung mechanics, and gas exchange. The two most commonly used parameters for determining surgical resectability are FEV_1 and DLCO. Surgical risk has little or no correlation with preoperative FEV_1 when lung function is relatively preserved. An observational study of patients categorized into either normal lung function (FEV_1 >80% predicted, mean = 92.2%) or reduced lung function (FEV_1 ≤80% predicted, mean = 64.2%) found no differences in the rates of air leaks >7 days, atelectasis, bleeding, contralateral pneumothorax, or atrial fibrillation.[16] However, the value of preoperative FEV_1 evaluation is more important with a greater reduction in pulmonary function. The risk of pulmonary resection increases substantially if the preoperative FEV_1 is less than 60% predicted.[17] In general, patients who fall below this mark need further testing with ventilation/perfusion scanning, which is used to determine preoperative split lung function and predicted postoperative FEV_1. DLCO is used to evaluate the integrity of the alveolar capillary membrane for gas exchange. Ferguson et al.[18] found in a retrospective study of 237 patients that preoperative DLCO predicted postoperative pulmonary complications in patients with acceptable FEV_1. They subsequently confirmed the importance of DLCO by showing that predicted postoperative DLCO is a predictor of morbidity and mortality independent of FEV_1.[19] In addition, patients with DLCO less than 60% for pneumonectomy and less than 50% for lobectomy have an increased risk of postoperative complications.[20] Although these factors are frequently utilized in the preoperative risk assessment, it should be noted that others have not found spirometric parameters such as FEV_1 or DLCO to be significant predictors of postoperative complications.[21,22] Others have successfully utilized spirometry in combination with exercise tolerance as a means of predicting pulmonary complications following resection.[23] Vital capacity, exercise induced hypoxemia (Δ PaO_2), low oxygen uptake/body weight (VO_2 max/BW), and Δ PaO_2/Δ VO_2 max/BW may be associated with an increased risk for complications.

After poor pulmonary reserve, the next most important factor contributing to risk of pulmonary resection is the presence of concomitant organ system dysfunction. In general, preoperative dysfunction of each of a particular organ system makes the risk of postoperative complications involving that organ system more likely. It is therefore essential to assess these organ systems preoperatively by history, physical exam, and special studies as needed.

INTRAOPERATIVE COMPLICATIONS

The most common, immediately life-threatening intraoperative complications of pulmonary resection not related to anesthesia management are massive hemorrhage, cardiac ischemia, arrhythmias, and contralateral pneumothorax. Common intraoperative complications that cause significant morbidity and mortality postoperatively are nerve injuries and injuries to the esophagus and thoracic duct.

Hemorrhage Massive intraoperative hemorrhage is usually the result of an injury to a pulmonary artery or vein branch sustained during dissection. The pulmonary artery and its branches are especially thin walled and easily injured during manipulation or traction employed to increase exposure. In contrast, the walls of the pulmonary vein are more resilient and withstand surgical manipulation much better. The risk of a difficult dissection and pulmonary artery injury can be anticipated in patients who have had induction chemotherapy or prior irradiation. In addition, patients with mediastinal granulomatosis or prior silica exposure will have regional bronchopulmonary lymph nodes densely adherent to branch pulmonary arteries. In such cases, it is prudent to begin the surgical dissection by encircling the ipsilateral main pulmonary artery and both pulmonary veins to obtain proximal and distal control in the event of vessel injury.

Because the pulmonary circulation is under low pressure, arterial and venous injury can usually be immediately controlled with local pressure at the injury site. It is necessary, when massive hemorrhage occurs, that the surgeon make an immediate analysis, knowing the site and magnitude of the injury, of what will be required to control the bleeding. This often requires calling for additional assistance in the operating room. With additional help and a good plan of attack, it is usually possible to readily obtain control, and perform a fine nonabsorbable suture. Rarely, injury to the main pulmonary artery, left atrium medial to the pulmonary vein, or superior or inferior vena cava will require cardiopulmonary bypass to control the situation for adequate repair.

In addition, injuries to bronchial arteries, parenchymal surfaces, pleural adhesions, as well as intercostal and internal mammary vessels can also lead to significant intraoperative blood loss if they go unnoticed. It is important to use careful dissection techniques at all times during the conduct of the operation to avoid injury to these structures and to control them quickly when they occur.

Ventilatory Complications A host of problems can occur and put the gas exchange of the patient at risk. If ventilation is established through a double-lumen endobronchial tube or a single-lumen tube with a bronchial blocking balloon, it is essential that the surgeon as well as the anesthesiologist be confident that it is in the correct position before starting the resection. The surgeon must also be aware of the presentation of tube displacement. High airway pressure and absent CO_2 in the ventilator circuit indicates that the bronchial cuff has herniated into the trachea producing an effective tracheal obstruction. Deflation of the cuff solves the problem and advancement of the tube prevents the problem from reoccurring. While conducting a right-sided resection with ventilation only on the left, persistent hypoxemia suggests that the left limb off the double-lumen tube has advanced too far and is occluding the left upper lobe orifice. This problem is sometimes first detected by the attentive surgeon, who recognizes that the usual ventilatory movement of the mediastinum is absent because of the progressively atelectatic left upper lobe. Withdrawal of the tube solves the problem.

Occasionally, it is necessary to change the endotracheal tube during resection. During resection of central T2 or T3 lesions, the endobronchial cuff may be injured or the tube may interfere with the bronchial resection or repair. The surgeon can assist with tube change by fixing a heavy suture to the distal end of the tube to be changed. After it is withdrawn, the anesthesiologist affixes the new tube to the suture. Traction on the suture by the surgeon helps guide the tube into position.

Patients undergoing thoracotomy for lung cancer resection as a rule are more susceptible to barotrauma pneumothorax because of preexisting bullous emphysema. Pneumothorax can occur at the time of induction and onset of positive pressure ventilation or, at any point, during the actual operation on the contralateral side. The surgeon should be aware of this development because airway pressures will increase, and the rhythmic movement of the mediastinum will be absent. Indeed, the mediastinum will sometimes balloon out toward the operative side. The problem is easily remedied by opening the mediastinal pleura.

Nerve Injury Nerve injuries occur in 1% to 2% of patients undergoing surgery for lung cancer. The recurrent laryngeal nerve as well as the phrenic nerve are generally considered the most important nerves encountered during lung cancer surgery. However, musculocutaneous nerves, such as the long thoracic nerve, can also be injured directly during dissection or by traction injuries during exposure. Injury to the phrenic nerve most often occurs when tumors are adherent or directly adjacent to the nerve with injury resulting in hemidiaphragm paralysis. Diaphragm plication may improve symptoms of dyspnea and breathlessness following phrenic nerve injury although the relative benefit remains controversial.[24]

The recurrent laryngeal nerve provides ipsilateral motor innervation to the intrinsic laryngeal muscles for vocalization. Injury to the nerve unilaterally may result in hoarseness or a weak voice, whereas bilateral nerve injury frequently results in a compromised airway with associated respiratory distress in the immediate postoperative period. The right recurrent laryngeal nerve can be injured during resection of apical tumors on the right as it originates from the vagus nerve at the level of the right subclavian artery medially. The left recurrent laryngeal nerve can be injured during mediastinoscopy as well as during dissection of level 5 and 6 lymph nodes or during dissection of tumors adjacent to the preaortic and subaortic region on the left side. Unilateral nerve injury significantly increases the risk of aspiration and pneumonia following lung resection. Direct laryngoscopy is diagnostic, and strict precautions should be undertaken to avoid aspiration when the diagnosis is made. Several surgical techniques are available to improve vocal cord function after injury if symptoms are debilitating or if they do not improve with speech therapy.

POSTOPERATIVE COMPLICATIONS

General Considerations

There are many complications that can arise after pulmonary resection, and some can be fatal if not recognized and managed early and aggressively. Attention to patient symptoms, clinical exam, and routine chest x-rays (CXR), in addition to a high level of suspicion during the postoperative period, will help the clinician identify complications and manage them effectively.

Airway Complications

Sputum Retention Poor airway hygiene is a significant life-threatening problem in the postthoracotomy patient. Factors such as postoperative pain and compromised mental status lead to inability to deep breathe and cough with subsequent retention of airway secretions. These airway secretions can go on to plug the airways causing atelectasis, lobar collapse, pneumonia, and respiratory failure. Specific patients at risk for postoperative sputum retention are current smokers and patients with a history of chronic obstructive pulmonary disease (COPD), cerebrovascular accident (CVA), or ischemic heart disease, and those without regional analgesia.[25] Prophylactic measures should be considered in these patients to reduce the incidence of sputum retention. An important maneuver to reduce this risk preoperatively is smoking cessation prior to elective thoracotomy. Vaporciyan et al.[26] demonstrated that patients undergoing pneumonectomy who continued to smoke within 1 month of operation were at increased risk for developing pneumonia and acute respiratory distress syndrome (ARDS). Chest physiotherapy, including coughing, early ambulation, incentive spirometry, and percussion with postural drainage, is the standard for postoperative prophylaxis and therapy for sputum retention. However, patients with recalcitrant sputum retention may require intermittent bronchoscopy to aspirate secretions and stimulate a more vigorous cough. Some surgeons recommend liberal use of minitracheostomy tubes in high-risk patients as a form of prophylaxis and treatment. The minitracheostomy tube allows immediate and repeated aspiration of the tracheobronchial tree. It is placed percutaneously through the cricothyroid membrane either at the time of surgery or at the bedside postoperatively. In a prospective randomized trial of 102 high-risk patients, Bonde et al.[27] found that prophylactic use of minitracheostomy tubes significantly lowered the incidence of sputum retention. Similarly, Au et al.[28] reported decreased need for suction bronchoscopy in patients who had undergone minitracheostomy tube placement.

Lobar Torsion Lobar torsion is a rotation of the remaining lobar bronchovascular pedicle with resultant airway obstruction, vascular compromise, and gangrene. This is a rare but life-threatening complication with an associated mortality of 12% to 16%.[29] The incidence of lobar torsion after pulmonary resection is 0.09% to 0.3%.[30–32] Lobar torsion after right upper lobe resections accounted for 70% of the cases in the literature, whereas 15% involved the left lower lobe following resection of the left upper lobe. The majority of lobar torsions involve the right middle lobe. As with most complications, prevention is the key. The surgeon should visualize the remaining lung fully inflated to ensure proper orientation after every pulmonary resection.

The presentation of lobar torsion may be dramatic, especially in the early postoperative period. Physical findings may include fever, tachycardia, sudden cessation of a previous air leak, and loss of breath sounds over the affected lung field. Computed tomography (CT) is more sensitive than CXR in the evaluation of these patients. Radiologic findings include rapid opacification or serial positional change of the affected lobe, complete opacification of the involved lung or inversion of the vascular pattern. However, immediate bronchoscopy is the most expedient diagnostic modality to confirm suspected lobar torsion. Bronchoscopy reveals a compressed bronchus with a fishmouth appearance.

Exploratory thoracotomy must be performed without delay. The involved lobe or lung is untwisted to assess its viability. If the diagnosis is made early, the involved lobe may be viable and fixation may be all that is necessary. However, when a gangrenous lobe or lung is rotated back into normal position, the airways may be flooded with serosanguineous fluid. It is, therefore, prudent to use a double-lumen endotracheal tube to prevent soilage of the remaining lung. Many times, the involved lobe or lung must be resected. The concern for lobar torsion has lead to the common practice of prophylactic fixation of the middle lobe to the lower lobe after right upper lobectomy if the oblique fissure is complete to prevent middle lobe torsion.

Bronchopleural Fistula After pulmonary resection, a communication between the airway and the pleural space can establish itself in the form of a bronchopleural fistula. This is a serious and potentially life-threatening complication that can occur after pulmonary resection. The incidence of bronchopleural fistula after pulmonary resection ranges from 1.6% to 6.2%.[33] A multivariate analysis of 1360 pulmonary resections demonstrated that risk factors for bronchopleural fistula include wider resection such as pneumonectomy, residual cancer at the bronchial stump, preoperative radiation therapy, and diabetes mellitus.[34] Subsequent mortality after bronchopleural fistula was 71%. It has also been noted that postpneumonectomy bronchopleural fistula is more likely to occur on the right side. Postlobectomy bronchopleural fistula is exceedingly uncommon except following bilobectomy involving the right middle and lower lobes. Other situations have been shown to predispose to the development of bronchopleural fistula (e.g., radical mediastinal lymphadenectomy, and resections for infectious or inflammatory disease).

Whether to staple or suture the bronchus at the time of resection is a continuing source of controversy in thoracic surgery. In experimental conditions, El-Gamel et al.[35] found that hand sutured bronchi tolerate higher inflation pressures compared with stapled ones before leaking air but at supraphysiologic pressures (200 vs. 105 mm Hg, respectively). Clinically, both manual suture[36] and stapled closure[37] have been found to be safe and reliable methods of bronchial stump closure. There has been no definitive study to show that one method is superior to the other. However, in cases in which close bronchial margins are likely, it is better to cut the bronchus with a scalpel and close the bronchial stump by suturing to avoid the possibility of residual cancer at the bronchial stump. In addition, patients with any of the previously described risk factors should have preventive pedicled flap coverage at the time initial resection.

During the early postoperative period (1 to 2 days), the most likely cause of bronchopleural fistula is technical failure. This usually manifests as a massive air leak from the chest tube and progressive increase in subcutaneous emphysema. These early fistulae should be repaired surgically and the bronchial stump securely covered with a viable pedicled flap. Bronchopleural fistula sustained later in the postoperative course are usually caused by bronchial stump ischemia secondary to extensive dissection, or the presence of infected pleural fluid with resulting rupture of the empyema through the bronchial stump closure. At this point, the patient will typically develop a cough with expectoration of serosanguineous, frothy fluid. Efforts to protect the contralateral lung should be instituted such as placing the operated side down and prompt drainage of the infected pleural space. The bronchopleural fistula, which occurs later than 2 weeks, is also likely secondary to an infected pleural space. However, the patient is more likely to present with sepsis, and the sputum is more likely to be purulent. In addition, these patients may have a more indolent presentation. In fact, patients may present with minimal symptoms yet demonstrate a fall in the air fluid level on radiographs, suggesting a fluid leak into the airway (Fig. 39.1). The diagnosis of bronchopleural fistula can be confirmed by bronchoscopy, bronchography, or radionuclide inhalation imaging.

Initial management of bronchopleural fistula involves drainage of the involved pleural space and dependent drainage of the operative side to prevent soiling of the uninvolved lung. Subsequent management is based on timing after surgery and the presence or absence of sepsis. An early bronchopleural fistula (first 7 days) is unlikely to have significant pleural space infection and is usually caused by a technical problem. These should be reexplored with bronchial stump closure and covered with a flap of muscle, pericardium, or omentum. A bronchopleural fistula, which develops later than the first week is less likely to be the result of a technical problem and should not be treated with immediate stump reclosure. A delayed bronchopleural fistula is usually associated with some degree of empyema and requires immediate chest tube drainage of the infected

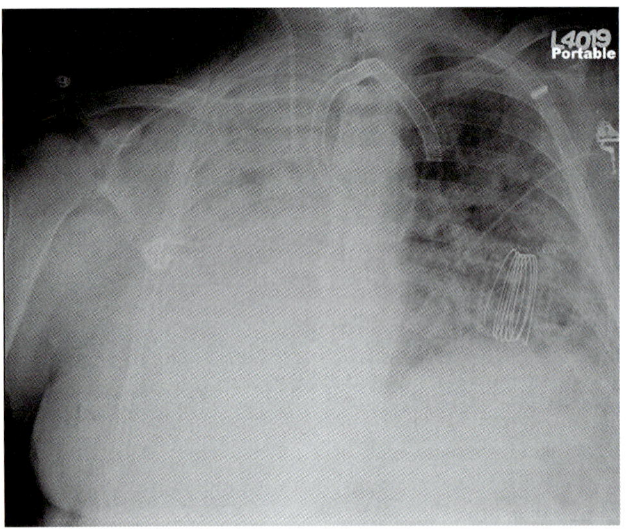

A

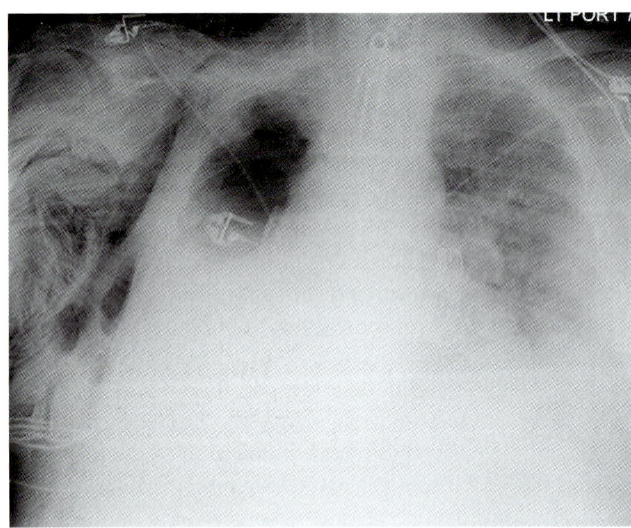
B

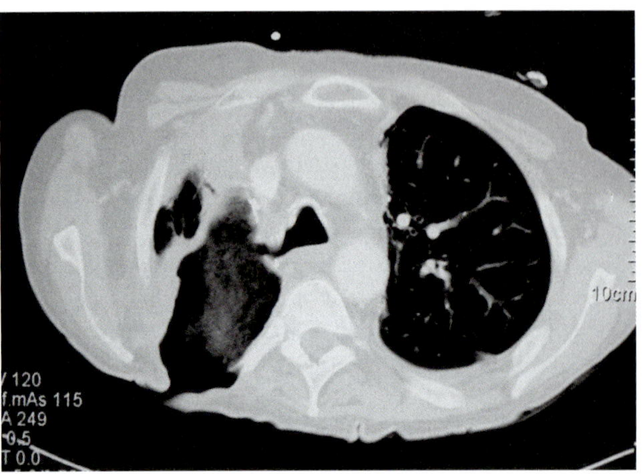

C

FIGURE 39.1 Bronchopleural fistula. **A:** Postoperative CXR following right pneumonectomy with diffuse infiltrative process of remaining left lung and opacification of right pleural space filled with fluid. **B:** CXR 2 days later with increased subcutaneous air and new air fluid level in right pleural cavity suggesting a new bronchopleural fistula. **C:** CT scan with visible right upper lobe bronchial stump defect.

space and appropriate antibiotic therapy. If the fistula is not large and there is remaining lung in the pleural space, spontaneous closure will often occur with this management alone.

A detailed discussion of the management of postpneumonectomy bronchopleural fistula is beyond the scope of this chapter. The traditional management approach involves three separate procedures; early open drainage, closure of the fistula, and subsequent closure of the cavity. Open window thoracoplasty such as Eloesser flap or Clagett window provides excellent drainage, prevents soilage of the contralateral lung, and creates a large opening for insertion of sterile packing. Ordinarily, a period of several weeks or months of intensive dressing changes are required to get the pleural cavity clean and covered with healthy granulation tissue. Indeed, depending on the overall status of the patient and the anticipated technical challenges of possible closure, the best option for the patient may be a permanent open-window thoracostomy.

The strategy for fistula repair depends on the location of the fistula. Direct dissection and primary repair of the bronchopleural fistula is usually impossible. Lobar fistulae can usually be successfully covered with a pedicled muscle flap or omentum. Depending on the bulk of the flap and the size of the pleural space, this coverage procedure may also serve to fill the cavity and achieve simultaneous closure of the cavity. For postpneumonectomy bronchopleural fistulae, there are several options for fistula closure. If there is some length of main bronchus proximal to the fistula, the main bronchus can be sealed and divided proximal to the fistula. A transsternal, transpericardial approach provides access to either main bronchus by retracting the superior vena cava and ascending aorta laterally. If there is inadequate bronchial length, closure of the fistula by muscle flap or omentum is the best option. In this circumstance, depending on bulk of flap and size of pleural space, the flap may completely fill the cavity. If not a subsequent rotation or free-flap procedure may be necessary to fill the cavity.

Postpneumonectomy Syndrome Tracheobronchial obstruction may occur after pneumonectomy associated with severe mediastinal shift. This is a rare complication most commonly seen after right pneumonectomy in which the left mainstem bronchus is displaced toward the side of the pneumonectomy resulting in its compression between the thoracic spine and the aorta or pulmonary artery (Fig. 39.2). It can also be seen after left pneumonectomy in patients with a right aortic arch. It has a late clinical presentation with findings of dyspnea on exertion, ineffective cough, expiratory stridor, difficulty clearing secretions, and recurrent pulmonary infections. Complete shift of the heart and mediastinum into a hemithorax devoid of fluid is usually seen on chest radiograph. Chest CT clearly demonstrates the mediastinal shift and cardiac rotation as well as compression of the mainstem bronchus between the vertebral body and the aorta or pulmonary artery.

Management of postpneumonectomy syndrome involves repositioning the mediastinum back toward the midline, thereby relieving the bronchial obstruction. This can be done with cardiopexy and placement of autologous tissue or an expandable prosthesis placed in the pneumonectomy space (Fig. 39.2).[38,39] Aortic division and bypass has been utilized for this problem with less favorable results. In some patients with longstanding airway compression, bronchomalacia can develop which significantly lowers the efficacy of mediastinal repositioning. Placement of bronchial stents has also been described for relief of postpneumonectomy airway obstruction.[40] This may prove useful for patients with associated bronchomalacia.

Parenchymal Complications

Postresection Pulmonary Edema Noncardiogenic pulmonary edema is a rare but lethal complication of major lung resection. The incidence is 2% to 5% after pneumonectomy (right more common than left) and 1% after lobectomy.[41,42] This complication is often fatal with mortality rates of 30% to 100%. Consistent findings include onset 24 to 72 hours after surgery, diffuse interstitial infiltration to frank alveolar edema on chest radiograph (Fig. 39.3) and CT scan, progressive hypoxia, and overall rapid clinical decline. These patients have no evidence of heart failure, pneumonia, pulmonary emboli, or fluid overload.

It has been thought that the edema is caused by intraoperative or postoperative fluid overload. In a retrospective study by Parquin et al.,[43] multivariate analysis identified prior radiotherapy, perfusion of the remaining lung of 55% or less and high intraoperative fluid load as independent risk factors for postpneumonectomy pulmonary edema. Zeldin et al.[44] as well as Verheijen-Breemhaar et al.[45] found overhydration to be a common precipitating factor in these cases. However, Turnage and Lunn[46] found no association between fluid balance and the development of edema. Other factors such as increased permeability and filtration pressure[12] and decreased lymphatic drainage from the affected lung are thought to play a more important role.

Given the rapid progression of this syndrome, therapy must be early and aggressive including early intubation and mechanical ventilation, aggressive diuresis to improve fluid balance, broad-spectrum antibiotic coverage, and aggressive pulmonary toilet such as bronchoscopy and frequent position changes of the patient (to include prone and lateral positioning during mechanical ventilation). Steroid therapy has been recommended by some but has no proven benefit. Mathisen et al.[47] found early use of inhaled nitric oxide to be a useful strategy in these patients.

As this condition most commonly occurs following right pneumonectomy, there is a distinct risk of bronchopleural fistula, if mechanical ventilation is required. This risk can be minimized by immediate tracheostomy and insertion of an endotracheal tube, which can be advanced into the left main bronchus to accomplish positive pressure ventilation without exposing the bronchial stump to positive pressure. Using this ventilatory strategy and the other techniques described previously, we have had success in salvaging some patients with this devastating problem.

Postoperative Pneumonia Postoperative pneumonia continues to be a significant cause of morbidity and mortality after major thoracic procedures. The incidence of pneumonia after

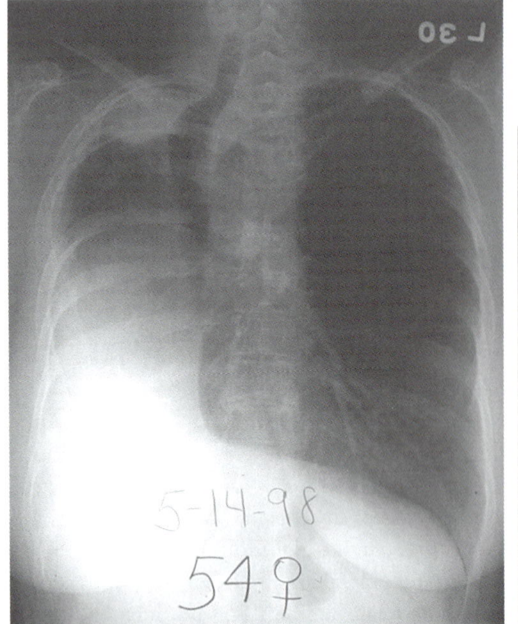

A

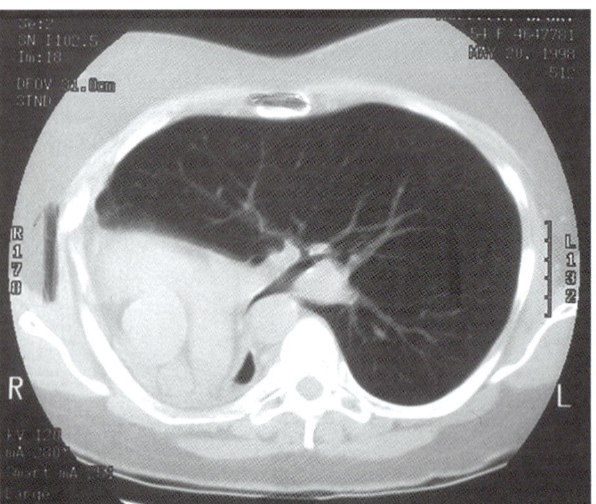

B

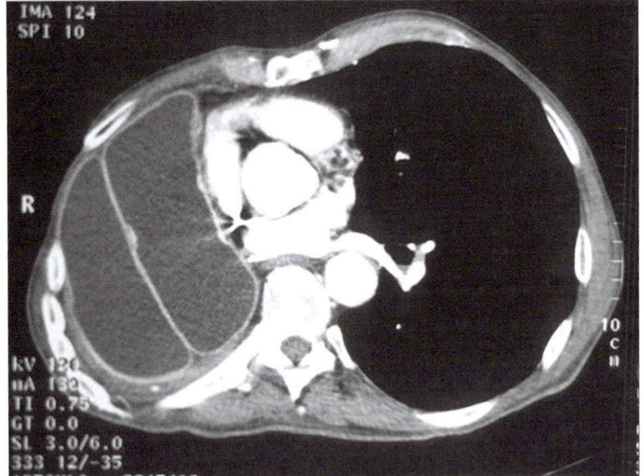

C

FIGURE 39.2 Postpneumonectomy syndrome. Chest radiograph showing mediastinal shift into pneumonectomy space **(A)**. Chest CT scan showing complete displacement of mediastinal structures with compression of the left mainstem bronchus against the vertebral column **(B)**. Chest CT scan showing expandable saline implants used to reposition the mediastinum back to midline **(C)**.

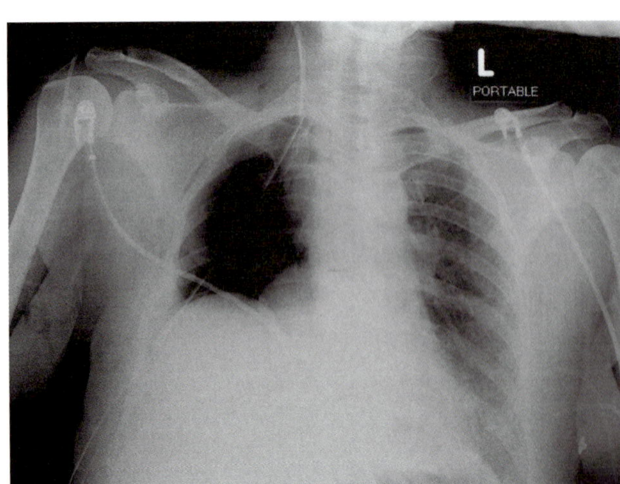

A

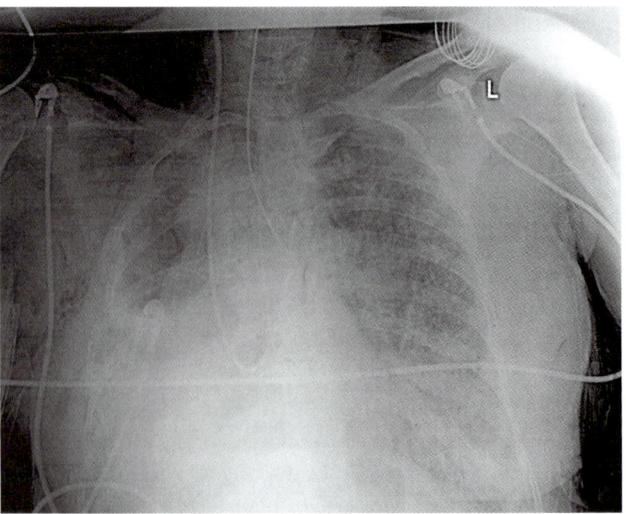

B

FIGURE 39.3 Postpneumonectomy pulmonary edema after right pneumonectomy. CXR on postoperative day 1 **(A)**. Several hours later, the patient was intubated for acute hypoxia. The endotracheal tube was advanced over a bronchoscope into the left main bronchus to protect the right pneumonectomy stump. The chest radiograph shows severe diffuse interstitial infiltrates of the remaining left lung **(B)**.

pulmonary resection is 5.3% to 11.7%.[9,31,48] In a retrospective study, Kutlu et al.[49] found pneumonia to be the cause of 5% of all deaths after pulmonary resection. Risk factors for the development of postoperative pneumonia include preoperative pneumonia, postoperative sputum retention, current smoking status, poor mental status, poor pain control, COPD, bronchitis, immunodeficiency, and prolonged ventilator support.

Prophylactic measures to avoid postoperative pneumonia include preoperative smoking cessation, good postoperative airway hygiene, and good postoperative pain control with routine epidural catheter use. The use of prophylactic antibiotics is controversial. Older reports have shown that prophylactic antibiotics do not protect against the development of pneumonia after pulmonary resection.[50,51] However, these studies assessed the efficacy of first-generation cephalosporins and penicillin, which may lack effectiveness against the common causes of pneumonia such as Gram-negative bacteria or *Staphylococcus aureus*. Other studies have shown the benefits of cephalosporins for wound infection.[52,53] Today, it is common practice to use first-generation cephalosporins for pulmonary resections, although the benefit for prevention of postoperative pneumonia is still lacking. In a randomized study of 212 patients, cephalothin was effective in reducing wound infections, although there was no statistically significant change in the rate of pulmonary infections.[53] In a prospective randomized study using broader coverage, sulbactam plus ampicillin was more effective than cefazolin in preventing postoperative pulmonary infections.[54] The initial dose should be administered such that levels are highest at the time of incision.

It is often difficult to determine the etiology of postoperative pneumonia as many patients may have some degree of postobstructive process preoperatively from the tumor. It can also be difficult to determine the difference between true infection and airway colonization associated with a chronic condition such as COPD and bronchitis. In general, postoperative patients with persistent fever, elevated white blood cell count, purulent sputum, pathogenic bacteria from endotracheal aspirate, and persistent infiltrate on CXR should be aggressively treated for pneumonia with appropriate antibiotic coverage, chest physiotherapy, and dependent drainage. The most common responsible organisms are Gram-negative rods and *S. aureus*. Although most pneumonias are bacterial in nature, the possibility of other causes such as viral, fungal, *Legionella* and *Mycoplasma* should be entertained in patients that do not respond to antibiotic therapy. The index of suspicion should be higher in patients who are immunocompromised. Antibiotic therapy should be adjusted on the basis of tracheobronchial culture results.

Pleural Space Problems

Residual Air Space and Prolonged Air Leaks During the normal conduct of partial lung resection for lung cancer, there can be small injuries to the visceral pleura resulting in air leaks. These small visceral pleural injuries can be minimized with meticulous technique. Normally, these small air leaks are impeded by apposition of pleural surfaces once the lung is reexpanded, resulting in termination of the leak. A residual air space exists when there is failure to fill the chest cavity after reexpansion of the lung. Greater amounts of parenchymal resection increase the risk of residual air space such that bilobectomies and lobectomies have a higher rate of residual air space than segmentectomies and wedge resections. Usually, the space is noted at the apex after upper lobectomy but can also be found at the base near the diaphragm after other types of resections. Although persistent residual air space is a common cause of persistent air leak, many patients will not suffer any other morbidity from this problem. The space gradually disappears over several weeks, secondary to reabsorption of gases within the space, further reexpansion of the lung, and pleural peel formation. When a residual air space is associated with symptoms such as pain, dyspnea, hemoptysis, or fever, a bronchopleural fistula should be suspected and requires appropriate intervention with thoracostomy tube placement.

Prolonged air leak is generally defined as an air leak that persists more than 7 days after surgery. It is the most common complication seen after pulmonary resection and the most common reason for prolonged hospital stay. Prolonged air leak occurs in 4% to 15% after partial lung resection.[51,55] It is responsible for approximately 25% of all morbidity after lung resection. It also increases patient discomfort, cost of care, and utilization of resources. The most consistent risk factor for prolonged air leak is severe obstructive pulmonary disease.[56,57] Other potential risk factors for prolonged air leak include advanced age, pleural adhesions, preoperative steroid use, and induction chemotherapy or radiation therapy.

Preoperative awareness of increased risk for prolonged air leaks should engender extra measures in addition to meticulous technique during the operation to help prevent them. The use of bovine pericardial strips as a buttress along the lung staple line to decrease air leaks was first described for lung volume reduction surgery.[58] However, their efficacy for completing fissures during lobectomy and segmentectomy is unclear. Previously, Venuta et al.[59] found that the use of pericardial strips to complete interlobar fissures for pulmonary lobectomy significantly reduced the duration of postoperative air leaks and hospital stay. More recently, in a randomized controlled group of 80 patients, Miller et al.[60] found a trend but no statistically significant improvement in prolonged air leak rate after lobectomy and segmentectomy when utilizing buttressed staple lines. The use of synthetic (polytetrafluoroethylene or vicryl) sleeves has also been described, but more data is needed to examine efficacy.

Other measures to reduce the incidence of prolonged air leak in the high-risk patient are maneuvers, which displace the potential residual space to an extrapleural position, thereby making apposition of pleural surfaces more likely. One common practice is the creation of a pleural tent. In a prospective randomized study of 200 patients undergoing upper lobectomy, Brunelli et al.[61] found that pleural tenting reduced the duration of air leaks and the hospital costs. Similarly, a randomized study by Okur et al.[62] and a retrospective study by Robinson and Preksto[63] showed that pleural tenting following lobectomy shortens the duration of chest tube drainage and hospital costs. A second way to limit the potential residual pleural air space is to elevate the diaphragm by insufflating air into the peritoneal cavity. Pneumoperitoneum has been described to treat air leaks and residual spaces after lung volume reduction surgery.[64] Subsequently, De Giacomo et al.[65] described its use after pulmonary resection. In a prospective randomized study of 16 patients undergoing bilobectomy, Cerfolio et al.[66] showed that intraoperative creation of pneumoperitoneum decreased the incidence of air leaks and shortened hospital stay without increasing morbidity.

A third measure, which has been used to lower the incidence of prolonged air leak, is the use of biologic sealants. Their effectiveness is controversial. Previously, it was shown that fibrin glue is not effective in reducing the duration of air leaks after lobectomy.[67,68] More recently, Fabian et al.[69] showed in a randomized study that fibrin glue reduced the rate of postoperative air leak from 15% to 2% after lung resection. Similarly, Wain et al.[70] found that the use of fibrin glue treated patients had a mean air leak time of 31 hours, whereas untreated patients had a mean air leak time of 52 hours. Although this difference was significant, there was no reduced time to chest tube removal and earlier hospital discharge. Further study is needed to determine patient selection and cost-effectiveness for the use of fibrin sealants to prevent prolonged air leak.

Despite preventive measures, many patients go on to develop prolonged air leak. Although this is the most common problem thoracic surgeons deal with in the postoperative period, there is no consensus on the management. Most surgeons believe that conversion from suction to water seal is an effective way of encouraging an air leak to seal. Development of a pneumothorax in the setting of an expiratory air leak is uncommon. This is supported by a study by Cerfolio et al.[71] in which 33 patients with postoperative air leak were randomized to continued suction versus water seal on postoperative day 2. In this study, 67% of the patients treated with water seal versus 7% of the patients that remained on suction had air leak resolution by postoperative day 3. Air leaks that do not resolve on water seal should be placed on a Heimlich valve once the fluid drainage is minimal. The patient can be discharged to home with the chest tube and Heimlich valve in place as long as there is no new or enlarging pneumothorax on chest radiograph. Outpatient chest tube management is well tolerated and desirable for the patient as it avoids prolonged hospitalization. Most air leaks stop after several days, and the chest tube can be removed at that time. The chest tube can usually be removed at 2 to 3 weeks even if the air leak is still present because the formation of pleural adhesions prevent further lung collapse and tension pneumothorax.

Postresection Empyema Although less common than in the early years of thoracic surgery, empyema still occurs in 2% to 12% of patients after pneumonectomy and 1% to 3% after lobectomy. This complication is often associated with a bronchopleural fistula, leading to a further increase in morbidity and mortality. In addition to the presence of bronchopleural fistula, other factors such as poor pulmonary function, lower preoperative serum hemoglobin, right pneumonectomy, completion pneumonectomy, and lack of bronchial stump reinforcement have been shown to be associated with the development of postresection empyema.[72] It is also believed that the use of neoadjuvant and adjuvant therapy also contribute to the development of postresection empyema. For postpneumonectomy empyema, the perioperative mortality rate is 12% to 40%.

The diagnosis of empyema is suspected in any patient with signs and symptoms of infection after lung resection. Development of serosanguinous sputum, purulent chest tube or wound drainage are also highly suspicious findings. Imaging studies consistent with empyema are pleural opacity with or without an air-fluid level after partial lung resection or a new or falling air fluid level after pneumonectomy (Fig. 39.1).

Once the diagnosis of postresectional empyema is made or strongly suspected, immediate management includes closed chest tube thoracostomy as well as appropriate antibiotic therapy. Once adequate drainage has been established and the patient is stabilized, the appropriate definitive management can be decided. Factors determining definitive management include presence or absence of bronchopleural fistula, partial lung resection versus pneumonectomy, stability of the patient and need for positive pressure ventilation. The traditional management approach involves three separate procedures as previously outlined for bronchopleural fistula management; early open drainage, closure of a fistula if present, and subsequent closure of the cavity as previously outlined. Several weeks of dressing changes are usually required to get the pleural cavity clean and covered with healthy granulation tissue. Patients deemed unsuitable for definitive closure can be managed with open window thoracostomy and dressing changes indefinitely. A more aggressive approach for management of postpneumonectomy empyema utilizes VATS techniques for debridement in conjunction with antibiotic irrigation. In a small series of patients with postpneumonectomy empyema with no evidence of bronchopleural fistula, this technique, using antibiotic irrigation for 10 days, was successful in the treatment of empyema with prevention of the need for open drainage in 89% (16/18) of patients.[73] Further data is needed to assess the efficacy of this technique in a larger group of patients.

Chylothorax The incidence of chylothorax after thoracotomy is less than 1%.[74,75] When untreated, the mortality from this complication can be as high as 50%. The additional morbidity is caused by the metabolic and mechanical insults of nutritional deficiency, dehydration from volume loss, immunosuppression from lymphocyte depletion, and pulmonary dysfunction.

The etiology of chylothorax involves injury to the thoracic duct or one of its tributaries. The thoracic duct carries intestinal lymph from the cisterna chyli to the venous system at the junction of the left internal subclavian veins. The fat contained in chyle is what gives it its characteristic appearance. The main cellular components of chyle are lymphocytes. Injury to the thoracic duct or one of its tributaries may occur while dividing the pulmonary ligament, mediastinal lymph node dissection, or pleural flap creation along the thoracic aorta. It can occur after upper or lower lobectomy and pneumonectomy on either side.

The diagnosis is suspected by the findings of high volume (500 to 1200 cc/day), milky chest drain output, or thoracentesis fluid postoperatively. Occasionally, a patient may have high-volume output but the fluid is not milky in character. In these cases, the diagnosis can be confirmed by giving the patient a fat challenge with cream by mouth. This will turn the chest drain output milky if chylothorax exists. Microscopic examination of the chest drainage will show the presence of fat globules that stain positive with Sudan-3. In addition, the chest drainage can be tested for triglyceride levels, which will be elevated in the case of chylothorax.

The initial management of postoperative chylothorax is maintenance of effective chest drainage, cessation of enteral feeds and implementation of central total parenteral nutrition. In approximately 50% of patients, the leak will stop with this therapy alone. There is no standard recommendation for the period of time to wait for spontaneous leak closure. However, most would agree that if the drainage remains greater than 500 cc per day for several days, then operative intervention is mandatory unless there is a contraindication to thoracotomy. Many groups recommend early reoperation and thoracic duct ligation in patients with higher chest tube outputs that increase or fail to respond to conservative management within 1 to 7 days.[76–78] Our technique of thoracic duct ligation involves a mass ligature technique, encircling all tissue between the azygos vein, esophagus, and aorta immediately above the diaphragm, and not at the fistula site. Other techniques described in the management of postoperative chylothorax include pleuroperitoneal shunting[79] and percutaneous catheterization with thoracic duct embolization.[80] In addition, somatostatin has proved useful for the conservative management of chylothorax of other causes and may be used as an adjunct but is rarely useful in a large volume chylothorax.[81] More data is needed to determine the benefit of these techniques over traditional reoperation and thoracic duct ligation.

Complications of Bronchoplastic Procedures

A worthwhile alternative to pneumonectomy for proximal lung tumors is sleeve lobectomy. In addition to preserving pulmonary function, these bronchoplastic procedures are associated with lower morbidity and mortality. However, bronchoplastic procedure complication rates exceed those of lesser resections. In a review of 1915 bronchoplastic procedures for malignancy, Tedder et al.[82] found the mortality rate to be 7.5%.

Patients tend to be particularly susceptible to sputum retention caused by edema at the bronchial anatomists in the early postoperative period after sleeve resection. Good postoperative airway hygiene is crucial in these patients. Liberal use of bronchoscopy or minitracheostomy can be very helpful. In addition, there are complications that are specific to bronchoplastic procedures such as bronchial anastomotic dehiscence (3.5%), bronchial stenosis (5.0%), bronchopleural fistula (3.5%), and bronchovascular fistula (2.6%). Similar to traditional pulmonary resections, comorbidities such as preexisting poor pulmonary function and cardiovascular disease significantly influence the postoperative complication rate. Bronchial anastomotic dehiscence is caused by impaired healing with resulting necrosis of the bronchial mucosa and subsequent bronchopleural fistula formation. These small areas of bronchopleural fistulae at the anastomosis usually heal over time. However, occasionally, these small defects can progress to complete dehiscence, especially in patients who require mechanical ventilation. Bronchoscopy can be used to assess the extent of bronchial wall necrosis in these patients. Hemoptysis after sleeve resection is concerning for erosion of the bronchial anastomosis into a nearby blood vessel, usually a branch of the pulmonary artery. The mortality of this complication is high and mandates immediate reexploration. Anastomotic stenosis is a late complication with an incidence between 2% and 5%. It can be caused by granulation tissue or an interrupted blood supply or anastomotic dehiscence with secondary healing and stricture formation. Management consists of bronchoscopic removal of the granulation tissue and repeated dilatation. Stents may be useful. In recalcitrant cases, re-resection with redo anastomosis or completion pneumonectomy may be necessary.

Cardiovascular Complications

General Considerations Given the high degree of associated mortality, cardiovascular complications are among the most concerning. Overall, noncardiac thoracic surgery is considered intermediate risk as a category of procedures by the American College of Cardiology and the American Heart Association with an overall risk of less than 5% for perioperative myocardial infarction (MI) and related mortality.[83] A comprehensive review of the recommendations for preoperative cardiac risk assessment has recently been updated by Eagle et al.[84] In general, the presence of preexisting heart disease is the greatest risk factor for the development of postoperative cardiovascular complications.

Cardiac Ischemia and Arrhythmias

Patients with preexisting cardiac disease are at greatest risk for perioperative cardiac ischemia and infarction. It is important to identify these patients based on history, physical exam, and preoperative testing to determine the need for prophylactic measures to avoid cardiac ischemia. For MI the importance of preexisting heart disease is characterized in a review of the literature by Herrington and Shumway[73,85] with a reported incidence of postoperative MI of 0.13% in patients with no prior history and between 2.8% and 17% for patients with a prior history of heart disease. Postoperative MI is associated with mortality as high as 32%.[86] Recently, the American College of Cardiology and the American Heart Association published recommendations for patients who should undergo preoperative evaluation with a cardiac stress test.[84] Under these guidelines, patients are categorized into one of three risk strata based on their medical history, cardiac symptoms, and exercise tolerance. Clinical factors that characterize the highest risk group that should not have an elective noncardiac operation are unstable angina, decompensated congestive heart failure (CHF), severe valvular disease, and significant arrhythmias. Intermediate risk factors that indicate the need for a preoperative stress test, depending on the planned operation and exercise tolerance are a history of prior MI, mild angina, compensated CHF, diabetes, renal insufficiency. Factors that place patients in the low-risk strata are old age, uncontrolled hypertension, history of stroke, low functional capacity, and an abnormal electrocardiogram (EKG). Patients in this group do not necessarily require preoperative testing under the current guidelines, unless they are unable to exercise at the level of four METs (metabolic equivalents). These guidelines help the clinician council patients about the risk of perioperative MIs and identify patients that will benefit from perioperative prophylactic measures or perhaps should have their planned operation delayed until coronary intervention is undertaken.

Perioperative MIs are thought to occur by one of two pathways that occur with an equal incidence. Patients with fixed high-grade coronary stenosis may have perioperative MI during times of cardiac stress associated with tachycardia. Other patients have perioperative MI as the result of relatively low-grade plaques that rupture and cause coronary thrombosis.[87] MIs that result from high-grade lesions tend to occur in the first 24 hours, following surgery and are tightly associated with episodes of tachycardia.[88] Patients having MIs as the result of plaque rupture occur with no particular peak incidence in the first 30 postoperative days.[87]

Perioperative heart rate control is critical for the prevention of MI occurring from high-grade coronary lesions. Several prospective randomized studies have shown a significant reduction in perioperative MI and death when β-blockers are used in patients with significant coronary risk factors.[89–91]

Indications for cardiac catheterization are similar to those in patients not being evaluated for surgery. They include evidence of ischemia on noninvasive testing, angina unresponsive to medical therapy, unstable angina, and equivocal noninvasive test results in patients at high-clinical risk. In general, patients found to have significant coronary artery disease amenable to vascular reconstruction should have an intervention; either at the time of the cardiac catheterization via percutaneous technique or coronary artery bypass grafting (CABG). The Coronary Artery Surgery Study (CASS) database evaluated almost 25,000 patients with known or suspected coronary disease and looked at outcomes after CABG versus medical therapy. Eagle et al.[92] looked at 1961 patients in this study who underwent major noncardiac surgery, including thoracic procedures. They found significantly lower rates of MI and perioperative death in the group that had known coronary artery disease managed with CABG rather than medical treatment. This data implies that percutaneous coronary interventions would also offer a benefit to these patients. Whether the benefit is greater than CABG because of lower morbidity and shorter recovery, time is unclear as patients who undergo percutaneous intervention are routinely placed on antiplatelet agents for at least 2 to 6 weeks, making lung resection unsafe immediately after percutaneous coronary interventions as well.

Cardiac Arrhythmias By far, the most common cardiac complication after thoracic surgery is supraventricular tachycardia (SVT). Ninety-five percent of SVT is atrial fibrillation with the rest being atrial flutter and multifocal atrial tachycardia. The incidence of SVT after thoracic surgical procedures ranges from 9% to 33%. Clinically significant ventricular arrhythmias are rare. Advanced age and the presence of COPD are the most common factors that predispose patients to develop SVT after lung resection for cancer. Other risk factors for the development of SVT include coronary artery disease, CHF, and valvular disease. Surgical risk factors for the development of SVT are increasing extent of resection (Table 39.3) and need for intrapericardial dissection. VATS procedures may be associated with a decrease in the incidence of postoperative SVT although others have suggested that the VATS approach does not alter the incidence compared to open resections.[93] Patients without preexisting cardiac dysfunction can also be exposed to intraoperative physiologic alterations that can cause intraoperative arrhythmias such as hypothermia, hypoxemia, hypokalemia,

TABLE 39.3 Incidence of Supraventricular Tachychardia according to Extent of Resection for Malignancy at Barnes-Jewish Hospital, 2003–2006

Lung (n = 695)	N	Dysrhythmia	%
Wedge	74	6	8.1%
Segmentectomy	30	4	13.3%
Lobectomy	398	78	19.6%
VATS Lobe	21	2	9.5%
Wedge & lobectomy	47	9	19.1%
Bilobectomy	33	7	21.2%
Sleeve	37	9	24.3%
Pneumonectomy	55	21	38.2%
TOTAL	**695**	**136**	**19.6%**

hyperkalemia, hypovolemia, and acidosis. These problems must be corrected as soon as possible when they occur.

Most patients who develop SVT after pulmonary resection do so by postoperative day 3. The consequences of SVT depend on the duration and frequency of the events. Patients who have a single episode of SVT, which is short in duration, may have very little or no consequences. Patients at the other end of the spectrum with prolonged or recurrent SVT have been shown to have a prolonged hospital stay.[94] In addition, it has been shown that patients who experience SVT have poorer survival after thoracic surgical procedures independent of advanced age, stage of disease, and extent of resection.[95]

Given its ubiquity and adverse effect upon the management and outcomes, there has been a great deal of interest in prophylaxis against the development of SVT. Agents that have been shown to have a prophylactic effect against the development of SVT after pulmonary resection include β-blockers,[96] calcium channel blockers,[97,98] magnesium sulfate,[99] and class I antiarrhythmics.[100] Unfortunately, adverse effects were also seen with the use of these agents such as hypotension and bradycardia for β-blockers and calcium channel blockers. Class I antiarrhythmics have significant proarrhythmic potential. Amiodarone, a class III antiarrhythmic agent, has been shown significant reduction in the incidence of SVT[101] in cardiac surgical patients. There has been apprehension for the use of amiodarone after pulmonary resection for lung cancer given the risk of lung toxicity in a patient population with smoking and surgically reduced pulmonary function. Randomized data are needed to determine clinical efficacy and toxicity after pulmonary resection.

When SVT occurs, its management depends on the acute clinical consequences, including symptoms, heart rate, and blood pressure. Occasionally, patients will develop chest discomfort or hypotension. These patients should undergo urgent electrical cardioversion. More commonly, patients will have a sensation of malaise and palpitations without chest discomfort or hypotension. This situation is less urgent and can be managed by rate control with β-blockers, calcium channel blockers, or digoxin. The use of amiodarone to chemically cardiovert these patients has become more widespread recently. In general, patients with persistent or recurrent SVT despite rate control or the use of amiodarone should undergo elective electrical cardioversion or anticoagulation to minimize the risk of thromboembolic sequelae. Although SVT is a common event after otherwise uncomplicated pulmonary resection, the clinician should keep in mind that SVT can also be a marker of the presence of other postoperative complications such as MI and pulmonary embolism. These complications should be investigated depending on clinical circumstances.

Cardiac Herniation Cardiac herniation is a rare complication of intrapericardial pneumonectomy. However, when it occurs, it is associated with 50% mortality. The herniation occurs through the pericardial defect (right more commonly than left). This complication usually occurs within the first 24 hours after surgery. The diagnosis is based on clinical suspicion and findings on chest radiograph. It is associated with sudden onset of hypotension, tachycardia, and cyanosis. Chest radiograph after right-sided herniation will show obvious mediastinal displacement (Fig. 39.4), whereas left herniation will have more subtle radiographic findings of subtle cardiac shift with a rounded opacity in left chest.

Factors thought to contribute to the development of cardiac herniation include placing the chest tube to suction and positive pressure ventilation. The pathophysiology of right and left cardiac herniation differs. Right herniation is associated with torsion of venous inflow at the superior and inferior vena cavae as well as distorted and compromised left ventricular outflow. Left herniation involves constriction of the left ventricle by the sharp edges of the pericardial defect with potential laceration of epicardial vessels resulting in myocardial ischemia, edema, and dysfunction.

A
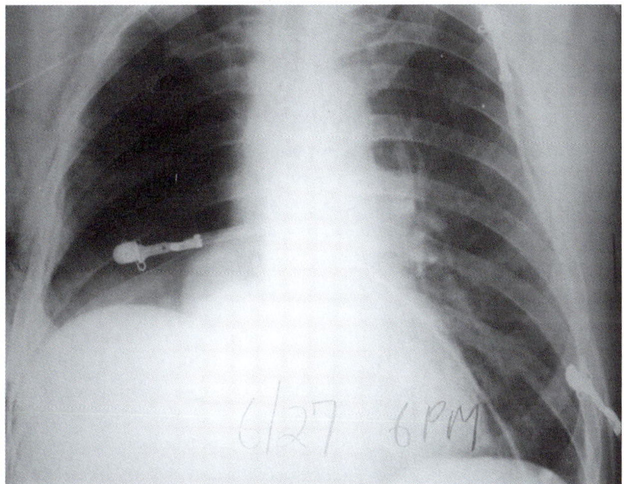

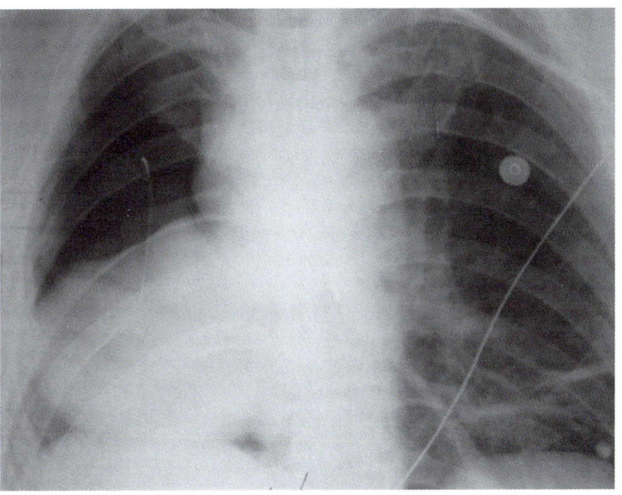
B

FIGURE 39.4 Cardiac herniation. Chest radiograph immediately following right pneumonectomy **(A)**. Chest radiograph repeated shortly thereafter for hemodynamic instability showing cardiac displacement into the right chest **(B)**.

Once cardiac herniation is recognized, the patient should be taken emergently back to the operating room or undergo bedside thoracotomy if severely unstable. Management of right cardiac herniation consists of reducing the heart and closure of the pericardium primarily or with a Dacron or polytetrafluoroethylene patch. Management of left herniation consists of opening the pericardium down to the diaphragm to eliminate cardiac strangulation.

ACKNOWLEDGMENT: *The authors thank Kathleen Atwater and Jennifer Zoole, RN, for their assistance with the preparation of this manuscript.*

REFERENCES

1. Allen MS, Darling GE, Pechet TT, et al. Morbidity and mortality of major pulmonary resections in patients with early-stage lung cancer: initial results of the randomized, prospective ACOSOG Z0030 trial. *Ann Thorac Surg* 2006;81:1013–1019.
2. Deslauriers J, Ginsberg RJ, Piantadosi S, et al. Prospective assessment of 30-day operative morbidity for surgical resections in lung cancer. *Chest* 1994;106(6 Suppl):329S–330S
3. Ferguson MK, Durkin AE. A comparison of three scoring systems for predicting complications after major lung resection. *Eur J Cardiothorac Surg* 2003;23:35–42.
4. Ginsberg RJ, Hill LD, Eagan RT, et al. Modern thirty-day operative mortality for surgical resections in lung cancer. *J Thorac Cardiovasc Surg* 1983;86:654–658.
5. Romano PS, Mark DH. Patient and hospital characteristics related to in-hospital mortality after lung cancer resection. *Chest* 1992;101:1332–1337.
6. Silvestri GA, Handy J, Lackland D, et al. Specialists achieve better outcomes than generalists for lung cancer surgery. *Chest* 1998;114:675–680.
7. Strand TE, Rostad H, Damhuis RA, et al. Risk factors for 30-day mortality after resection of lung cancer and prediction of their magnitude. *Thorax* 2007;62:991–997.
8. Wada H, Nakamura T, Nakamoto K, et al. Thirty-day operative mortality for thoracotomy in lung cancer. *J Thorac Cardiovasc Surg* 1998;115:70–73.
9. Harpole DH Jr, DeCamp MM Jr, Daley J, et al. Prognostic models of thirty-day mortality and morbidity after major pulmonary resection. *J Thorac Cardiovasc Surg* 1999;117:969–979.
10. Naunheim KS, Kesler KA, D'Orazio SA, et al. Lung cancer surgery in the octogenarian. *Eur J Cardiothorac Surg* 1994;8:453–456.
11. Pagni S, Federico JA, Ponn RB. Pulmonary resection for lung cancer in octogenarians. *Ann Thorac Surg* 1997;63:785–789.
12. Melendez JA, Carlon VA. Cardiopulmonary risk index does not predict complications after thoracic surgery. *Chest* 1998;114:69–75.
13. Brunelli A, Fianchini A, Xiume F, et al. Evaluation of the POSSUM scoring system in lung surgery. Physiological and Operative Severity Score for the enumeration of Mortality and Morbidity. *Thorac Cardiovasc Surg* 1998;46:141–146.
14. Melendez JA, Barrera R. Predictive respiratory complication quotient predicts pulmonary complications in thoracic surgical patients. *Ann Thorac Surg* 1998;66:220–224.
15. Pierce RJ, Copland JM, Sharpe K, et al. Preoperative risk evaluation for lung cancer resection: predicted postoperative product as a predictor of surgical mortality. *Am J Respir Crit Care Med* 1994;150:947–955.
16. Santambrogio L, Nosotti M, Baisi A, et al. Pulmonary lobectomy for lung cancer: a prospective study to compare patients with forced expiratory volume in 1 s more or less than 80% of predicted. *Eur J Cardiothorac Surg* 2001;20:684–687.
17. Bryant LR, Rams JJ, Trinkle JK, et al. Present-day risk of thoracotomy in patients with compromised pulmonary function. *Arch Surg* 1970;101:140–144.
18. Ferguson MK, Little L, Rizzo L, et al. Diffusing capacity predicts morbidity and mortality after pulmonary resection. *J Thorac Cardiovasc Surg* 1988;96:894–900.
19. Ferguson MK, Reeder LB, Mick R. Optimizing selection of patients for major lung resection. *J Thorac Cardiovasc Surg* 1995;109:275–281.
20. Bousamra M II, Presberg KW, Chammas JH et al. Early and late morbidity in patients undergoing pulmonary resection with low diffusion capacity. *Ann Thorac Surg* 1996;62:968–974.
21. Boysen PG, Block AJ, Moulder PV. Relationship between preoperative pulmonary function tests and complications after thoracotomy. *Surg Gynecol Obstet* 1981;152:813–815.
22. Stéphan F, Boucheseiche S, Hollande J, et al. Pulmonary complications following lung resection: a comprehensive analysis of incidence and possible risk factors. *Chest* 2000;118:1263–1270.
23. Matsuoka H, Nishio W, Sakamoto T, et al. Prediction of morbidity after lung resection with risk factors using treadmill exercise test. *Eur J Cardiothorac Surg* 2004;26:480–482.
24. Simansky DA, Paley M, Refaely Y, et al. Diaphragm plication following phrenic nerve injury: a comparison of paediatric and adult patients. *Thorax* 2002;57:613–616.
25. Bonde P, McManus K, McAnespie M, et al. Lung surgery: identifying the subgroup at risk for sputum retention. *Eur J Cardiothorac Surg* 2002;22:18–22.
26. Vaporciyan AA, Merriman KW, Ece F, et al. Incidence of major pulmonary morbidity after pneumonectomy: association with timing of smoking cessation. *Ann Thorac Surg* 2002;73:420–425.
27. Bonde P, Papachristos I, McCraith A, et al. Sputum retention after lung operation: prospective, randomized trial shows superiority of prophylactic minitracheostomy in high-risk patients. *Ann Thorac Surg* 2002;74:196–202.
28. Au J, Walker WS, Inglis D, et al. Percutaneous cricothyroidostomy (minitracheostomy) for bronchial toilet: results of therapeutic and prophylactic use. *Ann Thorac Surg* 1989;48:850–852.
29. Schuler JG. Intraoperative lobar torsion producing pulmonary infarction. *J Thorac Cardiovasc Surg* 1973;65:951–955.
30. Cable DG, Deschamps C, Allen MS, et al. Lobar torsion after pulmonary resection: presentation and outcome. *J Thorac Cardiovasc Surg* 2001;122:1091–1093.
31. Keagy BA, Lores ME, Starek PJ, et al. Elective pulmonary lobectomy: factors associated with morbidity and operative mortality. *Ann Thorac Surg* 1985;40:349–352
32. Larsson S, Lepore V, Dernevik L, et al. Torsion of a lung lobe: diagnosis and treatment. *Thorac Cardiovasc Surg* 1988;36:281–283.
33. Vester SR, Faber LP, Kittle CF, et al. Bronchopleural fistula after stapled closure of bronchus. *Ann Thorac Surg* 1991;52:1253–1257.
34. Asamura H, Naruke T, Tsuchiya R, et al. Bronchopleural fistulas associated with lung cancer operations. Univariate and multivariate analysis of risk factors, management, and outcome. *J Thorac Cardiovasc Surg* 1992;104:1456–1464.
35. El-Gamel A, Tsang GM, Watson DC. The threshold for air leak: stapled versus sutured human bronchi, and experimental study. *Eur J Cardiothorac Surg* 1999;15:7–10.
36. Hubaut JJ, Baron O, Al Habash O, et al. Closure of the bronchial stump by manual suture and incidence of bronchopleural fistula in a series of 209 pneumonectomies for lung cancer. *Eur J Cardiothorac Surg* 1999;16:418–423.
37. Asamura H, Kondo H, Tsuchiya R. Management of the bronchial stump in pulmonary resections: a review of 533 consecutive recent bronchial closures. *Eur J Cardiothorac Surg* 2000;17:106–110.
38. Birdi I, Bughai M, Wells FC. Surgical correction of postpneumonectomy stridor by saline breast implantation. *Ann Thorac Surg* 2001;71:1704–1706.
39. Grillo HC, Shepard JA, Mathisen DJ, et al. Postpneumonectomy syndrome: diagnosis, management, and results. *Ann Thorac Surg* 1992;54:638–650.
40. Cordova FC, Travaline JM, O'Brien GM, et al. Treatment of left pneumonectomy syndrome with an expandable endobronchial prosthesis. *Chest* 1996;109:567–570.

41. Slinger PD. Perioperative fluid management for thoracic surgery: the puzzle of postpneumonectomy pulmonary edema. *J Cardiothorac Vasc Anesth* 1995;9:442–451.
42. Waller DA, Keavey P, Woodfine L, et al. Pulmonary endothelial permeability changes after major lung resection. *Ann Thorac Surg* 1996;61:1435–1440.
43. Parquin F, Marchal M, Mehiri S, et al. Post-pneumonectomy pulmonary edema: analysis and risk factors. *Eur J Cardiothorac Surg* 1996;10:929–932.
44. Zeldin RA, Normandin D, Landtwing D, et al. Postpneumonectomy pulmonary edema. *J Thorac Cardiovasc Surg* 1984;87:359–365.
45. Verheijen-Breemhaar L, Bogaard JM, van den Berg B, et al. Postpneumonectomy pulmonary oedema. *Thorax* 1988;43:323–326.
46. Turnage WS, Lunn JJ. Postpneumonectomy pulmonary edema. A retrospective analysis of associated variables. *Chest* 1993;103:1646–1650.
47. Mathisen DJ, Kuo EY, Hahn C, et al. Inhaled nitric oxide for adult respiratory distress syndrome after pulmonary resection. *Ann Thorac Surg* 1998;66:1894–1902.
48. Duque JL, Ramos G, Castrodeza J, et al. Early complications in surgical treatment of lung cancer: a prospective, multicenter study. Grupo Cooperativo de Carcinoma Broncogénico de la Sociedad Española de Neumología y Cirugía Torácica. *Ann Thorac Surg* 1997;63:944–950.
49. Kutlu CA, Williams EA, Evans TW, et al. Acute lung injury and acute respiratory distress syndrome after pulmonary resection. *Ann Thorac Surg* 2000;69:376–380.
50. Frimodt-Møller N, Ostri P, Pedersen IK, et al. Antibiotic prophylaxis in pulmonary surgery: a double-blind study of penicillin versus placebo. *Ann Surg* 1982;195:444–450.
51. Truesdale R, D'Alessandri R, Manuel V, et al. Antimicrobial vs placebo prophylaxis in noncardiac thoracic surgery. *JAMA* 1979;241:1254–1256.
52. Bryant LR, Dillon ML, Mobin-Uddin K. Prophylactic antibiotics in noncardiac thoracic operations. *Ann Thorac Surg* 1975;19:670–676.
53. Ilves R, Cooper JD, Todd TR, et al. Prospective, randomized, double-blind study using prophylactic cephalothin for major, elective, general thoracic operations. *J Thorac Cardiovasc Surg* 1981;81:813–817.
54. Boldt J, Piper S, Uphus D, et al. Preoperative microbiologic screening and antibiotic prophylaxis in pulmonary resection operations. *Ann Thorac Surg* 1999;68:208–211.
55. Deslauriers J, Ginsberg RJ, Dubois P, et al. Current operative morbidity associated with elective surgical resection for lung cancer. *Can J Surg* 1989;32:335–339.
56. Abolhoda A, Liu D, Brooks A, et al. Prolonged air leak following radical upper lobectomy: an analysis of incidence and possible risk factors. *Chest* 1998;113:1507–1510.
57. Cerfolio RJ, Bass CS, Pask AH, et al. Predictors and treatment of persistent air leaks. *Ann Thorac Surg* 2002;73:1727–1730.
58. Cooper JD. Technique to reduce air leaks after resection of emphysematous lung. *Ann Thorac Surg* 1994;57:1038–1039.
59. Venuta F, Rendina EA, DeGiacomo T, et al. Technique to reduce air leaks after pulmonary lobectomy. *Eur J Cardiothorac Surg* 1998;13: 361–0364.
60. Miller JI Jr, Landreneau RJ, Wright CE, et al. A comparative study of buttressed versus nonbuttressed staple line in pulmonary resections. *Ann Thorac Surg* 2001;71:319–322.
61. Brunelli A, Al Refai M, Monteverde M, et al. Pleural tent after upper lobectomy: a randomized study of efficacy and duration of effect. *Ann Thorac Surg* 2002;74:1958–1962.
62. Okur E, Kir A, Halezeroglu S, et al. Pleural tenting following upper lobectomies or bilobectomies of the lung to prevent residual air space and prolonged air leak. *Eur J Cardiothorac Surg* 2001;20:1012–1015.
63. Robinson LA, Preksto D. Pleural tenting during upper lobectomy decreases chest tube time and total hospitalization days. *J Thorac Cardiovasc Surg* 1998;115:319–326.
64. Handy JR Jr, Judson MA, Zellner JL. Pneumoperitoneum to treat air leaks and spaces after a lung volume reduction operation. *Ann Thorac Surg* 1997;64:1803–1805.
65. De Giacomo T, Rendina EA, Venuta F, et al. Pneumoperitoneum for the management of pleural air space problems associated with major pulmonary resections. *Ann Thorac Surg* 2001;72:1716–1719.
66. Cerfolio RJ, Holman WL, Katholi CR. Pneumoperitoneum after concomitant resection of the right middle and lower lobes (bilobectomy). *Ann Thorac Surg* 2000;70:942–946
67. Fleisher AG, Evans KG, Nelems B, et al. Effect of routine fibrin glue use on the duration of air leaks after lobectomy. *Ann Thorac Surg* 1990;49:133–134.
68. Wong K, Goldstraw P. Effect of fibrin glue in the reduction of post-thoracotomy alveolar air leak. *Ann Thorac Surg* 1997 October;64(4): 979–981.
69. Fabian T, Federico JA, Ponn RB. Fibrin glue in pulmonary resection: a prospective, randomized, blinded study. *Ann Thorac Surg* 2003;75:1587–1592.
70. Wain JC, Kaiser LR, Johnstone DW, et al. Trial of a novel synthetic sealant in preventing air leaks after lung resection. *Ann Thorac Surg* 2001;71:1623–1628.
71. Cerfolio RJ, Bass C, Katholi CR. Prospective randomized trial compares suction versus water seal for air leaks. *Ann Thorac Surg* 2001;71: 1613–1617.
72. Deschamps C, Bernard A, Nichols FC III, et al. Empyema and bronchopleural fistula after pneumonectomy: factors affecting incidence. *Ann Thorac Surg* 2001;72:243–247.
73. Bagan P, Boissier F, Berna P, et al. Postpneumonectomy empyema treated with a combination of antibiotic irrigation followed by videothoracoscopic debridement. *J Thorac Cardiovasc Surg* 2006;132:708–710.
74. Sarsam MA, Rahman AN, Deiraniya AK. Postpneumonectomy chylothorax. *Ann Thorac Surg* 1994;57:689–690.
75. Sieczka EM, Harvey JC. Early thoracic duct ligation for postoperative chylothorax. *J Surg Oncol* 1996;61:56–60.
76. Cerfolio RJ, Allen MS, Deschamps C, et al. Postoperative chylothorax. *J Thorac Cardiovasc Surg* 1996;112:1361–1365.
77. Patterson GA, Todd TR, Delarue NC, et al. Supradiaphragmatic ligation of the thoracic duct in intractable chylous fistula. *Ann Thorac Surg* 1981;32:44–49.
78. Shimizu K, Yoshida J, Nishimura M, et al,. Treatment strategy for chylothorax after pulmonary resection and lymph node dissection for lung cancer. *J Thorac Cardiovasc Surg* 2002;124:499–502.
79. Milsom JW, Kron IL, Rheuban KS, et al. Chylothorax: an assessment of current surgical management. *J Thorac Cardiovasc Surg* 1985;89: 221–227.
80. Cope C, Salem R, Kaiser LR. Management of chylothorax by percutaneous catheterization and embolization of the thoracic duct: prospective trial. *J Vasc Interv Radiol* 1999;10:1248–1254.
81. Collard JM, Laterre PF, Boemer F, et al. Conservative treatment of postsurgical lymphatic leaks with somatostatin-14. *Chest* 2000;117: 902–905.
82. Tedder M, Anstadt MP, Tedder SD, et al. Current morbidity, mortality, and survival after bronchoplastic procedures for malignancy. *Ann Thorac Surg* 1992;54:387–391.
83. Kim MH, Eagle KA. Cardiac risk assessment in noncardiac thoracic surgery. *Semin Thorac Cardiovasc Surg* 2001;13:137–146.
84. Eagle KA, Berger PB, Calkins H, et al. ACC/AHA guideline update for perioperative cardiovascular evaluation for noncardiac surgery–executive summary a report of the American College of Cardiology/American Heart Association Task Force on Practice Guidelines (Committee to Update the 1996 Guidelines on Perioperative Cardiovascular Evaluation for Noncardiac Surgery). *Circulation* 2002;105:1257–1267.
85. Herrington CS, Shumway SJ. Myocardial ischemia and infarction post-thoracotomy. *Chest Surg Clin N Am* 1998;8:495–502.
86. von Knorring J. Postoperative myocardial infarction: a prospective study in a risk group of surgical patients. *Surgery* 1981;90:55–60.
87. Cohen MC, Aretz TH. Histological analysis of coronary artery lesions in fatal postoperative myocardial infarction. *Cardiovasc Pathol* 1999;8:133–139.

88. Landesberg G, Mosseri M, Zahger D, et al. Myocardial infarction after vascular surgery: the role of prolonged stress-induced, ST depression-type ischemia. *J Am Coll Cardiol* 2001;37:1839–1845.
89. Lindenauer PK, Pekow P, Wang K, et al. Perioperative beta-blocker therapy and mortality after major noncardiac surgery. *N Engl J Med* 2005;353:349–361.
90. Mangano DT, Layug EL, Wallace A, et al. Effect of atenolol on mortality and cardiovascular morbidity after noncardiac surgery. Multicenter Study of Perioperative Ischemia Research Group. *N Engl J Med* 1996;335:1713–1720.
91. Poldermans D, Boersma E, Bax JJ, et al. The effect of bisoprolol on perioperative mortality and myocardial infarction in high-risk patients undergoing vascular surgery. Dutch Echocardiographic Cardiac Risk Evaluation Applying Stress Echocardiography Study Group. *N Engl J Med* 1999;341:1789–1794.
92. Eagle KA, Rihal CS, Mickel MC, et al. Cardiac risk of noncardiac surgery: influence of coronary disease and type of surgery in 3368 operations. CASS Investigators and University of Michigan Heart Care Program. Coronary Artery Surgery Study. *Circulation* 1997;96: 1882–1887.
93. Park BJ, Zhang H, Rusch VW, et al. Video-assisted thoracic surgery does not reduce the incidence of postoperative atrial fibrillation after pulmonary lobectomy. *J Thorac Cardiovasc Surg* 2007;133: 775–779.
94. Polanczyk CA, Goldman L, Marcantonio ER, et al. Supraventricular arrhythmia in patients having noncardiac surgery: clinical correlates and effect on length of stay. *Ann Intern Med* 1998;129:279–285.
95. Amar D, Burt M, Reinsel RA, et al. Relationship of early postoperative dysrhythmias and long-term outcome after resection of non-small cell lung cancer. *Chest* 1996;110:437–439.
96. Jakobsen CJ, Bille S, Ahlburg P, et al. Andresen EB. Perioperative metoprolol reduces the frequency of atrial fibrillation after thoracotomy for lung resection. *J Cardiothorac Vasc Anesth* 1997;11:746–751.
97. Amar D, Roistacher N, Rusch VW, et al. Effects of diltiazem prophylaxis on the incidence and clinical outcome of atrial arrhythmias after thoracic surgery. *J Thorac Cardiovasc Surg* 2000;120:790–798.
98. Van Mieghem W, Tits G, Demuynck K, et al. Verapamil as prophylactic treatment for atrial fibrillation after lung operations. *Ann Thorac Surg* 1996;61:1083–1085.
99. Terzi A, Furlan G, Chiavacci P, et al. Prevention of atrial tachyarrhythmias after non-cardiac thoracic surgery by infusion of magnesium sulfate. *Thorac Cardiovasc Surg* 1996;44:300–303.
100. Borgeat A, Petropoulos P, Cavin R, Biollaz J, Munafo A, Schwander D. Prevention of arrhythmias after noncardiac thoracic operations: flecainide versus digoxin. *Ann Thorac Surg* 1991;51:964–967.
101. Daoud EG, Strickberger SA, Man KC, et al. Preoperative amiodarone as prophylaxis against atrial fibrillation after heart surgery. N Engl J Med 1997;337:1785–1791.
102. Licker MJ, Widikker I, Robert J, et al. Operative mortality and respiratory complications after lung resection for cancer: impact of chronic obstructive pulmonary disease and time trends. *Ann Thorac Surg* 2006; 81(5):1830–1837.
103. Dominguez-Ventura A, Allen MS, Cassivi SD, et al. Lung cancer in octogenarians: factors affecting morbidity and mortality after pulmonary resection. *Ann Thorac Surg* 2006;82(4):1175–1179.
104. Nagasaki F, Flehinger BJ, Martini N. Complications of surgery in the treatment of carcinoma of the lung. *Chest* 1982;82(1):25–29.
105. Weiss W. Operative mortality and five year survival rates in patients with bronchogenic carcinoma. *Am J Surg* 1974;128(6):799–804. No abstract available.

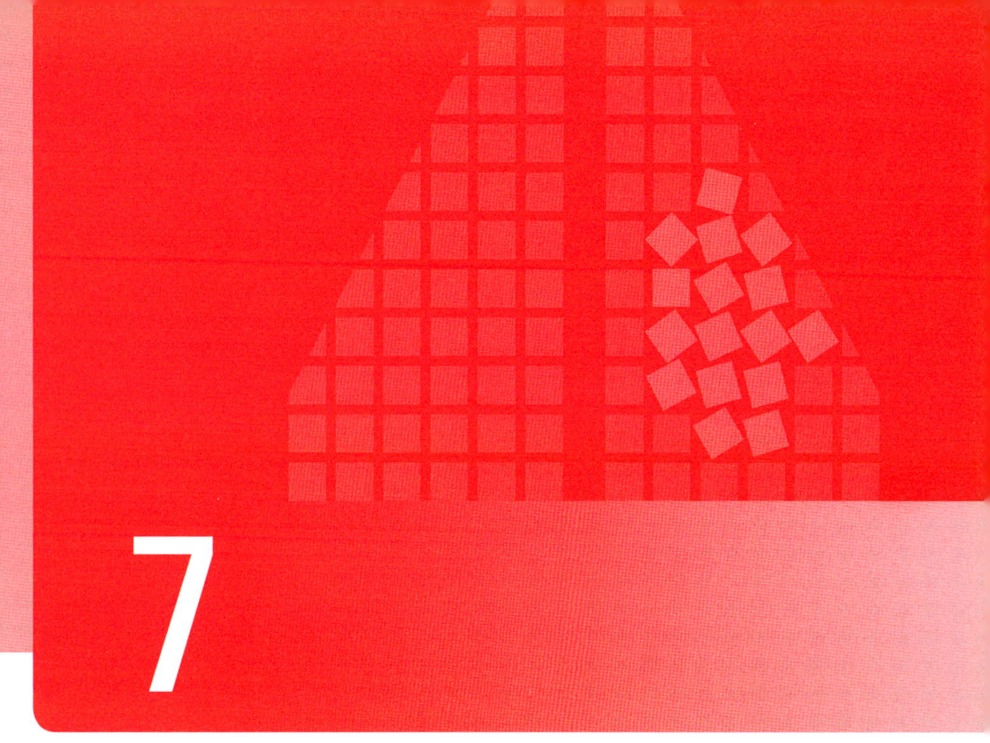

SECTION 7

Radiation Therapy and Lung Cancer

CHAPTER 40

Paul Keall
José Belderbos
Feng-Ming (Spring) Kong

Physical Basis of Modern Radiotherapy: Dose and Volume

About 60% of cancer patients receive radiation therapy (RT),[1] making radiation the most common "drug" (or more appropriately termed, *prodrug*) in cancer treatment. Radiation affects cell function by either directly ionizing intracellular targets or creating free radicals near the intracellular targets, which can then react with and disrupt normal cell processes. The most important and understood intracellular target is deoxyribonucleic acid (DNA), where single- and double-strand breaks can occur resulting in cell damage and cell death.

Radiotherapy is an example of individualized therapy. The delivery of the cytotoxic agent—radiation—varies from patient to patient as a result of the changing tumor and normal anatomy. Determining the appropriate dose and tumor volume to treat, choosing the appropriate beam shapes and energy for the treatment plan, and executing the treatment plan during radiation delivery involves a dedicated and coordinated effort by the treatment team, including the radiation oncologist, medical physicist, dosimetrist, and radiation therapist. Lung cancer is a particular challenge for radiotherapy given the number of radiation-sensitive tissues that ideally should be avoided—the lungs, esophagus, heart, spinal cord, mainstem bronchii, pulmonary vessels, brachial plexus and ribs, as well as the large changes in tissue density that challenge accurate calculation of dose to these structures.

This chapter describes the physical basis of dose and volume in radiotherapy and is divided into four main parts: imaging for volume delineation in RT, treatment planning, dose and fractionation, and treatment delivery. Although imaging, planning, and delivery have previously been three distinct processes in radiotherapy, with the emergence of image-guided therapy and adaptive therapy, the imaging–planning–delivery processes are merging.

IMAGING FOR VOLUME DELINEATION IN RADIATION THERAPY

Preparation In radiotherapy for lung cancer, it is important to keep geometrical uncertainties such as patient tumor delineation, organ motion, and setup variation to a minimum. The requirements on accuracy, dependent on the dose prescribed, are dictated by the purpose of the irradiation. In case a palliative treatment for lung cancer is prescribed, the requirements of the radiotherapy treatment preparation (traditional two dimensional [2D] using x-ray simulator) and delivery are relatively uncomplicated compared with three- or four-dimensional radiotherapy techniques used in radical or curative settings. Three-dimensional (3D) conformal radiotherapy is based on computed tomography (CT) scan treatment preparation and individualized treatment fields. Four-dimensional (4D) CT scans provide information on respiratory-induced tumor motion, which can be used for patient-specific treatment preparation.

Immobilization To reassure stable and reproducible patient positioning during treatment preparation and execution, the patient is placed (as comfortably as possible) on a flat couch with both hands stable above the head using immobilization devices (e.g., T-bar device, forearm support, alpha cradle, Wing Board, or vacuum mattress). These immobilization devices, sometimes personalized, will decrease the setup errors and reduce the daily setup uncertainty.[2] Available data support the use of an immobilization device to achieve stable and reproducible patient positioning during treatment planning and delivery.[3–5] The delivery of hypofractionated treatment fractions (stereotactic body irradiation; see Chapter 43) or gated treatments (irradiation to a restricted portion of the respiratory cycle) takes more beam-on and total machine time. For these treatments with prolonged treatment time, additional immobilization devices such as a stereotactic body frame and/or abdominal compression might be used to increase intrafraction stability or decrease respiratory tumor motion. Other devices such as head and knee cushions are frequently used to ensure maximum comfort and thus improve the position reproducibility. However, results of studies reveal that the setup accuracy (with respect to the bony anatomy) using a stereotactic body frame is of the same order (2 to 4 mm [1 standard deviation]) as without using such immobilization devices.[6,7]

The training and attention to detail of the treatment team is important in maintaining anatomic reproducibility throughout the treatment course.

Simulation For radiotherapy treatment preparation of a palliative schedule, an x-ray simulation session using a diagnostic x-ray generator (that has the same geometrical features of the linear accelerator) can be sufficient, although a growing number of centers are performing CT simulation for all patients, including those treated for palliation. During simulation the patient is in treatment position, and the radiation oncologist will determine the treatment field borders. Tumor motion information gathered during fluoroscopy in the cranial–caudal direction may be used. The anterior and lateral laser lines and/or the treatment field borders will be marked on the patient (sometimes using tattoos) to be used during daily patient setup.

For 3D conformal radiotherapy, a CT scan of the thorax in treatment position using a CT simulator is necessary. A CT simulator is a CT scanner with a laser system to align the patient and specific software. Laser lines will be marked on the patient, and the isocenter of the laser lines will be made visible on the planning CT scan. This so-called planning (or simulation) CT scan provides information on the 3D tumor extensions (and the normal tissues surrounding the tumor) and will be used to determine the optimal beam arrangements and calculate the dose distribution. An axial planning CT slice is shown in Figure 40.1. This planning CT is normally performed from middle/upper neck (the level of C2–C3) to middle abdomen (L2–L3), so that the whole lung is included for dosimetric estimation. Intravenous contrast is recommended for patients with tumors near the mediastinum and/or pathological lymph nodes. This is helpful for differentiating centrally located tumors and enlarged lymph nodes in the hilum and mediastinum from adjacent vessels.[8,9] The use of intravenous contrast may not be that critical if a recent contrast-enhanced diagnostic CT scan or positron emission tomography (PET)-CT simulation is available,[10,11] or for a peripherally located tumor without positive lymph nodes. CT scans with a slice thickness of 2 to 3 mm are recommended to enable accurate gross tumor volume (GTV) delineation, better recognition of nodal structures, and high-resolution digitally reconstructed radiographs (DRR) to be generated, which in turn may allow for the omission of a separate simulation step.[12] Study of a small patient series indicated that the impact of contrast on dose estimation is less than 2% to 3% of the prescription dose.[13]

Multiple laser setup points are placed on the patient to ensure that the patient is approximately in the same position each day for treatment. The distributions of treatment setup errors measured against DRRs obtained in the CT simulation are similar to previously obtained distributions measured against simulator films, and DRRs are well suited for setup verification. A verification simulation under conventional fluoroscopic simulator may be omitted.[12] However, the tumor motion should be checked for estimation of planning target volume (PTV) margin and adequate target coverage if the simulation and treatment were performed under free breathing (see section on "Motion Considerations" later in this chapter).

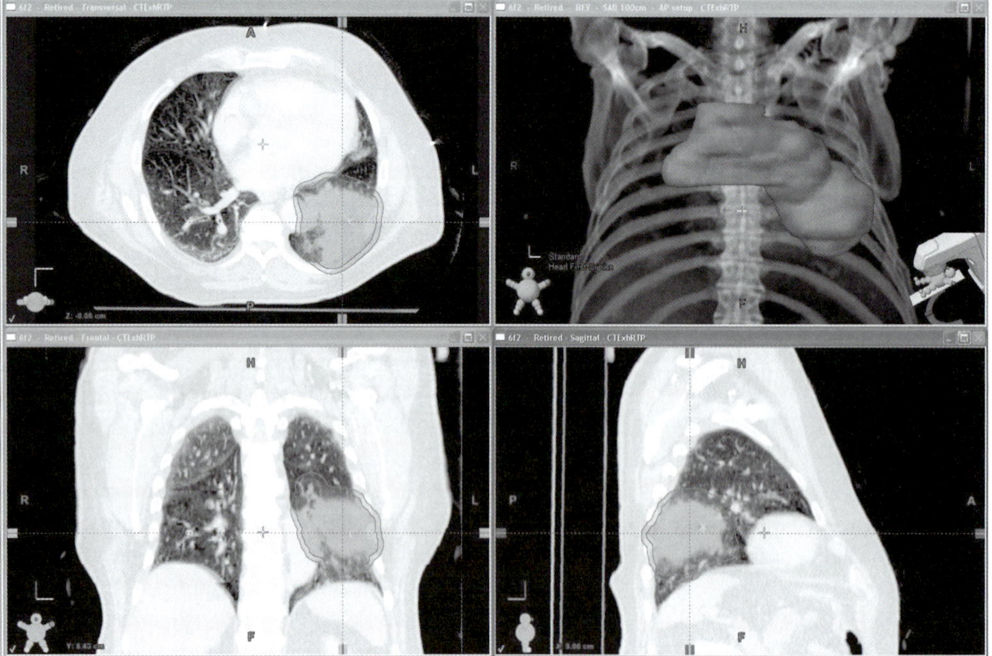

FIGURE 40.1 Views from a planning CT scan. Note the flat tabletop used for radiation therapy imaging, the absence of the patient's arms as they are above their head to avoid being radiated during treatment, and the foam mold surrounding the patient to assist with immobilization. The gross tumor volume (*red*) and planning target volume (*pink*) are shown. (See color plate.)

To minimize simulator setup errors, a treatment isocenter (preferably located within the treatment target) should be defined at the time of treatment planning. Volumetric information from spiral CT scans is superior for defining target volumes rather than data derived using axial CT scans.[14] However, it should be recognized that movement-induced artifacts for mobile organs or targets can arise during most CT scan techniques.[15] The possibility of time-related displacements and treatment-related changes of target volumes that had been defined prior to a 4- to 7-week course of radiotherapy has not been adequately studied,[16] and is an import topic of future research.

Determination of Treatment Volumes The modern 3D conformal radiation technique (CRT) requires precise definition of the treatment target and organs at risk. This is different from the traditional 2D practice. Definitions: the GTV includes the primary tumor (GTV-P) and the nodal GTV (GTV-N). The clinical target volume (CTV) accounts for microscopic (subclinical) disease. The PTV incorporates tumor delineation uncertainty, organ motion, setup variation, and intrafraction stability.

Lymphatic spread is an important pathway of progression of non–small cell lung cancer (NSCLC), along with local spread and distant metastasis. The probability of lymph node invasion is dependent on the site of the primary lung tumor, tumor stage, and histology. Before radiotherapy treatment starts, the extent of lymph node spread needs to be determined as correctly as possible. In the past, it was impossible to stage lymphatic spread accurately, and large radiation fields were used to encompass lymph node areas that were clinically and radiologically uninvolved. These large fields, called elective nodal irradiation (ENI), were covering, for example, the homolateral supraclavicular fossa, the hilar region, or the mediastinal lymph nodes. The use of these large irradiation fields increased the volume of normal tissues irradiated considerably, which led to more toxicity and prevented successful dose escalation. The influence of these large elective fields on treatment outcome was never established in randomized trials. Obviously, the extent and quality of the staging examinations performed pretreatment influences the need for ENI.

Delineation of Gross Tumor Volume Target delineation of GTV is essential for 3D CRT. The target volume definition should follow the guidelines of the International Commission of Radiation Units and Measurements (ICRU). The GTV includes the GTV-P, and the GTV-N; GTV-N includes any abnormally enlarged regional lymph node (hilar and/or mediastinal), as well as mediastinal and/or supraclavicular nodes enlarged 1 cm or more in the short axis,[12] unless metastases have been excluded by other means such as mediastinoscopy or ^{18}F-fluorodeoxyglucose (FDG)-PET scanning. GTV-N should also include lymph nodes that are not enlarged but have been documented by mediastinoscopy/endoscopic ultrasound (EUS)/endobronchial ultrasound (EBUS) as being pathologically involved or have higher FDG activity than the mediastinal blood pool. The measured diameter of tumors in lung parenchyma or mediastinum is highly dependent on the window width and level chosen during the delineating process.[17] Lung primary tumors should be outlined under the standard lung window, whereas the nodal disease and centrally located tumors are better contoured under mediastinum window/levels. The specific window widths and levels may vary with the CT scanner, software used, and the technique, with lung settings at W = 400 to 1600, L = −400 to −600, and mediastinum settings ranges W = 400 to 1000, L = 0 to 50.[17–19] One study found that the best concordance between measured and actual diameters and volumes was obtained with the following settings: W = 1600 and L = −600 for parenchyma, and W = 400 and L = 20 for mediastinum.[19] It is preferable that such parameters be specified in each center with the help of a radiologist, and be preset in treatment planning workstations, to improve consistency in contouring.

Depending on the tumor location, the adequate window and level setting should be viewed to delineate the GTV. For example, when the tumor is surrounded by lung tissue only, the lung level and window CT settings should be used. For lymph nodes and lung tumors invading the mediastinum or chest wall, only the window with mediastinum level and window settings should be viewed. The use of 4D CT scanning may reduce delineation uncertainties because of an improved visualization of the tumor shape (see section on "Motion Considerations").

Determination of Clinical Target Volume The CTV accounts for microscopic (subclinical) disease. This subclinical area may involve a region around the GTV as well as regional lymph node areas that were not documented to have adenopathy or proved by mediastinoscopy to be involved. It is controversial what this volume should include. It is extremely challenging to estimate the extent of CTV. Generally, the size of margin added to the GTV to account for microscopic extent has been arbitrary, ranging from 5 to 8 mm. Giraud et al.[19] examined NSCLC surgical specimens with adenocarcinoma (ADC) and squamous cell carcinoma (SCC) histology. The mean value of microscopic extension was 2.7 mm for ADC and 1.5 mm for SCC. A 5-mm margin covers 80% of the microscopic disease extension for ADC and 91% for SCC. To have 95% confidence that all tumor is included in the clinical target volume, a margin of 8 and 6 mm must be chosen for ADC and SCC, respectively. Grill et al.[20] analyzed microscopic disease extension in 35 cases and reported that in a GTV contoured using CT lung windows, the margin required to cover microscopic extension for 90% of the cases was 9 mm (9, 7, and 4 mm for grade 1 to 3, respectively).

The concept of nodal CTV includes CTV around the GTV-N and the microscopic disease within clinically normal nodes. Yuan et al.[21] studied extracapular extension (ECE) in 243 cases and concluded that ECE extent was related to lymph node size, stage, and differentiation. The extent of ECE was 3 mm in 95% of the nodes. It may be reasonable to recommend 3-mm CTV margins for pathologic lymph nodes (GTV-N) $<$20 mm and more generous margins for lymph nodes $\geq$20 mm. The microscopic disease extension to the clinically uninvolved nodal regions has been a topic of debate and has been evolving over the last several years. During the 1980s, this volume routinely included mediastinum, bilateral hilum, and the supraclavicular areas. Emami et al.[22] reported that inclusion of the contralateral hilum, the mediastinum, and supraclavicular lymph nodes in the field did not affect local control or survival. In the 1990s, most had eliminated the contralateral hilum and/or the supraclavicular areas. However, whether or not the ipsilateral hilum lymph node group was included per protocol did appear to affect local control and survival.[23] Recent results with 3D CRT without intentionally including these elective nodal regions showed a low incidence (0% to 7%) of isolated nodal failure in several dose escalation studies.[16,24–26]

There is lack of solid evidence currently existing for either pro or con ENI.[27] Although most of the published results from the cooperative groups used the elective radiation to most of the mediastinum regions, the newly activated protocols for NSCLC have a tendency to omit such radiation (Radiation Therapy Oncology Group [RTOG] 0617 and European Organisation for Research and Treatment of Cancer [EORTC] trials). If the treating physician believes an elective nodal area (primarily of the mediastinum or ipsilateral hilum) is indicated, it should be contoured and identified on CT scans. The atlas of nodal regions from University of Michigan is an important tool to determine the anatomic area of the lymph nodes involved.[28]

Determination of Planning Target Volume A range of geometrical uncertainties are associated with radiotherapy of lung cancer patients, such as target definition uncertainties, setup errors, organ motion, and anatomical changes. Errors (uncertainties) made during treatment preparation (e.g., target definition errors, or a nonrepresentative planning CT scan) will be made only once. In the absence of correction protocols, these errors will then be present during every treatment fraction. Errors made during treatment delivery of fractionated radiotherapy (e.g., misalignment of the patient), on the other hand, will be made several times and are likely to be different every day. Errors that are identical for every fraction are called *systematic errors*, whereas errors that vary day-by-day are called *random errors*. The dosimetric effect of systematic and random errors is different; random errors blur the cumulative dose distribution, whereas systematic errors shift the cumulative dose distribution.

To account for geometrical uncertainties, safety margins are applied around the CTV, thereby defining the PTV and thus irradiating a larger volume (Fig. 40.2). Often, separate margins are used for patient positioning uncertainty and for organ motion, called the *setup margin* (SM) and the *internal margin* (IM), respectively. As external error sources and internal error sources are generally not correlated, a linear addition of these margins, however, is not correct. Alternatively, the CTV is directly expanded to the PTV. Several margin recipes have been proposed in the literature with different objectives. For example, van Herk et al.[29] showed that the margin around the CTV for conventional fractionation should be 2.5 times the standard deviation of all the systematic error plus 0.7 times the standard deviation of all the

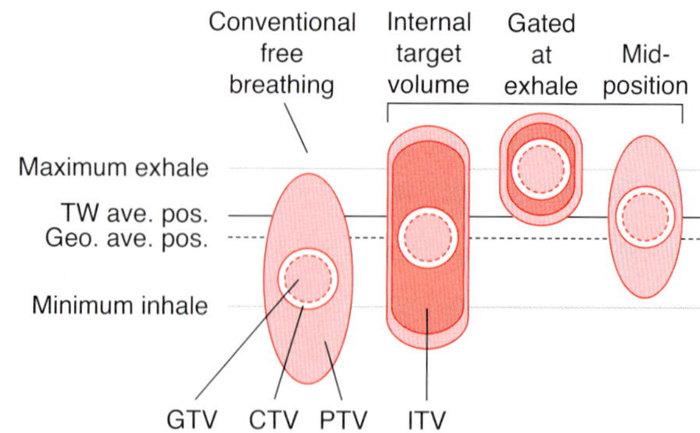

FIGURE 40.2 Schematic of the relationship of planning target volumes (PTVs) for various planning concepts: conventional free breathing, internal target volume, gating (at exhale), and midposition. *Ave.*, average; *CTV*, clinical target volume; *Geo.*, geometrical; *GTV*, gross tumor volume; *ITV*, internal target volume; *pos.*, position; *TW*, time-weighted.

random error to make sure that 90% of the patient's GTV will receive at least 95% of the dose. Note that the distribution of systematic and random uncertainties is institution dependent and, thus, need to be carefully evaluated for each department.

Traditionally, a uniform 7- to 10-mm margin was used to extend the CTV in all directions to form the PTV. However, because the respiratory induced tumor motion is nonuniform and patient dependent, the PTV should also be nonuniform and patient dependent. Moreover, detailed analysis of several sources of geometrical uncertainties[30–33] has revealed that such margins are too small in the absence of image guidance and associated correction strategies.

The use of 4D CT scanning technique allows for accurate estimation of tumor motion, although over a short time interval, and generates individualized margins. Various approaches for the incorporation of 4D CT scanning in treatment planning have been published recently.[34–37] In general, the use of 4D scanning in combination with gating, or the reconstruction of a time-averaged tumor position (midventilation CT scan), allows an important reduction of the PTV (Fig. 40.2) compared with the PTV for conventional free breathing CT scanning or the internal target volume (ITV). The ITV concept (note that the ITV is defined differently from the original ICRU definition) covers the entire tumor motion, in one breathing cycle, and therefore, may overestimate the influence of the motion on the tumor dose.[38] Additionally, critical normal tissues where knowledge of the radiation dose is important and/or dose should be minimized need to be carefully and consistently defined. An example of normal structure definition is shown in Figure 40.3.

The Role of the Positron Emission Tomography Scan on Target Delineation FDG-PET has had a significant impact on the delineation of the GTV for NSCLC, because it images metabolically active tumor cells, and identifies pathological lymph nodes more accurately than CT scanning.[39,40,54] A metaanalysis of 39 FDG–PET studies examined

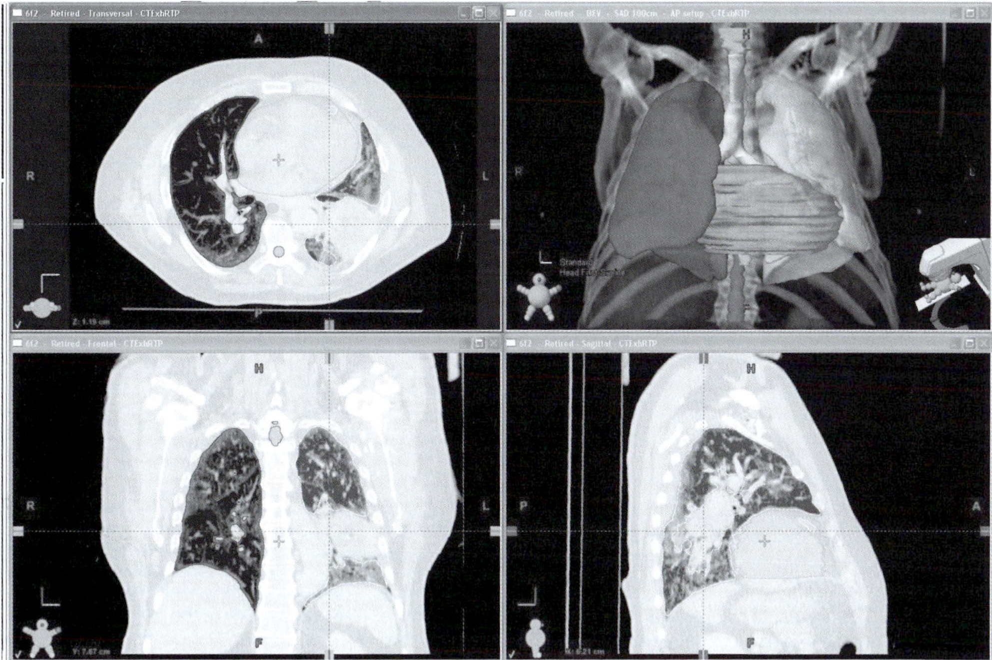

FIGURE 40.3 Dose-limiting normal tissues to avoid and/or limit radiation dose. Target volume delineation is performed on the entire 3D (or 4D) data set. Right lung: *blue*; left lung: *green*; heart: *pink*; esophagus: *green*; spinal cord: *brown*; main airways: *yellow*. The target volumes can be seen in Figure 40.1. (See color plate.)

the diagnostic accuracy of FDG–PET scanning in patients with NSCLC using stratification for mediastinal lymph node size on CT scan.[41] Based on this analysis, the sensitivity of the FDG–PET scan for enlarged mediastinal lymph nodes was 91% and 75% for not-enlarged lymph nodes. FDG-PET also improved the staging of solitary pulmonary lesions[42] and extrathoracic spread of the disease. Another advantage of FDG–PET scanning is the possibility to distinguish tumor from collapsed lung or mediastinal structures. In addition, evidence is accumulating that the standardized uptake value (SUV) of FDG–PET tracer in the primary tumor is an important prognostic factor for radiotherapy treatment outcome.[43–46]

The introduction of FDG-PET has a large influence on selecting patients for radical radiotherapy treatment. Several studies have demonstrated that FDG–PET scan implementation in radiotherapy treatment planning influenced the delineation of the GTV.[47–61] The most common findings of the studies have been changes of GTV and PTV based on the PET image, which subsequently might improve the estimated tumor control probability and normal-tissue complication probability.[55,56] PET imaging can provide a more accurate representation of the 3D volume-encompassing motion of model tumors and has the potential to provide patient-specific motion volumes for an individualized ITV.[57] For patients, the PET-delineated target volume seemed to be consistent with the ITV determined from all sets of gated-CT and regular spiral CT images. PET use in estimating the individual ITV is further addressed by Fernando et al.[58] Additionally, implementing matched CT-FDG-PET reduced interobserver and intraobserver variation in target delineation significantly with respect to CT only.[52,59]

Steenbakkers et al.[33] observed a reduction in the interobserver variability of more than 50% in the standard deviation of the GTV delineations if FDG–PET information coregistered with CT was used. Preferably, the tumor delineation should be based on a matched CT-FDG-PET scan (with both examinations in treatment position) and performed by a radiation oncologist experienced in lung cancer treatment in the presence of a detailed delineation protocol and adequate delineation software.[33]

It is clear that PET has significantly changed the treatment planning of NSCLC patients, and is considered to be a state-of-the-art technique. Images from a planning FDG-PET-CT scan are shown in Figure 40.4.

Issues remain, however, with the use of PET in target delineation, some of which were discussed in a recent journal editorial.[60] For example, the determination of the edges of the tumor in the metabolically active area on PET is not straightforward. Most of the studies that were mentioned used an arbitrary threshold value of the maximum intensity (30% to 50%) in the PET-avid area or a standardized uptake value (range: 2 to 5). This threshold, however, was generated from phantom studies of limited target size,[61] and is not correct for most patients with NSCLC.[62] Several phantom studies have attempted to determine optimal threshold values, with differing results. Researchers from Beaumont Hospital[63] performed a series of sphere phantom studies to determine an accurate and uniformly applicable method for defining a GTV with

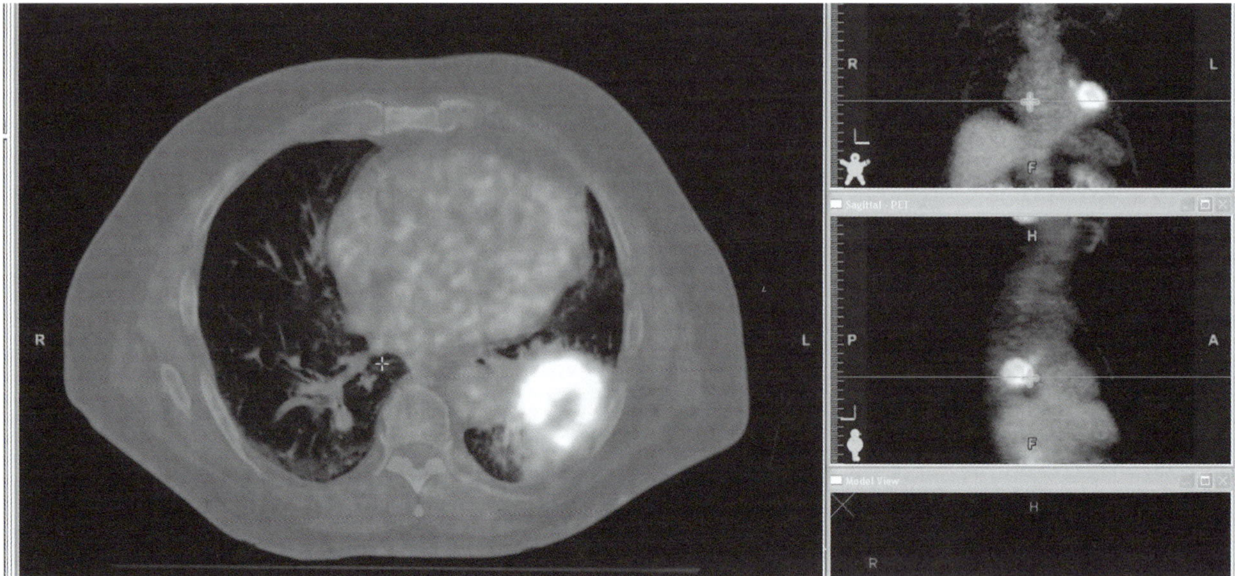

FIGURE 40.4 PET images overlaid on the CT scan from a treatment planning PET-CT simulation session. For radiation oncology, a critical step is the delineation of the tumor boundaries that are necessary for determining the shape of the radiation treatment beams. (See color plate.)

FDG-PET. They found a strong linear relationship between the threshold SUV and the mean target SUV. Recent studies from patients further confirmed that the threshold for the best match of CT-GTV averaged 20% to 25% (range: 10% to 50%) ITV 15% to 20% (range: 10% to 50%), depending on the tumor size, activity, and location.[58]

Unfortunately, FDG-PET has its limitations. Firstly, the spatial resolution of FDG–PET images is poor (4 to 6 mm) compared with CT scan images.[57,64] Therefore, the increased FDG uptake should be used for localization of the tumor, not for defining boundaries, except for the tumor-atelectasis region. In a study by Steenbakkers et al.[33] 10% of the lymph nodes with increased FDG uptake were missed by the radiation oncologists. One explanation might be that the FDG–PET report was not read accurately enough by the radiation oncologists. Furthermore, for some lymph nodes, the level and window settings of the FDG-PET had to be changed before they were visible.

Another challenging issue of using PET for treatment planning is to register the PET image accurately when a PET-CT simulator or hybrid PET-CT is not available. An ideal registration method, which uses the entire volume of image data (i.e., intensities of the image voxels) for matching of "mutual information" and displays the two modalities simultaneously, would significantly improve the accuracy of PET in target delineation.

Motion Considerations

Tumor motion caused by breathing and heartbeat is a topic of many investigations. Tumor motion could be rather substantial and heterogeneous, ranging from a few millimeters to 25 mm based on tumor location, size, and patient condition.[65–69] The greatest tumor motion is seen in the cranial–caudal direction. Information on the individual patient's lung tumor motion is necessary to determine individual margins.[66] It is critical to accurately estimate the motion for each tumor, so that the treatment planning is optimized for target coverage and normal-tissue sparing. With the advancement of imaging techniques, several strategies are now available to approach this goal. These include, but are not limited to, visualization under fluoroscopy, respiratory-gated CT simulation, and 4D CT simulation.

Tumor motion can be visualized under a conventional simulator with fluoroscopy, and the extent of motion can be estimated for each tumor.[70,71] With quiet respiration, the maximum tumor movement in the craniocaudal direction was 12 mm, and the mediolateral and dorsoventral direction was 5 mm in a study by Ekberg et al.[70] Other reported movements ranged from 0 to 12.8 mm in the superior–inferior direction, 0 to 3.2 mm in the lateral direction, and 0 to 4.4 mm in the anterior–posterior direction.[71] Large variation in GTV motion from patient to patient was observed, especially in the superior–inferior direction, for which interpatient variability was >10 mm.

Tumor motion seemed to be unique for each patient and in each dimension. A standard uniform PTV margin of 10 or 15 mm is inappropriate. Motion check under fluoroscopy can provide an estimation of the internal motion in each patient. This method is simple; however, it is limited by the facts that (a) some tumors can be difficult to visualize with fluoroscopy x-rays; (b) diaphragm motion may not correlate with tumor movement; and (c) the shape change of the tumor cannot be measured clearly. Additionally, fluoroscopy generally overestimates the mobility of visible lung tumors and may result in irradiation of unnecessarily large target volumes.[72] Even if an individualized margin is obtained from the fluoroscopy, an ideal PTV cannot be guaranteed from GTV because the free-breathing CT images can be taken in any phase of the breathing cycle when the target volume is scanned. For example, assume the target is scanned at the end of exhale (the target in the most superior position), a uniform expansion would include unnecessary normal tissue superiorly and would not cover the inferior part of the target adequately.

With the wide availability of CT simulation, techniques with modifications to the CT simulation procedure have been proposed to better define the treatment target. The most common of these is respiratory correlated 4D CT.[73–76] A multislice CT scanner is typically used for 4D CT. In the cine mode, the CT scanner scans the same table position for one or more whole respiratory cycles, and then moves to another table position. Computer programs then sort out the images according to the respiratory phases and reconstruct the 3D CT images at each phase. Usually, 10 sets of images of 10 different phases are obtained for one simulation.

An ITV can then be generated by combining the GTVs of different phases with a CTV margin. Theoretically, using 4D CT images should be the best way to approach ITV accurately. The challenge of this technique is the burden for the treatment planning computer to handle the large amount of data and for the radiation oncologists to delineate/check the target in each image set. Also, there are several artifacts found using current generation 4D CT scan technology[77–79] that could be improved through breathing training, improved acquisition techniques, and/or better post-acquisition reconstruction methods.

Another technique referred to as the mid-ventilation (MidV) CT scan generates a single 3D CT frame from 4D CT images representing the tumor closest to its mean tumor motion position.[37] Using this MidVCT scan, the systematic contribution caused by breathing motion can be reduced to nearly zero, permitting a reduction of the treatment margin. The expected dose-blurring effect of the respiration can be accounted for in the CTV to PTV margin. Because of the presence of the wide beam penumbra in lung, Engelsman et al.[80] and Witte et al.[81] reported that if a treatment plan is designed for the tumor in its (time-weighted) average position during the respiration cycle, a good dose coverage is still obtained even if the tumor is not fully within the PTV during a small part of the breathing cycle.

One or more phases of the 4D CT scan (e.g., the end exhale, or scans near and including end exhale) can be used for respiratory-gated treatment planning/delivery. Alternatively, a gated CT scan can be acquired by triggering the CT scanner to acquire imaging data when the patient's respiratory signal crosses a predetermined threshold (e.g., near end exhale).

To reduce tumor motion, several strategies have been developed and tested. These fall within two classes: abdominal compression and breath-hold techniques. Abdominal compression was originally developed for stereotactic irradiation of small lung and liver lesions by Lax and Blomgren[82–84] and has been used elsewhere.[6,85–91] The technique employs a frame with an attached plate that is pressed against the abdomen. The applied pressure to the abdomen reduces diaphragmatic excursions, while still permitting limited normal respiration. The accuracy and reproducibility of both the body frame and the pressure plate have been evaluated by several groups, with a comprehensive assessment reported by Negoro et al.[86] Abdominal compression has predominantly been applied to early stage lung and liver tumors without mediastinal involvement or nodal disease, although the technology is also applicable to conventional lung treatments.

The most widely used breath-hold methods are active breathing control (ABC) described by Wong et al.[92,93] and deep inspiration breath hold.[94–96] Using breath-hold devices, CT simulation and treatment delivery can be performed at the same fixed level of controlled breathing; thus, the target is considerably reduced during treatment planning and delivery. In addition to motion reduction, breath-hold techniques have the advantage that the lung volume is expanded by 30% to 50%, thus for a given beam aperture, the fraction of lung being irradiated is smaller. However, implementation of breath-hold techniques requires patient selection for compliance and increases the time of the imaging and treatment procedures.

Other motion management techniques, such as using gated treatment at a specifically defined phase window when the patient breathes freely, or tumor tracking (in which the radiation beam follows a measurement or estimate of the tumor motion) are clinically available and, with improved integration of image guidance with treatment delivery, are likely to become more widespread.

TREATMENT PLANNING

Aiming to maximize the radiation dose to the target volume while minimizing dose to surrounding normal tissues, the 3D CRT is now the standard technique of RT in lung cancer. Planning and delivery of RT is a multistep process that is individualized for each patient. Literature-based EORTC guidelines on each of these steps for 3D CRT in the setting of clinical practice and clinical trial have been published.[97] The process of RT planning includes dose/fractionation, immobilization/localization, target and normal-tissue delineation (including tumor and important normal structures), radiation beam design, and treatment delivery.

Beam Arrangements/Aids and 3D CRT The design of the radiation beam field or aperture depends on the treatment volume, with or without inclusion of ENI. With ENI, the beam selections are limited by the extensive volume of the target—often large fields aimed from the anterior and posterior (AP/PA) direction of the patient in parallel-opposed fashion. The AP/PA beam arrangement is limited by the tolerance dose of the cord, thus, one or more "off-cord" fields are always needed for radical treatment when a dose of 60 Gy or higher is needed. Although the nodal volume was traditionally determined by anatomical landmarks located on simulator radiographs or reconstructed coronal CT planes (as it was for 2D planning), the nodal regions should be contoured consistently, so the PTV can be defined and the plan of 3D CRT can be generated. This technique offers the potential advantage of improved dose delivery to a target volume (as opposed to a point dose calculation in 2D planning, historically).

Using 3D CRT with selective ENI or without ENI, the PTV is to be treated with any combination of coplanar or noncoplanar 3D conformal fields shaped to deliver the specified dose while restricting the dose to the normal tissues. Field arrangements are determined by 3D planning to produce the optimal conformal plan in accordance with volume definitions. Multiple coplanar or noncoplanar field arrangements are preferred, but AP/PA fields are still used, if appropriate, on an individual basis. The beam directions are selected by the use of the beam's eye view (BEV) tool. Target and normal structures are viewed from different directions in planes perpendicular to the beam's central axis using BEV. The beam shape is then modified by designing a block or a block substitute called a *multileaf collimator* (MLC) shaper, which will allow full dose to the PTV but minimize the dose to surrounding normal tissue. To cover the entire PTV with the prescription dose, an additional margin (block margin) should be added to each aperture. The block margin is to compensate the penumbra at each beam edge; and often 5 to 10 mm is needed for an adequate coverage at the peripheral part of PTV. It should be kept in mind that this margin width is dependent on the number and arrangement of fields and the specific technique used. For coplanar arrangement of multiple beams, smaller lateral margins are needed for adequate PTV coverage (i.e., relatively larger superior–inferior margins for each beam).

Once beam angles and shapes are designed, beam energy and beam aids need to be chosen for each individual beam. To select the appropriate energy for each beam, one should keep in mind the nature of low intensity of lung tissue. Photon energy of 6 megaelectron volts (MV) is preferred for beams passing through large volume of lower–density lung parenchyma to provide better PTV coverage; 15 to 18 MV may decrease the monitor unit (MU) and provide better dose homogeneity for AP/PA mediastinal beams. In the case of a large sloping contour, such as usually encountered when treating upper lobe tumors in large patients, beam aids such as wedge or compensating filters are recommended to improve the dose distribution. Dose calculations incorporate basic data that characterize the radiation beam energy and geometry, such as depth dose curves and isodose information for standard field sizes. Computerized algorithms have been developed to combine the dose distributions generated by combinations of beams, using individual patient information such as depth of the point of calculation, external body contour, and various densities of anatomical structures. Dose distributions are displayed with concentric curves for chosen dose levels (isodoses), which are displayed as overlays on anatomic structures. These curves are normalized to a reference dose, either at isocenter (ICRU point) or to the lowest isodose curve that encompasses the PTV.

The treatment plan can be evaluated whether it meets the objectives of PTV coverage and normal-tissue avoidance. The idealized, perfect plan would be 100% coverage of a tumor target with a minimal amount of dose heterogeneity or overdose to achieve that 100% minimum dose coverage. This is very often a quite difficult goal, as lung tumors are often surrounded by low density of the lungs or other critical structures. In practice, a 95% PTV coverage is acceptable for 3D RT. A set of criteria for normal-tissue tolerances (discussed in the next section) must be given to guide the treatment planning. Dose distributions for 3D volumes can be displayed and analyzed graphically with dose–volume histograms (DVH), which are generated for each structure. The cumulative form of the DVH is a plot of the volume of a given structure receiving a certain dose or higher as a function of dose. The DVH for normal lung is the addition of the dose distributions of both lungs but minus the dose distribution in the GTV. The GTV is selected instead of the PTV, because the PTV contains normal lung receiving a high dose, which influences the normal-tissue toxicity rate. A 3D conformal radiotherapy treatment plan is shown in Figure 40.5.

If the treatment plan does not meet the given dose–volume objectives, beam arrangements or other parameters are adjusted. This can include a change of beam energy, beam angle, or

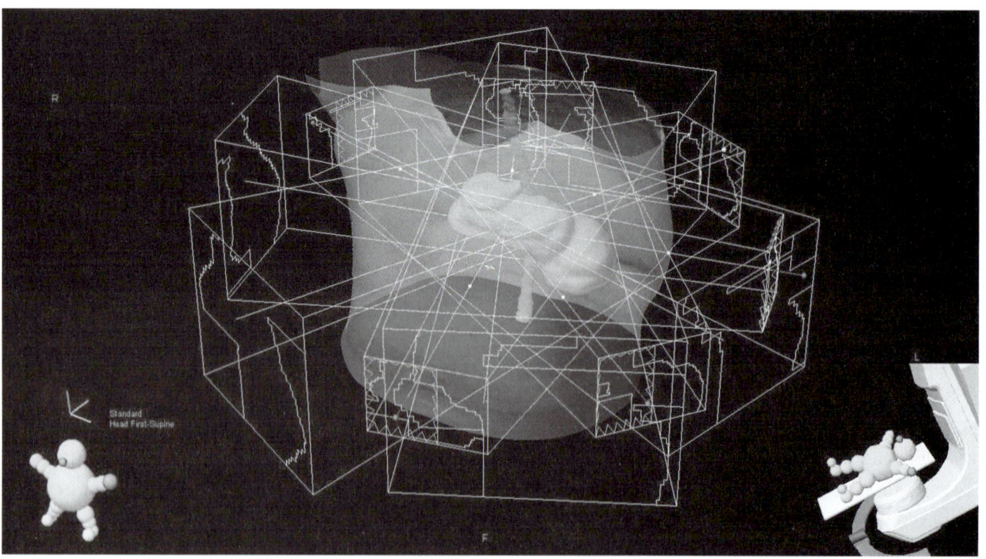

FIGURE 40.5 The beam arrangement for an intensity-modulated radiotherapy (IMRT) treatment of lung cancer. (See color plate.)

adjustment of the beam intensity. For conformal therapy, beam arrangements and adjustments are carried out manually, with changes made in an iterative fashion by the treatment planner.

Once the final beams are designed, radiographs in the form of DRRs are generated from the treatment planning CT to enhance the bony anatomy with high contrast, and are in the BEV plane. DRRs are used to compare with portal images taken before treatment, which are either films placed in the beam exiting the patient or with an electronic portal device. Verification of the radiation beam placement should be carried out pretreatment and at least weekly during the course of treatment so that patient position can be adjusted accordingly.

Intensity-Modulated Radiation Therapy Although radiation intensity is uniform across the beam/field for conventional 3D CRT, intensity-modulated radiation therapy (IMRT) adjusts the beam intensity across the beam width and length. The simplest modification of the intensity is a wedge-shaped filter or a physical compensator placed in the machine head. Modern machines can also use MLC movement to achieve the same goal. A slightly more complex method is to break the field aperture into segments with varying beam-on times. Currently, the most intricate form of intensity modulation achieves a checkerboard pattern with each square of a varying intensity. The modern concept of IMRT involves delivery of this type of pattern with a device called an MLC, which can be moved under computer control to shape segments of the field to deliver the intensity pattern. Because the intensity pattern is so complex, a different type of computerized treatment planning is used, called *inverse planning*. The treatment planner defines the dose to be delivered to a target volume and the limiting dose to the surrounding normal tissues, and beam angles. The computer determines the corresponding intensity profiles to achieve the desired dose distribution. There have been several theoretical treatment planning studies published, with findings that higher levels of tumor dose can be achieved while maintaining the same normal lung dose–volume indices.[98–102] Compared with 3D CRT, IMRT reduced the percentage of lung volume that received >20 Gy and the mean lung dose, with a median reduction of 8% and 2 Gy, respectively.[103] Treatment planning with IMRT under deep breath-hold results in lower V_{20} and lower-modeled pneumonitis rates,[104] allowing delivery of a higher dose to the target. IMRT can be used to reduce the irradiation of, for example, the esophagus (whose damage causes dysphagia) without deterioration of the target coverage. This might be particularly important for patients treated with concomitant chemoradiation regimes. Therefore, IMRT is of significant value (compared with 3D CRT) in node-positive cases with target volumes close to the esophagus.[98,105] For such patients, IMRT can deliver RT doses 125% to 130% greater than an optimized 3D CRT plan and 130% to 140% greater than a plan including ENI.[100] In a planning study by Schwarz et al.,[102] the increase in deliverable dose was 135% compared with the 3D CRT plan if IMRT and dose heterogeneity within the PTV was allowed. IMRT is of limited additional value (compared with 3D CRT) in node-negative patients.[100,102] IMRT is associated with increased lung volume exposed to low doses (<10 Gy) in some studies,[98] but Schwarz reported no increase of lung volume receiving (very) low doses, even down to 5 Gy. Additionally, IMRT delivers radiation through multiple small segments that do not cover the whole target, and may thus underdose parts of the target or overdose the adjacent normal tissue if the motion is not appropriately controlled. IMRT is in an early stage of clinical practice in the treatment of lung cancer and the clinical impact on lung toxicity is not yet completely known. An IMRT treatment plan is shown in Figure 40.6.

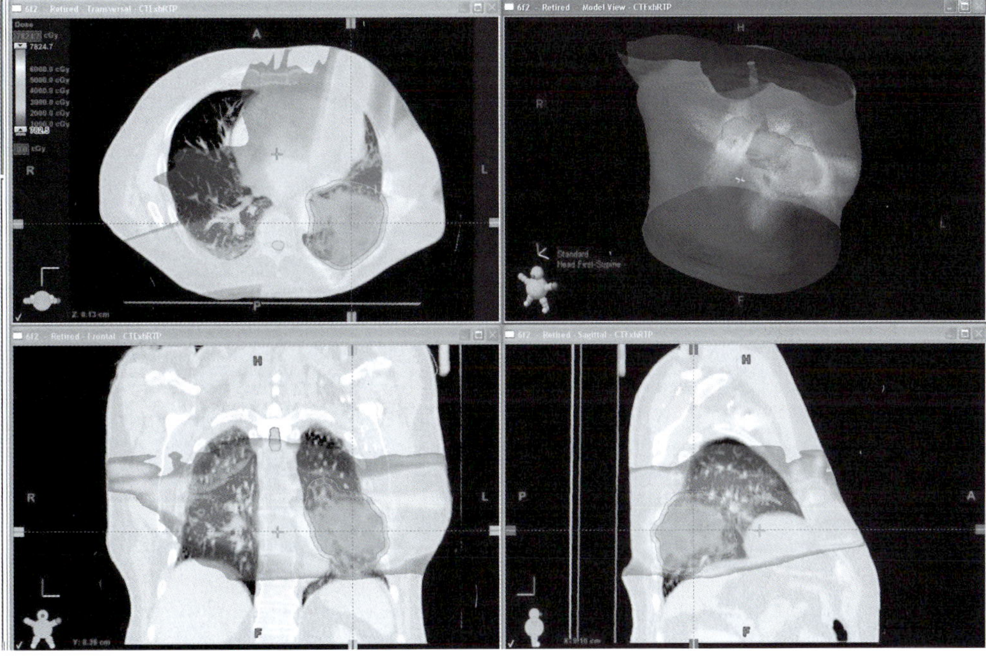

FIGURE 40.6 The dose distribution for an intensity-modulated radiotherapy (IMRT) treatment of lung cancer. (See color plate.)

Dose Calculation and Tissue Heterogeneity Correction With the availability of either superposition/convolution (SC) or Monte Carlo (MC) dose calculation algorithms on all major treatment planning systems, tissue heterogeneities (particularly those found for lung cancer radiotherapy treatment plans) can be accurately accounted for. Accurate dose calculation algorithms give the treatment team confidence that the planned dose is a valid estimate of the delivered dose, keeping in mind that there are several other uncertainties, such as target delineation, interfraction and intrafraction motion, and tumor response to radiation treatment. The challenge of dose calculation in the lung is that the reduced lung density (from 0.1 to 0.5 times that of surrounding muscle and tissue) means that photons and electrons will travel 2 to 10 times further in the lung tissue relative to the surrounding material. This increased particle range means that the beam edges become less sharply defined, and larger beam apertures may be necessary to ensure adequate coverage of the edge of the target volume. Secondary build up at the tumor-lung interface can also occur.

For lung cancer cases, SC and MC method–calculated dose distributions are characterized by reduced penetration and increased penumbra caused by larger secondary electron range in the low-density media compared with previously used correction methods (e.g., equivalent path length [EPL] methods). Based on the MC method, target dose was overestimated (though less than 10%), and the dose of adjacent lung was underestimated in the plans calculated by the EPL method.[106–108] This effect is more prominent around the tumor-lung boundary, less at the PTV-mediastinal boundary. The mean lung dose as determined by the CS and EPL algorithms differed on average by 17%, and the V_{20} differed on average by 12%.[106]

In general, tissue heterogeneity effects depend on the lung density, the lung length traversed, beam energy, and beam field size. In addition to altering PTV coverage, heterogeneity correction changes the ICRU prescription dose. Correction factors for 6 MV photon AP/PA beams in lung range from 1.05 to 1.13, which varies with dose calculation algorithms. The CS and MC methods provide very close estimation. When dose was measured in a benchmark test phantom to a point in between two lungs, there was increased dose ranging from 5% to 14% relative to a phantom of unit density. The effect decreases as the photon energy increases. The use of high-energy beams could be used to minimize the dose correction discrepancies. However, higher energy beams tend to "spare" the surface of the tumor when traversing through the lung. Higher energies will have an increased range of secondary electrons in lung tissue, which further spreads out the low isodoses relative to a water-equivalent tissue.[109] When a clinically relevant phantom study was performed,[110] the dose delivered to the PTV with 6 MV was within 5% of prediction, but low by 11% with the use of 18 MV. MC calculations showed that all target coverage indicators were significantly worse for 15 MV than for 6 MV, particularly the portion of the PTV receiving at least 95% of the prescription dose.[107]

Between SC and MC, MC is considered the most accurate algorithm as photons and electrons are individually transported through the patient using our best understanding of the laws of physics, although careful commissioning and implementation is required.[111] It is now the consensus of RTOG and the American Association of Physicists in Medicine (AAPM)[111,112] that tissue heterogeneity needs to be corrected for treatment planning of lung cancer and the most accurate dose calculation algorithm used for treatment.

DOSE AND FRACTIONATION

Dose and Fractionation in Non–Small Cell Lung Cancer

Dose and Fractionation for Definitive Radiation

DOSE FOR ADJUVANT RADIATION FOR PATIENTS WITH RESECTED NSCLC. A dose of 45 to 50 Gy in 1.8 to 2 Gy daily fractions is generally recommended for preoperative radiation. When postoperative RT is indicated, the mediastinum is commonly treated to 50 Gy in 25 fractions, and regions of extracapsular extension and/or bulky nodal disease boosted by an additional 10 Gy. Areas of gross residual disease may be treated to 66 to 70 Gy if the volume to the normal structure is limited. When T3N0 chest tumors with chest wall invasion are given postoperative RT, the regional nodal area does not require postoperative RT if it was adequately staged during surgery. However, the chest wall should receive up to 60 Gy postoperatively. (See also Chapter 41.)

DOSE AND DOSE ESCALATION FOR PATIENTS WITH INOPERABLE OR UNRESECTABLE NSCLC. The prescription dose for definitive RT depends on the presence of chemotherapy and the volume of the organ at risk. It is generally felt, and supported by a few studies, that if high doses of radiation could be delivered safely, treatment outcomes might improve. For definitive RT alone, the mediastinum or elective nodal area (if given) was traditionally treated to 45 to 50 Gy in conventional fractions (once-daily doses of 1.8 to 2.0 Gy), and the primary or gross tumor boosted to a total dose of 60 Gy or more. The tumor dose of 60 Gy was established as the standard of care in RTOG 73-01, the only randomized trial that reported intrathoracic failure rates of 52%, 42%, and 33% for 40, 50, and 60 Gy, respectively, at 3-year follow-up.[113,114] Although the study did not show an improved overall survival, review of the results from other RTOG trials led to the conclusion that local tumor control was significantly correlated with improved survival.[114] A dose of 60 Gy or slightly higher has since become a frequently employed prescription dose, but long-term tumor control and survival are generally poor. Evaluation by means of bronchoscopy and biopsy at 1 year after treatment completion revealed local control rates of only 15% to 17%,[115] with 5-year overall survival reported to be less than 10%.[116,117] For stage I NSCLC, retrospective studies from Duke University and Washington University reported that patients who received a dose of ≥70 Gy had local tumor control compared with those who had <70 Gy.[118,119] More than 64 Gy was associated with superior survival in patients with stage III NSCLC disease based on a recent retrospective review from the Memorial Sloan-Kettering Cancer Center.[120] Using 3D CT-based conformal RT techniques, several radiation dose escalation studies have shown much higher than 60 to 70 Gy to be feasible,[26,118,121–128] and higher doses appear to be associated with better local tumor control and survival in medically inoperable or unresectable NSCLC.[16,120]

Several phase I/II dose escalation trials were performed and the safety of radiotherapy doses above 100 Gy for patients with small tumor volumes was reported by researchers from the University of Michigan.[124] Most dose escalation trials entered patients into different risk groups to develop pulmonary toxicity based on the relative mean lung dose or the percentage of lung receiving more than a certain threshold dose. The RTOG 9311 trial escalated the dose to 83.8 Gy for patients with V_{20} <37.5% (the lung volume received >20 Gy), using daily fractions of 2.15 Gy.[121] Investigators from the Netherlands Cancer Institute reported that doses up to 94.5 Gy in 42 fractions within 6 weeks could be safely delivered in case the mean lung dose was less than 11.3 Gy (corresponding to 13.6 Gy in case a simple planning algorithm is used).[129] Investigators from Memorial Sloan-Kettering Cancer Center safely escalated to a dose of 84 Gy for normal-tissue complication probability (NTCP) of less than 25%.[122] The maximum tumor dose delivered in these dose escalation trials (using different fractionation schedules and overall treatment times) can be compared by the calculation of the time-corrected biologically effective dose (tBED)[130] (with $\alpha/\beta = 10$ Gy and proliferation starting at 28 days). Compared with the dose escalation trial of the University of Michigan (UM 9204) and the RTOG 93-11 trial, the tBED in the trial of the Netherlands Cancer Institute was the highest (108 Gy) because of the reduced overall treatment time of 6 weeks.

Higher doses significantly increased the failure-free interval for the total group of patients in multivariable analysis in this dose escalation trial.[129] Kong et al.[16] reported improved local control and survival in patients irradiated with doses above 74 Gy in the dose escalation trial from the University of Michigan. For patients with newly diagnosed or recurrent stage I to III disease, multivariate analysis of this dose escalation trial found the radiation dose to be the only significant factor for local tumor control and overall survival. This demonstrated a positive relationship between dose and local/regional control, as well as overall survival, when doses ranging from 63 to 103 Gy were used. An increase of 1 Gy was associated with a more than 1% improvement in the 5-year tumor control, and a 3% decrease in the risk of death. Higher radiation doses may, therefore, be beneficial to patients with inoperable/unresectable NSCLC. A recent secondary analysis from RTOG trials has demonstrated a 2% reduction of risk from death with each increase of 1 Gy biological equivalent dose.[131] Bogart et al.[126] used >2.25 Gy daily fractions to a total nominal dose up to 84 Gy (range: 60 to 84) and reported a promising overall tumor response rate of 88% (35% complete response and 53% partial response), actuarial median survival of 38 months, and 3-year overall survival of 60% in early stage medical inoperable NSCLC.

In the setting of concurrent chemoradiation therapy (ChemoRT), the group from the University of North Carolina reported safe dose escalation up to 90 Gy with 2 Gy daily fractions, and with concurrent cyclophosphamide (CP) chemotherapy.[132] Clinical trials are ongoing to confirm the efficacy of such high-dose radiation in patients receiving concurrent ChemoRT, an example of which is RTOG 0617/North Central Cancer Treatment Group [NCCTG] N0628/Cancer and Leukemia Group B [CALGB] 30609, a randomized phase III comparison of standard dose (60 Gy) versus high-dose (74 Gy) conformal radiotherapy with concurrent ChemoRT in patients with stage IIA/IIIB NSCLC.[133]

In summary, the dose of radiation should be individualized based on normal-tissue tolerance, particularly normal lung, and the use of concurrent chemotherapy. A dose of more than 70 Gy may be given with RT, or sequential ChemoRT, and when the lung volume to be irradiated is limited (see succeeding section for lung dose tolerance). For large tumors when normal lung irradiation is extensive, or concurrent chemotherapy is given, most patients are unable to tolerate higher radiation doses due to severe toxicity; the safe prescription dose may still be around 60 to 70 Gy.

Treatment Duration and Altered Fractionation

TREATMENT DURATION. Extension of treatment duration may allow tumor repopulation and decrease the probability of local tumor control and survival. In RTOG 83-11, the highest survival was found in patients who received 69.6 Gy. These patients often had extended treatment duration and delays caused by acute esophagitis. Indeed, survival at 2 and 5 years was significantly better in patients who completed treatment in the planned time, compared with those who had treatment interruptions (24% vs. 13% at 2 years and 10% vs. 3% at 5 years).[134] In a large phase III trial reported by Saunders et al.,[135] 563 patients were randomized into two groups treated with radiation alone: standard RT (60 Gy in 2 Gy fractions, Monday through Friday in 6 weeks), or continuous hyperfractionated accelerated RT (CHART)—54 Gy delivered over 12 consecutive days. Two-year survival was noted to be superior in the CHART arm (29% vs. 20%; $p = 0.008$), which could be caused by a reduction in the overall treatment time with CHART, as the biological equivalent dose (BED) was 72 and 62 Gy for the conventional arm and CHART regimen, respectively. The ECOG 2597 trial compared 64 Gy/32fx/6.5 weeks with hyperfractionated accelerated radiation therapy (HART) (57.6 Gy/36 fx/3 weeks) after induction chemotherapy in locally advanced stage III NSCLC, and reported a trend of improved survival with the accelerated arm.[136] An early analysis estimated that the tumor control probability of NSCLC decreases 1.6% per day after a 6-week duration of RT.[137] In a recent secondary analysis of three RTOG trials in patients with stage III NSCLC who were treated with immediate concurrent ChemoRT, prolonged treatment time was significantly associated with poorer survival.[131]

The latter translated into a 2% increase in the risk of death for each day of prolongation in therapy. It was estimated that the tumor control probability of NSCLC decreases 1.6% per day after a 6-week duration of RT.[137] Thus, every effort should be made to limit treatment duration and avoid treatment delays. Currently, there are investigative efforts to increase daily fraction size to escalate total radiation dose without extending the treatment duration. One approach involves dose escalation using 2.25 Gy daily fractions (once or twice daily) but limiting treatment duration to 6 weeks.[126] This approach was used to escalate radiation doses to 94.5 Gy in patients with limited lung volume.[129] Another approach is to use a higher fraction dose every day while limiting the treatment duration to 5 weeks.[130] The University of Michigan has an ongoing trial to limit the radiation to 6 weeks by escalating daily dose at the later part of the week (Thursday and Friday).

ALTERED FRACTIONATION. Hyperfractionated RT delivers multiple smaller fractions each day, and used to be an area of interest for clinical trials to prevent excessive late tissue toxicities such as radiation pneumonitis that result from large daily fractions. However, randomized clinical trials have not unequivocally shown an advantage for hyperfractionated RT.[134,138,139] With radiation alone, the RTOG 8311 trial tested multiple total tumor doses (60, 64.8, 69.6, 74.5, and 79.2 Gy) and showed superior results with 69.6 Gy in 1.2 Gy twice daily fractions, compared with 60 Gy in 2 Gy daily fractions with a similar BED and treatment duration.[134] Although there is no reduction of radiation pneumonitis, the apparent survival benefit in these phase I/II trials was used to justify the inclusion of a hyperfractionated arm in subsequent trials, such as RTOG 8808 and RTOG 9410.[138,139] In the setting of neoadjuvant chemotherapy, RTOG 8808 failed to show a significant advantage to using hyperfractionated radiation. Using concurrent ChemoRT, RTOG 9410 compared induction chemotherapy with vinblastine and cisplatin followed by standard, single daily fraction RT (day 50) versus either identical chemotherapy and radiation given concurrently on day 1, or a third arm incorporating hyperfractionated RT and concurrent cisplatin and oral etoposide. The hyperfractionated arm was associated with an increased incidence of esophagitis and inferior survival compared to the daily fractionated concurrent arm.[139] Using hyperfractionated and accelerated radiation, the aforementioned CHART and HART delivered 1.5 Gy in three fractions a day with or without continuous radiation during the weekend, was associated with increased mortality when it was delivered with concurrent chemotherapy, or resulted in a higher esophagitis rate (25% for HART vs. 16% for the conventional arm) with sequential ChemoRT. In summary, hyperfractionated schemes are not recommended because of the lack of significant survival benefit in phase III trials, increased acute esophagitis, especially with concurrent chemotherapy, and the burden to the patients and radiation departments. Although hyperfractionated accelerated RT may be an option for radiation alone, the "safe" fractionation prescription is still 1.8 to 2.0 Gy conventional fractionations, particularly when concurrent chemotherapy is given.

Dose and Fractionation in Small Cell Lung Cancer

Thoracic radiation for limited stage small cell lung cancer (LS-SCLC) should be delivered early and concurrently with cisplatin-based chemotherapy, with 45 Gy in 1.5 Gy twice-daily fractions. If hyperfractionation is not possible, a dose of at least 54 to 60 Gy in 2 Gy daily fractions should be given. If the chemotherapy has been given prior to the thoracic RT, 50 to 54 Gy in 1.8 to 2.0 Gy should be given to the complete responders and 60 Gy to partial responders. Current investigations within cooperative groups include dose escalation to 70 Gy using standard fractionation (such as CALGB) and 61.2 Gy using a concomitant boost scheme (such as RTOG). Accelerated hyperfractionated RT (45 Gy in 1.5 Gy twice-daily fractions) was based on a randomized phase III clinical trial, intergroup trial (INT) 0096.[140] This trial compared once daily (45 Gy in 1.8 Gy daily fractions) versus twice-daily RT (45 Gy given in twice daily 1.5-Gy fractions) in combination with concurrent cisplatin and etoposide therapy. An improved median survival time and 5-year survival rate was observed in the accelerated arm compared with the once-daily group, 23 months versus 19 months and 26% versus 16%, respectively ($p = 0.04$). One must note that the accelerated hyperfractionated RT was associated with increased toxicities. A dose of 45 Gy in 1.8 Gy daily fractions is not biologically equivalent to 45 Gy in 1.5 Gy twice daily. Treatment duration may also impact the outcome of SCLC treatment. Using a similar regimen of hyperfractionated RT with a treatment break of 2.5 weeks, the NCCTG failed to show a benefit of using hyperfractionated RT compared with conventional RT.[141,142] Nevertheless, 45 Gy in 30 fractions over 3 weeks concurrent with etoposide and cisplatin therapy generated superior results to other published reports and is the recommended regimen for the treatment of LS-SCLC. When twice-daily radiation is impossible, daily fractionation with higher dose (54 to 60 Gy in 2 Gy fractions) is an acceptable alternative.

Palliative Thoracic Radiation

Symptoms such as chest pain, hemoptysis, dysphagia, and dyspnea in NSCLC as well as in SCLC can be effectively palliated using different treatment regimes. The optimal dose for palliation remains controversial.[143] Several randomized trials were performed with sometimes controversial results. Comparing the trials reported next is difficult, because frequency and duration of measurements vary substantially. Another aspect is the need to analyze the sum of the palliative effect: the symptom reduction and symptoms induced by the treatment.

In the first Medical Research Council (MRC) trial reported in 1991,[144] no differences in palliative effect or in survival were seen between 10 × 3 Gy and 2 × 8.5 Gy. In a second MRC trial (1992),[145] no differences in survival were seen between 10 Gy single fraction and 2 × 8.5 Gy. In a study by Bezjak et al.,[146] however, 5 × 4 Gy and a single 10-Gy dose was favorable for the multifractionated treatment only in patients with good performance. For patients in poor general condition and/or exhibiting significant weight loss, the 10 × 3 Gy treatment was significantly better than the 2 × 8 Gy in a large Dutch randomized trial reference.[147] The palliative effect differed significantly over time between the treatment arms. In the 10 × 3 Gy arm, the onset of the palliative effect occurred later and persisted longer with less worsening symptoms than in 2 × 8 Gy. Furthermore, the 1-year survival in this trial was better in patients treated with 10 × 3 Gy. Based on a recent informal survey performed among RTOG lung committee members, a wide range of regimens are currently in use: once 10 Gy, 5 times 4 Gy, twice 8.5 Gy (with a week interval), 13 or 15 times 3 Gy daily, 2.5 Gy daily times 20, or even 2 Gy daily.[30]

A short treatment regimen such as 30 Gy in 10 daily fractions is frequently used in this patient population to achieve a quick palliation without the patient and family spending significant time traveling back and forth to the treatment center.[147–150] Although using this dose regimen does initially relieve symptoms, it may not have a sustained effect. Thus, in an effort to keep the amount of therapy to a minimum, but tailor the therapy to the needs of the patients, another short course of radiation may be considered after a 2-week break. Under such circumstances, the patients are reevaluated for overall status and tumor response. If they have improvement in their symptoms, and have continuing good performance status, an additional 20 Gy in 4 fractions to 30 Gy in 10 fractions with oblique fields may be given to these patients for a sustained palliative benefit while reducing the time commitment and minimizing the side effects during the course of treatment. If patients show evidence of disease progression, either locally or systemically, and their general condition is continuing to decline, no additional RT is given after the initial treatment. There is limited evidence showing that higher palliative dose thoracic irradiation is associated with improved survival (in patients with good performance status).[147,148]

Selection of regimen should be based on comprehensive consideration of age, performance status, tumor burden, and symptoms of each individual patient. Patients with poor performance status, and patients with large distant tumor burden (regardless of their performance status) should be treated by a short course of relatively low-dose radiotherapy. For patients with good performance status, the choice of the optimal radiation schedule could be between 30 and 45 Gy in 2.5 to 3.0 Gy fractions. A definitive dose of radiation with combined chemotherapy may be preferred for patients with good performance and limited distant disease (such as solitary brain metastasis).

Cranial Irradiation The standard dose prescription for prophylactic cranial irradiation (PCI; see also Chapters 57, 60, and 63) for LS-SCLC is 25 to 30 Gy in 2 to 2.5 Gy daily fractions over 12 to 14 days for patients in complete remission.[140,151] However, a review including 42 PCI trials with 4749 patients revealed the optimal total RT dose to be 30 to 35 Gy given as 2 Gy fractions.[152] A dose of 24 Gy in 3 Gy fractions also appeared safe based on data from a large randomized study. According to a comparison of four dose regimens: 8 Gy, 24 to 25 Gy, 30 Gy, and 36 to 40 Gy, higher doses of radiation appeared to be correlated with incremental decreases in the risk of brain metastasis (p for trend = 0.02), without significant impact on survival.[153] Meanwhile, high-dose radiation may be associated with impaired neurocognitive function. Thus, more efficacious and less toxic treatment regimens are being sought. A recent randomized phase III INT (RTOG 0212) compared different doses of PCI in LS-SCLC (25 Gy in 2.5 Gy daily vs. 36 Gy in 2.0 Gy daily vs. 36 Gy in 1.5 Gy twice-daily fractions). Initial results from this large trial revealed no significant change in quality of life caused by PCI compared with baseline, although longer follow-up is necessary.[154] For patients with extensive stage (ES) SCLC, PCI significantly reduced the incidence of symptomatic brain metastases and prolonged both disease-free and overall survival and should be part of standard care in SCLC patients who respond to chemotherapy.[155]

Normal-Tissue Dose Constraints The other important consideration in treatment planning is to limit the radiation to the normal tissue to avoid excess treatment toxicity. The critical structures for radiation of lung cancer are lung, esophagus, spinal cord, and heart. A set of criteria for normal-tissue tolerances should be established from published studies and adapted for local clinical use. A good starting point is the report by a National Cancer Institute–sponsored task force, which carried out an extensive literature search and presented updated information on tolerance of normal tissues, with emphasis on partial volume effects.[156] For uniform irradiation of normal lung, tolerance doses for a 5% chance of pneumonitis occurring within 5 years for uniform irradiation of one third of the lung was 45 Gy, two thirds was 30 Gy, and whole lung was 17.5 Gy. For the esophagus, the corresponding doses are 60 Gy (one third), 58 Gy (two third), and 55 Gy (whole) for an end point of clinical stricture/perforation. For the heart: 60 Gy (one third), 45 Gy (two third), and 40 Gy (whole) for the end point of pericarditis. The above Emami tolerance data summary was one of the early efforts toward the use of objective criteria in evaluating treatment plans. However, the tolerance doses given were based on limited volumetric dose data publications and are "guesstimates" based on clinical experience.

As 3D dose distributions became available, dosimetric parameters have been correlated with complication data. Although there is not sufficient toxicity data in spinal cord and heart tolerance to change the above criteria, toxicity data for esophagus and lungs are available and should be taken into consideration in the treatment planning. For example, of the lung, many dosimetric factors are associated with the occurrence of grade 2 to 3 radiation pneumonitis. As it was recently reviewed,[16] lung volumes receiving a certain dose (V_d), such as V_5, V_{13}, V_{20}, V_{25}, and V_{30}, are highly correlated with each other and associated with the incidence of pneumonitis in multiple series; similarly, the doses to a specific percentage of the lung volume (D_v such as D_{20}) are also associated with the incidence of pneumonitis. The problem with those point dosimetric factors is its dependency on the shape of the DVH, which vary with the beam arranging pattern of each individual practicing physician. Lung effective volume (V_{eff}, a "toxicity normalized" volume to a reference dose), mean lung dose, and model estimations of NTCP include the contributions of all parts of the dose distribution and may thus provide the most consistent prediction. Indeed, Seppenwoolde et al.[157] suggested that the mean lung dose model was significantly better than V_d models. Although it rarely occurs, radiation pneumonitis increases remarkably after mean lung dose reaching 15 to 20 Gy, and the curve is in agreement with the traditional sigmoid-shaped dose–response relationship, with increasing steepness in the slope after passing a threshold dose. Using a 20-Gy cutoff for mean lung dose, the probability of freedom from pneumonitis in patients treated with radiation alone or sequential ChemoRT is given in Kong et al.[16]; for concurrent ChemoRT, refer to Liao et al.[158] Despite the very attractive feature of NTCP models, it is generally observed that for these mostly conformal irradiation techniques, the NTCP correlates mean lung dose or V_{20}, and fails to show significant superiority in predicting either moderate pneumonitis or clinical fibrosis.[16] However, these NTCP models, because of their averaging (or weighting) of doses across the organ, have better potential for describing a wider realm of irradiation conditions, and may provide better prediction when the functional status of the organ are taken into consideration.

Although the lungs and the spinal cord are the primary organs of concern in limiting the dose and field of radiation, toxicities to other structures within the mediastinum, such as esophagitis and resultant dysphagia and odynophagia, are often the dose-limiting side effects of combined chemotherapy and radiotherapy to the chest. In practice, severe esophagitis ranges from 5% to 37%. Many dosimetric parameters are significantly associated with the occurrence of grade 2 and above esophageal toxicity. Such factors include, but are not limited to, the length of the irradiated esophagus, the surface area of receiving 55 Gy, the volume receiving more than 60 Gy, maximal dose, or volume of the organ treated beyond a threshold dose (40 to 70 Gy), NTCP of esophagus, and the use of concurrent chemotherapy. Bradley et al.[159] correlated the rate of ≥grade 2 acute esophagitis to radiation dose–volume parameters for patients treated with or without concurrent chemotherapy. The data suggests that the use of concurrent chemotherapy increases the risk of clinically relevant esophagitis significantly.[155,160] Hyperfractionation also significantly increases the esophageal toxicity.[161] The heart does not, except under rare circumstances, contribute to the acute toxicity. However, cardiac toxicity in the form of pericardial disease or pericardial effusions and later myocardial and coronary artery disease has been reported in long-term survivors, making it desirable to reduce the dose to the entire heart as much as possible. However, one must note that radiation heart toxicity in general is poorly studied in patients with lung cancer.

The University of Michigan's current ongoing trial sets constraints for dose to normal tissue for patients receiving concurrent ChemoRT as the following: the maximum dose to the spinal cord is a dose biologically equivalent to 50 Gy in 2 Gy fractions. The V_{eff} computed for the esophagus with a normalization dose biologically equivalent to 72 Gy in 2 Gy fractions must be less than one third. The V_{eff} for the heart with a normalization dose of 40 and 65 Gy must be less than 100% and 33%, respectively. The V_{eff} computed for both lungs minus the composite volume of inhale and exhale GTVs for the prescription dose must be generating less than 15% of NTCP, approximating a mean lung dose of 20 Gy. Current ongoing RTOG trials use V_{20} of 30% for lungs.[105,159–170]

TREATMENT DELIVERY

The Linear Accelerator The delivery of thoracic radiation treatment is almost exclusively delivered using a linear accelerator, although radioactive cobalt therapy units are still in use. Linear accelerators deliver x-ray beams with peak energies between 4 and 23 MeV. The x-ray beams have an energy spectrum with the mean energy typically one third of the maximum energy. Hence, the energy of these beams is often referred to as *MV* rather than MeV to recognize the beam spectrum. Typically, 6 MV is the most common energy used for lung cancer radiotherapy. Higher energy beams offer increased depth penetration at the cost of broader lateral radiation spread and underdosage of tumor target at the side of beam entry. Higher energy beams also require more shielding for radiation protection, and energies above 10 MV produce neutrons that are a dose concern. An IMRT planning study by Weiss et al.[171] found, on average, no clinically or statistically significant differences between treatment plans generated for low (6 MV) and high (18 MV) photon energies.

An example of a modern linear accelerator is shown in Figure 40.7. Modern linear accelerators have variable collimators, typically MLCs, to automatically create treatment fields for conformal radiotherapy and IMRT. Another feature of modern accelerators is the in-room imaging options provided by either the linear accelerator vendor or independent companies. These imaging systems may include the following:

- Electronic portal imaging devices (EPIDs) that image the radiation emitted from the treatment machine that has passed through the patient (shown in Fig. 40.7). The EPID

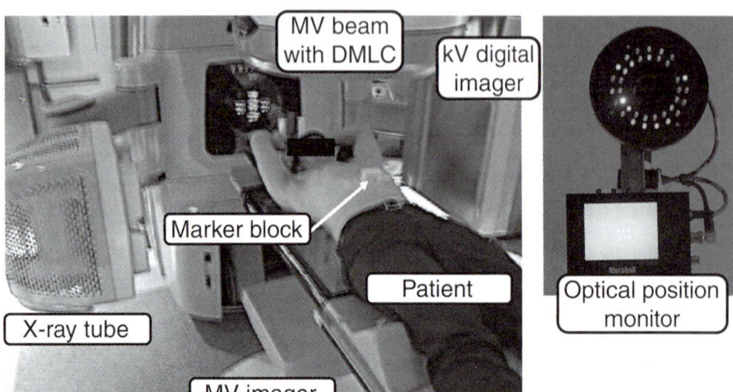

FIGURE 40.7 An example of a treatment setup in a modern linear accelerator for the radiotherapy treatment of lung cancer. Note the two x-ray imaging (kilovoltage and megavoltage) and optical device that can be used to monitor internal and external motion. *DMLC*, dynamic multileaf collimation; *kV*, kilovoltage; *MV*, megavoltage.

can be used to reduce setup errors, to acquire megavoltage CT scans,[172] monitor target position during radiation delivery,[173,174] and potentially be used to adjust the treatment delivery in real time.[175]

- Kilovoltage (kV) x-ray tubes and detectors that image the patient (shown in Fig. 40.7), provide superior soft-tissue visualization compared with megavolt imaging. For real-time tracking images, radiopaque markers are particularly useful. These radiopaque markers should be implanted into or near the tumor using either percutaneous or bronchoscopic techniques. These kV images can be used for pretreatment cone–beam CT acquisition,[176] fluoroscopic verification of motion at the time of treatment,[176] and respiratory-correlated (4D) cone beam CT.[177]
- Optical monitoring of a point (shown in Fig. 40.7) or points on the patient surface or the actual surface itself, which gives real-time information without giving extraradiation dose. The optical signals can be used to monitor respiration and patient motion for respiratory-gated radiotherapy,[178] and can also be combined with kV or MV imaging data to estimate internal target positions.[179,180]

MRI is a modality for in-room imaging currently under development by several groups and is promising because of its exquisite soft-tissue contrast that is very attractive for image-guided radiotherapy. Electromagnetic transponders, currently used for prostate radiotherapy, are another promising area under investigation for lung treatments.

These imaging systems facilitate image-guided radiotherapy (IGRT). There are strong similarities between image-guided surgery and IGRT, where in IGRT images of the patient acquired during a treatment fraction are used to measure or estimate the position of the patient's anatomy at a given time to drive the therapeutic instrument—the radiation treatment beam.

IGRT has the potential to considerably increase the precision of radiotherapy as lung tumors change between treatments because of changes in the functional reserve capacity, tumor shrinkage, and radiation-induced pulmonary changes. Lung tumors move during treatment because of respiration, cardiac, musculoskeletal, and gastrointestinal motion. Several authors (Borst, Erridge, van Sornsen, de Boer)[3,28,29,181] have studied interfraction patient setup error and reported systematic and random errors up to 4 and 3 mm (1 SD), respectively, in the absence of setup correction protocols. Using simple offline correction protocols (imaging approximately one third of the fractions), the systematic error can be reduced by a factor of 2 to 3. More recently, considerable day-to-day variation of the tumor relative to the bony anatomy (baseline shifts) were observed (Wulf,[6] Purdie,[6a] Sonke[30]), with systematic and random baseline variations up to 4 and 2 mm (1 SD), respectively. Soft-tissue visualization or accurate surrogates are required to correct for such baseline shifts. In the absence of such corrections, the application of gated treatment delivery is not recommended. Note that when an ITV is constructed to account for internal organ motion, baseline shifts need to be taken into account next to respiration. The type of correction strategy applied to reduce geometrical uncertainties is a balance between work load and precision, and depends on the fractionation scheme. For conventional fractionation using a large number of fractions, an offline correction strategy is generally considered adequate. Stereotactic body radiation therapy (SBRT), using a limited number of high-dose fractions, requires daily imaging and corrections based on soft-tissue guidance.

It is clear that regular observation and correction for patient setup is a necessity. Commonly, a margin of 5 to 7 mm should be added to the ITV for set-up error. However, special immobilization and image-guided devices can reduce the setup margin to 3 mm.

Quality Assurance The sensitivity of lung cancer and normal-tissue response to radiation, along with published errors in radiotherapy,[182,183] drives the need to establish and perform quality assurance procedures to facilitate patient safety and treatment accuracy. Imaging devices for optimal use require image quality assessment, dose measurement, and geometric fidelity tests. Because of their complexity, treatment planning systems, and by extension, the linear accelerators that they model, require a broad range of assessments as there are many variables that affect the dose distribution, such as the energy, field size, gantry angle, couch angle, collimator angle, beam-defining devices, patient position, and patient heterogeneities. Linear accelerators, and any additional in-room image devices, require alignment of the optical, laser, mechanical, and radiation coordinate systems to ensure radiation delivery accuracy. The output dose, under various different conditions, needs to be measured. The development of a quality assurance program, and oversight of its implementation is one of the tasks of the medical physicist.

For guidance, the AAPM have several freely available Task Group reports pertaining to quality assurance for imaging,[184] treatment planning,[185] and treatment delivery,[186] applicable to all radiotherapy, as well as reports on dose calculation,[111,187] and motion management[112] that are particularly important for lung cancer radiotherapy.

CONCLUSION

Modern lung cancer radiotherapy is a complex combination of many processes—imaging, treatment planning, and treatment delivery—to individualize the delivery of therapeutic radiation to each patient. It involves several dedicated personnel, including radiation oncologists, medical physicists, dosimetrists, and radiation therapists, as well as several peripheral specialists from biology, molecular imaging, medical oncology, pathology, pulmonology, radiology, and surgery.

Ongoing advances in imaging, treatment planning, image guidance, motion management, and adaptive radiotherapy strategies lead to a continued increase in complexity, together with the increased efficacy. The accuracy with which lung tumors can be targeted with radiation, and normal tissues spared the toxic effects of radiation, is constantly improving. Similarly, we are learning more about normal-tissue tolerances from clinical data during conventional and stereotactic regimens (see Chapter 43) and also in the concurrent chemoradiotherapy setting. It is expected that clinical outcomes, with time, will reflect the evolving technological improvements and clinical understanding of the effects of radiation in lung cancer.

ACKNOWLEDGMENT: *The authors wish to thank Elizabeth Roberts for assistance with the preparation and review of this manuscript, and Devon Murphy for careful editing. Grateful thanks to Dr. Annie Hsu for assistance with compiling the figures.*

REFERENCES

1. Garcia-Barros M, Paris F, Cordon-Cardo C, et al. Tumor response to radiotherapy regulated by endothelial cell apoptosis. *Science* 2003;300: 1155–1159.
2. Giraud P, De Rycke Y, Rosenwald JC, et al. Conformal radiotherapy planning for lung cancer: analysis of set-up uncertainties. *Cancer Invest* 2007;25:38–46.
3. de Boer HC, van Sörnsen de Koste JR, Senan S, et al. Analysis and reduction of 3D systematic and random setup errors during the simulation and treatment of lung cancer patients with CT-based external beam radiotherapy dose planning. *Int J Radiat Oncol Biol Phys* 2001;49: 857–868.
4. Halperin R, Roa W, Field M, et al. Setup reproducibility in radiation therapy for lung cancer: a comparison between T-bar and expanded foam immobilization devices. *Int J Radiat Oncol Biol Phys* 1999;43:211–216.
5. Samson MJ, van Sörnsen de Koste JR, de Boer HC, et al. An analysis of anatomic landmark mobility and setup deviations in radiotherapy for lung cancer. *Int J Radiat Oncol Biol Phys* 1999;43:827–832.
6. Wulf J, Hädinger U, Oppitz U, et al. Stereotactic radiotherapy of extracranial targets: CT-simulation and accuracy of treatment in the stereotactic body frame. *Radiother Oncol* 2000;57:225–236.

6a. Purdie TG, Bissonnette JP, Franks K, et al. Cone-beam computed tomography for on-line image guidance of lung stereotactic radiotherapy: localization, verification, and intrafraction tumor position. *Int J Radiat Oncol Biol Phys* 2007;68(1):243–252. Epub 2007 Feb 27.

7. Shioyama Y, Nakamura K, Anai S, et al. Stereotactic radiotherapy for lung and liver tumors using a body cast system: setup accuracy and preliminary clinical outcome. *Radiat Med* 2005;23:407–413.
8. Senan S, van Sörnsen de Koste J, Samson M, et al. Evaluation of a target contouring protocol for 3D conformal radiotherapy in non-small cell lung cancer. *Radiother Oncol* 1999;53:247–255.
9. Feng F, Kong FM, Quint LE, et al. Target delineation in radiation therapy of non-small cell lung cancer: a correlation study with local tumor failure. *Int J Radiat Oncol Biol Phys* 2005;63:S415–S416.
10. Cascade PN, Gross BH, Kazerooni EA, et al. Variability in the detection of enlarged mediastinal lymph nodes in staging lung cancer: a comparison of contrast-enhanced and unenhanced CT. *AJR Am J Roentgenol* 1998;170:927–931.
11. Patz EF Jr, Erasmus JJ, McAdams HP, et al. Lung cancer staging and management: comparison of contrast-enhanced and nonenhanced helical CT of the thorax. *Radiology* 1999;212:56–60.
12. van Sörnsen de Koste JR, Lagerwaard FJ, Nijssen-Visser MR, et al. Tumor location cannot predict the mobility of lung tumors: a 3D analysis of data generated from multiple CT scans. *Int J Radiat Oncol Biol Phys* 2003;56:348–354.
13. Lees L, Holloway L, Fuller M, et al. Effect of intravenous contrast on treatment planning system dose calculations in the lung. *Australas Phys Eng Sci Med* 2005;28:190–195.
14. Wormanns D, Diederich S, Lentschig MG, et al. Spiral CT of pulmonary nodules: interobserver variation in assessment of lesion size. *Eur Radiol* 2000;10:710–713.
15. Balter JM, Ten Haken RK, Lawrence TS, et al. Uncertainties in CT-based radiation therapy treatment planning associated with patient breathing. *Int J Radiat Oncol Biol Phys* 1996;36:167–174.
16. Kong FM, Ten Haken RK, Schipper MJ, et al. High-dose radiation improved local tumor control and overall survival in patients with inoperable/unresectable non-small-cell lung cancer: long-term results of a radiation dose escalation study. *Int J Radiat Oncol Biol Phys* 2005;63:324–333.
17. Harris KM, Adams H, Lloyd DC, et al. The effect on apparent size of simulated pulmonary nodules of using three standard CT window settings. *Clin Radiol* 1993;47:241–244.
18. de Koste JR, Lagerwaard FJ, de Boer HC, et al. Are multiple CT scans required for planning curative radiotherapy in lung tumors of the lower lobe? *Int J Radiat Oncol Biol Phys* 2003;55:1394–1399.
19. Giraud P, Antoine M, Larrouy A, et al. Evaluation of microscopic tumor extension in non-small-cell lung cancer for three-dimensional conformal radiotherapy planning. *Int J Radiat Oncol Biol Phys* 2000;48:1015–1024.
20. Grills IS, Fitch DL, Goldstein NS, et al. Clinicopathologic analysis of microscopic extension in lung adenocarcinoma: defining clinical target volume for radiotherapy. *Int J Radiat Oncol Biol Phys* 2007;69:334–341.
21. Yuan S, Meng X, Yu J, et al. Determining optimal clinical target volume margins on the basis of microscopic extracapsular extension of metastatic nodes in patients with non-small-cell lung cancer. *Int J Radiat Oncol Biol Phys* 2007;67:727–734.
22. Emami B. Management of hilar and mediastinal lymph nodes with radiation therapy in the treatment of lung cancer. *Front Radiat Ther Oncol* 1994;28:102–120.
23. Emami B, Mirkovic N, Scott C, et al. The impact of regional nodal radiotherapy (dose/volume) on regional progression and survival in unresectable non-small cell lung cancer: an analysis of RTOG data. *Lung Cancer* 2003;41:207–214.
24. Rosenzweig KE, Sim SE, Mychalczak B, et al. Elective nodal irradiation in the treatment of non-small-cell lung cancer with three-dimensional conformal radiation therapy. *Int J Radiat Oncol Biol Phys* 2001;50:681–685.
25. Bradley JD, Wahab S, Lockett MA, et al. Elective nodal failures are uncommon in medically inoperable patients with stage I non-small-cell lung carcinoma treated with limited radiotherapy fields. *Int J Radiat Oncol Biol Phys* 2003;56:342–347.
26. Chen M, Hayman JA, Ten Haken RK, et al. Long-term results of high-dose conformal radiotherapy for patients with medically inoperable T1-3N0 non-small-cell lung cancer: is low incidence of regional failure due to incidental nodal irradiation? *Int J Radiat Oncol Biol Phys* 2006;64:120–126.
27. Belderbos JS, Kepka L, Spring Kong FM, et al. Report from the International Atomic Energy Agency (IAEA) consultants' meeting on elective nodal irradiation in lung cancer: non-small cell lung cancer (NSCLC). *Int J Radiat Oncol Biol Phys* 2008;72(2):335–342.
28. Chapet O, Kong FM, Quint LE, et al. CT-based definition of thoracic lymph node stations: an atlas from the University of Michigan. *Int J Radiat Oncol Biol Phys* 2005;63(1):170–178.
29. van Herk M, Remeijer P, Lebesque JV. Inclusion of geometric uncertainties in treatment plan evaluation. *Int J Radiat Oncol Biol Phys* 2002;52:1407–1422.
30. Borst GR, Sonke JJ, Betgen A, et al. Kilo-voltage cone-beam computed tomography setup measurements for lung cancer patients; first clinical results and comparison with electronic portal-imaging device. *Int J Radiat Oncol Biol Phys* 2007;68:555–561.
31. Erridge SC, Seppenwoolde Y, Muller SH, et al. Portal imaging to assess set-up errors, tumor motion and tumor shrinkage during conformal radiotherapy of non-small cell lung cancer. *Radiother Oncol* 2003;66: 75–85.
32. Sonke JJ, Lebesque J, van Herk M. Variability of four-dimensional computed tomography patient models. *Int J Radiat Oncol Biol Phys* 2008;70: 590–598.

33. Steenbakkers RJ, Duppen JC, Fitton I, et al. Reduction of observer variation using matched CT-PET for lung cancer delineation: a three-dimensional analysis. *Int J Radiat Oncol Biol Phys* 2006;64:435–448.
34. Engelsman M, Sharp GC, Bortfeld T, et al. How much margin reduction is possible through gating or breath hold? *Phys Med Biol* 2005;50:477–490.
35. Keall PJ, Joshi S, Vedam SS, et al. Four-dimensional radiotherapy planning for DMLC-based respiratory motion tracking. *Med Phys* 951;32:942–951.
36. Rietzel E, Liu AK, Doppke KP, et al. Design of 4D treatment planning target volumes. *Int J Radiat Oncol Biol Phys* 2006;66:287–295.
37. Wolthaus JW, Schneider C, Sonke JJ, et al. Mid-ventilation CT scan construction from four-dimensional respiration-correlated CT scans for radiotherapy planning of lung cancer patients. *Int J Radiat Oncol Biol Phys* 2006;65:1560–1571.
38. Wolthaus JW, Sonke JJ, van Herk M, et al. Comparison of different strategies to use four-dimensional computed tomography in treatment planning for lung cancer patients. *Int J Radiat Oncol Biol Phys* 2008;70: 1229–1238.
39. de Langen AJ, Raijmakers P, Riphagen I, et al. The size of mediastinal lymph nodes and its relation with metastatic involvement: a meta-analysis. *Eur J Cardiothorac Surg* 2006;29:26–29.
40. Vansteenkiste J, Fischer BM, Dooms C, et al. Positron-emission tomography in prognostic and therapeutic assessment of lung cancer: systematic review. *Lancet Oncol* 2004;5:531–540.
41. Gould MK, Kuschner WG, Rydzak CE, et al. Test performance of positron emission tomography and computed tomography for mediastinal staging in patients with non-small-cell lung cancer: a meta-analysis. *Ann Intern Med* 2003;139:879–892.
42. Gould MK, Maclean CC, Kuschner WG, et al. Accuracy of positron emission tomography for diagnosis of pulmonary nodules and mass lesions: a meta-analysis. *JAMA* 2001;285:914–924.
43. Higashi K, Ueda Y, Arisaka Y, et al. 18F-FDG uptake as a biologic prognostic factor for recurrence in patients with surgically resected non-small cell lung cancer. *J Nucl Med* 2002;43:39–45.
44. Sasaki R, Komaki R, Macapinlac H, et al. [18F]fluorodeoxyglucose uptake by positron emission tomography predicts outcome of non-small-cell lung cancer. *J Clin Oncol* 2005;23:1136–1143.
45. Lee P, Weerasuriya DK, Lavori PW, et al. Metabolic tumor burden predicts for disease progression and death in lung cancer. *Int J Radiat Oncol Biol Phys* 2007;69:328–333.
46. Borst GR, Belderbos JS, Boellaard R, et al. Standardised FDG uptake: a prognostic factor for inoperable non-small cell lung cancer. *Eur J Cancer* 2005;41:1533–1541.
47. Nestle U, Walter K, Schmidt S, et al. 18F-deoxyglucose positron emission tomography (FDG-PET) for the planning of radiotherapy in lung cancer: high impact in patients with atelectasis. *Int J Radiat Oncol Biol Phys* 1999;44:593–597.
48. Vanuytsel LJ, Vansteenkiste JF, Stroobants SG, et al. The impact of (18)F-fluoro-2-deoxy-D-glucose positron emission tomography (FDG-PET) lymph node staging on the radiation treatment volumes in patients with non-small cell lung cancer. *Radiother Oncol* 2000;55:317–324.
49. Mah K, Caldwell CB, Ung YC, et al. The impact of (18)FDG-PET on target and critical organs in CT-based treatment planning of patients with poorly defined non-small-cell lung carcinoma: a prospective study. *Int J Radiat Oncol Biol Phys* 2002;52:339–350.
50. Erdi YE, Rosenzweig K, Erdi AK, et al. Radiotherapy treatment planning for patients with non-small cell lung cancer using positron emission tomography (PET). *Radiother Oncol* 2002;62:51–60.
51. Bradley J, Thorstad WL, Mutic S, et al. Impact of FDG-PET on radiation therapy volume delineation in non-small-cell lung cancer. *Int J Radiat Oncol Biol Phys* 2004;59:78–86.
52. De Ruysscher D, Wanders S, Minken A, et al. Effects of radiotherapy planning with a dedicated combined PET-CT-simulator of patients with non-small cell lung cancer on dose limiting normal tissues and radiation dose-escalation: a planning study. *Radiother Oncol* 2005;77:5–10.
53. Messa C, Ceresoli GL, Rizzo G, et al. Feasibility of [18F]FDG-PET and coregistered CT on clinical target volume definition of advanced non-small cell lung cancer. *Q J Nucl Med Mol Imaging* 2005;49:259–266.
54. Fox JL, Rengan R, O'Meara W, et al. Does registration of PET and planning CT images decrease interobserver and intraobserver variation in delineating tumor volumes for non-small-cell lung cancer? *Int J Radiat Oncol Biol Phys* 2005;62:70–75.
55. van Der Wel A, Nijsten S, Hochstenbag M, et al. Increased therapeutic ratio by 18FDG-PET CT planning in patients with clinical CT stage N2-N3M0 non-small-cell lung cancer: a modeling study. *Int J Radiat Oncol Biol Phys* 2005;61:649–655.
56. Ashamalla H, Rafla S, Parikh K, et al. The contribution of integrated PET/CT to the evolving definition of treatment volumes in radiation treatment planning in lung cancer. *Int J Radiat Oncol Biol Phys* 2005;63:1016–1023.
57. Caldwell CB, Mah K, Skinner M, et al. Can PET provide the 3D extent of tumor motion for individualized internal target volumes? A phantom study of the limitations of CT and the promise of PET. *Int J Radiat Oncol Biol Phys* 2003;55:1381–1393.
58. Fernando S, Kong FM, Kessler M, et al. Using FDG-PET to delineate gross tumor and internal target volumes. *Int J Radiat Oncol Biol Phys* 2005;63:S400–S401.
59. Steenbakkers RJ, Duppen JC, Fitton I, et al. Reduction of observer variation using matched CT-PET for lung cancer delineation: a three-dimensional analysis. *Int J Radiat Oncol Biol Phys* 2006;64:435–448.
60. Paulino AC, Johnstone PA. FDG-PET in radiotherapy treatment planning: Pandora's box?. *Int J Radiat Oncol Biol Phys* 2004;59:4–5.
61. Erdi YE, Mawlawi O, Larson SM, et al. Segmentation of lung lesion volume by adaptive positron emission tomography image thresholding. *Cancer* 1997;80:2505–2509.
62. Biehl K, Kong FM, Bradley JD, et al. Using FDG-PET for radiation treatment planning: is 40% threshold appropriate? *2004 Annual Meeting of American Radium Society.* Nappa Valley, CA.
63. Black QC, Grills IS, Kestin LL, et al. Defining a radiotherapy target with positron emission tomography. *Int J Radiat Oncol Biol Phys* 2004;60: 1272–1282.
64. Teräs M, Tolvanen T, Johansson JJ, et al. Performance of the new generation of whole-body PET/CT scanners: Discovery STE and Discovery VCT. *Eur J Nucl Med Mol Imaging* 2007;34:1683–1692.
65. Mageras GS, Pevsner A, Yorke ED, et al. Measurement of lung tumor motion using respiration-correlated CT. *Int J Radiat Oncol Biol Phys* 2004;60:933–941.
66. Shirato H, Seppenwoolde Y, Kitamura K, et al. Intrafractional tumor motion: lung and liver. *Semin Radiat Oncol* 2004;14:10–18.
67. Seppenwoolde Y, Shirato H, Kitamura K, et al. Precise and real-time measurement of 3D tumor motion in lung due to breathing and heartbeat, measured during radiotherapy. *Int J Radiat Oncol Biol Phys* 2002;53:822–834.
68. Langen KM, Jones DT. Organ motion and its management. *Int J Radiat Oncol Biol Phys* 2001;50:265–278.
69. Suh Y, Dieterich S, Cho B, et al. An analysis of thoracic and abdominal tumour motion for stereotactic body radiotherapy patients. *Phys Med Biol* 2008;53:3623–3640.
70. Ekberg L, Holmberg O, Wittgren L, et al. What margins should be added to the clinical target volume in radiotherapy treatment planning for lung cancer? *Radiother Oncol* 1998;48:71–77.
71. Sixel KE, Ruschin M, Tirona R, et al. Digital fluoroscopy to quantify lung tumor motion: potential for patient-specific planning target volumes. *Int J Radiat Oncol Biol Phys* 2003;57:717–723.
72. van der Geld YG, Senan S, van Sörnsen de Koste JR, et al. Evaluating mobility for radiotherapy planning of lung tumors: a comparison of virtual fluoroscopy and 4DCT. *Lung Cancer* 2006;53:31–37.
73. Ford EC, Mageras GS, Yorke E, et al. Respiration-correlated spiral CT: a method of measuring respiratory-induced anatomic motion for radiation treatment planning. *Med Phys* 2003;30:88–97.
74. Vedam SS, Keall PJ, Kini VR, et al. Acquiring a four-dimensional computed tomography dataset using an external respiratory signal. *Phys Med Biol* 2003;48:45–62.
75. Low DA, Nystrom M, Kalinin E, et al. A method for the reconstruction of four-dimensional synchronized CT scans acquired during free breathing. *Med Phys* 2003;30:1254–1263.

76. Rietzel E, Pan T, Chen GT. Four-dimensional computed tomography: image formation and clinical protocol. *Med Phys* 2005;32:874–889.
77. Abdelnour AF, Nehmeh SA, Pan T, et al. Phase and amplitude binning for 4D-CT imaging. *Phys Med Biol* 2007;52:3515–3529.
78. Mutaf YD, Antolak JA, Brinkmann DH. The impact of temporal inaccuracies on 4DCT image quality. *Med Phys* 2007;34:1615–1622.
79. Yamamoto T, Langner UW, Loo BW Jr, et al. Retrospective analysis of artifacts in the four-dimensional CT images of 50 patients. *Int J Radiat Oncol Biol Phys* 2008 Nov 15;72(4):1250–1258.
80. Engelsman M, Damen EM, De Jaeger K, et al. The effect of breathing and set-up errors on the cumulative dose to a lung tumor. *Radiother Oncol* 2001;60:95–105.
81. Witte MG, van der Geer J, Schneider C, et al. The effects of target size and tissue density on the minimum margin required for random errors. *Med Phys* 2004;31:3068–3079.
82. Blomgren H, Lax I, Näslund I, et al. Stereotactic high dose fraction radiation therapy of extracranial tumors using an accelerator. Clinical experience of the first thirty-one patients. *Acta Oncol* 1995;34:861–870.
83. Lax I. Target dose versus extratarget dose in stereotactic radiosurgery. *Acta Oncol* 1993;32:453–457.
84. Lax I, Blomgren H, Näslund I, et al. Stereotactic radiotherapy of malignancies in the abdomen. Methodological aspects. *Acta Oncol* 1994;33: 677–683.
85. McGarry RC, Papiez L, Williams M, et al. Stereotactic body radiation therapy of early stage non-small-cell lung carcinoma: Phase I study. *Int J Radiat Oncol Biol Phys* 2005;63:1010–1015.
86. Negoro Y, Nagata Y, Aoki T, et al. The effectiveness of an immobilization device in conformal radiotherapy for lung tumor: reduction of respiratory tumor movement and evaluation of the daily setup accuracy. *Int J Radiat Oncol Biol Phys* 2001;50:889–898.
87. Herfarth KK, Debus J, Lohr F, et al. Extracranial stereotactic radiation therapy: set-up accuracy of patients treated for liver metastases. *Int J Radiat Oncol Biol Phys* 2000;46:329–335.
88. Lohr F, Debus J, Frank C, et al. Noninvasive patient fixation for extracranial stereotactic radiotherapy. *Int J Radiat Oncol Biol Phys* 1999;45: 521–527.
89. Papiez L, Timmerman R, DesRosiers C, et al. Extracranial stereotactic radioablation: physical principles. *Acta Oncol* 2003;42:882–894.
90. Timmerman R, Papiez L, McGarry R, et al. Extracranial stereotactic radioablation: results of a phase I study in medically inoperable stage I non-small cell lung cancer. *Chest* 2003;124:1946–1955.
91. Timmerman R, Papiez L, Suntharalingam M. Extracranial stereotactic radiation delivery: expansion of technology beyond the brain. *Technol Cancer Res Treat* 2003;2:153–160.
92. Remouchamps VM, Letts N, Vicini FA, et al. Initial clinical experience with moderate deep-inspiration breath hold using an active breathing control device in the treatment of patients with left-sided breast cancer using external beam radiation therapy. *Int J Radiat Oncol Biol Phys* 2003;56:704–715.
93. Wong JW, Sharpe MB, Jaffray DA, et al. The use of active breathing control (ABC) to reduce margin for breathing motion. *Int J Radiat Oncol Biol Phys* 1999;44:911–919.
94. Mah D, Hanley J, Rosenzweig KE, et al. Technical aspects of the deep inspiration breath-hold technique in the treatment of thoracic cancer. *Int J Radiat Oncol Biol Phys* 2000;48:1175–1185.
95. Rosenzweig KE, Hanley J, Mah D, et al. The deep inspiration breath-hold technique in the treatment of inoperable non-small-cell lung cancer. *Int J Radiat Oncol Biol Phys* 2000;48:81–87.
96. Hanley J, Debois MM, Mah D, et al. Deep inspiration breath-hold technique for lung tumors: the potential value of target immobilization and reduced lung density in dose escalation. *Int J Radiat Oncol Biol Phys* 1999;45:603–611.
97. Senan S, De Ruysscher D, Giraud P, et al. Literature-based recommendations for treatment planning and execution in high-dose radiotherapy for lung cancer. *Radiother Oncol* 2004;71:139–146.
98. Derycke S, De Gersem WR, Van Duyse BB, et al. Conformal radiotherapy of Stage III non-small cell lung cancer: a class solution involving non-coplanar intensity-modulated beams. *Int J Radiat Oncol Biol Phys* 1998;41:771–777.
99. van Sörnsen de Koste J, Voet P, Dirkx M, et al. An evaluation of two techniques for beam intensity modulation in patients irradiated for stage III non-small cell lung cancer. *Lung Cancer* 2001;32:145–153.
100. Grills IS, Yan D, Martinez AA, et al. Potential for reduced toxicity and dose escalation in the treatment of inoperable non-small-cell lung cancer: a comparison of intensity-modulated radiation therapy (IMRT), 3D conformal radiation, and elective nodal irradiation. *Int J Radiat Oncol Biol Phys* 2003;57:875–890.
101. Marnitz S, Stuschke M, Bohsung J, et al. Intraindividual comparison of conventional three-dimensional radiotherapy and intensity modulated radiotherapy in the therapy of locally advanced non-small cell lung cancer a planning study. *Strahlenther Onkol* 2002;178:651–658.
102. Schwarz M, Alber M, Lebesque JV, et al. Dose heterogeneity in the target volume and intensity-modulated radiotherapy to escalate the dose in the treatment of non-small-cell lung cancer. *Int J Radiat Oncol Biol Phys* 2005;62:561–570.
103. Liu HH, Wang X, Dong L, et al. Feasibility of sparing lung and other thoracic structures with intensity-modulated radiotherapy for non-small-cell lung cancer. *Int J Radiat Oncol Biol Phys* 2004;58:1268–1279.
104. Manon RR, Jaradat H, Patel R, et al. Potential for radiation therapy technology innovations to permit dose escalation for non-small-cell lung cancer. *Clin Lung Cancer* 2005;7:107–113.
105. Chapet O, Kong FM, Lee JS, et al. Normal tissue complication probability modeling for acute esophagitis in patients treated with conformal radiation therapy for non-small cell lung cancer. *Radiother Oncol* 2005;77:176–181.
106. De Jaeger K, Hoogeman MS, Engelsman M, et al. Incorporating an improved dose-calculation algorithm in conformal radiotherapy of lung cancer: re-evaluation of dose in normal lung tissue. *Radiother Oncol* 2003;69:1–10.
107. Wang L, Yorke E, Chui CS. Monte Carlo evaluation of 6 MV intensity modulated radiotherapy plans for head and neck and lung treatments. *Med Phys* 2002;29:2705–2717.
108. Chetty IJ, Charland PM, Tyagi N, et al. Photon beam relative dose validation of the DPM Monte Carlo code in lung-equivalent media. *Med Phys* 2003;30:563–573.
109. Ekstrand KE, Barnes WH. Pitfalls in the use of high energy X rays to treat tumors in the lung. *Int J Radiat Oncol Biol Phys* 1990;18:249–252.
110. Klein EE, Morrison A, Purdy JA, et al. A volumetric study of measurements and calculations of lung density corrections for 6 and 18 MV photons. *Int J Radiat Oncol Biol Phys* 1997;37:1163–1170.
111. Chetty IJ, Curran B, Cygler JE, et al. Report of the AAPM Task Group No. 105: issues associated with clinical implementation of Monte Carlo-based photon and electron external beam treatment planning. *Med Phys* 2007;34:4818–4853.
112. Keall PJ, Mageras GS, Balter JM, et al. The management of respiratory motion in radiation oncology report of AAPM Task Group 76. *Med Phys* 2006;33:3874–3900.
113. Perez CA, Stanley K, Rubin P, et al. A prospective randomized study of various irradiation doses and fractionation schedules in the treatment of inoperable non-oat-cell carcinoma of the lung. Preliminary report by the Radiation Therapy Oncology Group. *Cancer* 1980;45:2744–2753.
114. Perez CA, Pajak TF, Rubin P, et al. Long-term observations of the patterns of failure in patients with unresectable non-oat cell carcinoma of the lung treated with definitive radiotherapy. Report by the Radiation Therapy Oncology Group. *Cancer* 1987;59:1874–1881.
115. Le Chevalier T, Arriagada R, Quoix E, et al. Radiotherapy alone versus combined chemotherapy and radiotherapy in unresectable non-small cell lung carcinoma. *Lung Cancer* 1994;10 Suppl 1:S239–244.
116. Dillman RO, Herndon J, Seagren SL, et al. Improved survival in stage III non-small-cell lung cancer: seven-year follow-up of cancer and leukemia group B (CALGB) 8433 trial. *J Natl Cancer Inst* 1996;88:1210–1215.
117. Sause W, Kolesar P, Taylor SI, et al. Final results of phase III trial in regionally advanced unresectable non-small cell lung cancer: Radiation Therapy Oncology Group, Eastern Cooperative Oncology Group, and Southwest Oncology Group. *Chest* 2000;117:358–364.

118. Bradley JD, Ieumwananonthachai N, Purdy NA, et al. Gross tumor volume, critical prognostic factor in patients treated with three-dimensional conformal radiation therapy for non-small-cell lung carcinoma. *Int J Radiat Oncol Biol Phys* 2002;52:49–57.
119. Sibley GS, Mundt AJ, Shapiro C, et al. The treatment of stage III non-small cell lung cancer using high dose conformal radiotherapy. *Int J Radiat Oncol Biol Phys* 1995;33:1001–1007.
120. Rengan R, Rosenzweig KE, Venkatraman E, et al. Improved local control with higher doses of radiation in large-volume stage III non-small-cell lung cancer. *Int J Radiat Oncol Biol Phys* 2004;60:741–747.
121. Bradley J, Graham MV, Winter K, et al. Toxicity and outcome results of RTOG 9311: a phase I-II dose-escalation study using three-dimensional conformal radiotherapy in patients with inoperable non-small-cell lung carcinoma. *Int J Radiat Oncol Biol Phys* 2005;61:318–328.
122. Rosenzweig KE, Fox JL, Yorke E, et al. Results of a phase I dose-escalation study using three-dimensional conformal radiotherapy in the treatment of inoperable nonsmall cell lung carcinoma. *Cancer* 2005;103: 2118–2127.
123. Hayman JA, Martel MK, Ten Haken RK, et al. Dose escalation in non-small-cell lung cancer using three-dimensional conformal radiation therapy: update of a phase I trial. *J Clin Oncol* 2001;19:127–136.
124. Narayan S, Henning GT, Ten Haken RK, et al. Results following treatment to doses of 92.4 or 102.9 Gy on a phase I dose escalation study for non-small cell lung cancer. *Lung Cancer* 2004;44:79–88.
125. Maguire PD, Marks LB, Sibley GS, et al. 73.6 Gy and beyond: hyperfractionated, accelerated radiotherapy for non-small-cell lung cancer. *J Clin Oncol* 2001;19:705–711.
126. Belderbos JS, De Jaeger K, Heemsbergen WD, et al. First results of a phase I/II dose escalation trial in non-small cell lung cancer using three-dimensional conformal radiotherapy. *Radiother Oncol* 2003;66:119–126.
127. Rosenzweig KE, Dladla N, Schindelheim R, et al. Three-dimensional conformal radiation therapy (3D-CRT) for early stage non-small-cell lung cancer. *Clin Lung Cancer* 2001;3:141–144.
128. Bogart JA, Alpert TE, Kilpatrick MC, et al. Dose-intensive thoracic radiation therapy for patients at high risk with early stage non-small-cell lung cancer. *Clin Lung Cancer* 2005;6:350–354.
129. Belderbos JS, Heemsbergen WD, De Jaeger K, et al. Final results of a Phase I/II dose escalation trial in non-small-cell lung cancer using three-dimensional conformal radiotherapy. *Int J Radiat Oncol Biol Phys* 2006;66:126–134.
130. Mehta M, Scrimger R, Mackie R, et al. A new approach to dose escalation in non-small-cell lung cancer. *Int J Radiat Oncol Biol Phys* 2001; 49:23–33.
131. Machtay M. Higher BED is associated with improved local-regional control and survival for NSCLC treated with chemoradiotherapy: an RTOG analysis. *Int J Radiat Oncol Biol Phys* 2005;63:S66.
132. Socinski MA, Morris DE, Halle JS, et al. Induction and concurrent chemotherapy with high-dose thoracic conformal radiation therapy in unresectable stage IIIA and IIIB non-small-cell lung cancer: a dose-escalation phase I trial. *J Clin Oncol* 2004;22:4341–4350.
133. A Randomized Phase III Comparison of Standard-Dose (60 Gy) Versus High-dose (74 Gy) Conformal Radiotherapy with Concurrent and Consolidation Carboplatin/Paclitaxel +/− Cetuximab (IND #103444) in Patients with Stage IIIA/IIIB Non-Small Cell Lung Cancer. RTOG 0617/NCCTG N0628/CALGB 30609/ECOG R0617. Available at Radiation Therapy Oncology Group Web site. http://rtog.org/members/protocols/0617/0617.pdf. Accessed November 11, 2009.
134. Cox JD, Azarnia N, Byhardt RW, et al. A randomized phase I/II trial of hyperfractionated radiation therapy with total doses of 60.0 Gy to 79.2 Gy: possible survival benefit with greater than or equal to 69.6 Gy in favorable patients with Radiation Therapy Oncology Group stage III non-small-cell lung carcinoma: report of Radiation Therapy Oncology Group 83-11. *J Clin Oncol* 1990;8:1543–1555.
135. Saunders M, Dische S, Barrett A, et al. Continuous, hyperfractionated, accelerated radiotherapy (CHART) versus conventional radiotherapy in non-small cell lung cancer: mature data from the randomised multicentre trial. CHART Steering committee. *Radiother Oncol* 1999;52:137–148.
136. Belani CP, Choy H, Bonomi P, et al. Combined chemoradiotherapy regimens of paclitaxel and carboplatin for locally advanced non-small-cell lung cancer: a randomized phase II locally advanced multi-modality protocol. *J Clin Oncol* 2005;23:5883–5891.
137. Fowler JF, Chappell R. Non-small cell lung tumors repopulate rapidly during radiation therapy. *Int J Radiat Oncol Biol Phys* 2000;46: 516–517.
138. Sause WT, Scott C, Taylor S, et al. Radiation Therapy Oncology Group (RTOG) 88–08 and Eastern Cooperative Oncology Group (ECOG) 4588: preliminary results of a phase III trial in regionally advanced, unresectable non-small-cell lung cancer. *J Natl Cancer Inst* 1995;87: 198–205.
139. Curran WJ, Scott CB, Langer CJ, et al. Long-term benefit is observed in a phase III comparison of sequential vs. concurrent chemo-radiation for patients with unresected stage III NSCLC: RTOG 9410 [abstract]. *Proc Am Soc Clin Oncol* 2003;22:621.
140. Turrisi AT III, Kim K, Blum R, et al. Twice-daily compared with once-daily thoracic radiotherapy in limited small-cell lung cancer treated concurrently with cisplatin and etoposide. *N Engl J Med* 1999;340: 265–271.
141. Bonner JA, Sloan JA, Shanahan TG, et al. Phase III comparison of twice-daily split-course irradiation versus once-daily irradiation for patients with limited stage small-cell lung carcinoma. *J Clin Oncol* 1999;17:2681–2691.
142. Schild SE, Bonner JA, Shanahan TG, et al. Long-term results of a phase III trial comparing once-daily radiotherapy with twice-daily radiotherapy in limited-stage small-cell lung cancer. *Int J Radiat Oncol Biol Phys* 2004;59:943–951.
143. Lester JF, MacBeth F, Toy E, et al. Palliative radiotherapy regimens for non-small cell lung cancer. Available at the Cochran Collaboration Web site. http://www.cochrane.org/reviews/en/ab002143.html. Published April 23, 2001; updated August 20, 2006.
144. Bleehen NM. Inoperable non-small-cell lung cancer (NSCLC): a Medical Research Council randomized trial of palliative radiotherapy with two fractions or ten fractions. *Br J Cancer* 1991;63:265.
145. Bleehen NM. A Medical Research Council (MRC) randomized trial of palliative radiotherapy with two fractions or a single fraction in patients with inoperable non-small-cell lung cancer (NSCLC) and poor performance status. *Br J Cancer* 1992;65:934–941.
146. Bezjak A, Dixon P, Brundage M, et al. Randomized phase III trial of single versus fractionated thoracic radiation in the palliation of patients with lung cancer (NCIC CTG SC.15). *Int J Radiat Oncol Biol Phys* 2002;54:719–728.
147. Kramer GW, Wanders SL, Noordijk EM, et al. Results of the Dutch National study of the palliative effect of irradiation using two different treatment schemes for non-small-cell lung cancer. *J Clin Oncol* 2005;23: 2962–2970.
148. Budach W, Belka C. Palliative percutaneous radiotherapy in non-small-cell lung cancer. *Lung Cancer* 2004;45 Suppl 2:S239–245.
149. Macbeth FR, Bolger JJ, Hopwood P, et al. Randomized trial of palliative two-fraction versus more intensive 13-fraction radiotherapy for patients with inoperable non-small cell lung cancer and good performance status. Medical Research Council Lung Cancer Working Party. *Clin Oncol (R Coll Radiol)* 1996;8:167–175.
150. Cross CK, Berman S, Buswell L, et al. Prospective study of palliative hypofractionated radiotherapy (8.5 Gy × 2) for patients with symptomatic non-small-cell lung cancer. *Int J Radiat Oncol Biol Phys* 2004;58:1098–1105.
151. Komaki R, Byhardt RW, Anderson T, et al. What is the lowest effective biologic dose for prophylactic cranial irradiation? *Am J Clin Oncol* 1985;8:523–527.
152. Sørensen JB. The role of prophylactic brain irradiation in small cell lung cancer treatment. *Monaldi Arch Chest Dis* 2003;59:128–133.
153. Aupérin A, Arriagada R, Pignon JP, et al. Prophylactic cranial irradiation for patients with small-cell lung cancer in complete remission. Prophylactic Cranial Irradiation Overview Collaborative Group. *N Engl J Med* 1999;341:476–484.

154. Le Pechoux C, Senan S, Quiox E, et al. Initial results from an intergroup phase III trial evaluating two different doses of prophylactic cranial irradiation (PCI) in patients with limited small cell cancer (SCLC) in complete remission (PCI99-01, IFCT 99-01, EORTC 22003-08004, RTOG 0212). *J Thorac Oncol* 2007;2:S389–S390.
155. Slotman B, Faivre-Finn C, Kramer G, et al. Prophylactic cranial irradiation in extensive small-cell lung cancer. *N Engl J Med* 2007:357: 664–672.
156. Emami B, Lyman J, Brown A, et al. Tolerance of normal tissue to therapeutic irradiation. *Int J Radiat Oncol Biol Phys* 1991;21:109–122.
157. Seppenwoolde Y, Lebesque JV, de Jaeger K, et al. Comparing different NTCP models that predict the incidence of radiation pneumonitis. *Int J Radiat Oncol Biol Phys* 2003;55:724–735.
158. Liao Z, Wang SL, Wei X, et al. Analysis of clinical and dosimetric factors associated with radiation pneumonitis (RP) in patients with non-small cell lung cancer (NSCLC) treated with concurrent chemotherapy (ConChT) and three dimensional conformal radiotherapy (3D-CRT). *Int J Radiat Oncol Biol Phys* 2005;63:S41.
159. Bradley J, Deasy JO, Bentzen S, et al. Dosimetric correlates for acute esophagitis in patients treated with radiotherapy for lung carcinoma. *Int J Radiat Oncol Biol Phys* 2004;58:1106–1113.
160. Singh AK, Lockett MA, Bradley JD. Predictors of radiation-induced esophageal toxicity in patients with non-small-cell lung cancer treated with three-dimensional conformal radiotherapy. *Int J Radiat Oncol Biol Phys* 2003;55:337–341.
161. Rosenman JG, Halle JS, Socinski MA, et al. Morris. High-dose conformal radiotherapy for treatment of stage IIIA/IIIB non-small-cell lung cancer: technical issues and results of a phase I/II trial. *Int J Radiat Oncol Biol Phys* 2002;54:348–356.
162. Maguire PD, Sibley GS, Zhou SM, et al. Clinical and dosimetric predictors of radiation-induced esophageal toxicity. *Int J Radiat Oncol Biol Phys* 1999;45:97–103.
163. Komaki R, Lee JS, Kaplan B, et al. Randomized phase III study of chemoradiation with or without amifostine for patients with favorable performance status inoperable stage II-III non-small cell lung cancer: preliminary results. *Semin Radiat Oncol* 2002:12:46–49.
164. Werner-Wasik M, Pequignot E, Leeper D, et al. Predictors of severe esophagitis include use of concurrent chemotherapy, but not the length of irradiated esophagus: a multivariate analysis of patients with lung cancer treated with nonoperative therapy. *Int J Radiat Oncol Biol Phys* 2000;48:689–696.
165. Ahn SJ, Kahn D, Zhou S, et al. Dosimetric and clinical predictors for radiation-induced esophageal injury. *Int J Radiat Oncol Biol Phys* 2005;61;335–347.
166. Takeda K, Nemoto K, Saito H, et al. Dosimetric correlations of acute esophagitis in lung cancer patients treated with radiotherapy. *Int J Radiat Oncol Biol Phys* 2005;62:626–629.
167. Hirota S, Tsujino K, Endo M, et al. Dosimetric predictors of radiation esophagitis in patients treated for non-small-cell lung cancer with carboplatin/paclitaxel/radiotherapy. *Int J Radiat Oncol Biol Phys* 2001;51:291–295.
168. Kahn D, Zhou S, Ahn SJ, et al. "Anatomically correct" dosimetric parameters may be better predictors for esophageal toxicity than are traditional CT-based metrics. *Int J Radiat Oncol Biol Phys* 2005;62:645–651.
169. Belderbos J, Heemsbergen W, Hoogeman M, et al. Acute esophageal toxicity in non-small cell lung cancer patients after high dose conformal radiotherapy. *Radiother Oncol* 2005;75:157–164.
170. Patel AB, Edelman MJ, Kwok Y, et al. Suntharalingam. Predictors of acute esophagitis in patients with non-small-cell lung carcinoma treated with concurrent chemotherapy and hyperfractionated radiotherapy followed by surgery. *Int J Radiat Oncol Biol Phys* 2004;60:1106–1112.
171. Weiss E, Siebers JV, Keall PJ. An analysis of 6-MV versus 18-MV photon energy plans for intensity-modulated radiation therapy (IMRT) of lung cancer. *Radiother Oncol* 2007;82:55–62.
172. Pouliot J, Bani-Hashemi A, Chen J, et al. Low-dose megavoltage cone-beam CT for radiation therapy. *Int J Radiat Oncol Biol Phys* 2005;61:552–560.
173. Berbeco RI, Hacker F, Ionascu D, et al. Clinical feasibility of using an EPID in CINE mode for image-guided verification of stereotactic body radiotherapy. *Int J Radiat Oncol Biol Phys* 2007;69:258–266.
174. Berbeco RI, Neicu T, Rietzel E, et al. A technique for respiratory-gated radiotherapy treatment verification with an EPID in cine mode. *Phys Med Biol* 2005;50:3669–3679.
175. Keall PJ, Todor AD, Vedam SS, et al. On the use of EPID-based implanted marker tracking for 4D radiotherapy. *Med Phys* 2004;31:3492–3499.
176. Jaffray DA, Drake DG, Moreau M, et al. A radiographic and tomographic imaging system integrated into a medical linear accelerator for localization of bone and soft-tissue targets. *Int J Radiat Oncol Biol Phys* 1999:45:773–789.
177. Sonke JJ, Zijp L, Remeijer P, et al. Respiratory correlated cone beam CT. *Med Phys* 2005;32:1176–1186.
178. Ohara K, Okumura T, Akisada M, et al. Irradiation synchronized with respiration gate. *Int J Radiat Oncol Biol Phys* 1989;17:853–857.
179. Berbeco RI, Jiang SB, Sharp GC, et al. Integrated radiotherapy imaging system (IRIS): design considerations of tumour tracking with linac gantry-mounted diagnostic x-ray systems with flat-panel detectors. *Phys Med Biol* 2004;49:243–255.
180. Cho B, Suh Y, Dieterich S, et al. A monoscopic method for real-time tumour tracking using combined occasional x-ray imaging and continuous respiratory monitoring. *Phys Med Biol* 2008;53:2837–2855.
181. Van Sornsen de Koste JR, de Boer HC, Schuchhard-Schipper RH, et al. Procedures for high precision setup verification and correction of lung cancer patients using CT-simulation and digitally reconstructed radiographs (DRR). *Int J Radiat Oncol Biol Phys* 2003:55:804–810.
182. ROSIS. Radiation Oncology Safety Information System. Available at http://www.clin.radfys.lu.se/ (2008). Accessed November 11, 2009.
183. IAEA. *Lessons Learned from Accidental Exposures in Radiotherapy*. Safety Reports Series No. 17, 2000.
184. Mutic S, Palta JR, Butker EK, et al. Quality assurance for computed-tomography simulators and the computed-tomography-simulation process: report of the AAPM Radiation Therapy Committee Task Group No. 66. *Med Phys* 2003;30:2762–2792.
185. Fraass B, Doppke K, Hunt M, et al. American Association of Physicists in Medicine Radiation Therapy Committee Task Group 53: quality assurance for clinical radiotherapy treatment planning. *Med Phys* 1998;25: 1773–1829.
186. Kutcher GJ, Coia L, Gillin M, et al. Comprehensive QA for radiation oncology: report of AAPM Radiation Therapy Committee Task Group 40. *Med Phys* 1994;21:581–618.
187. Report of Task Group No. 65 of the Radiation Therapy Committee of the American Association of Physicists in Medicine. *Tissue Inhomogeneity Corrections for Megavoltage Photon Beams*. AAPM Report No. 85. Madison, WI: Medical Physics Publishing, 2004. Web site available at http://aapm.org/pubs/reports/rpt_85.pdf.

CHAPTER 41

Dirk De Ruysscher
Vincent S. Khoo
Søren M. Bentzen

Biological Basis of Fractionation and Timing of Radiotherapy

THE BIOLOGY OF DOSE FRACTIONATION IN RADIOTHERAPY

Radiation biology is the study of the biological effects of ionizing radiation; clinical radiation biology is concerned with the clinical response of human tumors and normal tissues to the doses normally used in radiation therapy. Basic and clinical radiation biology together form the scientific basis for application of radiation as an anticancer agent and provide the framework for understanding dose-fractionation and dose–volume effects as well as the rational basis for combining radiation with cytotoxic or molecular targeted agents.

Although advances in molecular radiation biology of tumors[1,2] and normal tissue[3] play an increasingly important role in further developing the scientific basis for radiation therapy, the conceptual basis for dose fractionation is still, to a large extent, rooted in the target-cell hypothesis, that is, the hypothesis that the main biological effect of ionizing radiation on cells and tissues is direct cell killing and loss of proliferative capacity of surviving cells. Therefore, much of the current chapter describes dose-fractionation effects within the target-cell framework, often referred to as "classical radiobiology." However, the more recent thinking in the field will be brought in, where this is relevant for understanding some of the newer trends in radiation dose fractionation.

The Physical–Biological Interactions of Radiation

The basic interaction of radiation with matter has been well understood since the first third of the 20th century. When a radiation beam traverses through matter, energy is deposited along its path. Compton scattering is the dominating interaction for radiation beam energies used clinically (Fig. 41.1). The Compton effect is an inelastic scattering of photons by an electron (i.e., the photon loses some of its energy in the event), leading to ionization events either within the molecules of the critical cells (direct effect) or in adjacent water molecules (indirect effect).[4] These direct and indirect effects result in the formation of unstable and highly reactive free radicals that are responsible for the biological effects on DNA and tissues. Cellular damage and cell killing occurs when critical molecular target(s) such as DNA are damaged within the cell.[5] Cancer cell killing can be defined as the loss of the cell's reproductive ability. Most cells do not die immediately when they are critically damaged. They usually proceed to mitosis and either may fail to complete mitosis or may progress through one or more cycles before failing at a subsequent mitosis. However, some cell types, such as lymphocytes, die before reaching mitosis in a process called apoptosis or "programmed cell death."[6] In the apoptotic process, the radiation damage initiates signaling cascades, whereby preset mechanisms are evoked to cause cellular self-destruction. Characteristic histological features are seen in apoptotic cells such as blebbing and fragmentation of the nucleus.[7]

In addition to the "direct-targeted" effects of ionizing radiation on cells, there is increasing evidence for nontargeted effects of radiation such as bystander cell killing.[8] The therapeutic implications, if any, of this mode of cell killing are not well understood.

The Cell Survival Curves The target cell hypothesis postulates that the response of tumors and normal tissues to ionizing radiation is a direct result of the loss of reproductive ability of the irradiated cells. This can be assessed in vitro by the ability of cells in culture to continue sustained cellular division to form a colony. A plot of the colony-forming ability of cells as a function of dose is called a cell survival curve. The parameters that influence cell survival curves will be described later in this chapter. The cell survival curve was first described by Puck and Marcus[9] in 1956, who examined the survival of HeLa tumor cells as a function of radiation dose. The cell survival curve shape for early- and late-reacting tissues (see discussion that follows) is represented in Figure 41.2, in which the cell's survival fraction is plotted against dose on a semilogarithmic scale. In general, at very low radiation doses, the cell survival curve is relatively shallow, whereas at higher doses, the survival curve bends more, reflecting the greater cell kill per unit Gu as dose

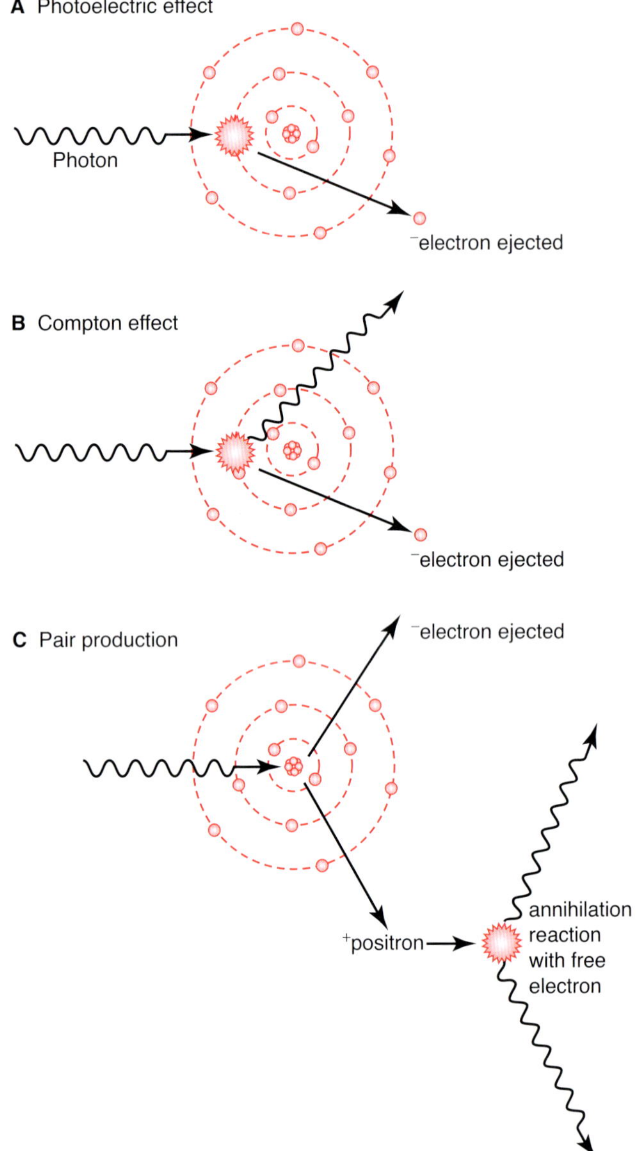

FIGURE 41.1 Radiation tissue interaction effects. **A:** The photoelectric effect occurs when the incident photon strikes one of the bound inner shell electrons around the atomic nucleus and transfers its entire energy to the electron, causing the electron to be ejected from its orbit. This electron may then collide with other orbiting electrons and result in a chain of further strikes, electron expulsion, ionization, and other collisions. The incident photon disappears when its energy is used up. **B:** Compton process differs from the photoelectric effect in that only a portion of the energy of the incident photon is used in ejecting the orbiting electron, and the remaining energy is emitted in a secondary photon of less energy. This secondary photon can subsequently cause further ionization either through the photoelectric or Compton process. **C:** Pair production process is the least common therapeutic method of energy absorption. This only occurs when an incident photon interacts with an atomic nucleus and its energy is completely transformed into two particles (a positron and an electron). These two particles do not come from the atom, so no single charged particle has been lost; therefore, there is no ionization of the atom. The positron can then react with an orbital electron of another atom resulting in an "annihilation" reaction producing two photons of 0.51 MeV. For this process to occur, the initial incident photon must have energy of least 1.02 MeV. A pair production chain reaction never results because the annihilation photons never have energy greater than 0.51 MeV. (From Khoo V, Bidmead M. Chapter 1. Physical basis of radiotherapy. In: Huddart RA, Murthy V, eds. *Cancer Radiotherapy: Methods and Protocols.* Clifton, New Jersey, Humana Press, 2007.)

increases. This shape of the cell survival curve with an initial shallow slope followed by a "broad-shoulder" curve is typical of low–linear energy transfer (LET) radiation (e.g., photons, which are commonly used for lung radiotherapy). In contrast, cell survival curves for high LET radiation, such as neutrons and ^{12}C-ions have very little "shoulder" but are approximately straight lines in semilogarithmic coordinates.

Several mathematical models have been devised to describe the cell survival curve shape. Of these models, the most widely adopted is the linear-quadratic model[10] that appears to provide the best description of cell survival within the range of doses used clinically. The linear-quadratic equation is expressed mathematically as follows:

$$S = e^{-\alpha \cdot \mathrm{d} - \beta \cdot \mathrm{d}^2}$$

where S = survival of a cell population after a dose of radiation (d) and where α and β are constants. Assuming that the effect per fraction is constant, it is easily shown that the effect of n fractions of size d is:

$$S = e^{-\alpha \cdot D - \beta \cdot d \cdot D}$$

where D = nd is the total dose after n fractions. It follows from this equation that a total dose D_1 delivered with dose per fraction d_1, will result in the same biological effect as a total dose D_2 delivered with dose per fraction d_2 if (and only if):

$$D_2 = D_1 \cdot \frac{d_1 + \frac{\alpha}{\beta}}{d_2 + \frac{\alpha}{\beta}}.$$

This equation is known as Withers' formula.[11] This formula can be interpreted operationally as a means of adjusting for dose per fraction—irrespective of any underlying mechanistic interpretation at the cellular level. It can be seen from the mathematical form of Withers formula that it is the ratio between α and β, rather than the parameter values themselves,

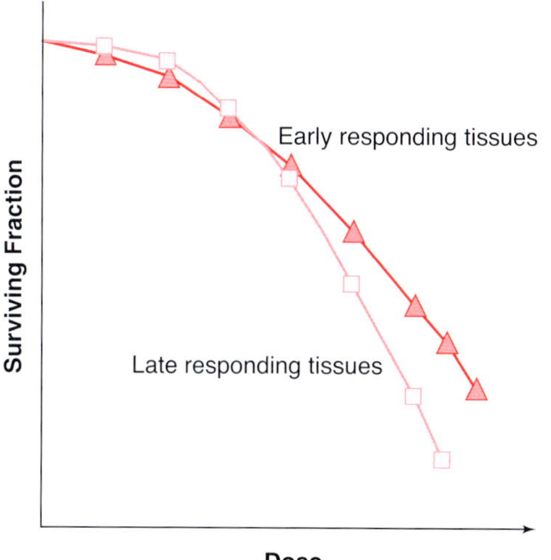

FIGURE 41.2 The dose–survival curves for early- and late-responding tissues. The cell survival curve for late-responding tissues is more "curvy" than for early-responding tissues and at least some cancer types. The α/β ratio is approximately 2 Gy for late-responding tissues and 10 Gy for some cancers or early-responding tissues.

which determines the change in total dose as a function of a change in dose per fraction that will be required to maintain the same level of biological effect.

The α/β ratio will be specific to different normal-tissue side effects and can be seen, as mentioned previously, as a measure of fractionation sensitivity of an end point.[12] Early side effects are generally characterized by a high α/β ratio, in the order of 10 Gy, and these occur, for example, in the gastrointestinal epithelium, skin, and bone marrow (Fig. 41.2). Late end points such as radiation myelopathy or radiation-induced fibrosis will typically have a low α/β ratio in the range from 1 to 5 Gy (Fig. 41.2). There are relatively sparse data on α/β for human tumors, but it is often assumed that it is in the same range as for early normal-tissue effects of radiation.

This differential in fractionation sensitivity between, at least, some human tumors and some types of late-occurring side effects of radiotherapy provides a rationale for dividing the total prescribed radiation dose into many smaller doses delivered over a period of time. This difference has been exploited by investigators using altered fractionation schemes to manipulate the therapeutic ratio in favor of improved tumor control while reducing damage to normal structures or late-responding tissues. A good example of this fractionation strategy is the development of the continuous hyperfractionated accelerated radiotherapy (CHART) regime in lung cancer.[13,14]

The Four R's of Radiotherapy Several biological parameters influence the response of both normal tissues and cancers cells to fractionated radiotherapy. Following Withers,[15] these are memorized as the four R's of radiotherapy: Repair, Redistibution, Repopulation, and Reoxygenation. All of these are processes taking place in the interval between fractions, and the differential between tumors and normal tissues in these four R's form the classical rationale for dose fractionation as well as the "Radiosensitivity" of cells/tissues. Steel[16] subsequently advocated to add this fifth R, namely Radiosensitivity, as a cofactor in determining cellular response to radiation. However, this R is clearly of a different nature than the original four R's. These R's of radiotherapy are summarized in Table 41.1 and will briefly be described in the following.

Repair Both normal and cancer cells show split-dose recovery, expressed as a higher in vitro cell survival if the same physical dose is split in two, with a sufficient time interval between irradiations. This phenomenon is thought to reflect chemical and enzymatic repair of DNA damage in the interval between doses.[17]

The clinical implication of this is that if multiple fractions are being given within a single day, then there must be an adequate time interval given between fractions (minimum 6 hours, preferably 8 or 10 hours) in order to permit repair of sublethal damage. As previously mentioned, the shoulder of the cell survival curve is repeated for each dose fraction as shown in Figure 41.3, provided that cellular recovery is complete between fractions. The broader the shoulder, the greater the repair capacity of the cells. This is in particular seen in late-responding tissues with low α/β ratios. These tissues can be spared from accumulating radiation DNA damage by fractionation.

In general, these repair processes will affect the response of both normal tissues and tumors to a course of radiation.

TABLE 41.1 The Four R's of Radiotherapy

	Radiobiological Effect
Repair	Cellular damage is repaired in the time interval between one fraction and the next. Sometimes referred to as "recovery" to avoid the impression that this reflects DNA damage repair only.
Redistribution	Progression of surviving cells from relatively more radioresistant to more sensitive phases of the cell cycle.
Repopulation	Repopulation, often referred to as accelerated repopulation, is the active proliferative response to a cytotoxic insult mounted by some tumors and (early-responding) normal tissues.
Reoxygenation	Hypoxic cells are more resistant to both radiation and chemotherapy. This means that surviving cells will preferentially be found in hypoxic regions of a tumor. As tumor cells are killed, the metabolic consumption of oxygen is reduced and this is thought to lead to reoxygenation of the remaining tumor cells, thus effectively increasing their sensitivity to subsequent dose fractions.

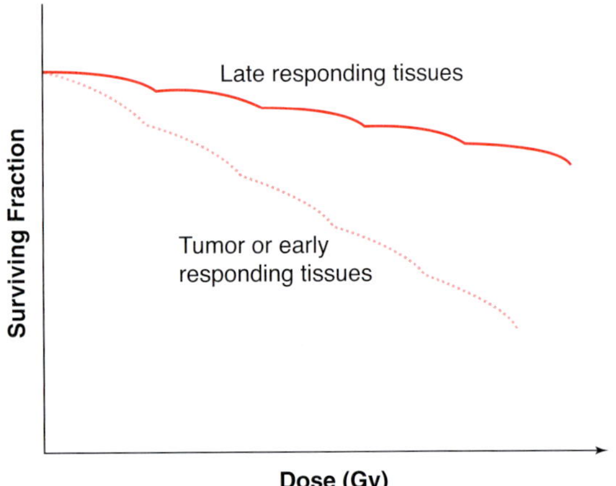

FIGURE 41.3 The target cell hypothesis and the rationale for low dose per fraction. The cell survival curve for late-responding tissues is more curved than that for tumors or early-responding tissues as shown in Figure 41.2. When radiation dose is fractionated, and provided that the interfraction interval is sufficiently long, the shoulder portion of the respective curves is repeated, following each fraction. Fractionation will tend to spare late-responding tissues such as spinal cord, heart, and kidney relative to the tumor or early-responding tissues such as skin or gastrointestinal cells. With increasing number of fractions, there is greater kill of tumor cells—with a possible added effect from redistribution and reoxygenation—but with a potential benefit being reduced by accelerated repopulation is the overall treatment time is extended. Late-responding tissues are less affected by the overall treatment time but are relatively more sensitive to fraction size, as reflected by their lower α/β ratio. Thus, if large dose per fraction is used, then the total dose needs to be reduced in order to maintain the same level of normal-tissue toxicity.

Using daily fractionation with time intervals of approximately 24 hours between fractions, there is adequate time for repair to occur. If the radiotherapy factions are too close together (i.e., less than 6 hours) then, unrepaired damage will accumulate. Although this may be beneficial for tumor cell killing, it can result in substantial normal-tissue damage and increase the rate of treatment-related complication, thereby reducing the potential therapeutic ratio.

Redistribution A general schema divides the biological cell cycle into four phases: (a) mitosis, or M phase; (b) G1 phase; (c) DNA synthesis, or the S phase; and (d) G2 phase. Cells in the late G2 and M phase of the cell cycle tend to be most sensitive to irradiation, whereas those in the mid-late S and early G2 phase are more radioresistant.[18] This means that after irradiating a population of proliferating cells, surviving cells will predominantly be in the radioresistant late S and early G2 phases. During a course of fractionated radiotherapy, these surviving cells will progress through the cell cycle and "redistribute" into more radiosensitive phases in the interval between fractions and will be "caught" in a relatively more sensitive phase by the next fraction of radiation.

Radiation blocks cell progression through the cell cycle at the G2-M and the G1-S checkpoints. These checkpoints are controlled by several genes. The radiation induced G1 block is p53 dependent,[19] but as many tumors are p53 deficient, the G2 block may be more important in tumors receiving radiation. The duration of the G2 block is dose dependent.[20,21]

Repopulation Cells in both normal tissues and tumors may respond to a cytotoxic insult by accelerated repopulation.[22,23] Early-reacting tissues, such as the gastrointestinal mucosa, have a high cellular repopulation capacity, and this is an important component of their response to chemotherapy and radiation therapy. A reduction in overall treatment time will reduce the time available for repopulation in these tissues and lead to more side effects. Late-reacting tissues proliferate slowly and show less of a proliferative response to cytotoxic therapy, thus changing the treatment intensity is less important for these tissues. Accelerated repopulation, as reflected by the overall time factor, has been demonstrated in many cancers. Most convincingly, this has been shown by the outcome of a large number of randomized controlled trials of intensified radiation therapy for squamous cell carcinoma of the head and neck.[24] In head and neck squamous cell carcinoma (HNSCC), there are relatively reliable estimates of the dose recovered (or lost) per day because of proliferation, and this is consistently estimated at around 0.6 Gy/day.[25] This represents the increased total dose required to compensate for tumor repopulation, resulting from a 1-day protraction of treatment. This implies that if 2 Gy/day was used, the effective dose would only be 1.4 Gy as 0.6 Gy would be lost to counteract the effect of tumor repopulation. The lag time before repopulation takes effect will vary between different tissues and tumors and likely between patients. This lag time period may be in the region of 2 to 3 weeks[24] for HNSCC.

Reoxygenation Human tumors often contain hypoxic regions, and it was hypothesized as early as the 1950s[26] that this may be associated with radiation resistance. Hypoxic radioresistance has been documented and extensively studied in cells in vitro as well as in small animal tumor models. Oxygen is thought to inhibit the cellular repair of DNA damage induced by free radicals thereby "fixing" the radiation damage. More recently, it has been shown that hypoxic tumors also have a poorer outcome after chemotherapy or surgery, and a link has been established between malignant progression and hypoxia.[27] Research has shown that tumor cells under hypoxic conditions switch on several survival pathways that let them survive in a hypoxic microenvironment and confer resistance against cytotoxic therapy. Reoxygenation refers to the process by which previously hypoxic cells become better supplied by oxygen as they are brought closer to well-perfused regions when tumor cells in these oxygenated areas die during a course of radiation.

The fact that tumor oxygenation assessed at baseline (i.e., before the start of any therapy, by means of polarographic), microelectrodes is associated with survival after fractionated radiotherapy in HNSCC proves that reoxygenation cannot completely offset the detrimental effect of hypoxia.[28] Whether this is because reoxygenation is not 100% efficient in countering radiobiological hypoxia or a result of the link between hypoxia and malignant, progression remains to be clarified.

HYPERFRACTIONATED AND ACCELERATED RADIOTHERAPY

Cancer radiotherapy was widely introduced in clinical practice in the early 20th century, and it soon became apparent that the way radiotherapy was delivered over time had a major influence on tumor and normal-tissue effects. Indeed, as discussed earlier in this chapter, fractionated radiotherapy was introduced as a method to take advantage of the differential in the four R's between (most) tumor histologies and dose-limiting normal tissues. Even in those early days, the overall treatment time (i.e., the time elapsed between the first and the last day of radiotherapy), was recognized as a factor determining side effects.

Most of the altered radiotherapy fractionation schedules have explored two types of modification: hyperfractionation (HFX) and accelerated fractionation (AF). There is no consensus as to the definition of these two concepts, and some authors have proposed definitions based on a more or less complicated link between the time–dose factors of a fractionated regime of radiotherapy, namely the dose per fraction, number of fractions, daily or weekly dose, overall treatment time, and total dose. This has led to some confusion regarding the classification of radiotherapy schedules, and there is a need to return to more general definitions, directly reflecting the different rationales underpinning nonconventional schedules.[29] Indeed, the concept of HFX is essentially linked to dose fraction size and not to time. Therefore, any schedule employing a dose per fraction of less than 1.8 Gy is classified as *hyperfractionated*. AF relates to the intensity of therapy over time and, therefore, a schedule in which the rate of dose accumulation exceeds 10 Gy/wk is classified as *accelerated*. This simple definition, besides its pedagogic character, has the advantage of being applicable to all altered fractionation schedules. In addition, it clearly separates the issues of dose/fraction from overall treatment time and total dose, which result from distinct radiobiological concepts. In a schedule using a dose per fraction different from 2 Gy, the rate of dose accumulation is estimated from the total dose converted into the biologically equivalent dose in 2-Gy fractions (EQD_2) using the linear-quadratic model with an assumed α/β of 10 Gy for non–small cell lung cancer (NSCLC). Similarly, a schedule employing a dose per fraction exceeding 2.2 Gy is classified as *hypofractionated*.

Hyperfractionation

The biological basis of HFX is to exploit the postulated different capacity of target cells in tumor tissue and late-responding normal tissue to recover from sublethal radiation damage, given that the time interval between the two fractions is sufficiently long. The latter condition is not entirely trivial as there are data suggesting that the recovery half-time in human tissues may be considerably longer, in the order of 4 to 8 hours, than what was derived from in vitro and experimental animal studies.[30–32] That HFX might be useful to improve the therapeutic ratio of radiotherapy relies on the putative difference in fractionation sensitivity between tumors and late effects. In patients with HNSCC, this rationale is supported by the results of randomized clinical trials.[33] Thus, from a radiobiological perspective, HFX with increased total dose compared to conventional fractionation appears to be a promising option to improve local control and survival in NSCLC, without increasing the risk of late normal-tissue damage.

Dose-escalated HFX was compared with conventional or moderate hypofractionation in three randomized trials in NSCLC.[34] A metaanalysis of these three trials found a significantly improved overall survival after HFX compared with conventional fractionation or hypofractionation, with an odds ratio (OR) for death of 0.69 (95% confidence interval [C.I.], 0.51 to 0.95; $p = 0.02$).

In summary, based on radiobiological data, there is good reason to believe that dose-escalated HFX may improve survival in NSCLC. However, there appears currently no strong evidence from randomized trials supporting this approach, possibly, because of the fact that only a relatively small number of patients were included in these trials.

Accelerated and Accelerated Hyperfractionated Radiotherapy

The biological rationale for AF is to counteract the so-called time factor of fractionated radiotherapy (i.e., the loss of local tumor control with increasing overall treatment time). This time factor is generally thought to reflect rapid repopulation of clonogenic tumor cells during treatment, although alternative mechanisms may contribute.[23,35] A significant time factor has so far been demonstrated in randomized clinical trials for NSCLC[36–39] and small cell lung cancer (SCLC).[40] In contrast to tumors, overall treatment time has no or little impact on classical late radiation damage such as lung fibrosis and spinal cord damage.[41] Short overall treatment times increase acute normal-tissue reactions such as esophagitis but also radiation pneumonitis.[41] From a radiobiological perspective, AF might increase the therapeutic ratio between local tumor control and late toxicity in NSCLC.

The combination of HFX with AF, leading to a short overall treatment time, resulted in the CHART schedule in which 54 Gy is delivered in 12 days (3 times 1.5 Gy/day). In a large phase III trial, CHART was subsequently compared to the conventional schedule of 60 Gy in 30 fractions.[38] In the CHART arm, the 3-year local tumor control was 17% versus 13% in the conventional arm, and the corresponding 3-year survival data were 20% versus 13% ($p = 0.008$). The CHART trial proves the concept that accelerated proliferation of tumor clonogens is an important reason for treatment failure.

In Eastern Cooperative Oncology Group (ECOG) 2597, patients were randomized after induction chemotherapy to conventional fractionation (64 Gy/6.5 wk) or hyperfractionated accelerated radiotherapy (HART) (57.5 Gy in

2.5 weeks).[37] This schedule delivered 1.5 Gy per fraction with three fractions per day, 5 days a week. This is a strongly accelerated schedule, delivering the equivalent dose in 2-Gy fractions of 22 Gy/wk. The HART trial closed prematurely after recruiting 144 of a planned 388 patients, resulting in a loss of statistical power to detect the hypothesized improvement in median survival from 14 to 21 months. The actual observed median survival was 14.9 and 20.3 months ($p = 0.28$) after conventional fractionation and HART, respectively.

SEQUENCING OF RADIATION AND CHEMOTHERAPY

In general, when radiotherapy is used with curative intent, it is delivered in relatively small daily doses, typically 1.8 to 2.0 Gy/day, 5 days per week. As described earlier, there are sound radiobiological arguments for doing so, resulting in relative sparing of normal tissues. Similarly, chemotherapy is often administered with intervals of about 3 weeks between each treatment. This is because many of these drugs cause damage to proliferating hematological precursor cells in the bone marrow. It typically takes about 3 weeks for adequate repopulation from bone marrow stem cells and their progeny to replenish the cellular damage from a cytotoxic insult.

Although protracting the overall treatment time allows increased repopulation of cells in normal tissues, surviving tumor cells will repopulate as well, leading to an increase in the number of tumor cells that must be eradicated. There is extensive experimental and clinical evidence, as reviewed previously, that the repopulation of tumor cells limits the effectiveness of radiation therapy, and that tumor cell repopulation might accelerate during a course of radiotherapy. However, tumor cell repopulation may also be triggered by chemotherapy (and possibly surgery) and occur during the time intervals between cycles of chemotherapy, and thereby limit its effectiveness.

Accelerated repopulation is consistently observed in rodent models after cytotoxic injury.[42–46] Less is known about repopulation in human tumors after chemotherapy. In these studies, tumor cell proliferation was assessed from biopsy samples taken at various intervals after the last course of chemotherapy. Bourhis et al.[47] found that in patients with oropharyngeal cancer, the estimated potential doubling time shortened after chemotherapy, indicative for accelerated repopulation, which was associated with a poor response to treatment. In contrast, in a small study of patients with ovarian cancer treated with platinum-based chemotherapy, Davis et al.[48] found that, at variable times after the last chemotherapy (mean 33 days), the percentage of Ki67 (a nuclear protein associated with proliferation) positive tumor cells was increased in 4 patients, reduced in 12, and unchanged in 5 patients.

It is clear that much more work has to be done to investigate accelerated proliferation in relation to chemotherapy, the importance of the effect and the associated molecular tumor characteristics.

The possible triggering of accelerated tumor cell proliferation by either chemotherapy or radiotherapy, as well as the potential for radiosensitization of the tumor, has been one of the theoretical advantages of delivering chemotherapy and radiotherapy concurrently instead of sequentially.[49] In many cancers, including head and neck and NSCLC, concurrent chemotherapy and radiotherapy has consistently lead to improved survival although a higher incidence and severity of early toxicity may become dose limiting for one or both modalities. Therefore, some investigators have tried to deliver radiotherapy during the last part of chemotherapy. Moreover, in lung cancer, both local tumor failure and distant metastases remain a clinical problem. Therefore, delaying local radiation could theoretically allow more adequate delivery of chemotherapy.

Timing of Chest Radiotherapy The issue of timing and sequencing of chemotherapy and radiotherapy has been subject to several randomized phase III trials, both in locally advanced NSCLC and limited disease small cell lung cancer (LD-SCLC).

In locally advanced NSCLC, only one phase III trial in which induction chemotherapy followed by concurrent chemoradiation was compared to chemoradiation alone has been published as a full-length article at the time of writing.[50] Readers are referred to Chapter 55 for the details. No differences were observed between both arms regarding overall survival or the incidence of distant metastases. However, more toxicity occurred in the induction arm.

In contrast to the paucity of data in NSCLC, many phase III studies have investigated the timing of chest radiation in LD-SCLC.[51,52] When all studies were considered, the delivery of early versus late thoracic irradiation did not influence the survival. However, when the most active chemotherapy regimen (platinum based) was administered concomitantly with chest radiotherapy, long-term survival was increased at the expense of a higher incidence of severe, though, transient esophagitis. Interestingly, lung toxicity was not different according to the timing of radiotherapy. Because a time interaction between chest radiation and chemotherapy was suspected, an integrated approach was proposed.[53] It was hypothesized that accelerated repopulation was triggered by the first dose of any effective cytotoxic agent and that in order to obtain local tumor control; the last tumor clonogen should be killed by the end of radiotherapy. It follows from these two assumptions that the long-term survival should decrease with increasing time between the start of *any* treatment to the end of radiotherapy (SER). A metaanalysis of published data showed superior long-term survival if the SER was kept less than 30 days in LD-SCLC (Fig. 41.4).

These results are consistent with accelerated proliferation of tumor clonogens triggered by radiotherapy and/or chemotherapy. As expected, accelerated treatments also cause more toxicity in rapidly proliferating tissues such as the esophageal mucosa.

In conclusion, for limited-stage SCLC, current evidence supports the early administration of thoracic radiotherapy with concurrent platinum-based chemotherapy. In locally advanced NSCLC, induction chemotherapy administered before

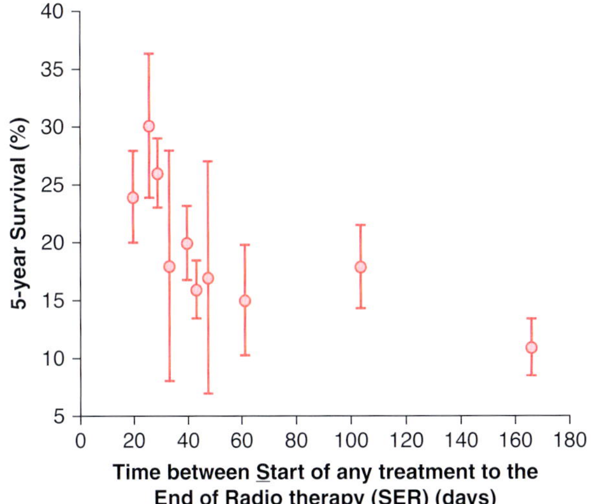

FIGURE 41.4 The survival at 5 years as a function of the SER (start of *any* treatment to the end of radiotherapy). Each dot represents a single trial ± S.E.

concurrent chemotherapy and radiotherapy seems not beneficial, but in view of the limited data, this conclusion should not be viewed as definitive.

Timing of Prophylactic Cranial Irradiation From a theoretical point of view, delaying prophylactic cranial irradiation (PCI) should reduce its potential benefit. Indeed, PCI is given because chemotherapy fails to achieve therapeutic concentrations in the brain because of the blood-brain barrier. Delaying PCI would reduce the probability that proliferating cells in micrometastases in the brain would be controlled. A metaanalysis based on individual patient data in LD-SCLC indeed found a significantly lower hazard ratio (HR) when patients were randomized to PCI within 4 months after the initiation of induction therapy.[54] The HRs with 95% CI for developing brain metastases were 0.27 (0.16, 0.46), 0.50 (0.35, 0.72), and 0.69 (0.44, 1.08) for delays after induction therapy of less than 4 months, between 4 and 6 months, and more than 6 months, respectively.

No data are available on PCI timing in NSCLC.

BIOLOGY OF TUMOR CELL REPOPULATION

Models of Repopulation

Radiotherapy As described in the previous sections, solid tumors have a high spontaneous rate of cell loss, which may be as high as 80% to 90% of the rate of cell production.[55] The potential doubling time of a tumor (see previous discussion) is therefore much shorter than its actual doubling time. In a model proposed by Fowler,[56] well-oxygenated cells in the vicinity of blood vessels die and are removed following radiotherapy. As a consequence, the nutritional and oxygen status of the remaining cells improves, with the result that the rate of spontaneous cell death decreases. This is magnified over a course of fractionated radiotherapy. The decrease in the spontaneous death of tumor cells is then the predominant factor, which leads to accelerated repopulation.

Other investigators have proposed a model based on proliferation and differentiation during the renewal of normal tissues.[57,58] In this model, tumor stem cells normally produce more of themselves as well as cells that undergo terminal differentiation. When repopulation occurs during radiotherapy, a larger proportion of the progeny of stem cells is assumed to retain clonogenic capacity. The rate of proliferation of clonogenic tumor cells might also be faster, with fewer aborted cell divisions. Alterations in the cellular microenvironment may also influence such mechanisms and may be relevant to both models.[59]

The molecular mechanisms that underlie accelerated repopulation during radiotherapy are being unraveled. Ionizing radiation has been shown to activate the epidermal growth factor receptor (EGFR) and other members of the ERBB family of tyrosine kinases, leading to activation of mitogen-activated protein kinase (MAPK) pathways and the stimulation of cellular proliferation.[60–64] In an experimental model, it was shown that radiotherapy induced the proliferation of human squamous cell carcinoma and that this response was mediated through EGFR autophosphorylation, which observed over a clinically relevant dose range.[65] The levels of EGFR and cyclin D1, a downstream effector of EGFR, were found to correlate with radiocurability of nine murine epithelial carcinoma cell lines.[66,67]

In humans, the prognostic and predictive value of EGFR expression is unclear in relation to the selection of patients who are likely to benefit from accelerated radiotherapy schedules and/or concurrent chemoradiation. An indication that high EGFR expression in the primary tumor may be predictive for a favorable outcome after accelerated radiotherapy comes from studies in head and neck cancer.[68] EGFR expression may thus be necessary for accelerated tumor repopulation. In contrast, Ki-67 expression did not predict a favorable outcome after accelerated radiotherapy in head and neck cancer.[69] EGFR inhibition is thus a logical way to combine with radiotherapy in order to decrease accelerated proliferation and has indeed been shown to produce a benefit when added to fractionated radiotherapy in HNSCC.[70] It is too early to evaluate the results of this strategy in NSCLC.

Chemotherapy Investigating the spatial origin of cells that contribute to accelerated repopulation after treatment of multicellular tumor spheroids by chemotherapy showed that there is a gradient of decreasing cell proliferation with increasing distance from the surface of spheroids, similar to that from tumor blood vessels.[71–73] Most anticancer drugs are preferentially toxic to proliferating cells, and many drugs have poor penetration into solid tissue.[74–76] Cells near to the periphery of spheroids are, therefore, more likely to be killed by chemotherapy, and subsequent repopulation occurs because of entry into the cell cycle of originally quiescent cells near the center of spheroids, probably because of improved nutrition. This mechanism was confirmed in a human colon cancer xenograft by measuring the uptake of bromodeoxyuridine (BrdU) after treatment with gemcitabine. Initially, gemcitabine inhibited the proliferation of most cancer cells, but repopulation was observed starting from cells that were more distant from tumor blood vessels, which had lower rates of proliferation before therapy.[77]

From the preceding discussion, it is likely that as a result of chemotherapy, tumor cells close to blood vessels are most likely to be killed because of their higher rate of proliferation (and resultant chemosensitivity) and better drug access. When these cells die or shut down their metabolism, nutrition of the more distant cells improves, death of the distal cells decreases, and the distal cells reenter the cell cycle and repopulate the tumor. This model provides a mechanism for the paradox that some cancer cells might survive that would have died in the absence of treatment.

The proliferation of tumor cells after chemotherapy depends ultimately on the activation of cyclin/cyclin-dependent kinase complexes that control the entry of cells into the cell cycle and their passage through the cell cycle. Like after radiotherapy, activation of these proteins might occur through signaling from receptors, such as the EGFR, but little is known about changes in activity of these pathways in tumors treated with chemotherapy.

CONCLUSION

Understanding the biological parameters that influence radiation response can provide opportunities for treatment optimization to improve the therapeutic ratio. Among these include strategies to increase radiation tumor kill, limit cellular repair by tumor, deal with tumor-related accelerated repopulation and hypoxia, and incorporation of targeted systematic therapies with radiotherapy.

As accelerated repopulation is one of the main reasons for treatment failure after radiotherapy and chemotherapy, strategies to inhibit this process are of obvious interest.

More recently, the delivery of external beam radiotherapy may be further optimized to exploit the radiobiological rationale for large dose per fraction or hypofractionation in order to provide improved tumor kill and minimize tumor cellular repair (see earlier discussion, "The Four R's of Radiotherapy"). The therapeutic ratio for hypofractionation can only be of benefit if late normal-tissue complications can be realistically minimized. Technically, in tumors that move considerably such as lung cancers caused by diaphragmatic excursions, hypofractionation should be best achieved through the use of respiratory-gated extracranial stereotactic radiotherapy treatments or tracking of lung tumors using implanted radiopaque fiducial markers within the target region and delivery of radiotherapy fractions when the target is within a predefined treatment zone. These recent radiotherapy strategies have been collectively termed image-guided radiotherapy (IGRT). The emphasis of IGRT is to ensure both improved tumor volume definition for the target as well as four-dimension (4D) (in which the fourth dimension represents the time during and in between each radiotherapy fraction) verification for quality assurance of any temporal–spatial uncertainties in treatment delivery.

Moreover, the molecular mechanisms underlying accelerated repopulation are being rapidly unraveled. Inhibition of repopulation should ideally be specific for cancer cells as otherwise no gain of the therapeutic ratio can be expected. Apart from accelerated radiotherapy schedules and the delivery of radiotherapy with chemotherapy, discussed in this chapter, the combination of targeted drugs together with radiotherapy or concurrent chemoradiation is a rational choice.

Examples of molecular-targeted agents include small molecule inhibitors and antibodies against specific proteins that are related to crucial cancer pathways such as proliferation. These agents should not only be used concurrently with chemotherapy and radiotherapy, but also in between courses of treatment. Because EGFR inhibitors have been introduced successfully in clinical trials and because this pathway plays a major role in accelerated repopulation, their combination with chemoradiation is being investigated actively.[70]

Besides EGFR inhibitors, agents that target the MAPK pathway have been found to modulate radiosensitivity in preclinical studies and are in early trial with radiotherapy.[78] The rapamycin analogue CCI-779 is a cytostatic agent that is active against tumors with mutation of the tumor suppressor gene phosphatase and tensin homologue (PTEN). Phase I trials demonstrate that it is feasible to combine these agents with radiation and cisplatin with in mouse models no increase of pulmonary toxicity.[79,80]

Targeted agents are primarily cytostatic, and as a consequence, tumor response (basically, shrinkage on CT scans) is relatively rare, and when it occurs, it is usually delayed. Delivering these agents concurrently with chemotherapy (with or without radiation) could, therefore, lead to disappointing results as the cytostatic effects of targeted agents might render tumor cells less sensitive to cycle-specific chemotherapy. Kim and Tannock[23] therefore suggested to give cytostatic agents between courses of chemotherapy to inhibit repopulation, with the stopping of such treatment before the next round of chemotherapy to allow cells to reenter the cycle and regain sensitivity to cycle-active drugs. This method would obviously also be applicable for concurrent chemoradiation.

Besides repopulation, hypoxia still remains an important area of research. Identifying hypoxic cells in human tumors has improved by the help of new imaging and physiologic techniques.[81] Indeed, surrogate noninvasive techniques to identify hypoxia, such as circulating osteopontin and positron emission tomography (PET) imaging with hypoxia tracers such as ^{18}F-misonidazole have enabled the selection of patients with head and neck cancer that have a better outcome with hypoxic cell sensitizers such as nimorazole and tirapazamine. An updated systematic review identified 10,108 patients in 86 randomized trials designed to modify tumor hypoxia in patients treated with curative attempted primary radiation therapy alone.[82] Overall modification of tumor hypoxia significantly improved the effect of radiotherapy, with an OR of

0.77 (95% CI, 0.71 to 0.86) for the outcome of locoregional control and with an associated significant overall survival benefit (OR = 0.87; 95% CI, 0.80 to 0.95). No significant influence was found on the incidence of distant metastases or on the risk of radiation-related complications.

Further trials will build on more insights of molecular biology, imaging, and physiology, all leading to a further increase of the efficiency of radiotherapy in the treatment of lung cancer.

REFERENCES

1. Gudkov AV, Komarova EA. The role of p53 in determining sensitivity to radiotherapy. *Nat Rev Cancer* 2003;3:117–129.
2. Sarkaria JN, Bristow RG. Overview of cancer molecular radiobiology. In: Bentzen SM, Harari PM, Tome W, et al., eds. *Radiation Oncology Advances*. New York: Springer, 2008:117–133.
3. Bentzen SM. Preventing or reducing late side effects of radiation therapy: radiobiology meets molecular pathology. *Nat Rev Cancer* 2006;6:702–713.
4. McMillan TJ, Steel GG. DNA damage and cell killing. In: Steel GG, ed. *Basic Clinical Radiobiology*. 3rd Ed. London: Hodder Arnold, 2002:1–74.
5. Warters RL, Hofer KG. Radionuclide toxicity in cultured mammalian cells. Elucidation of the primary site for radiation-induced division delay. *Radiat Res* 1977;69(2):348–358.
6. Kerr JF, Wyllie AH, Currie AR. Apoptosis: a basic biological phenomenon with wide-ranging implications in tissue kinetics. *Br J Cancer* 1972;26(4):239–257.
7. Wyllie AH, Kerr JF, Currie AR. Cell death: the significance of apoptosis. *Int Rev Cytol* 1980;68:251–306.
8. Prise KM, Schettino G, Folkard M, et al. New insights on cell death from radiation exposure. *Lancet Oncol* 2005;6:520–528.
9. Puck TT, Marcus PI. Action of x-rays on mammalian cells. *J Exp Med* 1956;103(5):653–666.
10. Hall EJ, Gross W, Dvorak RF, et al. Survival curves and age response functions for Chinese hamster cells exposed to x-rays or high LET alpha-particles. *Radiat Res* 1972;52(1):88–98.
11. Withers HR, Thames HD Jr, Peters LJ. A new isoeffect curve for change in dose per fraction. *Radiother Oncol* 1983;2:187–191.
12. Thames HD, Bentzen SM, Turesson I, et al. Time-dose factors in radiotherapy: a review of the human data. *Radiother Oncol* 1990;19:219–235.
13. Saunders MI, Dische S. Continuous, hyperfractionated, accelerated radiotherapy (CHART) in non-small cell carcinoma of the bronchus. *Int J Radiat Oncol Biol Phys* 1990;19(5):1211–1215.
14. Saunders MI, Dische S, Barrett A, et al. Randomised multicentre trials of CHART vs conventional radiotherapy in head and neck and non-small-cell lung cancer: an interim report. CHART Steering Committee. *Br J Cancer* 1996;73(12):1455–1462.
15. Withers HR. The four r's of radiotherapy. In: Lett JT, Adler H, eds. *Advances in Radiation Biology*. New York: Academic Press, 1975: 241–271.
16. Steel GG. Cell survival as a determinant of tumour response. In: Steel GG, ed. *Basic Clinical Radiobiology*. 3rd Ed. London: Hodder Arnold, 2002:61–62,
17. Elkind MM, Sutton H. X-ray damage and recovery in mammalian cells in culture. *Nature* 1959;184:1293–1295.
18. Sinclair WK, Morton RA. X-Ray and ultraviolet sensitivity of synchronized Chinese hamster cells at various stages of the cell cycle. *Biophys J* 1965;5:1–25.
19. Kastan MB, Onyekwere O, Sidransky D, et al. Participation of p53 protein in the cellular response to DNA damage. *Cancer Res* 1991; 51(23 Pt 1):6304–6311.
20. Terasima T, Tolmach LJ. Changes in x-ray sensitivity of HeLa cells during the division cycle. *Nature* 1961;190:1210–1211.
21. Terasima T, Tolmach LJ. Variations in several responses of HeLa cells to x-irradiation during the division cycle. *Biophys J* 1963;3:11–33.
22. Bentzen SM. Repopulation in radiation oncology: perspectives of clinical research. *Int J Radiat Biol* 2003;79:581–585.
23. Kim JJ, Tannock IF. Repopulation of cancer cells during therapy: an important cause of treatment failure. *Nat Rev Cancer* 2005;5:516–525.
24. Bernier J, Bentzen SM. Altered fractionation and combined radiochemotherapy approaches: pioneering new opportunities in head and neck oncology. *Eur J Cancer* 2003; 39:560–571.
25. Hendry JH, Bentzen SM, Dale RG, et al. A modelled comparison of the effects of using different ways to compensate for missed treatment days in radiotherapy. *Clin Oncol (R Coll Radiol)* 1996;8:297–307.
26. Gray LH, Conger AD, Ebert M, et al. The concentration of oxygen dissolved in tissues at the time of irradiation as a factor in radiotherapy. *Br J Radiol* 1953;26(312):638–648.
27. Harris AL. Hypoxia—a key regulatory factor in tumour growth. *Nat Rev Cancer* 2002;2:38–47.
28. Nordsmark M, Bentzen SM, Rudat V, et al. Prognostic value of tumor oxygenation in 397 head and neck tumors after primary radiation therapy. An international multi-center study. *Radiother Oncol* 2005;77:18–24.
29. Bentzen SM. Quantitative clinical radiobiology. *Acta Oncol* 1993;32: 259–275.
30. Bentzen SM, Ruifrok AC, Thames HD. Repair capacity and kinetics for human mucosa and epithelial tumors in the head and neck: clinical data on the effect of changing the time interval between multiple fractions per day in radiotherapy. *Radiother Oncol* 1996;38:89–101.
31. Bentzen SM, Saunders MI, Dische S. Repair halftimes estimated from observations of treatment-related morbidity after CHART or conventional radiotherapy in head and neck cancer. *Radiother Oncol* 1999;53:219–226.
32. Ang KK, Jiang GL, Guttenberger R, et al. Impact of spinal cord repair kinetics on the practice of altered fractionation schedules. *Radiother Oncol* 1992;25:287–294.
33. Bourhis J, Overgaard J, Audry H, et al. Meta-analysis of Radiotherapy in Carcinomas of Head and neck (MARCH) Collaborative Group. Hyperfractionated or accelerated radiotherapy in head and neck cancer: a meta-analysis. *Lancet* 2006;368:843–854.
34. Stuschke M, Thames HD. Hyperfractionated radiotherapy of human tumors: overview of the randomized clinical trials. *Int J Radiat Oncol Biol Phys* 1997;37:259–267.
35. Baumann M, Dörr W, Petersen C, et al. Repopulation during fractionated radiotherapy: much has been learned, even more is open. *Int J Radiat Biol* 2003;79:465–467.
36. Curran WJ, Scott CB, Langer CJ, et al. Long-term benefit is observed in a phase III comparison of sequential vs concurrent chemoradiation for patients with unresectable stage III nsclc: RTOG 94-10. *Proc Am Soc Clin Oncol* 2003;22:621a. (abstr 2499).
37. Belani CP, Wang W, Johnson DH, et al. Eastern Cooperative Oncology Group. Phase III study of the Eastern Cooperative Oncology Group (ECOG 2597): induction chemotherapy followed by either standard thoracic radiotherapy or hyperfractionated accelerated radiotherapy for patients with unresectable stage IIIA and B non-small-cell lung cancer. *J Clin Oncol* 2005;23:3760–3767.
38. Saunders M, Dische S, Barrett A, et al. Continuous, hyperfractionated, accelerated radiotherapy (CHART) versus conventional radiotherapy in non-small cell lung cancer: mature data from the randomised multicentre trial. CHART Steering committee. *Radiother Oncol* 1999;52:137–148.
39. Baumann M, Herrmann T, Koch R, et al. Continuous hyperfractionated accelerated radiotherapy - weekend less (CHARTWEL) versus conventionally fractionated (CF) radiotherapy in non-small-cell lung cancer (NSCLC): first results of a phase III randomised multicentre trial (ARO 971) ECCO 13, 2005. *Eur J Cancer* (Suppl) 2005;3:322.
40. Turrisi AT III, Kim K, Blum R, et al. Twice-daily compared with once-daily thoracic radiotherapy in limited small-cell lung cancer treated concurrently with cisplatin and etoposide. *N Engl J Med* 1999;340:265–271.

41. Bentzen SM, Skoczylas JZ, Bernier J. Quantitative clinical radiobiology of early and late lung reactions. *Int J Radiat Biol* 2000;76:453–462.
42. Malaise E, Tubiana M. Growth of the cells of an experimental irradiated fibrosarcoma in the C3H mouse. *Hebd Seances Acad Sci, Ser D Sci Nat* 1966;263:292–295.
43. Beck-Bornholdt HP, Omniczynski M, Theis E, et al. Influence of treatment time on the response of rat rhabdomyosarcoma R1H to fractionated irradiation. *Acta Oncol* 1991;30:57–63.
44. Milas L, Yamada S, Hunter N, et al. Changes in TCD_{50} as a measure of clonogen doubling time in irradiated and unirradiated tumours. *Int J Radiat Oncol Biol Phys* 1991;21:1195–1202.
45. Begg AC, Hofland I, Kummermehr J. Tumour cell repopulation during fractionated radiotherapy: correlation between flow cytometric and radiobiological data in three murine tumours. *Eur J Cancer* 1991;27:537–543.
46. Hessel F, Petersen C, Zips D, et al. Repopulation of moderately well-differentiated and keratinizing GL human squamous cell carcinomas growing in nude mice. *Int J Radiat Oncol Biol Phys* 2004;58:510–518.
47. Bourhis J, Wilson G, Wibault P, et al. Rapid tumour cell proliferation after induction chemotherapy in oropharyngeal cancer. *Laryngoscope* 1994;104:468–472 .
48. Davis AJ, Chapman W, Hedley DW, et al. Assessment of tumour cell repopulation after chemotherapy for advanced ovarian cancer: pilot study. *Cytometry* 2003;A51:1–6.
49. Bentzen SM, Harari PM, Bernier J. Exploitable mechanisms for combining drugs with radiation: concepts, achievements and future directions. *Nat Clin Pract Oncol* 2007;4:172–180.
50. Vokes EE, Herndon JE II, Kelley MJ, et al. Cancer and Leukemia Group B. Induction chemotherapy followed by chemoradiotherapy compared with chemoradiotherapy alone for regionally advanced unresectable stage III Non-small-cell lung cancer: Cancer and Leukemia Group B. *J Clin Oncol* 2007;25: 1698–1704.
51. Pijls-Johannesma M, De Ruysscher D, Vansteenkiste J, et al. Timing of chest radiotherapy in patients with limited stage small cell lung cancer: a systematic review and meta-analysis of randomised controlled trials. *Cancer Treat Rev* 2007;33:461–473.
52. Fried DB, Morris DE, Poole C, et al. Systematic review evaluating the timing of thoracic radiation therapy in combined modality therapy for limited-stage small-cell lung cancer. *J Clin Oncol* 2004;22:4837–4845.
53. De Ruysscher D, Pijls-Johannesma M, Bentzen SM, et al. Time between the first day of chemotherapy and the last day of chest radiation is the most important predictor of survival in limited-disease small-cell lung cancer. *J Clin Oncol* 2006;24:1057–1063.
54. Auperin A, Arriagada R, Pignon JP, et al. Prophylactic cranial irradiation for patients with small-cell lung cancer in complete remission. Prophylactic Cranial Irradiation Overview Collaborative Group. *N Engl J Med* 1999;341:476–484.
55. Steel GG. *Growth Kinetics of Tumours: Cell Population Kinetics in Relation to the Growth and Treatment of Cancer*. Oxford: Clarendon, 1977.
56. Fowler JF. Rapid repopulation in radiotherapy: a debate on mechanism. The phantom of tumour treatment—continually rapid proliferation unmasked. *Radiother Oncol* 1991;22:156–158.
57. Kummermehr J, Trott KR. *Tumour Stem Cells*. In: Potten CS, ed. London: Academic, 1997:363–399.
58. Dörr W. Three A's of repopulation during fractionated irradiation of squamous epithelia: asymmetry loss, acceleration of stem-cell divisions and abortive divisions. *Int J Radiat Biol* 1997;72:635–643.
59. Petersen C, Eicheler W, Frömmel A, et al. Proliferation and micromilieu during fractionated irradiation of human FaDu squamous cell carcinoma in nude mice. *Int J Radiat Biol* 2003;79:469–477.
60. Balaban N, Moni J, Shannon M, et al. The effect of ionizing radiation on signal transduction: antibodies to EGF receptor sensitize A431 cells to radiation. *Biochim Biophys Acta* 1996;1314:147–156.
61. Schmidt-Ullrich RK, Contessa JN, Dent P, et al. Molecular mechanisms of radiation-induced accelerated repopulation. *Radiat Oncol Investig* 1999;7:321–330.
62. Carter S, Auer KL, Reardon DB, et al. Inhibition of the mitogen activated protein (MAP) kinase cascade potentiates cell killing by low dose ionizing radiation in A431 human squamous carcinoma cells. *Oncogene* 1998;16:2787–2796.
63. Kavanagh BD, Dent P, Schmidt-Ullrich RK, et al. Calcium-dependent stimulation of mitogen-activated protein kinase activity in A431 cells by low doses of ionizing radiation. *Radiat Res* 1998;149:579–587.
64. Bowers G, Reardon D, Hewitt T, et al. The relative role of ErbB1–4 receptor tyrosine kinases in radiation signal transduction responses of human carcinoma cells. *Oncogene* 2001;20:1388–1397.
65. Schmidt-Ullrich RK, Mikkelsen RB, Dent P, et al. Radiation-induced proliferation of the human A431 squamous carcinoma cells is dependent on EGFR tyrosine phosphorylation. *Oncogene* 1997;15:1191–1197.
66. Akimoto T, Hunter NR, Buchmiller L, et al. Inverse relationship between epidermal growth factor receptor expression and radiocurability of murine carcinomas. *Clin Cancer Res* 1999;5:2884–2890.
67. Milas L, Akimoto T, Hunter NR, et al. Relationship between cyclin D1 expression and poor radioresponse of murine carcinomas. *Int J Radiat Oncol Biol Phys* 2002;52:514–521.
68. Bentzen SM, Atasoy BM, Daley FM, et al. Epidermal growth factor receptor expression in pretreatment biopsies from head and neck squamous cell carcinoma as a predictive factor for a benefit from accelerated radiation therapy in a randomized controlled trial. *J Clin Oncol* 2005;23:5560–5567.
69. Wilson GD, Saunders MI, Dische S, et al. Pre-treatment proliferation and the outcome of conventional and accelerated radiotherapy. *Eur J Cancer* 2006;42:363–371.
70. Bonner JA, Harari PM, Giralt J, et al. Radiotherapy plus cetuximab for squamous-cell carcinoma of the head and neck. *N Engl J Med* 2006;354:567–578.
71. Durand RE. Distribution and activity of antineoplastic drugs in a tumour model. *J. Natl Cancer Inst* 1989;81:146–152.
72. Lankelma J, Dekker H, Luque FR, et al. Doxorubicin gradients in human breast cancer. *Clin Cancer Res* 1999;5:1703–1707.
73. Jain RK. Delivery of molecular and cellular medicine to solid tumours. *Adv Drug Deliv Rev* 2001;46:149–168.
74. Tannock IF. Tumour physiology and drug resistance. *Cancer Metastasis Rev* 2001;20:123–132.
75. Tannock IF, Lee CM, Tunggal JK, et al. Limited penetration of anticancer drugs through tumour tissue: a potential cause of resistance of solid tumours to chemotherapy. *Clin Cancer Res* 2002;8:878–884.
76. Tredan O, Galmarini CM, Patel K, et al. Drug resistance and the solid tumor microenvironment. *J Natl Cancer Inst* 2007;99:1441–1454.
77. Huxham LA, Kyle AH, Baker JH, et al. Microregional effects of gemcitabine in HCT-116 xenografts. *Cancer Res* 2004;64:6537–6541.
78. Quick QA, Gewirtz DA. Enhancement of radiation sensitivity, delay of proliferative recovery after radiation and abrogation of MAPK (p44/42) signaling by imatinib in glioblastoma cells. *Int J Oncol* 2006;29:407–412.
79. Wu L, Birle DC, Tannock IF. Effects of the mammalian target of rapamycin inhibitor CCI-779 used alone or with chemotherapy on human prostate cancer cells and xenografts. *Cancer Res* 2005;65:2825–2831.
80. Sarkaria JN, Schwingler P, Schild SE, et al. Phase I trial of sirolimus combined with radiation and cisplatin in non-small cell lung cancer. *J Thorac Oncol* 2007;2:751–757.
81. Rischin D, Fisher R, Peters L, et al. Hypoxia in head and neck cancer: studies with hypoxic positron emission tomography imaging and hypoxic cytotoxins. *Int J Radiat Oncol Biol Phys* 2007;69(2 Suppl): S61–S63.
82. Overgaard J. Hypoxic radiosensitization: adored and ignored. *J Clin Oncol* 2007;25:4066–4074.

CHAPTER 42

Jason R. Pantarotto
Suresh Senan

Radiotherapy for Locally Advanced Lung Cancer: Stages IIIA and IIIB

THE SCOPE OF THE PROBLEM

Lung cancer is the leading cause of cancer deaths in the United States and non–small cell lung cancer (NSCLC) accounts for approximately 80% to 85% of all cases.[1] The 1997 revision of the lung cancer staging system[2] classifies stage IIIA as T1–3N2 and T3N1 disease, whereas stage IIIB includes either N3 or T4 disease. In the Surveillance, Epidemiology, and End Results (SEER) 2004 registry, 29.7% of new NSCLC cases presented with stage III disease, of which 12.1% were stage IIIA and 17.6% were stage IIIB.[3] The International Association for the Study of Lung Cancer (IASLC) Lung Cancer Staging Project database (see Chapter 30) of 67,725 cases of NSCLC revealed 5-year overall survival figures for clinically staged IIIA and IIIB disease of only 18% and 8%, respectively, and for pathologically staged IIIA and IIIB disease, it was 25% and 19%, respectively.[4] The poor outcomes observed are caused by locoregional failure rates between 30% and 55%, with distant failure rates in the range of 40% to 60%.[5]

TREATMENT STRATEGIES FOR STAGE III NSCLC

Staging Subsets of Stage III NSCLC Strategies to improve outcomes have centered on improved staging and tailoring aggressive treatment regimens to subcategories of stage III disease that are most likely to benefit. This population is heterogeneous in terms of presentation and outcomes—an issue that is being addressed in the forthcoming seventh edition of the TNM stage groupings.[4] This chapter will not address the treatment of three categories of patients with stage III disease, namely, (a) stage T3N1 that are generally resectable, (b) tumors of the superior sulcus where the addition of surgery is considered useful,[6,7] and (c) stage IIIB patients with malignant pleural effusions.

Improvements in staging modalities, such as positron emission tomography with ^{18}F-fluorodeoxyglucose (FDG-PET), multislice computed tomography (CT), and endoscopic techniques, have had a profound effect on the pretreatment evaluation of NSCLC. The routine use of PET is now recommended by the American College of Chest Physicians (ACCP) as a standard staging investigation for stages IB to IIIB prior to a curative treatment[8] (see Chapter 27). The false-positive and false-negative rates with CT scans alone are unacceptably high.[9–11] FDG-PET has a higher sensitivity of 84% and specificity of 89%, and the sensitivity improves to 93% and specificity to 95% when using combined PET-CT.[12–14] As false-positive rates range from 10% to 15%, it has been recommended that any positive PET findings should be confirmed by cytopathology in patients who are candidates for surgery.[14–16] However, the same approach can be taken for patients who are candidates for high-dose concurrent chemoradiotherapy (CRT).[17] Up to 30% of conventionally staged patients with stage III cancer referred for radical radiotherapy are excluded after a PET scan, mainly because of the detection of occult metastatic disease.[18] At least part of the incremental survival benefit seen in stage III NSCLC over the last decade may be a result of the migration of patients with otherwise occult metastases to stage IV. Although mediastinoscopy is still considered, the gold standard for confirming N2 disease,[19] only a minority of patients treated in nonsurgical trials have undergone this invasive procedure. In recent years, minimally invasive staging by techniques such as biopsy during endoscopic ultrasound (EUS-FNA) and transbronchial needle aspiration without (TBNA) or with endobronchial ultrasound guidance (EBUS-TBNA) are increasingly used to minimize invasive staging procedures[20–22] (see Chapters 28 and 29). Radiation oncologists with access to endoscopic staging can use this approach to optimally define nodal target volumes in patients with stage III disease.

Factoring in Tumor and Patient Characteristics An appropriate treatment strategy for stage III NSCLC can only be formulated once the extent of disease, any comorbidity, and general fitness of a patient has been fully characterized. The ACCP guidelines have chosen to classify N2 tumors into four subsets for the purpose of generating rational treatment guidelines.[23] Nodal metastases found either after or during a surgical resection are denoted as $IIIA_1$ and $IIIA_2$, respectively. Nodal disease identified preoperatively is $IIIA_3$, whereas bulky or fixed multistation N2 disease is classified as $IIIA_4$. Although there is no uniform definition of what constitutes "bulky" nodal disease, the ACCP recommendation includes nodes of 2 cm or larger in short-axis diameter as measured by chest CT, multistation nodal disease, and/or groupings of multiple positive smaller lymph nodes.[23]

Patients with lung cancer generally tend to have significant smoking-related comorbidities, suboptimal pulmonary function and impaired performance score. Each of these factors may impact on their ability to tolerate potentially curative treatment, and each is exacerbated with increasing age.[24] The median age of presentation for NSCLC cases from a SEER database analysis was 67,[3] and this is expected to rise in the future.

Primary Treatment The choice of optimal local treatment has been the topic of active research in the last 2 decades. Current guidelines recommend that platinum-based combination CRT should be the primary treatment in patients with stage IIIA NSCLC and ipsilateral mediastinal disease identified preoperatively.[23] The same strategy is also recommended for patients with stage IIIB NSCLC and a good performance score with minimal weight loss (≤5%).[25]

The role of surgery in stage III disease was evaluated in two large randomized trials, which concluded that the addition of surgery did not improve survival in comparison to either sequential chemoradiotherapy (CT-RT)[5] or concurrent CRT[26] alone (see Chapter 55). Subgroup analysis has suggested that surgical outcomes were more favorable in patients with "downstaged" N2 disease, and in whom a radical resection was achieved with a lobectomy rather than a pneumonectomy.[26] However, conditions that favor postsurgical survival are generally established only after a resection. The majority of patients with N2 disease will still have persistent disease despite induction therapy, and "gaps" in CRT, arising during mediastinal restaging risk exposing such patients to a poorer survival caused by longer overall treatment time.[27]

Radiotherapy alone is an inappropriate treatment for fit patients as an updated metaanalysis by the NSCLC Collaborative Group revealed a significant survival benefit for sequential CT-RT versus radiotherapy alone.[28] When concurrent CRT was compared to radiotherapy alone, a survival advantage was seen for the former (HR = 0.88; 95% CI, 0.81 to 0.95), with an absolute benefit of 3.2% (from 13.4% to 16.6%) at 3 years.[28] Concurrent CRT also improved the progression-free survival, and there was no evidence that any patient subgroup benefited more or less from concurrent CRT.

A second metaanalysis based on 6 trials and 1199 patients evaluated overall and progression-free survival after the concurrent administration of chemotherapy and radiation versus the sequential administration of both modalities.[29] At a median follow-up of 5 years, a significant survival benefit was observed for concurrent CRT with an absolute benefit of 6.6% (from 18.2% with sequential CT-RT to 24.8% with concurrent CRT) at 3 years. Concurrent CRT decreased locoregional progression (HR = 0.76; 95% CI, 0.62 to 0.94) but distant progression rates were similar. Concurrent CRT increased acute grade 3 and 4 esophageal toxicity from 3% to 18%, but no significant difference in acute pulmonary toxicity between both approaches was observed.

Choice of Systemic Agents with Concurrent Radiotherapy Platinum-based concurrent CRT regimens improve outcomes in several malignancies, including lung cancer.[29] A scheme widely used in recent phase III trials consists of cisplatin 50 mg/m^2 on days 1, 8, 29, and 36, and etoposide 50 mg/m^2 on days 1 through 5 and 29 to 33.[6,26] Cisplatin given at full dose provides both a radiosensitization effect within the irradiated volume, and an overall survival benefit related to reduced distant metastases, as demonstrated in the lung adjuvant cisplatin evaluation (LACE) metaanalysis.[30] Significant pathological response rates were observed using an induction scheme of cisplatin-etoposide for stage III NSCLC with only 45 Gy of concurrent radiation in INT 0139, with an 18% pathologic complete response (pT0N0) and 46% complete nodal response ($T_{any}N0$).[26]

Immunohistochemical analysis in resected NSCLC for excision repair cross-complementation group 1 (ERCC1) protein expression suggested that adjuvant cisplatin-based chemotherapy was only beneficial in ERCC1 negative tumors.[31] Studies are currently underway to prospectively validate this finding in the adjuvant setting, and the likely role of ERCC1 expression in selecting chemotherapy schemes in primary CRT remains to be elucidated.

Although the use of concurrent low-dose carboplatin-paclitaxel is widespread in the United States, the outcomes of some recent trials with this combination have been disappointing.[32] This finding may be explained by the fact that three randomized clinical trials of carboplatin plus radiotherapy have not been shown to be superior to radiotherapy alone.[33–35]

Adjuvant Management of Completely Resected Stage III NSCLC The adjuvant management of stage III disease consists of cisplatin-based chemotherapy[30,36,37]; however, locoregional failure rates of 20% to 40% persist in this setting.[36,37] In the Adjuvant Navelbine International Trialist Association (ANITA) trial, a nonrandomized subanalysis comparing 5-year overall survival in N2 patients who did or did not receive postoperative radiotherapy (PORT) found higher survival rates in patients receiving radiotherapy in both the observation and chemotherapy arms (21% vs. 17% and 47% vs. 34%, respectively).[36] A retrospective SEER study also reported superior survival rates associated with PORT in N2 disease.[38] This has renewed interest in adjuvant radiotherapy for resected patients—a strategy that fell out of favor after the PORT metaanalysis of 2128 patients with stage I to III disease reported a significant adverse effect of PORT on survival in 1998.[39] This metaanalysis has been criticized as many of the included trials used radiotherapy techniques that are now considered suboptimal, leading to higher morbidity and mortality rates than more recent studies.[40,41] A phase III European Intergroup trial (LungART), designed to address this issue, opened in 2007 and will compare three-dimensional (3D) conformal PORT to no PORT.[42] Present guidelines do not recommend adjuvant radiotherapy for completely resected stage IIIA disease[23,43] but do suggest PORT when the risk of nodal recurrence is elevated because of extranodal spread, close or microscopically positive resection margins, or involvement of multiple nodal stations.

Options for Poor Performance Status Patients

A significant proportion of patients with stage III cancer cannot tolerate aggressive CRT regimens because of considerable comorbidities. Decisions to withhold concurrent CRT in patients who are fit to receive cisplatin-containing regimens have to be made carefully, however, as every subgroup in the NSCLC Collaborative Group metaanalysis demonstrated a survival benefit as compared to sequential CT-RT.[29] In high-risk patients, sequential CT-RT remains a viable option.[44] Radiation oncologists have flexibility in tailoring treatment to a reduced dose and/or volume in patients who are deemed too frail. Postplanning assessment of a proposed treatment includes a calculation of the V_{20} (percentage volume of normal lung minus planning target volumes [PTV], which receives doses of 20 Gy or more).[45] Patients with a V_{20} in excess of 35% have not only an increased risk of high-grade radiation pneumonitis, but also a significantly poorer survival.[46] Large fields, often required in stage III disease, lead to a higher risk of esophagitis with CRT.[47]. Presentations such as extensive N2 involvement, bilateral hilar node disease, and a peripheral tumor in the lower lobe with contralateral upper mediastinal nodes are examples of cases where clinicians can assume a large V_{20} will result from any radiotherapy plan, and thus make alternate decisions regarding treatment up front.

TARGET DEFINITION IN STAGE III NSCLC

The last 2 decades has witnessed a dramatic shift from two-dimensional (2D) radiotherapy, where bony landmarks and planar images were used to guide field setup, to four-dimensional (4D) radiotherapy, where CT-contoured target volumes are modified to account for intrafraction motion. The use of 2D radiotherapy for lung cancer carries a risk for target miss in up to 15% of patients,[48] and may partly account for the poor local control rates seen in NSCLC trials performed to date. Target volumes drawn on CT images now represent the minimum standard of care.

Defining the Gross Tumor Volume for the Primary Lung Tumor Precise definition of the gross tumor volume (GTV) is important, as contouring errors are compounded when volumetric expansions are made to account for microscopic tumor spread, motion, and setup errors. The boundary between macroscopic tumor and the lung parenchyma is best defined when viewing CT images with proper window width and level settings. Distinguishing the tumor border is more difficult when atelectasis or pulmonary effusions are present, potentially leading to an overestimation of the GTV. Reviewing diagnostic scans in which intravenous contrast has been given, or using contrast for CT simulation, may be helpful. PET scans have been used to avoid atelectatic lung in the target volume,[49] but data to validate this approach are awaited.[50]

PET and PET-CT images (where functional and anatomical data are coregistered as a result of being obtained during the same procedure) may serve a far greater purpose in NSCLC delineation than crude tumor identification. Using PET for radiotherapy planning results in a reduction in interobserver contouring variability, and more consistent delineation of GTV.[51] Some groups have proposed using PET-CT for generating GTVs automatically by using a standardized uptake value (SUV) threshold,[50] an approach that may be confounded by factors, including (a) heterogeneous uptake of FDG within the tumor as a result of necrosis, hypoxia, or degree of tumor differentiation, (b) elevated SUV levels as a result of inflammatory processes, and (c) low SUVs from small tumors caused by partial volume effects.[52] It has been recommended that radiation oncologists should work closely with their nuclear medicine counterparts to interpret PET scans, and caution has been advised when using automatic delineation.[50]

Involved-Field Nodal Radiotherapy Radiotherapy fields have traditionally encompassed the radiologically normal mediastinum, and occasionally, the ipsilateral supraclavicular region, in order to treat potential subclinical disease. The presumed benefits of this approach, referred to as prophylactic or elective nodal irradiation (ENI),[53] have never been clearly demonstrated. Advances in the nonsurgical assessment of the mediastinal nodes, together with analyses of recurrence patterns following involved-field radiotherapy (IFRT) have called into question the need for routine ENI.

A growing body of data from patients with stage III NSCLC where ENI was omitted show that isolated nodal failures outside the PTV occur in less than 7% of patients[54–58] despite the fact that only one of these trials used information from PET scans for radiotherapy planning.[55] In a phase III study of CRT where patients were randomized between IFRT and ENI, significantly fewer IFRT patients had a V_{20} of greater than 20% and fewer experienced radiation pneumonitis.[58] Only 7% of patients randomized to the IFRT arm experienced elective nodal failure compared to 4% in the ENI arm at 5 years. IFRT is advocated on the basis of allowing dose escalation to improve local control while avoiding the toxicity experienced with larger fields (Fig. 42.1).[59]

An increasing number of patients with stage III NSCLC have pathologically confirmed N2 disease, but sampling often fails to evaluate all nodal stations. Definition of the nodal GTV is often based on CT imaging alone, with a short-axis diameter of 10 mm, commonly used to define the upper limit of normal.[60,61] The correlation between size and positivity is tenuous, however, as up to 44% of tumor-bearing nodes are less than 10 mm in size and 18% of patient with pathologically confirmed N2 disease do not have any nodes greater than 10 mm.[62] Data from the

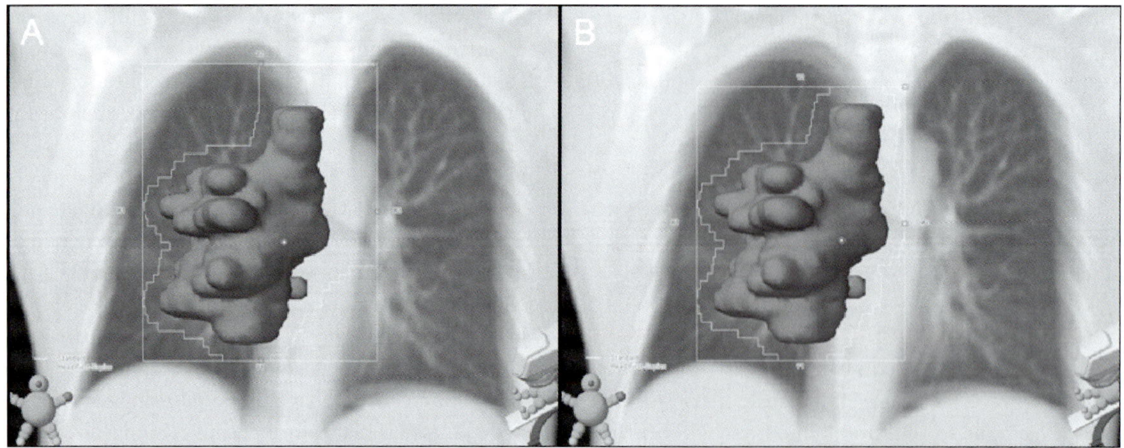

FIGURE 42.1 Treatment portals (*in yellow*) for an anterior field used in elective nodal irradiation **(A)** and involved-field radiotherapy **(B)** in the same patient. Uninvolved nodal regions, including the contralateral upper mediastinum, are routinely treated with the first approach, leading to higher doses to the contralateral lung and esophagus. (See color plate.)

surgical literature, in addition to trials investigating staging techniques such as PET, are very useful to the radiation oncologist in helping to define the nodal target volumes for IFRT.

The limitations of PET scans for defining nodal target volumes should be appreciated. European Society for Thoracic Surgery guidelines caution that invasive nodal staging should be carried out in patients with central tumors, bronchioalveolar carcinoma, hilar N1 disease seen on PET, and when large PET-negative lymph nodes (i.e., ≥16 mm) are present.[63] General guidelines for the inclusion of suspicious nodes are provided in Table 42.1, with supportive data obtained from surgical series.[64] Integrated PET-CT systems provide further improvements over visually correlated studies with excellent spatial resolution,[65] making it the preferred tool in radiotherapy planning. In the absence of contradictory histologic findings, PET-positive nodes should be included in the GTV with the understanding that the positive predictive value of PET is only in the range of 80%.

TABLE 42.1 Schema for Defining Mediastinal Nodal GTV in NSCLC

Nodal Diameter (Short Axis)	PET Status	Approach	Comment
<1 cm	Positive	Include in GTV	Positive predictive value higher for PET than CT, biopsy when possible
<1 cm	Negative	Exclude from GTV	High negative predictive value for PET, small probability of N2 disease[64]
>1 cm	Positive	Include in GTV unless representative cytology from the node is negative	Sensitivity for TBNA is inferior to EBUS or EUS-TBNA,[21] thus consideration of sampling method is required
1–1.5 cm (and no cytology available)	Negative	Exclude from GTV if primary tumor is PET positive, unless cytology or histology is positive	High negative predictive value for PET, small probability (5%) of N2 disease[64]
≥1.5 cm (and no cytology available)	Negative	Include in GTV	21% probability of N2 disease[64]

EBUS, endobronchial ultrasound; EUS, endoscopic ultrasound; GTV, gross tumor volume; NSCLC, non–small cell lung cancer; PET, positron emission tomography; TBNA, transbronchial needle aspiration.

Defining a Clinical Target Volume around the Primary Tumor Data from pathological specimens represent the "gold standard" for determining margins to be added for subclinical disease (i.e., GTV to clinical target volume [CTV] margins). A study performed on NSCLC surgical specimens recommended margins of 8 mm for adenocarcinomas, and 6 mm for squamous cell carcinomas in order to account for 95% of all microscopic extension.[66] A similar analysis in resected proximal tumors revealed microscopic bronchial extension of malignant cells in 24% of cases, and recommended a bronchial margin of 15 mm from macroscopic tumor in order to provide clear margins in 93% of all patients.[67]

Clinical Target Volume Margins around Nodal Disease Nodal extracapsular extension (ECE) has been shown to predict both recurrence and survival.[68,69] In one report of resected mediastinal nodes, ECE was found in 80% of nodes ≥1 cm but the majority of nodes studied were greater than 3 cm in size.[69] A similar analysis, limited to nodes less than 3 cm in size, found ECE in 41.6% of patients with a significant positive correlation with nodal size.[70] To ensure coverage of 95% of the ECE observed, the authors recommended a margin of 3 mm for nodes with a short-axis diameter of 20 mm or less, and an 8-mm margin for nodes greater than 20 mm.

Individualized Planning Target Volumes and Motion Management Radiotherapy planning based on scans acquired during quiet respiration can introduce motion artefacts that incorrectly characterize the geometric shape and extent of a tumor.[71] This may result in tumors being imaged in two or more distinct parts, with the axial slices being shuffled out of order. As even tumors adherent to the chest wall[72] and mediastinal lymph nodes[73–75] can move to a significant degree, plans based on a conventional CT scan may lead to inaccurate information on the actual dose distribution in these structures. Until recently, standard "safety" margins were added around tumors in order to ensure target coverage. Studies have shown that even these margins may be insufficient to account for extremes of mobility[76,77] and may increase the risks of toxicity to surrounding organs, which in turn limits the total dose that can be given. Patient-specific margins are required as no clear correlation exists between mobility and anatomical tumor location in the thorax.[78,79]

The addition of individualized margins to the CTV can be used to derive the internal target volume (ITV), as defined by the International Commission on Radiation Units and Measurements (ICRU). The ITV plus setup margin is used to derive the PTV.[80] A large analysis of respiration-induced tumor motion in mainly stage III NSCLC patients reported that the principal component of motion was in the superior–inferior (SI) direction, with 10.8% of tumors moving greater than 1 cm.[72] The proportion of tumors with motion of greater than 5 mm during normal breathing (the value at which a strategy for respiratory motion management was recommended by the American Association of Physicists in Medicine [AAPM] Task Force 76)[81] was 39.2%, 1.8%, and 5.4%, respectively, along the SI, lateral, and anterior–posterior axes.

Several 4D imaging techniques can be used to derive an ITV and determine an approach for motion management. During 4DCT (or respiration-correlated) scanning, spatial and temporal information on organ mobility are generated using cine scans, whereas the respiration waveform is synchronously recorded during imaging.[82,83] One approach involves recording respiratory signals using infrared-reflecting markers on the upper abdomen of the patient during quiet free breathing.[77] The markers are illuminated by infrared-emitting diodes surrounding a camera, which captures the motion of these markers. Generating a single 4DCT scan during quiet respiration is relatively simple, and it poses no problems to patients with poor pulmonary function. The 4DCT scanning procedure of the entire thorax takes about 90 seconds. Ten respiration-correlated 3D datasets are commonly derived from a single 4D dataset, and each represents the patient's anatomy during a single respiratory phase. Options for deriving ITVs from 4DCT scans include (a) contouring the GTV in all phases of the 4DCT, (b) contouring the GTV in only the extreme phases of respiration, and (c) using a maximum intensity projection (MIP) of all phases of the 4DCT.[84]

RADIOTHERAPY PLANNING AND DELIVERY TECHNIQUES THAT INCREASE THE THERAPEUTIC RATIO

A total dose ranging from 60 to 66 Gy, delivered in once-daily fractions of 1.8 to 2 Gy, has arguably been the most common scheme used with full-dose chemotherapy.[26,32,85–87] Phase I/II studies in selected patients assigned with stage III given concurrent chemotherapy have shown the feasibility of dose escalation to 74 Gy.[88,89] However, there is little evidence to support the routine use of a dose greater than 60 Gy when full-dose CRT is used, and the issue is being addressed in an ongoing Radiation Therapy Oncology Group (RTOG) study (0617) of 60 Gy versus 74 Gy.

Interest in altered fractionation regimens led to randomized clinical trials evaluating the radiobiologic hypothesis that radiation delivered over a shorter period of time can minimize the amount of accelerated tumor-cell repopulation observed once cytotoxic therapy is initiated.[90] In the setting of advanced NSCLC, daily doses are increased and usually divided into two or three treatments per day, with time allowed between each dose to minimize late radiation toxicity. A European phase III randomized trial tested the CHART regimen (continuous, hyperfractionated, accelerated radiation therapy) of 1.5 Gy tid to 54 Gy in 12 consecutive days versus a standard regimen of 60 Gy in 6 weeks. A 9% survival benefit for CHART was observed at 2 years.[91] Concurrent chemotherapy schemes have not been evaluated with CHART in phase III trials, and the CHART schedule has not been widely adopted because of high rates of acute mucosal toxicity in addition to the logistics required. In patients who are unfit for concurrent CRT, accelerated fractionated regimens have both radiobiological advantages and increased convenience for patients, when compared to conventional 1.8 to 2 Gy/day regimens. Data from a recent phase III study using once-daily fractions of 2.75 Gy after induction chemotherapy indicated that a dose of 66 Gy can safely be delivered in 5 weeks.[92]

Minimizing Toxicity of Chemoradiotherapy The target volume for stage III tumors lies in close proximity to several important organs at risk such as spinal cord, lung, heart, and esophagus. Therefore, dose intensification or adding concurrent chemotherapy accentuates the need to produce highly conformal radiotherapy plans that restrict high-dose regions to the PTV by varying beam arrangements, technique, fractionation, and dose. Radiation myelitis is rarely seen clinically, but is a potentially devastating complication. Therefore, a majority of radiation oncologists limit doses to the spinal cord to between 45 and 50 Gy. Attempts to deliver doses that exceed this amount will require beam arrangements that usually lead to increased dose deposition to the lungs. Cardiac dose is usually not a limiting factor as the majority of involved nodes lie above the atria, but can be a consideration in central or retrocardiac tumors. The esophagus is a mediastinal structure that usually runs the entire length of the PTV, resulting in a sixfold increase in grade 3 or greater esophagitis with concurrent CRT.[29] Management of acute esophagitis is therefore a key component of any stage III NSCLC radiotherapy treatment, but it is rarely dose limiting.

A few key developments in the technology of radiation planning and delivery have allowed radiotherapy departments to produce plans that are closer to the "ideal" than ever before. They include the availability of improved dose-calculation algorithms, respiratory-gated radiotherapy (RGRT), intensity-modulated radiotherapy (IMRT), and image acquisition during a course of treatment leading to the possibility of adaptive radiotherapy.

Improved Radiation Dose Calculation Good clinical decisions can only be made if the dose estimated by a treatment planning system accurately portrays reality. Corrections for density differences within the thorax results in more accurate dose distributions, with studies showing that previous lung plans that ignored density differences often delivered 5% to 10% in excess of the intended dose.[93] The AAPM Task Group 65 recommends that lung inhomogeneity correction always be used.[94] Not all modern treatment planning algorithms accurately perform this correction, however, and significant discrepancies may still exist.[95] Unfortunately, despite incorporating motion within a suitable treatment volume, planning systems that adjust dose calculations for 4D motion have not been released as of yet. Plans for mobile tumors are currently mainly based on a single intermediate phase of respiration.

Respiratory-Gated Radiotherapy Several strategies for mobility management are entering routine clinical practice, including full incorporation of target motion, freezing target motion, intercepting target motion, or tracking the tumor.[96] It is essential that a department first consider the accuracy, work load, patient tolerance, imaging dose, and resources required for the chosen approach.[97] The use of RGRT permits a reduction in field sizes as irradiation can be limited to phases in which the mobile target volume is in a predetermined position (Fig. 42.2). An analysis in stage III NSCLC suggested a potential benefit of RGRT using three consecutive phases at end-tidal expiration.[98] Specifically, gating reduced the V_{20} and mean lung dose by 5% and 3 Gy, respectively, and was most beneficial for the more mobile tumors located in the middle and lower lobes.

Intensity-Modulated Delivery of Radiotherapy IMRT abandons the traditional static, coplanar fields of conventional radiotherapy in order to give highly conformal dose delivery. The intensity of beams are modulated by moving small leaves in and out of the field aperture, resulting in individual fields that deliver a heterogeneous dose but when summed from a number of different directions deliver a homogenous dose to a target with excellent conformality. IMRT can be used to limit the amount of high-dose radiation to normal lung and to produce complex concavities in dose distributions that spare

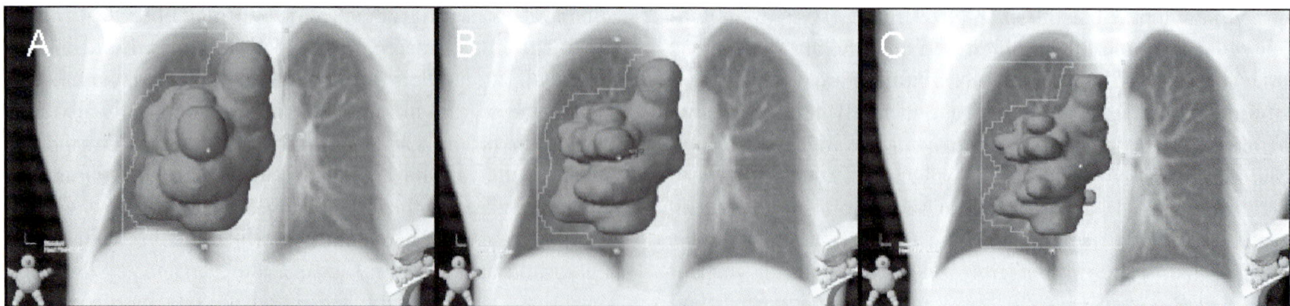

FIGURE 42.2 Planning target volumes (*red*) and corresponding treatment portals (*yellow*) for a patient with stage III NSCLC. **(A)** is derived from a single 3DCT scan with the addition of standard planning margins,[98] **(B)** is an internal target volume (ITV) encompassing all motion observed on 4DCT scan acquired during quiet respiration, and **(C)** is the ITV from motion in three phases at end inspiration for audio-coached gated radiotherapy. The amount of right lung tissue outside the portal is maximal with approach **C**. (See color plate.)

dose to structures like spinal cord and esophagus.[99] IMRT delivery is sensitive to target motion, however, based on the summation required to deliver a homogenous dose. Furthermore, the use of IMRT has led to an increase in the V_5 (percentage volume of normal lung receiving more than 5 Gy), which may in turn increase treatment-related pneumonitis rates.[100,101] IMRT combined with concurrent chemotherapy has yet to be compared to conventional radiotherapy with concurrent chemotherapy in randomized clinical trials.

Adaptive Radiotherapy The reproducibility of NSCLC volumes generated at time of simulation over an entire course of radiotherapy has been investigated by several groups[102–104] with the intent of potentially reducing the irradiated volume to treat a PTV that has potentially shrunk over time. In a group of stage I tumors treated with stereotactic radiotherapy,[105] repeat 4DCT showed no significant change in the ITV. Studies that have included patients with stage III cancer have shown conflicting results[106,107] and prospective data to show that reduced margins will not increase local recurrence rates secondary to inadequately treated microscopic disease are awaited.

CONCLUSION

Radiotherapy remains a key treatment modality for stage III NSCLC, with improvements in survival attributed mainly to combined treatment with cisplatin-containing chemotherapy. Locoregional control remains suboptimal, however, and recent efforts have been aimed at incorporating the technological advances in multimodality imaging and radiotherapy planning to further improve the therapeutic ratio.

REFERENCES

1. Jemal A, Siegel R, Ward E, et al. Cancer statistics, 2007. *CA Cancer J Clin* 2007;57:43–66.
2. Mountain CF. Revisions in the International System for Staging Lung Cancer. *Chest* 1997;111:1710–1717.
3. Wisnivesky JP, Yankelevitz D, Henschke CI. Stage of lung cancer in relation to its size: part 2. Evidence. *Chest* 2005;127:1136–1139.
4. Goldstraw P, Crowley J, Chansky K, et al. The IASLC Lung Cancer Staging Project: proposals for the revision of the TNM stage groupings in the forthcoming (seventh) edition of the TNM Classification of malignant tumours.[Article]. *J Thoracic Oncol* 2007;2:706–714.
5. van Meerbeeck JP, Kramer GW, Van Schil PE, et al. Randomized controlled trial of resection versus radiotherapy after induction chemotherapy in stage IIIA-N2 non-small-cell lung cancer. *J Natl Cancer Inst* 2007;99:442–450.
6. Rusch VW, Giroux DJ, Kraut MJ, et al. Induction chemoradiation and surgical resection for superior sulcus non-small-cell lung carcinomas: long-term results of Southwest Oncology Group Trial 9416 (Intergroup Trial 0160). *J Clin Oncol* 2007;25:313–318.
7. Eberhardt WE, Albain KS, Pass H, et al. Induction treatment before surgery for non-small cell lung cancer. *Lung Cancer* 2003;42(Suppl 1): S9–S14.
8. Silvestri GA, Gould MK, Margolis ML, et al. Noninvasive staging of non-small cell lung cancer: ACCP evidenced-based clinical practice guidelines (2nd edition). *Chest* 2007;132:S178–S201.
9. Naruke T, Suemasu K, Ishikawa S. Lymph node mapping and curability at various levels of metastasis in resected lung cancer. *J Thorac Cardiovasc Surg* 1978;76:832–839.
10. Wahl RL, Quint LE, Greenough RL, et al. Staging of mediastinal non-small cell lung cancer with FDG PET, CT, and fusion images: preliminary prospective evaluation. *Radiology* 1994;191:371–377.
11. Fernández-Esparrach G, Ginès A, Belda J, et al. Transesophageal ultrasound-guided fine needle aspiration improves mediastinal staging in patients with non-small cell lung cancer and normal mediastinum on computed tomography. *Lung Cancer* 2006;54:35–40.
12. Dwamena BA, Sonnad SS, Angobaldo JO, et al. Metastases from non-small cell lung cancer: mediastinal staging in the 1990s—meta-analytic comparison of PET and CT. *Radiology* 1999;213:530–536.
13. Line BR, White CS. Positron emission tomography scanning for the diagnosis and management of lung cancer. *Curr Treat Options Oncol* 2004;5:63–73.
14. Shah PL, Singh S, Bower M, et al. The role of transbronchial fine needle aspiration in an integrated care pathway for the assessment of patients with suspected lung cancer. *J Thorac Oncol* 2006;1:324–327.
15. Toloza EM, Harpole L, McCrory DC. Noninvasive staging of non-small cell lung cancer: a review of the current evidence. *Chest* 2003;123: S137S–S146.
16. Gupta NC, Tamim WJ, Graeber GG, et al. Mediastinal lymph node sampling following positron emission tomography with fluorodeoxyglucose imaging in lung cancer staging. *Chest* 2001;120:521–527.
17. Senan S. Staging nodal disease in non-small cell lung cancer: implications for radiation therapy. *J Thorac Oncol* 2007;2:585–587.
18. Mac Manus MP, Hicks RJ, Ball DL, et al. F-18 fluorodeoxyglucose positron emission tomography staging in radical radiotherapy candidates with nonsmall cell lung carcinoma: powerful correlation with survival and high impact on treatment. *Cancer* 2001;92:886–895.
19. Rusch VW. Mediastinoscopy: an endangered species? *J Clin Oncol* 2005;23:8283–8285.
20. Annema JT, Versteegh MI, Veseliç M, et al. Endoscopic ultrasound added to mediastinoscopy for preoperative staging of patients with lung cancer. *JAMA* 2005;294:931–936.
21. Yasufuku K, Nakajima T, Chiyo M, et al. Endobronchial ultrasonography: current status and future directions. *J Thorac Oncol* 2007;2:970–979.
22. Herth FJ, Rabe KF, Gasparini S, et al. Transbronchial and transoesophageal (ultrasound-guided) needle aspirations for the analysis of mediastinal lesions. *Eur Respir J* 2006;28:1264–1275.
23. Robinson LA, Ruckdeschel JC, Wagner H Jr, et al. Treatment of non-small cell lung cancer-stage IIIA: ACCP evidence-based clinical practice guidelines (2nd edition). *Chest* 2007;132:S243–S265.
24. Gridelli C, Langer C, Maione P, et al. Lung cancer in the elderly. *J Clin Oncol* 2007;25:1898–1907.
25. Jett JR, Schild SE, Keith RL, et al. Treatment of non-small cell lung cancer, stage IIIB: ACCP evidence-based clinical practice guidelines (2nd edition). *Chest* 2007;132:S266–S276.
26. Albain KS, Swann RS, Rusch VW, et al. Radiotherapy plus chemotherapy with or without surgical resection for stage III non-smallcell lung cancer: a phase III randomised controlled trial. *Lancet* 2009; 374:379–386.
27. Machtay M, Hsu C, Komaki R, et al. Effect of overall treatment time on outcomes after concurrent chemoradiation for locally advanced non-small-cell lung carcinoma: analysis of the Radiation Therapy Oncology Group (RTOG) experience. *Int J Radiat Oncol Biol Phys* 2005;63:667–671.
28. Rolland E, Le Chevalier T, Auperin A, et al. Sequential radio-chemotherapy (RT-CT) versus radiotherapy alone (RT) and concomitant RT-CT versus RT alone in locally advanced non-small cell lung cancer (NSCLC): Two meta-analyses using individual patient data (IPD) from randomised clinical trials (RCTs). *J Thorac Oncol* 2007;2:S309–S310.
29. Auperin A, Rolland E, Curran WJ, et al. Concomitant radio-chemotherapy (RT-CT) versus sequential RT-CT in locally advanced non-small cell lung cancer (NSCLC): A meta-analysis using individual patient data (IPD) from randomised clinical trials (RCTs). *J Thorac Oncol* 2007;2:S310.

30. Pignon JP, Tribodet H, Scagliotti GV, et al. Lung adjuvant cisplatin evaluation (LACE): A pooled analysis of five randomized clinical trials including 4,584 patients. *J Clin Oncol* 2006;24:S366.
31. Olaussen KA, Dunant A, Fouret P, et al. DNA repair by ERCC1 in non-small-cell lung cancer and cisplatin-based adjuvant chemotherapy. *N Engl J Med* 2006;355:983–991.
32. Vokes EE, Herndon JE II, Kelley MJ, et al. Induction chemotherapy followed by chemoradiotherapy compared with chemoradiotherapy alone for regionally advanced unresectable stage III Non-small-cell lung cancer: Cancer and Leukemia Group B. *J Clin Oncol* 2007;25: 1698–1704.
33. Clamon G, Herndon J, Cooper R, et al. Radiosensitization with carboplatin for patients with unresectable stage III non-small-cell lung cancer: a phase III trial of the Cancer and Leukemia Group B and the Eastern Cooperative Oncology Group. *J Clin Oncol* 1999;17:4–11.
34. Groen HJ, van der Leest AH, Fokkema E, et al. Continuously infused carboplatin used as radiosensitizer in locally unresectable non-small-cell lung cancer: a multicenter phase III study. *Ann Oncol* 2004;15: 427–432.
35. Gervais R, Ducolone A, Le chevalier T, et al. Conventional radiation (RT) with daily carboplatin (Cb) compared to RT alone after induction chemotherapy (ICT) [vinorelbine (Vr)-cisplatine (P)]: Final results of a randomized phase III trial in stage III unresectable non small cell lung (NSCLC) cancer. Study CRG/BMS/NPC/96 of the French Lung Cancer Study Group FNCLCC and IFCT. *J Clin Oncol* 2005; 23:S625.
36. Douillard JY, Rosell R, De Lena M, et al. Adjuvant vinorelbine plus cisplatin versus observation in patients with completely resected stage IB-IIIA non-small-cell lung cancer (Adjuvant Navelbine International Trialist Association [ANITA]): a randomised controlled trial. *Lancet Oncol* 2006;7:719–727.
37. Arriagada R, Bergman B, Dunant A, et al. Cisplatin-based adjuvant chemotherapy in patients with completely resected non-small-cell lung cancer. *N Engl J Med* 2004;350:351–360.
38. Lally BE, Zelterman D, Colasanto JM, et al. Postoperative radiotherapy for stage II or III non-small-cell lung cancer using the surveillance, epidemiology, and end results database. *J Clin Oncol* 2006;24: 2998–3006.
39. Postoperative radiotherapy in non-small-cell lung cancer: systematic review and meta-analysis of individual patient data from nine randomised controlled trials. PORT Meta-analysis Trialists Group. *Lancet* 1998;352:257–263.
40. Machtay M, Lee JH, Shrager JB, et al. Risk of death from intercurrent disease is not excessively increased by modern postoperative radiotherapy for high-risk resected non-small-cell lung carcinoma. *J Clin Oncol* 2001;19:3912–3917.
41. Wakelee HA, Stephenson P, Keller SM, et al. Post-operative radiotherapy (PORT) or chemoradiotherapy (CPORT) following resection of stages II and IIIA non-small cell lung cancer (NSCLC) does not increase the expected risk of death from intercurrent disease (DID) in Eastern Cooperative Oncology Group (ECOG) trial E3590. *Lung Cancer* 2005;48:389–397.
42. Le Péchoux C, Dunant A, Pignon JP, et al. Need for a new trial to evaluate adjuvant postoperative radiotherapy in non-small-cell lung cancer patients with N2 mediastinal involvement. *J Clin Oncol* 2007;25: E10–E11.
43. Pisters KM, Evans WK, Azzoli CG, et al. Cancer Care Ontario and American Society of Clinical Oncology adjuvant chemotherapy and adjuvant radiation therapy for stages I-IIIA resectable non small-cell lung cancer guideline. *J Clin Oncol* 2007;25:5506–5518.
44. Senan S, Lagerwaard FJ. The role of radiotherapy in non-small-cell lung cancer. *Ann Oncol* 2005;16(Suppl 2):II223–II228.
45. Graham MV, Purdy JA, Emami B, et al. Clinical dose-volume histogram analysis for pneumonitis after 3D treatment for non-small cell lung cancer (NSCLC). *Int J Radiat Oncol Biol Phys* 1999;45:323–329.
46. Kelly K, Chansky K, Gaspar LE, et al. Updated analysis of SWOG 0023: a randomized phase III trial of gefitinib versus placebo maintenance after definitive chemoradiation followed by docetaxel in patients with locally advanced stage III non-small cell lung cancer. *ASCO Meeting Abstracts* 2007;25:7513.
47. Ahn SJ, Kahn D, Zhou SM, et al. Dosimetric and clinical predictors for radiation-induced esophageal injury. *Int J Radiat Oncol Biol Phys* 2005;61:335–347.
48. Rosenman JG, Halle JS, Socinski MA, et al. High-dose conformal radiotherapy for treatment of Stage IIIA/IIIB non-small-cell lung cancer: technical issues and results of a phase I/II trial. *Int J Radiat Oncol Biol Phys* 2002;54:348–356.
49. Mah K, Caldwell CB, Ung YC, et al. The impact of (18)FDG-PET on target and critical organs in CT-based treatment planning of patients with poorly defined non-small-cell lung carcinoma: a prospective study. *Int J Radiat Oncol Biol Phys* 2002;52:339–350.
50. Nestle U, Kremp S, Grosu AL. Practical integration of [F-18]-FDG-PET and PET-CT in the planning of radiotherapy for non-small cell lung cancer (NSCLC): the technical basis, ICRU-target volumes, problems, perspectives. *Radiother Oncol* 2006;81:209–225.
51. Caldwell CB, Mah K, Ung YC, et al. Observer variation in contouring gross tumor volume in patients with poorly defined non-small-cell lung tumors on CT: the impact of (18)FDG-hybrid PET fusion. *Int J Radiat Oncol Biol Phys* 2001;51:923–931.
52. Greco C, Rosenzweig K, Cascini GL, et al. Current status of PET/CT for tumour volume definition in radiotherapy treatment planning for non-small cell lung cancer (NSCLC). *Lung Cancer* 2007;57:125–134.
53. Emami B. Three-dimensional conformal radiation therapy in bronchogenic carcinoma. *Semin Radiat Oncol* 1996;6:92–97.
54. Hayman JA, Martel MK, Ten Haken RK, et al. Dose escalation in non-small-cell lung cancer using three-dimensional conformal radiation therapy: update of a phase I trial. *J Clin Oncol* 2001;19:127–136.
55. Belderbos JS, De Jaeger K, Heemsbergen WD, et al. First results of a phase I/II dose escalation trial in non-small cell lung cancer using three-dimensional conformal radiotherapy. *Radiother Oncol* 2003;66: 119–126.
56. Senan S, Burgers S, Samson MJ, et al. Can elective nodal irradiation be omitted in stage III non-small-cell lung cancer? Analysis of recurrences in a phase II study of induction chemotherapy and involved-field radiotherapy. *Int J Radiat Oncol Biol Phys* 2002;54:999–1006.
57. Rosenzweig KE, Sim SE, Mychalczak B, et al. Elective nodal irradiation in the treatment of non-small-cell lung cancer with three-dimensional conformal radiation therapy. *Int J Radiat Oncol Biol Phys* 2001;50: 681–685.
58. Yuan S, Sun X, Li M, et al. A randomized study of involved-field irradiation versus elective nodal irradiation in combination with concurrent chemotherapy for inoperable stage III nonsmall cell lung cancer. *Am J Clin Oncol* 2007;30:239–244.
59. Senan S, De Ruysscher D, Giraud P, et al. Literature-based recommendations for treatment planning and execution in high-dose radiotherapy for lung cancer. *Radiother Oncol* 2004;71:139–146.
60. Glazer GM, Gross BH, Quint LE, et al. Normal mediastinal lymph nodes: number and size according to American Thoracic Society mapping. *AJR Am J Roentgenol* 1985;144:261–265.
61. Kiyono K, Sone S, Sakai F, et al. The number and size of normal mediastinal lymph nodes: a postmortem study. *AJR Am J Roentgenol* 1988;150:771–776.
62. Prenzel KL, Mönig SP, Sinning JM, et al. Lymph node size and metastatic infiltration in non-small cell lung cancer. *Chest* 2003;123: 463–467.
63. De Leyn P, Lardinois D, Van Schil PE, et al. ESTS guidelines for preoperative lymph node staging for non-small cell lung cancer. *Eur J Cardiothorac Surg* 2007;32:1–8.
64. de Langen AJ, Raijmakers P, Riphagen I, et al. The size of mediastinal lymph nodes and its relation with metastatic involvement: a meta-analysis. *Eur J Cardiothorac Surg* 2006;29:26–29.
65. Lardinois D, Weder W, Hany TF, et al. Staging of non-small-cell lung cancer with integrated positron-emission tomography and computed tomography. *N Engl J Med* 2003;348:2500–2507.

66. Giraud P, Antoine M, Larrouy A, et al. Evaluation of microscopic tumor extension in non-small-cell lung cancer for three-dimensional conformal radiotherapy planning. *Int J Radiat Oncol Biol Phys* 2000;48: 1015–1024.
67. Kara M, Sak SD, Orhan D, et al. Changing patterns of lung cancer; (3/4 in.) 1.9 cm; still a safe length for bronchial resection margin? *Lung Cancer* 2000;30:161–168.
68. Vansteenkiste JF, De Leyn PR, Deneffe GJ, et al. Survival and prognostic factors in resected N2 non-small cell lung cancer: a study of 140 cases. *Ann Thorac Surg* 1997;63:1441–1450.
69. Lee YC, Wu CT, Kuo SW, et al. Significance of extranodal extension of regional lymph nodes in surgically resected non-small cell lung cancer. *Chest* 2007;131:993–999.
70. Yuan S, Meng X, Yu J, et al. Determining optimal clinical target volume margins on the basis of microscopic extracapsular extension of metastatic nodes in patients with non-small-cell lung cancer. *Int J Radiat Oncol Biol Phys* 2007;67:727–734.
71. Balter JM, Ten Haken RK, Lawrence TS, et al. Uncertainties in CT-based radiation therapy treatment planning associated with patient breathing. *Int J Radiat Oncol Biol Phys* 1996;36:167–174.
72. Liu HH, Balter P, Tutt T, et al. Assessing respiration-induced tumor motion and internal target volume using four-dimensional computed tomography for radiotherapy of lung cancer. *Int J Radiat Oncol Biol Phys* 2007;68:531–540.
73. Piet AH, Lagerwaard FJ, Kunst PW, et al. Can mediastinal nodal mobility explain the low yield rates for transbronchial needle aspiration without real-time imaging? *Chest* 2007;131:1783–1787.
74. Donnelly ED, Parikh PJ, Lu W, et al. Assessment of intrafraction mediastinal and hilar lymph node movement and comparison to lung tumor motion using four-dimensional CT. *Int J Radiat Oncol Biol Phys* 2007;69:580–588.
75. Sher DJ, Wolfgang JA, Niemierko A, et al. Quantification of mediastinal and hilar lymph node movement using four-dimensional computed tomography scan: implications for radiation treatment planning. *Int J Radiat Oncol Biol Phys* 2007;69:1402–1408.
76. van Sörnsen de Koste JR, Lagerwaard FJ, Schuchhard-Schipper RH, et al. Dosimetric consequences of tumor mobility in radiotherapy of stage I non-small cell lung cancer—an analysis of data generated using 'slow' CT scans. *Radiother Oncol* 2001;61:93–99.
77. Underberg RW, Lagerwaard FJ, Cuijpers JP, et al. Four-dimensional CT scans for treatment planning in stereotactic radiotherapy for stage I lung cancer. *Int J Radiat Oncol Biol Phys* 2004;60:1283–1290.
78. Underberg RW, Lagerwaard FJ, Slotman BJ, et al. Benefit of respiration-gated stereotactic radiotherapy for stage I lung cancer: An analysis of 4DCT datasets. *Int J Radiat Oncol Biol Phys* 2005;62:554–560.
79. van Sörnsen de Koste JR, Lagerwaard FJ, Nijssen-Visser MR, et al. Tumor location cannot predict the mobility of lung tumors: a 3D analysis of data generated from multiple CT scans. *Int J Radiat Oncol Biol Phys* 2003;56:348–354.
80. International Commission on Radiation Units and Measurements. Prescribing, Recording and Reporting Photon Beam Therapy (supplement to ICRU Report 50). Bethesda, MD, 1999. ICRU Report 62.
81. Keall PJ, Mageras GS, Balter JM, et al. The management of respiratory motion in radiation oncology report of AAPM Task Group 76. *Med Phys* 2006;33:3874–3900.
82. Pan T, Lee TY, Rietzel E, et al. 4D-CT imaging of a volume influenced by respiratory motion on multi-slice CT. *Med Phys* 2004;31: 333–340.
83. Ford EC, Mageras GS, Yorke E, et al. Respiration-correlated spiral CT: a method of measuring respiratory-induced anatomic motion for radiation treatment planning. *Med Phys* 2003;30:88–97.
84. Underberg RW, Lagerwaard FJ, Slotman BJ, et al. Use of maximum intensity projections (MIP) for target volume generation in 4DCT scans for lung cancer. *Int J Radiat Oncol Biol Phys* 2005;63:253–260.
85. Fournel P, Robinet G, Thomas P, et al. Randomized phase III trial of sequential chemoradiotherapy compared with concurrent chemoradiotherapy in locally advanced non-small-cell lung cancer: Groupe Lyon-Saint-Etienne d'Oncologie Thoracique-Groupe Francais de Pneumo-Cancérologie NPC 95-01 Study. *J Clin Oncol* 2005;23: 5910–5917.
86. Senan S, Van Meerbeeck JP, Cardenal F, et al. 159: Treatment Compliance and Early Toxicity of 3D Involved-Field Radiotherapy (RT) and Chemotherapy (CT) in a Randomized Study Comparing Induction CT Followed by Concurrent CT-RT With Concurrent CT-RT Followed by Consolidation CT, in Non-Small-Cell Lung Cancer (NSCLC). *Int J Radiat Oncol Biol Phys* 2006;66:S89–S90.
87. Garrido P, Massuti T, Moran T, et al. Concomitant chemoradiation plus induction (I) or consolidation (C) chemotherapy (CT) with docetaxel (D) and gemcitabine (G) for unresectable stage III non-small cell lung cancer (NSCLC) patients (p). Results of the randomized SLCG 0008 phase II trial. *ASCO Meeting Abstracts* 2007;25:7620.
88. Bradley JD, Graham M, Suzanne S, et al. Phase I results of RTOG L-0117; a phase I/II dose intensification study using 3DCRT and concurrent chemotherapy for patients with Inoperable NSCLC. *ASCO Meeting Abstracts* 2005;23:7063.
89. Schild SE, McGinnis WL, Graham D, et al. Results of a phase I trial of concurrent chemotherapy and escalating doses of radiation for unresectable non-small-cell lung cancer. *Int J Radiat Oncol Biol Phys* 2006;65:1106–1111.
90. Mehta M, Scrimger R, Mackie R, et al. A new approach to dose escalation in non-small-cell lung cancer. *Int J Radiat Oncol Biol Phys* 2001; 49:23–33.
91. Saunders M, Dische S, Barrett A, et al. Continuous hyperfractionated accelerated radiotherapy (CHART) versus conventional radiotherapy in non-small-cell lung cancer: a randomised multicentre trial. CHART Steering Committee. *Lancet* 1997;350:161–165.
92. Belderbos J, Uitterhoeve L, van Zandwijk N, et al. Randomised trial of sequential versus concurrent chemo-radiotherapy in patients with inoperable non-small cell lung cancer (EORTC 08972-22973). *Eur J Cancer* 2007;43:114–121.
93. Orton CG, Chungbin S, Klein EE, et al. Study of lung density corrections in a clinical trial (RTOG 88-08). Radiation Therapy Oncology Group. *Int J Radiat Oncol Biol Phys* 1998;41:787–794.
94. American Association of Physicists in Medicine. *Tissue Inhomogeneity Corrections for Megavoltage Photon Beams*. Madison, WI: Medical Physics Publishing, 2004. AAPM Report No.85.
95. De Jaeger K, Hoogeman MS, Engelsman M, et al. Incorporating an improved dose-calculation algorithm in conformal radiotherapy of lung cancer: re-evaluation of dose in normal lung tissue. *Radiother Oncol* 2003;69:1–10.
96. Lagerwaard FJ, Senan S. Lung cancer: intensity-modulated radiation therapy, four-dimensional imaging and mobility management. *Front Radiat Ther Oncol* 2007;40:239–252.
97. Mageras GS. Introduction: management of target localization uncertainties in external-beam therapy. *Sem Radiat Oncol* 2005;15:133–135.
98. Underberg R, van Sörnsen de Koste JR, Lagerwaard F, et al. A dosimetric analysis of respiration-gated radiotherapy in patients with stage III lung cancer. *Radiat Oncol* 2006;1:8.
99. Derycke S, Van Duyse B, De Gersem W, et al. Non-coplanar beam intensity modulation allows large dose escalation in stage III lung cancer. *Radiother Oncol* 1997;45:253–261.
100. Yorke ED, Jackson A, Rosenzweig KE, et al. Correlation of dosimetric factors and radiation pneumonitis for non-small-cell lung cancer patients in a recently completed dose escalation study. *Int J Radiat Oncol Biol Phys* 2005;63:672–682.
101. Wang S, Liao Z, Wei X, et al. Analysis of clinical and dosimetric factors associated with treatment-related pneumonitis (TRP) in patients with non-small-cell lung cancer (NSCLC) treated with concurrent chemotherapy and three-dimensional conformal radiotherapy (3D-CRT). *Int J Radiat Oncol Biol Phys* 2006;66:1399–1407.
102. Kupelian PA, Ramsey C, Meeks SL, et al. Serial megavoltage CT imaging during external beam radiotherapy for non-small-cell lung cancer: observations on tumor regression during treatment. *Int J Radiat Oncol Biol Phys* 2005;63:1024–1028.

103. Siker ML, Tomé WA, Mehta MP. Tumor volume changes on serial imaging with megavoltage CT for non-small-cell lung cancer during intensity-modulated radiotherapy: how reliable, consistent, and meaningful is the effect? *Int J Radiat Oncol Biol Phys* 2006;66:135–141.
104. Ramsey CR, Langen KM, Kupelian PA, et al. A technique for adaptive image-guided helical tomotherapy for lung cancer. *Int J Radiat Oncol Biol Phys* 2006;64:1237–1244.
105. Haasbeek CJ, Lagerwaard FJ, Cuijpers JP, et al. Is adaptive treatment planning required for stereotactic radiotherapy of stage I non-small-cell lung cancer? *Int J Radiat Oncol Biol Phys* 2007;67:1370–1374.
106. Britton KR, Starkschall G, Tucker SL, et al. Assessment of gross tumor volume regression and motion changes during radiotherapy for non-small-cell lung cancer as measured by four-dimensional computed tomography. *Int J Radiat Oncol Biol Phys* 2007;68: 1036–1046.
107. Bosmans G, van Baardwijk A, Dekker A, et al. Intra-patient variability of tumor volume and tumor motion during conventionally fractionated radiotherapy for locally advanced non-small-cell lung cancer: a prospective clinical study. *Int J Radiat Oncol Biol Phys* 2006; 66:748–753.

CHAPTER 43

Robert D. Timmerman
Timothy D. Solberg
Brian D. Kavanagh
Simon S. Lo

Stereotactic Techniques for Lung Cancer Treatment

Historically, the term *stereotactic* is related to the correlation of tumor target position to reliable fiducials position that could be readily identified from various imaging platforms.[1] Radiation treatments guided by such fiducials were referred to as *stereotactic radiation therapy*. Fiducials define a coordinate system that can be used to target the tumor, orient the treatment planning process, and ultimately guide the therapy toward the intended location in the body. These fiducials were typically placed in a rigid frame outside the patient.[2] Today, with sophisticated real-time image guidance, the tumor itself can serve as the fiducial negating the need for external markers that have classically characterized stereotactic treatments. [3–6] In the end, modern stereotactic radiotherapy is a little about "stereotaxy" and a lot about dose fractionation, target definition, motion control (four-dimensional [4D] therapy), image guidance, conformal and compact dose distributions, and high levels of quality assurance in treatment conduct.[7] Irrespective of the current significance of the term "stereotaxy," modern treatments to lung tumors using such technology intensive techniques and giving less than five potent treatments are referred to as stereotactic body radiation therapy (SBRT).[8,9]

SBRT, or synonomously stereotactic ablative radiotherapy (SABR), is biologically unique from conventional fractionated radiation therapy (CFRT). Whereas CFRT is typically administered in small daily doses in the range of 1.8 to 2.0 Gy to total doses of 60 to 70 Gy, SBRT is intended to be ablative. These ablative treatments are very potent because considerably higher doses per fraction are applied, generally in the range of 10 to 20 Gy per fraction. Biologically, affected cells are both unable to divide and unable to perform intended cellular functions (e.g., secretion, transport oxygen, etc.). Such high doses per treatment were historically out of bounds because limitations in treatment delivery technology did not allow the radiation oncologist to avoid catastrophic toxicity when large volumes of normal tissues were exposed to so much radiation each treatment. With improvements in tumor imaging, image guidance, computerized dosimetry, and treatment delivery devices, such very large dose-per-fraction treatments are no longer out of bounds. Indeed, they are showing dramatic utility for their ability to safety eradicate cancer.

SBRT has been shown to be particularly effective in eradicating the primary tumor in early stage lung cancer.[10–17] SBRT offers an elegant, noninvasive, and highly efficient treatment option that is preferred by patients because of its convenience. SBRT has not been generally used in patients with lymph node metastases, however, because of difficulty in targeting the entire extent of tumor as well as toxicity concerns relating to the central chest. In metastatic lung cancer, SBRT may be used as an ablative or cytoreductive agent in selected patients.

Because of its normal-tissue dose sparing facilitated by the unique dose distribution and imaging technology, frail patients can tolerate the treatment surprisingly well. It is considered a standard treatment in such patients with stage I non–small cell lung cancer (NSCLC).[18] Despite its ability to treat the frailest patients, SBRT should still be viewed as the most potent radiation treatment with clinical experience in fighting gross tumor deposits. Local control with SBRT has been shown to be dramatically superior to historical controls using CFRT for early stage lung cancer. Indeed, local control with SBRT rivals surgical resection for most indications. Limitations definitely exist as will be discussed in this chapter. With careful clinical testing and implementation, SBRT is finding a prominent place within the cancer treatment arsenal.

DEVELOPMENT OF STEREOTACTIC BODY RADIATION THERAPY

The success of brain radiosurgery pioneered by Swedish neurosurgeon Lars Leksell[1] forms the basis of SBRT. Leksell not only developed what would become the modern day Gamma Knife, he departed from the current practice of the time to deliver radiation in a protracted fractionation schedule. With the newly developed technology, large dose-per-fraction treatments given in a single treatment at dose levels that would have historically resulted in considerable calamity were able to be routinely delivered in the dose intolerant brain. The new treatment conduct went to great lengths to avoid prescription level dose to normal tissues. Whatever normal tissue was included, either by being adjacent to the target or by inferior dosimetry, was likely damaged. However, if this damaged tissue was small in volume or noneloquent, the patient did not suffer clinically apparent toxicity, even as a late event. On the other hand, it is undeniable that the large dose-per-fraction treatments are biologically extremely potent by overwhelming repair mechanisms.[19] Targeted tumors are disabled and toxicity is avoided by simply missing most normal tissue.

Hamilton et al.[20] performed the earliest examples of treatments mimicking the stereotactic radiosurgery (SRS) treatments outside of the brain. These treatments employed the same rigid immobilization principles of SRS in the spine by screwing a frame to the spinous processes. Although reports were encouraging, the conduct of the treatment was not as gratifying as natural and inherent motion confounded accuracy. The brain can be practically immobilized by immobilizing the skull. Once the skull is immobilized, targets within the brain have very little additional movement. Such is not the case outside of the skull. Tumors in the body may be displaced as a function of time by forces exerted by muscle contraction, breathing, gastrointestinal peristalsis, cardiac activity, and many other important physiological processes. It is not possible to eliminate or account for all of these forces. As a result, SBRT is inherently less accurate than SRS.

As with the Gamma Knife, researchers again from Sweden, Ingmar Lax and Henric Blomgren, set out to overcome these problems by constructing a body frame that would both comfortably immobilize the patients torso as well as dampen the internal motion relating to respiration.[21,22] Subsequently, they treated patients with localized tumors using dosimetry plans that mimicked SRS.[23] The dosimetry was constructed using multiple noncoplanar beams with aperture dimensions on the order of the target dimensions. Each of the many beams carried relatively lower weight than with CFRT such that the target dose at the convergence could be dramatically escalated. Blomgren and Lax treated patients with mostly metastases initially. Local tumor control was better than expected, leading them to treat more limited stage cancer patients. Blomgren et al.[24] shared their results via publications and eventually trained others in this new technique.

Meanwhile, investigators from Japan were exploring radiosurgery-like treatments in the chest. Shirato et al.[25] pioneered investigation into characterization and accounting of respiratory motion. Initially, they used CFRT dose schedules, but the understanding of target motion control was very important for the ultimate feasibility of SBRT, as it currently exists. Uematsu et al.[26–28] again from Japan worked in the early 1990s on developing technologies for delivering multiple focused beams of radiation for extracranial targets. In addition, Uematsu's group treated patients with lung tumors primarily from primary non–small cell cancer.

Prospective testing of SBRT began with acquisition of the technology by the groups from the University of Heidelberg, University of Wurzburg, Kyoto University, and Indiana University.[11,14,29,30] Initially, dose-escalation toxicity studies were carried out in the liver and lung trying to find the most potent dose schedules for typically radioresistant primary and metastatic tumors. These prospective trials have been reported but are still maturing and will add a wealth of understanding for the use of SBRT. It is already clear that local tumor control will be higher with SBRT than has been observed with CFRT. SBRT is now a standard treatment for patients with peripheral tumors from early stage lung cancer with simultaneous medical problems precluding surgery. However, toxicity from large dose-per-fraction radiation schedules often appears quite "late" from time of treatment. Therefore, the total impact of treatment, good and bad, will require many years of follow-up to fully appreciate.

DEFINITIONS AND NOMENCLATURE OF STEREOTACTIC BODY RADIATION THERAPY

SBRT is best defined by its conduct. The proper performance of SBRT requires a team approach to carry out the following tasks[31]:

1. Secure yet comfortable immobilization avoiding patient movement for the typical long treatment sessions.
2. Accurate repositioning of the patient from planning sessions to each of the treatment sessions.
3. Proper accounting of inherent internal organ motion, including breathing motion consistently between planning and treatment.
4. Construction of dose distributions confidently covering tumor and yet falling off very rapidly to surrounding normal tissues. The dosimetry must be extremely conformal in relation to the prescription isodose line compared to the target outline but may allow very heterogeneous target dose ranges.
5. Registration of the patient's anatomy, constructed dosimetry, and treatment delivery to a three-dimensional coordinate system as referenced to fiducials. Fiducials are "markers" whose position can be confidently correlated to both the tumor target and the treatment delivery device. A "stereotactic" treatment is one directed by such fiducial references.
6. Biologically, potent dose prescriptions using a few (i.e., one to five) fractions of very high dose (e.g., generally a minimum of 6 Gy per fraction but often as high as 20 to 30 Gy per fraction).

A working group from the American College of Radiology and American Society for Therapeutic Radiology and Oncology had formulated guidelines for the conduct of SBRT.[8] In general, SBRT is used to treat well-demarcated visible gross disease up to 5 to 7 cm in dimension. It is not used for prophylactic (adjuvant) treatment, as the intent is to totally disrupt clonogenicity and likely disrupt all cellular functioning of the target tissues (i.e., the definition of an ablative therapy).[32–36]

Tissues exposed to the prescription dose level or nearby are likely to be ablated. Such a treatment, properly directed would constitute a most potent form of cancer therapy. In turn, if misdirected or used too liberally, SBRT could lead to debilitating toxicity. At any rate, SBRT is very different from conventionally fractionated radiation therapy (CFRT) in its conduct, toxicity, and ability to control cancer. To this end, it is clear that all forms of radiotherapy do not constitute a black box.

MOTION ISSUES FOR LUNG STEREOTACTIC BODY RADIATION THERAPY

Treatment plans are generally static with no specific accounting of motion that is typical in the treated patients. Still, the geometry and dose distribution from the radiation therapy treatment plan should be a reasonably true characterization of what is actually delivered to the patient. With the typical large volume of treatment and homogeneous dose-distributions characteristic of CFRT, such an emphasis on the proper correlation of the treatment plan and actual treatment is probably not so critical. However, for SBRT, claims regarding accuracy of equipment, quality of dose distributions, and dose tolerance should not be made based on the virtual computer simulation of the treatment plan; rather, on actual delivery of dose to treated patients. This is particularly true for predicting normal-tissue toxicity from SBRT where both heterogeneous dose and differential volume effects may equally affect outcome.

Although there is a general fascination within the radiotherapy community for electronic or sophisticated mechanical solutions to motion, passive immobilization can be extremely effective. Body frames, vacuum pillows, thermal plastic restraints, and other equipment have been used to try to achieve relocalization similar to the position of simulation,[22,37–49] Other systems will effectively relocate a reference position within the patient prior to each treatment, without the aid of frames or other immobilization devices (i.e., "frameless" systems).[27,50–52] Both approaches have advantages and disadvantages, and no clearly superior method has been identified in clinical practice. In the end, it is most critical to be practical. SBRT treatment sessions are longer than CFRT sessions. Hence, it is important that the positioning system be comfortable and avoids awkward positions or positions fighting against gravity. In addition, the system employed must be properly utilized. As such, staff training and properly administered quality assurance programs are more essential than using a particular brand of equipment.

To minimize treatment margins for coverage, tumor (and normal tissue) motion must be characterized, controlled, or compensated. Motion control accounting approaches fall into three general categories: (a) dampening, (b) gating, and (c) chasing. Within the category of dampening includes the systems of abdominal compression aimed at decreasing one of the largest contributors to respiratory motion related to the diaphragm.[22,41,44–46,49] Also included in this category are the systems employing breath-hold maneuvers to "freeze" the tumor in a reproducible stage of the respiratory cycle (e.g., deep inspiration).[53–56] Gating systems follow the respiratory cycle using a surrogate and employ an electronic beam activation trigger, allowing irradiation to only occur during a specific segment (e.g., end expiration).[50,57–59] Tracking systems literally move the radiation beam along the same path as the tumor from the beam's eye view.[25,60–63] Tracking may be accomplished by moving the entire accelerator, the aperture (e.g., with the multileaf collimator), or moving the patient on the couch counter to the motion of the tumor. In the case of gating and breath hold, the beam is triggered on and off, constituting a duty cycle avoided by the other systems. In any case, the acquisition of planning information must include the same consideration for motion accounting as the treatment to achieve accuracy. Despite available motion control equipment, some uncertainty continues to require that planning treatment volume (PTV) is larger than gross tumor volume (GTV). In general, for typical dose prescriptions, this enlargement should not be greater than 1.0 cm in the cranial caudal plane and 0.5 cm in the axial plane.

BIOLOGICAL ASPECTS OF STEREOTACTIC BODY RADIATION THERAPY

Tumor Biology The cell survival curve (logarithm of surviving fraction vs. dose) after exposure to sparsely ionizing radiation, such as photons and gamma rays, follows a characteristic shape starting with a curving portion called the "shoulder" and then becoming linear with increasing dose. With CFRT, daily treatment is given on the shoulder of the survival curve (daily dose range of 1.5 to 3.0 Gy), where cells are able to repair some of the inflicted damage. The survival data in this region can be mathematically "fit" by a second order polynomial to give a simple functional representation. The predictive model related to is called the linear-quadratic (LQ) model.[64–66] Although this formula had served the field of radiobiology quite well for decades, several authors have pointed out that this formalism is not applicable in the range of high doses applied with SBRT.[67–69] In effect, the LQ model grossly overestimates the potency of treatment for daily dose delivery beyond the shoulder (i.e., 6 to 8 Gy for most tumor cell lines) caused by erroneous extrapolation outside the area of fit. Guerrero and Li[69] have proposed modifying the LQ formula by incorporating features of the so-called lethal–potentially lethal (LPL) model. The LPL model differs from the LQ model primarily insofar as it accounts for ongoing radiation repair processes that occur *during* the radiation exposure. Marks[68] and Park et al.[67] have borrowed formalism from the older multitarget model[70] to determine a "single fraction equivalent dose" for hypofractionated treatments with daily dose levels greater than 7 to 10 Gy that avoids any use whatsoever of the erroneous LQ model. The net result of more appropriate estimation from tumor cell kill models is a substantial difference in the predicted tumor cell kill at SBRT-level doses. For example, for a dose of approximately 20 Gy, the LQ model would erroneously predict several orders of magnitude greater cell kill than the LPL model.[69]

This debate has practical clinical implications when trying to make comparisons to different dose-fractionation schemes for SBRT. In addition, proper modeling has an impact on the understanding of dose-rate effects. Benedict et al.[71] evaluated clonogenic survival in vitro doses in the range of 12 to 18 Gy, using a glioma cell line. For a dose of 18 Gy, increasing the length of treatment from approximately 1.5 to 2 hours corresponded to an order of magnitude decrement in cytotoxicity. Fowler et al.[72] have reviewed this topic of loss of biological effect with length individual treatment delivery and concluded that any treatment administration that lasts more than half an hour might be associated with a clinically significant loss of cytotoxicity.

Normal-Tissue Biology and Tolerance With large dose-per-fraction treatment given with SBRT, it is useful to define tissues according to their basic organizational structure. Linear or branching structures such as nerves, airways, and bowel passageways are called *serial* (borrowed from electrical circuit nomenclature), because damage at any point effects function downstream. In contrast, redundant repeating structures such as acini within glands, alveoli within the lung, and nephrons within the kidney are called *parallel*, because injury to one does not necessarily imply that neighbors will be affected. Within the lung itself, there are various tissues that possess unique radiation tolerance characteristics, namely, the airways (both large and small functioning as serial structures), vascular trunks and pedicles, following similar routes as the bronchial tree (functioning as serial structures), and the alveoli/capillary complexes (functioning as parallel structures).[73,74] In addition, the thoracic cavity includes the serially functioning esophagus, serially functioning nerve tissue (e.g., phrenic nerves, brachial plexus, etc.), heart, pericardium, and pleura (all difficult to categorize as parallel or serial), and the bones and musculature of the chest wall. All of these structures will have a unique mechanism of injury and tolerance after SBRT.

CFRT commonly causes large serially functioning airway irritation, such as cough, but, rarely, dose-limiting toxicity. In contrast, high-dose SBRT schemes may cause significant large airway damage by both mucosal injury and ultimate collapse of the airway. Along the routes of bronchial airways, a similar injury is experienced by blood vessels following a similar route. Altogether, this collective radiation injury appears to mostly affect oxygenation parameters including diffusing capacity of lung for carbon monoxide (DLCO), arterial oxygen tension (pressure) on room air (PO_2), and supplemental oxygen requirements (FIO_2).[29] Decline in spirometry indices, including forced expiratory volume in 1 second (FEV_1) and forced vital capacity (FVC), are less commonly observed. Because the degree of this airway injury toxicity is related to the proximity of the target to proximal trunks of the branching tubular lung structure, great care should be taken when considering treatment to tumors near the hilum or central chest.

Again, one can show dramatic differences in normal-tissue response between a similar dose of CFRT and SBRT. Although acute and, sometimes, severe esophageal toxicity is commonly seen after CFRT for lung cancer, most of the injury is self-limiting and resolves after treatment. After high-dose SBRT, esophageal strictures may form as a late effect. Another more unique toxicity from SBRT relates to pericardial injury. Pericardial effusions may result after SBRT treatment for tumors treated adjacent to the heart. Probably, by a similar mechanism, pleural effusions commonly develop after SBRT treatment of tumors treated adjacent to the chest wall. Usually, these fluid collections will reabsorb without intervention after several months of follow-up. Rarely, such fluid collections will need to be drained via thoracentesis in patients symptomatic with shortness of breath, pleurisy, or hypoxia.

The term *late effect* implies that it may not first manifest for long periods after delivery of the therapy. Most reports of SBRT do not include long-term follow-up data. As such, there may be unexpected toxicities that need to be recognized, monitored, and evaluated. Particularly, with large doses per fraction, there may be unexpected injury related to nerve tissue and vascular tissue. Ideally, dose to brachial plexus, spinal cord, phrenic nerves, and intercostal nerves will be kept low via prudent treatment planning. Furthermore, avoiding large blood vessels in the central chest would be reasonable as well. Neurovascular calamities including aneurysms, fistulae with bleeding, or neuropathies (including phrenic or vagal nerve palsies) have rarely been reported but may only manifest after many years of follow-up.

In contrast to large volume of irradiation CFRT, direct injury to pulmonary alveoli is considerably less with SBRT owing to the much smaller volumes that receive intermediate and high dose. However, toxicity related to serially functioning tissues is more predominant with SBRT, especially in the central chest. Ideally, SBRT should demonstrate a high degree of conformality between the prescription dose and the target. Lung within the target exceeds tolerance and is no longer functional after high-dose SBRT. A dose-falloff region exists outside of the target, the volume of which depends on the size of the target, the location of the target within the chest, the quality of the radiation dosimetry (e.g., number of beams, beam arrangements, radiation energy, etc.), and the type of radiation (e.g., photon vs. proton, etc.). This dose-falloff region, also called the gradient region, constitutes unintended radiation exposure and should be kept as small as possible.

PHYSICS AND DOSIMETRY OF STEREOTACTIC BODY RADIATION THERAPY

It is essential that the dosimetry for SBRT be highly conformal between the target margin and the high-dose distribution. In addition, it is essential that the dose outside the target falls off very rapidly, ideally in all directions. Both of these conditions generally require the use of multiple shaped beams.[75–77] Highly shaped beams are desired because high dose is best eliminated in normal tissues by sharp collimation of primary beam fluence outside of the target from the beam's-eye-view. Conversely, smaller nonshaped beams may be used to treat successive regions of the target.[78] Scatter dose is less easily controlled, even by highly shaped beams. Most modern SBRT treatments for lung targets use around 10 to 15 highly collimated beams. To avoid overlap dose between entrance and exit trajectories, these beams are ideally nonopposing and have as large hinge angles between them as possible. In addition and in an effort to assure that dose gradients fall off rapidly in all directions, the beams should generally be noncoplanar. Coplanar treatments such as those that are commonly utilized in CFRT particularly with IMRT result in low and intermediate dose "spillage" that surrounds the tumor in an annular fashion. Ideally, this spillage dose would be distributed in a geometry potentially capable of treating occult microscopic extension of tumor (even though not specifically accounted for in the target). Except, perhaps, for targets in the vertebral bodies of the spine, there is no reason based on anatomy, tissue function, or known patterns of tumor spread to construct such a predominantly axial dose distribution around the target. Collisions between the patient and accelerator head or the couch and accelerator head will limit the ability to create truly isotropically decreasing dose gradients around targets, but effort should be made to mimic such ideal distributions as much as possible.[78,79]

Unlike with CFRT, for SBRT it is assumed that the GTV is nearly identical to the clinical target volume (CTV) for conduct of the treatment. Because of target motion and setup inaccuracies, an additional margin must encompass the GTV/CTV target to avoid missing the intended target during part or all of the treatment session. This expanded target called the PTV constitutes the final target for high-dose conformal coverage. Some centers divide the addition margin in the PTV between margin needed to encompass tumor motion (called the internal target volume or ITV) and setup error. In addition to the PTV and its contents, ablation is likely to occur in the shell of normal tissue immediately outside of the target in the regions of intermediate to high dose. As such, side effects will or will not occur depending on (a) how essential this inner shell of tissue is for normal function of the organ and (b) the thickness or volume of this shell as it relates to the quality of the dosimetry. This *high-dose spillage* is likely the culprit in most of the toxicity related to serially functioning tissues like tubular structures in the lung, gastrointestinal tract, and liver, causing obliteration of the lumen and subsequent downstream effects. Furthermore, the quality of the dose distribution will affect the volume and geometry of low-to-intermediate dose distributions. This *intermediate-dose spillage* is characterized by the maximum dose at a defined distance away from the target (e.g., 2 to 3 cm) or by the volume of tissue encompassed by an intermediate isodose line (e.g., the 50% of prescription isodose line). Intermediate-dose spillage can affect the organ more globally, similar to the historically large fields associated with CFRT, damaging parallel functioning tissues, but may also cause focal organ injury if the prescription dose is high enough.

The degree to which the prescription isodose volume and the target volume are coincident is generally quantified by a conformality index and a percent coverage. The conformality index is the ratio of the prescription isodose volume to the PTV volume. Generally, this ratio should be kept below 1.2. Achieving this degree of conformality is easier with larger targets. The percent coverage indicates what percent of the volume of the PTV is covered by the prescription dose. The percent coverage should generally be 95% to 100%. Although CFRT results in mostly homogeneous target dose distributions, SBRT may have dramatic heterogeneity of dose. It must be insured that regions within the PTV target is not underdosed relative to the minimum prescription dose; however, overdosage is probably of no consequence and may even be advantageous in centrally hypoxic tumors. It is critical, however, that high-dose "hot spots" associated with this dose heterogeneity are not physically located outside of the PTV. This would be an extreme form of *high-dose spillage* and can generally be avoided by using additional highly shaped beams with unique entrance angles.

Organ exposure limits must be respected with SBRT. It has been known that radiation tolerance of specific organs is related to total dose (and fractionation), volume, and inherent radiosensitivity. However, most quoted tolerances are generally quantified as essentially dose limits. Such characterization is clearly inadequate for SBRT where toxicity is more often related to exceeding a specified volume of tissue receiving a given dose than the absolute dose level itself. Data is accumulating for dose–volume tolerances for specific organs affected by SBRT. Because volume effects are poorly understood, absolute point limits were implemented for critical organs like the spinal cord, esophagus, and major bronchial airways. One of the biggest benefits of enrolling SBRT patients on to multicenter prospective trials is the opportunity to collect dose, volume, and patient outcome data, so that the proper limits for SBRT fractionation might be determined with follow-up.

Particularly for targets within the lung, beams to travel through tissues of variable electronic density en route to the target. Ideally, then, the planning system would include algorithms for accurate accounting of tissue heterogeneity effects as it relates to dose deposition from both attenuation and scattering events. Some planning systems do a good job of modeling these effects; however, some do a very poor job.[80,81] Indeed, published reports show that using a primitive heterogeneity correction algorithm may lead to greater inaccuracies of dose representation at the edge of the PTV than using no correction at all.[82] As such, it seems most reasonable that either sophisticated heterogeneity corrections be implemented (e.g., collapsed cone) or that no heterogeneity corrections should be used for SBRT treatments in or near the lungs.

Beam arrangements for a typical SBRT treatment for treating a primary lung cancer is shown in Figure 43.1. The beam angles were chosen by first considering the realm of attainable beam angles for a tumor in this location, avoiding collisions with the accelerator head. Within this subset of attainable beam angles, a beam weight optimization algorithm was used

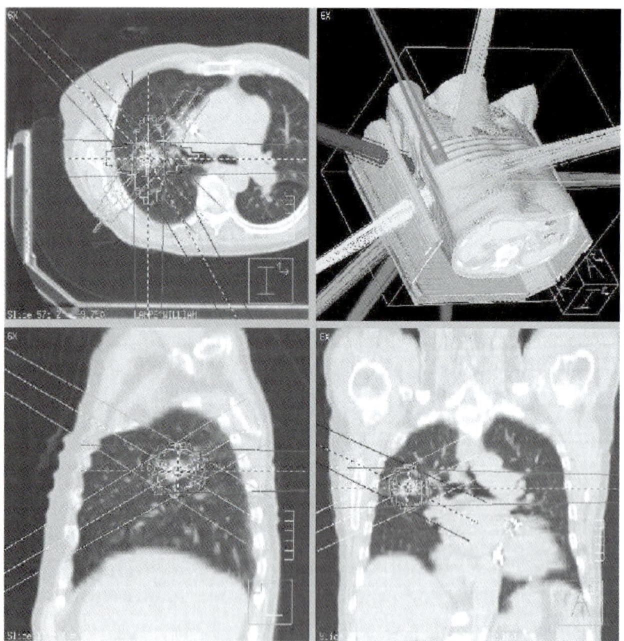

FIGURE 43.1 Typical beam arrangement for SBRT for primary early stage lung cancer. Ten nonopposing and noncoplanar beams coming from various incident directions converge on the demarcated tumor target. (See color plate.)

to select these particular 10 angles using the Radiation Therapy Oncology Group (RTOG) tolerances to construct avoidance structures.[31] In the end, the beams are noncoplanar, nonopposing, and are separated by fairly large hinge angles. Beam weights are divided fairly equal between all beams so as to spread out entrance dose. Figure 43.2 shows the dose–volume histogram for the optimized treatment plan. The PTV target receives a minimum of 95% coverage by the prescription line, which is 60 Gy in this case. Despite the high prescription dose, note that the volume of lung that receives 20 Gy or more is only 5% for this typical case. This is in striking contrast to the 20% to 30% levels commonly seen with CFRT for this parameter known to predict radiation pulmonary toxicity.

CLINICAL EXPERIENCE WITH STEREOTACTIC BODY RADIATION THERAPY

SBRT is a potent local modality and not particularly suitable for adjuvant or prophylactic therapy because of a high likelihood of serious collateral damage to normal tissues. In contrast, CFRT has been most successful as an adjuvant therapy capable of eradicating occult micrometastatic tumor deposits without catastrophic injury to the tissues, which bear these deposits. As SBRT is very effective at eradicating gross visible targeted tumor, diseases with demarcated tumor, the extent of which is mostly visible on available imaging such as CT scans, should be the ideal SBRT diseases. Diseases with high likelihood of regional or distant spread or for which staging is inaccurate should not be treated with SBRT, at least as a sole modality. As such, small cell lung cancer and advanced stages of non–small cell cancer are not ideal SBRT diseases. Early stage non–small cell cancer with no evidence of regional or distant spread would be much better clinical models for testing SBRT. In addition, limited lung metastases, especially in patients with otherwise good systemic control and longer disease free interval, would be reasonable diseases for SBRT. Indeed, these diseases have been studied prospectively using SBRT as will be outlined in this section.

Medically Inoperable Patients with Stage I Cancer Early retrospective experience using SBRT in lung cancer showed that tumor shrinkage early after therapy was very likely, even with more modest dose prescriptions. There was wide variability of both the number of fractions and the dose prescribed per fraction, even within a single institution experience. Some reports had very small numbers followed short periods of time, yet made strong conclusions regarding adequacy of dose and late effects. Of note, tumor recurrence after an effective therapy will occur much later than after an ineffective therapy because of population growth kinetics. Furthermore, toxicity of high dose-per-fraction therapy will likely occur quite late after therapy. Therefore, it is most rational to investigate the role of SBRT in NSCLC using clearly defined selection, consistent treatment, strict quality assurance measures, and uniform follow-up policy. In addition, follow-up should make mandatory that all patients are assessed and published reports await mature evaluation

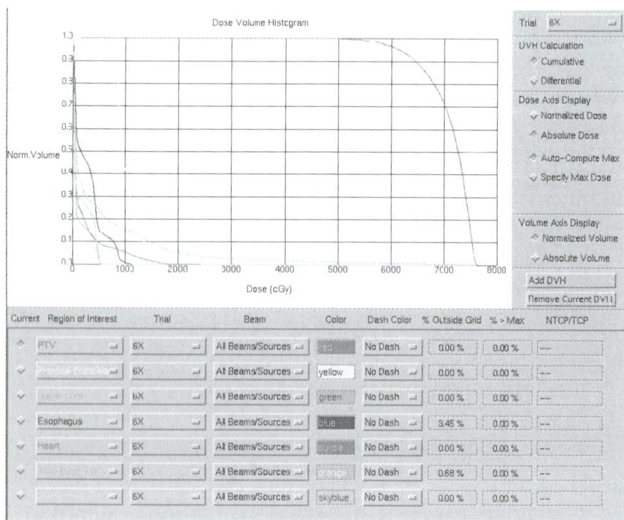

FIGURE 43.2 Dose–volume histogram for an optimized dosimetry plan using the beam arrangements from Figure 43.1. The red line is for the PTV, the yellow for the proximal bronchial tree, the green for the spinal cord, the dark blue for the esophagus, the purple for the heart, the orange for the total lung minus GTV, and the light blue for the proximal trachea. (See color plate.)

of outcome data. Such constraints can only be met by regimented prospective testing.

Indiana University performed a formal phase I dose escalation toxicity study with 47 patients with medically inoperable lung cancer.[29,83] The starting dose was 8 Gy per fraction times three, 24 Gy total. All patients were treated with three fractions at all dose levels. Independent dose escalation trials were carried out in three separate patient groups: patients with T1 tumor, patients with <5-cm T2 tumor, and patients with 5- to 7-cm T2 tumor. There was no restriction regarding the location of the tumor in the lung as both central and peripheral tumors were treated. Seven dose levels were tested. The maximum tolerated dose (MTD) was never reached for T1 tumors and T2 tumors less than 5 cm despite reaching 60 to 66 Gy in 3 fractions. For the largest tumors, dose was escalated all the way to 72 Gy in 3 fractions, which proved to be too toxic. Dose-limiting toxicity in that subset included pneumonia and pericardial effusion. Therefore, the MTD for tumors 5 to 7 cm in diameter was 66 Gy in 3 fractions, whereas the MTD for smaller tumors lies at an undetermined level beyond this dose. Classic radiation pneumonitis (fever, chest pain, shortness of breath, dry cough, and infiltrative x-ray findings), which had been erroneously predicted to be the dose-limiting toxicity, only occurred sporadically.

At the lower doses (i.e., 24 to 36 Gy in 3 fractions), very impressive tumor responses with little normal-tissue effects were observed by 3 months as indicated in Figure 43.3. Unfortunately, with longer follow-up, often past several years, many of these patients ultimately had tumor recurrence. As the dose was escalated beyond 42 to 48 Gy, striking imaging changes began to appear near the treated tumor by around 6 to 12 months. This seemed to be related to a bronchial toxicity, which was not commonly described with CFRT. Radiographic changes by themselves were not considered dose limiting, and most of these imaging changes were asymptomatic. In many cases, the radiographic changes mimic tumor recurrence.[84,85] With no salvage therapy in this population, patients were followed without treatment. Repeat positron emission tomography (PET) scans and biopsies showed no evidence of tumor recurrence in most patients treated at the higher dose levels. In the end, a dose of 60 to 66 Gy in 3 fractions was determined to be reasonably safe for enrolled medically inoperable NSCLC patients.

With a potent tumor dose confirmed to be reasonably tolerable from the phase I study, the Indiana group embarked on a 70-patient phase II study in the same population. The phase II study was aimed at validating toxicity in a larger patient population and determining efficacy (local control or survival) using a total dose of 60 Gy in 3 fractions for the small tumors and 66 Gy in 3 fractions for the large tumors (35 patients for each group). The target control rate for the statistical power calculation was 80%, which is dramatically higher than the typical 30% to 45% control seen with CFRT. All high-grade adverse events (e.g., emergency room visits, surgical procedures, hospitalizations, and deaths) were reviewed by an independent data safety monitoring panel to determine if the event was treatment related (i.e., treatment-related toxicity). In addition, this panel was responsible for final scoring of efficacy such as determining local recurrence.

The preliminary results of the phase II study were published early because of the discovery of a serious toxicity not appreciated in the phase I study.[86] The actuarial 2-year local control for this potent dose regimen is 95%, and isolated hilar or mediastinal nodal relapse is extremely rare despite clinical staging. The overall 2-year survival for this frail population is poor at 56%, with most of the deaths related to comorbid illness rather than disease progression or toxicity. The protocol placed no time limits on scoring treatment-related toxicity, and many late toxic events have been recorded. Fewer than 20% of patients have experienced high-grade toxicity confirming the phase I model. However, interim analysis showed that severe toxicity (grade 3 to 5) was significantly more likely in patients treated for tumors in the regions around the proximal bronchial tree or central chest region. In fact, the risk of severe toxicity is 11 times greater when treating central tumors as compared to peripheral tumors.

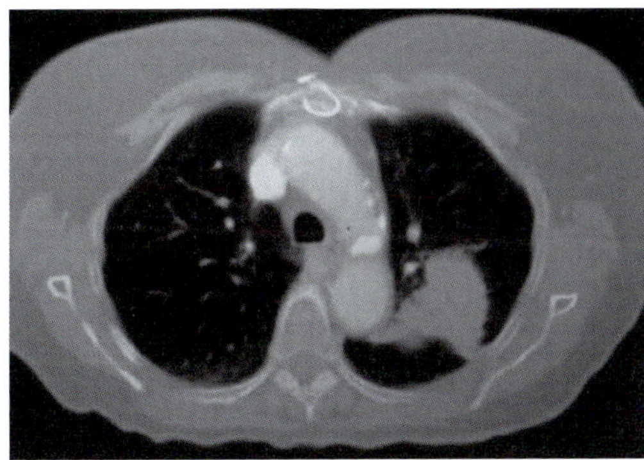

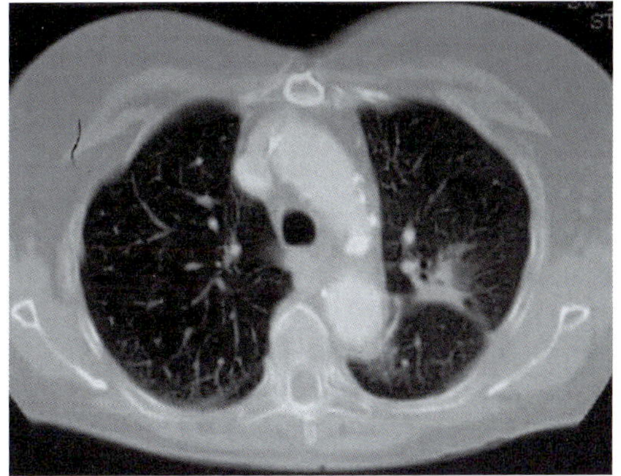

FIGURE 43.3 Patient with a solitary pulmonary nodule treated on the Indiana University phase I trial using SBRT. After just 3 months, the tumor has dramatically reduced in size, but a remnant remains.

TABLE 43.1 Local Control in Early Stage Non–Small Cell Lung Cancer

Author	Treatment	Local Control	Single Fraction Equivalent Dose (D_q = 2 Gy)[12]	Reference
Europe/North America				
Pennathur et al., 2007	20 Gy × 1	84% (crude)	20 Gy	104
Hof et al., 2007	19–24 Gy × 1	50% (2 yrs)	19–24 Gy	105
	26–30 Gy × 1	72% (2 yrs)	26–30 Gy	
Fritz et al., 2007	30 Gy × 1	81% (3 yrs)	30 Gy	15
Timmerman et al., 2006	20–22 Gy × 3	95% (2+ yrs)	56–62 Gy	86
Baumann et al., 2006	15 Gy × 3	80% (3 yrs)	41 Gy	17
Nyman et al., 2006	15 Gy × 3	80% (crude)	41 Gy	88
Zimmermann et al., 2005	12.5 Gy × 3	87% (3 yrs)	43.5 Gy	87
Timmerman et al., 2003	8–16 Gy × 3	60% (2 yrs)	20–44 Gy	29
	18–24 Gy × 3	90% (2 yrs)	50–68 Gy	
Asia				
Koto et al., 2007	15 Gy × 3 or 7.5 Gy × 6	T1 78%, T2 40% (3 yrs)	41–46 Gy	106
Xia et al., 2006	5 Gy × 10	95% (3 yrs)	32 Gy	107
Hara et al., 2006	30–34 Gy × 1	80% (3 yrs)	30–34 Gy	108
Nagata et al., 2005	12 Gy × 4	94% (3 yrs)	42 Gy	14

Similar experience relating to efficacy has been reported in Europe and Japan. Active groups from Sweden, Denmark, Germany, the Netherlands, and Italy have reported rates of local control and toxicity similar to the Indiana experience at similar dose levels.[17,87–89] Various dose and fractionation schemes have been used, however, generally fewer than five total fractions have been employed. As with the Indiana group, Wulf et al.[90] from Wurzburg have demonstrated a clear dose–response relationship with better control at higher dose levels. As shown in Table 43.1, clinical results are favorable for tumor control when single fraction equivalent dose (SFED) levels of 40 Gy or higher are used. SFED is a far more ideal method for comparing different SBRT fractionation schemes as compared to biologically equivalent dose (BED) because it does not grossly overestimate the potency of large dose-per-fraction treatments as BED comparisons based on the linear quadratic model (see previous discussion under "Biological Aspects of Stereotactic Body Radiation Therapy").[67,68] With SFED of 40 Gy, actuarial tumor control is consistently 75% to 80% at 2 to 3 years, whereas for SFED of 50 Gy or higher, tumor control consistently exceeds 90%. This level of primary tumor control rivals surgical lobectomy.

RTOG 0236 using SBRT for medically inoperable lung cancer in patients with peripherally situated tumors completed its accrual of 56 patients in 2006. This trial used SBRT to a dose of 60 Gy in 3 fractions for T1, T2, and peripheral T3 tumors less than 5 cm in diameter. Treatment dosimetry was carried out without the use of heterogeneity correction factors, and subsequent dosimetric analysis showed the actual dose for RTOG 0236 was around 54 Gy in 3 fractions. Extensive accreditation, conduct, and dosimetry constraints were developed in the RTOG Lung, Physics, and Image-Guided Therapy Committees to form a basis for meaningful quality assurance and consistent treatment for a multicenter trial. Three toxicity analyses were performed during the trial, which showed no excessive toxicity warranting trial closure. The first formal report of toxicity was presented at the American Society of Therapeutic Radiology and Oncology annual meeting in Los Angeles.[18] The rate of protocol defined severe toxicity was around 10%, whereas at time of analysis (median follow-up 13 months), only 1 patient out of 55 evaluable had a local recurrence. Another trial in patients with centrally situated tumors, RTOG 0813, is being planned that will use a more gentle fractionation scheme for medically inoperable patients.

The Japan Clinical Oncology Group (JCOG) 0413 trial is a phase II trial using SBRT for peripheral lesions in two groups: operable and medically inoperable patients with stage I cancer. The treatment dose is 48 Gy in 4 fractions to the isocenter based on the Kyoto experience. Accreditation was carried out for enrolling institutions.[91] Like RTOG 0236, quality assurance is being monitored through the Advanced Technology Consortium with a requirement that all institutions submit digital plans for review. The medically operable group enrolled quickly and those patients are being followed. The medically inoperable group is still enrolling.

Operable Patients with Stage I Cancer Surgery continues to be the standard of care for operable patients with stage I cancer. However, some patients are adverse to the idea of surgical resection and have opted to be treated with SBRT. Most of the work in this population has been carried out in Japan. Onishi et al.[13,92] performed a large retrospective chart review of patients treated at several Japanese centers using SBRT in early stage NSCLC. Although dose and number of fractions varied considerably, all patients were treated with small radiation fields under stereotactic guidance. This report included a large number of operable patients that were analyzed separately. For such patients who received dose levels such that the biological effective dose (BED) was greater than 100,[93] local control and survival rivaled best surgical series according to the authors. The 3-year overall survival in this group was 88%. This report, along with the experience from Kyoto, has formed the basis for enrolling patient with operable tumors onto a separate arm of the JCOG 0403 trial for peripheral T1N0 stage I patients. As noted previously, this trial completed enrollment and patients are being followed.

In the United States, very few patients with operable stage I NSCLC have been treated on clinical trials. That situation will change with the enactment of RTOG 0618 for operable patients. Based on best surgical literature from North America, it will be required that SBRT attain a local control rate of 90% or better to compete with lobectomy.[94] As such, very potent dose prescriptions will be required. RTOG 0618 is modeled after RTOG 0236 except eligibility is for healthier patients capable of tolerating thoracotomy. The potent prescription dose is 60 Gy in 3 fractions and frequent tumor status assessments are made to identify failure early and attempt surgical salvage.

CONCLUSION

Ablation of deadly lung tumors has been made possible by technological developments delivered to the clinic by important engineering and physics research. However, they serve to allow the utilization of the most potent biological form of radiotherapy delivered to date.[95] Ablation of tumor using total dose or dose per fraction well beyond conventional radiation promises in the end to serve to improve outcome. This new collaboration between technology innovators and biological researchers holds considerable promise for improving the outcome of a large population of patients with lung cancer.

At one time, it was felt that improvements in systemic therapy would lead to a decrease in utilization of local therapies like surgery and radiotherapy. Interestingly, the opposite has occurred. As systemic treatments become more effective, local disease becomes the prominent mode of failure. Radiotherapy will be used more selectively to target isolated deposits of gross disease.[96] Currently limited to treatment with curative intent in stage I to III disease, radiotherapy will likely be used more often in stage IV disease either as a measure for consolidation or to ablate cancer deposits resistant to systemic therapy. With exploitation of technology and biological understanding, this is an ideal role for radiotherapy as an effective and cost-effective modality for local control of gross disease.

Patients would be best served if their cancer therapy was customized according to the exact nature and threat of their specific tumor. The goal of technical, biological, and clinical research in radiation oncology as well as in collaboration with surgical and medical oncologists is to facilitate adaptive therapy.[97–99] In this paradigm, pretreatment diagnostic information including imaging, staging, tissue samples (proteomic, genomics, etc), and other predictive assays are integrated to make therapy selection.[100] Having chosen the correct approach, the patient is started on therapy while monitoring progress. Early assessments relating to accuracy of delivery, tumor response, metabolic changes, tolerance, and others can be used to change the therapy appropriately during therapy.[101–103] Soon after treatment, imaging and metabolic assessment may direct the need for adjuvant therapies or avoid toxicity. Rather than a "one-size-fits-all" cancer therapy, the adaptive process uses a tailored approach that constantly reevaluates and responds to redirect the therapy toward a better outcome. Until this goal is achieved, patients will continue to be enrolled onto well-designed prospective trials such that SBRT might be refined to its optimal potential.

REFERENCES

1. Leksell L. The stereotaxic method and radiosurgery of the brain. *Acta Chir Scand* 1951;102:316–319.
2. Murray B, Forster K, Timmerman R. Frame-based immobilization and targeting for stereotactic body radiation therapy. *Med Dosim* 2007; 32:86–91.
3. Purdie TG, Bissonnette JP, Franks K, et al. Cone-beam computed tomography for on-line image guidance of lung stereotactic radiotherapy: localization, verification, and intrafraction tumor position. *Int J Radiat Oncol Biol Phys* 2007;68:243–252.
4. Jaffray DA. Image-guided radiation therapy: from concept to practice. *Semin Radiat Oncol* 2007;17:243–244.
5. Franks KN, Bezjak A, Purdie TG, et al. Early results of image-guided radiation therapy in lung stereotactic body radiotherapy (SBRT). *Clin Oncol (R Coll Radiol)* 2007;19:S10.
6. Dawson LA, Jaffray DA. Advances in image-guided radiation therapy. *J Clin Oncol* 2007;25:938–946.
7. Timmerman R, Papiez L, Suntharalingam M. Extracranial stereotactic radiation delivery: expansion of technology beyond the brain. *Technol Cancer Res Treat* 2003;2:153–160.
8. Potters L, Steinberg M, Rose C, et al. American Society for Therapeutic Radiology and Oncology and American College of Radiology practice guideline for the performance of stereotactic body radiation therapy. *Int J Radiat Oncol Biol Phys* 2004;60:1026–1032.
9. Potters L, Timmerman R, Larson D. Stereotactic body radiation therapy. *J Am Coll Radiol* 2005;2:676–680.
10. Zimmermann FB, Geinitz H, Schill S, et al. Stereotactic hypofractionated radiotherapy in stage I (T1-2 N0 M0) non-small-cell lung cancer (NSCLC). *Acta Oncol* 2006;45:796–801.
11. Wulf J, Haedinger U, Oppitz U, et al. Stereotactic radiotherapy for primary lung cancer and pulmonary metastases: a noninvasive treatment approach in medically inoperable patients. *Int J Radiat Oncol Biol Phys* 2004;60:186–196.

12. Timmerman RD, Park C, Kavanagh BD. The North American experience with stereotactic body radiation therapy in non-small cell lung cancer. *J Thorac Oncol* 2007;2:S101–S112.
13. Onishi H, Shirato H, Nagata Y, et al. Hypofractionated stereotactic radiotherapy (HypoFXSRT) for stage I non-small cell lung cancer: updated results of 257 patients in a Japanese multi-institutional study. *J Thorac Oncol* 2007;2:S94–S100.
14. Nagata Y, Takayama K, Matsuo Y, et al. Clinical outcomes of a phase I/II study of 48 Gy of stereotactic body radiotherapy in 4 fractions for primary lung cancer using a stereotactic body frame. *Int J Radiat Oncol Biol Phys* 2005;63:1427–1431.
15. Fritz P, Kraus HJ, Blaschke T, et al. Stereotactic, high single-dose irradiation of stage I non-small cell lung cancer (NSCLC) using four-dimensional CT scans for treatment planning. *Lung Cancer* 2008; 60:193–199.
16. Brown WT, Wu X, Wen BC, et al. Early results of CyberKnife image-guided robotic stereotactic radiosurgery for treatment of lung tumors. *Comput Aided Surg* 2007;12:253–261.
17. Baumann P, Nyman J, Lax I, et al. Factors important for efficacy of stereotactic body radiotherapy of medically inoperable stage I lung cancer. A retrospective analysis of patients treated in the Nordic countries. *Acta Oncol* 2006;45:787–795.
18. Timmerman R, Paulus R, Galvin J, et al. Toxicity Analysis of RTOG 0236 using stereotactic body radiation therapy (SBRT) to treat medically inoperable early stage lung cancer patients. *Int J Radiat Oncol Biol Phys* 2007;69:S86.
19. Hall EJ, Astor M, Bedford J, et al. Basic radiobiology. *Am J Clin Oncol* 1988;11:220–252.
20. Hamilton AJ, Lulu BA, Fosmire H, et al. Preliminary clinical experience with linear accelerator-based spinal stereotactic radiosurgery. *Neurosurgery* 1995;36:311–319.
21. Lax I. Target dose versus extratarget dose in stereotactic radiosurgery. *Acta Oncol* 1993;32:453–457.
22. Lax I, Blomgren H, Naslund I, Svanstrom R. Stereotactic radiotherapy of malignancies in the abdomen. Methodological aspects. *Acta Oncol* 1994;33:677–683.
23. Blomgren H, Lax I, Näslund I, et al. Stereotactic high dose fraction radiation therapy of extracranial tumors using an accelerator. Clinical experience of the first thirty-one patients. *Acta Oncol* 1995;34:861–870.
24. Blomgren H, Lax I, Goranson H, et al. Radiosurgery for tumors in the body: clinical experience using a new method. *J Radiosurg* 1998;1:63–74.
25. Shirato H, Shimizu S, Shimizu T, et al. Real-time tumour-tracking radiotherapy. *Lancet* 1999;353:1331–1332.
26. Uematsu M, Shioda A, Tahara K, et al. Focal, high dose, and fractionated modified stereotactic radiation therapy for lung carcinoma patients: a preliminary experience. *Cancer* 1998;82:1062–1070.
27. Uematsu M, Shioda A, Suda A, et al. Intrafractional tumor position stability during computed tomography (CT)-guided frameless stereotactic radiation therapy for lung or liver cancers with a fusion of CT and linear accelerator (FOCAL) unit. *Int J Radiat Oncol Biol Phys* 2000;48:443–448.
28. Uematsu M, Shioda A, Suda A, et al. Computed tomography-guided frameless stereotactic radiotherapy for stage I non-small cell lung cancer: a 5-year experience. *Int J Radiat Oncol Biol Phys* 2001;51:666–670.
29. Timmerman R, Papiez L, McGarry R, et al. Extracranial stereotactic radioablation: results of a phase I study in medically inoperable stage I non-small cell lung cancer. *Chest* 2003;124:1946–1955.
30. Hof H, Herfarth KK, Münter M, et al. Stereotactic single-dose radiotherapy of stage I non-small-cell lung cancer (NSCLC). *Int J Radiat Oncol Biol Phys* 2003;56:335–341.
31. Timmerman R, Galvin J, Michalski J, et al. Accreditation and quality assurance for Radiation Therapy Oncology Group: Multicenter clinical trials using Stereotactic Body Radiation Therapy in lung cancer. *Acta Oncol* 2006;45:779–786.
32. Sloviter HA. The effect of complete ablation of thyroid tissue by radioactive iodine on the survival of tumor-bearing mice. *Cancer Res* 1951; 11:447–449.
33. Allen HC Jr. Subtotal ablation of the thyroid gland with a single dose of radioactive Iodine-131 for the treatment of thyrotoxicosis. *South Med J* 1956;49:1428–1440.
34. Lippincott SW, Lewallen CG, Shellabarger CJ. Pathology of radioisotopic ablation of the thyroid in the dog. *AMA Arch Pathol* 1957;63: 540–556.
35. Storaasli JP, Schoeniger EL, Hellerstein HK, et al. Thyroid ablation with I-131 in euthyroid cardiac patients, with special reference to preparation with antithyroid drugs. *Radiology* 1960;74:810–815.
36. Goolden AW, Davey JB. The ablation of normal thyroid tissue with iodine 131. *Br J Radiol* 1963;36:340–345.
37. Alheit H, Dornfeld S, Dawel M, et al. Patient position reproducibility in fractionated stereotactically guided conformal radiotherapy using the BrainLab mask system. *Strahlenther Onkol* 2001;177:264–268.
38. Bale RJ, Sweeney R, Vogele M, et al. [Noninvasive head fixation for external irradiation of tumors of the head and neck area]. *Strahlenther Onkol* 1998;174:350–354.
39. Fairclough-Tompa L, Larsen T, Jaywant SM. Immobilization in stereotactic radiotherapy: the head and neck localizer frame. *Med Dosim* 2001;26:267–273.
40. Fuss M, Salter BJ, Rassiah P, et al. Repositioning accuracy of a commercially available double-vacuum whole body immobilization system for stereotactic body radiation therapy. *Technol Cancer Res Treat* 2004;3: 59–67.
41. Herfarth KK, Debus J, Lohr F, et al. Extracranial stereotactic radiation therapy: set-up accuracy of patients treated for liver metastases. *Int J Radiat Oncol Biol Phys* 2000;46:329–335.
42. Hof H, Herfarth KK, Münter M, et al. The use of the multislice CT for the determination of respiratory lung tumor movement in stereotactic single-dose irradiation. *Strahlenther Onkol* 2003;179:542–547.
43. Lax I, Blomgren H, Larson D, et al. Extracranial stereotactic radiosurgery of localized targets. *J Radiosurg* 1998;1:135–148.
44. Lohr F, Debus J, Frank C, et al. Noninvasive patient fixation for extracranial stereotactic radiotherapy. *Int J Radiat Oncol Biol Phys* 1999; 45:521–527.
45. Nagata Y, Negoro Y, Aoki T, et al. [Three-dimensional conformal radiotherapy for extracranial tumors using a stereotactic body frame]. *Igaku Butsuri* 2001;21:28–34.
46. Negoro Y, Nagata Y, Aoki T, et al. The effectiveness of an immobilization device in conformal radiotherapy for lung tumor: reduction of respiratory tumor movement and evaluation of the daily setup accuracy. *Int J Radiat Oncol Biol Phys* 2001;50:889–898.
47. Nevinny-Stickel M, Sweeney RA, Bale RJ, et al. Reproducibility of patient positioning for fractionated extracranial stereotactic radiotherapy using a double-vacuum technique. *Strahlenther Onkol* 2004;180:117–122.
48. Takacs II, Kishan A, Deogaonkar M, et al. Respiration induced target drift in spinal stereotactic radiosurgery: evaluation of skeletal fixation in a porcine model. *Stereotact Funct Neurosurg* 1999;73:70.
49. Wulf J, Hädinger U, Oppitz U, et al. Stereotactic radiotherapy of extracranial targets: CT-simulation and accuracy of treatment in the stereotactic body frame. *Radiother Oncol* 2000;57:225–236.
50. Wang LT, Solberg TD, Medin PM, et al. Infrared patient positioning for stereotactic radiosurgery of extracranial tumors. *Comput Biol Med* 2001;31:101–111.
51. Uematsu M, Sonderegger M, Shioda A, et al. Daily positioning accuracy of frameless stereotactic radiation therapy with a fusion of computed tomography and linear accelerator (focal) unit: evaluation of z-axis with a z-marker. *Radiother Oncol* 1999;50:337–339.
52. Takai Y, Mituya M, Nemoto K, et al. [Simple method of stereotactic radiotherapy without stereotactic body frame for extracranial tumors]. *Nippon Igaku Hoshasen Gakkai Zasshi* 2001;61:403–407.
53. Yin F, Kim JG, Haughton C, et al. Extracranial radiosurgery: immobilizing liver motion in dogs using high-frequency jet ventilation and total intravenous anesthesia. *Int J Radiat Oncol Biol Phys* 2001;49:211–216.
54. O'Dell WG, Schell MC, Reynolds D, et al. Dose broadening due to target position variability during fractionated breath-held radiation therapy. *Med Phys* 2002;29:1430–1437.

55. Murphy MJ, Martin D, Whyte R, et al. The effectiveness of breath-holding to stabilize lung and pancreas tumors during radiosurgery. *Int J Radiat Oncol Biol Phys* 2002;53:475–482.
56. Kimura T, Hirokawa Y, Murakami Y, et al. Reproducibility of organ position using voluntary breath-hold method with spirometer for extracranial stereotactic radiotherapy. *Int J Radiat Oncol Biol Phys* 2004; 60:1307–1313.
57. Vedam SS, Keall PJ, Kini VR, et al. Determining parameters for respiration-gated radiotherapy. *Med Phys* 2001;28:2139–2146.
58. Kini VR, Vedam SS, Keall PJ, et al. Patient training in respiratory-gated radiotherapy. *Med Dosim* 2003;28:7–11.
59. Hara R, Itami J, Aruga T, et al. [Development of stereotactic irradiation system of body tumors under respiratory gating]. *Nippon Igaku Hoshasen Gakkai Zasshi* 2002;62:156–160.
60. Kitamura K, Shirato H, Seppenwoolde Y, et al. Tumor location, cirrhosis, and surgical history contribute to tumor movement in the liver, as measured during stereotactic irradiation using a real-time tumor-tracking radiotherapy system. *Int J Radiat Oncol Biol Phys* 2003;56: 221–228.
61. Kuriyama K, Onishi H, Sano N, et al. A new irradiation unit constructed of self-moving gantry-CT and linac. *Int J Radiat Oncol Biol Phys* 2003;55:428–435.
62. Schweikard A, Shiomi H, Adler J. Respiration tracking in radiosurgery. *Med Phys* 2004;31:2738–2741.
63. Sharp GC, Jiang SB, Shimizu S, et al. Prediction of respiratory tumour motion for real-time image-guided radiotherapy. *Phys Med Biol* 2004;49:425–440.
64. Hall EJ, Gross W, Dvorak RF, et al. Survival curves and age response functions for Chinese hamster cells exposed to x-rays or high LET alpha-particles. *Radiat Res* 1972;52:88–98.
65. Kellerer AM, Rossi HH. Dependence of RBE on neutron dose. *Br J Radiol* 1972;45:626.
66. Rossi HH, Kellerer AM. Radiation carcinogenesis at low doses. *Science* 1972;175:200–202.
67. Park C, Papiez L, Zhang S, et al. The universal survival curve and single fraction equivalent dose: useful tools in understanding the potency of ablative radiation therapy. *Int J Radiat Oncol Biol Phys* 2008 1;70(3):847–852.
68. Marks LB. Extrapolating hypofractionated radiation schemes from radiosurgery data: regarding Hall et al., IJROBP 21:819–824; 1991 and Hall and Brenner, IJROBP 25:381–385; 1993. *Int J Radiat Oncol Biol Phys* 1995;32:274–276.
69. Guerrero M, Li XA. Extending the linear-quadratic model for large fraction doses pertinent to stereotactic radiotherapy. *Phys Med Biol* 2004;49:4825–4835.
70. Hall EJ. *Radiobiology for the Radiologist*. 2nd Ed. Philadelphia, PA: Harper & Row Publishers, 1978.
71. Benedict SH, Lin PS, Zwicker RD, et al. The biological effectiveness of intermittent irradiation as a function of overall treatment time: development of correction factors for linac-based stereotactic radiotherapy. *Int J Radiat Oncol Biol Phys* 1997;37:765–769.
72. Fowler JF, Welsh JS, Howard SP. Loss of biological effect in prolonged fraction delivery. *Int J Radiat Oncol Biol Phys* 2004;59:242–249.
73. Yaes RJ, Kalend A. Local stem cell depletion model for radiation myelitis. *Int J Radiat Oncol Biol Phys* 1988;14:1247–1259.
74. Wolbarst AB, Chin LM, Svensson GK. Optimization of radiation therapy: integral-response of a model biological system. *Int J Radiat Oncol Biol Phys* 1982;8:1761–1769.
75. Cardinale RM, Wu Q, Benedict SH, et al. Determining the optimal block margin on the planning target volume for extracranial stereotactic radiotherapy. *Int J Radiat Oncol Biol Phys* 1999;45: 515–520.
76. Liu R, Buatti JM, Howes TL, et al. Optimal number of beams for stereotactic body radiotherapy of lung and liver lesions. *Int J Radiat Oncol Biol Phys* 2006;66:906–912.
77. Papiez L, Timmerman R, DesRosiers C, et al. Extracranial stereotactic radioablation: physical principles. *Acta Oncol* 2003;42:882–894.
78. Papiez L. On the equivalence of rotational and concentric therapy. *Phys Med Biol* 2000;45:399–409.
79. Hadinger U, Thiele W, Wulf J. Extracranial stereotactic radiotherapy: evaluation of PTV coverage and dose conformity. *Z Med Phys* 2002; 12:221–229.
80. Traberg Hansen A, Petersen JB, Høyer M, et al. Comparison of two dose calculation methods applied to extracranial stereotactic radiotherapy treatment planning. *Radiother Oncol* 2005;77:96–98.
81. Ding GX, Duggan DM, Lu B, et al. Impact of inhomogeneity corrections on dose coverage in the treatment of lung cancer using stereotactic body radiation therapy. *Med Phys* 2007;34:2985–2994.
82. Mayer R, Williams A, Frankel T, et al. Two-dimensional film dosimetry application in heterogeneous materials exposed to megavoltage photon beams. *Med Phys* 1997;24:455–460.
83. McGarry RC, Papiez L, Williams M, et al. Stereotactic body radiation therapy of early-stage non-small-cell lung carcinoma: phase I study. *Int J Radiat Oncol Biol Phys* 2005;63:1010–1015.
84. Takeda A, Kunieda E, Takeda T, et al. Possible misinterpretation of demarcated solid patterns of radiation fibrosis on CT scans as tumor recurrence in patients receiving hypofractionated stereotactic radiotherapy for lung cancer. *Int J Radiat Oncol Biol Phys* 2008; 70:1057–1065.
85. Matsuo Y, Nagata Y, Mizowaki T, et al. Evaluation of mass-like consolidation after stereotactic body radiation therapy for lung tumors. *Int J Clin Oncol* 2007;12:356–362.
86. Timmerman R, McGarry R, Yiannoutsos C, et al. Excessive toxicity when treating central tumors in a phase II study of stereotactic body radiation therapy for medically inoperable early-stage lung cancer. *J Clin Oncol* 2006;24:4833–4839.
87. Zimmermann FB, Geinitz H, Schill S, et al. Stereotactic hypofractionated radiation therapy for stage I non-small cell lung cancer. *Lung Cancer* 2005;48:107–114.
88. Nyman J, Johansson KA, Hultén U. Stereotactic hypofractionated radiotherapy for stage I non-small cell lung cancer—mature results for medically inoperable patients. *Lung Cancer* 2006;51:97–103.
89. Fritz P, Kraus HJ, Mühlnickel W, et al. Stereotactic, single-dose irradiation of stage I non-small cell lung cancer and lung metastases. *Radiat Oncol* 2006;1:30.
90. Wulf J, Baier K, Mueller G, et al. Dose-response in stereotactic irradiation of lung tumors. *Radiother Oncol* 2005;77:83–87.
91. Matsuo Y, Takayama K, Nagata Y, et al. Interinstitutional variations in planning for stereotactic body radiation therapy for lung cancer. *Int J Radiat Oncol Biol Phys* 2007;68:416–425.
92. Onishi H, Araki T, Shirato H, et al. Stereotactic hypofractionated high-dose irradiation for stage I nonsmall cell lung carcinoma: clinical outcomes in 245 subjects in a Japanese multiinstitutional study. *Cancer* 2004;101:1623–1631.
93. Fowler JF. The linear-quadratic formula and progress in fractionated radiotherapy. *Br J Radiol* 1989;62:679–694.
94. Ginsberg RJ, Rubinstein LV. Randomized trial of lobectomy versus limited resection for T1 N0 non-small cell lung cancer. Lung Cancer Study Group. *Ann Thorac Surg* 1995;60:615–622; discussion 622–623.
95. Timmerman RD, Story M. Stereotactic body radiation therapy: a treatment in need of basic biological research. *Cancer J* 2006;12:19–20.
96. Timmerman R, Papiez L, Review of Song, et al. Stereotactic body radiation therapy: rationale, techniques, applications, and optimization of an emerging technology. *Oncology* 2004;18:474–477.
97. Song W, Schaly B, Bauman G, et al. Image-guided adaptive radiation therapy (IGART): Radiobiological and dose escalation considerations for localized carcinoma of the prostate. *Med Phys* 2005;32:2193–2203.
98. Martinez AA, Yan D, Lockman D, et al. Improvement in dose escalation using the process of adaptive radiotherapy combined with three-dimensional conformal or intensity-modulated beams for prostate cancer. *Int J Radiat Oncol Biol Phys* 2001;50:1226–1234.
99. Bortfeld T, Paganetti H. The biologic relevance of daily dose variations in adaptive treatment planning. *Int J Radiat Oncol Biol Phys* 2006;65: 899–906.

100. Potti A, Mukherjee S, Petersen R, et al. A genomic strategy to refine prognosis in early-stage non-small-cell lung cancer. *N Engl J Med* 2006;355:570–580.
101. Yan D, Lockman D, Brabbins D, et al. An off-line strategy for constructing a patient-specific planning target volume in adaptive treatment process for prostate cancer. *Int J Radiat Oncol Biol Phys* 2000;48:289–302.
102. Wu C, Jeraj R, Olivera GH, et al. Re-optimization in adaptive radiotherapy. *Phys Med Biol* 2002;47:3181–3195.
103. Brahme A. Biologically optimized 3-dimensional in vivo predictive assay-based radiation therapy using positron emission tomography-computerized tomography imaging. *Acta Oncol* 2003;42:123–136.
104. Pennathur A, Luketich JD, Burton S, et al. Stereotactic radiosurgery for the treatment of lung neoplasm: initial experience. *Ann Thorac Surg* 2007;83:1820–1824; discussion 1824–1825.
105. Hof H, Muenter M, Oetzel D, et al. Stereotactic single-dose radiotherapy (radiosurgery) of early stage nonsmall-cell lung cancer (NSCLC). *Cancer* 2007;110:148–155.
106. Koto M, Takai Y, Ogawa Y, et al. A phase II study on stereotactic body radiotherapy for stage I non-small cell lung cancer. *Radiother Oncol* 2007;85:429–434.
107. Xia T, Li H, Sun Q, et al. Promising clinical outcome of stereotactic body radiation therapy for patients with inoperable Stage I/II non-small-cell lung cancer. *Int J Radiat Oncol Biol Phys* 2006;66: 117–125.
108. Hara R, Itami J, Kondo T, et al. Clinical outcomes of single-fraction stereotactic radiation therapy of lung tumors. *Cancer* 2006;106: 1347–1352.

CHAPTER 44

Zhongxing Liao
Elizabeth L. Travis
Ritsuko Komaki

Radiation Treatment–Related Lung Damage

More than 50% of patients with lung cancer receive radiation during case management. Because treatment sometimes requires that a large volume of lung be exposed to high doses of radiation, definitive radiation therapy requires total doses that can result in late sequelae: lung injury. These late sequelae were observed as early as the 1920s, less than 2 decades after the discovery of x-rays.[1] The two phases of lung damage—radiation pneumonitis and radiation fibrosis—were first described in 1925 by Evans and Leucutia,[2] who divided the damage into these now well-recognized sequelae of lung irradiation. Although almost a century of studies of patients and experimental models has provided a wealth of information on these two potentially fatal complications, we remain unable to circumvent these untoward reactions completely. Both continue to limit radiation's effectiveness against malignant tumors of the lung.

Since the third edition of this book was published, significant advances have been made in understanding the molecular and physical basis of radiation-induced lung damage and how genetic regulation functions within it. The radiation dose–volume effect in mouse lung has been clearly defined, and experimental findings have been substantiated by clinical studies. As three-dimensional (3D) conformal radiation therapy has become the norm for treating lung cancer, new methods of estimating the risk of pulmonary injury from dose–volume histograms (DVHs) and normal-tissue complication probability models (NTCPs) have been developed. The development of such advanced radiation therapy technologies as intensity-modulated radiation therapy (IMRT), image-guided radiation therapy (IGRT), and proton beam therapy (PBT) has reduced the risk and severity of radiation-induced lung damage and morbidity, and clinical outcomes have been promising. The radiotherapy target in lung cancer may be more carefully delineated and not necessarily include the large volumes of lung once thought necessary and standard. The goal of this chapter is to review information in these areas and to present new findings regarding the development of quantitative and easily accessible markers of lung damage and predictive assays of pulmonary radiosensitivity.

DAMAGE VERSUS MORBIDITY

The terms *damage* and *morbidity* are often used interchangeably, but they are quite different concepts. In clinical practice, some degree of radiation-induced lung damage, either pneumonitis or fibrosis, is considered acceptable because of the large functional reserve of this tissue. The whole organ does not fail to function if some part of it is destroyed. Morbidity, on the other hand, is a clinical term that describes how well an individual patient feels or how well a specific organ functions. The morbidity of treatment is determined by many factors, including the damage to the tissue, the effect of this damage on organ function, and the effect of both of these factors on the patient's well-being and lifestyle. Because of the functional reserve of the lung, structural damage is not necessarily reflected in clinical morbidity, assessed in terms of whole-lung function.

The dissociation between damage and morbidity in the lung reflects the organization of those anatomical units responsible for lung function.[3] Morbidity is a reflection of two parameters: (a) the survival of sufficient numbers of cells to maintain tissue function and (b) the organization of those cells into units that carry out tissue function. The spatial relationship between these functional subunits differs between tissues and is a critical determinant of the relationship between damage and any resultant morbidity.

Anatomically, the lung is a system of branching ducts and accompanying blood vessels that ultimately terminate in the alveoli, the site of gas exchange. The functional subunit in the lung is most likely the *acinus*, which is structurally well defined, beginning at the ramification of the terminal bronchiole to the respiratory bronchioles and terminating in the alveolar sacs, each of which bears numerous alveoli. Each acinus is a self-contained entity independent of its neighbor. Presumably, destruction of one acinus will have no measurable effect on lung function in a normal healthy lung, and functional damage, particularly total lung function, will be manifested only when a critical number of these units are destroyed. A useful analogy is a strand of sequential lights arranged in parallel.

When one burns out (damage), none of the others is affected, and the overall effect is not diminished; that is, the damage is below the threshold of the human eye to distinguish it (no morbidity). However, when sufficient numbers of lights burn out such that damage is noticeable (the threshold for damage detectable by the human eye is exceeded), the overall effect is diminished (morbidity occurs).

Many assays are available to quantify radiation-induced damage and morbidity in the lungs in experimental animals and in patients. In humans, regional pulmonary function or the extent of pneumonitis and fibrosis evident on radiographs can be quantified by using functional imaging modalities such as single photon emission computed tomography (SPECT), ^{18}F-fluorodeoxyglucose positron emission tomography (FDG-PET), and ventilation planning computed tomography (CT), thereby providing systems by which damage can be scored.[4–15] In rats and mice, the experimental animals most commonly used to study radiation- and drug-induced lung injury, measurements of regional lung function are difficult and pulmonary function tests most often assess total lung function, a measure of morbidity.[16–20] The diffusion capacity, measured as DLCO (diffusing capacity of lung for carbon monoxide) is the most useful clinical tool of functional lung oxygen exchange. When sufficient functional reserve units are destroyed, either as preexisting lung damage from smoking, or as new damage from treatment, this can be a sensitive measure of that injury. In patients, structural damage can be quantified by noninvasive methods, for example by CT scanning; in experimental animals, such damage is most often assessed in autopsy specimens. In this chapter, clear distinctions will be made between damage and morbidity and the assessment of each.

RADIATION-INDUCED LUNG DAMAGE

Pathophysiology Radiation-induced damage to the lung occurs in distinct phases characterized by differences in when after irradiation they occur and their histologic or molecular manifestations (Table 44.1).[21] Damage to the human lung has long been described as occurring in four clinical phases: a phase

TABLE 44.1 Principal Histopathologic Abnormalities after Irradiation of the Thorax in Animals

	Abnormalities after Irradiation		
Site	**Immediate and Early (0–2 mo)**	**Intermediate (2–9 mo)**	**Late (9+ mo)**
Capillaries	2 hr: Endothelial cell changes, increased capillary permeability	Marked capillary abnormalities with widespread obstruction caused by platelets, fibrin, and collagen	Loss of many capillaries, regeneration of new capillaries
	2–7 day: Marked endothelial cell changes and separation from basement membrane and sloughing, producing obstruction of lumen	Regeneration of capillaries; reduced capillary permeability	Reduced capillary permeability
	1+ mo: Many capillaries swollen and obstructed		
Type I pneumocytes	Degenerative changes or normal	Decreased number	Further decrease in number
Type II pneumocytes	Very early degenerative changes becoming more marked with time or normal	Large increase in size and number, abnormal appearance	Return to normal size and number
Basement membrane	Early swelling, indistinct, later very irregular	Folded and thickened	Folded and thickened
Interstitial space	Edema and debris, infiltrated with inflammatory cells and basophils; slight increase in connective tissue	Infiltrated with mononuclear cells, mast cells, inflammatory cells, and connective tissue	Few inflammatory cells; large increase in collagen
Alveolar space	Fibrin, hemorrhages, and debris; Increased number of alveolar macrophages	Becomes smaller	Small or absent, distortion of architecture
Bronchial epithelium	Early transient inflammatory reaction; cillary paralysis, increase in goblet cells or normal	Epithelial proliferation	—

Note: Changes are dependent on mouse strain

From Gross NJ. Pulmonary effects of radiation therapy. *Ann Intern Med* 1977;86:81–92, with permission.[21]

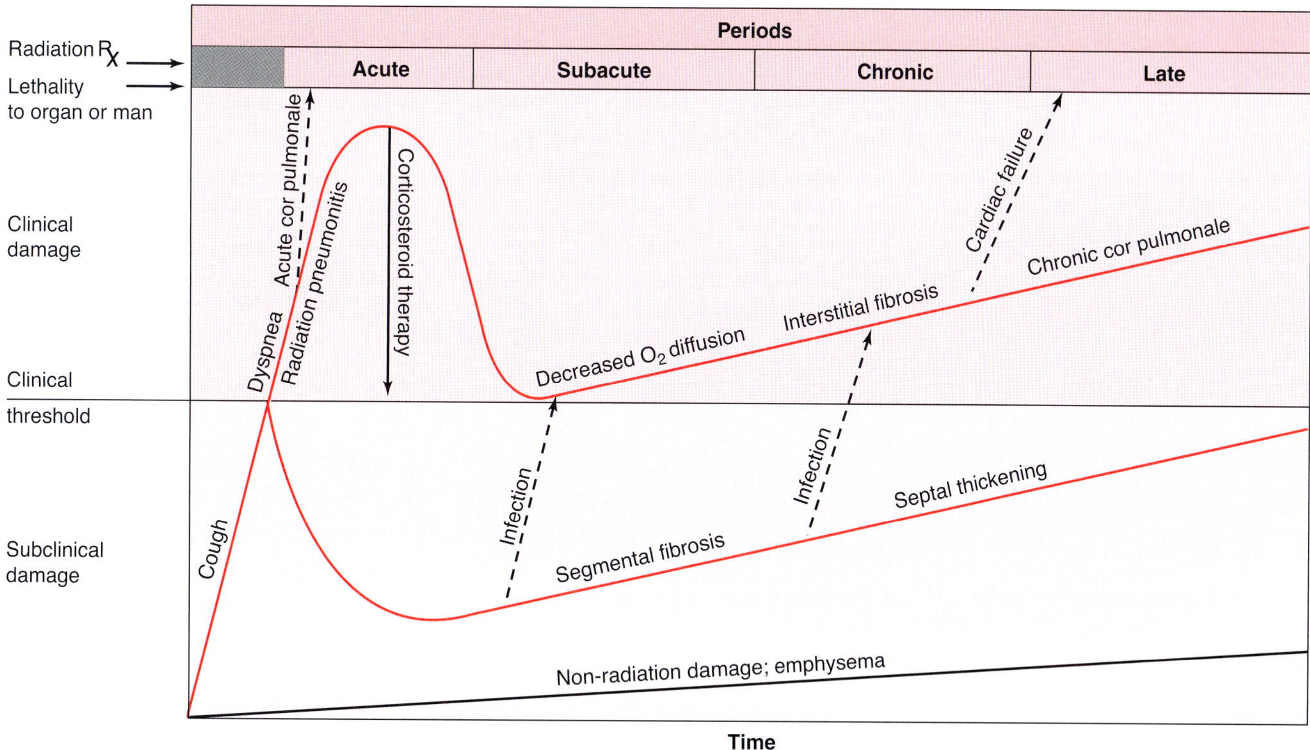

FIGURE 44.1 The clinical course of radiation-induced pulmonary damage consists of four phases, each having distinct pathologic and clinical signs and symptoms. These changes are dependent on dose, as depicted in the upper curve (high dose) and the lower curve (low dose). The changes in the acute phase after high doses are those generally associated with radiation pneumonitis, whereas those occurring during the chronic and late phase are associated with pulmonary fibrosis. After low doses, the pathologic changes are subtle, consisting mostly of interstitial fibrosis, which is usually not sufficiently severe to cause clinical symptoms.[26] (From Rubin P, Casarett GW. *Clinical Radiation Pathology*. Philadelphia: WB Saunders, 1968;459, with permission.)

of acute injury termed *radiation pneumonitis*, a subacute phase, a chronic phase characterized by lung fibrosis, and a late phase (Fig. 44.1).[22–26] Two of these phases are clearly separated in time: pneumonitis occurs from 3 to 6 months after the beginning of treatment, whereas fibrosis occurs from 1 year onward. Both pneumonitis and fibrosis have been well defined histopathologically under controlled conditions in animals. However, because animals can be sacrificed and studied at predetermined times after irradiation, an additional earlier, asymptomatic phase of damage has been defined—the latent phase.[26–28] The characteristics of radiation-induced lung damage during each of these five phases are described further in the following sections.

Latent Phase The weeks to months preceding the overt appearance of radiation pneumonitis is referred to as the "latent" period, because no overt histopathologic, radiographic, or clinical signs and symptoms of radiation damage can be observed. In most cases, overt pulmonary reactions are not expressed either clinically or histologically in humans or in animal models for the first 2 or 3 months after irradiation, regardless of the volume of lung irradiated. Although no changes can be observed at the light microscopy level during this latent period, electron microscopy reveals degranulation and loss of type II cells (with attendant loss of surfactant), loss of basal laminar proteoglycans (resulting in swelling of the basement membrane), and transudation of proteins into the alveolar spaces (indicating increased capillary permeability and suggesting a loss of endothelial cells) within the first month after whole-lung irradiation.[24,25,27] Endothelial cells themselves become vacuolated and pleomorphic and may slough, leading to denudation of the basement membrane and changes in capillary permeability.[29] Although these changes are dose related and diffuse throughout the lung, they are not in themselves sufficiently severe to result in death during this time. Deaths do not occur before overt histologic damage appears.

It was formerly assumed that during the latent phase, a series of biochemical events occurred later manifest as overt expression of damage during the next phase of lung injury (pneumonitis), although no such events had been identified. New molecular techniques and tools suggest that dramatic changes do occur during this period and, depending on the radiation dose, may resolve or may progress to the next phase, which is characterized by overt signs and symptoms of radiation pneumonitis. These molecular changes are discussed next.

Acute Phase: Classic Radiation Pneumonitis Evidence of structural changes in the lung appear within the first 6 months after irradiation of all or part of the lung of humans or experimental animals, resulting in diffuse alveolar damage.[1,26–28] Although this phase of damage occurs relatively long after the lung irradiation, histologically, it is an acute effect that is characterized by a prominent inflammatory cell infiltrate consisting of macrophages, lymphocytes, and mononuclear cells in the pulmonary interstitium, which is normally devoid of cells, and in the air sacs.[3,22,24–28] In animal models, neutrophils usually do not predominate in this inflammatory cell infiltrate. Although loosening and widening of the interstitium indicates interstitial edema, only after high doses is edema observed in the air spaces. When the whole of both lungs is irradiated in humans or experimental animals, the damage is diffuse and, if sufficiently severe, fatal.

This acute phase of damage in the lung is generally referred to as *pneumonitis*, a term that usually refers to an inflammatory reaction in the lung caused by local growth of bacteria, fungi, or parasites. In such situations, the cellular infiltrate contains polymorphonuclear leukocytes, a cell type rarely found in the "sterile" inflammatory infiltrate in the irradiated lungs of experimental animals. When present, these cells are indicative of a superimposed infection and the cause of death—radiation, infection, or both—is unclear. Perhaps a more appropriate term for this phase of diffuse alveolar damage after lung irradiation is *alveolitis*, which refers to an inflammatory reaction, in this case a pathological condition not caused by a microorganism.[30] Although an inflammatory cell infiltrate in the interstitium and the air sacs is a prominent component of radiation alveolitis, the relative contribution of these inflammatory events versus direct tissue injury from radiation in the pathogenesis of this syndrome is unclear.

In mice, pneumonitis begins at 3 months after radiation is administered and persists for up to 6 months, with most deaths occurring between 4 and 5 months posttreatment. The latency period for the appearance of damage depends on the radiation dose, appearing sooner after high doses than after low doses. To account for the dose-dependent difference in the latency period and to include all responders in the assay, researchers set the standard time for scoring deaths from pneumonitis in animal experiments between 3 and 7 months. Techniques used to quantify this phase of lung damage in experimental animals include functional assays such as breathing rate[16,18,20] and carbon monoxide uptake[17]; CT scans[19]; quantitative morphometry[28,31]; and, of course, lethality from the syndrome.[3] These measures provide steep dose–response curves from which estimates of an effect dose for a given severity of injury can be obtained. Generally, the dose that prompts a certain effect in 50% of animals (ED_{50}) or the dose that kills 50% of the population (LD_{50}) is used. In mice, estimates of the LD_{50} from radiation pneumonitis occurring between 3 and 6 months after whole-lung irradiation range from 9 Gy to greater than 16 Gy, depending on the mouse strain. In the clinic, the use of large single doses to the upper half of the body or to the whole body has provided information on radiation dose–response curves for radiation pneumonitis in humans.[32] When either the incidence of pneumonitis[33–36] or evidence of damage on CT scans[9,37] is used to quantify increases in lung density in patients, the shape of the resultant dose–response curves for lung damage in humans parallels those for mice. The ED_{50} for pneumonitis in humans, 9 to 10 Gy, is within the range of LD_{50}s for pneumonitis measured for different mouse strains, although on the low end of the range. In one study, the relationship between regional dose and radiation pneumonitis response was linear when pneumonitis was evaluated with FDG–PET/CT imaging.[14] Although treatment of lung cancer can involve irradiation of large volumes of lung, rarely is the whole lung irradiated, and thus, fatal pneumonitis is relatively uncommon, occurring in 1% to 4% of cases.[38,39] However, that the range in irradiated patients is 2% to 33% for severe pneumonitis,[38–42] and an even higher proportion (up to 77%) demonstrate CT scans lung changes consistent with pneumonitis.

Previously, diffuse alveolitis had been considered characteristic of the acute phase of radiation-induced lung damage in humans and animals, but the histopathologic differences between mouse pneumonitis and human pneumonitis could not be explained. For example, a characteristic histologic finding in irradiated human lung is the presence of hyaline membranes. Mice do not develop fibrosis during the pneumonitis phase, but focal areas of fibrosis have been reported in patients within the first month or two after lung irradiation, the time generally associated with the infiltrative, exudative lesions of radiation pneumonitis. These discrepancies between mice and humans have been partially resolved by the work of Sharplin and Franko,[43] who report that the pathology depends on the strain of mouse used. For example, mice of the C3H and CBA strains showed a classic diffuse alveolitis (pneumonitis) without evidence of fibrosis, whereas the C57B16 strain exhibited protein-rich edema, hyaline membranes, and focal fibrosis, with few of the changes characteristic of pneumonitis (Fig. 44.2). These findings indicate that the choice of mouse strain is critical in studies of radiation lung damage. In fact, mouse strains used to study pneumonitis would be different from those chosen to study fibrosis. Clearly, the mechanism of damage varies between strains, and the underlying mechanisms may vary in humans as well.

Intermediate (Subacute) Phase If the radiation dose is low, or if less than a critical volume of lung is irradiated, the acute pneumonitis phase resolves. Although few data are available on this phase in humans, irradiated mouse lung experiments

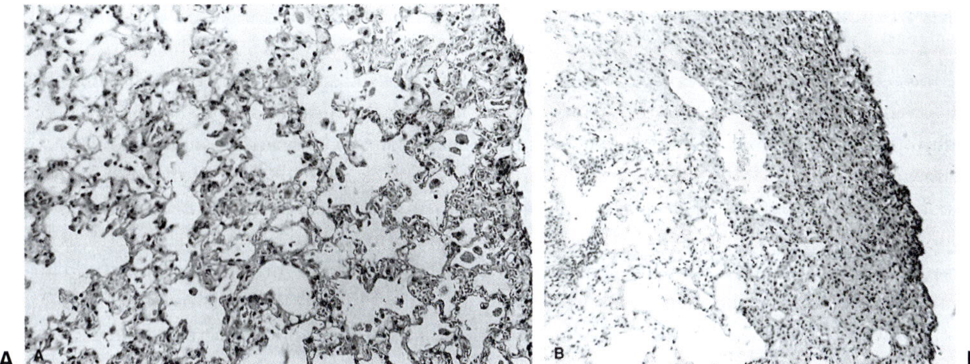

FIGURE 44.2 Characteristic changes in the lungs of C3Hf/Kam **(A)** mice and C57/BL6 **(B)** mice after equivalent single doses of radiation or cobalt-60 gamma rays to the whole thorax. The C3H mouse was sacrificed at 3.5 months because of overt signs of severe respiratory distress; the C57 mouse was sacrificed at 5 months. The lungs of the C3H mouse show a classic radiation alveolitis (pneumonitis), whereas the lungs of the C57 mouse show collapsed atelectatic alveoli with collagen. Superimposed alveolitis is not a feature.

provide a model.[18] In mice that survive the acute pneumonitis phase, lung function, as measured by breathing rate, improves. The lungs, though, are not totally normal, and foci of foamy macrophages with hyperplasia of type II epithelial cells in the air spaces are the dominant findings; however, no deaths occur during this phase of damage. Thus, this phase appears to be one of resolution of the early exudative alveolitis.

Late Phase: Radiation Fibrosis In contrast to the effects of acute alveolitis, the effects of radiation in humans that are chronic are observed from months to years later, even though biochemical and histologic changes occur months earlier. Pulmonary fibrosis develops insidiously and may stabilize after 1 to 2 years. Although numerous studies have attempted to elucidate the mechanism(s) leading to pulmonary fibrosis, the pathogenesis of this late lung response remains elusive and controversial.

Pulmonary fibrosis is the end stage of a complex process of abnormal repair of damage that may be preceded by an inflammatory response dominated by macrophages and lymphocytes. Radiation-induced lung fibrosis is generally thought to be the repair process that follows radiation pneumonitis or radiation alveolitis. Fibrosis of the pulmonary parenchyma may occur as a diffuse or focal lesion, but the designation of pulmonary fibrosis is usually reserved for diffuse or widespread multifocal collagen deposition involving the peripheral air spaces. Although often termed *interstitial fibrosis*, collagenous thickening of alveolar walls is often a consequence of the incorporation of intra-alveolar exudate into the interstitium and the subsequent reepithelialization, which leads to a revision of alveolar architecture. In fact, it is often suggested that severe exudative alveolitis of long-standing duration results in a generalized fibrotic thickening of the alveolar septa.[30,44] Loss of pulmonary function results from focal microcollapse of alveoli and apposition of alveolar walls, leading to irreversible remodeling of pulmonary architecture.

Although lung irradiation studies in mice indicate that pneumonitis and fibrosis are directly related,[28,45–47] other studies, also in murine models, show that these two sequelae of lung irradiation can be dissociated from each other. They also indicate that radiation-induced lung fibrosis can and does occur without a preceding inflammatory event.[48–50] These studies suggest that this phase of injury may result from different pathogenic mechanisms than those underlying pneumonitis.

In mice, the exact form of lung fibrosis that occurs after lung irradiation depends on the strain. In early studies of radiation-induced lung damage, mice were killed at 7 months after irradiation, when the pneumonitis phase of damage ended. However, in later studies, mice surviving to 7 months were followed for periods of up to a year after thoracic irradiation. A diffuse thickening of the alveolar septa characterized by collagen deposition was observed at necropsy in these long-surviving mice.[49,50] The air spaces were clear and patent, and pulmonary architecture was preserved, though the lungs were stiff. Sharplin and Franko[31,43] reported that radiation-induced lung fibrosis in mice was not always manifested as a diffuse thickening of the alveolar septa and that some strains exhibited atelectasis accompanied by collagen deposition in the collapsed area, resulting in a focal contracted scar. In this form of lung fibrosis, alveolar architecture is obliterated. We too have found a difference in the fibrotic lesions in irradiated mouse lung, with the C57B1/6J mice exhibiting collapsed atelectatic alveoli with superimposed collagen and the C3H strain showing a more diffuse fibrosis of the alveolar walls and small stellate scars surrounded by patent alveoli.[51] In C57B1/6J mice, the collagen appears in organized bundles, making it easily distinguishable on light microscopy with collagen-specific stains; in C3H mice, the initial deposition of the collagen as fine, wispy fibrils in the alveolar wall makes this type of fibrosis more difficult to resolve with light microscopy. In addition to these distinct histologic features, these two forms of fibrosis are distinguished further by the time at which they appear in the two strains after irradiation. Fibrosis in the C57B1/6J strain occurs within the first 6 months after irradiation, a period during which only pneumonitis is found in the C3H strain. In the C57B1/6J strain, fibrosis of the alveolar walls does not occur until 9 months (or later) after irradiation.

The suggestion from these mouse studies that the pathogenesis of radiation-induced pulmonary fibrosis may not be uniform across strains suggests that there may be three different pathways to lung fibrosis that may depend on the toxic agent: *luminal fibrosis*, in which granulation tissue buds into the air spaces; *mural fibrosis*, in which exudate is incorporated into the alveolar walls; and *atelectatic induration*, which involves partial or complete collapse of alveoli and permanent apposition of alveolar walls followed by fibrous tissue proliferation and collagen deposition in the area.[30] Franko et al.[52] have suggested from breeding studies in inbred strains of mice that radiation-induced lung fibrosis results from two independent pathways that may involve different genes. Further support for the hypothesis that pulmonary fibrosis can arise through several mechanisms comes from studies of the colon, in which two distinct types of fibrosis have been shown to occur after irradiation, possibly as a result of two distinct mechanisms.[53]

Most studies in mice involve irradiating the whole lung, which is not the standard procedure for radiation-based treatment of lung cancer in humans, in which limited volumes of lung are irradiated. Thus, the question remains as to how relevant findings from experimental animal models are to the radiation-based treatment of lung cancer in humans. For example, hemithoracic irradiation in mice and rats does not produce the same mortality and morbidity as that of whole-lung irradiation because of hypertrophy of the contralateral lung; however, the mechanisms of collapse and fibrosis of the irradiated lung may differ from those that occur after whole-lung irradiation. In studies of the kidney (a paired organ such as the lung), nephrectomy 1 day after bilateral kidney irradiation was found to induce a proliferative response in the remaining irradiated kidney that in turn resulted in partial restoration of kidney function compared with kidney function in irradiated nonnephrectomized mice.[54] Although these differences between animal experiments and radiation-based treatment of humans for lung cancer must be borne in mind, clinical observations indicate that similar-appearing damage occurs in humans and in mice after lung irradiation, supporting the use of these animal models for mechanistic studies. What is most important is that the studies in mice that identified the form and severity of radiation-induced lung fibrosis as being related to the strain of mouse suggest that this late consequence of lung irradiation may be genetically regulated. Identifying, mapping, and cloning the gene(s) for radiation-induced lung fibrosis could provide a means to identify "sensitive" individuals in the population before treatment commences.

Sporadic Radiation Pneumonitis Because one of the characteristic features of classic radiation pneumonitis is that the damage is confined to the irradiated area, it has been suggested that radiation damage that appears outside the irradiated field, anecdotal evidence of which has been available for more than 40 years,[55–58] represents a hypersensitivity pneumonitis. First suggested by Holt in 1964,[59] this syndrome has been given little attention for two reasons: first, it is rare, and second, in most cases the contralateral lung also received some dose, although the actual quantity was unknown. Three factors suggest that this clinical syndrome may be different from the classic form of radiation-induced lung damage: (a) it affects 10% to 15% of patients; (b) symptoms often resolve without sequelae; and (c) it often develops earlier than classic pneumonitis that is within 2 to 6 weeks after the completion of therapy. In an extensive study of four women treated for breast cancer who experienced bilateral changes after radiation confined solely to one lung, Gibson et al.[60] found marked lymphocytosis in bronchioalveolar lavage samples from both the irradiated and nonirradiated lungs. Gallium scanning confirmed these findings, indicating increased gallium uptake in both the irradiated and nonirradiated lungs. In all four patients, symptomatic improvement was prompt after corticosteroid administration. With these observations, these authors concluded that finding equal abnormalities in both the irradiated and nonirradiated fields was not consistent with simple direct radiation-induced damage but rather implied an immunologically mediated mechanism such as hypersensitivity pneumonitis.

More recently, several investigators have challenged the idea that bilateral radiation pneumonitis after unilateral lung irradiation is relatively uncommon.[61,62] These authors contend that the extreme dyspnea experienced by patients with radiation-induced pneumonitis seems to be out of proportion to the volume of lung irradiated and cannot be explained on the basis of localized tissue destruction. Calveley et al.[63] investigated the early activation of inflammatory cytokines and macrophages in different regions of the lung after partial volume irradiation and found evidence of an inflammatory response triggered by the partial volume irradiation in the whole rat lung at very early times after irradiation; that response is maintained in a cyclic pattern until later, when the onset of functional symptoms would be expected. The extent of elevation of cytokines and activated macrophages was similar both in the field of treatment and out of it, although more micronuclei were present in field than out of field. Reactive oxygen species induced by this response were thought to play an important role in the induction of both in-field and out-of-field DNA damage.[63] In a prospective study of 17 women with breast cancer, bronchioalveolar lavage analysis and gallium scanning showed diffuse lymphocytosis, increased gallium scan uptake, and decreased alveolar volume and vital capacity in both the irradiated and nonirradiated lungs. Further analysis of the lymphocyte infiltrate in a patient with clinical radiation pneumonitis showed that these cells were almost exclusively recently activated CD4+ helper T cells, cells that have been implicated in hypersensitivity pneumonitis after other insults. In a further analysis of these patients plus an additional five patients with clinical features of pneumonitis, these investigators found no statistically significant differences between bronchioalveolar findings on the irradiated and nonirradiated sides of the chest either before or after treatment or with or without clinical pneumonitis. Although bilateral lymphocytosis was found in 13 of the 17 patients (76.5%), only 2 had clinical features of radiation-induced pneumonitis. Symptoms resolved spontaneously in the other 11 patients. The other four patients did not demonstrate subclinical or clinical symptoms. Based on these findings, these authors suggested that bilateral involvement of both lungs after the irradiation of one lung represents an immune-mediated hypersensitivity pneumonitis that leads to clinical radiation pneumonitis in only 10% of the irradiated population. Because this syndrome seems to result from an entirely different pathogenetic mechanism than classic radiation pneumonitis, these authors suggested that this form of radiation-induced lung damage be distinguished from the classical form and be called "sporadic radiation pneumonitis." What distinguishes this type of lung damage from the classic type is that it occurs in an unpredictable manner and involves nonirradiated portions of the lung.

At this time, no animal model for sporadic radiation pneumonitis has been identified. However, in a study of CT changes after irradiation of only the right lung of rats, Geist and Trott[64] observed fluctuations in the radiologic density in the shielded left lung of the irradiated rats that were greater than those observed in control rats and parallel to those occurring in the irradiated right lung, similar to the sporadic pneumonitis in humans. However, a study of rabbits indicated that irradiation of one lung resulted in a decrease in the number of alveolar macrophages, but only in the irradiated lung.[65]

Pathogenesis

The Target Cell Concept It has been hypothesized that radiation depletes some critical "target" cells in the lung and that this depletion after a latent period, initiates late sequelae of pneumonitis and fibrosis.[66] The expression of radiation damage also is generally thought to require cell division. Therefore, in tissues like the lung in which damage is not overtly expressed for months after treatment is completed, the long latency period was thought to reflect slowly proliferating target cells. For these reasons, a major research effort has been mounted to identify the target cells with the intention of protecting them from radiation damage, and thereby preventing or at least minimizing the severity of radiation-induced pneumonitis and fibrosis without compromising tumor cell kill and tumor control. The two most likely candidate target cells were thought to be type II cells[26,67–74] and vascular endothelial cells.[26,75–84] Type II cells divide more frequently than do other types of lung parenchymal cells. They are responsible for synthesizing, storing, and secreting surfactant, the surface-active material that prevents alveolar collapse. Vascular endothelial cells also divide more quickly than do other cell types in the lung. Furthermore, edema, a consistent finding in the interstitium and air spaces after lung irradiation, indicates vascular leakage, which in turn implies the radiation-induced killing and depletion of vascular endothelial cells.

Type II Cells The first evidence to support the hypothesis that type II cells were the target cells for radiation pneumonitis was published in 1982 by Shapiro et al.,[69] who showed that in mice, local irradiation of both lungs with a range of single doses of x-rays produced dose-dependent changes in phospholipids in lung lavage fluid and in lung tissue as early as 24 hours after irradiation. These changes persisted for the first 4 weeks after irradiation, indicating that changes in the function of type II cells occurred long before tissue damage was perceivable with light microscopy. Although the relationship of these early events to the later incidence of pneumonitis and fibrosis was unclear, these findings were the first indication that the latent period was not really latent at all. These investigators then sought to identify biochemical markers of surfactant that could be assessed in patients during radiation therapy, before the onset of clinical and pathologic pneumonitis, with the aim of identifying patients at high risk of developing severe radiation pneumonitis.[85] Their discovery that surfactant apoprotein in the serum was an accurate predictor and marker of radiation pneumonitis in rabbits led to further testing in the context of a clinical trial for patients with lung cancer. In that trial, surfactant apoprotein was measured in serum from blood samples collected before treatment, weekly during treatment, and at 1 week after treatment, and the findings were compared with the incidence and severity of radiation pneumonitis and fibrosis assayed by CT scans every 3 months after treatment and by chest radiography at 1 year after treatment.

Endothelial Cells The suggestion that vascular damage was the underlying mechanism of radiation pneumonitis and fibrosis was based primarily on the hypothesis that the lung cell most likely to divide soon after irradiation was the capillary endothelial cell. The parenchymal cells, particularly the type II cells, were thought to divide more slowly than endothelial cells. This hypothesis was substantiated by pathologic findings in humans and experimental models that pneumonitis after irradiation was characterized by edema in the air spaces and interstitium and an inflammatory cell infiltrate. Among the many investigators attempting to elucidate the role of the vasculature in radiation-induced lung damage, Ward et al.[86–89] undertook comprehensive studies to correlate changes in four parameters of endothelial function (angiotensin-converting enzyme activity, plasminogen activator activity, and prostacyclin and thromboxane production) with histopathologic and ultrastructural changes in rat lungs irradiated with the same doses and with changes measured by arterial perfusion, a vascular functional assay. Those studies showed dose-dependent changes in all endothelial function parameters and good agreement between these functional changes and pathologic changes in the lungs of the rats. These findings suggest that changes in vasculature do occur after lung irradiation, but they do not necessarily implicate the endothelial cell as the target cell.

TABLE 44.2 Target Cells and Growth Factors Associated with Radiation-Induced Pneumonitis and Fibrosis

Pathophysiologic Target Cells	Biochemical Marker	Growth Factors	Lesion or Event
Type II pneumocyte	Surfactant released into alveolus	TGF-α TGF-β	Acute pneumonitis
Capillary endothelial cell	Surfactant protein enters into blood serum through altered permeability	FGF IL-1 PDGF	Acute pneumonitis and/or fibrosis
Macrophage	Surfactant persists for days or weeks because of decrease in macrophases essential to its removal	IL-1 PDGF TGF-α TGF-β	May protect against pneumonitis, increase septal fibrosis
Septal fibrocyte	Procollagen III appears preceding fibrosis buildup; also, metaloprotease appears, as does elastase and collagenase		

Abbreviations: TGF, transforming growth factor; FGF, fibroblast growth factor; IL, interleukin; PDGF, platelet-derived growth factor.

From Rubin P, Finkelstein J, Shapiro D. Molecular biology mechanisms in the radiation induction of pulmonary injury syndromes: interrelationship between the alveolar macrophage and the septal fibroblast. *Int J Radiat Oncol Biol Phys* 1992;24:93–101, with permission.[91]

BIOLOGICAL BASIS OF RADIATION-INDUCED LUNG DAMAGE

Changes in both the pulmonary parenchyma and pulmonary vasculature contribute to radiation pneumonitis and fibrosis (Table 44.2), and these sequelae of lung irradiation arise from dynamic interactions among different cell types, the major players being type II pneumocytes and endothelial cells, as well as fibroblasts, macrophages, and lymphocytes (Fig. 44.3).[90,91] However, the concept that one or more target cells are solely responsible for radiation-induced pneumonitis and pulmonary fibrosis has been replaced by the paradigm that it is not only cells but also the messages that those cells send that determine the final outcome.

Molecular and Tissue Responses during Radiation-Induced Lung Damage Radiation is but one of many insults that prompt the release of trophic factors that subsequently act through various signaling pathways to

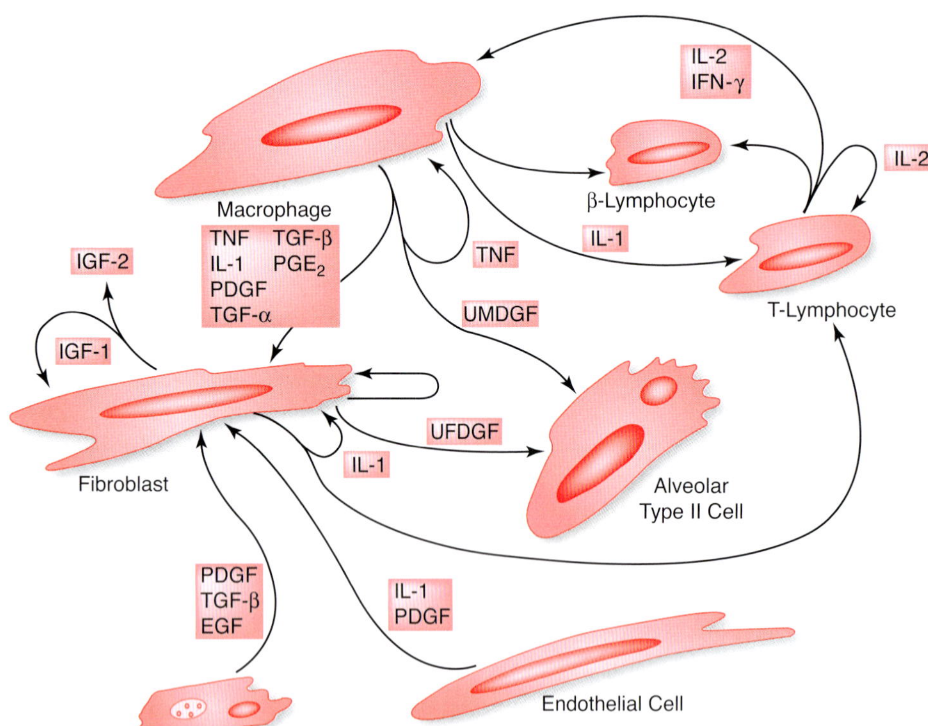

FIGURE 44.3 Diagram of hypothesized interaction of different lung target cells and cytokines and growth factors in the development of alveolitis and fibrosis. *EGF,* epidermal growth factor; *IGF,* insulin-like growth factor; *IFN,* interferon; *IL,* interleukin; *PDGF,* platelet-derived growth factor; *PGE,* prostaglandin E_2; *TGF,* transforming growth factor; *TNF,* tumor necrosis factor; *UFDGF,* unidentified fibroblast-derived growth factor; *UMDGF,* unidentified macrophage-derived growth factor. (From King RJ, Jones MB, Minoo P. Regulation of lung cell proliferation by polypeptide growth factors. *Am J Physiol* 1989; 257:L23–L38, with permission.)

produce the pathologic end results of radiation pneumonitis and fibrosis.[92–97] The messages are delivered via the diffusion of soluble mediators over short distances; such mediators may have been secreted by one population of cells and then act locally on either another population (paracrine stimulation) or the same population (autocrine stimulation), or they can interact with membrane-associated molecules that activate receptors on adjacent target cells (juxtacrine stimulation). These soluble mediators, known as cytokines or growth factors, are crucial in stimulating cells to overproduce the extracellular matrix components that characterize fibrosis.[23,92–94,98] After their initial contact with the cell surface, these molecules are postulated to activate intracellular signaling pathways, which in turn leads to activation of complex genetic programs characteristic of the fibrotic response.

Two concepts have been proposed to explain how cells read signals from cytokines.[93,99,100] In the first concept, cytokine signaling pathways are not insular or isolated paths or devices but rather are segments in a dense network that monitors itself through various crosstalk and feedback links and adjusts the activity of each constituent pathway. The nature of those adjustments, in turn, determines the nature and timing of the signals conveyed. In the second concept, the pathway provides the cell with information about the arrival of a certain cue but does not provide precise instructions. The cell, more than the pathway, determines the outcome of the signal.[100] In either event, cytokines are known to mediate the development of pneumonitis and fibrosis, both of which represent tissue responses to the damage induced by ionizing radiation. Several such cytokines, including transforming growth factor β (TGF-β), tumor necrosis factors (TNF-α and TNF-β), the interleukins, KL-6, and the intracellular adhesion molecule (ICAM)-1, are discussed further in the following paragraphs.

Transforming Growth Factor β The TGF-β cytokine family regulates the proliferation and differentiation of cells, embryonic development, wound healing, tumor progression, and angiogenesis[101,102] and can trigger a bewildering diversity of responses depending on the genetic makeup and environment of the target cells.[100] TGF-β regulates cellular process by binding to three high-affinity cell-surface receptors known as types I, II, and III (TGF-β: TGF-β1, TGF-β2, and TGF-β3). Each isoform is encoded by a distinct gene and is expressed in both a tissue-specific and a developmentally regulated fashion. The type I and II receptors contain serine-threonine protein kinases in their intracellular domains that initiate intracellular signaling by phosphorylating several transcription factors know as Smads (derived from the Sma and MAD gene homologues in *Caenorhabditis elegans* and *Drosophila melanogaster*). Of the 10 Smads, Smads 2 and 3 are phosphorylated by activated type I TGF-β receptors, whereas Smads 6 and 7 block the phosphorylation of Smads 2 and 3.[102] Deregulation of TGF-β signaling pathways has been implicated in the development of several major diseases, including cancer; atherosclerosis; fibrotic disease of the kidney, liver, and lung; and autoimmune diseases.[102] Mutations in the genes for TGF-β, its receptor, or intracellular signaling molecules associated with TGF-β are also important in the pathogenesis of disease, particularly cancer and hereditary hemorrhagic telangiectasia.[101]

TGF-β is an important mediator of tissue damage in various abnormal conditions associated with excess collagen production. TGF-β1 in particular is often associated with lung fibrosis in response to several types of toxic insult, including radiation.[23,98,103] The TGF-β signal is transduced to the nucleus through the activation of its receptors, which in turn activate one or more Smad transcription factors, which then act on one or more of many potential target genes (Fig. 44.4).[102,104]

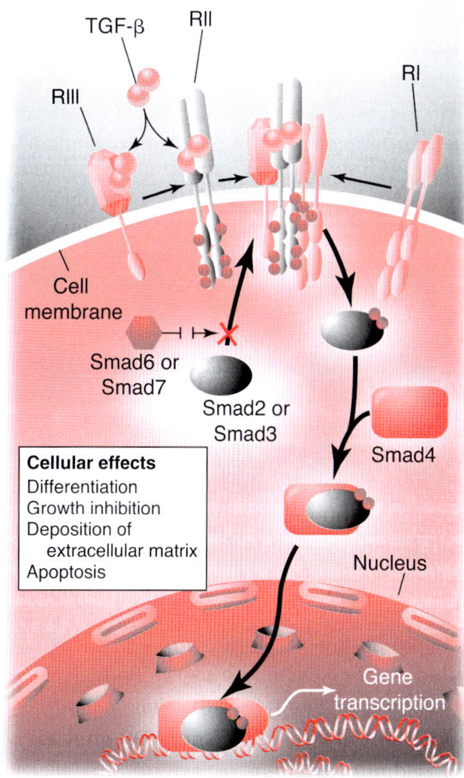

FIGURE 44.4 Mechanism of signal transduction mediated by transforming growth factor β (TGF-β). In the extracellular space, TGF-β binds either to the type III TGF-β receptor (RIII), which presents it to the type II receptor (RII), or directly to RII on the cell membrane. The binding of TGF-β to RII then leads to binding of the type I receptor (RI) to the complex and the phosphorylation of RI (*small spheres*). This phosphorylation activates the RI protein kinase, which then phosphorylates the transcription factor Smad2 or Smad3. Phosphorylated Smad2 or Smad3 binds to Smad4, the common Smad, and the resulting complex moves from the cytoplasm into the nucleus. In the nucleus, the Smad complex interacts in a cell-specific manner with various other transcription factors to regulate the transcription of TGF-β–responsive genes and mediate the effects of TGF-β at the cellular level. Inhibitory Smad6 and Smad7 lack the region normally phosphorylated by RI and thus interfere with the phosphorylation of Smad2 or Smad3 by RI.[102] (From Blobe GC, Schiemann WP, Lodish HF. Role of transforming growth factor beta in human disease. *N Engl J Med* 2000 May 4; 342[18]:1350–1358.)

In vivo, TGF-β stimulates the recruitment of lymphocytes and fibroblasts to sites of damage, promotes fibroblast proliferation, and stimulates the production of collagen and fibronectin—the effect being a net increase in extracellular matrix material, which eventually replaces the normal architecture of the tissue. TGF-β also increases the production of type I plasminogen activator inhibitor while simultaneously decreasing the production of plasminogen activators, resulting in not only an increase in the production of connective tissue but also a decrease in its breakdown, leading ultimately to maturation of this excess connective tissue and the formation of scars.[51,102]

Rubin et al.[91] were the first to report that alveolar macrophages obtained from bronchial lavage specimens from irradiated rabbits demonstrated increased production and release of TGF-β relative to macrophages from normal lungs. Those investigators suggested that the fibroblast proliferation and extracellular matrix production seen after irradiation resulted from the release of cytokines such as TGF-β from parenchymal cells. Johnston et al.[105] reported an increase in the expression of TGF-β1 messenger RNA (mRNA) in radiation-fibrosis–prone but not in radiation-fibrosis–resistant strains of mice. That increase in TGF-β mRNA correlated with an increase in extracellular matrix protein expression in the irradiated lung tissue. Finkelstein et al.[92] studied whether changes in early expression of collagen precursors or cytokines known to be involved in the fibrotic process were expressed during the latent period, before damage was manifested histologically. These investigators used two single whole-thorax radiation doses to C57B1/6J mice, a strain known to be sensitive to the fibrogenic effects of lung radiation. The lower dose (5 Gy) is well below the threshold known to induce clinical symptoms and pathologic changes of radiation pneumonitis and fibrosis, and the higher dose (12.5 Gy) is closer to the reported LD_{50} for radiation-induced lung damage in this strain, although this dose itself does not cause death from lung damage. The results showed that mRNAs for all three isoforms of TGF-β (i.e., TGF-β1, -β2, and -β3) were increased in the lungs of C57B1/6J mice at 14 days, but a consistent dose–response relationship was not found. Thus, radiation doses that cause neither clinical signs nor pathologic changes indicative of radiation lung damage can lead to changes in the expression of this fibrogenic cytokine before the onset of overt lung damage and may ultimately lead to the development of chronic fibrosis.

The importance of TGF-β1 in the development of radiation-induced lung damage has been underscored in human studies as well as in animal experiments.[106–109] The feasibility of using TGF-β1 levels to identify patients who can safely tolerate radiation dose escalation was tested in 38 patients with non–small cell lung cancer (NSCLC).[106,110] At the end of the initial radiation treatment, patients with TGF-β1 levels lower than pretreatment levels and patients with TGF-β1 levels of less than 7.5 ng/mL were selected for subsequent radiation dose escalation (86.4 vs. 73.6 Gy) to the primary tumor and enlarged lymph nodes. The predominant severe (grade $\geq$ 3) late toxicity in that study was not pulmonary but rather was esophageal, suggesting that monitoring plasma TGF-β1 levels might be useful for identifying patients resistant to both radiation-induced lung damage and esophageal toxicity.[106,107,110] In a later study, TGF-β1 levels were found to be elevated (>20 ng/mL) before treatment in 51% of 68 patients with NSCLC.[111] Plasma TGF-β1 levels after radiation therapy were associated with both pretreatment levels ($p = 0.001$) and with mean radiation dose to lung, and the mean ratio of plasma levels at weeks 4 to 6 of treatment to pretreatment levels predicted radiation pneumonitis, according to Southwest Oncology Group criteria ($p = 0.01$) but not that defined by other scoring systems. However, this study was criticized for its high TGF-β1 baseline values, which were thought to be artifacts from the methods of blood collection and processing.[111]

Inflammatory Cytokines Just as depletion of one type of target cell is unlikely to trigger the complex pathologic process of radiation pneumonitis and fibrosis, it is equally unlikely that the overexpression of a single cytokine initiates and promulgates the fibrogenic process in the lung. Much more likely is that the damage, repair, and restructuring of the lung after irradiation (as well as after other toxic insults) are the results of a cytokine network orchestrated by a few key cytokines, such as TNF-α/β and TGF-β. Several classes of cytokines can contribute to the risk of radiation pneumonitis, among which the interleukins, TNF-α, and TGF-β1 have been recognized to play major roles. At the core of the inflammatory response after radiation exposure is the production of such proinflammatory cytokines as TNF-α and interleukin-1 and interleukin-6 (IL-1 and IL-6) and macrophages, lymphocytes, and other lung cell types.[112–114] Thus, it may be the balance of a few positive profibrogenic cytokines and negative antifibrogenic cytokines generated from the interaction of several cytokines constituting these networks that may finally determine the outcome of lung injury and inflammation. Unfortunately, dissecting the specific role of any of these cytokines in lung damage and repair is not easy; however, one approach to determining the role of various cytokines in lung fibrosis is to take advantage of known differences in susceptibility to radiation-induced fibrosis among inbred mouse strains.

Johnston et al.[115] used the fibrosis-prone C57B1/6J mouse strain and the fibrosis-resistant C3H/HeJ mouse strain to show that the elevation of mRNA levels of several chemokines implicated in the recruitment of inflammatory cells to sites of pulmonary damage was not different between the two strains when assessed at 8 weeks after irradiation. However, by 26 weeks after irradiation, messages encoding transcripts produced predominantly by macrophages and lymphocytes were elevated only in the fibrosis-prone mice. These findings indicate that lymphocytic recruitment and activation are key components of radiation-induced fibrosis, but their role in the pathogenesis of this process remains unclear.

Clinical studies have shown that elevation of IL-1α, IL-6, and IL-10 are associated with the risk of radiation-induced lung damage.[116–118] In fact, IL-1α and IL-6 have been used as markers for the diagnosis or prediction of radiation pneumonitis.[118] TNF-α[119] vascular endothelial growth factor, and fibroblast growth factor (FGF) have also been shown to be associated with radiation lung injury.[120–122] Arpin et al.[116] found that IL-6 levels were significantly higher ($p = 0.047$) during 3D conformal radiation therapy in patients who later were diagnosed with radiation pneumonitis and that covariations of IL-6 and IL-10 levels during the first 2 weeks of that therapy were independently predictive of radiation pneumonitis ($p = 0.011$). Chen et al.[118] also confirmed the importance of IL-6 measurements for the prediction of radiation pneumonitis. These results suggest that levels of one or more cytokines could be useful as biomarkers to monitor tissue response during the early course of radiation therapy with the goal of identifying patients who may benefit from adaptive redesign of that therapy.

Patient smoking status has also been linked with the risk of radiation pneumonitis. An in vitro study showed that cigarette smoke extract augmented the release of IL-8 from bronchial epithelial cells in a concentration- and time-dependent manner.[123] That study also showed that IL-8 in bronchoalveolar lavage samples from smokers was higher than that in samples from nonsmokers.[123] Other work has shown that exposure to tobacco smoke suppressed the expression of proinflammatory cytokine mediators.[124] In 2005, Hart et al.[125] reported that pretreatment IL-8 levels were four times higher in patients who did not develop symptomatic radiation-induced lung damage than in patients who did, suggesting that the IL-8 level might be useful for predicting who may develop radiation pneumonitis before the treatment is begun.

KL-6 The antigen KL-6 is a mucinlike high–molecular weight glycoprotein that is expressed on type II pneumocytes and bronchiolar epithelial cells and has been used as a serum marker of interstitial pneumonitis. The group that discovered KL-6 noted that 60% of patients with various kinds of interstitial pneumonitis had abnormally high KL-6 levels and that serum KL-6 levels correlated with the degree of clinical disease activity, as measured by gallium-67 citrate scintigraphy and the clinical course.[126] KL-6 also seems to be a useful marker for detecting severe pneumonitis and estimating its prognosis.[126–128] In another study of patients who developed severe radiation pneumonitis, serum KL-6 levels tended to increase before or after the clinical diagnosis of extensive radiation pneumonitis outside the radiation fields, but no change was noted before or after localized radiation pneumonitis inside the radiation fields. Moreover, patients whose serum KL-6 levels rose more than 1.5 times higher than their pretreatment serum KL-6 level were at greater risk of developing severe radiation pneumonitis that was unresponsive to steroid hormones and resulted in death.[129] In a study of women undergoing adjuvant radiation therapy for breast cancer, posttreatment serum levels were significantly different between patients with radiation pneumonitis and those without radiation pneumonitis.[130] Other investigators studying patients with primary and metastatic lung tumors who had been given single-fraction stereotactic radiotherapy found that the ratio of serum KL-6 levels at 2 months after treatment and levels at baseline correlated with the occurrence of radiation pneumonitis.[131] This 1- to 2-month gap between the time at which predictive measurements are the most accurate and the diagnosis of radiation pneumonitis, however, limits the predictive value of KL-6 for this purpose.

Intercellular Adhesion Molecule–1 ICAM-1 is an intercellular adhesion molecule of the immunoglobulin supergene family involved in adherence of leukocytes to the endothelium and in leukocytic accumulation in pulmonary injury. ICAM-1 is upregulated in association with inflammation in response to numerous types of inducing factors. In normal lung tissue, the expression of ICAM-1 on alveolar type I epithelial cells is stronger than on alveolar macrophages and on endothelial cells.[132] Selective ICAM-1 expression was detected on the surface of type I alveolar epithelial cells and, to a lesser extent, on the pulmonary capillary endothelium and on alveolar macrophages. Bleomycin-induced lung fibrosis demonstrated altered ICAM-1 distribution at the alveolar epithelial surface, and soluble ICAM-1 was detected by Western blot analysis.[132] The expression of ICAM-1 on pulmonary endothelial cells after stimulus and subsequent binding of neutrophils is a first step leading to lung injury. A similar process may dictate the binding of tumor cells to the pulmonary endothelium during metastasis. TNF-α upregulates ICAM-1 expression in a dose- and treatment interval–dependent fashion.[80]

Expression of ICAM-1 can also be upregulated by gamma irradiation through the action of catalase. Furthermore, catalase, c-Jun N-terminal kinases (JNKs), and activator protein 1 (AP-1) activation induce ICAM-1 upregulation through a sequential process.[133] ICAM-1 and lymphocyte function–associated antigen–1 (LFA-1) expression on alveolar macrophages was significantly increased starting 1 week after irradiation, whereas their expression on lung tissue was not elevated up to 8 weeks after irradiation, suggesting that adhesion molecules play a role in the development of radiation-induced lung injury.[134] Using immunohistochemical assay for upregulation of adhesion molecules associated with recruitment, transendothelial migration, and proliferation of bronchoalveolar macrophages, researchers found significant upregulation of vascular cell adhesion molecule–1 (VCAM-1) and ICAM-1 at 100 days after 20 Gy to total lung irradiation with further increases up to the time of death. Increases were first detected in endothelin-positive endothelial cells. These data suggest an association between late irradiation-induced pulmonary fibrosis and the upregulation of adhesion molecules and disclose potential targets for intervention in the pulmonary vascular endothelium.[135]

Clinically, expression of human leukocyte–associated antigen (HLADR) and ICAM-1 on T cells in bronchoalveolar lavage fluid increased in patients who developed radiation pneumonitis after radiation for lung cancer. A significant association was seen between the incidence of ICAM-1 expression on T cells and the number of days from the initiation of radiotherapy to the onset of radiation pneumonitis.[136] In another study, 30 patients were irradiated with a total dose of approximately 60 Gy. Blood samples were taken before, midway, and after radiotherapy.

Bronchoalveolar lavage was also performed before and after radiation therapy in seven cases. A total of 12 out of 30 (40%) cases developed radiation pneumonitis. Serum levels of soluble ICAM-1 after radiation therapy were significantly elevated in patients who developed pneumonitis compared with those who did not. In some of the cases, sICAM-1 levels began to increase at an early phase of irradiation. These findings suggest that ICAM-1 may have an important role in the development of radiation pneumonitis and that sICAM-1 may be a useful marker for the early detection of radiation pneumonitis.[137]

Thus, despite abundant evidence that expression of a multitude of cytokines is elevated in radiation-induced pneumonitis and lung fibrosis, their actual in vivo role and the mechanism of their upregulation remain to be determined. Regardless of our lack of understanding of how these factors mediate damage and repair in the lung, it is clear that the latent phase preceding the overt expression of radiation damage in the lung is not a quiescent time. Molecular changes are occurring that may later ultimately result in the clinical and histopathologic picture of pneumonitis and fibrosis. The events that lead to the overt expression of radiation-induced lung damage involve several complex cellular and molecular processes, which explain why both the inflammatory responses and the triggering mechanism that induces the fibrotic response in the lung remain poorly understood.

Genetic Regulation

Animal Studies Animal studies, particularly those showing strain-dependent outcomes, indicate that genetics are implicated in vulnerability to pneumonitis and fibrosis. Twenty years ago, Steel et al.[138] reported an anomalous finding after irradiation of the whole thorax of C57B1 mice that the survival time of this inbred strain of mice was significantly longer than the standard 80 to 180 days reported in other strains with radiation pneumonitis. Subsequent studies by Down et al.[139,140] in several inbred mouse strains showed that the incidence of radiation pneumonitis and fibrosis was strain dependent. Although strain-dependent differences could result from several factors, genetics offers a plausible explanation. In an in-depth survey of the incidence of radiation pneumonitis and fibrosis in nine inbred mouse strains, Sharplin and Franko[43] showed that the strains could be categorized as fibrosing, nonfibrosing, or intermediate, based on quantitative histologic findings. Further studies by these authors showed that crossbreeding strains with different proneness to fibrosis produced hybrids with the same sensitivity of the parent least prone to fibrosis: the hybrid of a fibrosing and a nonfibrosing strain was uniformly nonfibrosing, whereas a cross of an intermediate with a fibrosing strain produced an intermediate hybrid,[141] suggesting that sensitivity to radiation-induced fibrosis is an autosomal recessive trait. Supporting this hypothesis is a report from Haston et al.[51] that one locus on chromosome 17 segregates with the fibrosing phenotype and that this locus, which is within the region containing the major histocompatibility locus (MHC), was linked to both bleomycin-induced lung fibrosis[142] and susceptibility to ozone-induced lung damage in mice.[143] These researchers also showed that a quantitative trait locus on chromosomes 17 influenced susceptibility to radiation-induced pulmonary fibrosis. Chromosome 6 (logarithm of the odds [LOD] = 4.6), which has an additional region containing a quantitative trait locus, showed linkage in female mice only. The evidence for linkage to chromosome 18 weakened when it was analyzed jointly with other markers. These loci—on chromosomes 1, 6, 17, and 18—were estimated to account for 70% of the genetic contribution to this trait, with chromosome 17 accounting for 28% and chromosome 1 for 24%. Furthermore, the quantitative trait locus on chromosome 17 for radiation-induced lung fibrosis is within the same region as a quantitative trait locus identified for lung damage after other insults (e.g., from bleomycin, ozone, and particle exposure) as well as from asthma, suggesting that this region of chromosome 17 may harbor a "universal" lung injury gene.[144] These findings suggest that although other loci have been shown to be insult dependent, at least one genetic factor regulating pulmonary fibrosis may be universal and independent of the etiology of that fibrosis.

Also supporting a genetic sensitivity theory is that other pathologic processes in the lung are known to be under genetic regulation. Pulmonary inflammation is well-known to be controlled by genes in the H-2 complex.[145–147] Mice with an H-2^k locus are high responders, and those with an H-2^b locus are low responders.[145,147,148] In the studies of Sharplin and Franko[43] and Down et al.,[140] pneumonitis was found to be strain dependent and related to the H-2 locus; that is, an inflammatory cell infiltrate was not a feature of pneumonitis in the highly fibrogenic strain, and, conversely, an inflammatory cell infiltrate was the most prominent characteristic of the pneumonitis phase in the weakly fibrogenic strain. Although these observations refute the hypothesis that immune-inflammatory processes usually precede fibrosis, they clearly indicate that pneumonitis after irradiation of mouse lung is genetically regulated. However, the strain sensitivity to radiation pneumonitis is exactly opposite for that of radiation-induced fibrosis.

Two forms of lung fibrosis have been described.[31] One form of fibrosis is a collagen deposition in the interstitium and air spaces, resulting in contracture and collapse of the alveoli, an obliteration of normal lung architecture, and an attendant loss of pulmonary function resulting in the death of the mouse. Another form of fibrosis is characterized by collagen deposited only in the interstitium, a process that maintains alveolar structure, and was largely ignored because it was suggested that this lesion alone would not produce sufficient functional impairment to cause death. The genetic regulation that controls these two forms of fibrotic processes may not be identical to that controlling interstitial fibrosis, although there may be overlap between the two. Furthermore, interstitial fibrosis in the lung[18] and colon[53] can result in death in animal studies.[139]

Evidence suggests that the fibrosis evident in mouse lung after exposure to radiation can arise through two independent mechanisms: one is controlled by two autosomal recessive determinants that act additively, and the other is regulated independently by two additional genes, one of which is X-linked.[45] Similar strain variations in pulmonary fibrosis after other kinds of insults have been reported. Particularly interesting are the results obtained after treatment with bleomycin, another DNA-damaging agent often used to induce lung fibrosis in model systems. The most striking observation after bleomycin treatment is that[149–152] the findings were remarkably similar to those observed after radiation. These findings, like those reported by Haston et al.,[144] suggest that genetic factors related to susceptibility to lung fibrosis may operate independently of the etiologic agent.

Clinical Evidence Intrinsic sensitivity to radiation is known to differ among individuals. Estimates indicate that, given the same standardized radiation dose, technical and clinical factors account for about one third of the interpatient variation in normal-tissue reactions, and genetic differences between patients account for the greater proportion of differences in sensitivity.[153] Certainly the severity of treatment-related complications, including the severity of radiation-induced pneumonitis and fibrosis after definitive radiation therapy for lung cancer, have been evident clinically for some time. Geara et al.[154] demonstrated considerable patient-to-patient heterogeneity in a group of 56 patients with limited small cell lung cancer treated with chemoradiation therapy, suggesting that the risk of lung fibrosis is strongly affected by inherent factors that vary among individuals.

Evidence is increasing that indicates that genetic variations in a few selected cellular pathways, such as those involved in DNA repair, cell cycle, and inflammation, may affect radiation sensitivity, treatment response, and toxicity.[155–162] For example, patients with the genetic syndromes of ataxia telangiectasia, Nijmegen breakage syndrome (NBS1), or Bloom syndrome (BLM) demonstrate hypersensitivity to radiation,[163–165] and genes that are defective in these syndromes (ataxia telangiectasia mutated [ATM], NBS1, or BLM, respectively) are known to play critical roles in DNA repair, particularly double-strand break repair. In vitro studies in cell lines that are hypersensitive to radiation have demonstrated that the repair genes for double-strand breaks, x-ray repair cross-complementing 1 gene (XRCC1) to x-ray repair cross-complementing 7 genes (XRCC7), are responsible for hypersensitivity. Patients with immune deficiencies arising from defects in double-strand break repair genes, such as defects in the DNA-dependent protein kinase catalytic subunit (DNA-PKcs) (XRCC7), Ku70 (XRCC6), and Ku86 (XRCC5) genes, exhibit high radiation sensitivity.[166–168]

Family studies also suggest a genetic predisposition to radiosensitivity. Roberts et al.[169] studied the heritability of radiation sensitivity in peripheral blood lymphocytes in families of patients with breast cancer. They found that 62% of the first-degree relatives of radiation-sensitive patients were also sensitive compared with 7% of the first-degree relatives of patients with normal sensitivity. Segregation analysis of 95 family members showed clear evidence of high heritability of radiation sensitivity.

PHYSICAL BASIS OF RADIATION-INDUCED LUNG DAMAGE

Fractionation, Volume, and Dose

Fractionation The sparing effects of fractionating dose in radiotherapy has been known since the experiments performed on rams' testicles in the 1920s and 1930s. Assuming that the testes were a model of a rapidly growing tumor and the skin of the scrotum was representative of normal tissues, researchers found that a ram could not be sterilized by a single dose of radiation without causing extensive damage to the skin; however, spreading the dose over several weeks resulted in sterilization without producing unacceptable skin reactions. The basis of fractionation lies in the understanding that dose fractionation spares normal-tissue reactions by allowing repair of sublethal damage and repopulation of target cells during treatment while increasing tumor cell kill by allowing reoxygenation and reassortment of cells into more sensitive parts of the cell cycle.[170–174] For years, the standard fractionation regimen consisted of radiation delivered in doses of 1.8 to 2.0 Gy per fraction over treatment times of 4 to 6 weeks. Modification of this conventional treatment schedule by increasing the dose per fraction in the treatment of lung cancer resulted in unacceptable sequelae in tissues such as the spinal cord. However, it was not until the early 1980s that radiation oncologists began to understand differences in normal tissues' fractionation sensitivity.

Lung is a *late-responding normal tissue*; that is, damage is not evident until weeks to months after completion of a standard course of radiotherapy. In contrast, tissues such as intestinal mucosa, which are acutely responding normal tissue, manifest damage during and shortly after completion of a course of treatment. An analysis of experimental data for a variety of both acutely and late-responding normal tissues by Thames et al.[175] demonstrated a clear and consistent difference between fractionation effects in these two categories of tissues. By plotting the total dose for an isoeffect specific to various tissues versus the dose per fraction, it was found that the total dose for a given effect in any late-responding normal tissue increased more rapidly as the dose per fraction was decreased than did the total dose for an effect in any acutely responding normal tissue. This pattern was observed consistently in all acutely and late-responding tissues analyzed and suggests that late-responding tissues such as the lung are more sensitive than acutely responding tissues to changes in dose per fraction. These data imply that decreasing the dose per fraction should spare late-responding tissues such as the lung more than acutely responding tissues as well as the tumor, if tumors respond like acutely responding normal tissues. It has been suggested that the difference in fractionation response for acutely and late-responding normal tissues is because of differences in the repair capacity or shoulder shape of the underlying dose–response curves for these two classes of tissues(the dose–response curve for the late-responding tissues is curvier [has a narrower shoulder] than that for acutely responding tissues).[175] One way of defining these differences is by the α/β ratio, which derives from the linear quadratic model of cell killing.[175–179] In brief, this model assumes that there are two components of cell killing by radiation, one that is proportional to dose and the second that is proportional to dose.[2] The α/β ratio, then, is the dose at which the linear and quadratic contributions to cell killing are equal. For late-responding tissues, such as the lung, the dose-response curve bends at lower doses than for acutely responding tissues, and therefore, the dose at which the α and β contribution to cell killing is equal is lower in late-responding than acutely responding tissues. In general, the α/β ratio is below 5 Gy for late-responding normal tissues and greater than 5 Gy for acutely responding normal tissues. For the lung, the α/β is about 3 Gy.[173,180–183] In clinical radiotherapy, then, significant sparing of normal lung damage can be gained by decreasing the dose per fraction.

A second factor in the sparing of normal tissues is repopulation of surviving cells during treatment. The lung's late response, occurring weeks to months after completion of treatment, means that repopulation does not occur during a conventional 4- to 6-week treatment schedule. Although retreatment studies in the lung suggest that this may not be totally correct and that repopulation may occur within the first 4 weeks after irradiation,[184] it remains a general axiom that conventional fractionation schedules extending for 6 weeks do not allow triggering of proliferation and subsequent repopulation in the lung. Therefore, prolonging overall clinical radiation treatment time will have little, if any, sparing effect on the lung.

Supporting this hypothesis are clinical data that demonstrate that lung fibrosis incidence increases with increasing total dose greater than a threshold of 30 to 35 Gy, with concurrent use of cisplatin and etoposide chemotherapy, with accelerated fractionation (Fig. 44.5).[185] Other support for this hypothesis comes from a meta analysis of 24 series that included 29 treatment groups and 1911 patients. Investigators evaluated such factors as the radiation dose per fraction, total radiation dose, fractionation scheme (split or continuous), type of chemotherapy and intended dose intensity, overall treatment time, histology (small cell lung cancer or NSCLC), and treatment schedule (concurrent or induction, sequential, or alternating chemotherapy). The median total dose of radiation used in the trials analyzed was 50 Gy (range, 25 to 63 Gy). The median daily fraction dose used was 2.0 Gy (range, 1.5 to 4.0 Gy). Nineteen series included 22 treatment groups and 1745 patients treated with single daily fractions. Among these patients, 136 received a daily fraction greater than 2.67 Gy. Five series used twice-daily radiation therapy and included 166 patients (fraction dose, 1.5 to 1.7 Gy). The incidence of radiation pneumonitis was 7.8%. In a multivariate analysis, only radiation dose per fraction, number of daily fractions, and total dose were significantly associated with the risk of radiation pneumonitis ($p < .0001$, $p < .018$, and $p < .003$, respectively). The use of a fraction dose greater than 2.67 Gy was the most significant factor associated with an increased risk of radiation pneumonitis. High total dose also seemed to be associated with an increased risk, but twice-daily irradiation seems to reduce

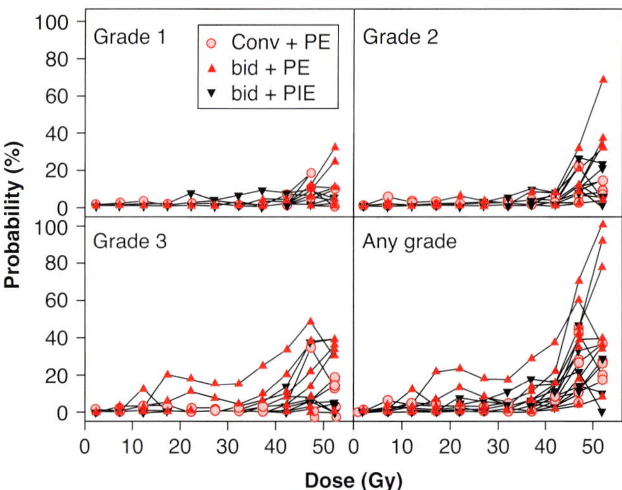

FIGURE 44.5 Fibrosis. Graphs show the average probability of physician-identified radiographic grade 1, 2, or 3 fibrosis or any fibrosis occurring as a function of dose for each fractionation and chemotherapy combination. For doses of 30 to 55 Gy and cisplatin and etoposide (PE) chemotherapy, the risk of fibrosis (any grade) with the accelerated fractionation schedule (bid, twice daily) was 2.01 ± 0.34 times higher than that with conventional (*conv*, i.e., once-daily) fractionation ($p < .005$). The probability of fibrosis with the PIE chemotherapy (cisplatin-etoposide [PE] plus ifosfamide) was not statistically significantly different from either of the other schedules (error bars, ±1 standard error).[185] (From Rosen II, Fischer TA, Antolak JA, et al. Correlation between lung fibrosis and radiation therapy dose after concurrent radiation therapy and chemotherapy for limited small cell lung cancer. *Radiology* 2001 Dec;221[3]:614–622, with permission.)

the risk expected had the same total daily dose been given as a single fraction (Fig. 44.6).[186] In a comparison of incidence of radiation pneumonitis for patients who received single daily fractions of ≤2.67 Gy, split doses in twice-daily treatment, or once-daily irradiation using fractions >2.67 Gy, patients who received daily doses exceeding 2.67 Gy had the highest incidence of radiation pneumonitis.[186] Hence, the size of the dose per fraction of radiation delivered to the lung is the dominant factor in determining lung damage, and overall treatment time has relatively little influence. The more important consideration is that prolonging treatment time may decrease tumor response because of the accelerated repopulation of surviving and proliferating tumor cells during treatment.[187–189]

These radiobiological findings have been translated into the clinical treatment of lung cancer using fractionation protocols that vary from the conventional protocols by reducing the size of the dose and giving more than one fraction per day while keeping the overall treatment time the same as in traditional schedules. To compensate for the loss of cell killing in the tumor by the reduction in dose per fraction, radiation oncologists give higher total doses. Thus, the goal is holding the lung damage constant by reducing dose per fraction while simultaneously increasing tumor control by giving a higher total dose. The fractionation schedule most commonly used

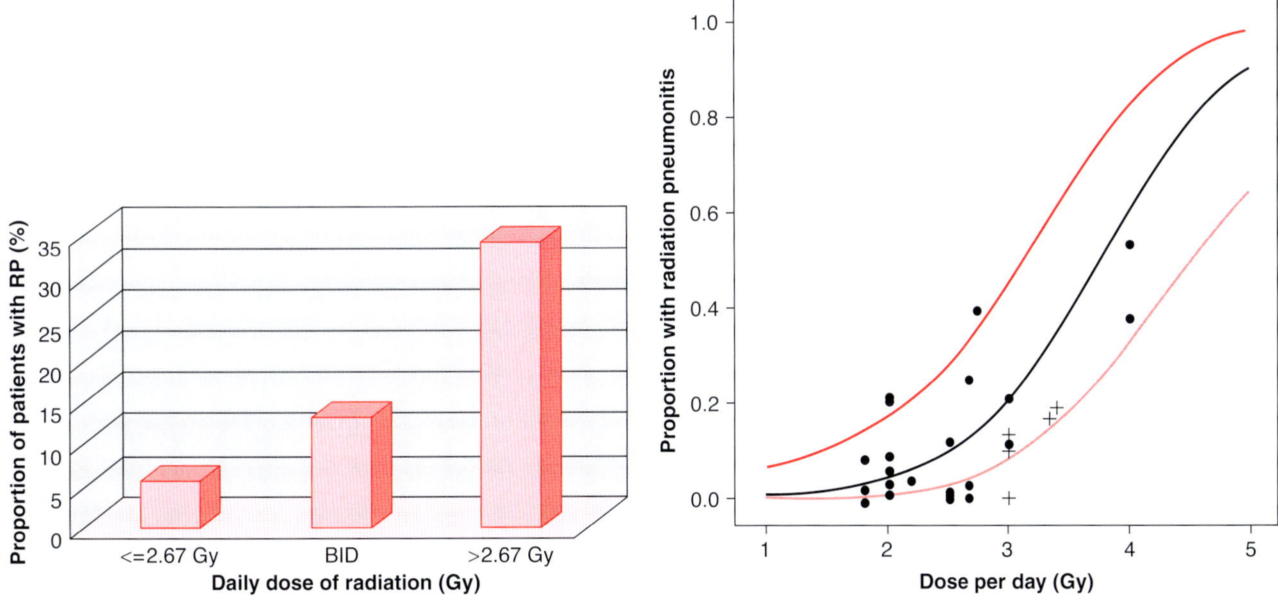

FIGURE 44.6 Relationship of dose per day and probability of radiation pneumonitis. Incidence of radiation pneumonitis for patients who received single daily fractions of ≤2.67 Gy, twice-daily treatment, or once-daily irradiation using fractions >2.67 Gy are shown in the bar graph (**left**). Patients who received a daily dose >2.67 Gy had the highest incidence of radiation pneumonitis. Curve (**right**) represents predicted proportion of patients who experienced radiation pneumonitis based on 27 treatment groups (+, studies with twice-daily fractions) and includes 95% confidence intervals. Curve was generated using the mean proportion as a function of daily dose, assuming a total dose of 48 Gy. Note a rapidly increasing incidence of radiation pneumonitis is predicted for daily fractions >2.5 Gy. Twice-daily irradiation was associated with a lower incidence than expected.[186] *BID*, twice daily; *RP*, radiation pneumonitis. (Adapted from Roach M III, Gandara DR, Yuo HS, et al. Radiation pneumonitis following combined modality therapy for lung cancer: analysis of prognostic factors. *J Clin Oncol* 1995 Oct;13(10):2606–2612, with permission.)

in this type of treatment, termed *hyperfractionation*, gives two doses of 1.2 Gy per day. In initial clinical trials, the total doses given ranged from 60 Gy, the same total dose given in conventional schedules using one fraction of 2 Gy per fraction, to 69.6 Gy.[190–192] The risk of both acute and late effects was found to be acceptable, and there was a dose response for survival, with survival significantly improved in patients receiving the highest total dose. In a second trial, total doses were escalated to a maximum of 79.2 Gy, but this increase in total dose did not result in a significant survival advantage, although lung toxicity remained acceptable.

Irradiated Lung Volume It is well accepted in radiation oncology that in addition to using and modifying fractionation, reducing the volume of normal lung irradiated is an effective technique for lowering morbidity. The use of 3D treatment planning and conformal radiation therapy has allowed the use of more than the traditional two to four opposing treatment fields, making it possible to tailor the treatment plan to the individual patient and tumor; however, the dose distributions in these nontraditional plans may be very different from those used in standard two- or three-field treatments. For example, some plans may deliver a small dose to a larger volume of lung than in opposed fields, making it difficult for the radiotherapist to extrapolate from experience a prediction of the probability of incurring morbidity. In addition, the lung is a paired organ and has a large functional reserve; thus, it is expected that it would exhibit a threshold volume, that is, a subvolume below, which irradiation causes no detectable injury, even at very high doses.[3,174,193,194] However, such useful information as the threshold volume or measures indicating the relationship of the volume of lung irradiated to dose and/or morbidity have not been defined because most experimental studies have been performed using whole-lung irradiation.

Volume Effect and Spatial Heterogeneity In the late 1990s, with the increasing use of conformal therapy and increasing questions from radiotherapists regarding the volume response of the lung, experimental mouse studies have been initiated in several laboratories to address these questions. Most of the data for partial lung irradiation have been obtained from hemithoracic irradiation studies in mice and rats. In these studies, single-dose irradiation of only one lung led to dose-dependent increases inbreathing rate but not in lethality (Travis, unpublished observations). The initial increase in breathing rate was followed by a decrease that was suggested to be coincident with compensatory hypertrophy of the nonirradiated lung and/or the formation of new alveoli that increased the surface area of the lung. Both breathing rate and lethality are indications of total lung function, both the irradiated half

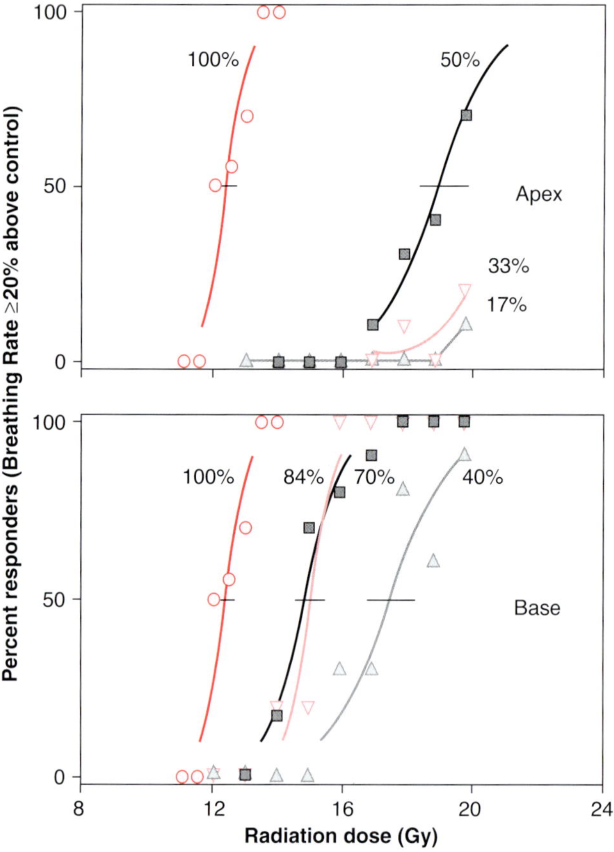

FIGURE 44.7 Dose–response curves of lethality after irradiation of two partial volumes of the lungs of C3H mice: 70% to 75% (**top**) or 50% (**bottom**), located in the apex or base of the lung. The dose–response curve for whole lung is shown for comparison. These data show a clear volume effect. The lethal dose that kills 50% of the population (LD_{50}) for irradiation of 50% in either the base or apex is higher than the irradiation of the larger volume of 75% in these same two sites. In addition, these data show that the LD_{50} is dependent on the site of the lung irradiated. The isoeffect dose is less for both volumes irradiated in the base than in the apex, suggesting that the base is more sensitive than the apex. These data indicate that the volume effect is dependent not only on the volume of lung irradiated but also on the site of the lung irradiated. (From Liao ZX, Travis EL, Tucker SL. Damage and morbidity from pneumonitis after irradiation of partial volumes of mouse lung. *Int J Radiat Oncol Biol Phys* 1995;32:1359–1370, with permission.)

and the nonirradiated half, and assays of both show clearly that the lung has a large functional reserve. Other studies using blood flow changes in mice and rats undergoing hemithoracic irradiation showed that vascular changes in the irradiated lung were similar to those after whole-lung irradiation.[79] Thus, this assay of regional function showed no difference between whole- versus partial-lung irradiation.

A series of mouse experiments has been undertaken to define the relationship of radiation dose and volume to lung damage, assessed histopathologically, and morbidity, assessed by two tests of total lung function—breathing rate and lethality.[195,196] In these studies, a range of lung volumes, from 20% to 100%, were irradiated. Matched volumes were also irradiated in the base or in the apex of the lung to test the hypothesis that the functional subunits were randomly and homogeneously distributed. Figure 44.7 shows the proportion of dead mice after irradiation of two of the matched volumes in the apex and base of the lung, 50% and 75%. Figure 44.8 shows breathing rate and lethality as a function of the percentage volume of lung irradiated in the apex or the

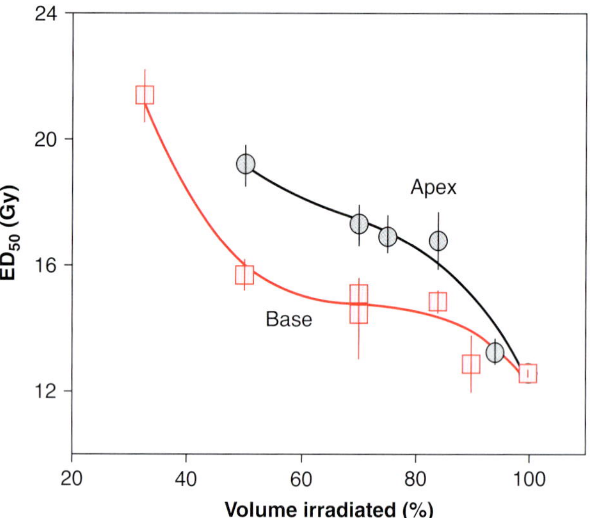

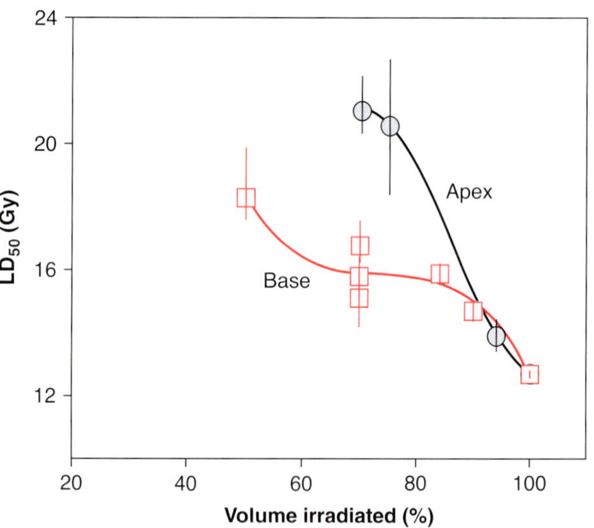

FIGURE 44.8 Breathing rate (ED_{50}) (**top**) and lethality (LD_{50}) (**bottom**) for radiation pneumonitis, plotted as a function of partial volume irradiated in the apex or base of the lung. The curves are second-order regression fits to the data. The curve for irradiation of a range of volumes in the base is consistently displaced below that for irradiation of the same volumes in the apex; that is, the isoeffect doses for both breathing rate and lethality are lower for all volumes irradiated in the base than in the apex. These data show clearly that the base is more sensitive than the same volume in the apex for the induction of radiation pneumonitis.[196] (From Travis EL, Liao ZX, Tucker SL. Spatial heterogeneity of the volume effect for radiation pneumonitis in mouse lung. *Int J Radiat Oncol Biol Phys* 1997;38:1045–1054, with permission.)

base of the lung.[196] These findings clearly show that for any given volume, the base of the lung is more sensitive than the same volume in the apex, that is, that the isoeffect doses for both breathing rate and lethality are lower for all irradiated volumes in the base than in the apex.

Although the underlying mechanism of this spatial heterogeneity in the response of the mouse lung to radiation is unknown, Travis et al.[196] suggested that the target cells or functional subunits are heterogeneously distributed in the lung because of the anatomy of the tracheobronchial tree. The alveoli are concentrated in the periphery of the lung, whereas the midregion of the lung is most occupied by conducting airways, which are not involved in gas exchange. Thus, the base of the lung is more sensitive because there is a higher concentration of alveoli and fewer conducting airways in this region, whereas a large portion of the midregion of the lung is occupied by large branching bronchi and bronchioles. Boersma et al.[197] suggested that these regional differences in the incidence of pneumonitis could be accounted for by differences in functionality of cells in the base and apex rather than to a difference in density. Khan et al.[198,199] ascribed these regional differences in the incidence of radiation pneumonitis to differences in the amount of DNA damage sustained by the cells in the apex and the base. They proposed that during irradiation the cells in the base sustain more DNA damage than those in the apex, whereas out-of-field effects are observed primarily in the upper lung (i.e., after lower lung irradiation). Interestingly, this differential in DNA damage between cells isolated from the apex or base of the lung disappears, whereas the left lung sustains more damage than the right lung when the whole lung is irradiated.[199]

Regardless of the mechanism underlying these regional differences, the morbidity of lung irradiation is related not only to the volume of lung irradiated but also to the location of the irradiated subvolume within the lung. These findings, then, would suggest that morbidity would be greater when the irradiation portal includes the base than when it includes the apex. These findings also suggest that the volume irradiated in the base in the course of conformal therapy be kept as small as possible.

Regardless of the mechanism of the heterogeneity of the lung's response to partial-volume irradiation, these findings influence the use of less conventional treatment techniques such as 3D conformal radiation therapy and, more recently, IMRT for the treatment of lung cancer. Both of these techniques treat larger volumes of normal lung than do conventional treatment techniques, although the normal lung would get a smaller dose. However, the question of whether giving a lot of radiation to a little volume (conventional treatment) is better or worse than a giving a little to a lot (3D and IMRT) has not been answered. Using the mouse data, Tucker et al.[200] calculated the incidence of pneumonitis for subvolumes of the lung irradiated with a fixed dose. The complication rate varied over the entire range of possible responses, from a 100% incidence after irradiation of the base to a 0% incidence after irradiation of the mid lung, with an intermediate incidence after irradiation of the apex (Fig. 44.9).[200] These data indicate that relatively small changes in the location of the irradiated subvolume in lung may

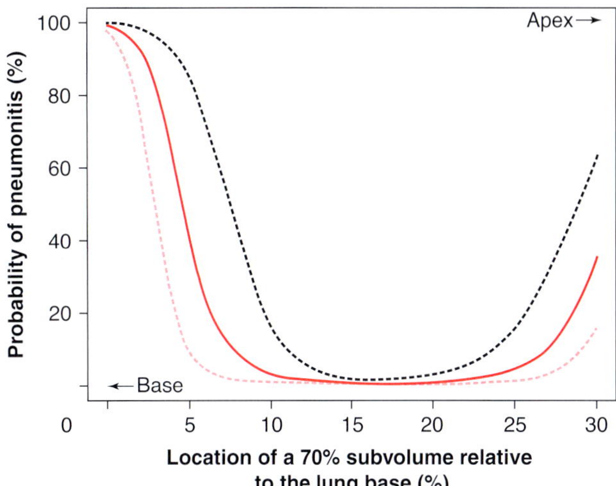

FIGURE 44.9 Effect of subvolume location on response calculated using estimates of cell density in different subvolumes of the lung. The *solid curve* shows the predicted incidence of pneumonitis in mice after irradiation of a subvolume of fixed size (70%) with a fixed dose (22 Gy), plotted as a function of the location in the lung of the irradiated subvolume. The complication rate varies over the entire range, from a 100% incidence rate after irradiation of the base to a 0% incidence after irradiation of the mid-lung to an intermediate incidence after irradiation of the apex. The 95% confidence band (*dashed curves*) around the predicted curve is based on the uncertainty in the estimated cell density parameters.[200] (From Tucker SL, Liao ZX, Travis EL. Estimation of the spatial distribution of target cells for radiation pneumonitis in mouse lung. *Int J Radiat Oncol Biol Phys* 1997;38:1055–1066, with permission.)

correspond to significantly greater changes in the incidence of pneumonitis than moderate changes in either the dose or the size of the irradiated subvolume. With the mouse data, Tucker et al.[200] used a constant integrated dose of 12.7 Gy and found that the risk of pneumonitis varied enormously depending on the site of the irradiated subvolume (Fig. 44.10), whereas for both the apex and the midregion of mouse lung, a little to a lot was found to be worse that a lot to a little, provided that the integrated dose (the product of volume and dose) was kept constant. However, a quite different picture emerges for the base, where irradiation of 50% to 70% of the lung is predicted to be worse than irradiation of either larger or smaller subvolumes, again provided that the integrated dose is kept constant. After volumes larger than 70%, the decrease in the probability of pneumonitis occurs because the increase in the number of cells irradiated is more than offset by the decrease in dose required to maintain the constant integrated dose. In terms of the threshold volume, that is, the volume below, which radiation causes no detectable injury even at very high doses, the predicted size of this volume depends on the region of lung irradiated and ranges from 10% in the base to 30% to 40% in the apex.

Interestingly, clinical studies[42,201–203] have found that the risk of pneumonitis in patients varies with the location of the irradiated site, just as had been observed in mouse lung. In a study of 60 patients treated with radiation and chemotherapy

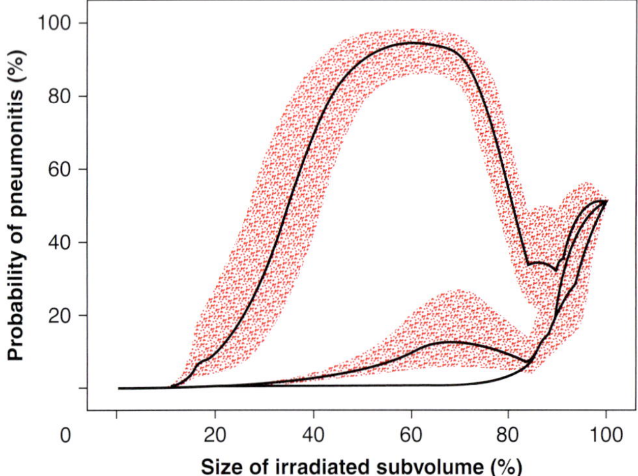

FIGURE 44.10 Predicted incidence of pneumonitis in mouse lung as a function of irradiated volume where the integrated dose (dose × volume) is kept fixed at 12.7 Gy, equal to the whole-lung LD_{50}. The upper, middle, and lower curves represent volumes in the base, apex, or midregion of the lung, respectively. Stippled regions around the curves represent the 95% confidence limits. It is clear that whether a lot to a little is better than a little to a lot is critically dependent on the location of the irradiated subvolume. In the base, the risk of pneumonitis is highest after irradiation of an intermediate subvolume with an intermediate dose, whereas in the apex, a little to a lot is generally worse than a lot to a little.[200] (From Tucker SL, Liao ZX, Travis EL. Estimation of the spatial distribution of target cells for radiation pneumonitis in mouse lung. *Int J Radiat Oncol Biol Phys* 1997;38:1055–1066, with permission.)

given either sequentially or concurrently for lung cancer, the site of irradiation was evaluated by dividing the whole lung into three-by-three areas, that is, the right and left lung were divided into three equal areas from upper to lower lung field. When the risk of pneumonitis was analyzed by irradiated site, it was found that when the lower lung field was irradiated, the incidence of pneumonitis was 70%, compared with 20% for other fields ($p < 0.01$). Multivariate analysis revealed a significant relationship between irradiated field and the risk of pneumonitis ($p = 0.0096$). In another study of 106 patients, registered chest CT and SPECT lung perfusion scans were obtained before curative or radical radiation therapy for NSCLC. The mean lung dose (MLD) was calculated. The SPECT perfusion data were used to weight the MLD with perfusion, resulting in a mean perfusion-weighted lung dose. In addition, the lungs were geometrically divided into different subvolumes. The mean dose for each region was calculated and weighted with the perfusion of each region to obtain a mean perfusion-weighted regional dose. The incidence of radiation pneumonitis correlated significantly with the MLD and mean regional dose of the posterior, caudal, ipsilateral, central, and peripheral lung subvolumes ($p \leq 0.05$). A statistically significant difference ($p = 0.01$) in the incidence of radiation pneumonitis was found between patients with cranial and caudal tumors (11% and 40%, respectively). When a dose-independent offset NTCP parameter for caudal tumors was included in the NTCP model, most correlations were significantly improved, confirming that patients with caudal tumors have a greater probability of developing radiation pneumonitis.[202] These results are consistent with those from mouse studies indicating that irradiation of the base of the lung is significantly associated with a higher risk of pneumonitis.

Clinical Evidence of a Volume Effect Animal studies have demonstrated conclusively that a low dose scattered over a large lung volume causes more early toxicity than an extreme dose confined to a small volume.[204] Since the introduction of 3D conformal radiation therapy, many clinical studies have reported an association between the volume of lung irradiated and the risk of radiation pneumonitis.[40,41,74,203,205,206] The dose–volume parameters thought to be crucial for the development of radiation pneumonitis have varied among investigators: Willner et al.[74] found rV10, V20, V30, and V40 to be the most important, whereas Fay et al.[205] found rV30, V40, and V50 and Wang et al.[41] found V5 to be the significant parameters. Clinical evidence supports the findings from animal studies that a little radiation to a lot of lung is not safe. In a study of 223 patients with NSCLC treated with concurrent chemoradiation, the rV5 was found to be the only independent factor associated with grade ≥3 radiation pneumonitis in multivariate analysis.[41] This finding suggested that damage to the lung, which has functional subunits arranged in parallel, may depend more on the volume irradiated than on the radiation dose. This finding is supported by Gopal et al.,[207] who observed a sharp loss in the diffusing capacity for carbon monoxide of normal lung exposed to as little as 13 Gy. The investigators concluded that a small dose of radiation to a large volume of lung could be much worse than a large dose to a small volume in functional lung damage. Yorke et al.[208] also reported that the risk of complications rises steeply above a MLD of 10 Gy, indicating a need to limit widespread irradiation of normal lung tissue, even at low doses. Furthermore, fatal pneumonitis was reported when a large volume of normal lung received low-dose irradiation.[209] Nonetheless, findings have not been uniform. Willner et al.[74] reported, in contrast, that logistic regression curves for V10, V20, V30, and V40 demonstrated sharper increases in risk of radiation pneumonitis at higher doses, and the investigators concluded that a small dose, such as 10 Gy, to a large volume of normal lung is preferable to a large dose, such as 40 Gy, to a small volume.

In contrast to the data from lung function tests, no volume effect was found for damage in the studies of Liao et al.[195] In their animal studies, a characteristic pneumonitis was found in all mice regardless of the volume of lung irradiated. These results illustrate the necessity to define whether damage or morbidity is being assessed in both clinical and animal studies, as different answers may be obtained. These findings also indicate that measures of total lung function that are a sum of the function in the irradiated volume and the function of normal lung in the nonirradiated volume will be different from regional lung function measures that assess damage only in the irradiated area.

Dose–Volume Relationship in Patients

Assessing Regional Lung Function: CT Density

Approximately 50% to 0% of patients who undergo lung irradiation will have radiographic or pulmonary function abnormalities following treatment; however, the significance of these changes in terms of morbidity varies from minimal to severe, depending on lung volume irradiated. A comprehensive study of radiation pneumonitis after partial volume fractionated irradiation in patients was conducted by Mah et al.[33] The end point was an increase in lung density observed within the irradiated volume on CT in the posttreatment period. The estimated single-dose equivalent (ED_{50}) was 10 ± 4 ED units, at the low end of the dose range for pneumonitis in various mouse strains (Fig. 44.11).[33] However, no information was obtained for the effect of these changes on pulmonary function. More recent studies by Boersma et al.[4,6] and Marks et al.[11] in which changes in regional lung function were quantified showed that the dose–effect curves for both functional parameters studied—perfusion and ventilation (Fig. 44.12)—were less steep than the dose–effect curve for structural changes as measured by density changes on CT published previously by Mah et al.[9,37] The lack of correlation between CT changes as a measure of structural damage and tests of regional lung function was clearly observed in one study by Boersma et al.,[4] in which all assays were performed in the same patients. These data suggest that lung density may be a different biological end point from perfusion and ventilation, the former representing the late phase of fibrosis, whereas the latter measure the ability of the irradiated lung within that area to perform gas exchange.

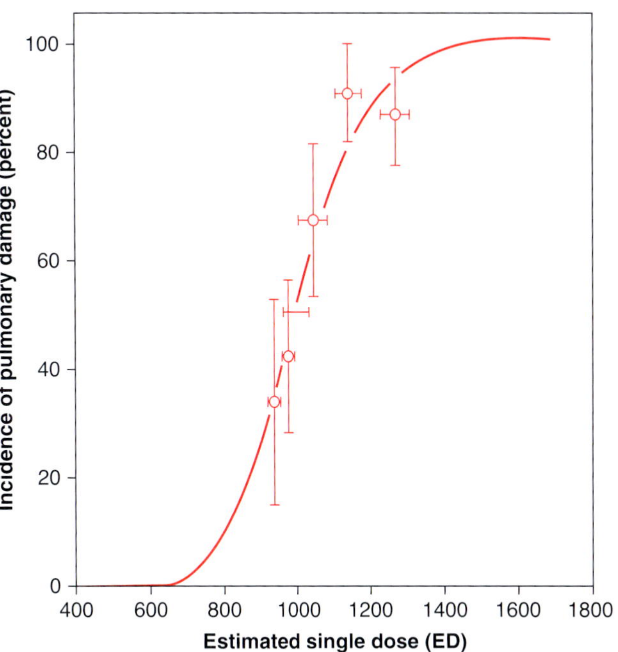

FIGURE 44.11 Dose–response curve for the incidence of acute radiation pneumonitis after fractionated radiation therapy of the whole lung in humans. The solid curve is the best fit sigmoid to the data points as determined by probit regression. An ED_{50} of 1000 ED units with a standard error of 40 ED units is predicted. Vertical error bars are the standard deviation of the points.[33] (From Mah K, Van Dyk J, Keane T, et al. Acute radiation-induced pulmonary damage: a clinical study on the response to fractionated radiation therapy. *Int J Radiat Oncol Biol Phys* 1987;13:179, with permission.)

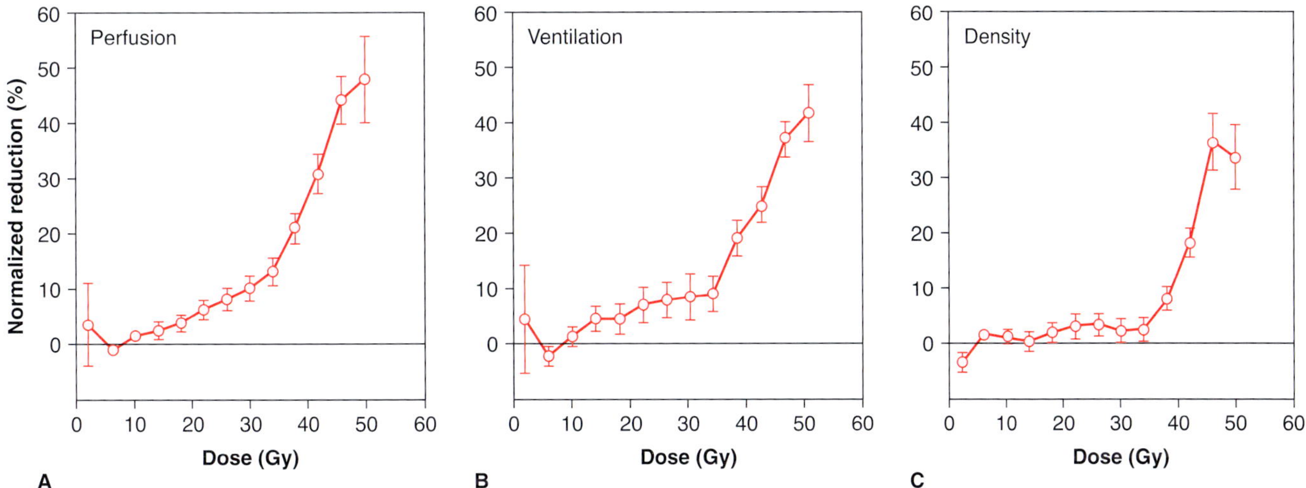

FIGURE 44.12 Dose–incidence curves for perfusion **(A)**, ventilation **(B)**, and lung-density changes **(C)** greater than 20%, indicating the fraction of patients with average local changes greater than 20%. The *solid lines* are logistic fits to the data points; the *error bars* on the points indicate the 68% confidence limits.[4] (From Boersma LJ, Damen EM, de Boer RW, et al. Dose-effect relations for local functional and structural changes of the lung after irradiation for malignant lymphoma. *Radiother Oncol* 1994;32:201–209, with permission.)

Assessing Regional Lung Function: SPECT Numerous studies in the literature describe changes in local lung function using several assays, such as those described previously and others such as SPECT scanning.[10,11,202,210–215] In a study of 184 patients who were treated before the 3D conformal therapy era, Marks et al.[216] calculated dose function–volume histograms by correlating pretreatment CT data with SPECT data. Within 6 months of radiation therapy, 80% of the radiation-induced symptoms were noted. Neither was there an association between the presence or absence of radiation-induced pulmonary symptoms and the frequency of radiation-induced radiographic changes, nor in the dose–response curve for radiation-induced reductions in regional perfusion, because these end points did not consider the volume of lung affected.[214] Another study that sought to correlate the changes in pulmonary function test results after radiation therapy with radiation dose, tumor regression, and changes in lung perfusion included 82 patients who were treated during the 3D conformal radiation therapy era (DVHs were available).[217] In a multivariate analysis, the total tumor dose and MLD were not associated with a reduction in pulmonary function. Tumor regression resulted in a significant improvement of forced expiratory volume in one second (FEV_1), but it was also associated with a reduction of total lung diffusion capacity (TL,COc). The mean perfusion-weighted lung dose (MpLD) and the predicted perfusion reduction showed a significant ($p \leq 0.04$) but low correlation ($r \leq 0.31$) with the reduction of both FEV_1 and TL,COc. The perfusion-related dose variables (the MpLD or the predicted perfusion reduction) are the best parameters for estimating pulmonary function after radiation therapy.[217]

In summary, prediction of radiation pneumonitis based on SPECT data DVHs was not superior to standard DVHs, nor was the overall predictability of radiation-induced lung damage improved when receiver operating characteristic curves, a plot of the true-positive rate versus the false-positive rate, were applied to evaluate SPECT perfusion-based dose-function histograms. Interestingly, in the subgroup of patients with pretreatment single-breath carbon monoxide diffusing capacity (DL_{CO}) >40%, SPECT-based dosimetric parameters were more predictive than the CT-based ones. [215] Despite the potential benefit of integrating SPECT into predictive models, the latter has not yet become a standard practice.

Assessing Regional Lung Function: FDG-PET FDG-PET can detect metabolic changes in regions of the normal tissue that have been irradiated.[14,218,219] Guerrero et al.[14] quantified the relationship between the local radiation dose received and the posttreatment PET/CT FDG uptake in the lung in 36 patients with esophageal cancer who were treated with preoperative concurrent chemoradiation. These patients provided a good clinical normal-lung model, because their lungs were not diseased and they had good lung function. Their treatment planning CT was registered with the restaging PET/CT. The median time between radiation therapy completion and FDG–PET imaging was 40 days (range, 26 to 70 days). The median of the mean standard uptake value in the lung that received 0 to 5 Gy was 0.63 (range, 0.36 to 1.27), 5 to 10 Gy was 0.77 (range, 0.40 to 1.35), 10 to 20 Gy was 0.80 (range, 0.40 to 1.72), and >20 Gy was 1.08 (range, 0.44 to 2.63). Statistical modeling found a linear relationship. The slope of this relationship varied over an order of magnitude, reflecting the range of the underlying biological response to radiation among the study population. (Fig. 44.13[14]) Furthermore, Hassaballa et al.[218] tried to determine whether acute changes in shielded lungs could be detected by FDG-PET in 16 patients with NSCLC. They found that 13 of 16 patients (81.3%) showed increased FDG uptake in shielded nonirradiated lung in four distinct patterns: contralateral peripheral pleural uptake, ipsilateral peripheral pleural uptake, bilateral peripheral pleural uptake, and bilateral diffuse background uptake. This last patient developed clinically evident radiation pneumonitis. The role of functional images, such as SPECT and FDG–PET scans, in predicting the risk of radiation pneumonitis is limited because the information for comparison and prediction is only available after the completion of radiation, when damage to the lung has been done, hence, defeating the purpose of prediction.

Quantifying the Dose–Volume Relationship However, what is critical in 3D conformal treatment in which both dose and volume are changing is the effect of these changes

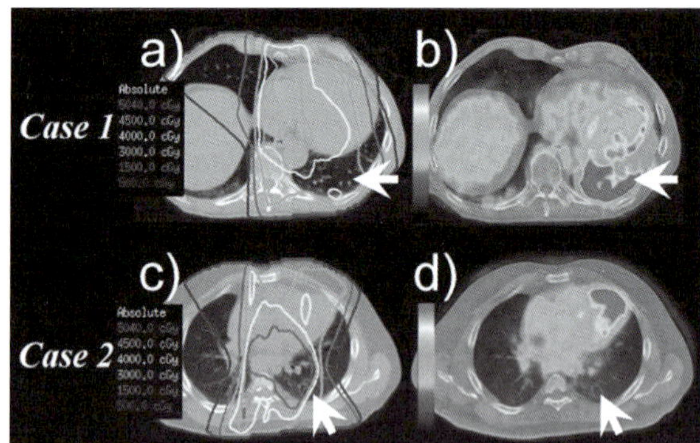

FIGURE 44.13 Radiation pneumonitis: local dose versus ^{18}F-fluorodeoxyglucose (FDG) uptake response in irradiated lung.[14] Radiation dose and FDG positron emission tomography (PET) response are illustrated for examples of high (case 1) and low (case 2) response. Case 1: **(A)** isodose distribution for patient with esophageal cancer shown overlaying single transaxial section from treatment planning computed tomography (CT) scan; **(B)** corresponding restaging FDG-PET scan (high response), after image registration, shown overlaying transaxial treatment planning CT scan. The pulmonary region with high FDG uptake is indicated by horizontal arrows. Case 2: **(C)** isodose distribution shown overlaying transaxial section from treatment planning CT scan; **(D)** corresponding restaging FDG–PET scan shown overlaying transaxial treatment planning CT scan. The pulmonary region of high dose and its corresponding PET region are indicated by diagonal arrows. These two cases represent the range of FDG uptake response found in all 36 cases evaluated.[14] (From Guerrero T, Johnson V, Hart J, et al. Radiation pneumonitis: local dose versus [18F]-fluorodeoxyglucose uptake response in irradiated lung. *Int J Radiat Oncol Biol Phys* 2007 Jul 15;68[4]:1030–1035.) (See color plate.)

in regional function and structure on whole-lung function. In other words, as the volume of normal lung irradiated increases, should the dose be decreased, and if so, by how much? Clearly, the correlation of clinical symptoms or changes in whole-lung function depends greatly on the volume of functioning lung remaining. What is well accepted is that there is a clear separation between whole organ and regional organ tolerance. The impact of changes in regional lung function and structure on whole-lung function will depend on the DVH.

Numerous studies have shown that the risk of radiation pneumonitis is strongly influenced by the distribution of radiation doses to normal lung. In particular, the MLD has been shown to be significantly associated with the incidence of radiation pneumonitis.[38,40,41,203,205,206,220–226] For example, Graham et al.[38] reported that when the MLD exceeds 20 Gy, the incidence of radiation pneumonitis is more than 20%. Many other studies have identified associations between the proportion of lung exposed to doses exceeding a threshold dose (V_{Dose}) and subsequent radiation pneumonitis incidence.[38,40,41,74,203,205,206,220–229] When multiple dose–threshold volumes are investigated (e.g., V_{10}, V_{20}, V_{30}, and V_{40}), all of the dose–volume parameters are typically found to be highly correlated with one another[41,202] making it challenging to determine the relative importance of the individual parameters[41,202] (Fig. 44.14, a correlation of dosimetric factors, from Wang et al.[41]).This observation also suggests that the shape of the DVH is perhaps more important than single points on the DVH curve, such as V_{20}, rV_5, or MLD, in predicting the probability of radiation pneumonitis. The ideal shape of the DVH would drop steeply in lung volume in the low-dose (5 Gy) region and be flattened in the moderate-dose (20 to 50 Gy) region. Most recently, a study from MD Anderson Cancer Center[230] demonstrated that if lung DVH met a set of "threshold" constraints (Fig. 44.15) (i.e., V_{20} ≤25%, V_{25} ≤20%, V_{35} ≤15%, and V_{50} ≤10% (curve A in Fig. 44.15), the incidence of treatment-related pneumonitis of grade 3 or higher was extremely low at only 2% at 1 year. When the constraints were relaxed by 10% each (i.e., V_{20} ≤35%, V_{25} ≤30%, V_{35} ≤25%, and V_{50} ≤20%) (curve B in Fig. 44.15), the incidence of pneumonitis of grade 3 or higher among patients meeting these constraints but not the more stringent constraints (group B) was 16% (Fig. 44.15). As the constraints were relaxed still further by another 10% (i.e., V_{20} ≤35%, V_{25} ≤30%, V_{35} ≤25%, and V_{50} ≤20%) (curve C in Fig. 44.15 [230]), the 1-year incidence of pneumonitis in patients whose DVHs met these constraints but not the previous ones (group C) was 25%. For those patients whose lung DVHs violated one or more of the constraints defined by curve C (group D), the rate of pneumonitis of grade 3 or higher at 1 year was 36% (Fig. 44.16).[230] Until the effects of different dose levels on lung toxicity are better understood, we propose using the shape of the DVH curve, rather than a single point on the DVH, as a guide to limiting incidence of treatment-related pneumonitis. [230] What is of importance is that these dosimetric factors useful for predicting who will experience radiation pneumonitis in response to radiation therapy,

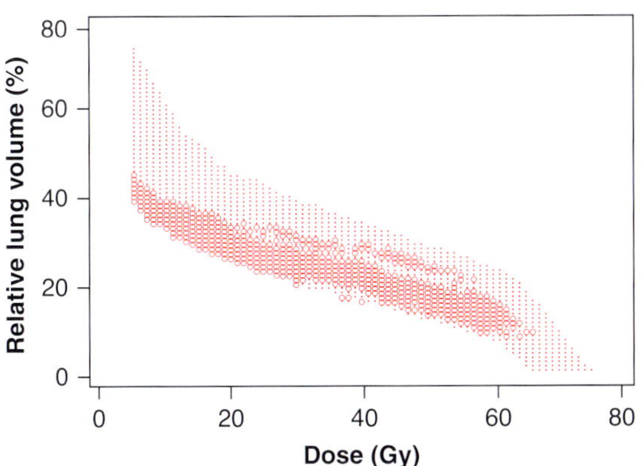

FIGURE 44.14 Correlation of dosimetric factors and treatment-related pneumonitis (TRP). Comparison of time to TRP of grade 3 or higher in patient subgroups divided according to magnitude (%) of relative volume of lung receiving more than a threshold dose (D) of radiation (dose, 5 to 80 Gy). Comparisons reported here are those for which each subset of the cohort included at least 10% of the patients (*small dots*) and comparisons for which the comparison of time to grade ≥3 TRP in the corresponding subgroups reached statistical significance ($p<0.05$) by log–rank test (*solid circles*).[41] (From Wang S, Liao Z, Wei X, et al. Analysis of clinical and dosimetric factors associated with treatment-related pneumonitis [TRP] in patients with non-small-cell lung cancer [NSCLC] treated with concurrent chemotherapy and three-dimensional conformal radiotherapy [3D-CRT]. *Int J Radiat Oncol Biol Phys* 2006 Dec 1;66[5]:1399–1407, with permission.)

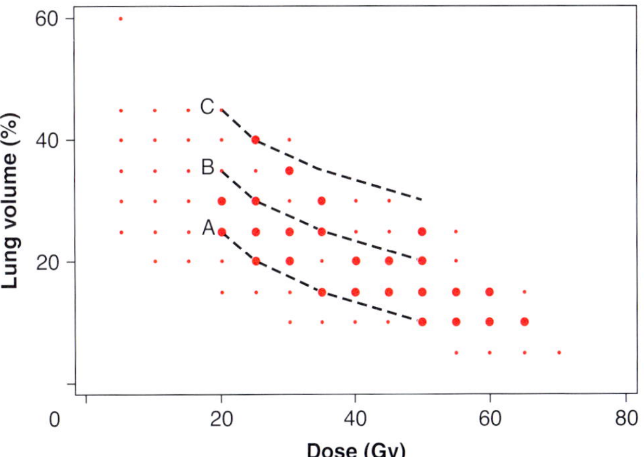

FIGURE 44.15 Dose–volume histogram (DVH) constraints. Three DVH constraints are compared: *curve A*, the most stringent set of lung DVH constraints, with V_{20} ≤25%, V_{25} ≤20%, V_{35} ≤15%, and V_{50} ≤10%; *curve B*, constraints of curve A relaxed by 10 percentage points each: V_{20} ≤35%, V_{25} ≤30%, V_{35} ≤25%, and V_{50} ≤20%; *curve C*, constraints of curve B relaxed by a further 10 percentage points each: V_{20} ≤45%, V_{25} ≤40%, V_{35} ≤35%, and V_{50} ≤30%.[230] (From Jin H, Tucker S, Liu H, et al. Dose–volume thresholds and smoking status for the risk of treatment-related related pneumonitis. *Radiother Oncol* 2009 Jun;91[3]:427–432.)

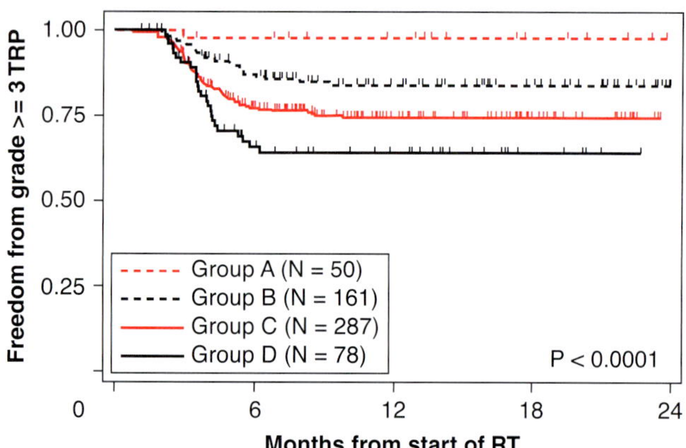

FIGURE 44.16 Freedom from treatment-related pneumonitis of grade 3 or higher in patients stratified by the lung dose–volume histogram (DVH) constraints defined by curves A to C defined in Figure 44.15. Four groups are compared: *group A*, patients with lung DVHs satisfying the constraints of curve A; *group B*, patients with DVHs satisfying the constraints of curve B but not of curve A; *group C*, patients with DVHs satisfying the constraints of curve C but not of curve B; *group D*, patients whose DVHs fail to meet one or more of the constraints of curve C.[230] *RT*, radiation therapy; *TRP*, treatment-related pneumonitis. (From Jin H, Tucker SL, Liu HH, et al. Dose–volume thresholds and smoking status for the risk of treatment-related pneumonitis in inoperable non-small cell lung cancer treated with definitive radiotherapy. *Radiother Oncol* 2009 Jun;91[3]:427–432.)

such as the percentage of the CT-defined total lung volume receiving >5, >20, and >30 GyE (Gray equivalent), and MLD, were not predictive for radiation pneumonitis after carbon-ion radiation therapy (Koto et al.[231] in Table 44.3).

RISK PREDICTION OF RADIATION-INDUCED LUNG DAMAGE

Methematical Modeling The dose distribution to normal tissues during radiation therapy for malignant disease is known to influence the incidence of radiation-induced complications. The modern knowledge of normal-tissue tolerance comes from a seminal publication by Emami et al.[232] These authors compiled tolerance dose values for uniform irradiation of 28 critical structures based on literature data and personal experience. In an accompanying article, Burman et al.[233] fit the tolerance dose data into a phenomenological NTCP model proposed by Lyman.[234]

The Lyman NTCP quantifies the probability of injury for a given uniform dose to an organ by the integral of a Gaussian probability function from $-\infty$ to the uniform dose.[234] The parameters defining the Gaussian function are the mean (the uniform dose for 50% probability of injury) and standard deviation (σ). Because the lung dose distribution is nonuniform, the equivalent uniform dose was approximated using the generalized equivalent uniform dose formulation as

$$\text{uniform dose} = (\Sigma_i V_i D_i^{\alpha} / \Sigma_i V_i)^{1/\alpha},$$

where V_i is the volume at dose D_i. Thus, the three unknown parameters are the uniform dose for 50% probability of injury, σ, and the generalized equivalent uniform dose exponent α. These three parameters are fitted to the data using the maximum likelihood estimation technique. Because the Lyman model is defined for uniform irradiation and normal tissues are rarely irradiated uniformly, several algorithms that convert a heterogeneous dose distribution into a uniform dose distribution resulting in the same NTCP have been designed. An effective volume method for DVH reduction proposed by Kutcher and Burman[235] is the most commonly used. The combined formalism is often referred to as the Lyman–Kutcher–Burman model in the literature. The Lyman model is the most widely used NTCP model and is implemented in many radiation treatment-planning systems.

NTCP models are most often fitted to binary data, in which each patient is scored yes or no according to whether or not the specified complication is observed; however, this approach can lead to false negatives, because some patients scored as no might have experienced the end point with longer follow-up. To limit the number of false negatives, investigators often restrict NTCP analyses to patients having a minimum follow-up time, based on the time interval during which the majority of complications are expected to occur. In the case of pneumonitis, a common requirement is that patients be followed for at least 6 months after the end of radiation therapy.[216,223] In some studies, patients having <6 months follow-up but experiencing radiation pneumonitis before 6 months are also included.[208,236] Moreover, the standard Lyman model does not incorporate nondosimetric risk factors such as comorbidities and other patient characteristics.

Radiation pneumonitis among patients with inoperable NSCLC is an example of a normal-tissue toxicity for which analysis with the standard Lyman model may not be appropriate. Severe radiation pneumonitis (grade 3 or higher), when it occurs, is observed within the first year after radiation therapy. Unfortunately, many patients with inoperable NSCLC succumb to disease during that same period. As improvements in treatment are developed that raise survival rates for these patients, cases of radiation pneumonitis are likely to occur that would otherwise have been masked by disease-related deaths. It would be desirable to have a model of radiation pneumonitis risk that remains accurate as improvements in disease control are made. Knowledge of accurate parameter estimates is essential for incorporating NTCP models into biologically based treatment planning. Several investigators have attempted to estimate the parameters for the Lyman NTCP model by using data from a single institution or by analyzing multi-institutional toxicity data for the lung and other organs.[215,237–242] Although many parameter estimates for different NTCP models and critical structures continue to appear in the literature, it is difficult to justify the use of any single parameter set obtained at a selected institution for the purposes of biologically based treatment planning. Parameters estimated based on cumulative experience at various institutions are thought to be more representative of the overall practice of radiation therapy and could be more confidently incorporated into clinical use.[223,240]

Considerable evidence suggests that the risk of radiation pneumonitis is influenced not just by dose–volume parameters but also by nondosimetric factors as well, including poor performance status,[243] poor pulmonary function before radiation therapy,[243] chronic obstructive pulmonary disease,[244] low partial pressure of oxygen (PaO_2) (>80 mm of mercury) before radiation therapy,[245] lower lobe tumor location,[42,202,236] neoadjuvant chemotherapy,[246–248] concurrent chemotherapy,[42] high total radiation dose, and high radiation dose per fraction.[186] Although when these clinical factors are analyzed together with dosimetric factors, the clinical factors lose their predictive value for radiation pneumonitis in most studies.[38,205,221,228,249,250] A few factors, such as smoking status,[206,230] a history of chronic obstructive pulmonary disease,[244,251] or induction chemotherapy with mitomycin,[244] have retained independent predictive value, suggesting that, besides dose–volume effect, other clinical and biologic factors play a role in pulmonary complications.

To improve predictive accuracy, thereby steepening the dose–response curves, investigators have found it important to incorporate additional covariates into the modeling. A recent analysis of data from 570 patients with lung cancer treated with radiation therapy suggested that the risk of radiation pneumonitis was significantly lower among smokers than among nonsmokers (1-year incidence, 14% vs. 39%), with an intermediate risk for former smokers (24%).[230] Moreover, smoking status was found to be independent of every dose–volume factor investigated.[230] To take the smoking status into consideration, Jin et al.[252] presented two alternatives to the standard Lyman NTCP model: a generalized Lyman model and a generalized log-logistic model. Both of these alternatives are suitable for predicting radiation pneumonitis and other end points that might be unobserved because of censoring. Whereas the standard Lyman model is fitted to binary (yes/no) event data, the generalized models are fitted to censored time-to-event data. The value of such a model is that it should remain more accurate in its NTCP predictions than the standard Lyman model as evolving treatment regimens lead to prolonged patient survival. Accordingly, the generalized model leads to higher NTCP estimates than the standard Lyman model (Fig. 44.17).

In another study, Das et al.[237] tried to augment the predictive capability of the parametric dose-based Lyman NTCP metric by combining it with weighted nonparametric decision trees that use dose and nondose inputs and by adding a decision tree using a "boosting" process that enhances the accuracy of prediction. A simplified model was developed that

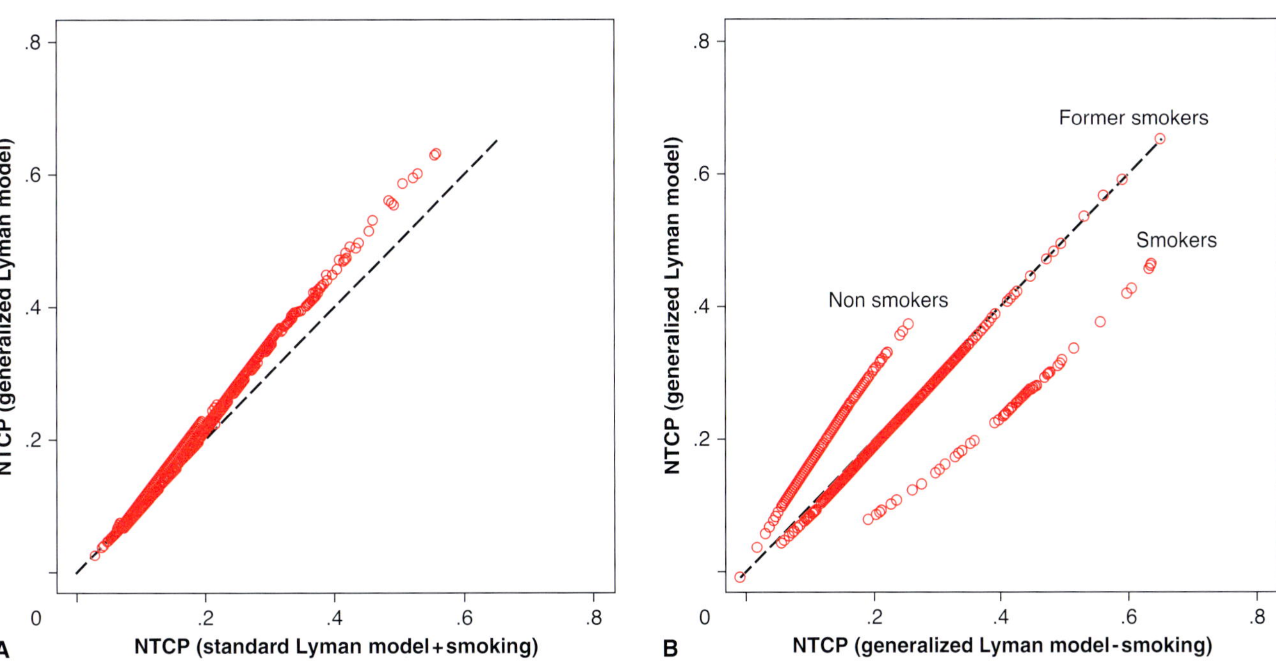

FIGURE 44.17 **A:** Comparison of NTCP values computed using the generalized Lyman model and those computed using the standard Lyman model with covariates added to reflect patient smoking status but with toxicities regarded as binary (yes/no) events. For both models, the volume parameter was fixed at n = 1, and patient smoking status was taken into account. Because the generalized model "anticipates" additional toxicities, it produces NTCP values that are, on average, higher than those from the standard model.[252] **B:** NTCP values computed using the generalized Lyman model, with or without covariates to represent smoking status, are compared. With smoking status included in the model, the generalized Lyman model produced NTCP values that were up to 18 percentage points lower for smokers and up to 12 percentage points higher for nonsmokers than the NTCP values obtained by omitting smoking status from the fit.[252] *NTCP*, normal-tissue complication probability. (From Tucker SL, Liu HH, Liao Z, et al. Analysis of radiation pneumonitis risk using a generalized Lyman. *Intl J Radiat Oncol Biol Phys*, 2008;72[2]:568–574.)

incorporated nondosimetric variables to produce a measure of injury: such as Lyman NTCP, sex, histologic type, chemotherapy schedule, and treatment schedule. For a given patient's radiation treatment plan, injury prediction was highest for the combination of preradiation chemotherapy, once-daily treatment, and being female and lowest for the combination of no preradiation chemotherapy and nonsquamous cell histologic type. Application of the simplified model to the example cases revealed that injury prediction for a given treatment plan can range from very low to very high, depending on the settings of the nondose variables.[237]

Several groups have also shown that the anatomic region of lung exposed to radiation, as previously mentioned, influences the risk of complications.[38,42,195,196,202,203,208,224,236,253] Others have noted the influence of patient and clinical factors, such as chronic obstructive pulmonary disease or use of chemotherapy.[244] A summary of the association of dosimetric, clinical, and biologic factors with radiation pneumonitis as reported in the literature is provided in Table 44.3.[11,38,40,41,74,203,206,221,223–225,228–231,244,254] Markers of individual susceptibility to radiation pneumonitis, such as genetic information or cytokine expression levels, are likely to improve the prediction of radiation pneumonitis risk.

TABLE 44.3 The Association of Dosimetric, Clinical, and Biologic Factors with Radiation Pneumonitis as Reported in the Literature

Author, Year (N)	Radiation Pneumonitis Criteria (Incidence)	Normal-Tissue Complication Probability Models		Mean Lung Dose		V_{dose}		Clinical Factors	TGF-β
		Subgroup	Rate (%)	Subgroup	Rate (%)	Subgroup	Rate (%)		
Martel et al., 1994[224] (n = 42)	G ≥1, SWOG (21%)	1st quart. 2nd quart. 3rd quart. 4th quart.	0 5 14 29	—	—		—	—	—
Oetzel et al., 1995[225] (n = 66)	G ≥1, RTOG (15%)	—	—	Ipsilateral ≤15 17.5–20 22.5–25 ≥27.5	0 13 21 43		—	—	—
Marks et al., 1997[324] (n = 67)	G ≥2, Duke University self-measure (22%)	1st quart. 2nd quart. 3rd quart. 4th quart. Good PFT	0 15 23 46	—	—	—	—	—	—
Armstrong et al., 1997[254] (n = 31)	G ≥3, SWOG (13%)	<12% ≥12%	0 29	—	—	V_{25} ≤30% >30%	— 4 38	—	—
Kwa et al., 1998[223] (n = 400)	G ≥2, SWOG (16%)	—	—	0–8 8–16 16–24 24–36	5 11 24 25	—	—	—	—
Graham et al., 1999[38] (n = 99)	G≥2, RTOG (14% at 6 months)	—	—			V_{20} <22 22–31 32–40 >40	— 0 7 13 36	NS	—
Fu et al., 2001[228] (n = 78)	G ≥1, SRILI (17% at 1 year)	—	—	—	—	V_{30}: 30% LR IR HR	—β 7 23 43	NS	S

TABLE 44.3 The Association of Dosimetric, Clinical, and Biologic Factors with Radiation Pneumonitis as Reported in the Literature *(continued)*

Author, Year (N)	Radiation Pneumonitis Criteria (Incidence)	Normal-Tissue Complication Probability Models		Mean Lung Dose		V_{dose}		Clinical Factors	TGF-β
		Subgroup	Rate (%)	Subgroup	Rate (%)	Subgroup	Rate (%)		
Hernando et al., 2001[206] (n = 201)	G ≥1, CTC 2.0 (19%)	1st quart. 2nd quart. 3rd quart. 4th quart.	10 18 16 33	<10 10–20 21–30 >30	10 16 27 44	V_{30} ≤18 >18	— 6 24	Ongoing smoking	—
Yorke et al., 2002[203] (n = 49)	G ≥3, RTOG (18%)	Lower lung	—	Total lung Ipsilateral lower lung	—	V20 Ipsilateral	—	—	—
Willner et al., 2003[74] (n = 49)	G ≥2, CTC 3.0 (37%)	—	—	Ipsilateral	—	V_{40} V_{30} V_{20} V_{10}	—	—	—
Tsujino et al., 2003[229] (n = 71)	G ≥2, CTC 2.0 (27% at 6 months)	—	—	—	—	V_{20} ≤20 21–25 26–30 ≥31	— 9 18 51 85	NS	—
Rancati et al., 2003[244] (n = 84)	G ≥2, SWOG (17%)	—	—	W/o COPD ($p = 0.082$)	—	NS	—	COPD in mitomycin	—
Claude et al., 2004[40] (n = 90)	G ≥1, Lent-Soma (44%)	—	—	Total ($p = 0.01$)	—	V_{20}:18% V_{30}:13% V_{40}:10%	33 56	Age	—
Kim et al., 2005[221] (n = 76)	G ≥3, RTOG (16%)	—	—	<10 10–14.9 ≥15	0 11 45	NS	—	NS	—
Wang et al., 2006[41] (n = 223)	G ≥3, CTC 3.0 (22% at 6 months)	—	—	<16.5 ≥16.5	13 36	V_5<42% V_5≥42%	3 36		
Koto et al., 2007[231]* (n = 80)	G ≥2, RTOG (10% within 6 months) G ≤1, RTOG (90% within 6 months)	—	—	Not predictive		V_5 V_{20} V_{30}			
Jin et al., 2008[230] (n = 576)	G ≥3, CTC 3.0	—	—	Dose region defined	—	—	—	Smoking	—

*Carbon–ion radiotherapy. Differences between those receiving equivalent measures of therapy to CT-defined total lung volume, but developing radiation pneumonitis of grade ≥2 or grade ≤1 were not statistically significant.

COPD, chronic obstructive pulmonary disease; CTC, National Cancer Institute Common Toxicity Criteria; G, grade; NS, not specified; pft, pulmonary function test; RTOG, Radiation Therapy Oncology Group; SRILI, symptomatic radiation-induced lung injury; SWOG, Southwest Oncology Group; TGF, transforming growth factor; quart., quarter; UT MDACC, University of Texas MD Anderson Cancer Center.

Radiation-Sensitivity Testing

Genetic Testing of Susceptibility to Radiation Pneumonitis by Analysis of Single-Nucleotide Polymorphisms

As discussed previously in this chapter, pathologic processes in the lung are known to be controlled genetically, and individuals differ in their intrinsic sensitivity to radiation. Therefore, genetic testing before radiation is a promising approach to identify a particular patient's risk of radiation pneumonitis. One genetic test relies on the detection of single-nucleotide polymorphisms (SNPs).

SNPs represent the most abundant type of sequence variation in the human genome. A great deal of research has been done to determine if this type of genetic germline variation influences a variety of oncology-related phenotypes, such as cancer susceptibility, disease outcome, and treatment response. The involvement of SNPs in normal-tissue complications after radiation therapy treatment is also being extensively studied.[255] The mechanisms by which SNPs affect phenotype and influence complex diseases vary according to their locations on the genes. Substitutions in coding regions may affect the amino acid sequences of predicted proteins, reducing or abolishing functions such as DNA binding, catalytic activity, and receptor-ligand contact. SNPs may interrupt the initiation or the termination codon or introduce errors in the reading frame shift, all with consequences for insufficient or prematurely truncated peptides. SNPs located in regulatory regions may influence gene expression, whereas SNPs in noncoding sequences may affect splicing or RNA cleavage, stability, and export.[256]

SNPs may be correlated with clinical normal-tissue radiosensitivity in patients.[257–259] SNPs in TGF-β1, DNA repair genes, and DNA damage response pathways have been linked with clinical radiosensitivity.[156,159,260–263] Many association studies have been published recently that implicate germline genetic variations in a few select cellular pathways (particularly those involved in DNA repair, cell cycle, and inflammation), and these may modify radiation sensitivity, treatment response, and toxicity.[155,157–162,260,262]

In parallel with this pharmacogenomic approach, a new term—*radiogenomics*—was coined to reflect the emerging field of predicting tumor and normal-tissue radiation therapy response using genetic biomarkers, particularly polymorphisms in critical pathways relevant to radiation action.[162,260,264] A broad international effort has been organized, comprising investigators from the United States, France, Switzerland, Denmark, and Israel, to create the Gene-PARE project (Genetic Predictors of Adverse Radiotherapy Effects). In the early stages of this project, which involves more than 2000 patients from five countries undergoing radiation therapy, a handful of selected functional polymorphisms in double-strand break repair (base excision repair, or BER) and inflammation pathways were screened for their association with radiosensitivity, and a few positive associations were identified, including polymorphisms in XRCC1, x-ray repair cross-complementing 3 gene (XRCC3), and TGF-β1 genes.[161] Preliminary findings from the Gene-PARE project, from other cancer risk association studies, and from pharmacogenetic studies strongly indicate that cancer risk and clinical outcome (e.g., radiosensitivity) are complex genetic traits that depend on the effect of multiple DNA sequence variants. Any one variant may not exert a dramatic effect, but the aggregation of multiple polymorphisms in the same or relevant pathways may amplify the effect of individual polymorphisms and produce higher risk estimates that may be clinically relevant.[265]

Of the particular importance are the polymorphisms in the TGF-β1 gene. TGF-β1 possesses a highly polymorphic, extensive regulatory region that likely has an impact on the pathogenesis of numerous TGF-β1–related diseases through altered TGF-β1 expression due to polymorphisms.[266] Comprehensive examination of function and diversity for the TGF-β1 promoter region and exon 1 (-2665 to $+423$) demonstrated that the TGF-β1 alleles clustered into three phylogenetic groups based on the common functional SNPs c.-1347C $>$ T (commonly known as -509C-T) and c.$+29$T $>$ C (commonly known as $+869$T-C), suggesting three phenotypic groups.[266] The common TGF-β1 promoter SNP c.-1347C $>$ T (-509C-T, rs1800469) has been linked to a nearly twofold difference in plasma levels among individuals and with risk, progression, and outcome of numerous diseases and it was suggested that the molecular mechanism for the difference in TGF-β1 plasma levels linked to -1347 is a result of transcriptional suppression by activator protein 1 binding to -1347C.[266] SNPs in TGF-β1 gene are associated with otosclerosis,[267] Alzheimer disease,[268] renal allograft rejection,[269] chronic obstructive pulmonary disease,[270,271] increased risk of lung cancer,[272] colorectal neoplasia,[273] invasive breast cancer,[264] and normal-tissue reactions and clinical toxicity in patients[156,262,263] with breast cancer and gynecologic cancer after radiation therapy.

Three recent studies demonstrated that polymorphisms in the TGF-β1 gene had strong associations with normal-tissue reactions and clinical toxicity in patients with breast cancer and gynecologic cancer after radiation therapy.[156,262,263] For example, Quarmby[263] found that the patients with the -509TT or $+869$CC genotypes were between 7 and 15 times more likely to develop severe fibrosis. Goitopoulos et al.[274] found that patients homozygous (TT) for the TGF-β1 C509T variant allele had a 15-fold increased risk of fibrosis after radiation therapy compared with patients with the homozygous (CC) variant. This association was most pronounced[259,261,263] when the mutant homozygous genotype was compared with the wild-type genotype, and a strong link between the -509C $>$ T and Leu10Pro polymorphisms was reported. However, the reported results have been controversial. Andreassen et al.[156,260] first reported a possible association between selected SNPs and the risk of subcutaneous fibrosis in 41 Danish breast cancer patients given postmastectomy radiation therapy and in 26 early stage breast cancer patients after breast conservation treatment, a confirmatory study of 120 patients by the same group failed to demonstrate any association between risk of radiation-induced subcutaneous fibrosis and SNPs in TGF-β1, XRCC1, XRCC3, SOD2 (manganese superoxide dismutase gene) or ATM genes after postmastectomy radiation therapy.[157]

Theoretically, using SNP for genetic testing of radiation sensitivity and risk of radiation pneumonitis is ideal, because the risk is known before the treatment begins. This type of biological marker should, if validated clinically, be able to increase the accuracy of the risk prediction models. However, the data in this area are quite sparse and more extensive research is warranted.

Radiosensitivity of Ex Vivo Lung Fibroblasts As discussed previously in this chapter, radiosensitivity varies in the same normal-tissue cell type from different individuals, suggesting that radiosensitivity is genetically regulated. Studies of patients with ataxia telangiectasia have established not only that these individuals are highly sensitive to ionizing radiation but also that in survival assays, fibroblasts isolated and cultured from these patients are more radiosensitive by several logs than are fibroblasts from unaffected individuals.[275–278] Even in the normal population, a wide range of radiosensitivities is known to exist. If normal-tissue radiosensitivity has a genetic component, then the radiosensitivity of cultured cells isolated from an individual should reflect the genetics of the individual.

Several studies have been done to determine the relationship between fibroblast radiosensitivity, as measured by the function of cells surviving a dose of 2 Gy (SF2 Gy), and late tissue damage in patients.[275,279,280] Although early studies reported variable results, more recent findings suggest that fibroblast radiosensitivity may be a useful predictor of late radiation damage in vasculoconnective tissues. However, most of these studies have been done with skin fibroblasts cultured from women with breast cancer. Fibroblast radiosensitivity as measured by SF2 has been compared with both acute and late end points; although no clear relationship was demonstrated between fibroblast radiosensitivity and chronic skin damage, the findings seemed nevertheless to be promising.[275]

In the case of patients with lung cancer, two issues must be resolved experimentally. First, is there a correlation between lung fibrosis and survival of cultured lung fibroblasts? Also, because it would be difficult to obtain biopsies of normal lung from patients with lung cancer before treatment, the second issue is whether the radiosensitivity of fibroblasts isolated from another tissue, for example skin, from the same patient will be similarly radiosensitive as lung fibroblasts. Both of these questions have been investigated using two inbred strains of mice with documented differences in radiation-induced lung fibrosis.

Dileto and Travis[281] determined the radiosensitivity of fibroblasts cultured from the lung and skin of the fibrosis-prone C57Bl/6 strain and the fibrosis-resistant C3Hf/Kam strains of mice. In these mouse models, lung fibroblast radiosensitivity was not different as measured by survival at 2.0 Gy (SF2), despite a more than 20-fold difference in fibrosis scores 5.1% and 0.2% in the fibrosis-prone and fibrosis-resistant strains, respectively. Similar SF2 values were obtained for skin fibroblasts from the two strains, indicating that the radiosensitivity of fibroblasts isolated from lung and skin of the same strain is the same. These data indicate that the in vitro radiosensitivity of lung fibroblasts as assayed by survival at 2 Gy does not correlate with the development of lung fibrosis, at least in the two strains of mice used in the studies of Dileto.[281] Thus, the usefulness of the fibroblast radiosensitivity as measured by SF2 for predicting lung fibrosis remains unclear.

Circulating Biomarkers A second approach to identifying at risk patients would be to identify the expression of cytokines, growth factors, or other factors during treatment that correlate with the later incidence of radiation induce lung damage. The underlying rationale of this approach is to identify and intervene in the early expression of gene products that may participate in the pathogenesis of radiation-induced lung damage. The goal would be to define factors that could be monitored regularly and routinely during treatment. The requirement of such a test would be that these factors be easily accessible for multiple sampling.

Transforming Growth Factor β As discussed previously in this chapter, TGF-β1 has a particularly important role in the development of radiation-induced lung injury.[106–109] In an animal study, a dose-dependent induction of TGF-β1 in the lung tissue of fibrosis-prone mice after radiation was reported,[282] and soluble TGF-β1 type II receptor gene therapy reduced the tissue level of active TGF-β1 and consequently ameliorated acute radiation-induced lung injury.[108] Anscher et al.[106,109,110,228] reported that a normal plasma TGF-β1 by the end of radiation therapy was more common in patients who did not develop radiation pneumonitis. A return of the plasma TGF-β1 to normal levels accurately identified patients who would not develop radiation pneumonitis, with a sensitivity and positive predictive value of 90%. Changes in plasma TGF-β1 levels during radiation therapy were found to be useful in identifying patients at low risk for complications in whom higher doses of radiation up to 86.4 Gy (1.6 Gy twice daily) could be safely delivered.[222] Furthermore, a trend of a decrease in plasma TGF-β1 concentration to below the pretreatment value during radiation treatment in patients who did not develop pulmonary complications after radiation therapy supports the use of this biomarker as a predictive factor.[283] However, De Jaeger et al.[111] did not find an association between increased levels of TGF-β1 at the end of radiation therapy and symptomatic radiation pneumonitis, although the TGF-β1 level at the end of radiation therapy was significantly associated with the MLD and the pretherapy level.

In an early study, Anscher et al.[284] measured the circulating levels of TGF-β in patients with breast cancer undergoing bone marrow transplantation and correlated these values with the later incidence of pulmonary fibrosis and hepatic venoocclusive disease, both of which are significant side effects of this treatment. TGF-β was determined initially after induction chemotherapy but before the administration of high-dose chemotherapy and subsequently after high-dose chemotherapy and transplantation. Hepatic venoocclusive disease and lung fibrosis were observed clinically between 1 and 3 weeks and

40 and 75 days after transplantation, respectively. Analysis of the TGF-β levels after induction chemotherapy with the later incidence of liver and pulmonary fibrosis in individual patients showed that plasma levels of TGF-β had a positive predictive value of more than 90% for the development of fibrosis in either of these organs in a given patient. Although plasma levels of TGF-β were not determined before any treatment, and thus, its usefulness in selecting patients more likely to develop lung damage before treatment begins is unknown, these data suggest that routine monitoring of plasma TGF-β in individual patients undergoing radiation or chemotherapy for lung cancer could be useful as a predictor of lung fibrosis. More recently, Anscher et al.[106] investigated in a prospective study the usefulness of TGF-β1 as a predictive marker for the development of radiation-induced lung damage. In this study, 73 lung cancer patients were treated with curative intent, and all treatment parameters were similar in this patient cohort. TGF-β1 levels were measured before, weekly during treatment, and at each follow-up to 6 months after the completion of radiation therapy, when the study was ended. The end point was the development of radiation pneumonitis at 6 months after treatment, which was defined by the National Cancer Institute Common Toxicity Criteria (http://ctep.cancer.gov/reporting/ctc.html). Only 15 (21%) of these patients developed symptomatic pneumonitis. In this study, a normal plasma TGF-β1 level by the end of radiation therapy was more common in patients who did not develop pneumonitis (Fig. 44.18). A return of TGF-β1 plasma levels to normal accurately identified with a positive predictive value of 90% patients who would not develop pneumonitis, indicating that the level of this cytokine may be useful in identifying patients at low risk for the development of radiation pneumonitis. These patients could then be considered for dose escalation.

However, results concerning the predictive value of TGF-β1 for the risk of radiation pneumonitis have been inconsistent.[111,285] Though some investigators have reported that a return of the plasma TGF-β1 value to normal levels identified with a sensitivity and positive predictive value of 90% patients who would not develop radiation pneumonitis,[106,110] others have failed to confirm this finding.[111,283,286,287] Moreover, TGF-β1 can be produced by both tumor and normal tissue, and numerous factors, including improper handling of the blood samples or inadequate centrifugation[285] can artificially increase the circulating TGF-β1 level. Such studies provide the impetus to search for other early markers of radiation- and drug-induced lung damage in the hope of preventing the potentially fatal complications associated with radiation pneumonitis.

Inflammatory Cytokines As discussed previously in this chapter, proinflammatory, profibrotic, and proangiogenic cytokines have been implicated in radiation lung damage.[94] Some of these cytokines have been considered as potential markers for radiation lung damage in humans including IL-1α, IL-6, IL-8, and IL-10.[95,116,125,288]

Chen et al.[289] was among the first to assess the IL-1α and IL-6 plasma levels prospectively in a series of 31 patients with lung cancer and thymoma. Negative predictive value of IL-1α, measured before and throughout radiation therapy, was ≤50%, whereas it was slightly higher for IL-6, with the highest negative predictive value of 54% for levels at 3 weeks of radiation therapy. These biomarkers were unable to distinguish patients at low risk of radiation lung damage who could benefit from dose

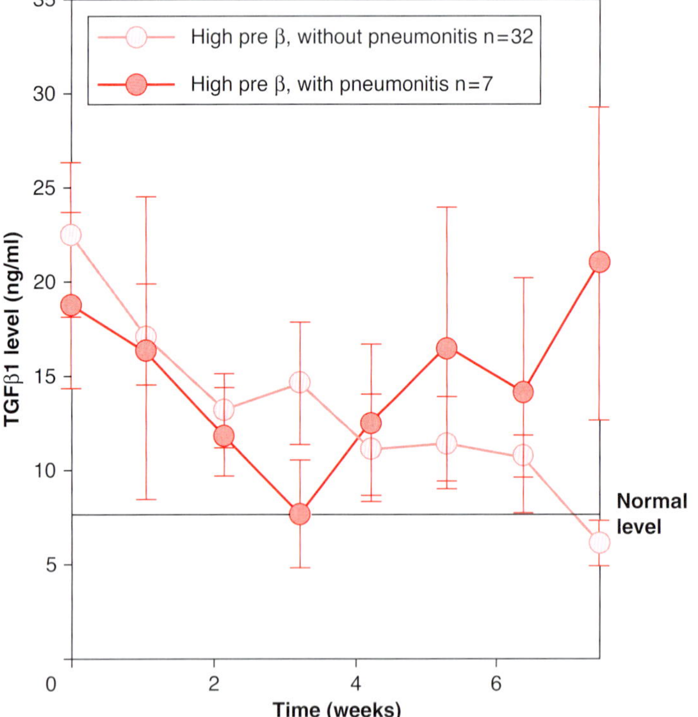

FIGURE 44.18 Plasma TGF-β levels as a function of time for patients with an elevated pretreatment plasma TGFβ level who did not (*open symbols*) or did (*closed symbols*) develop radiation pneumonitis. Although both groups experienced a reduction in TGF-β levels during treatment, in one group this decrease was transient, and the TGF-β levels returned to high levels. This group had a significantly higher risk of developing pneumonitis than those patients whose TGF-β levels remained within control values.[106] *TGF-β*, transforming growth factor β. (From Anscher MS, Kong FM, Andrews K, et al. Plasma transforming growth factor β1 as a predictor of radiation pneumonitis. *Int J Radiat Oncol Biol Phys* 1998;41:1029–1035, with permission.)

escalation. Arpin et al.[116] prospectively followed 90 patients with NSCLC with serial blood testing. Although changes in IL-6 plasma levels after 2 weeks of treatment were significantly correlated with the occurrence of radiation pneumonitis seen at 6 to 8 weeks after the end of radiotherapy, that correlation disappeared for radiation pneumonitis seen at 6 months, despite the putatively sustained character of radiation lung damage.

More recent studies have considered multiple cytokines. Hart et al.[125] reported a fourfold increase in median IL-8 plasma levels in patients without symptomatic radiation lung damage compared with those who did develop symptomatic lung damage or with healthy control subjects: 1.49 pg/mL versus 0.34 pg/mL and 0 pg/mL ($p < 0.001$), suggesting a negative predictive value of 91.1%. However, that study was limited by its retrospective nature, patient selection criteria (availability of plasma samples), and uncertainty between the authors' assumptions of incidence of symptomatic radiation lung damage and its actual incidence in the subset of studied patients (of 55 patients, 22 patients had symptomatic lung damage), preventing any conclusive statement about the correlation between IL-8 levels and the end point. Hartsell et al.[288] studied serum markers (surfactant apoprotein, procollagen type III, IL-1, IL-6, and TNF-α) in 127 patients with inoperable NSCLC treated on Radiation Therapy Oncology Group (RTOG) trial. The median survival time was 10.9 months, with 43% of patients living 1 year and 10% living 3 years. Elevated levels of serum IL-6 after 10 Gy of lung irradiation appear to predict acute lung toxicity of grade 2 or greater, and high serum levels of surfactant apoproteins at 20 Gy that correlated with late pulmonary toxicity of grade 2 or greater. These findings need to be confirmed but could be useful in a model to predict risk of pulmonary injury with high doses of radiation. For future studies, it is necessary to evaluate serum markers at multiple time points during treatment, and quality control is critical during the collection, storage, and analysis of these serum markers.[288]

Other Potential Biomarkers Molecules other than interleukins have also tested as predictors of radiation pneumonitis, including soluble ICAM-1 (sICAM-1), KL-6, the cytokeratin 19 fragment (CYFRA 21-1), and pulmonary surfactant proteins A (SP-A) and D (SP-D). However, to date most of the studies investigating the predictive role of circulating biomarkers have had small numbers of patients, discrepancies in the end points used, different treatment regimens, and no standard procedure for processing the blood samples. Until these issues are addressed, the use of circulating cytokine levels to predict risk of radiation lung damage and to identify which patients can tolerate radiation dose escalation remains investigational.

RISK REDUCTION AND PERSONALIZATION OF CANCER TREATMENT

Advanced Treatment Technologies for Reducing Lung Dose and Volume Because radiation pneumonitis is known to be strongly associated with lung dose–volume parameters, the possibility of using advanced radiation techniques to reduce lung exposure during radiation therapy has been explored. Murshed et al.[290] demonstrated dosimetric improvements with respect to tumor dose conformity and normal tissue sparing by using IMRT rather than 3D conformal radiation therapy in a treatment planning study. The results showed that, using IMRT, the median absolute reduction in the percentage of lung volume irradiated to >10 and >20 Gy was 7% and 10%, respectively. This corresponded to a decrease of >2 Gy in the total lung mean dose and a statistically significant decrease in the corresponding risk of radiation pneumonitis estimated with the Lyman NTCP model. The size of the estimated risk reduction depended on the choice of parameters for the Lyman model: using the parameters published by Burman et al.,[233] the median radiation pneumonitis risk would decrease from 36% with the 3D conformal plans to 9% with the intensity-modulated plans, whereas using the parameters of Hayman et al.,[291] the median radiation pneumonitis risk would decrease from 13% for the 3D conformal treatment to 7% with the intensity-modulated treatment. Based on the encouraging preclinical study described previously, during the past 4 years, IMRT has been adapted to treat thoracic malignancies. The first report of clinical experience included 68 patients with NSCLC whose disease extent was not amenable to treatment by 3D conformal radiation therapy (68%) or whose medical history indicated previous thoracic irradiation (14%), poor lung function (3%), or prior surgery (16%).[39] That retrospective study showed a significant reduction in radiation pneumonitis with the use of IMRT rather than 3D conformal radiation therapy. At 1 year after therapy, the rates of radiation pneumonitis of grade 3 or higher were 8% among patients treated with IMRT and 32% among patients treated with 3D conformal radiation therapy ($p = 0.002$). Compared with 3D conformal radiation therapy, use of IMRT led to significantly lower median volumes of normal lung treated with multiple dose levels, ranging from 15 to 65 Gy ($p < 0.01$). Recently, the same group further compared the effects of IMRT and 3D conformal radiation therapy on the end points of toxicity and disease outcomes in a subset of 496 patients treated with concomitant chemoradiation therapy between 1999 and 2006 (Fig. 44.19)[292] from our data set. Among these, 318 were treated with 3D conformal therapy using standard CT scans for planning, and 91 were treated with IMRT using 4D CT scans for planning. The end points for analysis were locoregional progression, distant metastasis, overall survival, and grade ≥3 radiation pneumonitis. The hazard ratios for 4D-CT/IMRT were <1 for all end points, and values were statistically significantly lower for overall survival and radiation pneumonitis, indicating IMRT's ability to reduce risk. Freedom from distant metastasis was nearly identical in the two groups, suggesting that stage migration did not play a major role in influencing the observed differences in the disease and treatment-related toxicity end points. These findings, therefore, suggest that the use of IMRT was associated with a real therapeutic gain, with increased survival and decreased radiation pneumonitis of grade 3 or higher. Such

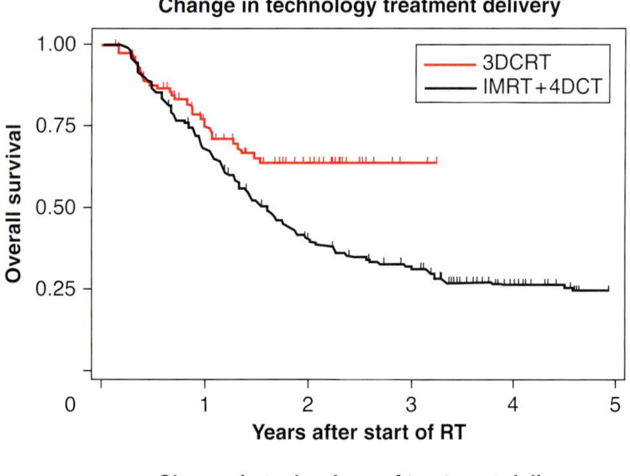

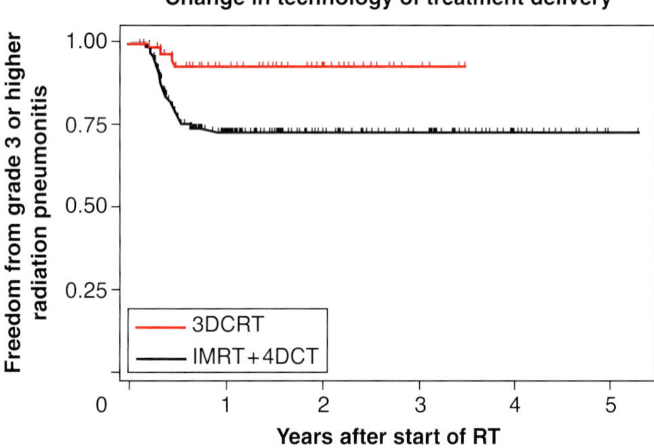

FIGURE 44.19 Pneumonitis risk reduction and overall survival rates using advanced technology. The curves compare the patients treated with 3D conformal radiation therapy (3D CRT) and those treated with intensity-modulated radiation therapy with four-dimensional computed tomography planning (IMRT + 4DCT). The latter was associated with significant reductions in radiation pneumonitis and significantly better overall survival rates.[292] (From Liao ZX, Komaki RR, Thames HD Jr, Liu et al. Influence of Technologic Advances on Outcomes in Patients With Unresectable, Locally Advanced Non-Small-Cell Lung Cancer Receiving Concomitant Chemoradiotherapy. *Int J Radiat Oncol Biol Phys* 2009.

an improvement in therapeutic ratio suggests that with IMRT, the radiotherapist has the ability to further increase dose to the tumor while staying within normal thoracic tissues' range of tolerance.[292] The results prompted a prospective clinical trial to confirm the clinical benefit of IMRT.

Wang et al.[41] showed that V_5 was a strong predictor of radiation pneumonitis in patients with locally advanced NSCLC receiving concurrent chemotherapy. Taking advantage of the physics characteristics of proton radiation with low entrance and exiting dose, these investigators explored the possibility of using this modality for 108 patients with locally advanced NSCLC treated with chemotherapy and proton therapy (31 patients) or IMRT (75 patients) from January 2003 to September 2007. Median dose was 74 cobalt Gy equivalent (CGE) (i.e., 1 CGE = 1 Gy) (range, 63 to 74 CGE) in the proton group, and 63 Gy (range, 60 to 76 Gy) in the IMRT group. Proton therapy significantly reduced V_5 ($p < 0.0001$), V_{10} ($p < 0.0001$), and V_{20} ($p = 0.005$) compared with IMRT. The rates of grade 2 to 5 radiation pneumonitis were 19.4% with proton radiation and 33% with IMRT ($p = 0.15$). No patients treated with proton radiation experienced grade 3 or greater radiation pneumonitis, but 9.3% of those undergoing IMRT did ($p = 0.07$). These results indicate that proton radiation is associated with a reduction in the frequency of radiation pneumonitis in spite of delivering a higher total cumulative dose than IMRT.[293] In a separate treatment planning study[294] in which the same investigators compared the effectiveness of proton therapy with that of IMRT in shaping dose distributions and in boosting the dose to the gross tumor volume (GTV), they found that the GTV dose could be increased from 66 to 84 CGE while maintaining the same level of doses to normal tissues. As the trends in preferred treatment technologies move from 3D conformal radiation therapy to IMRT to proton therapy, radiation oncologists are progressively gaining more capability to customize the radiation dose delivered to the lung tumor while protecting the surrounding normal tissues.

Biological Interventions for Radiation-Induced Lung Damage

Although changes in dose-fractionation schedules and information on the effect of irradiated volume on the incidence and severity of radiation pneumonitis and fibrosis have led to advances in the treatment of lung cancer, the challenge is to identify agents that either protect against lung damage or specifically intervene in the pathogenesis of pneumonitis or fibrosis. Although it has been generally thought that interventional techniques would not work, recent studies on the events occurring during the latent period could prove useful in designing compounds that specifically intervene in these processes.

Much information has been obtained at the cellular and molecular level on the biology of connective tissue formation and the pathophysiology of connective tissue diseases. The knowledge that pharmacologic interventions can be specifically targeted at varying strategic points in the life cycle of fibroproliferative processes has broadened considerably the realm of therapeutic modalities that might be investigated to control these processes. Numerous approaches designed to control collagen deposition remain untested in the lung. It would be useful to develop delivery methods that exploit the unique aspects of the lung to overcome the toxicity associated with collagen inhibitors. Collagen degradation, steroidal and nonsteroidal anti-inflammatory drugs, and cyclic nucleotides offer opportunities to control the accumulation of extracellular matrix in the lung.

Gene Therapy

Gene therapy has for almost 2 decades been considered a promising interventional approach to treat human disease and prevent therapeutic toxicities. Because TGF-β is closely involved in the process of radiation-induced lung damage, it seems a logical step to manipulate the TGF-β

gene as part of a therapeutic strategy to prevent this complication. Gene therapy strategies that used a recombinant human adenoviral vector that carried a soluble TGF-β1 type II receptor induced an increase in circulating levels of soluble receptors, reduced the tissue level of active TGF-β1, and consequently ameliorated acute radiation-induced lung damage histologically and functionally.[108,295] Furthermore, the adenoviral-mediated soluble TGF-β receptor may have potential as a therapeutic intervention for radiation-induced pulmonary damage,[296] because the expression of the exogenous Smad7 gene that blocked the signal transduction of TGF-β reduced the level of TGF-β, the level of type I collagen and type III collagen deposition in the lung, and the level of hydroxyproline.[297]

Radiation-induced apoptosis is thought to underlie the toxicity of radiation to normal tissues as well as to cancer cells. Bcl-2 is an antiapoptotic molecule that when expressed ectopically reduced radiation-induced apoptosis in normal cells including cells in lung (not in cancer cells).[298] Epperly et al.[299] reported that overexpression of superoxide dismutase (MnSOD) in the lungs of mice before irradiation prevents irradiation-induced acute and chronic damage evidenced by decreased levels of mRNA for IL-1, TNF-α, and TGF-β in the days immediately following irradiation and the decrease in the percentage of lung demonstrating fibrosis or organizing alveolitis at 132 days. Furthermore, MnSOD-PL administration before irradiation decreased both BrdU incorporation and delayed expression of VCAM-1 and ICAM-1, suggesting that late irradiation-induced pulmonary fibrosis is associated with the upregulation of adhesion molecules, and that potential targets for intervention may focus on the pulmonary vascular endothelium.[135]

Inhibition of Cellular Pathways Increasing evidence suggests that a few cellular signaling pathways, such as those involved in DNA repair, cell cycle, and inflammation, may affect radiation sensitivity, treatment response, and toxicity.[155,157–162,260] Therefore, interventions that regulate certain pathways might prove novel approaches in modulating normal-tissue toxicity. A few preclinical studies have tested this hypothesis.

Tumor Necrosis Factor α Radiation-induced lung toxicity limits the delivery of high-dose radiation to thoracic tumors. Zhang et al.[300] investigated the potential of inhibiting the TNF-α pathway as a novel radioprotection strategy for radiation-induced lung damage and found that radiation-induced lung TNF-α production correlates with early cell apoptosis and latent lung function damage. Inhibition of lung TNFR1 was selectively radioprotective for the lung without compromising tumor response. These findings support the development of a novel radioprotection strategy using inhibition of the TNF-α pathway.

Stem Cells Murine mesenchymal stem cells are capable of differentiating in vitro into different lineages under stimulation with certain cytokines, growth factors, and chemicals; however, the true capacity of these cells to contribute to different cell types in vivo is still unclear, especially under minimal injury conditions. Investigators have described a method of purifying murine mesenchymal stem cells from bone marrow and efficiently transducing them using a lentivirus vector expressing the enhanced green fluorescent protein (eGFP) reporter gene. In this experiment, lentivirus-transduced mesenchymal stem cells retained their in vitro ability to differentiate into adipocytes, osteocytes, and chondrocytes as well as into myocytelike and astrocytelike cells.

In brief, the eGFP mesenchymal stem cells were delivered systemically into minimally injured syngeneic mice. Tracking and tissue-specific differentiation were determined by polymerase chain reaction and immunohistochemical staining, respectively. We found donor-derived hepatocytes, lung epithelial cells, myofibroblasts, myofibers, and renal tubular cells in some of the recipient mice. Our findings indicate that even in the absence of substantial injury, phenotypically defined murine mesenchymal stem cells could acquire tissue-specific morphology and antigen expression and thus contribute to different tissue cell types in vivo.[301]

Cytokines It is well documented that radiation promotes the expression of cytokine genes in the lung after single and fractionated doses. The overexpression of cytokine genes has included mTNF-α, mIL-1α, mIL-1β, mIL-2, mIL-3, mIL-4, mIL-5, mIL-6, and mIFN-γ. IL-1β was the major cytokine induced in the lungs of C3H/HeJ mice within the first day after thoracic irradiation. Radiation doses as low as 1 Gy were effective. Responses to 20 Gy peaked within 4 to 8 hours and subsided by 24 hours. With the exception of IL-1α and TNF-α, the other cytokines that were investigated had undetectable pretreatment mRNA levels and could not be induced by radiation. Pretreatment with dexamethasone reduced basal and induced IL-1 levels, but complete inhibition was not achieved. Dexamethasone was also effective if given immediately after irradiation. Fractionated daily doses of radiation (4 Gy/day) helped to maintain cytokine gene expression for a longer period.[302] Studies of the events occurring during the latent phase of radiation lung injury have shown that several of these molecules and growth factors are activated during this time, some of which may be exploited interventionally.

Basic Fibroblast Growth Factor A cytokine investigators are proposing as useful in protecting against radiation pneumonitis in mice is basic fibroblast growth factor (bFGF). Fuks et al.[82,303,304] have shown that this cytokine protects against radiation-induced apoptosis in bovine arterial endothelial cells in vitro[303,304] as well as against apoptosis in endothelial cells in irradiated lungs and the central nervous system of mice.[82,305] They found bFGF also protected mice against the lethal effects of radiation pneumonitis.[82,305] However, neither the time of death nor the histologic changes observed were consistent with classic radiation pneumonitis. Hemorrhage and edema in the air spaces was a consistent finding at 8 to 10 weeks, when the mice were sacrificed because they were moribund. In a separate study in which bFGF was given after pneumonitis-inducing radiation to the whole lung, no protection against the classic form with bFGF was found.[306] Although the reason for the discrepancy between the findings in these two studies is not clear, it is possible that the higher doses used by Fuks et al.[82] produced sporadic pneumonitis, whereas the lower doses used in the study by Tee[306] induced a classic pneumonitis. Despite these unresolved differences, these studies do indicate the potential for intervening in these reactions. These studies also indicate our incomplete understanding of the events that occur after chest irradiation.

Interferon-γ The rationale for the use of interferon α in modulating radiation pneumonitis is that interferon-γ has been shown to reduce the severity of bleomycin-induced fibrosis in mouse lung[307] and to inhibit acute inflammation.[308,309] Thus, if radiation-induced fibrosis is a sequelae of an acute inflammatory response, that is, pneumonitis, then interferon-γ could potentially reduce the severity of lung fibrosis after irradiation. In a study in rats, Rosiello et al.[310] showed that interferon-γ markedly reduced the neutrophil influx and protein leak into the alveoli after irradiation of rat lung with a single dose of 15 Gy, suggesting that prophylactic administration of interferon-γ could reduce the severity of radiation pneumonitis in humans. However, long-term follow-up of these animals showed that although interferon-γ reduced early inflammatory events in irradiated lungs, the tissue response at 35 days, at the end of the study, showed that the number of cells and exudate in the irradiated lungs of the interferon-γ–treated rats was not different from that in rats only irradiated. Thus, it is unclear whether interferon-γ could be useful in modulating either radiation pneumonitis or fibrosis.

Antioxidants Pulmonary oxidant stress plays an important pathogenetic role in disease conditions, including acute lung injury/adult respiratory distress syndrome, hyperoxia, ischemia-reperfusion, sepsis, radiation injury, lung transplantation, chronic obstructive pulmonary disease, and inflammation. Reactive oxygen species released from activated macrophages and leukocytes or formed in the pulmonary epithelial and endothelial cells damage the lungs and initiate cascades of proinflammatory reactions propagating pulmonary and systemic stress. Diverse molecules, including small organic compounds (e.g., glutathione, tocopherol [vitamin E], flavonoids) serve as natural antioxidants that reduce oxidized cellular components, decompose reactive oxygen species, and detoxify toxic oxidation products. Antioxidant enzymes can either facilitate these antioxidant reactions (e.g., peroxidases using glutathione as a reducing agent) or directly decompose the reactive oxygen species (e.g., superoxide dismutases and catalase).

Many antioxidant agents are being tested for treatment of pulmonary oxidant stress. The administration of small antioxidants via the oral, intratracheal, and vascular routes for the treatment of short- and long-term oxidant stress has shown rather modest protective effects in animal and human studies. Intratracheal and intravascular administration of antioxidant enzymes is being currently tested for the treatment of acute oxidant stress. For example, intratracheal administration of recombinant human superoxide dismutase is protective in premature infants exposed to hyperoxia. However, animal and human studies show that more effective delivery of drugs to cells experiencing oxidant stress is needed to improve protection. Diverse delivery systems for antioxidants including liposomes, chemical modifications (e.g., attachment of masking PEGylated groups) and coupling to affinity carriers (e.g., antibodies against cellular adhesion molecules) are being employed and currently tested, mostly in animal and, to a limited extent, in humans, for the treatment of oxidant stress. Further studies are needed, however, to develop and establish effective applications of pulmonary antioxidant interventions useful in clinical practice. Although beyond the scope of this review, antioxidant gene therapies may eventually provide a strategy for the management of subacute and chronic pulmonary oxidant stress.[311]

Preventing Focal Scarring or Collagen Formation Because radiation damage in the lung is manifested as alveolitis followed by focal scarring with an attendant increase in collagen, many studies have focused on identifying drugs active against either one or both of these. One of the first drugs to be used clinically was the steroid prednisolone, which was hypothesized to modify radiation pneumonitis by reducing the inflammatory and exudative portion of lung injury. Both animal and human studies showed that prednisolone did protect against the early phase of pneumonitis. However, when drug administration was terminated, the alveolitis reappeared and in mice the LD_{50} for pneumonitis was not changed.

A second approach of these early studies was to attempt to intervene in the fibrotic process with collagen antagonists. Perhaps the most widely tested was D-penicillamine, a compound shown in experimental studies to inhibit collagen accumulation significantly in rat lung for up to 1 year after irradiation.[89,312] This biochemical effect translated into significant improvement in pulmonary function. Although shown to be effective in rats at a concentration that produced no deleterious side effects, D-penicillamine has not been widely tested clinically, perhaps because it requires continuous administration to be effective.

Endothelial dysfunction plays an important role in the pathogenesis of radiation-induced pneumonitis and fibrosis. A time- and dose-dependent decrease in angiotensin-converting enzyme activity, a marker of endothelial function, was observed after irradiation of either the whole thorax or hemithorax, a finding in good agreement with pulmonary perfusion scans.[86–88] Irradiation plus cyclophosphamide caused a chronic pneumonitis with septal fibrosis and vasculitis affecting, in particular, small caliber pulmonary arteries and arterioles, with markedly elevated concentrations of hydroxyproline, thromboxane (TxA_2), and prostaglandin (PGI_2) (two markers of pulmonary endothelial damage).[313–315] A significant increase in alpha actomyosin staining was also observed in vessels, septa, and macrophages of the same animals that also overexpressed

TGF-β. Supplementing the radiation plus cyclophosphamide treatment with the angiotensin type II receptor antagonist L 158809 or the angiotensin-converting enzyme inhibitors captopril and enalapril led to significant amelioration of the histologic damage as well as the overexpression of alpha-smooth muscle actin (SMA). Lung concentrations of hydroxyproline, PGI_2, TxA_2, and TGF-β were also observed in these animals so that the values of these compounds were closer to those measured in untreated control rats than to their radiation- and cyclophosphamide-treated counterparts. Angiotensin II plays an important role in the regulation of TGF-β and alpha-SMA, two proteins involved in the pathogenesis of pulmonary fibrosis. The finding that angiotensin-converting enzyme inhibitors or angiotensin II receptor blockers protect the lungs from radiation-induced pneumonitis and fibrosis reaffirms the involvement of angiotensin II in this inflammatory process and suggests an additional indication of treatment of this condition, thus opening a new potential pharmacologic use of these drugs.[315] However, clinical studies have yet to prove the value of these drugs for this indication.

CONCLUSION

Evidence promises improved local control and overall survival with increased radiation dose, but prescribed doses are limited by the risk of injury to surrounding normal tissues, particularly the lung and esophagus. Risk models have been developed to predict treatment-related toxicity based on radiation treatment parameters, and the potential to individualize treatment plans based on such models has been demonstrated. Delivery of such individualized plans can now be realized through such recent improvements in radiation treatment techniques as 3D conformal radiation therapy, IMRT, and proton therapy all becoming readily available.

Although intervening in the process that results in radiation-induced fibrosis is certainly one way of reducing the morbidity of thoracic irradiation for lung cancer, this approach would be reactive rather than proactive and would not necessarily facilitate tumor control by increasing the radiation dose to the tumor. The ultimate goal is to identify individuals who are at a higher risk of developing treatment-related pneumonitis and fibrosis before treatment begins. Clinically, a wide variation exists in the severity of lung fibrosis exhibited by individual patients treated similarly. These and other data in other normal tissues demonstrate that variations in radiosensitivity exist in the same normal-tissue cell type from different individuals. However, "tolerance" doses of both drugs and radiation are determined empirically from population averages and may be skewed by a genetically oversensitive minority. These data imply then that most patients could be treated with higher doses of either modality without exceeding their individual tolerance to the treatment. One approach to increasing tumor control while maintaining an acceptable level of lung morbidity is to be able to identify those sensitive individuals before treatment begins and to design treatment accordingly, creating so-called personalized radiation.

Personalized radiation therapy trials in general are investigating the feasibility of using an individualized total tumor dose to the limit of normal-tissue tolerance to achieve the highest therapeutic ratio.[316] Investigators found that the total tumor dose is most often limited by MLD and spinal cord exposure. Other studies investigated an individualized 3D margin, higher fraction dose,[317] and dose escalation based on normal-tissue dose constraints.[318,319] RTOG-93-11 was a radiation dose escalation study that used a threshold volume of lung receiving more than 20 Gy to stratify patients according to the risk of radiation lung toxicity and incorporated three dose categories for customizing the dose escalation. This trial identified an association between increasing gross tumor volume and poor progression-free survival.[320,321] Efforts to identify patients at risk for pneumonitis have focused on physical factors, such as dose and volume.[41,322] Recently, the underlying molecular biological mechanisms behind radiation-induced lung injury have come under study. Elevation of plasma TGF-β1 level after 4 weeks of radiation therapy was significantly predictive of radiation-induced lung toxicity,[109] and TGF-β1 genotypes had a role in mediating pulmonary dysfunction in patients with cystic fibrosis[323] and radiation fibrosis.[156] Improved knowledge of the molecular events associated with radiation-induced lung injury may translate into a better ability to individualize therapy.

Individual differences in susceptibility to radiation injury (which may be associated with genetic predisposition) are known to exist, and it is the most sensitive patients who limit the radiation doses used clinically, because standard doses are selected based on population-averaged toxicity. Thus, adding genetic factors to predictive models combining clinical and physical factors will likely strengthen risk assessment and improve its reliability. In addition, biomarkers, particularly cytokines, have been shown to mediate the process of radiation injury. Thus, cytokine measurement during treatment may provide an early warning for the onset of toxicity posttherapy. By proactively monitoring cytokines and updating the risk prediction during treatment, we can customize therapy in an ongoing manner using repeat imaging and treatment planning. This is the strategy that will allow us to tailor radiation therapy effectively to prevent the risk of major toxicity while pursuing and achieving curative individual radiation intervention.

REFERENCES

1. Groover TA, Christie AC, Merritt EA. Observations on the use of the copper filter in the roentgen treatment of deep seated malignancies. *South Med J* 1922;15:440–444
2. Evans WA, Leucutia T. Thoracic changes induced by heavy radiation. *AJR Am J Roentgenol* 1925;13:203.
3. Travis EL, Lung Morbidity of Radiotherapy. Oxford: Butterworth-Heineman, 1991:232–249.
4. Boersma LJ, Damen EM, de Boer RW, et al. Dose-effect relations for local functional and structural changes of the lung after irradiation for malignant lymphoma. *Radiother Oncol* 1994;32:201–209.

5. Mah K, Keane TJ, Van Dyk J, et al. Quantitative effect of combined chemotherapy and fractionated radiotherapy on the incidence of radiation-induced lung damage: a prospective clinical study. *Int J Radiat Oncol Biol Phys* 1994;28:563–574.
6. Boersma LJ, Damen EM, de Boer RW, et al. A new method to determine dose-effect relations for local lung-function changes using correlated SPECT and CT data. *Radiother Oncol* 1993;29:110–116.
7. Choi NC, Kanarek DJ, Kazemi H. Physiologic changes in pulmonary function after thoracic radiotherapy for patients with lung cancer and a role of regional pulmonary function studies in predicting post radiotherapy pulmonary function before radiotherapy. *Cancer Treat Symp* 1985;2:119–130.
8. Damen EM, Muller SH, Boersma LJ, et al. Quantifying local lung perfusion and ventilation using correlated SPECT and CT data. *J Nucl Med* 1994;35:784–792.
9. Mah K, Van Dyk J. Quantitative measurement of changes in human lung density following irradiation. *Radiother Oncol* 1988;11:169–179.
10. Marks LB, Spencer DP, Bentel GC, et al. The utility of SPECT lung perfusion scans in minimizing and assessing the physiologic consequences of thoracic irradiation. *Int J Radiat Oncol Biol Phys* 1993;23: 659–668.
11. Marks LB, Munley MT, Spencer DP, et al. Quantification of radiation-induced regional lung injury with perfusion imaging. *Int J Radiat Oncol Biol Phys* 1997;38:399–409.
12. Kwa S, Theuws J, van Herk M, et al, Automatic three-dimensional matching of CT-SPECT and CT-CT to localize lung damage after radiotherapy. *J Nucl Med* 1998;39:1074–1080.
13. Hebert ME, Lowe VJ, Hoffman JM, et al. Positron emission tomography in the pretreatment evaluation and follow-up of non-small cell lung cancer patients treated with radiotherapy: preliminary findings. *Am J Clin Oncol* 1996;19:416–421.
14. Guerrero T, Johnson V, Hart J, et al. Radiation pneumonitis: local dose versus [18F]-fluorodeoxyglucose uptake response in irradiated lung. *Int J Radiat Oncol Biol Phys* 2007;68:1030–1035.
15. Guerrero T, Sanders K, Noyola-Martinez J, et al. Quantification of regional ventilation from treatment planning CT. *Int J Radiat Oncol Biol Phys* 2005;62:630–634.
16. Travis EL, Vojnovic B, Davies EE, et al. A plethysmographic method for measuring function in locally irradiated mouse lung. *Br J Radiol* 1979;52:67–74.
17. Depledge MH, Collis CH, Barrett A. A technique for measuring carbon monoxide uptake in mice. *Int J Radiat Oncol Biol Phys* 1981;7: 485–489.
18. Travis EL, Down JD, Holmes SJ, et al. Radiation pneumonitis and fibrosis in mouse lung assayed by respiratory frequency and histology. *Radiat Res* 1980;84:133–143.
19. Nicholas D, Down JD. The assessment of early and late radiation injury to the mouse lung using X-ray computerised tomography. *Radiother Oncol* 1985;4:253–263.
20. Lockhart S, Hill D, King S. A semi-automated method for breathing rate measurement in the mouse. *Radiother Oncol* 1991;22:68–70.
21. Gross NJ. Pulmonary effects of radiation therapy. *Ann Intern Med* 1977; 86:81–92.
22. Marks LB. The pulmonary effects of thoracic irradiation. *Oncology (Williston Park)* 1994; 8:89–106.
23. McDonald S, Rubin P, Constine L. Biochemical markers as predictors for pulmonary effects of radiation. *Radiat Oncol Investig* 1995;3:56.
24. Nonn R, Gross N. Effectws of radiation on the lung. *Curr Opin Pulm Med* 1996;2:390.
25. Rosiello R, Merrill W. Radiation-induced lung injury. *Clin Chest Med* 1990;11:65.
26. Rubin P, Casarett GW. *Clinical Radiation Pathology*. Philadelphia: WB Saunders Company, 1968.
27. McDonald S, Rubin P, Phillips TL, et al. Injury to the lung from cancer therapy: Clinical syndromes, measurable endpoints, and potential scoring systems. *Int J Radiat Oncol Biol Phys* 1995;31:1187–1203.
28. Travis EL. The sequence of histological changes in mouse lungs after single doses of x-rays. *Int J Radiat Oncol Biol Phys* 1980;6:345–347.
29. Penney DP, Siemann DW, Rubin P, et al. Morphologic changes reflecting early and late effects of irradiation of the distal lung of the mouse: a review. *Scan Electron Microsc* 1982;(Pt 1):413–425.
30. Burkhardt A, Cottier H. Cellular events in alveolitis and the evolution of pulmonary fibrosis. B, cell pathology including molecular pathology. *Virchows Arch* 1989;58:1.
31. Sharplin J, Franko A. A quantitative histological study of strain-dependent differences in the effects of irradiation on mouse lung during the intermediate and late phases. *Radiat Res* 1989;119:15–31.
32. Schneider RA, Schultze J, Jensen JM, et al. Long-term outcome after static intensity-modulated total body radiotherapy using compensators stratified by pediatric and adult cohorts. *Int J Radiat Oncol Biol Phys* 2008;70:194–202.
33. Mah K, Van Dyk J, Keane T, et al. Acute radiation-induced pulmonary damage: a clinical study on the response to fractionated radiation therapy. *Int J Radiat Oncol Biol Phys* 1987;13:179.
34. Prato FS, Kurdyak R, Saibil EA, et al. The incidence of radiation pneumonitis as a result of single fraction upper half body irradiation. *Cancer* 1976;39:71–78.
35. Van Dyk J, Keane T, Kan S, et al. Radiation pneumonitis following large single dose irradiation: a re-evaluation based on absolute dose to lung. *Int J Radiat Oncol Biol Phys* 1981;7:461–467.
36. Van Dyk J, Mah K, Keane T. Radiation-induced lung damage: dose-time-fractionation considerations. *Radiother Oncol* 1989;14:55.
37. Mah K, Poon PY, Van Dyk J, et al. Assessment of acute radiation-induced pulmonary changes using computed tomography. *J Comput Assist Tomogr* 1986;10:736–743.
38. Graham MV, Purdy JA, Emami B, et al. Clinical dose-volume histogram analysis for pneumonitis after 3D treatment for non-small cell lung cancer (NSCLC). *Int J Radiat Oncol Biol Phys* 1999;45:323–329.
39. Yom SS, Liao Z, Liu HH, et al. Initial evaluation of treatment-related pneumonitis in advanced-stage non-small-cell lung cancer patients treated with concurrent chemotherapy and intensity-modulated radiotherapy. *Int J Radiat Oncol Biol Phys* 2007;68:94–102.
40. Claude L, Perol D, Ginestet C, et al. A prospective study on radiation pneumonitis following conformal radiation therapy in non-small-cell lung cancer: clinical and dosimetric factors analysis. *Radiother Oncol* 2004;71:175–181.
41. Wang S, Liao Z, Wei X, et al. Analysis of clinical and dosimetric factors associated with treatment-related pneumonitis (TRP) in patients with non-small-cell lung cancer (NSCLC) treated with concurrent chemotherapy and three-dimensional conformal radiotherapy (3D-CRT). *Int J Radiat Oncol Biol Phys* 2006;66:1399–1407.
42. Yamada M, Kudoh S, Hirata K, et al. Risk factors of pneumonitis following chemoradiotherapy for lung cancer. *Eur J Cancer* 1998;34:71–75.
43. Sharplin J, Franko A. Quantitative histological study of strain dependent differences in the effects of irradiation on mouse lung during the early phase. *Radiat Res* 1989;119:1–12.
44. Bachofen M, Weibel ER. Alterations of the gas exchange apparatus in adult respiratory insufficiency associated with septicemia. *Am Rev Respir Dis* 1977;116:589–615.
45. Franko A, Sharplin J. Development of fibrosis after lung irradiation in relation to inflammation and lung function in a mouse strain prone to fibrosis. *Radiat Res* 1994;140:347–355.
46. Travis E, Down J, Holmes S. Radiation pneumonitis and fibrosis in mouse lung assayed by respiratory frequency and histology. *Radiat Res* 1980 Oct;84(1):133–143.
47. Ullrich R, Casarett G. Interrelationship between the early inflammatory response and subsequent fibrosis after radiation exposure. *Radiat Res* 1977;72:107–121.
48. Pickrell J, Diel J, Slauson D, et al. Radiation-induced pulmonary fibrosis resolves spontaneously if dense scars are not formed. *Exper Mol Pathol* 1983;38:22–32.
49. Travis E, Down J. Repair in mouse lung after split doses of X rays. *Radiat Res* 1981;87:166–174.
50. Travis E, Meistrich M, Finch-Neimeyer M, et al. Late functional and biochemical changes in mouse lung after irradiation: differential effects of WR-2721. *Radiat Res* 1985;103:219–231.

51. Haston CK, Travis EL. Murine susceptibility to radiation-induced pulmonary fibrosis is influenced by a genetic factor implicated in susceptibility to bleomycin-induced pulmonary fibrosis. *Cancer Res* 1997;57:5286–291.
52. Franko A, Sharplin J, Ward W, et al. Evidence for two patterns of inheritance of sensitivity to induction of lung fibrosis in mice by radiation, one of which involves two genes. *Radiat Res* 1996;146:68–74.
53. Followill D, Kester D, Travis E. Histological changes in mouse colon after single- and split-dose irradiation. *Radiat Res* 1993;136:280–288.
54. Liao Z, Travis E. Unilateral nephrectomy 24 hours after bilateral kidney irradiation reduces damage to the function and structure of the remaining kidney. *Radiat Res* 1994;139:290–299.
55. Bennett D, Million R, Ackerman L. Bilateral radiation penumonitis, a complication of the radiotherapy of bronchogenic carcinoma. (Report and analysis of seven cases with autopsy). *Cancer* 1969;23:1001–1018.
56. Cohen Y, Gellei B, Robinson E. Bilateral radiation pneumonitis after unilateral lung and mediastinal irradiation. *Radiol Clin Biol* 1974;43:465–471.
57. Goldman AL, Enquist R. Hyperacute radiation pneumonitis. *Chest* 1975;67:613–615.
58. Smith J. Radiation pneumonitis: case report bilateral reaction after unilateral irradiation. *Am Rev Respir Dis* 1964;89:264–269.
59. Holt J. The acute radiation pneumonitis syndrome. *J Coll Radiol Australas* 1964;8:40–47.
60. Gibson P, Bryant D, Morgan G, et al. Radiation-induced lung injury: a hypersensitivity pneumonitis? *Ann InternMed* 1988;109:288–291.
61. Morgan GW, Pharm B, Breit SN. Radiation and the lung: A reevaluation of the mechanisms mediating pulmonary injury. *Int J Radiat Oncol Biol Phys* 1995;31:361–369.
62. Kawai S, Baba K, Tanaka H, et al. [A case of radiation pneumonitis with eosinophilia in bronchoalveolar lavage fluid]. *Nihon Kokyuki Gakkai Zasshi* 2008;46:44–49.
63. Calveley VL, Khan MA, Yeung IW, et al. Partial volume rat lung irradiation: temporal fluctuations of in-field and out-of-field DNA damage and inflammatory cytokines following irradiation. *Int J Radiat Biol* 2005;81:887–899.
64. Geist B, Trott K. Radiographic and function changes after partial lung irradiation in the rat. *Strahlenther Onkol* 1992;168:168.
65. Penney D, Rubin P. Specific early fine structural changes in the lung irradiation. *Int J Radiat Oncol Biol Phys* 1977;2:1123–1132.
66. Travis E, Tucker S. The relationship between functional assays of radiation response in the lung and target cell depletion. *Br J Cancer* 1986;53:304–319.
67. Rubin P, Shapiro D, Finklestein J, et al. The early release of surfactant following lung irradiation of alveolar type II cells. *Int J Radiat Oncol Biol Phys* 1980;6:75–77.
68. Rubin P, Siemann D, Shapiro D, et al. Surfactant release as an early measure of radiation pneumonitis. *Int J Radiat Oncol Biol Phys* 1983;9:1669–1673.
69. Shapiro D, Finkelstein J, Penney D, et al. Sequential effects of irradiation on the pulmonary surfactant system. *Int J Radiat Oncol Biol Phys* 1982;8:879–882.
70. Kasper M, Albrecht S, Grossmann H, et al. Monoclonal antibodies to surfactant protein D: evaluation of immunoreactivity in normal rat lung and in a radiation-induced fibrosis model. *Exp Lung Res* 1995;21:577–588.
71. Kasper M, Koslowski R, Luther T, et al. Immunohistochemical evidence for loss of ICAM-1 by alveolar epithelial cells in pulmonary fibrosis. *Histochem Cell Biol* 1995;104:397–405.
72. Kasper M, Muller M. Modulation of pan-cadherin expression in alveolar epithelial cells of mini pigs with pulmonary fibrosis. *Acta Histochem* 1994;96:439–444.
73. Kasper M, Rudolf T, Haase M, et al. Changes in cytokeratin, vimentin and desmoplakin distribution during the repair of irradiation-induced lung injury in adult rats. *Virchows Arch B Cell Pathol Mol Pathol* 1993;64:271–279.
74. Willner J, Jost A, Baier K, et al. A little to a lot or a lot to a little? An analysis of pneumonitis risk from dose-volume histogram parameters of the lung in patients with lung cancer treated with 3-D conformal radiotherapy. *Strahlenther Onkol* 2003;179:548–556.
75. Gross N. Experimental radiation pneumonitis. IV leakage of circulatory proteins onto the alveolar surface. *J Lab Clin Med* 1980;95:19–31.
76. Hopewell J. The importance of vascular damage in the development of late radiation effects in normal tissues. In: Meyn RE, Withers, HR, eds. *Radiation Biology in Cancer Research*. New York: Raven Press, 1980.
77. Law M. Radiation induced vascular injury and its relation to late effects in normal tissues. *Adv Radiat Biol* 1981;9:37.
78. Law M, Ahier R. Vascular and epithelial damage in the lung of the mouse after X-rays or neutrons. *Radiat Res* 1989;117:128–144.
79. Peterson L, Evans M, Graham M, et al. Vascular response to radiation injury in the rat lung. *Radiat Res* 1992;129:139–148.
80. Fingar VH, Taber SW, Buschemeyer WC, et al. Constitutive and stimulated expression of ICAM-1 protein on pulmonary endothelial cells in vivo. *Microvasc Res* 1997;54:135–144.
81. Fleckenstein K, Gauter-Fleckenstein B, Jackson IL, et al. Using biological markers to predict risk of radiation injury. *Semin Radiat Oncol* 2007;17:89–98.
82. Fuks Z, Persaud RS, Alfieri A, et al. Basic fibroblast growth factor protects endothelial cells against radiation-induced programmed cell death in vitro and in vivo. *Cancer Res* 1994;54:2582–2590.
83. Kwock L, Davenport WC, Clark RL, et al. The effects of ionizing radiation on the pulmonary vasculature of intact rats and isolated pulmonary endothelium. *Radiat Res* 1987;111:276–291.
84. Michel RP, Hakim TS, Freeman CR. Distribution of pulmonary vascular resistance in experimental fibrosis. *J Appl Physiol* 1988;65:1180–1190.
85. Rubin P, McDonald S, Maasilta P, et al. Serum markers for prediction of pulmonary radiation syndromes. Part I: Surfactant apo. *Int J Radiat Oncol Biol Phys* 1989;17:553–558.
86. Ts'ao C, Ward W, Port C. Radiation injury in rat lung. I. Prostacyclin (PGI2) production, arterial perfusion, and ultrastructure. *Radiat Res* 1983;96:284–293.
87. Ts'ao C, Ward W, Port C. Radiation injury in rat lung. III. Plasminogen activator and fibrinolytic inhibitor activities. *Radiat Res* 1983;96:301–308.
88. Ward W, Solliday N, Molteni A, et al. Radiation injury in rat lung. II. Angiotensin-converting enzyme activity. *Radiat Res* 1983;96:294–300.
89. Ward W, Solliday N, Molteni A, et al. Radiation injury in rat lung. IV. Angiotensin-converting enzyme activity. *Radiat Res* 1983;98:397.
90. King RJ, Jones MB, Minoo P. Regulation of lung cell proliferation by polypeptide growth factors. *Am J Physiology* 1989;257:L23–L38.
91. Rubin P, Finkelstein J, Shapiro D. Molecular biology mechanisms in the radiation induction of pulmonary injury syndromes: interrelationship between the alveolar macrophage and the septal fibroblast. *Int J Radiat Oncol Biol Phys* 1992;24:93–101.
92. Finkelstein JN, Johnston CJ, Baggs R, et al. Early alterations in extracellular matrix and transforming growth factor beta gene expression in mouse lung indicative of late radiation fibrosis. *Int J Radiat Oncol Biol Phys* 1994;28:621–631.
93. Martinet Y, Menard O, Vaillant P. Cytokines in human lung fibrosis. *Arch Toxicol* 1996;S18:127.
94. Rubin P, Johnston CJ, Williams JP, et al. A perpetual cascade of cytokines postirradiation leads to pulmonary fibrosis. *Int J Radiat Oncol Biol Phys* 1995;33:99–109.
95. Chen Y, Williams J, Ding I, et al. Radiation pneumonitis and early circulatory cytokine markers. *Semin Radiat Oncol* 2002;12:26–33.
96. Rube CE, Wilfert F, Uthe D, et al. Modulation of radiation-induced tumour necrosis factor alpha (TNF-alpha) expression in the lung tissue by pentoxifylline. *Radiother Oncol* 2002;64:177–187.
97. Rube CE, Wilfert F, Palm J, et al. Irradiation induces a biphasic expression of pro-inflammatory cytokines in the lung. *Strahlenther Onkol* 2004;180:442–448.
98. Franklin TJ. Therapeutic approaches to organ fibrosis. *Int J Biochem Cell Biol* 1997;29:79–89.

99. Massague J, Blain SW, Lo RS. TGFbeta signaling in growth control, cancer, and heritable disorders. *Cell* 2000;103:295–309.
100. Massague J, Chen YG. Controlling TGF-beta signaling. *Genes Dev* 2000;14:627–644.
101. Blobe GC, Liu X, Fang SJ, et al. A novel mechanism for regulating transforming growth factor beta (TGF-beta) signaling. Functional modulation of type III TGF-beta receptor expression through interaction with the PDZ domain protein, GIPC. *J Biol Chem* 2001;276:39608–39617.
102. Blobe GC, Schiemann WP, Lodish HF. Role of transforming growth factor beta in human disease. *N Engl J Med* 2000;342:1350–1358.
103. Grande JP. Role of transforming growth factor-beta in tissue injury and repair. *Proc Soc Exper Biol Med* 1997;214:27–40.
104. Hall A, Massague J. Cell regulation. *Curr Opin Cell Biol* 2008;20: 117–118.
105. Johnston CJ, Williams JP, Okunieff P, et al. Radiation-induced pulmonary fibrosis: examination of chemokine and chemokine receptor families. *Radiat Res* 2002;157:256–265.
106. Anscher MS, Kong FM, Andrews K, et al. Plasma transforming growth factor [beta]1 as a predictor of radiation pneumonitis. *Int J Radiat Oncol Biol Phys* 1998;41:1029–1035.
107. Anscher MS, Kong FM, Marks LB, et al. Changes in plasma transforming growth factor beta during radiotherapy and the risk of symptomatic radiation-induced pneumonitis. *Int J Radiat Oncol Biol Phys* 1997;37:253–258.
108. Rabbani ZN, Anscher MS, Zhang X, et al. Soluble TGFbeta type II receptor gene therapy ameliorates acute radiation-induced pulmonary injury in rats. *Int J Radiat Oncol Biol Phys* 2003;57:563–572.
109. Zhao L, Sheldon K, Chen M, et al. The predictive role of plasma TGF-beta1 during radiation therapy for radiation-induced lung toxicity deserves further study in patients with non-small cell lung cancer. *Lung Cancer* 2008;59:232–239.
110. Anscher MS, Kong FM, Jirtle RL. The relevance of transforming growth factor beta 1 in pulmonary injury after radiation therapy. *Lung Cancer* 1998;19:109–120.
111. De Jaeger K, Seppenwoolde Y, Kampinga HH, et al. Significance of plasma transforming growth factor-beta levels in radiotherapy for non-small-cell lung cancer. *Int J Radiat Oncol Biol Phys* 2004;58:1378–1387.
112. Holler E, Kolb H, Hintermeier-Knabe R, et al. Role of tumor necrosis factor alpha in acute graft-versus-host disease and complications following allogeneic bone marrow transplantation. *Transplant Proc* 1993; 25:1234–1236.
113. Holler E, Kolb HJ, Moller A, et al. Increased serum levels of tumor necrosis factor alpha precede major complications of bone marrow transplantation. *Blood* 1990;75:1011–1016.
114. Xun C, Thompson J, Jennings C, et al. Effect of total body irradiation, busulfan-cyclophosphamide, or cyclophosphamide conditioning on inflammatory cytokine release and development of acute and chronic graft-versus-host disease in H-2-incompatible transplanted SCID mice. *Blood* 1994;83:2360–2367.
115. Johnston C, Wright T, Rubin P, et al. Alterations in the expression of chemokine mRNA levels in fibrosis-resistant and -sensitive mice after thoracic irradiation. *Exper Lung Res* 1998;24:321–337.
116. Arpin D, Perol D, Blay JY, et al. Early variations of circulating interleukin-6 and interleukin-10 levels during thoracic radiotherapy are predictive for radiation pneumonitis. *J Clin Oncol* 2005;23:8748–8756.
117. Chen CI, Abraham R, Tsang R, et al. Radiation-associated pneumonitis following autologous stem cell transplantation: predictive factors, disease characteristics and treatment outcomes. *Bone Marrow Transplant* 2001;27:177–182.
118. Chen Y, Hyrien O, Williams J, et al. Interleukin (IL)-1A and IL-6: applications to the predictive diagnostic testing of radiation pneumonitis. *Int J Radiat Oncol Biol Phys* 2005;62:260–266.
119. Piguet PF. Is "tumor necrosis factor" the major effector of pulmonary fibrosis? *Eur Cytokine Netw* 1990;1:257–258.
120. Vujaskovic Z, Marks LB, Anscher MS. The physical parameters and molecular events associated with radiation-induced lung toxicity. *Semin Radiat Oncol* 2000;10:296–307.
121. Warburton D, Bellusci S. The molecular genetics of lung morphogenesis and injury repair. *Paediatr Respir Rev* 2004;5(Suppl A):S283–S287.
122. Ware LB, Matthay MA. Keratinocyte and hepatocyte growth factors in the lung: roles in lung development, inflammation, and repair. *Am J Physiol Lung Cell Mol Physiol* 2002;282:L924–L940.
123. Mio T, Romberger DJ, Thompson AB, et al. Cigarette smoke induces interleukin-8 release from human bronchial epithelial cells. *Am J Respir Crit Care Med* 1997;155:1770–1776.
124. Chen H, Cowan MJ, Hasday JD, et al. Tobacco smoking inhibits expression of proinflammatory cytokines and activation of IL-1R-associated kinase, p38, and NF-kappaB in alveolar macrophages stimulated with TLR2 and TLR4 agonists. *J Immunol* 2007;179:6097–6106.
125. Hart JP, Broadwater G, Rabbani Z, et al. Cytokine profiling for prediction of symptomatic radiation-induced lung injury. *Int J Radiat Oncol Biol Phys* 2005;63:1448–1454.
126. Kohno N, Hamada H, Fujioka S, et al. Circulating antigen KL-6 and lactate dehydrogenase for monitoring irradiated patients with lung cancer. *Chest* 1992;102:117–122.
127. Kohno N. Serum marker KL-6/MUC1 for the diagnosis and management of interstitial pneumonitis. *J Med Invest* 1999;46:151–158.
128. Matsuno Y, Satoh H, Ishikawa H, et al. Simultaneous measurements of KL-6 and SP-D in patients undergoing thoracic radiotherapy. *Med Oncol* 2006;23:75–82.
129. Goto K, Kodama T, Sekine I, et al. Serum levels of KL-6 are useful biomarkers for severe radiation pneumonitis. *Lung Cancer* 2001;34:141–148.
130. Tokiya R, Hiratsuka J, Yoshida K, et al. Evaluation of serum KL-6 as a predictive marker of radiation pneumonitis in patients with breast-conservation therapy. *Int J Clin Oncol* 2004;9:498–502.
131. Hara R, Itami J, Komiyama T, et al. Serum levels of KL-6 for predicting the occurrence of radiation pneumonitis after stereotactic radiotherapy for lung tumors. *Chest* 2004;125:340–344.
132. Kasper M, Behrens J, Schuh D, et al. Distribution of E-cadherin and Ep-CAM in the human lung during development and after injury. *Histochem Cell Biol* 1995;103:281–286.
133. Son EW, Rhee DK, Pyo S. Gamma-irradiation-induced intercellular adhesion molecule-1 (ICAM-1) expression is associated with catalase: activation of Ap-1 and JNK. *J Toxicol Environ Health A* 2006;69:2137–2155.
134. Kawana A, Shioya S, Katoh H, et al. Expression of intercellular adhesion molecule-1 and lymphocyte function-associated antigen-1 on alveolar macrophages in the acute stage of radiation-induced lung injury in rats. *Radiat Res* 1997;147:431–436.
135. Epperly MW, Sikora CA, DeFilippi SJ, et al. Pulmonary irradiation-induced expression of VCAM-I and ICAM-I is decreased by manganese superoxide dismutase-plasmid/liposome (MnSOD-PL) gene therapy. *Biol Blood Marrow Transplant* 2002;8:175–187.
136. Nakayama Y, Makino S, Fukuda Y, et al. Activation of lavage lymphocytes in lung injuries caused by radiotherapy for lung cancer. *Int J Radiat Oncol Biol Phys* 1996;34:459–467.
137. Ishii Y, Kitamura S. Soluble intercellular adhesion molecule-1 as an early detection marker for radiation pneumonitis. *Eur Respir J* 1999;13:733–738.
138. Steel G, Adams K, Peckham M. Lung damage in C57B1 mice following thoracic irradiation: enhancement by chemotherapy. *Br J Radiol* 1979;52:741–747.
139. Down J, Nicholas D, Steel G. Lung damage after hemithoracic irradiation: dependence on mouse strain. *Radiother Oncol* 1986;6:43–50.
140. Down J, Steel G. The expression of early and late damage after thoracic irradiation: a comparison between CBA and C57B1 mice. *Radiat Res* 1983;96:603–610.
141. Franko A, Sharplin J, Ward W, et al. The genetic basis of strain-dependent differences in the early phase of radiation injury in mouse lung. *Radiat Res* 1991;126:349–356.
142. Haston CK, Amos CI, King TM, et al. Inheritance of Susceptibility to Bleomycin-induced pulmonary fibrosis in the mouse. *Cancer Res* 1996;56:2596–2601.
143. Kleeberger S, Levitt R, Zhang L, et al. Linkage analysis of susceptibility to ozone-induced lung inflammation in inbred mice. *Nature Genetics* 1997;17:475–478.

144. Haston CK, Zhou X, Gumbiner-Russo L, et al. Universal and radiation-specific loci influence murine susceptibility to radiation-induced pulmonary fibrosis. *Cancer Res* 2002;62:3782–3788.
145. Rossi G, Hunninghake G, Kawanami O, et al. Motheaten mice—an animal model with an inherited form of interstitial lung disease. *Am Rev Respir Dis* 1985;131:150–158.
146. Vaz NM, Vaz EM, Levine BB. Relationship between Histocompatibility (H-2) genotype and immune responsiveness to low doses of ovalbumin in the mouse. *J Immunol* 1970;104:1572–1574.
147. Wilson BD, Sternick JL, Yoshizawa Y, et al. Experimental murine hypersensitivity pneumonitis: multigenic control and influence by genes within the I-B subregion of the H-2 complex. *J Immunol* 1982; 129:2160–2163.
148. Allen EM, Moore VL, Stevens JO. Strain variation in BCG-induced chronic pulmonary inflammation in mice: I. Basic model and possible genetic control by non-H-2 genes. *J Immunol* 1977;119:343–347.
149. Hoyt D, Lazo J. Bleomycin and cyclophosphamide increase pulmonary tupe IV procollagen MRNA ion mice. *J Physiol* 1988;246:765.
150. Hoyt D, Lazo J. Alterations in pulmonary MRNA encoding procollagens, fibronectin and transorming. *J Physiol* 1990;246:765.
151. Schrier D, Kunkel R, Phan S. The role of strain variation in murine bleomycin-induced pulmonary fibrosis. *Am Rev Respir Dis* 1983;127:63–66.
152. Mori H, Kawada K, Zhang P, et al. Bleomycin-induced pulmonary fibrosis in genetically mast cell-deficient WBB6F1-W/Wv mice and mechanism of the suppressive effect of tranilast, an antiallergic drug inhibiting mediator release from mast cells, on fibrosis. *Int Arch Allergy App Immunol* 1991;95:195–201.
153. Awwad H. Normal tissue radiosensitivity: prediction on deterministic or stochastic basis? *J Egypt Natl Canc Inst* 2005;17:221–230.
154. Geara FB, Komaki R, Tucker SL, et al. Factors influencing the development of lung fibrosis after chemoradiation for small cell carcinoma of the lung: evidence for inherent interindividual variation. *Int J Radiat Oncol Biol Phys* 1998;41:279–286.
155. Andreassen CN, Alsner J, Overgaard J. Does variability in normal tissue reactions after radiotherapy have a genetic basis—Where and how to look for it. *Radiother Oncol* 2002;64:131–140.
156. Andreassen CN, Alsner J, Overgaard J, et al. TGFB1 polymorphisms are associated with risk of late normal tissue complications in the breast after radiotherapy for early breast cancer. *Radiother Oncol* 2005;75:18–21.
157. Andreassen CN, Alsner J, Overgaard M, et al. Risk of radiation-induced subcutaneous fibrosis in relation to single nucleotide polymorphisms in TGFB1, SOD2, XRCC1, XRCC3, APEX and ATM—a study based on DNA from formalin fixed paraffin embedded tissue samples. *Int J Biol* 2006;82:577–586.
158. Andreassen CN, Overgaard J, Alsner J, et al. ATM sequence variants and risk of radiation-induced subcutaneous fibrosis after postmastectomy radiotherapy. *Int J Radiat Oncol Biol Phys* 2006;64:776–783.
159. De Ruyck K, Van Eijkeren M, Claes K, et al. Radiation-induced damage to normal tissues after radiotherapy in patients treated for gynecologic tumors: Association with single nucleotide polymorphisms in XRCC1, XRCC3, and OGG1 genes and in vitro chromosomal radiosensitivity in lymphocytes. *Int J Radiat Oncol Biol Phys* 2005;62:1140–1149.
160. Fernet M, Hall J. Genetic biomarkers of therapeutic radiation sensitivity. *DNA Repair* 2004;3:1237–1243.
161. Ho AY, Atencio DP, Peters S, et al. Genetic predictors of adverse radiotherapy effects: the gene-PARE project. *Int J Radiat Oncol Biol Phys* 2006;65:646–655.
162. West CML, McKay MJ, Hölscher T, et al. Molecular markers predicting radiotherapy response: report and recommendations from an International Atomic Energy Agency technical meeting. *Int J Radiat Oncol Biol Phys* 2005;62:1264–1273.
163. Crompton NEA, Shi YQ, Emery GC, et al. Sources of variation in patient response to radiation treatment. *Int J Radiat Oncol Biol Phys* 2001;49:547–554.
164. Jeggo PA, Carr AM, Lehmann AR. Splitting the ATM: distinct repair and checkpoint defects in ataxia-telangiectasia. *Trends in Genet* 1998; 14:312–316.
165. Rogers PB, Plowman PN, Harris SJ, et al. Four radiation hypersensitivity cases and their implications for clinical radiotherapy. *Radiother Oncol* 2000;57:143–154.
166. Blunt T, Finnie N, Taccioli G, et al. Defective DNA-dependent protein kinase activity is linked to V(D)J recombination and DNA repair defects associated with the murine scid mutation. *Cell* 1995;80: 813–823.
167. Gu Y, Seidl KJ, Rathbun GA, et al. Growth retardation and leaky SCID phenotype of Ku70-deficient mice. *Immunity* 1997;7:653–665.
168. Nussenzweig A, Chen C, da Costa Soares V, et al. Requirement for Ku80 in growth and immunoglobulin V(D)J recombination. *Nature* 1996;382:551–555.
169. Roberts SA, Spreadborough AR, Bulman B, et al. Heritability of cellular radiosensitivity: a marker of low-penetrance predisposition genes in breast cancer. *Am J Hum Gen* 1999;65:784–794.
170. Fowler JF. The eighteenth Douglas Lea lecture. 40 years of radiobiology: its impact on radiotherapy. *Phys Med Biol* 1984;29:97.
171. Withers H, Peters L, Kogelnik H. The pathobiology of late effects of irradiation. In: Meyn RE, Withers HR, eds. *Radiation Biology in Cancer Research*. New York: Raven Press, 1980.
172. Travis E, Parkins C, Down J, et al. Repair in mouse lung between multiple small doses of X rays. *Radiat Res* 1983;94:326–339.
173. Travis E, Thames HJ, Watkins T. The kinetics of repair in mouse lung after fractionated radiation. *In J Radiat Biol* 1987;52:903.
174. Withers H, Thames HJ, Peters L. Dose fractionation and volume effects in normal tissue and tumors. *Cancer Treat Symp* 1984;1:75.
175. Thames HJ Jr, Withers HR, Peters LJ, et al. Changes in early and late radiation responses with altered dose fractionation: implications for dose-survival relationships. I *Int J Radiat Oncol Biol Phys* 1982; 8:219–226.
176. Douglas BG, Fowler JF. The effect of multiple small doses of x-ray on skin reactions in the mouse and a basic interpretation. *Radiat Res* 1976; 66:401–426.
177. Fowler JF. The linear-quadratic formula and progress in fractionated radiotherapy. *Br J Cancer* 1989;62:679–694.
178. Peters L, Withers H, Thames HJ. Radiobiological bases for multiple daily fractionation. In: Kaercher KH, Kogelnik HD, Reiinartz G, eds. *Progress in Radio-oncology II*. New York: Raven Press, 1982.
179. Withers H, Thames HJ, Peters L. Normal tissue radio-resistance in clinical radiotherapy. In: Fletcher GH, Nervi C, Withers HR, eds. *Biological Bases and Clinical Implications of Tumor Radioresistance*. New York: Masson, 1983.
180. Down J, Easton D, Steel G. Repair in the mouse lung during low dose-rate irradiation. *Radiother Oncol* 1986;6:29–42.
181. Parkins C, Fowler J. Repair in mouse lung after multifraction X rays and neutrons: extension to 40 fractions. *Br J Radiol* 1985;58:1097–1103.
182. Parkins C, Fowler J, Maughan R, et al. Repair in mouse lung for up to 20 fractions of X rays or neutrons. *Br J Radiol* 1985;58:225–241.
183. Vegesna V, Withers HR, Thames HD Jr, et al. Multifraction radiation response of mouse lung. *Int J Radiat Biol Relat Stud Phys Chem Med* 1985;47:413–422.
184. Terry NH, Tucker SL, Travis EL. Residual radiation damage in mouse lung associated with pneumonitis. *Int J Radiat Oncol Biol Phys* 1988; 14: 929–938.
185. Rosen II, Fischer TA, Antolak JA, et al. Correlation between lung fibrosis and radiation therapy dose after concurrent radiation therapy and chemotherapy for limited small cell lung cancer. *Radiology* 2001;221:614–622.
186. Roach M III, Gandara DR, Yuo HS, et al. Radiation pneumonitis following combined modality therapy for lung cancer: analysis of prognostic factors. *J Clin Oncol* 1995;13:2606–2612.
187. Macijewski B, Withers HR, Taylor JM, et al. Dose fractionation and regeneration in radiotherapy for cancer of the oral cavity and oropharynx: tumor dose-response and repopulation. *Int J Radiat Oncol Biol Phys* 1989;16:831–843.
188. Withers HR, Maciejewski B, Taylor JM, et al. Accelerated repopulation in head and neck cancer. *Front Radiat Ther Oncol* 1988;22:105–110.

189. Withers HR, Taylor JM, Maciejewski B. The hazard of accelerated tumor clonogen repopulation during radiotherapy. *Acta Oncol* 1988; 27:131–146.
190. Cox JD, Azarnia N, Byhardt RW, et al. A randomized phase I/II trial of hyperfractionated radiation therapy with total doses of 60.0 Gy to 79.2 Gy: possible survival benefit with greater than or equal to 69.6 Gy in favorable patients with Radiation Therapy Oncology Group stage III non-small-cell lung carcinoma: report of Radiation Therapy Oncology Group 83-11. *J Clin Oncol* 1990;8:1543–1555.
191. Komaki R, Pajak T, Byhardt R, et al. Analysis of early and late deaths on RTOG non-small cell carcinoma of the lung trials: comparison with CALGB 8433. *Lung Cancer* 1993;10:189–197.
192. Shibamoto Y, Jeremic B, Acimovic L, et al. Influence of interfraction interval on the efficacy and toxicity of hyperfractionated radiotherapy in combination with concurrent daily chemotherapy in stage III non-small-cell lung cancer. *Int J Radiat Oncol Biol Phys* 2001;50:295–300.
193. Withers HR, Taylor JM, Maciejewski B. Treatment volume and tisse tolerance. *Int J Radiat Oncol Biol Phys* 1988;14:751–759.
194. Withers HR, Thames HD. Dose fractionation and volume effects in normal tussue and tumors. *Am J Clin Oncol* 1988;11:313–329.
195. Liao ZX, Travis EL, Tucker SL. Damage and morbidity from pneumonitis after irradiation of partial volumes of mouse lung. *Int J Radiat Oncol Biol Phys* 1995;32:1359–1370.
196. Travis EL, Liao ZX, Tucker SL. Spatial heterogeneity of the volume effect for radiation pneumonitis in mouse lung. *Int J Radiat Oncol Biol Phys* 1997;38:1045–1054.
197. Boersma LJ, Thews JC, Kwa SL, et al. Regional variation in functional subunit density in the lung: regarding Liao et al. IJEOBP 32(5):1359-1370; 1995. *Int J Radiat Oncol Biol Phys* 1996;34:1187–1188.
198. Khan M, Hill R, Van Dyk J. Partial volume rat lung irradiation: an evaluation of early DNA damage. *Int J Radiat Oncol Biol Phys* 1998; 40:467–476.
199. Khan MA, Van Dyk J, Yeung IW, et al. Partial volume rat lung irradiation; assessment of early DNA damage in different lung regions and effect of radical scavengers. *Radiother Oncol* 2003;66:95–102.
200. Tucker SL, Liao ZX, Travis EL. Estimation of the spatial distribution of target cells for radiation pneumonitis in mouse lung. *Int J Radiat Oncol Biol Phys* 1997;38:1055–1066.
201. Bradley JD, Hope A, El Naqa I, et al. A nomogram to predict radiation pneumonitis, derived from a combined analysis of RTOG 9311 and institutional data. *Int J Radiat Oncol Biol Phys* 2007;69:985–992.
202. Seppenwoolde Y, De Jaeger K, Boersma LJ, et al. Regional differences in lung radiosensitivity after radiotherapy for non-small-cell lung cancer. *Int J Radiat Oncol Biol Phys* 2004;60:748–758.
203. Yorke ED, Jackson A, Rosenzweig KE, et al. Dose-volume factors contributing to the incidence of radiation pneumonitis in non-small-cell lung cancer patients treated with three-dimensional conformal radiation therapy. *Int J Radiat Oncol Biol Phys* 2002;54:329–339.
204. Novakova-Jiresova A, van Luijk P, van Goor H, et al. Changes in expression of injury after irradiation of increasing volumes in rat lung. *Int J Radiat Oncol Biol Phys* 2007;67:1510–1518.
205. Fay M, Tan A, Fisher R, et al. Dose-volume histogram analysis as predictor of radiation pneumonitis in primary lung cancer patients treated with radiotherapy. *Int J Radiat Oncol Biol Phys* 2005;61:1355–1363.
206. Hernando ML, Marks LB, Bentel GC, et al. Radiation-induced pulmonary toxicity: a dose-volume histogram analysis in 201 patients with lung cancer. *Int J Radiat Oncol Biol Phys* 2001;51:650–659.
207. Gopal R, Tucker SL, Komaki R, et al. The relationship between local dose and loss of function for irradiated lung. *Int J Radiat Oncol Biol Phys* 2003;56:106–113.
208. Yorke ED, Jackson A, Rosenzweig KE, et al. Correlation of dosimetric factors and radiation pneumonitis for non-small-cell lung cancer patients in a recently completed dose escalation study. *Int J Radiat Oncol Biol Phys* 2005;63:672–682.
209. Allen AM, Czerminska M, Janne PA, et al. Fatal pneumonitis associated with intensity-modulated radiation therapy for mesothelioma. *Int J Radiat Oncol Biol Phys* 2006;65:640–645.
210. De Jaeger K, Hoogeman MS, Engelsman M, et al. Incorporating an improved dose-calculation algorithm in conformal radiotherapy of lung cancer: re-evaluation of dose in normal lung tissue. *Radiother Oncol* 2003;69:1–10.
211. Fan M, Marks LB, Lind P, et al. Relating radiation-induced regional lung injury to changes in pulmonary function tests. *Int J Radiat Oncol Biol Phys* 2001;51:311–317.
212. Goethals I, Dierckx R, De Meerleer G, et al. The role of nuclear medicine in the prediction and detection of radiation-associated normal pulmonary and cardiac damage. *J Nucl Med* 2003;44: 1531–1539.
213. Lind PA, Marks LB, Hollis D, et al. Receiver operating characteristic curves to assess predictors of radiation-induced symptomatic lung injury. *Int J Radiat Oncol Biol Phys* 2002;54:340–347.
214. Marks LB, Fan M, Clough R, et al. Radiation-induced pulmonary injury: symptomatic versus subclinical endpoints. *Int J Radiat Biol* 2000;76:469–475.
215. Nioutsikou E, Partridge M, Bedford JL, et al. Prediction of radiation-induced normal tissue complications in radiotherapy using functional image data. *Phys Med Biol* 2005;50:1035–1046.
216. Marks LB. Physiology-based studies of radiation-induced normal tissue injury. *Radiother Oncol* 1999;51:101–103.
217. De Jaeger K, Seppenwoolde Y, Boersma LJ, et al. Pulmonary function following high-dose radiotherapy of non-small-cell lung cancer. *Int J Radiat Oncol Biol Phys* 2003;55:1331–1340.
218. Hassaballa HA, Cohen ES, Khan AJ, et al. Positron emission tomography demonstrates radiation-induced changes to nonirradiated lungs in lung cancer patients treated with radiation and chemotherapy. *Chest* 2005;128:1448–1452.
219. Nestle U, Hellwig D, Fleckenstein J, et al. Comparison of early pulmonary changes in 18FDG-PET and CT after combined radiochemotherapy for advanced non-small-cell lung cancer: a study in 15 patients. *Frontiers Radiat Ther Oncol* 2002;37:26–33.
220. Kahan Z, Csenki M, Varga Z, et al. The risk of early and late lung sequelae after conformal radiotherapy in breast cancer patients. *Int J Radiat Oncol Biol Phys* 2007;68:673–681.
221. Kim TH, Cho KH, Pyo HR, et al. Dose-volumetric parameters of acute esophageal toxicity in patients with lung cancer treated with three-dimensional conformal radiotherapy. *Int J Radiat Oncol Biol Phys* 2005;62:995–1002.
222. Kong FM, Hayman JA, Griffith KA, et al. Final toxicity results of a radiation-dose escalation study in patients with non-small-cell lung cancer (NSCLC): predictors for radiation pneumonitis and fibrosis. *Int J Radiat Oncol Biol Phys* 2006;65:1075–1086.
223. Kwa SLS, Lebesque JV, Theuws JCM, et al. Radiation pneumonitis as a function of mean lung dose: an analysis of pooled data of 540 patients. *Int J Radiat Oncol Biol Phys* 1998;42:1–9.
224. Martel MK, Ten Haken RK, Hazuka MB,et al. Dose-volume histogram and 3-D treatment planning evaluation of patients with pneumonitis. *Int J Radiat Oncol Biol Phys* 1994;28:575–581.
225. Oetzel D, Schraube P, Hensley F,et al. Estimation of pneumonitis risk in three-dimensional treatment planning using dose-volume histogram analysis. *Int J Radiat Oncol Biol Phys* 1995;33:455–460.
226. Schallenkamp JM, Miller RC, Brinkmann DH, et al. Incidence of radiation pneumonitis after thoracic irradiation: dose-volume correlates. *Int J Radiat Oncol Biol Phys* 2007;67:410–416.
227. Armstrong JG, Zelefsky MJ, Leibel SA, et al. Strategy for dose escalation using 3-dimensional conformal radiation therapy for lung cancer. *Ann Oncol* 1995;6:693–697.
228. Fu XL, Huang H, Bentel G, et al. Predicting the risk of symptomatic radiation-induced lung injury using both the physical and biologic parameters V(30) and transforming growth factor beta. *Int J Radiat Oncol Biol Phys* 2001;50:899–908.
229. Tsujino K, Hirota S, Endo M, et al. Predictive value of dose-volume histogram parameters for predicting radiation pneumonitis after concurrent chemoradiation for lung cancer. *Int J Radiat Oncol Biol Phys* 2003;55:110–115.

230. Jin H, Tucker S, Liu H, et al. Dose-volume thresholds for the risk of treatment-related pneumonitis in inoperable non-small cell lung cancer treated with definitive radiotherapy. *Radiothera Oncol* 2009 Jun;91(3):427–432.
231. Koto M, Tsujii H, Yamamoto N, et al. Dosimetric factors used for thoracic X-ray radiotherapy are not predictive of the occurrence of radiation pneumonitis after carbon-ion radiotherapy. *Tohoku J Exp Med* 2007;213:149–156.
232. Emami B, Lyman J, Brown A, et al. Tolerance of normal tissue to therapeutic irradiation. *Int J Radiat Oncol Biol Phys* 1991;21:109–122.
233. Burman C, Kutcher GJ, Emami B, et al. Fitting of normal tissue tolerance data to an analytic function. *Int J Radiat Oncol Biol Phys* 1991;21:123–135.
234. Lyman J. Complication probability as assessed from dose-volume histograms. *Radiati Res Suppl* 1985;8:S13–S19.
235. Kutcher GJ, Burman C. Calculation of complication probability factors for non-uniform normal tissue irradiation: the effective volume method. *Int J Radiat Oncol Biol Phys* 1989;16:1623–1630.
236. Hope AJ, Lindsay PE, El Naqa I, et al. Modeling radiation pneumonitis risk with clinical, dosimetric, and spatial parameters. *Int J Radiat Oncol Biol Phys* 2006;65:112–124.
237. Das SK, Zhou S, Zhang J, et al. Predicting lung radiotherapy-induced pneumonitis using a model combining parametric Lyman probit with nonparametric decision trees. *Int J Radiat Oncol Biol Phys* 2007;68:1212–1221.
238. Deasy JO, El Naqa I. Image-based modeling of normal tissue complication probability for radiation therapy. *Cancer Treat Res* 2008;139: 215–256.
239. Rancati T, Wennberg B, Lind P, et al. Early clinical and radiological pulmonary complications following breast cancer radiation therapy: NTCP fit with four different models. *Radiother Oncol* 2007;82:308–316.
240. Semenenko VA, Li XA. Lyman-Kutcher-Burman NTCP model parameters for radiation pneumonitis and xerostomia based on combined analysis of published clinical data. *Phys Med Biol* 2008;53:737–755.
241. Tsougos I, Mavroidis P, Theodorou K, et al. Clinical validation of the LKB model and parameter sets for predicting radiation-induced pneumonitis from breast cancer radiotherapy. *Phys Med Biol* 2006;51:L1–L9.
242. Tsougos I, Nilsson P, Theodorou K, et al. NTCP modelling and pulmonary function tests evaluation for the prediction of radiation induced pneumonitis in non-small-cell lung cancer radiotherapy. *Phys Med Biol* 2007;52:1055–1073.
243. Robnett TJ, Machtay M, Vines EF, et al. Factors predicting severe radiation pneumonitis in patients receiving definitive chemoradiation for lung cancer. *Int J Radiat Oncol Biol Phys* 2000;48:89–94.
244. Rancati T, Ceresoli GL, Gagliardi G, et al. Factors predicting radiation pneumonitis in lung cancer patients: a retrospective study. *Radiother Oncol* 2003;67:275–283.
245. Inoue A, Kunitoh H, Sekine I, et al. Radiation pneumonitis in lung cancer patients: a retrospective study of risk factors and the long-term prognosis. *Int J Radiat Oncol Biol Phys* 2001;49:649–655.
246. Mao J, Kocak Z, Zhou S, et al. The impact of induction chemotherapy and the associated tumor response on subsequent radiation-related changes in lung function and tumor response. *Int J Radiat Oncol Biol Phys* 2007;67:1360–1369.
247. Saunders MI, Rojas A, Lyn BE, et al. Dose-escalation with CHARTWEL (continuous hyperfractionated accelerated radiotherapy week-end less) combined with neo-adjuvant chemotherapy in the treatment of locally advanced non-small cell lung cancer. *Clin Oncol (R Coll Radiol)* 2002;14:352–360.
248. Wang S, Liao Z, Wei X, et al. Association between systemic chemotherapy before chemoradiation and increased risk of treatment-related pneumonitis in esophageal cancer patients treated with definitive chemoradiotherapy. *J Thorac Oncol* 2008;3:277–282.
249. Sunyach MP, Falchero L, Pommier P, et al. Prospective evaluation of early lung toxicity following three-dimensional conformal radiation therapy in non-small-cell lung cancer: preliminary results. *Int J Radiat Oncol Biol Phys* 2000;48:459–463.
250. Tsuji H, Ishikawa H, Yanagi T, et al. Carbon-ion radiotherapy for locally advanced or unfavorably located choroidal melanoma: a Phase I/II dose-escalation study. *Int J Radiat Oncol Biol Phys* 2007;67: 857–862.
251. Moreno M, Aristu J, Ramos LI, et al. Predictive factors for radiation-induced pulmonary toxicity after three-dimensional conformal chemoradiation in locally advanced non-small-cell lung cancer. *Clin Translational Oncol* 2007;9:596–602.
252. Tucker SL, Liu HH, Liao Z, et al. Analysis of radiation pneumonitis risk using a generalized Lyman models. *Int J Radiat Oncol Biol Phys* 2008;72(2):568–574.
253. Moiseenko VV, Battista JJ, Hill RP, et al. In-field and out-of-field effects in partial volume lung irradiation in rodents: possible correlation between early DNA damage and functional endpoints. *Int J Radiat Oncol Biol Phys* 2000;48:1539–48.
254. Armstrong J, Raben A, Selefsky M, et al. Promising survival with three-dimensional conformal radiation therapy for non–small cell lung cancer. *Radiother Oncol* 1997;44:17–22.
255. Erichsen H, Chanock S. SNPs in cancer research and treatment. *Br J Cancer* 2004;90:747–751.
256. Wjst M. Target SNP selection in complex disease association studies. *BMC Bioinformatics* 2004:92.
257. Iannuzzi CM, Atencio DP, Green S, et al. ATM mutations in female breast cancer patients predict for an increase in radiation-induced late effects. *Int J Radiat Oncol Biol Phys* 2002;52:606–613.
258. Oppitz U, Bernthaler U, Schindler D, et al. Sequence analysis of the ATM gene in 20 patients with RTOG grade 3 or 4 acute and/or late tissue radiation side effects. *Int J Radiat Oncol Biol Phys*1999;44: 981–988.
259. Severin DM, Leong T, Cassidy B, et al. Novel DNA sequence variants in the hHR21 DNA repair gene in radiosensitive cancer patients. *Int J Radiat Oncol Biol Phys* 2001;50:1323–1331.
260. Andreassen CN, Alsner J, Overgaard M, et al. Prediction of normal tissue radiosensitivity from polymorphisms in candidate genes. *Radiother Oncol* 2003;69:127–135.
261. Angele S, Romestaing P, Moullan N, et al. ATMHaplotypes and cellular response to DNA damage: Association with breast cancer risk and clinical radiosensitivity. *Cancer Res* 2003;63:8717–8725.
262. De Ruyck K, Van Eijkeren M, Claes K, et al. TGF[beta]1 polymorphisms and late clinical radiosensitivity in patients treated for gynecologic tumors. *Int J Radiat Oncol Biol Phys* 2006;65:1240–1248.
263. Quarmby S, Fakhoury H, Levine E, et al. Association of transforming growth factor beta-1 single nucleotide polymorphisms with radiationi-induced damage to normal tissues in breast cancer patients. *Int J Radiat Oncol Biol Phys* 2003;79:137–143.
264. Dunning AM, Ellis PD, McBride S, et al. A transforming growth factorbeta1 signal peptide variant increases secretion in vitro and is associated with increased incidence of invasive breast cancer. *Cancer Res* 2003;63:2610–2615.
265. Wu X, Gu J, Wu T-T, et al. Genetic variations in radiation and chemotherapy drug action pathways predict clinical outcomes in esophageal cancer. *J Clin Oncol* 2006;24:3789–3798.
266. Shah R, Hurley CK, Posch PE. A molecular mechanism for the differential regulation of TGF-beta1 expression due to the common SNP -509C-T (c. -1347C > T). *Hum Genet* 2006;120:461–469.
267. Thys M, Schrauwen I, Vanderstraeten K, et al. The coding polymorphism T263I in TGF-beta1 is associated with otosclerosis in two independent populations. *Hum Mol Genet* 2007;16:2021–2030.
268. Dickson MR, Perry RT, Wiener H, et al. Association studies of transforming growth factor-beta 1 and Alzheimer's disease. *Am J Med Genet B Neuropsychiatr Genet* 2005;139B:38–41.
269. Park JY, Park MH, Park H, et al. TNF-alpha and TGF-beta1 gene polymorphisms and renal allograft rejection in Koreans. *Tissue Antigens* 2004;64:660–666.
270. Celedon JC, Lange C, Raby BA, et al. The transforming growth factor-beta1 (TGFB1) gene is associated with chronic obstructive pulmonary disease (COPD). *Hum Mol Genet* 2004;13:1649–1656.

271. Su ZG, Wen FQ, Feng YL, et al. Transforming growth factor-beta1 gene polymorphisms associated with chronic obstructive pulmonary disease in Chinese population. *Acta Pharmacol Sin* 2005;26:714–720.
272. Park KH, Lo Han SG, Whang YM, et al. Single nucleotide polymorphisms of the TGFB1 gene and lung cancer risk in a Korean population. *Cancer Genet Cytogenet* 2006;169:39–44.
273. Saltzman BS, Yamamoto JF, Decker R, et al. Association of genetic variation in the transforming growth factor beta-1 gene with serum levels and risk of colorectal neoplasia. *Cancer Res* 2008;68:1236–1244.
274. Giotopoulos G, Symonds RP, Foweraker K, et al. The late radiotherapy normal tissue injury phenotypes of telangiectasia, fibrosis and atrophy in breast cancer patients have distinct genotype-dependent causes. *Br J Cancer* 2007;96:1001–1007.
275. Brock WA, Tucker SL, Geara FB, et al. Fibroblast radiosensitivity versus acute and late normal skin responses in patients treated for breast cancer. *Int J Radiat Oncol Biol Phys* 1995;32:1371–1379.
276. Cole J, Arlett C, Green M, et al. Comparative human cellular radiosensitivity: II. The survival following gamma-irradiation of unstimulated (G0) T-lymphocytes, T-lymphocyte lines, lymphoblastoid cell lines and fibroblasts from normal donors, from ataxia-telangiectasia patients and from ataxia-telangiectasia heterozygotes. *Int J Radiat Biol* 1988;54:929–943.
277. Deschavanne P, Debieu D, Fertil B, et al. Re-evaluation of in- vitro radiosensitivity of human fibroblasts of different genetic origins. *Int J Radiat Biol Relat Stud Phys Chem Med* 1986;50:279–293.
278. Woods W, Byrne T, Kim T. Sensitivity of cultured cells to gamma radiation in a patient exhibiting marked in vivo radiation sensitivity. *Cancer* 1988;62:2341–2345.
279. Geara F, Peters L, Ang K, et al. Radiosensitivity measurement of keratinocytes and fibroblasts from radiotherapy patients. *Int J Radiat Oncol Biol Phys* 1992;24:287–293.
280. Geara F, Peters L, Ang K, et al. Prospective comparison of in vitro normal cell radiosensitivity and normal tissue reactions in radiotherapy patients. *Int J Radiat Oncol Biol Phys* 1993;27:1173–1179.
281. Dileto C, Travis E. Fibroblast radiosensitivity in vitro and lung fibrosis in vivo: comparison between a fibrosis-prone and fibrosis-resistant mouse strain. *Radiat Res* 1996;146:61–67.
282. Rube CE, Uthe D, Schmid KW, et al. Dose-dependent induction of transforming growth factor beta (TGF-beta) in the lung tissue of fibrosis-prone mice after thoracic irradiation. *Int J Radiat Oncol Biol Phys* 2000;47:1033–1042.
283. Novakova-Jiresova A, Van Gameren MM, Coppes RP, et al. Transforming growth factor-beta plasma dynamics and post-irradiation lung injury in lung cancer patients. *Radiother Oncol* 2004;71:183–189.
284. Anscher M, Crocker I, Jirtle R. Transforming growth factor-beta 1 expression in irradiated liver. *Radiat Res* 1990;122:77–85.
285. Kong F, Ao X, Wang L, et al. The use of blood biomarkers to predict radiation lung toxicity: a potential strategy to individualize thoracic radiation therapy. *Cancer Control* 2008;15:140–150.
286. Barthelemy-Brichant N, Bosquee L, Cataldo D, et al. Increased IL-6 and TGF-beta1 concentrations in bronchoalveolar lavage fluid associated with thoracic radiotherapy. *Int J Radiat Oncol Biol Phys* 2004;58:758–767.
287. Evans ES, Kocak Z, Zhou SM, et al. Does transforming growth factor-beta1 predict for radiation-induced pneumonitis in patients treated for lung cancer? *Cytokine* 2006;35:186–192.
288. Hartsell WF, Scott CB, Dundas GS, et al. Can serum markers be used to predict acute and late toxicity in patients with lung cancer? Analysis of RTOG 91-03. *Am J Clin Oncol* 2007;30:368–376.
289. Chen Y, Okunieff P, Ahrendt SA. Translational research in lung cancer. *Semin Surg Oncol* 2003;21:205–219.
290. Murshed H, Liu H, Liao Z, et al. Dose and volume reduction for normal lung using intensity-modulated radiotherapy for advanced-stage non-small-cell lung cancer. *Int J Radiat Oncol Biol Phys* 2004;58: 1258–1267.
291. Hayman JA, Martel MK, Ten Haken RK, et al. Dose escalation in non-small-cell lung cancer using three-dimensional conformal radiation therapy: update of a phase I trial. *J Clin Oncol* 2001;19:127–136.
292. Liao ZX, Komaki RR, Thames HD Jr, Liu et al. Influence of Technologic Advances on Outcomes in Patients With Unresectable, Locally Advanced Non-Small-Cell Lung Cancer Receiving Concomitant Chemoradiotherapy. *Int J Radiat Oncol Biol Phys* 2009.
293. Sejpal S, Komaki R, Wei X, et al. Does proton beam radiotherapy (PBT) reduce treatment related pneumonitis (TRP) compared to intensity modulated related radiation therapy (IMRT) in patients with locally advanced non-small-cell lung cancer (NSCLC) treated with concurrent chemotherapy? Presented at the *2008 Annual Meeting of the American Radium Society*. Laguna Beach, CA.
294. Dong L, Liao Z, Sahoo N, et al. Dosimetric advantages of proton simultaneous in-field boost (PSIB) technique for treating lung cancer. Presented at the *2008 Meeting of the Particle Therapy Cooperative Group*. Jacksonville, FL.
295. Haiping Z, Takayama K, Uchino J, et al. Prevention of radiation-induced pneumonitis by recombinant adenovirus-mediated transferring of soluble TGF-beta type II receptor gene. *Cancer Gene Ther* 2006; 13:864–872.
296. Nishioka A, Ogawa Y, Mima T, et al. Histopathologic amelioration of fibroproliferative change in rat irradiated lung using soluble transforming growth factor-beta (TGF-beta) receptor mediated by adenoviral vector. *Int J Radiat Oncol Biol Phys* 2004;58:1235–1241.
297. Wang L, Feng Y, Fu XL, et al. [Effects of gene therapy with replication-defective adenovirus ericlosing Egr-1 promoter and Smad7 cDNA on irradiation-induced pulmonary fibrosis: experiment with mice]. *Zhonghua Yi Xue Za Zhi* 2006;86:2847–2852.
298. Itamochi H, Yamasaki F, Sudo T, et al. Reduction of radiation-induced apoptosis by specific expression of Bcl-2 in normal cells. *Cancer Gene Ther* 2006;13:451–459.
299. Epperly MW, Bray JA, Krager S, et al. Intratracheal injection of adenovirus containing the human MnSOD transgene protects athymic nude mice from irradiation-induced organizing alveolitis. *Int J Radiat Oncol Biol Phys* 1999;43:169–181.
300. Zhang M, Qian J, Xing X, et al. Inhibition of the tumor necrosis factor-alpha pathway is radioprotective for the lung. *Clin Cancer Res* 2008;14:1868–1876.
301. Anjos-Afonso F, Siapati EK, Bonnet D. In vivo contribution of murine mesenchymal stem cells into multiple cell-types under minimal damage conditions. *J Cell Sci* 2004;117:5655–5664.
302. Hong JH, Chiang CS, Tsao CY, et al. Rapid induction of cytokine gene expression in the lung after single and fractionated doses of radiation. *Int J Radiat Biol* 1999;75:1421–1427.
303. Haimovitz-Friedman A, Balaban N, McLoughlin M, et al. Protein kinase C mediates basic fibroblast growth factor protection of endothelial cells against radiation-induced apoptosis. *Cancer Res* 1994;54: 2591–2597.
304. Haimovitz-Friedman A, Vlodavsky I, Chaudhuri A, et al. Autocrine effects of fibroblast growth factor in repair of radiation damage in endothelial cells. *Cancer Res* 1991;51:2552–2558.
305. Pena LA, Fuks Z, Kolesnick RN. Radiation-induced apoptosis of endothelial cells in the murine central nervous system: protection by fibroblast growth factor and sphingomyelinase deficiency. *Cancer Res* 2000;60:321–327.
306. Tee PG, Travis EL. Basic fibroblast growth factor does not protect against classical radiation pneumonitis in two strains of mice. *Cancer Res* 1995;55:298–302.
307. Giri SN, Hyde DM, Marafino BJ Jr. Ameliorating effect of murine interferon gamma on bleomycin-induced lung collagen fibrosis in mice. *Biochem Med Metabolic Biol* 1986;36:194–197.
308. Granstein RD, Deak MR, Jacques SL, et al. The systemic administration of gamma interferon inhibits collagen synthesis and acute inflammation in a murine skin wounding model. *J Invest Dermatol* 1989;93:18–27.
309. Granstein RD, Flotte TJ, Amento EP. Interferons and collagen production. *J Invest Dermatol* 1990;95:S75–S80.
310. Rosiello R, Merrill W, Rockwell S, et al. Radiation pneumonitis. Bronchoalveolar lavage assessment and modulation by a recombinant cytokine. *Am Rev Respir Dis* 1993;148:1671–1676.

311. Christofidou-Solomidou M, Muzykantov VR. Antioxidant strategies in respiratory medicine. *Treat Respir Med* 2006;5:47–78.
312. Ward WF, Shih-Hoellwarth A, Tuttle RD. Collagen accumulation in irradiated rat lung: modification by D-penicillamine. *Radiology* 1983; 146:533–537.
313. Molteni A, Moulder JE, Cohen EF, et al. Control of radiation-induced pneumopathy and lung fibrosis by angiotensin-converting enzyme inhibitors and an angiotensin II type 1 receptor blocker. *Int J Radiat Biol* 2000;76:523–532.
314. Molteni A, Ward WF, Ts'ao CH, et al. Cytostatic properties of some angiotensin I converting enzyme inhibitors and of angiotensin II type I receptor antagonists. *Curr Pharm Des* 2003;9:751–761.
315. Molteni A, Wolfe LF, Ward WF, et al. Effect of an angiotensin II receptor blocker and two angiotensin converting enzyme inhibitors on transforming growth factor-beta (TGF-beta) and alpha-actomyosin (alpha SMA), important mediators of radiation-induced pneumopathy and lung fibrosis. *Curr Pharm Des* 2007;13:1307–1316.
316. van Baardwijk A, Bosmans G, Bentzen SM, et al. Radiation dose prescription for non-small-cell lung cancer according to normal tissue dose constraints: an in silico clinical trial. *Int J Radiat Oncol Biol Phys* 2008;71:1103–1110.
317. Kim B, Ahn YC, Lim DH, et al. High-dose thoracic radiation therapy at 3.0 Gy/fraction in inoperable stage I/II Non-small cell lung cancer. *Japanese J Clin Oncol* 2008;38:92–98.
318. Kong FM, Zhao L, Hayman JA. The role of radiation therapy in thoracic tumors. *Hematol Oncol Clin North Am* 2006;20:363–400.
319. Liang SX, Zhu XD, Xu ZY, et al. Radiation-induced liver disease in three-dimensional conformal radiation therapy for primary liver carcinoma: the risk factors and hepatic radiation tolerance. *Int J Radiat Oncol Biol Phys* 2006;65:426–434.
320. Underwood LJ, Murray BR, Robinson DM, et al. An evaluation of forward and inverse radiotherapy planning using Helax-TMS (version 6.0) for lung cancer patients treated with RTOG 93-11 dose-escalation protocol. *Med Dosim* 2003;28:167–170.
321. Werner-Wasik M, Swann RS, Bradley J, et al. Increasing tumor volume is predictive of poor overall and progression-free survival: secondary analysis of the Radiation Therapy Oncology Group 93-11 phase I-II radiation dose-escalation study in patients with inoperable non-small-cell lung cancer. *Int J Radiat Oncol Biol Phys* 2008;70: 385–390.
322. Graham MV, Purdy JA, Emami B, et al. Preliminary results of a prospective trial using three dimensional radiotherapy for lung cancer. *Int J Radiat Oncol Biol Phys* 1995;33:993–1000.
323. Arkwright PD, Laurie S, Super M, et al. TGF-beta(1) genotype and accelerated decline in lung function of patients with cystic fibrosis. *Thorax* 2000;55:459–462.
324. Marks LB, Munley MT, Bentel GC, et al. Physical and biological predictors of changes in whole-lung function following thoracic irradiation. *Int J Radiat Oncol Biol Phys* 1997;39:563–570.

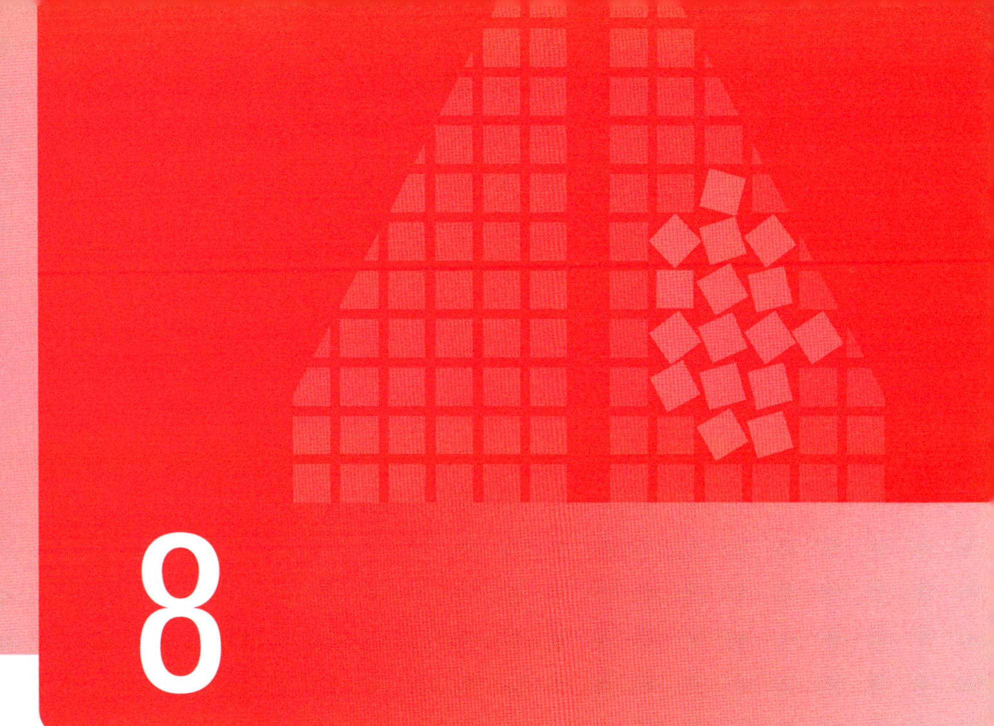

SECTION 8

Chemotherapy and Lung Cancer

CHAPTER 45

Leora Horn
Cesare Gridelli
Corey Langer
David H. Johnson

Chemotherapy for Advanced Non–Small Cell Lung Cancer

Lung cancer is the leading cause of cancer-related mortality worldwide.[1,2] In North America and Europe, an estimated 40% of all newly diagnosed non–small cell lung cancer (NSCLC) patients present with advanced-stage disease (stage IIIB with pleural effusion or stage IV). Moreover, a significant number of patients who present with early stage NSCLC will eventually relapse with extrathoracic metastases. When managed with supportive care alone, these patients experience a median survival of approximately 4 to 5 months and 1-year survival rates of around 10%.[3,4] For more than 6 decades, clinical investigators have labored to improve on these results with little success.[5,6] Early efforts were hampered by the use of relatively inactive cytotoxic agents.[7] Subsequent attempts to improve outcome were predicated on the supposition that combination therapies could increase antitumor activity while minimizing host toxicity.[8] However, with rare exception, the early clinical trials comparing combination chemotherapy to supportive care alone failed to yield a meaningful survival benefit. Although the negative outcome of these trials was commonly attributed to lack of efficacy of the available drugs, some experts posited the initial studies simply lacked adequate statistical power to detect a modest, but clinically important improvement in survival. To remedy this shortcoming, a metaanalysis of the extant data was undertaken in 1995.[9] This landmark study confirmed the lack of a survival benefit with chemotherapy regimens comprised of alkylating drugs or vinca alkaloids; however, NSCLC patients treated with cisplatin-based therapy were shown to have a survival advantage over those given supportive care alone (hazard ratio [HR] = 0.73; $p < 0.0001$). The survival advantage amounted to a 1.5-month increase in median survival and a 10% improvement in 1-year survival. Platinum-based chemotherapy was subsequently shown to be cost-effective and capable of improving quality of life.[10,11]

In a recent update of the 1995 metaanalysis, six randomized clinical trials (RCT) and an additional 1702 patients were added to the previously analyzed database.[12] In total, the updated analysis included 15 randomized studies involving 2666 patients. Eleven of the trials employed cisplatin-based chemotherapy, whereas four studies involved a comparison of single agents (etoposide, vinorelbine, gemcitabine, or paclitaxel) and supportive care alone. The results of the updated metaanalysis affirmed the previously identified survival benefit of chemotherapy (HR = 0.78; 95% CI, 0.71 to 0.84; $p < 0.000001$). Somewhat surprisingly, there was no apparent difference in the magnitude of effect between trials that used cisplatin-based regimens or the single agents. Moreover, there was also no evidence that any patient subgroup as defined by age, sex, stage, or histology benefited more or less from chemotherapy. The absolute survival benefit of chemotherapy at 1-year did vary according to World Health Organization (WHO)/Eastern Cooperative Oncology Group (ECOG) performance status (PS) 0 = 8% (from 26% to 34%), PS 1 = 8% (from 18% to 26%), PS 2 = 5% (from 6% to 11%), and PS 3 = 4% (from 5% to 9%). The updated metaanalysis suggests the effectiveness of newer agents such as vinorelbine, paclitaxel, and gemcitabine is similar to that of cisplatin combined with older agents such as vindesine or mitomycin (see succeeding discussion) and also reaffirms the substantial and consistent relative survival benefit of chemotherapy in advanced NSCLC.[12]

Although the improvement in the survival of patients with advanced NSCLC is caused, in part, by better chemotherapy, as outlined previously, changes in the natural history of NSCLC may have also played a role. Wakelee et al.[13] analyzed all advanced NSCLC ECOG trials conducted between 1981 and 2000. These investigators first assessed changes in demographic factors and treatment regimens and then correlated these findings with survival outcome among patients diagnosed between 1981 and 1990 compared to those diagnosed from 1991 to 2000. Survival was clearly better, in the trials conducted between 1991 and 2000, explained in part by favorable changes in eligibility criteria (e.g., more women and more favorable patterns of metastases). However,

TABLE 45.1 Phase III Trials of Third-Generation Drugs and BSC in Advanced NSCLC

				Survival	
Author	**CT**	**Pt No**	**RR**	**MST**	**1 Yr**
ELVIS [80]*	Vinorelbine	76	20%	6.5 mo	32%
	BSC	78	—	4.9 mo	14%
Anderson et al.[81]	Gemcitabine	150	18.5%	5.7 mo	25%
	BSC	150	—	5.9 mo	22%
Ranson et al.[15]	Paclitaxel	79	16%	6.8 mo	24%
	BSC	78	—	4.8 mo	23%
Roszkowski et al.[16]	Docetaxel	137	13%	6.0 mo	25%
	BSC	70	—	5.7 mo	16%

*In elderly patients.

BSC, best supportive care, CT, chemotherapy; RR, response rate; MST, median survival time; NSCLC, non–small cell lung cancer.

these investigators also observed a change in the natural history of the disease. For example, there was a longer time to progression suggesting that improved chemotherapy yielded improved survival in the post–1990 era. They also observed a longer interval between disease progression and death, suggesting second-line therapies and supportive care options improved after 1990. Although these observations are conceivably caused by the enrollment of patients with more indolent disease after 1990 or the earlier detection of less symptomatic, advanced NSCLC, this seems less likely. Regardless, the results of this retrospective analysis are consistent with the hypothesis that the improved survival observed over the past decade in patients with advanced NSCLC is indeed multifactorial.

THE EVOLUTION OF CHEMOTHERAPY IN ADVANCED NSCLC

In the latter part of the 20th century, a number of new cytotoxic agents, including vinorelbine, paclitaxel, docetaxel, gemcitabine, irinotecan, and pemetrexed, were found to possess single-agent activity in advanced NSCLC.[14] Collectively, these agents are known as third-generation drugs to distinguish them from older agents such as etoposide, ifosfamide, mitomycin, and vindesine, which are often referred to as second-generation drugs. In some cases, single-agent administration of these third-generation drugs has yielded a modest survival benefit when compared to supportive care (Table 45.1).[14–16] When a third-generation drug is combined with a platinum compound, objective response and survival rates are improved compared to the same third-generation drug used alone[17–20] (Table 45.2). Similarly, a third-generation drug combined with a platinum agent produces better responses and improved survival compared to single-agent cisplatin[21–23] (Table 45.3). Under either circumstance, however, the higher response rates and improved survival come at a cost of increased host toxicity albeit with no increase in treatment-related mortality.[20] In general, and most importantly, third-generation platinum-based doublet chemotherapy regimens tend to produce higher response rates and superior overall survival (OS) compared to second-generation platinum-based dou-

TABLE 45.2 Trials Comparing Third-Generation Doublets and Single Agents in NSCLC

				Survival	
Author	**CT**	**Pt No**	**RR**	**MST**	**1 Yr**
Georgoulias et al.[17]	CDDP/docetaxel	167	36%	10.5 mo	44%
	Docetaxel	152	22%	8.0 mo	43%
Lilenbaum et al.[18]	CBDCA/paclitaxel	284	30%	8.8 mo	37%
	Paclitaxel	277	17%	6.7 mo	32%
Sederholm et al.[19]	CBDCA/gemcitabine	164	30%	10.0 mo	40%
	Gemcitabine	170	11%	8.6 mo	32%

CDDP, cisplastin; CBDCA, carboplatin; CT, chemotherapy; RR, response rate; MST, median survival time; NSCLC, non–small cell lung cancer.

TABLE 45.3 Trials Comparing Third-Generation Doublets and Cisplatin in NSCLC

Author	CT	Pt No	RR	Survival MST	Survival 1 Yr
Wozniak et al.[21]	CDDP/vinorelbine	209	26%	8.0 mo	36%
	CDDP	206	12%	6.0 mo	20%
Gatzemeier et al.[22]	CDDP/paclitaxel	207	26%	8.1 mo	30%
	CDDP	207	17%	8.6 mo	36%
Sandler et al.[23]	CDDP/gemcitabine	260	30%	9.1 mo	39%
	CDDP	262	11%	7.6 mo	28%

CDDP, cisplastin; CT, chemotherapy; RR, response rate; MST, median survival time.

blet therapies[24–28] (Table 45.4). Interestingly, the survival improvement observed with some of the third-generation agents used alone is comparable to that achieved with platinum doublets employing second-generation drugs[29,30] (Table 45.4).

Following the development of third-generation platinum-based regimens, randomized trials were undertaken to compare their respective activities[31–37] (Table 45.5). Typical of these studies was a trial conducted by the ECOG (E1594) in which chemotherapy-naive patients with advanced NSCLC were randomized to receive cisplatin plus paclitaxel, considered a reference regimen based on an earlier ECOG trial,[26] or one of three regimens employing a third-generation drug: cisplatin plus gemcitabine, cisplatin plus docetaxel, or carboplatin plus paclitaxel.[31] Overall response rates and survival did not differ significantly between the reference regimen of cisplatin and paclitaxel and the three investigational arms. Comparable outcomes have been reported by others.[32–37] Although there were some modest differences in the responses rates and survival among these trials, they are almost certainly a result of subtle, although critical differences in the study population characteristics.[13] For example, the survival rates in the TAX-326 study appear superior to other trials[35]; however, approximately one third of the participants in TAX-326 had stage III disease, compared with just 13% of the patients enrolled in the ECOG study E1594.[31] In some cases, the toxicity profiles appear to be quite different, especially among studies carried out exclusively in Asia.[36] Most likely, the different toxicity profiles are caused by ethnic differences in drug metabolism.[38] Regardless, no truly clinically relevant survival differences have emerged among the commonly used third-generation platinum-based doublet regimens. Taken together, these data indicate that third-generation platinum-based doublets represent the current standard of care in patients with advanced NSCLC and good PS (PS 0 to 1).[4,14]

TABLE 45.4 Trials Comparing Second- and Third-Generation Doublets in NSCLC

Author	CT	Pt No	RR	Survival MST	Survival 1 Yr
Le Chevalier et al.[24]	CDDP/vinorelbine	206	30%	9.3 mo	34%
	CDDP/vindesine	200	19%	7.4 mo	27%
	Vindesine	206	14%	7.2 mo	30%
Giaccone et al.[25]	CDDP/paclitaxel	155	45%	9.9 mo	41%
	CDDP/teniposide	162	32%	9.7 mo	40%
Bonomi et al.[26]	CDDP/paclitaxel (HD)	201	28%	10.0 mo	40%
	CDDP/paclitaxel (LD)	198	25%	9.5 mo	37%
	CDDP/etoposide	200	12%	7.6 mo	32%
Negoro et al.[27]	CDDP/irinotecan	133	44%	11.6 mo	46%
	CDDP/vindesine	133	32%	10.6 mo	38%
	Irinotecan	132	20.5%	10.7 mo	42%
Kubota et al.[28]	CDDP/docetaxel	151	37%	11.3 mo	48%
	CDDP/vindesine	151	21%	9.6 mo	41%

CDDP, cisplastin; CT, chemotherapy; HD, high dose; LD, low dose; MST, median survival time; RR, response rate.

TABLE 45.5 Trials Comparing Third-Generation Platinum Doublets in Advanced NSCLC

				Survival	
Group	**CT**	**Pt No**	**RR**	**Median**	**1 Yr**
ECOG[31]	Paclitaxel/cisplatin	288	21%	7.8 mo	31%
	Gemcitabine/cisplatin	288	22%	8.1 mo	36%
	Docetaxel/cisplatin	289	17%	7.4 mo	31%
	Paclitaxel/carboplatin	290	17%	8.1 mo	34%
EORTC[32]	Paclitaxel/cisplatin	159	31%	8.1 mo	35%
	Gemcitabine/cisplatin	160	36%	8.8 mo	31%
	Gemcitabine/paclitaxel	161	27%	6.9 mo	26%
ILCP[33]	Vinorelbine/cisplatin	201	30%	9.5 mo	37%
	Gemcitabine/cisplatin	205	30%	9.8 mo	37%
	Paclitaxel/carboplatin	201	32%	9.9 mo	43%
SWOG[34]	Paclitaxel/carboplatin	206	25%	8.0 mo	38%
	Vinorelbine/cisplatin	202	28%	8.0 mo	36%
TAX-326[35]	Vinorelbine/cisplatin	394	25%	10.1 mo	41%
	Docetaxel/cisplatin	406	32%	11.3 mo	46%
	Docetaxel/carboplatin	404	24%	9.4 mo	38%
FACS[36]	Irinotecan/cisplatin	145	31%	13.9 mo	59%
	Paclitaxel/carboplatin	145	32%	12.3 mo	51%
	Gemcitabine/cisplatin	146	30%	14.0 mo	60%
	Vinorelbine/cisplatin	145	33%	11.4 mo	48%
H3H-MC-JMDB[37]	Gemcitabine/cisplatin	863	28%	10.3 mo	42%
	Pemetrexed/cisplatin	862	31%	10.3 mo	44%

ECOG, Eastern Cooperative Oncology Group; EORTC, European Organisation for Research and Treatment of Cancer; FACS, Four-Arm Cooperative Study; H3H-MC-JMDB, H3H-MC-Japanese Medical Database; ILCP, Italian Lung Cancer Project; SWOG, Southwest Oncology Group; TAX-326, Taxotere-326 Trial.

Triplet versus Doublet Platinum-Based Drug Combinations A time-honored strategy for improving the effectiveness of cytotoxic therapy is to combine multiple agents with different mechanisms of action and nonoverlapping toxicities.[39] Thus, adding a third active drug to the aforementioned third-generation platinum doublets has considerable theoretical appeal given their improved activity and favorable toxicity profiles.[40,41] In fact, triple-drug combinations have demonstrated good tolerability and excellent activity in both phase II and phase III trials.[29] However, in two separate metaanalyses of the extant data, improved overall response rates failed to result in an increase in OS[40,42] (Table 45.6). In addition, host toxicity is greater with triple drug therapy.[30,40] Together, these data indicate triplet drug chemotherapy is not appropriate for patients with advanced NSCLC outside the confines of a clinical trial.

Duration of Therapy The duration of initial chemotherapy administration in advanced NSCLC is a matter of some controversy.[30] American Society of Clinical Oncology (ASCO) practice guidelines recommend no more than six cycles in responding patients, the American College of Chest Physicians guidelines recommend no more than three to four cycles, whereas the National Comprehensive Cancer Network (NCCN) guidelines are basically noncommittal on this topic.[43–45] The lack of agreement among the various guidelines is perhaps not too surprising given the relative paucity of adequately powered prospective studies addressing this issue[46–49] (Table 45.7). Among the first to tackle this issue were Smith et al.[46] who randomized advanced NSCLC patients to three versus six cycles of mitomycin, vinblastine, and cisplatin. Median (6 vs. 7 months) and 1-year survival rates (22% vs. 25%; $p = 0.2$) as well as the median durations of symptom relief (4.5 months in both arms) were essentially identical in the two arms. Quality-of-life parameters also were the same or improved for patients randomized to only three courses, including a significant decrease in fatigue ($p = 0.03$) and a trend toward decreased nausea and vomiting ($p = 0.06$). von Plessen et al.[48] reported nearly identical results using carboplatin plus vinorelbine. Both studies employed relatively modest doses of platinum drug, which may have influenced the outcomes. However, there is little evidence for a cisplatin-dose response in NSCLC[50,51] rendering this potential criticism somewhat mute. Moreover, in patients

TABLE 45.6 Metaanalyses Addressing Number of Drugs in Advanced NSCLC

	Drugs	No. of Comparisons	Pts	Ratio*	*p* Value	Absolute Benefit
Response rate:						
	2 vs. 1	33	7175	0.42 (0.37–0.47)	<0.001	13%
	3 vs. 2	35	4814	0.66 (0.58–0.75)	0.06	8%
1-Year survival:						
	2 vs. 1	13	4125	0.80 (0.70–0.91)	<0.001	5%
	3 vs. 2	10	2249	1.01 (0.85–1.21)	0.59	0%
Median survival:						
	2 vs. 1	30	6022	0.83 (0.79–0.89)	<0.001	NA
	3 vs. 2	30	4550	1.00 (0.94–1.06)	0.97	NA

*Ratio is either an odds ratio or median ratio.

Adapted from Delbaldo C, Michiels S, Syz N, et al. Benefits of adding a drug to a single-agent or a 2-agent chemotherapy regimen in advanced non-small-cell lung cancer: a meta-analysis. *JAMA* 2004;292(4):470–484.

NA, not applicable; NSCLC, non–small cell lung cancer.

with stages IIIB or IV NSCLC, investigators at the University of North Carolina compared four cycles of standard doses of carboplatin and paclitaxel every 3 weeks to continuous treatment with these agents until disease progression.[47] Fifty-seven percent of patients allocated to four cycles completed the intended course of chemotherapy. Patients randomized to the continuous treatment arm received a median of four cycles of chemotherapy; 42% received ≥5 cycles of carboplatin and paclitaxel. Overall response rates (22% vs. 24%; $p = 0.80$), median survival (6.6. vs. 8.5 months), and 1-year survival rates (28% vs. 34%; log rank $p = 0.63$) were comparable and not statistically different. Hematologic and nonhematologic toxicity rates also were similar between the two arms, whereas neuropathy was more common in the continuous treatment arm (14% vs. 27%; $p = 0.02$). There were no differences in quality-of-life parameters. The frequency of patients who received second-line therapy was identical in the two groups as well (42% vs. 47%; $p = 0.42$).

The likely death knell for prolonged duration therapy came from a study conducted by the Korean Cancer Study Group.[49] Patients with advanced NSCLC who had not progressed after two induction courses of a third-generation platinum-based chemotherapy were subsequently randomized to four or six additional cycles of chemotherapy. The study population presumably represents a subset of patients with the highest probability of benefiting from extended duration of therapy because they had already demonstrated "platinum sensitivity." Nonetheless, there was no improvement in response rate (43% vs. 42%) or survival (15.9 vs. 14.9 months) with six additional cycles of chemotherapy although time to

TABLE 45.7 Phase III Trials: Duration of Chemotherapy in Advanced NSCLC

				Survival	
Author	CT	Pt No	RR	MST	1 Yr
Smith et al.[46]	MVP × 3	155	32%	6.0 mo	22%
	MVP × 6	153	38%	7.0 mo	25%
von Plessen et al.[48]	CbVin × 3	150	NR	6.5 mo	25%
	CbVin × 6	147	NR	7.4 mo	25%
Socinski et al.[47]	CbPac × 4	114	22%	6.6 mo	28%
	CbPac × >4	116	24%	8.5 mo	34%
Park et al.[49]	P-based × 2*	158	42%	14.9 mo†	59%†
	P-based × 4*	158	43%	15.9 mo†	62%†

*Treatment was continued treatment beyond initial 2 cycles of chemotherapy for non-progressing patients.

†Survival of non-progressing patients from time of initial diagnosis.

Cb, carboplatin; CT, chemotherapy; MST, median survival time; MVP, mitomycin, vinblastine, cisplatin; NR, not reported; NSCLC, non–small cell lung cancer; Pac, paclitaxel; RR, response rate; Vin, vinorelbine.

disease progression was improved. Moreover, patients randomly assigned to four cycles were more likely to receive second-line treatment, experienced less toxicity, and regained their functional status more rapidly than those patients randomly assigned to six cycles.

A recent metaanalysis including 13 trials and 2416 patients found a significant improvement in progression-free survival (PFS) (HR = 0.78; 95% CI, 0.72 to 0.86; p <0.0001) but no improvement in OS (HR = 0.94; 95% CI, 0.87 to 1.10; p = 0.1) as well as increased toxicity and decreased quality of life for longer duration chemotherapy[52] (Fig. 45.1). The improvement in PFS was greater for third-generation regimens (HR = 0.73 vs. 0.92; p = 0.02). Interestingly, when a trial of maintenance pemetrexed conducted by Ciuleanu et al.[53] (see next discussion) was added to the analysis there was a significant, albeit modest improvement in OS (HR = 0.92, 95% CI, 0.86 to 0.99; p = 0.03).[52] This trend is likely caused by the fact that the Ciuleanu study enrolled 663 patients, almost 3 times the number of all other studies included in the analysis, therefore, significantly influencing the study results. In addition, the addition of the Ciuleanu study to the metaanalysis is questionable as all other trials included in the analysis compared maintenance doublet chemotherapy to no further therapy, whereas the study by Ciuleanue et al. used maintenance single-agent therapy.

Collectively, these data indicate treatment beyond three to four cycles of platinum-based therapy is of limited to no benefit in patients with advanced NSCLC.[30,54,55] Rather than employing prolonged administration of a first-line platinum-based therapy, a more patient-friendly strategy would appear to be the attentive use of sequential single active agents after initial induction therapy.[56] Future research efforts should concentrate on diagnostic methodologies that would allow oncologists to select patients who are more likely to benefit from a particular therapy instead of continued efforts to *optimize* treatment duration with existing therapies.[56]

Maintenance Therapy Two large randomized controlled trials have demonstrated improvements in PFS[57,58] and OS[57] when chemotherapy, paclitaxel and carboplatin[57] or gemcitabine and cisplatin[58] were combined with bevacizumab, a monoclonal antibody targeting vascular endothelial growth factor (VEGF) in patients with nonsquamous NSCLC. Based on these results, Patel et al.[59] conducted a phase II trial of pemetrexed and carboplatin plus bevacizumab with maintenance pemetrexed and bevacizumab in patients with advanced nonsquamous NSCLC and found a response rate of 55% (95% CI, 51% to 69%) median PFS of 9.3 months and OS of 13.5 months (Table 45.8).

Ciuleanu et al.[53] conducted a randomized phase III trial in patients who had responded to four cycles of platinum-based chemotherapy comparing maintenance single-agent pemetrexed to best supportive care. Early treatment with pemetrexed was associated with a significant improvement in PFS (4.04 vs. 1.79 months; p <0.00001) and trend toward improvement in OS (13.0 vs. 10.2 months; p = 0.060). Similar to prior studies evaluating pemetrexed in NSCLC, the benefit was limited to patients with nonsquamous cell histology NSCLC.[37] It should be noted that in this trial, only 50% of patients receiving best supportive care received second-line chemotherapy of which only 11.2% received pemetrexed. It is not known how many patients in the best supportive care arm that received third-line chemotherapy, which was administered to 37% of pemetrexed-treated patients. Treatment with pemetrexed was associated with significantly more serious adverse events (4.3% vs. 0%) and grade 3 or 4 adverse events (14.3% vs. 3.6%; p <0.001).

Maintenance therapy with gefitinib after three cycles of chemotherapy was compared to continued platinum-doublet

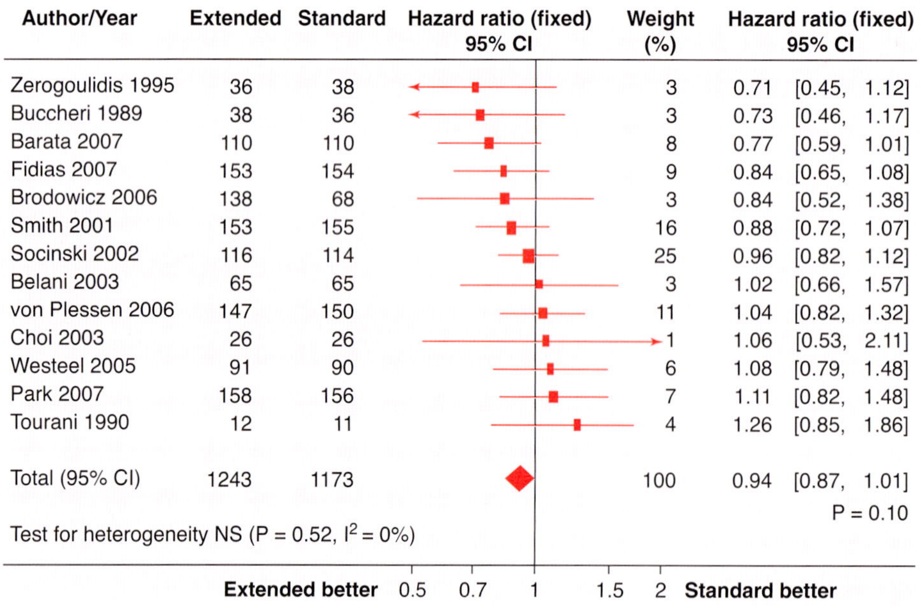

Author/Year	Extended	Standard	Weight (%)	Hazard ratio (fixed) 95% CI
Zerogoulidis 1995	36	38	3	0.71 [0.45, 1.12]
Buccheri 1989	38	36	3	0.73 [0.46, 1.17]
Barata 2007	110	110	8	0.77 [0.59, 1.01]
Fidias 2007	153	154	9	0.84 [0.65, 1.08]
Brodowicz 2006	138	68	3	0.84 [0.52, 1.38]
Smith 2001	153	155	16	0.88 [0.72, 1.07]
Socinski 2002	116	114	25	0.96 [0.82, 1.12]
Belani 2003	65	65	3	1.02 [0.66, 1.57]
von Plessen 2006	147	150	11	1.04 [0.82, 1.32]
Choi 2003	26	26	1	1.06 [0.53, 2.11]
Westeel 2005	91	90	6	1.08 [0.79, 1.48]
Park 2007	158	156	7	1.11 [0.82, 1.48]
Tourani 1990	12	11	4	1.26 [0.85, 1.86]
Total (95% CI)	1243	1173	100	0.94 [0.87, 1.01] P = 0.10

Test for heterogeneity NS (P = 0.52, I^2 = 0%)

Extended better 0.5 0.7 1 1.5 2 Standard better

FIGURE 45.1 Overall survival for extended versus standard chemotherapy.[52] The summary HR 0.94 (95% CI, 0.87 to 1.01; p = 0.10) suggests no benefit to extended chemotherapy. It should be noted when an additional study by presented by Cuilenau et al.[53] at the same meeting was included in the analysis the HR marginally improved to 0.92 (95% CI, 0.86 to 0.99; p = 0.03). *CI*, confidence interval. (From Soon Y, Stockler MR, Boyer M, Askie L. Duration of chemotherapy for advanced non-small cell lung cancer: An updated systematic review and meta-analysis. *ASCO Meeting Abstracts* 2008;26[15 Suppl]:8013.)

TABLE 45.8 Maintenance Therapy in Advanced NSCLC

Author	CT	Pt No	RR	Survival	
				PFS	MST
Patel et al.[59]	Pemetrexed + Bevacizumab	51	49%	7.2 mo TTP	14.0 mo
Ciuleanu et al.[53]	Pemetrexed	441		4.3 mo	13.0 mo
	Placebo	222		2.6 mo	10.2 mo
Hida et al.[60]	Gefitinib	300	34%	4.6 mo	13.7 mo
	Chemotherapy	298	29%	4.3 mo	12.9 mo

Chemotherapy regimens: carboplatin plus palitaxel, cisplatin plus irinotecan, cisplatin plus vinorelbine, cisplatin plus docetaxel, cisplatin plus gemcitabine.

CT, chemotherapy ; MST, median survival time; NSCLC, non–small cell lung cancer; PFS, progression-free survival; RR, response rate; TTP, time to progression.

chemotherapy, up to six cycles of carboplatin plus paclitaxel, cisplatin plus irinotecan, cisplatin plus vinorelbine, cisplatin plus docetaxel, or cisplatin plus gemcitabine in Asian patients with advanced NSCLC.[60] Chemotherapy was associated with a significantly higher incidence of anemia (22% vs. 13.3%), whereas rash and elevations in liver function tests occurred in 4% and 11% of gefitinib-treated patients, respectively. The median number of chemotherapy cycles was three in both treatment groups. There was a similar response rate between treatment groups. Patients treated with gefitinib had a significant, albeit, small improvement in PFS (4.6 vs. 4.3 months; $p < 0.001$) but no difference in OS (13.7 vs. 12.9 months; $p = 0.10$). In a prespecified subset analysis of patients with adenocarcinoma, approximately 80% of study patients, treatment with maintenance gefitinib was associated with a significant improvement in OS (15.4 vs. 14.3 months; $p = 0.03$). Although not significant, patients with nonadenocarcinoma receiving maintenance gefitinib had a worse OS compared to chemotherapy alone (7.7 vs. 9.2 months; $p = 0.24$). When patients were stratified by smoking status, never-smokers appeared to have a better OS regardless of therapy compared to smokers. Smokers with adenocarcinoma appeared to have an improvement in OS with maintenance gefitinib compared to chemotherapy alone (13.6 vs. 10.0 months; $p = 0.003$). Interestingly, although not significant, never-smokers receiving maintenance gefitinib appeared to have a worse OS compared to chemotherapy alone (21.6 vs. 23.5 months; $p = 0.72$). Therefore, it appears that maintenance gefitinib following platinum-based chemotherapy may be beneficial in a subset of patients with adenocarcinoma. A large randomized phase III trial, comparing maintenance erlotinib to placebo following treatment with carboplatin and paclitaxel with or without bevacizumab (ATLAS), has closed to accrual in North America and results are expected to be reported in late 2009.

Cisplatin versus Carboplatin Whether to use cisplatin or carboplatin as the platinum agent of choice in frontline therapy is another of the more enduring controversies surrounding the treatment of advanced NSCLC.[61,62] The controversy intensified with the publication of two prospective trials that demonstrated a superior survival in advanced NSCLC patients treated with cisplatin-based third-generation doublets as compared to carboplatin-based third-generation doublets[35,63] (Table 45.9).

Two recent metaanalyses have examined the clinical relevance of cisplatin versus carboplatin in frontline treatment for advanced NSCLC.[61,62] The first of these was a literature-based analysis of eight trials that directly compared cisplatin- and carboplatin-based doublets, five of which employed a third-generation doublet.[61] A total of 2948 patients were enrolled in these trials. Cisplatin-based chemotherapy produced a statistically significant higher response rate (OR = 1.36; 95% CI, 1.15 to 1.61; $p < 0.001$) but no survival advantage (HR = 1.050; 95% CI, 0.907 to 1.216; $p = 0.515$). However, in the subgroup of trials that employed third-generation drugs, cisplatin-based combinations yielded a survival benefit compared to carboplatin-based doublets (HR = 1.106; 95% CI, 1.005 to 1.218; $p = 0.039$).

The second metaanalysis, the so-called CISCA (CISplatin vs. CArboplatin) study,[62] was based on individual patient data from nine randomized trials that involved a total of 2968 patients.[31,35,63–68] The objective response rate was higher for patients treated with cisplatin than in the cohort treated with carboplatin (30% vs. 24%, respectively; OR = 1.37; 95%

TABLE 45.9 Cisplatin versus Carboplatin Chemotherapy in Advanced NSCLC

Author	CT	Pt No	RR	Survival	
				MST	1 Yr
Rosell et al.[63]	PPac	309	28%	9.8 mo	38%
	CbPac	309	25%	8.5 mo	33%
Fossella et al.[35]	PDoc	408	32%	11.3 mo	46%
	CbDoc	406	24%	9.4 mo	38%

Cb, carboplatin; CT, chemotherapy; Doc, docetaxel; MST, median survival time; NSCLC, non–small cell lung cancer; P, cisplatin; Pac, paclitaxel; RR, response rate.

CI, 1.16 to 1.61; $p < 0.001$). Notably, carboplatin treatment was associated with a nonstatistically significant increase in the hazard of mortality relative to treatment with cisplatin (HR = 1.07; 95% CI, 0.99 to 1.15; $p = 0.100$) (Fig. 45.2). Cisplatin-treated patients experienced a median survival and 1-year survival rate of 9.1 months and 37%, respectively, whereas carboplatin-treated patients had a median survival of 8.4 months and a 1-year survival rate of 34%. In patients with *nonsquamous* tumors and those treated with third-generation chemotherapy, carboplatin-based chemotherapy was associated with a statistically significant increase in mortality (HR = 1.12; 95% CI, 1.01 to 1.23 and HR = 1.11; 95% CI, 1.01 to 1.21, respectively). The authors opined that cisplatin-based third-generation regimens should remain the standard reference for the treatment of selected patients with advanced-stage NSCLC.[62] Parenthetically, it may be worth noting that the subset of patients who seemingly derived the greatest benefit from cisplatin is the same subset of patients that appear to benefit from the addition of bevacizumab to frontline chemotherapy (see succeeding discussion).

Taken together, these data suggest cisplatin is the preferred platinum compound in good PS patients with advanced NSCLC if survival benefit is the principal goal of therapy.[69] Relative to carboplatin-based therapy, cisplatin-based therapy imparts an approximate 3% to 4% improvement in 1-year survival, an increase that is roughly comparable to that achieved with the use of third-generation as opposed to a second-generation agents.[70,71] The incidence of treatment-related deaths is more or less equivalent (4% vs. 3%, respectively).[61,62] However, cisplatin-based chemotherapy is clearly associated with more severe nausea and vomiting and nephrotoxicity, whereas carboplatin-based chemotherapy is associated with more severe thrombocytopenia. Accordingly, it is reasonable to consider substituting carboplatin for cisplatin in selected circumstances where cisplatin toxicities could be particularly problematic (i.e., preexisting neuropathy, hearing difficulties, renal dysfunction, etc.). Of note, even after all these years of use, the optimal doses of cisplatin and carboplatin are not well defined although randomized trials have shown that higher doses of cisplatin (i.e., $\geq$100 mg/m^2) are not required to achieve the results outlined previously.[50] By contrast, a dose of cisplatin less than 60 mg/m^2 every 3 to 4 weeks appears to produce suboptimal outcome.[72] Comparable dose–response data for carboplatin are lacking.

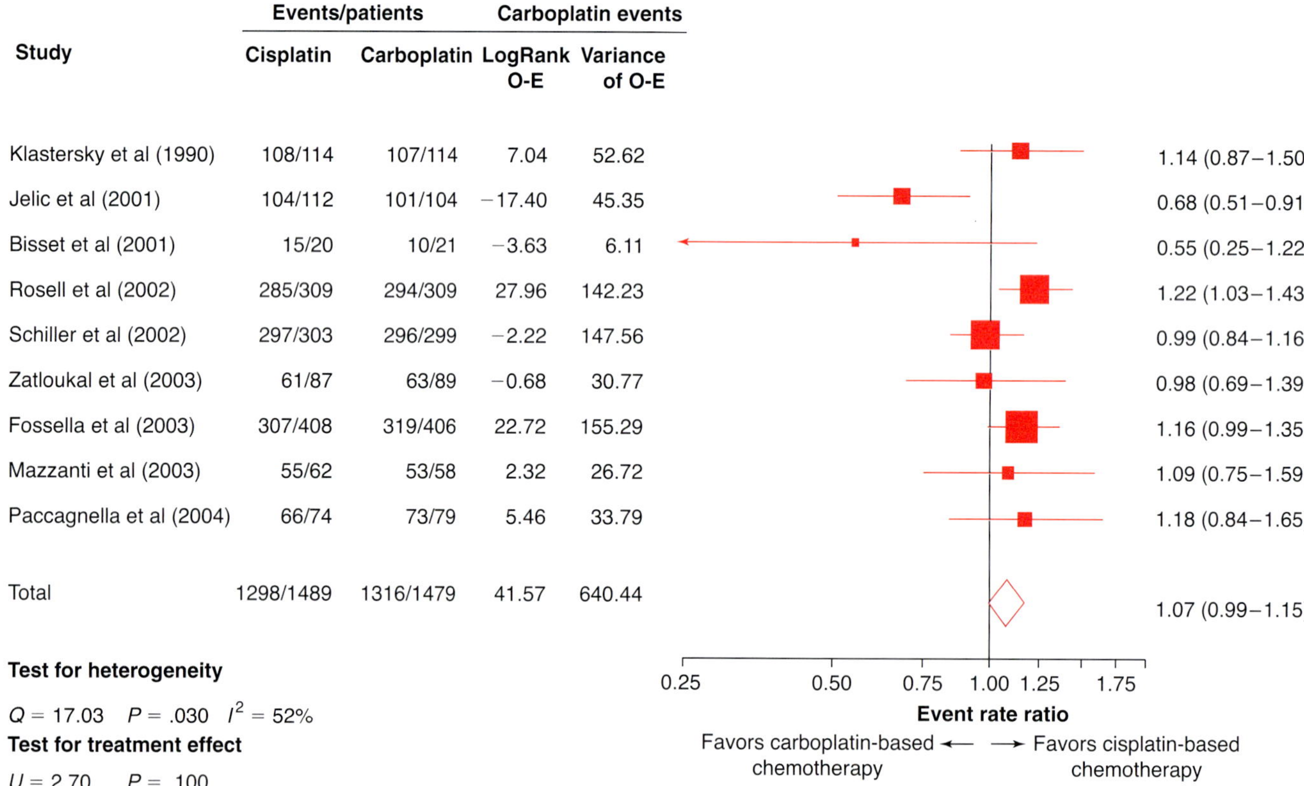

FIGURE 45.2 Overall survival of carboplatin- versus cisplatin-based chemotherapy. To describe the effect of carboplatin on mortality, the log-rank statistic (the observed minus the expected number of deaths) and its variance were computed for each trial. Combining these statistics, the event rate ratios of all trials and their weighted average were calculated with 95% confidence intervals (CIs). The test statistics U and Q were used for hypothesis testing about treatment difference and presence of heterogeneity across studies, respectively. The summary hazard ratio was 1.07 (95% CI, 0.99 to 1.15; $p = 0.100$). (From Ardizzoni A, Boni L, Tiseo M, et al. *J Natl Cancer Inst* 2007;99[11]:847–857.)

Platinum- versus Non–Platinum-Containing Chemotherapy Although improvement in survival is clearly a crucial factor in choosing a particular chemotherapy regimen, serious consideration also should always be given to other factors, such as tolerability, quality of life, convenience, and cost.[44] Accordingly, there has been considerable interest in developing non–platinum-based chemotherapy regimens.[73] As one recent example, Greek investigators found no difference in the response or survival rates in advanced NSCLC patients treated with gemcitabine plus docetaxel compared to the combination of cisplatin plus docetaxel.[74] Gemcitabine and docetaxel also possessed a superior toxicity profile suggesting that it was a reasonable alternative first-line regimen to platinum-based therapy. In spite of this encouraging report, however, other studies indicate non–platinum-based chemotherapy may be less efficacious than extant platinum-based regimens.[32]

To address this question, D'Addario et al.[75] performed a literature-based metaanalysis that compared the activity, efficacy and toxicity of platinum- and non–platinum-based chemotherapy in patients with advanced NSCLC. The analysis included data from 37 randomized phase II and phase III trials involving more than 7500 patients. Compared to nonplatinum therapies, platinum-based chemotherapy was associated with a 62% increase in the odds ratio for response (OR = 1.62; 1.46 to 1.8; $p < 0.0001$) and a 5% increase in 1-year survival rate (34% vs. 29%) (OR = 1.21; 1.09 to 1.35; $p = 0.0003$). This effect was also statistically significant for the comparison of platinum-based regimens versus single-agent nonplatinum therapy (1-year survival = 35% vs. 25%; $p = 0.0001$) and for platinum-based regimens compared to third-generation–based nonplatinum regimens (37% vs. 31%; $p = 0.0057$). However, when single-agent trials were excluded from the analysis, there was not a statistically significant increase in 1-year survival with platinum-based therapies as compared to third generation–based combination regimens (36% vs. 35% respectively; OR = 1.11; 0.96 to 1.28; $p = 0.17$). Platinum-based regimens had significantly higher hematologic toxicity, nephrotoxicity, and nausea and vomiting whereas neurotoxicity, rate of febrile neutropenia, and toxic death rates were similar. As the metaanalysis was literature-based and included some studies in which platinum-based therapy was compared with a nonplatinum single agent, some experts have questioned the value of these data. An accompanying editorial made the following observation: "By no means [does] the meta-analysis indicate that non–platinum-containing regimens are preferred for most patients. None of the randomized studies showed a significant survival advantage for the nonplatinum combinations, and in many the survival was slightly inferior in the nonplatinum arm. Noninferiority analyses were not conducted in these trials."[73]

A second literature-based metaanalysis excluded phase II data and included only randomized phase III trials that directly compared a platinum- to non–platinum-based chemotherapy as first-line chemotherapy.[71] Fourteen trials were included; experimental arms were gemcitabine/vinorelbine (n = 4), gemcitabine/taxane (n = 7), gemcitabine/epirubicin (n = 1), paclitaxel/vinorelbine (n = 1), and gemcitabine/ifosfamide (n = 1). The comparator was a doublet of a platinum compound plus a third-generation agent for all but two studies. The primary end point of this analysis was the 1-year survival rate. Patients treated with a platinum-based regimen benefited from a statically significant reduction in the risk of death at 1 year (OR = 0.88; 95% CI, 0.78 to 0.99; $p = 0.044$), equal to an approximate 3% survival improvement at 1-year (Fig. 45.3), and a lower risk of being refractory to chemotherapy (OR = 0.87; 0.73 to 0.99; $p = 0.049$). The risks of grades 3 and 4 gastrointestinal and hematological toxicities were substantially higher with platinum-based chemotherapies. There was also a nonsignificant increase in the risk of febrile neutropenia ($p = 0.063$) and a trend toward an increase in treatment-related deaths on the platinum-based regimens (1.9% vs. 1.3%; $p = 0.08$). The authors concluded platinum-containing regimens were associated with a statistically significant reduction in the risk of death when compared with platinum-free chemotherapy without a perceptible increase in risk of toxic death.[71] However, they also suggested that non–platinum-chemotherapy regimens were appropriate for patients in whom platinum-associated toxicities are a major concern; for the majority of good PS patients with advanced disease, however, platinum-based therapy remains the preferred initial treatment of choice.

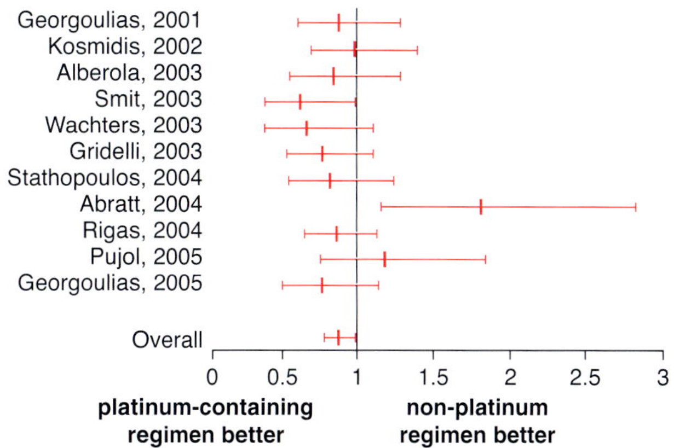

FIGURE 45.3 Overall 1-year survival with platinum-based versus non-platinum chemotherapy regimens. The summary odds ratio for the risk of death within 1 year was 0.88 (95% CI, 0.78–0.99, $p = 0.044$) indicating a 2.94% survival benefit at 1 year for patients treated with a platinum-based chemotherapy doublet. (From Pujol JL, Barlesi F, Daures JP. Should chemotherapy combinations for advanced non-small cell lung cancer be platinum-based? A meta-analysis of phase III randomized trials. *Lung Cancer* 2006;51[3]:335–345.)

Palliation of Tumor-Related Symptoms Advanced NSCLC is accompanied by various debilitating symptoms that may include incessant coughing, anorexia and weight loss, dyspnea, chest pain, hemoptysis, fatigue, among others.[76] More than 60 years ago, Karnofsky et al.[5] demonstrated that even the marginally active cytotoxic agent nitrogen mustard could ameliorate many of these symptoms. Indeed, symptom improvement with cytotoxic therapy may occur even in the absence of a classic tumor response[77,78] and is often achieved within the first two cycles of therapy.[5,77,79] However, some practitioners still prefer to avoid platinum-based chemotherapy for palliative purposes because of the known side effects of these agents. Fortunately, newer agents with favorable toxicity profiles such as gemcitabine, paclitaxel, docetaxel, and vinorelbine can be used with beneficial effects.[15,16,80,81] For example, in one study, patients treated with gemcitabine were far less likely to require palliative radiotherapy at 2 months compared to those treated with supportive care alone (7% vs. 42%).[81] The median time to initiation of palliative radiation therapy was 7 months for patients receiving gemcitabine versus 1 month for patients treated with supportive care. Duration of symptom relief achieved varied considerably but resulted in a median relief of 3 to 5 months for dyspnea, cough, and chest pain and 2 to 3 months for anorexia and hemoptysis.[82] It turns out that symptomatic relief derived from chemotherapy is not limited to first-line therapy. In patients with recurrent NSCLC, second-line docetaxel provided greater improvement in tumor-related symptoms, including asthenia, pain, pulmonary, and neurologic symptoms compared with supportive care as well as a survival benefit.[83]

SPECIAL POPULATIONS WITH ADVANCED NSCLC

Elderly Patients Lung cancer is primarily a disease of older individuals; the median age at diagnosis is 68 years and as many as 40% of patients may be 70 years at diagnosis.[84] Because older NSCLC patients tend to have substantial comorbidities, oncologists may be reticent to administer standard chemotherapy regimens fearing excessive toxicity.[84,85] However, when deciding a treatment strategy, the biological rather than the chronological age should be carefully assessed, and treatment should only be modified or withheld for very good reasons.[86] This applies equally to surgery and radiotherapy as well as chemotherapy as numerous prospective studies have clearly demonstrated the benefits of chemotherapy in the elderly. Randomized trials have confirmed the superiority of single-agent vinorelbine to supportive care and to combination therapy with vinorelbine and gemcitabine.[80,87] In addition, retrospective analyses of multiple cooperative group phase III studies indicate patients age 70 years and older experience survival and quality-of-life benefits of platinum-based chemotherapy similar to their younger counterparts.[18,31,35,88] However, the role of platinum-based chemotherapy needs to be investigated formally in phase III prospective randomized trials.

In general, little data exist regarding the outcome of chemotherapy in NSCLC patients aged 80 or more, a rapidly expanding, potentially vulnerable population cohort. In an age-specific subset analysis of trial ECOG 1594, investigators observed only nine patients more than 80 years of age (<1% of all enrollees).[89] It is notable that only one of these nine patients was able to complete four cycles of chemotherapy. Efficacy in this group was very poor with no objective responses noted and a median survival of just 4.2 months. These patients fared worse than patients aged 70 to 79 when treated with platinum-based combinations with time to progression and survival roughly half that observed in the much larger cohort of patients 70 to 79 years of age.[89]

A combined analysis of a trial conducted by the Southwest Oncology Group (SWOG; S0027) and a second investigator-initiated trial performed in elderly patients provides additional insight.[90] Both trials were confined to patients ≥70 years old. The SWOG trial employed sequential vinorelbine followed by docetaxel and included 23 patients aged 80 or older.[91] The second trial compared weekly docetaxel to every 3-week docetaxel, and enrolled 26 patients aged ≥80 years.[92] Tolerance to treatment was similar between patients aged 70 to 79 and those over 80 years. For patients with PS 0 to 1, median survival was actually shorter in the octogenarian group compared to patients aged 70 to 79 (7 months vs. 11 months). For PS 2 patients, survival was equally poor in both groups (4 months vs. 5 months). The authors concluded that these chemotherapy regimens were associated with an encouraging disease-control rate (54%) in patients 80 years or older with advanced NSCLC and were well tolerated. Thus, selected octogenarians with advanced NSCLC may benefit from single-agent chemotherapy. Clearly, more studies in this age group need to be conducted.

Recently, a panel of international experts in geriatric oncology was convened to develop guidelines for the treatment of elderly patients with NSCLC.[85] The panel recommended single-agent chemotherapy with a third-generation agent (vinorelbine, gemcitabine, docetaxel, or paclitaxel), as an option for elderly patients with advanced NSCLC. Several factors must be considered when selecting a particular drug including the expected toxicity profile of the agent, pharmacokinetics, organ function, and comorbidities as well as the patient's preferences. The expert panel also indicated that a platinum-based chemotherapy regimen represented a valid option in older patients with a good PS and adequate organ function.

Poor Performance Status Patients Poor PS (i.e., ECOG PS ≥2) is a strong negative prognostic factor in advanced NSCLC and administration of chemotherapy in this setting is controversial.[93,94] Although chemotherapy fails to improve survival in PS 2 patients, there is nevertheless a potential for an improved quality of life.[10,95,96] Accordingly, the approach taken in clinical practice is highly variable.[97] Many patients are desirous of treatment even when informed of the minimal survival benefits. In such settings, single-agent chemotherapy with one of the third-generation cytotoxic agents (e.g., vinorelbine, gemcitabine, or a taxane) or newer formulations of these agents (e.g., paclitaxel poliglumex [PPX]) may provide clinical benefit with minimal host toxicity.[94] However, some of the newer third-generation platinum-based combination regimens appear to improve survival modestly without engendering excessive host toxicity.[18,98] For example, in CALGB trial 9730, a randomized trial of single-agent paclitaxel versus carboplatin plus paclitaxel,

PS 2 patients had a significantly worse outcome compared with patients with PS 0 or 1 (median survival of 3.0 vs. 8.8 months and 1-year survival of 14% vs. 38%, respectively).[18] However, PS 2 patients treated with carboplatin plus paclitaxel had a better survival rate than those treated with paclitaxel alone (median survival 4.7 vs. 2.4 months; 1-year survival = 18% vs. 10%; $p = 0.016$) (Table 45.10).

Given the significance often attached to ECOG trial E1594, it is worth remembering that the study was initially designed to include patients with an ECOG PS of 0, 1, or 2. However, grade 3 to 4 hematologic toxicities occurred in more than half of the initial 68 PS 2 patients enrolled along with 5 deaths (7.4%). Only two of the deaths were clearly attributed to therapy, but the study was nonetheless amended to exclude PS 2 patients thereafter. The overall response rate for the 64 evaluable patients was 14%, and the overall median survival was 4.1 months. Notably, a nonsignificant trend toward increased median survival was observed with cisplatin plus gemcitabine and carboplatin plus paclitaxel. In addition, nonhematologic grade 3 to 4 toxicities occurred significantly less often in the paclitaxel and carboplatin arm ($p = 0.0032$). These observations prompted ECOG investigators to conduct a randomized phase II trial in which PS 2 patients were randomized to slightly modified regimens of cisplatin plus gemcitabine or the standard regimen of carboplatin plus paclitaxel every three weeks. The trial was designed to detect an absolute 10% increase in 1-year survival compared with historic controls. The 1-year survival rate of PS-2 patients enrolled onto ECOG 1594 was approximately 20%.[99] The toxicity of both regimens in this trial was deemed acceptable but was fairly substantial. Carboplatin plus paclitaxel featured substantially more grade 3 or higher neutropenia than did the cisplatin plus gemcitabine (59% vs. 33%); the relative incidence of grade 4 neutropenia was 34% and 10%, respectively. Carboplatin plus paclitaxel also featured significantly more grade 3 sensory neuropathy (10% vs. 0%) and grade 2 sensory neuropathy (16% vs. 2%). However, cisplatin plus gemcitabine resulted in significantly more grade 3 or higher thrombocytopenia (38% vs. 14%). It also yielded significantly more grade 3 nausea and emesis (23% vs. 6%), grade 3 fatigue (22% vs. 12%), and grade 1 or higher creatinine elevation (43% vs. 6%). Overall response was 23% with cisplatin plus gemcitabine and 14% with carboplatin and paclitaxel. Median and 1-year survival rates were 6.9 months and 25.5% and 6.2 months and 19.6%, respectively.

A randomized phase III trial Selected Targeted Efficacy in Lung Cancer to Lower Adverse Reactions 3 (STELLAR3) compared carboplatin plus paclitaxel to carboplatin plus PPX in chemotherapy naive PS 2 patients.[100] Although treatment with carboplatin plus paclitaxel had a significantly higher response rate (37% vs. 20%), there was no difference in time to progression (4.6 vs. 3.9 months) or OS (7.9 vs. 7.8 months). Treatment with PPX was associated with a significantly higher incidence of thrombocytopenia, neutropenia, and fatigue; 27% of PPX-treated patients discontinued treatment for adverse events compared to 20% of paclitaxel-treated patients. There was no difference in quality of life between treatment groups. In multivariate analysis, the presence of extrathoracic metastasis, weight loss $\geq$5% and lung cancer subscale (LCS) score $<$18 were associated with poorer outcome. A second randomized phase III trial (STELLAR4) compared single-agent PPX to vinorelbine or gemcitabine in the same patient population and found a similar response rate (11% and 15%) and OS (7.3 vs. 6.6 months; HR = 0.95; $p = 0.686$) between treatment groups.[101] Lilenbaum et al.[102] performed regression analysis pooling patient datasets from STELLAR 3 and 4 and identified four factors that were significant predictors of survival; albumin $<$3.5 gm, presence of extrathoracic metastases

TABLE 45.10 Chemotherapy in PS Two Patients

Author	CT	Pt No	RR	Survival	
				TTP	MST
Langer et al.[98]	CbPac	51	14%	4.2 mo	6.2 mo
	PGem	47	23%	4.8 mo	6.9 mo
Sweeney et al.[99]	CPac	18	17%	1.4 mo	7.0 mo
	PGem	13	23%	4.6 mo	7.9 mo
	PDoc	18	6%	1.4 mo	2.3 mo
	CbPac	15	13%	1.5 mo	4.6 mo
Langer et al.[100]	CbPac	201	37%	4.6 mo	8.0 mo
	CbPPX	199	20%	3.9 mo	7.9 mo
O'Brien et al.[101]	PPX	191	11%	2.8 mo	7.2 mo
	Vin or Gem	190	16%	3.5 mo	6.5 mo
Lilenbaum et al.[103]	Erlotinib	52	2%	(PFS) 1.9 mo	6.5 mo
	CbPac	51	12%	3.5 mo	9.7 mo

Cb, carboplatin; CT, chemotherapy; Doc, docetaxel; Gem, gemcitabine; MST, median survival time; P, cisplatin ; Pac, paclitaxel; PFS, progression-free survival available for all patients reported as hazard ratio (HR) by mutation status; PPX, paclitaxel poliglumex; PS, performance status; RR, response rate; TTP, time to progression; Vin, vinorelbine.

(excluding brain), >2 comorbid conditions and history of tobacco use. Patients with none of these factors had a median survival of 15.6 months, whereas patients with all four factors had a survival of 3.1 months. Outcome did not differ between single-agent and doublet chemotherapy

Finally, the favorable toxicity profile of the oral EGFR inhibitors gefitinib and erlotinib makes them an attractive option for PS 2 patients as well. However, a cautionary note is warranted. In a randomized phase II trial, PS 2 patients seemed to fare better with standard doublet chemotherapy than with erlotinib as initial therapy.[103] Hence, empiric use of a targeted agent in this setting with the assumption that it is automatically less toxic and therapeutically equivalent to conventional chemotherapy is not supported by the literature. There remains a critical need for novel therapeutic strategies for all patients with NSCLC and especially for those with a poor PS.

COMBINING CHEMOTHERAPY PLUS TARGETED THERAPIES

A casual perusal of the lay or scientific press will easily demonstrate the high level of enthusiasm for the burgeoning field of so-called targeted therapy in the management of multiple cancers including NSCLC.[104] The initial attempts to incorporate targeted agents into the treatment of NSCLC concentrated on patients with advanced, metastatic disease, which is not necessarily the optimal setting in which to test these drugs. However, this approach is a time-honored one and was based, in part, on data derived from preclinical studies indicating some targeted agents yielded additive or even synergistic cytotoxic activity when combined with chemotherapy.[105,106] Unfortunately, with one notable exception,[57] most of these initial efforts failed to demonstrate a survival improvement.[107–113]

Combination Chemotherapy plus EGFR Tyrosine Kinase Inhibitors The epidermal growth factor receptor (EGFR) is a receptor tyrosine kinase of the ErbB family that is abnormally activated in many epithelial tumors.[114] Several mechanisms lead to the receptor's aberrant activation in cancers, including receptor overexpression, mutation, ligand-dependent receptor dimerization, and ligand-independent activation.[114] More recently, point mutation or small in-frame deletions in specific EGFR gene exons such as those codifying for the tyrosine kinase domain (mostly exons 19 and 21) have been described in a subset of NSCLC as described in Chapters 5 and 49.[115,116] Two classes of anti-EGFR agents are currently FDA approved for the treatment of patients with cancer: gefitinib and erlotinib, oral, low–molecular weight, adenosine triphosphate-competitive inhibitors of the receptor's tyrosine kinase and cetuximab (Erbitux), a chimeric IgG1 monoclonal antibody directed at the extracellular domain of the receptor.[114,117] Gefitinib and erlotinib yielded antitumor activity in patients with refractory NSCLC and additive cytotoxicity when combined with cytotoxic drugs in preclinical studies.[105,106] Accordingly, several groups of investigators sought to combine gefitinib or erlotinib with standard front-line platinum-based chemotherapy in advanced NSCLC.[107–110] (Table 45.9). Unfortunately, none of the studies yielded a significant survival improvement. These studies were later criticized because of the lack of patient selection using such selection factors as EGFR expression, somatic mutations, or other putative markers of tyrosine kinase inhibitors (TKI) efficacy.[118,119] However, neither EGFR mutations nor amplification appeared to identify distinct subsets of NSCLC with an increased response to gefitinib in the phase II/III randomized trials nor did the combination of gefitinib with chemotherapy improve survival in patients with tumors expressing these particular molecular markers.[120] Parenthetically, a similar lack of correlation with these putative markers of EGFR TKI activity has been observed in second line therapy as well.[121] However, the lack of correlation may well be a result of technical differences in how these studies were carried out. Interestingly, never-smokers treated with erlotinib and chemotherapy seemed to experience an improvement in survival in one of these trials.[109] Never-smoking has been associated with a greater probability of response to EGFR TKIs and may represent a surrogate marker for the presence of EGFR mutations.[122] Some experts have speculated that these studies failed because EGFR inhibitors act mainly by reducing proliferation in wild-type EGFR tumor cells.[123] Because proliferating tumor cells are those most affected by chemotherapy, an antagonistic effect between EGFR TKIs and chemotherapy may occur. In any case, neither erlotinib nor gefitinib combined with standard chemotherapy regimens confers a survival advantage over chemotherapy alone in *unselected* chemo-naive patients with advanced NSCLC.[109]

IPASS was a large randomized phase III noninferiority trial conducted in Asia comparing first-line gefitinib to carboplatin plus paclitaxel in chemotherapy naive patients who were never or light ex-smokers with advanced NSCLC[124] (Table 45.11). Treatment with gefitinib was associated with a significant improvement in response rate (43% vs.

TABLE 45.11 IPASS Gefitinib versus Carboplatin Plus Paclitaxel in Advanced NSCLC

				Survival	
Author	**CT**	**Pt No**	**RR**	**PFS**	**MST**
All patients	Gefitinib	609	43%	5.7mo	18.6 mo
	CbPac	608	32%	5.8 mo	17.3 mo
EGFR +	Gefitinib	132	71%	HR = 0.48	
	CbPac	129	47%		
EGFR −	Gefitinib	91	1%	HR = 2.85	
	CbPac	85	24%		

Cb, carboplatin; CT, chemotherapy; EGFR, epidermal growth factor receptor; HR, hazard ratio; IPASS, Iressa Pan-Asia Study; MST, preliminary median survival time; NSCLC, non–small cell lung cancer; Pac, paclitaxel; PFS, progression-free survival available for all patients reported as HR by mutation status; RR, response rate.

32%, p = 0.0001) compared to chemotherapy. PFS initially favored chemotherapy-treated patients; however, 12-month PFS was superior for gefitinib-treated patients (25% vs. 7; p <0.0001). The final OS data is still pend[illegible] to be similar at this time, 18.6 months fo[illegible] patients compared to 17.3 mont[illegible] patients. On progression 38%[illegible] ceived carboplatin plus pacli[illegible] of carboplatin plus paclitaxel-treated patients received an EGFR TKI. Grade 3, 4, or 5 toxicities were more common for patients receiving carboplatin plus paclitaxel (57% vs. 17%). Quality of life favored treatment with gefitinib. Approximately one third of patients had samples available for EGFR expression, copy number and mutation analysis. EGFR mutation positive patients had a superior response to both gefitinib (71%) and chemotherapy (47%) compared to EGFR mutation negative patients of whom 1% responded to gefitinib and 23.5% responded to chemotherapy. As predicted, treatment with gefitinib was favored over chemotherapy in patients with a positive EGFR mutation (HR = 0.48; 95% CI, 0.36 to 0.64; p <0.0001), whereas chemotherapy was favored in patients with a negative EGFR mutation (HR = 2.85; 95% CI, 2.05 to 3.98; p <0.0001). The results of this trial suggest that gefitinib could be considered first line therapy in a subset of patients with advanced NSCLC who have a positive EGFR mutation.[124]

Combination Chemotherapy plus HER-1/2 Antibodies As noted previously, the EGFR is a receptor tyrosine kinase of the ErbB family that is abnormally activated in many epithelial tumors the activation of which is a common mechanism for autonomous, dysregulated cancer cell growth in many human epithelial cancers.[114] EGFR overexpression has been generally associated with advanced disease and poor prognosis and with the development of resistance to anticancer treatments.[125] Cetuximab (Erbitux) is a chimeric IgG1 monoclonal antibody directed at the extracellular domain of the receptor thereby preventing ligand binding and activation of the receptor.[117] The resultant blockage of the downstream signaling of EGFR results in impaired cell growth and proliferation. Cetuximab has also been shown to mediate antibody-dependent cellular cytotoxicity (ADCC). The observation that the addition of cetuximab to chemotherapy could seemingly overcome chemotherapy resistance in some patients with colon cancer or with head and neck cancer,[117] and promising phase II data suggesting a similar survival benefit in NSCLC,[126] prompted the initiation of a prospective multinational randomized phase III trial known as FLEX (for First-Line treatment for patients with EGFR-EXpressing advanced NSCLC) in patients with advanced NSCLC. In this trial, patients with stage IIIB with pleural effusion or stage IV NSCLC and immunohistochemical evidence of EGFR expression on tumor tissue were randomized to cisplatin plus vinorelbine and cetuximab, followed by maintenance cetuximab or cisplatin plus vinorelbine alone (Table 45.12). Treatment with chemotherapy and cetuximab resulted in no difference in PFS compared to placebo, there was, however, a significant increase in response rate (36% vs. 29%; p = 0.012) and OS (11.3 vs. 10.1 months) compared to placebo (HR = 0.87; 95% CI, 0.762 to 0.996; p = 0.044). A prespecified subset analysis showed no improvement in OS among patients of Asian ethnicity receiving cetuximab compared with placebo (17.6 vs. 20.4 months). However, fewer patients treated with cetuximab received poststudy treatment with EGFR TKI (50% vs. 73%). There was, however, a significant improvement in OS for white patients treated with chemotherapy plus cetuximab compared to placebo (10.5 vs. 9.1 months; p = 0.003); this appeared true regardless of histology. This data would suggest that chemotherapy with cisplatin and vinorelbine plus cetuximab is a reasonable alternative to patients with advanced NSCLC.[127]

HER-2/neu is also a member of the ErbB family of receptor tyrosine kinases. The knowledge that HER-2/neu plays a role in the pathogenesis and progression of lung cancer dates back to at least 1990 when Kern et al.[128] described a negative impact of HER-2/neu expression on the survival of patients with lung adenocarcinomas. Subsequently, these investigators found that a monoclonal antibody to HER-2 inhibited the growth of HER-2/neu-expressing lung cancer cell lines in a dose-dependent manner.[129] This important observation went more or less unexplored until nearly a decade later when several groups initiated phase II trials designed to assess the impact of trastuzumab on the response rate and survival of lung cancer patients.[130–133] Support for these trials came from preclinical studies indicating that trastuzumab could inhibit growth of lung cancer cell lines in vitro.[134] Moreover, a significant synergistic effect was seen when trastuzumab was combined with cytotoxic agents (i.e., gemcitabine, cisplatin, vinorelbine, and paclitaxel) in HER-2/neu positive cell lines.[134] Unlike the preclinical studies with EGFR, treatment effect was shown to correlate with the level of HER-2/neu expression.[134] However, in spite of these encouraging preclinical data, the results of the completed phase II studies are generally thought to be insufficient to carry forward into larger phase III studies, in large part, because of the low rate of HER-2/neu overexpression (only 6% to 8% of NSCLC tumors have 3+ overexpression).[135,136] Likewise, increased gene copy number as determined by fluorescence in situ hybridization (FISH) is quite rare.[136] Positive HER-2/neu expression is most often seen in adenocarcinomas but rarely in squamous cell carcinomas or large cell carcinomas, further limiting the population from which patients might be drawn for a large-scale study. Thus, to conduct a phase III trastuzumab trial in NSCLC potentially would require the screening of an extremely large number of patients to identify the relatively small percentage of patients with tumors overexpressing HER-2/neu. Many experts feel such a study would be logistically difficult, if not impossible. Nonetheless, the recent discovery of somatic mutations in HER-2/neu has rekindled interest in HER-2/neu as a potential target.[137,138] Stephens et al.[137] identified in-frame and missense mutations in the kinase domain of HER-2/neu in 4% of 120 primary lung tumors. This figure is remarkably similar to the

TABLE 45.12 Chemotherapy ± Targeted Therapy in Advanced NSCLC

				Survival	
Author	**CT**	**Pt No**	**RR**	**MST**	**1 Yr**
Giaccone et al.[107]	PGem	363	47%	10.9 mo	44%
	PGem + ↓Gefitinib	365	51%	9.9 mo	41%
	PGem + ↑Gefitinib	365	50%	9.9 mo	43%
Herbst et al.[108]	CbPac	345	29%	9.9 mo	42%
	CbPac + ↓Gefitinib	345	30%	9.8 mo	41%
	CbPac + ↑Gefitinib	347	30%	8.7 mo	37%
Herbst et al.[109]	CbPac	533	19%	10.5 mo	44%
	CbPac + Erlotinib	526	22%	10.6 mo	47%
Gatzemeier et al.[110]	PGem	50	36%	7.0 mo*	—
	PGem + Trastuzumab	51	41%	6.1 mo*	—
Bisset et al.[111]	PGem	181	26%	10.8 mo	38%
	PGem + Prinomastat	181	27%	11.5 mo	43%
Leighl et al.[112]	CbPac	387	34%	9.2 mo	32%
	CbPac + BMS-275291	387	26%	8.6 mo	30%
Pirker et al.[127]	PVin	568	29%	10.1 mo	42%
	PVin + Cetuximab	557	36%	11.3 mo	47%
Hirsh et al.[147]	CbPac	420	23%	10.3 mo	44%
	CbPac + PF-3512676	408	25%	10.2 mo	42%
Manegold et al.[148]	PGem	423	27%	10.7 mo	46%
	PGem + PF-3512676	416	29%	11.1 mo	47%
Karp et al.[151]	CbPac	53	41%	4.3 mo	—
	CbPac + CP-751 871	97	54%	3.6/5.0 mo†	—
Gatzemeier et al.[185]	PGem	536	20%	10.3 mo	42%
	PGem + Erlotinib	533	32%	10.0 mo	41%

*PFS, progression-free survival.

†10mg/kg/20 mg/kg.

BMS, best supportive care; Cb, carboplatin; CT, chemotherapy; ↓gefitinib = 250 mg; ↑gefitinib = 500 mg; Gem, gemcitabine; MST, median survival time; NSCLC, non–small cell lung cancer; P, cisplatin; Pac, paclitaxel; RR, response rate; Vin, vinorelbine.

aggregate number of 3+ HercepTest patients screened for the published clinical trials.[130–133] Collectively, these data suggest that inhibitors of HER-2/neu should be considered for retesting in NSCLC although in a more defined way. However, unlike previous studies, trastuzumab should probably be tested in the subset of lung adenocarcinomas that overexpress HER-2 protein, have an increased gene copy number or carry a HER-2/neu mutation. In support of such a trial, Gatzemeier et al.[132] noted an overall response rate of 83% and a median PFS of 8.5 months in HER-2/neu 3+ and FISH positive NSCLC patients when trastuzumab was combined with platinum-based chemotherapy. Although performing a phase III study in a population selected for a molecular abnormality that occurs in less than 5% of patients is a daunting challenge, it can be done efficiently under the right circumstances. Simon et al.[139] calculated that a randomized trial in as few as 138 patients could detect a 20% survival improvement over baseline, provided one has a validated molecular target and a means of testing for the presence of the target.

Combination Chemotherapy with Matrix Metalloproteinases Matrix metalloproteinases (MMPs) belong to a family of enzymes that digest extracellular matrix and basement membrane components, and facilitate tumor growth, metastasis, and angiogenesis.[140,141] Certain MMPs, including MMP-2 and MMP-9, are often upregulated in tumor tissue and are associated with a poor prognosis in NSCLC.[141] With the advent of MMP inhibitors, it was postulated that inhibition of these enzymes might slow tumor progression and improve survival in many tumors including NSCLC.[142] However, two large studies failed to demonstrate any evidence of survival improvement.[111,112] For example, BMS-275291 is a sulfhydryl-based second-generation MMP inhibitor that selectively inhibits MMP-1, MMP-2, MMP-8, MMP-9, and MMP-14. The combination of BMS-275291 with carboplatin and paclitaxel, however, failed to yield an improved response rate or OS in patients with advanced NSCLC compared to chemotherapy alone.[112] Similar negative results were observed with prinomastat, a synthetic hydroxamic acid derivative that inhibits MMP-2, MMP-9, MMP-13, and

MMP-14, when combined with cisplatin plus gemcitabine[111] (Table 45.12).

Combination Chemotherapy with Toll-like Receptor 9 Agonists The toll-like receptor 9 (TLR9) is part of the family of toll-like receptors that are involved in the immune systems detection and response to infectious challenges.[143] Droemann et al.[144] found that human lung cancer tissues express a functionally active TLR9, although there is only weak TLR9 expression in normal-lung tissue. Preclinical data showed promising activity for a TLR9-agonist in combination with chemotherapy in vitro.[145] A randomized phase II trial reported a median survival of 12.3 months with the addition of PF-3512676, an oligodeoxynucleotide TLR9 agonist, to platinum-taxane chemotherapy compared to 6.8 months with chemotherapy alone.[146] However, two large randomized phase III trials evaluating the addition of PF-3512676 to chemotherapy with paclitaxel plus carboplatin and cisplatin plus gemcitabine in patients with advanced NSCLC were closed early because of lack of efficacy and added toxicity compared to chemotherapy alone[147,148] (Table 45.12)

Combination Chemotherapy plus Insulin-like Growth Factor Receptor Inhibitors The insulin-like growth factor receptor 1 (IGFR-1) is a transmembrance protein involved in the growth and survival of cancer cells.[149] The binding of insulin-like growth factor (IGF) I and II to the extracellular domain of IGFR-1 triggers signal transduction through the Ras/Raf and phospoinositol-3-kinase (PI3K) transduction pathways.[150] Ludovini et al.[150] measured IGFR-1 and EGFR expression using immunohistochemistry in 125 patients with early stage NSCLC and found positive IGFR-1 expression (>10% of cells) in 36% of samples. Although IGFR-1 expression was more prominent in larger tumors, expression alone was not predictive of either overall or disease-free survival. High coexpression of IGFR-1 and EGFR was associated with worse disease-free survival (HR = 2.51; 95% CI, 1.21 to 5.12; p = 0.012) in all patients and a trend toward poorer OS in patients with stage I NSCLC (HR = 2.19; 95% CI, 0.86 to 5.56; p = 0.08). A randomized phase II trial compared standard chemotherapy with carboplatin plus paclitaxel to carboplatin plus paclitaxel and CP-751, 871 (10 mg/kg and 20 mg/kg), an antibody to the IGFR-1, in patients with advanced NSCLC[151] (Table 45.12). There was a higher incidence of neutropenia and hyperglycemia in patients treated with chemotherapy plus CP-751, 871. Chemotherapy plus CP-751, 871 was associated with a higher response rate (54% vs. 41%, p <0.00001); regardless of histology responses appeared to be highest at the 20 mg/kg dose level. There was a trend toward improved PFS for CP-751, 871 20 mg/kg compared to chemotherapy alone (5.0 vs. 4.3 months, p = 0.07). Patients with squamous cell histology appeared to derive the greatest benefit from treatment with CP-751, 871 with a response rate of 78% and PFS of 5.6 months. Studies of CP-751, 871 in combination with carboplatin and paclitaxel in patients with nonadenocarcinoma are currently underway.

Combination Chemotherapy plus Inhibitors of Vascular Endothelial Growth Factor Over the past decade, inhibition of angiogenesis has been a major thrust of new drug development in many solid tumors including lung cancer.[152–154] Drugs that target the VEGF pathway include bevacizumab, sunitinib, sorafenib, axitinib, AZD2171, ABT-869, AMG 706, and VEGF trap many of which are under active investigation in NSCLC.[155,156] In NSCLC, the most advanced of these drugs is bevacizumab, a recombinant humanized monoclonal antibody to the VEGF. In a randomized phase II trial, bevacizumab combined with carboplatin and paclitaxel improved both overall response rates and times to disease progression.[157] However, bevacizumab was associated with a high rate of life-threatening pulmonary hemorrhage, mainly in patients with squamous cell carcinomas. When an analysis was performed that excluded patients with squamous histology, the results looked even more promising with a numerically superior overall response and an improved time to progression. Median survival exceeded 18 months in a subset of patients with nonsquamous carcinomas. To confirm these preliminary results, ECOG undertook a phase III trial in which patients were randomized to chemotherapy with or without bevacizumab. The confirmatory trial was limited to patients with nonsquamous histology, an absence of significant hemoptysis (defined as ≤ 0.5 teaspoon at baseline) and no brain metastases.[57] Patients receiving bevacizumab experienced an improved response rate (35% vs. 15%; p <0.001), PFS (6.2 vs. 4.5 months; HR = 0.66; p <0.001) and OS (12.3 vs. 10.3 months; HR = 0.79; p = 0.003) (Table 45.13). The survival benefit was consistent among all prespecified stratification

TABLE 45.13 Chemotherapy ± Bevacizumab in Advanced NSCLC

Author	CT	Pt No	RR	Survival PFS	Survival MST	Survival 1 Yr
Sandler et al.[57]	CbPac	444	15%	4.5 mo	10.3 mo	44%
	CbPac + ↑Bev	434	35%	6.2 mo	12.3 mo	51%
Reck et al.[58]	PGem	347	20%	6.1 mo	—	—
	PGem + ↓Bev	345	34%	6.7 mo	—	—
	PGem + ↑Bev	351	30%	6.5 mo	—	—

↓ = 7.5 mg/kg; ↑ = 15 mg/kg; Bev, bevacizumab; Cb, carboplatin; CT, chemotherapy; Gem, gemcitabine; MST, median survival time; NSCLC, non–small cell lung cancer; P, cisplatin; Pac, paclitaxel; PFS, progression-free survival; Pac, paclitaxel; RR, response rate.

groups including measurable or nonmeasurable disease, prior radiation therapy or no prior radiation therapy, weight loss ≥5% or <5%, and stage IIIB disease with pleural effusion or stage IV disease, or recurrent disease. In an exploratory analysis of the treatment groups according to baseline characteristics, bevacizumab was beneficial in all subgroups with the possible exception of women (Fig. 45.4). Possible explanations for this finding including imbalances between the two groups with respect to known or unknown baseline prognostic factors, imbalances in the use of second- and third-line therapies, or a true sex-based difference. Given the lack of gender-specific bevacizumab-related survival differences in colon or breast cancers[158]; it is quite likely this observation represents a statistical aberration. These survival benefits came at a cost that included more treatment-related deaths (15 vs. 5 deaths; $p = 0.001$) and a higher rate of clinically significant bleeding (4.4% vs. 0.7%; $p < 0.001$) with bevacizumab. Nonetheless, the substantial improvement in OS indicates that bevacizumab plays a key role in the management of selected NSCLC patient with metastatic disease.

Confirmation of the ECOG data seemingly stems from a European trial (BO17704; also known as Avastin in Lung Cancer [AVAiL] trial) in which advanced NSCLC patients were randomized to one of two doses of bevacizumab (7.5 mg/kg or 15 mg/kg) or a placebo in combination with cisplatin and gemcitabine.[58] The study was designed to detect a 30% reduction in the risk of a PFS with bevacizumab compared with chemotherapy alone using a two-sided log-rank test (alpha = 2.5%) with 80% power. Both bevacizumab-containing arms

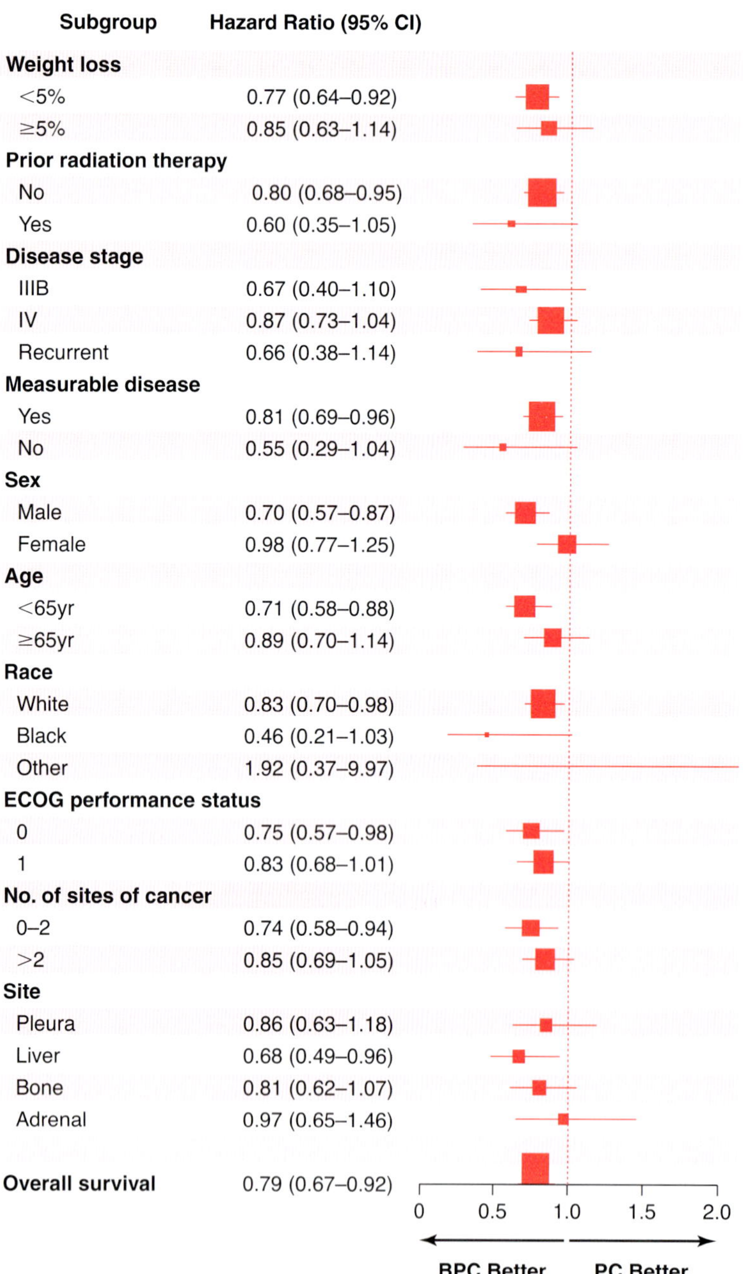

FIGURE 45.4 Hazard ratios for death, according to the subgroup analysis. The size of each square represents the number of patients, with larger squares indicating a greater number. Horizontal lines represent confidence intervals. BPC denotes paclitaxel and carboplatin plus bevacizumab, and PC paclitaxel and carboplatin alone. *CI*, confidence interval; *ECOG*, Eastern Cooperative Oncology Group. (From Sandler A, Gray R, Perry MC, et al. Paclitaxel-carboplatin alone or with bevacizumab for non-small-cell lung cancer. *N Engl J Med* 2006;355[24]:2542–2550.)

exhibited a statistically significant prolongation of PFS compared to chemotherapy alone (Table 45.13). However, the numeric difference in PFS among the three arms is minimal and the clinical significance is unknown in the absence of OS data. Of note, the PFS in the bevacizumab arms is consistent with that observed in the ECOG trial. What is striking, however, is the nearly 2-month difference in PFS in the ECOG study versus just 2- to 3-week difference in PFS in the European study. Also, although the PFS of 4.5 months with chemotherapy alone in the ECOG trial is consistent with previous ECOG studies employing carboplatin plus paclitaxel, these data are interesting in light of the possible inferiority of carboplatin vis-à-vis cisplatin in advanced NSCLC (see earlier discussion). Could it be that the ECOG trial yielded an OS benefit with bevacizumab simply because carboplatin-based therapy is inherently less effective than cisplatin-based therapy? In other words, did bevacizumab simply increase OS with carboplatin-based chemotherapy to what would be achieved with cisplatin-based therapy? This is an issue that warrants additional study. Finally, it should be noted that there was *not* a statistically significant increase in life-threatening bleeding in the bevacizumab-containing arms of the European trial compared to chemotherapy alone in this trial.

PERSONALIZING CHEMOTHERAPY IN ADVANCED NSCLC

Ideally, clinicians would prefer to develop customized treatment plans for each individual patient that improve survival and minimize toxicities. Fortunately, such an approach may be feasible in the not too distant future, as modern techniques have facilitated the identification of specific genetic factors that may play a role in disease progression and patient response to therapy.[159] For example, the nuclear excision repair (NER) pathway is highly specialized process for the repair of damage caused by polycyclic aromatic hydrocarbons, ultraviolet light, or exogenous chemicals that induce bulky DNA adducts.[160,161] Alkylating agents such as platinum components interfere in the DNA-replication process by inducing DNA adducts that lead to cell death.[162] As a consequence of their increased capacity of DNA repair, some cancer cells are resistant to the effects of chemotherapy.[163,164] The excision repair cross-complementation group 1 (ERCC1) enzyme plays a rate-limiting role in the NER pathway that can recognize and remove cisplatin-induced DNA adducts.[165] In vitro studies have linked platinum resistance to the expression of ERCC1 mRNA in various cell lines.[166] These data suggest knowledge of ERCC1 status may permit greater precision in selecting a chemotherapy regimen for advanced NSCLC patients. Toward that end, Spanish investigators performed a landmark trial in advanced NSCLC in which ERCC1 mRNA expression was determined by quantitative real-time reverse transcriptase PCR using RNA isolated from pretreatment biopsies.[167] Patients were randomized to either a control or genotypic arm (1:2 ratio) before ERCC1 assessment. In the genotypic arm, patients with low ERCC1 levels received docetaxel plus cisplatin and those with high levels received a nonplatinum regimen (docetaxel plus gemcitabine). Patients in the control arm all received standard docetaxel plus cisplatin. The primary end point was the objective response rate. The response rate in the control arm was 39% and 51% in the genotypic arm ($p = 0.02$). OS was not significantly different; nonetheless, these data strongly suggest that ERCC1 mRNA levels can predict response to platinum-based therapy. In fact, in resected early stage NSCLC, patients with tumors overexpressing ERCC1 protein did not appear to benefit from platinum-based adjuvant chemotherapy, whereas patients with ERCC1 negative tumors did.[168]

Ribonucleotide reductase M1 (RRM1) encodes the regulatory subunit of ribonucleotide reductase, the rate-limiting enzyme in DNA synthesis.[169] Ribonucleotide reductase converts ribonucleotide 5′-diphosphate to deoxyribonucleotide 5′-diphosphate. Notably, gemcitabine competes with ribonucleotide 5′-diphosphate for incorporation into DNA. Consequently, the overexpression of ribonucleotide reductase would be expected to interfere with the efficacy of gemcitabine. Preclinical studies[170] and two recently completed clinical studies support the potential predictive value of RRM1.[171,172] For example, among a group of NSCLC patients treated with cisplatin plus gemcitabine, Spanish investigators found low RRM1 mRNA expression levels were associated with a significantly longer median survival than those with high levels (13.7 vs. 3.6 months; 95% CI, 9.6 to 17.8 months; $p = 0.009$)[171] (RRM1 and ERCC1 mRNA was assessed in paraffin-embedded samples by real-time quantitative reverse transcription-PCR). Bepler et al.[169] reported that the levels of RRM1 expression was significantly ($p = 0.002$) and inversely correlated ($r = -0.498$) with disease response after two cycles of gemcitabine and carboplatin in patients with locally advanced NSCLC.

Beta-tubulin is one of the major components of microtubules.[173] Taxanes bind to beta-tubulin and produce growth arrest at the G2-M phase of the cell cycle. High levels of beta-tubulin, which exists as multiple isotypes, are associated with resistance to taxanes.[173] More specifically, high levels of class III beta-tubulin are associated with taxane resistance in lung cancer cell lines.[174] The clinical relevance of this observation has been highlighted by Sève et al.[175] who assessed the prognostic and predictive value of class III beta-tubulin in tumors taken from patients with locally advanced or metastatic NSCLC treated with paclitaxel-based or other nontubulin-binding agents. Tumor samples were obtained before treatment with a paclitaxel-based regimen or a nontubulin-binding agent. Treatment response, PFS, and OS were then correlated with the expression of class III beta-tubulin protein. The response rate was 37.5% among patients receiving paclitaxel. Patients whose tumors expressed low levels of class III beta-tubulin isotype had a better response rate ($p < 0.001$), longer PFS ($p = 0.004$), and OS ($p = 0.002$), whereas this variable was not found to be predictive in patients receiving regimens without tubulin-binding agents. Taking into account sex, age, histology, stage, and class III beta-tubulin a multivariate analysis confirmed that low-level class III beta-tubulin expression was independently correlated with PFS ($p = 0.003$) and OS ($p = 0.003$). These findings suggest that the expression levels

TABLE 45.14 Survival Based on Histology in H3H-MC-JMDB Trial

Histology	CT	MST	HR	*p* Value
Adenocarcinoma	Gemcitabine/cisplatin	10.9 mo	0.84	0.03
	Pemetrexed/cisplatin	12.6 mo		
Large cell carcinoma	Gemcitabine/cisplatin	6.7 mo	0.67	0.03
	Pemetrexed/cisplatin	10.4 mo		
Nonsquamous carcinoma	Gemcitabine/cisplatin	10.4 mo	0.81	0.005
	Pemetrexed/cisplatin	11.8 mo		
Squamous Carcinoma	Gemcitabine/cisplatin	10.8 mo	1.23	0.05
	Pemetrexed/cisplatin	9.4 mo		

Adapted from Scagliotti GV, Parikh P, von Pawel J, et al. Phase III study comparing cisplatin plus gemcitabine with cisplatin plus pemetrexed in chemotherapy-naive patients with advanced-stage non-small-cell lung cancer. *J Clin Oncol* 2008;26(21):3543–3551.

of class III beta-tubulin in tumor cells may predict response to therapy and survival toutcome in patients with advanced NSCLC receiving paclitaxel-based chemotherapy; however, expression level is not a general prognostic factor.

Thymidylate synthase (TS) catalyzes the methylation of dUMP to dTMP and is the rate limiting irreversible step in de novo DNA synthesis.[176] As the sole source of de novo thymidylate in the cell, it is an important target for chemotherapy drugs such as 5-fluorouracil (5-FU), methotrexate, capecitabine and other novel folate-based drugs such as pemetrexed.[177] TS expression has been shown to be an independent prognostic and predictive factor in several cancers, including lung cancers, and overexpression of TS has been linked to resistance to these drugs.[176,178–182] TS mRNA levels ($p < 0.0001$) and protein levels ($p = 0.027$) have been shown to be significantly higher in squamous cell carcinomas of the lung as compared with adenocarcinomas.[183] Keeping in mind that pemetrexed targets TS, the potential significance of this finding is highlighted by the results of a large phase III trial in which cisplatin plus pemetrexed was found to be more effective than cisplatin plus gemcitabine in adenocarcinomas and large cell carcinomas, whereas cisplatin plus gemcitabine was noted to yield a better survival in squamous carcinomas compared to the pemetrexed regimen[37] (Table 45.14). The observed survival difference may have been related to differences in intratumoral TS expression although no definitive data pertaining to intratumoral TS expression have yet been presented.

In summary, the available evidence clearly indicates that the identification and exploitation of genetic markers, predictive of response to specific cytotoxic drugs, is an achievable goal. Moreover, these early results indicate that the application of pharmacogenomics has the potential to profoundly influence outcomes and improve OS.

CONCLUSION

For much of the 20th century, advances in the systemic treatment of advanced NSCLC were modest at best.[3,184] In fact, in 1998, the noted oncologist B.J. Kennedy derisively opined on the "snail's pace" of progress in the management of late stage NSCLC.[6] Fortunately, much has changed since Dr. Kennedy's rather pessimistic commentary. It is now well established that modern chemotherapy can prolong survival of NSCLC patients with late stage disease as well as improve the symptoms and quality of life and do so in a cost-effective manner.[3,4] It is now well accepted that doublet platinum-based chemotherapy with a third-generation drug is the preferred treatment for physically fit patients with advanced NSCLC. No single regimen stands apart as the optimal program for all patients. Nonplatinum therapy is a reasonable alternative approach in selected circumstances where cisplatin or carboplatin is not appropriate. Subtle differences among the extant regimens allow clinicians flexibility to choose among toxicity profiles, convenience, and cost. For a subset of patients, namely those with adenocarcinoma, no brain metastases or hemoptysis, the addition of bevacizumab to chemotherapy appears to be warranted based on a significant improvement in OS. Whether the addition of bevacizumab to doublets other than carboplatin and paclitaxel is beneficial remains to be determined. The available data indicate that no more than three to four cycles of chemotherapy regimen are required to achieve optimal survival results and minimize host toxicity. Older patients who are not physically fit and patients with a poor initial PS may be candidates for monotherapy with a third-generation drug or possibly one of the newer so-called targeted agents (e.g., erlotinib). Finally, all therapy in the setting of metastatic disease is ultimately palliative. Consequently, treatment decisions need to be tempered by this very sobering reality.

REFERENCES

1. Jemal A, Siegel R, Ward E, et al. Cancer statistics, 2008. *CA Cancer J Clin* 2008;58(2):71–96.
2. Parkin DM, Bray F, Ferlay J, et al. Global cancer statistics, 2002. *CA Cancer J Clin* 2005;55(2):74–108.
3. Spiro SG, Silvestri GA. One hundred years of lung cancer. *Am J Respir Crit Care Med* 2005;172(5):523–529.

4. Molina JR, Adjei AA, Jett JR. Advances in chemotherapy of non-small cell lung cancer. *Chest* 2006;130(4):1211–1219.
5. Karnofsky DA, Abelmann WH, Craver LF, et al. The use of nitrogen mustards in the palliative treatment of carcinoma. With particular reference to bronchogenic carcinoma. *Cancer* 1948;1:634–656.
6. Kennedy BJ. The snail's pace of lung carcinoma chemotherapy. *Cancer* 1998;82(5):801–803.
7. Green RA, Humphrey E, Close H, et al. Alkylating agents in bronchogenic carcinoma. *Am J Med* 1969;46(4):516–525.
8. Breathnach OS, Freidlin B, Conley B, et al. Twenty-two years of phase III trials for patients with advanced non-small-cell lung cancer: sobering results. *J Clin Oncol* 2001;19(6):1734–1742.
9. Non-small Cell Lung Cancer Collaborative Group. Chemotherapy in non-small cell lung cancer: a meta-analysis using updated data on individual patients from 52 randomised clinical trials. *BMJ* 1995;311(7010): 899–909.
10. Cullen MH, Billingham LJ, Woodroffe CM, et al. Mitomycin, ifosfamide, and cisplatin in unresectable non-small-cell lung cancer: effects on survival and quality of life. *J Clin Oncol* 1999;17(10):3188–3194.
11. Dooms CA, Lievens YN, Vansteenkiste JF. Cost-utility analysis of chemotherapy in symptomatic advanced nonsmall cell lung cancer. *Eur Respir J* 2006;27(5):895–901.
12. Burdett S, Johnson DH, Stewart L, et al., on behalf of the NSCLC Collaborative Group. Supportive care and chemotherapy (CT) versus supportive care alone in advanced non-small cell lung cancer (NSCLC): A meta-analysis using individual patient data (IPD) from randomised controlled trials (RCTs). *J Thorac Oncol* 2007;2(8):S337.
13. Wakelee HA, Bernardo P, Johnson DH, et al. Changes in the natural history of nonsmall cell lung cancer (NSCLC)-comparison of outcomes and characteristics in patients with advanced NSCLC entered in Eastern Cooperative Oncology Group trials before and after 1990. *Cancer* 2006;106(10):2208–2217.
14. Baggstrom MQ, Stinchcombe TE, Fried DB, et al. Third-generation chemotherapy agents in the treatment of advanced non-small cell lung cancer: a meta-analysis. *J Thorac Oncol* 2007;2(9):845–853.
15. Ranson M, Davidson N, Nicolson M, et al. Randomized trial of paclitaxel plus supportive care versus supportive care for patients with advanced non-small-cell lung cancer. *J Natl Cancer Inst* 2000;92(13):1074–1080.
16. Roszkowski K, Pluzanska A, Krzakowski M, et al. A multicenter, randomized, phase III study of docetaxel plus best supportive care versus best supportive care in chemotherapy-naive patients with metastatic or non-resectable localized non-small cell lung cancer (NSCLC). *Lung Cancer* 2000;27(3):145–157.
17. Georgoulias V, Ardavanis A, Agelidou A, et al. Docetaxel versus docetaxel plus cisplatin as front-line treatment of patients with advanced non-small-cell lung cancer: a randomized, multicenter phase III trial. *J Clin Oncol* 2004;22(13):2602–2609.
18. Lilenbaum RC, Herndon JE, II, List MA, et al. Single-agent versus combination chemotherapy in advanced non-small-cell lung cancer: The Cancer and Leukemia Group B (study 9730). *J Clin Oncol* 2005;23(1):190–196.
19. Sederholm C, Hillerdal G, Lamberg K, et al. Phase III trial of gemcitabine plus carboplatin versus single-agent gemcitabine in the treatment of locally advanced or metastatic non-small-cell lung cancer: the Swedish Lung Cancer Study Group. *J Clin Oncol* 2005;23(33): 8380–8388.
20. Hotta K, Matsuo K, Ueoka H, et al. Addition of platinum compounds to a new agent in patients with advanced non-small-cell lung cancer: a literature based meta-analysis of randomised trials. *Ann Oncol* 2004;15(12): 1782–1789.
21. Wozniak AJ, Crowley JJ, Balcerzak SP, et al. Randomized trial comparing cisplatin with cisplatin plus vinorelbine in the treatment of advanced non-small-cell lung cancer: a Southwest Oncology Group study. *J Clin Oncol* 1998;16(7):2459–2465.
22. Gatzemeier U, von Pawel J, Gottfried M, et al. Phase III comparative study of high-dose cisplatin versus a combination of paclitaxel and cisplatin in patients with advanced non-small-cell lung cancer. *J Clin Oncol* 2000;18(19):3390–3399.
23. Sandler AB, Nemunaitis J, Denham C, et al. Phase III trial of gemcitabine plus cisplatin versus cisplatin alone in patients with locally advanced or metastatic non-small-cell lung cancer. *J Clin Oncol* 2000;18(1):122–130.
24. Le Chevalier T, Brisgand D, Douillard JY, et al. Randomized study of vinorelbine and cisplatin versus vindesine and cisplatin versus vinorelbine alone in advanced non-small-cell lung cancer: results of a European multicenter trial including 612 patients. *J Clin Oncol* 1994;12(2):360–367.
25. Giaccone G, Splinter TA, Debruyne C, et al. Randomized study of paclitaxel-cisplatin versus cisplatin-teniposide in patients with advanced non-small-cell lung cancer. The European Organization for Research and Treatment of Cancer Lung Cancer Cooperative Group. *J Clin Oncol* 1998;16(6):2133–2141.
26. Bonomi P, Kim K, Fairclough D, et al. Comparison of survival and quality of life in advanced non-small-cell lung cancer patients treated with two dose levels of paclitaxel combined with cisplatin versus etoposide with cisplatin: results of an Eastern Cooperative Oncology Group trial. *J Clin Oncol* 2000;18(3):623–631.
27. Negoro S, Masuda N, Takada Y, et al. Randomised phase III trial of irinotecan combined with cisplatin for advanced non-small-cell lung cancer. *Br J Cancer* 2003;88(3):335–341.
28. Kubota K, Watanabe K, Kunitoh H, et al. Phase III randomized trial of docetaxel plus cisplatin versus vindesine plus cisplatin in patients with stage IV non-small-cell lung cancer: the Japanese Taxotere Lung Cancer Study Group. *J Clin Oncol* 2004;22(2):254–261.
29. Bunn PA, Jr. Chemotherapy for advanced non-small-cell lung cancer: who, what, when, why? *J Clin Oncol* 2002;20(18 Suppl):S23–S33.
30. Socinski MA. Cytotoxic chemotherapy in advanced non-small cell lung cancer: a review of standard treatment paradigms. *Clin Cancer Res* 2004;10(12 Pt 2):S4210–S4214.
31. Schiller JH, Harrington D, Belani CP, et al. Comparison of four chemotherapy regimens for advanced non-small-cell lung cancer. *N Engl J Med* 2002;346(2):92–98.
32. Smit EF, van Meerbeeck JP, Lianes P, et al. Three-arm randomized study of two cisplatin-based regimens and paclitaxel plus gemcitabine in advanced non-small-cell lung cancer: a phase III trial of the European Organization for Research and Treatment of Cancer Lung Cancer Group–EORTC 08975. *J Clin Oncol* 2003;21(21):3909–3917.
33. Scagliotti GV, De Marinis F, Rinaldi M, et al. Phase III randomized trial comparing three platinum-based doublets in advanced non–small-cell lung cancer. *J Clin Oncol* 2002;20(21):4285–4291.
34. Kelly K, Crowley J, Bunn PA Jr, et al. Randomized phase III trial of paclitaxel plus carboplatin versus vinorelbine plus cisplatin in the treatment of patients with advanced non–small-cell lung cancer: a Southwest Oncology Group trial. *J Clin Oncol* 2001;19(13):3210–3218.
35. Fossella F, Pereira JR, von Pawel J, et al. Randomized, multinational, phase III study of docetaxel plus platinum combinations versus vinorelbine plus cisplatin for advanced non-small-cell lung cancer: the TAX 326 study group. *J Clin Oncol* 2003;21(16):3016–3024.
36. Ohe Y, Ohashi Y, Kubota K, et al. Randomized phase III study of cisplatin plus irinotecan versus carboplatin plus paclitaxel, cisplatin plus gemcitabine, and cisplatin plus vinorelbine for advanced non-small-cell lung cancer: Four-Arm Cooperative Study in Japan. *Ann Oncol* 2007;18(2):317–323.
37. Scagliotti GV, Parikh P, von Pawel J, et al. Phase III study comparing cisplatin plus gemcitabine with cisplatin plus pemetrexed in chemotherapy-naive patients with advanced-stage non-small-cell lung cancer. *J Clin Oncol* 2008;26(21):3543–3551.
38. Gandara DR, Kawaguchi T, Crowley JJ, et al. Pharmacogenomic (PG) analysis of Japan-SWOG common arm study in advanced stage non-small cell lung cancer (NSCLC): A model for testing population-related pharmacogenomics. *J Clin Oncol* 2007;25(18S):S385.
39. Skipper HE. The forty-year-old mutation theory of Luria and Delbrück and its pertinence to cancer chemotherapy. *Adv Cancer Res* 1983;40: 331–363.
40. Delbaldo C, Michiels S, Syz N, et al. Benefits of adding a drug to a single-agent or a 2-agent chemotherapy regimen in advanced non-small-cell lung cancer: a meta-analysis. *JAMA* 2004;292(4):470–484.

41. Delbaldo C, Michiels S, Rolland E, et al. Second or third additional chemotherapy drug for non-small cell lung cancer in patients with advanced disease. *Cochrane Database Syst Rev*; 2007;(4):CD004569.
42. Baggstrom MQ, Socinski MA, Hensing TA, et al. Addressing the optimal number of cytotoxic agents in stage IIIB/IV non-small cell lung cancer (NSCLC): a meta-analysis of the published literature. *Proc Am Soc Clin Oncol* 2003;22:624.
43. Ettinger DS, Akerley W, Bepler G, et al. Non-small cell lung cancer clinical practice guidelines in oncology. *J Natl Compr Canc Netw* 2006;4(6): 548–582.
44. Pfister DG, Johnson DH, Azzoli CG, et al. American Society of Clinical Oncology treatment of unresectable non-small-cell lung cancer guideline: update 2003. *J Clin Oncol* 2004;22(2):330–353.
45. Socinski MA, Crowell R, Hensing TE, et al. Treatment of non-small cell lung cancer, stage IV: ACCP evidence-based clinical practice guidelines (2nd edition). *Chest* 2007;132(3 Suppl):277S-289S.
46. Smith IE, O'Brien ME, Talbot DC, et al. Duration of chemotherapy in advanced non-small-cell lung cancer: a randomized trial of three versus six courses of mitomycin, vinblastine, and cisplatin. *J Clin Oncol* 2001;19(5):1336–1343.
47. Socinski MA, Schell MJ, Peterman A, et al. Phase III trial comparing a defined duration of therapy versus continuous therapy followed by second-line therapy in advanced-stage IIIB/IV non-small-cell lung cancer. *J Clin Oncol* 2002;20(5):1335–1343.
48. von Plessen C, Bergman B, Andresen O, et al. Palliative chemotherapy beyond three courses conveys no survival or consistent quality-of-life benefits in advanced non-small-cell lung cancer. *Br J Cancer* 2006;95(8): 966–973.
49. Park JO, Kim S-W, Ahn JS, et al. Phase III trial of two versus four additional cycles in patients who are nonprogressive after two cycles of platinum-based chemotherapy in non small-cell lung cancer. *J Clin Oncol* 2007;25(33):5233–5239.
50. Gandara DR, Crowley J, Livingston RB, et al. Evaluation of cisplatin intensity in metastatic non-small-cell lung cancer: a phase III study of the Southwest Oncology Group. *J Clin Oncol* 1993;11(5): 873–878.
51. Klastersky J, Sculier JP, Ravez P, et al. A randomized study comparing a high and a standard dose of cisplatin in combination with etoposide in the treatment of advanced non-small-cell lung carcinoma. *J Clin Oncol* 1986;4(12):1780–1786.
52. Soon Y, Stockler MR, Boyer M, et al. Duration of chemotherapy for advanced non-small cell lung cancer: An updated systematic review and meta-analysis. *ASCO Meeting Abstracts* 2008;26(15 Suppl):8013.
53. Ciuleanu T, Brodowicz T, Zielinski C, et al. Maintenance pemetrexed plus best supportive care versus placebo plus best supportive care for non-small-cell lung cancer: a randomised, double-blind, phase 3 study. *Lancet* 2009;374(9699):1432–1440.
54. Socinski MA, Baggstrom MQ, Hensing TA. Duration of therapy in advanced, metastatic non-small-cell lung cancer. *Clin Adv Hematol Oncol* 2003;1(1):33–38.
55. Westeel V, Quoix E, Moro-Sibilot D, et al. Randomized study of maintenance vinorelbine in responders with advanced non-small-cell lung cancer. *J Natl Cancer Inst* 2005;97(7):499–506.
56. Socinski MA, Stinchcombe TE. Duration of first-line chemotherapy in advanced non small-cell lung cancer: less is more in the era of effective subsequent therapies. *J Clin Oncol* 2007;25(33):5155–5157.
57. Sandler A, Gray R, Perry MC, et al. Paclitaxel-carboplatin alone or with bevacizumab for non-small-cell lung cancer. *N Engl J Med* 2006;355(24):2542–2550.
58. Reck M, von Pawel J, Zatloukal P, et al. Phase III trial of cisplatin plus gemcitabine with either placebo or bevacizumab as first-line therapy for nonsquamous non-small-cell lung cancer: AVAil. *J Clin Oncol* 2009;27(8):1227–1234.
59. Patel JD, Hensing TA, Rademaker F, et al. Pemetrexed and carboplatin plus bevacizumab with maintenance pemetrexed and bevacizumab as first-line therapy for advanced non-squamous non-small cell lung cancer (NSCLC). *J Clin Oncol (Meeting Abstracts)*. 2008;26(15 Suppl): abstract 8044.
60. Hida T, Okamoto I, Kashii T, et al. Randomized phase III study of platinum-doublet chemotherapy followed by gefitinib versus continued platinum-doublet chemotherapy in patients (pts) with advanced non-small cell lung cancer (NSCLC): results of West Japan Thoracic Oncology Group trial (WJTOG) [abstract LBA8012]. *Proc Am Soc Clin Oncol* 2008.
61. Hotta K, Matsuo K, Ueoka H, et al. Meta-analysis of randomized clinical trials comparing cisplatin to carboplatin in patients with advanced non-small-cell lung cancer. *J Clin Oncol* 2004;22(19):3852–3859.
62. Ardizzoni A, Boni L, Tiseo M, et al. Cisplatin- versus carboplatin-based chemotherapy in first-line treatment of advanced non-small-cell lung cancer: An individual patient data meta-analysis. *J Natl Cancer Inst* 2007;99(11):847–857.
63. Rosell R, Gatzemeier U, Betticher DC, et al. Phase III randomised trial comparing paclitaxel/carboplatin with paclitaxel/cisplatin in patients with advanced non-small-cell lung cancer: a cooperative multinational trial. *Ann Oncol* 2002;13(10):1539–1549.
64. Klastersky J, Sculier JP, Lacroix H, et al. A randomized study comparing cisplatin or carboplatin with etoposide in patients with advanced non-small-cell lung cancer: European Organization for Research and Treatment of Cancer Protocol 07861. *J Clin Oncol* 1990;8(9): 1556–1562.
65. Jelic S, Mitrovic L, Radosavljevic D, et al. Survival advantage for carboplatin substituting cisplatin in combination with vindesine and mitomycin C for stage IIIB and IV squamous-cell bronchogenic carcinoma: a randomized phase III study. *Lung Cancer* 2001;34(1):1–13.
66. Zatloukal P, Petruzelka L, Zemanova M, et al. Gemcitabine plus cisplatin vs. gemcitabine plus carboplatin in stage IIIb and IV non-small cell lung cancer: a phase III randomized trial. *Lung Cancer* 2003;41(3):321–331.
67. Mazzanti P, Massacesi C, Rocchi MB, et al. Randomized, multicenter, phase II study of gemcitabine plus cisplatin versus gemcitabine plus carboplatin in patients with advanced non-small cell lung cancer. *Lung Cancer* 2003;41(1):81–89.
68. Paccagnella A, Favaretto A, Oniga F, et al. Cisplatin versus carboplatin in combination with mitomycin and vinblastine in advanced non small cell lung cancer. A multicenter, randomized phase III trial. *Lung Cancer* 2004;43(1):83–91.
69. Azzoli CG, Kris MG, Pfister DG. Cisplatin versus carboplatin for patients with metastatic non-small-cell lung cancer—an old rivalry renewed. *J. Natl. Cancer Inst* 2007;99(11):828–829.
70. Pujol JL, Carestia L, Daures JP. Is there a case for cisplatin in the treatment of small-cell lung cancer? A meta-analysis of randomized trials of a cisplatin-containing regimen versus a regimen without this alkylating agent. *Br J Cancer* 2000;83(1):8–15.
71. Pujol JL, Barlesi F, Daures JP. Should chemotherapy combinations for advanced non-small cell lung cancer be platinum-based? A meta-analysis of phase III randomized trials. *Lung Cancer* 2006;51(3): 335–345.
72. Rapp E, Pater JL, Willan A, et al. Chemotherapy can prolong survival in patients with advanced non-small-cell lung cancer—report of a Canadian multicenter randomized trial. *J Clin Oncol* 1988;6(4):633–641.
73. Bunn PA Jr. Platinums in Lung Cancer: Sufficient or Necessary? *J Clin Oncol* 2005;23(13):2882–2883.
74. Georgoulias V, Papadakis E, Alexopoulos A, et al. Platinum-based and non-platinum-based chemotherapy in advanced non-small-cell lung cancer: a randomised multicentre trial. *Lancet* 2001;357(9267): 1478–1484.
75. D'Addario G, Pintilie M, Leighl NB, et al. Platinum-based versus non-platinum-based chemotherapy in advanced non-small-cell lung cancer: a meta-analysis of the published literature. *J Clin Oncol* 2005;23(13): 2926–2936.
76. Beckles MA, Spiro SG, Colice GL, et al. Initial evaluation of the patient with lung cancer: symptoms, signs, laboratory tests, and paraneoplastic syndromes. *Chest* 2003;123:97–104.
77. Ellis PA, Smith IE, Hardy JR, et al. Symptom relief with MVP (mitomycin C, vinblastine and cisplatin) chemotherapy in advanced non-small-cell lung cancer. *Br J Cancer* 1995;71(2):366–370.

78. Stinnett S, Williams L, Johnson DH. Role of chemotherapy for palliation in the lung cancer patient. *J Support Oncol* 2007;5(1):19–24.
79. Tummarello D, Graziano F, Isidori P, et al. Symptomatic, stage IV, non-small-cell lung cancer (NSCLC): response, toxicity, performance status change and symptom relief in patients treated with cisplatin, vinblastine and mitomycin-C. *Cancer Chemother Pharmacol* 1995;35(3):249–253.
80. The Elderly Lung Cancer Vinorelbine Italian Study Group. Effects of vinorelbine on quality of life and survival of elderly patients with advanced non-small-cell lung cancer. *J Natl Cancer Inst* 1999;91(1): 66–72.
81. Anderson H, Hopwood P, Stephens RJ, et al. Gemcitabine plus best supportive care (BSC) vs BSC in inoperable non-small cell lung cancer—a randomized trial with quality of life as the primary outcome. UK NSCLC Gemcitabine Group. Non-Small Cell Lung Cancer. *Br J Cancer* 2000;83(4):447–453.
82. Thatcher N, Anderson H, Betticher DC, et al. Symptomatic benefit from gemcitabine and other chemotherapy in advanced non-small cell lung cancer: changes in performance status and tumour-related symptoms. *Anticancer Drugs* 1995;6(Suppl 6):39–48.
83. Shepherd FA, Dancey J, Ramlau R, et al. Prospective randomized trial of docetaxel versus best supportive care in patients with non-small-cell lung cancer previously treated with platinum-based chemotherapy. *J Clin Oncol* 2000;18(10):2095–2103.
84. Ramsey SD, Howlader N, Etzioni RD, et al. Chemotherapy use, outcomes, and costs for older persons with advanced non-small-cell lung cancer: evidence from surveillance, epidemiology and end results-Medicare. *J Clin Oncol* 2004;22(24):4971–4978.
85. Gridelli C, Aapro M, Ardizzoni A, et al. Treatment of advanced non-small-cell lung cancer in the elderly: results of an international expert panel. *J Clin Oncol* 2005;23(13):3125–3137.
86. Booton R, Jones M, Thatcher N. Lung cancer 7: management of lung cancer in elderly patients. *Thorax* 2003;58(8):711–720.
87. Gridelli C, Perrone F, Gallo C, et al. Chemotherapy for elderly patients with advanced non-small-cell lung cancer: the Multicenter Italian Lung Cancer in the Elderly Study (MILES) phase III randomized trial. *J Natl Cancer Inst* 2003;95(5):362–372.
88. Langer CJ, Manola J, Bernardo P, et al. Cisplatin-based therapy for elderly patients with advanced non-small-cell lung cancer: implications of Eastern Cooperative Oncology Group 5592, a randomized trial. *J Natl Cancer Inst* 2002;94(3):173–181.
89. Langer CJ, Vangel M, Schiller JH, et al. Age-specific subanalysis of ECOG 1594: Fit elderly patients (70–80 YRS) with NSCLC do as well as younger pts (< 70). *Proc Am Soc Clin Oncol.* 2003;22:639.
90. Hesketh PJ, Lilenbaum RC, Chansky K, et al. Chemotherapy in patients > or = 80 with advanced non-small cell lung cancer: combined results from SWOG 0027 and LUN 6. *J Thorac Oncol* 2007;2(6):494–498.
91. Hesketh PJ, Chansky K, Lau DH, et al. Sequential vinorelbine and docetaxel in advanced non-small cell lung cancer patients age 70 and older and/or with a performance status of 2: a phase II trial of the Southwest Oncology Group (S0027). *J Thorac Oncol* 2006;1(6):537–544.
92. Lilenbaum R, Rubin M, Samuel J, et al. A randomized phase II trial of two schedules of docetaxel in elderly or poor performance status patients with advanced non-small cell lung cancer. *J Thorac Oncol* 2007;2(4):306–311.
93. Brundage MD, Davies D, Mackillop WJ. Prognostic factors in non-small cell lung cancer : A decade of progress. *Chest* 2002;122(3):1037–1057.
94. Gridelli C, Ardizzoni A, Le Chevalier T, et al. Treatment of advanced non-small-cell lung cancer patients with ECOG performance status 2: results of an European Experts Panel. *Ann Oncol* 2004;15(3): 419–426.
95. Billingham LJ, Cullen MH. The benefits of chemotherapy in patient subgroups with unresectable non-small-cell lung cancer. *Ann Oncol* 2001;12(12):1671–1675.
96. Blackhall FH, Bhosle J, Thatcher N. Chemotherapy for advanced non-small cell lung cancer patients with performance status 2. *Curr Opin Oncol* 2005;17(2):135–139.
97. Lilenbaum RC. Treatment of patients with advanced lung cancer and poor performance status. *Clin Lung Cancer* 2004;6(Suppl 2): S71–S74.
98. Langer C, Li S, Schiller J, et al. Randomized phase II trial of paclitaxel plus carboplatin or gemcitabine plus cisplatin in Eastern Cooperative Oncology Group performance status 2 non-small-cell lung cancer patients: ECOG 1599. *J Clin Oncol* 2007;25(4):418–423.
99. Sweeney CJ, Zhu J, Sandler AB, et al. Outcome of patients with a performance status of 2 in Eastern Cooperative Oncology Group Study E1594: a Phase II trial in patients with metastatic nonsmall cell lung carcinoma. *Cancer* 2001;92(10):2639–2647.
100. Langer CJ, O'Byrne KJ, Socinski MA, et al. Phase III trial comparing paclitaxel poliglumex (CT-2103, PPX) in combination with carboplatin versus standard paclitaxel and carboplatin in the treatment of PS 2 patients with chemotherapy-naive advanced non-small cell lung cancer. *J Thorac Oncol* 2008;3(6):623–630.
101. O'Brien ME, Socinski MA, Popovich AY, et al. Randomized phase III trial comparing single-agent paclitaxel Poliglumex (CT-2103, PPX) with single-agent gemcitabine or vinorelbine for the treatment of PS 2 patients with chemotherapy-naive advanced non-small cell lung cancer. *J Thorac Oncol* 2008;3(7):728–734.
102. Lilenbaum R, Bandstra B, Langer C, et al. Single agent versus combination therapy in advanced NSCLC patients with performance status 2: Results from a regression analysis of STELLAR 3 and 4: B2-04. *Journal of Thoracic Oncology* 2008;2(8):S337–S338.
103. Lilenbaum R, Axerold R, Thomas S, et al. Randomized phase II trial of single agent erlotinib vs. standard chemotherapy in patients with advanced non-small cell lung cancer (NSCLC) and performance status (PS) of 2. *J Clin Oncol, Proc ASCO* 2006;24(18S) abst# 7022.
104. Sun S, Schiller JH, Spinola M, Minna JD. New molecularly targeted therapies for lung cancer. *J Clin Invest* 2007;117(10):2740–2750.
105. Ciardiello F, Caputo R, Bianco R, et al. Antitumor effect and potentiation of cytotoxic drugs activity in human cancer cells by ZD-1839 (Iressa), an epidermal growth factor receptor-selective tyrosine kinase inhibitor. *Clin Cancer Res* 2000;6(5):2053–2063.
106. Sirotnak FM, Zakowski MF, Miller VA,. et al. Efficacy of cytotoxic agents against human tumor xenografts is markedly enhanced by coadministration of ZD1839 (Iressa), an inhibitor of EGFR tyrosine kinase. *Clin Cancer Res* 2000;6(12):4885–4892.
107. Giaccone G, Herbst RS, Manegold C, et al. Gefitinib in combination with gemcitabine and cisplatin in advanced non-small-cell lung cancer: a phase III trial—INTACT 1. *J Clin Oncol* 2004;22(5):777–784.
108. Herbst RS, Giaccone G, Schiller JH, et al. Gefitinib in combination with paclitaxel and carboplatin in advanced non-small-cell lung cancer: a phase III trial—INTACT 2. *J Clin Oncol* 2004;22(5):785–794.
109. Herbst RS, Prager D, Hermann R, et al. TRIBUTE: a phase III trial of erlotinib hydrochloride (OSI-774) combined with carboplatin and paclitaxel chemotherapy in advanced non-small-cell lung cancer. *J Clin Oncol* 2005;23(25):5892–5899.
110. Gatzemeier U, Pluzanska A, Szczesna A, et al. Phase III study of erlotinib in combination with cisplatin and gemcitabine in advanced non-small-cell lung cancer: the Tarceva Lung Cancer Investigation Trial. *J Clin Oncol* 2007;25(12):1545–1552.
111. Bissett D, O'Byrne KJ, von Pawel J, et al. Phase III study of matrix metalloproteinase inhibitor prinomastat in non-small-cell lung cancer. *J Clin Oncol* 2005;23(4):842–849.
112. Leighl NB, Paz-Ares L, Douillard JY, et al. Randomized phase III study of matrix metalloproteinase inhibitor BMS-275291 in combination with paclitaxel and carboplatin in advanced non-small-cell lung cancer: National Cancer Institute of Canada-Clinical Trials Group Study BR.18. *J Clin Oncol* 2005;23(12):2831–2839.
113. Manegold C, von Pawel J, Zatloukal P, et al. Randomised, double-blind multicentre phase III study of bevacizumab in combination with cisplatin and gemcitabine in chemotherapy-naïve patients with advanced or recurrent non-squamous non-small cell lung cancer (NSCLC): BO17704. *J Clin Oncol* 2007;25(18S Part I of II):388s.

114. Mendelsohn J, Baselga J. Epidermal growth factor receptor targeting in cancer. *Semin Oncol* 2006;33(4):369–385.
115. Lynch TJ, Bell DW, Sordella R, et al. Activating mutations in the epidermal growth factor receptor underlying responsiveness of non-small-cell lung cancer to gefitinib. *N Engl J Med* 2004;350(21):2129–2139.
116. Paez JG, Jänne PA, Lee JC, et al. EGFR mutations in lung cancer: correlation with clinical response to gefitinib therapy. *Science* 2004;304(5676):1497–1500.
117. Galizia G, Lieto E, De Vita F, et al. Cetuximab, a chimeric human mouse anti-epidermal growth factor receptor monoclonal antibody, in the treatment of human colorectal cancer. *Oncogene* 2007;26(25):3654–3660.
118. Hirsch FR, Varella-Garcia M, Bunn PA Jr, et al. Molecular predictors of outcome with gefitinib in a phase III placebo-controlled study in advanced non-small-cell lung cancer. *J Clin Oncol* 2006;24(31):5034–5042.
119. Hirsch FR, Varella-Garcia M, Cappuzzo F, et al. Combination of EGFR gene copy number and protein expression predicts outcome for advanced non-small-cell lung cancer patients treated with gefitinib. *Ann Oncol* 2007;18(4):752–760.
120. Bell DW, Lynch TJ, Haserlat SM, et al. Epidermal growth factor receptor mutations and gene amplification in non-small-cell lung cancer: molecular analysis of the IDEAL/INTACT gefitinib trials. *J Clin Oncol* 2005;23(31):8081–8092.
121. Douillard J-Y, Kim E, Hirsh V, et al. Gefitinib (IRESSA) versus docetaxel in patients with locally advanced or metastatic non-small-cell lung cancer pre-treated with platinum based chemotherapy: a randomized, open-label Phase III study (INTEREST). *J Thorac Oncol* 2007;2(8):S305.
122. Miller VA, Kris MG, Shah N, et al. Bronchioloalveolar pathologic subtype and smoking history predict sensitivity to gefitinib in advanced non-small-cell lung cancer. *J Clin Oncol* 2004; 22(6):1103–1109.
123. Johnson DH. Targeted therapies in combination with chemotherapy in non-small cell lung cancer. *Clin Cancer Res* 2006;12(14 Pt 2):S4451–S4457.
124. Mok TS, Wu YL, Thongprasert S, et al. Gefitinib or carboplatin-paclitaxel in pulmonary adenocarcinoma. *N Engl J Med* 2009;361(10):947–957.
125. Yarden Y, Sliwkowski MX. Untangling the ErbB signalling network. *Nat Rev Mol Cell Biol* 2001;2(2):127–137.
126. Morgensztern D, Govindan R. Is there a role for cetuximab in non small cell lung cancer? *Clin Cancer Res.* 2007;13(15):S4602–S4605.
127. Pirker R, Szczesna A, von Pawel J, et al. FLEX: A randomized, multicenter, phase III study of cetuximab in combination with cisplatin/vinorelbine (CV) versus CV alone in the first-line treatment of patients with advanced non-small cell lung cancer (NSCLC). *ASCO Meeting Abstracts.* 2008;26(15 Suppl): abstract 3.
128. Kern JA, Schwartz DA, Nordberg JE, et al. p185neu expression in human lung adenocarcinomas predicts shortened survival. *Cancer Res* 1990;50(16):5184–5187.
129. Kern JA, Torney L, Weiner D, et al. Inhibition of human lung cancer cell line growth by an anti-p185HER2 antibody. *Am J Respir Cell Mol Biol* 1993;9(4):448–454.
130. Langer CJ, Stephenson P, Thor A, et al. Trastuzumab in the treatment of advanced non-small-cell lung cancer: is there a role? Focus on Eastern Cooperative Oncology Group study 2598. *J Clin Oncol* 2004;22(7):1180–1187.
131. Zinner RG, Glisson BS, Fossella FV, et al. Trastuzumab in combination with cisplatin and gemcitabine in patients with Her2-overexpressing, untreated, advanced non-small cell lung cancer: report of a phase II trial and findings regarding optimal identification of patients with Her2-overexpressing disease. *Lung Cancer* 2004;44(1):99–110.
132. Gatzemeier U, Groth G, Butts C, et al. Randomized phase II trial of gemcitabine-cisplatin with or without trastuzumab in HER2-positive non-small-cell lung cancer. *Ann Oncol* 2004;15(1):19–27.
133. Clamon G, Herndon J, Kern J, et al. Lack of trastuzumab activity in nonsmall cell lung carcinoma with overexpression of erb-B2: 39810: a phase II trial of Cancer and Leukemia Group B. *Cancer* 2005;103(8):1670–1675.
134. Bunn PA Jr, Helfrich B, Soriano AF, et al. Expression of Her-2/neu in human lung cancer cell lines by immunohistochemistry and fluorescence in situ hybridization and its relationship to in vitro cytotoxicity by trastuzumab and chemotherapeutic agents. *Clin Cancer Res* 2001;7(10):3239–3250.
135. Hirsch FR, Franklin WA, Veve R, et al. HER2/neu expression in malignant lung tumors. *Semin Oncol.* 2002;29(1 Suppl 4):51–58.
136. Hirsch FR, Varella-Garcia M, Franklin WA, et al. Evaluation of HER-2/neu gene amplification and protein expression in non-small cell lung carcinomas. *Br J Cancer* 2002;86(9):1449–1456.
137. Stephens P, Hunter C, Bignell G, et al. Lung cancer: intragenic ERBB2 kinase mutations in tumours. *Nature* 2004;431(7008):525–526.
138. Shigematsu H, Takahashi T, Nomura M, et al. Somatic mutations of the HER2 kinase domain in lung adenocarcinomas. *Cancer Res* 2005;65(5):1642–1646.
139. Simon R, Maitournam A. Evaluating the efficiency of targeted designs for randomized clinical trials. *Clin Cancer Res* 2004;10(20):6759–6763.
140. Nelson AR, Fingleton B, Rothenberg ML, et al. Matrix metalloproteinases: biologic activity and clinical implications. *J Clin Oncol* 2000;18(5):1135–1149.
141. Coussens LM, Fingleton B, Matrisian LM. Matrix metalloproteinase inhibitors and cancer: trials and tribulations. *Science* 2002;295(5564):2387–2392.
142. Pavlaki M, Zucker S. Matrix metalloproteinase inhibitors (MMPIs): the beginning of phase I or the termination of phase III clinical trials. *Cancer Metastasis Rev* 2003;22(2–3):177–203.
143. Krieg AM. Toll-like receptor 9 (TLR9) agonists in the treatment of cancer. *Oncogene* 2008;27(2):161–167.
144. Droemann D, Albrecht D, Gerdes J, et al. Human lung cancer cells express functionally active Toll-like receptor 9. *Respir Res* 2005;6:1.
145. Vicari AP, Luu R, Zhang N, et al. Paclitaxel reduces regulatory T cell numbers and inhibitory function and enhances the anti-tumor effects of the TLR9 agonist PF-3512676 in the mouse. *Cancer Immunol Immunother* 2009;58(4):615–628.
146. Manegold C, Gravenor D, Woytowitz D, et al. Randomized phase II trial of a toll-like receptor 9 agonist oligodeoxynucleotide, PF-3512676, in combination with first-line taxane plus platinum chemotherapy for advanced-stage non-small-cell lung cancer. *J Clin Oncol* 2008;26(24):3979–3986.
147. Hirsh V, Boyer M, Rosell R, et al. Randomized phase III trial of paclitaxel/carboplatin with or without PF-3512676 as first line treatment of advanced non-small cell lung cancer (NSCLC). *ASCO Meeting Abstracts.* 2008;26(15 Suppl): abstact 8016.
148. Manegold C, Thatcher N, Benner RJ, et al. Randomized phase III trial of gemcitabine/cisplatin with or without PF-3512676 as first line treatment of advanced non-small cell lung cancer (NSCLC). *ASCO Meeting Abstracts.* 2008;26(15 Suppl): abstact 8017.
149. Cappuzzo F, Toschi L, Tallini G, et al. Insulin-like growth factor receptor 1 (IGFR-1) is significantly associated with longer survival in non-small-cell lung cancer patients treated with gefitinib. *Ann Oncol* 2006;17(7):1120–1127.
150. Ludovini V, Bellezza G, Pistola L, et al. High coexpression of both insulin-like growth factor receptor-1 (IGFR-1) and epidermal growth factor receptor (EGFR) is associated with shorter disease-free survival in resected non-small-cell lung cancer patients. *Ann Oncol* 2009;20(5):842–849.
151. Karp DD, Paz-Ares LG, Novello S, et al. High activity of the anti-IGF-IR antibody CP-751,871 in combination with paclitaxel and carboplatin in squamous NSCLC. *ASCO Meeting Abstracts.* 2008;26(15 Suppl): abstact 8015.
152. Cascone T, Troiani T, Morelli MP, et al. Antiangiogenic drugs in non-small cell lung cancer treatment. *Curr Opin Oncol* 2006;18(2):151–155.
153. Folkman J. Angiogenesis: an organizing principle for drug discovery? *Nat Rev Drug Discov* 2007;6(4):273–286.
154. Cabebe E, Wakelee H. Role of anti-angiogenesis agents in treating NSCLC: Focus on bevacizumab and VEGFR tyrosine kinase inhibitors. *Curr Treat Options Oncol* 2007;8(1):15–27.

155. Gridelli C, Maione P, Del Gaizo F, et al. Sorafenib and sunitinib in the treatment of advanced non-small cell lung cancer. *Oncologist* 2007;12(2):191–200.
156. Giaccone G. The potential of antiangiogenic therapy in non-small cell lung cancer. *Clin Cancer Res* 2007;13(7):1961–1970.
157. Johnson DH, Fehrenbacher L, Novotny WF, et al. Randomized phase II trial comparing bevacizumab plus carboplatin and paclitaxel with carboplatin and paclitaxel alone in previously untreated locally advanced or metastatic non-small-cell lung cancer. *J Clin Oncol* 2004;22(11):2184–2191.
158. Hurwitz H, Fehrenbacher L, Novotny W, et al. Bevacizumab plus irinotecan, fluorouracil, and leucovorin for metastatic colorectal cancer. *N Engl J Med* 2004;350(23):2335–2342.
159. Bepler G. Pharmacogenomics: a reality or still a promise? *Lung Cancer* 2006;54(Suppl 2):S34–S37.
160. Furuta T, Ueda T, Aune G, et al. Transcription-coupled nucleotide excision repair as a determinant of cisplatin sensitivity of human cells. *Cancer Res* 2002;62(17):4899–4902.
161. Hoeijmakers JH. Genome maintenance mechanisms for preventing cancer. *Nature* 2001;411(6835):366–374.
162. Reed E. Platinum-DNA adduct, nucleotide excision repair and platinum based anti-cancer chemotherapy. *Cancer Treat Rev* 1998;24(5):331–344.
163. Wei Q, Frazier ML, Levin B. DNA repair: a double-edged sword. *J Natl Cancer Inst* 2000;92(6):440–441.
164. Simon GR, Ismail-Khan R, Bepler G. Nuclear excision repair-based personalized therapy for non-small cell lung cancer: from hypothesis to reality. *Int J Biochem Cell Biol* 2007;39(7–8):1318–1328.
165. Reed E. ERCC1 and clinical resistance to platinum-based therapy. *Clin Cancer Res* 2005;11(17):6100–6102.
166. Olaussen KA, Mountzios G, Soria JC. ERCC1 as a risk stratifier in platinum-based chemotherapy for nonsmall-cell lung cancer. *Curr Opin Pulm Med* 2007;13(4):284–289.
167. Cobo M, Isla D, Massuti B, et al. Customizing cisplatin based on quantitative excision repair cross-complementing 1 mRNA expression: A phase III trial in non-small-cell lung cancer. *J Clin Oncol* 2007; 25(19):2747–2754.
168. Olaussen KA, Dunant A, Fouret P, et al. DNA repair by ERCC1 in non-small-cell lung cancer and cisplatin-based adjuvant chemotherapy. *N Engl J Med* 2006;355(10):983–991.
169. Bepler G, Kusmartseva I, Sharma S, et al. RRM1 modulated in vitro and in vivo efficacy of gemcitabine and platinum in non-small-cell lung cancer. *J Clin Oncol* 2006;24(29):4731–4737.
170. Shepherd FA, Rosell R. Weighing tumor biology in treatment decisions for patients with non-small cell lung cancer. *J Thorac Oncol* 2007; 2(Suppl 2):S68–S76.
171. Rosell R, Danenberg KD, Alberola V, et al. Ribonucleotide reductase messenger RNA expression and survival in gemcitabine/cisplatin-treated advanced non-small cell lung cancer patients. *Clin Cancer Res* 2004;10(4): 1318–1325.
172. Simon G, Sharma A, Li X, et al. Feasibility and efficacy of molecular analysis-directed individualized therapy in advanced non-small-cell lung cancer. *J Clin Oncol* 2007;25(19):2741–2746.
173. Burkhart CA, Kavallaris M, Band Horwitz S. The role of beta-tubulin isotypes in resistance to antimitotic drugs. *Biochim Biophys Acta* 2001; 1471(2):O1–O9.
174. Sève P, Isaac S, Trédan O, et al. Expression of class III {beta}-tubulin is predictive of patient outcome in patients with non-small cell lung cancer receiving vinorelbine-based chemotherapy. *Clin Cancer Res* 2005; 11(15):5481–5486.
175. Sève P, Mackey J, Isaac S, et al. Class III beta-tubulin expression in tumor cells predicts response and outcome in patients with non-small cell lung cancer receiving paclitaxel. *Mol Cancer Ther* 2005;4(12):2001–2007.
176. Marsh S. Thymidylate synthase pharmacogenetics. *Invest New Drugs* 2005;23(6):533–537.
177. Chattopadhyay S, Moran RG, Goldman ID. Pemetrexed: biochemical and cellular pharmacology, mechanisms, and clinical applications. *Mol Cancer Ther* 2007;6(2):404–417.
178. Jensen SA, Vainer B, Sorensen JB. The prognostic significance of thymidylate synthase and dihydropyrimidine dehydrogenase in colorectal cancer of 303 patients adjuvantly treated with 5-fluorouracil. *Int J Cancer* 2007;120(3):694–701.
179. Miyoshi T, Kondo K, Toba H, et al. Predictive value of thymidylate synthase and dihydropyrimidine dehydrogenase expression in tumor tissue, regarding the efficacy of postoperatively administered UFT (tegafur+uracil) in patients with non-small cell lung cancer. *Anticancer Res* 2007;27(4C):2641–2648.
180. Rosell R, Cuello M, Cecere F, et al. Usefulness of predictive tests for cancer treatment. *Bull Cancer* 2006;93(8):E101–E108.
181. Nakagawa T, Tanaka F, Otake Y, et al. Prognostic value of thymidylate synthase expression in patients with p-stage I adenocarcinoma of the lung. *Lung Cancer* 2002;35(2):165–170.
182. Meropol NJ, Gold PJ, Diasio RB, et al. Thymidine phosphorylase expression is associated with response to capecitabine plus irinotecan in patients with metastatic colorectal cancer. *J Clin Oncol* 2006; 24(25):4069–4077.
183. Ceppi P, Volante M, Saviozzi S, et al. Squamous cell carcinoma of the lung compared with other histotypes shows higher messenger RNA and protein levels for thymidylate synthase. *Cancer* 2006;107(7):1589–1596.
184. Silvestri GA, Spiro SG. Carcinoma of the bronchus 60 years later. *Thorax* 2006;61(12):1023–1028.
185. Gatzemeier U, Pluzanska A, Szczesna A, et al. Results of a phase III trial of erlotinib (OSI-774) combined with cisplatin and gemcitabine (GC) chemotherapy in advanced non-small cell lung cancer (NSCLC). *J Clin Oncol* 2004;22:617.

CHAPTER 46

Peter M. Ellis
Frances A. Shepherd

Chemotherapy for Recurrent or Refractory Advanced Non–Small Cell Lung Cancer

Publication of the Non–Small Cell Lung Cancer (NSCLC) Collaborative Group metaanalysis in 1995 established that first-line platinum-based chemotherapy is associated with a modest improvement in survival for patients with metastatic disease.[1] In general, most patients experience disease progression within a short time, with a median time to progression of approximately 4 months.[2–4] However, at the time of progression, many patients maintain a good performance status (PS) and may be candidates for further systemic therapy. Even as recently as 1997 though, guidelines for the management of NSCLC stated, "there is no current evidence that either confirms or refutes that second-line chemotherapy improves survival in patients with advanced NSCLC."[5]

Fortunately, substantial progress has been made over the last decade, and currently, numerous systemic therapeutic options are available for the treatment of advanced and metastatic NSCLC (Table 46.1). Several chemotherapeutic agents have been evaluated in the second-line setting. More recently, molecularly targeted agents have also shown benefit in this group of patients. Agents targeting the epidermal growth factor receptor (EGFR) and vascular endothelial growth factor (VEGF) have been widely investigated. As a result, multiple options now exist for second and subsequent lines of therapy for these patients.

This chapter will examine the available evidence for second-line treatment options for patients with NSCLC, progressing after first-line chemotherapy. Recommendations are based on data from randomized trials examining second-line treatment options for NSCLC. Published data were identified from a literature search using MEDLINE, as well as review of conference proceedings from meetings of the American Society of Clinical Oncology (ASCO), the International Association for the Study of Lung Cancer (IASLC), European Society of Medical Oncology (ESMO), and European Conference on Clinical Oncology (ECCO).

DOES SECOND-LINE CHEMOTHERAPY IMPROVE SURVIVAL AND/OR QUALITY OF LIFE?

Studies of second-line therapy in NSCLC are summarized in Table 46.2. The TAX 317 trial represents a milestone in the recent approach to second-line therapy for NSCLC.[6] This was a randomized trial of docetaxel versus best supportive care (BSC) for patients who previously had been treated with a platinum-containing (cisplatin or carboplatin) chemotherapy regimen. BSC could include treatment with antibiotics, analgesics, blood transfusions, and palliative radiation. Patients could have received more than one prior chemotherapy regimen, but were not eligible if they had received a prior taxane including paclitaxel. The study included patients with Eastern Cooperative Oncology Group (ECOG) PS 0 to 2. The primary outcome of TAX 317 was overall survival. Secondary outcomes included response rate, response duration, time to disease progression, and quality of life (QOL) (measured by the Lung Cancer Symptom Scale in North America and European Organization for Research and Treatment of Cancer quality of life questionnaire in Europe). In patients with measurable disease, response was assessed using bidimensional response criteria.

The planned dose of docetaxel was initially 100 mg/m^2. However, an interim safety analysis by the Data Safety and Monitoring Committee identified five toxic deaths among 49 patients randomized to docetaxel 100 mg/m^2 (D100). As a result, the protocol was amended and the dose of docetaxel was reduced to 75 mg/m^2 (D75) in the second half of the study. The two dose levels of docetaxel were analyzed together in the primary analysis. Patients randomized to docetaxel could continue to receive chemotherapy until disease progression was documented, or there was unacceptable toxicity.

There were 204 patients randomized on the trial (BSC = 100; D100 = 49; D75 = 55). Baseline characteristics were generally well balanced between the groups. The TAX 317

TABLE 46.1 Major Advances in Second-Line Treatment of NSCLC over the Past Decade and a Half

Year	Advance
1995	Metaanalysis showed first-line therapy improves survival[1]
2000	Docetaxel shown to improve survival in two randomized phase III trials[6,7]
2004	Pemetrexed shown to be noninferior to docetaxel[27]
2005	Erlotinib shown to improve survival in second- and third-line setting[52]
2007	Gefitinib shown to be noninferior to docetaxel[60]

trial demonstrated that docetaxel significantly improved survival compared to BSC, in patients who had received prior platinum containing chemotherapy ($p = 0.047$). The median and 1-year survival for patients randomized to docetaxel were 7 months (95% confidence interval [CI], 5.5 to 9.0) and 29%, respectively, compared with 4.6 months (95% CI, 3.7 to 6.0) and 19% for patients randomized to BSC (Fig. 46.1). The magnitude of this difference was slightly greater for patients randomized during the second phase of the trial to D75 or BSC (7.5 vs. 4.6; 1-year survival = 37% vs. 12%, $p = 0.01$).

Hematological toxicities occurred commonly in patients receiving docetaxel. Grade 3 or 4 neutropenia was seen in 76% of patients, with febrile neutropenia occurring in 11.5% of patients overall, but only 1.8% of patients in the 75-mg/m^2 group. Nearly 11% of patients had grade 3 or 4 anemia, but interestingly, a similar rate was observed among BSC patients. The predominant nonhematological toxicities occurring in the docetaxel group included asthenia, fever, infection, diarrhea, fluid retention, nausea, stomatitis, and neurologic. However, asthenia and infection were common adverse effects in the BSC group as well.

Supportive evidence that docetaxel is an effective second-line therapy for patients with NSCLC comes from the TAX 320 trial reported by Fossella et al.[7] In this trial, patients were randomized to receive D100, D75, or a control arm (vinorelbine/ifosfamide [V/I]) of either ifosfamide (2 gm/m^2 days 1 to 3 every 21 days) or vinorelbine (30 mg/m^2 day 1, 8, and 15 every 21 days). In the docetaxel 100-mg/m^2 group, granulocyte colony-stimulating factor (G-CSF) was used in subsequent cycles to manage prolonged neutropenia, or febrile neutropenia. As in the Tax 317 trial, participants could have received one or more prior therapy and the trial included patients with PS 0 to 2. However, unlike the trial by Shepherd et al.[6] participants could have received prior paclitaxel. QOL was measured using the Lung Cancer Symptom Scale.

TABLE 46.2 Summary of Trials of Second-Line Chemotherapy: Baseline Characteristics

Reference	Treatment	Number of Patients	Treatment Line 2nd/3+	Prior Platinum	Prior Taxane	PD with Prior CT	Stage III/IV (%)	PS 0-1 / 2	Response Rate OR/SD/PD	TTP	Median Survival	1-Year Survival	Overall Survival *p* Value
Shepherd et al.[6]	Docetaxel 100 or 75	104	74/26	100	0	18	23/77	76/24	5.8/43/33*	10.6 wk	7.0 mo	29%	0.047
	BSC	100	76/24	100	0	20	19/81	75/25	NA	6.7 wk	4.6 mo	19%	
Fossella et al.[7]	Doc 100	125	65/35	100	31	33	14/86	83/17	10.8/33/56	8.4 wk	5.5 mo	21%	>0.05
	Doc 75	125	74/26	100	42	24	10/90	82/18	6.7/36/57	8.5 wk	5.7 mo	32%	
	Vin/Ifos	122	71/29	100	41	32	9/91	85/15	0.8/31/68	7.9 wk	5.6 mo	19%	
Hanna[27]	Docetaxel	288	100	90	28	31	25/75	88/12	8.8/46/45	3.5 mo	7.9 mo	29.7%	>0.05
	Pemetrexed	283	100	93	26	27	25/75	89/11	9.1/46/45	3.4 mo	8.3 mo	29.7%	
Cullen et al.[32]	Pem 500	295	100	100	NR	NR	23/77	87/13	7.1/51/36	2.6 mo	6.7 mo	NR	0.893
	Pem 900	293	100	100			23/77	88/12	4.3/53/37	2.8 mo	6.9 mo		
Ramlau et al.[33]	Docetaxel	415	100	98	0	NR	28/72	84/16	5/36/44*	13 wk	31 wk	29%	0.0568
	Topotecan	414	100	95	0		26/74	86/14	5/27/49	11 wk	28 wk	25%	
Krzakowski et al.[35]	Docetaxel	277	100	100	21	NR	25/60	88/12	5.5/40/51	2.3 mo	7.2 mo	NR	0.96
	Vinflunine	274	100	100	20	NR	24/61	89/11	4.4/36/49	2.3 mo	6.7 mo	NR	

*May not total 100% as the trial allowed patients with non-measurable disease.

BSC, best supportive care; CT, chemotherapy; Doc, docetaxel; Ifos, ifosphamide; NA, not applicable; NR, not recorded; OR, objective response; PD, progressive disease; Pem, pemetrexed; PS, performance status; SD, stable disease; TTP, time to progression; Vin, vinorelbine.

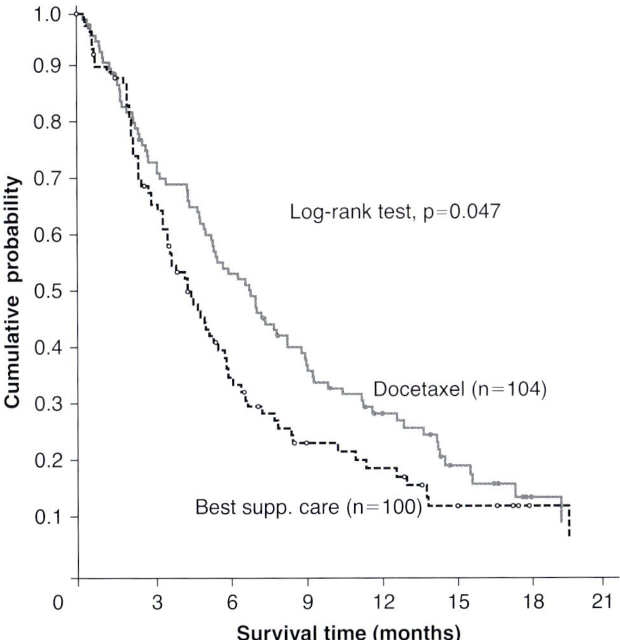

FIGURE 46.1 Overall survival of docetaxel versus best supportive care (BSC; Tax 317). (From Shepherd FA, Dancey J, Ramlau R, et al. Prospective randomized trial of docetaxel versus BSC in patients with non-small-cell lung cancer previously treated with platinum-based chemotherapy. *J Clinic Oncol* 2000;18[10]:2095–2103.)

A total of 373 patients were randomized (D75 = 125; D100 = 125, V/I = 123). Compared to TAX 317, the patients were more heavily pretreated. A greater number of patients had received two or more prior chemotherapy regimens and more patients had disease progression as the best response to their last therapy. Between 31% and 42% of patients had received prior paclitaxel. Patients in the D75 group received more cycles of chemotherapy than those in the D100 group (median number of cycles 10 vs. 6). Both docetaxel groups had a significantly higher response rate than the V/I group (D100 = 10.8%, $p = 0.001$; D75 = 6.7%, $p = 0.036$; V/I = 0.8%). The response rate for patients who received prior paclitaxel was similar to the response rate for all patients. The median time to progression was similar among the three groups. However, progression-free survival (PFS) at 26 weeks favored the docetaxel groups (D100 = 19%, $p = 0.013$; D75 = 17%, $p = 0.031$; V/I = 8%). There were no significant differences in overall survival (median survival D100 = 5.5 months; D75 = 5.7 months; V/I = 5.6 months). However, there was a significant improvement in 1-year survival rate for the D75 group (D100 = 21%; D75 = 32%, $p = 0.025$; V/I = 19%). The observed toxicity was similar to that seen in the TAX 317 trial.

QOL was assessed in both TAX 317 and TAX 320,[8,9] with the results demonstrating improvements in symptom scales in patients randomized to docetaxel. Dancey et al.[8] reported a significant improvement in pain scores favoring docetaxel over BSC. Trends were also noted in favor of docetaxel for overall LCSS score, fatigue, and appetite. Mean overall QOL scores declined less in the docetaxel group than the BSC group.

These two landmark studies established the survival and QOL benefit from second-line chemotherapy with docetaxel for patients with NSCLC. These data are reflected in the 2003 updated ASCO guidelines for the treatment of unresectable NSCLC, which now recommend the use of docetaxel as second-line therapy for patients with adequate PS who have progressed following platinum-based chemotherapy.[10] Increasingly though, the decision to implement treatment guidelines has incorporated economic arguments in addition to data on therapeutic efficacy. As such, Leighl et al.[11] performed an economic evaluation of the TAX 317 trial to determine the cost-effectiveness of docetaxel versus BSC in the Canadian environment. Costs were determined from resource utilization for patients entered on the trial from one tertiary academic center. Given the short survival overall for this group of patients, discounting was not employed. Efficacy data were taken from the overall trial results. The incremental cost of docetaxel was $57,749 per life year gained. However, the cost-effectiveness of D75 was only $31,776 per life year gained. In comparison to other health interventions, this is within a range of expenditure generally considered reasonable.

WHAT ARE THE APPROPRIATE DOSE AND SCHEDULE OF ADMINISTRATION OF DOCETAXEL?

The trials by Shepherd et al.[6] and Fossella et al.[7] established D75 administered every 21 days as the standard of care for second-line therapy for NSCLC. Over recent years, various investigators have explored alternate schedules of docetaxel in an attempt to improve the therapeutic ratio (Table 46.3). Nonrandomized comparisons of D100 and D75 in the TAX 317 trial showed no difference in efficacy and significantly more toxicity.[6] Quiox et al.[12] evaluated this question in a randomized phase II trial. Patients were randomized to D75 (n = 94) or D100 (n = 89). The response rate (7.4% vs. 7.6%) was similar as was the rate of disease control (45.7% vs. 57%). There were no significant differences in time to progression (D75 = 1.5 months; 95% CI, 1.3 to 2.0 months vs. D100 = 2.1 months; 95% CI, 1.3 to 2.7 months), or overall survival (D75 = 4.7 months; 95% CI, 3.8 to 5.9 months vs. D100 = 6.7 months; 95% CI, 4.8 to 7.1 months). More grade 3 and 4 neutropenia (72.7% vs. 44%) and asthenia (19.1% vs. 8.6%) were observed with the higher dose of docetaxel. However, there was no difference in the rate of febrile neutropenia (6.8% vs. 6.7%). The rates of other nonhematological toxicities were similar between the two groups. The authors conclude that D75 every 3 weeks is the preferred dose because of a more favorable toxicity profile.

TABLE 46.3 Trials Comparing Alternate Doses and Schedules of Docetaxel

Reference	N	Treatment (dose in mg/m²)	Response Rate OR/SD/PD (%)	TTP	Median Survival	1-Year Survival	Overall Survival *p* Value
Fossella et al.[7]	125	Doc 75	6.7/36/57	8.5 wk	5.7 mo	32%	NA
	125	Doc 100	10.8/33/56	8.4 wk	5.5 mo	21%	
Quoix et al.[12]	94	Doc 75	8.6/37/54	1.5 mo	4.7 mo	NR	>0.05
	89	Doc 100	7.6/49/43	2.1 mo	6.7 mo		
Schuette et al.[23]	107	Doc 75	12.6/38/45	3.4 mo	6.3 mo	27%	0.07
	108	Doc 35 D1, 8,15 q28d	10.5/33/46	3.3 mo	9.3 mo	39%	
Camps et al.[19]	129	Doc 75	9.3/34/48	2.7 mo	6.6 mo	27%	0.076
	125	Doc 36 q1w × 6 q8w	8.4/27/51	2.9 mo	5.4 mo	22%	
Gridelli et al.[22]	110	Doc 75	2.7/NR/NR	NR	29 wk	21%	0.80
	110	Doc 33.3 q1w × 6 q8w	5.5/ NR/NR		25 wk	31%	
Gervais et al.[21]	62	Doc 75	4.8/28/67	2.1 mo	5.8 mo	18%	>0.05
	63	Doc 40 q1w × 6 q8w	3.2/22/76	1.8 mo	5.5 mo	6%	
Chen et al.[20]	33	Doc 75	6.1/54/33	2.8 mo	9.5 mo	29%	0.437
	64	Doc 35 D1,8,15 q4w	17.2/50/25	4.2 mo	8.4 mo	33%	
	64	Doc 40 D1,8 q3w	10.9/53/33	3.5 mo	7.2 mo	32%	

Doc 33, Docetaxel 33.3 mg/m² weekly for 6 weeks followed by 2-week rest; Doc 35, Docetaxel 35 mg/m² days 1,8,15, every 28 days; Doc 36, Docetaxel 36 mg/m² weekly for 6 weeks followed by 2-week rest; Doc 40, Docetaxel 40 mg/m² days 1 and 8 every 21 days, or weekly for 6 weeks followed by 2-week rest; Doc 75, Docetaxel 75 mg/m² day 1 every 21 days; NA, not applicable; NR, not recorded; OR, objective response; PD, progressive disease; SD, stable disease; TTP, time to progression.

Some variation exists in the dose of docetaxel. In Japan, the dose of docetaxel routinely used is 60 mg/m² every 3 weeks. This is based on data from a phase I clinical trial in which the maximum tolerated dose of docetaxel was found to be 70 mg/m² every 3 weeks.[13] As a result several Japanese phase II trials evaluated docetaxel at a dose of 60 mg/m².[14–16] Response rates, survival, and toxicity all appear comparable to the observed efficacy of docetaxel at a dose of 75 mg/m² every 3 weeks in western populations. It is postulated that pharmacogenomic differences may exist between Japanese and North American populations to account for this difference.[17,18]

Five trials have evaluated docetaxel given in a weekly schedule versus the standard three weekly schedule.[19–23] Di Maio et al.[24] recently published an individual patient metaanalysis of these trials.[24] The five trials randomized 865 patients to three weekly docetaxel (n = 433), or a weekly schedule (n = 432). Doses of docetaxel, in the weekly schedule, ranged from 33.3 mg/m² to 40 mg/m² weekly, either for 6 weeks followed by a 2-week rest, or for 3 weeks followed by a 1-week rest. There was no difference in survival between the two schedules of docetaxel (hazard ratio [HR] = 1.09; 95% CI, 0.94 to 1.26). The median survival for patients treated with three weekly docetaxel was 27.4 weeks compared with 26.1 weeks for patients treated with a weekly schedule. One- and two-year survival rates were 24.8% versus 27% and 10.3% versus 6.8%, respectively. Response rates were similar between the two groups (8.1% vs. 6.7%; $p = 0.43$). Weekly docetaxel was associated with significantly less grade 3 and 4 neutropenia (18% vs. 5%) and febrile neutropenia (6% vs. <1%). The available data suggest, therefore, that both the three weekly and weekly schedules of docetaxel can be used as second-line therapy for NSCLC. The toxicity advantages of weekly docetaxel may be counterbalanced by the increased frequency of treatment visits and associated increased resource utilization.

ALTERNATIVE CHEMOTHERAPY OPTIONS TO DOCETAXEL

Pemetrexed is a multitargeted antifolate with a broad spectrum of activity. It inhibits thymidine synthase, which is important in pyrimidine synthesis, as well as dihydrofolate reductase and glycinamide ribonucleotide formyltransferase, which are important enzymes in purine synthesis. Phase II trials have demonstrated activity of pemetrexed in NSCLC.[25,26] Based on the phase II activity of pemetrexed, Hanna et al.[27] conducted a randomized phase III trial of second-line therapy in NSCLC comparing pemetrexed to docetaxel.

The JMEI trial randomized patients to a standard arm of D75 every 21 days, or pemetrexed 500 mg/m² every 21 days.[27] Patients on the pemetrexed arm all received vitamin supplementation with folic acid and vitamin B_{12} based on data from a trial of pemetrexed in malignant pleural mesothelioma.[28] Dexamethasone premedication was used in both arms of the trial. Patients were excluded if they had received more than one prior chemotherapy for advanced disease, had prior docetaxel or pemetrexed, weight loss ≥10% in preceding 6 weeks, significant peripheral neuropathy (≥ grade 3), were unable to interrupt nonsteroidal anti-inflammatory drugs, or had uncontrolled pleural effusions (not further defined). The last two criteria relate to concerns about pemetrexed clearance. The study was designed to show that overall survival of patients randomized to pemetrexed was noninferior to that of docetaxel.

Five hundred and seventy-one patients were randomized (pemetrexed 283, docetaxel 288). The groups were well balanced regarding baseline characteristics. No differences were seen in any of the outcomes. The response rates (9.1% vs. 8.8%) and rates of disease stability (45.8% vs. 46.4%) were almost identical for pemetrexed and docetaxel, respectively. Prior paclitaxel therapy did not predict for any differential response. There were no differences in the PFS of pemetrexed compared with docetaxel (median PFS = 2.9 months vs. 2.9 months; HR = 0.97; 95% CI, 0.82 to 1.16). Median survival (8.3 months vs. 7.9 months) and 1-year survival (29.7% vs. 29.7%) of patients randomized to pemetrexed was not statistically different to that of docetaxel (HR = 0.99; 95% CI, 0.8 to 1.20; Fig. 46.2). The assumption of noninferiority was assessed using two methods. Using the percent retention method, the trial met its primary outcome of noninferiority. The alternate method of noninferiority defined pemetrexed as ≤10% worse than docetaxel. The trial did not meet this outcome of noninferiority as the upper limit of the 95% CI exceeded an HR of 1.11. Although this has created issues with some regulatory authorities, pemetrexed is generally considered to be an equally effective alternative to docetaxel as second-line therapy for NSCLC.

Although there were no differences in any of the efficacy parameters, there were some differences observed between the toxicities of pemetrexed compared with docetaxel. There was more hematological toxicity in patients receiving docetaxel compared with pemetrexed, and the rates of grade 3 and 4 neutropenia (40.2% vs. 5.3%) and febrile neutropenia (12.7% vs. 1.9%) were significantly higher in the docetaxel group. This resulted in a higher rate of hospitalization and G-CSF use. There were differences in nonhematological toxicities as well with more alopecia (37.7% vs. 6.4%), diarrhea (24.3% vs. 12.8%), and neurosensory toxicity (15.9% vs. 4.9%) among patients receiving docetaxel, but more nausea (16.7% vs. 30.9%), rash (6.2% vs. 14%), and liver enzyme abnormalities (1.4% vs. 7.9%) among patients receiving pemetrexed. Interestingly, despite these differences in toxicity, there were no differences in QOL between the two treatment groups.

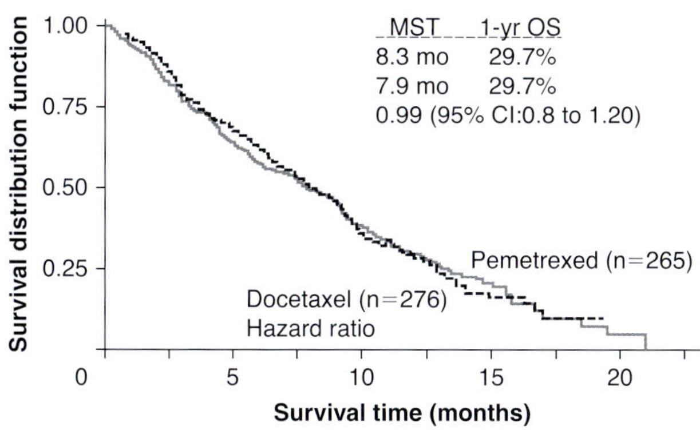

Pts at risk					
Pemetrexed	283	189	78	16	0
Docetaxel	288	177	78	19	1

FIGURE 46.2 Overall survival of docetaxel versus pemetrexed (JMEI). (From Hanna N, Shepherd FA, Fossella FV, et al. Randomized phase III trial of pemetrexed versus docetaxel in patients with non-small-cell lung cancer previously treated with chemotherapy. *J Clin Oncol* 2004;22[9]:1589–1597.)

A retrospective analysis of this trial was undertaken to explore predictors of survival for patients in the second-line setting.[29] In univariate analyses, the following variables demonstrated associations with survival: sex (females = 9.4 months vs. males = 7.2 months, p = 0.001); stage at diagnosis (stage III = 9.5 months vs. stage IV = 7.8 months, p = 0.036); histology (adenocarcinoma = 9.1 months vs. squamous carcinoma = 6.5 months vs. other = 7.8 months, p = 0.004); PS (PS 0 = 12.7 months vs. PS 1 = 8.3 months vs. PS 2 = 2.6 months, p <0.001); best response to prior therapy (complete response [CR]/partial response [PR] = 15.8 months vs. stable disease [SD] = 10.5 months vs. progressive disease [PD] = 4.6 months, p <0.001); time from first-line to second-line therapy (≤3 months = 6.9 months vs. 3 to 6 months = 9.2 months vs. ≥6 months = 9.3 months, p = 0.001); and first-line regimen (platinum-gemcitabine = 9.1 months vs. platinum-taxane = 7.4 months vs. other = 7.8 months, p = 0.63). The authors conclude that these variables should be used as stratification variables in future randomized trials. However, given the retrospective nature of these analyses, these variables should not be used to select between docetaxel and pemetrexed.

A further retrospective analysis of the JMEI trial suggested that there may be a difference in the effectiveness of pemetrexed compared with docetaxel based on histology.[30] Previous research has suggested thymidine synthase expression may be higher in squamous carcinoma compared with other histological subtypes.[31] This is postulated to reduce the sensitivity of squamous carcinoma to pemetrexed. Peterson et al.[30] reported that survival of patients with squamous carcinoma treated with pemetrexed was less than that of patients treated with docetaxel (6.2 months vs. 7.4 months; HR = 1.563; 95% CI, 1.079 to 2.264). Interestingly, they also observed an improvement in survival for patients with nonsquamous histology treated with pemetrexed (9.3 months vs. 8.0 months; HR = 0.778; 95% CI, 0.607 to 0.997).

As a result of the JMEI trial, pemetrexed is considered a reasonable option to docetaxel for second-line therapy of metastatic NSCLC. It is considered to be a less toxic chemotherapy option than docetaxel by many physicians. It is unclear whether histology should be used to select between pemetrexed and docetaxel. However, there are substantial cost differences between the two agents. There are no published economic analyses comparing pemetrexed to docetaxel, but economic considerations should be considered in the choice of second-line chemotherapy.

The maximum tolerated dose of pemetrexed was established prior to the routine implementation of supplementation with vitamin B_{12} and folic acid. As a result of the routine use of vitamin supplementation, it became apparent that the dose of pemetrexed could be increased beyond 500 mg/m^2. Cullen et al.[32] undertook a randomized trial comparing a standard dose of pemetrexed with pemetrexed 900 mg/m^2. A total of 588 patients were randomized (pemetrexed 500 = 295, pemetrexed 900 = 293). Escalating the dose of pemetrexed did not result in any improvement in efficacy. The median survival for patients randomized to pemetrexed 500 mg/m^2 was similar to that of pemetrexed 900 mg/m^2 (6.7 months vs. 6.9 months; HR = 1.013; 95% CI, 0.837 to 1.226). There were no differences in time to progression (2.6 months vs. 2.8 months), or response rate (7.1% vs. 4.3%). Patients receiving the higher dose of pemetrexed received slightly fewer cycles of treatment (mean 4.3 cycles vs. 3.5 cycles) and required more dose reductions (4.2% vs. 1.1%). There was more grade 3 and 4 neutropenia (7.9% vs. 3.4%), anemia (5.8% vs. 4.5%), thrombocytopenia (5.4% vs. 2.8%), and elevated aspartate aminotransferase (AST) (1.3% vs. 0%) among patients randomized to the higher dose of pemetrexed. Based on these data, the standard dose of pemetrexed should remain 500 mg/m^2 every 3 weeks.

Another chemotherapeutic agent that has been evaluated as second-line therapy for NSCLC is oral topotecan.[33] A phase II trial of oral topotecan demonstrated response and survival data consistent with docetaxel.[34] Based on these data, Ramlau et al.[33] conducted a randomized trial of oral topotecan 2.3 mg/m^2 day 1 to 5 every 21 days versus D75. Dose escalation in subsequent cycles of topotecan was allowed in the absence of any grade 3 toxicity. The design of this trial was similar to that of other second-line chemotherapy trials except that patients who had received prior taxane were excluded. The trial had a noninferiority design assuming that the 1-year survival of oral topotecan was ≤10% worse than docetaxel. A total of 414 patients were randomized to receive topotecan and 415 to receive docetaxel. The objective response rate for both groups was 5%. The study met its primary outcome of noninferiority as the difference in 1-year survival was −3.6% (95% CI, 9.6% to 2.5%). However, there was a trend toward improved overall survival in favor of docetaxel (log rank p = 0.0568). Furthermore, after adjustment for stratification variables, there was a significant improvement in survival for patients randomized to docetaxel (HR = 1.23; 95% CI, 1.06 to 1.44).

The available data suggest that oral topotecan may not be as effective as docetaxel. Despite demonstrating noninferiority in 1-year survival, trends in the overall survival favor docetaxel. Although the option of an oral agent has appeal, the efficacy concerns preclude widespread adoption of oral topotecan as second-line chemotherapy for NSCLC.

One additional trial compared second-line vinflunine, a vinca alkaloid, with docetaxel.[35] Vinflunine was administered at a dose of 320 mg/m^2 intravenously every 3 weeks, compared with D75 every 3 weeks. The trial was designed to show the PFS of vinflunine was noninferior to docetaxel (lower limit of 95% CI HR >0.755). All patients had received prior platinum-based chemotherapy and were stratified for type of prior chemotherapy (vinka alkaloid vs. paclitaxel vs. other), PS (0/1 vs. 2), and stage at diagnosis (IIIB vs. IV vs. other). Baseline characteristics were well balanced.

A total of 551 patients were randomized (vinflunine 274, docetaxel 277). The trial met its primary outcome of noninferiority for PFS of vinflunine compared with docetaxel (2.3 months vs. 2.3 months; HR = 1.004; 95% CI, 0.841 to 1.199; p = 0.965). There were no differences between vinflunine and docetaxel in response rates (4.4% vs. 5.5%), or overall survival (6.7 months vs. 7.2 months; HR = 0.973; 95% CI, 0.805 to 1.176). There were differences observed in toxicity between the two arms. Patients randomized to vinflunine had more anemia, neutropenia, nausea, abdominal pain, and constipation, but less alopecia, nail changes, edema, and diarrhea than patients randomized to docetaxel. Although vinflunine provides another choice of second-line chemotherapy for NSCLC, its toxicity profile does not offer any clear advantages over existing second-line options, and it is unlikely to have a major impact on practice.

COMBINATION CHEMOTHERAPY IN THE SECOND-LINE SETTING

In the *first-line* treatment of metastatic NSCLC, multiple trials have examined two-drug combinations versus single-agent chemotherapy. Metaanalyses of these trials demonstrate that the addition of a second agent improves response rates and overall survival.[36,37] Given these data, several investigators have evaluated the addition of a second chemotherapy drug for second-line therapy in NSCLC (Table 46.4).[38–43] As a rule, these trials have failed to demonstrate superiority of a two-drug combination over docetaxel.

Irinotecan combinations have been evaluated in five trials.[39–43] Two randomized phase II trials evaluated the addition of irinotecan to docetaxel.[42,43] Wachters et al.[43] randomized patients to receive D75, or docetaxel 60 mg/m^2 and irinotecan 200 mg/m^2 day 1 followed by lenograstim 150 mg/m^2 day 2 to 12, every 21 days. Pectasides et al.[42] used the standard schedule of docetaxel compared with docetaxel 30 mg/m^2 and irinotecan 60 mg/m^2 both on days 1 and 8, every 21 days. Neither trial showed an advantage to the combination arm. There were no differences in response, time to progression, or overall survival. Furthermore, both trials showed additional toxicity from the addition of irinotecan. This was predominantly more diarrhea in the combination arm. Therefore, the addition of irinotecan to docetaxel does not improve the therapeutic ratio of docetaxel and cannot be recommended.

TABLE 46.4 Trials Evaluating Combination Second-Line Therapy in NSCLC

Reference	N	Treatment	Response Rate OR/SD/PD (%)	TTP	Median Survival	1-Year Survival	Overall Survival *p* Value
Wachters et al.[43]*	56	Docetaxel	16/45/36	18 wk	32 wk	26%	0.49
	52	Docetaxel + irinotecan	10/42/35	15 wk	27 wk	30%	
Pectasides et al.[42]†	65	Docetaxel	14/35/NR	5.6 mo	6.5 mo	37%	0.49
	66	Docetaxel + irinotecan	20/37NR	4.8 mo	6.4 mo	34%	
Georgoulias et al.[40]‡	75	Irinotecan	4.2/25/70	5 mo	7 mo	29%	0.589
	79	Irinotecan + gemcitabine	18.4/26/55	7.5 mo	9 mo	24%	
Georgoulias et al.[39]§	73	Cisplatin	7/29/63	2.1 mo	8.8 mo	32%	0.934
	74	Cisplatin + irinotecan	22/15/62	2.6 mo	7.8 mo	34%	
Lilenbaum et al.[41]ll	34	ID + CBX	2.9/25/46	NR	6.4 mo	20%	>0.05
	35	ID	6.3/20/52		8.8 mo	41%	
	33	IG + CBX	3/21/52		6.3 mo	24%	
	31	IG	6/24/46		9 mo	36%	
Takeda et al.[44]¶	65	Docetaxel	NR	2.1 mo	10.1 mo	38%	0.69
	65	Docetaxel + gemcitabine		3.1 mo	11.3 mo	47%	
Fannucchi et al.[38]#	75	Bortezomib	8/21/56	1.5 mo	7.4 mo	39%	>0.05
	80	Bortezomib + docetaxel	9/45/35	4 mo	7.8 mo	33%	

*Docetaxel 75 mg/m^2 vs. Docetaxel 60 mg/m^2 + Irinotecan 200 mg/m^2 day 1 every 21 days.

†Docetaxel 75 mg/m^2 vs. Docetaxel 30 mg/m^2 + Irinotecan 60 mg/m^2 day 1 and 8 every 21 days.

‡Irinotecan 300 mg/m^2 day 1 every 21 days vs. Irinotecan 300 mg/m^2 day 1 + gemcitabine 1000 mg/m^2 day 1 and 8 every 21 days.

§Cisplatin 80 mg/m^2 day 1 vs. Cisplatin 80 mg/m^2 day 1 + Irinotecan 100 mg/m^2 day 1 and 8 every 21 days.

llIrinotecan 60 mg/m^2 + docetaxel 35 mg/m^2 day 1 and 8 vs. Irinotecan 100 mg/m^2 + gemcitabine 1000 mg/m^2 day 1 and 8 every 21 days ± celecoxib 400 mg bid.

¶Docetaxel 60 mg/m^2 vs. Docetaxel 60 mg/m^2 + gemcitabine 800 mg/m^2.

#Bortezomib 1.5 mg/m^2 days 1, 4, 8, & 11 vs. Bortezomib 1.3 mg/m^2 days 1, 4, 8, and 11 + docetaxel 75 mg/m^2 day 1 every 21 days.

CBX, celecoxib; ID, irinotecan docetaxel; IG, irinotecan gemcitabine; NR, not recorded; OR, objective response; PD, progressive disease; SD, stable disease; TTP, time to progression.

One randomized trial of first-line therapy for NSCLC showed marginal superiority for a docetaxel and cisplatin combination.[2] Therefore, in some parts of the world, docetaxel is routinely used in first-line chemotherapy combinations. The Helenic Oncology Research Group (HORG) has conducted two trials of second-line chemotherapy combinations in patients previously treated with docetaxel.[39,40] One trial randomized patients previously treated with cisplatin and docetaxel to receive irinotecan and gemcitabine, or irinotecan alone.[40] The second trial randomized patients previously treated with a taxane and gemcitabine to receive irinotecan and cisplatin, or irinotecan alone.[39] Gemcitabine plus irinotecan resulted in a significantly higher response rate than irinotecan alone. However, there was no improvement in survival in the combination arm of either trial. Neither of these trials included a control arm previously demonstrated to improve survival in the second-line setting; therefore, they do not add to the available second-line chemotherapy options for NSCLC.

In a phase II study, Lilenbaum et al.[41] randomized patients to receive docetaxel and irinotecan, or gemcitabine and irinotecan, with or without celecoxib. Survival in patients randomized to chemotherapy plus celecoxib was numerically *inferior* to chemotherapy alone (median 8.99 vs. 6.31 months, 1-year survival 36% vs. 24%). Survival in both the chemotherapy combination arms was similar to that expected from single-agent docetaxel or pemetrexed, suggesting little incremental benefit from the addition of irinotecan. Takeda et al.[44] evaluated the addition of gemcitabine to docetaxel in Japanese patients. They observed a high rate of interstitial lung disease (ILD) in the combination arm, with a 5% death rate from ILD. There was a slight numeric advantage for the combination arm in both response rate and overall survival, but this appeared to be too toxic a regimen to evaluate further in this population.

One additional trial evaluated the proteosome inhibitor bortezomib.[38] This trial randomized patients to bortezomib 1.5 mg/m^2 days 1, 4, 8, and 11, every 21 days versus D75 and bortezomib 1.3 mg/m^2 days 1, 4, 8, and 11, every 21 days. One hundred and fifty-five patients were included (bortezomib = 75, docetaxel and bortezomib = 80). Response rates were similar (8% vs. 9%), but there was a longer median time to progression for patients receiving the combination of bortezomib plus docetaxel (4.0 months vs. 1.5 months). Overall survival for the two groups was similar (median 7.8 vs. 7.4 months; 1-year survival 33.1% vs. 38.7%). There was more hematological toxicity associated with the combination arm, but the rate of nonhematological toxicity was similar between the groups. It is difficult to comment about the role of bortezomib as a second-line treatment option for NSCLC as this trial did not include a standard arm of docetaxel alone. However, the results for the combination arm are similar to that expected from docetaxel alone, suggesting that bortezomib does not add significantly to the therapeutic efficacy of docetaxel. Therefore, for the present time, bortezomib remains an investigational treatment for NSCLC.

WHAT IS THE ROLE OF EPIDERMAL GROWTH FACTOR RECEPTOR INHIBITORS AS SECOND-LINE THERAPY?

The trials described previously demonstrate a modest improvement in survival from second-line chemotherapy. Although second-line therapy with either docetaxel or pemetrexed improves outcomes for patients with NSCLC, there remains a need for additional treatment options for this group of patients. A greater understanding of the molecular abnormalities associated with NSCLC has led to the evaluation of new therapeutic targets for NSCLC. The EGFR is one targeted commonly overexpressed in NSCLC.[45–47] Early phase clinical trials showed that receptor tyrosine kinase inhibitors (TKIs) of the EGFR such as gefitinib and erlotinib had antitumor activity, and this prompted further evaluation in advanced NSCLC (Table 46.5) (see Chapter 49).[48]

Two randomized phase II trials were undertaken comparing two dose levels of gefitinib (250 vs. 500 mg daily) in patients considered not to be candidates for further chemotherapy.[49,50] The Iressa Dose Evaluation in Advanced Lung Cancer (IDEAL) 1 trial was conducted in Japan, Europe, South Africa, and Australia,[49] whereas the IDEAL 2 trial was

TABLE 46.5 Summary of Trials Evaluating Targeted Agents in Second-Line Therapy

Reference	Treatment	Number of Patients	Treatment Line 2nd/3+ (%)	Prior Platinum	Prior Taxane	PD with Prior CT	Stage III/IV (%)	PS 0-1/2	Response Rate OR/SD/PD	TTP	Median Survival	1-Year Survival	Overall Survival *p* Value
Fukuoka et al.[49]	Gefitinib 250	104	66/44	100	NR	NR	22/88	88/12	18.4/36/41	2.7 mo	7.6 mo	35%	>0.05
	Gefitinib 500	106	67/33	100			17/83	87/13	19/32/42	2.8 mo	8 mo	29%	
Kris et al.[50]	Gefitinib 250	102	0/100	100	NR	NR	15/85	81/19	12/-/-	NR	7 mo	27%	0.54
	Gefitinib 500	114	0/100	100			8/92	80/20	9/-/-		6 mo	24%	
Shepherd et al.[52]	Erlotinib	488	51/49	92	NR	28	NR	66/34*	8.9/36/45	2.2 mo	6.7 mo	31	<0.001
	BSC	243	50/50	91		28		68/32*	NA/27/57	1.8 mo	4.7 mo	21	
Thatcher et al.[54]	Gefitinib	1129	49/51	96	27	38	21/79	49/51†	8/32/37	3 mo	5.6 mo	27%	0.087
	BSC	563	49/51	96	28	40	20/80	49/51†	1/31/48	2.6 mo	5.1 mo	21%	
Cufer et al.[59]	Docetaxel	73	98/2	96	0	NR	NR	71/29	13.7/45/15	3.4 mo	7.1 mo	NR	0.88
	Gefitinib	68	97/3	91	0			63/37	13.2/50/19	3 mo	7.5 mo		
Niho et al.[61]	Docetaxel	244	82/17	100	NR	15	20/80	96/4	12.8/21/66	2 mo	14 mo	54	0.33
	Gefitinib	245	87/13	100		17	19/81	96/4	22.5/12/66	2 mo	11.5 mo	48%	
Douillard et al.[60]	Docetaxel	733	83/17	100	18	25	13/87	88/12	7.6/NR/NR	2.7 mo	8 mo	34%	>0.05
	Gefitinib	733	84/16	100	19	26	14/86	88/12	9.1/NR/NR	2.2 mo	7.6 mo	32%	
Herbst et al.[67]‡	Chemo	41	100	100	NR	37	NR	98/2	12.2/27/61	3 mo	8.6 mo	33%	>0.05
	Chemo + bevacizumab	40	100	100		18		100/0	12.5/40/48	4.8 mo	12.6 mo	54%	
	Erlotinib + bevacizumab	39	100	100		33		100/0	17.9/33/49	4.4 mo	13.7 mo	57%	
Heymach et al.[68]	Docetaxel	41	100	100	NR	NR	31/69	100	12/44/37	12 wk	13.4 mo	NR	>0.05
	Docetaxel + vandetanib 100	42	100	100			31/69	100	26/57/10	18.7 wk	13.1 mo		
	Docetaxel + vandetanib 300	44	100	100			21/79	100	18/45/27	17 wk	7.9 mo		

*Includes PS 3 patients (8.6% in each arm).

†Includes PS 3 patients (1% in each arm).

‡Chemotherapy could be either docetaxel or pemetrexed at investigators discretion.

NR, not recorded; OR, objective response; PD, progressive disease; SD, stable disease; TTP, time to progression.

conducted primarily in the United States.[50] Very similar results were observed in both trials. There were no differences in the response rates for the 250- and 500-mg doses. Disease control rates as high as 54% were observed, and approximately 40% of patients demonstrated improvement in disease-related symptoms. The most significant improvements were observed in pulmonary symptoms such as shortness of breath, cough, and chest tightness.[51] The toxicity profile of gefitinib was different to that commonly seen with chemotherapy. The most common side effects included skin rash, pruritis, and diarrhea, but treatment was seldom discontinued for toxicity.

Around this same time, another EGFR TKI, erlotinib, was evaluated as a second- or third-line therapy for NSCLC. This phase III trial, conducted by the National Cancer Institute of Canada Clinical Trials Group (BR.21), randomized patients to erlotinib or placebo.[52] The intent of the trial was to evaluate erlotinib as a third-line treatment option for NSCLC, but also allowed patients who were not candidates for second-line docetaxel. Therefore, patients were eligible if they had received one or two prior chemotherapy regimens if they were not considered eligible for further chemotherapy. A total of 731 patients were randomized in a 2:1 ratio (488 erlotinib, 243 placebo). Approximately 50% of patients had received only one previous therapy prior to trial entry. In general, treatment was well tolerated. The side effects occurring significantly more commonly in the erlotinib arm compared with placebo were rash (76% vs. 17%), diarrhea (55% vs. 19%), anorexia (69% vs. 56%), stomatitis (19% vs. 3%), and infection (34% vs. 21%). The response rate to erlotinib was 8.9%. Erlotinib significantly improved the time to disease progression compared with placebo (2.2 months vs. 1.8 months; HR = 0.61; 95% CI, 0.51 to 0.74). A significant improvement in survival was also observed for patients receiving erlotinib (6.7 months vs. 4.7 months; HR = 0.70; 95% CI, 0.58 to 0.85; Fig. 46.3). Subgroup analyses of these data suggest that there were no subgroups in which a survival benefit was not apparent. The benefit was similar for patients receiving erlotinib as second- or third-line therapy. Additionally, a benefit was seen in patients with poor PS as well as good PS. In a multivariate analysis, variables associated with improved survival in addition to therapy with erlotinib included adenocarcinoma histology, Asian origin and never having smoked.

QOL analyses demonstrate that patients randomized to erlotinib experienced improved QOL compared with the placebo group.[53] QOL was assessed with the European Organisation for Research and Treatment of Cancer (EORTC) QLQ30 and the EORTC QLQ-LC13. The primary QOL analysis examined time to symptom deterioration. Patients randomized to erlotinib had significantly longer time to deterioration in cough (4.9 vs. 3.7 months, $p = 0.04$), dyspnea (4.7 vs. 2.9 months; $p = 0.04$), and pain (2.8 vs. 1.9 months; $p = 0.03$). Statistically significant differences favoring erlotinib were seen for physical functioning, pain, cough, dyspnea, and constipation. Patients achieving an objective response to therapy were more likely to demonstrate QOL improvements.

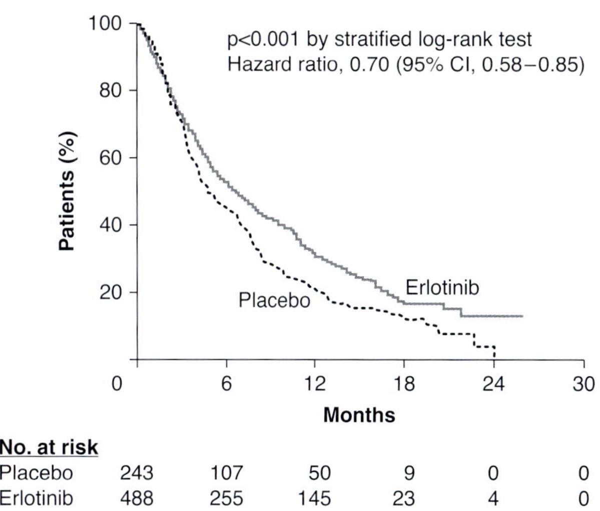

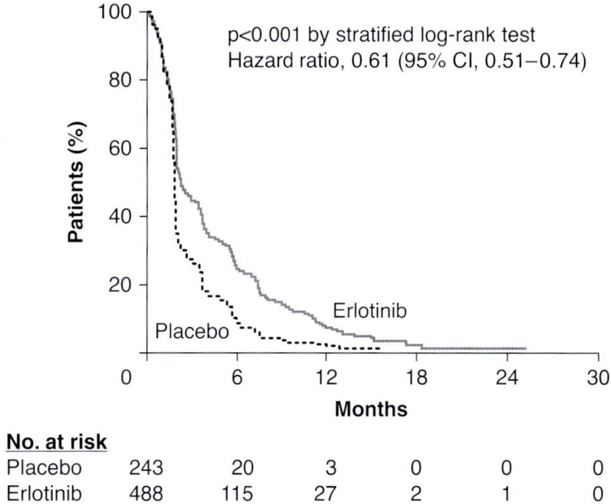

FIGURE 46.3 Overall **(A)** and progression-free **(B)** survival of erlotinib versus best supportive care (NCIC CTG BR.21). (From Shepherd FA, Rodrigues Pereira J, Ciuleanu T, et al. Erlotinib in previously treated non-small-cell lung cancer. *N Engl J Med* 2005;353[2]:123–132.)

The results of the IDEAL 1 and 2 trials resulted in regulatory approval of gefitinib in many countries including the United States. However, the Food and Drug Administration (FDA) requested additional postmarketing studies, including a placebo-controlled randomized trial to assess the survival advantage of gefitinib in the second- and third-line setting. The ISEL trial randomized patients who had received one or two prior chemotherapy regimens to gefitinib 250 mg daily or placebo.[54] The inclusion criteria were similar to the National Cancer Institute of Canada Clinical Trials Group (NCIC CTG) BR.21 trial with the exception that patients were required to be refractory to (progressed within 90 days), or intolerant of their last chemotherapy. ISEL randomized 1692 patients (gefitinib 1129, placebo 563). The trial failed to demonstrate a significant improvement in survival for patients randomized to gefitinib (Fig. 46.4). The median survival for gefitinib was 5.6 months versus 5.1 months for control (HR = 0.89; 95% CI, 0.77 to 1.02). There was a slightly greater benefit in the predefined subpopulation of patients with adenocarcinoma, although this difference still did not achieve statistical significance (HR = 0.84; 95% CI, 0.68 to 1.03). Subgroup analyses did, however, show significant improvements in survival among patients of Asian origin (HR = 0.66; 95% CI, 0.48 to 0.91; p = 0.01)[55] and never-smokers (HR = 0.67; 95% CI, 0.49 to 0.92; p = 0.012).

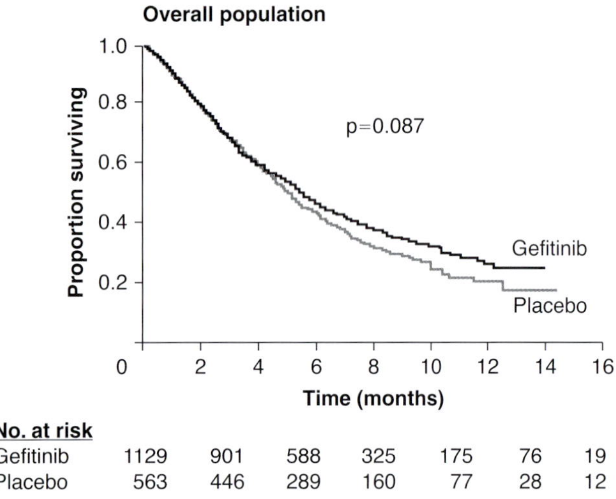

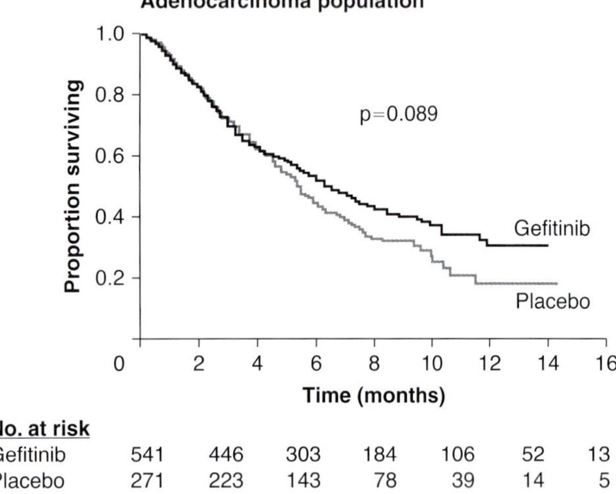

FIGURE 46.4 Survival in overall population and in patients with adenocarcinoma for gefitinib versus best supportive care (ISEL). (From Thatcher N, Chang A, Parikh P, et al. Gefitinib plus best supportive care in previously treated patients with refractory advanced non-small-cell lung cancer: results from a randomised, placebo-controlled, multicentre study [Iressa Survival Evaluation in Lung Cancer]. *Lancet* 2005;366[9496]:1527–1537.)

Different interpretations have been made of results from the ISEL trial. One interpretation is that gefitinib is less effective than erlotinib given it did not improve survival in the second- and third-line setting of NSCLC. Others have suggested that the outcome may have been better had a higher dose of gefitinib been used. However, the results of the two IDEAL trials do not support this hypothesis. An alternative explanation is that the differences in outcomes between the NCIC CTG BR.21 and ISEL trials may have resulted from differences in the inclusion criteria between the two trials. Limiting the ISEL trial to refractory patients only, may have inadvertently selected a group of patients less likely to benefit from any therapeutic intervention. Nevertheless, following release of the ISEL data, several regulatory authorities, including the U.S. FDA modified gefitinib's licence, effectively removing the drug from the market.

Patient and tumor characteristics associated with improved *response* to EGFR TKIs include female gender, adenocarcinoma histology, Asian origin, and absence of smoking history. However, there is not a direct correlation between clinical factors associated with response to treatment and factors associated with improved *survival*, and patients without these characteristics (males, smokers, squamous cell carcinoma) can also respond to EGFR inhibition, as seen in the BR.21.[52] There has also been extensive translational research to better understand the molecular predictors of response and survival in patients treated with EGFR TKIs. This topic is covered in more details in Chapter 49. At the laboratory level, EGFR status, whether defined as EGFR protein expression, *EGFR* gene copy number or *EGFR* mutation status, has been shown to influence response and survival benefit in patients treated with erlotinib and gefitinib.[56–58] More recently, markers of resistance have also been identified including the T790M mutation on *EGFR* exon 20 and the presence of *KRAS* mutations.

In conclusion, erlotinib represents a third option for treatment of NSCLC after failure of platinum-based chemotherapy, and is approved as a second- or third-line therapy in many countries worldwide. It is important to emphasize that in both of the large randomized trials of erlotinib and gefitinib, patients who were treated as second-line therapy were considered unsuitable for further chemotherapy. By definition, this is a more restrictive population of patients that were included in the trial of second-line docetaxel and pemetrexed. Although the magnitude of benefit from erlotinib is similar to that of second-line docetaxel or pemetrexed, there are methodological issues that limit the ability to make direct comparisons between trials with the available data. Direct comparisons are needed to help identify the best way in which to sequence chemotherapy and EGFR TKI therapy and to determine whether it is appropriate to use EGFR TKIs as second-line treatment in patients who are fit for chemotherapy. The selection of patients for therapy based on molecular characteristics awaits prospective biomarker validation trials.

COMPARISON OF SECOND-LINE CHEMOTHERAPY AND EGFR TKI

Several second-line therapy trials comparing an EGFR TKI with docetaxel have recently been reported.[59–61] As a result, the issue of sequencing of therapy following failure of platinum-based chemotherapy is much clearer. Cufer et al.[59] reported the results of a randomized phase II trial comparing D75 with gefitinib 250 mg daily. The SIGN trial was a multicenter trial whose primary outcome evaluated symptom improvement using the Lung Cancer Subscale (LCS) of the Functional Assessment of Cancer Therapy–Lung (FACT-L). Additional outcomes included total scores measured by FACT-L, response rate and overall survival. Patients who received prior taxane therapy were ineligible. A total of 68 patients were randomized to gefitinib and 73 to docetaxel. Compliance in completing QOL questionnaires was more than 85%. Symptom improvement on the LCS was defined as >2 point increase in scores. More patients randomized to gefitinib demonstrated symptom improvement assessed by LCS (38.8% vs. 26%). Similar differences were seen with the overall FACT-L scores. Response rates for gefitinib were similar to docetaxel (13.2% vs. 13.7%), and there were no differences seen in overall survival (median 7.5 months vs. 7.1 months). There were fewer drug-related adverse events for patients receiving gefitinib (51.5% vs. 78.9%).

The SIGN trial suggested that gefitinib was similarly effective and associated with better QOL. However, it was underpowered to make firm conclusions about the relative effectiveness of an EGFR TKI and second-line chemotherapy. Two phase III trials of similar design were reported in 2007.[60,61] The V-15-32[61] trial in Japan and Iressa Non–small cell lung cancer Trial Evaluating REsponse and Survival against Taxotere (INTEREST)[60] trial done internationally were both phase III noninferiority trials comparing gefitinib with docetaxel. In the V-15-32 trial, 489 Japanese patients were randomized to gefitinib 250 mg daily (n = 245) or docetaxel 60 mg/m^2 every 21 days (n = 244). The predefined criterion for noninferiority was an HR ≤1.25. Patients randomized to gefitinib demonstrated a significantly higher response rate (22.5% vs. 12.8%, $p = 0.009$). PFS for gefitinib was similar to docetaxel (2 vs. 2 months; HR = 0.90; 95% CI, 0.72 to 1.12). However, the median survival of docetaxel was 14 months compared with 11.5 months for gefitinib and the trial failed to demonstrate noninferiority in the overall survival of gefitinib compared with docetaxel (HR = 1.12; 95% CI, 0.89 to 1.40). Significantly, more patients randomized to gefitinib demonstrated symptom improvement assessed by FACT-L (23.4% vs. 13.9%; $p = 0.023$). An important distinction in the V-15-32 trial is that there were differences in the rate of further therapy following disease progression. Fifty-three percent of patients randomized to docetaxel received gefitinib at the time of progression, whereas only 36% of patients randomized to gefitinib received docetaxel on progression. This difference may explain the small difference in overall survival observed between the groups.

The INTEREST trial[60] presented at the 2007 IASLC World Conference provides a clearer answer to the question of second-line EGFR TKI or chemotherapy. This trial randomized 1466 patients to receive gefitinib or placebo. The trial was designed to demonstrate that the survival of patients randomized to gefitinib was not inferior to that of docetaxel (HR <1.154). Based on emerging data from translational research, a coprimary outcome was added that gefitinib was superior to docetaxel in patients who had high EGFR gene copy number as measured by fluorescent in situ hybridization (FISH). Baseline characteristics were well matched between the groups. The likelihood of response to therapy was similar for gefitinib and docetaxel (9.1% vs. 7.6%; $p = 0.33$). PFS was also very similar for the two groups (2.2 vs. 2.7 months; HR = 1.04; 95% CI, 0.93 to 1.18). The trial met its primary outcome of noninferiority for survival. The median survival for gefitinib was 7.6 months compared with 8.0 months for docetaxel (HR = 1.02; 95% CI, 0.905 to 1.150). One-year survival was almost identical for the two groups (32% vs. 34%). There was no subgroup in which survival favored gefitinib over docetaxel including patients who were EGFR-FISH positive.

Differences were observed in QOL measures between the two groups. A greater proportion of patients randomized to gefitinib demonstrated improvement in total FACT-L scores (25.1% vs. 14.7%; $p < 0.001$), and the trial outcome index (17.3% vs. 10.3%; $p = 0.0026$). More patients showed improvement in the LCS (20.4% vs. 16.8%; $p = 0.13$) but this did not achieve statistical significance. Patients on gefitinib experienced more rash and diarrhea, whereas patients on docetaxel experienced more hematological toxicity, asthenia, alopecia, and neurotoxicity.

However, INTEREST did not show superiority for gefitinib in the coprimary outcome. EGFR gene copy number was assessed centrally in patients with available tissue. Among patients with high EGFR gene copy number, there were no significant differences between gefitinib and docetaxel patients in PFS (HR = 0.84; 95% CI, 0.59 to 1.19) or overall survival (HR = 1.09; $p = 0.62$). There was no evidence of any differential effect on survival between gefitinib and docetaxel for any of the biomarkers examined (EGFR-FISH, EGFR protein expression, *EGFR* mutations, *KRAS* mutations).

Unlike the V-15-32 trial, the proportion of patients receiving further therapy following progression of their disease was similar between the two groups. Just over half of patients received no further therapy upon progression. Among patients randomized to docetaxel, 37% received an EGFR TKI upon progression and 31% of patients randomized to gefitinib received docetaxel at the time of progression. This balance in subsequent therapy may explain the nearly identical survival in INTEREST in comparison with the Japanese trial.

Based on the results of the INTEREST trial, we now have direct evidence that second-line therapy of NSCLC with an EGFR TKI will result in survival outcomes similar to that achieved with second-line chemotherapy. Available data do not support the use of clinical characteristics (females, adenocarcinoma, Asian origin, never-smokers) to select therapy. The important lesson inferred from the comparison of INTEREST and the Japanese trial is that the sequence of therapy is probably not as important as maximizing the delivery of third-line therapy as well. Therefore, second-line therapy with an EGFR TKI should not be thought of as a means of avoiding further chemotherapy, except for patients whose clinical condition declines to a point where further therapy is unlikely to produce meaningful benefit.

COMBINATIONS OF TARGETED AGENTS WITH CHEMOTHERAPY

Combining EGFR TKIs with chemotherapy in the second-line therapy is not an appealing strategy. Four trials have evaluated either erlotinib or gefitinib in combination with first-line chemotherapy and failed to show any improvement in progression or survival outcomes.[62–65] However, inhibition of VEGF in combination with first-line chemotherapy has shown improvement in survival.[66] Evaluation of this approach is, therefore, also warranted in the second-line treatment of NSCLC. Initial investigation of this approach has shown promise. Two randomized phase II trials have shown improvements in intermediate outcomes.[67,68] Heymach et al.[68] undertook a randomized phase II trial of docetaxel alone, or in combination with two dose levels of vandetanib. Vandetanib is an oral receptor TKI known to inhibit both EGFR and VEGFR. Patients received standard doses of docetaxel, docetaxel plus vandetanib 100 mg daily, or docetaxel plus vandetanib 300 mg daily. One hundred and twenty-seven patients were randomized. Higher response rates were seen with the combination of docetaxel and vandetanib 100 mg (26%) or vandetanib 300 mg (18%) than with docetaxel alone (12%). The primary outcome of this phase II trial was PFS. PFS was longer in the vandetanib 100-mg arm (18.7 weeks) and 300-mg arm (17 weeks) than docetaxel alone (12 weeks). Based on the results of this trial, a randomized phase III trial of docetaxel versus docetaxel plus vandetanib 100 mg daily has been conducted. A total of 1391 patients were randomized (D = 694, DV = 697). There was a significant improvement in response rate (17% vs. 10%; $p < 0.001$) and PFS (HR = 0.79; 97% CI, 0.70–0.90; $p < 0.001$). There was no significant improvement in overall survival (HR = 0.91; 97% CI, 0.78–1.07, $p = 0.20$).[69]

An additional randomized phase II trial has evaluated bevacizumab in combination with second-line therapies. Bevacizumab is a monoclonal antibody against circulating VEGF-A. It has been shown to improve activity of first-line chemotherapy.[66] Herbst et al.[67] conducted a randomized phase II trial of docetaxel alone, docetaxel plus bevacizumab, and erlotinib plus bevacizumab. One hundred and twenty-two patients were randomized. The combination of bevacizumab with docetaxel, or bevacizumab with erlotinib appeared more active than docetaxel alone. The median PFS for docetaxel (3.0 months) was less than docetaxel plus bevacizumab (4.8 months) or erlotinib plus bevacizumab (4.4 months). Similar differences were seen for overall survival (8.6 vs. 12.6 vs. 13.7 months). This trial has also moved on to a confirmatory phase III comparison. The BETA trial randomized patients to erlotinib plus bevacizumab, or erlotinib plus placebo. There were 636 patients randomized. A significant improvement in PFS was observed in favour of the combination therapy (3.4 vs. 1.7 months; $p < 0.0001$; HR = 0.62; 95% CI, 0.52–0.75). However, the results from this trial did not confirm the survival analysis from the randomized phase II trial. No differences were observed in overall survival between the two groups (9.3 months [B + E] vs. 9.2 months [E]; $p = 0.75$; HR = 0.97; 95% CI, 0.80–1.18).[70]

Although the addition of drugs inhibiting VEGF, or VEGFR holds promise for improved efficacy of second-line treatment approaches, these agents have toxicities not typically associated with cytotoxic agents. Common adverse events include hypertension, hemorrhage, fatigue, and diarrhea. As these agents gain greater use in the treatment of NSCLC, oncologists will need to carefully consider these differing toxicities in selecting patients for appropriate therapy.

CONCLUSION

The last decade has seen a rapid expansion of second-line therapies in NSCLC. We have moved from a situation where there was insufficient information to recommend the routine use of second-line therapy, to one where there are now multiple agents available, with survival gains demonstrated for second as well as third-line options. Docetaxel, pemetrexed, and erlotinib are all approved for use in NSCLC in many countries. Data exist for the use of gefitinib as well; however, this agent is not currently available in many non-Asian parts of the world. The important issue for oncologists treating NSCLC is to select patients appropriately to ensure that as many patients as possible have the opportunity to consider both second- and third-line treatment options. Treatment decisions should reflect careful consideration of the toxicity profile of the agents together with individual patient preferences. The importance of economic considerations varies from region to region, but the issue should not be avoided given the cost of many of these new agents.

Therapeutic options following progression from platinum-based chemotherapy is an area of intense clinical trial activity. Multiple classes of agents are under evaluation. Oncologists should be encouraged to seek out clinical trial opportunities to ensure that we continue to advance the treatment of second and subsequent lines of therapy for NSCLC over the next decade.

REFERENCES

1. Chemotherapy in non-small cell lung cancer: a meta-analysis using updated data on individual patients from 52 randomised clinical trials. Non-small Cell Lung Cancer Collaborative Group [see comments]. *BMJ* 1995;311(7010):899–909.
2. Fossella F, Pereira JR, von Pawel J, et al. Randomized, multinational, phase III study of docetaxel plus platinum combinations versus vinorelbine plus cisplatin for advanced non-small-cell lung cancer: the TAX 326 study group. *J Clin Oncol* 2003;21(16):3016–3024.

3. Scagliotti GV, De Marinis F, Rinaldi M, et al. Phase III randomized trial comparing three platinum-based doublets in advanced non-small-cell lung cancer. *J Clin Oncol* 2002;20(21):4285–4291.
4. Schiller JH, Harrington D, Belani CP, et al. Comparison of four chemotherapy regimens for advanced non-small-cell lung cancer. *N Engl J Med* 2002;346(2):92–98.
5. Clinical practice guidelines for the treatment of unresectable non-small-cell lung cancer. Adopted on May 16, 1997 by the American Society of Clinical Oncology. *J Clin Oncol* 1997;15(8):2996–3018.
6. Shepherd FA, Dancey J, Ramlau R, et al. Prospective randomized trial of docetaxel versus best supportive care in patients with non-small-cell lung cancer previously treated with platinum-based chemotherapy. *J Clin Oncol* 2000;18(10):2095–2103.
7. Fossella FV, DeVore R, Kerr RN, et al. Randomized phase III trial of docetaxel versus vinorelbine or ifosfamide in patients with advanced non-small-cell lung cancer previously treated with platinum-containing chemotherapy regimens. The TAX 320 Non-Small Cell Lung Cancer Study Group.[erratum appears in *J Clin Oncol* 2004 Jan 1;22(1):209]. *J Clin Oncol* 2000;18(12):2354–2362.
8. Dancey J, Shepherd FA, Gralla RJ, et al. Quality of life assessment of second-line docetaxel versus best supportive care in patients with non-small-cell lung cancer previously treated with platinum-based chemotherapy: results of a prospective, randomized phase III trial. *Lung Cancer* 2004;43(2):183–194.
9. Miller V, Fossella F,DeVore R, et al. Docetaxel (D) benefits lung cancer symptoms and quality of life (qol) in a randomized phase III study of non-small cell lung cancer (NSCLC) patients previously treated with platinum based therapy. *J Clin Oncol* 1999;18:A1895. 1999 ASCO Annual Meeting Proceedings.
10. Pfister DG, Johnson DH, Azzoli CG, et al. American Society of Clinical Oncology treatment of unresectable non-small-cell lung cancer guideline: update 2003. *J Clin Oncol* 2004;22(2):330–353.
11. Leighl NB, Shepherd FA, Kwong R, et al. Economic analysis of the TAX 317 trial: docetaxel versus best supportive care as second-line therapy of advanced non-small-cell lung cancer. *J Clin Oncol* 2002; 20(5):1344–1352.
12. Quoix E, Lebeau B, Depierre A, et al. Randomised, multicentre phase II study assessing two doses of docetaxel (75 or 100 mg/m2) as second-line monotherapy for non-small-cell lung cancer. *Ann Oncol* 2004;15(1):38–44.
13. Taguchi T, Furue H, Niitani H, et al. Phase I clinical trial of RP 56976 (docetaxel) a new anticancer drug. *Gan To Kagaku Ryoho* 1994 Sep;21(12):1997–2005.
14. Kunitoh H, Watanabe K, Onoshi T, et al. Phase II trial of docetaxel in previously untreated advanced non-small-cell lung cancer: a Japanese cooperative study. *J Clin Oncol* 1996;14(5):1649–1655.
15. Mukohara T, Takeda K, Miyazaki M, et al. Japanese experience with second-line chemotherapy with low-dose (60 mg/M2) docetaxel in patients with advanced non-small-cell lung cancer. *Cancer Chemother Pharmacol* 2001;48(5):356–360.
16. Yokoyama A, Kurita Y, Watanabe K, et al. Early phase II clinical study of RP56976 (Docetaxel) in patients with primary pulmonary cancer. *Gan To Kagaku Ryoho* 1994 Nov;21(15):2609–2616.
17. Gandara DR, Kawaguchi T, Crowley JJ, et al. Pharmacogenomic (PG) analysis of Japan-SWOG common arm study in advanced stage non-small cell lung cancer (NSCLC): A model for testing population-related pharmacogenomics. *J Clin Oncol* 2007 25;(18Supp):7500. ASCO Annual Meeting Proceedings Part I, 2007.
18. Lara P, Redman M, Lenz,H, et al. Cisplatin (Cis)/etoposide (VP16) compared to cis/irinotecan (CPT11) in extensive-stage small cell lung cancer (E-SCLC): Pharmacogenomic (PG) and comparative toxicity analysis of JCOG 9511 and SWOG 0124. *J Clin Oncol* 2007;25(18Supp):7524. ASCO Annual Meeting Proceedings Part I, 2007.
19. Camps C, Massuti B, Jimenez A, et al. Randomized phase III study of 3-weekly versus weekly docetaxel in pretreated advanced non-small-cell lung cancer: a Spanish Lung Cancer Group trial. *Ann Oncol* 2006;17(3):467–472.
20. Chen YM, Shih JF, Perng RP, et al. A randomized trial of different docetaxel schedules in non-small cell lung cancer patients who failed previous platinum-based chemotherapy. *Chest* 2006;129(4):1031–1038.
21. Gervais R, Ducolone A, Breton JL, et al. Phase II randomised trial comparing docetaxel given every 3 weeks with weekly schedule as second-line therapy in patients with advanced non-small-cell lung cancer (NSCLC). *Ann Oncol* 2005;16(1):90–96.
22. Gridelli C, Gallo C, Di Maio M, et al. A randomised clinical trial of two docetaxel regimens (weekly vs 3 week) in the second-line treatment of non-small-cell lung cancer. The DISTAL 01 study. *Br J Cancer* 2004;91(12):1996–2004.
23. Schuette W, Nagel S, Blankenburg T, et al. Phase III study of second-line chemotherapy for advanced non-small-cell lung cancer with weekly compared with 3-weekly docetaxel. *J Clin Oncol* 2005;23(33): 8389–8395.
24. Di Maio M, Perrone F, Chiodini P, et al. Individual patient data meta-analysis of docetaxel administered once every 3 weeks compared with once every week second-line treatment of advanced non-small-cell lung cancer. *J Clin Oncol* 2007;25(11):1377–1382.
25. Rusthoven JJ, Eisenhauer E, Butts C, et al. Multitargeted antifolate LY231514 as first-line chemotherapy for patients with advanced non-small-cell lung cancer: A phase II study. National Cancer Institute of Canada Clinical Trials Group. *J Clin Oncol* 1999;17(4):1194.
26. Smit EF, Mattson K, von Pawel J, et al. ALIMTA (pemetrexed disodium) as second-line treatment of non-small-cell lung cancer: a phase II study. *Ann Oncol* 2003;14(3):455–460.
27. Hanna N, Shepherd FA, Fossella FV, et al. Randomized phase III trial of pemetrexed versus docetaxel in patients with non-small-cell lung cancer previously treated with chemotherapy. *J Clin Oncol* 2004;22(9):1589–1597.
28. Vogelzang NJ, Rusthoven JJ, Symanowski J, et al. Phase III study of pemetrexed in combination with cisplatin versus cisplatin alone in patients with malignant pleural mesothelioma. *J Clin Oncol* 2003;21(14): 2636–2644.
29. Weiss G.J, Rosell R, Fossella F, et al. The impact of induction chemotherapy on the outcome of second-line therapy with pemetrexed or docetaxel in patients with advanced non-small-cell lung cancer. *Ann Oncol* 2007;18(3):453–460.
30. Peterson P, Park K, Fossella F, et al. Is pemetrexed more effective in adenocarcinoma and large cell lung cancer than in squamous cell carcinoma? A retrospective analysis of a phase III trial of pemetrexed vs docetaxel in previously treated patients with advanced non-small cell lung cancer (NSCLC). 12th World Conference on Lung Cancer; pp. P2–328. abstract.
31. Ceppi P, Volante M, Saviozzi S, et al. Squamous cell carcinoma of the lung compared with other histotypes shows higher messenger RNA and protein levels for thymidylate synthase. *Cancer* 2006;107(7): 1589–1596.
32. Cullen M, Zatloukal P, Sörenson S, et al. Pemetrexed in advanced non-small cell lung cancer: A randomized trial of 500 mg/m2 vs 900 mg/m2 in 588 patients who progressed after platinum-containing chemotherapy. *J Clin Oncol*, 2007 25;18S(Supp):LBA7727. ASCO Annual Meeting Proceedings Part I, 2007.
33. Ramlau R, Gervais R, Krzakowski M, et al. Phase III study comparing oral topotecan to intravenous docetaxel in patients with pretreated advanced non-small-cell lung cancer. *J Clin Oncol* 2006;24(18):2800–2807.
34. White SC, Cheeseman S, Thatcher N, et al. Phase II study of oral topotecan in advanced non-small cell lung cancer. *Clin Cancer Res* 2000; 6(3):868–873.
35. Krzakowski M, Douillard J, Ramlau R, et al. Phase III study of vinflunine versus docetaxel in patients (pts) with advanced non-small cell lung cancer (NSCLC) previously treated with a platinum-containing regimen. *J Clin Oncol,* 2007 25;(18Supp):7511. ASCO Annual Meeting Proceedings Part I, 2007.
36. Hotta K, Matsuo K, Ueoka H, et al. Addition of platinum compounds to a new agent in patients with advanced non-small-cell lung cancer: a literature based meta-analysis of randomised trials. *Ann Oncol* 2004;15(12):1782–1789.

37. Delbaldo C, Michiels S, Syz N, et al. Benefits of adding a drug to a single-agent or a 2-agent chemotherapy regimen in advanced non-small-cell lung cancer: a meta-analysis. *JAMA* 2004;292(4):470–484.
38. Fannucchi MP, Fossella FV, Belt R, et al. Randomized phase II study of bortezomib alone and bortezomib in combination with docetaxel in previously treated advanced non-small cell lung cancer. *J Clin Oncol* 2007;24(31):5025–5033.
39. Georgoulias V, Agelidou A, Syrigos K, et al. Second-line treatment with irinotecan plus cisplatin vs cisplatin of patients with advanced non-small-cell lung cancer pretreated with taxanes and gemcitabine: a multicenter randomised phase II study. *Br J Cancer* 2005;93(7):763–769.
40. Georgoulias V, Kouroussis C, Agelidou A, et al. Irinotecan plus gemcitabine vs irinotecan for the second-line treatment of patients with advanced non-small-cell lung cancer pretreated with docetaxel and cisplatin: a multicentre, randomised, phase II study. *Br J Cancer* 2004; 91(3):482–488.
41. Lilenbaum R, Socinski MA, Altorki NK, et al. Randomized phase II trial of docetaxel/irinotecan and gemcitabine/irinotecan with or without celecoxib in the second-line treatment of non-small-cell lung cancer. *J Clin Oncol* 2006;24(30):4825–4832.
42. Pectasides D, Pectasides M, Farmakis D, et al. Comparison of docetaxel and docetaxel-irinotecan combination as second-line chemotherapy in advanced non-small-cell lung cancer: a randomized phase II trial. *Ann Oncol* 2005;16(2):294–299.
43. Wachters FM, Groen HJ, Biesma B, et al. A randomised phase II trial of docetaxel vs docetaxel and irinotecan in patients with stage IIIb-IV non-small-cell lung cancer who failed first-line treatment. *Br J Cancer* 2005;92(1):15–20.
44. Takeda K, Negoro S, Tamura T, et al, Docetaxel (D) versus docetaxel plus gemcitabine (DC) for second line treatment of non-small cell lung cancer (NSCLC): Results of a JCOG randomized trial (JCOG0104). *J Clin Oncol* 2004 ASCO Meeting Proceedings, 2004. 22(14S (July 15 Suppl)):7034.
45. Volm M, Rittgen W, and Drings P. Prognostic value of ERBB-1, VEGF, cyclin A, FOS, JUN and MYC in patients with squamous cell lung carcinomas.[erratum appears in *Br J Cancer* 1998 Apr;77(7):1198]. *Br J Cancer* 1998;77(4):663–669.
46. Fujino S, Enokibori T, Tezuka N, et al. A comparison of epidermal growth factor receptor levels and other prognostic parameters in non-small cell lung cancer. *Eur J Cancer* 1996;32A(12):2070–2074.
47. Pavelic K, Banjac Z, Pavelic J, et al. Evidence for a role of EGF receptor in the progression of human lung carcinoma. *Anticancer Res* 1993; 13(4):1133–1137.
48. Ranson M, Hammond LA, Ferry D, et al. ZD1839, a selective oral epidermal growth factor receptor-tyrosine kinase inhibitor, is well tolerated and active in patients with solid, malignant tumors: results of a phase I trial. *J Clin Oncol* 2002;20(9):2240–2250.
49. Fukuoka M, Yano S, Giaccone G, et al. Multi-institutional randomized phase II trial of gefitinib for previously treated patients with advanced non-small-cell lung cancer (The IDEAL 1 Trial) [corrected][erratum appears in *J Clin Oncol* 2004 Dec 1;22(23):4811]. *J Clin Oncol* 2003; 21(12):2237–2246.
50. Kris MG, Natale RB, Herbst RS, et al, Efficacy of gefitinib, an inhibitor of the epidermal growth factor receptor tyrosine kinase, in symptomatic patients with non-small cell lung cancer: a randomized trial. *JAMA* 2003;290(16):2149–2158.
51. Cella D, Herbst RS, Lynch TJ, et al, Clinically meaningful improvement in symptoms and quality of life for patients with non-small-cell lung cancer receiving gefitinib in a randomized controlled trial. *J Clin Oncol* 2005;23(13):2946–2954.
52. Shepherd FA, Rodrigues Pereira J, Ciuleanu,T, et al. Erlotinib in previously treated non-small-cell lung cancer. *N Engl J Med* 2005;353(2): 123–132.
53. Bezjak A, Tu D, Seymour L, et al, Symptom improvement in lung cancer patients treated with erlotinib: quality of life analysis of the National Cancer Institute of Canada Clinical Trials Group Study BR.21. *J Clin Oncol* 2006;24(24):3831–3837.
54. Thatcher N, Chang A, Parikh P, et al. Gefitinib plus best supportive care in previously treated patients with refractory advanced non-small-cell lung cancer: results from a randomised, placebo-controlled, multicentre study (Iressa Survival Evaluation in Lung Cancer). *Lancet* 2005;366(9496):1527–1537.
55. Chang A, Parikh P, Thongprasert S, et al. Gefitinib (IRESSA) in patients of Asian origin with refractory advanced non-small cell lung cancer: subset analysis from the ISEL study. *J Thorac Oncol*: Official Publication of the International Association for the Study of Lung Cancer 2006;1(8):847–855.
56. Hirsch FR, Varella-Garcia M, Bunn PA Jr, et al. Molecular predictors of outcome with gefitinib in a phase III placebo-controlled study in advanced non-small-cell lung cancer. *J Clin Oncol* 2006; 24(31): 5034–5042.
57. Shepherd FA, and Rosell R. Weighing tumor biology in treatment decisions for patients with non-small cell lung cancer. *J Thorac Oncol* 2007; 2 Suppl 2:S68–76.
58. Tsao MS, Sakurada A, Cutz JC, et al. Erlotinib in lung cancer—molecular and clinical predictors of outcome. [erratum appears in N Engl J Med. 2006 Oct 19;355(16):1746]. *N Engl J Med* 2005; 353(2):133–144.
59. Cufer T, Vrdoljak E, Gaafar R, et al. Phase II, open-label, randomized study (SIGN) of single-agent gefitinib (IRESSA) or docetaxel as second-line therapy in patients with advanced (stage IIIb or IV) non-small-cell lung cancer. Anti-Cancer Drugs 2006;17(4):401–409.
60. Kim ES, Hirsh V, Mok T, et al. Gefitinib versus docetaxel in previously treated non-small-cell lung cancer (INTEREST): a randomised phase III trial [see comment]. *Lancet* 2008;372(9652):1809–1818.
61. Maruyama R, Nishiwaki Y, Tamura T, et al. Phase III study, V-15-32, of gefitinib versus docetaxel in previously treated Japanese patients with non-small-cell lung cancer [see comment]. *J Clin Oncol* 2008;26(26): 4244–4252.
62. Gatzemeier U, Pluzanska A, Szczesna A, et al. Phase III study of erlotinib in combination with cisplatin and gemcitabine in advanced non-small-cell lung cancer: the Tarceva Lung Cancer Investigation Trial. *J Clin Oncol* 2007;25(12):1545–1552.
63. Giaccone G, Herbst RS, Manegold C, et al. Gefitinib in combination with gemcitabine and cisplatin in advanced non-small-cell lung cancer: a phase III trial—INTACT 1. *J Clin Oncol* 2004;22(5):777–784.
64. Herbst RS, Giaccone G, Schiller JH, et al. Gefitinib in combination with paclitaxel and carboplatin in advanced non-small-cell lung cancer: a phase III trial—INTACT 2. *J Clin Oncol* 2004;22(5):785–794.
65. Herbst RS, Prager D, Hermann R, et al. TRIBUTE: a phase III trial of erlotinib hydrochloride (OSI-774) combined with carboplatin and paclitaxel chemotherapy in advanced non-small-cell lung cancer. *J Clin Oncol* 2005;23(25):5892–5899.
66. Sandler A, Gray R, Perry MC, et al. Paclitaxel-carboplatin alone or with bevacizumab for non-small-cell lung cancer. *N Engl J Med* 2006; 355(24):2542–2550.
67. Herbst RS, O'Neill VJ, Fehrenbacher L, et al. Phase II study of efficacy and safety of bevacizumab with chemotherapy or erlotinib compared with chemotherapy alone for treatment of recurrent or refractory non-small cell lung cancer. *J Clin Oncol* 2007;25(30):4743–4750.
68. Heymach JV, Johnson BE, Prager D, et al. Randomized, placebo-controlled phase II study of vandetanib plus docetaxel in previously treated non small-cell lung cancer. *J Clin Oncol* 2007;25(27): 4270–4277.
69. Herbst RS, Sun Y, Korfee S, et al. Vandetanib plus docetaxel versus docetaxel as second-line treatment for patients with advanced non-small cell lung cancer (NSCLC): A randomized, double-blind phase III trial (ZODIAC). *J Clin Oncol* 2009;27(18S):CRA8003.
70. Hainsworth J, Herbst R. A Phase III, Multicenter, Placebo-controlled, Double-blind, Randomized Clinical Trial to Evaluate the Efficacy of Bevacizumab (Avastin®) in Combination With Erlotinib (Tarceva®) Compared With Erlotinib Alone for Treatment of Advanced Non-small Cell Lung Cancer after Failure of Standard First-line Chemotherapy (BETA). *J Thorac Oncol* 2008;3(11[Suppl 4]):S302.

CHAPTER 47

Oliver Gautschi
Philip C. Mack
David R. Gandara
Rafael Rosell

Pharmacogenomics in Lung Cancer: Predictive Biomarkers for Chemotherapy

Commonly used platinum-based chemotherapy regimens have shown comparable activity in randomized studies of advanced stage non–small cell lung cancer (NSCLC) patients.[1–3] In a similar fashion, both platinum/etoposide and platinum/irinotecan are highly active in the frontline treatment of small cell lung cancer (SCLC).[4,5] However, outcomes vary greatly among individual patients with the same histology, ranging from a best response of complete remission (CR) to that of progressive disease (PD). Despite the introduction of new chemotherapy drugs and molecular targeted agents in recent years, therapeutic outcomes in lung cancer patients remain poor; thus, there is a critical need for development of predictive factors to optimize selection of chemotherapy regimens for both NSCLC and SCLC and in advanced and early stages. Equally important, predictive molecular biomarkers of efficacy and toxicity could also reduce chemotherapy-related toxicity by eliminating those patients least likely to benefit, as well as those predicted to have unacceptable levels of toxicity.

Although clinical prognostic factors for lung cancer are well established, they do not provide the basis for selection of chemotherapy in individual patients. A pooled analysis by Mandrekar et al.[6] of 1053 patients with advanced-stage NSCLC undergoing first-line chemotherapy showed that gender, age, performance status, and hematologic parameters were significant predictors of severe adverse events. In another analysis, the incidence of grade 3 and 4 neutropenia was associated with advanced age (odds ratio = 7), low baseline white blood cell count (odds ratio = 5), and chronic hepatitis B or C virus infection (odds ratio = 3) in patients with advanced NSCLC undergoing second-line chemotherapy with docetaxel.[7] Thus, clinical parameters such as performance status or age are commonly used by the practicing oncologist to decide which patients may not be suitable for standard chemotherapy approaches or who may need upfront dose reduction. On the other hand, when Borges et al.[8] analyzed the potential predictive value of 22 clinical factors, including tumor histology, to predict tumor response following first-line chemotherapy in 1052 patients with NSCLC, none of the clinical factors accurately predicted response. Pursuing an alternative approach, Shaw et al.[9] prospectively collected tumor tissue from 165 patients with NSCLC and SCLC, tested the chemosensitivity of tumor cells in vitro, and assigned individualized therapy based on these results. Despite efficient specimen collection (viable tumor specimens were available for 98% of the patients) and state-of-the-art culture methodology, only 28% of the patients received individualized chemotherapy based on laboratory results. This disappointing result precluded the comparison between treatment arms as well as the correlation between in vitro and clinical response to specific drugs. Although other groups have reported more optimistic results, in vitro drug sensitivity testing remains challenging and is not broadly accepted for clinical application at present.[10–12]

Conversely, a biomolecular approach to individualized chemotherapy, attempting to exploit individual patient differences in underlying tumor or host biology, is emerging as a more promising strategy for personalizing therapy (Fig. 47.1). The field of pharmacogenomics originated from the observation that inheritance plays an important role in individual variation in drug metabolism and disposition. In a broader sense, pharmacogenomics incorporates the entirety of molecular factors that modify drug activity and toxicity in individual patients. The development of this field occurred in parallel with recent advances in genomic science.[13,14] Although the principle of individualizing chemotherapy for lung cancer patients is not new, the tools available to implement such an approach have previously been limited. Unfortunately, although clinical characteristics can give some insight into likelihood of response (i.e., the associations between female gender and good performance status with a higher response rate), they cannot reliably predict an individual patient's response to chemotherapy. Similarly, past attempts at in vitro drug sensitivity testing have identified significant problems with the feasibility and reproducibility of this approach. Recent advances in genomic technologies and our understanding of the molecular mechanisms of chemotherapy, however, have brought forward several promising biomarkers with prognostic and/or predictive potential. Also, significant contributions toward a comprehensive understanding of the genetic variations underlying individual differences in drug metabolism have been made. In the near future, these advances

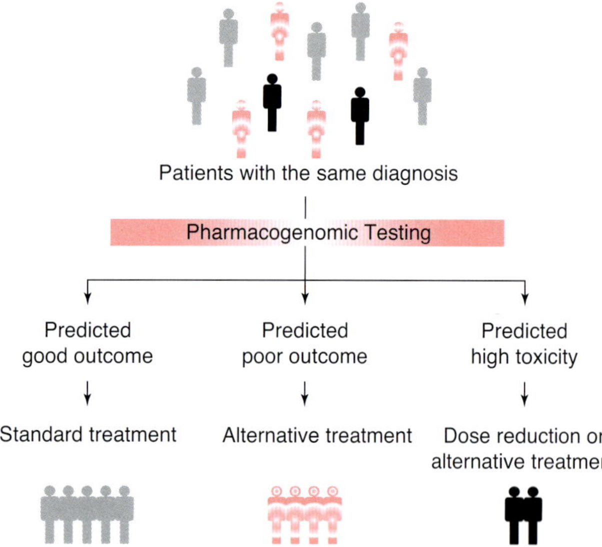

FIGURE 47.1 Concept of individualized chemotherapy. Activity and tolerability of chemotherapy varies among individual patients. Pharmacogenomic testing has the potential to predict who is likely to benefit from a specific drug (or drug combination) and who will have no benefit or may even be harmed by this treatment. Customized therapy may thus ultimately improve patient outcome.

are expected to impact on clinical decision making and ultimately improve the outcome of patients with lung cancer.

In this chapter, two distinct aspects of pharmacogenomics are reviewed: (a) tumor-related factors including molecular drug targets that regulate the biochemical and physiological effects of drugs and their mechanisms of action and (b) host-related factors including metabolizing enzymes and transporters that regulate drug metabolism and disposition.

TUMOR-RELATED FACTORS: SINGLE-GENE BIOMARKERS

Biomarkers of Platinum Resistance The backbone of systemic treatment for both NSCLC and SCLC remains platinum-based chemotherapy.[5,15] Among the platinum compounds, cisplatin (cis-diammine-dichloro-platinum, CDDP) is reported to have superior activity over carboplatin in NSCLC, in terms of response rate and, in patients with nonsquamous tumors, survival.[16] The mode of action for cisplatin relates to the aquation equilibrium, a process by which a chloride ligand of cisplatin is displaced with water, allowing cisplatin to cross-link DNA via displacement of its second chloride ligand.[17] The leaving ligand for carboplatin (cis-1,1-cyclobutanedicarboxylato-diammineplatinum[II]) is bidentate cyclobutane dicarboxylate (CBDCA); whether there are consequences of this difference for biomarker development remains to be determined. Cross-linked DNA activates the nucleotide excision repair (NER) machinery, which includes a large complex consisting of at least 30 proteins, including ERCC1 (excision repair cross-complementing rodent repair deficiency, group 1), XPA (xeroderma pigmentosa group A), XPB/ERCC3, XPC, XPD/ERCC2, XPF/ERCC4, XPG/ERCC5, Cockayne syndrome protein A (CSA/ERCC8), CSB/ERCC6, and others (Fig. 47.2).[18,19] If repair proves inadequate, NER triggers apoptosis. Thus, it is the balance between DNA damage and repair that determines the fate of cancer cells exposed to platinum. ERCC1, which forms a heterodimer with XPF, appears to be the rate-limiting step in NER, hence, its implication in platinum resistance. In preclinical models, ERCC1 levels correlated with the removal capacity of the cisplatin-induced DNA adducts as well as the relative cisplatin resistance.[20–22] ERCC1-knockout cells were highly sensitive to DNA cross-linking agents, and transfection with ERCC1 exhibited an increase in the DNA repair capacity and cisplatin resistance.[23,24]

In view of these preclinical data, ERCC1 has emerged as an attractive single gene target in biomarker development for platinum-based chemotherapy. Indeed, clinical translation of these findings is highlighted by results in both advanced-stage NSCLC as well as in the adjuvant chemotherapy setting. In 2002, Lord et al.[25] first reported that ERCC1 messenger RNA (mRNA) expression was significantly associated with response to cisplatin/gemcitabine chemotherapy in patients with advanced-stage NSCLC.

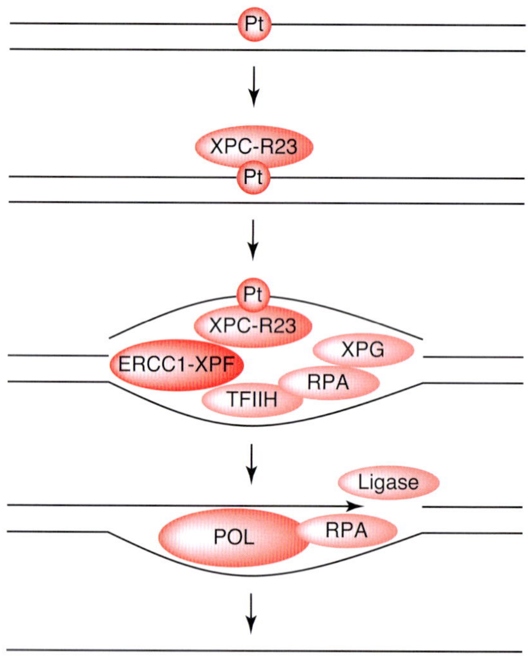

FIGURE 47.2 Molecular mechanisms of nucleotide excision repair (NER). DNA cross-linking by cisplatin (Pt) is recognized by XPC-R23, which recruits other proteins to form the active NER-complex. Only a few of these proteins are depicted here. For example, TFIIH unwinds the DNA, and ERCC1-XPF plus XPG cut out the damaged DNA strand. The gap is filled by polymerases (POL) and the ends are connected by ligases. These events restore the configuration of the damaged DNA strand. *ERCC1*, excision repair cross-complementing 1; *POL*, polymerase; *RPA*, replication protein A; *TFIIH*, transcription factor IIH; *XP*, xeroderma pigmentosum.

The genomic international lung trial (GILT) of customized chemotherapy by the Spanish Lung Cancer Group also demonstrated the predictive value of ERCC1 for platinum-based chemotherapy but tested the role of nonplatinum chemotherapy as well.[26] In this prospective phase III trial of individualized chemotherapy, 444 patients with previously untreated advanced NSCLC were randomized in a 1:2 ratio to either a control arm of docetaxel/cisplatin or a genotypic arm in which treatment was assigned based on the level of tumor ERCC1 mRNA expression, quantified by real-time reverse transcription polymerase chain reaction (RT-PCR). Patients in the genotypic arm, with tumors expressing ERCC1 mRNA levels lower than the median, received docetaxel plus cisplatin, whereas those with higher levels received docetaxel plus gemcitabine. With a significantly better response rate in the genotypic arm compared with the control arm (51.2% vs. 39.3%; $p = 0.02$), the study reached its primary end point. In multivariate analysis, low ERCC1 was an independent predictor of tumor response to cisplatin (Fig. 47.3). Neither median progression-free survival (PFS) (6.1 vs. 5.2 months; hazard ratio [HR] = 0.9; $p = 0.30$), nor overall survival (OS) was significantly different between the control and genotypic arm overall. However, there were interesting differences in outcomes between ERCC1-negative and -positive patients within the genotypic arm. Although response rates in the genotypic arm were relatively similar between ERCC1-negative patients treated with docetaxel/cisplatin (53%) versus the ERCC1-positive group receiving docetaxel-gemcitabine (47%), both PFS (6.7 vs. 4.7 months) and OS (10.3 vs. 9.4 months) were numerically higher in the ERCC1-negative group. These results suggest that although ERCC1-negative patients do well with platinum-based therapy, alternatives may be needed for the ERCC1-positive group, which extend beyond currently available nonplatinum regimens, such as that, used in this trial. The prognostic and predictive value of ERCC1 protein expression, assessed by immunohistochemistry, was reported by the International Adjuvant Lung Cancer Trial Biologic Program (IALT-Bio), a correlative science component of the IALT phase III trial testing adjuvant chemotherapy in early stage NSCLC reported (Fig. 47.4).[27] The previously reported prognostic value of ERCC1 expression was confirmed in the control arm of IALT (surgery only), where ERCC1 positivity was associated with longer survival

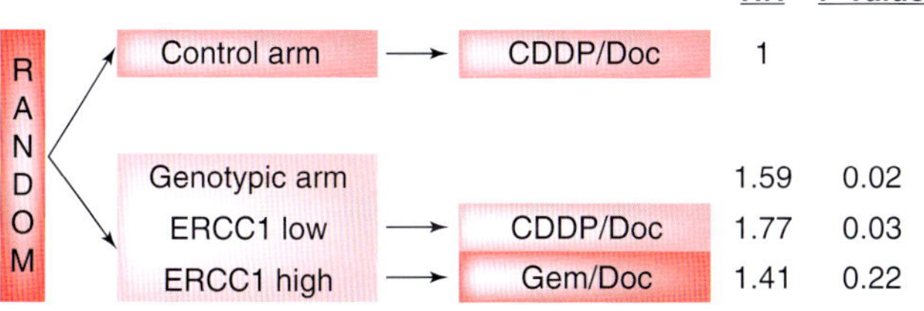

FIGURE 47.3 Genomic international lung trial (GILT). Trial design and results of the multivariate analysis for response according to tumor ERCC1 expression. See text for details. *CDDP*, cisplatin; *Doc*, docetaxel; *ERCC1*, excision repair cross-complementing 1; *Gem*, gemcitabine; *HR*, hazard ratio (for tumor response).

(HR = 0.66; 95% CI, 0.49 to 0.90; $p = 0.009$) compared with ERCC1 negativity. In the chemotherapy arm of IALT, only patients with ERCC1-negative tumors benefited from treatment (ERCC1-negative tumors: HR = 0.65; 95% CI, 0.50 to 0.86; $p = 0.002$), demonstrating the predictive value of this biomarker (ERCC1-positive tumors: HR = 1.14; 95% CI, 0.84 to 1.55; $p = 0.40$). These findings raise the question of whether patients with ERCC1-positive tumors would benefit from alternative therapies, such as nonplatinum-based chemotherapy regimens, or whether they would be best served by receiving no chemotherapy at all.

Ribonucleotide reductase M1 (RRM1) is the regulatory subunit of ribonucleotide reductase, which provides deoxyribonucleotides for de novo DNA synthesis and DNA repair. Gemcitabine, a nucleoside analogue that replaces cytidine during DNA replication, inhibits RRM1. High expression levels of RRM1 have been associated with gemcitabine resistance in NSCLC cell lines.[28] Thus, RRM1 and ERCC1 may cooperate in resistance to platinum-based chemotherapy, especially platinum–gemcitabine combinations. In a study of 70 patients with advanced NSCLC, mRNA expression levels of ERCC1 and RRM1 ($r = 0.624$; $p < 0.001$) were strongly correlated, and for the 33 patients treated with cisplatin plus gemcitabine, concomitant low levels of ERCC1 and RRM1 were predictive of better survival (14.9 vs. 10.0 months; $p = 0.03$).[29] Bepler et al.[30] in advanced NSCLC demonstrated that RRM1 mRNA expression correlated with tumor response from carboplatin plus gemcitabine. A prospective phase II trial (MADEIT) conducted by Simon et al.[31] tested the feasibility and efficacy of patient selection for chemotherapy based on tumor ERCC1 and RRM1 mRNA levels. Median expression values were used to separate patients into four groups and patients were treated accordingly, with gemcitabine plus carboplatin (RRM1 low, ERCC1 low), gemcitabine plus docetaxel (RRM1 low, ERCC1 high), docetaxel plus carboplatin (RRM1 high, ERCC1 low), or docetaxel plus vinorelbine (RRM1 high, ERCC1 high). A median survival of 13.3 months was achieved, comparing favorably with previous results at the same institution and suggesting the clinical applicability of this approach. Zheng et al.[32] used a newly developed fluorescence staining methodology for automated quantitative protein expression analysis (AQUA) to evaluate both ERCC1 and RRM1 protein in 187 patients with surgically resected NSCLC. RRM1 and ERCC1 expression were significantly correlated ($r = 0.3$; $p = 0.001$). With a median survival of 120 months, the 55 patients with concomitant high levels of RRM1 and ERCC1 lived significantly longer than other subgroups ($p = 0.02$). Based on the data reviewed previously, the Southwest Oncology Group will investigate the prognostic and predictive role of ERCC1 and RRM1 assessed by AQUA for adjuvant chemotherapy in patients with resected stage I NSCLC in a feasibility study, S0720.[33] Patients with concomitantly high tumor levels of ERCC1 and RRM1 will receive no adjuvant chemotherapy, based on a good prognosis and predicted poor outcome from platinum chemotherapy, whereas all other patients will receive adjuvant chemotherapy with gemcitabine and cisplatin. Because adjuvant chemotherapy is not standard of care in stage I disease, this group is appropriate for such a study.[34]

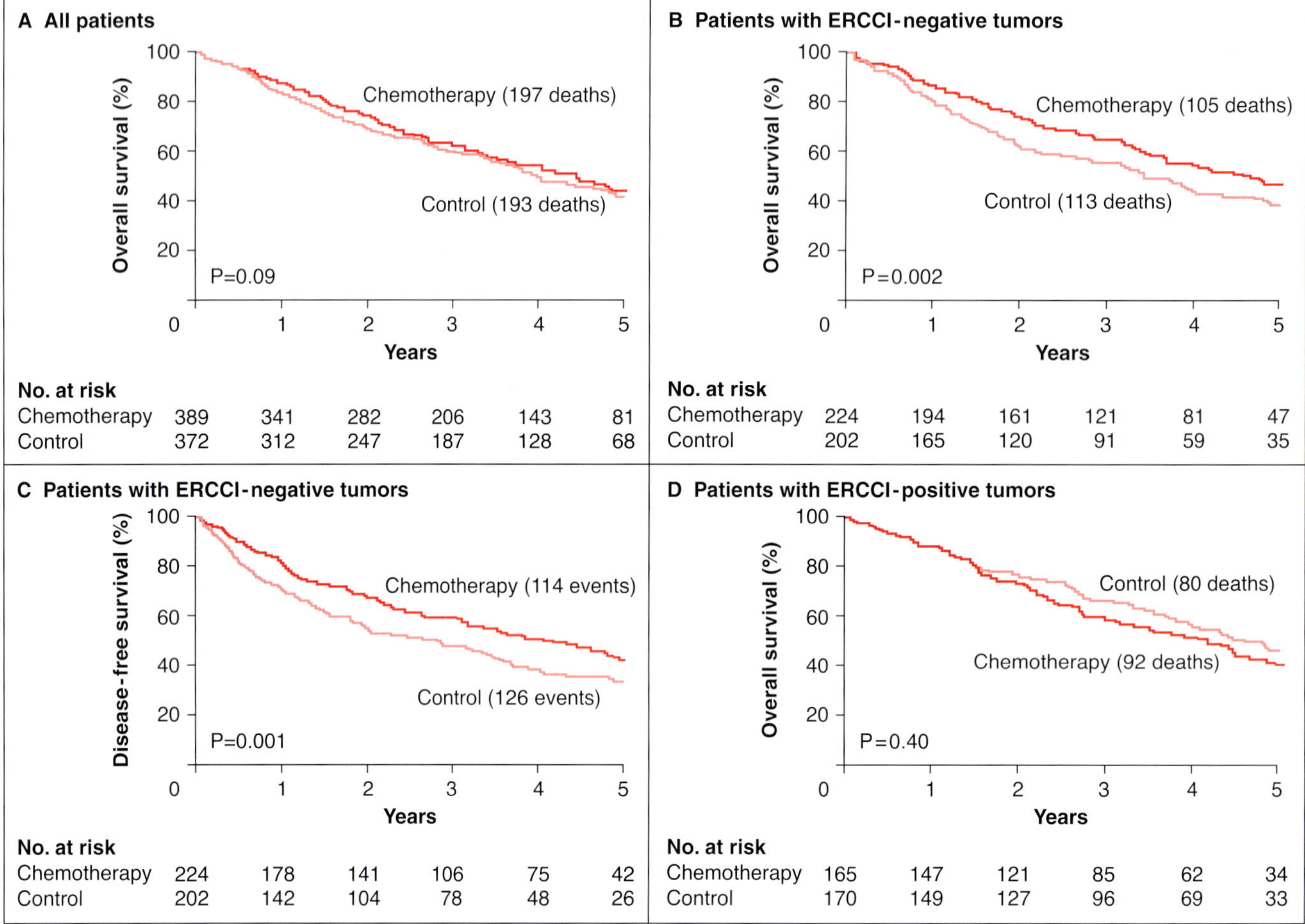

FIGURE 47.4 Kaplan–Meier curves of patients eligible for ERCC1 immunohistochemistry in the International Adjuvant Lung Trial (IALT). **A:** Overall survival according to treatment in 761 eligible patients. **B:** Overall survival according to treatment in patients with ERCC1-negative tumors. **C:** Disease-free survival according to treatment in patients with ERCC1-negative tumors. **D:** Overall survival according to treatment in patients with ERCC1-positive tumors. (From Olaussen KA, Dunant A, Fouret P, et al. DNA repair by ERCC1 in non-small-cell lung cancer and cisplatin-based adjuvant chemotherapy. *N Engl J Med* 2006;355[10]:983–991. Copyright ©2006 Massachusetts Medical Society. All rights reserved.)

The primary end point is feasibility, gauged by the percentage of patients in which a tumor specimen can be collected in a group-wide setting, assessed by AQUA, and results applied for treatment assignment.

Another emerging factor in platinum resistance is BRCA1 (breast cancer 1, early onset). Although the involvement of BRCA1 in hereditary breast cancer and other malignancies is well known, other functions of this gene are still incompletely understood. A particular feature of BRCA1-deficient cells, as well as many cells showing a defect in homologous recombination, is sensitivity to the DNA cross-linking agents.[35] In breast cancer cells, the absence of BRCA1 results in high sensitivity to cisplatin; conversely, BRCA1 expression increased sensitivity to antimicrotubule agents.[36] Based on these findings, Taron et al.[37] used real-time quantitative PCR (RTqPCR) to measure BRCA1 expression in 55 surgically resected tumors of patients with NSCLC who had received neoadjuvant gemcitabine/cisplatin chemotherapy. In this study, patients with low BRCA1 expression levels had better outcomes than those with high levels. More recently, Rosell et al.[38] studied the prognostic impact of BRCA1 expression in 126 specimens of resected early stage NSCLC. In this study, patients with high tumor expression of BRCA1 had significantly poorer survival. These results, taken together, led the Spanish Lung Cancer Group to initiate a pilot study of customized adjuvant chemotherapy based on BRCA1 mRNA levels in resected stage II to IIIA NSCLC patients, where adjuvant chemotherapy was customized based on BRCA1 mRNA levels in 84/100 completely resected N1 and N2 NSCLC patients. A total of 11 with high BRCA1 levels received docetaxel (doc); 29 patients with intermediate BRCA1 levels received doc/cisplatin (cis); 44 patients with low BRCA1 levels received cis/gemcitabine (gem). As of American Society of Clinical Oncology (ASCO) 2008, median survival had not been reached in patients with high or intermediate BRCA1 levels, although it was 25.6 months (m) in patients with low levels ($p = 0.04$). In a multivariate analysis for survival in all 84 patients, the HR were 5.23 for patients with high BRCA1 levels ($p = 0.07$) and 3.57 for patients with tumor size >4 cm ($p = 0.07$). In the multivariate

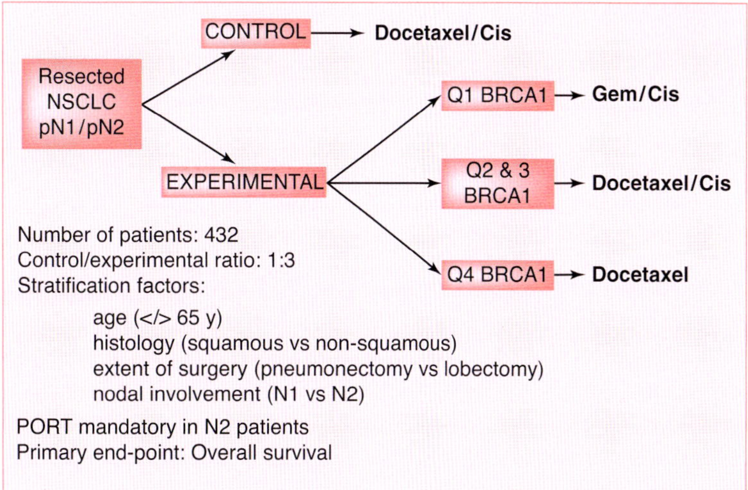

FIGURE 47.5 Schema for the SCAT (Spanish customized adjuvant treatment in completely resected N1 and N2 non–small cell lung cancer) trial showing customized BRCA1 adjuvant treatment. See text for details. *BRCA1*, breast cancer 1; *Cis*, cisplatin; *Gem*, gemcitabine; *NSCLC*, non–small cell lung cancer; *PORT*, postoperative radiation therapy.

analysis of 42 N2 patients, the HRs were 0.13 for 18 patients receiving postoperative radiotherapy ($p = 0.04$) and 22 for 15 patients with intermediate or high BRCA1 levels ($p = 0.01$). These interim analyses were interpreted to reveal that single-agent doc had no detrimental effect on survival in comparison with doc/cis. In addition, high BRCA1 mRNA expression could be a poor prognostic marker.[39]

These encouraging results led the Spanish Lung Cancer Group to initiate the ongoing Spanish customized adjuvant trial (SCAT) study. This phase III randomized study is testing the concept of customized adjuvant chemotherapy based on BRCA1 mRNA levels in completely resected stages II to IIIA NSCLC patients. (Fig. 47.5)

In summary, ERCC1, RRM1, and BRCA1 are, at present, the most promising single predictive biomarkers for patients with NSCLC planning to undergo platinum-based chemotherapy (Table 47.1).[25–27,29–31,37,40–46] At least in the adjuvant setting, additional testing for the cell cycle regulator

TABLE 47.1 Markers for Platinum Resistance in NSCLC

Marker	Stage	Chemotherapy	Correlation	N	Method
ERCC1	IIIB/IV	Cis/gem[25]	Low ERCC1 and good survival	56	RTqPCR
	IIIB/IV	Cis/gem[46]	None	33	IHC
	I–IIIA	Adjuvant platinum based (IALT)[27]	Low ERCC1 and survival benefit with chemotherapy	761	IHC
	Recurrence after surgery	Platinum based[41]	Low ERCC1 and good survival	67	IHC
	IIIB/IV	Platinum based[42]	None	66	RTqPCR
	III	Neoadjuvant platinum based[43]	Low ERCC1 and tumor response	35	IHC
	IV	Customized (GILT)[26]	Low ERCC1 and tumor response	444	RTqPCR
ERCC1 +RRM1	IIIB/IV	Gem based[44]	Low RRM1/ERCC1 and good survival	100	RTqPCR
	IIB–IIIB	Neoadjuvant cis/gem[45]	Low RRM1 and tumor response	67	RTqPCR
	IIIB/IV	Cis/gem[29]	Low RRM1/ERCC1 and good survival	70	RTqPCR
	IIIB/IV	Customized (MADE IT)[31]	RRM1 and ERCC1 coexpression	55	RTqPCR
RRM1	Inoperable II–III	Gem/carb[30]	Low RRM1 and tumor response	40	RTqPCR
$p27^{KIP1}$	I–IIIA	Adjuvant platinum based (IALT)[47]	Low $p27^{KIP1}$ and survival benefit with chemotherapy	778	IHC
BRCA1	III	Neoadjuvant cis/gem[37]	Low BRCA1 and poor survival	55	RTqPCR
p53	IB–II	Adjuvant cis/vin (BR.10)[48]	High p53 and greater survival benefit with chemotherapy	253	IHC

Modified from Gautschi O, Mack PC, Davies AM, et al. Pharmacogenomic approaches to individualizing chemotherapy for non-small cell lung cancer: current status and future directions. *Clin Lung Cancer* 2008;9(Suppl 3):S129–S138.

BRCA1, breast cancer 1, early onset; carb, carboplatin; cis, cisplatin; ERCC1, excision repair cross-complementing rodent repair deficiency complementation group 1; gem, gemcitabine; GILT, genomic international lung trial; IALT, International Adjuvant Lung Cancer Trial; IHC, immunohistochemistry; RTqPCR, reverse transcription quantitiative polymerase chain reaction; RRM1, ribonucleotide reductase M1; vin, vinorelbine.

p27[KIP1] and for p53 may provide further important information, as suggested by IALT and JBR.10 trial results.[47,48] Thus, future efforts should focus on the integration of these markers into robust predictive models.

Biomarkers for Antimitotic Drugs Paclitaxel and docetaxel bind to the beta subunit of tubulins, block microtubule disassembly, and lead to mitotic arrest and cell death.[49] Conversely, vinca alkaloids bind tubulin but prevent microtubule polymerization, promote depolymerization, and lead to metaphase blockade.[50] In humans, at least six distinct beta-tubulin classes (I, II, III, IVa, IVb, and VI) exist. Expression of class III beta tubulin (TUBBIII) is specific to neurons, testis cells, and some types of cancer, including NSCLC. In vitro studies demonstrate that TUBBIII overexpression lowers the affinity of paclitaxel for microtubules, suggesting that TUBBIII may be a natural antagonist for this class of drug.[51] Following this line of reasoning, high tumor TUBBIII expression has been correlated with resistance to paclitaxel and vinorelbine in patients with advanced NSCLC.[52,53] The adjuvant JBR.10 trial provided an interesting basis for testing the prognostic and predictive value of TUBBIII.[54] Tumor specimens from 265 patients were available for immunohistochemical analysis of TUBBIII protein expression. In the control arm (surgery only), TUBBIII positivity was associated with poor relapse-free survival (HR = 1.92; 95% CI, 1.16 to 3.18; $p = 0.01$) and poor overall survival (HR, 1.72; 95% CI, 1.02 to 2.88; $p = 0.04$). TUBBIII-positive patients showed a benefit from chemotherapy in terms of relapse-free survival (HR = 0.45; 95% CI, 0.27 to 0.75; $p = 0.002$). This was contrary to the expected result, and the authors speculated a differential predictive value of TUBBIII in early versus advanced NSCLC. Thus, the predictive value of TUBBIII as a single-gene biomarker in NSCLC remains unclear. A similar conclusion can be made with regard to tubulin mutations. Although mutations of class I beta tubulin clearly are observed in preclinical models, clinical data have shown mixed results, and the clinical relevance of true beta-tubulin mutations may apply to only a small patient subset.[55–57]

In breast adenocarcinomas, the microtubule-associated protein Tau is expressed at higher levels in docetaxel-sensitive tumors than in docetaxel-resistant ones.[58] Rouzier et al.[59] demonstrated that in patients with breast cancer undergoing neoadjuvant chemotherapy with paclitaxel, tumors with pathologic complete remission (pCR) had significantly lower Tau mRNA levels. Small interfering RNA to downregulate Tau increased sensitivity to paclitaxel in vitro, and incubation of tubulin with Tau resulted in decreased paclitaxel binding and reduced paclitaxel-induced microtubule polymerization. It was thus speculated that low Tau expression may be used as a marker to select patients for paclitaxel therapy, and that Tau inhibition might be exploited as a therapeutic strategy to increase sensitivity to paclitaxel. These data led Dumontet et al.[60] to study Tau expression in NSCLC. Although Tau protein was expressed in 9 out of 18 (50%) NSCLC samples, no correlation with patient outcome after taxane-based chemotherapy was observed. An analysis of Southwest Oncology Group (SWOG) data revealed strong Tau positivity in only 5% of the NSCLC specimens tested and no association with response to mitotic drugs (unpublished data). Aside from promising BRCA1 data described previously, these studies illustrate the current lack of predictive biomarkers for antimitotic drugs and the need for more translational work in this important area.

Multiparameter Models and Gene Signatures In view of the heterogeneity and complex tumor biology underlying NSCLC, a multiparameter approach to individualizing chemotherapy may offer significant advantages.[61] Kwiatkowski et al.[62] first described the value of a multivariate model, including p53, KRAS and HRAS, for determining prognosis in stage I resected NSCLC. Mack et al.[63] subsequently demonstrated that a score derived from five markers (ERCC1, TUBBIII, p53, p27KIP1, and Ki-67) predicted survival in patients with advanced NSCLC undergoing platinum-based chemotherapy, whereas each marker failed when used alone. Recently, with the broad availability of gene expression microarrays, it has became possible to explore the potential prognostic and predictive value of gene expression profiles.[64] Potti et al.[65] reported a genomics prognostic model, the lung metagene score (LMS), which correlated with recurrence in a training cohort of 89 surgically resected NSCLC patients and in two subsequent validation cohorts. The LMS outperformed recognized clinical prognostic factors, and was accurate in all early stages of NSCLC. Cancer and Leukemia Group B (CALGB) has proposed a clinical trial (C30506) for patients with resected stage I NSCLC 2 to 4 cm in size, a group not routinely recommended for adjuvant chemotherapy. Patients with a low LMS, who are felt to be at low risk for recurrence, are observed, whereas those with unfavorable score are randomized to either adjuvant chemotherapy or to standard observation. The two primary objectives of the trial are to validate the positive prognostic value for survival of a low LMS and to determine if a survival advantage exists for adjuvant chemotherapy in patients with a high LMS. As discussed in a recent review by Minna et al.,[66] this powerful methodology is also being utilized to identify gene expression profiles that correlate with drug sensitivity. In lung cancer, Oshita et al.[67] carried out genome-wide complementary DNA (cDNA) microarray screening and correlated gene expression profiles with chemoresistance in 37 patients with advanced NSCLC and SCLC. Transbroncheal biopsy specimens of tumors were obtained before chemotherapy, and the expression levels of 1176 genes were analyzed. Allogenic inflammatory factor, human leukocyte antigen DR (HLA-DR)–associated invariant subunit and major histocompatibility complex (MHC) class II HLA-DR-beta precursor were independently associated with chemoresistance in the multivariate analysis. In a separate study using in vitro drug sensitivity data coupled with microarray data, Hsu et al.[68] developed gene expression signatures to predict sensitivity to cisplatin and pemetrexed. Signatures were then validated using 59 samples from patients previously treated with cisplatin. Interestingly, ERCC1 was part of the signature for cisplatin resistance, and an inverse correlation was seen between cisplatin and pemetrexed sensitivity in vitro and in patient samples. Based on this finding, a clinical trial has been proposed in which tumors from patients with metastatic NSCLC will be screened for platinum sensitivity by microarray.[69] Patients with predicted platinum-sensitive tumors will receive cisplatin plus gemcitabine, whereas patients with predicted platinum-resistant tumors will receive pemetrexed and gemcitabine. Inherent in these studies is the question of broad applicability, for example, the quality of fresh frozen biopsies obtained in the clinical setting, and whether similar results may be obtained with microarrays using paraffin-embedded tissue.

HOST-RELATED FACTORS

A completely independent paradigm for personalizing chemotherapy exploits interindividual differences that are host related rather than tumor related. Single nucleotide polymorphisms (SNPs), substitutions of a single base in a DNA sequence, account for approximately 90% of genetic variation in humans. It is estimated that SNPs occur as frequently as every 100 to 300 bases, and, by definition, must be present in at least 1% of the population. SNPs are found in both coding and noncoding sequences and may alter DNA transcription rates, RNA splicing, translation efficiency, and protein function.

Chemotherapy metabolism and detoxification are influenced by a large number of SNPs.[70] As a key example, polymorphisms in the UGT1A1 gene (uridine diphosphate glucuronosyltransferase 1A1) have a significant effect on gastrointestinal and myelosuppressive toxicity accompanying treatment with irinotecan by altering the glucuronidation rate of its active metabolite SN-38.[71,72] Polymorphic variance in cytochrome P450 (CYP) proteins are also recognized as a determinant of chemotherapy activity and toxicity. This large and diverse family of enzymes catalyzes the metabolism of xenobiotics, including many anticancer agents.[73] CYP3A members are the most abundant type of CYP in the small intestine and liver, with substantial interindividual and interracial variation in expression attributed to SNPs.[74,75] CYP3A expression affects the pharmacokinetic disposition of multiple drugs and may impact on the metabolism of environmental procarcinogens, thus influencing an individual's predisposition toward cancer. The role of SNPs in drug metabolism and disposition is complex, and efforts to define their utility for personalized medicine are underway.[76,77]

Interindividual differences in host DNA repair capacity may also affect response to chemotherapy. Multiple SNPs have been identified in genes involved in NER, double-strand DNA break repair, nucleotide synthesis, and other DNA repair processes[78,79] Decreased DNA repair capacity resulting from SNPs appears to contribute to lung cancer risk, particularly in patients who are young, female, and light smokers or nonsmokers.[80] However, reduced DNA repair has also been associated with improved survival following platinum-based therapies.[81–83]

Although such host-related differences are typically viewed on an individual patient basis, in a broader sense, genotyping studies may help to explain differences in patient outcomes based on ethnic or racial background (i.e., population-related pharmacogenomics). For example, variations in taxane metabolism between Japanese and white populations have been reported and purported to account for differences in patient outcome from taxane-based chemotherapy.[84] To address this question, joint studies between Japanese and U.S. investigators have been designed to identify population-related differences in drug pharmacogenomics using a "common arm" approach.[85] In such studies, separate phase III trials evaluating paclitaxel-carboplatin in advanced-stage NSCLC incorporated similar study criteria for patient eligibility and treatment. In a preliminary report, differences in allelic distribution for genes involved in paclitaxel disposition or DNA repair were observed between Japanese and U.S. patients. Genotype-associated correlations with clinical outcomes were observed for PFS with CYP3A4*1B and for response with ERCC2 K751Q. This research strategy may assist in determining whether the significant differences in efficacy and toxicity observed between Japanese and U.S. patients are attributable to population-related genetic variance.

The recent development of high-throughput genomic arrays should facilitate incorporation of SNP analysis into multiparameter predictive models, which could be tested internationally. The recent availability of highly sensitive methods to detect SNPs, as well as tumor-derived DNA mutations, in peripheral blood, now provides the opportunity for the noninvasive molecular analysis and serial monitoring of patients.[86–90] This promising methodology will require additional validation and prospective confirmation in appropriately designed clinical trials.

FUTURE DIRECTIONS

Contrary to prior reports showing no strong correlations between tumor histology and response to chemotherapy, a recent randomized clinical trial suggested that histology may indeed have implications for tumor response to chemotherapy, at least in the case of pemetrexed, an antifolate drug that inhibits several enzymes, including thymidylate synthase (TS), dihydrofolate reductase (DHFR), and glycinamide ribonucleotide formyl transferase (GARFT).[91] In this large phase III trial in advanced-stage NSCLC, Scagliotti et al.[92] compared the activity of pemetrexed plus cisplatin versus gemcitabine plus cisplatin. In a preplanned subset analysis, patients with nonsquamous carcinomas had significantly better survival in the pemetrexed arm compared with the gemcitabine arm. Correlative science results from this study are awaited with great interest, to see whether any potential biomarkers for pemetrexed, platinum, or gemcitabine match with the histology-based results. In line with these data, Ceppi et al.[93] previously reported higher mRNA and protein levels for TS in squamous cell lung carcinomas compared with other histotypes. Thus, TS is one of several candidate predictive markers in the differential response of lung cancers to pemetrexed. In vitro drug sensitivity testing with freshly isolated tumor specimens demonstrated that the expression levels of DHFR and GARFT correlated with chemosensitivity to pemetrexed.[94] Because the drug classification for pemetrexed is that of a multitargeted antifolate compound, it would not be unexpected that a number of factors may be related to pemetrexed activity, as suggested by gene expression microarray data detailed previously.

Transcriptional profiling can only reveal gene expression at the mRNA level, which does not always correlate with the protein level, as demonstrated for ERCC1.[32] Proteomics is a promising approach to more directly and globally address current biological and pharmacological issues related to drug sensitivity.[95] Ma et al.[96] determined whether proteomic signatures of untreated cancer cells were sufficient to predict drug response in vitro. The authors used the databases at the National Cancer Institute on the proteomic profiles of the NCI-60 cell line panel and the activity of 118 drugs tested. By combining the two databases, the feasibility of using proteomic approaches for predicting chemosensitivity was shown. Although EGFR pathways are discussed in detail elsewhere in this text, we note the work of Taguchi et al.,[97] who reported the value of proteomic profiling in patient serum to predict survival benefit from EGFR tyrosine kinase inhibition in NSCLC. The predictive value of the serum proteomic profile in this study was restricted to erlotinib and gefitinib, but offers promise that a similar approach will prove useful in predicting tumor response to chemotherapeutic agents in individual patients.

CONCLUSION

In the past 5 years, significant progress has been made in the identification of prognostic and predictive single biomarkers and gene expression profiles for lung cancer. Although individualized chemotherapy for lung cancer remains investigational at this point, it is anticipated that clinical applicability will be established for at least some biomarkers in the near future. The results of the ongoing prospective trials designed to personalize therapy for lung cancer patients are awaited with great interest.

REFERENCES

1. Kelly K, Crowley J, Bunn PA Jr, et al. Randomized phase III trial of paclitaxel plus carboplatin versus vinorelbine plus cisplatin in the treatment of patients with advanced non–small-cell lung cancer: a Southwest Oncology Group trial. *J Clin Oncol* 2001;19(13):3210–3218.
2. Scagliotti GV, De Marinis F, Rinaldi M, et al. Phase III randomized trial comparing three platinum-based doublets in advanced non-small-cell lung cancer. *J Clin Oncol* 2002;20(21):4285–4291.
3. Schiller JH, Harrington D, Belani CP, et al. Comparison of four chemotherapy regimens for advanced non-small-cell lung cancer. *N Engl J Med* 2002;346(2):92–98.
4. Noda K, Nishiwaki Y, Kawahara M, et al. Irinotecan plus cisplatin compared with etoposide plus cisplatin for extensive small-cell lung cancer. *N Engl J Med* 2002;346(2):85–91.
5. Simon GR, Turrisi A. Management of small cell lung cancer: ACCP evidence-based clinical practice guidelines (2nd edition). *Chest* 2007;132(3 suppl):S324–S339.
6. Mandrekar SJ, Northfelt DW, Schild SE, et al. Impact of pretreatment factors on adverse events: a pooled analysis of North Central Cancer Treatment Group advanced stage non-small cell lung cancer trials. *J Thorac Oncol* 2006;1(6):556–563.
7. Chen JP, Lo Y, Yu CJ, et al. Predictors of toxicity of weekly docetaxel in chemotherapy-treated non-small cell lung cancers. *Lung Cancer* 2008; 60:92–97.
8. Borges M, Sculier JP, Paesmans M, et al. Prognostic factors for response to chemotherapy containing platinum derivatives in patients with unresectable non-small cell lung cancer. (NSCLC). *Lung Cancer* 1996;16(1):21–33.
9. Shaw GL, Gazdar AF, Phelps R, et al. Individualized chemotherapy for patients with non-small cell lung cancer determined by prospective identification of neuroendocrine markers and in vitro drug sensitivity testing. *Cancer Res* 1993;53(21):5181–5187.
10. Higashiyama M, Kodama K, Yokouchi H, et al. Cisplatin-based chemotherapy for postoperative recurrence in non-small cell lung cancer patients: relation of the in vitro chemosensitive test to clinical response. *Oncol Rep* 2001;8(2):279–283.
11. Lang DS, Droemann D, Schultz H, et al. A novel human ex vivo model for the analysis of molecular events during lung cancer chemotherapy. *Respir Res* 2007;8:43.
12. Pirnia F, Frese S, Gloor B, et al. Ex vivo assessment of chemotherapy-induced apoptosis and associated molecular changes in patient tumor samples. *Anticancer Res* 2006;26(3A):1765–1772.
13. Johnson JA. Pharmacogenetics: potential for individualized drug therapy through genetics. *Trends Genet* 2003;19(11):660–666.
14. Weinshilboum R, Wang L. Pharmacogenomics: bench to bedside. *Nat Rev Drug Discov* 2004;3(9):739–748.
15. D'Addario G, Pintilie M, Leighl NB, et al. Platinum-based versus non-platinum-based chemotherapy in advanced non-small-cell lung cancer: a meta-analysis of the published literature. *J Clin Oncol* 2005;23(13): 2926–2936.
16. Ardizzoni A, Boni L, Tiseo M, et al. Cisplatin- versus carboplatin-based chemotherapy in first-line treatment of advanced non-small-cell lung cancer: an individual patient data meta-analysis. *J Natl Cancer Inst* 2007;99(11):847–857.
17. Rosenberg B. Anticancer activity of cis-dichlorodiammineplatinum(II) and some relevant chemistry. *Cancer Treat Rep* 1979;63(9–10):1433–1438.
18. Friedberg EC. How nucleotide excision repair protects against cancer. *Nat Rev Cancer* 2001;1(1):22–33.
19. Reed E. Platinum-DNA adduct, nucleotide excision repair and platinum based anti-cancer chemotherapy. *Cancer Treat Rev* 1998;24(5):331–344.
20. Britten RA, Liu D, Tessier A, et al. ERCC1 expression as a molecular marker of cisplatin resistance in human cervical tumor cells. *Int J Cancer* 2000;89(5):453–457.
21. Dabholkar M, Vionnet J, Bostick-Bruton F, et al. Messenger RNA levels of XPAC and ERCC1 in ovarian cancer tissue correlate with response to platinum-based chemotherapy. *J Clin Invest* 1994;94(2):703–708.
22. Lee KB, Parker RJ, Bohr V, et al. Cisplatin sensitivity/resistance in UV repair-deficient Chinese hamster ovary cells of complementation groups 1 and 3. *Carcinogenesis* 1993;14(10):2177–2180.
23. Chang IY, Kim MH, Kim HB, et al. Small interfering RNA-induced suppression of ERCC1 enhances sensitivity of human cancer cells to cisplatin. *Biochem Biophys Res Commun* 2005;327(1):225–233.
24. Larminat F, Bohr VA. Role of the human ERCC-1 gene in gene-specific repair of cisplatin-induced DNA damage. *Nucleic Acids Res* 1994;22(15):3005–3010.
25. Lord RV, Brabender J, Gandara D, et al. Low ERCC1 expression correlates with prolonged survival after cisplatin plus gemcitabine chemotherapy in non-small cell lung cancer. *Clin Cancer Res* 2002;8(7):2286–2291.
26. Cobo M, Isla D, Massuti B, et al. Customizing cisplatin based on quantitative excision repair cross-complementing 1 mRNA expression: a phase III trial in non-small-cell lung cancer. *J Clin Oncol* 2007;25(19):2747–2754.

27. Olaussen KA, Dunant A, Fouret P, et al. DNA repair by ERCC1 in non-small-cell lung cancer and cisplatin-based adjuvant chemotherapy. *N Engl J Med* 2006;355(10):983–991.
28. Davidson JD, Ma L, Flagella M, et al. An increase in the expression of ribonucleotide reductase large subunit 1 is associated with gemcitabine resistance in non-small cell lung cancer cell lines. *Cancer Res* 2004; 64(11):3761–3766.
29. Ceppi P, Volante M, Novello S, et al. ERCC1 and RRM1 gene expressions but not EGFR are predictive of shorter survival in advanced non-small-cell lung cancer treated with cisplatin and gemcitabine. *Ann Oncol* 2006;17(12):1818–1825.
30. Bepler G, Kusmartseva I, Sharma S, et al. RRM1 modulated in vitro and in vivo efficacy of gemcitabine and platinum in non-small-cell lung cancer. *J Clin Oncol* 2006;24(29):4731–4737.
31. Simon G, Sharma A, Li X, et al. Feasibility and efficacy of molecular analysis-directed individualized therapy in advanced non-small-cell lung cancer. *J Clin Oncol* 2007;25(19):2741–2746.
32. Zheng Z, Chen T, Li X, et al. DNA synthesis and repair genes RRM1 and ERCC1 in lung cancer. *N Engl J Med* 2007;356(8):800–808.
33. Bepler G. Phase II pharmacogenomics-based adjuvant therapy trial in patients with non-small-cell lung cancer: Southwest Oncology Group Trial 0720. *Clin Lung Cancer* 2007;8(8):509–511.
34. Wakelee H, Dubey S, Gandara D. Optimal adjuvant therapy for non-small cell lung cancer—how to handle stage I disease. *Oncologist* 2007;12(3): 331–337.
35. Moynahan ME, Cui TY, Jasin M. Homology-directed dna repair, mitomycin-c resistance, and chromosome stability is restored with correction of a Brca1 mutation. *Cancer Res* 2001;61(12):4842–4850.
36. Quinn JE, Kennedy RD, Mullan PB, et al. BRCA1 functions as a differential modulator of chemotherapy-induced apoptosis. *Cancer Res* 2003;63(19):6221–6228.
37. Taron M, Rosell R, Felip E, et al. BRCA1 mRNA expression levels as an indicator of chemoresistance in lung cancer. *Hum Mol Genet* 2004; 13(20):2443–2449.
38. Rosell R, Skrzypski M, Jassem E, et al. BRCA1: a novel prognostic factor in resected non-small cell lung cancer. *PLoS One* 2007;2(11): E1129.
39. Cobo M, Massuti B, Morán T, et al. Spanish customized adjuvant trial (SCAT) based on BRCA1 mRNA levels. *J Clin Oncol* 2008;26(suppl): abstract 7533.
40. Gautschi O, Mack PC, Davies AM, et al. Pharmacogenomic approaches to individualizing chemotherapy for non-small-cell lung cancer: current status and future directions. *Clin Lung Cancer* 2008;9(Suppl 3): S129–S138.
41. Azuma K, Komohara Y, Sasada T, et al. Excision repair cross-complementation group 1 predicts progression-free and overall survival in non-small cell lung cancer patients treated with platinum-based chemotherapy. *Cancer Sci* 2007;98(9):1336–1343.
42. Booton R, Ward T, Ashcroft L, et al. ERCC1 mRNA expression is not associated with response and survival after platinum-based chemotherapy regimens in advanced non-small cell lung cancer. *J Thorac Oncol* 2007;2(10):902–906.
43. Fujii T, Toyooka S, Ichimura K, et al. ERCC1 protein expression predicts the response of cisplatin-based neoadjuvant chemotherapy in non-small-cell lung cancer. *Lung Cancer* 2008;59:377–384.
44. Rosell R, Danenberg KD, Alberola V, et al. Ribonucleotide reductase messenger RNA expression and survival in gemcitabine/cisplatin-treated advanced non-small cell lung cancer patients. *Clin Cancer Res* 2004;10(4):1318–1325.
45. Rosell R, Felip E, Taron M, et al. Gene expression as a predictive marker of outcome in stage IIB-IIIA-IIIB non-small cell lung cancer after induction gemcitabine-based chemotherapy followed by resectional surgery. *Clin Cancer Res* 2004;10(suppl 12, pt 2):S4215–S4219.
46. Wachters FM, Wong LS, Timens W, et al. ERCC1, hRad51, and BRCA1 protein expression in relation to tumour response and survival of stage III/IV NSCLC patients treated with chemotherapy. *Lung Cancer* 2005;50(2):211–219.
47. Filipits M, Pirker R, Dunant A, et al. Cell cycle regulators and outcome of adjuvant cisplatin-based chemotherapy in completely resected non-small-cell lung cancer: the International Adjuvant Lung Cancer Trial Biologic Program. *J Clin Oncol* 2007;25(19):2735–2740.
48. Tsao MS, Aviel-Ronen S, Ding K, et al. Prognostic and predictive importance of p53 and RAS for adjuvant chemotherapy in non small-cell lung cancer. *J Clin Oncol* 2007;25(33):5240–5247.
49. Schiff PB, Fant J, Horwitz SB. Promotion of microtubule assembly in vitro by taxol. *Nature* 1979;277(5698):665–667.
50. Noble RL. The discovery of the vinca alkaloids–chemotherapeutic agents against cancer. *Biochem Cell Biol* 1990;68(12):1344–1351.
51. Kamath K, Wilson L, Cabral F, et al. BetaIII-tubulin induces paclitaxel resistance in association with reduced effects on microtubule dynamic instability. *J Biol Chem* 2005;280(13):12902–12907.
52. Sève P, Isaac S, Trédan O, et al. Expression of class III {beta}-tubulin is predictive of patient outcome in patients with non-small cell lung cancer receiving vinorelbine-based chemotherapy. *Clin Cancer Res* 2005; 11(15):5481–5486.
53. Sève P, Mackey J, Isaac S, et al. Class III beta-tubulin expression in tumor cells predicts response and outcome in patients with non-small cell lung cancer receiving paclitaxel. *Mol Cancer Ther* 2005;4(12):2001–2007.
54. Sève P, Lai R, Ding K, et al. Class III beta-tubulin expression and benefit from adjuvant cisplatin/vinorelbine chemotherapy in operable non-small cell lung cancer: analysis of NCIC JBR.10. *Clin Cancer Res* 2007;13(3):994–999.
55. Giannakakou P, Sackett DL, Kang YK, et al. Paclitaxel-resistant human ovarian cancer cells have mutant beta-tubulins that exhibit impaired paclitaxel-driven polymerization. *J Biol Chem* 1997;272(27):17118–17125.
56. Monzó M, Rosell R, Sánchez JJ, et al. Paclitaxel resistance in non-small-cell lung cancer associated with beta-tubulin gene mutations. *J Clin Oncol* 1999;17(6):1786–1793.
57. Sale S, Sung R, Shen P, et al. Conservation of the class I beta-tubulin gene in human populations and lack of mutations in lung cancers and paclitaxel-resistant ovarian cancers. *Mol Cancer Ther* 2002;1(3):215–225.
58. Veitia R, Bissery MC, Martinez C, et al. Tau expression in model adenocarcinomas correlates with docetaxel sensitivity in tumour-bearing mice. *Br J Cancer* 1998;78(7):871–877.
59. Rouzier R, Rajan R, Wagner P, et al. Microtubule-associated protein tau: a marker of paclitaxel sensitivity in breast cancer. *Proc Natl Acad Sci U S A* 2005;102(23):8315–8320.
60. Dumontet C, Isaac S, Souquet PJ, et al. Expression of class III beta tubulin in non-small cell lung cancer is correlated with resistance to taxane chemotherapy. *Bull Cancer* 2005;92(2):E25–E30.
61. Gautschi O, Mack P, Heighway J, et al. Cellular and molecular biology of lung cancer as the basis for targeted therapy. In: Pandya K, Brahmer J, Hidalgo M, eds. *Lung Cancer: translational and other emerging therapies.* New York: Taylor and Francis, 2007.
62. Kwiatkowski DJ, Harpole DH Jr, Godleski J, et al. Molecular pathologic substaging in 244 stage I non-small-cell lung cancer patients: clinical implications. *J Clin Oncol* 1998;16(7):2468–2477.
63. Mack PC, Galvin IV, Kimura T, et al. Molecular abnormalities of DNA damage and anti-microtubule response pathways in non-small cell lung carcinomas (NSCLC) from patients on the Southwest Oncology Group (SWOG) 9509 trial. *Proc Am Soc Clin Oncol* 2003;22:(abstr 2569).
64. Chen HY, Yu SL, Chen CH, et al. A five-gene signature and clinical outcome in non-small-cell lung cancer. *N Engl J Med* 2007;356(1):11–20.
65. Potti A, Mukherjee S, Petersen R, et al. A genomic strategy to refine prognosis in early-stage non-small-cell lung cancer. *N Engl J Med* 2006; 355(6):570–580.
66. Minna JD, Girard L, Xie Y. Tumor mRNA expression profiles predict responses to chemotherapy. *J Clin Oncol* 2007;25(28):4329–4336.
67. Oshita F, Ikehara M, Sekiyama A, et al. Genomic-wide cDNA microarray screening to correlate gene expression profile with chemoresistance in patients with advanced lung cancer. *J Exp Ther Oncol* 2004;4(2):155–160.
68. Hsu DS, Balakumaran BS, Acharya CR, et al. Pharmacogenomic strategies provide a rational approach to the treatment of cisplatin-resistant patients with advanced cancer. *J Clin Oncol* 2007;25(28):4350–4357.

69. Hsu DS, Balakumaran BS, Acharya CR, et al. Pharmacogenomic strategies provide a rational approach to the treatment of cisplatin-resistant patients with advanced cancer. *J Clin Oncol* 2007;25(28):4350–4357.
70. Camps C, Sirera R, Iranzo V, et al. Gene expression and polymorphisms of DNA repair enzymes: cancer susceptibility and response to chemotherapy. *Clin Lung Cancer* 2007;8(6):369–375.
71. Innocenti F, Undevia SD, Iyer L, et al. Genetic variants in the UDP-glucuronosyltransferase 1A1 gene predict the risk of severe neutropenia of irinotecan. *J Clin Oncol* 2004;22(8):1382–1388.
72. Iyer L, Das S, Janisch L, et al. UGT1A1*28 polymorphism as a determinant of irinotecan disposition and toxicity. *Pharmacogenomics J* 2002;2(1):43–47.
73. Kivistö KT, Kroemer HK, Eichelbaum M. The role of human cytochrome P450 enzymes in the metabolism of anticancer agents: implications for drug interactions. *Br J Clin Pharmacol* 1995;40(6):523–530.
74. Koch I, Weil R, Wolbold R, et al. Interindividual variability and tissue-specificity in the expression of cytochrome P450 3A mRNA. *Drug Metab Dispos* 2002;30(10):1108–1114.
75. Kuehl P, Zhang J, Lin Y, et al. Sequence diversity in CYP3A promoters and characterization of the genetic basis of polymorphic CYP3A5 expression. *Nat Genet* 2001;27(4):383–391.
76. Giacomini KM, Brett CM, Altman RB, et al. The pharmacogenetics research network: from SNP discovery to clinical drug response. *Clin Pharmacol Ther* 2007;81(3):328–345.
77. Henningsson A, Marsh S, Loos WJ, et al. Association of CYP2C8, CYP3A4, CYP3A5, and ABCB1 polymorphisms with the pharmacokinetics of paclitaxel. *Clin Cancer Res* 2005;11(22):8097–8104.
78. Ford BN, Ruttan CC, Kyle VL, et al. Identification of single nucleotide polymorphisms in human DNA repair genes. *Carcinogenesis* 2000;21(11):1977–1981.
79. Kiyohara C, Yoshimasu K. Genetic polymorphisms in the nucleotide excision repair pathway and lung cancer risk: a meta-analysis. *Int J Med Sci* 2007;4(2):59–71.
80. Rosell R, Cecere F, Santarpia M, et al. Predicting the outcome of chemotherapy for lung cancer. *Curr Opin Pharmacol* 2006;6(4):323–331.
81. Gurubhagavatula S, Liu G, Park S, et al. XPD and XRCC1 genetic polymorphisms are prognostic factors in advanced non-small-cell lung cancer patients treated with platinum chemotherapy. *J Clin Oncol* 2004;22(13):2594–2601.
82. Ryu JS, Hong YC, Han HS, et al. Association between polymorphisms of ERCC1 and XPD and survival in non-small-cell lung cancer patients treated with cisplatin combination chemotherapy. *Lung Cancer* 2004;44(3):311–316.
83. de las Peñas R, Sanchez-Ronco M, Alberola V, et al. Polymorphisms in DNA repair genes modulate survival in cisplatin/gemcitabine-treated non-small-cell lung cancer patients. *Ann Oncol* 2006;17(4):668–675.
84. Sekine I, Nokihara H, Yamamoto N, et al. Common arm analysis: one approach to develop the basis for global standardization in clinical trials of non-small cell lung cancer. *Lung Cancer* 2006;53(2):157–164.
85. Gandara DR, Kawaguchi T, Crowley J, et al. Japanese-US common-arm analysis of paclitaxel plus carboplatin in advanced non-small-cell lung cancer: a model for assessing population-related pharmacogenomics. *J Clin Oncol* 2009;27(21):3540–3546.
86. Gautschi O, Bigosch C, Huegli B, et al. Circulating deoxyribonucleic acid as prognostic marker in non-small-cell lung cancer patients undergoing chemotherapy. *J Clin Oncol* 2004;22(20):4157–4164.
87. Gautschi O, Huegli B, Ziegler A, et al. Origin and prognostic value of circulating KRAS mutations in lung cancer patients. *Cancer Lett* 2007;254(2):265–273.
88. Kimura T, Holland WS, Kawaguchi T, et al. Mutant DNA in plasma of lung cancer patients: potential for monitoring response to therapy. *Ann N Y Acad Sci* 2004;1022:55–60.
89. Ramirez JL, Rosell R, Taron M, et al. 14-3-3sigma methylation in pretreatment serum circulating DNA of cisplatin-plus-gemcitabine-treated advanced non-small-cell lung cancer patients predicts survival: the Spanish Lung Cancer Group. *J Clin Oncol* 2005;23(36):9105–9112.
90. Sozzi G, Conte D, Leon M, et al. Quantification of free circulating DNA as a diagnostic marker in lung cancer. *J Clin Oncol* 2003;21(21):3902–3908.
91. Shih C, Habeck LL, Mendelsohn LG, et al. Multiple folate enzyme inhibition: mechanism of a novel pyrrolopyrimidine-based antifolate LY231514 (MTA). *Adv Enzyme Regul* 1998;38:135–152.
92. Scagliotti GV, Parikh P, von Pawel J, et al. Phase III study comparing cisplatin plus gemcitabine with cisplatin plus pemetrexed in chemotherapy-naive patients with advanced-stage non-small-cell lung cancer. *J Clin Oncol* 2008;26(21):3543–3551.
93. Ceppi P, Volante M, Saviozzi S, et al. Squamous cell carcinoma of the lung compared with other histotypes shows higher messenger RNA and protein levels for thymidylate synthase. *Cancer* 2006;107(7):1589–1596.
94. Hanauske AR, Eismann U, Oberschmidt O, et al. In vitro chemosensitivity of freshly explanted tumor cells to pemetrexed is correlated with target gene expression. *Invest New Drugs* 2007;25(5):417–423.
95. Chung CH, Levy S, Chaurand P, et al. Genomics and proteomics: emerging technologies in clinical cancer research. *Crit Rev Oncol Hematol* 2007;61(1):1–25.
96. Ma Y, Ding Z, Qian Y, et al. Predicting cancer drug response by proteomic profiling. *Clin Cancer Res* 2006;12(15):4583–4589.
97. Taguchi F, Solomon B, Gregorc V, et al. Mass spectrometry to classify non-small-cell lung cancer patients for clinical outcome after treatment with epidermal growth factor receptor tyrosine kinase inhibitors: a multicohort cross-institutional study. *J Natl Cancer Inst* 2007;99(11):838–846.

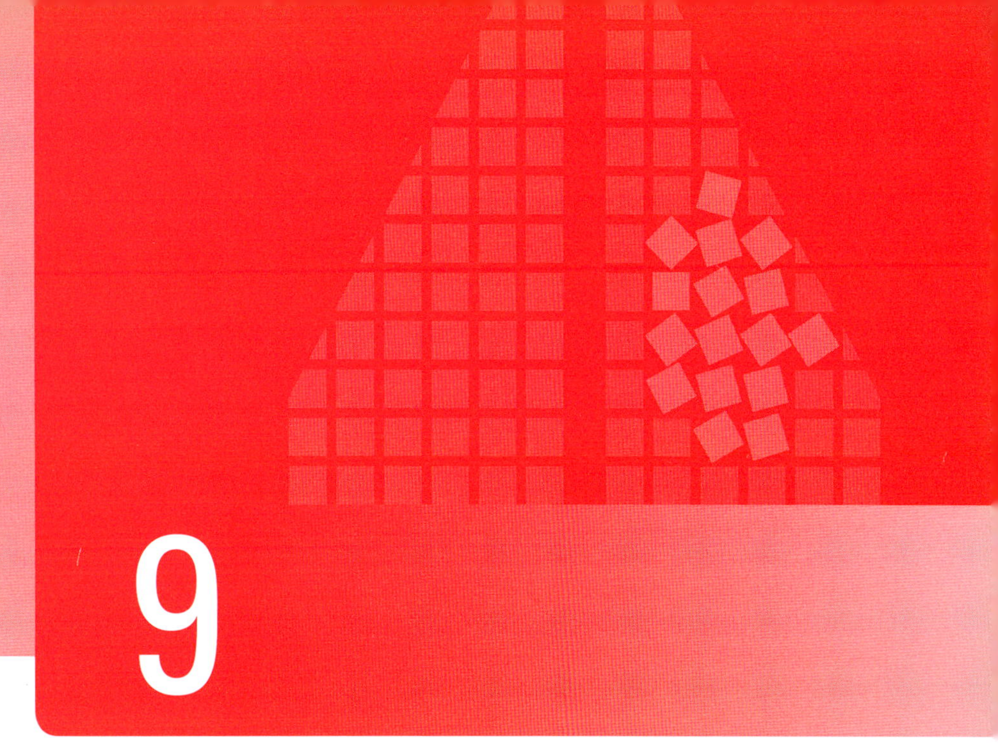

SECTION 9

Novel Targeted Agents and Lung Cancer

CHAPTER 48

Christian Manegold
Leora Horn
Alan Sandler

Antiangiogenic Agents

ROLE OF ANGIOGENESIS IN SOLID TUMORS

Tumor development is a multistep and complex process, requiring the transformation of a normal cell into a tumor cell through the accumulation of genetic alterations and the expansion of cell populations that have acquired growth and invasion advantages. However, in addition to the genetic and epigenetic alterations of transformation, another discrete process is required to allow tumor growth and metastasis—the induction of tumor vasculature known as the "angiogenic switch" (see also Chapter 8). Small tumors with a diameter <2 mm are dormant, receiving oxygen and nutrients by diffusion. Malignant growth and metastatic progression requires the tumor to develop an independent capillary network through two distinct processes, vasculogenesis and angiogenesis.[1] In vasculogenesis, new blood vessels are formed when endothelial precursor cells (angioblasts) migrate and differentiate in response to stimuli such as growth factors. These nascent vascular trees are then remodeled and extended through angiogenesis. During tumor growth, circulating endothelial progenitor cells (derivatives of stem cells) can contribute to neovascularization.[2] In contrast to vasculogenesis, angiogenesis is the formation of new blood vessels from preexisting vasculature.

Like many other physiological processes, angiogenesis is tightly orchestrated, regulated by a dynamic balance of proangiogenic and antiangiogenic molecules that drive and inhibit angiogenesis, respectively. The primary factor controlling angiogenesis is a lack of oxygen (hypoxia). Low oxygen tension triggers the secretion of proangiogenic factors and stimulates new vessel formation to increase oxygen supply. Tumor progression relies on tipping the balance in favor of molecules that drive angiogenesis. To achieve this, tumors undergo an angiogenic switch, creating an imbalance between the proangiogenic and antiangiogenic factors, resulting in increased angiogenesis and subsequent tumor progression and metastasis.[3,4] The timing of this angiogenic switch during tumor progression is influenced by various factors including tumor type and environment.

Angiogenesis in tumors is aberrant, and tumor blood vessels have multiple structural and functional abnormalities. They are unusually dynamic and naturally undergo sprouting, proliferation, remodeling, or regression. The vessels are irregularly shaped and lack the normal architectural arrangement of arterioles, capillaries, and venules. Endothelial cells in tumors have abnormalities in gene expression, require growth factors for survival, and have defective barrier function to plasma proteins. Pericytes are relatively undifferentiated cells associated with the walls of physiologically normal small blood vessels and are also important elements of the vascular support structure of tumors, regulating endothelial cell survival and directing capillary growth.[5] Pericytes on tumor vessels are also abnormal and, together with aberrant endothelial cells, generate a defective basement membrane. The effects of agents that inhibit factors involved in angiogenesis include stopping the growth of tumor vasculature, modifying existing vessels, and normalizing surviving vessels,[6] indicating that tumor vasculature is reliant on continued expression of these factors for growth and survival.

Proangiogenic molecules that promote proliferation and migration are mainly receptor tyrosine kinase ligands, such as vascular endothelial growth factor (VEGF), fibroblast growth factors, platelet-derived growth factor (PDGF), and epidermal growth factor, but can also be of very different origin, such as lysophosphatic acid. Antiangiogenic molecules include statins such as angiostatin (a fragment of plasminogen that binds adenosine triphosphate [ATP] synthase and annexin II), endostatin, tumstatin, and canstatin (fragments of collagens that bind to integrins). Table 48.1 lists the known proangiogenic and antiangiogenic molecules. Changes in the balance of these proangiogenic and antiangiogenic molecules mediate the angiogenic switch.[4] The precise role of many of these factors remains unclear; it is likely that ongoing and future research will attempt to further define the roles of these factors.

TABLE 48.1 List of Known Proangiogenic and Antiangiogenic Molecules and Agents

List of Known Angiogenic Growth Factors	List of Known Angiogenesis Inhibitors in the Body
Angiogenin	Angioarrestin
Angiopoietin-1	Angiostatin (plasminogen fragment)
Del-1	Antiangiogenic antithrombin III
Fibroblast growth factors: acidic (aFGF) and basic (bFGF)	Cartilage-derived inhibitor (CDI)
Follistatin	CD59 complement fragment
Granulocyte colony-stimulating factor (G-CSF)	Endostatin (collagen XVIII fragment)
Hepatocyte growth factor (HGF)/scatter factor (SF)	Fibronectin fragment
Interleukin 8 (IL-8)	Gro-β
Leptin	Heparinases
Midkine	Heparin hexasaccharide fragment
Placental growth factor	Human chorionic gonadotropin (hCG)
Platelet-derived endothelial cell growth factor (PD-ECGF)	Interferon $\alpha/\beta/\gamma$
Platelet-derived growth factor-BB (PDGF-BB)	Interferon-inducible protein (IP-10)
Pleiotrophin (PTN)	Interleukin 12 (IL-12)
Progranulin	Kringle 5 (plasminogen fragment)
Proliferin	Metalloproteinase inhibitors (TIMPs)
Transforming growth factor α (TGF-α)	2-methoxyestradiol
Transforming growth factor β (TGF-β)	Placental ribonuclease inhibitor
Tumor necrosis factor α (TNF-α)	Plasminogen activator inhibitor
Vascular endothelial growth factor (VEGF)/ vascular permeability factor (VPF)	Platelet factor-4 (PF4)
	Prolactin 16kD fragment
	Proliferin-related protein (PRP)
	Retinoids
	Tetrahydrocortisol-S
	Thrombospondin-1 (TSP-1)
	Transforming growth factor β (TGF-β)
	Vasculostatin
	Vasostatin (calreticulin fragment)

From Understanding angiogenesis. Angiogenesis Foundation Web site. http://www.angio.org/understanding/understanding.html.

Angiogenesis does occur normally in the human body at specific times in development and growth; for example, it is an integral part of fetal development in utero. However, angiogenesis has a limited physiological role in healthy adults, where its functions are restricted to wound healing and the female menstrual cycle for a few days each month as new blood vessels form in the lining of the uterus. Inhibiting angiogenesis, therefore, has minimal adverse effects on normal physiological processes. As angiogenesis is essential for tumor growth, it is a rational therapeutic target. Agents targeting the effects of VEGF, one of the most important proangiogenic factors, and its downstream signaling pathways have been developed for the first-line treatment of patients with advanced non–small cell lung cancer (NSCLC) as well as other solid tumors, including metastatic colorectal, breast, and renal cell carcinoma.

VEGF: THE KEY MEDIATOR OF ANGIOGENESIS

VEGF directly stimulates angiogenesis and is a key protein for sustaining tumor growth. VEGF is first synthesized inside tumor cells and then secreted into the surrounding tissue. When the VEGF ligand encounters endothelial cells, it binds to its main cell surface receptor, VEGF receptor 2. Ligand-receptor binding activates the endothelial cell and sets in motion a cascade of events that lead to the creation of new blood vessels (Fig. 48.1).[7] First, the activated endothelial cell produces matrix metalloproteinases, a special class of degradative enzymes. These enzymes are released from the endothelial cell into the surrounding tissue where they degrade the extracellular matrix, allowing the migration of endothelial cells. As they migrate into the surrounding tissues, activated endothelial

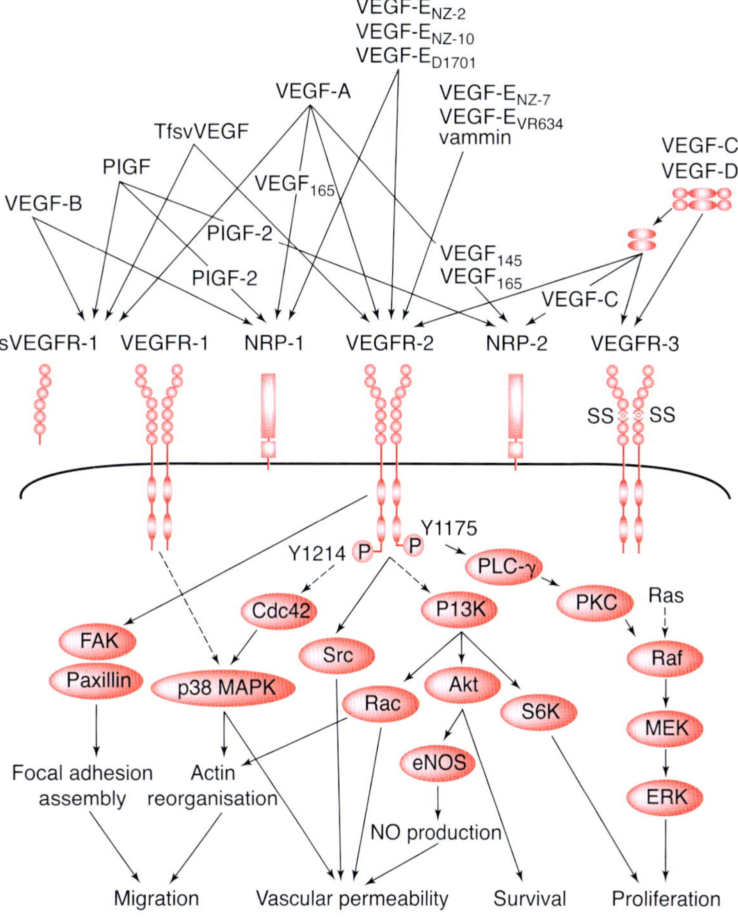

FIGURE 48.1 The vascular endothelial growth factor (VEGF) signaling pathway.[7] *AKT*, AKT8 virus oncogene homologue; *CDC42*, cell division control protein 42; *ERK*, extracellular signal-regulated kinase; *FAK*, focal adhesion kinase; *MAPK*, mitogen-activated protein kinase; *MEK*, MAPK/Erk kinase; *NRP*, neuropilin; *PI3K*, phosphatidylenositol 3 kinase; *PKC*, protein kinase C; *PLC*, phospholipase C; *PIGF*, placenta growth factor; *Src*, rous sarcoma oncogene cellular; *VEGFR*, vascular endothelial growth factor receptor.

cells begin to divide, organize into hollow tubes, and gradually evolve into a mature network of blood vessels.[8,9]

VEGF and the VEGF signaling pathway have been the focus of an increasing number of studies as cancer targets. VEGF is expressed by many solid tumors, including melanoma,[10] gastrointestinal,[11] breast,[12] central nervous system (CNS),[13] ovarian,[14] cervical,[15] lung,[16] hepatic,[17] head and neck,[18] and kidney[19] carcinomas. Analysis of microvessel density can provide an indirect measure of angiogenesis. In many studies, VEGF levels have been shown to correlate with microvessel density, which is higher in advanced tumors compared with early stage tumors.[20–24] A study of 105 patients with NSCLC demonstrated a significant association between VEGF expression and new vessel formation ($p < 0.0001$), overall survival ($p = 0.00003$), and disease-free survival ($p = 0.0004$).[21] In another study of specimens from 223 patients with operable NSCLC, 46.6% of cases had high VEGF expression. VEGF positivity was associated with high vascular grade disease ($p = 0.009$) and was prognostic for poor survival ($p = 0.02$).[20] Several other studies have now confirmed a strong association between VEGF positivity and tumor grade and prognosis in NSCLC: Prognosis for patients with VEGF-positive tumors has been consistently shown to be significantly worse than that for patients with VEGF-negative tumors ($p = 0.003$[22] and $p = 0.019$[23]).

VEGF exists in at least seven isoforms that result from alternative patterns of splicing of VEGF mRNA.[8,9] One study evaluating the correlation between the expression of four different VEGF mRNA isoforms suggests that expression of $VEGF_{189}$ mRNA isoform shows a greater correlation with survival and postoperative relapse time than expression of $VEGF_{121}$, $VEGF_{165}$, and $VEGF_{206}$ mRNA isoforms.[24] High $VEGF_{189}$ mRNA isoform expression was associated with short survival (<24 months; $p = 0.001$) and early postoperative relapse (<12 months; $p = 0.001$), whereas no correlation was seen with $VEGF_{165}$ and $VEGF_{206}$, suggesting that only expression of certain VEGF isoforms may be prognostic indicators for NSCLC.[24]

Structurally, VEGF (sometimes referred to as VEGF-A or vascular permeability factor[25]) belongs to the platelet-derived growth factor (PDGF) family of cystine-knot growth factors.[8] Other closely related proteins have been discovered (placenta growth factor [PlGF], VEGF-B, VEGF-C, and VEGF-D), and together these comprise the VEGF subfamily of growth factors.[8] Several VEGF-related proteins are produced by viruses (VEGF-E) and in the venom of some snakes (VEGF-F).

VEGF growth factor ligands have specific VEGF receptors to which they bind to produce their physiological effects. VEGF-A binds to both VEGF receptor 1 (Flt-1) and

2 (KDR/Flk-1), but VEGF receptor 2 is believed to mediate almost all known cellular responses to VEGF.[8] The function of VEGF receptor 1 is less well defined, although it is thought to modify VEGF receptor 2 signaling.[8] Another function of VEGF receptor 1 may be to act as a decoy receptor, sequestering VEGF from VEGF receptor 2 binding, and this may be particularly important during embryonic vasculogenesis.[26] A third receptor has been discovered (VEGF receptor 3), but VEGF-A is not a ligand for this receptor. VEGF receptor 3 mediates lymphangiogenesis in response to VEGF-C and VEGF-D binding.[8,9,16]

The biological effects of VEGF are thus initialized primarily through binding to VEGF receptor 2,[27] which is expressed predominantly on vascular endothelial cells.[28] VEGF receptor 2 is similar in structure to other tyrosine kinase receptors. It consists of seven extracellular immunoglobulin-like domains, a transmembrane region, and an intracellular domain with tyrosine kinase activity.[29,30] VEGF binding to VEGF receptor 2 and subsequent receptor homodimerization are essential for stimulation of VEGF receptor 2-induced intracellular signaling, which is in turn essential to the VEGF signaling pathway.

MECHANISM OF ACTION OF ANTIANGIOGENIC AGENTS

Neutralizing the biological activity of VEGF reduces tumor vascularization and consequently inhibits tumor growth.[6,31] A nonspecific tyrosine kinase inhibitor of the VEGF receptor prevented migration of endothelial cells, blocked capillary-like tubule formation, and prevented tumor blood vessel formation.[31] Inhibition also prevented the formation of lung metastases and slowed progression of tumor growth. Importantly, for a potential therapeutic target, VEGF receptor inhibition had minimal effects on established blood vessels or blood flow. These findings indicate that a potent therapeutic role for VEGF inhibitors may be to prevent the formation of new blood vessels. Inhibition of VEGF signaling by blocking VEGF receptor 2 also inhibits angiogenesis, tumor growth, and invasion. VEGF receptor 2 blockade causes vessel regression and normalization as well as stromal maturation, resulting in a reversion to a noninvasive tumor phenotype. Importantly, this study suggests a crucial role for the stromal microenvironment (see Chapter 50) in regulating tumor phenotype and thus maintained and continuous VEGF inhibition may be essential for prolonged tumor suppression, which, in the clinical setting, may translate to prolonged progression-free survival (PFS).[32–34]

"Ghosts" or "tracks" of basement membrane and accompanying pericytes left behind after endothelial cells degenerate may provide a "scaffold" for microvascular regrowth in the absence of inhibition of angiogenesis. Given the transient and reversible effects of VEGF inhibition on tumors, with revascularization documented within weeks of withdrawal of inhibition,[32–34] eradication of pericytes and ghosts of basement membrane may augment and prolong VEGF-inhibitor activity by decreasing the potential for vascular regrowth.[34] Preclinical data suggest that dual targeting of pericytes and endothelial cells may be a more effective antiangiogenic strategy than anti-endothelial cell targeting alone.[5]

Antiangiogenic Approaches

As discussed, the evidence for the central role of VEGF-regulated angiogenesis in tumor growth and progression has provided a strong rationale for the development of agents that exert their antitumor effects through inhibition of various stages of the VEGF pathway. As such, the majority of antiangiogenic approaches to date have focused on the inhibition of this key proangiogenic factor. Of these, the most promising approaches are monoclonal antibodies directed at VEGF ligand and small molecule tyrosine kinase inhibitors that block the VEGF receptor(s) (Fig. 48.2).

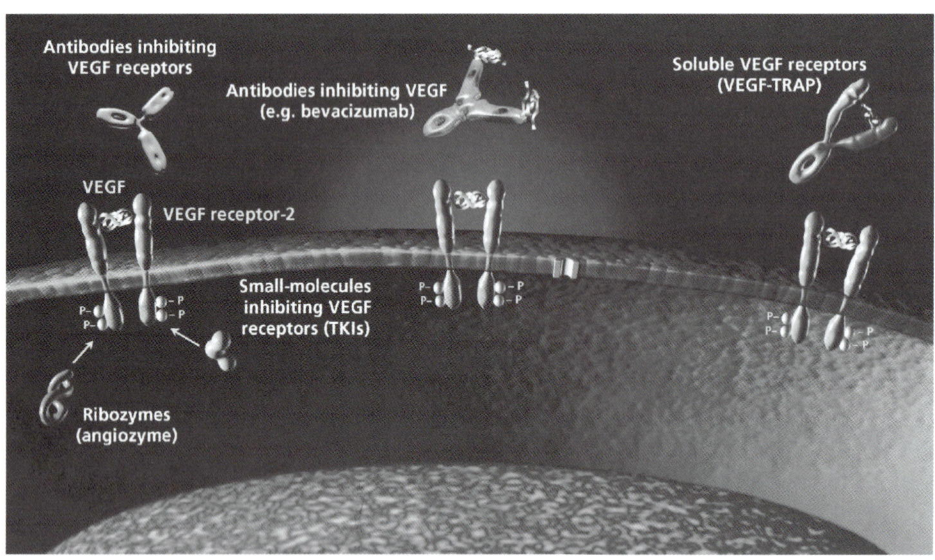

FIGURE 48.2 Agents targeting the vascular endothelial growth factor (VEGF) pathway. *TKIs*, tyrosine kinase inhibitors; *VEGF*, vascular endothelial growth factor.

Anti-VEGF Antibodies

Bevacizumab Bevacizumab, developed from the murine antihuman antibody A4.6.1, is a monoclonal antibody with a high affinity for VEGF.[35,36] A4.6.1 was shown to potently suppress neovascularization and tumor growth and was humanized by site-directed mutagenesis to facilitate therapeutic use. The recombinant humanized antibody, bevacizumab, was able to bind VEGF with similar affinity to that of the original murine antibody and inhibit VEGF-induced proliferation of endothelial cells in vitro and tumor growth in vivo with potency and efficacy similar to A4.6.1. Bevacizumab exerts its antiangiogenic effects by binding to free, circulating VEGF, thereby inhibiting the binding of VEGF to its receptors, preventing VEGF ligand-receptor downstream signaling.[36] To date, first-line bevacizumab combined with standard platinum-based chemotherapy has demonstrated clinical activity in a phase II trial[37] and two phase III trials in patients with NSCLC.[38,39]

In the phase II trial, bevacizumab in combination with carboplatin and paclitaxel improved overall response and time to progression in patients with untreated advanced or recurrent NSCLC.[37] In this trial, 99 patients were randomized to carboplatin/paclitaxel every 3 weeks (n = 32) or carboplatin/paclitaxel with bevacizumab 7.5 mg/kg (n = 32) or 15 mg/kg (n = 35) every 3 weeks. Patients with progressive disease who had received chemotherapy alone went on to receive single-agent bevacizumab. The combination of bevacizumab 15 mg/kg with carboplatin/paclitaxel increased response rate (31.5% vs. 18.8%) and prolonged time to progression (median 7.4 vs. 4.2 months; $p = 0.023$) with a 46% reduction in the risk of progression during treatment. With bevacizumab 7.5 mg/kg, there was a modest increase in response rate (28.1% vs. 18.8%) but no difference in time to progression (median 4.3 vs. 3.2 months). One-year survival was 47% for patients (n = 19) receiving chemotherapy alone who progressed and went on to receive single-agent bevacizumab. Bleeding was the most prominent adverse event (AE), mainly evident as minor mucocutaneous hemorrhage and major hemoptysis. Severe pulmonary hemorrhage was observed in six patients (9.1%) and led to four fatalities. An exploratory analysis identified increased risk of bleeding in patients with squamous cell histology, tumor necrosis and cavitation, and disease location close to major blood vessels.[40] Further analysis excluding patients with squamous histology suggested that both doses of bevacizumab increased response rate, time to progression, and survival compared with chemotherapy alone and with only a small increased risk of bleeding (~4%).[37]

Based on the positive results of the phase II trial, a randomized phase III trial of bevacizumab-based first-line therapy was conducted by the Eastern Cooperative Oncology Group (ECOG).[38] In the E4599 trial, 878 patients with recurrent or advanced NSCLC (stage IIIB or IV) were randomized to bevacizumab 15 mg/kg with carboplatin/paclitaxel (n = 434) or carboplatin/paclitaxel alone (n = 444) every 3 weeks for six cycles until disease progression or unacceptable toxicity.[38] The 15 mg/kg dose was chosen based on its activity in the phase II trial and based on exploratory analyses from the phase II trial, patients with squamous histology were excluded from E4599. Patients with brain metastases or clinically significant hemoptysis were also excluded. The primary end point was overall survival.

A survival advantage was demonstrated for bevacizumab-based first-line therapy compared with conventional chemotherapy alone. Median overall survival was 12.3 months for bevacizumab-based therapy compared with 10.3 months for chemotherapy alone (hazard ratio [HR] = 0.79; $p = 0.003$). Median PFS was 6.2 and 4.5 months, respectively (HR = 0.66; $p < 0.001$), with corresponding response rates of 35% and 15% ($p < 0.001$). Exclusion of patients with squamous cell histology resulted in a reduction in the rates of clinically significant bleeding compared with the earlier phase II trial.[37] Notably, the incidence of severe pulmonary hemorrhage in E4599 was reduced when compared with the patients with nonsquamous histology in the phase II trial (1.9% vs. 4%, respectively). There were 15 treatment-related deaths among patients receiving bevacizumab-based therapy, including five from pulmonary hemorrhage. VEGF levels before treatment were measured and found not to correlate with overall survival. An exploratory analysis found that despite improvements in PFS, there was no improvement in overall survival for women treated with bevacizumab-based therapy compared with chemotherapy alone (13.3 vs. 13.1 months). This was not true for men (11.7 vs. 8.7 months). The reasons for this are not clear.

In a pre-planned subset analysis of patients in E4599 with adenocarcinoma histology, bevacizumab-based therapy extended median overall survival to 14.2 months compared with 10.3 months for chemotherapy alone (HR = 0.69, a 31% reduction in the risk of death).[41] A retrospective subset analysis of elderly patients (≥70 years of age), representing 26% of study patients, found a trend toward higher response rates (17% vs. 29%) and PFS (4.9 vs. 5.9 months) but no difference in overall survival (12.1 vs. 11.3 months) for paclitaxel/carboplatin versus paclitaxel/carboplatin plus bevacizumab, respectively. Paclitaxel/carboplatin plus bevacizumab was also associated with a significantly higher incidence of grade 3 to 5 toxicities than paclitaxel/carboplatin (61% vs. 87%; $p < 0.001$).[42]

The improved outcome for bevacizumab-based first-line therapy in NSCLC has recently been confirmed in a second randomized phase III trial of bevacizumab in combination with cisplatin/gemcitabine. In the Avastin in lung (AVAiL; BO17704) trial, the combination of bevacizumab with cisplatin/gemcitabine improved PFS when compared with the platinum-based regimen alone.[39] In this trial, 1043 patients with advanced or recurrent nonsquamous NSCLC were randomized to receive cisplatin/gemcitabine for up to six cycles plus bevacizumab 7.5 mg/kg (n = 345), bevacizumab 15 mg/kg (n = 351), or placebo (n = 347) every 3 weeks until disease progression or unacceptable toxicity. As in E4599, patients with squamous cell histology, baseline hemoptysis, or brain metastases were excluded to minimize toxicity. In this trial, patients with tumors in proximity to or abutting major vessels were also excluded. Following the positive survival results of the E4599 trial for bevacizumab-based therapy versus chemotherapy alone, the primary end point of AVAiL was amended from overall survival to PFS.

Both doses of bevacizumab-based therapy demonstrated a significant PFS benefit compared with chemotherapy alone. Median PFS for bevacizumab 7.5 mg/kg and 15 mg/kg versus placebo was 6.7 versus 6.1 months (HR = 0.75; p = 0.003) and 6.5 versus 6.1 months (HR = 0.82; p = 0.03), respectively. Objective response rates were 34.1%, 30.4%, and 20.1% for bevacizumab 7.5 mg/kg, 15 mg/kg, and placebo, respectively. The PFS benefit did not translate into a significant overall survival benefit, possibly due to the high use of efficacious second-line therapies in the trial. Median overall survival for bevacizumab 7.5 mg/kg and 15 mg/kg versus placebo was 13.6 versus 13.1 months (HR 0.93; p = 0.420) and 13.4 versus 13.1 months (HR 1.03; p = 0.761), respectively.[43] The majority of AEs were grade 1 or 2 and the incidence of grade ≥3 AEs was similar across arms. Although 9% of patients received therapeutic anticoagulation, severe pulmonary hemorrhage rates were ≤1.5% for all arms, highlighting the role of patient selection in managing the risk of bleeding. The AE fatality rate (from any cause) was similar across treatment groups (4% to 5%). Although the AVAiL trial was not powered to compare the two bevacizumab doses directly, efficacy and safety data were similar for both doses. Table 48.2 presents a summary of results for the clinical trials of bevacizumab-based first-line therapy in NSCLC.

In addition to the two phase III trials, E4599 and AVAiL, the safety and clinical activity of bevacizumab-based therapy is being investigated in the Safety of Avastin in lung (SAiL; MO19390) trial. SAiL is a large (n = >2,100 patients are expected), open-label, multicentre, single-arm trial that is being conducted to generate further safety and efficacy data for bevacizumab combined with a range of standard first-line chemotherapy regimens in a broad 'real-life' clinical population of patients with advanced non-squamous NSCLC. The primary objective is to evaluate the safety profile of bevacizumab-based therapy. Interim results show that no new safety signals have been reported in this large study and that the safety profile of bevacizumab-based therapy is consistent with that reported in previous phase III trials.[44] Interim results from SAiL further confirm the safety profile of bevacizumab when used in combination with a wide range of chemotherapies. Final data, including efficacy outcomes, are anticipated in 2010. The clinical potential and therapeutic advance offered by bevacizumab are being evaluated further in an ongoing clinical research program. The majority of these (approximately 80%) are phase II trials with most evaluating the potential benefit of the addition of bevacizumab to different chemotherapy regimens, including pemetrexed/oxaliplatin,[45,46] pemetrexed/carboplatin,[47–49] docetaxel/carboplatin,[50] oxaliplatin/gemcitabine,[51] and gemcitabine/carboplatin.[52] However, many trials are combining bevacizumab not only with standard chemotherapy but with other biological therapies, most notably erlotinib in almost one quarter of trials listed. More creative approaches are also being studied, including novel combinations with targeted therapies and improved prognostic profiling to identify those patients most likely to benefit from specific therapeutic interventions. The increasing sophistication of clinical trials reflects the number of innovative agents available or in development, and our improved understanding of the underlying pathogenesis and tumorigenic processes that allow for rational combination of therapies with potentially complementary antitumor activity. Several of the significant ongoing bevacizumab trials, including trials in the neoadjuvant setting and trials in specific patient populations, deserve a special mention and are summarized later.

Combining Bevacizumab with Other Targeted Agents The concept of using two novel agents, such as an epidermal growth factor receptor (EGFR) inhibitor and an anti-VEGF agent, is intriguing. As discussed, the angiogenesis pathway is crucial in lung cancer development. Data have also demonstrated the significant therapeutic involvement of the

TABLE 48.2 Summary of Phase II and III Data for Bevacizumab-Based Therapy[37–39,43]

			Bevacizumab		
Trial	**Outcome**	**Control**	**7.5 mg/kg**	**15 mg/kg**	$p<0.05$*
Phase II[37]	ORR (%)	18.8	28.1	31.5	N/G
	Median PFS (mo)	4.2*	4.3	7.4*	✓
	Median OS (mo)	14.9	11.6	17.7	✗
E4599[38]	ORR (%)	15*	N/A	35*	✓
	Median PFS (mo)	4.5*	N/A	6.2*	✓
	Median OS (mo)	10.3*	N/A	12.3*	✓
AVAiL[39,43]	ORR (%)	20.1*	34.1*	30.4*	✓
	Median PFS (mo)	6.1*	6.7*	6.5*	✓
	Median OS (mo)	13.1	13.6	13.4	✗

*p values significant (<0.05) relative to control for asterisked values.

N/A, not applicable; N/G, not given; ORR, overall response rate; OS, overall survival; PFS, progression-free survival.

EGFR pathway in tumorigenesis.[53] Therefore, inhibiting both pathways to exert a greater combined antitumor effect, but with fewer nonspecific toxicities than chemotherapy,[54] represents a rational therapeutic approach.

Erlotinib (Tarceva), an oral HER-1 (human epidermal receptor 1)/EGFR tyrosine kinase inhibitor has shown a survival benefit in the treatment of lung cancer in phase III trials and is approved for the treatment of locally advanced or metastatic NSCLC in patients failing at least one prior chemotherapy regimen.[55] A phase I/II trail of 40 patients with advanced, nonsquamous NSCLC who had failed at least one prior chemotherapy regimen demonstrated a 20% response rate, 6.2 months PFS, 12.6 months overall survival, and no grade III/IV toxicity when bevacizumab (15 mg/kg) was combined with erlotinib (150 mg daily).[56] These results led to a randomized phase II trial comparing chemotherapy alone (docetaxel 75 mg/m^2 or pemetrexed 500 mg/m^2 every 3 weeks) to chemotherapy plus bevacizumab (15 mg/kg) or bevacizumab plus erlotinib (150 mg daily) in 120 patients with nonsquamous NSCLC who had progressed following platinum-based chemotherapy. Grade 3/4 toxicities were greater in the chemotherapy treatment arms with a higher proportion of patients discontinuing treatment caused by AEs (24% for chemotherapy alone vs. 28% for chemotherapy plus bevacizumab and 13% for erlotinib plus bevacizumab). The response rate was higher for the erlotinib plus bevacizumab combination (18%), versus 12% for chemotherapy alone and 13% for chemotherapy plus bevacizumab. Compared with chemotherapy alone, patients who received chemotherapy plus bevacizumab and erlotinib plus bevacizumab had superior outcomes, respectively, in terms of median PFS (3.0 vs. 4.8 vs. 4.4 months), overall survival (8.6 vs. 12.6 vs. 13.7 months), and 1-year survival (33% vs. 53.8% vs. 57.4%).[57]

Based on these results, the BeTa lung trial (OSI3364g/NCT00130728) has opened. This phase III trial will compare erlotinib with erlotinib plus bevacizumab in 655 patients with nonsquamous NSCLC who have progressed following standard first-line therapy. The primary end point is overall survival; secondary end points are PFS, response rate, and response duration. ATLAS (AVF3671g/NCT00257608) is another phase III trial assessing the efficacy and safety of maintenance bevacizumab with or without erlotinib following chemotherapy (carboplatin/paclitaxel, cisplatin/gemcitabine, or carboplatin/docetaxel) plus bevacizumab before randomization to bevacizumab with or without erlotinib, in 1150 previously untreated patients. The primary end point is PFS and secondary end points include safety of bevacizumab during the chemotherapy phase (by chemotherapy regimen) and safety of bevacizumab plus erlotinib versus bevacizumab plus placebo. Of note, patients with squamous cell histology and brain metastases are excluded from this trial.

Given that bevacizumab is administered until disease progression, a key issue to address is when it is appropriate to add erlotinib, which is approved in the second- or third-line settings. The value of earlier versus delayed initiation of erlotinib should be assessed, as should the optimal timing of bevacizumab/erlotinib therapy in the disease pathway.

A two-stage phase II trial evaluating up-front administration of erlotinib (150 mg daily) with bevacizumab (15 mg/kg every 21 days) is currently ongoing. Preliminary data from 33 patients indicate major toxicities (>10% of patients) to be rash and diarrhea. The primary end point of nonprogression at 6 weeks has been met in 75% of patients. With a median follow up of 6.3 months, the median time to progression is 5.5 months.[58] More mature data with correlative studies are pending.

These studies will shed light on how biologically active therapies can be best combined and possibly also identify subgroups of patients who derive most benefit from these interventions.

Bevacizumab in the Adjuvant Setting Based on results of the E4599 study, ECOG is conducting a phase III randomized trial in 1500 patients, evaluating the addition of bevacizumab to standard chemotherapy (cisplatin/gemcitabine, cisplatin/vinorelbine, or cisplatin/taxotere) in the adjuvant setting. Carboplatin/paclitaxel is not being utilized after the lung adjuvant cisplatin evaluation (LACE) metaanalysis demonstrated superior outcomes for patients treated with cisplatin-based regimens in the adjuvant setting.[59] Patients receive bevacizumab every 3 weeks for up to 1 year. The primary end point for this trial is overall survival and secondary end points are disease-free survival and toxicity. Analysis of tissue and blood samples for identification of predictive factors and evaluation of outcome according to smoking status is also planned.

Bevacizumab in the Neoadjuvant Setting Three trials are evaluating the potential of bevacizumab in the neoadjuvant setting. If effective, this approach may reduce tumor burden and either facilitate or negate the need for resection. The first of these is the randomized phase II BEACON study (NCT00130780) in patients (n = 70) with resectable (stage IB to IIIA) NSCLC. Patients are randomized based on histology, tumor, and patient factors. Patients with adenocarcinoma will receive presurgical treatment with bevacizumab (15 mg/kg) for 2 weeks followed by bevacizumab plus docetaxel/cisplatin, whereas patients with squamous cell histology, central tumor location, or recent hemoptysis will receive presurgical docetaxel/cisplatin alone. All patients receive adjuvant bevacizumab for 1 year following surgical resection. The primary goal of the study is to assess whether the addition of bevacizumab improves the rate of pathologic downstaging, defined as any decrease in the final pathologic stage compared with the clinical stage before induction therapy. Secondary end points include combined overall survival for both groups. Preliminary analyses show a similar rate of downstaging in both groups (5/9 patients in the bevacizumab treatment group and 5/8 patients in the chemotherapy-alone treatment group) and a low incidence of significant AEs (one patient developed hemoptysis preoperatively, and one patient had an upper gastrointestinal bleed postoperatively). Single-agent bevacizumab can regress tumors after 2 weeks and can be safely administered in the neoadjuvant and adjuvant setting.[60]

In another phase II neoadjuvant trial (NCT00025389), bevacizumab is being combined with carboplatin/paclitaxel in approximately 29 patients with resectable (stage IB to IIIA)

NSCLC. End points are clinical and pathologic response rate, resectability rate, and safety. This study, led by the National Cancer Institute, has now completed accrual. A final study (NCT00293332) combines bevacizumab with docetaxel/carboplatin in 50 patients. The primary end point is clinical response rate. Secondary end points include pathologic response rate, resectability rate, overall survival, time to treatment failure, and safety. Analysis of VEGF levels before and after treatment and/or resection is also planned.

Trials of bevacizumab in the neoadjuvant setting should elucidate the risks of bleeding and wound-healing complications in patients with NSCLC when bevacizumab is administered prior to surgery. In accordance with the recommendations in the Avastin Summary of Product Characteristics, elective major surgery should be delayed for at least 28 days following the last bevacizumab dose.[61] The administration of bevacizumab >28 days after major surgery appears to be feasible and safe in patients with colorectal cancer.[62] Of note, in the BEACON study, surgery occurs at least 42 days after the last bevacizumab administration, whereas in the NCT00025389 trial, patients underwent surgical resection 4 to 6 weeks after receiving two cycles of bevacizumab in combination with chemotherapy. Given the clear rationale for the use of bevacizumab in the neoadjuvant setting, it is important to obtain further information on the safety profile of neoadjuvant bevacizumab in patients with NSCLC.

Bevacizumab in Specific Patient Populations: Squamous Cell Histology Based on phase II data and the increased incidence of severe pulmonary hemorrhage in patients with squamous cell histology,[37] later phase III trials have generally excluded these patients[38,39] and bevacizumab is not indicated in patients with predominantly squamous histology. The precise reason for the increased risk of bleeding in particular patient subsets remains unknown. What makes squamous cell tumors particularly susceptible to bleeding with anti-VEGF therapy? These tumors tend to be more centrally located[63] and perhaps associated with increased local invasion. Large central lesions, which may undergo early cavitation, may increase the risk for bleeding complications. Furthermore, of all bronchogenic carcinomas, squamous cell carcinoma is the most likely to cavitate (about 15% of cases).[64] It is also possible that these tumors might form an integral component of the pulmonary arterial wall or be adjacent to another vital vascular structure. Finally, it is possible that bleeding complications are caused by an anti-VEGF class effect or a profound tumor response.

However, following preliminary positive efficacy data from an exploratory subgroup analysis of bevacizumab-based therapy in patients with squamous cell histology in the phase II trial AVF0757g,[37] the safety and efficacy of bevacizumab in these patients is now being specifically evaluated in further phase II studies. BRIDGE (AVF3744g/NCT00318136) is a pilot study of first-line bevacizumab in combination with carboplatin/paclitaxel (n = 40). The rate of grade ≥3 bleeding is the primary end point and rate of other AEs and PFS are secondary end points.

Bevacizumab in Specific Patient Populations: Brain Metastases Exclusion of patients with brain metastases from trials of bevacizumab in NSCLC[37–39] was a conservative approach based, in part, on the occurrence of a severe cerebrovascular bleeding event in a patient with hepatocellular carcinoma treated with single-agent bevacizumab in a phase I study (n = 25).[65] As trials to date have excluded patients with brain metastases, the balance between potential risk and potential benefit for bevacizumab-based therapy in this patient population remains to be assessed. Two ongoing phase II trials are evaluating the safety and efficacy of bevacizumab in combination with pemetrexed in the second-line setting (n = 40; NCT00227019) and in combination with first- or second-line chemotherapy (n = 110; PASSPORT trial; NCT00312728). The primary end point for both trials is the incidence of cerebrovascular bleeding, with other AEs and survival (PFS or overall) as secondary end points. Results from these trials are awaited. Based on safety data showing that the risk of bleeding in patients with untreated brain metastases is similar for patients who receive bevacizumab and those who do not,[66] the European Medicines Agency in March 2009 removed the restriction on the use of bevacizumab in patients with untreated brain metastases. No such restriction has ever existed in the USA. Data from ongoing phase IV trials of bevacizumab, in combination with a range of commonly used chemotherapy regimens involving 2000 (NCT00451906; SAiL) and 6000 (NCT00388206; ARIES) patients, should help to identify patient populations most suitable for, or likely to derive most benefit from, bevacizumab-based therapy.

Although bevacizumab is the first anti-VEGF therapy to be approved for NSCLC, other approaches are in rapid development. Table 48.3 provides an overview of drugs currently in development that target the VEGF pathway. The most promising of these approaches are reviewed in the remainder of this chapter.

Bevacizumab in Specific Patient Populations: Small Cell Lung Cancer Microvessel count (MVC), as a measure of angiogenesis, is a significant predictor of increased risk of metastatic disease and worse overall survival in patients with NSCLC.[67,68] The median MVC in SCLC is higher than seen in NSCLC. Elevated MVC and VEGF expression are associated with a worse prognosis in SCLC.[69] ECOG conducted a phase II trial (E3501) in 64 patients with chemotherapy-naive extensive stage SCLC. In this trial, bevacizumab (15 mg/kg) was added to standard chemotherapy with cisplatin (60 mg/m^2 on day 1) and etoposide (120 mg/m^2 on days 1 to 3) for four cycles.[70] Patients without disease progression continued on bevacizumab until progression or unacceptable toxicity. The most common grade 3/4 toxicities (>10% of patients) were neutropenia, thrombocytopenia, fatigue, hypertension, febrile neutropenia, and dehydration; two patients experienced grade 5 toxicities (hypertension and infection with grade 3/4 neutropenia). There was 69% response rate. PFS was 4.7 months and overall survival was 11.1 months.[70] CALGB conducted a similar phase II study (CALGB 30306) in which bevacizumab (15 mg/kg) was combined with cisplatin (30 mg/m^2 on days 1 and 8) and irinotecan (85 mg/m^2

TABLE 48.3 Clinical Status of Drugs that Target the Vascular Endothelial Growth Factor Pathway and Are Currently Approved or in Development for the Treatment of Non–Small Cell Lung Cancer

Drug	Target	Route of Administration	Frequency of Administration	Clinical Status
Bevacizumab	VEGF ligand	iv	Every 3 weeks	Approved
Sorafenib	Raf, Kit, Flt-3, VEGFR-2, VEGFR-3, PDGFR-β	po	Twice daily	Phase III
Vandetanib	VEGFR-2, VEGFR-3, RET, EGFR	po	Daily	Phase III
Sunitinib	VEGFR-1, VEGFR-2, VEGFR-3, PDGFR-α, PDGFR-β, Flt-3, c-kit	po	Twice daily	Phase III
Cediranib	VEGFR-2, VEGFR-1, VEGFR-3, c-kit, Flt-3	po	Daily	Phase III
Motesanib	VEGFR-1, VEGFR-2, VEGFR-3, PDGFR, RET, kit	po	Daily	Phase III
Axitinib	VEGFR-1, VEGFR-2, VEGFR-3, PDGFR-β, kit	po	Twice daily	Phase II
Pazopanib	VEGFR-2, VEGFR-2, VEGFR-3, PDGFR-α, PDGFR-β, c-kit	po	Daily	Phase II
XL647	VEGFR-2, EGFR, erbB2, EphB4	po	Daily/twice daily	Phase II

EphB4, Eph receptor B4; erbB2, v-erb-b2 erythroblastic leukemia viral oncogene homolog 2; Flt-3, FMS-like tyrosine kinase 3; iv, intravenous; po, per oral; PDGFR, platelet-derived growth factor receptor; VEGFR, vascular endothelial growth factor receptor.

on days 1 and 8) in 72 chemotherapy-naive patients with extensive stage SCLC. Grade 3/4 toxicities included cytopenias, hypertension, fatigue, diarrhea, nausea, bowel perforation, infection, and heart failure. One patient died from hemorrhage secondary to a stroke. Compared with findings of the ECOG E3501 study of etoposide/cisplatin plus bevacizumab,[70] response rate (75%) was greater and PFS (7.1 months) was longer, but overall survival was similar (11.7 vs. 11.1 months).[71] A third phase II trial of 50 patients with extensive stage SCLC is evaluating the benefits of maintenance bevacizumab (10 mg/kg) for 6 months in patients who do not progress following initial chemotherapy with carboplatin (area under the curve [AUC] = 4 on day 1) and irinotecan (60 mg/m^2 on days 1, 8, and 15) for four to six cycles. Preliminary data indicates the regimen is well tolerated; the most common grade 3/4 toxicities (>10% of patients) include diarrhea, fatigue, and neutropenia. Survival data is immature.[72] Based on these results, a randomized phase II study of cisplatin/etoposide with or without bevacizumab is planned.

A multicenter phase II trial evaluated the role of bevacizumab in patients with limited-stage SCLC.[73] In this trial, 57 patients with limited-stage SCLC received combined modality therapy: 61.2 Gy of radiation therapy, and chemotherapy with carboplatin (AUC = 5) and irinotecan (50 mg/m^2 on days 1 and 8) for four cycles. Those patients without progressive disease went on to receive consolidation treatment with bevacizumab (10 mg/kg) every 2 weeks for 10 doses. Major grade 3/4 toxicities (>10% of patients) included neutropenia, thrombocytopenia, and vomiting during combined modality treatment. Less than 10% of patients receiving bevacizumab alone experienced grade 3/4 toxicities. There were two treatment-related deaths, both caused by respiratory failure. The response rate of 80%, the 1- and 2-year PFS rates of 63% and 54%, respectively, and the 1- and 2-year overall survival rates of 71% and 29%, respectively, are similar to outcomes seen with traditional chemotherapy with cisplatin/etoposide.[73–75]

Small Molecule Kinase Inhibitors Tyrosine kinase activity is intrinsic to the signaling activity of many membrane-bound receptors, including VEGF receptors. Activity is mediated by ligand binding to the extracellular region of the receptor, which stimulates tyrosine phosphorylation of the intracellular domain via ATP binding and subsequently activates intracellular signaling cascades.[25] Tyrosine kinase inhibitors block or compete with ATP binding, thus inhibiting the intracellular signaling cascade stimulated by a receptor or several receptors. As such, they are involved in many cellular processes such as proliferation, metabolism, survival, and apoptosis. Evidence suggests that several tyrosine kinases are activated in cancer cells and drive tumor growth and progression. Therefore, blocking tyrosine kinase activity represents a rational approach to cancer therapy.

VEGF receptor tyrosine kinase inhibitors exert their effects by inhibiting downstream signaling from VEGF receptors following stimulation by VEGF. By blocking the activity of VEGF receptors, and potentially other receptors, it might be suggested that these tyrosine kinase inhibitors have the potential to exert broader activity than VEGF inhibitors targeting a single ligand. However, VEGF is the ligand for several receptors (VEGF receptors 1 and 2, neuropilin-1 [NRP-1]) with several targets each. Therefore, VEGF-ligand inhibition limits further paracrine and autocrine stimulation via VEGF, and also prevents further downstream activation of the VEGF-mediated angiogenesis pathways. The clinical relevance of multiple receptor inhibition will be discussed. A summary of the clinical activity of these small molecule kinase inhibitors can be found following discussion of the individual agents in Table 48.4.[76–91]

Sorafenib Sorafenib (Bay 43-9006; Nexavar) is an oral multikinase inhibitor targeting both tumor proliferation via inhibition of Raf, stem cell factor receptor (c-kit), fms-like tyrosine kinase-3 (Flt-3), and angiogenesis by targeting VEGF receptors 2 and 3 and PDGF-receptor (PDGFR)-β.[92–94] In preclinical models,

TABLE 48.4 Summary of Clinical Data for Small Molecule Kinase Inhibitors in Patients with Non–Small Cell Lung Cancer

Author	Treatment	Pt no	PFS	RR
Liu et al.[72]	Sorafenib 400 mg bid	11	N/R	40%
Gatzemeier et al.[73]	Sorafenib 400 mg bid	54	2.7 mo	29%
Adjei et al.[74]	Sorafenib (200–400 mg bid) + gefitinib 250 mg daily	31	N/R	3.25%
Schiller et al.[75]	Sorafenib + CBDCA+pac*	15	7.9 mo	29%
Scagliotti et al.[76]	Sorafenib + CBDCA+pac*	464	10.7 mo	30%
	Placebo + CBDCA+pac*	462	10.6 mo	24%
Natale et al.[77]	Vandetanib 300 mg daily	83	2.5 mo	8%
	Gefitinib 250 mg daily	85	1.9 mo	1%
Heymach et al.[78,79]	Vandetanib 100 mg + docetaxel	42	4.4 mo	
	Vandetanib 300 mg + docetaxel	44	3.9 mo	N/R
	Docetaxel	41	2.8 mo	
Heymach et al.[80]	CBDCA+pac*	52	5.3 mo	25%
	Vandetanib + CBDCA+pac*	56	5.5 mo	32%
Arnold et al.[81]	Vandetanib	107	2.7 mo	
	Placebo		2.8 mo	
Socinski et al.[82]	Sunitinib 50 mg daily†	64	11.3 wks	9.5%
Brahmer et al.[83]	Sunitinib 37.5 mg daily‡	47	12.3 wks	2%
Reck et al.[84]	Sunitinib (37.5 or 50 mg daily) + CDDP + gem§	13	N/R	23%
Laurie et al.[85]	Cediranib (30 or 45 mg daily) + CBDCA+pac*	15	N/R	40%
Goss et al.[86]	Cediranib + CDDP + gem§	14	N/R	N/R
Schiller et al.[87]	Axitinib	32	5.8 mo	9.4%

*Carboplatin and paclitaxel.

†Sunitinib administered daily for 4 weeks of 6-week cycle.

‡Sunitinib administered daily for 4 weeks of 4-week cycle.

§Cisplatin and gemcitabine.

bid, twice daily; CBDCA, carboplatin; CDDP, cisplatin; NR, not reported; PFS, progression-free survival; RR, response rate.

sorafenib has been found to inhibit tumor growth, including NSCLC, when administered alone and/or in combination with vinorelbine, cisplatin, or gefitinib.[95,96] Phase I studies, which have included patients with NSCLC, determined sorafenib 400 mg twice daily to be safe and well tolerated.[97,98] Clinical studies in patients with solid tumors, including NSCLC, demonstrated disease stabilization following treatment with single-agent sorafenib, regardless of prior chemotherapy regimen.[76,77,97,98]

SINGLE-AGENT SORAFENIB. In a multicenter, uncontrolled phase II trial, 54 patients with relapsed or refractory NSCLC received sorafenib (400 mg twice daily continuously for 28-day cycle). Patients with a history of significant bleeding in the previous month were excluded from the trial, although patients with squamous cell histology and asymptomatic brain metastases were included. Median PFS was 2.7 months and overall survival was 6.8 months. Although there were no confirmed partial responses in the 51 evaluable patients, disease tumor shrinkage was observed in 29% of patients, whereas 59% of patients had stable disease. The most common toxicities (>25% of patients) were diarrhea, hand–foot syndrome, fatigue, and nausea. Hypertension was also observed in 2% of patients. In many cases, hypertension is amenable to management with standard antihypertensive therapy; however, severe or persistent hypertension or hypertensive crisis despite institution of antihypertensive therapy may require permanent discontinuation. Less common sorafenib-related events that may require interruption or termination of therapy include bleeding and cardiac ischemia. In this phase II trial, four patients had a bleeding event thought to be associated with treatment with sorafenib. Of these, three patients had epistaxis and one patient with a central cavitary lesion and squamous cell histology had a fatal pulmonary hemorrhage (30 days after stopping treatment with sorafenib).[77] In a two-stage design phase II trial, patients who had failed one prior chemotherapy regimen were treated with sorafenib (400 mg twice daily continuously for 28-day cycle). Response was evaluated by dynamic contrast-enhanced magnetic resonance imaging (DCE-MRI). Five patients were assessable for response and six for toxicity. Best response was one partial response (41% tumor reduction at week 8, sustained to week 28). Additional responses included one partial response (unconfirmed at week 3), two stable disease (16 and 19 weeks), and one progressive disease after 8 weeks of treatment. Toxicities included those previously mentioned in addition to anemia, hyponatremia, keratoacanthoma, and vasculitis. DCE-MRI of one patient showed decrease in tumor permeability and size; however, this was not observed in two other patients responding to therapy.[76] Single-agent sorafenib does not appear to adversely affect health-related quality of life in patients with advanced NSCLC.[99] In a first-line study, 25 patients with stage IIIB (pleural effusion) or IV NSCLC were treated with sorafenib (400 mg twice daily continuously for 28-day cycle) prior to receiving standard chemotherapy. Although the study did not meet stage I efficacy criteria (only one confirmed partial response in the first 20 patients), the authors concluded that the median survival of 8.8 months and objective response rate of 12% suggests single-agent sorafenib achieves similar activity compared with two-drug combinations and should be considered for combination studies with standard chemotherapy regimens.[100]

COMBINATION THERAPY. In a phase I dose-escalation trial of 31 patients, 12 patients with locally advanced or recurrent NSCLC were treated with sorafenib (200 or 400 mg twice daily) plus gefitinib (250 mg daily). An additional 20 patients were treated with single-agent sorafenib or gefitinib for 21 days followed by a 7-day washout period with crossover to the other agent for 21 days, followed by a 7-day washout period and the combination of sorafenib (400 mg twice daily) and gefitinib (250 mg daily for 28-day cycle). No dose-limiting toxicities were observed at the sorafenib 200 mg daily dose level. One dose-limiting toxicity (elevated alanine transaminase [ALT]) was observed at the sorafenib 400 mg daily dose level, the dose selected for phase B of the study. The most common AEs included dermatologic effects, diarrhea, and elevated ALT, with the latter two being the most common grade 3/4 AEs. Serious AEs each occurring in one patient included dyspnea, fever, elevated ALT, and diarrhea. Although gefitinib had no effect on sorafenib pharmacokinetics, sorafenib did effect the pharmacokinetics of gefitinib. There was one partial response and 20 stable disease of ≥4 months' duration. Sorafenib 400 mg twice daily and gefitinib 250 mg daily oral is the recommended dose for future studies.[78,101]

In a phase I/II trial, carboplatin (AUC = 6)/paclitaxel (225 mg/m^2 intravenously [iv] on day 1) were combined with sorafenib (100, 200, or 400 mg twice daily on days 2 to 18 of a 21-day cycle) in patients with advanced NSCLC. An encouraging median PFS of 8.5 months was achieved in addition to a 79% disease control rate (29% partial response and 50% stable disease). The most common adverse reactions were similar to single-agent treatment (rash, hand–foot syndrome, and gastrointestinal symptoms). Grade 1/2 bleeding events were seen in three patients.[79] Based on these results, the ESCAPE trial was opened. This was a randomized phase III trial evaluating sorafenib (400 mg twice daily on days 2 to 19) in combination with carboplatin (AUC = 6)/paclitaxel (200 mg/m^2 every 21 days for six to eight cycles), in 926 newly diagnosed patients with stage IIIB/IV NSCLC. Patients with squamous cell histology were eligible for this trial. Patients were ineligible if they had a history of brain metastases, uncontrolled hypertension, and anticoagulation. The primary end point was overall survival. Secondary end points included tumor response, duration of response, patient reported outcomes, and biological correlates. Major grade 3/4 toxicities (>10% of patients) were neutropenia, thrombocytopenia, infection, and fatigue. There were two cases of fatal hemorrhage (one in each treatment group). Patients receiving chemotherapy plus sorafenib had similar PFS (5.1 vs. 5.4 months) and overall survival (10.6 vs. 10.7 months) compared with patients receiving chemotherapy alone. Interestingly, patients with squamous cell histology appeared to do significantly worse when sorafenib was added to chemotherapy compared with those receiving chemotherapy alone (PFS: 4.4 vs. 5.8 months; overall survival: 8.9 vs. 13.6 months). There was no difference in survival for those with nonsquamous cell histology.[80]

A search for sorafenib and NSCLC on the http://www.ClinicalTrials.gov database identifies 15 clinical trials involving approximately 2700 patients (as of January 23, 2008).[102] One of these studies, NEXUS, is a large phase III trial investigating first-line sorafenib in combination with standard platinum-based doublet therapy (carboplatin/paclitaxel; gemcitabine/cisplatin). Another phase III trial, which investigated sorafenib in combination with carboplatin/paclitaxel, was closed early after an independent data monitoring committee determined that the trial would not meet its primary end point of improving overall survival. Phase I and II trials in chemonaive patients with locally advanced or metastatic disease are investigating sorafenib added to pemetrexed/carboplatin or carboplatin/paclitaxel/bevacizumab regimens. Further phase I/II studies in inoperable stage III disease are ongoing to assess sorafenib as part of a multimodality approach administered concomitantly with radiotherapy or as consolidation therapy following induction with cisplatin/etoposide/radiotherapy. The application of single-agent sorafenib in the treatment of patients with recurrent, refractory, or progressive disease (second line) is also being further examined. A phase II trial has been opened in chemotherapy-naive patients with NSCLC who are either ≥70 years of age and ECOG performance status (PS) 0 to 2 or <70 years of age and ECOG PS 2. In this trial, sorafenib (400 mg twice daily) will be administered in combination with gemcitabine 1200 mg/m^2 (days 1 and 8 every 21 days for maximum six cycles) or erlotinib (150 mg daily oral until disease progression).[103]

Vandetanib Vandetanib (AZD6474, Zactima) is an oral inhibitor of angiogenesis targeting VEGF receptors 2 and 3 as well as tumor growth with activity against RET, and EGFR/HER-1.[104,105] Vandetanib has been shown to be active against a wide range of tumor cells in preclinical studies.[106] In phase I studies, single-agent vandetanib was well tolerated in patients with various solid tumors including NSCLC.[107–109] The recommended daily dose is 300 mg.

SINGLE-AGENT VANDETANIB. Therapy with vandetanib (100, 200, or 300 mg daily) was evaluated in a randomized double-blind phase II dose-finding study of 53 Japanese patients with NSCLC. Toxicities included rash, diarrhea, and asymptomatic QTc prolongation. One patient died from treatment-related interstitial lung disease. An 11% partial response and 51%

disease control rate were observed.[110] In a randomized phase II trial of 168 patients, single-agent vandetanib (300 mg daily) was compared with gefitinib (250 mg daily) in patients after failure of first- or second-line platinum-based therapy. Of note, patients with hemoptysis, thromboses, squamous cell carcinoma, and brain metastases were permitted to enter this trial. Median PFS was 2.5 months for vandetanib compared with 1.9 months for patients receiving gefitinib. Objective responses were seen in 8% of vandetanib patients compared with 1% of gefitinib-treated patients, with disease control achieved in 37/83 (45%) versus 29/85 (34%) of patients, respectively. The most common toxicities (>10% of patients) seen in patients treated with vandetanib included nausea, diarrhea, rash, headache, dizziness, hypertension, and asymptomatic QTc prolongation. On progression, patients were allowed to switch to the alternative regimen after a 4-week washout period. In patients who switched therapies, disease control >8 weeks was seen in 16/37 (43%) patients who switched to vandetanib and 7/29 (24%) patients who switched to gefitinib. Overall survival was not significantly different between treatment arms (6.1 months for vandetanib and 7.4 months for gefitinib-treated patients).[81]

COMBINATION THERAPY. In a phase II randomized, placebo-controlled trial of 127 patients with stage IIIB/IV NSCLC, who had failed platinum-based chemotherapy, treatment with daily vandetanib (100 or 300 mg) plus docetaxel (75 mg/m^2 every 3 weeks) was compared with docetaxel alone. Patients with squamous cell histology were permitted to enter the trial, as were patients with clinically stable, previously treated brain metastases (without steroid treatment for 1 week at study entry). Patients in the run-in phase of this trial received vandetanib 100 mg/day or 300 mg/day plus docetaxel and were then randomized to receive further treatment with either vandetanib (100 or 300 mg/day) with docetaxel or placebo with docetaxel. Preliminary results reported an improvement in PFS with combination therapy, 4.4 and 3.9 months, for vandetanib 100 and 300 mg, respectively, compared with 2.8 months for docetaxel alone. However, no statistically significant difference in overall survival was noted between the three arms. AEs were similar to those mentioned previously. Nonfatal hemoptysis was reported in four patients with squamous cell histology.[82,111,112] The results of this study have led to a phase III trial comparing vandetanib plus docetaxel with docetaxel alone as a second-line treatment option for patients with advanced NSCLC. In a randomized phase II trial of 181, chemotherapy-naive patients with IIIB/IV NSCLC, treatment with single-agent vandetanib (300 mg daily) was compared with vandetanib plus paclitaxel (200 mg/m^2 iv) and carboplatin (AUC = 6 every 3 weeks)/paclitaxel and carboplatin alone. Patients with CNS metastases and squamous cell histology were permitted to enter this trial. The vandetanib monotherapy arm was stopped early after a planned interim analysis met the criterion for discontinuation. Combination therapy with vandetanib with carboplatin and paclitaxel prolonged PFS compared with carboplatin and paclitaxel alone (5.5 vs. 5.3 months). Overall survival was not significantly different. The objective response rates were 7% for vandetanib alone, 32% for combination therapy, and 25% for chemotherapy alone. Toxicities, although more common with vandetanib-treated patients were similar to those seen with single-agent therapy.[84,113]

A phase II randomized trial in patients with SCLC (limited or extensive disease) compared maintenance vandetanib (300 mg daily) with placebo in patients who had responded to platinum-based chemotherapy (complete or partial response) and completed radiation therapy (thoracic and prophylactic cranial). There was no significant difference in PFS or overall survival for patients treated with vandetanib compared with placebo, 2.7 versus 2.8 months and 10.6 versus 11.9 months, respectively. Patients treated with vandetanib were more likely to experience toxicities (gastrointestinal and rash) requiring dose reductions. In a planned subgroup analysis, a significant interaction was noted in patients based on disease extent; patients with limited disease randomized to vandetanib had a longer overall survival (HR = 0.45; one-sided p value 0.07), whereas those with extensive disease treated with vandetanib had a shorter overall survival (HR = 2.27; one-sided p value 0.996).[85]

The ongoing clinical trial program is further examining the clinical application of vandetanib in the first-, second-, and third-line settings. A search of the http://www.ClinicalTrials.gov database for vandetanib and NSCLC identifies 11 clinical trials involving approximately 4350 patients (as of January 23, 2008).[102] Three phase III trials are ongoing to examine vandetanib either in combination (pemetrexed or docetaxel) or as monotherapy (vs. erlotinib) in the second- or third-line settings, with data expected during 2009. An additional large, phase III trial in a planned 930 patients is evaluating vandetanib versus best supportive care in the second- or third-line setting. Smaller phase II trials are investigating vandetanib with carboplatin/paclitaxel as neoadjuvant treatment and in combination with standard chemotherapy regimens as a first-line treatment option.

Sunitinib Sunitinib (SU11248, Sutent) is a novel, multitargeted, small molecule inhibitor of the receptor tyrosine kinases involved in tumor proliferation and angiogenesis, including VEGF receptors 1, 2, and 3, PDGF receptor-α and -β, Flt-3, c-kit, and the receptor encoded by the *ret* proto-oncogene (RET; rearranged during transfection), and Flt-3.[114] Of note, it has been suggested that combined inhibition of PDGF receptor and VEGF receptor 2-mediated signaling may be particularly potent in the inhibition of angiogenesis.[115] Sunitinib demonstrated antitumor activity against several tumor cell lines including NSCLC in preclinical studies.[116,117] The recommended dose of sunitinib is 50 mg daily for 4 consecutive weeks of a 6-week cycle. The 2-week rest period is required because of the long half-life of sunitinib (80 hours for the active metabolite), which causes drug accumulation. However, in the clinical setting, this administration schedule may also allow some vascular regrowth.

SINGLE-AGENT SUNITINIB. A phase II trial of 64 patients evaluated sunitinib (50 mg daily for 4 weeks in a 6-week cycle) as second- or third-line therapy in patients with advanced NSCLC. Patients with recent grade 3 hemorrhage or recent gross hemoptysis, brain metastases, uncontrolled hypertension, or patients who had received surgery within 4 weeks of study entry were excluded from this trial. Patients with squamous cell histology were eligible, although a history of cardiac disease, cerebrovascular accident, or pulmonary embolism precluded patients from entering this trial. Treatment with sunitinib resulted in a 9.5% partial response and 42.9% stable disease. Median duration of response was 12.2 weeks. Median PFS was 2.6 months and overall survival was 5.5 months. Major toxicities included fatigue/asthenia, pain/myalgia, nausea and vomiting, dyspnea, and stomatitis/mucosal inflammation. There were two incidences of pulmonary hemorrhage (in patients with squamous cell histology, although only one event was believed to be sunitinib related) and one cerebral hemorrhage.[86] A subsequent phase II study evaluated 47 patients with previously treated stage IIIB/IV NSCLC treated with sunitinib (37.5 mg daily continuously for 4-week cycles). Patients with brain metastases and significant hemoptysis were excluded. One patient had a confirmed partial response and nine patients had stable disease. Median PFS was 2.8 months and overall survival was 8.6 months. AEs were similar to those mentioned previously in addition to congestive heart failure, hypomagnesemia, and hypoxic respiratory failure.[87] The results of these studies supports further investigation for sunitinib in combination with other treatments for NSCLC.

COMBINATION THERAPY. A phase I study in untreated patients with stage IIIB/IV NSCLC evaluated sunitinib (37.5 or 50 mg daily for 14 days) in combination with cisplatin (100 mg/m^2 iv on day 1)/gemcitabine (1000 mg/m^2 or 1250 mg/m^2 iv on days 1 and 8 of a 21-day cycle). No dose-limiting toxicities were seen with sunitinib 37.5 mg, whereas two were noted (neutropenia and infection) at the 50-mg dose. Additional grade 3/4 toxicities included anemia, neutropenia, and thrombocytopenia. Three patients achieved a partial response at the 50-mg dose level. Sunitinib 37.5 mg appears to be the recommended dose with this chemotherapy combination. Studies with the higher dose of gemcitabine and sunitinib administration on a continuous dosing schedule are currently ongoing.[88] A second phase I study in 37 patients with advanced solid tumors evaluated sunitinib (20, 37.5, or 50 mg daily for 4 weeks in a 6-week cycle or 2 weeks in a 3-week cycle) in combination with docetaxel (60 or 75 mg/m^2 iv every 3 weeks). Thirteen patients with NSCLC were enrolled. Neutropenia (with or without fever) was seen in five patients. One patient had pulseless electrical activity and pulmonary hemorrhage. With greater than 50% stable disease seen at both dose levels, the combination of sunitinib 37.5 mg daily for 2 weeks of a 3-week cycle and docetaxel 75 mg/m^2 iv has been recommended with ongoing pharmacokinetic and efficacy studies to determine the utility of further evaluation of this regimen.[118]

Searching the http://www.ClinicalTrials.gov database using the terms sunitinib and NSCLC identifies eight clinical trials involving approximately 1500 patients (as of January 23, 2008).[102] A phase III trial is evaluating sunitinib in combination with erlotinib versus erlotinib alone in 956 patients in the second- or third-line settings. Phase I and II trials are ongoing to investigate sunitinib added to standard first-line regimens (carboplatin/paclitaxel; carboplatin/paclitaxel/bevacizumab; carboplatin or cisplatin/pemetrexed; gemcitabine/cisplatin).

Cediranib Cediranib (AZD2171, Recentin) is a potent inhibitor of both VEGF receptors 1 and 2, it also has activity against c-kit, PDGFR-β, and Flt-4 at nanomolar concentrations, but is selective against other serine/threonine kinases studied. Cediranib has been shown to inhibit VEGF signaling with once-daily oral dosing. Cediranib 45 mg once daily has been shown to be well tolerated in patients with a broad range of solid tumors.[102] Most common toxicities include diarrhea, dysphonia, and hypertension.[119]

COMBINATION THERAPY. Cediranib (20, 30, or 45 mg daily) has been evaluated in phase I studies in combination with various chemotherapy regimens, including pemetrexed (500 mg/m^2 every 3 weeks) and docetaxel (75 mg/m^2 every 3 weeks), two agents commonly employed in the treatment of patients with NSCLC. In this group of heavily pretreated patients with advanced solid tumors, the safety profile of cediranib was similar to that observed in single-agent cediranib studies with the most common grade 3 toxicities including diarrhea, fatigue, and hypertension. Response rates were promising, and cediranib did not appear to effect the pharmacokinetic profile of either agent.[120] A second phase I study in patients with previously treated advanced solid tumors evaluated cediranib (20, 30, or 45 mg daily) in combination with gefitinib (250 mg daily). Cediranib 30 mg or lower appeared to be well tolerated. The most common toxicities were diarrhea, rash, abdominal pain, and hypertension, with only the latter side effect attributed to cediranib.[121] A phase I study in stage IIIB/IV chemotherapy-naive NSCLC patients evaluated cediranib (30 or 45 mg daily on day 2) in combination with carboplatin (AUC = 6)/paclitaxel (200 mg/m^2 day 1) every 3 weeks. Patients with prior hemoptysis or bleeding were ineligible for this trial. One patient at each of the 30 and 45 mg doses experienced a dose-limiting toxicity, grade 3 ALT, and febrile neutropenia with mucositis, respectively. Hypertension grade ≥ 2 was seen in six patients, prompting the institution of a standard algorithm to manage this expected toxicity. Other toxicities included fatigue, anorexia, mucositis, and diarrhea. Of the 15 patients evaluable for response, there were six patients with a partial response and eight with stable disease.[89] A second phase I study in the same population evaluated cediranib (30 or 45 mg) in combination with gemcitabine (1250 mg/m^2 on days 1 and 8) and cisplatin (80 mg/m^2 on day 1 every 3 weeks). A total of 14 patients were enrolled: five patients at the 30-mg dose and nine patients at the 45-mg dose. Toxicities including diarrhea, fatigue, hypertension, and voice changes were seen at both levels. Grade 4 toxicities included one patient with reversible ischemia and another with fatigue. Cediranib did not appear to affect gemcitabine pharmacokinetics. Responses were seen at both dose levels. Further testing of this combination has been recommended with 30-mg cediranib as the recommended dose level.[90]

In addition to those studies mentioned previously, searching the http://www.ClinicalTrials.gov database for NSCLC trials of cediranib identifies six clinical trials involving approximately

1000 patients (as of January 23, 2008).[102] However, the National Cancer Institute of Canada recently closed BR-24, a phase II/III trial of cediranib in combination with carboplatin/paclitaxel as the planned end of phase II efficacy and tolerability analysis by the study's Data Safety Monitoring Committee revealed an imbalance in toxicity. A phase II trial in 74 patients is investigating cediranib in combination with pemetrexed for the second-line treatment of NSCLC. A further phase I trial is evaluating cediranib plus gefitinib in patients with NSCLC or head and neck cancer.

Motesanib Motesanib (AMG 706) is a potent, oral, multikinase inhibitor with activity against VEGF receptors 1, 2, and 3, PDGF receptor, kit, and RET. Preclinical studies demonstrated inhibition of VEGF-induced angiogenesis and inhibition of tumor growth in vivo.[122] A phase I study evaluated motesanib (continuously for 3 weeks of a 4-week cycle) by DCE-MRI in 65 patients with advanced solid tumors. The most frequent toxicities (>10% of patients) were hypertension, fatigue, diarrhea, nausea, vomiting, and headache. Most events were mild to moderate in severity and reversible. Of note, early trials suggested that there was cause for concern with some patients who had received motesanib developing cholecystitis and gallbladder enlargement. Ongoing studies have continued to gather data on this issue, subject to protocol amendments to ensure that physicians are aware of the possibility that these conditions might occur. However, latest reports suggest that these events are manageable. Of 56 evaluable patients, there was a 4% partial response and 61% stable disease rate. DCE-MRI showed reductions up to 61% in AUC on day 21 of treatment. Motesanib 125 mg daily was well tolerated and has been recommended for phase II studies.[123]

COMBINATION THERAPY. A phase I trial evaluated motesanib (50 or 125 mg daily or 75 mg twice daily) in combination with gemcitabine (1000 mg/m^2 weekly for 7 of 8 weeks, then 3 of 4 weeks for up to 11 cycles) in 26 patients, including two patients with NSCLC. Motesanib pharmacokinetics did not appear to be affected by the schedule of gemcitabine administration. There were two dose-limiting toxicities: grade 4 neutropenia and grade 3 deep vein thrombosis. Other toxicities (>10% of patients) included lethargy, fatigue, headache, nausea, and diarrhea. Two unconfirmed partial responses and seven cases of stable disease were noted. Further testing of this regimen has been recommended.[124] In another phase I study, motesanib (50, 75, 100, 125 mg daily and 75 mg twice daily) was combined with panitumumab (9 mg/kg on day 1) plus cisplatin (75 mg/m^2 on day 1)/gemcitabine (1250 mg/m^2 on days 1 and 8 of a 21-day cycle) in 36 patients with advanced solid tumors, including 19 patients with NSCLC. Of the patients included in this trial, 42% had received one prior line of chemotherapy. There was a 39% rate of thromboembolism, one grade 5 pulmonary embolism was seen. Additional toxicities (>25% of patients) included nausea, fatigue, and hypertension. Of the 29 evaluable patients, there was one complete response with a partial response rate of 31% (including six cases seen in patients with NSCLC) and 59% of patients had stable disease. Motesanib pharmacokinetics at a daily dose of 125 mg were not affected by other therapies. Although this combination appears to be effective, the rate of thromboembolism needs to be compared with treatment with cisplatin/gemcitabine alone.[125,126]

The largest motesanib phase III, multicenter, placebo-controlled, double-blind trial, was planned to randomize 1240 patients to receive first-line motesanib with carboplatin/paclitaxel or placebo with carboplatin/paclitaxel. Patients with untreated or symptomatic CNS metastases, a history of pulmonary hemorrhage or gross hemoptysis (approximately 3 mL of bright red blood or more) within 6 months prior to randomization, or uncontrolled hypertension are not eligible to enter this trial. However, patients with squamous cell histology are eligible. The primary end point for this trial was overall survival; secondary end points include PFS, objective tumor response rate, and duration of response. Enrollment in the trial was suspended in November 2008, following a planned safety data review of 600 patients by the study's independent Data Monitoring Committee (DMC), which revealed higher early mortality rates in the motesanib group compared to the placebo group. In addition, the DMC recommended that the patients with squamous NSCLC immediately discontinue motesanib therapy based on an observation of a higher incidence of hemoptysis. The DMC did not recommend discontinuation of motesanib therapy for the patients with nonsquamous NSCLC.

A phase II head-to-head trial with bevacizumab to evaluate the difference in objective response rates between first-line motesanib plus carboplatin/paclitaxel and bevacizumab plus carboplatin/paclitaxel is also currently recruiting patients. Eligibility criteria for this trial reflect the bevacizumab eligibility profile (i.e., nonsquamous NSCLC, no history of or current CNS metastases, no history of pulmonary hemorrhage or gross hemoptysis, and no uncontrolled hypertension).

Axitinib (AG-013736) Axitinib is a small molecule tyrosine kinase inhibitor of VEGF receptors 1, 2, and 3, PDG receptor-β, and c-kit. A phase I dose escalation study evaluated axitinib (5 to 30 mg orally daily for 28-day cycle) in 36 patients with solid tumors (including NSCLC) who were refractory to standard therapy. The maximum-tolerated dose and the recommended dose for phase II/III trials is 5 mg twice daily. Three confirmed partial responses were observed with other evidence of antitumor activity. Dose-limiting toxicities (>10% of patients) associated with axitinib therapy included hypertension, fatigue, nausea, vomiting, diarrhea, headache, stomatitis, and erythema; however, the complete AE profile is not yet known. Cavitation of lung lesions was observed in the two patients with NSCLC, both subsequently died from hemoptysis (one was believed to be axitinib related). Similar treatment effects have been seen in patients treated with bevacizumab and may be a marker of antiangiogenic activity.[127] A phase II trial evaluated the activity and safety of axitinib (5 mg twice daily) in 32 patients with stage IIIB/IV NSCLC. Patients may have had prior chemotherapy, radiation therapy, or surgery, 13% of patients were treatment naive. Median duration of response was 9.4 months, PFS was 5.8 months, and overall survival was 12.8 months. Three responses were noted. Toxicities (occurring in 5% of patients) included fatigue, diarrhea, hypertension, and hyponatremia.[79]

The clinical trial program for axitinib in NSCLC is in development; a search of the http://www.ClinicalTrials.gov database for NSCLC trials of axitinib identifies only two clinical trials (as of January 23, 2008).[102] However, the first, a phase II study of new agents with and without docetaxel, was withdrawn prior to beginning recruitment. The second, a phase II trial of second- or third-line axitinib in patients with advanced NSCLC, is expected to report data during 2008.

Other Therapies Pazopanib (GW786034) is an oral, small molecule tyrosine kinase inhibitor targeting VEGF receptors 1, 2, and 3, PDGF receptor-α and -β, and c-kit. A phase I study in 43 patients with advanced solid tumors (including NSCLC). The most common AEs were nausea, diarrhea, fatigue, hypertension, anorexia, and vomiting. Hair depigmentation was observed at higher doses. Tumor shrinkage was noted in patients with renal cell cancer. One patient with NSCLC was included in the six patients with stable disease who remained on therapy for 6 months or more.[128] The clinical trial program for pazopanib in NSCLC is still in its infancy; searching the http://www.ClinicalTrials.gov database for NSCLC trials of pazopanib identifies only two ongoing/planned clinical trials (as of January 23, 2008).[102] A phase II trial evaluated the safety and efficacy of pazopanib in the neoadjuvant setting as presurgical therapy in patients with stage IA/B, resectable NSCLC. This open label, multicenter, phase II study was designed to assess the activity of pazopanib when given to 35 treatment-naive patients with stage I to II NSCLC prior to surgery. Pretreatment and posttreatment high-resolution computed tomography (HRCT) scans measuring tumor size showed that 30 patients (86%) had experienced a tumor volume reduction. Overall, patients experienced changes in tumor size ranging from a reduction of 86% to an increase of 17%. After an initial biopsy, 35 eligible patients had received 800 mg of pazopanib orally, once daily for 2 to 6 weeks, followed by a treatment free period of 7 days prior to scheduled surgery to allow the administered drug to be eliminated from the body. The median duration of pazopanib therapy was 16 days. Grade 3 toxicities were seen in five patients while participating in study. These toxicities included elevated liver enzymes (2), hypertension (1), shortness of breath (1), pneumonia (1), urinary tract infection (1), reduced white blood cell count (1), potassium increase (1), and rash (1). One grade 4 toxicity of a pulmonary embolus was seen in a patient in relation to surgery, 18 days after finishing pazopanib treatment. One patient discontinued treatment because of AEs. Twelve patients required adjustment or initiation of antihypertensive medication during the study.

A second phase II trial (n = 40) is investigating the safety and efficacy of single-agent pazopanib in the second- and third-line treatment settings.

XL647 is another oral, small molecule tyrosine kinase inhibitor with activity against VEGF receptor 2, EGFR, erbB2/HER-2, and EphB4. Initial phase I studies administered XL647 daily for 5 days in a 14-day schedule to 41 patients with advanced solid tumors. The maximum tolerated dose was 350 mg daily for 5 days. One patient with NSCLC had a partial response and an additional 14 patients had stable disease. Toxicities include diarrhea, fatigue, rash, and QTc prolongation.[129,130] In a second phase I study by the same group, XL647 was administered on a continuous daily schedule to patients with advanced solid tumors. To date, 12 patients have been evaluated; 300 mg daily is the highest dose administered with no dose-limiting toxicities. Four patients have stable disease beyond 3 months.[131] A modest clinical development program is ongoing for the development of XL647 in NSCLC, with two phase II clinical trials identified in a search of the http://www.ClinicalTrials.gov database (as of January 23, 2008).[102] Both monotherapy trials will enroll a planned ~40 patients each. One trial will evaluate the efficacy and safety of XL647 in the first-line setting, whereas the other will assess XL647 in patients who have relapsed NSCLC following failure of gefitinib or erlotinib.

CONCLUSION

Despite improvements in cytotoxic chemotherapy, it remains nonspecific, targeting rapidly dividing normal and tumor cells. Thus, chemotherapy is widely associated with several toxic side effects. A therapeutic plateau has been reached with chemotherapy in terms of efficacy with no recent improvements in survival and unpredictable tumor response. Realization of a new generation of molecular targeted therapies that interfere with factors intrinsic to tumor growth and metastases offers a highly specific approach with more acceptable toxicity. As such, these agents are being combined with standard chemotherapy regimens, improving patient outcomes.

Angiogenesis remains a rational therapeutic target in NSCLC and novel approaches include the development of anti-VEGF ligand and anti-VEGF receptor strategies. Specific and highly selective antibodies have been designed, binding only to the VEGF ligand. By binding all free circulating VEGF, these antibodies prevent VEGF ligand/receptor interaction at all binding sites (VEGF receptors 1 and 2 and the NRP-1 coreceptor). Synthetic soluble receptors currently in development, such as VEGF-Trap, also bind directly to the VEGF ligand; however, they have a much shorter half-life than antibodies directed against the VEGF ligand. These receptors may be less specific; binding other VEGF family members, including VEGF-B and PlGF. To date, little is known about the effects of inhibiting PlGF and VEGF-B functions. However, VEGF mediates its effects through stimulation of VEGF receptor 2 in an exclusive fashion (i.e., only VEGF binding to VEGF receptor 2 stimulates effects such as endothelial cell growth and vascular permeability).[3] Related molecules such as PlGF cannot stimulate these effects.[26] In conclusion, the proangiogenic effects of VEGF mediated through all of the receptors to which it binds can be inhibited by targeting VEGF.

Agents targeting VEGF receptors include small molecule inhibitors, antibodies, and ribozymes. Antibodies and ribozymes are highly specific, targeting a single receptor. As a result, VEGF signaling through a single receptor may be completely blocked; however, ligand interactions with other receptors will not be inhibited. Small molecule kinase inhibitors have the potential to inhibit the kinase activity of several receptors. As such, these molecules are not highly specific or selective and may inhibit activity mediated by receptors other than VEGF receptors 1 and 2.

Both the VEGF ligand and VEGF receptors are viable and promising targets for anticancer therapy, each with possible benefits and limitations. Leading the way are the positive data from phase III trials with the humanized anti-VEGF ligand monoclonal antibody bevacizumab, which has proven benefit as a first-line therapy in NSCLC.[38,39,41,43] Data for bevacizumab have made the first steps toward the future of antiangiogenic therapy, proving that the concept that antiangiogenesis in general, and VEGF inhibition in particular, is an effective anticancer option, adding to the efficacy of chemotherapy without overlapping toxicity.

The clinical relevance of multiple receptor inhibition remains under evaluation and several agents have demonstrated promising efficacy. These molecules are not as specific as antibodies developed against the VEGF ligand as they inhibit several tyrosine kinase receptors, including VEGF receptors 1 and 2. Although, as the influence of VEGF and other proangiogenic factors changes with disease progression, the relative nonspecificity of multitargeted tyrosine kinase inhibitors may be beneficial, conveying continued activity late in disease. However, with these broader actions, it is not clear whether all intended targets are inhibited equally at the therapeutic dose. For example, the tyrosine kinase inhibitor vandetanib has affinity for VEGF receptor 2 and EGFR, with higher affinity for VEGF receptor 2.[132] Therefore, depending on the dose used, the EGFR pathway may remain active, compensating for lost VEGF receptor 2 signaling. In addition, their broader activity leads to increased off-target AEs, similar to, and sometimes overlapping those seen with cytotoxic chemotherapy. In addition to those AEs widely accepted as being associated with antiangiogenic therapy (e.g., bleeding, hypertension, proteinuria, neutropenia), their toxicity profile also includes fatigue, rash, hand–foot syndrome, and diarrhea. Other dose-limiting toxicities of note include heart failure and QTc interval prolongation. Whether these agents can be safely combined with chemotherapy with acceptable toxicity profiles is being further evaluated in ongoing clinical trials.

The number of agents and approaches currently in clinical development and the large number of ongoing clinical trials are testimony to the considerable research into the application of antiangiogenic therapy and the commitment to transform the future of NSCLC care.

ACKNOWLEDGMENTS: *We thank Gardiner-Caldwell Communications for medical writing assistance; this assistance was funded by F. Hoffmann-La Roche Ltd.*

REFERENCES

1. Carmeliet P, Jain RK. Angiogenesis in cancer and other diseases. *Nature* 2000;407(6801):249–257.
2. Yancopoulos GD, Davis S, Gale NW, et al. Vascular-specific growth factors and blood vessel formation. *Nature* 2000;407(6801):242–248.
3. Ferrara N, Davis-Smyth T. The biology of vascular endothelial growth factor. *Endocr Rev* 1997;18(1):4–25.
4. Bergers G, Benjamin LE. Tumorigenesis and the angiogenic switch. *Nat Rev Cancer* 2003;3(6):401–410.
5. Bauman JE, Eaton KD, Martins RG. Antagonism of platelet-derived growth factor receptor in non small cell lung cancer: rationale and investigations. *Clin Cancer Res* 2007;13(suppl 15, pt 2):S4632–S4636.
6. Baluk P, Hashizume H, McDonald DM. Cellular abnormalities of blood vessels as targets in cancer. *Curr Opin Genet Dev* 2005;15(1):102–111.
7. Takahashi H, Shibuya M. The vascular endothelial growth factor (VEGF)/VEGF receptor system and its role under physiological and pathological conditions. *Clin Sci (Lond)* 2005;109(3):227–241.
8. Ferrara N, Gerber HP, LeCouter J. The biology of VEGF and its receptors. *Nat Med* 2003;9(6):669–676.
9. Ferrara N. Vascular endothelial growth factor: basic science and clinical progress. *Endocr Rev* 2004;25(4):581–611.
10. Ugurel S, Rappl G, Tilgen W, et al. Increased serum concentration of angiogenic factors in malignant melanoma patients correlates with tumor progression and survival. *J Clin Oncol* 2001;19(2):577–583.
11. Brown LF, Berse B, Jackman RW, et al. Expression of vascular permeability factor (vascular endothelial growth factor) and its receptors in adenocarcinomas of the gastrointestinal tract. *Cancer Res* 1993;53(19): 4727–4735.
12. Brown LF, Berse B, Jackman RW, et al. Expression of vascular permeability factor (vascular endothelial growth factor) and its receptors in breast cancer. *Hum Pathol* 1995;26(1):86–91.
13. Huang H, Held-Feindt J, Buhl R, et al. Expression of VEGF and its receptors in different brain tumors. *Neurol Res* 2005;27(4):371–377.
14. Boocock CA, Charnock-Jones DS, Sharkey AM, et al. Expression of vascular endothelial growth factor and its receptors Flt and KDR in ovarian carcinoma. *J Natl Cancer Inst* 1995;87(7):506–516.
15. Guidi AJ, Abu-Jawdeh G, Berse B, et al. Vascular permeability factor (vascular endothelial growth factor) expression and angiogenesis in cervical neoplasia. *J Natl Cancer Inst* 1995;87(16):1237–1245.
16. O'Byrne KJ, Koukourakis MI, Giatromanolaki A, et al. Vascular endothelial growth factor, platelet-derived endothelial cell growth factor and angiogenesis in non-small-cell lung cancer. *Br J Cancer* 2000;82(8): 1427–1432.
17. Suzuki K, Hayashi N, Miyamoto Y, et al. Expression of vascular permeability factor/vascular endothelial growth factor in human hepatocellular carcinoma. *Cancer Res* 1996;56(13):3004–3009.
18. Eisma RJ, Spiro JD, Kreutzer DL. Vascular endothelial growth factor expression in head and neck squamous cell carcinoma. *Am J Surg* 1997; 174(5):513–517.
19. Jacobsen J, Rasmuson T, Grankvist K, et al. Vascular endothelial growth factor as prognostic factor in renal cell carcinoma. *J Urol* 2000;163(1): 343–347.
20. Fontanini G, Faviana P, Lucchi M, et al. A high vascular count and overexpression of vascular endothelial growth factor are associated with unfavourable prognosis in operated small cell lung carcinoma. *Br J Cancer* 2002;86(4):558–563.
21. Fontanini G, Vignati S, Boldrini L, et al. Vascular endothelial growth factor is associated with neovascularization and influences progression of non-small cell lung carcinoma. *Clin Cancer Res* 1997;3(6):861–865.
22. Imoto H, Osaki T, Taga S, et al. Vascular endothelial growth factor expression in non-small-cell lung cancer: prognostic significance in squamous cell carcinoma. *J Thorac Cardiovasc Surg* 1998;115(5):1007–1014.
23. Volm M, Koomägi R, Mattern J. Prognostic value of vascular endothelial growth factor and its receptor Flt-1 in squamous cell lung cancer. *Int J Cancer* 1997;74(15):64–68.
24. Yuan A, Yu CJ, Kuo SH, et al. Vascular endothelial growth factor 189 mRNA isoform expression specifically correlates with tumor angiogenesis, patient survival, and postoperative relapse in non-small-cell lung cancer. *J Clin Oncol* 2001;19(2):432–441.
25. Dvorak HF. Vascular permeability factor/vascular endothelial growth factor: a critical cytokine in tumor angiogenesis and a potential target for diagnosis and therapy. *J Clin Oncol* 2002;20(21):4368–4380.

26. Park JE, Chen HH, Winer J, et al. Placenta growth factor. Potentiation of vascular endothelial growth factor bioactivity, in vitro and in vivo, and high affinity binding to Flt-1 but not to Flk-1/KDR. *J Biol Chem* 1994;269(41):25646–25654.
27. Risau W. Mechanisms of angiogenesis. *Nature* 1997;386(6626):671–674.
28. Shibuya M, Ito N, Claesson-Welsh L. Structure and function of vascular endothelial growth factor receptor-1 and -2. *Curr Top Microbiol Immunol* 1999;237:59–83.
29. Shibuya M, Yamaguchi S, Yamane A, et al. Nucleotide sequence and expression of a novel human receptor-type tyrosine kinase gene (Flt) closely related to the fms family. *Oncogene* 1990;5(4):519–524.
30. Terman BI, Carrion ME, Kovacs E, et al. Identification of a new endothelial cell growth factor receptor tyrosine kinase. *Oncogene* 1991;6(9):1677–1683.
31. Osusky KL, Hallahan DE, Fu A, et al. The receptor tyrosine kinase inhibitor SU11248 impedes endothelial cell migration, tubule formation, and blood vessel formation in vivo, but has little effect on existing tumor vessels. *Angiogenesis* 2004;7(3):225–233.
32. Kamba T, Tam BY, Hashizume H, et al. VEGF-dependent plasticity of fenestrated capillaries in the normal adult microvasculature. *Am J Physiol Heart Circ Physiol* 2006;290(2):H560–H576.
33. Vosseler S, Mirancea N, Bohlen P, et al. Angiogenesis inhibition by vascular endothelial growth factor receptor-2 blockade reduces stromal matrix metalloproteinase expression, normalizes stromal tissue, and reverts epithelial tumor phenotype in surface heterotransplants. *Cancer Res* 2005;65(4):1294–1305.
34. Mancuso MR, Davis R, Norberg SM, et al. Rapid vascular regrowth in tumors after reversal of VEGF inhibition. *J Clin Invest* 2006;116(10):2610–2621.
35. Ferrara N, Hillan KJ, Gerber HP, et al. Discovery and development of bevacizumab, an anti-VEGF antibody for treating cancer. *Nat Rev Drug Discov* 2004;3(5):391–400.
36. Presta LG, Chen H, O'Connor SJ, et al. Humanization of an anti-vascular endothelial growth factor monoclonal antibody for the therapy of solid tumors and other disorders. *Cancer Res* 1997;57(20):4593–4599.
37. Johnson DH, Fehrenbacher L, Novotny WF, et al. Randomized phase II trial comparing bevacizumab plus carboplatin and paclitaxel with carboplatin and paclitaxel alone in previously untreated locally advanced or metastatic non-small-cell lung cancer. *J Clin Oncol* 2004;22(11):2184–2191.
38. Sandler A, Gray R, Perry MC, et al. Paclitaxel-carboplatin alone or with bevacizumab for non-small-cell lung cancer. *N Engl J Med* 2006;355:2542–2550.
39. Reck M, von Pawel J, Zatloukal P, et al. Phase III trial of cisplatin plus gemcitabine with either placebo or bevacizumab as first-line therapy for nonsquamous non-small-cell lung cancer: AVAiL. *J Clin Oncol* 2009;27(8):1227–1234.
40. Novotny WF, Holmgren E, Griffing S, et al. Identification of squamous cell histology and central, cavitary tumors as possible risk factors for pulmonary hemorrhage (PH) in patients with advanced NSCLC receiving bevacizumab (BV). *Proc Am Soc Clin Oncol* 2001;20:1318.
41. Sandler AB, Kong G, Strickland D, et al. Treatment outcomes by tumor histology in Eastern Cooperative Group (ECOG) study E4599 of bevacizumab (BV) with paclitaxel/carboplatin (PC) for advanced non-small cell lung cancer (NSCLC). *J Thorac Oncol* 2008;3 (4 suppl): S283 (Abstract 133).
42. Ramalingam SS, Dahlberg SE, Langer CJ, et al. Outcomes for elderly, advanced-stage non small-cell lung cancer patients treated with bevacizumab in combination with carboplatin and paclitaxel: analysis of Eastern Cooperative Oncology Group Trial 4599. *J Clin Oncol* 2008;26(1):60–65.
43. Reck M, von Pawel J, Zatloukal P, et al. Overall survival with cisplatin/gemcitabine and bevacizumab or placebo as first-line therapy for non-squamous non-small cell lung cancer: results from a randomised phase III trial (AVAiL). *Ann Oncol* 2009, in press.
44. Crinò L, Mezger J, Griesinger F, et al. MO19390 (SAiL): safety and efficacy of first-line bevacizumab (Bv)-based therapy in advanced non-small cell lung cancer (NSCLC). *J Clin Oncol* 2009;27(15S suppl):417s(Abstract 8043).
45. Waples JM, Auerbach M, Boccia R, et al. A phase II study of oxaliplatin and pemetrexed plus bevacizumab in advanced non-squamous non-small cell lung cancer. *J Clin Oncol* 2007;25(18 suppl):18025.
46. Heist RS, Fidias P, Huberman M, et al. Phase II trial of oxaliplatin, pemetrexed, and bevacizumab in previously-treated advanced non-small cell lung cancer (NSCLC). *J Clin Oncol* 2007;25(18 suppl):7700.
47. Patel JD, Hensing TA, O'Keeffe P, et al. Pemetrexed and carboplatin plus bevacizumab as first-line therapy for advanced non-squamous non-small cell lung cancer: preliminary safety results of a phase II trial. *J Clin Oncol* 2006;24(18 suppl):17111.
48. Patel JD, Hensing TA, Villafor V, et al. Pemetrexed and carboplatin plus bevacizumab for advanced non-squamous non-small cell lung cancer (NSCLC): preliminary results. *J Clin Oncol* 2007;25 (18 suppl):7601.
49. Dalsania CJ, Hageboutros A, Harris E, et al. Phase II trial of bevacizumab plus pemetrexed and carboplatin in previously untreated advanced nonsquamous non-small cell lung cancer. *J Clin Oncol* 2007;25(18 suppl):18163.
50. William WN Jr, Kies MS, Fossella FV, et al. Phase II study of bevacizumab in combination with docetaxel and carboplatin in patients with metastatic non-small cell lung cancer (NSCLC). *J Clin Oncol* 2007;25(18 suppl):18098.
51. Davila E, Lilenbaum R, Raez L, et al. Phase II trial of oxaliplatin and gemcitabine with bevacizumab in first-line advanced non-small cell lung cancer (NSCLC). *J Clin Oncol* 2006;24(18 suppl):17009.
52. Kraut MJ. Phase II study of gemcitabine and carboplatin plus bevacizumab for stage III/IV non-small cell lung cancer: preliminary safety data. *J Clin Oncol* 2006;24(18 suppl):17091.
53. Shepherd FA, Pereira J, Ciuleanu TE, et al. A randomized placebo-controlled trial of erlotinib in patients with advanced non-small cell lung cancer (NSCLC) following failure of 1st line or 2nd line chemotherapy. A National Cancer Institute of Canada Clinical Trials Group (NCIC CTG) trial. *J Clin Oncol* 2004;22(15 suppl):S622 (abstract 7022).
54. Sandler A, Herbst R. Combining targeted agents: blocking the epidermal growth factor and vascular endothelial growth factor pathways. *Clin Cancer Res* 2006;12(14):4421–4425.
55. Shepherd FA, Rodrigues Pereira J, Ciuleanu T, et al. Erlotinib in previously treated non-small-cell lung cancer. *N Engl J Med* 2005; 353(2):123–132.
56. Herbst RS, Johnson DH, Mininberg E, et al. Phase I/II trial evaluating the anti-vascular endothelial growth factor monoclonal antibody bevacizumab in combination with the HER-1/epidermal growth factor receptor tyrosine kinase inhibitor erlotinib for patients with recurrent non-small-cell lung cancer. *J Clin Oncol* 2005;23(11):2544–2555.
57. Herbst RS, O'Neill VJ, Fehrenbacher L, et al. Phase II study of efficacy and safety of bevacizumab in combination with chemotherapy or erlotinib compared with chemotherapy alone for treatment of recurrent or refractory non small-cell lung cancer. *J Clin Oncol* 2007;25(30):4743–4750.
58. Groen HJ, Smit EF, Dingemans A. A phase II study of erlotinib (E) and bevacizumab (B) in patients (pts) with previously untreated stage IIIB/IV non-small cell lung cancer (NSCLC). *J Clin Oncol* 2007;25 (18 suppl):7625.
59. Pignon JP, Tribodet H, Scagliotti GV, et al. Lung adjuvant cisplatin evaluation (LACE): a pooled analysis of five randomized clinical trials including 4,584 patients. *J Clin Oncol* 2006;24(18 suppl):7008.
60. Rizvi NA, Rusch V, Zhao B, et al. Single agent bevacizumab and bevacizumab in combination with docetaxel and cisplatin as induction therapy for resectable IB-IIIA non-small cell lung cancer. *J Clin Oncol* 2007;25(18 suppl):18045.
61. F Hoffmann-La Roche. Avastin (bevacizumab) Summary of Product Characteristics. Available at: http://www.emea.europa.eu/humandocs/PDFs/EPAR/avastin/emea-combined-h582en.pdf. Accessed 12 October, 2009.
62. Scappaticci FA, Fehrenbacher L, Cartwright T, et al. Surgical wound healing complications in metastatic colorectal cancer patients treated with bevacizumab. *J Surg Oncol* 2005;91(3):173–180.

63. Sokhandon F, Sparschu RA, Furlong JW. Best cases from the AFIP: bronchogenic squamous cell carcinoma. *Radiographics* 2003;23(6):1639–1643.
64. Jain NK, Madan A, Sharma TN, et al. Bronchogenic carcinoma. A study of 109 cases. *J Assoc Physicians India* 1989;37(6):379–382.
65. Gordon MS, Margolin K, Talpaz M, et al. Phase I safety and pharmacokinetic study of recombinant human anti-vascular endothelial growth factor in patients with advanced cancer. *J Clin Oncol* 2001;19(3):843–850.
66. Rohr UP, Augustus S, Lasserre SF, et al. Safety of bevacizumab in patients with metastases to the central nervous system. *J Clin Oncol* 2009;27(15 suppl):88s(Abstract 2007).
67. Fontanini G, Bigini D, Vignati S, et al. Microvessel count predicts metastatic disease and survival in non-small cell lung cancer. *J Pathol* 1995;177(1):57–63.
68. Fontanini G, Lucchi M, Vignati S, et al. Angiogenesis as a prognostic indicator of survival in non-small-cell lung carcinoma: a prospective study. *J Natl Cancer Inst* 1997;89(12):881–886.
69. Lucchi M, Mussi A, Fontanini G, et al. Small cell lung carcinoma (SCLC): the angiogenic phenomenon. *Eur J Cardiothorac Surg* 2002;21(6):1105–1110.
70. Sandler A, Szwaric S, Dowlati A, et al. A phase II study of cisplatin (P) plus etoposide (E) plus bevacizumab (B) for previously untreated extensive stage small cell lung cancer (SCLC) (E3501): A trial of the Eastern Cooperative Oncology Group. *J Clin Oncol* 2007;25(18 suppl):7564.
71. Ready N, Dudek AZ, Wang XF, et al. CALGB 30306: a phase II study of cisplatin (C), irinotecan (I) and bevacizumab (B) for untreated extensive stage small cell lung cancer (ES-SCLC). *J Clin Oncol* 2007;25 (18 suppl):7563.
72. Spigel DR, Hainsworth JD, Yardley DA, et al. Phase II trial of irinotecan, carboplatin, and bevacizumab in patients with extensive-stage small cell lung cancer. *J Clin Oncol* 2007;25(18 suppl):18130.
73. Patton JF, Spigel DR, Greco FA, et al. Irinotecan (I), carboplatin (C), and radiotherapy (RT) followed by maintenance bevacizumab (B) in the treatment (tx) of limited-stage small cell lung cancer (LS-SCLC): update of a phase II trial of the Minnie Pearl Cancer Research Network. *J Clin Oncol* 2006;24(18 suppl):7085.
74. Zubkus JD, Spigel DR, Greco FA, et al. Phase II trial of irinotecan, carboplatin, and bevacizumab in patients with limited-stage small cell lung cancer. *J Clin Oncol* 2007;25(18 suppl):18133.
75. Sundstrøm S, Bremnes RM, Kaasa S, et al. Cisplatin and etoposide regimen is superior to cyclophosphamide, epirubicin, and vincristine regimen in small-cell lung cancer: results from a randomized phase III trial with 5 years' follow-up. *J Clin Oncol* 2002;20(24):4665–4672.
76. Liu B, Barrett T, Choyke P, et al. A phase II study of BAY 43-9006 (sorafenib) in patients with relapsed non-small cell lung cancer (NSCLC). *J Clin Oncol* 2006;24(18 suppl):17119.
77. Gatzemeier U, Blumenschein G, Fosella F, et al. Phase II trial of single-agent sorafenib in patients with advanced non-small cell lung carcinoma. *J Clin Oncol* 2006;24(18 suppl):7002.
78. Adjei AA, Molina JR, Mandrekar SJ, et al. Phase I trial of sorafenib in combination with gefitinib in patients with refractory or recurrent non-small cell lung cancer. *Clin Cancer Res* 2007;13(9):2684–2691.
79. Schiller JH, Flaherty KT, Redlinger M, et al. Sorafenib combined with carboplatin/paclitaxel for advanced non-small cell lung cancer: a phase I subset analysis. *J Clin Oncol* 2006;24(18 suppl):7194.
80. Scagliotti G, von Pawel J, Reck M, et al. Sorafenib plus carboplatin/paclitaxel in chemonaive patients with stage IIIB-IV non-small cell lung cancer (NSCLC): interim analysis (IA) results from the phase III, randomized, double-blind, placebo-controlled, ESCAPE (Evaluation of Sorafenib, Carboplatin, and Paclitaxel Efficacy in NSCLC) trial. 1st European Lung Cancer Conference 2008; Late breaking abstract.
81. Natale RB, Bodkin D, Govindan R, et al. ZD6474 versus gefitinib in patients with advanced NSCLC: final results from a two-part, double-blind, randomized phase II trial. *J Clin Oncol* 2006;24 (18 suppl):7000.
82. Heymach JV, Johnson BE, Prager D, et al. A phase II trial of ZD6474 plus docetaxel in patients with previously treated NSCLC: follow-up results. *J Clin Oncol* 2006;24(18 suppl):7016.
83. Heymach JV, Johnson BE, Prager D, et al. Randomized, placebo-controlled phase II study of vandetanib plus docetaxel in previously treated non small-cell lung cancer. *J Clin Oncol* 2007;25(27):4270–4277.
84. Heymach JV, Paz-Ares L, de Braud F, et al. Randomized phase II study of vandetanib (VAN) alone or in combination with carboplatin and paclitaxel (CP) as first-line treatment for advanced non-small cell lung cancer (NSCLC). *J Clin Oncol* 2007;25(18 suppl):7544.
85. Arnold AM, Smylie M, Ding K, et al. Randomized phase II study of maintenance vandetanib (ZD6474) in small cell lung cancer (SCLC) patients who have a complete or partial response to induction therapy: NCIC CTG BR.20. *J Clin Oncol* 2007;25(18 suppl):7522.
86. Socinski MA, Novello S, Sanchez JM, et al. Efficacy and safety of sunitinib in previously treated, advanced non-small cell lung cancer (NSCLC): Preliminary results of a multicenter phase II trial. *J Clin Oncol* 2006;24(18 suppl):7001.
87. Brahmer JR, Govindan R, Novello S, et al. Efficacy and safety of continuous daily sunitinib dosing in previously treated advanced non-small cell lung cancer (NSCLC): results from a phase II study. *J Clin Oncol* 2007;25(18 Suppl):7542.
88. Reck M, Frickhofen N, Gatzemeier U, et al. A phase I dose escalation study of sunitinib in combination with gemcitabine + cisplatin for advanced non-small cell lung cancer (NSCLC). *J Clin Oncol* 2007;25 (18 suppl):18057.
89. Laurie SA, Arnold A, Gauthier I, et al. Final results of a phase I study of daily oral AZD2171, an inhibitor of vascular endothelial growth factor receptors (VEGFR), in combination with carboplatin (C) + paclitaxel (T) in patients with advanced non-small cell lung cancer (NSCLC): a study of the National Cancer Institute of Canada Clinical Trials Group (NCIC CTG). *J Clin Oncol* 2006;24(18 suppl):3054.
90. Goss GD, Laurie S, Shepherd F, et al. IND.175: phase I study of daily oral AZD2171, a vascular endothelial growth factor receptor inhibitor (VEGFRI), in combination with gemcitabine and cisplatin (G/C) in patients with advanced non-small cell lung cancer (ANSCLC): a study of the NCIC Clinical Trials Group. *J Clin Oncol* 2007;25 (18 suppl):7649.
91. Schiller JH, Larson T, Ou SI, et al. Efficacy and safety of axitinib (AG-013736; AG) in patients (pts) with advanced non-small cell lung cancer (NSCLC): a phase II trial. *J Clin Oncol* 2007;25(18 suppl):7507.
92. Ahmad T, Eisen T. Kinase inhibition with BAY 43-9006 in renal cell carcinoma. *Clin Cancer Res* 2004;10(suppl 18, pt 2):S6388–S6392.
93. Wilhelm SM, Carter C, Tang L, et al. BAY 43-9006 exhibits broad spectrum oral antitumor activity and targets the RAF/MEK/ERK pathway and receptor tyrosine kinases involved in tumor progression and angiogenesis. *Cancer Res* 2004;64(19):7099–7109.
94. Murphy DA, Makonnen S, Lassoued W, et al. Inhibition of tumor endothelial ERK activation, angiogenesis, and tumor growth by sorafenib (BAY43-9006). *Am J Pathol* 2006;169(5):1875–1885.
95. Carter CA, Chen C, Brink C, et al. Sorafenib is efficacious and tolerated in combination with cytotoxic or cytostatic agents in preclinical models of human non-small cell lung carcinoma. *Cancer Chemother Pharmacol* 2007;59(2):183–195.
96. Wilhelm S, Chien DS. BAY 43-9006: preclinical data. *Curr Pharm Des* 2002;8(25):2255–2257.
97. Awada A, Hendlisz A, Gil T, et al. Phase I safety and pharmacokinetics of BAY 43-9006 administered for 21 days on/7 days off in patients with advanced, refractory solid tumours. *Br J Cancer* 2005;92(10):1855–1861.
98. Minami H, Kawada K, Ebi H, Kitagawa K, Kim YI, Araki K, et al. A phase I study of BAY 43-9006, a dual inhibitor of Raf and VEGFR kinases, in Japanese patients with solid cancers. *J Clin Oncol* 2005; 23(16 suppl):3062.
99. Gondek K, Dhanda R, Simantov R, et al. Health-related quality of life measures in advanced non-small cell lung cancer patients receiving sorafenib. *J Clin Oncol* 2006;24(18 suppl):17085.
100. Adjei AA, Molina JR, Hillman SL, et al. A front-line window of opportunity phase II study of sorafenib in patients with advanced non-small cell lung cancer: a North Central Cancer Treatment Group study. *J Clin Oncol* 2007;25(18 suppl):7547.

101. Adjei AA, Mandrekar S, Marks RS, et al. A phase I study of BAY 43-9006 and gefitinib in patients with refractory or recurrent non-small-cell lung cancer (NSCLC). *J Clin Oncol* 2005;23(16 suppl):3067.
102. Results from the US National Institutes of Health ClinicalTrials.gov website. Available at: www.clinicaltrial./gov. Assessed January 23, 2008.
103. Gridelli C, Rossi A, Mongillo F, et al. A randomized phase II study of sorafenib/gemcitabine or sorafenib/erlotinib for advanced non-small-cell lung cancer in elderly patients or patients with a performance status of 2: treatment rationale and protocol dynamics. *Clin Lung Cancer* 2007;8(6):396–398.
104. Carlomagno F, Vitagliano D, Guida T, et al. ZD6474, an orally available inhibitor of KDR tyrosine kinase activity, efficiently blocks oncogenic RET kinases. *Cancer Res* 2002;62(24):7284–7290.
105. Wedge SR, Ogilvie DJ, Dukes M, et al. ZD6474 inhibits vascular endothelial growth factor signaling, angiogenesis, and tumor growth following oral administration. *Cancer Res* 2002;62:4645–4655.
106. Ciardiello F, Bianco R, Caputo R, et al. Antitumor activity of ZD6474, a vascular endothelial growth factor receptor tyrosine kinase inhibitor, in human cancer cells with acquired resistance to antiepidermal growth factor receptor therapy. *Clin Cancer Res* 2004;10(2):784–793.
107. Hurwitz H, Holden SN, Eckhardt SG, et al. Clinical evaluation of ZD6474, an orally active inhibitor of VEGF signaling, in patients with solid tumors. *Proc Am Soc Clin Oncol* 2002;21:(Abstract 325).
108. Minami H, Ebi H, Tahara M, et al. A phase I study of an oral VEGF receptor tyrosine kinase inhibitor ZD6474, in Japanese patients with solid tumors. *Proc Am Soc Clin Oncol* 2003;22:(Abstract 778).
109. Holden SN, Eckhardt SG, Basser R, et al. Clinical evaluation of ZD6474, an orally active inhibitor of VEGF and EGF receptor signaling, in patients with solid, malignant tumors. *Ann Oncol* 2005;16(8):1391–1397.
110. Nakagawa K, Kiura K, Shinkai T, et al. A randomized double-blind phase IIa dose-finding study of ZD6474 in Japanese patients with NSCLC. *J Clin Oncol* 2006;24(18 suppl):7067.
111. Heymach JV, Johnson BE, Rowbottom JA, et al. A randomized, placebo-controlled phase II trial of ZD6474 plus docetaxel, in patients with NSCLC. *J Clin Oncol* 2005;23(16 suppl):3023.
112. Heymach JV, Dong RP, Dimery I, et al. ZD6474, a novel antiangiogenic agent, in combination with docetaxel in patients with NSCLC: results of the run-in phase of a two-part, randomized phase II study. *J Clin Oncol* 2004;22(14 suppl):S207 (Abstract 3051).
113. Johnson BE, Ma P, West H, et al. Preliminary phase II safety evaluation of ZD6474, in combination with carboplatin and paclitaxel, as 1st-line treatment in patients with NSCLC. *J Clin Oncol* 2005;23 (16 suppl):7102.
114. Abrams TJ, Lee LB, Murray LJ, et al. SU11248 inhibits KIT and platelet-derived growth factor receptor beta in preclinical models of human small cell lung cancer. *Mol Cancer Ther* 2003;2(5):471–478.
115. Cabebe E, Wakelee H. Role of anti-angiogenesis agents in treating NSCLC: focus on bevacizumab and VEGFR tyrosine kinase inhibitors. *Curr Treat Options Oncol* 2007;8(1):15–27.
116. Mendel DB, Laird AD, Xin X, et al. In vivo anti-tumor and mechanism of action studies of SU11248, a potent and selective inhibitor of the VEGF and PDGF receptors. *Proc Am Assoc Cancer Res* 2002;43:(Abstract 5349).
117. Potapova O, Laird AD, Nannini MA, et al. Contribution of individual targets to the antitumor efficacy of the multitargeted receptor tyrosine kinase inhibitor SU11248. *Mol Cancer Ther* 2006;5(5):1280–1289.
118. Robert F, Sandler A, Schiller JH, et al. A phase I dose-escalation and pharmacokinetic (PK) study of sunitinib (SU) plus docetaxel (D) in patients (pts) with advanced solid tumors (STs). *J Clin Oncol* 2007;25 (18 suppl):3543.
119. Drevs J, Siegert P, Medinger M, et al. Phase I clinical study of AZD2171, an oral vascular endothelial growth factor signaling inhibitor, in patients with advanced solid tumors. *J Clin Oncol* 2007;25(21):3045–3054.
120. LoRusso PM, Heath E, Valdivieso M, et al. Phase I evaluation of AZD2171, a highly potent and selective inhibitor of VEGFR signaling, in combination with selected chemotherapy regimens in patients with advanced solid tumors. *J Clin Oncol* 2006;24(18 suppl):3034.
121. van Cruijsen H, Voest EE, van Herpen CML, et al. Phase I clinical evaluation of AZD2171 in combination with gefitinib, in patients with advanced tumors. *J Clin Oncol* 2005;23(16 suppl):3030.
122. Polverino A, Coxon A, Starnes C, et al. AMG 706, an oral, multikinase inhibitor that selectively targets vascular endothelial growth factor, platelet-derived growth factor, and kit receptors, potently inhibits angiogenesis and induces regression in tumor xenografts. *Cancer Res* 2006;66(17):8715–8721.
123. Rosen L, Kurzrock R, Jackson E, et al. Safety and pharmacokinetics of AMG 706 in patients with advanced solid tumors. *J Clin Oncol* 2005;23(16 suppl):3013.
124. Price TJ, Lipton L, Williams J, et al. Safety and pharmacokinetics (PK) of AMG 706 in combination with gemcitabine for the treatment of patients (pts) with solid tumors. *J Clin Oncol* 2007;25(18 suppl):14005.
125. Blumenschein G Jr, Sandler A, O'Rourke T, et al. Safety and pharmacokinetics (PK) of AMG 706, panitumumab, and carboplatin/paclitaxel (CP) for the treatment of patients (pts) with advanced non-small cell lung cancer (NSCLC). *J Clin Oncol* 2006;24 (18 suppl):7119.
126. Crawford J, Burris H, Stephenson J Jr, et al. Safety and pharmacokinetics (PK) of AMG 706 in combination with panitumumab and gemcitabine-cisplatin in patients (pts) with advanced cancer. *J Clin Oncol* 2007;25(18 suppl):14057.
127. Rugo HS, Herbst RS, Liu G, et al. Phase I trial of the oral antiangiogenesis agent AG-013736 in patients with advanced solid tumors: pharmacokinetic and clinical results. *J Clin Oncol* 2005;23(24):5474–5483.
128. Hurwitz H, Dowlati A, Savage S, et al. Safety, tolerability and pharmacokinetics of oral administration of GW786034 in pts with solid tumors. *J Clin Oncol* 2005;23(16 suppl):3012.
129. Wakelee H, Adjei AA, Keer H, et al. A phase I dose-escalation and pharmacokinetic (PK) study of a novel multiple-targeted receptor tyrosine kinase (RTK) inhibitor, XL647, in patients with advanced solid malignancies. *J Clin Oncol* 2005;23(16 suppl):3142.
130. Wakelee HA, Adjei AA, Halsey J, et al. A phase I dose-escalation and pharmacokinetic (PK) study of a novel spectrum selective kinase inhibitor, XL647, in patients with advanced solid malignancies (ASM). *J Clin Oncol* 2006;24(18 suppl):3044.
131. Wakelee HA, Molina JR, Fehling JM, et al. A phase I study with exploratory pharmacodynamic endpoints of XL647, a novel spectrum selective kinase inhibitor, administered orally daily to patients (pts) with advanced solid malignancies. *J Clin Oncol* 2007;25 (18 suppl):14044.
132. Morabito A, De ME, Di MM, et al. Tyrosine kinase inhibitors of vascular endothelial growth factor receptors in clinical trials: current status and future directions. *Oncologist* 2006;11(7):753–764.

CHAPTER 49

Fred R. Hirsch
Tetsuya Mitsudomi
Pasi A. Jänne

Anti-EGFR Therapies: How to Select Patients

Epidermal growth factor receptor (EGFR) inhibitors have proven effective in some patients with advanced non–small cell lung cancer (NSCLC) previously untreated and/or treated with chemotherapy.[1] Most data are published on the EGFR tyrosine kinase inhibitors (TKIs) gefitinib and erlotinib. Objective response rates in phase II studies with gefitinib and erlotinib are 10% to 18% in western populations and up to 27% in Asian populations.[2–8] In addition, a substantial fraction of NSCLC patients, who failed previous chemotherapy, achieve long-term stable disease (SD), leading to disease control rate (DCR) exceeding 50% of patients and often associated with symptomatic improvement and prolonged survival. Thus, developing a biomarker capable of predicting DCR is equally if not more important than one predicting only those who have objective response.

Two large placebo controlled randomized studies were performed with EGFR TKIs as second- or third-line therapy.[6,7] The BR.21 study with erlotinib showed for the first time a survival benefit for a targeted therapy in NSCLC, whereas the Iressa Survival Evaluation in Lung Cancer (ISEL) study with gefitinib did not demonstrate a significant survival advantage, although subset analysis in the latter study did show survival benefit in certain clinical subgroups (i.e., never-smokers and Asians).[7] In both studies, clinical effect of EGFR TKIs on survival was seen also in patients with "unfavorable" clinical characteristics (e.g., men, smokers, and patients with tumors of squamous histology).[7,8] Thus, clinical features appear insufficient for identifying those patients who would and would not have survival benefit from these new agents.

After encouraging results of EGFR TKIs in relapsed patient categories, it was natural to test these drugs in combination with standard first-line chemotherapy of advanced NSCLC. In large prospective randomized studies, standard chemotherapy doublets were given in combination with EGFR TKIs or placebo, followed by maintenance with active drugs or placebo.[9–12] No benefit from adding EGFR TKIs to standard chemotherapy was observed in any of the four studies, and again clinical characteristics (except for never-smoking status in the TRIBUTE study) could not identify subsets of patients who benefited from combination therapy.

Thus, the search for other measures (i.e., biomarkers) for selection of patients for the EGFR TKIs was mandatory.

The use of monoclonal antibodies, mainly cetuximab has been studied in NSCLC, and most recently the results from the FLEX (**F**irst Line in **L**ung Cancer with **E**rbitu**X**) study, which is a comparison of cisplatin/vinorelbine with or without cetuximab in EGFR immunohistochemistry (IHC) positive was presented (see later).[13] The latter study showed a survival benefit for patients having cetuximab added to the chemotherapy in first-line therapy for advanced NSCLC patients with EGFR protein-expressing tumors. Although the survival benefit (median survival, 11.3 vs. 10.1 months; hazard ratio [HR] = 0.87) was statistically significant, the efficacy seems not to be dramatically improved, and the study calls for a better biomarker selection of patients to this type of therapy. Another study (BMS 099), which compared chemotherapy with or without cetuximab as first-line therapy in advanced unselected NSCLC did not meet the primary end point of prolonged progression-free survival (PFS).[14] Thus, selection of NSCLC patients to EGFR inhibitors based on EGFR markers might be crucial for outcome both with EGFR TKIs as well as with monoclonal antibodies. Potential clinical and molecular biomarkers for selection of patients to EGFR inhibitors for NSCLC is discussed later.

CLINICAL FACTORS

Early Clinical Trials

In the phase I trials of gefitinib, tumor response was exclusively seen in NSCLC (4/16 in NSCLC and 0/48 in other types of cancer in United States/European study, 5/23 in NSCLC and 0/8 in other types of cancer in Japanese study).[2,3] Especially in Japanese study, all four responders were with adenocarcinoma and three fourths were female patients.[2]

Two phase II trials of gefitinib, Iressa Dose Evaluation in Advanced Lung Cancer (IDEAL) 1 and 2, showed that certain patient subgroups appeared to have a higher response rate, namely women, adenocarcinoma, and Japanese.[4,5] In IDEAL 1 conducted in Japan and European countries, 210 patients with one or two prior chemotherapy regimens were randomly assigned either to have 250 or 500 mg of gefitinib. Objective tumor response rate was similar between the two groups (18.4% and 19.0% for 250- and 500-mg group, respectively). In contrast, adverse events were more common in the 500-mg group. In the 250-mg group, 15.5% of the patients had AEs requiring a short-treatment interruption, and none required a dose reduction, 28.3% and 10.4% of the patients in the 500-mg group required a treatment interruption and a dose reduction, respectively. Response rate was higher for Japanese patients than non-Japanese patients (27.5% vs. 10.4%; $p = 0.0023$). Multivariate analysis revealed that performance status (PS), sex, histology, and prior immuno/hormonal therapy were significant predictive factors at the 10% significance level. A similarly designed randomized phase II trial conducted in the United States (IDEAL 2) revealed that overall response rate was 10% (12% in 250-mg group and 9% in 500- mg group). In this trial, patients with stage IIIB/IV diseases, for which they had received at least two chemotherapy regimens, were eligible. Response rate was again higher in women (19%) than in men (3%), in adenocarcinomas (13%) than other histologic types (4%).

Miller et al.[15] were the first to report that smoking history as well as bronchioloalveolar pathologic subtypes predict sensitivity to gefitinib. Overall, a partial radiographic response was observed in 21 (15%) of 139 patients with advanced NSCLC. Never-smokers have a significantly higher response rate than former/current smokers (36% vs. 8%; $p < 0.001$).[15] In addition, adenocarcinoma with bronchioloalveolar features had higher response rate (38%) than other adenocarcinomas (14%, $p < 0.001$).[5] Multivariate analysis confirmed that these two factors were independent predictors of response ($p = 0.006$ and 0.004, respectively). However, gender was not identified as a significant predictor in both univariate and multivariate analyses. The authors speculated that this was because of comigration of smoking and gender.[15]

Subsequent Studies Following this observation, various groups confirmed that response to gefitinib or erlotinib very much affected patients' clinical backgrounds. In observation of over 4000 patients taken from previously published literature (Table 49.1), TKI response was dependent on smoking history (never-smokers 38% vs. former/current smokers 10%), gender (men 13% vs. women 36%), histologic type (adenocarcinoma 27% vs. nonadenocarcinoma 7%), and ethnicity (East Asians 29% vs. others 8%).

Several authors further showed that higher response rate was linked to longer survival in each patient subset. For example, Ando et al.[16] showed that median survival time (MST) after gefitinib treatment was 16.6 and 7.7 months in female and male patients, 15.6 and 7.6 months in never-smokers and former/current smokers, and 12.1 and 6.3 months in patients with adenocarcinoma and with other histologic types, respectively. In addition, multivariate analysis by the Cox regression model revealed that women, no smoking history, adenocarcinoma as well as absence of metastatic disease, good PS, previous chest surgery are independent prognostic factors.[16]

Clinical Predictors in Randomized Phase III Trials Aforementioned trends were also seen in randomized controlled clinical trials. In four randomized trials comparing TKI plus platinum doublet chemotherapy versus platinum doublet chemotherapy, namely Iressa NSCLC Trial Assessing Combination Treatment (INTACT) 1 and 2 using gefitinib, TALENT and TRIBUTE using erlotinib, addition of TKI did not yield survival advantage over platinum doublet.[9–12] However, subgroup analysis of TRIBUTE showed that addition of erlotinib to carboplatin plus paclitaxel confer an advantage in overall survival in patients who reported never smoking (MST, 23 vs. 10 months; HR, 0.49; 95% confidence interval [CI], 0.28 to 0.85).[12] None of other factors including gender, race, PS, or histology were predictive for overall survival.[12] The favorable predictive role of never smoking was also demonstrated for patients with bronchioloalveolar carcinomas (BAC).[17]

In a randomized, placebo-controlled trial to determine whether erlotinib prolongs survival in NSCLC patients after the failure of first- or second-line chemotherapy (BR.21), erlotinib significantly prolongs survival with MST of 6.7 versus 4.7 months (HR, 0.70; $p < 0.001$).[6] In this trial, tumor response was significantly better in never-smokers than former/current smokers (25% vs. 4%; $p < 0.001$).[12] Furthermore, smoking history was an independent prognostic factor ($p = 0.048$), as well as erlotinib treatment ($p = 0.002$), Asian ethnicity ($p = 0.01$), and adenocarcinoma histology ($p = 0.004$). In their exploratory subgroup analyses, a benefit from erlotinib was dependent on smoking history, with HR of 0.9 ($p = 0.14$) in former/current smokers and 0.4 ($p < 0.001$) in never-smokers.[6]

In contrast, similar placebo-controlled randomized trial using gefitinib in place of erlotinib, ISEL trial, failed to show overall survival advantage in gefitinib treatment group (median survival, 5.6 vs. 5.1 months; $p = 0.087$).[7] However, gefitinib prolongs survival in never-smokers (MST, 8.9 vs. 6.1 months; $p = 0.012$) as well as in Asian patients (MST, 9.5 vs. 5.5 months; $p = 0.010$) in preplanned subset analyses.[7]

The results of two randomized phase II trials comparing gefitinib with docetaxel were recently reported. V15-32 conducted in Japan failed,[18] but similarly designed Iressa Non–small cell lung cancer Trial Evaluating REsponse and Survival against Taxotere (INTEREST)[19] was able to show noninferiority of gefitinib to docetaxel in patients with NSCLC having been treated with one or two chemotherapy regimens. None of clinical parameters such as sex, PS, smoking status, age, ethnicity (INTEREST only) significantly affected overall survival in the both trials.[18,19] These somewhat unexpected observations are at least partly attributed to high crossover rate especially in V15-32, that is, 53% of patients with docetaxel arm received gefitinib upon progression and 36% of patients with gefitinib

TABLE 49.1 Relationship between Tumor Response and Clinical Parameters in Patients with Lung Cancer Treated with EGFR TKI

Author Year	TKI	Design	Overall N	Overall CR+PR	Overall RR	Smoking	Smoking N	Smoking CR+PR	Smoking RR	Gender	Gender N	Gender CR+PR	Gender RR	Histology	Histology N	Histology CR+PR	Histology RR	Ethnicity	Ethnicity N	Ethnicity CR+PR	Ethnicity RR
Fukuoka et al. 2003[4]	G	Rand P-II	208	38	18 %		N/A					N/A				N/A		Asian	102	29	28 %
																		Other	108	11	10 %
Kris et al. 2003[5]	G	Rand P-II	216	22	10 %		N/A			Male	123	4	3 %	Adeno	146	19	13 %				
										Female	93	18	19 %	Other	70	3	4 %				
Perez-Soler 2004[8]	E	P-II	57	7	12 %									Adeno	35	4	11 %				
														Other	22	3	14 %				
Takano et al. 2004[158]	G	Retro	98	32	33 %	NS	32	20	63 %	Male	66	15	23 %	Adeno	81	31	38 %	Asian	98	32	33 %
						S	66	12	18 %	Female	32	17	53 %	Other	17	1	6 %				
Kaneda et al. 2004[30]	G	Retro	101	20	20 %	NS	55	15	33 %	Male	64	6	9 %	Adeno	81	20	25 %	Asian	101	20	20 %
						S	46	5	9 %	Female	37	14	38 %	Other	20	0	0 %				
Huang et al. 2004[68]	G	Retro	16	9	56 %	NS	12	7	58 %	Male	4	2	50 %	Adeno	15	9	60 %	Asian	16	9	56 %
						S	4	2	50 %	Female	12	5	42 %	Other	1	0	0 %				
Miller et al. 2004[15]	G	Retro	139	21	15 %	NS	36	13	36 %	Male	48	4	8 %	Adeno	108	21	19 %				
						S	103	8	8 %	Female	91	17	19 %	Other	31	0	0 %	Other	139	21	15 %
Kris et al. 2004[17]	E	Retro	59	15	25 %	NS	19	7	37 %												
						S	21	4	19 %												
Lim 2005[154]	G	Retro	110	35	32 %	NS	66	31	47 %	Male	52	10	19 %					Asian	110	35	47 %
						S	44	4	%	Female	58	25	43 %								
Shepherd et al. 2005[6]	E	P-III	427	38	9 %	NS	93	23	25 %	Male	281	17	6 %	Adeno	209	29	14 %	Asian	53	10	19 %
						S	311	12	4 %	Female	146	21	14 %	Other	218	9	4 %	Other	374	28	8 %
Kim et al. 2005[31]	G	Retro	80	20	25 %	NS	17	10	59 %	Male	61	12	20 %	Adeno	39	16	41 %	Asian	80	20	25 %
						S	63	10	16 %	Female	19	8	42 %	Other	41	4	10 %				
Lee et al. 2005[20]	G	P-II	36	25	69 %	NS	36	25	69 %	Male	3	1	33 %	Adeno	36	25	69 %	Asian	36	25	69 %
						S	0	0	0 %	Female	33	24	73 %	Other			%				
Mitsudomi et al. 2005[67]	G	Retro	50	26	52 %	NS	25	17	68 %	Male	27	11	41 %	Adeno	43	25	58 %	Asian	50	26	52 %
						S	25	9	36 %	Female	23	15	65 %	Other	7	1	14 %				
Takano et al. 2005[61]	G	Retro	66	35	53 %	NS	43	28	65 %	Male	40	17	43 %	Adeno	62	34	55 %	Asian	66	35	53 %
						S	23	7	30 %	Female	26	18	69 %	Other	4	1	25 %				
Cappuzzo et al. 2005[40]	G	Prospective plus EAP	102	14	14 %	NS	15	6	40 %	Male	67	4	6 %	Adeno	63	11	17 %				
						S	87	8	9 %	Female	35	10	29 %	Other	39	3	8 %	Other	102	14	14 %
Han et al. 2005[70]	G	Retro	90	22	24 %	NS	43	15	35 %	Male	54	8	15 %	Adeno	58	20	34 %	Asian	90	22	24 %
						S	47	7	15 %	Female	36	14	39 %	Other	32	2	6 %				
Zhang et al. 2005[159]	G	Retro	98	31	32 %	NS	58	25	43 %	Male	56	11	20 %	Adeno	75	31	41 %	Asian	98	31	32 %
						S	37	6	16 %	Female	39	20	51 %	Other	20	0	0 %				

(continues)

TABLE 49.1 Relationship between Tumor Response and Clinical Parameters in Patients with Lung Cancer Treated with EGFR TKI *(continued)*

Author Year	TKI	Design	Overall N	Overall CR+PR	Overall RR	Smoking	Smoking N	Smoking CR+PR	Smoking RR	Gender	Gender N	Gender CR+PR	Gender RR	Histology	Histology N	Histology CR+PR	Histology RR	Ethnicity	Ethnicity N	Ethnicity CR+PR	Ethnicity RR
Tokumo et al.	G	Retro	21	10	48 %	NS	8	6	75 %	Male	13	6	46 %	Adeno	15	9	60 %	Asian	21	10	48 %
2005[69]						S	13	4	31 %	Female	8	4	50 %	Other	6	1	17 %				
Thatcher et al.	G	P-III	959	77	8 %	NS	204	37	18 %	Male			5 %	Adeno			11.9 %	Asian	209	26	12 %
2005[7]						S	755	40	5.3 %	Female			15 %	Other			4.8 %	Other	750	51	7 %
Tomizawa et al.	G	Retro	20	14	70 %	NS	11	10	91 %	Male	9	5	56 %	Adeno	18	13	72 %	Asian	20	14	70 %
2005[155]						S	9	4	44 %	Female	11	9	82 %	Other	2	1	50 %	Other	0	0	0 %
Ando et al.	G	Retro	1713	348	20 %	NS	653	225	35 %	Male	1086	126	12 %	Adeno	1288	311	24 %	Asian	20	14	70 %
2006[16]						S	1012	116	12 %	Female	627	222	35 %	Other	414	34	8 %	Other	0	0	0 %
Niho et al.	G	P-II	40	12	30 %	NS	8	6	75 %	Male	24	3	13 %	Adeno	30	11	37 %	Asian	40	12	30 %
2006[160]		first line				S	32	6	19 %	Female	16	9	56 %	Other	10	1	10 %				
Suzuki et al.	G	P-II	34	9	27 %	NS	11	5	46 %	Male	21	2	10 %	Adeno	25	7	28 %	Asian	34	9	27 %
2006[156]		first line				S	23	4	17 %	Female	13	7	54 %	Other	9	2	22 %				
Satouchi et al.	G	Retro	221	54	24 %	NS	89	37	42 %	Male	142	20	14 %	Adeno	196	52	27 %	Asian	221	54	24 %
2007[157]						S	131	17	13 %	Female	79	34	43 %	Other	25	2	8 %	Other	0	0	0 %
Tamura et al.	E	P-II	106	30	28 %	NS			51 %	Male			17 %	Adeno				Asian	106	30	28 %
2007[34]						S			14 %	Female			50 %	Other				Other	0	0	0 %
Total			4232	964	23 %	NS	1515	561	37 %	Male	2241	284	13 %	Adeno	2623	698	26.6 %	Asian	1571	463	29 %
						S	2852	285	10 %	Female	1434	511	36 %	Other	988	68	7 %	Other	1473	125	8 %

CR, complete response; E, erlotinib; EAP, expanded access program; G, gefitinib; N/A, not applicable; NS, non-smoker; P-II, phase II study; P-III, phase III study; PR, partial response; Rand P-II, randomized phase II study; RR, response rate; S, smokers; TKI, tyrosine kinase inhibitor.

arm received docetaxel,[18] whereas the rates were 31% and 37% in INTEREST,[19] respectively. Other concern was that rates of nonsmokers were not equal in V15-32 (i.e., 29% of gefitinib arm were nonsmokers, whereas 36% of docetaxel arm were nonsmokers).[18]

Clinical Trials for Patients Selected by Clinical Factors Prompted by these observations, Lee et al.[20] conducted phase II trial to evaluate the efficacy of gefitinib as a first-line therapy in never-smokers with advanced or metastatic adenocarcinoma in Korea. Out of 36 patients who were assessable for response, 25 patients (69%) had partial response and 4 (19%) had stable disease, yielding 88% of disease control rate.[16] This amazingly high rate could be achieved possibly because patients had a combination of three predictors of good response. Interestingly, they did not see difference in response between adenocarcinoma with bronchioloalveolar features (3/7, 43%) and that without bronchioloalveolar features (22/29, 76%) ($p = 0.16$).[20]

Although the contribution of each factor to the positive results is unknown, this study clearly supports the further study of EGFR TKI as a first-line therapy in certain subsets of NSCLC patients. This was prospectively investigated in Iressa Pan-Asia Study (IPASS), a phase III trial investigating gefitinib versus carboplatin/paclitaxel doublet chemotherapy as first-line treatment in selected subjects with stage IIIB/IV adenocarcinoma having no or light smoking history in East and South East Asia.[21] The result was recently reported to be positive and details were discussed later in this chapter.

Histology As shown in Tables 49.1, response rate for patients with adenocarcinoma was 27% compared with 7% in patients with other histologic types. As discussed earlier, Miller et al.[15] reported that patients with bronchioloalveolar histologic type predict sensitivity to gefitinib. Out of 139 NSCLC patients they reviewed, 21 (15%; 95% CI, 9% to 21%) experienced a partial radiographic response. In this study, the authors defined NSCLC of bronchioloalveolar subtype as adenocarcinoma with bronchioloalveolar features, bronchioloalveolar carcinoma with focal invasion, or pure bronchioloalveolar cancer. However, this definition of bronchioloalveolar features are not strictly followed to World Health Organization (WHO) criteria in which bronchioloalveolar cell carcinoma is defined as noninvasive, in situ carcinoma.[15] However, these observations do not preclude patients with nonadenocarcinoma histology from candidates of EGFR-TKI therapy. In aforementioned BR.21 trial comparing erlotinib with best supportive care, patients with nonadenocarcinoma histology also had a survival benefit with an HR of 0.8 ($p = 0.07$).[6]

Adenosquamous carcinoma is defined as having components of both squamous cell carcinoma and adenocarcinoma with each comprising at least 10% of the tumor. Although the majority of patients with this histologic type are smokers, several investigators reported similar incidence of EGFR mutation in adenosquamous cell carcinoma, one of putative predictive markers as discussed later. For example, Kang et al.,[22] Toyooka et al.,[23] and Sasaki et al.[24] reported that EGFR mutation was present in 11/25, 3/11, and 4/26 adenosquamous carcinomas, respectively. Although most patients were not treated with EGFR TKI, patients with adenosquamous histology harboring EGFR mutation can be candidates for EGFR-TKI therapy. Interestingly, these authors agree in that identical EGFR mutation is present in both squamous and adenocarcinoma components in the same adenosquamous tumor.[22–24] In addition, at least a part of patients with squamous cell carcinoma who responded to EGFR TKI in the literature may, in fact, be those with squamous cell carcinoma with adenocarcinoma component with EGFR mutation.

Similarly, Fukui et al.[25] reported that one of six patients with combined small cell carcinoma and adenocarcinoma of the lung had EGFR L858R mutation. This mutation was again present in both small cell and adenocarcinoma components.

Skin Toxicity Skin toxicity is most common adverse event relating to EGFR-TKI therapy. For example, during treatment with gefitinib 250 mg/day or erlotinib 150 mg/day, skin toxicity occurred in 62%[4] and 75% of the patients.[26] In a phase II trial of erlotinib, skin rash correlated with tumor response and overall survival. MSTs for patients without rash, those with grade 1, and those with grade 2 or 3 were 1.5, 8.5, and 19.6 months, respectively.[8] Similarly, Jänne et al.[27] reported a correlation between skin rash and survival in patients on an expanded access study. MST for patients with skin toxicity of any grade was 10 months that was significantly longer than 4.5 months for patients without skin toxicity ($p = 0.0001$).[27]

In general, data from multiple studies with cetuximab and erlotinib show a consistent relationship between rash and response/survival in NSCLC as well as other tumor types.[28] However, this relationship is less consistent for gefitinib, reason for this discrepancy is currently not known.[28]

Other Clinical Factors Related to Efficacy of EGFR TKIs Several other factors are reported to be associated with response/survival of patients treated with gefitinib or erlotinib. These included absence of metastatic disease,[16] good performance status,[4,16,26,27,29,30] previous chest surgery,[16] younger age,[7,13] presence of prior platinum chemotherapy.[6]

Interstitial Lung Disease In Japan, considerable fraction of patients with gefitinib treatment suffer from fatal interstitial lung disease (ILD).[32] Large multi-institutional retrospective analysis conducted by West Japan Clinical Oncology Group (WJOG) revealed that 70 (3.5%) cases and 31 deaths (1.6%) from gefitinib induced ILD among 1976 patients.[16] In a prospective study conducted by AstraZeneca Japan, incidence of ILD was 5.81% (193/3322) and 83 died of disease (2.5% mortality).[33] In combined analysis of two phase II studies of erlotinib monotherapy in Japan, ILD was observed 5 of 108 (4.6%).[34] In WJOG study, gefitinib-induced ILD was significantly associated with male sex, smoking history, and coincidence of interstitial pneumonia.[16] In AstraZeneca study, poor PS, smoking history, preexisting ILD, and prior history of chemotherapy were independently associated with ILD.[33]

However, incidence of ILD appears to be lower in other Asian countries than Japan except Taiwan. Chiu et al.[35] from Taiwan reported that four patients with NSCLC having brain metastases out of 76 patients (5.8%) developed ILD. In contrast, ILD was observed in 3/485 patients treated with erlotinib compared with 3/242 patients in the placebo group in BR.21 study in which about 13% of patients are of Asian ethnicity.[6] Similarly, the number of patients experiencing ILD as higher in Asian population than in the overall population; however, no difference was observed between the gefitinib and placebo groups (3% vs. 4%) in ISEL study in which about 20% of patients are of Asian ethnicity.[7] From Korea, no cases of gefitinib-related ILD was observed in 111 patients with advanced NSCLC on expanded access program.[29] It is difficult to understand difference of incidence of ILD among countries especially among several East Asian countries. However, variability in the criteria for ILD should exist making it difficult to estimate true incidence of gefitinib or erlotinib induced ILD among different countries. Therefore, eliminating patients with multiple risk factors for ILD from candidates of EGFR-TKI therapy is important for patient selection at least in several East Asian countries including Japan.

EGFR GENE COPY NUMBER

In breast cancer patients, amplification of the *HER-2* gene (HER-2 is a member of the EGFR family) detected by fluorescence in situ hybridization (FISH) is a strong predictive factor for treatment benefit from anti-HER-2 monoclonal antibody, trastuzumab, and recommended for use in clinical practice.[36] EGFR is an important signaling pathway for lung carcinogenesis[37] and was demonstrated to have a negative prognostic impact.[38,39] Thus, it was hypothesized that genomic gain of *EGFR* is a factor contributing to growth advantage of NSCLC cells and may be an important biomarker of sensitivity to EGFR TKIs. Investigators from the University of Colorado Cancer Center developed an original scoring system for *EGFR* gene copy number assessed by FISH in which tumors were classified into six categories, based on ascending number of gene copies per cell.[40] FISH-negative samples were classified as those with no or low genomic gain (≥ four copies of the gene per cell in <40% of cells), and FISH-positive samples were defined as tumors with high gene copy number (≥ four copies of the gene per cell in ≥40% of cells) or gene amplification (tight gene clusters and a ratio of gene/chromosome per cell ≥2, or ≥15 gene copies per cell in ≥10% of the cells). To date, several major studies have addressed the association between *EGFR* gene copy number by FISH and treatment outcome to EGFR TKIs. All the published studies demonstrated clinically important treatment benefit in patients with high *EGFR* gene copy number with EGFR TKIs versus placebo, and this test is now being validated in prospective clinical studies in enriched population of NSCLC patients.

Association between EGFR FISH and Outcome with EGFR TKIs as Second-Line Therapy

Cappuzzo et al.[40] analyzed 102 gefitinib-treated patients according to EGFR protein expression, phospho-Akt expression, *EGFR* gene copy number by FISH, and *EGFR* mutations. Patients who were FISH positive had significantly higher response rate (36% vs. 3% in FISH-negative patients), median time-to-progression (9.0 vs. 2.5 months, respectively) and median overall survival (18.7 vs. 7.0 months, respectively). The association of FISH positivity and superior survival was confirmed in multivariate survival analysis. Evaluation of *EGFR* gene copy number by FISH was also performed in tumor samples from 81 participants of the Southwest Oncology Group (SWOG) 0126 study, which assessed the role of gefitinib in bronchioloalveolar carcinoma and adenocarcinoma with bronchioloalveolar features. In this study, FISH-positive patients had about 50% reduction in the risk of death as compared with FISH-negative patients.[41] Data evaluating FISH in the ISEL trial are based on a subset of 370 patients, representing the largest evaluation of this biomarker in the study of EGFR TKIs in advanced NSCLC, and favor *EGFR* gene–copy number assessment by FISH as a clinically useful predictor of treatment benefit from gefitinib versus placebo.[42] The response rate in FISH-positive patients was 16% as compared with 3% in FISH-negative patients, and the median survival was almost doubled (8.3 in gefitinib treated FISH-positive patients vs. 4.5 months in FISH-positive patients treated with placebo, corresponding to an HR of 0.61). Patients with high *EGFR* copy number treated with placebo had slightly inferior survival when compared with patients with low *EGFR* gene copy number (4.5 vs. 6.2 months, respectively), indicating that increased *EGFR* gene copy number by FISH is purely predictive for the benefit from EGFR TKI and not a prognostic indicator. The lack of prognostic value of EGFR FISH is also supported by the results of *EGFR* gene copy number assessment from surgically treated NSCLC patients,[38] and in NSCLC patients treated with chemotherapy alone.[43] Molecular analysis of tumor samples from the BR.21 trial was performed using FISH according to the same criteria, although at a different institution. Although FISH result could be obtained only in 125 out of 221 samples (57%), the subset of FISH-positive patients achieved significant treatment benefit from erlotinib (20% response rate and an HR of 0.44), whereas this benefit was modest in FISH-negative patients (2% response rate and an HR of 0.85).[44]

Although the ISEL study and the BR.21 studies both compared EGFR TKI with placebo, randomized studies comparing EGFR TKIs with standard chemotherapy in the second-line setting were presented. The largest of these studies was the INTEREST study, which compared gefitinib with docetaxel as second-line treatment.[19] The trial included more than 1400 patients, and the results met the primary end point of noninferiority in the overall survival between the two arms. EGFR FISH analysis was included as a clinical end point; however, EGFR FISH results were available only for 26% of overall study population. No difference in outcome was seen between the FISH-positive and -negative patients between the treatment arms. Based on the previous published retrospective data, it would be expected that the EGFR FISH–positive patients would perform better with gefitinib as compared with docetaxel. One reason for the lack of expected result in the FISH-positive patients is that this particular subset of patients has a poor prognosis without any systemic therapy, which has been reported by our group,[38] and that this poor overall survival would be improved by chemotherapy per se. Although, the same classification for EGFR FISH assessment was used in the INTEREST study as in previous studies technical differences from one laboratory to another cannot be ruled out on this stage.

Association between EGFR FISH and Outcome with EGFR TKIs as First-Line Therapy EGFR TKIs have been studied in combination with standard chemotherapy as first-line treatment in patients with advanced NSCLC (outlined in the introduction). Neither of the four studies could demonstrate any survival advantage of adding a EGFR TKI to standard chemotherapy. EGFR FISH analysis has only been performed in the TRIBUTE study, and preliminary data have been presented.[45] Although no difference in the overall population could be demonstrated, the FISH-positive patients had a statistically significant longer PFS compared with the FISH-negative patients. Interestingly, this difference in PFS emerged after 6 months, which is the time when the patients stopped chemotherapy and continued with erlotinib alone. Furthermore, a lower response rate was seen in the EGFR FISH–positive group receiving chemotherapy and erlotinib as compared with those receiving chemotherapy and placebo (11.6% vs. 29.8%; $p = 0.495$). The immediate interpretation of these results and the raised hypothesis are that during the treatment with the combination of chemotherapy and EGFR TKI, the agents are acting antagonistic. This hypothesis remains in agreement with observation previously raised by the investigators from the University of California at Davis.[46] An EGFR-TKI therapy results in a G1-phase cell-cycle arrest and makes the activity of the G2/M phase-specific chemotherapy suboptimal. Based on this hypothesis, a pharmacodynamic separation between the chemotherapy and the EGFR TKI would be more optimal and this hypothesis is today studied in prospective clinical trials.[47]

Data from three phase II clinical studies were recently presented with EGFR FISH as a predictive marker for gefitinib monotherapy in chemonaive patients. In the INSTEP study, 201 chemonaive NSCLC patients with poor performance status (PS 2 to 3) were randomized to gefitinib versus placebo.[48] Consistently with previous observations, a subset analysis from patients with available tumor biopsies demonstrated that FISH-positive patients had an HR = 0.44 for survival compared with HR = 1.02 in the FISH-negative patient category. In the INVITE study, 196 chemonaive NSCLC patients ≥70 years old were randomized to gefitinib versus vinorelbine. In this trial, the HR for PFS in the FISH-positive patients was 3.13 compared with 0.93 in the FISH-negative category.[49] These results, together with the results of previously discussed INTERST trial,[19] indicate that EGFR FISH does not appear to predict who should be treated with EGFR TKIs versus who should be treated with chemotherapy, either in the first- or second-line setting. More data on this important issue are urgently needed.

Gefitinib was also tested in a phase II clinical trial (ONCOBELL Study) involving 42 untreated NSCLC patients with at least two of the following criteria: never-smoking history, EGFR FISH positivity, or phospho-Akt positivity by immunohistochemistry.[50] Patients who were EGFR FISH positive had higher response rate (68% vs. 9%), longer median time-to-progression (7.6 vs. 2.7 months), and a trend to longer survival as compared with EGFR FISH–negative patients. Although these results are encouraging, small patient numbers, multiple selection criteria, and lack of control group do not allow us to assess predictive value of EGFR FISH based on this trial.

Association between EGFR FISH and Outcome with Anti-EGFR Monoclonal Antibodies Although most of the studies performed in NSCLC patients with EGFR antagonists utilized orally available small molecule TKI, anti-EGFR monoclonal antibodies have shown promising results in phase II trials,[51–54] but no definitive predictive marker for outcome and selection of patients has so far been identified. Several new compounds are currently actively investigated, but most clinical data available are for cetuximab. SWOG recently presented preliminary results from the phase II study 0342, in which the patients were randomized in between chemotherapy and cetuximab given either concomitantly or sequentially. EGFR FISH analysis was done in biopsies from the subset of patients who participated in this study. A doubling of PFS from 3 to 6 months and of median overall survival from 7 to 15 months was seen for FISH-negative and -positive patients, respectively.[51] Thus, these data indicate that EGFR FISH might also be strongly associated with outcome after the cetuximab therapy. Interestingly, the best outcome in the FISH-positive patients was seen in the concurrent arm with a median survival of 16 months compared with 7 months in the FISH-negative group. Thus, the concurrent therapy with monoclonal antibody and chemotherapy seems to give the expected synergistic effect in the FISH-positive patients, in contrast to the combination of chemotherapy and EGFR TKIs, where antagonistic effect is observed.

Two large prospective randomized studies with cetuximab in patients with advanced NSCLC have just been reported. The BMS 099 study comparing carbotaxel/cisplatin with or without cetuximab was performed in unselected NSCLC patients and did not meet the primary end point of superiority in overall survival in the experimental arm.[14] The other study, the FLEX trial (first-line treatment for patients with EGFR-expressing advanced NSCLC), compared cisplatin/vinorelbine with and without cetuximab in EGFR immunohistochemistry–positive patients. The results from the latter study showed significantly better survival by adding cetuximab.[13] In light of contradictory results of two studies described previously, selection of patients for cetuximab therapy based on molecular criteria seems to be crucial. Studies with other anti-EGFR antibodies in NSCLC have not reported on EGFR FISH status.[55,56]

Prognostic Association of EGFR Gene Copy Number in NSCLC The predictive value of EGFR gene copy number for outcome to EGFR inhibitors cannot be determined without knowledge about the prognostic association independent of any therapy. Unfortunately, very few studies have addressed this question. Hirsch et al.,[38] studied tumors from about 200 surgically resected NSCLC patients and found a tendency, but not statistically significant, shorter survival for patients with tumors being EGFR FISH positive compared with the patients with EGFR FISH tumors.[38] Thus, similar to several publications showing an unfavorable prognosis associated to increased EGFR protein expression by IHC, increased EGFR gene copy number seems to be associated with an unfavorable prognosis without treatment with EGFR inhibitors, but data are not conclusive.

For advanced NSCLC patients treated with chemotherapy alone, no difference in outcome were observed between EGFR FISH+ and FISH patients.[43]

Ongoing Prospective Studies Validating EGFR FISH as a Predictive Marker for EGFR Inhibitors in NSCLC To prospectively validate EGFR gene copy number detected by FISH as a predictive marker for EGFR inhibitors in NSCLC, several prospective studies have been launched: in a U.S. Intergroup study initiated by National Cancer Institute, United States and the CPATH Institute (Critical Pathology Institute in the United States), and in collaboration with the U.S. Food and Drug Administration (FDA), a prospective randomized study for second-line therapy for advanced NSCLC comparing erlotinib with pemetrexed has been launched, in which a prospective validation of several biomarkers, but primarily EGFR FISH, is the primary goal. The study is called the MARVEL study (**MAR**ker **V**alidation of **E**GFR in **L**ung Cancer). All patients with tumor tissue available for EGFR FISH testing will be randomized to either erlotinib or pemetrexed. The study will include about 1000 patients, and the EGFR FISH assay is standardized and centralized. Two other prospective studies are also validating the role of the EGFR FISH assay. One study initiated by OSI Pharmaceuticals is a prospective randomized phase II study for advanced NSCLC patients comparing erlotinib versus chemotherapy and erlotinib in EGFR-postive patients as first-line therapy. The study has completed accrual and results from about 150 will be presented in 2009. The other study, the RADIANT study, is an adjuvant phase III study comparing erlotinib with placebo in EGFR-positive patients. The study is international and planned to include about 1200 patients.

To further validate EGFR FISH as a predictive marker for cetuximab based on the results from the SWOG 0342 study,[51] a prospective randomized phase III study is planned by the SWOG, which will compare chemotherapy (carboplatin/pclitaxel with or without bevacizumab depending on bevacizumab eligibility) with or without cetuximab in patients with advanced NSCLC. The study will include about 500 patients.

Methodological Considerations

EGFR gene copy number may be heterogeneous within different areas of the same tumor and between the primary and metastatic site, influencing the result of the FISH analysis.[58] Clinical significance of tumor heterogeneity with regard to sensitivity to EGFR TKIs is presently unknown. Other techniques of gene copy number assessment include quantitative polymerase chain reaction (qPCR) and chromogenic in situ hybridization (CISH). In the former method, copy number of the gene of interest is usually compared with that of the housekeeping gene, and expressed as a relative ratio. Direct comparison of *EGFR* gene copy number assessment by FISH and qPCR in 82 advanced NSCLC patients showed no significant association between FISH-positivity and qPCR results.[59] In this study, *EGFR* gene copy number by qPCR was not associated with outcome of gefitinib-treated patients. Molecular analysis of IDEAL (phase II) and INTACT (phase III studies comparing chemotherapy and gefitinib vs. chemotherapy and placebo) demonstrated no predictive value of *EGFR* gene amplification by qPCR for treatment outcome.[60] In a study from Japan on 66 gefitinib-treated patients, increased *EGFR* gene copy number by qPCR was linked to higher response rate and increased time to progression, but not overall survival.[61] At present, we need more definitive data to explain why the results of *EGFR* gene copy number quantification by FISH and qPCR are different with respect to its predictive value for EGFR TKI treatment benefit. Quantification of gene copy number by FISH is possible in individual tumor cells, whereas qPCR techniques assess gene copy number in a pool of cells, which may also contain inflammatory and stromal components. Tumor microdissection may help to ensure that the assessment is carried out in areas abundant in tumor cells, but this procedure significantly increases the assay cost. In qPCR technique, quantification of the reference gene copy number presents additional challenge because of the possibility of its deletion or amplification in tumor cells. CISH technique implements an enzymatic reaction to detect the DNA probe hybridized to the gene of interest. The main advantage of this technology is the use of light instead of fluorescent microscope enabling the reader to score the signals in histological sections. Data on CISH gene copy number evaluation and sensitivity to EGFR TKIs are sparse. In a group of 44 NSCLC patients treated with gefitinib or erlotinib, *EGFR* gene copy number by CISH did not associate with response rate.[62] A comparison study between CISH and FISH is currently ongoing.

In summary, retrospective studies have shown a significant survival benefit in pretreated NSCLC patients with high *EGFR* gene copy number evaluated by FISH, as demonstrated in several studies involving almost 700 patients. Several prospective clinical studies with patient selection based on FISH or combination of FISH and other biomarkers are currently underway in the adjuvant, first- and second-line setting. The value of EGFR FISH for the prediction of clinical outcome to EGFR TKIs compared with first- or second-line chemotherapy is not yet established. Ongoing large prospective adjuvant studies with EGFR TKIs (i.e., the RADIANT study) in selected patients based on EGFR expression will further shed light to the use of EGFR FISH for selection of NSCLC patients to adjuvant therapy. The association of EGFR FISH and outcome of NSCLC patients treated with chemotherapy and anti-EGFR monoclonal antibodies is compelling and will be further prospectively studied.

EGFR Protein Expression EGFR protein expression detected by IHC was initially thought to be a good predictor for response and outcome to EGFR inhibitors. However, clinical studies in NSCLC have not been able to demonstrate that IHC should be better than other measures. Some association to outcome was seen both in BR.21 study (HR = 0.68; p = 0.02) and the ISEL study with gefitinib (HR = 0.77; p = 0.13).[42,44] Most recently, however, results from the European FLEX study was presented (chemotherapy ± cetuximab as first-line therapy), which was based on EGFR IHC–positive patients as defined by one positive cell.[13] The study demonstrated superior survival for cetuximab treated patients, whereas the other similar study in the United States (BMS/Imclone 099 study) in unselected NSCLC patients did not meet the primary end point of superior PFS for cetuximab-treated patients.[14] Whether the IHC selection was crucial for the difference in outcome or other factors played a role are not yet clarified as PFS was not superior for cetuximab in the FLEX trial either.

Methodological aspects of EGFR IHC assessments are still to be solved. More specific EGFR antibodies have to be developed. Several scoring systems for EGFR IHC assessments have been applied. However, a comparison between different scoring systems and "cutoff" levels for positive and negative results did not show significant difference between the use of H-score (e.g., Hybrid score), which is defined by intensity (0 to 4) times frequency of IHC-positive cells (0% to 100%) or the more commonly used "DAKO scoring system."[63] The role of phosphorylated EGFR protein expression has been less studied because of the instability of the phosphorylated antibodies and its variability to various fixation procedures (Table 49.2).

TABLE 49.2 Epidermal Growth Factor Receptor Gene Copy Number and Sensitivity to Epidermal Growth Factor Receptor Tyrosine Kinase Inhibitors in Non–Small Cell Lung Cancer

Study	Number of Patients	Drug (Dose)	Method of Gene Copy Number Evaluation (Cutpoint)	Proportion Positive	Response Rates: Positive vs. Negative	Survival Hazard Ratio (95% CI)
Cappuzzo et al.[40]	102	Gefitinib (250 mg)	FISH (high polysomy and gene amplification)	32.3%	36% vs. 3%	0.44* (0.23–0.82)
Hirsch et al.[41] - SWOG 0126	81	Gefitinib (500 mg)	FISH (high polysomy and gene amplification)	32.0%	26% vs. 11%	0.50*¶ (0.25–0.97)
Tsao et al.[44] - BR.21	125	Erlotinib (150 mg) vs. placebo	FISH (high polysomy and gene amplification)	45%	20% vs. 2%	0.44‡ (0.23–0.82)
Hirsch et al.[42] - ISEL	370	Gefitinib (250 mg) vs. placebo	FISH (high polysomy and gene amplification)	30.8%	16.4% vs. 3%	0.61‡ (0.36–1.04)
Douillard et al.[19] - INTEREST	374	Gefitinib (250 mg) vs. docetaxel	FISH (high polysomy and gene amplification)	47%	13.0% vs. 7.4%ll	1.09§ (0.78–1.51)
Crino et al.[49] - INVITE	158	Gefitinib (250 mg) vs. vinorelbine	FISH (high polysomy and gene amplification)	34%	NR	2.88§ (1.21–6.83)
Goss et al.[48] - INSTEP	84	Gefitinib (250 mg) vs. placebo	FISH (high polysomy and gene amplification)	38%	NR	0.44‡ (0.17–1.12)
Bell et al.[60]		Gefitinib (250 and 500 mg)	Quantitative PCR (>4)			
- IDEAL	90			8%	29% vs. 15%	NR
- INTACT	453			7%	56% vs. 53%†	2.03‡ (0.67–6.13)
Dziadziuszko et al.[59]	82	Gefitinib (250 mg)	Quantitative PCR (> median)	51%	12% vs. 10%	1.04* (0.61–1.76)
Takano et al.[61]	66	Gefitinib (250 mg)	Quantitative PCR (≥3)	44%	72% vs. 38%	0.80* (0.42–1.50)

*Comparison between patients with high versus low *EGFR* gene copy number.

†Comparison between patients receiving chemotherapy and gefitinib versus chemotherapy and placebo.

‡Comparison between EGFR tyrosine kinase inhibitor versus placebo in patients with high *EGFR* gene copy number.

§Comparison between EGFR tyrosine kinase inhibitor versus chemotherapy in patients with high *EGFR* gene copy number.

llResponse rates to gefitinib versus placebo in patients with high *EGFR* gene copy number.

¶Hazard ratio was recalculated from original publication for consistency in the table.

CI, confidence interval; FISH, fluorescence in situ hybridization; IDEAL, Iressa Dose Evaluation in Advanced Lung Cancer; INSTEP, Iressa NSCLC Trial Evaluating Poor Performance Patients; INTACT, Iressa NSCLC Trial Assessing Combination Treatment; INTEREST, Iressa Non–small cell lung cancer Trial Evaluating REsponse and Survival against Taxotere; INVITE, Iressa in NSCLC vs. Vinorelbine Investigation in The Elderly; ISEL, Iressa Survival Evaluation in Lung Cancer; NR, not reported; PCR, polymerase chain reaction; SWOG, Southwest Oncology Group.

EGFR MUTATIONS IN NSCLC

Identification of EGFR Mutations

The phase II and III clinical studies of EGFR TKIs gefitinib and erlotinib demonstrate that the patients who are most likely to achieve radiographic responses included women, those with adenocarcinoma, never-smokers, and patients from Japan.[4,6,15] These clinical observations and the dramatic nature of occasional clinical responses to gefitinib led several investigators to sequence *EGFR* from patient's tumors and led to the identification of somatic *EGFR* activating mutations.[64–66] The initial descriptions of the correlation of *EGFR* mutations with response to gefitinib examined a series of 14 patients who had dramatic clinical and/or radiographic responses to gefitinib.[64,65] A total of 13 out of the 14 patients had *EGFR* mutations, whereas none of the 11 patients who progressed on gefitinib treatment had mutations. The association between *EGFR* mutations and clinical response to gefitinib and erlotinib was subsequently been documented around the world. Soon after the initial studies, reports from other institutions in the United States, Japan, Taiwan, and Korea have confirmed that more than 70 of the 87 patients (80%) with clinical responses to gefitinib and erlotinib had detectable somatic mutations of *EGFR*.[64–70]

Somatic mutations in *EGFR* are found in 10% to 15% of whites and in 30% to 40% of Asian NSCLC patients. *EGFR* mutations are present more frequently in never-smokers, women, those with adenocarcinoma, and in patients of East Asian ethnicity.[71] These are the clinical features of patients previously identified as most likely to benefit from gefitinib or erlotinib.[4,6,17] The reason behind the ethnic variation in *EGFR* mutation frequency is currently not understood. It is estimated that up to 20,000 to 25,000 of newly diagnosed NSCLCs in the United States will harbor *EGFR*-activating mutations. As lung cancer is such a common disease, there are more *EGFR* mutant NSCLC patients diagnosed annually in the United States than those with chronic myeloid leukemia (CML) and gastrointestinal stromal tumors (GISTs) combined.[72] Only one familial report of inherited *EGFR* mutations has so far been described.[73] Members of this family possessed a germline mutation in *EGFR* (EGFR T790M), associated with resistance to gefitinib and erlotinib, and were predisposed to the development of lung cancers.[73] Interestingly, the actual lung cancers in these patients also contained an *EGFR*-activating mutation in addition to *EGFR* T790M.

Clinically significant *EGFR* mutations are found in the first four exons[40,61,75,76] of the tyrosine kinase domain of EGFR. The mutations reported thus far have been predominantly of two types: ~45% are deletions involving at least 12 nucleotides in exon 19, eliminating a conserved LRE motif, and ~40% are a single-point mutation in exon 21 (L858R) (Fig. 49.1). In addition, rare point mutations in exons 18, 20, and 21 and insertion/duplications in exon 20 have been reported.[40,64,66,68,71,74] The common exon 19 deletions and L858R are also the ones that have been most extensively evaluated to date and are most closely linked to in vitro and in vivo sensitivity to gefitinib and erlotinib.

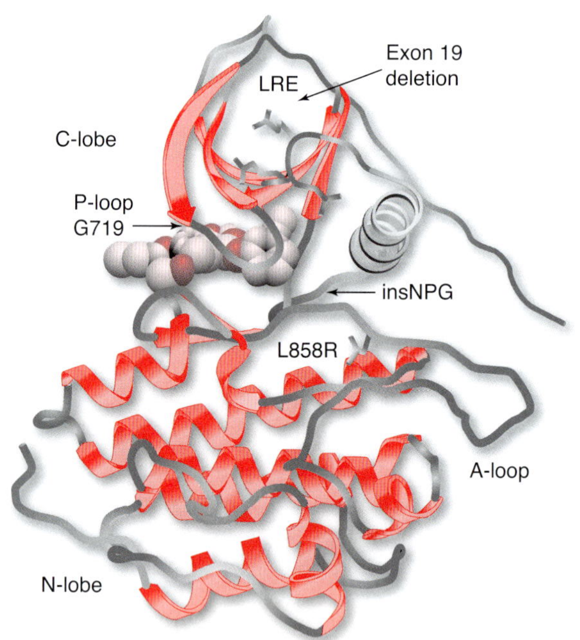

FIGURE 49.1 Schematic representation of EGFR with gefitinib bound to the ATP-binding pocket. The locations of the common exon 19 (deletion mutations) and 21 (L858R) are demonstrated. *insNPG*, insertion asparagine proline glycine; *LRE*, leucine-arginine-glutamic acid. (Courtesy of Dr. Michael Eck, Dana Farber, Cancer Institute, Boston, MA.)

EGFR-mutant tumors also often contain a concurrent increase in *EGFR* copy number.[40,61,75,76] Several studies to date suggest that in these cancers, there is preferential amplification of the *EGFR* mutation containing allele.[75,77] The clinical and biologic significance of the impact of a concurrent copy number gain is currently not well defined. Additional studies are needed to further define whether there are any clinical differences in *EGFR*-mutant lung cancers compared with those without a concurrent *EGFR* copy number gain. Furthermore, the relationship between a concurrent copy number gain and the specific subtype of an *EGFR* mutation (exon 19 deletion or L858R) has not been determined.

EGFR Mutations versus Clinical Factors

As discussed previously, adenocarcinoma histology, smoking history, and female gender are a good predictor of response as well as survival for patients treated with EGFR TKIs. Are patient clinical characteristics just as good in predicting the response to EGFR TKIs as knowing the *EGFR* mutation status? To address these matters, investigators from three institutions in Japan established a large-scale database and evaluated the factors that were related to clinical outcome of lung adenocarcinoma patients treated with gefitinib.[78] In 408 Japanese patients treated with gefitinib, 362 were adenocarcinoma, 200 were men and 170 were never-smokers. Survival curves according to gender and *EGFR* mutation (Fig. 49.2A), or smoking status and *EGFR* mutation (Fig. 49.2B) are shown.[78] It is clear that *EGFR* mutation is far superior to gender or smoking status

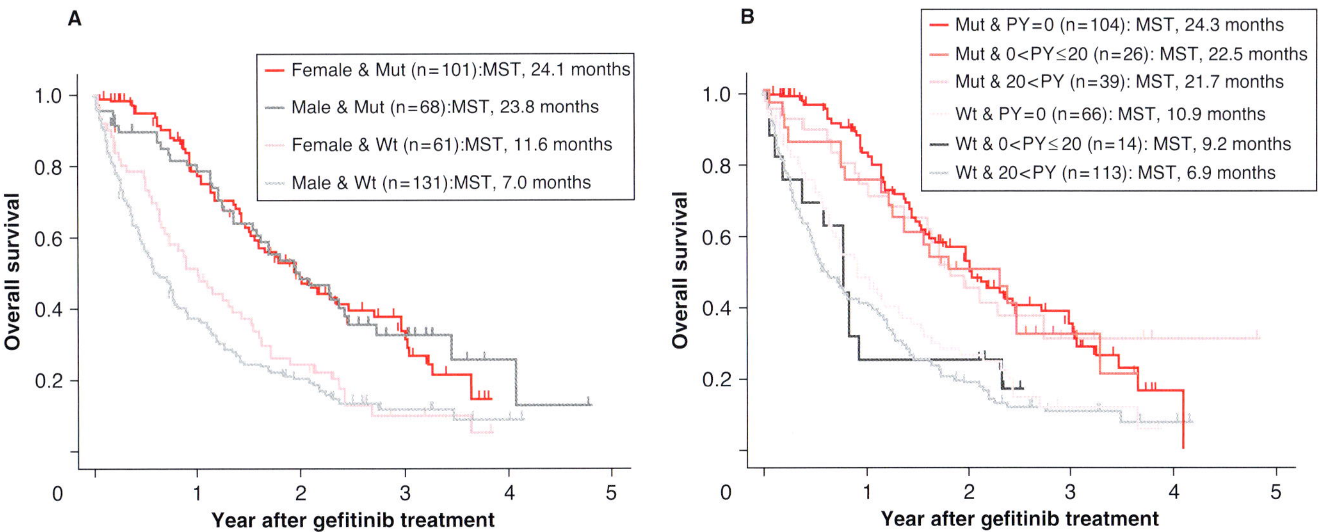

FIGURE 49.2 Survival curves of patients who were treated with gefitinib according to gender and *EGFR* mutational status **(A)** and according to smoking history and *EGFR* mutational status **(B)**. *MST*, median survival time; *Mut*, EGFR mutation positive; *PY*, pack year; *Wt*, EGFR wild-type. (From Toyooka S, Takano T, Kosaka T, et al. Epidermal growth factor receptor mutation, but not sex and smoking, is independently associated with favorable prognosis of gefitinib-treated patients with lung adenocarcinoma. *Cancer Sci* 2008;99:303–308.)

for predicting longer survival. Multivariate analysis revealed that EGFR mutation was the only significant prognostic factor (HR = 0.48; $p < 0.001$), but female gender (HR = 1.0; $p = 0.98$) and smoking status (HR = 0.81 for light smoker to heavy smoker, HR = 0.33 for never-smokers to heavy smokers, p for trend = 0.61).[78] These findings would suggest that genotype rather than phenotype is a better marker of benefit from EGFR TKIs.

The Biology of EGFR Mutations

Mutant *EGFR* is a bona fide oncogene. Mutant *EGFR* causes transformation and anchorage independent growth of NIH-3T3 cells in soft agar.[79] This occurs in a ligand-independent process, whereas wild-type *EGFR* is not transforming in the absence of ligand.[79] Similarly, *EGFR* mutations lead to interleukin 3 (IL-3) independent growth of Ba/F3 cells.[80] Furthermore, mutant *EGFR* alone is sufficient to lead to the development lung adenocarcinomas when expressed in the alveolar epithelium of mice.[81,82]

Several *EGFR*-mutant NSCLC cell lines harboring the common *EGFR* mutations found in NSCLC patients have also been identified and extensively characterized.[75,83,84] Laboratory-based studies using these cell lines as well as model systems harboring *EGFR* mutations have been invaluable to the understanding of the differences in EGFR signaling in *EGFR*-mutant compared with wild-type cancers. *EGFR*-mutant tumors are dependent or "addicted" to EGFR signaling for their growth and survival.[83,85,86] Studies to date suggest that, in these cancers, several (if not all) of the critical downstream signaling pathways including the PI3K/AKT, STAT, and ERK 1/2 pathways are solely controlled by EGFR. Thus, when these tumors are exposed to EGFR inhibitors, these intracellular pathways are turned off, and the cancer cells undergo apoptosis.[75,83–85] In contrast, EGFR does not singularly regulate these pathways in most other lung cancers, including in most *EGFR* wild-type lung cancer cell lines, and in such cancers, EGFR inhibitors are marginally, if at all, effective.

The PI3K/Akt-signaling pathway is the most critical of the downstream signaling pathways for the efficacy of EGFR kinase inhibitors. PI3K/Akt signaling must be turned off in order for gefitinib or erlotinib to be effective in an *EGFR*-mutant cancer. In fact, ectopic activation of PI3K/Akt signaling *alone* is sufficient to render resistance to gefitinib in vitro.[87] The detailed molecular events that lead to activation of EGFR and downstream signaling, including PI3K/Akt signaling, are beginning to be understood. EGFR is one of a family of four ERBB family members, and two other family members, HER-2 and ERBB3, are highly implicated in promoting EGFR activation of downstream signaling. ERBB3 is a unique member of this family in that is believed to be "kinase dead" (Fig. 49.3A). However, upon heterodimerization with other ERBB family members, it is phosphorylated on tyrosines and serves as a scaffold to activate downstream signaling. In lung cancers that are sensitive to EGFR inhibitors, PI3K/AKT is activated by binding to phosphorylated ERBB3.[34] In contrast, cancers that are not sensitive to EGFR inhibitors primarily use non-ERBB3 mechanisms for activating PI3K.[88] There are now several studies reporting a correlation between gefitinib sensitivity and ERBB3 expression in NSCLC cell lines and at least one clinical study that identified ERBB3 expression as a predictor of clinical benefit from EGFR inhibitors.[75,88–90]

There are two main reasons why gefitinib and erlotinib are effective therapies against *EGFR*-mutant cancers. The first, as discussed previously, is a biologic dependence or addiction to EGFR signaling in *EGFR*-mutant cancers.[86] The second is a

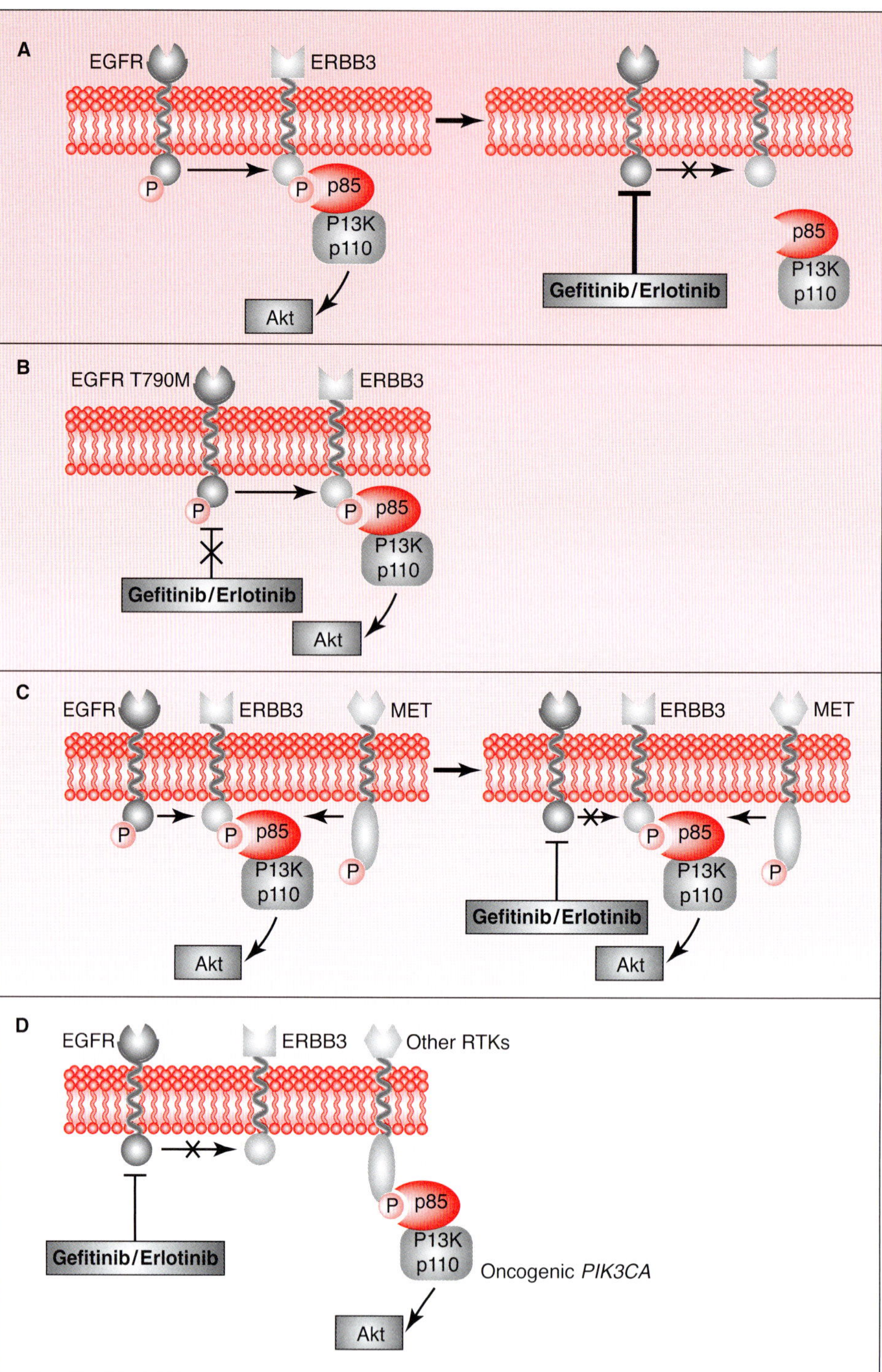

FIGURE 49.3 EGFR signaling in gefitinib/erlotinib sensitive and resistant EGFR-mutant NSCLCs. **A:** EGFR phosphorylates ERBB3 to activate PI3K/Akt signaling in gefitinib-/erlotinib-sensitive NSCLCs. In such cancers, following gefitinib/erlotinib treatment, EGFR, ERBB3 and Akt phosphorylation are turned off. **B:** Gefitinib and erlotinib are unable to inhibit EGFR phosphorylation in the presence of *EGFR* T790M. EGFR signaling persists in the presence of gefitinib/erlotinib leading to persistent ERBB3 and Akt phosphorylation. **C:** MET can also activate PI3K/Akt signaling through ERBB3. In NSCLCs with *MET* amplification, gefitinib/erlotinib can still inhibit EGFR phosphorylation but not ERBB3 phosphorylation. This leads to persistent activation of PI3K/Akt signaling via ERBB3 in an EGFR-independent manner. **D:** Other potential mechanisms of gefitinib/erlotinib resistance. These potential mechanisms include alternative ways of maintaining PI3K/Akt signaling such as by an oncogenic *PIK3CA* or by other receptor tyrosine kinases that could activate PI3K/Akt signaling in an ERBB3 independent fashion. In such cancers, gefitinib/erlotinib would be expected to inhibit EGFR and ERBB3 phosphorylation but not Akt phosphorylation. *AKT*, AKT8 virus oncogene homologue; *EGFR*, epidermal growth factor receptor; *ERBB3*, v-erb-b2 erythroblastic leukemia viral oncogene homologue 3; *MET*, mesenchymal-epidermal transection factor; *PI3K*, phosphatidylinositol 3 kinase. (Adapted from Arteaga CL. HER3 and mutant EGFR meet MET. *Nat Med* 2007;13:675–677, copyright 2007, Macmillan Publishers.)

pharmacologic advantage that occurs in the context of an *EGFR* mutation. The wild-type EGFR can adopt an inactive or an active conformation (when ligand activated). *EGFR* mutations promote the formation of the active conformation, and gefitinib and erlotinib preferentially bind the active conformation of EGFR.[91] The affinity of gefitinib for the mutant EGFR is ~30 times greater than for a wild-type EGFR.[91] Consequently, in *EGFR*-mutant cell line models, 10 to 100 times less gefitinib or erlotinib is required to completely inhibit phosphorylation of EGFR and downstream Akt and ERK 1/2 than is required to inhibit NSCLC cell lines with wild-type *EGFR*.[64,75,83]

EGFR Mutations and Relationship to Cigarette Smoking The initial clinical observations suggested that gefitinib and erlotinib had their greatest effect in never-smokers with NSCLC.[6] The subsequent molecular studies demonstrated that *EGFR* mutations were more frequent in never-smokers with NSCLC.[71,92–94] The highest frequencies of

EGFR mutations are found in both Asian (~60% to 70%) and white (30% to 50%) never-smokers,[71,92–94] with increasing cigarette smoke exposure, the frequency of an *EGFR*-mutant lung cancer decreases. However, some ethnic differences have also emerged. Even in never-smokers, the EGFR mutation frequency is significantly higher in Asian lung cancer patients compared with white lung cancer patients. Similarly, in white current smokers, the *EGFR* mutation frequency is <5%, whereas in Japanese patients, it is 22%.[92,93] Collectively, these findings raise the possibility that etiologies other than cigarette smoke are responsible for the genesis of *EGFR* mutant NSCLC. The apparent negative correlation between incidence of EGFR mutation and smoking dosage is a result of diluting the number of tumors with EGFR mutations with an increased number of tumors with wild-type EGFR as smoking dose increases. Indeed, this was suggested in our recent case-control study.[94] It will be critical to determine the other potential causes of NSCLC in never-smokers and their relationship to *EGFR* mutations as that may lead to the identification of another (in addition to smoking) preventable cause of lung cancer. Furthermore, as mentioned previously in this chapter, given that not all never-smokers with NSCLC, especially white patients, harbor *EGFR* mutations, assessment of smoking status alone may not be an adequate surrogate for clinical benefit from gefitinib or erlotinib.

EGFR-Targeted Agents and Their Efficacy in EGFR-Mutant Cancers Many EGFR-targeted agents have been developed, and several of them have been evaluated preclinically or clinically in *EGFR*-mutant cancers. The EGFR-targeted agents fall into several major categories (Table 49.3). Gefitinib and erlotinib are examples of reversible ATP mimetics and compete for ATP binding in the EGFR kinase domain. Irreversible EGFR inhibitors are similar in that they are also ATP mimetics but in addition covalently bind Cys-797 of EGFR. Many of these agents are also effective inhibitors of ERBB2 and ERBB4.[95–97] There are also now several multitargeted EGFR kinase inhibitors that have a broader spectrum of activity not solely against EGFR but against other kinases outside the ERBB family (Table 49.3). Several EGFR-targeted antibodies have also been developed and either interfere with ligand binding to EGFR (cetuximab and panitumumab) or effect EGFR dimerization (matuzumab).[98]

TABLE 49.3 Summary of Different Classes of EGFR Inhibitors

Reversible Inhibitor	Irreversible Inhibitor	Multitargeted Inhibitor	Antibody
Gefitinib	CI-1033	Vandetanib	Cetuximab
Erlotinib	EKB-569	XL647	Panitumumab
Lapatinib	HKI-272	BMS-690514	Matuzumab
	CI-387,785		
	PF00299804		
	BIBW2992		
	AV412		

Gefitinib and erlotinib are most effective against the common EGFR exon 19 deletion and L858R mutant forms for the receptor.[75,83,84] This has been extensively studied in vitro and clinically in NSCLC patients. However, they are not effective against all types of *EGFR*-activating mutations. One example is the exon 20 insertion mutations that make up 2% to 3% of all EGFR mutations.[71] Although these are *EGFR*-activating mutations, they confer resistance to gefitinib and erlotinib in preclinical models and in NSCLC patients.[50,79,99] Lapatinib, which is a better ERBB2 inhibitor than gefitinib or erlotinib, also inhibits EGFR. However, it appears to be less effective against mutant EGFR likely because unlike gefitinib or erlotinib, it binds the inactive conformation of EGFR.[91,100] The irreversible EGFR inhibitors are, in general, more effective than gefitinib or erlotinib against all classes of *EGFR*-activating mutations.[95,96,101] However, some specific differences have also emerged in vitro. HKI-272, BIWB2992, and PF00299804 are all more effective against EGFR L858R than gefitinib or erlotinib. Similarly, BIBW2992 and PF00299804 also more effectively inhibit the growth of models harboring EGFR exon 19 deletions.[95,96,101] However, HKI-272 is less effective in vitro against many of the exon 19 deletion variants than erlotinib. Whether these in vitro differences will ultimately translate into clinical differences remains to be determined. All of the irreversible EGFR inhibitors tested to date effectively inhibit the growth and EGFR phosphorylation of cell line models harboring the exon 20 insertion mutations.[95,96,101] Thus, these agents may also be clinically effective in NSCLC patients harboring EGFR exon 20 insertion mutations. In addition to inhibiting EGFR, the irreversible EGFR inhibitors are effective against lung cancer models harboring either amplification or somatic mutations in ERBB2.[95,97] These genomic alterations are detected in 2% to 5% of NSCLC patients and irreversible EGFR inhibitors may be effective therapies in this patient population.[102,103]

The multitargeted EGFR inhibitors have also been evaluated in some *EGFR*-mutant models. As vandetanib, XL647, and BMS-690514 inhibit VEGR2, the full potential of these agents is difficult to evaluate in vitro.[104,105] In vitro, these agents appear to have similar effects on models harboring *EGFR*-activating mutations as gefitinib or erlotinib.[104,105] In contrast, the EGFR-directed antibodies may be less effective against *EGFR*-mutant cancers. Cetuximab has been most extensively evaluated in models harboring *EGFR* mutations. Cetuximab has several potential effects in *EGFR*-mutant cancers. First, it can bind the ligand-binding site of EGFR. Second, it can lead to internalization or degradation of EGFR. In vitro, cetuximab is less effective at inhibiting the growth of NSCLC cell lines harboring *EGFR* mutations than gefitinib.[84] This is a result of the inability to turn off EGFR phosphorylation. In both xenograft and transgenic mouse models, cetuximab has been found to be effective against some models with *EGFR*-activating mutations. In these models, cetuximab leads to degradation of EGFR, and hence to tumor shrinkage, because these cancers are EGFR dependent.[81,106,107] However, as discussed later, the limited experience to date suggests that cetuximab is not effective in NSCLC patients harboring EGFR mutations.[84]

EGFR Mutations, Prognosis, and the Clinical Efficacy of EGFR-Targeted Therapies

Prognostic Significance In addition to being a predictive marker of efficacy of EGFR kinase inhibitors, *EGFR* mutations also confer some prognostic significance. That is, NSCLC patients whose cancers harbor an *EGFR* mutations likely have a better prognosis independent of EGFR inhibitor therapy. This has been examined both in surgically resected NSCLC patients as well as those with advanced NSCLC. The prognostic role of *EGFR* mutations is mixed when it has been examined in surgically resected tumor specimens. Some studies suggest that patients with *EGFR* mutations have a better outcome, whereas others suggest that it is similar to those whose tumors are *EGFR* wild-type.[71,108,109] However, many are limited by small patient numbers and future studies may be difficult to interpret as many patients would ultimately go on to receive EGFR inhibitor–based therapies. The impact of *EGFR* mutations in advanced NSCLC has been studied including in randomized phase III clinical trials.[44,60,110,111] In the phase III BR.21 trial of erlotinib compared with placebo, patients in the placebo arm with *EGFR* mutations had a longer median survival (9.1 vs. 3.5 months) than *EGFR* wild-type patients.[44] The prognostic role of EGFR mutations was also examined in the phase III clinical trials of chemotherapy with or without gefitinib (INTACT-1 and INTACT-2) or erlotinib (TRIBUTE).[12,60] In the INTACT-1 and -2 studies, NSCLC patients mutations had a better outcome when treated with chemotherapy-alone compared with *EGFR* wild-type patients (19.4 vs. 9.2 months; HR = 0.48; 95% CI, 0.29 to 0.82). In the TRIBUTE trial, the median survival of *EGFR* wild-type patients treated with chemotherapy alone was approximately 10 months, whereas it had not been reached (>15 months) for *EGFR*-mutant patients at the time of the analysis.[111] When the treatment arms (chemotherapy alone or with erlotinib) were combined, the median survival of patients that were *EGFR* wild-type was 10 months and had not been reached in patients with *EGFR* mutations ($p < 0.001$). Together, these studies suggest that in addition to conferring a predictive role, sensitivity to EGFR kinase inhibitors, *EGFR* mutations also confer a prognostic role. This needs to be considered in the design and interpretation of end points in clinical studies involving patients with known *EGFR* mutations or populations of patients known to harbor a high frequency of *EGFR* mutations such as East Asian NSCLC patients.

Detection of EGFR Mutations The initial studies that identified *EGFR* mutations used direct sequencing of EGFR exons 18 to 24 from patients' tumor specimens.[64–66] These studies were feasible only in a limited number of patients, because only a limited number of patients with advanced NSCLC have sufficiently sized tumor specimens available for direct DNA sequencing. Many patients with advanced NSCLC are diagnosed by bronchoscopy or by a fine needle aspirate. These methods are sufficient for the diagnosis of lung cancer but are often too small to be used for molecular diagnostic studies. This limitation has prompted the development of alternative nonsequencing-based mutation detection methods. Such methods include, variations of allele-specific PCR, a DNA heteroduplex analysis combined with a DNA endonuclease (Surveyor), and mass spectrometry.[112–118] Many of these methods have been examined in clinical settings or validated against direct DNA sequencing–based methods. An additional advantage of such methods is that they do not require microdissection or macrodissection of tumor material (which is often needed for DNA sequencing), and they are often more sensitive than direct DNA sequencing.[119] In addition to tumor-based studies, several investigators have pursued noninvasive genotyping methods using either tumor-derived DNA isolated from plasma or circulating tumor cells.[119–121] These techniques also hold the promise of being able to in a noninvasive manner sample the tumor multiple times during the course of a patient's treatment.

Prospective Phase II Trials of EGFR Inhibitors in EGFR-Mutant NSCLC The observations linking the sensitivity of *EGFR* mutations with EGFR kinase inhibitors were from retrospective studies of patients treated with either gefitinib or erlotinib.[64–66] Several prospective phase II clinical trials have been initiated and have now been published or presented (Table 49.4). These trials have all patients screened for the presence or absence of an *EGFR* mutation and then treated only the *EGFR*-mutant patients, either those that are chemotherapy naive or those that have failed one prior systemic therapy, with either gefitinib or erlotinib. The collective findings from these trials is remarkably similar (Table 49.4). The radiographic response rates range from 55% to 82% and the median times to progression from 8.9 to 13.3 months. These findings are substantially different than what is usually observed with cytotoxic chemotherapy and has prompted the initiation of randomized phase III clinical trials.[122] Furthermore, even though Asian lung cancer patients have a significantly higher frequency of *EGFR* mutations, the outcome of Asian lung cancer patients with *EGFR* mutations is also similar to white lung cancer patients with *EGFR* mutations. These findings suggest that it is the presence of the *EGFR* mutation, not ethnicity, that is the key determinant of the efficacy of EGFR kinase inhibitors.

There are no prospective clinical trials of second-generation EGFR inhibitors or of the multitargeted EGFR inhibitors in patients with *EGFR* mutations. Many such trials are currently underway. The relationship of EGFR mutations and cetuximab has also been examined. Only on phase II clinical trial of single-agent cetuximab has been

TABLE 49.4 Summary of Prospective Phase II Clinical Trials of Gefitinib or Erlotinib in NSCLC Patients with *EGFR* Mutations

Shown are the countries where the trial was performed, the number of patients screened, the number of *EGFR* mutant patients treated, the agent used in the study, and the clinical outcome.

Author	Country	Patients Screened	EGFR Mutants	Agent	Response Rate	TTP
Chemotherapy naive						
Inoue et al.[149]	Japan	99	16	Gefitinib	75%	9.7 months
Paz-Ares et al.[126]	Spain	1047	43	Erlotinib	82%	13.3 months
Tamura et al.[150]	Japan	118	32	Gefitinib	75%	11.5 months
Asahina et al.[151]	Japan	8ç2	16	Gefitinib	75%	8.9 months
Sequist et al.[124]	United States	98	31	Gefitinib	55%	11.4 months
Second-line therapy						
Sutani et al.[152]	Japan	107	23	Gefitinib	74%	9.4 months

EGFR, epidermal growth factor receptor; TTP, time to progression.

conducted.[123] In this clinical trial, the radiographic response rate was 4.5%.[123] Tumor analysis of the responding patients demonstrated that they were all *EGFR* wild-type. Some of the patients with either stable disease or progressive disease had *EGFR* mutations.[123] In addition, a small case series examined *EGFR*-mutant NSCLC patients treated sequentially with single-agent cetuximab and gefitinib.[84] Although cetuximab treatment led to stable disease, all of the patients achieved a partial response when treated with gefitinib. Collectively, these studies suggest that at least as a single agent, cetuximab has limited if any clinical efficacy in *EGFR* mutant NSCLC.

Ongoing and Completed Phase III Clinical Trials

The impressive findings from the prospective phase II clinical trials of treating EGFR mutant NSCLC patients with EGFR TKIs has prompted the initiation of several randomized clinical trials. These trials are either comparing the efficacy of an EGFR TKI with chemotherapy or the addition of chemotherapy to an EGFR TKI. Three phase III clinical trials are evaluating the efficacy of an EGFR TKI compared with chemotherapy. The first, IPASS (Iressa Pan-Asian Study), randomized 1217 chemotherapy-naive lung cancer patients to either gefitinib or carboplatin/paclitaxel. The eligibility for this Asian trial required the patients to be either never (<100 cigarettes/lifetime) or former (quit at least 15 years) light (≤10 pack-years) cigarette smokers with adenocarcinoma. The median age of these patients was younger[57] than that seen in the West, and included 79% women, and 94% never-smokers. Thirty-six percent of the trial population were able to have EGFR mutation results reported. The primary end point is PFS. Even though this is not a trial specifically for *EGFR* mutant patients, the clinical enrichment would predict that at least 60% of the patients will harbor *EGFR* mutations.[21] First-line gefitinib proved superior to paclitaxel and carboplatin, with 25% versus 7% of the respective treatment groups progression free at 1 year. (Fig. 49.4A)

PFS was higher for chemotherapy initially but subsequently was higher for gefitinib from about 5 months until the end of the study period. The PFS rate was higher among gefitinib-treated patients with an EGFR mutation compared with those receiving chemotherapy only: 27% versus 14% (Fig. 49.4B).

Overall, about 60% (201 patients) of a sample of 437 patients evaluated for EGFR mutations tested positive. Patients without EGFR mutations fared worse on gefitinib (PFS rate of 2% vs. 13% for those treated with carboplatin and paclitaxel). The objective response rates were significantly higher for gefitinib than chemotherapy—43% versus 32%. In patients positive for EGFR mutation, the rates were 71% for gefitinib and 47% for carboplatin and paclitaxel. In patients who did not have the EGFR mutation, the objective response rates were 1% for gefitinib but 23.5% for carboplatin/paclitaxel (Fig. 49.4C).

A second trial, conducted in Spain, is specifically randomizing (n = 146) chemotherapy-naive patients with known *EGFR* mutations (exon 19 deletion and L858R) to either erlotinib or to chemotherapy (cisplatin/gemcitabine or cisplatin/docetaxel). The primary end point of this trial is also PFS. Two additional trials, both being conducted in Japan, are asking a similar question. The first, conducted by the West Japan Oncology Group, is randomizing (n = 200) *EGFR*-mutant (exon 19 deletion or L858R) patients with postoperative recurrence to either gefitinib alone or to cisplatin/docetaxel (WJTOG 3405 trial). The second, conducted by the North East Japan Group, is randomizing (n = 300) patients with *EGFR* mutations (exon 19 deletions, L858R G719X, and L861Q) to either gefitinib or carboplatin/paclitaxel (NEJ 002 trial). The primary end point of both trials is PFS. The results of these two Japanese trials were recently reported.[123a,123b]

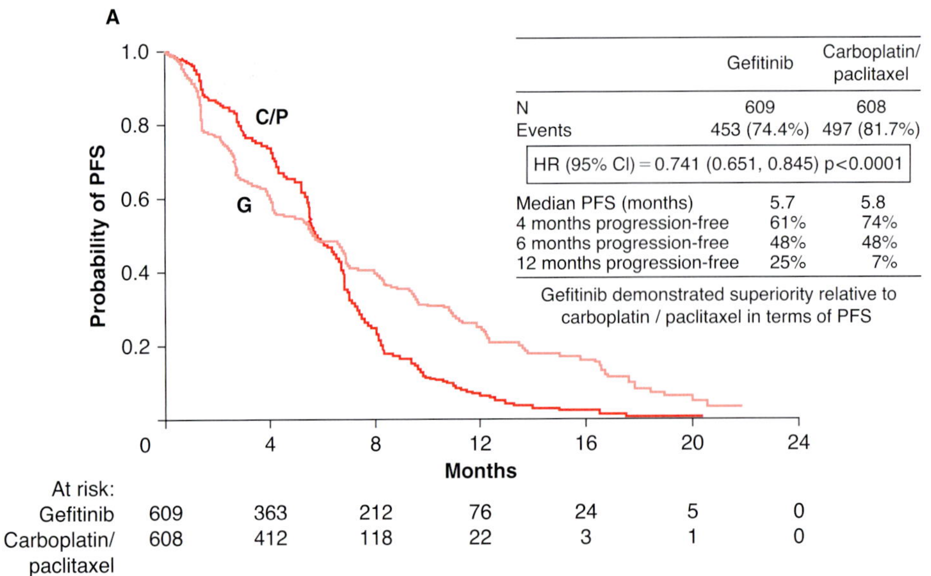

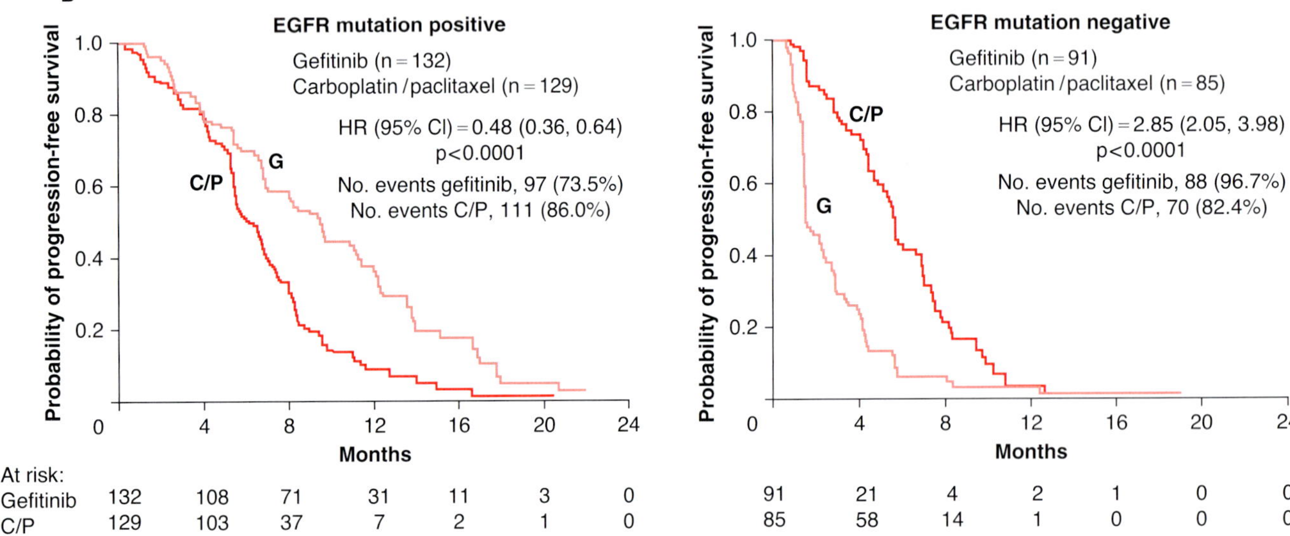

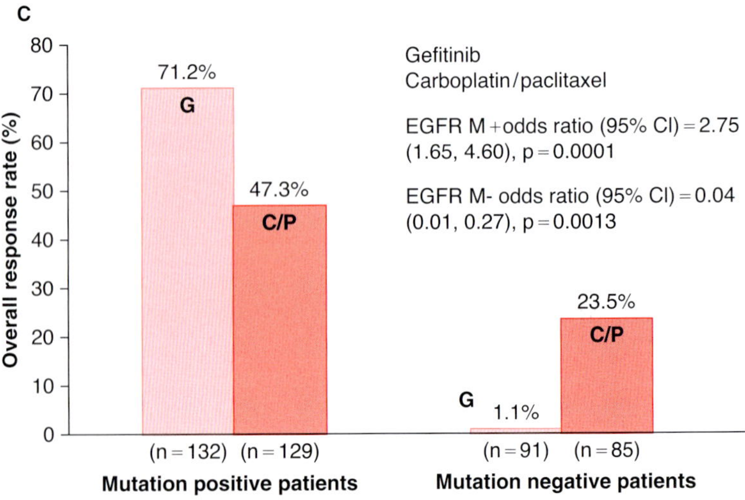

FIGURE 49.4 Gefitinib *(G)* versus carboplatin/paclitaxel *(C/P)*. **A:** Progression-free survival in intent-to-treat (ITT) population. Primary Cox analysis with covariates. HR <1 implies a lower risk of progression on gefitinib. **B:** Progression-free survival in EGFR mutation–positive and –negative ITT patients. Treatment by subgroup interaction test. $p<0.0001$ by Cox analysis of covariates. **C:** Objective response rate in EGFR mutation–positive and –negative patients. Odds ratio >1 implies greater chance of response on gefitinib. *EGFR*, epidermal growth factor receptor; *HR*, hazard ratio; *PFS*, progression-free survival.

PFS of patients with EGFR mutation treated with gefitinib in NEJ 002 and WJTOG 3405 were 10.4 and 9.2 months, while PFS of those treated with platinum-doublet therapy were 5.5 and 6.3 months, respectively.[123a,123b] HR of these studies were 0.357(95% CI, 0.25 to 0.51) and 0.489 (95% CI, 0.336 to 0.710), respectively.[123a,123b]

These studies clearly confirmed that the determinant of clinical efficacy of gefitinib is a presence of EGFR mutations and not clinical background of patients.

Another clinical question that is being evaluated is the impact of chemotherapy in addition to erlotinib. The hypothesis is based on a subset analysis of the phase III clinical trial (TRIBUTE) of chemotherapy-positive or -negative erlotinib. Although there were no differences in the treatment arms (chemotherapy alone vs. chemotherapy/erlotinib) when all patients were examined, an analysis of never-smokers revealed remarkable differences.[12] When never-smokers were treated with erlotinib in addition to the same chemotherapy regimen, the median survival increased to 22.5 months ($p = 0.01$). The response rate to chemotherapy with erlotinib was also higher than when the never-smoking patients were treated with chemotherapy alone (30%; 95% CI, 20% to 43% for erlotinib vs. 11%; 95% CI, 4% to 25% for placebo) ($p = 0.02$).[12] This clinical observation has prompted the initiation of a randomized phase II clinical trial being conducted through the Cancer and Leukemia Group B (CALGB). NSCLC patients who are never ($\leq$100 cigarettes/lifetime) or former light ($\leq$10 pack-years and quit $\geq$1 year ago) smokers are randomized to receive either erlotinib alone or carboplatin/paclitaxel/erlotinib in combination. *EGFR* mutation status will be examined in all patients. This trial will prospectively compare the efficacy of erlotinib alone or in combination with chemotherapy in *EGFR* mutant and *EGFR* wild-type patients.

These ongoing prospective clinical trials will provide additional information on the predictive and prognostic nature of *EGFR* mutations. Furthermore, they will provide a formal comparison to the standard of care (chemotherapy) and determine whether EGFR TKIs should be the treatment of choice for *EGFR* mutant chemotherapy-naive NSCLC patients with advanced disease.

Genotype/Phenotype Correlations

The two common *EGFR* mutations, exon 19 deletions and L858R, account for ~80% to 85% of all *EGFR* mutations. Whether these mutations confer the same degree of benefit from EGFR TKIs has been examined in both retrospective and prospective clinical trials. Two retrospective studies demonstrated that NSCLC patients with *EGFR* exon 19 deletion mutations treated with gefitinib or erlotinib had a significantly longer time to progression (24 vs. 10 months [$p = 0.04$] and 12 vs. 5 months [$p = 0.01$], exon 19 deletion vs. L858R, respectively) and survival (38 vs. 17 months [$p = 0.04$] and 34 vs. 8 months [$p = 0.01$], exon 19 deletion vs. L858R, respectively) times.[124,125] These findings have also been observed in some but not all prospective clinical trials of erlotinib and gefitinib.[126,127] This clinical observation may be caused by a pharmacologic effect, as analyses using purified intracellular EGFR kinase–domain constructs demonstrate that erlotinib is 20-fold less effective at inhibiting L858R compared with the exon 19 deletion.[128] This also raises the possibility that some of the second-generation EGFR inhibitors (irreversible EGFR inhibitors) may be more effective against the *EGFR* L858R mutation. Conformation of this hypothesis awaits findings from the ongoing clinical trials.

RESISTANCE MECHANISMS TO EGFR-TARGETED THERAPIES

The prospective phase II clinical trials have demonstrated that gefitinib and erlotinib are effective therapies for *EGFR*-mutant NSCLC. However, *all* patients will ultimately develop resistance (acquired resistance) to these agents.[153] It will be critical to understand the mechanisms of acquired resistance because it may lead to the development of effective therapies for patients who clinically develop acquired resistance to gefitinib or erlotinib. It is important to note that the mechanisms of acquired resistance to date have been identified in *EGFR*-mutant NSCLC patients. Whether these same mechanisms are responsible for resistance that develops in *EGFR* wild-type patients that benefit from gefitinib or erlotinib remains to be determined.

Two main mechanisms of acquired resistance have been identified in *EGFR*-mutant NSCLC patients. The first is a secondary *EGFR* mutation, T790M, that renders gefitinib and erlotinib ineffective inhibitors of EGFR kinase activity (Fig. 49.3B).[129,130] *EGFR* T790M has been detected both from tumors of *EGFR*-mutant NSCLC patients who have developed clinical resistance to gefitinib or erlotinib and from in vitro gefitinib-resistant *EGFR*-mutant cell lines.[87,129–133] To date, the *EGFR*-T790M mutation is found in 50% of tumors (93/116) from patients that have developed acquired resistance to gefitinib or erlotinib.[131,132,134] The mechanisms by which *EGFR* T790M causes gefitinib/erlotinib resistance was originally thought to be through steric hindrance analogous to the T315I mutation in the ABL kinase, which effects imatinib binding.[135,136] However, more recent studies have revealed that gefitinib can still effectively bind *EGFR* T790M but that the mutation alters the affinity of the receptor to bind ATP.[137] *EGFR* T790M is typically found on the same allele as the original *EGFR*-activating mutation, and together the two mutations increase EGFR kinase active compared with either mutation alone.[138,139] Gefitinib- or erlotinib-resistant cancers harboring *EGFR* T790M are still EGFR dependent for their growth that has prompted the search for alternative ways of inhibiting EGFR. The class of irreversible EGFR inhibitors are able to inhibit the growth and EGFR phosphorylation in model systems harboring *EGFR* T790M.[95,96] These agents are now in clinical development in patients that have developed acquired resistance to gefitinib or erlotinib. In addition, inhibitors of heat shock protein (HSP)90 are effective in preclinical models of *EGFR* T790M and are also undergoing clinical evaluation.[140] EGFR is an HSP90 client protein, and the mutant EGFR is degraded more effectively than wild-type EGFR.[140,141]

The second known mechanism of gefitinib/erlotinib resistance is amplification of the *MET* oncogence.[134,142] This was originally identified in an *EGFR*-mutant lung cancer cell line that had been made resistant to gefitinib in vitro. MET is a unique resistance mechanisms, because MET is not the immediate or downstream target of gefitinib or erlotinib. In fact, MET causes resistance because it creates a bypass signaling track and activates PI3K signaling through ERBB3 in the presence of gefitinib (Fig. 49.3C). This "redundant" activation of ERBB3 permits the cells to transmit the same downstream signaling in the presence of EGFR inhibitors. Thus, unlike for *EGFR* T790M, concomitant inhibition of *both* EGFR and MET is required to kill MET-amplified gefitinib- or erlotinib-resistant cells. The combination therapeutic approach of MET inhibitors with erlotinib are being evaluated in clinical trials. *MET* amplification has been detected in ~20% of *EGFR*-mutant NSCLC patients that have developed acquired resistance to gefitinib or erlotinib. Intriguingly, *MET* amplification and *EGFR* T790M are not mutually exclusive. In fact, resistant NSCLC patients have been identified harboring both *EGFR* T790M and *MET* amplification.[134,142] They have been detected in the same resistant tumor specimen and have been found to occur independently in different metastatic sites in the *same* patient.[134,142] Thus, a therapeutic strategy aimed solely at inhibiting *EGFR* T790M or *MET* amplification may not be very effective or lead only to regression of a subset of metastases that contain the particular mechanism of resistance. A more comprehensive and potentially effective strategy may be a combination of an irreversible EGFR and a MET kinase inhibitor. Alternatively, strategies such as HSP90 inhibitors may also be effective because both EGFR and MET are known HSP90 client proteins.[141,143]

EGFR T790M and *MET* amplification account for approximately 60% to 70% of all known causes of acquired resistance to gefitinib or erlotinib. Thus, other mechanisms of acquired resistance are likely to be discovered. The understanding of EGFR signaling both in gefitinib-sensitive and -resistant models has helped define how the likely additional resistance mechanisms will arise. Future resistance mechanisms are likely to lead to maintenance of PI3K/Akt signaling in the presence of gefitinib/erlotinib. This could occur through ERBB3 (such as for *EGFR* T790M or *MET* amplification) or by an ERBB3-independent mechanism (Fig. 49.3D). One recently identified mechanisms is the activation of insulin-like growth factor receptor (IGFR) signaling, which was identified in an EGFR wild-type gefitinib- or erlotinib-sensitive cell line model.[144] However, this mechanisms has not yet been validated in acquired resistant NSCLC patient specimens. It will be important to continue to study preclinical models and tumors from NSCLC patients that have developed gefitinib/erlotinib resistance to uncover novel resistance mechanisms.

KRAS Mutations It has been hypothesized that KRAS mutation is a good "negative" predictive marker for therapy with EGFR inhibitors in NSCLC. In contrast to colorectal cancer (CRC), in which KRAS mutations occurs in 40% to 50% and has demonstrated to be associated with lack of response and shortened survival,[145] the situation for NSCLC might be different. KRAS mutations in codons 12 to 13 occur in about 15% to 20% of unselected NSCLC patients, somewhat higher in adenocarcinomas (25% to 30%) and significantly less frequent in tumors with squamous histology (5% to 10%). It has been demonstrated in several studies that KRAS mutations in NSCLC are associated with poor prognosis independent of given therapy.[111,146]

It has been shown in several studies in patients with NSCLC treated with EGFR TKIs, that those with tumors harboring KRAS mutations most likely will not respond to EGFR inhibitors, and they have a dismal prognosis. However, it is not clear yet whether the negative association between KRAS mutations and outcome is only caused by the poor prognostic association and/or an inherent resistance to the EGFR TKIs. In the BR.21 study, an update of the biomarker analysis showed for patients with tumors having KRAS a median survival of 7.5 months with erlotinib and 3.4 months with placebo (HR = 0.69; $p = 0.03$), whereas patients having KRAS mutations had median survival of 3.7 months with erlotinib versus 7.0 months with placebo (HR = 1.67; $p = 0.3$).[147]

Serum Proteomics Investigators from Colorado and Vanderbilt Universities have developed a proteomic profile, which in several retrospective studies have demonstrated to classify NSCLC patients in a "bad" and "good" outcome group after EGFR TKI therapy, both as second-line therapy as well as first-line therapy.[148] The 11-peak proteomic profile is now commercialized by Biodesix (Steamboat Spring, Colorado) under the name Veristat® and is currently prospectively validated in several prospective studies in NSCLC.

REFERENCES

1. Dancey JE. Epidermal growth factor receptor inhibitors in non-small cell lung cancer. *Drugs* 2007;67(8):1125–1138.
2. Nakagawa K, Tamura T, Negoro S, et al. Phase I pharmacokinetic trial of the selective oral epidermal growth factor receptor tyrosine kinase inhibitor gefitinib (IRESSA, ZD1839) in Japanese patients with solid malignant tumors. *Ann Oncol* 2003;14:922–930.
3. Ranson M, Hammond LA, Ferry D, et al. ZD1839, a selective oral epidermal growth factor receptor-tyrosine kinase inhibitor, is well tolerated and active in patients with solid, malignant tumors: results of a phase I trial. *J Clin Oncol* 2002;20:2240–2250.
4. Fukuoka M, Yano S, Giaccone G, et al. Multi-institutional randomized phase II trial of gefitinib for previously treated patients with advanced non-small-cell lung cancer. *J Clin Oncol* 2003;21:2237–2246.
5. Kris MG, Natale RB, Herbst RS, et al. Efficacy of gefitinib, an inhibitor of the epidermal growth factor receptor tyrosine kinase, in symptomatic patients with non-small cell lung cancer: a randomized trial. *JAMA* 2003;290:2149–2158.
6. Shepherd FA, Rodrigues Pereira J, Ciuleanu T, et al. Erlotinib in previously treated non-small-cell lung cancer. *N Engl J Med* 2005;353:123–132.
7. Thatcher N, Chang A, Parikh P, et al. Gefitinib plus best supportive care in previously treated patients with refractory advanced

non-small-cell lung cancer: results from a randomised, placebo-controlled, multicentre study (Iressa Survival Evaluation in Lung Cancer). *Lancet* 2005;366:1527–1537.

8. Perez-Soler R. Phase II clinical trial data with the epidermal growth factor receptor tyrosine kinase inhibitor erlotinib (OSI-774) in non-small-cell lung cancer. *Clin Lung Cancer* 2004;6 Suppl 1:S20–S23.
9. Gatzemeier U, Pluzanska A, Szczesna A, et al. Phase III study of erlotinib in combination with cisplatin and gemcitabine in advanced non-small-cell lung cancer: the Tarceva Lung Cancer Investigation Trial. *J Clin Oncol* 2007;25:1545–1552.
10. Giaccone G, Herbst RS, Manegold C, et al. Gefitinib in combination with gemcitabine and cisplatin in advanced non-small-cell lung cancer: a phase III trial—INTACT 1. *J Clin Oncol* 2004;22:777–784.
11. Herbst RS, Giaccone G, Schiller JH, et al. Gefitinib in combination with paclitaxel and carboplatin in advanced non-small-cell lung cancer: a phase III trial—INTACT 2. *J Clin Oncol* 2004;22:785–794.
12. Herbst RS, Prager D, Hermann R, et al. TRIBUTE: a phase III trial of erlotinib hydrochloride (OSI-774) combined with carboplatin and paclitaxel chemotherapy in advanced non-small-cell lung cancer. *J Clin Oncol* 2005;23:5892–5899.
13. Pirker R, Pereira JR, Szczesna A, et al. Cetuximab plus chemotherapy in patients with advanced non-small-cell lung cancer (FLEX): an open-label randomised phase III trial. Lancet 2009;373(9674):1525–1531.
14. Lynch TJ, Patel T, Dreisbach L, et al. A randomized multicenter phase III study of cetuximab (Erbitux) in combination with Taxane/Carboplatin versus Taxane/Carboplatin alone as first-line treatment for patients with advanced /metastatic non-small cell lung cancer (NSCLC). *J Thorac Oncol* 2007;2(Suppl 4):S340 (Abstr. B3-03).
15. Miller VA, Kris MG, Shah N, et al. Bronchioloalveolar pathologic subtype and smoking history predict sensitivity to gefitinib in advanced non-small-cell lung cancer. *J Clin Oncol* 2004;22:1103–1109.
16. Ando M, Okamoto I, Yamamoto N, et al. Predictive factors for interstitial lung disease, antitumor response and survival in non-small-cell lung cancer patients treated with gefitinib. *J Clin Oncol* 2006; 24:2549–2556.
17. Kris MG, Sandler A, Miller V, et al. Cigarette smoking history predicts sensitivity to erlotinib: results of a phase II trial in patients with bronchioloalveolar carcinoma (BAC). *J Clin Oncol* 2004;22:S631, abstract no. 7062.
18. Niho S, Ichinose Y, Tamura T, et al. Results of a randomized phase III study to compare the overall survival of gefitnib (IRESSA) versus docetaxel in Japanese patients with pretreted advanced NSCLC. *J Clin Oncol* 2007;25:S387.
19. Douillard JY, Kim ES, Hirsh V, et al. Gefitinib (IRESSA) versus docetaxel in patients with locally advanced or metastatic non-small cell lung cancer pre-treated with platinum-based chemotherapy: a randomized, open label phase III study (INTEREST). *J Thorac Oncol* 2007;2:305.
20. Lee DH, Han JY, Lee HG, et al. Gefitinib as a first-line therapy of advanced or metastatic adenocarcinoma of the lung in never-smokers. *Clin Cancer Res* 2005;11:3032–3037.
21. Mok TS, Wu YL, Thongprasert S, et al. Gefitinib or carboplatin-paclitaxel in pulmonary adenocarcinoma. *N Engl J Med* 2009;361(10): 947–957.
22. Kang SM, Kang HJ, Shin JH, et al. Identical epidermal growth factor receptor mutations in adenocarcinomatous and squamous cell carcinomatous components of adenosquamous carcinoma of the lung. *Cancer* 2007;109:581–587.
23. Toyooka S, Yatabe Y, Tokumo M, et al. Mutations of epidermal growth factor receptor and K-ras genes in adenosquamous carcinoma of the lung. *Int J Cancer* 2006;118:1588–1590.
24. Sasaki H, Endo K, Yukiue H, et al. Mutation of epidermal growth factor receptor gene in adenosquamous carcinoma of the lung. *Lung Cancer* 2007;55:129–130.
25. Fukui T, Tsuta K, Furuta K, et al. Epidermal growth factor receptor mutation status and clinicopathological features of combined small cell carcinoma with adenocarcinoma of the lung. *Cancer Sci* 2007;98:1714–1719.
26. Pérez-Soler R, Chachoua A, Hammond LA, et al. Determinants of tumor response and survival with erlotinib in patients with non--small-cell lung cancer. *J Clin Oncol* 2004;22:3238–3247.
27. Jänne PA, Gurubhagavatula S, Yeap BY, et al. Outcomes of patients with advanced non-small cell lung cancer treated with gefitinib (ZD1839, "Iressa") on an expanded access study. *Lung Cancer* 2004;44:221–230.
28. Pérez-Soler R, Saltz L. Cutaneous adverse effects with HER1/EGFR-targeted agents: is there a silver lining? *J Clin Oncol* 2005;23:5235–5246.
29. Park J, Park BB, Kim JY, et al. Gefitinib (ZD1839) monotherapy as a salvage regimen for previously treated advanced non-small cell lung cancer. *Clin Cancer Res* 2004;10:4383–4388.
30. Kaneda H, Tamura K, Kurata T, et al. Retrospective analysis of the predictive factors associated with the response and survival benefit of gefitinib in patients with advanced non-small-cell lung cancer. *Lung Cancer* 2004;46:247–254.
31. Kim KS, Jeong JY, Kim YC, et al. Predictors of the response to gefitinib in refractory non-small cell lung cancer. *Clin Cancer Res* 2005; 11:2244–2251.
32. Inoue A, Saijo Y, Maemondo M, et al. Severe acute interstitial pneumonia and gefitinib. *Lancet* 2003;361:137–139.
33. Yoshida S. The results of gefitinib prospective investigation. *Med Drug J* 2005;41:772–789.
34. Tamura K, Nishiwaki Y, Watanabe K, et al. Evaluation of efficacy and safety of erlotinib as monotherapy for Japanese patients with advanced non-small cell lung cancer: integrated analysis of two Japanese phase II studies. *J Thorac Oncol* 2007;2(Suppl 4):S742.
35. Chiu CH, Tsai CM, Chen YM, et al. Gefitinib is active in patients with brain metastases from non-small cell lung cancer and response is related to skin toxicity. *Lung Cancer* 2005;47:129–138.
36. Bast RC Jr, Ravdin P, Hayes DF, et al. 2000 update of recommendations for the use of tumor markers in breast and colorectal cancer: clinical practice guidelines of the American Society of Clinical Oncology. *J Clin Oncol* 2001;19:1865–1878.
37. Hirsch FR, Scagliotti GV, Langer CJ, et al. Epidermal growth factor family of receptors in preneoplasia and lung cancer: perspectives for targeted therapies. *Lung Cancer* 2003;41(Suppl 1):S29–S42.
38. Hirsch FR, Varella-Garcia M, Bunn PA Jr, et al. Epidermal growth factor receptor in non-small-cell lung carcinomas: correlation between gene copy number and protein expression and impact on prognosis. *J Clin Oncol* 2003;21:3798–3807.
39. Meert AP, Martin B, Delmotte P, et al. The role of EGF-R expression on patient survival in lung cancer: a systematic review with meta-analysis. *Eur Respir J* 2002;20:975–981.
40. Cappuzzo F, Hirsch FR, Rossi E, et al. Epidermal growth factor receptor gene and protein and gefitinib sensitivity in non-small-cell lung cancer. *J Natl Cancer Inst* 2005;97:643–655.
41. Hirsch FR, Varella-Garcia M, McCoy J, et al. Increased epidermal growth factor receptor gene copy number detected by fluorescence in situ hybridization associates with increased sensitivity to gefitinib in patients with bronchioloalveolar carcinoma subtypes: a Southwest Oncology Group Study. *J Clin Oncol* 2005;23: 6838–6845.
42. Hirsch FR, Varella-Garcia M, Bunn PA Jr, et al. Molecular predictors of outcome with gefitinib in a phase III placebo-controlled study in advanced non-small-cell lung cancer. *J Clin Oncol* 2006;24: 5034–5042.
43. Dziadziuszko R, Holm B, Skov BG, et al. Epidermal growth factor receptor gene copy number and protein level are not associated with outcome of non-small-cell lung cancer patients treated with chemotherapy. *Ann Oncol* 2006;18:447–452.
44. Tsao MS, Sakurada A, Cutz JC, et al. Erlotinib in lung cancer - molecular and clinical predictors of outcome. *N Engl J Med* 2005;353:133–144.
45. Hirsch, FR, Varella-Garcia, M, Bunn, PA, et al. Fluorescence in situ hybridization subgroup analysis of TRIBUTE, a phase III clinical trial of erlotinib plus carboplatin and paclitaxel in non-small cell lung cancer. *Clin Cancer Res* 2008;1;14:6317–6323.

46. Gandara DR, Davies AM, Gautschi O, et al. Epidermal growth factor receptor inhibitors plus chemotherapy in non-small-cell lung cancer: biologic rationale for combination strategies. *Clin Lung Cancer* 2007;8(Suppl 2):S61–S67.
47. Davies AM, Ho C, Lara PN Jr, et al. Pharmacodynamic separation of epidermal growth factor receptor tyrosine kinase inhibitors and chemotherapy in non-small-cell lung cancer. *Clin Lung Cancer* 2006; 7:385–388.
48. Goss G, Ferry D, Wierzbicki R, et al. Randomized phase II study of gefitinib compared with placebo in chemotherapy-naive patients with advanced non-small-cell lung cancer and poor performance status. *J Clin Oncol* 2009;27(13):2253–2260.
49. Crinò L, Cappuzzo F, Zatloukal P, et al. Gefitinib versus vinorelbine in chemotherapy-naive elderly patients with advanced non-small-cell lung cancer (INVITE): a randomized, phase II study. *J Clin Oncol* 2008;26(26):4253–4260.
50. Cappuzzo F, Ligorio C, Janne PA, et al. Prospective study of gefitinib in epidermal growth factor receptor fluorescence in situ hybridization-positive/phospho-Akt-positive or never smoker patients with advanced non-small-cell lung cancer: the ONCOBELL trial. *J Clin Oncol* 2007;25:2248–2255.
51. Hirsch FR, Herbst RS, Olsen C, et al. Increased EGFR gene copy number detected by FISH predicts ourcome in non-small cell lung cancer patients treated with cetuximab and chemotherapy. *J Clin Oncol* 2008 Jul 10;26(20):3351–3357.
52. Robert F, Blumenschein G, Herbst RS, et al. Phase I/IIa study of cetuximab with gemcitabine plus carboplatin in patients with chemotherapy-naive advanced non-small-cell lung cancer. *J Clin Oncol* 2005; 23:9089–9096.
53. Rosell R, Daniel C, Ramlau R, et al. Randomized phase II study of cetuximab in combination with cisplatin (C) and vinorelbine (V) vs. CV alone in the first-line treatment of patients (pts) with epidermal growth factor receptor (EGFR)-expressing advanced non-small-cell lung cancer (NSCLC). *J Clin Oncol* 2004;22:7012.
54. Thienelt CD, Bunn PA Jr, Hanna N, et al. Multicenter phase I/II study of cetuximab with paclitaxel and carboplatin in untreated patients with stage IV non-small-cell lung cancer. *J Clin Oncol* 2005; 23:8786–8793.
55. Crawford J, Swanson P, Prager D, et al. Panitumumab, a fully human antibody, combined with paclitaxel and carboplatin versus paclitaxel and carboplatin alone for first line treatment of advanced non-small cell lung cancer (NSCLC): a primary analysis. Paper presented at the European Cancer Conference, 2005, Paris, France.
56. Kollmannsberger C, Schittenhelm M, Honecker F, et al. A phase I study of the humanized monoclonal anti-epidermal growth factor receptor (EGFR) antibody EMD 72000 (matuzumab) in combination with paclitaxel in patients with EGFR-positive advanced non-small-cell lung cancer (NSCLC). *Ann Oncol* 2006;17:1007–1013.
57. Hirsch FR, Varella- Garcia M, Cappuzzo F, et al. Combination of EGFR gene copy number and protein expression predicts outcome for advanced non-small-cell lung cancer patients treated with gefitinib. *Ann Oncol* 2007 Apr;18(4):752–760. Epub 2007 Feb 22.
58. Italiano A, Vandenbos FB, Otto J, et al. Comparison of the epidermal growth factor receptor gene and protein in primary non-small-cell-lung cancer and metastatic sites: implications for treatment with EGFR-inhibitors. *Ann Oncol* 2006;17:981–985.
59. Dziadziuszko R, Witta SE, Cappuzzo F, et al. Epidermal growth factor receptor messenger RNA expression, gene dosage, and gefitinib sensitivity in non-small cell lung cancer. *Clin Cancer Res* 2006;12:3078–3084.
60. Bell DW, Lynch TJ, Haserlat SM, et al. Epidermal growth factor receptor mutations and gene amplification in non-small-cell lung cancer: molecular analysis of the IDEAL/INTACT gefitinib trials. *J Clin Oncol* 2005;23:8081–8092.
61. Takano T, Ohe Y, Sakamoto H, et al. Epidermal growth factor receptor gene mutations and increased copy numbers predict gefitinib sensitivity in patients with recurrent non-small-cell lung cancer. *J Clin Oncol* 2005;23:6829–6837.
62. Miller VA, Zakowski M, Riely GJ, et al. EGFR mutation, immunohistochemistry (IHC) and chromogenic in situ hybridization (CISH) as predictors of sensitivity to erlotinib and gefitinib in patients (pts) with NSCLC. *J Clin Oncol* 2005;23(Suppl 16S):7031.
63. Hirsch FR, Dziadziuszko R, Thatcher N, et al. Epidermal growth factor receptor immunohistochemistry: comparison of antibodies and cutoff points to predict benefit from gefitinib in a phase 3 placebo-controlled study in advanced nonsmall-cell lung cancer. *Cancer* 2008; 112(5):1114–1121.
64. Paez JG, Jänne PA, Lee JC, et al. EGFR mutations in lung cancer: correlation with clinical response to gefitinib therapy. *Science* 2004; 304:1497–1500.
65. Lynch TJ, Bell DW, Sordella R, et al. Activating mutations in the epidermal growth factor receptor underlying responsiveness of non-small-cell lung cancer to gefitinib. *N Engl J Med* 2004;350:2129–2139.
66. Pao W, Miller V, Zakowski M, et al. EGF receptor gene mutations are common in lung cancers from "never smokers" and are associated with sensitivity of tumors to gefitinib and erlotinib. *Proc Natl Acad Sci U S A* 2004;101:13306–13311.
67. Mitsudomi T, Kosaka T, Endoh H, et al. Mutations of the epidermal growth factor receptor gene predict prolonged survival after gefitinib treatment in patients with non-small-cell lung cancer with postoperative recurrence. *J Clin Oncol* 2005;23:2513–2520.
68. Huang SF, Liu HP, Li LH, et al. High frequency of epidermal growth factor receptor mutations with complex patterns in non-small cell lung cancers related to gefitinib responsiveness in Taiwan. *Clin Cancer Res* 2004;10:8195–8203.
69. Tokumo M, Toyooka S, Kiura K, et al. The relationship between epidermal growth factor receptor mutations and clinicopathologic features in non-small cell lung cancers. *Clin Cancer Res* 2005;11: 1167–1173.
70. Han SW, Kim TY, Hwang PG, et al. Predictive and prognostic impact of epidermal growth factor receptor mutation in non-small-cell lung cancer patients treated with gefitinib. *J Clin Oncol* 2005;23:2493–2501.
71. Shigematsu H, Lin L, Takahashi T, et al. Clinical and biological features associated with epidermal growth factor receptor gene mutations in lung cancers. *J Natl Cancer Inst* 2005;97:339–346.
72. Jemal A, Siegel R, Ward E, et al. Cancer statistics, 2007. *CA Cancer J Clin* 2007;57:43–66.
73. Bell DW, Gore I, Okimoto RA, et al. Inherited susceptibility to lung cancer may be associated with the T790M drug resistance mutation in EGFR. *Nat Genet* 2005;37:1315–1316.
74. Marchetti A, Martella C, Felicioni L, et al. EGFR mutations in non-small-cell lung cancer: analysis of a large series of cases and development of a rapid and sensitive method for diagnostic screening with potential implications on pharmacologic treatment. *J Clin Oncol* 2005; 23:857–865.
75. Amann J, Kalyankrishna S, Massion PP, et al. Aberrant epidermal growth factor receptor signaling and enhanced sensitivity to EGFR inhibitors in lung cancer. *Cancer Res* 2005;65:226–235.
76. Miller VA, Riely GJ, Zakowski MF, et al. Molecular characteristics of bronchioloalveolar carcinoma and adenocarcinoma, bronchioloalveolar carcinoma subtype, predict response to erlotinib. *J Clin Oncol* 2008; 26:1472–1478.
77. Nomura M, Shigematsu H, Li L, et al. Polymorphisms, mutations, and amplification of the EGFR gene in non-small cell lung cancers. *PLoS Med* 2007;4:E125.
78. Toyooka S, Takano T, Kosaka T, et al. Epidermal growth factor receptor mutation, but not sex and smoking, is independently associated with favorable prognosis of gefitinib-treated patients with lung adenocarcinoma. *Cancer Sci* 2008;99(2):303–308.
79. Greulich H, Chen TH, Feng W, et al. Oncogenic transformation by inhibitor-sensitive and -resistant EGFR mutants. *PLoS Med* 2005;2:E313.
80. Jiang J, Greulich H, Janne PA, et al. Epidermal growth factor-independent transformation of Ba/F3 cells with cancer-derived epidermal growth factor receptor mutants induces gefitinib-sensitive cell cycle progression. *Cancer Res* 2005;65:8968–8974.

81. Ji H, Li D, Chen L, et al. The impact of human EGFR kinase domain mutations on lung tumorigenesis and in vivo sensitivity to EGFR-targeted therapies. *Cancer Cell* 2006;9:485–495.
82. Politi K, Zakowski MF, Fan PD, et al. Lung adenocarcinomas induced in mice by mutant EGF receptors found in human lung cancers respond to a tyrosine kinase inhibitor or to down-regulation of the receptors. *Genes Dev* 2006;20:1496–1510.
83. Tracy S, Mukohara T, Hansen M, et al. Gefitinib induces apoptosis in the EGFRL858R non-small-cell lung cancer cell line H3255. *Cancer Res* 2004;64:7241–7244.
84. Mukohara T, Engelman JA, Hanna NH, et al. Differential effects of gefitinib and cetuximab on non-small-cell lung cancers bearing epidermal growth factor receptor mutations. *J Natl Cancer Inst* 2005;97: 1185–1194.
85. Sordella R, Bell DW, Haber DA, et al. Gefitinib-sensitizing EGFR mutations in lung cancer activate anti-apoptotic pathways. *Science* 2004; 305:1163–1167.
86. Weinstein IB. Cancer. Addiction to oncogenes—the Achilles heal of cancer. *Science* 2002;297:63–64.
87. Engelman JA, Mukohara T, Zejnullahu K, et al. A. Allelic dilution obscures detection of a biologically significant resistance mutation in EGFR-amplified lung cancer. *J Clin Invest* 2006;116:2695–2706.
88. Engelman JA, Jänne PA, Mermel C, et al. ErbB-3 mediates phosphoinositide 3-kinase activity in gefitinib-sensitive non-small cell lung cancer cell lines. *Proc Natl Acad Sci U S A* 2005;102:3788–3793.
89. Ono M, Hirata A, Kometani T, et al. Sensitivity to gefitinib (Iressa, ZD1839) in non-small cell lung cancer cell lines correlates with dependence on the epidermal growth factor (EGF) receptor/extracellular signal-regulated kinase 1/2 and EGF receptor/Akt pathway for proliferation. *Mol Cancer Ther* 2004;3:465–472.
90. Fujimoto N, Wislez M, Zhang J, et al. High expression of ErbB family members and their ligands in lung adenocarcinomas that are sensitive to inhibition of epidermal growth factor receptor. *Cancer Res* 2005; 65:11478–11485.
91. Yun CH, Boggon TJ, Li Y, et al. Structures of lung cancer-derived EGFR mutants and inhibitor complexes: mechanism of activation and insights into differential inhibitor sensitivity. *Cancer Cell* 2007;11: 217–227.
92. Kosaka T, Yatabe Y, Endoh H, et al. Mutations of the epidermal growth factor receptor gene in lung cancer. *Cancer Res* 2004; 64:8919–8923.
93. Pham D, Kris M, Riely G, et al. Use of cigarette-smoking history to estimate the likelihood of mutations in epidermal growth factor receptor gene exons 19 and 21 in lung adenocarcinomas. *J Clin Oncol* 2006;24(11):1700–1704.
94. Matsuo K, Ito H, Yatabe Y, et al. Risk factors differ for non-small-cell lung cancers with and without EGFR mutation: assessment of smoking and sex by a case-control study in Japanese. *Cancer Sci* 2006;98(1):96–101.
95. Engelman JA, Zejnullahu K, Gale CM, et al. PF00299804, an irreversible pan-ERBB inhibitor, is effective in lung cancer models with EGFR and ERBB2 mutations that are resistant to gefitinib. *Cancer Res* 2007;67:11924–11932.
96. Li D, Ambrogio L, Shimamura T, et al. BIBW2992, an irreversible EGFR/HER2 inhibitor highly effective in preclinical lung cancer models. *Oncogene* 2008;27(34):4702–4711.
97. Minami Y, Shimamura T, Shah K, et al. The major lung cancer-derived mutants of ERBB2 are oncogenic and are associated with sensitivity to the irreversible EGFR/ERBB2 inhibitor HKI-272. *Oncogene* 2007; 26:5023–5027.
98. Schmiedel J, Blaukat A, Li S, et al. Matuzumab binding to EGFR prevents the conformational rearrangement required for dimerization. *Cancer Cell* 2008;13:365–373.
99. Sasaki H, Endo K, Takada M, et al. EGFR exon 20 insertion mutation in Japanese lung cancer. *Lung Cancer* 2007;58(3):324–328.
100. Gilmer TM, Cable L, Alligood K, et al. Impact of common epidermal growth factor receptor and HER2 variants on receptor activity and inhibition by lapatinib. *Cancer Res* 2008;68:571–579.
101. Yuza Y, Glatt KA, Jiang J, et al. Allele-dependent variation in the relative cellular potency of distinct EGFR inhibitors. *Cancer Biol Ther* 2007;6(5):661–667.
102. Shigematsu H, Takahashi T, Nomura M, et al. F. Somatic mutations of the HER2 kinase domain in lung adenocarcinomas. *Cancer Res* 2005; 65:1642–1646.
103. Stephens P, Hunter C, Bignell G, et al. Inhibition of the T790M gatekeeper mutant of the epidermal growth factor receptor by EXEL-7647. *Clin Cancer Res* 2007;13:3713–3723.
105. de La Motte Rouge T, Galluzzi L, Olaussen KA, et al. A novel epidermal growth factor receptor inhibitor promotes apoptosis in non-small cell lung cancer cells resistant to erlotinib. *Cancer Res* 2007; 67:6253–6262.
106. Doody JF, Wang Y, Patel SN, et al. Inhibitory activity of cetuximab on epidermal growth factor receptor mutations in non small cell lung cancers. *Mol Cancer Ther* 2007;6:2642–2651.
107. Perez-Torres M, Guix M, Gonzalez A, et al. Epidermal growth factor receptor (EGFR) antibody down-regulates mutant receptors and inhibits tumors expressing EGFR mutations. *J Biol Chem* 2006; 281:40183–40192.
108. Marks JL, Broderick S, Zhou Q, et al. Prognostic and therapeutic implications of EGFR and KRAS mutations in resected lung adenocarcinoma. *J Thorac Oncol* 2008;3:111–116.
109. Na II, Rho JK, Choi YJ, et al. The survival outcomes of patients with resected non-small cell lung cancer differ according to EGFR mutations and the P21 expression. *Lung Cancer* 2007;57:96–102.
110. Hotta K, Kiura K, Toyooka S, et al. Clinical significance of epidermal growth factor receptor gene mutations on treatment outcome after first-line cytotoxic chemotherapy in Japanese patients with non-small cell lung cancer. *J Thorac Oncol* 2007;2:632–637.
111. Eberhard DA, Johnson BE, Amler LC, et al. Mutations in the epidermal growth factor receptor and in KRAS are predictive and prognostic indicators in patients with non-small-cell lung cancer treated with chemotherapy alone and in combination with erlotinib. *J Clin Oncol* 2005;23:5900–5909.
112. Thomas RK, Baker AC, Debiasi RM, et al. High-throughput oncogene mutation profiling in human cancer. *Nat Genet* 2007;39: 347–351.
113. Takano T, Ohe Y, Tsuta K, et al. Epidermal growth factor receptor mutation detection using high-resolution melting analysis predicts outcomes in patients with advanced non small cell lung cancer treated with gefitinib. *Clin Cancer Res* 2007;13:5385–5390.
114. Sasaki H, Endo K, Konishi A, et al. EGFR mutation status in Japanese lung cancer patients: genotyping analysis using LightCycler. *Clin Cancer Res* 2005;11:2924–2929.
115. Nagai Y, Miyazawa H, Huqun TT, et al. Genetic heterogeneity of the epidermal growth factor receptor in non-small cell lung cancer cell lines revealed by a rapid and sensitive detection system, the peptide nucleic acid-locked nucleic acid PCR clamp. *Cancer Res* 2005; 65:7276–7282.
116. Yatabe Y, Hida T, Horio Y, et al. A rapid, sensitive assay to detect EGFR mutation in small biopsy specimens from lung cancer. *J Mol Diagn* 2006;8:335–341.
117. Thomas RK, Nickerson E, Simons JF, et al. Sensitive mutation detection in heterogeneous cancer specimens by massively parallel picoliter reactor sequencing. *Nat Med* 2006 Jul;12(7):852–855.
118. Jänne PA, Borras AM, Kuang Y, et al. A rapid and sensitive enzymatic method for epidermal growth factor receptor mutation screening. *Clin Cancer Res* 2006;12:751–758.
119. Kimura H, Kasahara K, Kawaishi M, et al. Detection of epidermal growth factor receptor mutations in serum as a predictor of the response to gefitinib in patients with non-small-cell lung cancer. *Clin Cancer Res* 200612:3915–3921.
120. Kimura H, Suminoe M, Kasahara K, et al. Evaluation of epidermal growth factor receptor mutation status in serum DNA as a predictor of response to gefitinib (IRESSA). *Br J Cancer* 2007;97: 778–784.

121. Nagrath S, Sequist LV, Maheswaran S, et al. Isolation of rare circulating tumour cells in cancer patients by microchip technology. *Nature* 2007;450:1235–1239.
122. Schiller JH, Harrington D, Belani CP, et al. Comparison of four chemotherapy regimens for advanced non-small-cell lung cancer. *N Engl J Med* 2002;346:92–98.
123. Hanna N, Lilenbaum R, Ansari R, et al. Phase II trial of cetuximab in patients with previously treated non-small-cell lung cancer. *J Clin Oncol* 2006;24:5253–5258.
123a. Kobayashi K, Inoue A, Maemondo M, et al. First-line gefitinib versus first-line chemotherapy by carboplatin (CBDCA) plus paclitaxel (TXL) in non-small cell lung cancer (NSCLC) patients (pts) with EGFR mutations: A phase III study (002) by North East Japan Gefitinib Study Group. *J Clin Oncol* 2009;27:15S(suppl; abstr 8016).
123b. Tsurutani J, Mitsudomi T, Mori S, et al. A phase III, first-line trial of gefitinib versus cisplatin plus docetaxel for patients with advanced or recurrent non-small cell lungcancer (NSCLC) harboring activating mutation of the epidermal growthfactor receptor (EGFR) gene: a preliminary results of WJTOG 3405. *Eur J Cancer* 2009;7(Suppl):505(suppl; abstr O-9002).
124. Jackman DM, Yeap BY, Sequist LV, et al. Exon 19 deletion mutations of epidermal growth factor receptor are associated with prolonged survival in non-small cell lung cancer patients treated with gefitinib or erlotinib. *Clin Cancer Res* 2006;12:3908–3914.
125. Riely GJ, Pao W, Pham D, et al. Clinical course of patients with non-small cell lung cancer and epidermal growth factor receptor exon 19 and exon 21 mutations treated with gefitinib or erlotinib. *Clin Cancer Res* 2006;12:839–844.
126. Paz-Ares L, Sanchez JM, García-Velasco A, et al. A prospective phase II trial of erlotinib in advanced non-small cell lung cancer (NSCLC) patients (p) with mutations in the tyrosine kinase (TK) domain of the epidermal growth factor receptor (EGFR). *J Clin Oncol (Meeting Abstracts)*. 2006;24(18S):7020.
127. Sequist LV, Martins RG, Spigel D, et al. First-line gefitinib in patients with advanced non-small-cell lung cancer harboring somatic EGFR mutations. *J Clin Oncol* 2008;26:2442–2449.
128. Carey KD, Garton AJ, Romero MS, et al. Kinetic analysis of epidermal growth factor receptor somatic mutant proteins shows increased sensitivity to the epidermal growth factor receptor tyrosine kinase inhibitor, erlotinib. *Cancer Res* 2006;66:8163–8171.
129. Kobayashi S, Boggon TJ, Dayaram T, et al. EGFR mutation and resistance of non-small-cell lung cancer to gefitinib. *N Engl J Med* 2005; 352:786–792.
130. Pao W, Miller VA, Politi KA, et al. Acquired resistance of lung adenocarcinomas to gefitinib or erlotinib is associated with a second mutation in the EGFR kinase domain. *PLoS Med* 2005;2:1–11.
131. Kosaka T, Yatabe Y, Endoh H, et al. Analysis of epidermal growth factor receptor gene mutation in patients with non-small cell lung cancer and acquired resistance to gefitinib. *Clin Cancer Res* 2006;12:5764–5769.
132. Balak MN, Gong Y, Riely GJ, et al. Novel D761Y and common secondary T790M mutations in epidermal growth factor receptor-mutant lung adenocarcinomas with acquired resistance to kinase inhibitors. *Clin Cancer Res* 2006;12:6494–6501.
133. Ogino A, Kitao H, Hirano S, et al. Emergence of epidermal growth factor receptor T790M mutation during chronic exposure to gefitinib in a non small cell lung cancer cell line. *Cancer Res* 2007;67:7807–7814.
134. Engelman JA, Zejnullahu K, Mitsudomi T, et al. MET amplification leads to gefitinib resistance in lung cancer by activating ERBB3 signaling. *Science* 2007;316:1039–1043.
135. Shah NP, Nicoll JM, Nagar B, et al. Multiple BCR-ABL kinase domain mutations confer polyclonal resistance to the tyrosine kinase inhibitor imatinib (STI571) in chronic phase and blast crisis chronic myeloid leukemia. *Cancer Cell* 2002;2:117–125.
136. Weisberg E, Manley PW, Cowan-Jacob SW, et al. Second generation inhibitors of BCR-ABL for the treatment of imatinib-resistant chronic myeloid leukaemia. *Nat Rev Cancer* 2007;7:345–356.
137. Yun CH, Mengwasser KE, Toms AV, et al. The T790M mutation in EGFR kinase causes drug resistance by increasing the affinity for ATP. *Proc Natl Acad Sci U S A* 2008;105:2070–2075.
138. Godin-Heymann N, Bryant I, Rivera MN, et al. Oncogenic activity of epidermal growth factor receptor kinase mutant alleles is enhanced by the T790M drug resistance mutation. *Cancer Res* 2007;67:7319–7326.
139. Vikis H, Sato M, James M, et al. EGFR-T790M is a rare lung cancer susceptibility allele with enhanced kinase activity. *Cancer Res* 2007;67: 4665–4670.
140. Shimamura T, Shapiro GI. Heat shock protein 90 inhibition in lung cancer. *J Thorac Oncol* 2008;3:S152–S159.
141. Shimamura T, Lowell AM, Engelman JA, et al. Epidermal growth factor receptors harboring kinase domain mutations associate with the heat shock protein 90 chaperone and are destabilized following exposure to geldanamycins. *Cancer Res* 2005;65:6401–6408.
142. Bean J, Brennan C, Shih JY, et al. MET amplification occurs with or without T790M mutations in EGFR mutant lung tumors with acquired resistance to gefitinib or erlotinib. *Proc Natl Acad Sci U S A* 2007;26;104(52):20932–20937.
143. Maulik G, Kijima T, Ma PC, et al. Modulation of the c-Met/hepatocyte growth factor pathway in small cell lung cancer. *Clin Cancer Res* 2002;8:620–627.
144. Guix M, Faber AC, Wang SE, et al. Acquired resistance to EGFR tyrosine kinase inhibitors in cancer cells is mediated by loss of IGF-binding proteins. *J Clin Invest* 2008;118:2609–2619.
145. Van Cutsem E, Lang I, D'haens G, et al. KRAS status and efficacy in the first-line treatment of patients with metastatic colorectal cancer (mCRC) treated with FOLFIRI with or without cetuximab: the CRYSTAL experience. *J Clin Oncol* 2008;26:(suppl)(abstr. 2).
146. Gautschi O, Huegli B, Ziegler A, et al. Origin and prognostic value of circulating KRAS mutations in lung cancer patients. *Cancer Lett* 2007 Sep 8;254(2):265–273.
147. Zhu CQ, Santos G, Ding K et al. Role of KRAS and EGFR as biomarkers for response to erlotinib in National Cancer Institute of Canada Clinical Trials Group study BR-21. *J Clin Oncol* 2008 Sep 10;26(26):4268–4275.
148. Taguchi F, Solomon B, Grecorg V, et al. Mass spectrometry to classify non-small cell lung cancer patients for clinical outcome after treatment with epidermal growth factor receptor tyrosine kinase inhibitors: a multicohort cross-institutional study. *J Natl Cancer Inst* 2007;99: 838–846.
149. Inoue A, Suzuki T, Fukuhara T, et al. Prospective phase II study of gefitinib for chemotherapy-naive patients with advanced non-small-cell lung cancer with epidermal growth factor receptor gene mutations. *J Clin Oncol* 2006;24:3340–3346.
150. Tamura K, Okamoto I, Kashii T, et al. Multicentre prospective phase II trial of gefitinib for advanced non-small cell lung cancer with epidermal growth factor receptor mutations: results of the West Japan Thoracic Oncology Group trial (WJTOG0403). *Br J Cancer* 2008;98:907–914.
151. Asahina H, Yamazaki K, Kinoshita I, et al. A phase II trial of gefitinib as first-line therapy for advanced non-small cell lung cancer with epidermal growth factor receptor mutations. *Br J Cancer* 2006;95:998–1004.
152. Sutani A, Nagai Y, Udagawa K, et al. Gefitinib for non-small-cell lung cancer patients with epidermal growth factor receptor gene mutations screened by peptide nucleic acid-locked nucleic acid PCR clamp. *Br J Cancer* 2006;95:1483–1489.
153. Engelman JA, Jänne PA. Mechanisms of acquired resistance to epidermal growth factor receptor tyrosine kinase inhibitors in non-small cell lung cancer. *Clin Cancer Res* 2008;14:2895–2899.
154. Lim, Y. Mining the tumor phosphoproteome for cancer markers. *Clin Cancer Res* 2005;11:3163–3169.
155. Tomizawa Y, Iijima H, Sunaga N, et al. Clinicopathologic significance of the mutations of the epidermal growth factor receptor gene in patients with non–small cell lung cancer. *Clin Cancer Res* 2005;11:6816–6822.
156. Suzuki R, Hasegawa Y, Baba K, et al. A phase II study of single-agent gefitinib as first-line therapy in patients with stage IV non-small-cell lung cancer. *Br J Cancer* 2006;94(11):1599–1603.

157. Satouchi M, Negoro S, Funada Y, et al. Predictive factors associated with prolonged survival in patients with advanced non-small-cell lung cancer (NSCLC) treated with gefitinib. *Br J Cancer* 2007;96(8):1191–1196.
158. Takano T, Ohe Y, Kusumoto M, et al. Risk factors for interstitial lung disease and predictive factors for tumor response in patients with advanced non-small cell lung cancer treated with gefitinib. Lung Cancer 2004;45:93–104.
159. Zhang XT, Li LY, Mu XL, et al. The EGFR mutation and its correlation with response of gefitinib in previously treated Chinese patients with advanced non-small-cell lung cancer. Ann Oncol 2005;16:1334–1342.
160. Niho S, Kubota K, Goto K, et al. First-line single agent treatment with gefitinib in patients with advanced non-small-cell lung cancer: a phase II study. J Clin Oncol 2006;24:64–69.

CHAPTER 50

Alex A. Adjei

Other Signal Transduction Agents

Cancer represents a multitude of diseases characterized by uncontrolled cellular proliferation and is the second most common cause of death in Western society.[1] Despite advances in diagnosis and treatment, overall survival (OS) remains poor.[2] Radiotherapy and chemotherapy are relatively nonspecific, affecting normal cells as well as rapidly proliferating tumor cells,[3] and cause toxicities that limit their long-term utility. Tumor responses from cytotoxic chemotherapy are usually transient and unpredictable.[4] Furthermore, resistance to chemotherapy is common in all malignancies.

Novel targeted agents that represent improvements over traditional treatments are therefore needed. These agents would ideally have high specificity toward tumor cells, resulting in minimal side effects.[5] Increased understanding of molecular mechanisms underlying tumor growth, progression, and metastasis over the past decade have identified promising anticancer targets; in particular, protein kinases—enzymes that modify cellular proteins by catalyzing the transfer of phosphate from adenosine triphosphate (ATP) to either serine/threonine or tyrosine amino acid residues.[6] Approximately 90 tyrosine kinases, of the transmembrane receptor type or the cytoplasmic nonreceptor type,[7] which regulate pivotal signaling pathways that control normal cellular function and development,[6,8] have been identified. Their activity is normally tightly controlled and highly regulated.[7] Dysregulated kinase activity, resulting from oncogenic gene mutation or overexpression, has a major role in carcinogenesis.[6] For example, overactivation of these enzymes increases tumor cell proliferation and growth, induces antiapoptotic effects, and promotes angiogenesis and metastasis.[4]

In this chapter, we discuss the discovery, biology, signaling pathways, and pharmacology of protein kinase targets (Fig. 50.1) as a well as a few nonkinase targets involved in cell proliferation, metastasis, and apoptosis. These targets include receptor tyrosine kinases (RTKs) with roles in proliferation—insulin-like growth factor receptor 1 (IGFR-1), mesenchymal-epithelial transition factor (c-Met), c-Kit, Flt-3, and RET (rearranged during transfection); and cytoplasmic nonreceptor kinases involved in proliferation and/or prevention of apoptosis—the serine/threonine kinases Raf, MEK, mammalian target of rapamycin (mTOR) and Aurora kinases, and tyrosine kinases Bcr-Abl and Src.

The kinases involved in angiogenic signaling as well as the epidermal growth factor receptor (EGFR) signaling are discussed elsewhere in this volume.

PROLIFERATIVE RECEPTOR TYROSINE KINASES

IGFR/PI3-Kinase Pathway The phosphatidyl-inositol 3 kinase (PI3K) pathway is one of the most important oncogenic pathways, with estimates suggesting that activating mutations in the p110α catalytic subunit occurs in up to 30% of all human cancer, although this is uncommon in non–small cell lung cancer (NSCLC). The most common mechanism of its aberrant activation though is the loss of the regulatory phosphatase and tensin homologue (PTEN) lipid phosphatase, which occurs frequently in NSCLC. PI3K is activated by Ras and RTKs such as EGFR, c-met, and IGF receptor pathway. Autocrine production of IGF as well as overexpression of its cognate receptor, IGF-1R, are well documented in NSCLC, with downstream signaling chiefly mediated by the PI3K–Akt pathway.

Regardless of the mechanism of its dysregulation, Akt is the chief mediator of downstream signaling through various targets. One key target is the mTOR, a serine/threonine kinase that serves as a key component regulating transcriptional and translational proteins that control cell growth, angiogenesis, apoptosis, as well as amino acid and glucose metabolism. This pathway has been implicated in mediating resistance to cytotoxic chemotherapy as well as resistance to novel agents such as the EGFR tyrosine kinase inhibitors (EGFR TKIs).

IGF Receptor The IGFs help regulate normal cell metabolism, growth, proliferation, differentiation, cell–cell and cell–matrix adhesion, and survival.[9] The IGF-1R is expressed in most cells, has ligand-activated tyrosine kinase activity,[10] and

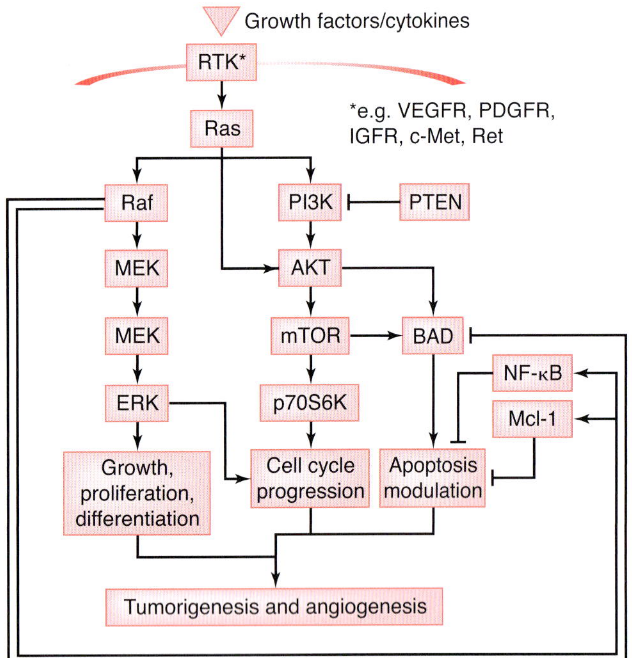

FIGURE 50.1 Overview of the key protein kinase signaling pathways involved in tumorigenesis. *AKT*, AKT8 virus oncogene homologue; *BAD*, Bcl2-antagonist of cell death; *c-Met*, growth factor receptor c-met; *ERK*, extracellular signal regulated kinase; *IGFR*, insulin-like growth factor 1 receptor; *Mcl-1*, myeloid cell leukemia sequence 1; *MEK*, MAPK/Erk kinase; *mTOR*, mechanistic target of rapamycin; *NF-κB*, nuclear factor kappa-light-chain-enhancer of activated B cells; *PDGFR*, platelet-derived growth factor receptor; *PI3K*, phosphatidylinositol 3-kinase; *PTEN*, phosphatase and tensin homologue; *Raf*, root abundant factor; *Ras*, ras protein; *Ret*, ret oncogene; *RTK*, receptor tyrosine kinase; *VEGFR*, vascular endothelial growth factor receptor.

activates several downstream signaling pathways, including Raf/MEK/extracellular signal-regulated kinase (ERK).[9] IGF bioactivity is influenced by a family of six IGF-binding proteins (IGFBPs) that sequester IGFs, thereby preventing excessive cell growth and/or promoting apoptosis.[11] Increased circulating levels of IGF, or an increased ratio of IGF to IGFBP, are implicated in the development of several types of tumors, including breast,[12] prostate,[13] lung,[14] and colon carcinomas.[15] Several monoclonal antibodies (MoAbs) and small molecule inhibitors of IGF-1R are in clinical testing.

CP-751,871 is a fully humanized IgG2 MoAb antagonist of IGF-1R with preclinical anticancer activity.[16] The MoAb interrupts the binding of IGF-I to IGF-1R, IGF-1R autophosphorylation and induces downregulation of IGF-1R in vitro and in tumor xenograft models. In a phase I study, CP-751,871 was administered intravenously every 21 days in advanced solid tumor patients.[17] CP-751,871 was escalated to the maximally feasible dose (based on duration of infusion) of 20 mg/kg without any dose-limiting toxicities (DLTs). The correlative studies revealed increased expression of serum insulin and human growth factor hormone, presumably, through a negative feedback loop. The most common adverse events were hyperglycemia, anorexia, nausea, elevated liver transaminases, hyperuricemia, and fatigue. In an exploratory assay, IGF-1R-expressing circulating cancer cells (CTCs) were analyzed. Three patients with detectable IGF-1R expressing CTCs at baseline were reported to have decreased level of CTCs following CP-751,871 administration that rebounded at the end of the 21-day period.[17,18] Preliminary phase II results of a randomized first-line advanced NSCLC phase II study of paclitaxel and carboplatin plus/minus CP751,871 were presented at American Society of Clinical Oncology (ASCO) 2007. A total of 46% of patients in the experimental arm achieved objective responses (22/48 patients) versus 32% (8/25 patients) in the control arm.[19] An unplanned subgroup analysis by histology has suggested a greater benefit in patients with squamous histology within this trial, but the mature results with additional patient numbers remain to be published. Based on these promising phase studies of CP-751,871 in combination with paclitaxel and carboplatin, phase III studies comparing this combination with chemotherapy alone as frontline therapy in NSCLC has commenced. In addition, a phase III trial of erlotinib with or without CP-751,871 is also ongoing, as are studies in multiple myeloma and other tumor types.[20–23]

AMG-479 is a fully humanized anti-IGF-1R MoAb with broad preclinical antitumor activity. The agent showed potent inhibition of the PI3k/Akt axis with increased antitumor effect when combined with anti-EGFR therapies in pancreatic cancer xenograft models.[24] In phase I testing of AMG-479, 16 patients with advanced solid tumors received escalating dose of the agent intravenously.[25] At 20 mg/kg every 2 weeks, one patient experienced grade 3 dose-limiting thrombocytopenia. No greater than grade 2 hyperglycemia was observed. The agent is currently being tested in non-Hodgkin lymphoma, Ewing sarcoma, and desmoplastic small round cell tumors.[26,27] Phase I studies in combination with gemcitabine or panitumumab, as well as phase I/II studies in combination with irinotecan and panitumumab in colorectal cancer are being planned at the time of writing.[28]

Other anti-IGF-1R agents under phase I/II evaluation include the MoAbs IMC-A12, R-1507, and BIIB022. As well as the oral small molecule inhibitors, XL-288, OSI-906, and nordihydrohuareacetic acid are also being tested.

mTOR mTOR is a serine/threonine kinase, acting downstream of PI3K/AKT.[29] The PI3K pathway is activated by Ras, which is often overstimulated in tumors where it contributes to cell cycle progression, inhibits apoptosis, and increases metastatic potential.[30] mTOR promotes RTK-induced cell growth, proliferation, and prolongs cell survival via its target, P70S6 kinase, which binds to mitochondrial membranes and inactivates the pro-apoptotic molecule Bcl2-antagonist of cell death (BAD).[31]

Overactivation of mTOR can also arise through inactivating mutations of the tumor suppressor PTEN gene, resulting in overstimulation of the PI3K/AKT signaling pathway. Loss of the PTEN gene is associated with poor prognosis, resistance to chemotherapy, and various solid tumors, including glioblastoma multiforme,[32] melanoma,[33] thyroid,[33] breast,[34] ovarian, and prostate carcinoma.[29] Dysregulation of mTOR signaling is also important in hematologic malignancies, including mantle cell lymphoma.[35]

The mTOR protein was discovered in the 1990s when the mechanism of action of rapamycin was investigated.[36] Rapamycin (sirolimus) is a macrolide isolated from *Streptomyces hygroscopicus*, a bacterial species native to Easter Island, and has been used widely as an immunosuppressant in organ transplantation.[37] Rapamycin has been evaluated orally as an anticancer agent in solid tumors and pancreatic cancer.[38,39] mTOR complexes with raptor (regulatory-associated protein of mTOR) and rictor (rapamycin-insensitive companion of mTOR) to form mTOR complex-1 (mTORC1) and mTORC2, respectively. mTORC1 is downstream to Akt and is susceptible to inhibition by rapamycin and its analogs, whereas mTORC2 is an upstream regulator of Akt and the activity is upregulated in certain circumstances as a compensatory response to mTORC1 inhibition.[40,41] Interestingly, recent evidence refuted the belief that mTORC2 is rapamycin resistant. It has been demonstrated that mTORC2 can, in fact, be inhibited by rapamycin and its analogs in a time- and cell line–dependent manner.[42,43]

Temsirolimus (CCI779) is a water-soluble synthetic rapamycin ester available in oral and intravenous formulations.[44] The drug is the first of the class to receive Food and Drug Administration (FDA) approval for the treatment of poor-risk untreated advanced renal cell carcinoma (RCC) patients.[45,46] In the pivotal randomized trial, temsirolimus was superior to interferon-α alone or in combination with interferon-α in prolonging survival. The most common grade 3 or 4 toxicities were asthenia, anemia, and dyspnea. The recommended dose of temsirolimus for this indication is 25 mg weekly intravenous administration. The drug is currently under testing in various tumor types either alone or in combination therapy.[46–49] A cohort of patients with NSCLC treated with temsirolimus as first-line therapy was assessed in a phase II study conducted by the North Central Cancer Treatment Group (trial 0323).[50] In a report of 50 evaluable patients primarily with stage IV disease, partial response (PRs) were observed in four patients (8%) and stable disease for a minimum of 56 days was observed in 15 patients (30%), suggesting an overall clinical benefit rate of 38%. Median progression-free survival (PFS) and OS were 2.3 and 6.6 months, respectively. Temsirolimus was noted to be well tolerated in this population of patients. A phase II study assessed the effect of temsirolimus alone as consolidation treatment in patients with extensive-stage small cell lung cancer (SCLC) in complete remission.[51] Temsirolimus was administered until the time of progression and in 85 evaluated patients, the median OS was 8 months. These results have prompted several studies of temsirolimus in combination with chemotherapy in SCLC.

Everolimus (RAD001) is an oral mTOR inhibitor with similar antineoplastic activity as other rapalogs.[52,53] In a phase I study in solid tumor patients, the optimal biologic dose for everolimus was determined as 20 mg weekly. This dose achieved pharmacokinetic and pharmacodynamic changes correlated with antineoplastic effects in animal models. Toxicities at this dose were mild and include anorexia, fatigue, rash, mucositis, headache, hyperlipidemia, and gastrointestinal disturbances.[54] When administered on a daily continuous manner, everolimus was well tolerated at a 10-mg dose in patients with refractory or relapsed hematological malignancies. No DLTs were reported and activity was seen in patients with myelodysplastic syndrome.[55] The dose of 5 mg/m^2 was the maximum tolerated dose (MTD) in pediatric solid tumor patients and DLTs (included diarrhea, mucositis, and elevation of alanine transaminase).[56] No objective tumor responses were observed. Everolimus was further tested in a clinical trial exclusively enrolling patients with NSCLC.[57] Patients in this phase II trial had an Eastern Cooperative Oncology Group (ECOG) performance status (PS) of ≤2 and had failed ≤2 cycles of platinum-based therapy (arm 1) or ≤2 cycles of platinum-based therapy with an EGFR antagonist (arm 2). Patients were treated with everolimus at a dose of 10 mg daily. In a preliminary report including 85 patients (42 patients on arm 1; 43 patients on arm 2), everolimus was administered as first- or second-line therapy in 64.3% of patients. With response data available for 74 patients in arms 1 and 2, a best response of PR was experienced in 5.3% and 2.8% of patients, respectively. Median PFS was 11.3 and 9.7 weeks on arms 1 and 2, respectively. The most frequent adverse events observed in the study were stomatitis/mucositis, cough, and dyspnea. Although therapy with everolimus was generally well tolerated, the limited antitumor activity led to discontinuation of the study.

A separate phase II study examined the efficacy of everolimus in the setting of refractory SCLC.[58] Patients enrolled in this trial had relapsed disease after 1 to 2 previous regimens, no evidence of brain metastases, and ECOG PS of ≤2. Everolimus was administered at a dose of 10 mg daily until disease progression or unacceptable toxicity. At an interim analysis in which 16 evaluable patients had been assessed, three patients had stable disease as a best response, whereas 81% of patients had progressive disease. Similar to the outcome in the aforementioned trial in patients with NSCLC, everolimus was well tolerated but showed limited efficacy in the setting of SCLC. The agent is being tested in non–small cell lung, kidney, prostate, colorectal, and breast cancers as either single-agent or combination therapies.[59–64]

Deforolimus (AP-23573) is the other mTOR inhibitor currently under clinical testing.[65–67] During phase I testing, the MTD was 18.75 mg/day and mouth sores was the DLT. Antitumor activity was seen in NSCLC, carcinosarcoma, RCC, and Ewing sarcoma. Phase II studies in sarcoma are ongoing.

Combination of Motor Inhibitors with Other Agents for Treatment of Lung Cancer A phase I study of gefitinib and everolimus therapy in 10 enrolled patients resulted in 2 DLT (grade 5 hypotension and grade 3 stomatitis), and 2 PRs were observed in 8 evaluable patients.[68] A phase II trial in previous smokers with stage IIIB/IV NSCLC[69] enrolled 2 cohorts of patients including previously untreated patients and patients with previous therapy with a platinating agent and docetaxel. Partial responses were observed in 4 of 23 evaluable patients (17%). This observed response rate in a group of smokers, for whom gefitinib has lessened antitumor activity, was encouraging. Frequently encountered toxicities with the regimen included diarrhea, rash, and mucosal ulcerations.

A phase I clinical trial combining everolimus with erlotinib[70] in patients with advanced NSCLC who had failed ≤2 chemotherapy regimens with an ECOG PS of ≤2 revealed 1 complete response and 3 PRs in 38 evaluable patients.

PKC Inhibitors Overexpression and increased activity of protein kinase C-β (PKC-β) have been implicated in transformation and tumorigenesis in NSCLC,[71–73] and recent evidence suggests a link between the PKC and protein kinase B/AK transforming (AKT) pathways.[74,75]

Enzastaurin, an oral serine/threonine kinase inhibitor, targets the PKC and AKT pathways and so inhibits phosphorylation of glycogen synthase kinase-3β and S^6kinase.[76] In a phase I dose–escalation study of daily oral enzastaurin (20 to 750 mg), four patients with advanced lung cancer had stable disease for 3 to 12 months.[77]

A phase II trial of enzastaurin to determine the 6-month PFS rate in 55 patients with advanced, metastatic NSCLC did not achieve its primary end point of a 20% PFS rate; however, 13% of the patients had PFS for ≥6 months.[78]

Akt Inhibitors Akt, also known as protein kinase B (PK-B), is a serine/threonine kinase upstream to mTORC1 and is implicated in the formation and maintenance of malignancies.[79] Akt is an attractive target as mTOR because of its role in several important cellular functions, including cell cycle progression, protein translation and transcription, apoptosis, and cellular metabolism. The side effects from Akt inhibition could theoretically be more severe than mTOR, given its key role in the axis, and the fact that its upstream of mTOR. The development of this class of agents has been challenging and disappointing so far.

Perifosine, a lipid-based derivative of miltefosine, is perhaps the best-characterized Akt inhibitor in clinical development now. The compound inhibits Akt translocation to the cell membrane and exhibits in vitro antiproliferative effects in several cancer cell lines.[80] It should be noted, however, that perifosine is a relatively nonspecific AKT inhibitor, and that by interrupting with cell membrane biology, pleiotropic effects on several signaling pathways and molecules are seen. Perifosine was tested as a daily oral dose on a 3-week cycle in patients with advanced solid tumors.[81] The patients reported dose-dependent gastrointestinal adverse events, such as nausea, diarrhea, and vomiting, which led to early therapy discontinuation in increasing number of patients at higher dose levels. The MTD was determined at 200 mg/day. An alternative loading/maintenance dosing schedule was tested in patients with advanced solid tumors.[82] The MTD was a loading dose of 150 mg every 6 hours for 4 doses followed by 100 mg once daily for maintenance. The DLTs during the loading period were nausea, diarrhea, dehydration, and fatigue and were manageable with prophylactic antiemetics. However, the side effects were more difficult to manage during the maintenance period. Despite encouraging evidence in preclinical studies, perifosine failed to demonstrate significant single-agent anticancer activity in sarcoma, melanoma, pancreatic, and head and neck cancers during phase II testings.[83–93] Perifosine continues to be evaluated as single-agent or combination therapies. GSK690693 is another Akt inhibitor planned for phase I testing.[94] Several lipid- and peptide-based Akt inhibitors are being evaluated preclinically.[95]

Currently, there is limited clinical experience with inhibitors of PI3k and 3-phosphoinositide-dependent protein kinase-1 (PDK-1). The ***PI3k inhibitors*** undergoing phase I evaluation include PI-103, BGT-226, BEZ-235, XL-765, and XL-147.[96–100] Current ***PDK-1 inhibitors*** are derivatives of staurosporin and celecoxib.[95] UCN-01 is a staurosporin derivative that inhibits multiple kinases including PDK-1 and has in vitro pro-apoptotic activity.[101,102] The drug is synergistic with cytotoxic agents in preclinical studies but the pro-apoptotic activity seemed to be from the inhibition of checkpoint homologue (Chk1), a cell cycle checkpoint kinase.[103] UCN-01 can be administered intravenously as an initial 72-hour continuous infusion on a monthly schedule or short infusion over 3 hours every 28 days with the second and subsequent doses at 50% of the first.[104,105] However, the clinical activity of UCN-01 was not associated with PI3k/Akt/mTOR pathway inhibition and its role as a PDK-1 inhibitor remains ambiguous. OSU-03012 is a celecoxib derivative that inhibits PDK-1 and induced apoptosis in rhabdomyosarcoma cell lines.[106] This drug is currently still under preclinical evaluation.

c-Met The protein product of *c-Met* proto-oncogene is a transmembrane RTK that is activated by the multifunctional cytokine hepatocyte growth factor (HGF)/scatter factor (SF),[107] which increases signaling through the Raf/MEK/ERK pathway.[108] HGF/SF mediates epithelial cell morphogenesis, migration, invasion, and differentiation.[107] HGF/SF is produced predominantly by mesenchymal cells, whereas c-Met is expressed primarily in epithelial cells.

Overexpression of c-Met is implicated in several tumor types, including glioblastomas, RCC,[109] hepatocellular carcinoma (HCC),[110] pancreatic adenocarcinomas,[111] thyroid carcinomas,[112] melanoma,[113] breast,[107] gastric,[114] pancreatic,[115] prostate, and lung cancers.[116,117]

There are currently several HGF/c-MET inhibitors under clinical evaluation. AMG-102 is a fully humanized immunoglobulin G2 (IgG2) MoAb against HGF with antitumor activity in preclinical models.[118] The interim result of the phase I study was reported at American Society of Clinical Oncology (ASCO) annual meeting in 2007.[119] The agent was administered intravenously at 0.5-, 1-, 3-, 5-, 10-, or 20-mg/kg dose levels. Patients with advanced solid tumors received a single dose followed by a 4-week treatment free period to assess safety and pharmacokinetic profile. The treatment was subsequently resumed at a 2 weekly schedule. Thirty-one patients were treated at doses up to 20 mg/kg. DLTs include dyspnea/hypoxia (at 0.5-mg/kg dose) and gastrointestinal bleed (at 1-mg/kg dose). Common treatment-related side effects include fatigue, constipation, anorexia, nausea, and vomiting. Pharmacokinetic analysis showed a linear relationship in the dose range of 0.5- to 20-mg/kg and no anti-AMG-102 antibodies were detected following administration. The 20-mg/kg dose was deemed tolerable and safe and the agent is being tested in RCC and malignant glioma.[120,121]

XL-880 is an oral small molecule inhibitor of c-MET and has activity against vascular endothelial growth factor receptor 2 (VEGFR2), PDGFR-β, kit, FLT3, Tie-2, and Ron. The interim result of the phase I study was presented at ASCO 2007 and two schedules were tested: a "5-day on/ 9-day off" schedule and a daily fixed-dose schedule.[122] Fifty-one solid tumor patients were enrolled and hypertension was universally observed. The DLTs with the first schedule were proteinuria and elevated lipase and liver enzymes. The MTD was 3.6 mg/kg and the MTD for the second schedule was not reached at the time of analysis, and common side effects include hypertension and fatigue. Correlative studies showed inhibition of c-MET, RON, Erk, Akt, and increased apoptosis at dose levels less than MTD. The agent is being evaluated in papillary RCC gastric and head and neck cancers.[123–125]

ARQ-197 and PF-02341066 are similar oral small-molecule c-Met inhibitors that are in early phase trials.[126] The recommended phase II dose for ARQ-197 was determined to be 120 mg twice daily. Common side effects include fatigue, diarrhea and constipation, and grade 3 elevated liver enzymes were the more severe toxicity.[127] Compounds with activity against the HGF/c-MET axis in the preclinical pipeline include MGCD-265, SU-11274, and MGCD-265.[128–131]

c-Kit Stem cell factor signaling through its transmembrane RTK c-Kit is essential for development of erythrocytes, melanocytes, germ cells, and mast cells. Cellular responses mediated by the c-Kit RTK include proliferation, survival, adhesion, secretion, and differentiation.[132] Overexpression of the c-Kit proto-oncogene results in the development of tumors,[133,134] including oncocytomas and chromophobe RCC,[135] SCLC,[136] uveal melanoma,[137,138] acute myeloid leukemia (AML),[139] colorectal cancer (CRC),[140] gastrointestinal stromal tumor (GIST),[141] and HCC.[142] Overactivation of c-Kit protects colon carcinoma cells against apoptosis and enhances their invasive potential.[143]

Flt-3 The growth factor ligand Flt-3 stimulates proliferation of hematopoietic progenitor cells of lymphoid and myeloid origin[144] and helps modulate cell proliferation and hematopoiesis.[145] Overexpression of Flt-3 leading to its constitutive activation increases proliferation and prolongs cell survival of leukemic blasts in AML. Activating internal tandem duplication (ITD) mutations of the Flt-3 (Flt-3-ITD) gene are the most frequent molecular abnormalities in AML, occurring in ~30% of cases,[146,147] and are associated with poor OS.[148]

RET The RET proto-oncogene encodes a transmembrane RTK that contains several internal autophosphorylation sites, which can activate the Raf/MEK/ERK, PI3K/AKT, p38, or c-Jun N-terminal kinase signaling pathways.[149]

Oncogenic RET promotes invasion and metastasis by increasing cell survival through AKT-mediated nuclear factor kappa-light-chain-enhancer of activated B cells (NF-κB) activation, BAD inactivation, and cyclin D1-mediated cell cycle progression.[150] RET mutations are responsible for the development of familial medullary thyroid carcinoma (MTC), papillary thyroid carcinoma (PTC), and multiple endocrine neoplasia 2A and 2B, which share clinical features of MTC.[151] Somatic chromosomal rearrangements of RET occur in 5% to 30% of sporadic and 60% to 70% of radiation-associated PTCs.[151] Somatic mutations constitutively activate RET to upregulate expression of the chemokine receptor CXCR4 in metastatic MTC.[152] Vandetanib is a novel, selective inhibitor of RET kinases, VEGFRs 2 and 3, and EGFR. Laboratory studies in human lung cancer cell line models demonstrated that vandetanib is comparable to other EGFR inhibitors in causing regression of established HCC827 xenografts.[153]

Vandetanib also was effective in cell lines with acquired resistance to EGFR inhibition (T790M mutation) and in cell lines with overexpression of K-ras.

Two phase I clinical trials with vandetanib established that daily oral doses up to 300 mg were generally well tolerated, with the most common adverse events consisting of mild-to-moderate rash, diarrhea, and asymptomatic QTc prolongation.[154,155]

Moreover, in Tamura's study, there were objective responses in four of nine Japanese patients with advanced NSCLC. A phase II, randomized, double-blind comparison of vandetanib and gefitinib in previously treated patients with advanced or metastatic NSCLC revealed that patients in the vandetanib arm achieved a statistically significant improvement in PFS compared with the gefitinib arm with a hazard ratio of 0.69 (95% confidence interval [CI], 0.50 to 0.96) and a two-sided p value of 0.025. Vandetanib achieved disease control in 16 of 37 patients (43%) who were initially treated with gefitinib. However, gefitinib achieved disease control in only 7 of 29 patients (24%) initially treated with vandetanib. A run-in feasibility study of docetaxel combined with vandetanib followed by a 3-armed phase II randomized trial of docetaxel, 75 mg/m^2 every 3 weeks alone or combined with 100 mg/day or 300 mg/day of vandetanib 5. One hundred twenty-seven patients were entered into the trial, and both vandetanib arms produced an improvement in PFS compared with the docetaxel control arm, but only the 100-mg dose level of vandetanib combined with docetaxel achieved the study end point, with a hazard ratio of 0.64 (95% CI, 0.38 to 1.05).[156] A phase III trial of second-line alimta compared to vandetanib has completed accrual.

Proliferative and Anti-apoptotic Cytoplasmic Nonreceptor Kinases

Raf Kinase Raf is a serine/threonine kinase member of the Raf/MEK/ERK signaling pathway,[157] which regulates many cellular processes, including growth, proliferation, differentiation, motility, and survival, in response to growth factors and cytokines.[157] Activation of Raf is initiated by association with

Ras-GTP, which then phosphorylates MEK, resulting in activation of ERK.[158] There are three functional isoforms of Raf (A-Raf, B-Raf, and Raf-1 [C-Raf]); B-Raf has the highest basal kinase activity; Raf-1 is ubiquitously expressed in tissues.

Dysregulated signaling through Raf is associated with several solid tumor types, including RCC,[159] HCC,[160] CRC,[161] and thyroid cancer.[162] Activating Ras mutations that increase Raf activity are present in ~30% of human cancers.[163] Oncogenic-activating B-Raf mutations are associated with ~60% of malignant melanomas[164] and are found in PTC,[165] colorectal,[166] pancreatic,[167] ovarian carcinomas,[168] and some cases of NSCLC.[164] Approximately 90% of B-Raf mutations involve a Glu-for-Val substitution at residue 599 (V599E, now termed V600E), which upregulates the kinase activity leading to constitutive activation of ERK.[158] Raf-1 can directly prolong cell survival independently of MEK/ERK by upregulating the anti-apoptotic proteins NF-κB[169] and Mcl-1, or directly inhibiting pro-apoptotic proteins, such as BAD,[170] apoptosis signal-regulating kinase,[171] and MST-2.[172]

Inactivating mutations within the von-Hippel Lindau (VHL) tumor suppressor gene, leading to overexpression of hypoxia-regulated genes, including VEGF, PDGF-β, and transforming growth factor α (TGF-α), results in uncontrolled stimulation of Raf-1.[173] VHL mutations are associated with various tumors, including RCC,[174] eye and CNS hemangioblastomas, and pheochromocytoma.[175]

Sorafenib (BAY43-9006) is an oral dual inhibitor of Raf and VEGFR. The molecule demonstrated preclinical antineoplastic activity against a wide spectrum of human cancers.[176] It has potent in vitro inhibitory effects against Raf-1, B-Raf, VEGFR2, PDGFR, and VEGFR3.[177,178] Sorafenib is approved by FDA for the treatment of advanced RCC and HCC.[177,179] The DLTs reported during phase I development were diarrhea, fatigue, and skin rashes.[180] The recommended dose is 400 mg twice daily on continuous basis. Rash, diarrhea, fatigue, and hand–foot syndrome were the common side effects during phase II and III studies.[181,182] Correlative studies showed mitogen-activated protein kinase (MAPK) pathway inhibition in peripheral lymphocytes with a sorafenib dose above 200 mg, indicating the potential usefulness of this pharmacodynamic assay in the development of Raf inhibitors.[180]

However, the contribution of Raf inhibition to sorafenib's clinical efficacy is difficult to assess. The success of bevacizumab and sunitinib in RCC indicated that the drug's anticancer effects may be related more to its antiangiogenic effects.[183,184] The real benefit of Raf inhibition in cancer therapy will perhaps only be answered by specific Raf inhibitors. A discussion of sorafenib lung cancer trials is found in Chapter 48.

XL-281 and PLX-4032 are oral inhibitors that are, reportedly, highly selective against Raf currently in phase I testing.[185–187] RAF-265 (CHIR-265) is another oral inhibitor of Raf and VEGFR in early phase trial.[188,189]

MEK Raf/MEK/ERK cascades form a three-kinase signaling module involved in transmitting membrane signals to the cell nucleus; MAPK (ERK) activated by MAP/ERK kinase (MEK, MAPKK), which, in turn, is activated by a MEK kinase (Raf, MEKK, MAPKKK).[190] Stimulation of MEK results in phosphorylation and activation of ribosomal S6 kinase and transcription factors, such as *c-Jun*, *c-Myc*, and *c-Fos*, resulting in the switching on of genes associated with proliferation.[157,191] MEK has roles in gene regulation,[156,190] promoting G1 cell cycle progression before DNA replication,[192] and spindle assembly during both meiotic and mitotic cell division.[193] Overactivation of the Raf/MEK/ERK pathway, through oncogenic mutations, can result in cellular transformation tumorigenesis.[194,195]

The Ras/Raf/MEK/ERK pathway is constitutively activated in various tumor cell lines and primary human tumor types.[196] Although MEK has not been identified as an oncogene product, it is the focal point of many mitogenic signaling pathways that are hyperactivated by oncogenes. MEK can also be hyperactivated by autocrine signaling through VEGFR, PDGFR, or EGFR in tumor cells. Inhibition of MEK inhibits several cellular processes, including proliferation, differentiation, apoptosis, and angiogenesis.[197]

CI-1040 is one of the first MEK inhibitors to be developed clinically. The oral agent demonstrated encouraging preclinical effects on tumor proliferation, survival, invasion, and angiogenesis.[198] Phase I study showed that the drug had poor metabolic stability and bioavailability that high doses had to be administered in phase II trials.[199,200] The encouraging antitumor activity seen in phase I development was not seen in phase II studies, leading to the termination of the agent's development. Despite this, correlative studies from phase I trial showed adequate target inhibition with CI-1040 and subsequent research effort was focused on improving on CI-1040.

PD0325901 is a second-generation MEK inhibitor that is structurally related to CI-1040. PD0325901 has a higher potency, better bioavailability, and induces more sustained MEK inhibition than CI-1040. Preclinical studies showed antitumor activities against a broad spectrum of human cancer cell lines.[201] The DLTs reported during phase I development include acneiform rash, syncope, and elevated liver enzymes.[202] Visual disturbances such as halos, spots, and decreased acuity were also reported. Antitumor effects were seen in melanoma, colon, and NSCLC. Phase II trials in melanoma, breast, lung, and colon cancers had ceased enrolling patients at the time of writing.[203,204]

AZD-6244 (ARRY-142886) is another second-generation, highly selective MEK inhibitor. The drug inhibited Erk phosphorylation, and was associated with growth inhibition in cell lines containing B-Raf and Ras mutations, and tumor regression in preclinical xenograft models.[205] The DLTs during phase I development were hypoxia, rash, and diarrhea, and common adverse events include nausea, fatigue, peripheral edema, altered taste, and blurred vision.[206] The recommended phase II dose was determined to be 200 mg twice daily. The best response was stable disease observed in three melanoma and one NSCLC patients. AZD6244 is being tested in phase II trials of various cancers, including lung, liver, colorectal, pancreas, and ovary.[207–210] Other MEK inhibitors under phase I testing include XL-518 and RDEA-119.[211,212]

Aurora Kinases Aurora kinases are microtubule-associated serine/threonine kinases that help control cell division. The three family members of the mammalian serine/threonine Aurora kinases, Aurora-A, -B, and -C, have roles in regulating the mitotic processes required for genome stability.[213] The Aurora-A gene is located on chromosome 20q13.2–13.3. Aurora-A localizes to centrosomes/spindle poles, facilitates assembly of the mitotic spindle,[213] and can promote neoplastic transformation. Overexpression of Aurora-A may result in abnormal mitosis because of the inability of chromosomes to orientate correctly on the mitotic spindle.[214] In cells with functional p53, this results in cell cycle arrest and apoptosis.[214] However, in cells lacking functional p53, Aurora-A overexpression leads to uncontrolled cell cycle progression, with abnormal segregation of the chromosomes and aneuploidy.[214] This can result in the overexpression of oncogenes, loss of tumor suppressor genes, and development of a malignant phenotype.[214] MLN8054 is a novel small molecule oral Aurora A kinase inhibitor, which has demonstrated specificity and potency against its Aurora kinase and also demonstrated broad activity both in vitro and in vivo at doses that were well tolerated. Phase I trials with the molecule are underway.

The Aurora-B gene is located on chromosome 17p13. Aurora-B is a chromosome passenger protein required for phosphorylation of histone H3, chromosome segregation, and cytokinesis.[213] Dysregulation of Aurora-B can also lead to aneuploidy.[215] Aurora-C also appears to act as a chromosome passenger that cooperates with Aurora-B,[216] localizing to the spindle poles during late-stage mitosis.[217] Overexpression of Aurora-A and/or -B has been reported in breast,[218] colon,[219] ovarian,[220] bladder,[221] and gastric tumors.[222] Furthermore, Aurora-B is overexpressed in human androgen-independent prostate cancer cells.[223]

Bcr-Abl The fusion protein Bcr-Abl is a nonreceptor tyrosine kinase created by the translocation of the "bcr" gene (chromosome 22) to the "abl" gene (chromosome 9), which generates the characteristic Philadelphia (Ph) chromosome and leads to the formation of the "bcr-abl" oncogene.[7] Bcr-Abl is constitutively active and overstimulates mitogenic pathways that promote cell division and oncogenesis. Whereas Abl can translocate to the nucleus to induce apoptosis, Bcr-Abl is retained in the cytoplasm and has no pro-apoptotic effect. The Ph chromosome is found in most cases of chronic myelogenous leukemia (CML) and many cases of adult acute lymphoblastic leukemia.[224]

Src The product of the SRC proto-oncogene, c-Src, is a nonreceptor tyrosine kinase that regulates cell division, adhesion, migration, invasion, resistance to apoptosis, and angiogenesis.[225–227] c-Src is associated with cancers of the breast,[228] colorectum,[229] lung (NSCLC),[230] stomach, pancreas, brain, and blood, and, to a lesser extent, melanomas.[227] Protein levels of c-Src are elevated 2- to 50-fold relative to normal tissue in ~70% of breast tumors.[228,231,232] c-Src may also promote tumor growth by augmenting signaling pathways initiated by oncogenes or growth factors, such as EGF.[233]

Accumulating data suggest that Src plays an important role in affecting cancer cell mitosis, adhesion, invasion, motility, and progression.[234] Src mediates the mitogenic signals between growth factor receptors, such as EGFR, c-Met, and IGF-1R, and downstream signaling cascades, such as focal adhesion kinase (FAK), MAPK, and PI3k/Akt/mTOR.[235,236] Dysregulated Src activity has been implicated in the development and progression of several human cancers, including breast, colorectal, lung, ovary, and hematological malignancies.[237,238] As such, much interest exists in developing Src-targeting compounds for cancer therapy.

Dasatinib (BMS-354825) is an orally available dual-specific Src and Abl kinase inhibitor with antiproliferative activity against a broad spectrum of hematological and solid cancer cell lines.[239] The compound has less stringent conformational requirement for Abl kinase inhibition than imatinib, dasatinib is active against many imatinib-resistant Bcr/Abl mutants in preclinical models.[240–242] Dasatinib was granted accelerated approval by FDA in 2006 for treatment of chronic phase, accelerated phase, or myeloid or lymphoid blast phase CML with resistance or intolerance to prior imatinib therapy following the pivotal large randomized trial.[243,244] In addition, dasatinib was approved for Ph chromosome-positive acute lymphoblastic leukemia. The toxicities include superficial edema, pleural effusion, constitutional and gastrointestinal and hematological events. Bleeding was reported in 40% of patients, of which 14% had gastrointestinal bleed. The recommended dosing schedules include 70 mg twice daily and 100 mg once daily. As a multikinase inhibitor, dasatinib is being evaluated in breast, lung, colorectal, and pancreatic cancers.[245–249] The effect of dasatinib on NSCLC cells is cell line dependent and includes cell cycle arrest, apoptosis, and/or reduced invasion. EGFR status/independency seems to be predictive of response. A phase II study of 13 chemonaive NSCLC patients performed at MD Anderson Cancer Center using oral dasatinib 100 mg twice daily (bid) revealed one partial response and five stable disease effects as of February 2008. A phase II trial of progressive NSCLC after EGFR TKI failure is presently accruing patients at Memorial Sloan-Kettering Cancer Center in New York.

Bosutinib (SKI-606) is another potent oral Src inhibitor, with anti-Abl activities. The compound demonstrated antitumor activities in preclinical models and clinical development in hematological and solid malignancies are underway.[250–252] AZD-0530, XL-999, and XL-228 are other Src inhibitors undergoing early phase testing.[253,254] Most of these small molecules have activities against other kinases as well.

CONCLUSION

In recent years, advances in the understanding of the cellular signaling pathways involved in tumorigenesis have led to the discovery of novel molecular targets for therapeutic intervention.[5] In particular, protein kinases are important regulators of intracellular signal–transduction pathways and have critical roles in modulating growth-factor signaling. Dysregulation of these enzymes is associated with the pathogenesis and progression of tumors.[6] Targeted inhibition of protein kinases is an attractive anticancer strategy and represents an advance in the management of advanced refractory tumors.[255] Targeted therapy has the potential to reduce the problems of toxicity associated with cytotoxic chemotherapy. At present, the most successful approach to inhibiting cell signaling appears to be the utilization of agents inhibiting multiple kinase targets (sorafenib, sunitinib) and MoAbs against these targets (bevacizumab, cetuximab, panitumumab).

It will become important to identify biomarkers to help predict the success of targeted agents and aid selection of patients most likely to respond to these therapies. For example, overactive Bcr-Abl tyrosine kinase is critical to the pathogenesis of CML.[223] c-Kit mutations are pivotal in GIST, and evaluation of the c-Kit gene may have prognostic and therapeutic significance.[140]

REFERENCES

1. Kumar CC, Madison V. Drugs targeted against protein kinases. *Expert Opin Emerg Drugs* 2001;6:303–315.
2. Stewart BW, Kelihues P. World Cancer Report. Lyon, France: IARC Press, 2003.
3. Segota E, Bukowski RM. The promise of targeted therapy: cancer drugs become more specific. *Cleve Clin J Med* 2004;71:551–560.
4. Arora A, Scholar EM. Role of tyrosine kinase inhibitors in cancer therapy. *J Pharmacol Exp Ther* 2005;315:971–979.
5. Adjei AA, Rowinsky EK. Novel anticancer agents in clinical development. *Cancer Biol Ther* 2003;2:S5–S15.
6. Krause DS, Van Etten RA. Tyrosine kinases as targets for cancer therapy. *N Engl J Med* 2005;353:172–187.
7. Blume-Jensen P, Hunter T. Oncogenic kinase signalling. *Nature* 2001;411:355–365.
8. Adjei AA, Hidalgo M. Intracellular signal transduction pathway proteins as targets for cancer therapy. *J Clin Oncol* 2005;23:5386–5403.
9. Jerome L, Shiry L, Leyland-Jones B. Deregulation of the IGF axis in cancer: epidemiological evidence and potential therapeutic interventions. *Endocr Relat Cancer* 2003;10:561–578.
10. Mauro L, Salerno M, Morelli C, et al. Role of the IGF-I receptor in the regulation of cell-cell adhesion: implications in cancer development and progression. *J Cell Physiol* 2003;194:108–116.
11. Rajah R, Khare A, Lee PD, et al. Insulin-like growth factor-binding protein-3 is partially responsible for high-serum-induced apoptosis in PC-3 prostate cancer cells. *J Endocrinol* 1999;163:487–494.
12. Ibrahim YH, Yee D. Insulin-like growth factor-I and breast cancer therapy. *Clin Cancer Res* 2005;11:S944–S950.
13. Chan JM, Stampfer MJ, Giovannucci E, et al. Insulin-like growth factor I (IGF-I), IGF-binding protein-3 and prostate cancer risk: epidemiological studies. *Growth Horm IGF Res* 2000;10 Suppl A: S32–S33.
14. Yu H, Spitz MR, Mistry J, et al. Plasma levels of insulin-like growth factor-I and lung cancer risk: a case-control analysis. *J Natl Cancer Inst* 1999;91:151–156.
15. Davies M, Gupta S, Goldspink G, et al. The insulin-like growth factor system and colorectal cancer: clinical and experimental evidence. *Int J Colorectal Dis* 2006;21:201–208.
16. Cohen BD, Baker DA, Soderstrom C, et al. Combination therapy enhances the inhibition of tumor growth with the fully human anti-type 1 insulin-like growth factor receptor monoclonal antibody CP-751,871. *Clin Cancer Res* 2005;11:2063–2073.
17. Haluska P, Shaw HM, Batzel GN, et al. Phase I dose escalation study of the anti insulin-like growth factor-I receptor monoclonal antibody CP-751,871 in patients with refractory solid tumors. *Clin Cancer Res* 2007;13:5834–5840.
18. de Bono JS, Attard G, Adjei A, et al. Potential applications for circulating tumor cells expressing the insulin-like growth factor-I receptor. *Clin Cancer Res* 2007;13:3611–3616.
19. Karp DD, Paz-Ares LG, Blakely LJ, et al. Efficacy of the anti-insulin like growth factor I receptor (IGF-IR) antibody CP-751871 in combination with paclitaxel and carboplatin as first-line treatment for advanced non-small cell lung cancer (NSCLC). *J Clin Oncol ASCO Annual Meeting Proceedings Part I* 2007;25(18S):7506.
20. Lacy M, Alsina M, Melvin CL, et al. Phase 1 first-in-human dose escalation study of cp-751,871, a specific monoclonal antibody against the insulin like growth factor 1 receptor. *J Clin Oncol. 2006 ASCO Annual Meeting Proceedings Part I* 2006;24:18S(June 20 Supplement). 7609.
21. Carboplatin and Paclitaxel With or Without CP-751, 871 (An IGF-1R Inhibitor) For Advanced NSCLC Of Squamous, Large Cell And Adenosquamous Carcinoma Histology. Available at: http://www.ClinicalTrials.gov/ct2/show/NCT00596830. ClinicalTrials.gov identifier: NCT00596830. Accessed October 10, 2009.
22. Study of CP-751,871 in Combination With Cisplatin and Gemcitabine in Chemotherapy-naïve Patients With Advanced Non-Small Cell Lung Cancer. Available at: http://www.ClinicalTrials.gov/ct2/show/NCT00560573. ClinicalTrials.gov identifier: NCT00560573. Accessed October 10, 2009.
23. Attard G, Fong PC, Molife R, et al. Phase I trial involving the pharmacodynamic (PD) study of circulating tumour cells, of CP-751,871 (C), a monoclonal antibody against the insulin-like growth factor 1 receptor (IGF-1R), with docetaxel (D) in patients (p) with advanced cancer. *J Clin Oncol, 2006 ASCO Annual Meeting Proceedings Part I* 2006;24:18S(June 20 Supplement). 3023.
24. Beltran PJ, Mitchell P, Moody G, et al. AMG-479, a fully human anti IGF-1 receptor antibody, inhibits PI3K/Akt signaling and exerts potent antitumor effects in combination with EGF-R inhibitors in pancreatic xenograft models. *2007 Gastrointestinal Cancers Symposium*. San Francisco, CA. Abstract No. 208.
25. Tolcher A, Rothenberg M, Rodon J, et al. A phase I pharmacokinetic and pharmacodynamic study of AMG 479, a fully human monoclonal antibody against insulin-like growth factor type 1 receptor (IGF-1R), in advanced solid tumors. *J Clin Oncol 2007 ASCO Annual Meeting Proceedings Part I* 2007;2518S(June 20 Supplement). 3002.
26. AMG-479 in Treating Patients With Advanced Solid Tumors or Non-Hodgkin Lymphoma. Available at: http://www.ClinicalTrials.gov/ct2/show/NCT00562380. ClinicalTrials.gov identifier: NCT00562380. Accessed October 10, 2009.
27. A Phase 2 Study of AMG 479 in Relapsed or Refractory Ewing's Family Tumor and Desmoplastic Small Round Cell Tumors. Available at: http://www.ClinicalTrials.gov/ct2/show/NCT00563680. ClinicalTrials.gov identifier: NCT00563680. Accessed October 10, 2009.
28. Amgen Product Pipeline: AMG 479. Available at: http://www.amgen.com/science/pipe_AMG479.html. Accessed March 03, 2008.
29. Vignot S, Faivre S, Aguirre D, et al. mTOR-targeted therapy of cancer with rapamycin derivatives. *Ann Oncol* 2005;16:525–537.
30. Paez J, Sellers WR. PI3K/PTEN/AKT pathway. A critical mediator of oncogenic signaling. *Cancer Treat Res* 2003;115:145–167.
31. Li B, Desai SA, MacCorkle-Chosnek RA, et al. A novel conditional Akt 'survival switch' reversibly protects cells from apoptosis. *Gene Ther* 2002;9:233–244.
32. Chang SM, Wen P, Cloughesy T, et al. Phase II study of CCI-779 in patients with recurrent glioblastoma multiforme. *Invest New Drugs* 2005;23:357–361.
33. Janus A, Robak T, Smolewski P. The mammalian target of the rapamycin (mTOR) kinase pathway: its role in tumourigenesis and targeted anti-tumour therapy. *Cell Mol Biol Lett* 2005;10:479–498.
34. DeGraffenried LA, Fulcher L, Friedrichs WE, et al. Reduced PTEN expression in breast cancer cells confers susceptibility to inhibitors of the PI3 kinase/Akt pathway. *Ann Oncol* 2004;15:1510–1516.

35. Hipp S, Ringshausen I, Oelsner M, et al. Inhibition of the mammalian target of rapamycin and the induction of cell cycle arrest in mantle cell lymphoma cells. *Haematologica* 2005;90:1433–1434.
36. Staunton J, Wilkinson B. Biosynthesis of Erythromycin and Rapamycin. *Chem Rev* 1997;97:2611–2630.
37. Augustine JJ, Bodziak KA, Hricik DE. Use of sirolimus in solid organ transplantation. *Drugs* 2007;67:369–391.
38. Jimeno A, Kulesza P, Cusati G, et al. Pharmacodynamic-guided, modified continuous reassessment method (mCRM)-based, dose finding study of rapamycin in adult patients with solid tumors. *J Clin Oncol, 2006 ASCO Annual Meeting Proceedings Part I* 2006;24:18S(June 20 Supplement). 3020.
39. Ma WW, Hidalgo M. Exploiting novel molecular targets in gastrointestinal cancers. *World J Gastroenterol* 2007;13:5845–5856.
40. Sarbassov DD, Guertin DA, Ali SM, et al. Phosphorylation and regulation of Akt/PKB by the rictor-mTOR complex. *Science* 2005;307: 1098–1101.
41. Sabatini DM. mTOR and cancer: insights into a complex relationship. *Nat Rev Cancer* 2006;6:729–734.
42. Jacinto E, Loewith R, Schmidt A, et al. Mammalian TOR complex 2 controls the actin cytoskeleton and is rapamycin insensitive. *Nat Cell Biol* 2004;6:1122–1128.
43. Sarbassov DD, Ali SM, Sengupta S, et al. Prolonged rapamycin treatment inhibits mTORC2 assembly and Akt/PKB. *Mol Cell* 2006;22:159–168.
44. Ma WW, Jimeno A. Temsirolimus. *Drugs Today (Barc)* 2007;43:659–669.
45. FDA Approval for Temsirolimus. Available at: http://www.nci.nih.gov/cancertopics/druginfo/fda-temsirolimus. Accessed March 15, 2008.
46. Hudes G, Carducci M, Tomczak P, et al. Temsirolimus, interferon alfa, or both for advanced renal-cell carcinoma. *N Engl J Med* 2007;356:2271–2281.
47. Sorafenib and Temsirolimus in Treating Patients with Metastatic, Recurrent, or Unresectable Melanoma. Available at: http://clinicaltrials.gov/ct/show/NCT00349206. ClinicalTrials.gov identifier: NCT00349206. Accessed October 10, 2009.
48. Bevacizumab, Sorafenib, and Temsirolimus in Treating Patients With Metastatic Kidney Cancer. Available at: http://clinicaltrials.gov/ct/show/NCT00378703. ClinicalTrials.gov identifier: NCT00378703. Accessed October 10, 2009.
49. Temsirolimus (CCI-770, Torisel) Combined With Cetuximab in Cetuximab-Refractory Colorectal Cancer. Available at: http://www.ClinicalTrials.gov/ct2/show/NCT00593060. ClinicalTrials.gov identifier:NCT00593060. Accessed October 10, 2009.
50. Molina JR, Mandrekar SJ, Rowland K, et al. A phase II NCCTG "Window of Opportunity Front-line" study of the mTOR inhibitor, CCI-779 (temsirolimus) given as a single agent in patients with advanced NSCLC. J Thor Oncol 2007; 2(suppl):s413 (abstract D7-07).
51. Pandya K, Dahlberg S, Hidalgo M, et al. A randomized, phase ii trial of two dose levels of temsirolimus (CCI-779) in patients with extensive-stage small-cell lung cancer who have responding or stable disease after induction chemotherapy: a trial of the Eastern Cooperative Oncology Group (E1500). *J Thorac Oncol* 2007;2:1036–1041.
52. Combination CCI-779 (Temsirolimus) and Bortezomib (Velcade) in Relapsed and/or Relapsed/Refractory Multiple Myeloma. Available at: http://www.ClinicalTrials.gov/ct2/show/NCT00483262. ClinicalTrials.gov identifier:NCT00483262. Accessed October 10, 2009.
53. A Phase I Study of CCI-779 (Temsirolimus) in Combination With Topotecan in Patients With Gynecologic Malignancies. Available at: http://www.ClinicalTrials.gov/ct2/show/NCT00523432. ClinicalTrials.gov identifier: NCT00523432. Accessed October 10, 2009.
54. Boulay A, Zumstein-Mecker S, Stephan C, et al. Antitumor efficacy of intermittent treatment schedules with the rapamycin derivative RAD001 correlates with prolonged inactivation of ribosomal protein S6 kinase 1 in peripheral blood mononuclear cells. *Cancer Res* 2004;64:252–261.
55. Lane H, Tanakam C, Kovarik J, et al. Preclinical and clinical pharmacokinetic/pharmacodynamic (PK/PD) modeling to help define an optimal biological dose for the oral mTOR inhibitor, RAD001, in oncology. *Proc Am Soc Clin Oncol* 2003:22 (abstract 951).
56. O'Donnell A, Faivre S, Judson I, et al. A phase I study of the oral mTOR inhibitor RAD001 as monotherapy to identify the optimal biologically effective dose using toxicity, pharmacokinetic (PK) and pharmacodynamic (PD) endpoints in patients with solid tumours. *Proc Am Soc Clin Oncol* 2003:22 (abstract 803).
57. Papadimitrakopoulou V, Soria JC, Douillard JY, et al. A phase II study of RAD001 (R) (everolimus) monotherapy in patients (pts) with advanced non-small cell lung cancer (NSCLC) failing prior platinum-based chemotherapy (C) or prior C and EGFR inhibitors (EGFR-I). *J Clin Oncol* 2007; 25(18 suppl):406s (abstract 7589).
58. Owonikoko TK, Stoller RG, Petro D, et al. Phase II study of RAD001 (everolimus) in previously treated small cell lung cancer (SCLC). *J Clin Oncol* 2008; 26(15 suppl):707s (abstract 19017).
59. Yee KW, Zeng Z, Konopleva M, et al. Phase I/II study of the mammalian target of rapamycin inhibitor everolimus (RAD001) in patients with relapsed or refractory hematologic malignancies. *Clin Cancer Res* 2006;12:5165–5173.
60. Fouladi M, Laningham F, Wu J, et al. Phase I study of everolimus in pediatric patients with refractory solid tumors. *J Clin Oncol* 2007;25:4806–4812.
61. Rosenberg J, Weinberg V, Claros C, et al. Phase I study of sorafenib and RAD001 for advanced clear cell renal cell carcinoma. *2008 Genitourinary Cancers Symposium*. San Francisco, CA. Abstract No. 356.
62. Milton DT, Riely GJ, Azzoli CG, et al. Phase 1 trial of everolimus and gefitinib in patients with advanced nonsmall-cell lung cancer. *Cancer* 2007;110:599–605.
63. Gridelli C, Rossi A, Morgillo F, et al. A randomized phase II study of pemetrexed or RAD001 as second-line treatment of advanced non-small-cell lung cancer in elderly patients: treatment rationale and protocol dynamics. *Clin Lung Cancer* 2007;8:568–571.
64. George DJ, Armstrong AJ, Creel P, et al. A phase II study of RAD001 in men with hormone-refractory metastatic prostate cancer (HRPC). *2008 Genitourinary Cancers Symposium*. San Francisco, CA. Abstract No. 181.
65. Gold PJ, Iriarte D, Arthur J, et al. Phase II trial of RAD001 in patients with refracory metastatic colorectal cancer. *2008 Gastrointestinal Cancers Symposium*. Orlando, FL, 2008. Abstract No. 513.
66. Ellard SG, K. A., Chia S, Clemons M, et al. A randomized phase II study of two different schedules of RAD001C in patients with recurrent/metastatic breast cancer. Journal of Clinical Oncology, *2007 ASCO Annual Meeting Proceedings Part I* 2007;25:18S(June 20 Supplement). 3513.
67. Mita MM, Mita AC, Chu QS, et al. Phase I trial of the novel mammalian target of rapamycin inhibitor deforolimus (AP23573; MK-8669) administered intravenously daily for 5 days every 2 weeks to patients with advanced malignancies. *J Clin Oncol* 2008;26:361–367.
68. Milton DT, Riely GJ, Azzoli CG, et al. Phase 1 trial of everolimus and gefitinib in patients with advanced nonsmall-cell lung cancer. *Cancer* 2007;110:599–605.
69. Kris MG, Riely GJ, Azzoli CG, et al. Combined inhibition of mTOR and EGFR with everolimus (RAD001) and gefitinib in patients with non-small cell lung cancer who have smoked cigarettes: A phase II trial. *J Clin Oncol* 2007;25(18 suppl):403s (Abstract 7575).
70. Papadimitrakopoulou V, Blumenschein GR, Leighl NB, et al. A phase 1/2 study investigating the combination of RAD001 (R) (everolimus) and erlotinib (E) as 2nd and 3rd line therapy in patients (pts) with advanced non-small cell lung cancer (NSCLC) previously treated with chemotherapy (C): phase 1 results. *J Clin Oncol* 2008;26(15 suppl):436s (Abstract 8051).
71. Clark AS, West KA, Blumberg PM, et al. Altered protein kinase C (PKC) isoforms in non-small cell lung cancer cells: PKC-delta promotes cellular survival and chemotherapeutic resistance. *Cancer Res* 2003;63:780–786.
72. Lahn M, McClelland P, Ballard D, et al. Immunohistochemical detection of protein kinase C-beta (PKC-beta) in tumour specimens of patients with non-small cell lung cancer. *Histopathology* 2006;49:429–431.
73. Barr LF, Campbell SE, Baylin SB. Protein kinase C-beta 2 inhibits cycling and decreases c-myc-induced apoptosis in small cell lung cancer cells. *Cell Growth Differ* 1997;8:381–392.

74. Balendran A, Hare GR, Kieloch A, et al. Further evidence that 3-phosphoinositide-dependent protein kinase-1 (PDK1) is required for the stability and phosphorylation of protein kinase C (PKC) isoforms. *FEBS Lett* 2000;484:217–223.
75. Partovian C, Simons M. Regulation of protein kinase B/Akt activity and Ser473 phosphorylation by protein kinase C-alpha in endothelial cells. *Cell Signal* 2004;16:951–957.
76. Graff JR, McNulty AM, Hanna KR, et al. The protein kinase C-beta-selective inhibitor, enzastaurin (LY317615.HCl), suppresses signaling through the AKT pathway, induces apoptosis, and suppresses growth of human colon cancer and glioblastoma xenografts. *Cancer Res* 2005;65:7462–7469.
77. Carducci MA, Musib L, Kies MS, et al. Phase I dose escalation and pharmacokinetic study of enzastaurin, an oral protein kinase C beta inhibitor, in patients with advanced cancer. *J Clin Oncol* 2006;24: 4092–4099.
78. Oh Y, Herbst RS, Burris H, et al. Enzastaurin, an oral serine/threonine kinase inhibitor, as second- or third-line therapy of non-small-cell lung cancer. *J Clin Oncol* 2008 Mar 1;26(7):1135–1141.
79. Colombo N, McMeekin S, Schwartz P, et al. A phase II trial of the mTOR inhibitor AP23573 as a single agent in advanced endometrial cancer. *J Clin Oncol, 2007 ASCO Annual Meeting Proceedings Part I* 2007;25;18S(June 20 Supplement). 5516.
80. Chawla SP, Tolcher A, Staddon A, et al. Survival results with AP23573, a novel mTOR inhibitor, in patients (pts) with advanced soft tissue or bone sarcomas: Update of phase II trial. *J Clin Oncol, 2007 ASCO Annual Meeting Proceedings Part I* 2007;25:18S(June 20 Supplement). 10076.
81. Kondapaka SB, Singh SS, Dasmahapatra GP, Sausville EA, Roy KK. Perifosine, a novel alkylphospholipid, inhibits protein kinase B activation. *Mol Cancer Ther.* 2003;2:1093–1103.
82. Crul M, Rosing H, de Klerk GJ, et al. Phase I and pharmacological study of daily oral administration of perifosine (D-21266) in patients with advanced solid tumours. *Eur J Cancer* 2002;38:1615–1621.
83. Van Ummersen L, Binger K, Volkman J, et al. A phase I trial of perifosine (NSC 639966) on a loading dose/maintenance dose schedule in patients with advanced cancer. *Clin Cancer Res* 2004;10:7450–7456.
84. Knowling M, Blackstein M, Tozer R, et al. A phase II study of perifosine (D-21226) in patients with previously untreated metastatic or locally advanced soft tissue sarcoma: A National Cancer Institute of Canada Clinical Trials Group trial. *Invest New Drugs* 2006;24:435–439.
85. Chee KG, Longmate J, Quinn DI, et al. The AKT inhibitor perifosine in biochemically recurrent prostate cancer: a phase II California/Pittsburgh cancer consortium trial. *Clin Genitourin Cancer* 2007;5:433–437.
86. Perifosine and Docetaxel in Patients With Relapsed Epithelial Ovarian Cancer. Available at: http://www.clinicaltrial.gov/ct2/show/NCT00431054. ClinicalTrials.gov Identifier:NCT00431054. Accessed October 10, 2009.
87. Argiris A, Cohen E, Karrison T, et al. A phase II trial of perifosine, an oral alkylphospholipid, in recurrent or metastatic head and neck cancer. *Cancer Biol Ther* 2006;5:766–770.
88. Bailey HH, Mahoney MR, Ettinger DS, et al. Phase II study of daily oral perifosine in patients with advanced soft tissue sarcoma. *Cancer* 2006;107:2462–2467.
89. Phase I/II Study of Safety & Efficacy of Perifosine & Bortezomib With or Without Dexamethasone for Multiple Myeloma Patients. Available at: http://www.clinicaltrial.gov/ct2/show/NCT00401011. ClinicalTrials.gov identifier:NCT00401011. Accessed October 10, 2009.
90. Clinical and Molecular-Metabolic Phase II Trial of Perifosine for Recurrent/Progressive Malignant Gliomas. Available at: http://www.ClinicalTrials.gov/ct2/show/NCT00590954. ClinicalTrials.gov identifier:NCT00590954. Accessed October 10, 2009.
91. Ernst DS, Eisenhauer E, Wainman N, et al. Phase II study of perifosine in previously untreated patients with metastatic melanoma. *Invest New Drugs* 2005;23:569–575.
92. A Phase 1/2 Trial of Perifosine in the Treatment of Non-Small Cell Lung Cancer. Available at: http://www.clinicaltrial.gov/ct2/show/NCT00399789. ClinicalTrials.gov identifier:NCT00399789. Accessed October 10, 2009.
93. Marsh Rde W, Rocha Lima CM, Levy DE, et al. A phase II trial of perifosine in locally advanced, unresectable, or metastatic pancreatic adenocarcinoma. *Am J Clin Oncol* 2007;30:26–31.
94. Hedley D, Moore M J, Hirte H, et al. A Phase II trial of perifosine as second line therapy for advanced pancreatic cancer. A study of the Princess Margaret Hospital [PMH] Phase II Consortium. *J Clin Oncol 2005 ASCO Annual Meeting Proceedings Part I* 2005;23:16S(June 1 Supplement). abstract 4166.
95. Open-Label Study to Investigate the Safety, Tolerability, PK, and Pharmacodynamics of the AKT Inhibitor GSK690693. Available at: http://www.ClinicalTrials.gov/ct2/show/NCT00493818. ClinicalTrials.gov identifier:NCT00493818. Accessed October 10, 2009.
96. Fan QW, Cheng CK, Nicolaides TP, et al. A dual phosphoinositide-3-kinase alpha/mTOR inhibitor cooperates with blockade of epidermal growth factor receptor in PTEN-mutant glioma. *Cancer Res* 2007;67:7960–7965.
97. A Phase I/II Study of BGT226 in Adult Patients With Advanced Solid Malignancies Including Patients With Advanced Breast Cancer. Available at: http://www.clinicaltrial.gov/ct2/show/NCT00600275. ClinicalTrials.gov identifier:NCT00600275. Accessed October 10, 2009.
98. A Phase I/II Study of BEZ235 in Patients With Advanced Solid Malignancies Enriched by Patients with Advanced Breast Cancer. Available at: http://www.clinicaltrial.gov/ct2/show/NCT00620594. ClinicalTrials.gov Identifier:NCT00620594. Accessed October 10, 2009.
99. Study of the Safety and Pharmacokinetics of XL765 in Adults with Solid Tumors. Available at: http://www.clinicaltrial.gov/ct2/show/NCT00485719. ClinicalTrials.gov identifier:NCT00485719. Accessed October 10, 2009.
100. Study of the Safety and Pharmacokinetics of XL147 in Adults With Solid Tumors. Available at: http://www.clinicaltrial.gov/ct2/show/NCT00486135. ClinicalTrials.gov identifier:NCT00486135. Accessed October 10, 2009.
101. Sato S, Fujita N, Tsuruo T. Interference with PDK1-Akt survival signaling pathway by UCN-01 (7-hydroxystaurosporine). *Oncogene* 2002;21:1727–1738.
102. Wan X, Yokoyama Y, Shinohara A, et al. PTEN augments staurosporine-induced apoptosis in PTEN-null Ishikawa cells by downregulating PI3K/Akt signaling pathway. *Cell Death Differ* 2002;9:414–420.
103. Graves PR, Yu L, Schwarz JK, et al. The Chk1 protein kinase and the Cdc25C regulatory pathways are targets of the anticancer agent UCN-01. *J Biol Chem* 2000;275:5600–5605.
104. Sausville EA, Arbuck SG, Messmann R, et al. Phase I trial of 72-hour continuous infusion UCN-01 in patients with refractory neoplasms. *J Clin Oncol* 2001;19:2319–2333.
105. Dees EC, Baker SD, O'Reilly S, et al. A phase I and pharmacokinetic study of short infusions of UCN-01 in patients with refractory solid tumors. *Clin Cancer Res* 2005;11:664–671.
106. Cen L, Hsieh FC, Lin HJ, et al. PDK-1/AKT pathway as a novel therapeutic target in rhabdomyosarcoma cells using OSU-03012 compound. *Br J Cancer* 2007;97:785–791.
107. Nagy J, Clark JS, Cooke A, et al. Expression and loss of heterozygosity of c-met proto-oncogene in primary breast cancer. *J Surg Oncol* 1995;60:95–99.
108. Jeffers M, Fiscella M, Webb CP, et al. The mutationally activated Met receptor mediates motility and metastasis. *Proc Natl Acad Sci U S A* 1998;95:14417–14422.
109. Inoue K, Karashima T, Chikazawa M, et al. Overexpression of c-met proto-oncogene associated with chromophilic renal cell carcinoma with papillary growth. *Virchows Arch* 1998;433:511–515.
110. Ueki T, Fujimoto J, Suzuki T, et al. Expression of hepatocyte growth factor and its receptor c-met proto-oncogene in hepatocellular carcinoma. *Hepatology* 1997;25:862–866.
111. Di Renzo MF, Poulsom R, Olivero M, et al. Expression of the Met/hepatocyte growth factor receptor in human pancreatic cancer. *Cancer Res* 1995;55:1129–1138.
112. de Luca A, Arena N, Sena LM, et al. Met overexpression confers HGF-dependent invasive phenotype to human thyroid carcinoma cells in vitro. *J Cell Physiol* 1999;180:365–371.

113. Natali PG, Nicotra MR, Di Renzo MF, et al. Expression of the c-Met/HGF receptor in human melanocytic neoplasms: demonstration of the relationship to malignant melanoma tumour progression. *Br J Cancer* 1993;68:746–750.
114. Kaji M, Yonemura Y, Harada S, et al. Participation of c-met in the progression of human gastric cancers: anti-c-met oligonucleotides inhibit proliferation or invasiveness of gastric cancer cells. *Cancer Gene Ther* 1996;3:393–404.
115. Ebert M, Yokoyama M, Friess H, et al. Coexpression of the c-met proto-oncogene and hepatocyte growth factor in human pancreatic cancer. *Cancer Res* 1994;54:5775–5778.
116. Birchmeier W, Brinkmann V, Niemann C, et al. Role of HGF/SF and c-Met in morphogenesis and metastasis of epithelial cells. *Ciba Found Symp* 1997;212:230–240.
117. Birchmeier C, Birchmeier W, Gherardi E, et al. Met, metastasis, motility and more. *Nat Rev Mol Cell Biol* 2003;4:915–925.
118. Burgess T, Coxon A, Meyer S, et al. Fully human monoclonal antibodies to hepatocyte growth factor with therapeutic potential against hepatocyte growth factor/c-Met-dependent human tumors. *Cancer Res* 2006;66:1721–1729.
119. Gordon MS, Mendelson D, Sweeney C, et al. Interim results from a first-in-human study with AMG102, a fully human monoclonal antibody that neutralizes hepatocyte growth factor (HGF), the ligand to c-Met receptor, in patients (pts) with advanced solid tumors. *J Clin Oncol, 2007 ASCO Annual Meeting Proceedings Part I.* 2007;25:18S(June 20 Supplement)2007. 3551.
120. A Phase II Study to Treat Subjects With Advanced Renal Cell Carcinoma. Available at: http://www.ClinicalTrials.gov/ct2/show/NCT00422019. ClinicalTrials.gov identifier: NCT00422019. Accessed October 10, 2009.
121. A Phase II Study to Treat Advanced Malignant Glioma. Available at: http://www.ClinicalTrials.gov/ct2/show/NCT00427440. ClinicalTrials.gov identifier: NCT00427440. Accessed October 10, 2009.
122. Eder JP, Heath E, Appleman L, et al. Phase I experience with c-MET inhibitor XL880 administered orally to patients (pts) with solid tumors. *J Clin Oncol 2007 ASCO Annual Meeting Proceedings Part I* 2007;25:18S(June 20 Supplement). 3526.
123. Ross RW, Stein M, Sarantopoulos J, et al. A phase II study of the c-Met RTK inhibitor XL880 in patients (pts) with papillary renal-cell carcinoma (PRC). *J Clin Oncol 2007 ASCO Annual Meeting Proceedings Part I* 2007;25:18S(June 20 Supplement):15601.
124. Study of XL880 in Subjects With Gastric Cancer. Available at: http://www.ClinicalTrials.gov/ct2/show/NCT00415480. ClinicalTrials.gov identifier: NCT 00415480. Accessed October 10, 2009.
125. Study of XL880 in Adults with Squamous Cell Cancer of the Head and Neck. Available at: http://www.ClinicalTrials.gov/ct2/show/NCT00482326. ClinicalTrials.gov identifier: NCT00482326. Accessed October 10, 2009.
126. A Study of Oral PF-02341066, a c-Met/Hepatocyte Growth Factor Tyrosine Kinase Inhibitor, in Patients With Advanced Cancer. Available at: http://www.ClinicalTrials.gov/ct2/show/NCT00585195. ClinicalTrials.gov identifier: NCT00585195. Accessed October 10, 2009.
127. Garcia AA, Rosen L, Cunningham CC, et al. Phase 1 study of ARQ 197, a selective inhibitor of the c-Met RTK in patients with metastatic solid tumors reaches recommended phase 2 dose. *J Clin Oncol 2007 ASCO Annual Meeting Proceedings Part I* 2007;25:18S(June 20 Supplement). 3525.
128. Available at: http://www.methylgene.com/content.asp?node=227. Accessed December 24, 2007.
129. Sattler M, Pride YB, Ma P, et al. A novel small molecule met inhibitor induces apoptosis in cells transformed by the oncogenic TPR-MET tyrosine kinase. *Cancer Res* 2003;63:5462–5469.
130. Berthou S, Aebersold DM, Schmidt LS, et al. The Met kinase inhibitor SU11274 exhibits a selective inhibition pattern toward different receptor mutated variants. *Oncogene* 2004;23:5387–5393.
131. Ma PC, Schaefer E, Christensen JG, et al. A selective small molecule c-MET Inhibitor, PHA665752, cooperates with rapamycin. *Clin Cancer Res* 2005;11:2312–2319.
132. Kissel H, Timokhina I, Hardy MP, et al. Point mutation in kit receptor tyrosine kinase reveals essential roles for kit signaling in spermatogenesis and oogenesis without affecting other kit responses. *EMBO J* 2000;19:1312–1326.
133. Kitamura Y, Hirotab S. Kit as a human oncogenic tyrosine kinase. *Cell Mol Life Sci* 2004;61:2924–2931.
134. Demetri GD. Targeting c-kit mutations in solid tumors: scientific rationale and novel therapeutic options. *Semin Oncol* 2001;28:19–26.
135. Krüger S, Sotlar K, Kausch I, et al. Expression of KIT (CD117) in renal cell carcinoma and renal oncocytoma. *Oncology* 2005;68:269–275.
136. Naeem M, Dahiya M, Clark JI, et al. Analysis of c-kit protein expression in small-cell lung carcinoma and its implication for prognosis. *Hum Pathol* 2002;33:1182–1187.
137. All-Ericsson C, Girnita L, Müller-Brunotte A, et al. c-Kit-dependent growth of uveal melanoma cells: a potential therapeutic target? *Invest Ophthalmol Vis Sci* 2004;45:2075–2082.
138. Lefevre G, Glotin AL, Calipel A, et al. Roles of stem cell factor/c-Kit and effects of Glivec/STI571 in human uveal melanoma cell tumorigenesis. *J Biol Chem* 2004;279:31769–31779.
139. Advani AS. C-kit as a target in the treatment of acute myelogenous leukemia. *Curr Hematol Rep* 2005;4:51–58.
140. Bellone G, Silvestri S, Artusio E, et al. Growth stimulation of colorectal carcinoma cells via the c-kit receptor is inhibited by TGF-beta 1. *J Cell Physiol* 1997;172:1–11.
141. Liu XH, Bai CG, Xie Q, et al. Prognostic value of KIT mutation in gastrointestinal stromal tumors. *World J Gastroenterol* 2005;11:3948–3952.
142. Chung CY, Yeh KT, Hsu NC, et al. Expression of c-kit protooncogene in human hepatocellular carcinoma. *Cancer Lett* 2005;217:231–236.
143. Bellone G, Carbone A, Sibona N, et al. Aberrant activation of c-kit protects colon carcinoma cells against apoptosis and enhances their invasive potential. *Cancer Res* 2001;61:2200–2206.
144. Dong J, McPherson CM, Stambrook PJ. Flt-3 ligand: a potent dendritic cell stimulator and novel antitumor agent. *Cancer Biol Ther* 2002;1:486–489.
145. Rathnasabapathy R, Lancet JE. Management of acute myelogenous leukemia in the elderly. *Cancer Control* 2003;10:469–477.
146. Yokota S, Kiyoi H, Nakao M, et al. Internal tandem duplication of the FLT3 gene is preferentially seen in acute myeloid leukemia and myelodysplastic syndrome among various hematological malignancies. A study on a large series of patients and cell lines. *Leukemia* 1997;11:1605–1609.
147. Meshinchi S, Woods WG, Stirewalt DL, et al. Prevalence and prognostic significance of Flt3 internal tandem duplication in pediatric acute myeloid leukemia. *Blood* 2001;97:89–94.
148. Levis M, Murphy KM, Pham R, et al. Internal tandem duplications of the FLT3 gene are present in leukemia stem cells. *Blood* 2005;106:673–680.
149. Hayashi H, Ichihara M, Iwashita T, et al. Characterization of intracellular signals via tyrosine 1062 in RET activated by glial cell line-derived neurotrophic factor. *Oncogene* 2000;19:4469–4475.
150. Pützer BM, Drosten M. The RET proto-oncogene: a potential target for molecular cancer therapy. *Trends Mol Med* 2004;10:351–357.
151. Kodama Y, Asai N, Kawai K, et al. The RET proto-oncogene: a molecular therapeutic target in thyroid cancer. *Cancer Sci* 2005;96:143–148.
152. Castellone MD, Guarino V, De Falco V, et al. Functional expression of the CXCR4 chemokine receptor is induced by RET/PTC oncogenes and is a common event in human papillary thyroid carcinomas. *Oncogene* 2004;23:5958–5967.
153. Briggs A, Molofsky D, Wang A, et al. Sensitivity of NSCLC cell lines bearing wild type and mutated EGFR to the VEGFR/EGFR inhibitor ZD6474. *Proc Am Assoc Can Res* 2005. abstract 5833.
154. Holden SN, Eckhardt SG, Basser R, et al. Clinical evaluation of ZD6474, an orally active inhibitor of VEGF and EGF receptor signaling, in patients with solid, malignant tumors. *Ann Oncol* 2005;16:1391–1397.
155. Tamura T, Minami H, Yamada Y, et al. A phase I dose-escalation study of ZD6474 in Japanese patients with solid, malignant tumors. *J Thorac Oncol* 2006;1:1002–1009.

156. Heymach JV, Johnson BE, Prager D, et al. Randomized, placebo-controlled phase II study of vandetinib plus docetaxel in previously treated non-small cell lung cancer. *J Clin Oncol* 2007;25:4270–4277.
157. Kolch W. Meaningful relationships: the regulation of the Ras/Raf/MEK/ERK pathway by protein interactions. *Biochem J* 2000;351:289–305.
158. Wan PT, Garnett MJ, Roe SM, et al. Mechanism of activation of the RAF-ERK signaling pathway by oncogenic mutations of B-RAF. *Cell* 2004;116:855–867.
159. Oka H, Chatani Y, Hoshino R, et al. Constitutive activation of mitogen-activated protein (MAP) kinases in human renal cell carcinoma. *Cancer Res* 1995;55:4182–4187.
160. Feng DY, Zheng H, Tan Y, et al. Effect of phosphorylation of MAPK and Stat3 and expression of c-fos and c-jun proteins on hepatocarcinogenesis and their clinical significance. *World J Gastroenterol* 2001;7:33–36.
161. Fang JY, Richardson BC. The MAPK signalling pathways and colorectal cancer. *Lancet Oncol* 2005;6:322–327.
162. Williams SF, Smallridge RC. Targeting the ERK pathway: novel therapeutics for thyroid cancer. *Curr Drug Targets Immune Endocr Metabol Disord* 2004;4:199–220.
163. Dancey JE. Agents targeting ras signaling pathway. *Curr Pharm Des* 2002;8:2259–2267.
164. Brose MS, Volpe P, Feldman M, et al. BRAF and RAS mutations in human lung cancer and melanoma. *Cancer Res* 2002;62:6997–7000.
165. Kimura ET, Nikiforova MN, Zhu Z, et al. High prevalence of BRAF mutations in thyroid cancer: genetic evidence for constitutive activation of the RET/PTC-RAS-BRAF signaling pathway in papillary thyroid carcinoma. *Cancer Res* 2003;63:1454–1457.
166. Nagasaka T, Sasamoto H, Notohara K, et al. Colorectal cancer With mutation in BRAF, KRAS, and wild-type with respect to both oncogenes showing different patterns of DNA methylation. *J Clin Oncol* 2004;22:4584–4594.
167. Ishimura N, Yamasawa K, Karim Rumi MA, et al. BRAF and K-ras gene mutations in human pancreatic cancers. *Cancer Lett* 2003;199:169–173.
168. Singer G, Oldt R III, Cohen Y, et al. Mutations in BRAF and KRAS characterize the development of low-grade ovarian serous carcinoma. *J Natl Cancer Inst* 2003;95:484–486.
169. Baumann B, Weber CK, Troppmair J, et al. Raf induces NF-kappaB by membrane shuttle kinase MEKK1, a signaling pathway critical for transformation. *Proc Natl Acad Sci U S A* 2000;97:4615–4620.
170. Zhong J, Troppmair J, Rapp UR. Independent control of cell survival by Raf-1 and Bcl-2 at the mitochondria. *Oncogene* 2001;20:4807–4816.
171. Chen J, Fujii K, Zhang L, et al. Raf-1 promotes cell survival by antagonizing apoptosis signal-regulating kinase 1 through a MEK-ERK independent mechanism. *Proc Natl Acad Sci U S A* 2001;98:7783–7788.
172. O'Neill E, Rushworth L, Baccarini M, et al. Role of the kinase MST2 in suppression of apoptosis by the proto-oncogene product Raf-1. *Science* 2004;306:2267–2270.
173. Kaelin WG Jr.. Molecular basis of the VHL hereditary cancer syndrome. *Nat Rev Cancer* 2002; 2:673–682.
174. Brauch H, Weirich G, Brieger J, et al. VHL alterations in human clear cell renal cell carcinoma: association with advanced tumor stage and a novel hot spot mutation. *Cancer Res* 2000;60:1942–1948.
175. Ling H, Cybulla M, Schaefer O, et al. When to look for Von Hippel-Lindau disease in gastroenteropancreatic neuroendocrine tumors? *Neuroendocrinology* 2004;80(suppl 1):39–46.
176. Wilhelm SM, Carter C, Tang L, et al. BAY 43-9006 exhibits broad spectrum oral antitumor activity and targets the RAF/MEK/ERK pathway and receptor tyrosine kinases involved in tumor progression and angiogenesis. *Cancer Res* 2004;64:7099–7109.
177. Kane RC, Farrell AT, Saber H, et al. Sorafenib for the treatment of advanced renal cell carcinoma. *Clin Cancer Res* 2006;12:7271–7278.
178. Baccarini M. An old kinase on a new path: Raf and apoptosis. *Cell Death Differ* 2002;9:783–785.
179. FDA approves Nexavar for patients with inoperable liver cancer. Available at: http://www.fda.gov/bbs/topics/NEWS/2007/NEW01748.html. Accessed December 19, 2007.
180. Strumberg D, Richly H, Hilger RA, et al. Phase I clinical and pharmacokinetic study of the Novel Raf kinase and vascular endothelial growth factor receptor inhibitor BAY 43-9006 in patients with advanced refractory solid tumors. *J Clin Oncol* 2005;23:965–972.
181. Abou-Alfa GK, Schwartz L, Ricci S, et al. Phase II study of sorafenib in patients with advanced hepatocellular carcinoma. *J Clin Oncol* 2006;24:4293–4300.
182. Escudier B, Eisen T, Stadler WM, et al. Sorafenib in advanced clear-cell renal-cell carcinoma. *N Engl J Med* 2007;356:125–134.
183. Motzer RJ, Hutson TE, Tomczak P, et al. Sunitinib versus interferon alfa in metastatic renal-cell carcinoma. *N Engl J Med* 2007;356:115–124.
184. Escudier B, Pluzanska A, Koralewski P, et al. Bevacizumab plus interferon alfa-2a for treatment of metastatic renal cell carcinoma: a randomised, double-blind phase III trial. *Lancet* 2007;370:2103–2111.
185. Exelixis Pipeline: XL281. Available at: http://www.exelixis.com/pipeline_xl281.shtml. Accessed March 20, 2008.
186. Plexxikon Oncology: PLX4032. Available at: http://www.plexxikon.com/oncology.html. Accessed March 20, 2008.
187. Safety Study of PLX4032 in Patients With Solid Tumors. Available at: http://www.clinicaltrial.gov/ct2/show/NCT00405587. ClinicalTrials.gov identifier: NCT00405587. Accessed October 10, 2009.
188. NCI Drug Dictionary: CHIR-265. Available at: http://www.cancer.gov/Templates/drugdictionary.aspx?CdrID=484456. Accessed March 20, 2008.
189. A Study to Evaluate RAF265, an Oral Drug Administered to Subjects With Locally Advanced or Metastatic Melanoma. Available at: http://www.clinicaltrial.gov/ct2/show/NCT00304525. ClinicalTrials.gov identifier: NCT00304525. Accessed October 10, 2009.
190. Seger R, Krebs EG. The MAPK signaling cascade. *FASEB J* 1995;9:726–735.
191. Kolch W, Kotwaliwale A, Vass K, et al. The role of Raf kinases in malignant transformation. *Expert Rev Mol Med* 2002:1–18.
192. Ussar S, Voss T. MEK1 and MEK2, different regulators of the G1/S transition. *J Biol Chem* 2004;279:43861–43869.
193. Tong C, Fan HY, Chen dY, et al. Effects of MEK inhibitor U0126 on meiotic progression in mouse oocytes: microtuble organization, asymmetric division and metaphase II arrest. *Cell Res* 2003;13:375–383.
194. Cowley S, Paterson H, Kemp P, et al. Activation of MAP kinase is necessary and sufficient for PC12 differentiation and for transformation of NIH 3T3 cells. *Cell* 1994;77:841–852.
195. Mansour SJ, Matten WT, Hermann AS, et al. Transformation of mammalian cells by constitutively active MAP kinase kinase. *Science* 1994;265:966–970.
196. Hoshino R, Chatani Y, Yamori T, et al. Constitutive activation of the 41-/43-kDa mitogen-activated protein kinase signaling pathway in human tumors. *Oncogene* 1999;18:813–822.
197. Sebolt-Leopold JS. Development of anticancer drugs targeting the MAP kinase pathway. *Oncogene* 2000;19:6594–6599.
198. Sebolt-Leopold JS, Dudley DT, Herrera R, et al. Blockade of the MAP kinase pathway suppresses growth of colon tumors in vivo. *Nat Med* 1999;5:810–816.
199. Allen LF, Sebolt-Leopold J, Meyer MB. CI-1040 (PD184352), a targeted signal transduction inhibitor of MEK (MAPKK). *Semin Oncol* 2003;30:105–116.
200. Rinehart J, Adjei AA, Lorusso PM, et al. Multicenter phase II study of the oral MEK inhibitor, CI-1040, in patients with advanced non-small-cell lung, breast, colon, and pancreatic cancer. *J Clin Oncol* 2004;22:4456–4462.
201. Sebolt-Leopold JS, Herrera R. Targeting the mitogen-activated protein kinase cascade to treat cancer. *Nat Rev Cancer* 2004;4:937–947.
202. Messersmith WA, Hidalgo M, Carducci M, Eckhardt SG. Novel targets in solid tumors: MEK inhibitors. *Clin Adv Hematol Oncol* 2006;4:831–836.
203. MEK Inhibitor PD-325901 to Treat Advanced Non-Small Cell Lung Cancer. Available at: http://www.clinicaltrial.gov/ct2/show/NCT00174369. ClinicalTrials.gov identifier: NCT00174369. Accessed October 10, 2009.

204. MEK Inhibitor PD-325901 To Treat Advanced Breast Cancer, Colon Cancer, And Melanoma. Available at: http://www.clinicaltrial.gov/ct2/show/NCT00147550. ClinicalTrials.gov Identifier: NCT00147550. Accessed October 10, 2009.
205. Yeh TC, Marsh V, Bernat BA, et al. Biological characterization of ARRY-142886 (AZD6244), a potent, highly selective mitogen-activated protein kinase kinase 1/2 inhibitor. *Clin Cancer Res* 2007;13:1576–1583.
206. Chow L, Eckhardt S, Reid A. A first in human dose-randing study to assess the pharmacokinetic, pharmacodynamics, and toxicities of the MEK inhibitor, ARRY-142886 (AZD6244) in patients with advanced solid malignancies. Proc AACR-EORTC-NCI Targeted Ther Conference. 2005:C162 (abstract).
207. A Phase 2 Study of AZD6244 in Hepatocellular Carcinoma. http://www.clinicaltrial.gov/ct2/show/NCT00604721. ClinicalTrials.gov Identifier: NCT00604721.
208. AZD6244 Versus Pemetrexed (Alimta®) in Patients With Non-Small Cell Lung Cancer, Who Have Failed One or Two Prior Chemotherapy Regimen. Available at: http://www.clinicaltrial.gov/ct2/show/NCT00372788. ClinicalTrials.gov identifier: NCT00372788. Accessed October 10, 2009.
209. AZD6244 vs. Capecitabine (Xeloda®) in Patients With Advanced or Metastatic Pancreatic Cancer, Who Have Failed First Line Gemcitabine Therapy. Available at: http://www.clinicaltrial.gov/ct2/show/NCT00372944. ClinicalTrials.gov identifier: NCT00372944. Accessed October 10, 2009.
210. AZD6244 in Treating Woman With Recurrent Low-Grade Ovarian Ca ncer. Available at: http://www.clinicaltrial.gov/ct2/show/NCT00551070. ClinicalTrials.gov identifier: NCT00551070. Accessed October 10, 2009.
211. Study of XL518 in Adults With Solid Tumors. Available at: http://www.clinicaltrial.gov/ct2/show/NCT00467779. ClinicalTrials.gov identifier: NCT00467779. Accessed October 10, 2009.
212. Phase 1 Dose-Escalation PK/PD Trial in Advanced Cancer Patients. Available at: http://www.clinicaltrial.gov/ct2/show/NCT00610194. ClinicalTrials .gov identifier: NCT00610194. Accessed October 10, 2009.
213. Keen N, Taylor S. Aurora-kinase inhibitors as anticancer agents. *Nat Rev Cancer* 2004;4:927–936.
214. Katayama H, Brinkley WR, Sen S. The Aurora kinases: role in cell transformation and tumorigenesis. *Cancer Metastasis Rev* 2003;22:451–464.
215. Nguyen HG, Chinnappan D, Urano T, et al. Mechanism of Aurora-B degradation and its dependency on intact KEN and A-boxes: identification of an aneuploidy-promoting property. *Mol Cell Biol* 2005;25:4977–4992.
216. Li X, Sakashita G, Matsuzaki H, et al. Direct association with inner centromere protein (INCENP) activates the novel chromosomal passenger protein, Aurora-C. *J Biol Chem* 2004;279:47201–47211.
217. Chen HL, Tang CJ, Chen CY, et al. Overexpression of an Aurora-C kinase-deficient mutant disrupts the Aurora-B/INCENP complex and induces polyploidy. *J Biomed Sci* 2005;12:297–310.
218. Tanaka T, Kimura M, Matsunaga K, et al. Centrosomal kinase AIK1 is overexpressed in invasive ductal carcinoma of the breast. *Cancer Res* 1999;59:2041–2044.
219. Bischoff JR, Anderson L, Zhu Y, et al. A homologue of Drosophila aurora kinase is oncogenic and amplified in human colorectal cancers. *EMBO J* 1998;17:3052–3065.
220. Gritsko TM, Coppola D, Paciga JE, et al. Activation and overexpression of centrosome kinase BTAK/Aurora-A in human ovarian cancer. *Clin Cancer Res* 2003;9:1420–1426.
221. Sen S, Zhou H, Zhang RD, et al. Amplification/overexpression of a mitotic kinase gene in human bladder cancer. *J Natl Cancer Inst* 2002;94:1320–1329.
222. Kamada K, Yamada Y, Hirao T, et al. Amplification/overexpression of Aurora-A in human gastric carcinoma: potential role in differentiated type gastric carcinogenesis. *Oncol Rep* 2004;12:593–599.
223. Chieffi P, Cozzolino L, Kisslinger A, et al. Aurora B expression directly correlates with prostate cancer malignancy and influence prostate cell proliferation. *Prostate* 2006;66:326–333.
224. Chalandon Y, Schwaller J. Targeting mutated protein tyrosine kinases and their signaling pathways in hematologic malignancies. *Haematologica* 2005;90:949–968.
225. Alper O, Bowden ET. Novel insights into c-Src. *Curr Pharm Des* 2005;11:1119–1130.
226. Bhatt AS, Erdjument-Bromage H, Tempst P, et al. Adhesion signaling by a novel mitotic substrate of src kinases. *Oncogene* 2005;24:5333–5343.
227. Summy JM, Gallick GE. Src family kinases in tumor progression and metastasis. *Cancer Metastasis Rev* 2003;22:337–358.
228. Biscardi JS, Ishizawar RC, Silva CM, et al. Tyrosine kinase signalling in breast cancer: epidermal growth factor receptor and c-Src interactions in breast cancer. *Breast Cancer Res* 2000;2:203–210.
229. Bolen JB, Veillette A, Schwartz AM, et al. Analysis of pp60c-src in human colon carcinoma and normal human colon mucosal cells. *Oncogene Res* 1987;1:149–168.
230. Johnson FM, Saigal B, Talpaz M, et al. Dasatinib (BMS-354825) tyrosine kinase inhibitor suppresses invasion and induces cell cycle arrest and apoptosis of head and neck squamous cell carcinoma and non-small cell lung cancer cells. *Clin Cancer Res* 2005;11: 6924–6932.
231. Ottenhoff-Kalff AE, Rijksen G, van Beurden EA, et al. Characterization of protein tyrosine kinases from human breast cancer: involvement of the c-src oncogene product. *Cancer Res* 1992;52:4773–4778.
232. Verbeek BS, Vroom TM, Adriaansen-Slot SS, et al. c-Src protein expression is increased in human breast cancer. An immunohistochemical and biochemical analysis. *J Pathol* 1996;180:383–388.
233. Maa MC, Leu TH, McCarley DJ, et al. Potentiation of epidermal growth factor receptor-mediated oncogenesis by c-Src: implications for the etiology of multiple human cancers. *Proc Natl Acad Sci U S A* 1995; 92:6981–6985.
234. Frame MC. Src in cancer: deregulation and consequences for cell behaviour. *Biochem Biophys Acta* 2002;1602:114–130.
235. Parsons JT, Parsons SJ. Src family protein tyrosine kinases: cooperating with growth factor and adhesion signaling pathways. *Curr Opin Cell Biol* 1997;9:187–192.
236. Lu Y, Yu Q, Liu JH, et al. Src family protein-tyrosine kinases alter the function of PTEN to regulate phosphatidylinositol 3-kinase/AKT cascades. *J Biol Chem* 2003;278:40057–40066.
237. Summy JM, Gallick GE. Src family kinases in tumor progression and metastasis. *Cancer Metastasis Rev* 2003;22:337–358.
238. Irby RB, Yeatman TJ. Role of Src expression and activation in human cancer. *Oncogene* 2000;19:5636–5642.
239. Laird AD, Li G, Moss KG, et al. Src family kinase activity is required for signal tranducer and activator of transcription 3 and focal adhesion kinase phosphorylation and vascular endothelial growth factor signaling in vivo and for anchorage-dependent and -independent growth of human tumor cells. *Mol Cancer Ther* 2003;2:461–469.
240. Burgess MR, Skaggs BJ, Shah NP, et al. Comparative analysis of two clinically active BCR-ABL kinase inhibitors reveals the role of conformation-specific binding in resistance. *Proc Natl Acad Sci U S A* 2005;102:3395–3400.
241. Carter TA, Wodicka LM, Shah NP, et al. Inhibition of drug-resistant mutants of ABL, KIT, and EGF receptor kinases. *Proc Natl Acad Sci U S A* 2005;102:11011–11016.
242. Shah NP, Tran C, Lee FY, et al. Overriding imatinib resistance with a novel ABL kinase inhibitor. *Science* 2004;305:399–401.
243. National Cancer Institute. FDA Approval for Dasatinib. Available at: http://www.cancer.gov/cancertopics/druginfo/fda-dasatinib. Accessed March 3, 2008.
244. Talpaz M, Shah NP, Kantarjian H, et al. Dasatinib in imatinib-resistant Philadelphia chromosome-positive leukemias. *N Engl J Med* 2006;354:2531–2541.
245. Johnson FM, Chiappori A, Burris H, et al. A phase I study (CA180021-Segment 2) of dasatinib in patients (pts) with advanced solid tumors. *J Clin Oncol, 2007 ASCO Annual Meeting Proceedings Part I* 2007;25: 18S(June 20 Supplement). 14042.
246. A Phase I/Expansion Study of Dasatinib (GD/GDE). Available at: http://www.ClinicalTrials.gov/ct2/show/NCT00598091. ClinicalTri als.gov identfier: NCT00598091. Accessed October 10, 2009.

247. Kopetz S, Wolff R, Golver K, et al. Phase I study of Src inhibition with dasatinib in combination with 5-fluoruracil, leucovorin, oxaliplatin (FOLFOX), and cetuximab in metastatic colorectal cancer. *2008 Gastrointestinal Cancers Symposium*. Orlando, FL. Abstract No. 273.
248. Phase II Study Evaluating The Safety And Response To Neoadjuvant Dasatinib In Early Stage Non-Small Cell Lung Cancer. Available at: http://www.ClinicalTrials.gov/ct2/show/NCT00564876. ClinicalTrials.gov: NCT00564876. Accessed October 10, 2009.
249. Study of Dasatinib (BMS-354825) in Patients With Advanced Estrogen/Progesterone Receptor-Positive (ER+/PR+) or Her2/Neu-Positive (Her2/Neu+) Breast Cancer. Available at: http://www.ClinicalTrials.gov/ct2/show/NCT00371345. ClinicalTrials.gov identifier: NCT00371345. Accessed October 10, 2009.
250. Gambacorti-Passerini C, Brummendorf T, Kantarjian HM, et al. Bosutinib (SKI-606) exhibits clinical activity in patients with Philadelphia chromosome positive CML or ALL who failed imatinib. *J Clin Oncology 2007 ASCO Annual Meeting Proceedings Part I* 2007;25:18S(June 20 Supplement). 7006.
251. Messersmith W, Krishnamurthi S, Hewes BA, et al. Bosutinib (SKI-606), a dual Src/Abl tyrosine kinase inhibitor: Preliminary results from a phase 1 study in patients with advanced malignant solid tumors. *J Clin Oncology 2007 ASCO Annual Meeting Proceedings Part I* 2007;25:18S(June 20 Supplement). 3552.
252. Study Evaluating SKI-606 in Subjects With Breast Cancer. Available at: http://www.ClinicalTrials.gov/ct2/show/NCT00319254. ClinicalTrials.gov identifier: NCT00319254. Accessed October 10, 2009.
253. Tabernero J, Cervantes A, Hoekman K, et al. Phase I study of AZD0530, an oral potent inhibitor of Src kinase: First demonstration of inhibition of Src activity in human cancers. *J Clin Oncology 2007 ASCO Annual Meeting Proceedings Part I* 2007;25:18S(June 20 Supplement). 3520.
254. Cripe L, McGuire W, Wertheim M, et al. Integrated report of the phase 2 experience with XL999 administered IV to patients (pts) with NSCLC, renal cell CA (RCC), metastatic colorectal CA (CRC), recurrent ovarian CA, acute myelogenous leukemia. *J Clin Oncol* 2007;25:18(suppl). 3591.
255. Dancey J, Sausville EA. Issues and progress with protein kinase inhibitors for cancer treatment. *Nat Rev Drug Discov* 2003;2:296–313.

CHAPTER 51

Nevin Murray
Robert Eager
John Nemunaitis

Lung Cancer Vaccines

Anecdotal observations of spontaneous regression of tumors in patients with cancer provided the initial evidence of the presence of an inborn antitumor immune response. Additionally, the observation of paraneoplastic autoimmunity that can accompany occult malignancies indicates the existence of immunologic activity. Historically, the first reports of therapeutic immune induced tumor regression came over a century ago when William Coley treated cancer patients by nonspecifically activating the immune system with inoculations of live bacterial cultures. However, little progress was made until the 1980s, when Rosenberg et al.[1] studied the use of high doses of interleukin 2 (IL-2) in individuals with metastatic kidney cancer or melanoma and achieved objective cancer regressions in 15% to 20% of treated patients.

Classic prophylactic vaccines that have had great success in the prevention of infectious diseases have relied mainly on generation of high titers of neutralizing antibodies. This chapter discusses therapeutic vaccines that elicit an active specific immune response. These vaccines aim at inducing strong antigen-specific T-cell responses. The requirements for therapeutic vaccine development are different and far more complex than those of prophylactic vaccines. The first important issue in vaccine design is that of antigen delivery. Therapeutic vaccines are divided into subunit vaccines or cell-based vaccines (Table 51.1). The subunit vaccine approach is based on the selection of well-defined antigens as targets. The term *subunit vaccine* may include a gene or gene product, representing part of or an entire polypeptide fragment carrying an antigen recognized by T cells. These include plasmid DNA, messenger RNA, peptides, recombinant proteins, or bacterial/viral vectors carrying gene inserts coding for tumor antigens. Cellular vaccines rely on the approach of using whole tumor cells for vaccination. Either irradiated tumor cells or lysates have been used. Tumor cells may be modified by gene transfer to express cytokines that may enhance their overall immunogenicity.

The focus of most lung cancer vaccines has been the generation of a T-cell response against antigens expressed by tumors. Cancer vaccination is based on the premise that an effective antitumor response can be elicited by the induction of major histocompatibility complex (MHC) class I-restricted cytotoxic T lymphocytes (CTLs), capable of recognizing and lysing tumor cells. Gene-modified tumor vaccines (GMTV) and dendritic cell vaccines (DCV), the two main classes of cellular vaccines investigated in lung cancer, utilize this approach.

GMTV use gene transfer technology to transduce tumor cells with genes encoding cytokines or other immunogenic proteins. DCV utilize antigen modification of autologous dendritic cells (DCs) to elicit a specific T-cell activation against cancer cells. Experimental studies of xenografted animals demonstrated that these vaccines considerably increased the immunogenicity of tumor cells, which, in many cases, induced tumor rejection and regression.[1a,2–4] Several GMTV platforms have been evaluated for cytokine and gene delivery. These include autologous tumor vaccines, allogeneic tumor vaccines, and bystander vaccines. Autologous tumor cell vaccines involve surgically harvested tumor cells that are genetically modified to increase immune recognition. More commonly, allogeneic vaccines are made up of tumor cell lines that express tumor-associated antigens (TAAs) and are genetically modified to express immunogenic cytokines and proteins. A bystander vaccine is a hybridization of both aforementioned approaches. It utilizes autologous tumor cell antigens, "bystander" cells, in combination with cytokine-secreting allogeneic tumor cells to recruit and activate immune effector cells.

The role of DCs in cell-mediated immunity has been extensively investigated.[1a,5–8] DCs have been found to play a central role in the induction of antitumor immunity in tumor-bearing host by a process of antigenic cross-presentation and have displayed activity in non–small cell lung cancer (NSCLC)[2] They efficiently display antigens on major histocompatibility complexes (MHC II) ultimately stimulating proliferation and activation of CD4+ and CD8+ T cells. CD4+ cells further augment the activity of natural killer (NK) cells and macrophages, in addition to amplifying antigen-specific immunity by local secretion of cytokines.[3,4,9–11] These attributes make DCs a central component in therapeutic strategies of many current immune-based therapies in NSCLC.

TABLE 51.1 Approaches to Lung Cancer Vaccines and Immunotherapy

Design	Characteristics	Examples
Intent	Prophylactic Therapeutic	Nicotine, HPV Antigen vaccine
Immune response	Nonspecific Specific	BCG Dendritic cell
Immunity	Passive antibody Active	Cetuximab Antigen vaccine
Active component	Noncellular Cellular	Tumor peptide CTL, dendritic
Material	Tumor peptide Cancer cells	MUC-1, MAGE-3 GVAX, Lucanix

BCG, Bacillus Calmette-Guérin; CTL, cytotoxic T lymphocyte; HPV, human papillomavirus; MAGE, melanoma antigen E; MUC, mucin.

Despite progress made in understanding the molecular biology behind carcinogenesis and advancements in our technical proficiency, clinical application of immune-based cancer vaccines have yielded modest results. There are several hypotheses to explain potential lack of activity, including ineffective priming of tumor-specific T cells, lack of high avidity of primed tumor-specific T cells, and physical or functional disabling of primed tumor-specific T cells by the primary host and or tumor-related mechanism. For example, in NSCLC, a high proportion of the tumor-infiltrating lymphocytes are immunosuppressive T-regulatory cells (CD4+ CD25+) that secrete transforming growth factor β (TFG-β) and express a high level of CTL antigen-4.[12,13] These cells have been shown to impede immune activation by facilitating T-cell tolerance to TAAs rather than cross-priming CD8+ T cells, resulting in the nonproliferation of killer T cells that recognize the tumor and will not attack it.[12–18] Elevated levels of IL-10 and TFG-β are found in patients with NSCLC. Animal models have shown immune suppression is mediated by these cytokines serving as a defense for malignant cells against the body's immune system.[19–28]

As our understanding of the pathogenesis of cancer steadily evolves, researchers are continuously developing novel therapies designed to overcome each new challenge. This chapter will discuss recent vaccine therapeutic strategies in lung cancer, focusing on clinical trials that have contributed to our overall understanding of the immune system and its utilization in the treatment of lung cancer.

NON–SMALL CELL LUNG CANCER CELLULAR VACCINES

Lucanix Lucanix is a nonviral gene-based allogeneic vaccine that incorporates the TFG-β2 antisense gene into a cocktail of four different NSCLC cell lines.[29] Elevated levels of TFG-β2 are linked to immunosupression in cancer patients.[30–35] Systemic levels of TFG-β are inversely correlated with prognosis in patients with NSCLC.[36] TFG-β2 has an antagonistic effect on NK cells, lymphokine-activated killer cells, and DCs.[21,25,26,37–39] Using an antisense gene to inhibit TFG-β2, several researchers have demonstrated an inhibition of cellular TFG-β2 expression resulting in an increased immunogenicity of gene-modified cancer cells.[40–48]

In a recent phase II study involving 75 early stage (n = 4) and late stage (n = 61) patients, a dose-related effect of Lucanix was defined. Twenty-nine patients were randomized to one of the three-dose cohorts (1.25×10^7, 2.5×10^7, or 5×10^7 cells/injection $\times$ 16 injections). Injections were administered one time each month or every other month until progressive disease criteria were fulfilled. Treatment was well tolerated with only one grade 3 toxic event attributed to the vaccine (arm swelling). A significant survival advantage at dose levels $\geq 2.5 \times 10^7$ cells/injection compared with the low dose level of 1.25×10^7 cells/injection was demonstrated with an estimated 2-year survival of 47% (Tables 51.2 and 51.3). This also compared favorably with the historical 2-year survival rate of <20% of comparable stage IIIB or IV NSCLC patients.[49–54] Furthermore, a correlation of positive outcome with induction of immune enhancement of tumor antigen recognition was observed. Immune function was explored in the 61 advanced stage IIIB or IV patients. Patients who achieved stable disease or better had increased frequency in the production of cytokines (interferon-γ [INF-γ], $p = 0.006$; IL-6, $p = 0.004$; IL-4, $p = 0.007$) and positive clinical outcomes were correlated with development of human leukocyte antigen (HLA)-antibody response to the vaccine. A total of 11 out of 20 patients with stable disease or better-developed novel HLA-antibody reactivity to one or more allotypes of the vaccinating cell lines compared with 2 of 16 progressive disease patients ($p = 0.014$). It was concluded that further phase III investigation of Lucanix is justified and warranted.

GVAX Lung Given the histological heterogeneity of NSCLC and the relative absence of information on the relevant immunodominant antigens in this disease, in initial trials, autologous tumor cells were selected as the source of tumor antigens in NSCLC.[55] The first pilot study of autologous GVAX Lung was conducted by Glenn Dranoff at the Dana-Faber Cancer Institute using a first-generation adenoviral vector and recombinant human granulocyte-macrophage colony-stimulating factor (GM-CSF).[56] A total of 35 patients underwent tumor harvest and 33 patients received vaccine treatment at three different dose levels. The vaccine was administered weekly for 2 weeks then biweekly until the supply was exhausted. Vaccines were well tolerated with the most common toxicity being local, self-limited vaccine site reactions and mild flulike symptoms in a minority of patients. Antitumor immunity was demonstrated by induction of delayed-type hypersensitivity (DTH) reaction to injections of irradiated, genetically unmodified autologous tumor cells in 82% of patients as well as the presence of inflammatory infiltrates in metastatic tumor biopsies. In addition, one patient demonstrated evidence of tumor regression (mixed response) and two others have remained recurrence

TABLE 51.2 Demographics for Recent Vaccine Trials in NSCLC

Vaccine	Vaccine Administration	Number of Patients	Stage	Reference
Lucanix	1.25 × 107 − 5 × 107 c/i q m or qo m × 16	75	II–IV	29
GVAX Ad autologous	1 × 106 − 10 × 106 c/i q wk × 3 then qo wk	35	IV	56
GVAX Ad autologous	5 × 106 − 10 × 107 c/i qo wk × 6	43	IB/II/IIIB/IV	57
GVAX bystander	5 × 106 − 80 × 106 autologus cells + 2.5 × 106 − 40 × 106 allogeneic GM-CSF secreting cells qo wk × 3–12	49	IIIB/IV	58
L523S	pVAX/L523S 8 mg day 0 and 14 then Ad/L523S at 1, 20, and 400 × 109 vp/i on day 28 and 56	13	IB/II	61
L-BLP-25	20 or 200 μg sc wk 0, 9, 5, 9	17	IIIB/IV	77
L-BLP-25	1000 mg q wk × 8 then q 6 wk	88	IIIB	78
EP2101	5 mg q 3 wk × 5 then qo m × 4 then q 3 m × 4.	135	IIIB/IV	
B7.1	5 × 107 id c/l qo wk	19	IIIB/IV	69
EGFR	20 pts 50 μg im i on days 0, 7, 14, 21, and 51; 20 pts 200-mg cyctoxan d -3 then 50 μg im i on d 0, 7, 14, 21, and 51	40	IIIB/IV	96
EGFR	71 or 142 mg im q wk × 4 then q m × 1	43	IIIB/IV	94
MAGE-3	300 mg id × 4 q 3 wk × 4 cycles	17	I/II	109
MAGE-3	5 vaccinations q 3 wk	182	IB/II	109a
Telomerase GV 1001 and HR2822	112 or 560 mg of GV 1001, 68 mg HR2822 and 30− or 75-μg GM-CSF id 3/wk during wk 1–4, 6, and 10	26	I, III A/B, IV	116
Dexosomes	1.3 × 1013 MHC II/injection ss/id q wk × 4	13	IIIB/IV	123
a(1, 3)-Galactosyltransferase	q 4 wks × 4	7	IV	125
Cyclophilin B	1 mg or 3 mg sc peptide or modified peptide qo wk × 3	16	IIIa–IV	129
Dendritic cells	prime 9.1 × 107 c/i boost 8.2 × 107 c/l	16	IA–IIIB	6

EGFR, epidermal growth factor receptor; GM-CSF, granulocyte monocyte colony-stimulating factor; id, intradermal; im, intramuscular; MAGE, melanoma antigen E; NSCLC, non–small cell lung cancer; q, every; qo, every other; sc, subcutaneous.

free for more than 5 years following resection of isolated metastatic sites for vaccine preparation.

The subsequent study was a multicenter phase I/II trial investigating again an autologous NSCLC tissue vaccine. Manufacturing processes were modified in this trial to enable more rapid commercial development. This study also involved both patients with early and advanced stage disease.[57] Patients were enrolled in two cohorts. Cohort A included patients with stage IB or II NSCLC with planned primary surgical resection and no preoperative or postoperative chemotherapy or radiotherapy. Patients in cohort B had surgically nonresectable stage III or IV NSCLC with an accessible tumor to harvest for vaccine processing.

Vaccines were administered subcutaneously every 2 weeks for a total of three to six vaccinations. The vaccine dose was individualized on the basis of yield, and each dose contained 5×10^6 to 10×10^6 cells per vaccination, 10×10^6 to 30×10^6 cells per vaccination, and 30×10^6 to 100×10^6 cells per vaccination (Tables 51.2 and 51.3).

A total of 83 patients underwent tumor harvest (20 in cohort A, 63 in cohort B) and 43 initiated vaccine treatment (10 in cohort A, 33 in cohort B). All 10 patients in cohort A completed vaccine treatment. The median number of vaccines in cohort B was five. The median number of days from tumor harvest to vaccine release was 31 and that from harvest to initiation of vaccine treatment was 49 days. Vaccines were successfully manufactured in 80% of patients in cohort A and 81% of patients in cohort B. The majority of manufacturing failures resulted from an insufficient number of tumor cells.

The most common vaccine-related adverse events were local vaccine injection site reactions (93%); followed by fatigue (16%), nausea (12%), and pain; arthralgia, and upper respiratory infection (each at 5%). Two grade 4 (pericardial effusion) and six grade 3 (dyspnea, fatigue, injection site reaction, hypokalemia, malignant ascites, and pulmonary embolism) possibly related events were reported. There was no association between vaccine dose and the total number of adverse events or grade 3 and 4 adverse events.

Vaccine reaction size (skin induration) was positively associated with level GM-CSF secretion from the transfected autologous malignant cells used as the product. Analysis of vaccine site biopsy specimen showed dense infiltration with CD4+ and CD8+ T cells, CD1a+ DCs, and eosinophils.

Three patients in cohort B achieved durable, complete tumor regressions lasting 6, 18, and 22 months. In addition, there was one minor response (30% decrease in a lung nodule)

TABLE 51.3 Results of Recent Vaccine Trials in NSCLC

Vaccine	Side Effects	Median Survival	1-Year Survival	Response	Reference
Lucanix	Grade 3: arm swelling (n = 1)	441 days (IIIB/IV only)	54%	6 PR	29
GVAX Ad autologous	Grade 1–2: erythema, induration, fatigue, flulike symptoms	NA	NA	5 SD, 1 MR	56
GVAX Ad autologous	Grade 1–2: erythema, induration, fatigue, nausea, dyspnea	12 mo	44%	3 CR, 6 SD	57
GVAX bystander	Grade 1–2: injection site pain, fatigue, nausea, fever, dyspnea	7 mo	31%	7 SD	58
L523S	Grade 1–2: erythema, injection site pain, flulike symptoms, nausea, HTN	NA	100%	2 PD <1 yr	61
L-BLP-25	Grade 1–2: injection site reaction, fever, nausea	5.4 (20 μg); 14.6 (200 μg) mo	NA	4 SD	77
L-BLP-25	Grade 1–2: injection site reaction, flulike symptoms	17.4 mo	NA	NA	78
EP2101	Dyspnea, injection site reaction/pain, nausea	583 days	55%	NA	
B7.1	Minor skin erythema	18 mo	52%	1 PR; 5 SD	69
EGFR	Grade 2: chills, fever, vomiting, nausea, HTN, HA, dizziness, flushing, injection site pain	8.17 mo	NA	12 SD	96
EGFR	Grade 1–2; fever, chills, nausea, vomiting, tremors, anorexia, pain	GAR 11.87 mo	NA	15 (39.5%) GAR	94
MAGE-3	NA	NA	NA	10 MAGE Ab+	109
MAGE-3	NA	NA	33%	NA	109a
Telomerase GV 1001 and HR2822	Mild induration and erythema at injection site, chills, fever	8.5 mo	36%	NA	116
Dexosomes	Grade 1–2: injection site reaction, flulike symptoms, edema, and pain	NA	NA	3 MAGE Ab+	123
a(1,3)-Galactosyltransferase	Grade 1–2: injection pain, erythema, fatigue, HTN, bradycardia, cough, diarrhea, dyspnea, HA, nausea, vomiting, pleural effusion	NA	NA	4 SD	125
Cyclophilin B	Grade 1: local skin reaction	67+ wks np; 29+ wks mp	NA	2 SD	129
Dendritic cells	Minor skin erythema and fatigue	NA	NA	6 ag response	6

CR, complete response; EGFR, epidermal growth factor receptor; GAR, good antibody response; HA, headache; HTN, hypertension; MAGE, melanoma antigen E; MR, minor response; NA, not applicable; NSCLC, non–small cell lung cancer; PD, progression; PR, partial response; SD, stable disease.

and two mixed responses; seven patients had stable disease with a mean duration of 7.7 months. Correlation of dose to survival was demonstrated to be significant at a threshold of 40 ng of GM-CSF per 10^6 cells per 24 hours expressed from an aliquot of the vaccine prior to the first injection. Long-term follow-up of two of the patients (stage IV refractory disease to prior cytotoxic therapy) achieving complete response reveals continued disease-free survival now more than 5 years after initial GVAX vaccination (unpublished data).

Salgia et al.[56] also conducted the first phase I trial of GVAX in NSCLC using an autologous vaccine strategy. A total of 37 patients with stage IIB to IV NSCLC were enrolled and 34 vaccines were successfully manufactured at three different dose levels (1×10^6, 4×10^6, 1×10^7 cells). The vaccines were administered weekly for 2 weeks then biweekly until the supply of vaccine was exhausted. Of these patients, 25 received ≥6 vaccinations. Toxicities were limited to grade 1 to 2 erythema and induration at the injection site, as well as fatigue and flu-like symptoms (Tables 51.2 and 51.3).

A total of 18 out of 25 patients who received six vaccinations showed significant local reactions. At the vaccination site, these 18 patients showed infiltration of DCs, macrophages, eosinophils, neutrophils, and lymphocytes. The intensity and frequency of the reaction was related to the dosage administered. Five patients showed stable disease after 33, 19, 12, 10, and 3 months (Tables 51.2 and 51.3). Based on the outcomes of the study, Salgia et al. concluded that GVAX enhances antitumor immunity in some patients with metastatic NSCLC.

In an effort to remove the requirement for genetic transduction of individual tumors and to optimize GM-CSF transgene expression (given that this correlated with improved survival), a second approach was developed called bystander GVAX, which is a vaccine composed of autologous tumor cells mixed with an allogeneic GM-CSF–secreting cell line (K562 cells)[58] and a phase I/II trial of this vaccine in advanced stage NSCLC was conducted. Tumors were harvested from 86 patients, tumor cell processing was successful in 76 patients, and 49 proceeded to vaccination. Serum GM-CSF pharmacokinetics were consistent with secretion of GM-CSF from vaccine cells for ≤4 days, with associated transient leukocytosis confirming the bioactivity of vaccine-secreted GM-CSF. Evidence of vaccine-induced immune activation was demonstrated. However, objective tumor responses were not seen despite a 25-fold higher GM-CSF secretion concentration with the bystander GVAX vaccine (Tables 51.2 and 51.3). The frequency of vaccine site reactions, tumor response, time to progression, and survival were all less favorable to autologous GVAX, although results were similar to historical cytotoxic therapy for second-line NSCLC.

Overall, these results suggest that autologous malignant tissue transfection with adenovirus-delivered GM-CSF is superior to the bystander approach, despite variability of GM-CSF expression levels and practical limitations inherent to surgically harvested tumor tissue.

L523S Vaccine L523S is a lung cancer antigen originally identified through screening of genes differentially expressed in cancer cells versus normal tissue.[59,60] L523S is shown to be expressed in approximately 80% of NSCLC cell lines.[59,60] In preclinical studies, the immunogenicity of L523S in humans was initially shown by detecting the presence of existent antibody and CD4+ T cell responses to L523S in patients with lung cancer. Subsequent studies further validated L523S's immunogenicity, demonstrating that human CTLs could specifically recognize and kill cells that express L523S. It has demonstrated preclinical safety when the gene is injected intramuscularly as an expressive plasmid (pVAX/L523S) and when delivered by E1B-deleted adenovirus (Ad/L523S).

A phase I clinical trial of 13 stage IB, IIA, and IIB NSCLC patients was conducted using a prime/boost vaccination strategy first with pVAX/ L523S at a dose of 8 mg on days 0 and 14 then Ad/ L523S at three dosing cohorts of 1, 20, and 400 $\times 10^9$ viral particles on days 28 and 56 (Tables 51.2 and 51.3).[61] No significant toxic effects related to the vaccination were reported. Although, all but one patient demonstrated at least a twofold increase in antiadenovirus antibodies, only one patient demonstrated a significant immune response to L523S. The reasons for the minimal detection of immune response are unknown, but suggest that alternate formulations and/or regimens need to be considered in addition to other surrogate immune function parameters. Two patients developed disease recurrence, and all patients were alive after the 290-day follow-up. The significance of the disease-free survival cannot be assessed because of the small sample size, however, one cannot exclude the possibility that the vaccine may induce a T-cell response that is below the threshold of detection in peripheral blood. The results of this trial suggest an excellent safety profile, but limited evidence of L523S-directed immune activation.

B7.1 Vaccine B7.1 (CD80+) is a costimulator molecule associated with induction of a T-cell and NK cell response.[62–65] Tumor cells transfected with B7.1, and HLA molecules have been shown to stimulate an avid immune response by direct antigen presentation and direct activation of T cells, in addition to allowing cross-presentation.[66–68] In a phase I trial, Raez et al.[69] used an allogeneic NSCLC tumor cell line (AD100) transfected with B7.1 and HLA-A1 or A2 to generate CD8+ CTL responses. Patients who were HLA-A1 or -A2 allotype received the corresponding HLA-matched vaccine. A total of 19 patients with stage IIIb or IV NSCLC were treated, and most had received prior chemotherapy. Patients who were neither HLA-A1 nor -A2 received the HLA-A1–transfected vaccine. Each patient received three intradermal vaccinations of 5×10^7 cells every 2 weeks. If the disease remained stable and toxicity was low, treatment was continued.

A total of 18 patients received at least one full course (three vaccinations) of treatment. One patient was removed before the completion of the first course caused by a serious adverse event not associated with the vaccine. Three more patients experienced serious adverse events, which were also not associated with the vaccine. Side effects associated with the vaccine included minimal skin erythema in four of the patients (Tables 51.2 and 51.3).

All but one patient had a measurable CD8+ response after three vaccinations. There was no statistically significant difference in CD8+ response depending in weather or not the patients were HLA matched. One patient showed a partial response for 13 months, and five patients had stable disease ranging from 1.6 to >52 months.[69,70] Based on the six surviving patients, the tumor vaccine appears to elevate immune response for at least 150 weeks. Overall, the Kaplan-Meier estimate for the median survival of 19 patients was 18 months. One-year survival was estimated at 52% (Tables 51.2 and 51.3). The low toxicity and good survival in this study suggested benefit from clinical vaccination. Further clinical investigation is ongoing.

NON–SMALL CELL LUNG CANCER SUBUNIT VACCINES

L-BLP-25 Liposomal Vaccine Mucin (MUC) 1 is a high–molecular weight integral membrane protein on the apical surface of MUC-secreting epithelial cells. The extracellular domain of MUC1 contains a heavily glycosylated peptide core composed of a tandemly repeating sequence of 20 amino acids.[71] It is expressed in many cancers, including NSCLC.[72] Although the MUC1 glycoprotein is expressed on the cell surface of many normal epithelial tissues and carcinomas, it has been selected as a target because of its high levels of overexpression and aberrant glycosylation patterns on carcinoma cells over normal cells, thereby conferring potentially high immunogenicity.[73] Recent studies have identified that MUC1 is associated with cellular transformation, as demonstrated by tumorigenicity,[74] and can confer resistance to genotoxic agents.[75] Both the oligosaccharide portion and the tandem repeat of the MUC extracellular domain have the potential for immunotherapeutic activity.

Clinical testing of an MUC1-directed vaccine called L-BLP-25 (Stimuvax) is ongoing. The L-BLP-25 vaccine consists of a synthetic lipopeptide with a sequence matching a part of the peptide core of the mucinous glycoprotein MUC1, immunoadjuvant, monophosphoryl lipid-A, and three lipids: cholesterol, dimyristoyl phosphatidylglycerol, and dipalmitoylphosphatidylcholine. Upon reconstitution with saline, lipopeptide and monophosphoryl lipid A associate with the lipid bilayer of liposomes. The vaccine is injected into four anatomical sites to stimulate an increased number of lymph nodes to increase the likelihood of an immune response.

Trials of the L-BLP-25 vaccine in stage III and IV NSCLC patients showed the vaccine to be safe but did not demonstrate a statistically significant survival benefit.[76,77] A phase I dose–comparison trial of 20- and 200-μg vaccine demonstrated that the agent could be administered safely. The relative safety and potential for efficacy found in phase I trials lead to the initiation of a randomized phase IIB study of L-BLP-25 in 171 advanced stage NSCLC patients.[78] Patients with Eastern Cooperative Oncology Group (ECOG) performance status of 0 to 2, stable or responding stage IIIB or IV NSCLC following standard first-line chemotherapy were randomized to either L-BLP-25 plus best supportive care (n = 88) or best supportive care (n = 83). Patients on the L-BLP-25 arm received a single dose of cyclophosphamide 300 mg/m^2 intravenously followed by 8 weekly subcutaneous immunizations with 1000 μg of L-BLP-25 (Tables 51.2 and 51.3). Maintenance immunizations (same dose) were given at 6-week intervals.

The overall survival results indicate a 4.4 month longer median survival for patients on the L-BLP-25 arm (17.4 vs. 13 months); however, this did not reach statistical significance (Tables 51.2 and 51.3). In a retrospective analysis searching for a potential subset of patients with greater therapeutic benefit, a closer look was given to the patients with stage IIIB disease without pleural effusions. With a median follow-up of 53 months, patients on the L-BLP-25 arm had a median survival of 30.6 months compared to 13.3 months for the control group $p = 0.16$ (n = 75). A favorable toxicity profile was evident in all trials of L-BLP-25 with modest erythema at the injection site and mild flulike symptoms.

Although this study failed to demonstrate a statistically significant survival difference between the L-BLP-25 and control arms in advanced NSCLC, the survival trend in stage III disease may be of clinical benefit in this subgroup that have been downstaged by chemotherapy and thoracic irradiation. A phase III multicenter (North America, Europe, Australia, and Asia) randomized, double-blind, placebo-controlled safety/efficacy study of Stimuvax in unresectable stage III NSCLC patients will evaluate patients who have shown stable disease or an objective clinical response after completing first-line chemoradiotherapy, either sequentially or concurrently. The primary end point is survival with a planned enrollment of 1322 patients and an expected completion date of 2011.

EP2101 EP2101 is a peptide-based vaccine designed to induce CTLs directed against carcinoembryonic antigen (CEA), p53, human epidermal growth factor receptor 2 (HER-2/neu), and melanoma antigen E (MAGE)-2/3 tumor-associated antigens.[79–87] These are frequently overexpressed in NSCLC. Analogue peptides have been shown to be capable of generating CTLs that are able to recognize wild-type epitopes expressed on tumor cell lines.[88–90] EP2101 has demonstrated immunogenicity in HLA-A2.1/k transgenic mice models.[91–93] It contains 10 lung cancer epitopes (p53, CEA, HER-2/neu, and MAGE), of which 9 out of 10 are restricted by HLA-A2.1. This potentially enables vaccination of approximately 45% of the NSCLC population in the United States.

Two phase I clinical trials examined the safety and immunogenicity of the EP2101 vaccine in patients with stage III colon cancer or stage IIA or IIIB NSCLC who were rendered disease free by standard therapy. A total of 24 patients were enrolled, 16 of whom completed 6 injections over 18 weeks. No significant toxicity was observed, and analysis of CTL response from 15 out of 16 patients who completes treatment with EP2101 indicated that the vaccine was immunogenic and effective at inducing strong and broad CTL responses in a high frequency of patients, as measured by the INF-γ enzyme-linked immunosorbent spot assay (presented in IND #10802). A phase II study of EP2101 in 135 patients (64 HLA-A2^{pos} and 71 HLA-A2^{neg}) with stage IIIB or IV disease has recently been completed. EP2101 was administered every 3 weeks for the first 15 weeks of the study, then every 2 months through year 1, then quarterly through year 2, for a total of 13 doses. Each injection contained 5 mg (0.5 mg of each peptide) of peptide. The study compared the survival rate of HLA-A2.1 positive patients when treated with EP2101 versus HLA-A2–negative patients who underwent standard treatment. The vaccine was well tolerated, and immune responses were seen in most patients. However, 1-year survival of HLA-A2^{pos} patients (55%) versus HLA-A2^{neg} patients (46%) and the median survival of 583 days (HLA-A2^{pos}) and 349 days (HLA-A2^{neg}) did not reach statistical significance (Tables 51.2 and 51.3).

Epidermal Growth Factor Vaccine Overexpression of epidermal growth factor receptor (EGFR) and its ligand, epidermal growth factor (EGF), has been linked with the promotion of cell proliferation, survival, and mortality. EGF transduces signaling through EGFR following binding to this cell surface receptor, ultimately resulting in cell proliferation. The immunotherapy developed by Ramos et al.[94] induces an immune response against self-produced EGF. This vaccine is a human protein from *Nisseria* *meningitides*. Several pilot studies have been completed.[94–96] Results from these demonstrated that vaccination with EGF is immunogenic and appears to be well tolerated.

In one trial, 43 patients with stage IIIB or IV NSCLC randomly received either a single or a double dose.[94] The patients were given 4 weekly dose followed by monthly immunizations. Side effects were mild to moderate, including mainly fever (42%), chills (47%), nausea (44%), vomiting (40%), tremors (44%), anorexia (35%), and pain (49%). Slightly higher toxic percentages were seen in the patients who received double dosages of the vaccine (Tables 51.2 and 51.3).

Tumor responses against EGF were measured in 38 out of 43 patients, 15 achieved a good antibody response (GAR) against EGF following vaccination. Kaplan-Meier analysis, separating patients by dose, predicted a median estimated life expectancy of 6.4 months for patients who received the single dose and 8.4 months for the patients who received the double dose (Tables 51.2 and 51.3). Based on immune response, however, patients classified as GARs had an average survival estimated at 12 months, whereas those who had a less favorable GAR had an average survival of 7 months, thereby identifying a potentially responsive treatment population of NSCLC patients.

Two other studies conducted by Gonzalez et al.[95–97] compared the effect of different adjuvants on patients' antibody response. In the first trial, 20 patients with stage IIIB or IV NSCLC were randomly vaccinated with either EGF-p64K absorbed to alum (n = 10) or emulsified in montanide ISA 51 (n = 10). In the second trial, 20 stage IIIB or IV patients were similarly randomized, but all received a single dose of cyclophosphamide 3 days prior to the first vaccination. The vaccine consisted of EGF conjugated to a P64K *N. meningitides* carrier protein. Patients were vaccinated intramuscularly on days 0, 7, 14, 21, and 51. The patients were revaccinated when antibody titers decreased to at least 50% of their peak titer at the induction phase.

No patients experienced severe toxicity. Side effects consisted of grade 2 fever, chills, nausea, vomiting, hypertension, headache, dizziness, flushing, pain at the injection site, bone pain, mouth dryness, and hot flashes (Tables 51.2 and 51.3).

The combined data of the two Gonzalez trials suggested that higher antibody responses were obtained when the vaccine was emulsified in montanide ISA 51 or when low-dose cyclophosphamide was administered before the vaccination; however, because of the small sample size, the difference was not statistically significant. Percentages of GAR were significantly higher when montanide ISA 51 was used as an adjuvant in both trials compared with alum groups. More than 90% of all vaccinated patients were seroconverted and GAR was achieved by approximately 50% of vaccinated patients. Median survival of GAR patients was 9.1 months, whereas poor antibody responding patients had survival of 4.5 months. The median survival of all vaccinated patients was 8.2 months. In addition, patients with ≥60 days response duration showed a significant increase in survival times compared with the corresponding groups with <60 days response duration (Tables 51.2 and 51.3). These data as well as the recent approval of EGFR inhibitors gefitinib and erlotinib justify further investigation in targeting EGF by vaccination strategy.

Melanoma-Associated Antigen E-3 Vaccine (MAGE-3) MAGE-AE is a 361 amino acid protein, which belongs to the category of cancer/testis tumor antigens. In normal tissue, MAGE-3 is expressed only by testicular germ cells; however, it is aberrantly expressed in a wide variety of tumors, including about 35% of NSCLC.[98] Several CD8+ T-cell epitopes of MAGE-3 have been identified in vitro,[88,89,99–105] including HLA-A1-restricted epitope 168 to 176[106] and HLA-A2-restricted epitope 271 to 279.[107] Based on these findings, synthetic peptides corresponding to these epitopes have been introduced into clinical vaccination studies in which they were associated with regression of melanoma in individual cases.[108] Clinical vaccination studies, using full-length recombinant proteins, have the advantage that this antigen potentially includes the full range of epitopes for CD4+ and CD8+ T cells. In addition, it is likely that protein vaccination leads to presentation of epitopes in the context of various HLA alleles and therefore, this type of vaccine should be applicable to any patient regardless of HLA restriction.[109] Atanackovic et al.[109] used a MAGE-3 protein as a vaccine to induce CD4+ T cells in patients with stage I or II NSCLC. All patients had undergone surgical resection of the primary lung tumor and had no evidence of disease at the onset of the study. A total of 9 of 17 total patients received 300 μg of the MAGE-3 protein alone, and 8 patients received the MAGE-3 protein combined with AS02B (Adjuvant System 2B; GlaxoSmithKline). Patients were given four intradermal injections every 3 weeks.

Of the nine patients who received the MAGE-3 protein alone, three developed an increase in antibodies against MAGE-3 protein and one had a CD8+ T-cell response. By comparison, of the eight patients who received MAGE-3 antigen combined with the adjuvant, seven showed an increase in serum concentrations of anti-MAGE-3 and four had a CD4+ response to HLA-DP4-restricted peptide.

Based on these results, further testing in a larger randomized phase II trial was conducted,[109a] involving 182 stage Ib or II completely resected NSCLC MAGE-A3+ patients (122 vaccine and 60 placebo). Patients received five vaccinations at 3-week intervals. A total of 1609 vaccinations were administered and no serious toxicities were attributed to the vaccine after preliminary analysis (Tables 51.2 and 51.3). After a median follow-up of 28 months, 30.6% had recurrence in the vaccine group versus 43.3% in the control group. The hazard ratio for progression-free survival was 0.73 (95% confidence interval [CI], 0.45 to 1.16; one-sided log-rank $p = 0.093$). For overall survival, the hazard ratio was 0.66 (95% CI, 0.36 to 1.20; one-sided log-rank $p = 0.088$).

Phase III investigation is underway with the MAGRIT study (MAGE A3 as Adjuvant Non-small cell lunG canceR ImmunoTherapy). This ambitious project will screen over 10,000 resected NSCLC patients for 2270 patients positive for MAGE-A3 immunohistochemistry. Eligible patients may or may not have received adjuvant chemotherapy and will be randomized between MAGE-A3 immunotherapeutic versus placebo.

Transcriptase Catalytic Subunit Antigen Vaccine It has been established that human T cells recognize telomerase as a TAA.[110–113] Although telomerase is also expressed in some normal tissue, such as bone marrow, and in crypts of the gastrointestinal epithelium,[114] it is highly expressed in most cancer cell lines. GV1001 is a unique peptide corresponding to a sequence of transcriptase catalytic subunit human telomerase reverse transcriptase (hTERT) derived from its active site. It contains the 611–626 sequence of hTERT and is capable of binding to molecules encoded by multiple alleles of all three loci of HLA class II.[115] HR2822 is a second peptide corresponding to sequences 540–548 of hTERT. Brunsvig et al.[116] initiated a phase I/II trial of GV1001 (112 or 560 μg), HR2822 68 mg, and GM-CSF (30 or 75 μg). A total of 26 patients with stage III or IV NSCLC were given 4 to 21 intradermal injections of the vaccine. No clinically significant toxicities were attributed to the investigational regimen including gastrointestinal or bone marrow toxicities. Side effects were considered mild consisting mainly of flulike symptoms.

A total of 24 out of 26 patients enrolled were considered evaluable having received a minimum of 4 weeks of treatment. A total of 14 patients completed the study, whereas 10 patients were taken off the study because of disease progression. Eleven patients demonstrated an immune response against GV1001, and two patients demonstrated a response to HR2822. After receiving booster vaccinations, two additional patients converted to immune responders. One patient with stage IIIA NSCLC had a complete response and developed GV1001-specific CTLs that could be cloned from peripheral blood. The median survival time for all 26 patients was 8.5 months (Tables 51.2 and 51.3). This trial demonstrated GV1001 and HR2882 to a lesser extent are immunogenic targets and warrant further investigation.

Dexosomes Dexosomes are DC-derived lipid vesicles that express high levels of a narrow spectrum of cell proteins, which have been shown to play a role in the activation of immune response.[117–121] In vitro, dexosomes have the capacity to present antigen to naive CD8+ cytotoxic T cells and CD4+ T cells.[117,122] Purified dexosomes were shown to be effective in both suppressing tumor growth and eradicating an established tumor in murine models.[119] Morse et al.[123] developed a vaccine using DC-derived dexosomes loaded with MAGE tumor antigens. The phase I trial enrolled 13 patients with stage IIIB or IV NSCLC demonstrating MAGE-3A or A4 expression. Autologous DCs were harvested to produce dexosomes. They were peptide pulsed with MAGE-3A, 4A, 10A, and −3DPG4 antigens. Dexosome vaccinations were administered to nine patients at a dose of 1.3 × 1013 MHC II class molecules in a volume of 3 mL via subcutaneous and intradermal injection weekly for 4 weeks.

Patients experienced grade 1 and 2 toxicities including injection site reactions, flulike symptoms, edema, and pain. Three patients exhibited DTH reactions against MAGE peptides. Only one had detectable increases in T-cell precursors frequency to MAGE-A10. Disease progression time ranges from 30 to 429 days and survival was in the range of 52 to 665 days. The study concluded that production of dexosome was feasible. The vaccine is well tolerated and produced long-term stable disease in some patients, and activation of immune effectors could be induced.

α(1,3)-Galactosyltransferase α(1,3)-Galactosyltransferase (agal) epitopes present on the surface of most nonhuman mammalian cells are the primary antigen source inductive of hyperactive xenographt rejection. Agal directs the addition of agal to N-acetyl glucosamine residues in humans. Expression of agal epitopes after gene transfer of agal (using retroviral vector) in human A375 melanoma cells prevented tumor formation in nude mice.[124]

Preliminary results by Morris et al.[125] using three irradiated lung cancer cell lines genetically altered to express xenotransplantation antigens by retroviral transfer of the murine agal gene, were recently described in seven patients with stage IV, recurrent or refractory NSCLC. Intradermal injections were given at doses of 3×10^6, 10×10^6, 30×10^6, or 100×10^6 cells/vaccine once every 4 weeks spanning a total of four doses. Only four patients received all four vaccinations, two patients received three vaccinations, and one patient received two vaccinations at the abstract was published. Toxicity involved grades 1 and 2 pain at the injection site, local skin reactions, fatigue, and hypertension. Four patients had stable disease for >16 months. Morris et al. concluded that the agal vaccine was feasible and safe. Full analysis is awaiting completion of this trial.

Dendritic Cell Vaccines DCs are potent antigen-presenting cells.[1a,2–5] As part of a phase II study, Hirschowitz et al.[2] recently produced a DC vaccine from CD14+ precursors, which were pulsed with apoptotic antibodies from an allogeneic NSCLC cell line that overexpressed HER-2/neu, CEA, WH1, MAGE-2, and survivin. A total of 16 patients with stage IA to IIIB NSCLC were vaccinated. The patients were immunized twice, 1 month apart.

There were 10 patients who experienced skin reaction at the injection site and 4 patients experienced minor fatigue. No patients experienced a serious adverse event. Five patients showed no antigen-independent response and six patients showed an antigen-specific response. The study concluded that the vaccine was safe and demonstrated immunologic activity. Further work is ongoing.

Cyclophilin B Cyclophilin-B (CypB) is a ubiquitous protein playing an important role in protein folding[126,127] and is expressed in both normal and cancerous cells. CypB-derived peptides are recognized by HLA-A24 restricted CTLs isolated from lung adenocarcinoma. CypB peptides induce CTLs from leukemic patients, but failed to induce an immune response in cells isolated from patients with epithelial cancer or normal donors. Modification of a single amino acid of the CypB gene increases its immunogenicity and results in CTL activation in both cancer patients and healthy donors.[128]

TABLE 51.4 Demographics for Recent Vaccine Trials in SCLC

Vaccine	Vaccine Administration	Number of Patients	Stage	Reference
Fucosyl GM1	30 μg sc q wk × 4 then q4 × 2	13	9ES, 4LS	133
Fucosyl GM1	30, 10, or 3 μg id q wk × 4 then q4 wk × 2	16	6ES, 10LS	134
BEC2	2.5 mg sc qo wk × 4 then q 4 wk × 1	15	8ES, 7LS	140
PolySA	30 μg q wk × 4 then q4 × 2	13	8ES, 5LS	148
p53	id qo wk × 3	29	ES	155

ES, extensive stage; id, intradermal; LS, limited stage; sc, subcutaneous; q, every; qo, every other.

Gohara et al.[129] investigated the immune response in advanced stage lung cancer patients treated with CypB vaccine. 16 HLA-A24+ patients, 15 with NSCLC, and 1 with SCLC, were treated with CypB or modified CypB peptide vaccine following completion of chemotherapy. All patients had stable disease at 5-week follow-up. Following vaccination, IFN-γ production by peripheral blood mononuclear cells isolated from patient sera were elevated in 3 of 12 patients. The median time to progression of patients vaccinated with CypB peptide or modified CypB peptide was 25 or 8 weeks, respectively. Overall survival for NSCLC patients receiving CypB or modified CypB vaccine was 67+ and 28+ weeks, respectively. One patient with SCLC was not evaluable for response.

SMALL CELL LUNG CANCER

Fucosyl GM-1 The ganglioside fucosyl-GM1 is a carbohydrate molecule present in most cases of small cell lung cancer (SCLC),[130,131] but absent in normal lung tissue. Immunostaining has demonstrated the presence of fucosyl-GM1 in culture media from SCLC cell lines, in tumor extracts and in serum of mouse xenografts.[132] Fucosyl-GM1 was detected in the serum of 4 of 20 SCLC patients with extensive-stage disease, but was not present in the serum of 12 patients with NSCLC or in 20 healthy volunteers.[132] The specificity of fucosyl-GM1 to SCLC makes it a potential target for immunotherapy.

Dickler et al.[133] treated 13 patients were with Fuc-GM1 isolated from bovine thyroid tissue; 10 patients completed the study and were evaluable.. All 10 patients demonstrated high titers of immunoglobulin M (IgM) and IgG antibodies to Fuc-GM1, despite recent chemotherapy and radiation. The most common toxicity was local skin reaction, lasting 2 to 5 days. Other adverse effects include transient flulike symptoms, fatigue, diarrhea, and worsening of sensory neuropathy (six patients). Three of six patients who completed the entire course of vaccinations remained relapse free at 18, 24, and 30 months from diagnosis. Krug et al.[134] administered synthetic fucosyl-GM1 following completion of conventional therapy to 17 patients. Patients were randomized to receive vaccine doses of 30, 10, or 5 μg. Five of six patients at the 30-μg dose demonstrated increased levels of antifucosyl GM1 IgM. Three of six patients receiving 10-μg doses showed antifucosyl GM1 IgM production, and none of five patients at the 3-μg dose level showed elevated IgM levels. The IgM titers for patients receiving 30- or 10-μg doses were similar to levels reached with patients treated with bovine fucosyl-GM1, whereas IgG levels were lower. Toxicities were minimal and included injection site reaction, mild flulike symptoms, myalgias, and sensory neuropathy (19%) (Tables 51.4 and 51.5).

TABLE 51.5 Results of Recent Vaccine Trials in SCLC

Vaccine	Side Effects	Median Survival	1-Year Survival	Response	Reference
Fucosyl GM1	Grade 1–3: local skin reaction, flulike symptoms, sensory neuropathy	NA	NA	NA	133
Fucosyl GM1	Grade 1–2: local skin reaction, myalgia, sensory neuropathy	17.5 mo from 1st vaccination	69%	NA	134
BEC2	Grade 1–3: local skin reaction, fever	20.5 mo from diagnosis	NA	NA	140
PolySA	Grade 1–4: local skin reaction, peripheral neuropathy	22 mo from 1st vaccination	61%	NA	148
p53	Grade 2: fatigue, arthralgia	11.8 mo from 1st vaccination	11%	1 PR, 7 SD	155

NA, not available; PR, partial response; SCLC, small cell lung cancer; SD, stable disease.

BEC2 Ganglioside GD3 is a cell surface glycosphingolipid whose expression in normal tissue is limited to cells of neuroectodermal origin and a subset of T lymphocytes.[135–137] High levels of expression have been demonstrated in SCLC tumors and cell lines.[138] Because GD3 is present at low levels in normal tissues, it is poorly immunogenic. BEC2, an anti-idiotypic IgG2b mouse antibody that is structurally similar to GD3, demonstrates strong immunogenic properties in patients with melanoma.[139]

Grant et al.[140] treated 15 SCLC patients, 8 with extensive-stage disease, and 7 with limited-stage disease, with BEC2 vaccination. Thirteen patients were evaluable for response; all developed IgM antibodies to BEC2, and three developed IgG antibodies. Duration of antibody production was variable, with at least one patient demonstrating measurable antibody production 1 year following treatment. Median survival was 20.5 months from diagnosis, and patients with measurable anti-GD3 antibodies showed the longest relapse-free intervals (Tables 51.4 and 51.5). When compared to SCLC patients treated with conventional therapy alone, the authors found patients treated with BEC2 vaccine to have longer than expected survival time, though not statistically significant. Significant toxicity was minimized to local skin irritation. There was no evidence of toxicity related to normal tissue destruction, despite the fact that GD3 is expressed by some normal tissues.

PolySA Polysialic acid (polySA) is found on the surface of Gram-negative bacteria (such as group B meningococcus), embryonic neural crest cells, and some malignancies of neural crest origin.[141,142] The large size and negative charge of this molecule inhibit binding of cell adhesion molecules, and it is this property that is believed to contribute to its role in neural crest cell migration and early metastasis of malignant cells.[143,144] PolySA has been shown to be expressed abundantly by SCLC tissues,[145–147] making it a potentially viable target for SCLC vaccine therapy.

Krug et al.[148] investigated the immunogenicity of polySA vaccination in 11 SCLC patients following conventional therapy. Two forms of polySA were administered to patients. Five patients received vaccination with polySA, and six patients received polySA manipulated by N-propionylation (NP-polySA), which has been shown to boost the IgG response in mice.[149] One of five patients treated with unmodified polySA demonstrated an IgM response. Of the six patients vaccinated with NP-polySA, all produced measurable IgM antibody responses. In five of the six cases, these antibodies cross-reacted with unmodified polySA. Flow cytometry confirmed the presence of IgM antibodies reactive to SCLC cell lines. Despite the demonstrable production of IgM antibodies to polySA, complement-dependent lysis of polySA-positive tumor cells with human complement could not be demonstrated. Common adverse effects were minimal and included injection site reaction and flulike symptoms lasting 2 to 4 days (Tables 51.4 and 51.5). Four patients reported sensory neuropathy.

p53 The tumor suppressor gene p53 plays a key role in cell cycle regulation and is mutated in 90% of SCLC.[150,151] In normal tissue, the p53 protein is present in low levels because of its brief half-life. Mutant p53 in cancer cells has a prolonged half-life and is therefore present at much higher levels in these tissues. When induced, anti-p53 CTLs attack tumor tissues while sparing normal tissue in preclinical studies.[152–154]

DCs activated by p53-producing adenovirus were administered to 29 patients with extensive-stage SCLC.[155] There were 57.1% of patients who showed significant p53-specific immune responses (Tables 51.4 and 51.5). Although only one patient showed an objective clinical response following vaccination, 61.9% of the 21 patients treated with second-line chemotherapy demonstrated clinical responses, compared to 2% to 5% response in nonvaccinated patients.

WT1 The Wilms' tumor gene (*WT1*) is responsible for Wilms' tumor, a pediatric renal cancer, and encodes a protein involved in cell proliferation and differentiation, apoptosis, and organ development.[156–158] WT1 is overexpressed in several hematological malignancies as well as various solid tumors, including lung, breast, thyroid, and colorectal cancers.[159,160] WT1-specific CTL lyse WT1 expressing tumor cells in vitro without damaging normal tissues that express WT1 physiologically.[161,162]

Oka et al.[163] treated 26 patients, including 10 lung cancer patients (histological type not specified), with WT1 vaccine following completion of conventional therapy. Three patients showed decreased serum levels of tumor markers (CEA or SLX) following vaccination; one patient also showed a decrease in tumor size radiographically. One patient had stable disease at follow-up; four patients developed progressive disease, and two were unevaluable. Three patients demonstrated increased activity of WT1-specific CTL activity. A correlation (p = 0.0397) between immunological and clinical response was observed for all study patients. Toxicities were limited to injection site inflammation. Despite the fact that WT1 is expressed in many normal tests, routine laboratory investigation did not reveal damage to these tissues following vaccine administration.

CONCLUSION

The poor overall survival of patients with advanced lung cancer, combined with the toxicity associated with many treatment modalities, mandates novel approaches to clinical management of lung cancer. Traditional approaches for management of advanced stage lung cancer have likely reached a plateau with respect to survival and response advantage to singlet, doublet, or triplet cytotoxic therapy combinations. Recent data of combinations of cytotoxic therapies with angiogenesis inhibitors and/or EGFR inhibitors appear encouraging in subsets of patients. Results summarized in this review suggest immune-based therapies may also "soon" provide sufficient validation to be considered as part of the therapeutic armetarium for lung cancer. Both "targeted" peptide and gene-transduced cell-based vaccines demonstrate the ability to activate and direct adaptive immune effecter cells to recognize and attack cancer. The activity of Lucanix, L-BLP-25, and MAGE-A3 in particular has lead to the conduct of phase III trials and the data generated from these trials will potentially serve to guide direction of these novel therapeutic modalities over the next several years. Yet, more remains to be discovered.

This chapter summarizes the current evidence of the clinical activity of immune-based vaccines in lung cancer. Through enhancement of tumor antigen recognition and immune activation, these vaccines may, one day, provide patients with a highly tolerable therapy to use in combination with traditional approaches. However, this treatment strategy is relatively new and will require continued development to determine its ultimate role in the treatment of lung cancer.

REFERENCES

1. Rosenberg SA, Lotze MT, Muul LM, et al. A progress report on the treatment of 157 patients with advanced cancer using lymphokine-activated killer cells and interleukin-2 or high-dose interleukin-2 alone. *N Engl J Med* 1987;316(15):889–897.

1a. Cranmer LD, Trevor KT, Hersh EM. Clinical applications of dendritic cell vaccination in the treatment of cancer. *Cancer Immunol Immunother* 2004;53(4):275–306.

2. Hirschowitz EA, Foody T, Kryscio R, et al. Autologous dendritic cell vaccines for non-small-cell lung cancer. *J Clin Oncol* 2004;22(14):2808–2815.

3. Banchereau J, Briere F, Caux C, et al. Immunobiology of dendritic cells. *Annu Rev Immunol* 2000;18:767–811.

4. Germain RN. MHC-dependent antigen processing and peptide presentation: providing ligands for T lymphocyte activation. *Cell* 1994; 76(2):287–299.

5. Gilboa E, Nair SK, Lyerly HK. Immunotherapy of cancer with dendritic-cell-based vaccines. *Cancer Immunol Immunother* 1998;46(2):82–87.

6. Timmerman JM, Levy R. Dendritic cell vaccines for cancer immunotherapy. *Annu Rev Med* 1999;50:507–529.

7. Conrad C, Nestle FO. Dendritic cell-based cancer therapy. *Curr Opin Mol Ther* 2003;5(4):405–412.

8. Keilholz U, Weber J, Finke JH, et al. Immunologic monitoring of cancer vaccine therapy: results of a workshop sponsored by the Society for Biological Therapy. *J Immunother* 2002;25(2):97–138.

9. McAdam AJ, Schweitzer AN, Sharpe AH. The role of B7 co-stimulation in activation and differentiation of CD4+ and CD8+ T cells. *Immunol Rev* 1998;165:231–247.

10. Pulendran B, Smith JL, Caspary G, et al. Distinct dendritic cell subsets differentially regulate the class of immune response in vivo. *Proc Natl Acad Sci U S A* 1999;96(3):1036–1041.

11. Akbari O, DeKruyff RH, Umetsu DT. Pulmonary dendritic cells producing IL-10 mediate tolerance induced by respiratory exposure to antigen. *Nat Immunol* 2001;2(8):725–731.

12. Woo EY, Chu CS, Goletz TJ, et al. Regulatory CD4(+)CD25(+) T cells in tumors from patients with early-stage non-small cell lung cancer and late-stage ovarian cancer. *Cancer Res* 2001;61(12):4766–4772.

13. Woo EY, Yeh H, Chu CS, et al. Cutting edge: regulatory T cells from lung cancer patients directly inhibit autologous T cell proliferation. *J Immunol* 2002;168(9):4272–4276.

14. Neuner A, Schindel M, Wildenberg U, et al. Cytokine secretion: clinical relevance of immunosuppression in non-small cell lung cancer. *Lung Cancer* 2001;34 Suppl 2:S79–S82.

15. Neuner A, Schindel M, Wildenberg U, et al. Prognostic significance of cytokine modulation in non-small cell lung cancer. *Int J Cancer* 2002; 101(3):287–292.

16. Dohadwala M, Luo J, Zhu L, et al. Non-small cell lung cancer cyclo-oxygenase-2-dependent invasion is mediated by CD44. *J Biol Chem* 2001;276(24):20809–20812.

17. Schwartz RH. Models of T cell anergy: is there a common molecular mechanism? *J Exp Med* 1996;184(1):1–8.

18. Lombardi G, Sidhu S, Batchelor R, et al. Anergic T cells as suppressor cells in vitro. *Science* 1994;264(5165):1587–1589.

19. Hirte HW, Clark DA, O'Connell G, et al. Reversal of suppression of lymphokine-activated killer cells by transforming growth factor-beta in ovarian carcinoma ascitic fluid requires interleukin-2 combined with anti-CD3 antibody. *Cell Immunol* 1992;142(1):207–216.

20. Smith KA. Interleukin-2: inception, impact, and implications. *Science* 1988;240(4856):1169–1176.

21. Ruffini PA, Rivoltini L, Silvani A, et al. Factors, including transforming growth factor beta, released in the glioblastoma residual cavity, impair activity of adherent lymphokine-activated killer cells. *Cancer Immunol Immunother* 1993;36(6):409–416.

22. Roszman T, Elliott L, Brooks W. Modulation of T-cell function by gliomas. *Immunol Today* 1991;12(10):370–374.

23. Smith KA. Lowest dose interleukin-2 immunotherapy. *Blood* 1993; 81(6):1414–1423.

24. Tigges MA, Casey LS, Koshland ME. Mechanism of interleukin-2 signaling: mediation of different outcomes by a single receptor and transduction pathway. *Science* 1989;243(4892):781–786.

25. Rook AH, Kehrl JH, Wakefield LM, et al. Effects of transforming growth factor beta on the functions of natural killer cells: depressed cytolytic activity and blunting of interferon responsiveness. *J Immunol* 1986;136(10):3916–3920.

26. Tsunawaki S, Sporn M, Ding A, et al. Deactivation of macrophages by transforming growth factor-beta. *Nature* 1988;334(6179):260–262.

27. Fontana A, Frei K, Bodmer S, et al. Transforming growth factor-beta inhibits the generation of cytotoxic T cells in virus-infected mice. *J Immunol* 1989;143(10):3230–3234.

28. Ranges GE, Figari IS, Espevik T, et al. Inhibition of cytotoxic Tcell-development by transforming growth factor beta and reversal by recombinant tumor necrosis factor alpha. *J Exp Med* 1987;166(4):991–998.

29. Nemunaitis J, Dillman RO, Schwarzenberger PO, et al. Phase II study of belagenpumatucel-L, a transforming growth factor beta-2 antisense gene-modified allogeneic tumor cell vaccine in non-small-cell lung cancer. *J Clin Oncol* 2006;24(29):4721–4730.

30. Border WA, Ruoslahti E. Transforming growth factor-beta in disease: the dark side of tissue repair. *J Clin Invest* 1992;90(1):1–7.

31. Sporn MB, Roberts AB, Wakefield LM, et al. Transforming growth factor-beta: biological function and chemical structure. *Science* 1986; 233(4763):532–534.

32. Massagué J. The TGF-beta family of growth and differentiation factors. *Cell* 1987;49(4):437–438.

33. Bodmer S, Strommer K, Frei K, et al. Immunosuppression and transforming growth factor-beta in glioblastoma. Preferential production of transforming growth factor-beta 2. *J Immunol* 1989;143(10): 3222–3229.

34. Jakowlew SB, Mathias A, Chung P, et al. Expression of transforming growth factor beta ligand and receptor messenger RNAs in lung cancer cell lines. *Cell Growth Differ* 1995;6(4):465–476.

35. Constam DB, Philipp J, Malipiero UV, et al. Differential expression of transforming growth factor-beta 1, -beta 2, and -beta 3 by glioblastoma cells, astrocytes, and microglia. *J Immunol* 1992;148(5):1404–1410.

36. Kong F, Jirtle RL, Huang DH, et al. Plasma transforming growth factor-beta1 level before radiotherapy correlates with long term outcome of patients with lung carcinoma. *Cancer* 1999;86(9):1712–1719.

37. Hirte H, Clark DA. Generation of lymphokine-activated killer cells in human ovarian carcinoma ascitic fluid: identification of transforming growth factor-beta as a suppressive factor. *Cancer Immunol Immunother* 1991;32(5):296–302.

38. Kasid A, Bell GI, Director EP. Effects of transforming growth factor-beta on human lymphokine-activated killer cell precursors. Autocrine inhibition of cellular proliferation and differentiation to immune killer cells. *J Immunol* 1988;141(2):690–698.

39. Naganuma H, Sasaki A, Satoh E, et al. Transforming growth factor-beta inhibits interferon-gamma secretion by lymphokine-activated killer cells stimulated with tumor cells. *Neurol Med Chir (Tokyo)* 1996; 36(11):789–795.

40. Kettering JD, Mohamedali AM, Green LM, et al. IL-2 gene and antisense TGF-beta1 strategies counteract HSV-2 transformed tumor progression. *Technol Cancer Res Treat* 2003;2(3):211–221.
41. Fakhrai H, Mantil JC, Liu L, et al. Phase I clinical trial of a TGF-beta antisense-modified tumor cell vaccine in patients with advanced glioma. *Cancer Gene Ther* 2006;13(12):1052–1060.
42. Liau LM, Fakhrai H, Black KL. Prolonged survival of rats with intracranial C6 gliomas by treatment with TGF-beta antisense gene. *Neurol Res* 1998;20(8):742–747.
43. Fakhrai H, Dorigo O, Shawler DL, et al. Eradication of established intracranial rat gliomas by transforming growth factor beta antisense gene therapy. *Proc Natl Acad Sci U S A* 1996;93(7):2909–2914.
44. Dorigo O, Shawler DL, Royston I, et al. Combination of transforming growth factor beta antisense and interleukin-2 gene therapy in the murine ovarian teratoma model. *Gynecol Oncol* 1998;71(2):204–210.
45. Tzai TS, Shaiu AL, Liu LL, et al. Immunization with TGF-beta antisense oligonucleotide-modified autologous tumor vaccine enhances the antitumor immunity of MBT-2 tumor-bearing mice through upregulation of MHC class I and Fas expressions. *Anticancer Res* 2000; 20(3A):1557–1562.
46. Tzai TS, Lin CI, Shiau AL, et al. Antisense oligonucleotide specific for transforming growth factor-beta 1 inhibit both in vitro and in vivo growth of MBT-2 murine bladder cancer. *Anticancer Res* 1998;18(3A): 1585–1589.
47. Marzo AL, Fitzpatrick DR, Robinson BW, et al. Antisense oligonucleotides specific for transforming growth factor beta2 inhibit the growth of malignant mesothelioma both in vitro and in vivo. *Cancer Res* 1997; 57(15):3200–3207.
48. Park JA, Wang E, Kurt RA, et al. Expression of an antisense transforming growth factor-beta1 transgene reduces tumorigenicity of EMT6 mammary tumor cells. *Cancer Gene Ther* 1997;4(1):42–50.
49. Shepherd FA, Rodrigues Pereira J, Ciuleanu T, et al. Erlotinib in previously treated non-small-cell lung cancer. *N Engl J Med* 2005;353(2):123–132.
50. Hanna N, Shepherd FA, Fossella FV, et al. Randomized phase III trial of pemetrexed versus docetaxel in patients with non-small-cell lung cancer previously treated with chemotherapy. *J Clin Oncol*, 2004; 22(9):1589–1597.
51. Tsao MS, Sakurada A, Cutz JC, et al. Erlotinib in lung cancer - molecular and clinical predictors of outcome. *N Engl J Med* 2005;353(2):133–144.
52. Kris MG, natale RB, Herbst RS, et al. Efficacy of gefitinib, an inhibitor of the epidermal growth factor receptor tyrosine kinase, in symptomatic patients with non-small cell lung cancer: a randomized trial. *JAMA* 2003;290(16):2149–2158.
53. Shepherd FA, Dancey J, Ramlau R, et al. Prospective randomized trial of docetaxel versus best supportive care in patients with non-small-cell lung cancer previously treated with platinum-based chemotherapy. *J Clin Oncol* 2000;18(10):2095–2103.
54. Fossella FV, DeVore R, Kerr RN, et al. Randomized phase III trial of docetaxel versus vinorelbine or ifosfamide in patients with advanced non-small-cell lung cancer previously treated with platinum-containing chemotherapy regimens. The TAX 320 Non-Small Cell Lung Cancer Study Group. *J Clin Oncol* 2000;18(12):2354–2362.
55. Hege KM, Carbone DP. Lung cancer vaccines and gene therapy. *Lung Cancer* 2003;41(Suppl 1):S103–S113.
56. Salgia R, Lynch T, Skarin A, et al. Vaccination with irradiated autologous tumor cells engineered to secrete granulocyte-macrophage colony-stimulating factor augments antitumor immunity in some patients with metastatic non-small-cell lung carcinoma. *J Clin Oncol* 2003;21(4):624–630.
57. Nemunaitis J, Sterman D, Jablons D, et al. Granulocyte-macrophage colony-stimulating factor gene-modified autologous tumor vaccines in non-small-cell lung cancer. *J Natl Cancer Inst* 2004;96(4):326–331.
58. Nemunaitis J, Jahan T, Ross H, et al. Phase 1/2 trial of autologous tumor mixed with an allogeneic GVAX vaccine in advanced-stage non-small-cell lung cancer. *Cancer Gene Ther* 2006;13(6):555–562.
59. Mueller-Pillasch F, Pohl B, Wilda M, et al. Expression of the highly conserved RNA binding protein KOC in embryogenesis. *Mech Dev* 1999;88(1):95–99.
60. Aguiar JC, Hedstrom RC, Rogers WO, et al. Enhancement of the immune response in rabbits to a malaria DNA vaccine by immunization with a needle-free jet device. *Vaccine* 2001;20(1–2):275–280.
61. Nemunaitis J, Meyers T, Senzer N, et al. Phase I Trial of sequential administration of recombinant DNA and adenovirus expressing L523S protein in early stage non-small-cell lung cancer. *Mol Ther* 2006;13(6):1185–1191.
62. Antonia SJ, Seigne J, Diaz J, et al. Phase I trial of a B7-1 (CD80) gene modified autologous tumor cell vaccine in combination with systemic interleukin-2 in patients with metastatic renal cell carcinoma. *J Urol* 2002;167(5):1995–2000.
63. Hörig H, Lee DS, Conkright W, et al. Phase I clinical trial of a recombinant canarypoxvirus (ALVAC) vaccine expressing human carcinoembryonic antigen and the B7.1 co-stimulatory molecule. *Cancer Immunol Immunother* 2000;49(9):504–514.
64. Hull GW, Mccurdy MA, Nasu Y, et al. Prostate cancer gene therapy: comparison of adenovirus-mediated expression of interleukin 12 with interleukin 12 plus B7-1 for in situ gene therapy and gene-modified, cell-based vaccines. *Clin Cancer Res* 2000;6(10):4101–4109.
65. von Mehren M, Arlen P, Tsang KY, et al. Pilot study of a dual gene recombinant avipox vaccine containing both carcinoembryonic antigen (CEA) and B7.1 transgenes in patients with recurrent CEA-expressing adenocarcinomas. *Clin Cancer Res* 2000;6(6):2219–2228.
66. Johnston JV, Malacko AR, Mizuno MT, et al. B7-CD28 costimulation unveils the hierarchy of tumor epitopes recognized by major histocompatibility complex class I-restricted CD8+ cytolytic T lymphocytes. *J Exp Med* 1996;183(3):791–800.
67. Liu B, Podack ER, Allison JP, et al. Generation of primary tumor-specific CTL in vitro to immunogenic and poorly immunogenic mouse tumors. *J Immunol* 1996;156(3):1117–1125.
68. Nabel GJ, Gordon D, Bishop DK, et al. Immune response in human melanoma after transfer of an allogeneic class I major histocompatibility complex gene with DNA-liposome complexes. *Proc Natl Acad Sci U S A* 1996;93(26):15388–15393.
69. Raez LE, Cassileth PA, Schlesselman JJ, et al. Allogeneic vaccination with a B7.1 HLA-A gene-modified adenocarcinoma cell line in patients with advanced non-small-cell lung cancer. *J Clin Oncol* 2004;22(14):2800–2807.
70. Raez LE, Santos ES, Mudad R, et al. Clinical trials targeting lung cancer with active immunotherapy: the scope of vaccines. *Expert Rev Anticancer Ther* 2005;5(4):635–644.
71. Kufe D, Inghirami G, Abe M, et al. Differential reactivity of a novel monoclonal antibody (DF3) with human malignant versus benign breast tumors. *Hybridoma* 1984;3(3):223–232.
72. Burchell J, Gendler S, Taylor-Papadimitriou J, et al. Development and characterization of breast cancer reactive monoclonal antibodies directed to the core protein of the human milk mucin. *Cancer Res* 1987; 47(20):5476–5482.
73. Gendler SJ, Lancaster CA, Taylor-Papadimitriou J, et al. Molecular cloning and expression of human tumor-associated polymorphic epithelial mucin. *J Biol Chem* 1990;265(25):15286–15293.
74. Li Y, Liu D, Chen D, et al. Human DF3/MUC1 carcinoma-associated protein functions as an oncogene. *Oncogene* 2003;22(38):6107–6110.
75. Ren J, Agata N, Chen D, et al. Human MUC1 carcinoma-associated protein confers resistance to genotoxic anticancer agents. *Cancer Cell* 2004;5(2):163–175.
76. Morse MA. Technology evaluation: BLP-25, Biomira Inc. *Curr Opin Mol Ther* 2001;3(1):102–105.
77. Palmer M, Parker J, Modi S, et al. Phase I study of the BLP25 (MUC1 peptide) liposomal vaccine for active specific immunotherapy in stage IIIB/IV non-small-cell lung cancer. *Clin Lung Cancer* 2001;3(1):49–57; discussion 58.
78. Butts C, Murray N, Maksymiuk A, et al. Randomized phase IIB trial of BLP25 liposome vaccine in stage IIIB and IV non-small-cell lung cancer. *J Clin Oncol* 2005;23(27):6674–6681.
79. Knutson KL, Schiffman K, Disis ML. Immunization with a HER-2/neu helper peptide vaccine generates HER-2/neu CD8 T-cell immunity in cancer patients. *J Clin Invest* 2001;107(4):477–484.
80. Marshall JL, Hoyer RJ, Toomey MA, et al. Phase I study in advanced cancer patients of a diversified prime-and-boost vaccination protocol

using recombinant vaccinia virus and recombinant nonreplicating avipox virus to elicit anti-carcinoembryonic antigen immune responses. *J Clin Oncol* 2000;18(23):3964–3973.

81. Rosenwirth B, Kuhn EM, Heeney JL, et al. Safety and immunogenicity of ALVAC wild-type human p53 (vCP207) by the intravenous route in rhesus macaques. *Vaccine* 2001;19(13–14):1661–1670.
82. Ferriès E, Connan F, Pagès F, et al. Identification of p53 peptides recognized by CD8(+) T lymphocytes from patients with bladder cancer. *Hum Immunol* 2001;62(8):791–798.
83. Tartaglia J, Bonnet MC, Berinstein N, et al. Therapeutic vaccines against melanoma and colorectal cancer. *Vaccine* 2001;19(17–19):2571–2575.
84. van der Bruggen P, Traversari C, Chomez P, et al. A gene encoding an antigen recognized by cytolytic T lymphocytes on a human melanoma. *Science* 1991;254(5038):1643–1647.
85. Coulie PG, Karanikas V, Colau D, et al. A monoclonal cytolytic T-lymphocyte response observed in a melanoma patient vaccinated with a tumor-specific antigenic peptide encoded by gene MAGE-3. *Proc Natl Acad Sci U S A* 2001;98(18):10290–10295.
86. Slamon DJ, Godolphin W, Jones LA, et al. Studies of the HER-2/neu proto-oncogene in human breast and ovarian cancer. *Science* 1989; 244(4905):707–712.
87. Disis ML, Calenoff E, McLaughlin G, et al. Existent T-cell and antibody immunity to HER-2/neu protein in patients with breast cancer. *Cancer Res* 1994; 54(1):16–20.
88. Kawashima I, Hudson SJ, Tsai V, et al. The multi-epitope approach for immunotherapy for cancer: identification of several CTL epitopes from various trumor-associated antigens expressed on solid epithelial tumors. *Hum Immunol* 1998;59:1–14.
89. Keogh E, Fikes J, Southwood S, et al. Identification of new epitopes from four different tumor-associated antigens: recognition of naturally processed epitopes correlates with HLA-A*0201-binding affinity. *J Immunol* 2001;167(2):787–796.
90. Zaremba S, Barzaga E, Zhu M, et al. Identification of an enhancer agonist cytotoxic T lymphocyte peptide from human carcinoembryonic antigen. *Cancer Res* 1997;57(20):4570–4577.
91. Wentworth PA, Vitiello A, Sidney J, et al. Differences and similarities in the A2.1-restricted cytotoxic T cell repertoire in humans and human leukocyte antigen-transgenic mice. *Eur J Immunol* 1996; 26(1):97–101.
92. Vitiello A, Marchesini D, Furze J, et al. Analysis of the HLA-restricted influenza-specific cytotoxic T lymphocyte response in transgenic mice carrying a chimeric human-mouse class I major histocompatibility complex. *J Exp Med* 1991;173(4):1007–1015.
93. McKinney DM, Skvoretz R, Qin M, et al. Characterization of an in situ IFN-gamma ELISA assay which is able to detect specific peptide responses from freshly isolated splenocytes induced by DNA minigene immunization. *J Immunol Methods* 2000;237(1–2):105–117.
94. Ramos TC, Vinageras EN, Ferrer MC, et al. Treatment of NSCLC patients with an EGF-based cancer vaccine: report of a phase I trial. *Cancer Biol Ther* 2006;5(2):145–149.
95. González G, Crombet T, Catalá M, et al. A novel cancer vaccine composed of human-recombinant epidermal growth factor linked to a carrier protein: report of a pilot clinical trial. *Ann Oncol* 1998;9(4):431–435.
96. Gonzalez G, Crombet T, Torres F, et al. Epidermal growth factor-based cancer vaccine for non-small-cell lung cancer therapy. *Ann Oncol* 2003;14:461–466.
97. Gonzalez G, Crombet T, Neninger E, et al. Therapeutic vaccination with epidermal growth factor (EGF) in advanced lung cancer: analysis of pooled data from three clinical trials. *Hum Vaccin* 2007;3(1):8–13.
98. Van den Eynde BJ, van der Bruggen P. T cell defined tumor antigens. *Curr Opin Immunol* 1997;9(5):684–693.
99. Herman J, van der Bruggen P, Luescher IF, et al. A peptide encoded by the human MAGE3 gene and presented by HLA-B44 induces cytolytic T lymphocytes that recognize tumor cells expressing MAGE3. *Immunogenetics* 1996;43(6):377–383.
100. Fleischhauer K, Fruci D, Van Endert P, et al. Characterization of antigenic peptides presented by HLA-B44 molecules on tumor cells expressing the gene MAGE-3. *Int J Cancer* 1996;68(5):622–628.
101. Tanaka F, Fujie T, Tahara K, et al. Induction of antitumor cytotoxic T lymphocytes with a MAGE-3-encoded synthetic peptide presented by human leukocytes antigen-A24. *Cancer Res* 1997;57(20):4465–4468.
102. Oiso M, Eura M, Katsura F, et al. A newly identified MAGE-3-derived epitope recognized by HLA-A24-restricted cytotoxic T lymphocytes. *Int J Cancer* 1999;81(3):387–394.
103. Tanzarella S, Russo V, Lionello I, et al. Identification of a promiscuous T-cell epitope encoded by multiple members of the MAGE family. *Cancer Res* 1999;59(11):2668–2674.
104. Russo V, Tanzarella S, Dalerba P, et al. Dendritic cells acquire the MAGE-3 human tumor antigen from apoptotic cells and induce a class I-restricted T cell response. *Proc Natl Acad Sci U S A* 2000;97(5):2185–2190.
105. Schultz ES, Chapiro J, Lurguin C, et al. The production of a new MAGE-3 peptide presented to cytolytic T lymphocytes by HLA-B40 requires the immunoproteasome. *J Exp Med* 2002;195(4):391–399.
106. Gaugler B, Van den Eynde B, van der Bruggen P, et al. Human gene MAGE-3 codes for an antigen recognized on a melanoma by autologous cytolytic T lymphocytes. *J Exp Med* 1994;179(3):921–930.
107. van der Bruggen P, Bastin J, Gajewski T, et al. A peptide encoded by human gene MAGE-3 and presented by HLA-A2 induces cytolytic T lymphocytes that recognize tumor cells expressing MAGE-3. *Eur J Immunol* 1994;24(12):3038–3043.
108. Marchand M, van Baren N, Weynants P, et al. Tumor regressions observed in patients with metastatic melanoma treated with an antigenic peptide encoded by gene MAGE-3 and presented by HLA-A1. *Int J Cancer* 1999;80(2):219–230.
109. Atanackovic D, Altorki NK, Stockert E, et al. Vaccine-induced $CD4^+$ T cell responses to MAGE-3 protein in lung cancer patients. *J Immunol* 2004;172:3289–3296.
109a. Halmos BH. Lung Cancer II. ASCO Annual Meeting Summaries, 2006:156–160.
110. Vonderheide RH, Hahn WC, Schultze JL, et al. The telomerase catalytic subunit is a widely expressed tumor-associated antigen recognized by cytotoxic T lymphocytes. *Immunity* 1999;10(6):673–679.
111. Vonderheide RH, Anderson KS, Hahn WC, et al. Characterization of HLA-A3-restricted cytotoxic T lymphocytes reactive against the widely expressed tumor antigen telomerase. *Clin Cancer Res* 2001;7(11):3343–3348.
112. Scardino A, Gross DA, Alves P, et al. HER-2/neu and hTERT cryptic epitopes as novel targets for broad spectrum tumor immunotherapy. *J Immunol* 2002;168(11):5900–5906.
113. Schroers R, Shen L, Rollins L, et al. Human telomerase reverse transcriptase-specific T-helper responses induced by promiscuous major histocompatibility complex class II-restricted epitopes. *Clin Cancer Res* 2003;9(13):4743–4755.
114. Uchida N, Otsuka T, Shigematsu H, et al. Differential gene expression of human telomerase-associated protein hTERT and TEP1 in human hematopoietic cells. *Leuk Res* 1999;23(12):1127–1132.
115. Tahara H, Yasui W, Tahara E, et al. Immuno-histochemical detection of human telomerase catalytic component, hTERT, in human colorectal tumor and non-tumor tissue sections. *Oncogene* 1999;18(8):1561–1567.
116. Brunsvig PF, Aamdal S, Gjertsen MK, et al. Telomerase peptide vaccination: a phase I/II study in patients with non-small cell lung cancer. *Cancer Immunol Immunother* 2006;55(12):1553–1564.
117. Théry C, Duban L, Segura E, et al. Indirect activation of naive CD4+ T cells by dendritic cell-derived exosomes. *Nat Immunol* 2002; 3(12):1156–1162.
118. Denzer K, van Eijk M, Kleijmeer MJ, et al. Follicular dendritic cells carry MHC class II-expressing microvesicles at their surface. *J Immunol* 2000;165(3):1259–1265.
119. Zitvogel L, Regnault A, Lozier A, et al. Eradication of established murine tumors using a novel cell-free vaccine: dendritic cell-derived exosomes. *Nat Med* 1998;4(5):594–600.
120. Théry C, Regnault A, Garin J, et al. Molecular characterization of dendritic cell-derived exosomes. Selective accumulation of the heat shock protein hsc73. *J Cell Biol* 1999;147(3):599–610.
121. Raposo G, Nijman HW, Stoorvogel W, et al. B lymphocytes secrete antigen-presenting vesicles. *J Exp Med* 1996;183(3):1161–1172.

122. Hsu DH, Paz P, Villaflor G, et al. Exosomes as a tumor vaccine: enhancing potency through direct loading of antigenic peptides. *J Immunother* 2003;26(5):440–450.
123. Morse MA, Garst J, Osada T, et al. A phase I study of dexosome immunotherapy in patients with advanced non-small cell lung cancer. *J Transl Med* 2005;3(1):9.
124. Link CJ Jr, Seregina T, Atchinson R, et al. Eliciting hyperacute xenograft response to treat human cancer: alpha(1,3) galactosyltransferase gene therapy. *Anticancer Res* 1998;18(4A):2301–2308.
125. Morris JC, Vahanian N, Janik JE. Phase I study of an antitumor vaccination using α(1,3)galactosyltransferase expressing allogeneic tumor cells in patients (Pts) with refractory or recurrent non-small cell lung cancer (NSCLC). *J Clin Oncol* 2005 *ASCO Annual Meeting Proceedings* 2005. 23(No. 16S, Part I of II (June 1 Supplement): p. 2586.
126. Price ER, Zydowsky LD, Jin MJ, et al. Human cyclophilin B: a second cyclophilin gene encodes a peptidyl-prolyl isomerase with a signal sequence. *Proc Natl Acad Sci U S A* 1991;88(5):1903–1907.
127. Bergsma DJ, Eder C, Gross M, et al. The cyclophilin multigene family of peptidyl-prolyl isomerases. Characterization of three separate human isoforms. *J Biol Chem* 1991;266(34):23204–23214.
128. Gomi S, Nakao M, Niiya F, et al. A cyclophilin B gene encodes antigenic epitopes recognized by HLA-A24-restricted and tumor-specific CTLs. *J Immunol* 1999;163(9):4994–5004.
129. Gohara R, Imai N, Rikimaru T, et al. Phase 1 clinical study of cyclophilin B peptide vaccine for patients with lung cancer. *J Immunother* 2002;25(5):439–444.
130. Brezicka FT, Olling S, Nilsson O, et al. Immunohistological detection of fucosyl-GM1 ganglioside in human lung cancer and normal tissues with monoclonal antibodies. *Cancer Res* 1989;49(5):1300–1305.
131. Brezicka T, Bergman B, Olling S, et al. Reactivity of monoclonal antibodies with ganglioside antigens in human small cell lung cancer tissues. *Lung Cancer* 2000;28(1):29–36.
132. Vangsted AJ, Clausen H, Kjeldsen TB, et al. Immunochemical detection of a small cell lung cancer-associated ganglioside (FucGM1) antigen in serum. *Cancer Res* 1991;51(11):2879–2884.
133. Dickler MN, Ragupathi G, Liu NX, Musselli C, et al. Immunogenicity of a fucosyl-GM1-keyhole limpet hemocyanin conjugate vaccine in patients with small cell lung cancer. *Clin Cancer Res* 1999;5(10):2773–2779.
134. Krug LM, Ragupathi G, Hood C, et al. Vaccination of patients with small-cell lung cancer with synthetic fucosyl GM-1 conjugated to keyhole limpet hemocyanin. *Clin Cancer Res* 2004;10(18 Pt 1): 6094–6100.
135. Graus F, Cordon-Cardo C, Houghton AN, et al. Distribution of the ganglioside GD3 in the human nervous system detected by R24 mouse monoclonal antibody. *Brain Res* 1984;324(1):190–194.
136. Dippold WG, Dienes HP, Knuth A, et al. Immunohistochemical localization of ganglioside GD3 in human malignant melanoma, epithelial tumors, and normal tissues. *Cancer Res* 1985;45(8):3699–3705.
137. Welte K, Miller G, Chapman PB, et al. Stimulation of T lymphocyte proliferation by monoclonal antibodies against GD3 ganglioside. *J Immunol* 1987;139(6):1763–1771.
138. Fuentes R, Allman R, Mason MD. Ganglioside expression in lung cancer cell lines. *Lung Cancer* 1997;18(1):21–33.
139. McCaffery M, Yao TJ, Williams L, et al. Immunization of melanoma patients with BEC2 anti-idiotypic monoclonal antibody that mimics GD3 ganglioside: enhanced immunogenicity when combined with adjuvant. *Clin Cancer Res* 1996;2(4):679–686.
140. Grant SC, Kris MG, Houghton AN, et al. Long survival of patients with small cell lung cancer after adjuvant treatment with the anti-idiotypic antibody BEC2 plus Bacillus Calmette-Guerin. *Clin Cancer Res* 1999;5(6):1319–1323.
141. Rutishauser U. Polysialic acid at the cell surface: biophysics in service of cell interactions and tissue plasticity. *J Cell Biochem* 1998;70(3):304–312.
142. Finne J, Finne U, Deagostini-Bazin H, et al. Occurrence of alpha 2-8 linked polysialosyl units in a neural cell adhesion molecule. *Biochem Biophys Res Commun* 1983;112(2):482–487.
143. Rutishauser U, Landmesser L. Polysialic acid in the vertebrate nervous system: a promoter of plasticity in cell-cell interactions. *Trends Neurosci* 1996;19(10):422–427.
144. Daniel L, Trouillas J, Renaud W, et al. Polysialylated-neural cell adhesion molecule expression in rat pituitary transplantable tumors (spontaneous mammotropic transplantable tumor in Wistar-Furth rats) is related to growth rate and malignancy. *Cancer Res* 2000;60(1):80–85.
145. Komminoth P, Roth J, Lackie PM, et al. Polysialic acid of the neural cell adhesion molecule distinguishes small cell lung carcinoma from carcinoids. *Am J Pathol* 1991;139(2):297–304.
146. Lantuejoul S, Moro D, Michalides RJ, et al. Neural cell adhesion molecules (NCAM) and NCAM-PSA expression in neuroendocrine lung tumors. *Am J Surg Pathol* 1998;22(10):1267–1276.
147. Zhang S, Cordon-Cardo C, Zhang HS, et al. Selection of tumor antigens as targets for immune attack using immunohistochemistry: I. Focus on gangliosides. *Int J Cancer* 1997;73(1):42–49.
148. Krug LM, Ragupathi G, Ng KK, et al. Vaccination of small cell lung cancer patients with polysialic acid or N-propionylated polysialic acid conjugated to keyhole limpet hemocyanin. *Clin Cancer Res* 2004; 10(3):916–923.
149. Jennings HJ, Roy R, Gamian A. Induction of meningococcal group B polysaccharide-specific IgG antibodies in mice by using an N-propionylated B polysaccharide-tetanus toxoid conjugate vaccine. *J Immunol* 1986;137(5):1708–1713.
150. Bodner SM, Minna JD, Jensen SM, et al. Expression of mutant p53 proteins in lung cancer correlates with the class of p53 gene mutation. *Oncogene* 1992;7(4):743–749.
151. D'Amico D, Carbone D, Mitsudomi T, et al. High frequency of somatically acquired p53 mutations in small-cell lung cancer cell lines and tumors. *Oncogene* 1992;7(2):339–346.
152. Ishida T, Chada S, Stipanov M, et al. Dendritic cells transduced with wild-type p53 gene elicit potent anti-tumour immune responses. *Clin Exp Immunol* 1999;117(2):244–251.
153. Mayordomo JI, Loftus DJ, Sakamoto H, et al. Therapy of murine tumors with p53 wild-type and mutant sequence peptide-based vaccines. *J Exp Med* 1996;183(4):1357–1365.
154. Nikitina EY, Clark JI, Van Beynen J, et al. Dendritic cells transduced with full-length wild-type p53 generate antitumor cytotoxic T lymphocytes from peripheral blood of cancer patients. *Clin Cancer Res* 2001;7(1):127–135.
155. Antonia SJ, Mirza N, Fricke I, et al. Combination of p53 cancer vaccine with chemotherapy in patients with extensive stage small cell lung cancer. *Clin Cancer Res* 2006;12(3 Pt 1):878–887.
156. Drummond IA, Madden SL, Rohwer-Nutter P, et al. Repression of the insulin-like growth factor II gene by the Wilms tumor suppressor WT1. *Science* 1992;257(5070):674–678.
157. Goodyer P, Dehbi M, Torban E, et al. Repression of the retinoic acid receptor-alpha gene by the Wilms' tumor suppressor gene product, wt1. *Oncogene* 1995;10(6):1125–1129.
158. Hewitt SM, Hamada S, McDonnell TJ, et al. Regulation of the proto-oncogenes bcl-2 and c-myc by the Wilms' tumor suppressor gene WT1. *Cancer Res* 1995;55(22):5386–5389.
159. Oji Y, Miyoshi S, Maeda H, et al. Overexpression of the Wilms' tumor gene WT1 in de novo lung cancers. *Int J Cancer* 2002;100(3):297–303.
160. Miyoshi Y, Ando A, Egawa C, et al. High expression of Wilms' tumor suppressor gene predicts poor prognosis in breast cancer patients. *Clin Cancer Res* 2002;8(5):1167–1171.
161. Oka Y, Elisseeva OA, Tsuboi A, et al. Human cytotoxic T-lymphocyte responses specific for peptides of the wild-type Wilms' tumor gene (WT1) product. *Immunogenetics* 2000;51(2):99–107.
162. Ohminami H, Yasukawa M, Fujita S. HLA class I-restricted lysis of leukemia cells by a CD8(+) cytotoxic T-lymphocyte clone specific for WT1 peptide. *Blood* 2000;95(1):286–293.
163. Oka Y, Tsuboi A, Taguchi T, et al. Induction of WT1 (Wilms' tumor gene)-specific cytotoxic T lymphocytes by WT1 peptide vaccine and the resultant cancer regression. *Proc Natl Acad Sci U S A* 2004; 101(38):13885–13890.

CHAPTER 52

David Raben
Amanda Schwer
Paul Van Houtte

Targeted Therapies and Radiation in Lung Cancer

The use of targeted drugs—those that attempt to render specific aspects of the cancer cell–signaling pathway ineffective—have moved forward, although slowly, in the management of advanced non–small cell lung cancer (NSCLC). Erlotinib is currently Food and Drug Administration (FDA) approved for chemorefractory NSCLC.[1] Response rates for epidermal growth factor receptor (EGFR) inhibitors are in the range of 9% to 26%,[2,3] and recent reports demonstrate that gefitinib has similar activity to docetaxel for second-line treatment in NSCLC.[4] These agents fall under the category of drugs that disrupt the EGFR-signaling pathway. Bevacizumab, an intravenously administered humanized monoclonal antibody (MAb), competes with vascular endothelial growth factor (VEGF) and is also active alone or with chemotherapy in advanced NSCLC.[5,6] Caution was emphasized when using bevacizumab in patients with central lesions and squamous histology because of increased risk of bleeding. Clinical trials incorporating agents that block VEGF receptor signaling also appear promising when compared to conventional chemotherapeutics.[7] So where are we with locally advanced lung cancer and molecularly selective drugs? Have we successfully integrated novel drugs to enhance radiation cytotoxicity? Have we increased toxicity or the therapeutic ratio?

Approaches for stage IIIA to IIIB disease typically include concurrent chemoradiation, which has been found to be superior to radiation alone or sequential chemotherapy and radiation.[8,9] Recent evidence suggests that we can indeed push the envelope so to speak and safely deliver much higher doses of radiation (in the range of 74 Gy) when we use extremely conformal techniques.[10] When we use conformal intensity-modulated radiation techniques (IMRT) with concurrent chemotherapy, we are reaching median survival rates in the 22-month range.[11–13] The Radiation Therapy Oncology Group (RTOG) is currently conducting a randomized phase III study (RTOG 0617) that will definitively answer the question of dose escalation by comparing 60 to 74 Gy, both arms incorporating concurrent chemotherapy.

Returning back to targeted agents, we have initiated a host of clinical trials combining EGFR inhibitors or antiangiogenic inhibitors with radiation or chemoradiation. The goals are to see if we can improve survival further without damaging the therapeutic ratio with increased overlapping toxicity. This chapter will review the current and recently completed studies utilizing newer generation molecularly targeted drugs with radiation. Our search for improved outcomes will begin with a review of past and recently published preclinical studies that are driving translational efforts with radiation. Finally, we will take an opportunity to discuss promising agents beyond EGFR and VEGF antagonism, which might also be rationally combined with radiation for lung cancer. A complete review of every study is beyond the scope of this chapter. Rather, we hope to provide some concepts to the reader that may enlighten and/or provoke thought in the area of molecularly targeted agents and radiation for lung cancer.

PRECLINICAL STUDIES WITH MOLECULARLY TARGETED AGENTS AND RADIATION

EGFR Inhibitors and Radiation Why combine EGFR inhibitors with radiation in the first place? We have learned over the past decade or so that there are many reasons to explain the beneficial effects of this combination as seen in preclinical studies. These include cell cycle shifts into phases such as early G1, modest increases in apoptosis, and reduced angiogenesis in vivo. Remember also that ionizing radiation is supposed to damage DNA irrevocably, both through indirect production of free radicals and direct photon interaction with various parts of the DNA matrix, including the base pairs. Cancer cells, however, have a remarkable capacity to repair themselves, and we know that radiation can actually induce this process as well. The hope is that, with the proper amounts of radiation in a clinical setting, through carefully fractionated doses, the cancer cells will be unable to repair all of the damage incurred. Thus, after several cell divisions, repair necessary for mitosis will be incapacitated and the cancer cell will die. EGFR inhibitors also interfere with the repair process, as we will discuss later, and thus contribute to the enhanced radiosensitization seen with combination therapy.

MAbs with competing activity against EGFR activation have been evaluated extensively in various disease sites. To understand progress to date, we need to review briefly early preclinical studies from over a decade ago starting with anti-EGFR MAbs. We had learned that radiocurability of human tumor xenografts in nude mice expressing EGFR was more difficult than in those without EGFR expression.[14] This finding generated a hypothesis that by preventing EGFR activation through prevention of extracellular EGFR dimerization, we might improve radioresponse. Studies performed soon thereafter did find that this was, in fact, the case in tumors expressing EGFR. By combining single or fractionated radiation with concurrent administration of EGFR antibodies, investigators found that they could reduce tumor growth in aerodigestive tract tumors.[15,16] These experiments incorporated cetuximab (C225), a human–mouse chimeric MAb, with selective and competitive binding affinity to the extracellular domain of the human EGFR. Investigators began to derive the mechanisms to explain why EGFR interference worked to enhance radiation effects—these included strategic cell cycle blocks at early G1, reduced DNA repair, and modest increases in apoptosis.[17] In this same model in vivo, angiogenic abrogation was observed as well. In 2003, further evidence confirming the rationale for blocking EGFR with radiation was evidenced by increased radioresistance observed when an EGFR expression vector was cloned into cancer cells. There was a direct correlation with the level of EGFR expression in the stable clones and radioresistance as measured by clonogenic assays by a factor of 1.28 to 1.6. Cetuximab counteracted this effect by both reducing the levels of EGFR and decreasing phosphorylation of EGFR-related AKT and mitogen-activated protein kinases (MAPK).[18]

In NSCLC models, there has been only modest exploration of antibodies against EGFR with radiation. Studies at the University of Colorado included evaluation of the EGFR status on NSCLC lines by flow cytometry—little was done at that time with fluorescence in situ hybridization (FISH) to look at EGFR gene amplification—which we have since learned, may be important in predicting response to these agents.[19–21] Cetuximab monotherapy demonstrated cytostatic effects on some, but not all, NSCLC cell lines with EGFR expression, an effect that appeared to be dose dependent. Cell cycle shifts were noted into the G1 phase, although no effect was seen in cell lines that did not express EGFR. Interestingly, cetuximab actually increased phosphorylated EGFR (pEGFR) in cell lines not stimulated with EGF in cell lines expressing EGFR; however, peak EGF-induced increases in pEGFR were reduced by cetuximab in the cetuximab-sensitive lines. Combination studies in vivo demonstrated cooperative effects between radiation and cetuximab, again only in cell lines sensitive to cetuximab alone, cell lines that did not express EGFR did not demonstrate advantages to combination therapy (Fig. 52.1). Small molecule

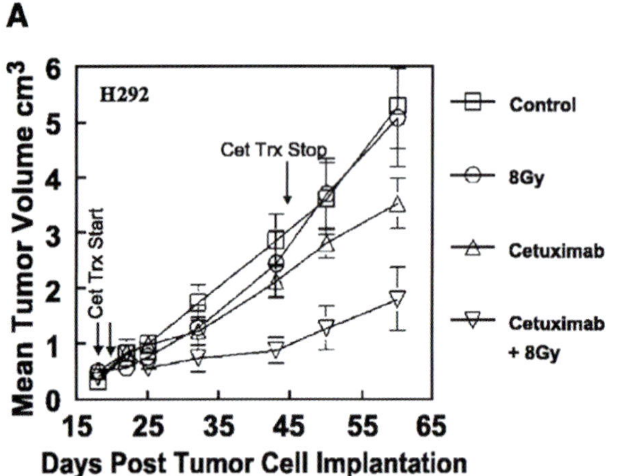

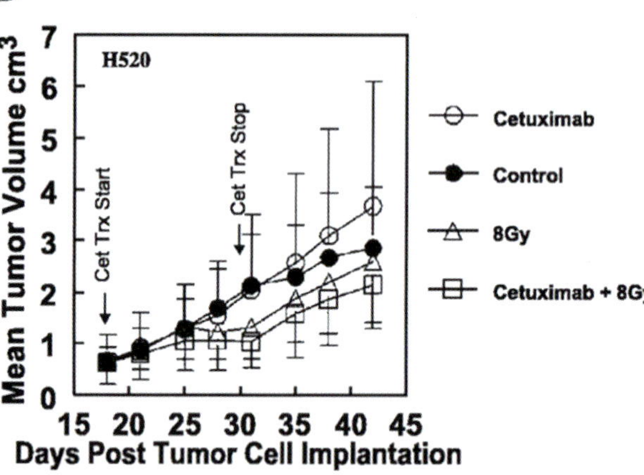

FIGURE 52.1 Mouse models bearing human NSCLC xenografts sensitive (H292; **A**) and insensitive (H520; **B**) to EGFR inhibition with cetuximab alone and in combination with single-fraction radiation. Treatment began when tumors had reached approximately 3 cm^3. Treatments were cetuximab alone (1 mg/animal twice a week for 2 weeks), ionizing radiation (5 Gy each Monday for 2 weeks), cisplatin (8 mg/kg twice a week for 2 weeks), and combinations of cetuximab plus radiation, cisplatin plus radiation, and cetuximab plus cisplatin plus radiation treatments. Tumor volume ± SE are shown. On day 93, the H292 mean tumor volume was 4.4 cm^3 in control animals, 2.2 cm^3 in animals treated with irradiation alone ($p = 0.049$), 1.8 cm^3 in animals treated with cisplatin plus radiation ($p = 0.024$), 1.5 cm^3 in animals treated with cetuximab plus radiation ($p = 0.012$), and 1.2 cm^3 in animals treated with cetuximab plus cisplatin and radiation ($p = 0.004$). The combinations produced a significant reduction in tumor volume compared with controls. Although the combination of all three agents produced the greatest reduction in tumor volume, the differences were not significant compared with cetuximab plus radiation ($p = 0.79$) or cisplatin plus radiation ($p = 0.54$). In the H520 xenografts, cetuximab alone and in combination with radiation, cisplatin or the triple combination did not significantly inhibit tumor growth. (From Raben D, Helfrich B, Chan DC, et al. The effects of cetuximab alone and in combination with radiation and/or chemotherapy in lung cancer. *Clin Cancer Res* 2005;11:795–805.)

inhibitors against EGFR-activated tyrosine kinase inhibitors (EGFR TKIs), including gefitinib and erlotinib, have also shown activity in NSCLC and head and neck squamous cell carcinoma (HNSCC) models. Explanations for their activity include competitive binding with adenosine triphosphate (ATP) to the intracellular tyrosine kinase domain of the EGFR, resulting in reduced receptor phosphorylation and activation.[22–24] Downstream interference with various pathways ensues, including the Ras-Raf-MAPK and the PI3K/Akt pathways.

In vitro combinations of radiation and erlotinib have resulted in an additive increase in apoptosis in H226 (NSCLC) cells with evidence of increased poly (adenosine diphosphate[ADP]-ribose) polymerase (PARP) cleavage. Erlotinib appeared to subdue radiation-induced pEGFR activation, which might account for rapid repopulation during radiation therapy. Adding to the story was the downregulation of Rad51, an important component of the DNA repair pathway, when erlotinib was added to H226 cells prior to radiation.[25] Inhibition of Rad51 has been shown to enhance radiosensitization. Further, erlotinib was also found to augment the effects of suboptimal fractionated radiation in animals bearing H226 flank xenografts.

The EGFR mutation story has received considerable attention over the past several years in regard to small molecule EGFR TKIs.[26,27] Specific mutations within the EGFR-binding domain that encode the ATP-binding region, located in exons 18 to 21, have been reported as more prevalent in tumors with adenocarcinoma histology, patients of Asian background, females, and never-smokers.[28] Do these same mutations also predict sensitivity or resistance to radiation in lung cancer? Recent evidence suggests that, indeed, mutant EGFR NSCLC cells have dramatically reduced survival rates measured by clonogenic assay compared with wild-type (WT) EGFR NSCLC cells in vitro.[29,30] The authors point out that the underlying reasons for this increase in radiosensitivity include delayed DNA repair kinetics. It is theorized that this select group of patients presenting with locally advanced NSCLC could be treated simply with induction EGFR inhibition followed by continued inhibition and radiation.

Adding to the molecular selection story for targeted agents and radiation is the role Kras mutations may play in determining the optimal EGFR-dependent or -independent pathway to block. Lung cancer cells with mutated Kras may drive radioresistance in different ways through EGFR-independent activation of anti-apoptotic pathways (PI3K-Akt), thus requiring different targeted agents to effectively enhance radiation cytotoxicity.[31] In this regard, blocking AKT signaling appears to enhance radiosensitivity in Kras mutated NSCLC cells primarily through reduced activation of DNA repair pathways, including interference with DNA double-strand break repair.[32,33] This certainly provides food for thought in regard to how we might design future clinical trials in locally advanced-stage NSCLC patients with Kras mutations—phase I clinical trials utilizing inhibitors of the AKT pathway with chemoradiation in these patients is the first step.

Angiogenic Inhibitors and Radiation in NSCLC

The use of antiangiogenic agents in advanced NSCLC has been validated and accepted by the oncology community. The benefits have been observed primarily in combination studies with chemotherapy[34,35] and the gains, although statistically significant, have been modest. As readers may recall, the Eastern Cooperative Oncology Group (ECOG) conducted a randomized phase III study in which 878 patients with recurrent or advanced NSCLC (stage IIIB or IV) were assigned to chemotherapy with paclitaxel and carboplatin alone or with bevacizumab, a humanized antibody against VEGF. This trial was limited only to nonsquamous histologies and patients without brain metastasis caused by bleeding episodes seen in the smaller phase II study. A survival advantage was seen in the bevacizumab arm (12.3 vs. 10.3 months; hazard ratio [HR] for death $= 0.79$; $p = 0.003$).[35]

Is this a valid strategy for radiation therapy for unresectable, locally advanced disease or earlier stage disease patients deemed medically inoperable? The concept of interfering with angiogenesis and the potential benefits and pitfalls with radiation has been explored for many years. The reader is directed toward several reviews that summarize nicely the underlying mechanisms and sequencing issues surrounding the use of antiangiogenics to enhance radiation therapy.[36–38]

Preclinical evidence appears promising at first glance. Whereas bevacizumab competitively binds VEGF, small molecules have been developed that attack the VEGF receptor tyrosine kinases (RTKs), thus functioning to inhibit VEGF signaling. The VEGF RTK VEGF receptor 2 (VEGFR2)/fetal liver kinase 1 (Flk-1)/kinase insert domain receptor (KDR) is associated with an important role in regulating VEGF-induced angiogenesis and is expressed within the endothelial cells that nurture growing cancers.[39,40] A variety of these small molecules against VEGFR2 or the family of VEGFR receptors include agents such as ZD6474, PTK787, SU11248, YM-359445, and AZD2171. We will focus on agents that have been combined with radiotherapy in lung cancer.

Vandetanib or ZD6474 is an orally bioavailable agent that has activity against VEGFR as well as EGFR.[41] Frederick et al.[42] has recently summarized some of the pertinent studies in which ZD6474 is combined with radiation. In earlier NSCLC xenograft studies, both sequential and concurrent administration of ZD6474 and fractionated radiation were superior to either ZD6474 or radiotherapy alone, with the sequential strategy demonstrating the longest growth delays.[43] Interestingly, this was seen in the Calu-6 human NSCLC line that displays resistance to EGFR inhibitors and Kras mutations. One of the underlying reasons to block angiogenic signaling is related to the observation that VEGFR2 along with basic fibroblast growth factor (bFGF) expression markedly increase after radiation therapy in orthotopic lung tumors. The ability of ZD6474 to prevent radiation-induced VEGFR2 and EGFR activation and bFGF expression explains, in part, the additive to synergistic responses seen. Shibuya et al.[44] have recently demonstrated impressive tumor growth inhibition with the combination of radiation and ZD6474, with rates of apoptosis greater than combination paclitaxel and radiation. In addition, in an orthotopic model, reduced angiogenesis and pleural

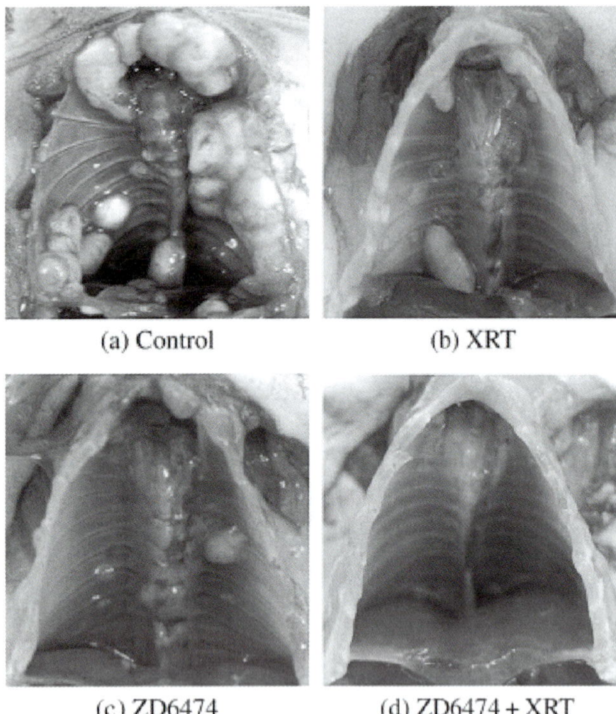

FIGURE 52.2 Effects of radiation (XRT), ZD6474, and combination ZD6474 plus fractionated radiation on pleural and lymph node metastasis in an orthotopic mouse model bearing human Calu-6 NSCLC tumors. (From Shibuya K, Komaki R, Shintani T, et al. Targeted therapy against VEGFR and EGFR with ZD6474 enhances the therapeutic efficacy of irradiation in an orthotopic model of human non-small-cell lung cancer. *Int J Radiat Oncol Biol Phys* 2007;69:1534–1543.)

effusion were seen with this combination (Fig. 52.2). This particular compound is being further evaluated both alone, and in combination with chemotherapy, in phase II and III clinical trials in lung cancer. Results of these studies are expected in mid-2008.

In small cell lung cancer (SCLC), overall results with ZD6474 were disappointing in a randomized phase II trial where eligible patients with complete response (CR) or partial response (PR) to combination chemotherapy (+/− thoracic or prophylactic cranial radiation) received maintenance oral ZD6474 at 300 mg/day or matched placebo for up to 2 years. Interestingly, however, when patients with limited-stage SCLC were evaluated in a planned subset analysis, a survival benefit was observed (HR = 0.45; $p = 0.07$).[45]

AZD2171 has shown promise when combined with radiation in lung cancer models. Radiation appears to activate Flk-1 signaling. In a recent study by Cao et al.,[46] AZD2171 demonstrated the ability to sensitize human umbilical vein endothelial cells (HUVEC) to radiation and thus favorably interact with it in a human NSCLC xenograft model. From a sequencing standpoint, it was encouraging to see that AZD2171 contributed to significant tumor growth delays in a Calu-6 xenograft model regardless of it being given prior to each radiation dose or after completion of fractionated radiation.[47]

Studies with PTK787, a VEGFR-TKI, suggest that the concept of antiangiogenesis makes sense based on the effects radiation has upon the surrounding vessels associated with tumor growth. Using an aerodigestive cancer model with FaDu squamous cell xenografts, Zips et al.[48] were able to show that, when tumors were implanted into irradiated tissue, growth was much slower than in unirradiated controls because of stromal changes. In addition, PTK787 was markedly more effective in inhibiting tumor growth through increased necrosis. PTK787 was essentially inactive when administered at 50 mg/kg in animals bearing FaDu tumors implanted into unirradiated tissue. This suggests that sequencing VEGFR TKIs may be critical and perhaps more effective when given later during, and possibly even after, a radiotherapy course for lung cancer patients.

Do we have any clinical data in 2008 with oral TKIs against angiogenic signaling? AE-941 is currently the only agent that has been tested in a large phase III trial. Depending on the center, patients were treated with an induction program of carboplatin-paclitaxel or cisplatin-vinorelbine followed by concurrent chemoradiotherapy using the same drugs. Patients were randomized to receive the drug or a placebo. The drug was administered orally twice daily during all the treatment and as maintenance therapy. There were 384 patients who were included in the study and 379 were eligible. AE-941 failed to improve survival: median survival times were 14.4 and 15.6 months for the drug and placebo groups, respectively.[49]

What about the potential deleterious effects of hypoxia caused by antiangiogenic agents? The cytotoxic effects of radiation are typically reduced twofold to threefold in hypoxic conditions compared to normoxic conditions. Studies by Reisterer et al.[50] indicate, in fact, that radiation abrogates the hypoxic effects of VEGFR TKIs such as PTK787. Elegant use of positron emission tomography (PET) imaging in their preclinical work showed that in contrast to PTK787 alone, adding radiation to animals bearing mammary carcinoma xenografts resulted in reduced expression or uptake of the hypoxia markers glucose transporter-1 (GLUT-1), and fluoromisonidazole (FMISO) (nitroimidazole derivative). Recurrent tumors after radiation also appear more sensitive to antiangiogenic therapy, which may again argue for giving these types of drugs at a minimum after definitive radiation. DC-101, an anti-VEGFR murine antibody, when administered to animals bearing recurrent and previously irradiated tumors, was more effective than when applied to animals bearing nonirradiated tumors. This finding is perhaps caused by increased VEGFR2 expression in previously irradiated vasculature leading to an alteration in tumor vasculature, the presence of which may work to the advantage of antiangiogenic agents.[51]

Combinations of Targeted Agents and Radiation in NSCLC Classic approaches to treating locally advanced NSCLC involve concurrent chemoradiation. Newer strategies are evaluating combinations of targeted agents and chemoradiation. Perhaps another intriguing approach would be to combine molecularly targeted agents against several pathways to improve radiation response even further, with an additional opportunity to reduce toxic effects if the combinations prove effective enough to supplant traditional chemotherapy drugs. We have clearly had difficulties with local control in this disease site and have essentially reached our limits of effective radiation dose at ~74 Gy (although this is dependent on the percentage of the total lung volume that receives >20 Gy with the treatment plan (V20) and can potentially be pushed higher with radiation alone when the V20 is <25%.).[52]

There are many redundant signaling pathways that may enable a cancer cell to escape a selected pathway blockade. We have already touched on the use of dual targeted agents to block multiple pathways simultaneously. What about combinations of different molecularly selective drugs? As an example, improved tumor growth inhibition was realized in NSCLC flank xenografts with combinations of fractionated radiation, an EGFR TKI (gefitinib) and a vascular-targeting agent (ZD6126). The results were superior to radiation alone and better than gefitinib + radiation or ZD6126 and radiation.[53]

Providing further support for the rationale to attack multiple molecular pathways is the fact that tumors that become resistant to EGFR inhibitors express angiogenic signaling factors including VEGF and cyclooxygenase-2 (COX-2).[54] Dual inhibition of COX-2 and EGFR in NSCLC lines were, for the most part, additive or synergistic and triple combination therapy was favorable with blockage of G2 checkpoint controls.[55]

Clinical Trials with Targeted Agents and Radiation in NSCLC Success was realized in a phase III randomized trial in locally advanced head and neck cancer when cetuximab was combined with radiation therapy with superior outcomes in local control, disease-free survival and overall survival over radiation alone.[56] Have we made any progress clinically in NSCLC with biologic agents and radiation? Three trials have evaluated cetuximab (C225) with either concurrent radiotherapy or concurrent chemoradiotherapy for patients with locally advanced NSCLC. In an RTOG phase II trial (RTOG 0324), including 93 patients (87 evaluable), C225 was given on day 1 at the dosage of 400 mg/m^2 and after weekly at a reduced dosage of 250 mg/m^2 for the next 17 weeks. Chemotherapy included carboplatin and paclitaxel for four cycles (during and after radiotherapy to a dose of 63 Gy). With a 21.6 median follow-up at the time of this report at American Society of Clinical Oncology (ASCO) 2008, the median survival reached 22.7 months. The reported response rate was 62% (n = 54), and the overall survival at 2 years was 49.3%. The authors reported 20% (n = 17) of patients experienced grade 4 hematologic toxicities, 8% (n = 7) grade 3 esophagitis, and 7% (n = 6) grade 3 to 4 pneumonitis. There were 5 G 5 events as well.[57] A subset analysis has since correlated the expression of EGFR with the outcome and the pattern of failure finding that tumors with a lower EGFR level had less primary failures but more metastases; the reverse of which was seen for tumors with higher EGFR.[58] Plans are underway in the RTOG to study this in a phase III fashion.

In the Cancer and Leukemia Group B (CALGB), a randomized phase II study of thoracic radiation (70 Gy) with concurrent intravenous carboplatin (area under the curve [AUC] = 5) and pemetrexed 500 mg/m^2 on day 1 was administered for four cycles (every 21 days; arm A) with or without cetuximab with a loading dose of 400 mg/m^2 followed a week later by 250 mg/m^2 weekly for additional 6 weeks (arm B). All patients went onto receive consolidation pemetrexed (500 mg/m^2 every 21 days for 4 cycles).[59] Early toxicity data was presented at ASCO 2008. A total of 106 patients were enrolled and preliminary grade 3 or greater toxicity data included neutropenia (36% in arm A; 37% in arm B); febrile neutropenia (5% in arm A; 7% in arm B); and thrombocytopenia (30% in arm A; 34% in arm B). Esophagitis was higher in arm A without cetuximab (35% vs. 22% in arm B) and as expected, skin rash was significantly higher in arm B (23% vs. 3% in arm A). One patient reportedly died of fatal hemoptysis. In two other already reported trials, cetuximab was given concurrently with radiation at a dosage of 250 mg/m^2 weekly; reported toxicity concerns included mainly fatigue and skin rash.[60,61] One of these, (the Synchronous Cetuximab Radiation Therapy and Chemotherapy [SCRATCH] study) incorporated induction chemotherapy followed by cetuximab and radiation, whereas the other incorporated IMRT with cetuximab and chemotherapy (Non-small cell lung cancer, Erbitux And Radiotherapy [NEAR] trial-NCT00115518). It appears in 2008 that combinations of cetuximab and radiation or chemoradiation appear tolerable without increases in expected toxicity over and above that with chemoradiation approaches.

Can we predict response to cetuximab in NSCLC to select patients most appropriate for this type of therapy? Recently, Hirsch et al.[62] confirmed for the first time that EGFR FISH was predictive of outcomes in patients with advanced, stage IV NSCLC treated with concurrent or sequential chemotherapy and cetuximab in a randomized phase II selection trial through the Southwest Oncology Group (SWOG 0342). Patients with FISH-positive tumors had a superior median progression-free survival time of 6 months compared with 3 months for FISH-negative patients ($p = 0.0008$). Remarkably, patients in the FISH-positive group experienced a median survival time more than double (15 months) that of the patients who were FISH negative (7 months; $p = 0.04$). It remains to be seen if EGFR FISH will be important in determining response to radiation and cetuximab in patients with locally advanced disease.

Data with small molecule EGFR TKIs such as gefinitib are primarily derived from two phase I trials, which combined a taxane-based chemotherapy approach with concurrent radiotherapy. Those trials were designed to escalate the dose of the cytotoxic agents, whereas gefinitib was given orally at a dosage of 250 mg/m^2 daily.[63,64] In one study, paclitaxel could be increased to 45 mg/m^2 weekly (carboplatin was given at an AUC of 2) with fixed-dose gefitinib at 250 mg daily. In the other, docetaxel was increased to 25 mg/m^2 with radiation and gefitinib and then followed by consolidative docetaxel and gefitinib. One patient experienced a grade V interstitial pneumonia, believed to be related to the gefitinib.[63] The recently reported results of SWOG 0023, a randomized phase III of maintenance gefitinib or placebo after concurrent chemoradiation followed by docetaxel consolidation gives one

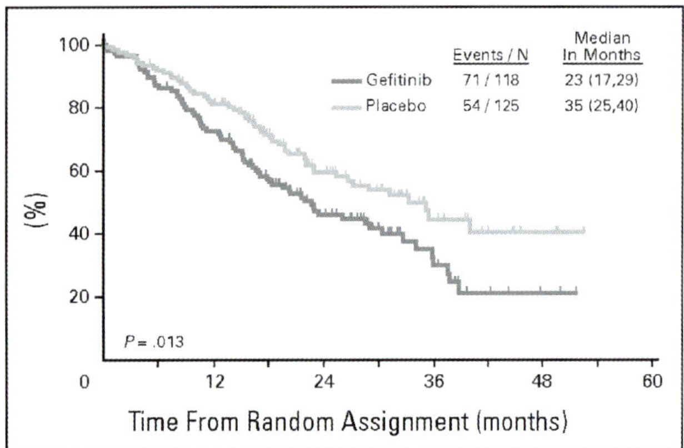

FIGURE 52.3 Overall survival results for patients with stage III NSCLC randomized to receive maintenance gefitinib or placebo after concurrent cisplatin-etoposide and radiation (61 Gy) followed by three cycles of docetaxel. Patients treated with gefitinib had a median overall survival of 23 months compared to 35 months for patients treated with placebo (Borrowed with permission from Kelly K, Chansky K, Gaspar LE, et al. Phase III trial of maintenance gefitinib or placebo after concurrent chemoradiotherapy and docetaxel consolidation in inoperable stage III non-small-cell lung cancer: SWOG S0023. *J Clin Oncol* 2008;26:2450–2456.)

room for pause and caution (Fig. 52.3).[65] Maintenance gefitinib did not improve overall survival and in fact, with a median follow-up time of 27 months, median overall survival time was 23 months for gefitinib (n = 118) and 35 months for placebo (n = 125; two-sided $p = .013$). The authors concluded that deaths were primarily related to disease progression and not toxicity from gefitinib (2% toxic death rate). The results were somewhat perplexing, and perhaps smoking history, a predictor of response to EGFR TKIs and a factor, which was not captured in SWOG 0023, might have contributed to survival differences. The authors added that additional factors not initially captured, which might also have impacted on the inferior overall survival results, include K-ras mutations and additional therapies offered to patients after progression. It is worth mentioning that survival times in both arms were superior when compared to other published randomized phase III NSCLC clinical trials.

In a study by Choong et al.,[66] erlotinib was given daily with weekly carboplatin and paclitaxel or with cisplatin and etoposide, using the classical SWOG schedule with radiation delivered conventionally. In both instances, a dose escalation was possible from 50 to 150 mg with only minor toxicities reported (primarily skin). The group at the University of North Carolina at Chapel Hill has tested the association of erlotinib (150 mg/m^2 twice weekly) and bevacizumab (10 mg/m^2 every 2 weeks) induction together with carboplatin and paclitaxel × two cycles followed by carboplatin and paclitaxel given weekly during radiation with bevacizumab initially and later with erlotinib and bevacizumab. Both squamous and nonsquamous histologies were allowed with early stopping rules incorporated for safety. In 20 patients enrolled in the phase I portion of the trial, there was one grade 3 pulmonary hemorrhage requiring stoppage of bevacizumab. In addition, the authors reported one grade 3 interstitial pneumonitis. A majority were able to receive the 74 planned dose. Esophagitis was most prevalent radiation induced complication with 5/15 with esophagitis (33%) having grade 3 toxicity. One grade 5 late hemorrhage occurred in a patient presenting with squamous histology. The trial is currently accruing in the phase II portion with 100 mg of erlotinib as the maximum tolerated dose (MTD). Evolving and current cooperative group trials are now including esophageal volume dose constraints in IMRT planning to reduce upper gastrointestinal toxicity further.[67]

Is there any information on alternative approaches to targeting specific pathways? Of interest has been the use of COX-2 inhibitors such as celecoxib to improve radiotherapy outcomes. A phase I trial has defined the safe dose of celecoxib given concurrently with radiation. In this cohort of 47 patients, the dose was escalated from 200 to 800 mg/day given in two equally divided doses without reaching the MTD.[68] The toxicity reported included a case of uncontrolled hypertension and two patients with hemorrhagic episodes. Soon thereafter, De Ruysscher et al.[69] tried to launch a randomized phase II trial, but it was terminated after the enrollment of only 41 patients because of poor recruitment and apparent toxicity problems with the drug.

CONCLUSION

We have pushed the envelope with concurrent chemoradiation and have probably reached a plateau in regard to further benefits in survival with classic approaches, even with state-of-the-art radiation techniques. Our intent with this chapter was to introduce the reader to some of the promising preclinical and clinical studies that suggest potential benefits of using agents that selectively interfere with tumor growth and angiogenic signaling. The current available data suggest that many of those targeted agents may be safely used with concurrent radiotherapy or chemoradiotherapy. We are at the first of many crossroads now in the development of these strategies and need to wait for the results of ongoing phase III trials to see if there may be some benefit demonstrated. In the interim, preclinical studies are pointing us toward newer directions beyond just EGFR targeting. It is safe to say that personalized cancer care is the next step with treatment decisions made based primarily on a patient's individual tumor molecular characteristics or gene abnormalities such as mutant Kras, Akt, EGFR FISH, and ligand expression, DNA repair expression, angiogenic-related signaling molecules such as VEGFR and insulin-like growth factor receptor expression to name a few.

REFERENCES

1. Shepherd FA, Rodrigues Pereira J, Ciuleanu T, et al. Erlotinib in previously treated non-small-cell lung cancer. *N Engl J Med* 2005;353:123–132.
2. Kris MG, Natale RB, Herbst RS, et al. Efficacy of gefitinib, an inhibitor of the epidermal growth factor receptor tyrosine kinase, in symptomatic patients with non-small cell lung cancer: a randomized trial. *JAMA* 2003;290:2149–2158.

3. Fukuoka M, Yano S, Giaccone G, et al. Multi-institutional randomized phase II trial of gefitinib for previously treated patients with advanced non-small-cell lung cancer (The IDEAL 1 Trial). *J Clin Oncol* 2003;21: 2237–2246.
4. Douillard JY, Kim E, Hirsh V, et al. Gefitinib (IRESSA) versus docetaxel in patients with locally advanced or metastatic non-small-cell lung cancer pre-treated with platinum-based chemotherapy: a randomized, open-label phase III study (INTEREST) [Abstract]. *J Thorac Oncol* 2007;2(suppl 4):S305–S306.
5. Herbst RS, Johnson DH, Mininberg E, et al. Phase I/II trial evaluating the anti-vascular endothelial growth factor monoclonal antibody bevacizumab in combination with the HER-1/epidermal growth factor receptor tyrosine kinase inhibitor erlotinib for patients with recurrent non-small-cell lung cancer. *J Clin Oncol* 2005;23(11):2544–2555.
6. Sandler A, Gray R, Perry MC, et al. Paclitaxel-carboplatin alone or with bevacizumab for non-small-cell lung cancer. *N Engl J Med* 2006; 355(24):2542–2550.
7. Heymach JV, Johnson BE, Prager D, et al. Randomized, placebo-controlled phase II study of vandetanib plus docetaxel in previously treated non small-cell lung cancer. *J Clin Oncol* 2007;25(27):4270–4277.
8. Furuse K, Fukuoka M, Kawahara M, et al. Phase III study of concurrent versus sequential thoracic radiotherapy in combination with mitomycin, vindesine, and cisplatin in unresectable stage III non-small-cell lung cancer. *J Clin Oncol* 1999;17:2692–2699.
9. Curran WJ, Scott CB, Langer CJ, et al. Long-term benefit is observed in a phase III comparison of sequential v. concurrent chemo-radiation for patients with unresectable stage III NSCLC: RTOG 9410 [Abstract]. *Proc Am Soc Clin Oncol* 2003;22:621.
10. Bradley J, Graham M, Suzanne S, et al. Phase II results of RTOG L-0117: a phase I/II dose intensification study using 3dCRT and concurrent chemotherapy for patients with inoperable NSCLC [Abstract]. *J Clin Oncol* 2005;23(Suppl 16):636.
11. Socinski MA, Rosenman JG, Halle J, et al. Dose-escalating conformal thoracic radiation therapy with induction and concurrent carboplatin/ paclitaxel in unresectable stage IIIA/B non-small cell lung carcinoma: A modified phase I/II trial. *Cancer* 2006;92:1213–1223.
12. Socinski MA, Blackstock AW, Bogart JA, et al. Randomized phase II trial of induction chemotherapy followed by concurrent chemotherapy and dose-escalated thoracic conformal radiotherapy (74 Gy) in stage III non-small-cell lung cancer: CALGB 30105. *J Clin Oncol* 2008;26(15):2457–2463.
13. Schild S, McGinnis WL, Graham D, et al. Results of a phase I/II trial of concurrent chemotherapy and escalating doses of radiation for unresectable non small cell lung cancer. *Int J Radiat Oncol Biol Phys* 2006;65:1106–1111.
14. Akimoto T, Hunter NR, Buchmiller L, et al. Inverse relationship between epidermal growth factor receptor expression and radiocurability of murine carcinomas. *Clin Cancer Res* 1999;5(10):2884–2890.
15. Huang SM, Bock JM, Harari PM. Epidermal growth factor receptor blockage with C225 modulates proliferation, apoptosis and radiosensitivity in squamous cell carcinomas of the head and neck. *Cancer Res* 1999;59(8):1935–1940.
16. Milas L, Mason K, Hunter N, et al. In vivo enhancement of tumor radioresponse by C225 antiepidermal growth factor receptor antibody. *Clin Cancer Res* 2000;6(2):701–708.
17. Huang SM, Harari PM. Modulation of radiation response after epidermal growth factor receptor blockade in squamous cell carcinomas: inhibition of damage repair cell cycle kinetics, and tumor angiogenesis. *Clin Cancer Res* 2000;6(6):2166–2174.
18. Liang K, Ang KK, Milas L, et al. The epidermal growth factor receptor mediates radioresistance. *Int J Radiat Oncol Biol Phys* 2003;57:246–254.
19. Raben D, Helfrich B, Chan DC, et al. The effects of cetuximab alone and in combination with radiation and/or chemotherapy in lung cancer. *Clin Cancer Res* 2005;11:795–805.
20. Hirsch FR, Varrella-Garcia M, Bunn PA Jr, et al. Molecular predictors of outcome with gefitinib in a phase III placebo-controlled study in advanced non-small-cell lung cancer. *J Clin Oncol* 2006;24(31):5034–5042.
21. Cappuzzo F, Hirsch FR, Rossi E, et al. Epidermal growth factor receptor gene and protein and gefitinib sensitivity in non-small-cell lung cancer. *J Natl Cancer Inst* 2005;97(9):643–655.
22. Wakeling AE, Barker AJ, Davies DH, et al. Specific inhibition of epidermal growth factor receptor tyrosine kinase by 4-anilinoquinazolines. *Breast Cancer Res Treat* 1996;38:67–73.
23. Levitzki A, Gazit A. Tyrosine kinase inhibitors: an approach to drug development. *Science* 1995;267:1782–1788.
24. Lidhtner RB, Menrad A, Sommer A, et al. Signaling-inactive epidermal growth factor receptor/ligand complexes in intact carcinoma cells by quinazoline tyrosine kinase inhibitors. *Cancer Res* 2001;61(15):5790–5795.
25. Chinnaiyan P, Huang S, Vallabhaneni G, et al. Mechanisms of enhanced radiation response following epidermal growth factor receptor signaling inhibition by erlotinib (Tarceva). *Cancer Res* 2005;65(8):3328–3335.
26. Paez JG, Jänne PA, Lee JC, et al. EGFR mutations in lung cancer: correlation with clinical response to gefitinib therapy. *Science* 2004; 304(5676):1497–1500.
27. Lynch TJ, Bell DW, Sordella R, et al. Activating mutations in the epidermal growth factor receptor underlying responsiveness of non-small-cell lung cancer to gefitinib. *N Engl J Med* 2004;350:2129–2139.
28. Johnson BE, Janne PA. Epidermal growth factor receptor mutations in patients with non-small cell lung cancer. *Cancer Res* 2005;65:7525–7529.
29. Das AK, Sato M, Story MD, et al. Non-small-cell lung cancers with kinase domain mutations in the epidermal growth factor receptor are sensitive to ionizing radiation. *Cancer Res* 2006;66(19):9601–9608.
30. Das AK, Chen BP, Story MD, et al. Somatic mutations in the tyrosine kinase domain of epidermal growth factor receptor (EGFR) abrogate EGFR-mediated radioprotection in non-small cell lung carcinoma. *Cancer Res* 2007;67(11):5267–5274.
31. Toulany M, Dittmann K, Krüger M, et al. Radioresistance of K-Ras mutated human tumor cells is mediated through EGFR-dependent activation of PI3K-AKT pathway. *Radiother Oncol* 2005;74:143–150.
32. Toulany M, Kasten-Pisula U, Brammer I, et al. Blockage of epidermal growth factor receptor-phosphatidylinositol 3-kinase-AKT signaling increases radiosensitivity of K-RAS mutated human tumor cells in vitro by affecting DNA repair. *Clin Cancer Res* 2006;12(13):4119–4126.
33. Toulany M, Kehlbach R, Florczak U, et al. Targeting of AKT1 enhances radiation toxicity of human tumor cells by inhibiting DNA-PKcs-dependent DNA double-strand break repair. *Mol Cancer Ther* 2008;7(7):1772–1781.
34. Johnson DH, Fehrenbacher L, Novotny WF, et al. Randomized phase II trial comparing bevacizumab plus carboplatin and paclitaxel with carboplatin and paclitaxel alone in previously untreated locally advanced or metastatic non-small-cell lung cancer. *J Clin Oncol* 2004;22(11): 2184–2191.
35. Sandler A, Gray R, Perry MC, et al. Paclitaxel-carboplatin alone or with bevacizumab for non-small-cell lung cancer. *N Engl J Med* 2006; 355(24):2542–2550.
36. Wachsberger P, Burd R, Dicker AP. Tumor response to ionizing radiation combined with antiangiogenesis or vascular targeting agents: exploring mechanisms of interaction. *Clin Cancer Res* 2003;9(6):1957–1971.
37. Jain RK. Normalization of tumor vasculature: an emerging concept in antiangiogenic therapy. *Science* 2005;307(5706):58–62.
38. Duda DG, Jain RK, Willett CG. Antiangiogenics: the potential role of integrating this novel treatment modality with chemoradiation for solid cancers. *J Clin Oncol* 2007;25(26):4033–4042.
39. Millauer B, Wizigmann-Voos S, Schnürch H, et al. High affinity VEGF binding and developmental expression suggest Flk-1 as a major regulator of vasculogenesis and angiogenesis. *Cell* 1993;72:835–846.
40. Quinn TP, Peters KG, De Vries C, et al. Fetal liver kinase 1 is a receptor for vascular endothelial growth factor and is selectively expressed in vascular endothelium. *Proc Natl Acad Sci U S A* 1993;90:7533–7537.
41. Sathornsumetee S, Rich JN. Vandetanib, a novel multitargeted kinase inhibitor, in cancer therapy. *Drugs Today (Barc)* 2006;42(10):657–670.
42. Frederick B, Gustafson D, Bianco C, et al. ZD6474, an inhibitor of VEGFR and EGFR tyrosine kinase activity in combination with radiotherapy. *Int J Radiat Oncol Biol Phys* 2006;64:33–37.

43. Williams KJ, Telfer BA, Brave S, et al. ZD6474, a potent inhibitor of vascular endothelial growth factor signaling, combined with radiotherapy: schedule-dependent enhancement of anti-tumor activity. *Clin Cancer Res* 2004;10(24):8587–8593.
44. Shibuya K, Komaki R, Shintani T, et al. Targeted therapy against VEGFR and EGFR with ZD6474 enhances the therapeutic efficacy of irradiation in an orthotopic model of human non-small-cell lung cancer. *Int J Radiat Oncol Biol Phys* 2007;69(5):1534–1543.
45. Arnold AM, Seymour L, Smylie M, et al. Phase II study of vandetanib or placebo in small-cell lung cancer patients after complete or partial response to induction chemotherapy with or without radiation therapy: National Cancer Institute of Canada Clinical Trials Group Study BR.20. *J Clin Oncol* 2007;25(27):4278–4284.
46. Cao C, Albert JM, Geng L, et al. Vascular endothelial growth factor tyrosine kinase inhibitor AZD2171 and fractionated radiotherapy in mouse models of lung cancer. *Cancer Res* 2006;66(23):11409–11415.
47. Williams KJ, Telfer BA, Shannon AM, et al. Combining radiotherapy with AZD2171, a potent inhibitor of vascular endothelial growth factor signaling: pathophysiologic effects and therapeutic benefit. *Mol Cancer Ther* 2007;6(2):599–606.
48. Zips D, Eicheler W, Geyer P, et al. Enhanced susceptibility of irradiated tumor vessels to vascular endothelial growth factor receptor tyrosine kinase inhibition. *Cancer Res* 2005;65(12):5374–5379.
49. Lu C, Lee JJ, Komaki R, et al. A phase III trial study of AE-941 with induction chemotherapy (IC) and concomitant chemoradiotherapy (CRT) for stage III non-small cell lung cancer (NSCLC) (NCI T99-0046, RTOG 02-70, MDA 99-303) [Abstract]. *J Clin Oncol* 2007; 25(suppl 18):7527.
50. Reisterer O, Honer M, Jochum W, et al. Ionizing radiation antagonizes tumor hypoxia induced by antiangiogenic treatment. *Clin Cancer Res* 2006;12(11):3518–3524.
51. Kozin SV, Winkler F, Garkavtsev I, et al. Human tumor xenografts recurring after radiotherapy are more sensitive to anti-vascular endothelial growth factor receptor-2 treatment than treatment-naive tumors. *Cancer Res* 2007;67(11):5076–5082.
52. Bradley J, Graham MV, Winter K, et al. Toxicity and outcome results of RTOG 9311: a phase I-II dose-escalation study using three-dimensional conformal radiotherapy in patients with inoperable non-small-cell lung carcinoma. *Int J Radiat Oncol Biol Phys* 2005;61(2):318–328.
53. Raben D, Bianco C, Damiano V, et al. Antitumor activity of ZD6126, a novel vascular-targeting agent, is enhanced when combined with ZD1839, an epidermal growth factor receptor tyrosine kinase inhibitor, and potentiates the effects of radiation in a human non-small cell lung cancer xenograft model. *Mol Cancer Ther* 2004;3(8):977–983.
54. Ciardiello F, Bianco R, Caputo R, et al. Antitumor activity of ZD6474, a vascular endothelial growth factor receptor tyrosine kinase inhibitor, in human cancer cells with acquired resistance to antiepidermal growth factor receptor therapy. *Clin Cancer Res* 2004;10(2):784–793.
55. Park JS, Jun HJ, Cho MJ, et al. Radiosensitivity enhancement by combined treatment of celecoxib and gefitinib on human lung cancer cells. *Clin Cancer Res* 2006;12(16):4989–4999.
56. Bonner JA, Harari PM, Giralt J, et al. Radiotherapy plus cetuximab for squamous-cell carcinoma of the head and neck. *N Engl J Med* 2006; 354(6):567–578.
57. Blumenschein GR, Paulus R, Curran WJ, et al. A phase II study of cetuximab (C225) in combination with chemoradiation (CRT) in patients (pts) with stage III A/B non-small cell lung cancer (NSCLC): a report of the 2 year and median survival (MS) for the RTOG 0324 trial. *J Clin Oncol* 2008:26(May 20 suppl; abstr 7516).
58. Komaki R, Moughan J, Ang K, et al. RTOG 0324: a phase II study of Cetuximab (C225) in combination with chemoradiation (CRT) in patients with stage IIIA/B non-small cell lung cancer (NSCLC): correlation between EGFR and the patients'outcome [Abstract]. *Int J Radiat Oncol Biol Phys* 2007;69(3):S57–S58.
59. Govindan R, Bogart J, Wang X, et al. A phase II study of pemetrexed, carboplatin and thoracic radiation with or without cetuximab in patients with locally advanced unresectable non-small cell lung cancer: CALGB 30407—Early evaluation of feasibility and toxicity. *J Clin Oncol* 2008:26(May 20 suppl; abstr 7518)
60. Hughes S, Liong J, Miah A, et al. A brief report on the safety study of induction chemotherapy followed by synchronous radiotherapy and cetuximab in stage III non-small cell lung cancer (NSCLC): SCRATCH study. *J Thorac Oncol* 2008;3(6):648–651.
61. Jensen AD, Münter MW, Bischoff HG, et al. IMRT and cetuximab in stage 3 non-small cell lung cancer: the NEAR trial (NCT00115518) [Abstract]. *J Clin Oncol* 2007;25(suppl 18):18168.
62. Hirsch FR, Herbst RS, Olsen C, et al. Increased EGFR gene copy number detected by fluorescent in situ hybridization predicts outcome in non-small-cell lung cancer patients treated with cetuximab and chemotherapy. *J Clin Oncol* 2008;26(20):3351–3357.
63. Blackstock A, Petty J, Oaks T, et al. Gefinitib (ZD-1839) with concurrent docetaxel and conformal three-dimensional thoracic radiation followed by consolidative docetaxel/gefinitib for patients with stage III NSCLC: a phase I study [Abstract]. *J Clin Oncol* 2007;25(suppl 18):18165.
64. Ball D, Burmeister B, Mitchell P, et al. Phase I trial of gefinitib in combination with concurrent carboplatin, paclitaxel and radiation therapy in patients with stage III non-small cell lung cancer ("CRITICAL") [Abstract]. *J Thorac Oncol* 2007;2(suppl 4):S633–S634.
65. Kelly K, Chansky K, Gaspar LE, et al. Phase III trial of maintenance gefitinib or placebo after concurrent chemoradiotherapy and docetaxel consolidation in inoperable stage III non-small-cell lung cancer: SWOG S0023. *J Clin Oncol* 2008;26:2450–2456.
66. Choong N, Mauer A, Lester E, et al. Phase I trial of erlotinib-based multimodality therapy for inoperable stage III non-small cell lung cancer: (C3-01) [Abstract]. *J Thorac Oncol* 2007;2(suppl 4):S364–S365.
67. Socinski M, Morris D, Stinchcombe T, et al. Incorporation of bevacizumab (B) and erlotinib (Er) with induction (I) and concurrent (C) carboplatin (Cb) paclitaxel (P) and 74 Gy of thoracic radiotherapy in stage III non-small cell lung cancer (NSCLC). *J Clin Oncol* 2008:26 (May 20 suppl; abstr 7517).
68. Liao Z, Komaki R, Milas L, et al. A phase I clinical trial of thoracic radiotherapy and concurrent celecoxib for patients with unfavorable performance status inoperable/unresectable non-small cell lung cancer. *Clin Cancer Res* 2005;11(9):3342–3348.
69. De Ruysscher D, Bussink J, Rodrigus P, et al. Concurrent celecoxib versus placebo in patients with stage II-III non-small cell lung cancer: a randomised phase II trial. *Radiother Oncol* 2007;84(1):23–25.

SECTION 10

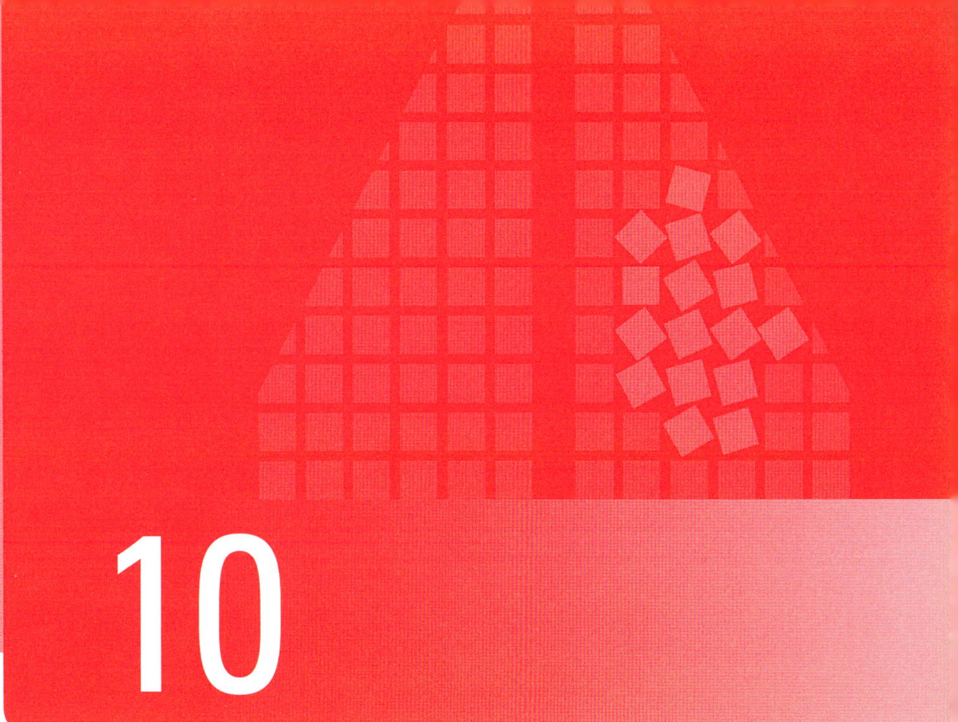

Adjuvant and Neoadjuvant Approaches for Non–Small Cell Lung Cancer

CHAPTER 53

Giorgio V. Scagliotti
Everett E. Vokes

Adjuvant Chemotherapy in Completely Resected Non–Small Cell Lung Cancer

Ninety percent of lung cancers are related to tobacco smoking, and the primary prevention of lung cancer by smoking cessation remains the primary goal of any physician involved in the field of diagnosis and treatment of lung cancer. However, given the rising trend in worldwide tobacco consumption and the fact that former smokers still have higher lung cancer risk than nonsmokers (in the United States, more than 50% of lung cancers occur in former smokers),[1] lung cancer will continue to globally represent a huge social health problem for a long period of time.

Lung cancer is the most common fatal malignancy among men and women in most countries throughout the world.[2,3] Non–small cell lung cancer (NSCLC) represents more than 80% of all newly diagnosed cases of lung cancer. The reference treatment for early stage disease (from stage IA to IIB) is surgery; specific groups of patients with stage III disease may also benefit from pulmonary resection, usually in combination with other treatment modalities. Globally, the proportion of newly diagnosed NSCLC that can benefit from radical resection does not exceed 25% to 30% of the total number of cases.

The use of a systemic therapy in completely resected NSCLC is reasonably justified by follow-up studies after radical resection that have shown the predominance of distant failures over local recurrences and on some clinical and pathologic evidence of early microdissemination of the disease at the time of surgery.

Long-term survival in NSCLC following surgical resection is stage related, but even in stage IA, one third of patients will relapse and die of their disease within 5 years.[4] Most of these relapses are distant metastases, whereas the risk of a local recurrence after complete resection is less than 10%. The central nervous system is the most common site of metastatic recurrence followed closely by bone, ipsilateral and contralateral lung, liver, and adrenals. More than 80% of recurrences occur within 2 years from the time of radical surgery.

The rate of recurrence for patients with stage II disease is higher than in stage I; more than 50% of resected stage II can be expected to relapse and, again, most recurrences are distant. The pattern of recurrence may differ by histology with more local recurrences seen for patients with squamous cell carcinoma and more distant metastases seen in patients with adenocarcinoma (Table 53.1).[5–8]

Positron emission tomography (PET) has been progressively implemented in the diagnostic workup for resectable NSCLC. Current experience indicates that metastatic disease will be found in 11% to 14% of the cases otherwise cleared for resection by conventional screening methods. In addition to distant metastases, almost all of these studies have demonstrated an increase in the rate of detection of unsuspected mediastinal and hilar nodal disease [9–11] (see Chapter 27).

Dissemination of cancer cells at much lower levels than those detected by any currently available imaging techniques, including PET scanning, seem to affect the prognosis of patients with clinical early stage NSCLC. Immunohistochemical and real-time polymerase chain reaction estimation of lymph node micrometastatic disease has been investigated in small retrospective studies evaluating the positivity for cytokeratins and carcinoembryonic antigen. Overall, the detection of positive findings in otherwise morphologically normal lymph nodes was almost invariably associated with an adverse outcome when compared with that of patients without occult micrometastatic disease.[12–15]

Quantification of free circulating DNA has also been proposed as a potential additional diagnostic tool for resected patients to detect persisting neoplastic disease.[16]

Although these studies are highly suggestive, additional confirmatory data are urgently needed to confirm the scientific hypothesis.

In addition to primary lung cancer prevention through smoking cessation campaigns, the detection of early stage disease through screening procedures represents the ultimate goal to defeat lung cancer. Unfortunately, this strategy remains investigational at this time and has not yet been proven to improve survival. Chest x-rays, analysis of cells contained in the sputum, and standard fiberbronchoscopy have shown limited effectiveness in early lung cancer detection. Newer tests

TABLE 53.1 Rates and Patterns of Relapse following Radical Resection for NSCLC

Author	Stage	Number of Patients	Pattern of Relapse, %	
			Locoregional Only	Distant Only
Feld et al.[5]	T1 N0	162	9	17
	T2 N0	196	11	30
	T1 N1	32	9	22
Martini et al.[6]	T1–T2 N1 (S)	93	16	31
	T1–T2 N1 (A)	114	8	54
	T2–T3 N2 (S)	46	13	52
	T2–T3 N2 (A)	103	17	61
Pairolero et al.[7]	T1 N0	170	6	15
	T2 N0	158	6	23
	T1 N1	18	28	39
Thomas and Rubenstein[8]	T1 N0 (S)	226	5	7
	T1 N0 (NS)	346	9	17

A, adenocarcinoma; S, squamous; NS, nonsquamous; NSCLC, non–small cell lung cancer.

such as low-radiation, high-resolution helical computed tomography (CT) scan and molecular markers in sputum have been demonstrated to lead to earlier detection of lung cancers. However, their ability to increase survival rates of affected patients has not yet been fully accepted. Nonrandomized studies of high-resolution helical CT scan indicate an increase in the rate of detection of small resectable lung cancers, usually adenocarcinomas, and thus the frequency of lung surgery (see Chapters 15 and 16). However, as previously shown for chest x-ray screening, there may be neither a meaningful reduction in the number of advanced cancers being diagnosed nor a reduction in the number of individuals who die of lung cancer.[17] This is because of the fact that CT screening can detect small nodules that may not be malignant or represent a group of slow-growing cancers that would not interfere with a patient's life expectancy if they remained unnoticed.

Molecular markers are needed to identify tiny malignant nodules, which may be present among many nodules, often benign, that can be visualized by helical CT. Biomarkers are also needed for central lesions that cannot be identified by CT techniques, to indicate which patients should have bronchoscopic explorations to identify tiny intraepithelial central lesions. Automated, reliable, high-throughput sputum biomarker tests will ultimately replace cytomorphological techniques.

The Rationale for Adjuvant Treatments Following complete resection, tumor load, if any, is theoretically minimal. The relatively small number of residual neoplastic cells present in micrometastatic disease should contain few chemotherapy- or radiation-resistant clones. The Gompertzian model of tumor growth and regression fits experimental and clinical data of most human solid cancers. If the assumption is correct, when the tumor is clinically undetectable, its growth rate should be at its largest and, although the numerical reduction induced by cytotoxic chemotherapy is small, the fractional cell kill from an effective dose of chemotherapy should be higher. In addition, pathological staging allows better prediction of prognosis and facilitates the comparison of treatment results between different trials.

How should the more appropriate treatment to be used in the adjuvant setting be selected? Realistically, no definitive rules have been established but, at least, the chosen treatment (or regimen) should be proven active in advanced disease, associated with good tolerability[18]; in the case of cytotoxic chemotherapy, it should be platinum based, initiated sufficiently early after radical surgery and administered for not less than three to four cycles.[19]

The Role of Adjuvant Radiotherapy For a long period of time, postoperative thoracic radiation therapy was the preferred adjuvant treatment. Results regarding its potential role have been reported from a large number of retrospective and prospective studies. Nine of these studies, collecting individual data from 2128 patients have been included in the Postoperative Radiation Therapy (PORT) metaanalysis and indicated postoperative radiotherapy as a treatment with significant detrimental effect on survival, especially in stages I and II.[20] These results have been further confirmed by a Cochrane systematic review and metaanalysis originally published in 2000 and substantially updated in 2004.[21] The results of this recent update indicate a significant adverse effect of PORT on survival with a hazard ratio (HR) of 1.18 or 18% relative increase in the risk of death. This is equivalent to an absolute detriment of 6% at 2 years

(95% CI, 2% to 9%) reducing overall survival from 58% to 52%. Exploratory subgroup analyses suggest that this detrimental effect was most pronounced for patients with stage I/II, whereas for patients with stage III, N2, there was no clear evidence of an adverse effect.

Most of the studies included in these two metaanalyses incorporated patients treated with older technology (cobalt-60) and different dosimetry, and these outdated parameters may be partially responsible for the higher mortality rate observed in the radiotherapy group and attributed to an excess of intercurrent deaths. The use of newer technologies and improved dosimetry may prove to be effective as more recently suggested in a retrospective review.[22] In addition, there were no sufficient data on the use of mediastinal lymph node dissection and surgical procedures, which differed from one study to the other and from one center to another. A more recent large scale analysis of PORT has been reported by Lally et al.[23] To investigate the association between survival and PORT in patients with resected NSCLC, 7465 patients coded as receiving PORT or observation with stage II or III NSCLC who underwent a lobectomy or pneumonectomy were selected within the Surveillance, Epidemiology, and End Results (SEER) database. Patients who survived less than 4 months were excluded. Median follow-up time was 3.5 years for patients still alive. Predictors for the use of PORT included age younger than 50 years, higher American Joint Committee on Cancer stage, T3 and T4 tumor stage, larger tumor size, advanced node stage, greater number of lymph nodes involved, and a ratio of lymph nodes involved to lymph nodes sampled approaching 1. On multivariate analysis, older age, T3 and T4 tumor stage, N2 node stage, male sex, fewer-sampled lymph nodes, and greater number of involved lymph nodes had a negative impact on survival. Overall, the use of PORT did not have a significant impact on survival. However, in subset analysis for patients with N2 nodal disease (HR = 0.855; 95% CI, 0.762 to 0.959; $p = 0.0077$), PORT was associated with a significant increase in survival. For patients with N0 (HR = 1.176; 95% CI, 1.005 to 1.376; $p = 0.0435$) and N1 (HR = 1.097; 95% CI, 1.015 to 1.186; $p = 0.0196$) nodal disease, PORT was associated with a significant decrease in survival. Hence, in this population-based SEER cohort, PORT use was associated with an increase in survival in patients with N2 nodal disease but not in patients with N1 and N0 nodal disease. A new large multi-institutional European phase III trial, Lung Adjuvant Radiotherapy Trial (Lung ART), compares three-dimensional conformal PORT to no PORT, and will include patients who have proven N2 disease and a complete resection irrespective of whether adjuvant or neoadjuvant chemotherapy was used.[24] Seven hundred patients will be included to show a 10% difference in terms of 3-year disease-free survival (bilateral test, power = 80%, alpha error = 5%, from 30% to 40% at 3 years), which is the primary end point. With a longer follow-up period (median of 5 years), this sample size could also show a difference in survival rate of 9% at 5 years. The secondary end points will be overall survival, patterns of relapse, local failure, secondary cancers, and treatment-related toxicity. This project is being studied by the Intergroupe Francophone de Cancérologie Thoracique (IFCT), the European Organisation for Research and Treatment of Cancer (EORTC Radiation Oncology Group and Lung Group), and the Lung Adjuvant Radiotherapy Spanish Group.

Early Studies of Adjuvant Chemotherapy The history of adjuvant chemotherapy in completely resected NSCLC initiated in the early 1960s and 1970s with earlier trials testing the role of alkylating agents and nonspecific immunotherapies (mainly levamisole and Bacillus Calmette-Guérin [BCG]) that uniformly failed to demonstrate any survival benefit and, occasionally, a detrimental effect was observed.[25] All the drugs used in these studies had shown very limited or at all no activity in advanced NSCLC.

Subsequently, the potential role of cisplatin-based chemotherapy was extensively tested in all the stages of resectable NSCLC. All but one of these studies failed to show clinical benefit from adjuvant therapies.[26–32]

Common findings in both of these groups of studies include the overestimation of the potential benefit of adjuvant chemotherapy in the calculation of the sample size, in some trials, the unbalance in patients and treatment characteristics (for instance, incomplete mediastinal lymph node dissection), and, in most of these studies, the impossibility to reach the planned accrual. This probably reflects the negative attitude of thoracic surgeons toward adjuvant chemotherapy and the modern multidisciplinary approach to the patient with early NSCLC may be a way to overcome this problem.

In addition, most of the trials dose delivery including both dose and dose intensity were very often reported inadequate with an average of 50% of the patients receiving the full course of treatment.

In 1995, a metaanalysis overviewed eight cisplatin-based adjuvant chemotherapy studies, including all of the aforementioned studies, and demonstrated a 13% reduction of the risk of death, which was close to the borderline of statistical significance ($p = 0.08$). Similarly, there was a 6% reduction in the risk of death in patients treated with postoperative radiotherapy and cisplatin-based chemotherapy compared with patients who received only postoperative radiotherapy ($p = 0.46$). Conversely, adjuvant chemotherapy with long-term alkylating agents was significantly detrimental.[33]

These findings failed to impact on clinical practice not because the absolute gain was too small, but because such an estimate was still imprecise, ranging from 1% detriment to a 10% benefit. In addition, the heterogeneity of surgical procedures, specific chemotherapy regimens, difference in the staging modalities, and absence of a single large prospective trial truly demonstrating increased survival as a result of the use of chemotherapy limited the applicability of the results of this metaanalysis. However, these data strongly supported additional prospective testing of adjuvant chemotherapy, and new trials using state-of-the-art chemotherapy were initiated.

Recent Platinum-Based Adjuvant Chemotherapy Trials The aforementioned metaanalysis generated enthusiasm to prompt the planning of several prospective randomized phase III studies, all platinum based (positive/negative thoracic radiotherapy), evaluating the role of modern platinum-based regimens in all resectable stages of NSCLC.

The North American Intergroup trial evaluated the efficacy of four cycles of postoperative cisplatin/etoposide plus concomitant thoracic radiotherapy (total dose of 50 Gy) in comparison with PORT alone in stage II and IIIA NSCLC. A total of 463 patients were included with no significant difference between the two arms in terms of median time to progression. The relative likelihood of survival among patients assigned to receive chemotherapy plus radiotherapy, as compared with those assigned to receive radiotherapy alone, was 0.93 (95% CI, 0.74 to 1.18).[34] Toxicity of radiation caused by the concomitant administration of cytotoxic agents may explain the lack of efficacy (more striking in stage II). Biological correlative studies evaluating differential expression of p53 and K-ras did not show any relationship with outcome.[35] This study was unique in its routine use of PORT. All other studies primarily tested the efficacy of adjuvant chemotherapy versus observation alone in completely resected NSCLC, with the optional administration of sequential PORT in some of them according to an investigator choice (Table 53.2).

From 1994 to 1999, a joint effort from Adjuvant Lung Project Italy (ALPI) and EORTC enrolled 1209 patients with completely resected stage I, II, or IIIA NSCLC.[36] Patients were randomly assigned to receive chemotherapy with mitomycin, vindesine, and cisplatin (MVP) for three cycles or observation. A total of 69% completed three cycles of MVP, with half of those patients requiring dose reduction. Radiotherapy was given according to the policy of individual centers: 43% of patients received PORT. No significant difference in overall survival was seen with an HR of death of 0.96. Median overall survival was 55 months in the chemotherapy arm and 48 months in the surgery arm. Subset analysis by stage showed that HR was 0.80 (95% CI, 0.60 to 1.06) for stage II versus 0.97 (0.71 to 1.33) and 1.06 (0.82 to 1.38) for stages I and III, respectively. It is remarkable that in the subgroup of patients with stage II NSCLC, although the hazard ratio was not statistically significant, a 10% survival advantage at 5 years for chemotherapy-treated patients was reported.

TABLE 53.2 Main Baseline and Treatment Characteristics of Patients Enrolled in the Recently Concluded Adjuvant Studies

	ALPI[36]	IALT[37]	BLT[41]	NCIC-BR 10[43]	CALGB[44]	ANITA[42]
Regimen	Cisplatin/ vinblastine/ mitomycin × 3 cycles	Cisplatin and vindesine or vinblastine or vinorelbine or etoposide × 3–4 cycles	Cisplatin and vindesine or vinorelbine or vinblastine/ mitomycin or mitomycin and ifosfamide × 3 cycles	Cisplatin/ vinorelbine × 4 cycles	Carboplatin/ paclitaxel × 4 cycles	Cisplatin/ vinorelbine × 4 cycles
Sequential RT allowed	Yes	Yes	Yes	No	No	Yes
Number of Patients enrolled/planned	1209/1300	1867/3300	381/500	482/450	344/384*	840/800
Median age	61	59	61	61	61	59
Male/female ratio	86/14	81/19	65/35	66/34	65/35	85/14
Stage, %						
I	39	37	29	46	100 (all IB)	36
II	31	24	37	54		22
IIIA	29	37	27	NT		41
Histology, %						
Squamous	51	47	48	37	35	59
Nonsquamous	45	46	52	65	NR	40
Pneumonectomy rate	26%	35%	NR	25%	11%	38%

*Original sample size was 500 patients, subsequently emended. The study was closed early based on the recommendation of the Data Safety Monitoring Board.

ALPI, Adjuvant Lung Project Italy; ANITA, Adjuvant Navelbine International Trial Association; BLT, Big Lung Trial; CALGB4, Cancer and Leukemia Group B; IALT, International Adjuvant Lung Cancer Trial; NCIC-BR10, National Cancer Institute of Canada Clinical Trials Group; NR, not reported; NT, not tested; RT, radiotherapy.

Although the incidence of grades 3 and 4 hematological and nonhematological toxicities related to chemotherapy did not differ quantitatively and qualitatively from those commonly reported in advanced NSCLC, the marginal reduction in survival observed in the MVP arm in the first year after randomization could potentially reflect a toxicity effect. This is also indirectly confirmed by the lower percentage of patients in the MVP arm who completed subsequent thoracic radiotherapy (65% vs. 81% in the control arm).

No statistically significant association between p53 or Ki67 expression and stage or histology was found. An analysis of K-ras mutation status and survival was performed in adenocarcinomas and large cell carcinomas: mutations were found in 22% of the 117 considered samples with no relationship to survival.

The International Adjuvant Lung Cancer Trial (IALT) collaborative group was the first large study to show a significant benefit in favor of adjuvant chemotherapy. A total of 1867 completely resected NSCLC patients were randomized to chemotherapy (a doublet of cisplatin plus vindesine, vinblastine, vinorelbine, or etoposide) or observation.[37] All stages were represented, with approximately 10% having stage IA disease, 27% stage IB, 24% stage II, and 39% stage III. In the chemotherapy arm, 74% of patients received at least 240 mg/m^2 of cisplatin, 27% of patients received PORT. Toxicity of grades 3 and 4 was experienced by 23% of patients (0.8% of toxic deaths). Survival was significantly longer in the chemotherapy arm with an HR of 0.86 (95% CI, 0.76 to 0.98; $p < 0.03$): 5-year survival rates were 44.5% and 40.4%, and median survival was 50.8 and 44.4 months in the chemotherapy group and in the control group, respectively, whereas median disease-free survival was 40.2 and 30.5 months.

Some methodological aspects regarding the final analysis of the IALT study raise concerns: in clinical trials in which a long follow-up is required, the difference between treatments may depend on the follow-up time. That implies that in the early phase of the study, there is the potential for a biased estimate of the treatment effect. In the IALT study, the accrual was prematurely interrupted when less than 60% of expected patients had been enrolled. The follow up continued until about 65% of expected events had been observed. If the study had continued until the planned number of events was reached, the conditional power to detect, under the null hypothesis, a statistically significant difference would have been less than 50%. Moreover, the adoption of a Bayesian approach that may be more appropriate for interpreting results, when early analysis shows a potential positive treatment effect, would have suggested to prolong follow-up.[38] Bayesian analysis to determine if the IALT results were convincing enough to change clinical practice were presented at the American Society of Clinical Oncology (ASCO) 2004 and the preponderance of evidence supported at least a 3% survival advantage for adjuvant therapy.[39] Of interest, however, is that the results of the IALT study, initially reported with a 4.7-year follow-up (ASCO 2003), were recently updated (ASCO 2008) with 3 additional years of follow-up.[40] Median follow-up was 7.5 years at the cutoff date of September 1, 2005. The survival status was known for 1807 patients. Results showed a beneficial effect of adjuvant chemotherapy on overall survival (HR = 0.91; 95% CI, 0.81 to 1.02; $p = 0.10$) and on disease-free survival (HR = 0.88; 95% CI, 0.78 to 0.98; $p = 0.02$). However, there was a significant difference between the results of overall survival before and after 5 years (HR = 0.86; CI, 0.76 to 0.97; $p = 0.01$ vs. HR = 1.45; CI, 1.02 to 2.07; $p = 0.04$); p value for interaction was 0.006. Disease-free survival benefit was also different according to the follow-up duration (p value for interaction: 0.04; global, first 5 years, HR = 0.85, $p = 0.006$; after 5 years, HR = 1.33, $p = 0.16$). The analysis of non–lung cancer deaths for the whole period showed an HR of 1.34 (CI, 0.99 to 1.81; $p = 0.06$). These results confirmed the efficacy of chemotherapy for the first 5 years after surgery. The difference in results between less than and more than 5 years of follow-up may suggest possible late adjuvant chemotherapy-related overmortality. This potential effect underscores the need for the long-term follow-up of adjuvant lung cancer trials in order to evaluate results in terms of treatment benefits and long-term hazards.

The Big Lung Trial (BLT) was designed to evaluate the role of cisplatin-based chemotherapy across all NSCLC stages. Within the study, resected stage I to III NSCLC patients were randomly assigned to three cycles of postoperative chemotherapy (doublet of cisplatin with either vindesine or vinorelbine or a triplet with mitomycin and ifosfamide or MVP) or surgery alone. A total of 381 patients were randomized: three cycles of chemotherapy were completed in 64% of patients, with 40% of patients requiring dose reductions. PORT was given to only 14% of cases. No significant differences in terms of survival were seen in the two groups, even if this trial was underpowered to answer to the adjuvant chemotherapy benefit question, had a short follow-up of 29 months and 15% of patients with incompletely resected disease.[41]

The Adjuvant Navelbine International Trial Association (ANITA) trial randomized 840 resected stage IB to IIIA NSCLC patients to cisplatin 100 mg/m^2 every 4 weeks and vinorelbine 30 mg/m^2 weekly versus observation: 301 (36%) patients had stage IB disease, 203 (24%) had stage II disease, and 325 (39%) had stage IIIA disease. After a median follow-up of 76 months, median survival was 65.7 months in the chemotherapy group and 43.7 months in the observation group. Chemotherapy significantly reduced the risk for death (HR = 0.80; 95% CI, 0.66 to 0.96; $p = 0.017$) with a survival advantage of 8.6% at 5 years, which was maintained at 7 years (8.4%).[42] Grade 3 and 4 neutropenia was documented in 85% of patients, febrile neutropenia in 9%, and severe infections in 11%. Among the nonhematological toxicities, the most commonly reported were asthenia (28%), nausea and vomiting (27%), and anorexia (15%).

As in many of the previously reported adjuvant studies, PORT was administered according to the policy of individual centers. A descriptive analysis from this study showed that radiotherapy could benefit patients with N2 status and could be harmful when combined with chemotherapy in patients with N1 status. These data are in contrast with the data from North American Intergroup Group study reported previously where no benefit from concurrent use of cisplatin/etoposide and radiotherapy in patients with stages II and IIIA disease, possibly because 42% of the patients had stage II.

Differently from ALPI, IALT, BLT, and ANITA, which considered every stage of resectable NSCLC, two additional studies investigated the role adjuvant chemotherapy in very early stages (I and II).

The National Cancer Institute of Canada Clinical Trials Group (NCIC-BR10) limited enrolment to patients with stage IB-II disease. Patients were randomized to receive four cycles of cisplatin (50 mg/m^2, days 1 and 8 every 4 weeks) and vinorelbine 25 mg/m^2 weekly for 16 weeks versus observation alone. Patients did not receive PORT and were stratified by nodal status (N0 vs. N1) and K-Ras mutation (24% with mutations). The study was powered to detect a 10% improvement in 3 years' survival, and 482 resected stages IB and II (excluding T3N0) NSCLC patients were enrolled and randomized. Overall survival was significantly longer in the chemotherapy arm (94 vs. 73 months; HR = 0.69 (95% CI, 0.52 to 0.91; p = 0.0009), as was recurrence-free survival (not reached vs. 47 months); 5-year survival rates were 69% and 54%, respectively, with an absolute gain of 15% at 5 years. The subset analysis by stage showed a greater benefit at 5 years for stage II (20%) than for stage I (7% not statistically significant); notably at 6 years, the benefit for stage I disappeared, and survival was greater in the control group.

Fifty-eight percent of randomized and treated patients (n = 231) received three courses of cisplatin/vinorelbine. Two patients (0.8%) died because of treatment-related toxicity, grades 3 and 4 neutropenia was documented in 73% of patients and febrile neutropenia in 7%. Nineteen percent of patients required hospitalization for medical problems related to the toxicity of chemotherapy. Quality-of-life analysis demonstrated a reversible reduction in quality of life for the treatment group.[43]

NCIC-BR10 and ANITA, two largely positive studies, unfortunately adopted doses and schedules that are not routinely used in current clinical practice. The commonest dose of cisplatin currently used is 75 mg/m^2 on day 1, and the cisplatin administration on days 1 and 8 (as in the BR10) is quite unusual. In addition, weekly administration of vinorelbine is quite rarely adopted in clinical practice and associated with a higher toxicity.

Cancer and Leukemia Group B (CALGB) 9633 further narrowed the adjuvant group only to patients with resected stage IB disease and was the only trial using the carboplatin–paclitaxel regimen. The study accrued slowly because of its limited range of eligible patients leading to a reduction in planned overall accrual cohort. In addition, it was closed early by its data-safety-monitoring committee because of a positive interim analysis with 90% of patients recruited based on the revised estimates. The study was powered to detect a 13% improvement in overall survival at 5 years. At the time of closure to accrual, 344 patients had been entered and randomly assigned to receive carboplatin area under the curve (AUC) 6 and paclitaxel 200 mg/m^2 every 3 weeks for a total of four cycles: an early report after a follow-up time of 34 months detected a 12% absolute improvement in overall survival at 4 years (71% vs. 59%; HR = 0.62; p = 0.028).[44]

The delivery of chemotherapy was excellent with nearly 85% of patients who received four cycles of chemotherapy. Toxicity in this group of patients was minimal, with only 36% of patients having grades 3 and 4 myelosuppression. There were no treatment-related deaths, which is an important aspect of an adjuvant study.

Unfortunately, a recently updated analysis could not confirm such favorable outcome after an extended follow-up (54 months) and showed only a trend toward survival improvement (59% vs. 57%) that lost significance (HR = 0.80; p = 0.10).[45] It should be noted that the small sample size did not allow for adequate power to detect small differences in survival. The 3-year failure-free survival (66% vs. 57%) and the 3-year survival (79% vs. 70%; p = 0.045) continued to favor the chemotherapy group. The real role of prolonging disease-free survival has not been well quantified in the adjuvant setting, and it is not known to necessarily translate into a permanent advantage in overall survival. A subgroup analysis, also presented at the follow-up at ASCO revealed that further dividing patients in CALGB 9633 into those with tumors smaller than 4 cm versus those greater than or equal to 4 cm identified a higher-risk group for which chemotherapy may be beneficial. In an unplanned subset analysis, patients in CALGB 9633 with tumors of at least 4 cm (close to 100 patients in each arm) retained an overall survival advantage (HR = 0.66; p <0.04). The 74 patients in each arm with tumors smaller than 4 cm did not differ in survival (HR = 1.02; p = 0.51).[46]

Overall, three studies showed a positive impact of adjuvant chemotherapy in resectable NSCLC with a survival benefit ranging from 4.1% (IALT) to 15% (NCIC- BR10) (Table 53.3). Why are there such huge difference in survival among these studies? First, there was a huge difference in the sample size calculations from one study to another (from less than 500 patients to 3300 according to the planned sample sizes) to assess a similar expected therapeutic effect in a similar patient population. The only two studies designed to observe an estimated survival advantage in an unrestricted population of early stage patients (stages I to III) in the range of that reported in the 1995 metaanalysis were the ALPI and the IALT studies that, not surprisingly, demonstrated a survival benefit relatively close to each other (3% for ALPI vs. 4.1% for IALT).

Second, in most of these studies, no information is available on the proportion of patients who, during surgical resection, underwent systematic lymph nodal dissection (SND) or mediastinal lymph node sampling (MLS). In a randomized clinical study, SND was found to significantly influence survival in every stage of resectable NSCLC.[47]

Third, lung cancer patients frequently suffer from comorbidities, including chronic obstructive pulmonary disease and cardiovascular diseases that were found to affect survival

TABLE 53.3 Overall and According to Clinical Stage Hazard Ratios for Survival in the Adjuvant Studies in which Currently Used Platinum Regimens Were Tested

	Hazard Ratio for Survival (95% CI)			
Study	**Overall**	**Stage I**	**Stage II**	**Stage III**
ALPI[36]	0.96 (0.81–1.13) $p = 0.59$	0.97 (0.71–1.33)	0.80 (0.60–1.06)	1.06 (0.82–1.38)
IALT[37]	0.86 (0.76–0.98) $p<0.03$	0.95 (0.74–1.23)	0.93 (0.72–1.20)	0.79 (0.66–0.95)
BLT[41]	1.02 (0.77–1.35) $p = 0.90$	NA	NA	NA
NCIC-BR10[43]	0.69 (0.52–0.91) $p =$ p.04	0.94	0.59 (0.42–0.85)	Not tested
CALGB[44] Early Data*	0.62 (0.41–0.95) $p = 0.028$	0.62 (0.41–0.95) $p = 0.028$	Not tested	Not tested
CALGB[45] Follow-up Data	0.80 (0.60–1.07) $p = 0.1$	0.80 (0.60–1.07) $p = 0.1$	Not tested	Not tested
ANITA[42]	0.80 (0.66–0.96) $p = 0.017$	1.14 (0.83–1.57)	0.67 (0.47–0.94)	0.60 (0.44–0.82)

*After a median follow-up time of 34 months.

NA, not available.

significantly.[48,49] Additionally, an unbalance in the proportion of patients who potentially quit smoking after radical surgery may potentially account for survival differences as shown in two retrospective studies in which smoking status was found to highly influence survival of resected NSCLC patients.[50,51]

One common feature of most of these studies, with the exclusion of the carboplatin-based CALGB 9633, is the less than optimal compliance to adjuvant regimens. The feasibility of three cycles of adjuvant chemotherapy (including delays and dose reductions) ranged between 58% and 74% of the cisplatin-based studies. Reasons for reduced therapeutic compliance may be related to the need of a longer time to fully recover from the surgical procedure itself for lung cancer patients in comparison with that needed for breast cancer patients. For instance, in some of these studies, the pneumonectomy rate was far exceeding that of consecutive surgical series and a specific subset analysis about tolerability of chemotherapy in this specific subgroup of patients (ALPI = 26%, IALT = 35%, ANITA = 41%) has not been performed.

Although the role of delivering the planned total dose of cytotoxic agents has not been fully evaluated in all the these studies, in adjuvant breast cancer, survival benefit was more striking in those patients receiving >85% of the intended total dose of chemotherapy.[52]

Adjuvant Studies with Oral Chemotherapy Agents

A single randomized study tested the efficacy of oral ubenimex versus placebo administered continuously for 2 years after radical resection. This agent is a potent inhibitor of aminopeptidases and is believed to have immunomodulatory activity. Four hundred patients with completely resected stage I squamous cell carcinoma were randomized, and 5-year survival rate favored the experimental arm (81% vs. 74%; $p = 0.02$).[53]

Uracil-tegafur (UFT), an oral fluoropyrimidine combining uracil and tegafur, has been extensively studied in Japan as adjuvant single agent or combined with other intravenous agents. The largest trial of postoperative UFT therapy in resected NSCLC randomly assigned 979 patients with completely resected stage I adenocarcinoma to either oral UFT 250 mg/m^2 for 2 years or observation. The overall survival favored the UFT arm with an HR of 0.71 (95% CI, 0.52 to 0.98; $p = 0.04$) and a 5-year survival of 88% in the UFT group and 85% in the control group. Subset analyses found the greatest benefit in the T2N0 subgroup (n = 263; HR = 0.48; 95% CI, 0.29 to 0.81; $p = 0.005$) but not in T1N0 (n = 716; HR = 0.97; 95% CI, 0.64 to 1.46; $p = 0.87$) . Compliance was limited at 74% at 12 months and only 61% at 24 months.[54] One questionable point in this trial is the absence of any advantage in disease-free survival for UFT-treated arm, and this clearly contrasts with all the positive, cisplatin-based adjuvant studies (IALT, NCIC-BR10, ANITA) where improvement in overall survival for patients receiving adjuvant chemotherapy was invariably associated with a similar or greater magnitude in disease-free survival.

Results in three other fully published studies of adjuvant UFT in smaller sample size of patients were inconsistent with the previously reported study.[55–57] In addition, there is no confirmatory data concerning the use of UFT in the adjuvant setting outside Japan. The concept of relatively mild, low-dose continuous adjuvant therapy is attractive, but the absence of confirmatory adjuvant UFT studies outside Japan strongly limit the applicability of these data into clinical practice. Additionally, questions regarding a peculiar genetic sensitivity to UFT in the Japanese population remain unanswered.

The West Japan Thoracic Oncology Group in December 2005 finished enrolling 607 patients in a phase III study comparing in stage IB to III adjuvant UFT 250 mg/m^2 daily for 1 year versus single-agent gemcitabine 1000 mg/m^2 days 1 to 8 every 3 weeks for 6 cycles. Final analysis is expected in 2010.

Systematic Reviews and Metaanalyses

Recently, several systematic reviews and metaanalyses have confirmed the value of adjuvant cisplatin- or UFT-based chemotherapy in resectable NSCLC[58–63] (Table 53.4). All of these reports consistently showed a benefit from adjuvant chemotherapy with HRs ranging from 0.72 for adjuvant UFT to 0.89 for cisplatin-based chemotherapy.

The largest systematic review included 7200 patients from 19 randomized adjuvant trials (12 trials with cisplatin-based therapy and 7 trials with UFT): cisplatin-based postoperative chemotherapy showed an 11% relative reduction in mortality, whereas UFT yielded a 17% reduction when compared with surgery alone.[59]

Two of these metaanalyses are based on individual patient data rather than published study reports. In a metaanalysis comparing the outcome of 2003 patients treated with adjuvant oral UFT as a single agent or in combination with other cytotoxic agents from six different studies, UFT significantly improved overall survival (HR = 0.74; 95% CI, 0.61 to 0.88), corresponding to a 4.6% benefit at 5 years ($p = 0.001$) and 7% at 7 years ($p = 0.001$).[58]

The Lung Adjuvant Cisplatin Evaluation (LACE) pooled analysis reported data from individual cases on 4584 patients from the five randomized adjuvant clinical trials (ALPI, ANITA, BLT, IALT, and BR10) and detected a significantly positive effect of chemotherapy in terms of overall survival (HR = 0.89; 95% CI, 0.82 to 0.96), disease-free survival (HR = 0.84; 95% CI, 0.78 to 0.90) with a relative reduction of the risk of death of 11% (HR = 0.89; 95% CI, 0.82 to 0.96) (Fig. 53.1). In stages II and III NSCLC, overall survival gain was 5.3% at 5 years (48.8% vs. 43.3%; HR = 0.83; 95% CI, 0.83 to 0.95). A small but not significant survival gain was also evident in stage IB (HR = 0.92; 95% CI, 0.78 to 1.10), but a detrimental effect was seen in stage IA (HR = 1.41; 95% CI, 0.96 to 2.1). The most active regimen seems to be cisplatin/vinorelbine mainly due to the higher number of patients treated (1888 patients, HR = 0.80) and to higher cisplatin total doses administered in combination with vinorelbine (320 to 400 mg/m^2).[62]

Adjuvant Chemotherapy in the Elderly

The consistent data on efficacy of adjuvant chemotherapy bring every

TABLE 53.4 Systematic Reviews and Metaanalysis or Individual Patient Data Metaanalyses of Cisplatin-based and UFT-based Adjuvant Trials

Author	Comparisons Surgery vs. Surgery plus Chemotherapy	Number of Studies	Number of Patients	Survival	
				Hazard Ratio	95% CI
Hotta et al.[58]	Cisplatin-based CT	8	3786	0.89	0.81–0.97
	Single-agent UFT	5	1751	0.79	0.67–0.96
Sedrakyan et al.[59]	Cisplatin-based CT	12	7200 in total	0.89	0.82–0.96
	Single-agent UFT	7		0.83	0.73–0.95
Berghmans et al.[60]	Cisplatin-based CT	16	7644 in total	0.86	0.80–0.92
	Single-agent UFT	6		0.72	0.61–0.85
Bria et al.[61]	Cisplatin-based CT	12	6494	0.93*	0.89–0.95
Hamada et al.[62]†	UFT-based CT	6	2003	0.74	0.61–0.88
Pignon et al.[63]†	Cisplatin-based CT	5	4584	0.89	0.82–0.96

*Expressed a risk ratio.

†Individual patient data metaanalyses.

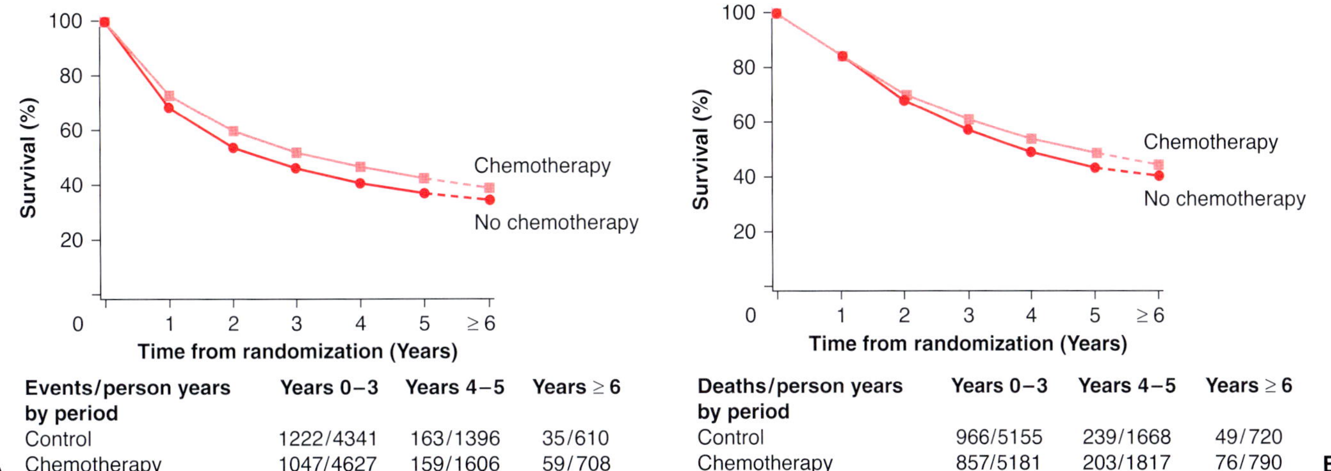

FIGURE 53.1 The Lung Adjuvant Cisplatin Evaluation (LACE) pooled analysis. Disease-free survival **(A)** and overall survival **(B)** curves (see text). (From Pignon JP, Tribodet H, Scagliotti GV, et al. Lung Adjuvant Cisplatin Evaluation [LACE]: a pooled analysis of five randomized clinical trials including 4,584 patients LACE meta-analysis. *J Clin Oncol* 2008;26:3552–3559.)

clinician to face a growing fraction of elderly patients who underwent surgery for NSCLC. More than 50% of lung cancer cases are diagnosed in patients older than 65 years, and approximately 30% are diagnosed in those older than 70.[63] The age cutoff to define elderly patients is usually established at 70 years, although it would be preferable to precisely assess the biological and not the chronological age.

Available data from younger patients do not automatically translate into a benefit in the elderly counterpart. It is well known that elderly patients tolerate chemotherapy poorly because of comorbidities and organ failure, especially the declining renal function altering drug pharmacodynamics. The prevalence of comorbidities, mainly respiratory and cardiovascular diseases, typical of heavy smokers, is higher in this subgroup of patients. Moreover, after a demanding surgery as in lobectomy or pneumonectomy, there is a higher risk of chemotherapy-induced toxicity. Higher toxicity or reduced compliance could vanish the potential survival benefit obtained with adjuvant chemotherapy. As a consequence, data are not conclusive because of the fact that elderly are generally excluded from clinical trials. Modified schedules or attenuated doses of platinum-containing chemotherapy should be investigated by specifically designed trials in the adjuvant setting.[64]

A retrospective analysis evaluated the influence of age on survival, chemotherapy compliance, and toxicity in the NCIC-BR10 study. Data from 327 young and 155 elderly patients (65 years or older) were evaluated. Histology showed a prevalence of adenocarcinoma and better performance status in younger patients. Elderly patients received significantly fewer doses of chemotherapy with no significant differences in toxicities. Overall survival in elderly patients remained significantly better with chemotherapy than with observation (HR = 0.61; p = 0.04) but in the few patients who are more than 75 years old (n = 23) had a significantly shorter survival than those aged 66 to 75.[65] These data suggest that in clinical practice, elderly patients fit to receive platinum-based chemotherapy should not be denied adjuvant chemotherapy.

Targeted Therapy In advanced NSCLC erlotinib, an epidermal growth factor receptor tyrosine-kinase inhibitor (EGFR TKI), as single agent in second/third line and bevacizumab, a monoclonal antibody against the isoform A of vascular endothelial growth factor (VEGF), as front-line treatment in combination with cytotoxic chemotherapy improve survival significantly.

Current clinical experience with EGFR TKIs in the adjuvant setting is limited and still evolving.

A pivotal Japanese phase III study planned to administer adjuvant gefitinib, another EGFR TKI, 250 mg/day or placebo to randomized patients with completely resected NSCLC (stages IB to IIIA) 4 to 6 weeks following surgery, for 2 years, until recurrence/withdrawal. However, recruitment was stopped after the randomization of 38 patients, because interstitial lung disease (ILD)-type events were being increasingly reported in Japan in the advanced disease setting leading to safety concerns in this population of potentially cured patients. Safety data for 38 recruited patients (18 gefitinib and 20 placebo) showed no unexpected adverse drug reactions, with the most common being grades 1 and 2 gastrointestinal and skin disorders in 12 and 16 patients receiving gefitinib and in five and six patients receiving placebo, respectively. Grades 3 and 4 adverse events occurred in four patients receiving gefitinib and one patient receiving placebo. ILD-type events were reported in one patient receiving gefitinib (concomitantly with other ILD-inducing drugs) who died and two patients receiving placebo. Adverse events associated with surgical complications were reported for six patients receiving gefitinib and four patients receiving placebo.[66]

In the same patient population, another phase III study from the National Cancer Institute of Canada (NCIC BR19) compared gefitinib versus placebo after four courses of cisplatin-based chemotherapy, but it was prematurely closed after the inclusion of 503 patients as consequence of the negative outcome of other phase III studies (SWOG 0139 in stage IIIB, which tested gefitinib versus placebo in nonprogressive patients following concurrent chemoradiotherapy and maintenance docetaxel[67] and a second-line study of gefitinib versus placebo, the ISEL study.[68] An analysis of the 503 entered patients is pending at this time.

Currently, an ongoing study is testing adjuvant erlotinib versus placebo after adjuvant platinum-based chemotherapy in stage IB to III NSCLC patients positive for EGFR expression (evaluated by immunohistochemistry and/or fluorescence in situ hybridization [FISH]). Potential limitations of this study are related to the current absence of established important predictive molecular selection factors, especially the still unproven role of FISH in early stages, and the role of secondary resistance mechanisms to EGFR inhibitors such as secondary mutations or induction of other signaling pathways (mesenchymal-epithelial transition factor [c-met]). The simple quantification of the presence of the EGFR receptor as a target on tumor cells could not be shown to be sufficiently predictive of response because of the variability of the activation state of the target and heterogeneity of pathways involved in the mechanism of action.

Exploratory studies selecting patients based on EGFR mutational testing most likely will occur in the near future but also retrospective studies could be helpful in this matter. An ongoing Japanese study in completely resected stage IIIA NSCLC with EGFR mutation is assessing the efficacy of gefitinib 250 mg/day for 1 year versus the combination of carboplatin/paclitaxel administered for four courses. The planned sample size is 150 patients and the primary end point of the study is progression-free survival.

The crucial role of angiogenesis in lung cancer development is very well documented, and it is an integral part of a preneoplastic lesion described as angiogenic squamous dysplasia.[69] Although other angiogenic factors have been identified, VEGF is the most potent and specific, with a well-defined role in normal and pathologic angiogenesis. VEGF stimulates proliferation of vascular endothelial cells and its expression is substantially increased in a majority of human tumors including lung cancer, when compared with the surrounding tumor-free tissues. A correlation has been noted between the degree of tumor vascularization and the level of VEGF messenger ribonucleic acid (mRNA) expression and in virtually all specimens examined, VEGF mRNA is expressed in tumor cells but not endothelial cells, whereas mRNAs for the two VEGF receptors, Flt-1 and kinase insert domain protein receptor (KDR), are upregulated in endothelial cells associated with the tumor.[70]

VEGF is a strong prognostic indicator in NSCLC and is associated with early postoperative relapse and decreased survival.[71]

The Eastern Oncology Cooperative Group (ECOG) and the U.S. Intergroup is conducting a multicenter randomized phase III trial of adjuvant chemotherapy alone (cisplatin/vinorelbine or cisplatin/gemcitabine or cisplatin/docetaxel) versus the same chemotherapy plus bevacizumab, in radically resected stage IB to IIIA NSCLC patients (ECOG 1505). An accrual of 1500 subjects is planned.

Genetic Predictive and Prognostic Factors In lung cancer, the choice of the cytotoxic chemotherapy is currently based on tumor (histology and disease extent) and clinical features, such as age and performance status, and it is often adjusted by considering both efficacy and toxicity. To individualize chemotherapy (i.e., to more specifically assign an effective treatment to individual patients who will likely benefit and avoid undue toxic effects to those who likely will not), a better definition of the prognostic or predictive implications of the tumors' genetic makeup as well as of the tumors' or patient's (germline) pharmacogenetic variations (the so called single-nucleotide polymorphisms) are needed. In early stage patients who undergo surgery, it is increasingly feasible to gather both kinds of indications through an extensive molecular characterization of the tumor and nonmalignant cells because of the availability of large amounts of resected neoplastic tissue and, at the same time, the easy availability of peripheral blood cells.

In the past, a large biomarker study retrospectively performed in 515 cases of resected stage I NSCLC failed to show any significant association between survival and the expression of an extensive panel of biomarkers, including EGFR, HER-2/neu, bcl-2, p53, and angiogenesis.[72]

The advent of the human genome–sequencing project and the concurrent development of many genomic-based technologies, including expression microarrays, have allowed translational researchers to explore the possibility of using expression profiles to better tune prognosis and predict tumor drug sensitivity or resistance.

Among epigenetic changes, aberrant gene promoter methylation is increasingly recognized as an extremely common event occurring early during carcinogenesis. An increasing number of genes that play a role in critical steps such as cell cycle control, DNA damage repair, growth factor regulation, invasion, and metastasis have been found highly methylated and altered very early in the carcinogenesis process.[73,74] More interestingly from a clinical perspective, patients with tumors harboring gene promoter hypermethylation have significantly worse prognosis.[75–77] This prognostic information needs to be validated prospectively with an adequate number of patients.

Several candidate signatures involving multigene expression profiles have been put forward as predictive of recurrence and survival for resected NSCLC, but these signatures need to be harmonized and crossvalidated before being used to select patients for therapy.[78–80] In one of these studies, researchers looked at 89 patients with early stage NSCLC. Gene-expression profiles (the lung metagene model) that predicted the risk of recurrence were evaluated in two independent groups of 25 and 84 patients, respectively. The lung metagene model predicted recurrence for individual patients significantly better than did clinical prognostic factors, and it was consistent across all early stages of NSCLC. When applied to other two cohorts, the model had an overall predictive accuracy of 72% and 79%.

The predictor also identified a subgroup of patients with stage IA disease who were at high risk for recurrence.[78] As a consequence of these results, the CALGB is currently planning a large randomized study in which patients who undergo surgery will then have their tumor tissue characterized by gene expression analysis and then assigned a predicted outcome of low or high risk. Low-risk patients will be only observed, whereas high-risk patients will be randomized to either observation, according to standard practice for stage IA NSCLC, or receive adjuvant chemotherapy.

Exploratory studies in advanced disease demonstrated an association between high level of mRNA expression of the excision repair cross-complementation group 1 (ERCC1) gene and cisplatin resistance[81,82] or ribonucleotide reductase M1 (RRM1) gene and gemcitabine resistance.[83]

Unfortunately, most of genetic markers are carrying on predictive and prognostic information.[84–86] In a retrospective study, RRM1 and ERCC1 expression as evaluated through a quantitative immunohistochemistry method was found to have a prognostic impact on survival after surgical treatment of early stage NSCLC. The overall survival was more than 120 months for patients with tumors with high expression of RRM1 versus 60 months for those with low expression of RRM1. Among these 187 patients, the survival advantage was limited to the 30% of patients with tumors that had a high expression of both RRM1 and ERCC1.[86] Another large retrospective study called Bio-IALT analyzed 761 tumor specimens and showed that the benefit of adjuvant chemotherapy was exclusively observed in the subgroup of tumors that were ERCC1 negative by immunohistochemistry. Thus, the low expressors are predicted to do worse without chemotherapy but to have better benefit from chemotherapy than the high expressors. In this study, the genetic marker was both prognostic and predictive.[87]

Subsequently, the expression of $p27^{Kip1}$, $p16^{INK4A}$, cyclin D1, cyclin D3, cyclin E, and Ki-67 was immunohistochemically assessed in tumor specimens of 778 patients from the IALT adjuvant study. Among patients with $p27^{Kip1}$-negative tumors, cisplatin-based chemotherapy resulted in longer overall survival compared with controls (adjusted HR for death = 0.66; 95% CI, 0.50 to 0.88; $p = 0.006$). In patients with $p27^{Kip1}$-positive tumors, overall survival was not different between patients treated with cisplatin-based chemotherapy and controls (adjusted HR for death = 1.09; 95% CI, 0.82 to 1.45; $p = 0.54$). The other cell cycle regulators and Ki-67 did not predict benefit of adjuvant cisplatin-based chemotherapy.[88]

Overexpression of class I and class III β-tubulin play a significant role in the acquisition of paclitaxel resistance.[89] Class III β-tubulin expression is also correlated with patient outcome in NSCLC patients treated with vinorelbine-based regimens.[90] The role of class III β-tubulin was assessed in the NCIC-BR10 study on 265 out of 482 patients enrolled in the trial. Higher class III β-tubulin expression was seen in women, in nonsquamous histology, in patients with Ras mutations, in patients <60 years and in performance status 1 (PS1) patients. Overexpression of class III β-tubulin was associated with worse overall survival in the observation arm (HR = 1.72; 95% CI, 1.02 to 2.88; $p = 0.04$) but not in the chemotherapy arm. A greater benefit from adjuvant chemotherapy was seen in patients with high expression of class III β-tubulin, whereas in the setting of advanced disease, the opposite was evident.[91] Such data need larger confirmatory studies but could be useful to design experimental trials to select patients and chemotherapy regimens based on a genomic profile.

Even if both of these markers have not yet fully validated, and the used techniques (quantitative real time polymerase chain reaction [qRT-PCR] and immunohistochemistry) are not yet fully standardized, the possibility to prospectively validate this experimental hypothesis generated from retrospective studies represents a high priority.

CONCLUSION

Phase III prospective randomized trials and metaanalyses have conclusively demonstrated that cisplatin-based adjuvant chemotherapy has a positive impact on disease-free and overall survival in postoperative stages II and III NSCLC. The efficacy of oral UFT continuously administered for 2 years has been shown only in Japanese studies and mainly in adenocarcinoma and stage I disease. The number of patients who will benefit from adjuvant treatment, however, represent a small proportion of all completely resected NSCLC patients (Fig. 53.2). Genome-wide and candidate gene approaches

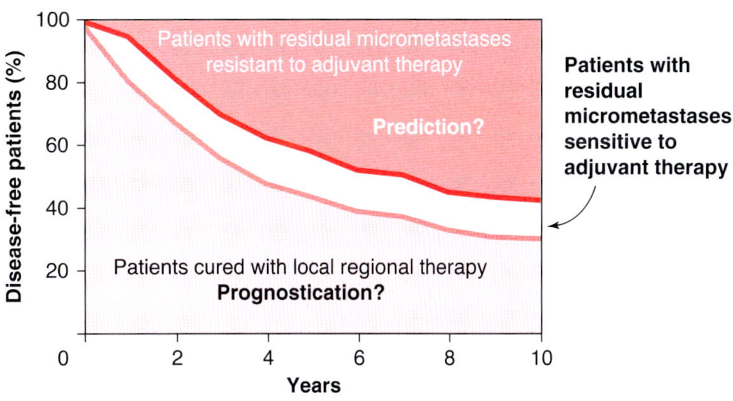

FIGURE 53.2 Graph indicating how much limited is the proportion of patients who really benefit from adjuvant treatments. Most are still cured by surgery alone or they have micrometastatic disease already resistant to empirical systemic treatments.

have already shown through retrospective studies the potential for refining and individualizing the treatment of early stage NSCLC and improving the efficacy of cytotoxic chemotherapy. These hypothesis generating findings need to be verified in prospective studies as well as the role of molecular-targeted therapies.

REFERENCES

1. Khuri JM, Spitz MR, Hong WK. Lung chemoprevention: targeting former rather than current smokers. *Cancer Prev In* 1995;2:55.
2. Levi F, Lucchini F, Negri E, et al. Cancer mortality in Europe 1990–1994, and overview of trends from 1955 to 1994. *Eur J Cancer* 1999;35:1477–1516.
3. Parkin DM, Pisani P, Ferlay J. Estimates of the worldwide incidence of 25 major cancers in 1990. *Int J Cancer* 1999;80:827–841.
4. Nesbitt JC, Putnam JB Jr, Walsh GL, et al. Survival in early-stage non-small cell lung cancer. *Ann Thorac Surg* 1995;60:466–472.
5. Feld R, Rubenstein I, Weisenberger T, et al. Sites of recurrence in resected stage I non-small cell lung cancer: a guide for future studies. *J Clin Oncol* 1984;2:1352–1358.
6. Martini N, Flehinger B, Zaman M, et al. Prospective study of 445 lung carcinomas with mediastinal lymph node metastases. *J Thorac Cardiovasc Surg* 1980;80:390–397.
7. Pairolero P, Williams D, Bergstralh M, et al. Post-surgical stage I bronchogenic carcinoma. Morbid implications of recurrent disease. *Ann Thorac Surg* 1984;38:331–338.
8. Thomas P, Rubenstein I. The Lung Cancer Study Group. Cancer recurrence after resection T1N0 non-small cell lung cancer. *Ann Thorac Surg* 1990;48:242–247.
9. Pieterman RM, van Putten JW, Meuzelaar JJ, et al. Preoperative staging of non-small-cell lung cancer with positron-emission tomography. *N Engl J Med* 2000;343:254–261.
10. Gupta NC, Graeber GM, Rogers JS II, et al. Comparative efficacy of positron emission tomography with FDG and computed tomographic scanning in preoperative staging of non-small cell lung cancer. *Ann Surg* 1999;229:286–291.
11. Weder W, Schmid RA, Bruchhaus H, et al. Detection of extrathoracic metastases by positron emission tomography in lung cancer. *Ann Thorac Surg* 1998;66:886–892.
12. Passlick B, Izbicki JR, Kubuschok B, et al. Detection of disseminated lung cancer cells in lymph nodes: impact on staging and prognosis. *Ann Thorac Surg* 1996;61–177.
13. Gu CD, Osaki T, Oyama T, et al. Detection of micrometastatic tumor cells in pN0 lymph nodes of patients with completely resected non small cell lung cancer: impact on recurrence and Survival. *Ann Surg* 2002;235(1):133–139.
14. D'Cunha J, Corfits AL, Herndon JE II, et al. Molecular staging of lung cancer: real-time polymerase chain reaction estimation of lymph node micrometastatic tumor cell burden in stage I non-small cell lung cancer—preliminary results of Cancer and Leukemia Group B Trial 9761. *J Thorac Cardiovasc Surg* 2002;123(3):484–491.
15. Maeda J, Inoue M, Okumura M, et al. Detection of occult tumor cells in lymph nodes from non-small cell lung cancer patients using reverse transcription-polymerase chain reaction for carcinoembryonic antigen mRNA with the evaluation of its sensitivity. *Lung Cancer* 2006;52:235–240.
16. Sozzi G, Conte D, Leon ME, et al. Quantification of free circulating DNA as a diagnostic marker in lung cancer. *J Clin Oncol* 2003;21:3902–3908.
17. Bach PB, Jett JR, Pastorino U, et al. Computed tomography screening and lung cancer outcomes. *JAMA* 2007;297(9):953–961.
18. Schabel FM Jr. Rationale for adjuvant chemotherapy. *Cancer* 1977;39(Suppl 6):2875–2882.
19. Ihde D, Ball D, Arriagada R, et al. Postoperative adjuvant therapy for non-small cell lung cancer: a consensus report. *Lung Cancer* 1994;11(Suppl 3)S15–S17.
20. PORT Meta-analysis Trialists Group. Postoperative radiotherapy in non-small-cell lung cancer: systematic review and meta-analysis of individual patient data from nine randomized controlled trials. *Lancet* 1998;352:257–263.
21. PORT Meta-analysis Trialists Group. Postoperative radiotherapy for non-small cell lung cancer. *Cochrane Database of Systematic Reviews* 2000, Issue 2. In The Cochrane Database of Systematic Reviews 2007 Issue 4, 2007 The Cochrane Collaboration. Published by John Wiley and Sons, Ltd. DOI: 10.1002/14651858.CD002142.pub.
22. Machtay M, Lee JH, Shrager JB, et al. Risk of death from intercurrent disease is not excessively increased by modern postoperative radiotherapy for high-risk resected non-small cell lung carcinoma. *J Clin Oncol* 2001;19:3912–3917.
23. Lally BE, Zelterman D, Colasanto JM, et al. Postoperative radiotherapy for stage II or III non-small-cell lung cancer using the surveillance, epidemiology, and end results database. *J Clin Oncol* 2006;24(19): 2998–3006.
24. Le Péchoux C, Dunant A, Pignon JP, et al. Need for a new trial to evaluate adjuvant postoperative radiotherapy in non-small-cell lung cancer patients with N2 mediastinal involvement. *J Clin Oncol* 2007;25(7): E10–E11.
25. Wagner H Jr, Bonomi P. Preoperative and postoperative therapy for non-small cell lung cancer. In: Roth JA, Ruckdeschel JC, Weisenburger TH, eds. *Thoracic Oncology*. 2nd ed. Philadelphia: WB Saunders, 1995:147–163.
26. Holmes EC, Gail M. Surgical adjuvant therapy for stage II and stage III adenocarcinoma and large-cell undifferentiated carcinoma. *J Clin Oncol* 1986;4(5):710–715.
27. The Lung Cancer Study Group. The benefit of adjuvant treatment for resected locally advanced non-small cell lung cancer. *J Clin Oncol* 1986;4:710–715.
28. Niiranen A, Niitamo-Korhonen S, Kouri M, et al. Adjuvant chemotherapy after radical surgery for non-small-cell lung cancer: a randomized study. *J Clin Oncol* 1992;10:1927–1932.
29. Feld R, Rubinstein L, Thomas PA. Adjuvant chemotherapy with cyclophosphamide, doxorubicin, and cisplatin in patients with completely resected stage I non-small-cell lung cancer. The Lung Cancer Study Group. *J Natl Cancer Inst* 1993;85:299–306.
30. Ohta M, Tsuchiya R, Shimoyama M, et al. Adjuvant chemotherapy for completely resected stage III non-small-cell lung cancer. Results of a randomized prospective study. The Japan Clinical Oncology Group. *J Thorac Cardiovasc Surg* 1993;106:703–708
31. Figlin RA, Piantodosi S. A phase 3 randomized trial of immediate combination chemotherapy vs delayed combination chemotherapy in patients with completely resected stage II and III non-small cell carcinoma of the lung. *Chest* 1994;106(6 Suppl):S310–S312.
32. Dautzenberg B, Chastang C, Arriagada R, et al. Adjuvant radiotherapy versus combined sequential chemotherapy followed by radiotherapy in the treatment of resected non-small cell lung carcinoma. A randomized trial of 267 patients. GETCB (Groupe d'Etude et de Traitement des Cancers Bronchiques). *Cancer* 1995;76(5):779–786.
33. Non-small Cell Lung Cancer Collaborative Group. Chemotherapy in non-small cell lung cancer: a meta-analysis using updated data on individual patients from 52 randomised clinical trials. *Br Med J* 1995;311:899–909.
34. Keller SM, Adak S, Wagner H, et al. A randomized trial of postoperative adjuvant therapy in patients with completely resected stage II or IIA non-small cell lung cancer. *N Engl J Med* 2000;343, 1217–1222.
35. Schiller JH, Adak S, Feins RH, et al. Lack of prognostic significance of p53 and K-ras mutations in primary resected non-small cell lung cancer on E4592: a laboratory ancillary study on an Eastern Cooperative Oncology Group prospective randomized clinical trial of postoperative adjuvant therapy. *J Clin Oncol* 2001;19:448–457.

36. Scagliotti GV, Fossati R, Torri V, et al. Randomized study of adjuvant chemotherapy for completely resected stage I, II or IIIA non-small cell lung cancer. *J Natl Cancer Inst* 2003;95:1453–1461.
37. Arriagada R, Bergman B, Dunant A, et al. Cisplatin-based adjuvant chemotherapy in patients with completely resected non-small cell lung cancer. *N Engl J Med* 2004;350:351–360.
38. Fayers PM, Ashby D, Parmar MK. Tutorial in biostatistics Bayesian data monitoring in clinical trials. *Stat Med* 1997;16:1413–1430.
39. Miksad RA, Roberts TG, Gonen RM, et al. Bayesian analysis of the International Adjuvant Lung Trial (IALT): should it change practice? *J Clin Oncol 2004 ASCO Annual Meeting Proceedings* (Post-Meeting Edition) 2004;22(14S), Abstract 6038.
40. Le Chevalier T, Dunant A, Arriagada R. Long-term results of the International Adjuvant Lung Cancer Trial (IALT) evaluating adjuvant cisplatin-based chemotherapy in resected non-small cell lung cancer (NSCLC). *J Clin Oncol* 2008;26(May 20 suppl). abstr 7507.
41. Waller D, Peake MD, Stephens RJ, et al. Chemotherapy for patients with non-small cell lung cancer. The surgical setting of the Big Lung Trial. *Eur J Cardio Thorac Surg* 2004;26,173–182.
42. Douillard JY, Rosell R, Delena M, et al. Adjuvant vinorelbine plus cisplatin versus observation in patients with completely resected stage IB-IIIA non-small-cell lung cancer (Adjuvant Navelbine International Trialist Association [ANITA]): a randomised controlled trial. *Lancet Oncol* 2006;7:719–727.
43. Winton T, Livingston R, Johnson D, et al. Vinorelbine plus cisplatin vs. observation in resected non-small-cell lung cancer. *N Engl J Med* 2005;352:2589–2597.
44. Strauss GM, Herndon J, Maddaus MA, et al. Randomized clinical trial of adjuvant chemotherapy with paclitaxel and carboplatin following resection in stage IB non-small cell lung cancer (NSCLC): report of Cancer and Leukemia Group B (CALGB) Protocol 9633. *J Clin Oncol* 2004;22(14S),7019.
45. Strauss GM, Herndon J, Maddaus MA, et al. Adjuvant chemotherapy in stage IB non-small cell lung cancer (NSCLC): update of Cancer and Leukemia Group B (CALGB) Protocol 9633. *J Clin Oncol* 2006;24(18S):7007.
46. Strauss GM, Herndon JE, Maddaus MA. Adjuvant chemotherapy in stage IB non-small cell lung cancer (NSCLC): update on Cancer and Leukemia Group B (CALGB) protocol 9633 [abstract]. *J Clin Oncol* 2006;24:S365.
47. Wu Y, Huang Z, Wang S, et al. A randomised trial of systematic nodal dissection in resectable non-small cell lung cancer. *Lung Cancer* 2002;36:1–6.
48. Ambrogi V, Pompeo E, Elia S, et al. The impact of cardiovascular comorbidity on the outcome of surgery for stage I and II non-small cell lung cancer. *Eur J Cardiovasc Surg* 2003;23:811–817.
49. Pastorino U, Valente M, Bedini V, et al. Effect of chronic cardiopulmonary disease on survival after resection for stage Ia lung cancer. *Thorax* 1982;37:680–683.
50. Wu Y, Lin CJ, Hsu W, et al. Long-term results of pathological stage I non-small cell lung cancer: validation of using the number of totally removed lymph nodes as a staging system. *Eur J Cardiovasc Surg* 2003;24:994–1001.
51. Toh CK, Gao F, Lim WT, et al. Never-smokers with lung cancer: epidemiologic evidence of a distinct disease entity *J Clin Oncol* 2006:2245–2251.
52. Bonadonna G, Valagussa P, Moliterni A, et al. Adjuvant cyclophosphamide, methotrexate, and fluorouracil in node-positive breast cancer: the results of 20 years of follow-up. *N Engl J Med* 1995;332: 901–906.
53. Kato H, Konaka C, Tsuboi M, et al. A randomised phase III study comparing ubeminex (Bestatin) versus placebo as post-operative adjuvant treatment in patients with stage I squamous cell lung cancer. *Proc Am Soc Clin Oncol* 2001;20:307a(abstr. 1225).
54. Kato H, Ichinose Y, Ohta M, et al. A randomized trial of adjuvant chemotherapy with uracil-tegafur for adenocarcinoma of the lung. *N Engl J Med* 2004;350:1713–1721.
55. Wada H, Hitomi S, Teramatsu T. The West Japan Study Group for Lung Cancer Surgery. Adjuvant chemotherapy after complete resection in non-small-cell lung cancer. *J Clin Oncol* 1996;14:1048–1054.
56. Endo C, Saito Y, Iwanami H, et al. A randomized trial of postoperative UFT therapy in p stage I, II non-small cell lung cancer: Northeast Japan Study Group for Lung Cancer Surgery. *Lung Cancer* 2003;40:181–186.
57. Imaizumi M. Postoperative adjuvant cisplatin, vindesine, plus uracil tegafur chemotherapy increased survival of patients with completely resected p-stage I non-small cell lung cancer. *Lung Cancer* 2005;49:85–94.
58. Hotta K, Matsuo K, Ueoka H, et al. Role of adjuvant chemotherapy in patients with resected non-small cell lung cancer: reappraisal with a meta-analysis of randomized controlled trials. *J Clin Oncol* 2004;22:3860–3867.
59. Sedrakyan A, van Der Meulen J, O'Byrne K, et al. Postoperative chemotherapy for non-small cell lung cancer: a systematic review and meta-analysis. *J Thorac Cardiovasc Surg* 2004;128:414–419.
60. Berghmans T, Paesmans M, Meert AP, et al. Survival improvement in resectable non-small cell lung cancer with (neo)adjuvant chemotherapy: results of a meta-analysis of the literature. *Lung Cancer* 2005;49:13–23.
61. Bria E, Gralla R, Raftopoulos H, et al. Does adjuvant chemotherapy improve survival in non small cell lung cancer (NSCLC)? A pooled-analysis of 6494 patients in 12 studies, examining survival and magnitude of benefit. *J Clin Oncol* 2005;23:A7140.
62. Hamada C, Tanaka F, Ohta M, et al. Meta-analysis of postoperative adjuvant chemotherapy with tegafur-uracil in non-small-cell lung cancer. *J Clin Oncol* 2005;23:4999–5006.
63. Pignon JP, Tribodet H, Scagliotti GV, et al. Lung Adjuvant Cisplatin Evaluation (LACE): a pooled analysis of five randomized clinical trials including 4,584 patients LACE meta-analysis. *J Clin Oncol* 2008 Jul 20;26(21):3552–3559.
64. Gridelli C, Perrone F, Monfardini S. Lung cancer in the elderly. *Eur J Cancer* 1997;33:2313–2314.
65. Pepe C, Hasan B, Winton T, et al. Adjuvant vionrelbine and cisplatin in elderly patients: National Cancer Institute of Canada and Intergroup Study JBR.10. *J Clin Oncol* 2007;25:1553–1561.
66. Tsuboi M, Kato H, Nagai K, et al. Gefitinib in the adjuvant setting: safety results from a phase III study in patients with completely resected non-small cell lung cancer. *Anticancer Drugs* 2005;16:1123–1128.
67. Kelly K, Chansky K, Gaspar LE, et al. Updated analysis of SWOG 0023: a randomized phase III trial of gefitinib versus placebo maintenance after definitive chemoradiation followed by docetaxel in patients with locally advanced stage III non-small cell lung cancer. *J Clin Oncol* 2007;25(suppl):388S(abst 7513).
68. Thatcher N, Chang A, Parikh P, et al. Gefitinib plus best supportive care in previously treated patients with refractory advanced non-small-cell lung cancer: results from a randomised, placebo-controlled, multicentre study (Iressa Survival Evaluation in Lung Cancer). *Lancet* 2005;366:1527–1537.
69. Keith RL, Miller YE, Gemmil RM, et al. Angiogenic squamous dysplasia in bronchi of individuals at high risk for lung cancer. *Clin Cancer Res* 2000;6:1616–1625.
70. Mattern J, Koomagi R, Volm M. Association of vascular endothelial growth factor expression with intratumoral microvessel density and tumour cell proliferation in human epidermoid lung carcinoma. *Br J Cancer* 1996;73:931–934.
71. Yuan A, Yu CJ, Kuo SH, et al. Vascular endothelial growth factor 189 mRNA isoform expression specifically correlates with tumor angiogenesis, patient survival, and postoperative relapse in non-small-cell lung cancer. *J Clin Oncol* 2001;19:432–441.
72. Pastorino U, Andreola S, Tagliabue E, et al. Immunocytochemical markers in stage I lung cancer: relevance to prognosis. *J Clin Oncol* 1997;15:2858–2865.
73. Robertson KD. DNA methylation, methyltransferases and cancer. *Oncogene* 2001;20:3139–3155.
74. Zochbauer-Muller S, Fong KM, Virmani AK, et al. Aberrant promoter methylation of multiple genes in non-small cell lung cancers. *Cancer Res* 2001;61:249–255.

75. Herbst RS, Yano S, Kuniyasu H, et al. Differential expression of E-cadherin and type IV collagenase genes predicts outcome in patients with stage I non-small cell lung carcinoma. *Clin Cancer Res* 2000;6:790–797.
76. Tang X, Khuri Fr, Lee JJ, et al. Hypermethylation of the death-associated protein kinase promoter and aggressiveness in stage I non-small cell lung cancer. *J Natl Cancer Inst* 2000;92:1511–1516.
77. Chang YS, Wang L, Liu D, et al. Correlation between insulin-growth factor-binding protein-3 promoter methylation and prognosis of patients with stage I non-small cell lung cancer. *Clin Cancer Res* 2002;8:3669.
78. Potti A, Mukherjee S, Petersen R, et al. A genomic strategy to refine prognosis in early stage non-small cell lung cancer. *N Engl J Med* 2006;355;570–580.
79. Chen HY, Yu SL, Chen CH, et al. A five-gene signature and outcome in non-small cell lung cancer. *N Engl J Med* 2007;356;11–20.
80. Seike M, Yanaihara N, Bowman ED, et al. Use of a cytokine gene expression signature in lung adenocarcinoma and the surrounding tissue as a prognostic classifier. *J Natl Cancer Inst* 2007;99:16:1257–1269.
81. Lord RVN, Brabender J, Gandara D, et al. Low ERCC1 expression correlates with prolonged survival after cisplatin plus gemcitabine chemotherapy in non-small-cell lung cancer. *Clin Cancer Res* 2002;8:2286–2291.
82. Ceppi P, Volante M, Novello S, et al. ERCC1 and RRM1 gene expressions but not EGFR are predictive of shorter survival in advanced non-small-cell lung cancer treated with cisplatin and gemcitabine. *Ann Oncol* 2006;17:1818–1825.
83. Bepler G, Kusmartseva I, Sharma S, et al. RRM1-modulated in vitro and in vivo efficacy of gemcitabine and platinum in non-small-cell lung cancer. *J Clin Oncol* 2006;24,4731–437.
84. Bepler G, Gautam A, McIntyre LM, et al. Prognostic significance of molecular genetic aberrations on chromosome segment 11p15.5 in non-small-cell lung cancer. *J Clin Oncol* 2002;20:1353–1360.
85. Bepler G, Sharma S, Cantor A, et al. RRM1 and PTEN as prognostic parameters for overall and disease-free survival in patients with non-small-cell lung cancer. *J Clin Oncol* 2004;22:1878–1885.
86. Zheng Z, Chen T, Li X, et al. DNA synthesis and repair genes RRM1 and ERCC1 in lung cancer. *N Engl J Med* 2007;356:800–808.
87. Olaussen KA, Dunant A, Fouret P, et al. DNA repair by ERCC1 in non–small-cell lung cancer and cisplatin-based adjuvant chemotherapy. *N Engl J Med* 2006;355:983–991.
88. Filipits M, Pirker R, Dunant A, et al. Cell cycle regulators and outcome of adjuvant cisplatin-based chemotherapy in completely resected non–small-cell lung cancer: the International Adjuvant Lung Cancer Trial Biologic Program. *J Clin Oncol* 2007;25:2735–2740.
89. Dumontet C, Sikic BI. Mechanisms of action and resistance to antitubulin agents: microtubule dynamics, drug transport and cell death. *J Clin Oncol* 1999;17:1061–1070.
90. Kamath K, Wilson L, Cabral F, et al. β III-tubulin induces paclitaxel resistance in association with reduced effects on microtubule dynamic instability. *J Biol Chem* 2005;280:12902–2907.
91. Seve P, Isaac S, Tredan O, et al. Expression of class III β-tubulin is predictive of patient outcome in patients with non-small cell lung cancer receiving vinorelbine-based chemotherapy. *Clin Cancer Res* 2005;11:5481–5486.

CHAPTER 54

Jan P. van Meerbeeck
Katherine M. Pisters

Preoperative Chemotherapy for Early Stage Non–Small Cell Lung Cancer

BACKGROUND

Surgery remains the cornerstone of treatment for patients with early stage non–small cell lung cancer (NSCLC) and provides the best hope for cure. Operable patients with stages IA through IIIA disease are candidates for complete resection with curative intent. Patients diagnosed with these stages represent approximately one third of all lung cancer cases.[1] However, despite complete surgical resection, a large number of patients will relapse after surgery. Five-year survival rates in patients with completely resected NSCLC average 78% and 58% for stages IA and IB, 46% and 36% for stages IIA and B, and 24% for stage IIIA, respectively.[2] The most frequent cause of death for patients with NSCLC after complete resection is the development of distant metastases. Although the frequency of intrathoracic recurrence averages 10% to 15% across stages, the frequency of distant metastasis as site of first relapse increases from 15% in stage IA over 40% in stage II to 60% in stage IIIA.[3–6] Relapse at distant sites is thought to be a result of occult micrometastatic disease, undetected at the time of preoperative staging.

Eradication of early metastatic disease by chemotherapy may theoretically translate into a decreased incidence of recurrence in distant sites, and thereby improve survival. This chemotherapy can be administered before (neoadjuvant or induction) or after (postoperative or adjuvant) surgery. Several randomized trials and metaanalyses have recently demonstrated an overall survival benefit with adjuvant platinum-based chemotherapy in early stage NSCLC.[7–9] These results have lead to the adoption of surgery and adjuvant chemotherapy as the new standard of care in selected patients.[10] This chapter will focus on the administration of chemotherapy prior to surgery as an alternate approach to adjuvant chemotherapy in early stage resectable NSCLC.

RATIONALE FOR NEOADJUVANT CHEMOTHERAPY

The term *neoadjuvant chemotherapy* was coined by Frei[11] to refer to the specific strategy of using a drug treatment at the earliest time possible. Neoadjuvant chemotherapy has several potential advantages over immediate surgery and adjuvant therapy. The most important is the systemic treatment of occult microscopic metastatic disease at the earliest possible time, with an improved progression-free and overall survival as compared to the local treatment only. The former is thought to be the result of a better control of the cytokines released by the wound repair, the latter by an improved sterilization of the occult metastases. Besides its potential systemic effects, chemotherapy induces cytotoxic effects at the level of the primary tumor, resulting in clinical and even pathological remissions. A reduction in the primary tumor mass may theoretically lead to less extensive surgery and possibly renders borderline unresectable lesions resectable (e.g., by downstaging of involved mediastinal lymph nodes). Another potential advantage of neoadjuvant chemotherapy is its better compliance. Only 45% to 60% of the patients are able to complete the adjuvant chemotherapy without dose reductions or delays, whereas the induction chemotherapy was shown to be administrated in more than 80% of the patients in most phase II induction trials.[12] Other potential advantages include the in vivo assessment of tumor chemosensitivity, a lower risk of developing drug resistance, and the selection of responsive patients, as patients with disease progression on chemotherapy will most likely not benefit from surgery.

The potential disadvantages of neoadjuvant chemotherapy include a delay in potentially curative surgery, less accurate staging—as the pathological staging is confounded by the induction treatment—and increased surgical morbidity and mortality after chemotherapy with decrease in quality of life. Lastly, a benefit of neoadjuvant chemotherapy is well established for the treatment of invasive bladder cancer and endothoracic esophageal cancer.[13,14]

EARLY STUDIES

Enthusiasm for the use of neoadjuvant chemotherapy for treating early stage NSCLC was generated by positive survival results from two small randomized studies in patients with stage IIIA. Roth et al.[15] randomized patients with potentially resectable clinical stage IIIA NSCLC between perioperative chemotherapy followed by surgery and a control arm of surgery alone. Patients allocated to chemotherapy were to receive three cycles of chemotherapy with cyclophosphamide, etoposide, and cisplatin before surgery; an additional three cycles were given after surgery to patients with preoperative radiographic response. Following an interim analysis, the trial was closed after 60 patients had been accrued because of a clinically meaningful survival benefit in favor of the induction chemotherapy arm. Long-term follow-up of this trial, after a median time from randomization of 82 months, confirmed the beneficial effect of induction chemotherapy. Median and 5-year survival rates were 21 months and 36% versus 14 months and 15% for surgery alone.[16]

In a similar randomized trial conducted by Rosell et al.,[17] clinical stage I to IIIA NSCLC patients were randomized to immediate surgery or surgery preceded by three cycles of mitomycin, ifosfamide, and cisplatin chemotherapy. Both treatment groups received postoperative mediastinal radiation therapy to 50 Gy. Interim analysis after 24 months follow-up with 60 eligible patients showed a significant difference in survival favoring induction chemotherapy and enrollment was stopped. Reassessment with 7-year follow-up found median and 5-year survival rates of 22 months and 17% in the chemotherapy arm compared to 10 months and 0% in the surgery-alone arm.[18] The outcome of patients treated with immediate surgery was, however, disappointingly low.

Pass et al.[19] randomized 27 patients between surgical resection either preceded by cisplatin–etoposide chemotherapy or followed by radiotherapy and observed median survival rates of 29 versus 16 months. The results of this trial are, however, difficult to interpret because of the asymmetry in randomization. Four other small randomized series did not observe a difference in outcome between an approach with or without preoperative chemotherapy.[20–23]

These earlier trials have a number of weaknesses in their design: (a) a variable use of adjuvant chemotherapy and radiotherapy; (b) the use of first- and second-generation drugs, of which some have been associated with a detrimental effect on survival[24]; and (c) the use of the 1986 staging classification, in which stage III is even more heterogenous than in the present one.[25]

In 2001, the results of a French phase III randomized trial of induction mitomycin, ifosfamide, cisplatin chemotherapy in resectable stages IB, II, and IIIA were reported.[26] Three hundred fifty-five eligible patients were randomized to surgery alone or combined modality therapy consisting of two cycles of chemotherapy followed by surgery. Responding patients (radiographically or pathologically) received two additional cycles of adjuvant chemotherapy. The arms were well balanced for patient characteristics with the exception that less clinical N2-assigned patients were assigned to the surgery-only arm (28% vs. 40%; $p = 0.65$). A nonsignificant excess of postoperative morbidity in the chemotherapy arm was seen (24/167 vs. 22/171). Postoperative mortality was 6.7% in the chemotherapy arm and 4.5% in the surgery arm ($p = 0.38$). Median survival was improved by 11 months (37 vs. 26 months) and at 4 years, there was an 8.6% increase in survival in the chemotherapy arm, but this did not achieve statistical significance. In a subset analysis, the benefit of chemotherapy was confined to patients with N0 and N1 disease with a relative risk of death of 0.68 ($p = 0.027$). After a nonsignificant excess of deaths in the combined modality arm during the treatment period, the effect of induction chemotherapy was favorable on survival. No difference was seen in local recurrence rates. A significant decrease in distant metastases was observed, favoring the chemotherapy arm with a relative risk of 0.54 ($p = 0.01$). Follow-up data on this trial, when minimal follow-up exceeded 60 months, showed that the 3- to 5-year survival differences were stable around 10% ($p = 0.04$ at 3 years and $p = 0.06$ at 5 years).[27] Statistically significant benefits in the N0–1 subgroup were confirmed with 5-year survival rates of 49% compared to 34% in the N2 subgroup ($p = 0.02$)

SURGICAL MORBIDITY AND MORTALITY AFTER INDUCTION THERAPY

The use of preoperative chemotherapy may increase surgical complication rates. Several large retrospective series have addressed this issue. Siegenthaler et al.[28] reported data from 335 patients undergoing lobectomy or greater resection for NSCLC, of whom 76 received induction chemotherapy. The use of preoperative chemotherapy did not significantly affect morbidity or mortality overall, based on clinical stage, postoperative stage, or extent of resection. No significant differences in overall or subset mortality or morbidity, including pneumonia, acute respiratory distress syndrome, reintubation, tracheostomy, wound complication, or length of hospitalization, were seen.

Four hundred and seventy patients treated with induction chemotherapy and surgery from 1993 through 1999 at Memorial Sloan-Kettering Cancer Center were reviewed.[29] Univariate and multivariate methods for logistic regression model were used to identify predictors of adverse events. Overall, a surgical mortality rate of 3.8% was observed, which compared favorably to other primary surgery studies. Total morbidity and major complication rates were 38% and 27%, similar to previous primary surgery studies. The authors concluded that overall morbidity rates were not significantly affected by the use of induction therapy. They did find an operative mortality rate of 24% for patients undergoing right pneumonectomy following induction therapy. This number was higher than previous mortality rates seen in trials wherein patients did not have induction therapy. The authors recommended that right pneumonectomy after induction therapy be performed very selectively and only when no alternative resection is possible.

A third French series reviewed 114 patients who underwent thoracotomy following induction chemotherapy.[30] In this series, there was only one death following pneumonectomy in 55 patients. Overall morbidity rate was 29%, similar to other surgical series. The authors concluded that preoperative chemotherapy did not increase postoperative morbidity and mortality.

The conclusion from these series is that induction chemotherapy is likely to be a feasible and safe procedure, not impacting on complication and hospitalization rates, with the possible exception of right-sided pneumonectomy.

RECENT EVIDENCE

The feasibility and safety of preoperative chemotherapy using third-generation drugs in early stage NSCLC, classified according to the 1997 staging classification, was prospectively established in the Bimodality Lung Oncology Team (BLOT) trial.[31] This phase II trial enrolled two sequential cohorts of patients with clinical stage IB, II, and IIIA patients. Clinical staging was defined by computed tomography (CT) imaging, and all patients were required to undergo mediastinoscopy. Positron emission tomography (PET) imaging was not routinely performed in this study. Patients with mediastinoscopy proven N2 disease or superior sulcus tumors were excluded from this trial. Patients were treated with paclitaxel and carboplatin before and after surgery (number of cycles in cohort I: 2 pre and 3 post; cohort 2: 3 pre and 4 post). For the two cohorts combined, the radiographic response rate was 51%, complete resection rate was 86%, and pathologic complete response rate was 5%. Three- and five-year survival rates were 61% and 45%, respectively, and comparable with historical series.[2,27] There were no significant differences in patient characteristics or outcome between the two cohorts. A detailed analysis of the radiological and pathological responses showed a lack of correlation between both, with 50% of, patients who were found to have equivalent or more extensive disease at surgery, having major chemotherapy responses. Two postoperative deaths occurred. A total of 96% of patients received the planned preoperative chemotherapy versus 45% receiving postoperative chemotherapy.

At least five randomized trials have since explored the issue of neoadjuvant chemotherapy. A common feature of these trials is that they all have been confronted with accrual problems, leading in some studies to their early closure, when the results of randomized trials showing a benefit of adjuvant chemotherapy were published. Table 54.1 details the patient, tumor and treatment characteristics of the two trials whose mature results are available.

The Southwest Oncology Group trial S9900 was a phase III randomized study comparing induction paclitaxel/carboplatin chemotherapy for three cycles followed by surgery to surgery alone in clinical stage IB, II, and IIIA NSCLC (excluding superior sulcus and N2 disease). Mediastinoscopy was performed whenever the mediastinal lymph node size exceeded 1 cm. PET imaging was not required. As such, the study built on the previously mentioned BLOT data and called for 600 patients to detect a 33% increase in median survival or 10% increase in 5-year survival. The rationale for the trial was to assess whether preoperative chemotherapy with paclitaxel and carboplatin for three cycles improves survival compared to surgery alone in previously untreated patients with clinical stage IB, II, and selected IIIA NSCLC and to compare operative mortality and other toxicities in the two study arms. Other specific aims included the evaluation of response rates (confirmed and unconfirmed, complete and partial) and the toxicities associated with the combination of paclitaxel and carboplatin.

This trial prematurely closed in June of 2004, when new evidence demonstrated the superiority of adjuvant chemotherapy over surgery alone, making continued accrual to the control arm of S9900 untenable. At the time of study closure, 336 of the planned 600 eligible patients had been enrolled representing one of the largest preoperative randomized trials in early stage NSCLC. Preoperative chemotherapy was well tolerated with 79% of patients receiving all three cycles. Objective responses were documented in 41% and 7% had progressive disease. Seven postoperative deaths were seen in the chemotherapy arm versus four deaths in the surgery-alone arm. With a median follow-up of 53 months, median and 5-year survival rates were 75 versus 46 months, and 50% versus 43% for the chemotherapy/surgery and surgery-alone arms, respectively. Although the use of chemotherapy was associated with a 19% reduction in the risk of death (hazard ratio [HR] = 0.81; $p = 0.19$), this difference did not achieve statistical significance. Progression-free survival trended in favor of neoadjuvant chemotherapy, with a median of 33 months vs. a median of 21 months for immediate surgery ($p = 0.07$; Fig. 54.1). Results have been presented in abstract form only to date.[32] Patient characteristics were well balanced between the two groups.

In the European Intergroup trial MRC-LU 22 EORTC-08012 NVALT-2, 519 patients with resectable early stage NSCLC were randomized to either surgery alone or three cycles of platinum-based chemotherapy followed by surgery. Choice of chemotherapy regimen was at investigator's choice, as was the intensity of preoperative staging, resulting in only one fourth of the patients being staged with mediastinoscopy and/or PET scan. Their characteristics were equally well balanced between both arms. This trial was also prematurely closed for slowing accrual and its results reported.[33] Of the patients randomized to chemotherapy, 75% completed three cycles of chemotherapy, 49% had radiographic response, and 81% had complete resection. Seventy-nine percent of patients on the control arm had a complete resection. With a median follow-up of 41 months, median and 5-year survival rates were 54 versus 55 months, and 44% versus 45% for the chemotherapy/surgery and surgery-alone arms, respectively. A peculiar finding is the inaccuracy of clinical staging, whereas 18% of the patients who were resected without neoadjuvant chemotherapy actually had a lower pathological than clinical stage, and 41% were likewise "upstaged." Patient's quality of life seemed not to suffer from the use of chemotherapy and the delayed resection.

Besides their low power and accrual, both trials have two further weaknesses in common: the survival in both control arms treated with immediate surgery is better than initially

TABLE 54.1 Summary Characteristics of Two Randomized Trials Comparing Neoadjuvant Chemotherapy to Immediate Surgery

	SWOG 9900[32]		European Intergroup Trial[33]	
	Immediate Surgery	**Neoadjuvant Chemotherapy**	**Immediate Surgery**	**Neoadjuvant Chemotherapy**
No. of patients	167	169	261	258
Accrual interval		1997–2005		1999–2004
Chemotherapy				
Regimen(s)		100% Paclitaxel 225 mg/m^2 Carboplatin AUC 6		Cisplatin-vinorelbin (45%) Cisplatin-gemcitabine (25%) Carboplatin-docetaxel (12%) Mitomycin-vindesin-cisplatin (12%) Mitomycin-ifosfamide-cisplatin (7%)
Frequency		Q 3 w × 3		Q 3–4 w × 3
Compliance (%)		79		75
Patient and tumor characteristics				
Age (median)	64	65	63	62
Female gender (%)	32	36	28	28
Stage I (%)	67	68	59	64
Stage II (%)	32	33	35	28
Stage IIIA (%)	NA	NA	6	8
Squamous cell (%)	42	34	48	51
Response on chemotherapy				
Clinical objective response (%)		41 (CR: 3)		49 (CR: 4)
Parkinson disease during chemotherapy (%)		7*		6
Pathological CR (%)		<10		4
Safety of chemotherapy				
Neutropenia (grade 3–4)		48%		NA
Myalgia/arthralgia (grade 3–4)		6%:7%		NA
Mortality		3%		1%
Surgical results				
Operated on (%)	96	97	93	91
Downstaging	NA	NA	18	31
Complete resection (%)	89	94	79	81
Pneumonectomy rate (%)	25	24	33	28
p stage I (%)	NA	NA	47	59
Pathological complete remission (%)		<10		4
Operative mortality (%)	2.3	4	2	2
Outcome				
Progression-free survival, median (m)	21	33	25	26
Overall survival, m	46	75	55	54
Overall survival, 5 yrs (%)	43	50	45	44
Hazard ratio (95% CI)	0.81 (0.6–1.1)		1.02 (0.8–1.3)	
p value	0.19		0.86	

AUC, area under the curve; CI, confidence interval; CR, complete response; NA, data not available; SWOG, Southwest Oncology Group.

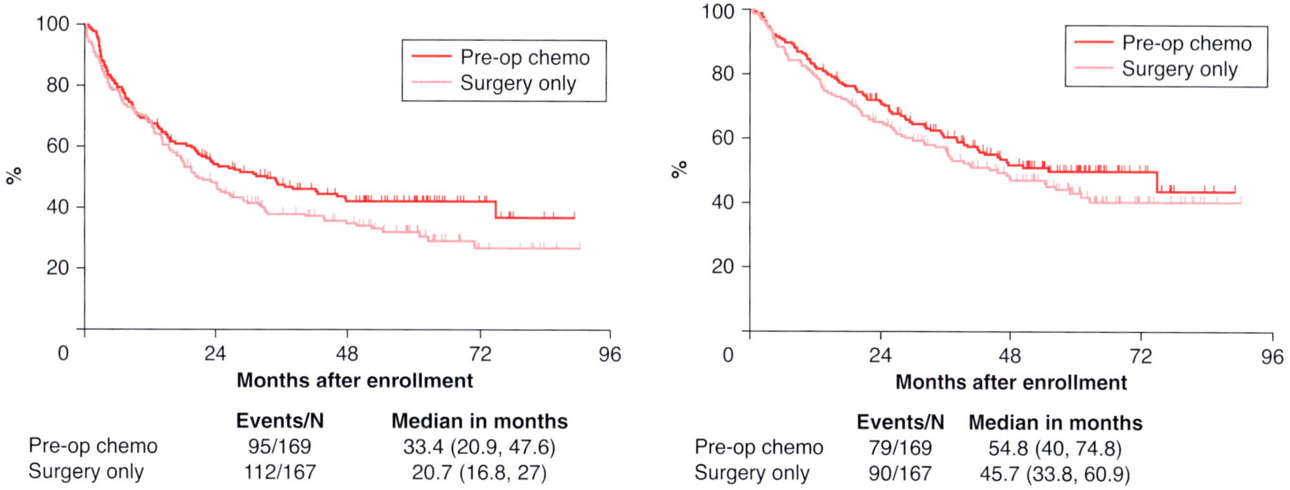

FIGURE 54.1 Surgery alone (*bottom line*) or surgery plus preoperative paclitaxel/carboplatin chemotherapy (*top line*) in early stage NSCLC. **A:** Progression-free survival. **B:** Overall survival. (From Pisters KM, E. Vallieres E, Bunn PA, et al. S9900: Surgery alone or surgery plus induction (ind) paclitaxel/carboplatin [PC] chemotherapy in early stage non-small cell lung cancer [NSCLC]: Follow-up on a phase III trial. *J Clin Oncol* 2007;25[18S]:7520.)

estimated, compounding the underpowering caused by the early closure of these trials, and stage I (clinical or pathological) accounted for more than 50% of the enrollment to both trials. The accumulated evidence in the adjuvant setting has not found a statistically significant survival benefit for postoperative chemotherapy in stage I disease.[9] The implication of this finding in the neoadjuvant setting might imply that a possible benefit for higher stages was diluted.

Mature result of three more trials are awaited. In the European chest trial, prematurely closed in August 2004, 270 patients with stages 1B to IIIA (T3N1) NSCLC were randomized to either surgery alone (141) or three cycles of cisplatin and gemcitabine (129) followed by surgery.[34] Eighty-six percent of the patients in the chemotherapy arm received all three cycles. The response rate was 35% (complete response [CR] = 3%; partial response [PR] = 32%) and 6% of the patients progressed through chemotherapy. A total of 97% of the patients in the surgery group received surgery, whereas 85% went onto surgery in the chemotherapy group. Causes for no surgery included patient refusal, progression, and lost to follow-up. There was a significant difference in progression-free survival favoring the chemotherapy group (HR = 0.71; CI, 0.50 to 0.98; $p = 0.011$). The benefit was greatest for the IIB and IIIA groups. Overall survival favored the chemotherapy group (HR = 0.63; 95% CI, 0.42 to 0.89; $p = 0.005$). The benefit was again greatest for the IIB and IIIA groups.

Three more European randomized trials comparing surgery with or without neoadjuvant chemotherapy have recently been presented as abstracts, with contradictory results. A Spanish trial found no outcome difference at 5 years,[35] a Scandinavian an HR of 0.89,[36] and an Italian an HR of 0.63 at 3 years,[37] both in favor of neoadjuvant chemotherapy.

SYSTEMATIC REVIEWS AND METAANALYSES

Two systematic reviews from published summary data of randomized chemotherapy trials in early stage NSCLC have been published.[8,37] These metaanalyses should be interpreted with caution, as they were not based on individual patient data (IPD), but on data extracted from abstracts and manuscripts. An IPD metaanalysis is considered vastly superior to one based on abstracted or pooled data, as it allows verification of randomization and patient data, updates the data, and is highly reliable. Drawbacks to the IPD metaanalysis are its increased cost and length of time required. Furthermore, most literature-based systematic reviews appear to be good proxy's of their ensuing IPD metaanalysis. The metaanalysis by Berghmans et al.[9] reported six randomized trials, including 590 patients, published between 1990 and 2003. The overall fixed-effect HR on survival was 0.69 (95% CI, 0.57 to 0.84), in favor of the addition of neoadjuvant chemotherapy to surgery. A less extreme result was seen in the publication by Burdett et al.[38] Data from seven randomized trials (published between 1990 and 2005), including 988 patients were combined in a systematic review and metaanalysis. Preoperative chemotherapy improved survival with an HR of 0.82 (95% CI, 0.69 to 0.97), equivalent to an absolute benefit of 6% at 5 years. They, furthermore, found an incremental benefit by stage (stage IA = +4%; stage IB = 6%; stage II to III = +7%) but did not observe any interaction between the kind of platinum-containing regimen or the kind of adjuvant treatment (chemotherapy or radiotherapy). The exploratory nature of these subgroup analyses warrants an IPD approach, which is ongoing. Gilligan et al.[33] added the mature results of the European Intergroup trial to the previous metaanalysis and observed a shift of the HR to

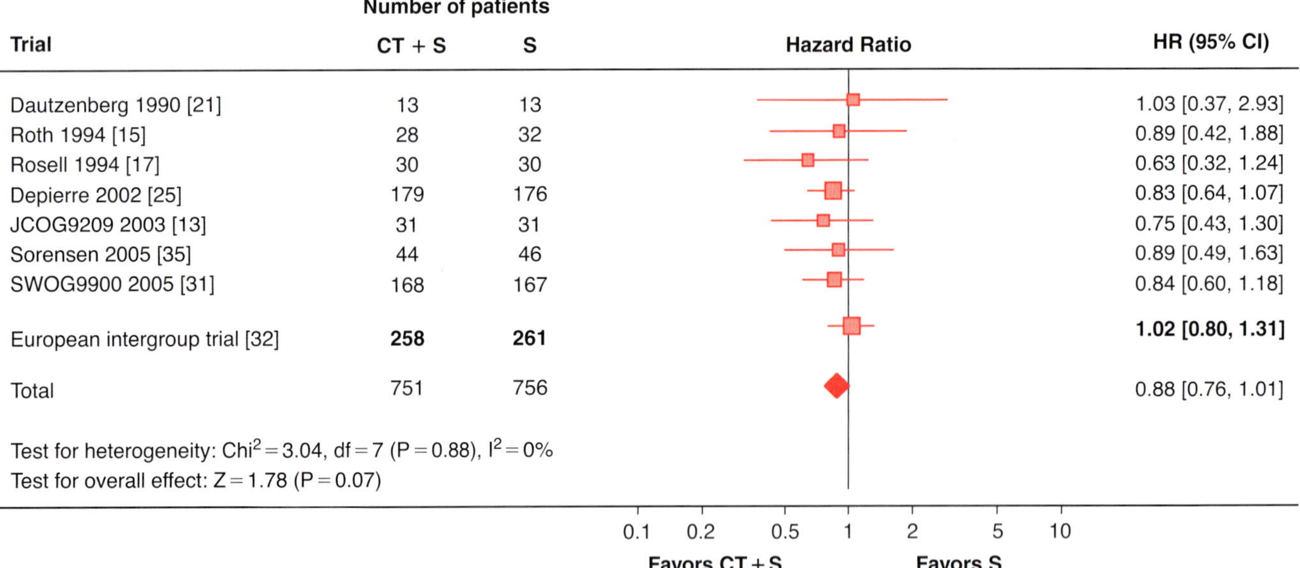

FIGURE 54.2 Hazard ratio plot for overall survival. Each individual trial is represented by a *square*, the center of which denotes the hazard ratio for that trial. The extremities of the *horizontal bars* denote the 99% CIs and the *inner bars* mark the 95% CIs. The size of the *square* is directly proportional to the amount of information in the trial. The *filled diamond* at the bottom of the plot gives an overall hazard ratio for the combined results of all trials. The center of the *diamond* denotes the hazard ratio for all trials and the extremities the 95% CIs. Trials are ordered chronologically by the age of the trial, with the oldest listed first. *95% CI*, 95% confidence intervals; *CT*, chemotherapy; *df*, degree of freedom; *HR*, hazard ratio; *S*, surgery. (Adapted from Gilligan D, Nicolson M, Smith I, et al. Preoperative chemotherapy in patients with resectable non-small cell lung cancer: results of the MRC LU22/NVALT 2/EORTC 08012 multicentre randomised trial and update of systematic review. *Lancet* 2007;369:1929–1937.)

0.87 (95% CI, 0.76 to 1.01), with loss of the significance of the improvement in outcome (Fig. 54.2, Table 54.2).

CONCLUSION

Do the observed results of neoadjuvant therapy in NSCLC match with the expectations?

The available outcome data trend in favor of neoadjuvant therapy, but the majority of individual trials did not find a statistically significant benefit. This can be a result of the underpowering of the individual studies or contamination of the outcome by the use of adjuvant therapy in some of them. The data of both systematic reviews, on the other hand, show an overall effect that is significantly in favor of neoadjuvant treatment. The size of the observed effect is comparable to the one described in a similar metaanalysis of adjuvant chemotherapy[9] (Table 54.2). One must keep in mind that both patient populations are different, as only selected patients are offered adjuvant chemotherapy, after pathological staging. The lack of clinicopathological correlation observed in the BLOT and European Intergroup trial illustrates the heterogeneity of patients enrolled on neoadjuvant trials.

TABLE 54.2 Metaanalysis of Outcome of Perioperative Platinum-Based Chemotherapy in NSCLC

Hazard Ratios (95% Confidence Intervals)	Adjuvant Chemotherapy	Neoadjuvant Chemotherapy
Early evidence[8]	0.86 (0.80–0.92)	0.66 (0.48–0.93)
Recent evidence	0.89 (0.82–0.96)[9]	0.88 (0.76–1.01)[33]

As the standard of care in resected NSCLC has since shifted to the selective use of adjuvant chemotherapy, the focus for further research might be redirected toward comparing neoadjuvant and adjuvant chemotherapy. It is, however, dubious whether this issue will ever be adequately addressed, as large number of patients will have to be included in such an undertaking. A randomized trial addressing this issue was recently closed secondary to poor patient accrual. The introduction of novel biological adjuvant approaches and the renewed interest for postoperative radiotherapy will confound and interfere with the results of any strategy aiming at the sole use of chemotherapy.

Neoadjuvant chemotherapy results in a clinical downstaging in approximately 40% to 60% of the patients and a pathological complete response rate in 5% to 10%. As expected, compliance is better with neoadjuvant chemotherapy compared to adjuvant treatment: more than 70% of the patients are able to complete all three cycles of neoadjuvant chemotherapy, whereas the full planned adjuvant chemotherapy could only be administrated in 45% to 60% of patients. Compliance with adjuvant chemotherapy may improve in the future now that it has proven effective in prolonging survival.

The feasibility and safety of preoperative chemotherapy has been established in several trials. Surgical concerns regarding neoadjuvant chemotherapy can be eased, as it does not result in an increased length of hospital stay or a significantly increased rate of perioperative complications, when compared to immediate surgery. One possible exception to this is increased mortality seen in patients undergoing right pneumonectomy following induction therapy. Induction chemotherapy also does not negatively influence patient's quality of life.

With the present status of knowledge, neoadjuvant regimens should be platinum-based, and at least three cycles of chemotherapy should be administered. As in advanced NSCLC, a two-drug combination of platinum and a third-generation drug seems preferable. The role of nonplatinum-containing regimens has not been explored up to now and remains an area of future research.

In conclusion, the current data favor the use of adjuvant (postoperative) chemotherapy in patients with resectable NSCLC. The neoadjuvant trials lend further support to the role of systemic therapy in operable lung cancer patients, but the data for its use is not as strong as it is in adjuvant therapy. At this time, preoperative therapy should not be offered outside of a clinical trial.

REFERENCES

1. Jemal A, Siegel R, Ward E, et al. Cancer statistics, 2007. *CA Cancer J Clin* 2007;57;43–66.
2. Goldstraw P, Crowley JJ, Chansky K, et al. and the International Association for the Study of Lung Cancer International Staging Committee and Participating Institutions. The IASLC Lung Cancer Staging Project: proposals for the revision of the TNM stage groupings in the forthcoming (seventh) edition of the TNM Classification of malignant tumours. *J Thorac Oncol* 2007;2:705–714.
3. Martini N, Flehinger BJ, Zaman MB, et al. Prospective study of 445 lung carcinomas with mediastinal lymph node metastases. *J Thorac Cardiovasc Surg* 1980;80(3):390–399.
4. Feld R, Rubinstein LV, Weisenberger TH. Sites of recurrence in resected stage I non-small-cell lung cancer: a guide for future studies. *J Clin Oncol* 1984;2(12):1352–1358.
5. Pairolero PC, Williams DE, Bergstralh EJ, et al. Postsurgical stage I bronchogenic carcinoma: morbid implications of recurrent disease. *Ann Thorac Surg* 1984;38(4):331–338.
6. Thomas P, Rubinstein L. Cancer recurrence after resection: T1 N0 non-small cell lung cancer. Lung Cancer Study Group. *Ann Thorac Surg* 1990;49(2):242–246.
7. Hotta K, Matsuo K, Ueoka H, et al. Role of adjuvant chemotherapy in patients with resected non-small-cell lung cancer: reappraisal with a meta-analysis of randomized controlled trials. *J Clin Oncol* 2004;22:3860–3867.
8. Berghmans T, Paesmans M, Meert AP, et al. Survival improvement in resectable non-small cell lung cancer with (neo)adjuvant chemotherapy: results of a meta-analysis of the literature. *Lung Cancer* 2005;49(1):13–23.
9. Pignon JP, Tribodet H, Scagliotti GV, et al. Lung adjuvant cisplatin evaluation (LACE): A pooled analysis of five randomized clinical trials including 4,584 patients. *J Clin Oncol* 2006;24(Suppl 18):7008(Abst).
10. Pisters KM, Evans KW, Azzolli CG, et al. Cancer Care Ontario and American Society of Clinical Oncology Adjuvant Chemotherapy and Adjuvant Radiation Therapy for Stages I-IIIA Resectable Non–Small-Cell Lung Cancer Guideline. *J Clin Oncol* 2007;25(34):5506–18.
11. Frei E III. Clinical cancer research: an embattled species. *Cancer* 1982;50:1979–1992.
12. Alam N, Shepherd FA, Winton T, et al. Compliance with post-operative adjuvant chemotherapy in non-small cell lung cancer. An analysis of National Cancer Institute of Canada and intergroup trial JBR.10 and a review of the literature. *Lung Cancer* 2005;47(3):385–394.
13. Advanced Bladder Cancer (ABC) Meta-analysis Collaboration. Neoadjuvant chemotherapy in invasive bladder cancer: update of a systematic review and meta-analysis of individual patient data advanced bladder cancer (ABC) meta-analysis collaboration. *Eur Urol* 2006;48:202–205; discussion 205–206.
14. Malthaner R, Fenlon D. Preoperative chemotherapy for resectable thoracic esophageal cancer. *Cochrane Database Syst Rev* 2003;4:CD001556.
15. Roth JA, Fosella F, Komaki R, et al. A randomized trial comparing perioperative chemotherapy and surgery with surgery alone in resectable stage IIIA non-small cell lung cancer. *J Natl Cancer Inst* 1994;86:673–680.
16. Roth JA, Atkinson EN, Fossella F, et al. Long-term follow-up of patients enrolled in a randomized trial comparing perioperative chemotherapy and surgery with surgery alone in resectable stage IIIA non-small-cell lung cancer. *Lung Cancer* 1998;21:1–6.
17. Rosell R, Gómez-Codina J, Camps C, et al. A randomized trial comparing preoperative chemotherapy plus surgery with surgery alone in patients with non-small-cell lung cancer. *N Engl J Med* 1994;330:153–158.
18. Rosell R, Gómez-Codina J, Camps C, et al. Preresectional chemotherapy in stage IIIA non-small-cell lung cancer: a 7-year assessement of a randomized controlled trial. *Lung Cancer* 1999;26:7–14.
19. Pass HI, Pogrebniak HW, Steinberg SM, et al. Randomized trial of neoadjuvant therapy for lung cancer: interim analysis. *Ann Thorac Surg* 1992;53:992–998.
20. Nagai K, Tsuchiya R, Mori T, et al. A randomized trial comparing induction chemotherapy followed by surgery with surgery alone for patients with stage IIIA N2 non-small cell lung cancer (JCOG 9209). *J Thorac Cardiovasc Surg* 2003;125:254–260.
21. Dautzenberg B, Benichou J, Allard P, et al. Failure of the perioperative PCV neoadjuvant polychemotherapy in resectable bronchogenic non-small cell carcinoma. Results from a randomized phase II trial. *Cancer* 1990;65:2435–2441.
22. Waller D, Peake MD, Stephens RJ, et al. Chemotherapy for patients with non-small cell lung cancer: the surgical setting of the Big Lung Trial. *Eur J Cardiothorac Surg* 2004;26:173–182.
23. Nagai K, Tsuchiya R, Mori T, et al. A randomised trial comparing induction chemotherapy followed by surgery with surgery alone for patients with stage IIIa N2 non-small cell lung cancer. *J Thorac Cardiovasc Surg* 2003;125:254–260.
24. NSCLC Collaborative Group. Chemotherapy in non-small cell lung cancer: a meta-analysis using updated data on individual patients from 52 randomised clinical trials. *Brit Med J* 1995;311:899–909.
25. Mountain CF. Revisions in the International System for Staging Lung Cancer. *Chest* 1997;111:1710–1717.
26. Depierre A, Milleron B, Moro-Sibilot D, et al. Preoperative chemotherapy followed by surgery compared with primary surgery in resectable stage I (except T1N0), II, and IIIA non-small-cell lung cancer. *J Clin Oncol* 2002:20:247–253.
27. Depierre A, Westeel V, Milleron B, et al. 5-year results of the French randomized study comparing preoperative chemotherapy followed by surgery and primary surgery in resectable stage I (except T1N0), II, and IIIA non-small cell lung cancer. *Lung Cancer* 2003;41(suppl 2):S62.

28. Siegenthaler MP, Pisters KM, Merriman KW, et al. Preoperative chemotherapy for lung cancer does not increase surgical morbidity. *Ann Thorac Surg* 2001:71:1105–1111; discussion 1111–1112.
29. Martin J, Ginsberg RJ, Abolhoda A, et al. Morbidity and mortality after neoadjuvant therapy for lung cancer: the risks of right pneumonectomy. *Ann Thorac Surg* 2001;72:1149–1154.
30. Perrot E, Guibert B, Mulsant P, et al. Preoperative chemotherapy does not increase complications after nonsmall cell lung cancer resection. *Ann Thorac Surg* 2005;80:423–427.
31. Pisters KM, Ginsberg RJ, Giroux DJ, et al. Induction chemotherapy before surgery for early-stage lung cancer: a novel approach. Bimodality Lung Oncology Team. *J Thorac Cardiovasc Surg* 2000;119:429–439.
32. Pisters KM, Vallieres E, Bunn PA, et al. S9900: Surgery alone or surgery plus induction (ind) paclitaxel/carboplatin (PC) chemotherapy in early stage non-small cell lung cancer (NSCLC): follow-up on a phase III trial. *J Clin Oncol* 2007;25(18S):7520.
33. Gilligan D, Nicolson M, Smith I, et al. Preoperative chemotherapy in patients with resectable non-small cell lung cancer: results of the MRC LU22/NVALT 2/EORTC 08012 multicentre randomised trial and update of systematic review. *Lancet* 2007;369:1929–1937.
34. Scagliotti GV on behalf of Ch.E.S.T. Investigators. Preliminary results of Ch.E.S.T.: A phase III study of surgery alone or surgery plus preoperative gemcitabine-cisplatin in clinical early stages non-small cell lung cancer (NSCLC). *J Clin Oncol* 2006;24S:LBA7023.
35. Felip E, Massutti B, Alonso G, et al. Surgery Alone, or Surgery Followed by Adjuvant (adj) Paclitaxel/Carboplatin (PC) Chemotherapy (CT) or Preoperative (preop) PC Followed by Surgery, in Early Stage Non-Small Cell Lung Cancer: Results of the Multicenter, Randomized, Phase III NATCH Trial. *J Clin Oncol* 2009;27(15S): abstract 7500 (382s).
36. Sorensen JB, Riska H, Ravn J, et al. Scandinavian phase III trial of neoadjuvant chemotherapy in NSCLC stages IB-IIIA/T3. *Proc Am Soc Clin Oncol* 2006;24S:7146.
37. Scagliotti GV, Pastorino U, Vansteenkiste J, et al. A phase III randomized study of surgery alone plus preoperative gemcitabinecisplatin in early stage NSCLC: follow up data of Ch.E.S.T. *J Clin Oncol* 2008;26(15S): abstract 7508 (399s).
38. Burdett S, Stewart LA, Rydzewska L, et al. A systematic review and meta-analysis of the literature: chemotherapy and surgery verus surgery alone in non-small cell lung cancer. *J Thorac Oncol* 2006;1:611–621.

CHAPTER 55

Brian E. Lally
Harvey I. Pass
Kathy S. Albain

Preoperative Chemotherapy/Radiation Therapy for Early Stage and Locally Advanced Non–Small Cell Lung Carcinoma

Surgery remains the cornerstone of management for patients with non–small cell lung cancer (NSCLC). Unfortunately, at the time of initial diagnosis, approximately half of all patients have localized disease and less than a third are candidates for surgical exploration. Despite complete resection, 5-year survival rates are disappointing, ranging from 73% for T1N0 disease to 24% for patients with T1–3N2 based on the proposed International Association of the Study of Lung Cancer staging recommendations (Table 55.1).[1] The ability of a patient to undergo a surgical resection of their lung cancer is associated with an improved survival, but this is the result of many factors. Despite complete resection, many patients develop local and distant recurrence and die as a result of uncontrolled lung cancer.

Efforts at improving survival for patients with resectable NSCLC, as well as those with potentially resectable, more advanced local disease, examined the use of chemotherapy or radiation in the postoperative (adjuvant) or preoperative (neoadjuvant or induction) settings. Postoperative therapy is discussed in Chapter 53. This chapter will focus on the use of chemotherapy and/or radiation in the preoperative setting. In approaching this topic, the reader must understand that this is one of the most controversial topics in the management of potentially resectable NSCLC. Some of the more contentious inquiries include: (a) whether it is justified to consider induction therapy in patients who, at presentation, can have a definitive (R0) resection of all disease; (b) whether a surgical resection should ever be performed after combined modality treatment in stage IIIA/B disease; (c) what (if any) pretreatment patient characteristics help determine the optimal method of local control; (d) what prescription for the timing of the local and systemic therapy best maximizes treatment effect with a minimum of complications; and (e) what specific cytotoxic chemotherapy combinations should be used. For patients with locally advanced disease, the current standard of care is concurrent chemotherapy and radiotherapy (chemoRT), and the long-term survival results in reported randomized phase III trials are between 8% and 15%. The limitations of this approach include persistent local disease, which is reported to be as high as 83% after treatment with chemotherapy and full-dose RT, and very high distant failure rates, primarily in the brain. Moreover, persistence of local disease after completion of treatment portends an especially poor prognosis, not only as a result of the local effects of the uncontrolled tumor but also hypothetically as a potential source of metastatic seeding. Those advocating a surgical removal of residual disease hypothesize that this method for local control could render a proportion of these patients disease free.

The pros and cons of how to orchestrate chemotherapy, RT, and surgery for locally advanced lung cancer revolve around the optimization of dose intensity, toxicity, and efficacy. Patients have better tolerance of adjunctive therapies prior to thoracotomy, resulting in improved delivery of planned doses of chemotherapy and RT. The ability to actually monitor the sensitivity of the tumor to the therapy at a time when micrometastatic disease may be lowest, while also cytoreducing the local tumor burden (possibly leading to improved resectability and a potential for less pneumonectomies) are appealing hypotheses for an induction strategy. Arguments against a neoadjuvant approach revolve around the impact of the therapy on the presurgical, nutritional, and immunological status of the patient, possibly leading to a delay of definitive surgery, early tumor progression, technically challenging surgery (especially if RT is incorporated in the induction program) and poor postoperative healing.

The most significant argument against the use of preoperative chemotherapy may be that the benefit associated with chemotherapy use in NSCLC has been rather extensively demonstrated in the postoperative setting.[2–4] This benefit appears to increase with more advanced disease. The investigations into adjuvant chemotherapy were based on a metaanalysis suggesting a potential benefit.[5] With more trials of preoperative chemotherapy having been completed over time, similar analyses have recently been performed, with results suggesting a possible survival benefit.[6–8] Given the heterogeneous populations that represent the patients with lung cancer clinically, some patients will benefit more from adjuvant therapy, whereas other patients may benefit more from induction therapy.

TABLE 55.1 Survival Rates for Early Stage NSCLC Based on Clinical and Pathologic Staging

		Overall Survival			
		Clinical		Pathologic	
Stage	TNM Classification	MST	5-Year	MST	5-Year
IA	T1a/bN0M0	60	50%	119	73%
IB	T2aN0M0	43	43%	81	58%
IIA	T2bN0M0 or T1/T2aN1M0	34	36%	49	46%
IIB	T2bN1M0 or T3/T4N0M0	18	25%	31	36%
IIIA	T1/2N2M0 or T3/T4N1/2M0	14	19%	22	24%
IIIB	T4N2M0 or TanyN3M0	10	7%	13	9%

Overall survival, expressed as median survival time (MST) and 5-year survival by clinical and pathologic stage using the proposed International Association of the Study of Lung Cancer recommendations.[1]

INDUCTION THERAPY FOR LOCALLY ADVANCED LUNG CANCER (STAGES IIIA AND IIIB)

First-Generation Induction Trials

Radiation Therapy as the Sole Induction Modality The initial trials of preoperative RT from the 1950s to the early 1970s were conducted without the benefit of modern staging technologies[9–12] and before effective cytotoxic chemotherapies for NSCLC existed. Pathologic complete responses (pCRs) were reported in up to 27% of patients, but operative morbidity rates rose with RT doses greater than 40 Gy. A large randomized study published in 1975, however, found no difference in overall survival (OS),[12] and a subsequent study from the Lung Cancer Study Group (LCSG 881)[13] for patients with pathologic stage IIIA (N2) disease given 44 Gy before surgery had disappointing results, with only one pCr and a median survival of 12 months. The last randomized trial that used RT alone as induction treatment was Cancer and Leukemia Group B (CALGB 9134).[14] This trial closed early because of poor accrual, and long-term results were not encouraging. Thus, based on more recent studies, RT is no longer recommended as the sole induction modality prior to surgery.

Early Phase II Studies of Induction Chemotherapy with or without Radiotherapy In the 1980s, a series of phase II induction trials of first-generation cisplatin-based chemotherapy were performed with or without sequential RT prior to surgery.[15–19] These were small trials with staging heterogeneity, and broad variability in both the amount of low- versus high-volume disease and in the percentage of biopsy-proven N2 disease. Three trials employed the CAP regimen (cyclophosphamide, doxorubicin, and low-dose cisplatin), whereas two studies used cisplatin plus etoposide-based preoperative chemotherapy. The study designs and outcomes of these trials are outlined in Table 55.2.[15–19] Response rates (RR) from the induction therapy were 39% to 82%, resection rates (percent of original number accrued) were 14% to 88%, and the survivals were highly variable. Staging and volume of tumor differences within these trials preclude conclusions about efficacy or comparisons across trials; however, these pivotal studies demonstrated the general safety of surgery after induction therapy and in some instances, provided intriguing survival data.

Therefore, larger, second-generation trials were designed that enrolled more restricted stage subsets, and required, in most instances, pathologic documentation of nodal disease. The following sections review the major categories of second-generation studies and long-term survival from selected trials.

Second-Generation Phase II Studies of Induction Chemotherapy as the Sole Induction Modality

Five phase II second-generation studies of induction therapy tested preoperative chemotherapy. These trials are described in Table 55.3.[13,20–25] Although all studies required pathologic documentation of N2 disease, tumors with a wide range of disease bulk were accrued. The LCSG 881 trial was a two-arm phase II randomized trial, in which one arm was assigned preoperative chemotherapy and the other received preoperative RT.[13] The results were reported for the entire group of patients and not separately for each treatment arm. Four of the studies utilized preoperative vinblastine and cisplatin with or without mitomycin C (MVP, VP [etoposide + cisplatinum]), and the fifth trial tested continuous infusion cisplatin and 5-fluorouracil (5-FU) with leucovorin rescue. The RT was variably given (intraoperative, postoperative, or not at all), and information on why RT was either given or withheld was not provided in detail for some of the studies. Thus, lack of concordance on the disease bulk and RT utilization variables makes comparison of results among the studies difficult.

Resection rates (based on the entire denominator) were 51% to 68%. Postoperative mortality ranged from 0% to 18%. The causes of death were predominantly pulmonary or

TABLE 55.2 Early Phase II Studies of Induction Chemotherapy with or without Radiotherapy

Investigators	Volume	Treatment Program	Patients	Biopsy-Proven N2/N3 Disease (%)	Response Rate (%)	Resection Rate (% Original N)	Median	Long-Term Survival
Dana-Farber I[15]	T3 or low-volume stage III (N2)	CAP × 2 → RT → surgery → RT → CAP × 3	41	68	43	88	32	31%, 3 yrs
LCSG 831[16]	T3 or low-volume stage III (N2)	CAP × 3 with split RT → surgery	39	51	51	33	11	8%, 2 yrs
University of Chicago[17]	High-volume T3 or T4N2 or N3	VdEP × 2 → surgery → RT	21	100	70	14	8	34%, 1 yr
Dana-Farber II[18]	T1–3N2 (mixed low and high volume)	CAP × 4 + RT → surgery → RT	54	94	39	56	18	22%, 5 yrs
Perugia[19]	T1–3N2 (clinically high tumor volume)	EP × 2– 3 → surgery → variable RT	42	0	82	72	24	24%, 3 yrs

Median survival in months.

A, doxorubicin; C, cyclophosphamide; E, etoposide; LCSG, Lung Cancer Study Group; P, cisplatin; RT, radiotherapy; Vd, vindesine.

TABLE 55.3 Second-Generation Phase II Studies of Induction Chemotherapy as the Sole Induction Modality

Investigators	N	Disease Burden	Treatment Schedule	Response Rate (%)*	Complete Resection Rates (%)*	Treatment-Related Mortality (%)†	Operative Mortality (%)*	pCR‡ Rates (%)	pCR† in Mediastinal Nodes (%)*	Median Survival (mo)
LCSG 881[13]	26	High volume	MVP × 2 → surgery or 44 Gy → surgery	65	68	14.5	18	4	Not stated	12
Memorial[24]	136	Mixed volume	MVP × 2 – 3 → surgery → radiotherapy for persistent N2	78	65	5	5	14	32	19
Toronto[20,21]	65	Mixed volume	MVP × 2 → surgery → MVP × 2 for responders	68	53	12	5	5	Not stated	19
Dana-Farber[22]	34	Mixed volume	PFL (continuous infusion) × 3 → surgery → radiotherapy	65	62	0	0	15	44	18
CALGB 8935[23,25]	74	High volume	VP × 2 → surgery → VP × 2 → radiotherapy	64§	62	2.7	3.2	0	12	15

*Percent of all enrolled patient.

†Pathological complete response.

‡Percent of patients subjected to surgery.

§Includes stable disease.

CALGB, Cancer and Leukemia Group B; F, 5-fluorouracil; L, leucovorin; LCSG, Lung Cancer Study Group; M, mitomycin C; P, cisplatin; pCR, pathologic complete response; V, vinblastine.

cardiopulmonary. Pulmonary complications attributable to mitomycin C in the Memorial Sloan-Kettering study, including the three lethal ones, all occurred after the cumulative dose of 24 mg/m^2. The studies that did not use mitomycin C had lower perioperative death rates. pCR rates ranged from 0% to 15%. Postoperative RT did not provide additional benefit in the Memorial Sloan-Kettering study ($p = 0.24$); however, the selection of patients receiving RT was based on unfavorable response to neoadjuvant chemotherapy, not by randomized assignment. In the Dana-Farber study, all mediastinal downstaging to N0 or N1 occurred in patients with low-volume disease. The CALGB study noted that persistent N2 disease following induction chemotherapy is unfavorable. Although there was no correlation between radiographic response to the induction regimen and pathological downstaging at the time of surgery, patients with a pCR in N2 nodes were felt to potentially benefit from surgical resection. Survival outcomes were highly variable, with median survival ranging from 12 to 21 months, because of differences in the study eligibility and design, as reviewed previously. In the Dana-Farber study and CALGB trial 8935, 15% and 41% of first relapses occurred in the brain, respectively.

Second-Generation Phase II Studies of Induction Chemoradiotherapy before Surgery

Trial Designs and Results The other major category of second-generation induction studies utilized concurrent chemoRT induction therapy in which the RT began on day 1 of the chemotherapy. These phase II trials are described in Table 55.4.[26–30] The RT varied in schedule (continuous to split course) and in total dose (30 to 59 Gy, single fractionation). All induction chemotherapy was cisplatin-based, with the addition of either etoposide, 5-FU, vinblastine, or some combination of these drugs. The treatment prescribed after surgical resection was not uniform among these five studies. There was no therapy after surgery in the Rush-Presbyterian and LCSG 852 trials; two cycles of additional chemotherapy plus 14 Gy of RT were given in the Southwest Oncology Group (SWOG) 8805 study (if residual disease in chest or mediastinum); and one cycle of chemotherapy plus 30 Gy of RT was used in the CALGB trial (all patients). The Tufts investigators initially gave etoposide plus cisplatin postoperatively, but later in the trial allowed use of the carboplatin plus paclitaxel regimen.

TABLE 55.4 Second-Generation Phase II Studies of Induction Chemotherapy before Surgery

Investigators	N	Disease Burden	IIIA (N2) (%)	T3N0–1/T4 or N3 (%)	Treatment Schema	Response Rate (%)*	Complete Resection Rate (%)*	Treatment-Related Mortality (%)	Operative Mortality (%)†	pCR (%)	pCR in N2 (%)	Median Survival (mo)
SWOG 8805[26]	126	High volume	60	0/40	EP × 2 + 45 Gy → surgery → EP × 2 + 14 Gy if persistent N2/incomplete resection	59	71	10	8	15	38	15
LCSG 852[30]	85	High volume	85	0/13	PF × 2 + 30 Gy → surgery	56	52	8	7	9	NS	13
Rush Presbyterian[27]	85	Mixed volume	73	21/6	PF or PEF + 40 Gy (split course) → surgery	92*	71	3.5	5	20	26	22
CALGB I[29]	41	Mixed volume	80	20/0	PVF × 2 + 30 Gy → surgery → PVF × 1 + 30 Gy	64‡	61	15	10	17	NS	16
Tufts[28]	42	High volume	66	2/45	EP × 2 + 59.4 Gy → surgery → PE × 4 or carbo T × 4	69*	79	0	0	21	59	30

*Percent of original number.

†Percent of patients subjected to surgery.

‡Includes stable disease.

CALGB, Cancer and Leukemia Group B; Carbo, carboplatin; E, etoposide; F, 5-fluorouracil; Gy, gray; LCSG, Lung Cancer Study Group; NS, not stated; P, cisplatin; SWOG, Southwest Oncology Group; T, paclitaxel; V, vinblastine.

Eligibility criteria for the five second-generation chemoRT induction trials were more varied than for the studies of induction chemotherapy alone. Biopsy documentation of N2 disease or T4 status was required only in the SWOG, LCSG, and CALGB trials, and the SWOG trial was unique in this regard because pathologic proof of N2, T3, or N3 disease was mandated. A broad range of stage subsets were included across trials, so that stage IIIA (N2) accounted for 47% to 87% of patients per trial. Two studies included T3N0 or T3N1 (21% and 20% in the Rush-Presbyterian and CALGB studies, respectively), whereas all patients with stage IIIA disease in the SWOG 8805, LCSG 852, and Tufts trials had N2 nodal involvement. The stage IIIB subsets of T4 and/or N3 were allowed in all trials except the CALGB study and accounted for 6% to 53% of patients per trial. The SWOG 8805 and Tufts trials were designed for bulky disease, whereas the others allowed a mix of minimal and bulky presentations.

Response or "response plus stable" (one study) rates were 56% to 92%, and 52% to 76% of the total number of patients accrued to each study had a complete resection at thoracotomy. Twenty-six of the thirty patients with stable disease as their "best" response to induction chemoRT underwent a complete resection of tumor in the SWOG 8805 trial.[26] The pCR rates were 16%, 21%, and 27% in the LCSG, SWOG, and Rush-Presbyterian trials, respectively.[26,27,30] An additional 37% had rare microscopic foci of tumor cells as the sole residual disease in the SWOG trial. It was demonstrated that postinduction assessment of nonresponse by computed tomography (CT) scan is often misleading because 46% of the 26 patients with resectable stable disease in the SWOG study had pCR or only rare microscopic foci.[26]

The operative mortalities were predominantly pulmonary related, as observed in the induction chemotherapy trials. The cause of death often resembled the adult respiratory distress syndrome (ARDS) to be considered in more detail in the morbidity and mortality section of this chapter. The Tufts trial was unique in that postoperative ARDS was not observed, despite the high total dose of induction RT.[28] A rigid protocol to minimize fluids, transfusions, and the fraction of inspired oxygen (Fi02) was employed in this study. The Tufts trial also utilized a higher dose of preoperative RT, a prescription similar to those used for standard concurrent chemoRT without surgery. Thus, most of the allowable dose of RT was given upfront without a break. In the other trials, truncation of the RT occurred at around 45 to 50 Gy to plan for the surgery. Thus, patients with residual disease or unresectable disease could only receive full-dose RT via an interruption of several to many weeks, depending on time to recovery from surgery.

The median survival for the two studies that excluded T3N0–1 tumors and required pathologic staging were 15 and 13 months.[26,30] In contrast, the other three trials included this better prognostic subset and did not require biopsy proof of the T and N substages. For these studies, the median survivals were 22, 16, and 20 months.[27–29] Patterns of first recurrence in the SWOG 8805 trial were 11% (locoregional only) and 61% (distant alone).[26] There was no difference in the sites of relapse between those patients with negative mediastinal nodes at the time of operation (but originally positive) versus those who had persistent involvement of the mediastinal nodes. A significant number of the distant first relapses (and in many cases, the only relapse or the sole cause of mortality) occurred in the brain.[26] The LCSG investigators noted that in patients who had complete resection, 28% of first recurrence sites were in the brain, in contrast to only 7% in patients who did not undergo surgery. In patients who experienced a recurrence in the brain, in almost one third that was the sole site of recurrence. Similar findings were noted by the SWOG 8805 study. The CALGB protocol called for prophylactic cranial irradiation (PCI) in patients with nonsquamous histologies who completed all the treatment, but about one third of eligible patients did not receive it. None of 13 patients who received PCI developed brain metastases, compared to 1 out of 7 who were eligible but did not receive it. The Tufts investigators also reported a very high rate of isolated brain metastases, all of which occurred within the first 32 months of follow-up.[28]

The Stage IIIB Subgroup in Second-Generation (and Subsequent) Studies of Chemoradiotherapy Induction Trials From a subset of these second-generation chemoRT trials, data are available regarding the role of induction therapy followed by surgery in selected stage IIIB subsets. The LCSG 852 trial and the Rush-Presbyterian study included 13% "minimal T4" and 6% "selected T4" lesions (clinically staged), respectively.[27,30] Separate survival data for this subset were not provided. Of note, two groups of investigators had reported equivalence in outcome of clinical stage IIIA and IIIB disease in combined modality trials with no surgery.[31,32] However, these authors suggested that the clinical T4N0 subset may have a better outcome than the other subsets and perhaps should be removed from the IIIB category, just as the T3N0 subset had been reassigned to stage IIB instead of its former designation of IIIA.[33] Based on this observation in chemoRT-alone trials, the SWOG 8805 study was designed prospectively to include a sufficient sample of the stage IIIB subgroup to allow independent assessment of outcome.

The SWOG 8805 trial was unique among the other chemoRT trials in that it included stage IIIB disease. Pathologic documentation of T4 or N3 disease was required and outcome was analyzed separately for this subset.[26,34] The Tufts investigators also reported outcome separately for the IIIB group, but the staging requirements were radiographic rather than pathologic.[28] The resection rates in these two studies for stage IIIA(N2) were 76% and 76%, and 63% and 50% for stage IIIB, respectively.

The median, 2- and 3-year survivals were identical for the IIIA (N2) versus the IIIB group in the SWOG 8805 study (27%, 24%).[26] This phenomenon was not seen in the Tufts trial where the 3-year survivals were 73% and 32% for the clinical IIIA (N2) and IIIB subsets, respectively, possibly because of the aforementioned staging requirements leading to inaccuracies. Of note, in the SWOG 8805 study, the T4N0–1 subset had an outcome identical to the T1N2 substage and achieved a 2-year survival of 64%. This substage variable was the only independent predictor of favorable outcome from the time of registration to the study in a multivariate analysis.[26] Exploratory survival analyses were conducted within the N3 subset of the SWOG trial, of which 27 patients were accrued. The 2-year survival for the contralateral nodal N3 subgroup was zero, whereas it was 35% for the supraclavicular N3 subset. However, the resection rate in this latter group was only 39%. An update of SWOG 8805 provided 6-year survival statistics: IIIA (N2), 20%; T4N0–1, 49%; and N2 or N3, 18%.[35]

A follow-up trial to SWOG 8805 for pathologic stage IIIB disease was conducted by the SWOG (SWOG 9019). Identical induction chemoRT was utilized as in SWOG 8805, but no surgery was given; instead, the RT was continued without a break to 61 Gy and two additional cycles of EP were given.[36] The OS in this study was identical to that observed for the stage IIIB group in SWOG 8805. This suggested that in an identically staged patient population, chemoRT with definitive-dose RT may achieve the same benefit as surgical resection after induction chemoRT (and lower RT total dose). However, in the SWOG 9019 trial (chemoRT alone), the 2-year survival was only 33% for the T4N0–1 subset, compared to 64% in 2-year and 49% in 6-year survival in the surgical study, SWOG 8805.[35,36] This historical comparison of these two consecutive trials in pathologically staged IIIB disease suggests *that surgery for stage IIIB tumors might be beneficial only in the select substage of T4N0–1*.

Based on these results, the Spanish Lung Cancer Group performed a phase II trial of induction chemotherapy with a cisplatin-based triplet follow by surgery for stage IIIA N2 and selected stage IIIB (T4N0–1).[37] A total of 136 patients were entered onto the study; the clinical RR in 129 assessable patients was 56%. Completely resected stage IIIA and IIIB patients (68.9% of those eligible for surgery) had an impressive median survival time of 48.5 months, with a 5-year survival rate of 41.4%. For completely resected stage IIIB patients, median survival time was 60.6 months, and 5-year survival rate was 53.2%. In the absence of mediastinal lymph nodes, median survival time for these patients was not reached, and 5-year survival rate was 57%. Still, a prospective randomized study is needed to validate these findings.

Additional studies have commented on the role of induction therapy for stage IIIB disease. Grunenwald et al.[38] prospectively studied 40 patients with stage IIIB disease, of whom 30 had T4 disease and 18, N3. Five patients had T4N0 tumors and one had T4N1. All patients underwent pretreatment surgical staging. Induction treatment consisted of 5-FU, cisplatin, and vinblastine for two cycles. A total of 42 Gy of external RT was given split in two 21 Gy courses, 1.5 Gy bid, with 10 days of rest between the courses. Patients who responded to the induction regimen underwent thoracotomy. A clinical response was obtained in 73% of patients and in 60% resection was performed. The resection was complete in all but one patient who underwent thoracotomy. Four patients (10%) had complete pathological response and 30% had complete mediastinal clearance. There were five treatment-related deaths and seven additional patients suffered serious morbidity. Median survival was 15 months and 5-year OS was 19%. Thirty percent of overall patient number had locoregional relapse and 50% had distant relapse. Pathological mediastinal nodal downstaging was the only significant favorable prognostic factor in a multivariate analysis (5-year survival 42% for postinduction N0/N1 vs. 12 % for postinduction N2/N3 for resected patients). All long-term survivors had persistent viable tumor cells in the primary tumor but six of seven were postinduction N0–1.

Pitz et al.[39] treated patients with stage IIIB NSCLC with neoadjuvant gemcitabine and cisplatin without RT, followed by surgery in responding patients. There was an RR of 66%, resection rate of 44%, and perioperative mortality of 2.4%. Median survival for all patients was 15.1 months and 3-year survival was 15%. The investigators found no difference in outcome between T4N0 and N2/N3 subsets. However, only patients with a response after induction chemotherapy were considered for surgical resection.

These trials highlight that the T4N0/N1 substage as a group does particularly well with trimodality therapy.

Second-Generation Induction Trials: Long-Term Survival and Predictors of Outcome

Mature Survival Data Long-term survival data were reported in several of the trials of induction chemotherapy and induction chemoRT (Table 55.5). Several of the trials suggest that a plateau emerges on the tails of the survival curves, as 5- to 7-year survival of 17% to 34% were reported. Despite differences in methodology and patient populations, the long-term outcomes were encouraging and provided support for subsequent phase III trials.

Factors that Predict Favorable Outcome The seven phase II trials of induction chemotherapy or chemoRT depicted in Table 55.5 also analyzed predictors of long-term survival. Favorable outcome predictors included postinduction pCR, complete resection, T3N0 or T3N1 disease, T4N0 or N1 disease, and pathologic clearance of initial N2 or N3 involvement (nodal downstaging). The significance of these predictive factors varied across trials, but all factors were not uniformly assessed in each study. Nevertheless, in most trials, a factor related to the *efficacy* of the induction therapy was important. It was suggested that the inclusion of RT in the induction removes the possible importance of pCR as a predictor observed in chemotherapy-only induction programs. However, the Memorial Sloan-Kettering Cancer Center trial of MVP alone did not report statistical significance to pCR.[24,40] Response to induction therapy was not an important predictive factor in some trials, most likely because of the mandate in those studies to resect disease even if "stable" was the best response.[26] This observation underscores the inability of standard CT scanning to detect those patients with major postinduction responses.

The SWOG 8805 trial analysis showed that nodal downstaging was an independent favorable prognostic impact of intermediate (2- to 3-year) survival is of interest, and was the

TABLE 55.5 Long-Term Survival in Selected Second-Generation Phase II Induction Trials in NSCLC

Investigators	Disease Burden	Included T3N0 or N1?	Biopsy Proof of N2 Status Required?	Selected Stage IIIB Included?	Long-Term Survival
Memorial[24]	Mixed volume	No	Yes	No	28%, 3 yrs; 17%, 5 yrs
Toronto[20,21]	Mixed volume	No	Yes	No	26%, 3 yrs
SWOG 8805[26]	High volume	No	Yes	Yes	27%, 3 yrs; 20%, 6 yrs, stage IIIA (N2); 24%, 3 yrs; 22%, 6 yrs, stage IIIB
CALGB II[22]	High volume	Yes	No	No	28%, 3 yrs; 22%, 7(+) yrs
CALGB 8935[25]	High volume	No	Yes	No	23%, 3 yrs
Rush-Presbyterian[27]	Mixed volume	Yes	No	Yes	40%, 3 yrs
Tuft[28]	High volume	Yes	No	Yes	37%, 5 yrs

CALGB, Cancer and Leukemia Group B; NSCLC, non–small cell lung cancer; SWOG, Southwest Oncology Group.

only significant factor in a multivariate model that included complete resection rate, pCR, and multiple other factors.[26] This variable was also the most important univariate discriminant of 6-year survival, although complete resection emerged as a long-term survival predictor as well.[35] The survivals 3 and 6 years after thoracotomy for patients with uninvolved nodes at surgery were 41% and 33%, respectively, versus only 11% and 11% if there was persistent mediastinal disease. Unfortunately, the prognostic impact of nodal downstaging was not assessed in multivariate models for any other study with second-generation therapy.

Implications of the nodal downstaging observation are that lack of residual disease in the mediastinum may be a surrogate marker for eradication of distant chemotherapy-sensitive micrometastases, implying that these patients may be the optimal candidates for additional postoperative chemotherapy. Conversely, persistent N2 or N3 disease may predict the presence of distant resistant disease. Thus, one wonders whether surgery is necessary for those cases with nodal downstaging, or are these patients the best candidates for maximal local control with surgery? If postinduction mediastinal status is clearly of prognostic value, then there would be a critical role for a second mediastinal assessment after induction, even though, in some cases, this would be technically difficult. How to assess the mediastinum after induction therapy remains an enigma, and the role of positron emission tomography (PET) scanning in this regard as well as the use of new bronchoscopic techniques are discussed in Chapters 27 and 28.

Third-Generation Phase II Studies of Induction Chemotherapy plus Concurrent Hyperfractionated Radiotherapy Four phase II induction trials used platinum-based chemotherapy and hyperfractionated RT either with a planned break or with radiation intensification by delivering it in an accelerated fashion. These trials are summarized in Table 55.6. The Massachusetts General Hospital (MGH) study enrolled 42 patients with histologically confirmed N2 disease to a preoperative regimen consisting of split course, hyperfractionated RT concurrent with chemotherapy.[41] The volume of mediastinal disease among patients was mixed in this study with 33% of patients having mediastinal lymph nodes smaller than 1 cm on a pretreatment CT, and 19% having lymph nodes that were greater than 2 cm. Twelve gray of postoperative RT was given for either complete response or microscopic disease only, and 18 Gy for residual disease or positive margins, concurrent with chemotherapy.

The West German Cancer Center (WGCC) study used three cycles of induction chemotherapy, followed by continuous hyperfractionated accelerated RT concurrent with chemotherapy.[42–44] Patients eligible for enrollment had to have either surgically unresectable disease, or more than one ipsilateral mediastinal lymph node involved, or positive contralateral mediastinal lymph nodes. This study mandated repeat mediastinoscopy at the completion of induction treatment. Only those patients whose mediastinal tumor burden was downstaged (defined as a negative mediastinal biopsy or only one positive lymph node) were offered surgical resection. Thus, not all patients with stable disease were mandated to proceed to thoracotomy, and the patients who did not undergo resection of residual disease were given additional RT to a total of 60 Gy. These investigators reported a high incidence of isolated brain relapse and introduced PCI in the third year of the study. The PCI dose was 30 Gy in 2 Gy fractions over 3 weeks, starting 1 day after the last chemotherapy administration.

The German Lung Cancer Cooperative Group (GLCCG) trial accrued 54 patients to a regimen that consisted of two cycles of induction chemotherapy, followed by hyperfractionated accelerated RT concurrent with chemotherapy, followed by resection.[45] Eligibility criteria included either biopsy-proven N2 disease or clinical T4 or N3 disease. Patients who had a tumor

TABLE 55.6 Third-Generation Phase II Trials of Concurrent Induction Chemotherapy with Hyperfractionation in NSCLC

Investigators	Stage Subset(s)/ No. Patients	Disease Burden	Chemotherapy	Radiotherapy	Resection Rates (%)*	Treatment-Related Mortality (%)*	Operative Mortality (%)†	Survival	Predictors of Favorable Outcome
MGH[41]	Biopsy-proven stage IIIA (N2) N = 42	Mixed volume	PVF × 2 concurrent with RT → surgery → VF × 1 concurrent with RT	42 Gy split (1.5 bid × 7 → 10-day rest → 1.5 bid × 7); postoperative 12 − 18 Gy 1.5 bid)	93	7	5	37%, 5 yrs	Downstaging to N0 (79%, 5-yr survival) • Complete resection
WGCC[42]	Mediastinoscopy required: n = 6, advanced T3 N0/1 n = 46, 2 or more N2 nodes n = 42, IIIB (T4) or contralateral (N3) N = 94	High volume	EP × 3 → reduced dose EP × 1 with RT → surgery	45 Gy (1.5 Gy bid over 3 wks); PCI later in trial	53* (60 IIIA, 45 IIIB)	6	7	28%, 4 yrs (31% IIIA, 26% IIIB)	4-yr survival from registration • Complete resection‡ 46% vs. 11%, $p = 0.0001$ • N2/3 → N0 38% vs. 15%, $p = 0.11$ • LDH ≤ 240 or not 37% vs. 0%, $p = 0.003$ • PCI decrease in first brain metastases, $p = 0.005$
German GLCCG[45]	N2, n = 25 All biopsy-proven T4 or N3, n = 29; N = 54	High Volume	ICE × 2 → PVd × 1 + RT →surgery	45 Gy (1.5 Gy bid over 3 wk)	63 (R0)	9	8	30%, 3 yrs	> 90% histological regression (3-yr survival 48% vs. 9%, $p = 0.007$) complete resection ($p = 0.009$)
Cleveland Clinic[46]	Mediastinoscopy required: 105 patients with stage pIIIA (n = 78) or pIIIB (n = 27)	High Volume	CT × 1 + RT → surgery → CT × 1 + RT	30 Gy (1.5 Gy bid) for both pre-op and post-op	79	2	1	32%, 5 yrs	Nodal status, advancing age, squamous histologic type, and higher pT predicted poorer survival.

*Percent of original number of patients.

†Percent of patients subjected to surgery.

‡Resection not mandated if persistent T4 or N2/N3 disease.

bid, twice a day; C, carboplatin; CR, complete response; E, etoposide; F, 5-fluorouracil; GLCCG, German Lung Cancer Cooperative Group; Gy, gray; I, ifosfamide; MGH, Massachusetts General Hospital; NSCLC, non–small cell lung cancer; P, cisplatin; PCI, prophylactic cranial irradiation; RT, radiotherapy; T, Paclitaxel; V, vinblastine; Vd, vindesine; WGCC, West German Cancer Center.

response or stable disease were eligible for surgery. Patients who did not have complete resection received additional 16 Gy of RT.

The Cleveland Clinic trial enrolled 105 patients with pathologically proven IIIA (n = 78) or IIIB (n = 27) NSCLC to a study of accelerated multimodality therapy, consisting of hyperfractionated RT with concurrent chemotherapy (paclitaxel and cisplatin) followed by resection.[46] All patients then underwent postoperative chemoradiation.

The results of these trials are presented in Table 55.6. Treatment-related mortality was 7%, 6%, 9%, and 2% and postoperative mortality 5%, 7%, 8%, and 1% (of patients who underwent thoracotomy) in the MGH, WGCC, GLCCG, Cleveland Clinic trials, respectively. The main perioperative complication seen in both WGCC and GLCCG trials was bronchial stump insufficiency, most often after right-sided resections. After both groups started reinforcing bronchial stumps with tissue later in each trial, the incidence of this problem dropped to zero.

A complete resection with negative margins was accomplished in 81% of all patients in the MGH trial. The median survival was 25 months and OS was 66%, 37%, and 37% at 2, 3, and 5 years, respectively. Of interest, the preoperative size of mediastinal nodes (≤1 vs. >1 cm) did not influence the survival, but the sample size was very small. Four patients had pCR, three of whom showed only a partial response on postinduction CT. Five-year survival was 79% if the nodes were downstaged to N0.

Sixty-four percent of patients entered on the WGCC study were eligible for surgery after the induction regimen, and 53% had complete resection with negative margins. A total of 24 (26%) had complete pathological response. Among 29 patients with radiographically stable disease after the induction treatment, about a third was completely resected and 3 had pathological complete response. Median survival was 20 and 18 months and 3-year survival were 36% and 31% for stages IIIA and IIIB, respectively (no statistical difference). No differences were observed for the different TNM categories and T (T1/T2 vs. T3/T4) and N (N0/N1 vs. N2/N3) subgroups. The complete resection rates were 60% for IIIA and 45% for IIIB. Of eight patients with T4N0–1, six were able to have a complete resection. PCI markedly reduced the incidence of brain relapse, but the difference in median survival (26 months with PCI and 20 months without) did not reach statistical significance, possibly because the follow-up period for the first group was shorter.

A complete resection with negative margins was achieved in 63% of patients enrolled on the GLCCG trial. Over a half of these exhibited a major histological response, defined as necrosis or fibrosis of more than 90% of tumor cells. Seven (13%) had pathological complete response. Preoperative assessment of response (complete/partial) did not correlate with the degree of tumor regression. Approximately 25% of patients who relapsed had only a local recurrence, whereas 35% had a distant-only relapse. The median survival for the whole group was 20 months, with 2- and 3-year survival of 40% and 30%, respectively. Median survivals for stages IIIA and IIIB (25 vs. 17 months) showed no statistical significance, as did 2- and 3-year survivals (52% and 35% vs. 30% and 26%).

In the Cleveland Clinic trial, all patients completed induction therapy in 12 days (100%). Ninety-eight patients (93%) were operative candidates. Among the seven inoperable cases, four patients had locoregional progression, two had new distant metastatic disease, and one was considered medically unfit for surgery. Eighty-three patients (79%) underwent curative resection. There were no clinically determined complete responses, probably because of the brief interval between induction therapy and reassessment. A total of 62% of patients had a measurable partial response, defined as a more than 50% reduction in the sum of the crossed diameters of measurable tumor. The 5-year survival for all patients from commencement of therapy was 30%; for the 81 patients who completed multimodality, the 5-year survival was 39%.

The MGH study and the Cleveland Clinic study had higher resection rates and OS than the two German studies but also enrolled patients with less advanced disease. The two German trials had similar patient populations, treatment, and outcome. The authors of those studies credit the accelerated radiation schedule for the fact that many of their patients with advanced, high-volume disease were able to undergo resection. However, second-generation trials with concurrent chemoRT in patients with high-volume tumor burdens (described previously, e.g., SWOG 8805) also achieved high resection rates.

COMPLETED RANDOMIZED TRIALS OF SURGERY ALONE VERSUS INDUCTION THERAPY FOLLOWED BY SURGERY IN MIXED-STAGE, RESECTABLE DISEASE

As mentioned briefly earlier in this chapter, four small randomized studies and three large phase III trial of induction chemotherapy for NSCLC were conducted for patients with a surgery-alone arm as the control. These trials are summarized in Table 55.7.[6,47–55] Although surgery alone (with or without some RT) was deemed acceptable for the control arms of these trials, the eligibility criteria regarding degree of homogeneity in the T and N subsets, volume of disease and mandate for pathologic staging varied among the studies. Patients with more advanced disease were enrolled in the National Cancer Institute (NCI) and Japan Clinical Oncology Group (JCOG) trials.[53–54] The NCI trial was the most homogeneous in the stage subsets accrued. However, neither the MD Anderson nor the Spanish studies required microscopic N2 disease and mediastinal node biopsy was not mandated if the CT scan was negative.[47,48,51,52] In fact, in the surgical control arm of the MD Anderson trial, 40% of cases were actually stage IIIB or IV at time of operation. Thus, the treatment groups of the small MD Anderson and Spanish studies had heterogeneous stage subset distributions. The same stage mix issues exist in the large French Thoracic Cooperative Group (FTCG) trial reported by Depierre et al.,[49]

TABLE 55.7 Reported Phase III Trials of Surgery with or without Induction Therapy Resectable NSCLC

Investigators	Stage Subset(s)	Disease Bulk	Chemotherapy	Radiotherapy	N	2–3 Year Survival No Cht	ChT	*p*
National Cancer Institute[53]	IIIA (N2) by biopsy	High volume	EP 2 cycles preoperative EP 4 cycles postoperative	Postoperative in no-ChT arm only (54–60 Gy)	28	21%	46%	0.12
JCOG 9209[54]	IIIA (N2) by biopsy	High volume	VdP preoperative	None	62	26%	23%	NS
MD Anderson[48,51]	IIIA (N2) not required; node biopsy not required; some IIIB	Low volume	CEP preoperative and postoperative	Postoperative only if residual disease	60	15%	56%	<0.05
Spain[47,52]	IIIA (N2) not required; node biopsy not required	Low volume	PIM preoperative	Postoperative for both arms	60	0%	30%	<0.05
French Thoracic Cooperative Group[49]	Clinical T2N0, II, IIIA	Low volume	MIP × 2 preoperative; also postoperative, if objective response	Postoperative to 60 Gy, if pT3 or pN2 for both arms	355	41%	52%	0.15
Scandinavian Trial[55]	IB, II, IIIA/T3	Low volume	AT × 3 then surgery	None	44	24%	36%	NS (5-yr survival)
SWOG 9900[50]	Clinical T2N0, T1–2N1, T3N0–1	Low volume	AT × 3 then surgery	None	354	57%	62%	NS
MRC LU22 / NVALT 2/ EORTC 08012[6]	Clinical T2N0, II, IIIA	Low volume	Platinum-based doublet × 3 then surgery	None	519	45%	44%	NS (5-yr survival)

A, Carboplatin; C, cyclophosphamide; ChT, chemotherapy; E, etoposide; EORTC, European Organisation for Research and Treatment of Cancer; I, ifosfamide; JCOG, Japan Clinical Oncology Group; M, mitomycin; MRC, Medical Research Council; NS, not significant; NSCLC, non–small cell lung cancer; NVALT, Dutch Society of Pulmonologist; P, cisplatin; SWOG, Southwest Oncology Group; T, paclitaxel; V, vinblastine; Vd, vindesine.

with some imbalance of stage subsets between the two arms ($p = 0.07$). Furthermore, clinical staging alone was accepted and documentation of N2 status was not required in the FTCG study. The largest of the induction trials was actually a successful collaboration between Medical Research Council (MRC), Dutch Society of Pulmonologist (NVALT), and European Organisation for Research and Treatment of Cancer (EORTC) known as the LU22 trial.[6] In the LU22 trial, 519 patients were randomized between immediate surgery or an induction regimen. The majority of these patients were early stage disease (stage I = 61%, stage II = 31%, and stage III = 7%). N2 status was not documented; for the patients treated with surgery alone, 41% were upstaged by pathological finding. In contrast, both the Scandinavian trial[55] and SWOG 9900[50] required documentation that the mediastinum was not involved prior to enrollment.

The induction chemotherapy regimens for these trials were platinum-based and were also variably given after surgery, depending on the study design. Some of the trials utilized RT if N2 involvement was demonstrated. For the trials that utilized RT, it was employed either postoperatively in the nonchemotherapy arm only of one trial or postoperatively for all patients. Although the use of RT is different in a few trials, several other trials did investigate a question of "pure" induction chemotherapy followed by surgery versus surgery alone.

Most of these trials closed before the target accrual goal was met. The MD Anderson and Spanish studies were stopped early because of large survival differences by data monitoring committees. The others closed because of slow accrual or the inappropriateness of a surgery-alone control arm based on postoperative chemotherapy data. The NCI investigators found no statistical difference between the two arms, but the *p* value decreased with longer follow-up to 0.11 in favor of the chemotherapy arm.[53] There were differences in recurrence patterns by arm in the NCI trial in that less distant but more local disease was observed in the induction chemotherapy group. In the JCOG trial,[54] both arms had survival comparable to the surgery-alone arm of the NCI study. However, both of these trials were small in number with very heterogeneous populations.

Two small randomized trials were stopped early because of strongly positive results in favor of the induction chemotherapy arms. With additional follow-up of the MD Anderson trial cohort (median follow-up, 81 months), 32% of patients were alive in the induction chemotherapy group versus 16% in the surgery-alone arm ($p = 0.06$).[48,51] The *p* value became significant if only deaths caused by cancer were considered. The update of the Spanish trial has revealed that no patients survived in the surgery group, whereas 16% were long-term survivors in the induction chemotherapy arm.[47,52]

These MD Anderson and Spanish trials generated extensive discussion and debate. The consensus was that these results were provocative but not definitive. There were many aspects of the design and outcome of the studies that clearly called for larger, confirmatory trials in more homogeneously staged subsets subsequently conducted or are ongoing. The major concern was the marked substage heterogeneity within these two trials. It is not clear if early stopping rules for these very small trials accounted for the strong potential influence of even slight substage or molecular prognostic factor imbalances between the two arms. Minor shifts of these factors between arms would have a major impact on the survival differences because of the small sample sizes. Furthermore, the surgical control arms fared poorly, possibly a result of substage imbalances. There were a large number of patients with unexpected stage IIIB/IV disease at time of surgery in the control arm of the MD Anderson trial. The Spanish trial control arm had 37% patients with N0 or N1 disease, but this arm contained more tumors with k-ras mutations and aneuploid DNA, both potential adverse prognostic factors. Small differences in unstratified prognostic factors such as k-ras could potentially affect the results.

These results prompted the initiation of a larger trial, the FTCG trial that enrolled patients with stage IB to IIIA disease.[49] All patients were judged to have resectable disease before any induction treatment. Staging was clinical (radiographic), and presurgery mediastinoscopy was not required. An excess of patients with N2 disease was accrued to the chemotherapy arm (12%), but the difference was not statistically significant ($p = 0.065$). Complete resection rate was 92% in the induction chemotherapy arm, and 86% in surgery-alone arm. Postoperative RT to 60 Gy was delivered for pathologic T3 or N2 status, or if the resection was incomplete. A total of 41% of patients in surgery alone arm and 23% in induction chemotherapy arm received postoperative RT. The 1-, 2-, 3-, and 4-year survivals were 77%, 71%, 59%, and 44%, respectively, in the induction chemotherapy arm and 73%, 52%, 41%, and 35% in the surgery-alone arm. The difference did not reach statistical significance ($p = 0.15$). Stage-adjusted relative risk of death was 0.80 in the chemotherapy arm ($p = 0.089$). In a subset analysis, there was a benefit to induction for patients with N0–1 disease (RR = 0.68; $p = 0.027$), but not for patients with N2 (RR = 1.04; $p = 0.85$). There was excess risk of deaths within the first 5 months after the surgery in the induction chemotherapy arm (RR = 1.32; $p = 0.37$), but the curves crossed at 5 months and the RR in the induction chemotherapy arm decreased to 0.74 after these first 5 months. There was a nonsignificant excess of mortality (10% vs. 5%) in the induction chemotherapy arm, consisting of pneumonia, emphysema, fistula, and pulmonary embolism. Induction chemotherapy reduced the risk of distant relapse (RR = 0.54; $p = 0.01$). Locoregional relapses were not significantly different between the treatment arms.

An additional three trials have been reported involving induction chemotherapy. All three are very similar in that they asked a primary induction chemotherapy question in patients with low burden of disease, of which two trials documented lack of N2 involvement. Also, all three failed to meet their accrual goal. Both the Scandinavian trial and SWOG 9900 utilize an induction paradigm of three cycles of carboplatin/paclitaxel. LU22 allowed three cycles of a platinum-based doublet. Collectively, these trials showed that chemotherapy was tolerable and resulted in a radiographic response in 70% to 80%. Still the resection rates were very good, ranging in the 70%'s for the Scandinavian trial and LU22 to the 90%'s for SWOG 9900. Induction chemotherapy consistently resulted in a slightly higher but nonsignificant resection rate. Lastly, induction chemotherapy in these three trials resulted in improved trends for both OS and disease-free survival.

Recently, several of the phase III trials have been analyzed as part of a metaanalysis.[7,8] The results suggest that, overall, some patients do benefit from induction chemotherapy. In light of the positive evidence in support of adjuvant chemotherapy, it is likely that some future clinical trials will ask the question, which is better, adjuvant or induction chemotherapy? Still, a more thoughtful question might be, which patients benefit from induction chemotherapy and which patients benefit from adjuvant chemotherapy?

RADIOTHERAPY AS A COMPONENT OF THE INDUCTION REGIMEN

There is debate regarding the role of RT in multimodality induction regimens. Proponents hypothesize that RT increases the rate of downstaging and resectability and plays a role in sterilizing microscopic mediastinal disease that cannot be completely removed during the surgery. Still, nodal downstaging is likely an important predictor of long-term survival. In a retrospective analysis from the University of Toronto, Uy et al.[56] showed that chemoradiation before pulmonary resection in carefully selected patients with surgically resectable stage IIIA (N2) NSCLC can lead to improved overall and disease-free survival.

Whether RT is needed as part of an induction regimen for patients with microscopic N2 disease remains an unanswered question. The only randomized trial to date that addressed the necessity of RT in an induction regimen for high-volume IIIA disease was that of Fleck et al.,[57] conducted in Brazil and reported only in abstract format. Ninety-six patients with either clinically bulky or biopsy-proven stage IIIA(N2) and T4 IIIB disease were randomized between chemoRT followed by surgery versus chemotherapy alone followed by surgery. Two programs commonly employed at the time were compared, cisplatin, and 5-FU plus RT versus the MVP regimen. At the 1994 abstract presentation, survival was significantly better in the chemoRT arm. More neutropenia and neurologic toxicity were observed in the MVP arm, whereas there was a higher rate of mucositis in the chemoRT group. Updated results were provided during a 1997 meeting presentation but are not published at this writing. The 5-year survival was 31% in the chemoRT arm but was only 15% in the MVP arm ($p = 0.05$). However, this study enrolled mixed volume disease with some, but not all, cases pathologically staged.

It is generally agreed that to definitively determine the worth of induction RT, additional studies are needed in a homogeneously staged population, probably with minimally bulky or microscopically involved mediastinal nodes, who receive identical induction chemotherapy on both arms. Moreover, controversy exists regarding the optimal timing of RT with respect to chemotherapy and surgery, as well as the dose of RT. An RT dose prescription of 40 to 45 Gy is generally used in induction regimens because it is efficacious but does not result in excessive perioperative and postoperative morbidity. Somewhat higher rates of postoperative complications were reported in trials that used higher doses of RT, especially in association with pneumonectomy.[58–60] One exception is the Tufts study that did not report any deaths after a neoadjuvant regimen that included 59.4 Gy of RT.[28] The optimal sequence of RT relative to surgery is also an unresolved issue. Patients with large, locally advanced tumors will likely have improved respectability when preoperative RT synergizes with chemotherapy, and there is a greater chance of receiving the entire planned RT dose when it is given preoperatively. Nevertheless, postoperative RT can be given to a higher dose, which may be important in patients for whom a complete resection is not possible. With chemoRT induction protocols, eligibility for surgical resection must be determined before fibrosis sets in, usually 6 to 8 weeks after the completion of the induction with "noncurative" RT doses. This break in therapy, especially for the patients with unresectable disease, may be associated with a detriment in survival.[61,62] This reassessment "break" time must be put in context when considering that many patients receiving postresection RT do not complete the planned treatment.[25]

The schedule of RT in trimodality programs also remains undefined. The hyperfractionated accelerated schedule intensifies the effect of RT, which may be important in locally advanced tumors. This schedule has been well tolerated and has not been associated with excessive rate of perioperative complications in three prospective phase II trials.[41,42,63] A recently completed phase III German trial built upon the phase II results randomized patients with stage IIIA disease after three cycles of cisplatin/etoposide to either hyperfractionated RT (45 Gy = 2 × 1.5 Gy/day) with concurrent carboplatin/vindesine, then surgery and, if no or R1/2 resection, additional preoperative hyperfractionated radiotherapy (hfRT; 24 Gy = 2 × 1.5 Gy/day) or surgery and postoperative RT (54 Gy or, if no or R1/2 resection, 68.4 Gy = 1.8 Gy/day).[64,65] Because both of the arms included RT, this trial does not test whether RT is necessary for improved survival. Regardless of therapy, the 3-year rate for OS and progression-free survival were 25% and 18% (p = ns). Treatment-related mortality was approximately 5% for both treatment arms. As mentioned, the timing and fraction of the RT as well as the chemotherapy drugs differed between the arms of this trial. A critique of this study includes its low resection rates, suboptimal chemotherapy, and a design that did not contain a control arm with any RT.[66] When published, this trial will also provide important information on the impact of RT on the pathologic RR, nodal downstaging, morbidity, and resectability.

PHASE III TRIALS OF CHEMORADIOTHERAPY WITH OR WITHOUT SURGERY

Several prospective, randomized trials involving trimodality therapy have been conducted in stage III NSCLC, and all but one closed early without reaching the planned accrual target. They are summarized in Table 55.8. A small NCI Canada study[67] that investigated the efficacy of induction chemotherapy followed by surgery versus RT alone was halted after a CALGB randomized trial showed the superiority of combined chemoRT over RT alone as definitive treatment of stage III NSCLC.[68] A CALGB trial[14] compared induction chemotherapy versus induction RT but closed early because of poor accrual. There was no difference in survival between the arms (median 24 months in RT induction vs. 18 months in chemotherapy induction; $p = 0.46$).

The Radiation Therapy Oncology Group (RTOG) 8901 study attempted to define the role of surgery by comparing whether definitive chemoRT alone to induction chemoRT followed by surgery. The original accrual goal was 244 patients, but the trial closed early because of poor accrual of only 73 patients, revealing no differences in median survival (19.4 vs. 17.4 months) or in 1-, 2-, or 4-year survival (70% vs. 66%, 48% vs. 34%, 22% vs. 22%, respectively).[69] Although patient accrual to this trial made its results inconclusive, several observations are notable. In this trial, histologic confirmation of N2 disease in the surgical and nonsurgical arms eliminated the usual biases from clinical staging. In this setting, local control and survival were essentially equal between the surgical and RT arms. The 3- and 5-year survival rates of nonsurgical therapy were comparable to published surgical trials of N2 disease.

The North American Intergroup trial 0139, chaired by RTOG, is the largest phase III trial to date that addressed the

TABLE 55.8 Reported Phase III Induction Trials of Chemotherapy for NSCLC

Investigators	Stage Subset	Question	Study Design	N	Outcome Comment
National Cancer Institute Canada[67]	Biopsy-proven stage IIIA (N2)	Postinduction surgery vs. RT?	PV → surgery vs. RT	31	Closed early because of radiotherapy-alone arm; survival curves superimposed at 2 yrs
RTOG 8901[69]	Biopsy-proven stage IIIA (N2)	Postinduction surgery vs. RT?	MVP or VP ↓ Surgery vs. RT ↓ MVP or VP	73	Closed early because of slow accrual; $p = 0.62$ for overall survival; 4-yr: 22% for surgery vs. 22% for RT
CALGB[14]	Biopsy-proven stage IIIA (N2)	Induction RT of chemo?	RT → surgery → RT vs. PV → surgery → PV → RT	57	Closed early because of slow accrual; median survival 24 mo (RT/S/RT) and 18 mo (CT/S/CT) ($p = 0.4$)
INT 0139[70]	Biopsy-proven stage IIIA (N2)	Postinduction surgery vs. chemoRT alone?	PE/RT → surgery → PE vs. PE/RT → RT → PE	392	CT/RT/S — CT/RT — *p*
					5-yr OS — 27.2% — 20.3% — 0.24
					Med OS — 23.6 mo — 22.2 mo
					3-yr PFS — 22.4% — 11.1% — 0.017
					Med PFS — 12.8 mo — 10.5 mo

CALGB, Cancer and Leukemia Group B; INT, North American Intergroup; M, mitomycin C; E, etoposide; NSCLC, non–small cell lung cancer; OS, overall survival; P, cisplatin; PFS, progression-free survival; RT, radiotherapy; RTOG, Radiation Therapy Oncology Group; S, surgery; V, vinblastine.

potential value of surgery in stage IIIA (N2) NSCLC.[71,72] The entry criteria for this study included T1-3 primary tumor, pathologically confirmed N2 disease, feasible resection from a surgical standpoint, and medical ability to undergo resection. Patients were stratified by performance status, T1 to T2 versus T3, and whether contralateral mediastinal nodes required biopsy or not (mandated if nodes visible on CT scan), and randomized between the trimodality versus the bimodality arm. The induction regimen was identical in both arms: 45 Gy of external RT given in once-daily fraction, concurrent with day 1 of induction chemotherapy, which was cisplatin, 50 mg/m^2 on days 1, 8, 29, 36 and etoposide, 50 mg/m^2 days 1 to 5 and 29 to 33. Patients were reevaluated by a CT scan 2 to 4 weeks after completion of the induction regimen in the surgical arm, and in the RT arm, a week before completion of treatment. Those patients with no progression proceeded with their assigned treatment. In the surgical arm, the treatment consisted of resection of all known disease and mediastinal nodal sampling. In the RT arm, the RT continued to 61 Gy without a break. In both arms, consolidation chemotherapy (two cycles of cisplatin and etoposide) was given to all patients. The study initially was designed to accrue 510 patients, but the Data Safety and Monitoring Board recommended closure at 429 patients because of sufficient events based on the slower than anticipated accrual. The second interim results were presented at the ASCO 2005 meeting.[71] At a median follow-up for all patients of 22.5 months (range: 0.9 to 125.1 months) and 69.3 months (range: 6.2 to 125.1 months) for patients still alive, 396 patients were analyzable. Induction treatment was delivered as per the protocol equally in both arms. In the surgical arm, 164 (81.2%) underwent thoracotomy. A complete resection was accomplished in 144 patients (71.3%), incomplete resection in 11 (5.4%), and no resection in 9 (4.5%). There were 18% pathologic complete responses (T0N0) and 46% with pathologic nodal clearance. The chemoRT toxicity was similar in both arms, with the exception of grades 3 and 4 esophagitis, which was more common in the chemoRT alone arm (23% vs. 10%; $p = 0.0006$). Consolidation chemotherapy was not administered to 44% of patients undergoing surgery and 25% of those not having undergone surgery ($p < 0.0001$), reiterating the difficulty of delivering chemotherapy after "definitive" surgical treatment for lung cancer. Conversely, RT was delivered according to protocol in 79% on the chemoRT arm versus 96% on the surgery arm ($p < 0.0001$). Four patients (2.1%) in chemoRT arm and 16 (7.9%) patients in chemoRT-surgery arm died from treatment-related toxicity. In the latter group, 10 of these deaths were caused by postoperative complications. All but two postoperative deaths followed a pneumonectomy (especially right sided), and the most frequent cause of death was ARDS.

Median progression-free survival was 12.8 and 10.5 months in the chemoRT-surgery arm and chemoRT arm, respectively. Five-year progression free survival was 22.4% in chemoRT-surgery arm versus 11.1% in chemoRT arm (log-rank $p = 0.017$). The median OS was 23.6 versus 22.2 months and the 5-year survival was 27.2% versus 20.3% in the chemoRT-surgery and chemoRT arms, respectively (log-rank $p = 0.51$). The OS curves cross over and begin to separate at 22 months. In 5 years, there was a 7% absolute survival benefit in the surgical arm, but the confidence intervals (CI) are wide and overlap. More patients died of treatment complications in the surgical arm, but more are alive without progression in the same treatment arm. Sites of relapse were also analyzed: 10% of patients in chemoRT-surgery arm had locoregional relapse only versus 22% in the chemoRT arm ($p = 0.002$). Relapse in the primary site was seven times more common in the nonsurgical arm. Brain was common site of first relapse in both arms (11% vs. 15 % in the chemoRT and chemoRT-surgery arm, respectively; $p = 0.29$). Pretreatment factors predictive of favorable outcome were female sex, less than 5% weight loss, and number of N2 stations positive. Age, Karnofsky performance status (KPS), T stage, lactate dehydrogenase (LDH), and histology did not reach statistical significance. After the induction treatment, patients who achieved complete response in the mediastinal nodes had median survival of 34 months and 5-year survival of about 41%, regardless of the response in the primary tumor. For the patients who achieved a T0N0 (pCR), the median survival was 40 months and the 5-year survival was 42%. Thus sterilization of the mediastinum can have significant prognostic importance.

The influence of type of resection on the results of this trial was performed in an unplanned, exploratory matching analysis. OS was significantly improved on the surgical arm if a lobectomy was performed compared to the matched cohort in the chemoRT arm. Median survivals were 33.6 versus 21.7 months, log-rank $p = 0.002$, with 5-year survival of 36.1% versus 17.8%. There was a nonsignificant trend toward worse survival for the pneumonectomy group versus a matched cohort in the chemoRT arm with median survivals of 18.9 versus 29.4 months, 3-year survival of 36.3% versus 45.0%, and 5-year survival of 21.9% versus 23.6%, respectively.

The authors of this study concluded that trimodality therapy increased the 5-year progression-free survival with a trend for increased 5-year OS and that N0 status at surgery significantly predicted a greater survival. Nevertheless, the trimodality approach was not optimal when a pneumonectomy was required because of high mortality risk. Thus, conventional wisdom for trimodality therapy in locally advanced IIIA disease dictates that surgical resection after chemoRT should only be considered for fit patients if a lobectomy is feasible.

PHASE II TRIALS OF INDUCTION REGIMENS THAT INCORPORATED THIRD-GENERATION CHEMOTHERAPY AGENTS

Third-generation chemotherapy agents were recently tested in phase II induction therapy protocols in stage III disease, similar to those reviewed earlier in this chapter for stage I, II, and selected early stage III presentations. Selected studies with larger numbers of patients are presented later (Table 55.9), but any comparisons among studies as well as conclusions regarding an improvement over second-generation induction programs are premature. In fact, studies with newer agents and concurrent RT as induction were often problematic with respect to excessive toxicity. The Swiss Group for Clinical Cancer Research (SAKK) enrolled 90 potentially operable stage IIIA patients with biopsy-proven ipsilateral mediastinal nodal involvement.[73,74] The induction regimen consisted of cisplatin 40 mg/m^2 on days 1 to 2 plus docetaxel 85 mg/m^2 on day 1 for three cycles. In all, 75 patients underwent tumor resection after three cycles of chemotherapy, with positive resection margin in 16% of patients. Interestingly, the median overall cisplatin dose-intensity in patients with negative

TABLE 55.9 Design and Results of Completed Phase II Trials Using Third-Generation Chemotherapy Drugs within Induction Regimen

Investigators	Stage Subset	Study Design	N	Response Rate (%)	Resection Rate (R0)* (%)	pCR	Survival
SAKK[73,74]	IIIA (pN2), mixed bulk	PD × 3 → surgery → variable RT	90	66	48	16	33%, 3 yrs
De Marinis et al.[75]	IIIA (pN2), bulky	GTP × 3 → surgery→ variable RT	49	74	55	16	Median 23 mo
ILCP[76]	IIIA, IIIB (clin) bulky	GTP × 4 → surgery→ variable RT	129	62	29	2	Median 19 mo
EORTC 08941[77]	IIIA (pN2)	C or P doublet → surgery/RT→variable PORT	579	57	86	5	Median 16 mo
EORTC 08955[78]	IIIA (pN2)	GC → surgery/RT	47	70	71	NR	69%, 1 yr
EORTC 08958[79]	IIIA (pN2)	TC → surgery/RT	52	64	80	NR	69%, 1 yr
EORTC 08984[80]	IIIA (pN2)	PD → surgery/RT	46	39	NR	NR	65%, 1 yr

*Of the original number of patients.

C, carboplatin; D, docetaxel; EORTC, European Organisation for Research and Treatment of Cancer; G, gemcitabine; ILCP, Italian Lung Cancer Project; NR, not reported; P, cisplatin; pCR, pathologic complete response; RT, radiotherapy; SAKK, Swiss Group for Clinical Cancer Research; T, paclitaxel.

resection margin was higher than that in patients with positive margin (96 vs. 80 mg/m^2/cycle; $p = 0.034$). Perioperative morbidity and mortality were low (17% and 3%, respectively). Complete pathological response was seen in 19% of resected patients. No postoperative chemotherapy was given and 33 patients (44%) received postoperative RT, with median total dose 60 Gy (range, 22 to 70). Of these, 23 patients were treated per protocol (i.e., for a positive margin and/or involvement of the upper lymph node). Nine patients who were due to receive postoperative RT did not actually receive this treatment.

After a median observation time of 5 years, the median OS was 35 months and the median event free survival was 15 months. Of 47 patients who died, 42 were caused by lung cancer. The median time to death caused by tumor was 43 months. At 3 years after initiation of trial therapy (a follow-up time that all patients reached), 27 patients (36%) were alive and free of disease.

Univariate analysis assessing the impact of baseline patient and tumor characteristics identified only multilevel involvement of mediastinal lymph nodes as a poor prognostic factor for OS. Among surgery characteristics, only complete resection was significantly associated with better OS and event-free survival. All aspects of chemotherapy activity (clinical response, pathological response, mediastinal downstaging, and clearance of the uppermost mediastinal lymph node) were significantly associated with improved OS and event-free survival. Pathological response (percentage of necrosis and fibrosis) was the most important feature of the chemotherapy activity on the primary tumor. Similar associations were seen when patients who died from non-NSCLC causes were censored. The prognostic impacts of complete tumor resection, mediastinal downstaging, and pathological response on OS and event-free survival were confirmed in multivariate analyses.

In another recent trial, three preoperative cycles of gemcitabine, paclitaxel, and cisplatin were delivered to 49 patients biopsy-documented N2 disease patients.[75] Patients with at least stable disease after the induction regimen underwent attempted surgical resection. Patients whose disease did not respond received RT alone, and the patients whose disease responded but did not undergo thoracotomy received three more cycles of the same chemotherapy followed by RT. Postoperative RT was delivered for patients with persistent N2 disease or incomplete resection. There was one death during the induction. An RR of 73.5% based on radiographic criteria was recorded, and a complete resection was performed in 55% of patients. Mediastinal nodal disease clearance occurred in 35% of cases, and complete pathological response in 16%. Median and progression-free survival were 23 and 18 months, respectively, and the brain was the most common metastatic site (16%).

The Italian Lung Cancer Project (ILCP) completed a phase II trial in 129 unresectable, locally advanced stage IIIA and IIIB NSCLC patients.[76] The induction regimen consisted of four cycles of gemcitabine 1000 mg/m^2 on days 1 and 8, and cisplatin 70 mg/m^2 on day 2. The RR was 80%, but the resectability rate was only 29%. There was no perioperative mortality and minimal morbidity. Postoperative RT was given for positive mediastinal lymph nodes and was continued to 60 Gy if the disease was unresectable. The median progression-free survival was 11 months and median survival was 20 months.

The EORTC 08941 was a phase III trial in clinical stage IIIA (N2) disease where all patients received induction chemotherapy with either cisplatin- (100 mg/m^2) or carboplatin- (400 mg/m^2) based chemotherapy and then where randomly assigned to surgery or radiation if at least a partial response was achieved.[77] This study closed to accrual on December 2002, with a total of 333 patients randomly assigned, and final results were recently reported (to be discussed shortly). Several phase II trials were embedded within this larger phase III trial as feasibility studies of three third-generation chemotherapy regimens.

The first study was EORTC 08955.[78] Gemcitabine 1000 mg/m^2 on days 1, 8, and 15 and cisplatin 100 mg/m^2 on day 2, were given every 4 weeks for three cycles. A total of 47 patients were enrolled, of whom 33 (70.2%) had objective responses, and 17 patients underwent thoracotomy, of whom 71% had complete resections. The second embedded pilot study (EORTC 08958) tested carboplatin (area under the curve [AUC] 6) and paclitaxel (200 mg/m^2) every 21 days for three cycles.[79] Fifty-two patients were accrued, of whom thirty-three (64%) had objective responses; twelve underwent surgery, two of these patients had mediastinal nodal clearance. In the third phase II trial (EORTC 08984),[80] cisplatin (40 mg/m^2 days 1 and 2) and docetaxel (85 mg/m^2 day 1) were given every 3 weeks for three cycles before surgery. Forty-six patients were enrolled, with eighteen (39%) patients who had objective responses. None of these embedded phase II studies planned to report survival outcomes, but instead established feasibility and efficacy for preoperative third-generation chemotherapy.

As mentioned, the parent phase III trial, EORTC 08941, was recently published in the literature.[77] Induction chemotherapy resulted in an RR of 61% (95% CI, 57% to 65%) among the 579 eligible patients. Only patients who demonstrated at least a "minor" response were subsequently randomized; a total of 167 patients were allocated to resection and 165 to RT. Thus this trial selected the "best of the best" patients for analysis. Of the 154 (92%) patients who underwent surgery, 14% had an exploratory thoracotomy, 50% a radical resection, 42% a pathologic downstaging, and 5% a pathologic complete response; 4% died after surgery. Among the 154 (93%) irradiated patients, overall compliance to the RT prescription was 55%, and grade 3 and 4 acute and late esophageal and pulmonary toxic effects occurred in 4% and 7%; one patient died of radiation pneumonitis. Median and 5-year OS for patients randomly assigned to resection versus RT were 16.4 versus 17.5 months and 15.7% versus 14%, respectively (hazard ratio = 1.06; 95% CI, 0.84 to 1.35). Rates of progression-free survival were also similar in both groups. The results maybe partially explained by the high number of pneumonectomies, especially because postoperative RT was administered to 62 (40%) patients in the surgery arm. This trial will be thoroughly parsed by surgeons, radiation oncologists, and medical oncologists alike to asses how each specialty's contribution might be improved and the negative aspects minimized.[81]

TREATMENT-RELATED MORBIDITY AND MORTALITY IN COMBINED MODALITY INDUCTION TRIALS

The morbidity from combined modality therapy that includes surgery is not insignificant. It is often difficult to attribute a particular toxicity to just one modality because the entire "package" affects patient tolerance and the treatment-related mortality. All combined modality induction programs were tested in the "fittest" patients who were fully ambulatory and had general medical conditions that permitted the rigors of this therapy. Eligibility criteria were of necessity quite strict in these trials. It may be dangerous to offer this type of treatment outside of a clinical trial, especially to patients who have a poor performance status and/or major comorbidities, because the literature will underestimate the extent of morbidity and mortality in this group. Clinical trials designed for the large group of patients ineligible for these aggressive approaches are needed. But for patients who match the eligibility criteria of published studies, the literature provides some information on the expected morbidity and mortality during induction therapy, the postoperative period, the late or posterior chemotherapy, or RT, and after all treatment is completed.

Morbidity/Mortality during Induction Therapy

The most common toxicity reported among all trials during the presurgery induction phase is myelosuppression from chemotherapy. This is usually short-lived and, in most studies, did not result in admissions for neutropenic fever. Other drug-specific side effects such as nausea and emesis, diarrhea, mucositis, and cisplatin-related malaise are variably reported. In fact, nausea and emesis are now quite infrequent compared to the rates reported in the initial trials because of the expanded number of compounds effective against this toxicity. Esophagitis is more often observed after induction chemoRT than chemotherapy alone, although severe events occurred in less than 10% of patients in most series with single fractionation RT.[26–30] The two-third generation trials with hyperfractionated RT reported severe esophagitis rates of 6% and 14%.[41,42] In a report phase I to II high-dose concurrent chemoRT protocol from the University of Maryland, patients with stage IIA or IIB were treated with induction concurrent carboplatin (area under the plasma concentration–time curve 1), vinorelbine (5 to 15 mg/m^2), and hyperfractionated RT (69.6 Gy) followed by consolidation chemotherapy (carboplatin area under the plasma concentration–time curve 6, vinorelbine 25 mg/m^2, docetaxel 75 mg/m^2) or surgery ($n = 19$) plus consolidation chemotherapy.[82] A low pretherapy body mass index and percentage of esophagus volume treated to >50 Gy were significantly associated with acute grade 2 or worse esophagitis.

Pneumonitis during induction therapy is quite rare, except that the risk of septic deaths from postobstructive pneumonia may be greater with the MVP regimen in one large series.[20,21] Overall, most second-generation induction regimens were fully managed in an outpatient setting. A significant proportion of patients who enter induction therapy with symptoms related to bulk disease in the chest report a gradual improvement in sense of well-being and performance status as treatment is ongoing. However, formal quality-of-life (QOL) studies have not been conducted for this group of patients.

In the previously mentioned GLCCG study,[64] after receiving induction therapy, patients were randomized to preoperative versus postoperative RT. The fractionation as well as the concomitant chemotherapy differed between the arms. Interestingly, grades 3 and 4 esophagitis was more frequent with preoperative RT (19% vs. 3%; $p = 0.0001$), whereas the incidence of pneumonitis grades 3 and 4 was higher with postoperative RT (1% vs. 6%; $p = 0.004$). QOL was assessed throughout therapy using the EORTC QLQ-C30 and EORTC QLQ-LC.[83] Of 126 eligible patients, 54 completed treatment. For patients in both treatment arms, physical functioning decreased, whereas dyspnea, fatigue, and pain increased from beginning to the end of treatment. For self-assessed QOL, no statistically significant effect was found in or between the two treatment arms. The combined modality approach with preoperative chemoRT proved to be feasible in treating locally advanced NSCLC patients without decreasing their subjective QOL.

Mortality/Morbidity during the 30-Day Postoperative Time Period

Despite the wealth of clinical trials that follow algorithms that lead to eventual exploration and resection after induction therapy, there is no consensus as to what constitutes expected or acceptable postinduction surgical morbidity and mortality. This lack of consensus is caused by the marked heterogeneity of induction regimens (as reviewed in preceding sections); the lack of consistency across trials in the adequate reporting of surgical complications; different criteria for preoperative eligibility regarding pulmonary function, comorbidities, and conditioning; and variable experience of the surgeon in dealing with postinduction surgical scenarios at the time of thoracotomy and in providing the required supportive care during the postoperative time period.

Several publications document the risk of pulmonary resection in the noninduction situation. The modern 30-day mortality for pneumonectomy is 3% to 6.2%, and the mortality of a standard lobectomy is 1% to 2%.[84–86] Surgical issues, in association with neoadjuvant therapy, have been reviewed.[87] It is generally agreed that postinduction resections usually pose a greater technical challenge and require more vigilance in postoperative care. More recent data suggest the possibility that the potential adverse effect of induction chemotherapy on postoperative mortality may have been over estimated.[88] Specific recommendations for patients undergoing postinduction resection include restriction of intravenous fluids perioperatively, reinforcing bronchial stumps with tissue, pain control via epidural/paravertebral catheter, early use of broad-spectrum antibiotics, aggressive pulmonary toilet, and monitoring/prevention of supraventricular tachycardia.

Acute surgical morbidities appear to be similar regardless of the type of induction, unless RT is given and too much time is allowed to elapse so that extensive fibrosis is encountered.

Fibrotic reaction from RT may obliterate resection planes. To minimize the effect of fibrotic reaction, surgery should be performed within 4 to 6 weeks after completion of induction regimen. Whether drugs that rarely cause pulmonary reactions during induction therapy increase the rates of these types of postoperative complications is not clear.

Pulmonary complications and deaths because of pulmonary causes during the postoperative time period are the greatest concern after induction therapy and collectively rates are probably greater than reported in the literature after surgery alone. In particular, events such as extensive pneumonitis, usually culture-negative, ARDS, and bronchopleural fistula have a high mortality in the postoperative period. Pulmonary morbidity and mortality rates are often quoted to be greater after induction regimens with chemoRT than after induction chemotherapy alone. However, a careful review of all the literature available discloses great variability. Postoperative mortality rates from 3.1% to 17% were reported after MVP- or VP-containing induction chemotherapy (including some cases of ARDS), from 4% to 15% after second-generation induction chemoRT, and 5% to 7% after induction chemoRT with hyperfractionation.

The specific type of mortal postoperative event may differ according to whether RT was included with induction chemotherapy or not although this issue is not fully resolved. For example, complicated stump insufficiency was the most common cause of postoperative death in the WGCC experience with twice-daily RT in the induction,[42] whereas ARDS may be the most common cause of postoperative deaths after single fractionation chemoRT in multiple series. The presence of RT in the induction regimen, however, may not be the sole explanation for greater pulmonary-related mortality, especially ARDS, after certain induction regimens. For the most part, many of the patients treated with concurrent chemoRT induction approaches had advanced, central disease that required a pneumonectomy after induction. Pulmonary-related postoperative mortality rates are expected to be much higher in this population with advanced disease.[26,27] So far, there has been no difference in overall postoperative mortality rates compared to the surgery-alone control arms in trials with induction chemotherapy for early, more minimal bulk disease.[47,48,51–53]

Serious pulmonary complications in the postoperative period clearly result from a combination of causes in addition to the type of induction therapy.[59,89–91] Although higher doses of RT than 45 Gy have been implicated,[59] the occurrence of ARDS in trials with no induction RT and the lack of an excess rate of ARDS in other trials with higher-dose RT or altered fraction RT[28,41,42] underscore that the tolerance of lymphatic sump disruption and postpneumonectomy shunts is variable after both induction chemotherapy and induction chemoRT. The type of complication may also vary based on schedule of the RT, with perhaps more events of serious stump insufficiency but less ARDS after hyperfractionated versus single-fraction RT. Moreover, stump problems can usually be eliminated when the surgeons incorporate a bronchial stump protection protocol for all patients.

Morbidity/Mortality after the Postoperative Time Period Many induction program algorithms recommend additional chemotherapy with or without RT after the patient has recovered from surgery. Usually, the spectrum of toxicities from posterior chemotherapy is similar to those observed during induction[26] although it may be more difficult to complete a boost dose of RT.[25] Patients are at greater risk for pneumonitis, either from prior RT or because of infectious causes, beyond the postoperative period, especially if the prior surgery was a pneumonectomy. Data on this issue is rarely reported in the induction therapy literature.[26] Prompt attention to symptoms of infection with broad-spectrum antibiotic coverage is critical to minimize the risk of mortality.

The other major morbidity experienced by many patients after induction therapy followed by surgery is a posttreatment constitutional syndrome. This consists of a constellation of symptoms including thoracotomy pain, malaise, anorexia, and poor pulmonary reserve. This syndrome probably occurs at a greater frequency than with radiation or surgery alone, but its rate is grossly underreported.[26] It often resolves within a year after treatment although its lingering presence is clearly discouraging to the patient and caregiver. Prospective QOL analyses and active rehabilitation protocols for this population are needed. Patients also continue to experience problems from their comorbid diseases long after treatment is completed, especially cardiovascular disease and noncancer pulmonary events. Competing cause of death reporting is rare, and often death certificates attribute cause to "lung cancer" even when the disease has never recurred. This was documented in the SWOG 8805 trial. Although cancer accounted for 64% of all deaths, 20% were caused by various other causes such as late pneumonia long after the end of treatment, myocardial infarction, pulmonary embolus, cerebrovascular accidents, trauma, ulcer, or second primaries.[26]

Strategies to Reduce Radiotherapy-Related Morbidity Induction RT likely helps improve resection rates, especially in locally advanced tumors, but at the same time, contributes to surgical morbidity and mortality. Two well-recognized morbid effects of RT are radiation pneumonitis (usually occurring within 6 months from completion of radiation) and late fibrosis. These complications are likely to be more devastating in patients who undergo a lobectomy or pneumonectomy. The occurrence of clinical radiation pneumonitis has been correlated with the volume of lung receiving over 20 Gy (V20).[92] Although there has been significant literature investigating correlation of lung volume and dose to predict pneumonitis, a V20 less than 30% to 35% is standard in most treatment plans.[93] However, impairment of diffusion capacity and perfusion can and do occur at lower doses.[94–97] By fitting patient data into a mathematical model, Gopal et al.[94] suggested a sharp loss in local diffusing capacity of the lung for carbon monoxide (DLCO) occurring with radiation doses above 13 Gy. These data suggest that it is prudent to limit the volume of lung receiving even low-dose radiation.

There are several strategies that can be used to limit the radiation effect on the normal lung; however, none have been studied in the context of a trimodality approach. Technical improvements in the application of thoracic radiation therapy for lung cancer, particularly with the integration of CT-based treatment planning, have greatly improved our ability to identify tumors and, relevant to this report, to delineate normal tissues. Three-dimensional conformal RT technique can ensure adequate radiation dose to the tumor and areas of risk and limit the irradiation of the healthy tissue. Limiting the mediastinal target volume to only those areas positive on PET scan will reduce the volume of irradiated lung and should be considered for future studies. Irradiation of contralateral uninvolved lung should be avoided to the maximum extent possible, especially in patients who are likely to require pneumonectomy. Ideally, the irradiated volume should include as little lung outside the area destined to be resected as possible. Also of note, the main source of death from intercurrent disease associated specifically with the postoperative use of RT is heart disease mortality.[98] A recent population-based study suggested that postoperative-associated heart disease mortality has decreased over time, particularly for patients who have tumors located where heart irradiation is more likely to occur.[99] Thus, it would appear that our ability has improved to deliver RT to the operative patient with minimal damage to the normal tissues.

WORLDWIDE PHASE III TRIALS: ONGOING AND PLANNED

The EORTC has just completed accrual to a phase III trial (EORTC 08941) of induction chemotherapy followed by either RT or surgery.[53] The trial enrolled patients with stage IIIA (N2) NSCLC, considered unresectable pretreatment with positive N2 nodal biopsy or ipsilateral vocal cord or diaphragm paralysis. Patients were given any combination chemotherapy regimen that contained cisplatin at 100 mg/m^2 or carboplatin at 400 mg/m^2. Upon completion, patients were reassessed for response, and those achieving either complete or partial response are randomized to either radical RT or surgical resection. Postoperative RT was given either for positive surgical margins of persistent N2 disease at surgery. This trial was opened in 1994 and first survival results are anticipated soon.

The German/French consortium has opened a new phase III trial based on encouraging pilot data of a novel trimodality regimen (see Chapter 56). Patients with advanced stage III disease (two or more N2 levels involved, large-volume N2 disease, selected IIIB subsets) are treated with induction cisplatin plus paclitaxel followed by (if no progression) hyperfractionated RT plus concurrent cisplatin plus vinorelbine. Upon restaging, patients with operable disease are randomized to either surgical resection or to a boost chemoRT program of cisplatin plus vinorelbine plus single daily fraction RT to 75 Gy.

A phase III Nordic trial is ongoing for patients with biopsy-proven N2 disease. The randomization is to either carboplatin plus paclitaxel for three cycles followed by RT to 60 Gy (single daily fraction) or to the same induction therapy followed by surgical resection and then followed by RT to 60 Gy (single daily fraction).

Other studies are planned to examine the role of RT in the induction regimen in patients with low-volume N2 disease that is proven by biopsy and with resectable primary tumors. A SAKK trial prescribes phase III trial is designed to give three cycles of cisplatin plus docetaxel, followed by restaging. If a response or stable disease occurs, patients will be randomized to either surgical resection or to daily RT (with a novel hyperfractionated imbedded boost) followed then by surgical resection. The North American Intergroup (RTOG0412/S0332) planed to also test induction cisplatin and docetaxel, but the randomization will be to concurrent daily RT or not. Both arms then receive surgical resection, followed by additional chemotherapy in all patients. Unfortunately, this trial closed early as a result of poor accrual.

CONCLUSION

Despite reported results of multiple clinical trials reviewed herein, the debate regarding combined modality therapy that involves surgery continues, and it must be concluded that there is no consensus whether neoadjuvant chemotherapy for early stage NSCLC results in improved survival or whether chemoRT in high-volume, advanced stage III NSCLC should be followed by surgical resection. In 2003, a consensus statement from the International Association for the Study of Lung Cancer (IASLC) reaffirmed surgical resection alone and chemoradiation alone as standards of care for early and locally advanced NSCLC, respectively.[100] However, the National Comprehensive Cancer Network's (NCCN) current clinical practice guidelines recommends either induction chemotherapy with or without radiation therapy, followed by surgery for patients with T1 to T2, N2-positive disease, or definitive chemoradiation.[101] For patients with T3N2 disease, the treatment recommended by the NCCN is chemoradiation, although no prospective trial specifically addresses this issue.

However, critical data emerged since these consensus recommendations were published and recent Evidence-based Clinical Practice Guidelines from the American College of Chest Physicians suggest considering induction therapy only in the context of a clinical trial.[102–104] Furthermore, the recent Cancer Care Ontario and American Society of Clinical Oncology recommend adjuvant for selected stage IB and all stage IIA to IIIA NSCLC. Some impact will be felt on the ability to complete large trials in stage I and II disease designed to test the role of induction chemotherapy. That is, the surgery-alone arms are now substandard therapy, which suggests that what remains to test is whether the chemotherapy is best given in an induction setting or as postoperative adjuvant therapy. For patients with patients with high-volume, mediastinal nodal positive disease, chemotherapy alone as induction may be problematic, since the complete resection rates are generally lower when the tumor burden is higher. The first report of the large North American Intergroup trial 0139 showed that surgical resection in this group of patients after induction chemoRT increases disease-free survival, but at the cost of increased noncancer mortality, ultimately resulting in same OS.[71] Longer follow-up will be necessary to determine whether this advantage in disease-free survival will translate into an OS improvement. Hence, until more data are available, trimodality treatment should not be routinely offered to this patient population outside a clinical trial without a detailed, informed discussion of risks and benefits. However, for patients with T4N0/1 disease, data collectively suggest that surgical resection markedly improves the long-term outcome for this subgroup, with 5-year survival of almost 50%. A phase III trial to validate these observations ideally should be done, but most likely will not be feasible. Thus, routine use of a published trimodality program in this uncommon subset appears to be reasonable as a present standard of care. However, as we develop a greater appreciation for the molecular mechanisms responsible for response and resistance to the various therapeutic options, we will be able to utilize molecular markers identifying which patients will benefit from induction versus adjuvant therapy. Such will also detail which agents to use and their sequence with respect to surgery. Paradigms investigating such will hopefully form the basis of the next generation of clinical trials.

REFERENCES

1. Goldstraw P, Crowley J, Chansky K, et al. The IASLC Lung Cancer Staging Project: proposals for the revision of the TNM stage groupings in the forthcoming (seventh) edition of the TNM Classification of malignant tumours. *J Thorac Oncol* 2007;2(8):706–714.
2. Arriagada R, Bergman B, Dunant A, et al. Cisplatin-based adjuvant chemotherapy in patients with completely resected non-small-cell lung cancer. *N Engl J Med* 2004;350(4):351–360.
3. Douillard JY, Rosell R, De Lena M, et al. Adjuvant vinorelbine plus cisplatin versus observation in patients with completely resected stage IB-IIIA non-small-cell lung cancer (Adjuvant Navelbine International Trialist Association [ANITA]): a randomised controlled trial. *Lancet Oncol* 2006;7(9):719–727.
4. Winton T, Livingston R, Johnson D, et al. Vinorelbine plus cisplatin vs. observation in resected non-small-cell lung cancer. *N Engl J Med* 2005;352(25):2589–2597.
5. Non-small Cell Lung Cancer Collaborative Group. Chemotherapy in non-small cell lung cancer: a meta-analysis using updated data on individual patients from 52 randomised clinical trials. *BMJ* 1995; 311(7010):899–909.
6. Gilligan D, Nicolson M, Smith I, et al. Preoperative chemotherapy in patients with resectable non-small cell lung cancer: results of the MRC LU22/NVALT 2/EORTC 08012 multicentre randomised trial and update of systematic review. *Lancet* 2007;369(9577):1929–1937.
7. Burdett SS, Stewart LA, Rydzewska L. Chemotherapy and surgery versus surgery alone in non-small cell lung cancer. *Cochrane Database Syst Rev* 2007;(3):CD006157.
8. Burdett S, Stewart LA, Rydzewska L. A systematic review and meta-analysis of the literature: chemotherapy and surgery versus surgery alone in non-small cell lung cancer. *J Thorac Oncol* 2006;1(7): 611–621.
9. Bromley LL, Szur L. Combined radiotherapy and resection for carcinoma of the bronchus; experiences with 66 patients. *Lancet* 1955;269(6897):937–941.
10. Bloedorn FG, Cowley RA, Cuccia CA, et al. Preoperative irradiation in bronchogenic carcinoma. *Am J Roentgenol Radium Ther Nucl Med* 1964;92:77–87.
11. Shields TW, Higgins GA Jr, Lawton R, et al. Preoperative x-ray therapy as an adjuvant in the treatment of bronchogenic carcinoma. *J Thorac Cardiovasc Surg* 1970;59(1):49–61.
12. Warram J. Preoperative irradiation of cancer of the lung: final report of a therapeutic trial. A collaborative study. *Cancer* 1975;36(3): 914–925.
13. Wagner H Jr, Lad T, Piantadosi S, et al. Randomized phase 2 evaluation of preoperative radiation therapy and preoperative chemotherapy with mitomycin, vinblastine, and cisplatin in patients with technically unresectable stage IIIA and IIIB non-small cell cancer of the lung. LCSG 881. *Chest* 1994;106(6 Suppl):S348–S354.
14. Elias AD, Kumar P, Herndon J III, et al. Radiotherapy versus chemotherapy plus radiotherapy in surgically treated IIIA N2 non-small-cell lung cancer. *Clin Lung Cancer* 2002;4(2):95–103.
15. Skarin A, Jochelson M, Sheldon T, et al. Neoadjuvant chemotherapy in marginally resectable stage III M0 non-small cell lung cancer: long-term follow-up in 41 patients. *J Surg Oncol* 1989;40(4):266–274.
16. Eagan RT, Ruud C, Lee RE, et al. Pilot study of induction therapy with cyclophosphamide, doxorubicin, and cisplatin (CAP) and chest irradiation prior to thoracotomy in initially inoperable stage III M0 non-small cell lung cancer. *Cancer Treat Rep* 1987;71(10):895–900.
17. Bitran JD, Golomb HM, Hoffman PC, et al. Protochemotherapy in non-small cell lung carcinoma. An attempt to increase surgical resectability and survival. A preliminary report. *Cancer* 1986;57(1):44–53.
18. Elias AD, Skarin AT, Gonin R, et al. Neoadjuvant treatment of stage IIIA non-small cell lung cancer. Long-term results. *Am J Clin Oncol* 1994;17(1):26–36.
19. Darwish S, Minotti V, Crinò L, et al. Neoadjuvant cisplatin and etoposide for stage IIIA (clinical N2) non-small cell lung cancer. *Am J Clin Oncol* 1994;17(1):64–67.
20. Burkes RL, Ginsberg RJ, Shepherd FA, et al. Induction chemotherapy with mitomycin, vindesine, and cisplatin for stage III unresectable non-small-cell lung cancer: results of the Toronto phase II Trial. *J Clin Oncol* 1992;10(4):580–586.
21. Burkes RL, Shepherd FA, Blackstein ME, et al. Induction chemotherapy with mitomycin, vindesine, and cisplatin for stage IIIA (T1-3, N2) unresectable non-small-cell lung cancer: final results of the Toronto phase II trial. *Lung Cancer* 2005;47(1):103–109.
22. Elias AD, Skarin AT, Leong T, et al. Neoadjuvant therapy for surgically staged IIIA N2 non-small cell lung cancer (NSCLC). *Lung Cancer* 1997;17(1):147–161.
23. Jaklitsch MT, Herndon JE II, DeCamp MM Jr, et al. Nodal downstaging predicts survival following induction chemotherapy for stage IIIA (N2) non-small cell lung cancer in CALGB protocol #8935. *J Surg Oncol* 2006;94(7):599–606.
24. Martini N, Kris MG, Flehinger BJ, et al. Preoperative chemotherapy for stage IIIa (N2) lung cancer: the Sloan-Kettering experience with 136 patients. *Ann Thorac Surg* 1993;55(6):1365–1373.
25. Sugarbaker DJ, Herndon J, Kohman LJ, et al. Results of cancer and leukemia group B protocol 8935. A multiinstitutional phase II trimodality trial for stage IIIA (N2) non-small-cell lung cancer. Cancer and Leukemia Group B Thoracic Surgery Group. *J Thorac Cardiovasc Surg* 1995;109(3):473–483.
26. Albain KS, Rusch VW, Crowley JJ, et al. Concurrent cisplatin/etoposide plus chest radiotherapy followed by surgery for stages IIIA (N2) and IIIB non-small-cell lung cancer: mature results of Southwest Oncology Group phase II study 8805. *J Clin Oncol* 1995;13(8):1880–1892.
27. Faber LP, Kittle CF, Warren WH, et al. Preoperative chemotherapy and irradiation for stage III non-small cell lung cancer. *Ann Thorac Surg* 1989;47(5):669–675.
28. Law A, Karp DD, Dipetrillo T, et al. Emergence of increased cerebral metastasis after high-dose preoperative radiotherapy with chemotherapy in patients with locally advanced nonsmall cell lung carcinoma. *Cancer* 2001;92(1):160–164.

29. Strauss GM, Herndon JE, Sherman DD, et al. Neoadjuvant chemotherapy and radiotherapy followed by surgery in stage IIIA non-small-cell carcinoma of the lung: report of a Cancer and Leukemia Group B phase II study. *J Clin Oncol* 1992;10(8):1237–1244.
30. Weiden PL, Piantadosi S. Preoperative chemotherapy (cisplatin and fluorouracil) and radiation therapy in stage III non-small cell lung cancer. A phase 2 study of the LCSG. *Chest* 1994;106(6 Suppl): S344–S347.
31. Bonomi PD, Gale M, Faber LP, et al. Prognostic importance of subdividing clinically staged IIIa and IIIb patients with non-small-cell lung cancer. *J Clin Oncol* 1991;9(2):357–359.
32. Curran WJ Jr, Stafford PM. Lack of apparent difference in outcome between clinically staged IIIA and IIIB non-small-cell lung cancer treated with radiation therapy. *J Clin Oncol* 1990;8(3):409–415.
33. Mountain CF. Revisions in the International System for Staging Lung Cancer. *Chest* 1997;111(6):1710–1717.
34. Rusch VW, Albain KS, Crowley JJ, et al. Neoadjuvant therapy: a novel and effective treatment for stage IIIb non-small cell lung cancer. Southwest Oncology Group. *Ann Thorac Surg* 1994;58(2):290–294.
35. Albain KS, Rusch VW, Crowley J. Long-Term Survival After Concurrent Cisplatin/Etoposide (PE) Plus Chest Radiotherapy (RT) Followed By Surgery in Bulky, Stages IIIA(N2) and IIIB Non-Small Cell Lung Cancer (NSCLC): 6-Year Outcomes from Southwest Oncology Group Study 8805. *Proc Am Soc Clin Oncol* 1999;18:A467.
36. Albain KS, Crowley JJ, Turrisi AT III, et al. Concurrent cisplatin, etoposide, and chest radiotherapy in pathologic stage IIIB non-small-cell lung cancer: a Southwest Oncology Group phase II study, SWOG 9019. *J Clin Oncol* 2002;20(16):3454–3460.
37. Garrido P, González-Larriba JL, Insa A, et al. Long-term survival associated with complete resection after induction chemotherapy in stage IIIA (N2) and IIIB (T4N0-1) non small-cell lung cancer patients: the Spanish Lung Cancer Group Trial 9901. *J Clin Oncol* 2007;25(30):4736–4742.
38. Grunenwald DH, André F, Le Péchoux C, et al. Benefit of surgery after chemoradiotherapy in stage IIIB (T4 and/or N3) non-small cell lung cancer. *J Thorac Cardiovasc Surg* 2001;122(4):796–802.
39. Pitz CC, Maas KW, Van Swieten HA, et al. Surgery as part of combined modality treatment in stage IIIB non-small cell lung cancer. *Ann Thorac Surg* 2002;74(1):164–169.
40. Pisters KM, Kris MG, Gralla RJ, et al. Pathologic complete response in advanced non-small-cell lung cancer following preoperative chemotherapy: implications for the design of future non-small-cell lung cancer combined modality trials. *J Clin Oncol* 1993;11(9): 1757–1762.
41. Choi NC, Carey RW, Daly W, et al. Potential impact on survival of improved tumor downstaging and resection rate by preoperative twice-daily radiation and concurrent chemotherapy in stage IIIA non-small-cell lung cancer. *J Clin Oncol* 1997;15(2):712–722.
42. Eberhardt W, Wilke H, Stamatis G, et al. Preoperative chemotherapy followed by concurrent chemoradiation therapy based on hyperfractionated accelerated radiotherapy and definitive surgery in locally advanced non-small-cell lung cancer: mature results of a phase II trial. *J Clin Oncol* 1998;16(2):622–634.
43. Eberhardt W, Stamatis G, Stuschke M, et al. Prognostically orientated multimodality treatment including surgery for selected patients of small-cell lung cancer patients stages IB to IIIB: long-term results of a phase II trial. *Br J Cancer* 1999;81(7):1206–1212.
44. Eberhardt WE, Albain KS, Pass H, et al. Induction treatment before surgery for non-small cell lung cancer. *Lung Cancer* 2003;42(Suppl 1): S9–S14.
45. Stuschke M, Eberhardt W, Pöttgen C, et al. Prophylactic cranial irradiation in locally advanced non-small-cell lung cancer after multimodality treatment: long-term follow-up and investigations of late neuropsychologic effects. *J Clin Oncol* 1999;17(9):2700–2709.
46. DeCamp MM, Rice TW, Adelstein DJ, et al. Value of accelerated multimodality therapy in stage IIIA and IIIB non-small cell lung cancer. *J Thorac Cardiovasc Surg* 2003;126(1):17–27.
47. Rosell R, Gómez-Codina J, Camps C, et al. Preresectional chemotherapy in stage IIIA non-small-cell lung cancer: a 7-year assessment of a randomized controlled trial. *Lung Cancer* 1999;26(1):7–14.
48. Roth JA, Atkinson EN, Fossella F, et al. Long-term follow-up of patients enrolled in a randomized trial comparing perioperative chemotherapy and surgery with surgery alone in resectable stage IIIA non-small-cell lung cancer. *Lung Cancer* 1998;21(1):1–6.
49. Depierre A, Milleron B, Moro-Sibilot D, et al. Preoperative chemotherapy followed by surgery compared with primary surgery in resectable stage I (except T1N0), II, and IIIa non-small-cell lung cancer. *J Clin Oncol* 2002;20(1):247–253.
50. Pisters KM, Vallieres E, Bunn PA Jr, et al. S9900: Surgery alone or surgery plus induction (ind) paclitaxel/carboplatin (PC) chemotherapy in early stage non-small cell lung cancer (NSCLC): Follow-up on a phase III trial. *Proc Am Soc Clin Oncol* 2007;25(18S):7520.
51. Roth JA, Fossella F, Komaki R, et al. A randomized trial comparing perioperative chemotherapy and surgery with surgery alone in resectable stage IIIA non-small-cell lung cancer. *J Natl Cancer Inst* 1994;86(9):673–680.
52. Rosell R, Gómez-Codina J, Camps C, et al. A randomized trial comparing preoperative chemotherapy plus surgery with surgery alone in patients with non-small-cell lung cancer. *N Engl J Med* 1994;330(3):153–158.
53. Pass HI, Pogrebniak HW, Steinberg SM, et al. Randomized trial of neoadjuvant therapy for lung cancer: interim analysis. *Ann Thorac Surg* 1992;53(6):992–998.
54. Nagai K, Tsuchiya R, Mori T, et al. A randomized trial comparing induction chemotherapy followed by surgery with surgery alone for patients with stage IIIA N2 non-small cell lung cancer (JCOG 9209). *J Thorac Cardiovasc Surg* 2003;125(2):254–260.
55. Sorensen J, Riska H, Ravn J, Hansen O, Palshof T, Rytter C, et al. Scandinavian phase III trial of neoadjuvant chemotherapy in NSCLC stages IB-IIIA/T3. *Proc Am Soc Clin Oncol* 2005;23(16S):7146.
56. Uy KL, Darling G, Xu W, et al. Improved results of induction chemoradiation before surgical intervention for selected patients with stage IIIA-N2 non-small cell lung cancer. *J Thorac Cardiovasc Surg* 2007;134(1):188–193.
57. Fleck J, Camargo J, Godoy D. Chemordiation therapy versus chemotherapy alone as a neoadjuvant treatment for stage III nonsmall cell lung cancer. Preliminary report of a Phase III prospective randomized trial. *Proc Am Soc Clin Oncol* 1994;12:333.
58. Yashar J, Weitberg AB, Glicksman AS, et al. Preoperative chemotherapy and radiation therapy for stage IIIa carcinoma of the lung. *Ann Thorac Surg* 1992;53(3):445–448.
59. Fowler WC, Langer CJ, Curran WJ Jr, et al. Postoperative complications after combined neoadjuvant treatment of lung cancer. *Ann Thorac Surg* 1993;55(4):986–989.
60. Deutsch M, Crawford J, Leopold K, et al. Phase II study of neoadjuvant chemotherapy and radiation therapy with thoracotomy in the treatment of clinically staged IIIA non-small cell lung cancer. *Cancer* 1994;74(4):1243–1252.
61. Jeremic B, Shibamoto Y, Milicic B, et al. Impact of treatment interruptions due to toxicity on outcome of patients with early stage (I/II) non-small-cell lung cancer (NSCLC) treated with hyperfractionated radiation therapy alone. *Lung Cancer* 2003;40(3):317–323.
62. Cox JD, Pajak TF, Asbell S, et al. Interruptions of high-dose radiation therapy decrease long-term survival of favorable patients with unresectable non-small cell carcinoma of the lung: analysis of 1244 cases from 3 Radiation Therapy Oncology Group (RTOG) trials. *Int J Radiat Oncol Biol Phys* 1993;27(3):493–498.
63. Thomas M, Rübe C, Semik M, et al. Impact of preoperative bimodality induction including twice-daily radiation on tumor regression and survival in stage III non-small-cell lung cancer. *J Clin Oncol* 1999;17(4):1185.
64. Rube C, Riesenbeck D, Semik M, et al. Neoadjuvant chemotherapy followed by preoperative radiochemotherapy (hfRTCT) plus surgery or surgery plus postoperative radiotherapy in stage III non-small

cell lung cancer: Results of a randomized phase III trial of the German lung cancer cooperative group. *Int J Radiat Oncol Biol Phys* 60(S1), S130. 2004.

65. Thomas M, Macha HN, Ukena D, et al. Cisplatin / etoposide (PE) followed by twice-daily chemoradiation (hfRT/CT) versus PE alone before surgery in stage III non-small cell lung cancer (NSCLC): A randomized phase III trial of the German Lung Cancer Cooperative Group (GLCCG). *Proc Am Soc Clin Oncol* 2004;22(14S):7004.
66. Farray D, Mirkovic N, Albain KS. Multimodality therapy for stage III non-small-cell lung cancer. *J Clin Oncol* 2005;23(14):3257–3269.
67. Shepherd FA, Johnston MR, Payne D, et al. Randomized study of chemotherapy and surgery versus radiotherapy for stage IIIA non-small-cell lung cancer: a National Cancer Institute of Canada Clinical Trials Group Study. *Br J Cancer* 1998;78(5):683–685.
68. Dillman RO, Herndon J, Seagren SL, et al. Improved survival in stage III non-small-cell lung cancer: seven-year follow-up of cancer and leukemia group B (CALGB) 8433 trial. *J Natl Cancer* Inst 1996;88(17):1210–1215.
69. Johnstone DW, Byhardt RW, Ettinger D, et al. Phase III study comparing chemotherapy and radiotherapy with preoperative chemotherapy and surgical resection in patients with non-small-cell lung cancer with spread to mediastinal lymph nodes (N2); final report of RTOG 89-01. Radiation Therapy Oncology Group. *Int J Radiat Oncol Biol Phys* 2002;54(2):365–369.
70. Albain KS, Swann RS, Rusch VW, et al. Radiotherapy plus chemotherapy with or without surgical resection for stage III non-small-cell lung cancer: a phase III randomised controlled trial. *Lancet* 2009;374(9687): 379–386.
71. Albain KS, Swann RS, Rusch VW, et al. Phase III study of concurrent chemotherapy and radiotherapy (CT/RT) vs CT/RT followed by surgical resection for stage IIIA(pN2) non-small cell lung cancer (NSCLC): Outcomes update of North American Intergroup 0139 (RTOG 9309). *Proc Am Soc Clin Oncol* 2005;23(16S):7014.
72. Albain KS, Scott CB, Rusch VW, et al. Phase III comparison of concurrent chemotherapy plus radiotherapy (CT/RT) and CT/RT followed by surgical resection for stage IIIA(pN2) non-small cell lung cancer (NSCLC): Initial results from intergroup trial 0139 (RTOG 93-09). *Proc Am Soc Clin Oncol* 2003;22:621.
73. Betticher DC, Hsu Schmitz SF, Tötsch M, et al. Mediastinal lymph node clearance after docetaxel-cisplatin neoadjuvant chemotherapy is prognostic of survival in patients with stage IIIA pN2 non-small-cell lung cancer: a multicenter phase II trial. *J Clin Oncol* 2003;21(9):1752–1759.
74. Betticher DC, Hsu Schmitz SF, Tötsch M, et al. Prognostic factors affecting long-term outcomes in patients with resected stage IIIA pN2 non-small-cell lung cancer: 5-year follow-up of a phase II study. *Br J Cancer* 2006;94(8):1099–1106.
75. De Marinis F, Nelli F, Migliorino MR, et al. Gemcitabine, paclitaxel, and cisplatin as induction chemotherapy for patients with biopsy-proven Stage IIIA(N2) nonsmall cell lung carcinoma: a Phase II multicenter study. *Cancer* 2003;98(8):1707–1715.
76. Cappuzzo F, Selvaggi G, Gregorc V, et al. Gemcitabine and cisplatin as induction chemotherapy for patients with unresectable Stage IIIA-bulky N2 and Stage IIIB nonsmall cell lung carcinoma: an Italian Lung Cancer Project Observational Study. *Cancer* 2003;98(1):128–134.
77. van Meerbeeck JP, Kramer GW, Van Schil PE, et al. Randomized controlled trial of resection versus radiotherapy after induction chemotherapy in stage IIIA-N2 non-small-cell lung cancer. *J Natl Cancer Inst* 2007;99(6):442–450.
78. van Zandwijk N, Smit EF, Kramer GW, et al. Gemcitabine and cisplatin as induction regimen for patients with biopsy-proven stage IIIA N2 non-small-cell lung cancer: a phase II study of the European Organization for Research and Treatment of Cancer Lung Cancer Cooperative Group (EORTC 08955). *J Clin Oncol* 2000;18(14):2658–2664.
79. O'Brien ME, Splinter T, Smit EF, et al. Carboplatin and paclitaxol (Taxol) as an induction regimen for patients with biopsy-proven stage IIIA N2 non-small cell lung cancer. an EORTC phase II study (EORTC 08958). *Eur J Cancer* 2003;39(10):1416–1422.
80. Biesma B, Manegold C, Smit HJ, et al. Docetaxel and cisplatin as induction chemotherapy in patients with pathologically-proven stage IIIA N2 non-small cell lung cancer: a phase II study of the European organization for research and treatment of cancer (EORTC 08984). *Eur J Cancer* 2006;42(10):1399–1406.
81. Johnson DH, Rusch VW, Turrisi AT. Scalpels, beams, drugs, and dreams: challenges of stage IIIA-N2 non-small-cell lung cancer. *J Natl Cancer Inst* 2007;99(6):415–418.
82. Patel AB, Edelman MJ, Kwok Y, et al. Predictors of acute esophagitis in patients with non-small-cell lung carcinoma treated with concurrent chemotherapy and hyperfractionated radiotherapy followed by surgery. *Int J Radiat Oncol Biol Phys* 2004;60(4):1106–1112.
83. Schumacher A, Riesenbeck D, Braunheim M, et al. Combined modality treatment for locally advanced non-small cell lung cancer: preoperative chemoradiation does not result in a poorer quality of life. *Lung Cancer* 2004;44(1):89–97.
84. Ginsberg RJ, Hill LD, Eagan RT, et al. Modern thirty-day operative mortality for surgical resections in lung cancer. *J Thorac Cardiovasc Surg* 1983;86(5):654–658.
85. Harpole DH, Liptay MJ, DeCamp MM Jr, et al. Prospective analysis of pneumonectomy: risk factors for major morbidity and cardiac dysrhythmias. *Ann Thorac Surg* 1996;61(3):977–982.
86. Mitsudomi T, Mizoue T, Yoshimatsu T, et al. Postoperative complications after pneumonectomy for treatment of lung cancer: multivariate analysis. *J Surg Oncol* 1996;61(3):218–222.
87. Liptay MJ, Fry WA. Complications from induction regimens for thoracic malignancies. Perioperative considerations. *Chest Surg Clin N Am* 199;9(1):79–95.
88. Mansour Z, Kochetkova EA, Ducrocq X, et al. Induction chemotherapy does not increase the operative risk of pneumonectomy! *Eur J Cardiothorac Surg* 2007 Feb;31(2):181–185.
89. Zeldin RA, Normandin D, Landtwing D, et al. Postpneumonectomy pulmonary edema. *J Thorac Cardiovasc Surg* 1984;87(3):359–365.
90. Roach M III, Gandara DR, Yuo HS, et al. Radiation pneumonitis following combined modality therapy for lung cancer: analysis of prognostic factors. *J Clin Oncol* 1995;13(10):2606–2612.
91. Mathru M, Blakeman B, Dries DJ, et al. Permeability pulmonary edema following lung resection. *Chest* 1990;98(5):1216–1218.
92. Graham MV, Purdy JA, Emami B, et al. Clinical dose-volume histogram analysis for pneumonitis after 3D treatment for non-small cell lung cancer (NSCLC). *Int J Radiat Oncol Biol Phys* 1999;45(2): 323–329.
93. Marks LB, Ma J. Challenges in the clinical application of advanced technologies to reduce radiation-associated normal tissue injury. *Int J Radiat Oncol Biol Phys* 2007;69(1):4–12.
94. Gopal R, Tucker SL, Komaki R, et al. The relationship between local dose and loss of function for irradiated lung. *Int J Radiat Oncol Biol Phys* 2003;56(1):106–113.
95. Marks LB, Munley MT, Spencer DP, et al. Quantification of radiation-induced regional lung injury with perfusion imaging. *Int J Radiat Oncol Biol Phys* 1997;38(2):399–409.
96. Seppenwoolde Y, Muller SH, Theuws JC, et al. Radiation dose-effect relations and local recovery in perfusion for patients with non-small-cell lung cancer. *Int J Radiat Oncol Biol Phys* 2000;47(3):681–690.
97. Theuws JC, Kwa SL, Wagenaar AC, et al. Dose-effect relations for early local pulmonary injury after irradiation for malignant lymphoma and breast cancer. *Radiother Oncol* 1998;48(1):33–43.
98. Wakelee HA, Stephenson P, Keller SM, et al. Post-operative radiotherapy (PORT) or chemoradiotherapy (CPORT) following resection of stages II and IIIA non-small cell lung cancer (NSCLC) does not increase the expected risk of death from intercurrent disease (DID) in Eastern Cooperative Oncology Group (ECOG) trial E3590. *Lung Cancer* 2005;48(3):389–397.
99. Lally BE, Detterbeck FC, Geiger AM, et al. The risk of death from heart disease in patients with nonsmall cell lung cancer who receive postoperative radiotherapy: analysis of the Surveillance, Epidemiology, and End Results database. *Cancer* 2007;110(4):911–917.

100. Eberhardt WE, Albain KS, Pass H, et al. Induction treatment before surgery for non-small cell lung cancer. *Lung Cancer* 2003;42(Suppl 1): S9–S14.
101. Ettinger DS, Bepler G, Bueno R, et al. Non-small cell lung cancer clinical practice guidelines in oncology. *J Natl Compr Canc Netw* 2006;4(6):548–582.
102. Jett JR, Schild SE, Keith RL, et al. Treatment of non-small cell lung cancer, stage IIIB: ACCP evidence-based clinical practice guidelines (2nd edition). *Chest* 2007;132(3 Suppl):S266–S276.
103. Robinson LA, Ruckdeschel JC, Wagner H Jr, et al. Treatment of non-small cell lung cancer-stage IIIA: ACCP evidence-based clinical practice guidelines (2nd edition). *Chest* 2007 Sep;132(3 Suppl): S243–S265.
104. Scott WJ, Howington J, Feigenberg S, et al. Treatment of non-small cell lung cancer stage I and stage II: ACCP evidence-based clinical practice guidelines (2nd edition). *Chest* 2007 Sep;132(3 Suppl): S234–S242.

CHAPTER 56

Wilfried E.E. Eberhardt
Paul E. Van Schil
Walter Curran, Jr.
Mark A. Socinski

Stage IIIB Non–Small Cell Lung Cancer

Radiation therapy approaches remain the cornerstone of management for patients with stage IIIB advanced non–small cell lung cancer (NSCLC). Radiation therapy alone, however, is today only rarely given as a single treatment modality. Historically, combined modality trials have demonstrated that induction chemotherapy prior to radiation already improves long-term results by improvement of systemic control.[1,2] Progress has been made significantly with concurrent application of platinum-based chemotherapy to radiation treatment. This concurrent chemoradiotherapy strategy significantly increases local control and thus long-term results. At this time point, a concurrent chemoradiotherapy strategy—whenever possible—represents the standard of care for a large number of patients in this stage.[3] Platinum-based combinations have emerged as typical partners of radiation, but adequate coverage of systemic risks of the patients has to be taken into account. Different strategies have either tried to give consolidation chemotherapy following a combined chemoradiation protocol. An alternate possibility looks at an induction chemotherapy strategy followed by the definitive concurrent chemoradiation protocol. The optimal combination strategy has not yet been established so far. The reader will learn to evaluate different multimodality regimens regarding their local and systemic efficiency. At the end of this chapter, the reader should in concert with the other chapters dealing with radiotherapy delivery and application be able to (a) learn that the patient population subsumed under the IIIB stage grouping represents a very heterogeneous patient group; (b) define the different risk factors of the individual patients including their local, locoregional, and systemic risks; (c) identify the small group of patients in whom surgery still represents a valuable strategy to include in this disease subset (e.g., T4N0 to N1); (d) group comorbidity profiles of the patients concerning their impact and relevance on the choice of the treatment protocol; (e) be critically aware of the results with typical chemoradiation protocols based on either cisplatinum combinations as well as carboplatinum combinations; (f) know about the differences of radiation delivery protocols including different dosing schedules as well as dose fractionation issues; (g) learn that new ways to improve this treatment design include a possible integration of molecular-targeted agents into this setting of definitive chemoradiation; (h) identify the toxicity profiles of typical definitive chemoradiation protocols both concerning their acute toxicities as well as possible late toxicities and their proper management; and (i) lead the interdisciplinary discussion in the individual patient based on his existing risks and define the aims of a multidisciplinary treatment strategy, including systemic treatments (medical oncology), radiation therapy, and surgery in selected cases. This knowledge of the possible pros and cons of individual treatment approaches will help to critically discuss these issues with the patient and finally, following this open discussion, generate an individualized treatment strategy for each patient. At the end of this chapter, the reader will also learn possible future innovative strategies to optimize the therapeutic management of patients with stage IIIB NSCLC.

HETEROGENEITY OF PATIENTS WITH STAGE IIIB NSCLC

The International Staging System includes into stage IIIB disease different patient groups with T4 tumors as well as involvement of contralateral mediastinal nodes at the N3 position.[4] Permutations of these factors lead to different TN groupings—from T4N0 to T1N3 or even more unfavorable T4N3 categories. Recently, the proposals by the International Association for the Study of Lung Cancer (IASLC) staging committee have regrouped ipsilateral pulmonary metastases outside the involved lobe as stage T4 disease and ipsilateral pulmonary metastases inside the primarily involved lobe as T3 disease[5] (see Chapter 30). Pleural effusion and pleural metastases are now considered to be M1 disease, thus reflecting the already known separation of this group outside of any combined modality approach including radiation therapy. The newly proposed stage groupings (especially the T4 subsets) have, so far, not been implemented into the clinical trials performed with multimodality treatment in NSCLC. Future trials for patients with stage IIIB should keep this in mind and should carefully give the individual subsets included into their patient selection. The T factor represents a very different number of clinical situations with important implications on possible surgical measures. T4 disease can include potentially resectable situations as involvement of the main carina, parts of the atrium, one or two segments of trachea, vertebral body, superior vena cava infiltration, or involvement of central parts of the pulmonary artery. Other subsets include those with esophageal, thoracic aorta, or extensive cardiac involvement. These represent definitively irresectable subsets. Even in the very few potentially resectable T4 indications, surgery is today usually performed within a clearly defined multimodality setting, taking care of the increased systemic risks of these patients. Besides the stage groupings and subsets, different other prognostic factors should be recognized for these patients, but some of them are not well defined yet (Table 56.1).[6] These include histopathology (e.g., neuroendocrine, rare histopathological subsets) or tumor differentiation (G3 vs. G1), serum-lactate dehydrogenase (LDH) as an unspecific marker of tumor burden, gender (female vs. male), performance status (0,1 vs. 2), pretreatment weight loss, and patient age. Besides prognostic factors, major comorbidities have to be taken into account for development of individual treatment plans. These include pulmonary function and significant pulmonary diseases (e.g., chronic obstructive pulmonary disease [COPD], emphysema, pulmonary hypertension), cardiovascular diseases (e.g., myocardial infarction, myocardial insufficiency), cardiovascular diseases (e.g., cerebral infarction), peripheral vascular problems, or other major organ dysfunctions (renal insufficiency, hepatic insufficiency, etc.). With most patients with lung cancer being at the age older than 60 years, these factors represent significant influences for the decision making in the individual patient. A valid denominator to make the comorbidity profiles of the patients objectively measurable are different Geriatric Assessment Scores in clinical use such as the Charlson Comorbidity Index.[7] Thus, a significant heterogeneity of the patient population with stage IIIB is the natural consequence. Besides impact on potential operability of patients, comparable criteria exist concerning eligibility to intensive, definitive chemoradiation protocols, and administration of effective platinum-based chemotherapy regimen. With chemotherapy, radiotherapy, and (rarely) surgery being the major partners in multimodality treatment approaches, significant experience with handling of these modalities requires multidisciplinary treatment groups based on medical oncologists, pulmonologists, and radiation oncologists together with dedicated lung cancer surgeons. With increasing experience in the dedicated treatment center, toxicities and adverse effects of treatment can be significantly reduced, last but not the least from learning effects over time.

TABLE 56.1 Factors with Potential Influence on Prognosis of Patients with Stage IIIB NSCLC

Factors
TNM Stage (T4N0 vs. any N)
Performance status
Pretreatment weight loss
Pretreatment serum LDH
Gender
Histopathology
Tumor size and volume (for radiotherapy)
Pretreatment FEV_1 (for radiotherapy)
Pretreatment serum Hb (for radiotherapy)

FEV_1, forced expiratory volume in 1 second; LDH, lactate dehydrogenase; Hb, hemoglobin; NSCLC, non–small cell lung cancer.

Impact of Diagnostic Investigations to Define Different Subsets and Risk Groups in Stage IIIB

The small subset of patients with stage IIIB in whom surgery is being considered (T4N0) is typically staged extensively including thoracic computed tomography (CT) scans with vascular imaging studies based on adequate contrast media bolus-tracking techniques. Recently, positron emission tomography (PET) scanning has become an important addendum to the staging investigations, mainly for ruling out systemic metastases as well as mediastinal lymph node involvement.[8] Cervical, parasternal, or extended mediastinocopy are typically performed to rule out extensive mediastinal lymph node involvement (N2, N3) that represents a major adverse prognostic factor in this patient group.[9] It can be used to verify positive findings from PET studies, and sometimes thoracoscopic techniques may be added to clarify unequivocal findings from imaging investigations. Recently, endoscopic ultrasound techniques (EUS) or endobronchial ultrasound techniques (EBUS) have become an interesting alternative to extend initial staging investigations to pathologic staging of solid tumors and mediastinal and hilar lymph nodes based on fine-needle biopsies guided by ultrasound.[10] However, these patients with intensive, surgically or endoscopically based staging investigations still represent a very selective and small subset of the population with stage IIIB. If definitive chemoradiation protocols with curative intent are planned, mostly imaging investigations only are performed including CT studies. This also holds true for most clinical phase II trials or phase III studies of multimodality treatment (chemoradiation) that will be mentioned and discussed later. Recently, PET and PET-CT investigations have been included into initial staging for a better definition of the treatment fields in three-dimensional (3D) radiotherapy treatment planning.[11] Functional PET imaging studies may also be used for identifying response to multimodality treatment on induction protocols but with limited impact once radiation therapy is included into the protocol.[12] Inflammatory and stromal response to radiation treatment significantly hamper interpretation of these investigations, especially during the postradiotherapy inflammatory pneumonitis phase. It is not yet clear, whether repeated EUS- or

EBUS-guided biopsies during or following multimodality protocols may help to identify selected high-risk treatment groups or low-risk patient groups with improved prognosis following multimodality treatment. Furthermore, some investigators have proposed redo-mediastinoscopy following induction protocols to select patients with upfront involvement of the mediastinal nodes properly for definitive local treatment following their response to initial treatment.[13,14]

Surgical Indications in Selected Stage IIIB NSCLC Patients as Part of Multimodality Protocols

Biologically, patients with T4N0 stage of NSCLC represent a small but selective subgroup of patients in this stage with more locally invasive tumors and probably, a lower risk of distant metastases. This may be the background for improved results with extensive surgical approaches that have been reported within several small phase II trials in this setting. Here, we will only give the selection criteria typically used in some of the reported trials. Following extensive surgical staging that has excluded mediastinal lymph node involvement, the final aim is complete resection, which can be achieved by extensive surgical procedures including simple and intrapericardial pneumonectomies, sleeve pneumonectomies, bilobectomies, pericardectomies, cardiosurgical techniques for the left atrium, plastic vascular surgical techniques involving the pulmonary artery, its branches and superior vena cava, carinal resections, resections of one to two tracheal rings, or vertebral body resections. Long-term survival has been reported in all of these subgroups. Unfortunately, most of these clinical trials have not employed chemotherapeutic integration within induction or adjuvant treatment protocols. Some of the multimodality trials that have looked at induction chemotherapy and radiotherapy protocols also had T4N0 patients among their patient selection (Table 56.2) (Fig. 56.1). The largest ones are probably the Southwest Oncology Group (SWOG) 8805 study,[15] the West German Cancer Center trial,[16] an Italian study,[17] and a Spanish study.[18] They tested definitive surgery following chemotherapy or complex chemoradiation induction protocols. In the SWOG 8805 study, 19 patients were included with T4N0 to N1 tumors.[15] A subset analysis showed that this group had an excellent median survival of 28 months. The West German Cancer Center Study included 10 patients with T4N0 to N1 treated with induction chemotherapy followed by chemoradiotherapy and definitive surgery.[16] The median survival of this selected subgroup of patients was found to be 26.5 months with a 5-year survival rate of 37.5%. An Italian study looked at an induction chemotherapy only protocol of two cycles of cisplatinum-based chemotherapy in 43 patients with T4 disease, but this included patients with N0 as well as N1 and N2 nodal status.[17] Four-year survival rates of this selected T4 group were 19.5%, proving that long-term survival is possible with aggressive induction and surgical strategies among these patient groups. In the phase II 9901 trial of the Spanish Lung Cancer Group, selected stage IIIA-N2 and T4N0–N1 tumors were included. Patients were treated by induction chemotherapy only, followed by surgical resection.[18] Overall response rate

TABLE 56.2 Selected Phase-II Trials with Surgery as Part of a Combined Modality Approach to NSCLC Stage IIIB (T4, N3)

Investigators	Stage Subsets TNM	Treatment Program	Number of Patients	Survival (mo)	5 -Yr Survival (%)
Albain et al. [15]	T4N0–N1	PE × 2 cc RT → surgery	19	28	6 yr: 50
Eberhardt et al. [16]	T4N0–N1	PE × 3 → PE cc HF-RT → surgery	10	26.5	37.5
Rendina et al. [17]	T4Nx	PVbIM × 3 → surgery	57 R0: 36	1 yr: 61.4%	4 yr:19.5
Garrido et al. [18]	T4N0–N1	PGD × 3 → surgery	7 R0: 29	16.8	R0: 53.2
Albain et al. [15]	T1–T3N3	PE × 2 cc RT → surgery	27	NR	Cl med N3: 0 Scl N3: 35
Stamatis et al. [19]	T1–T4N3	PE × 3 → PE cc HF-RT → surgery	32	20	28
Grunenwald et al. [20]	TxN3	PVbIFU × 2 cc HF-RT → surgery	18	20	17
DeCamp et al. [21]	TxN3	PT × 2 → cc RT → surgery	20	NR	2 yr: 15

cc RT, concurrent radiotherapy; cl med, contralateral mediastinal; HF-RT, hyperfractionated accelerated RT; NR, not reported; PE, cisplatin and etoposide; PVbIM, cisplatin and vinblastine and mitomycin; PGD, cisplatinum and gemcitabine and docetaxel; PT, cisplatinum and paclitaxel; PVbIFU, cisplatin and vinblastine and 5-fluorouracil; R0, complete (R0-) resection; RT, radiotherapy; scl, supraclavicular.

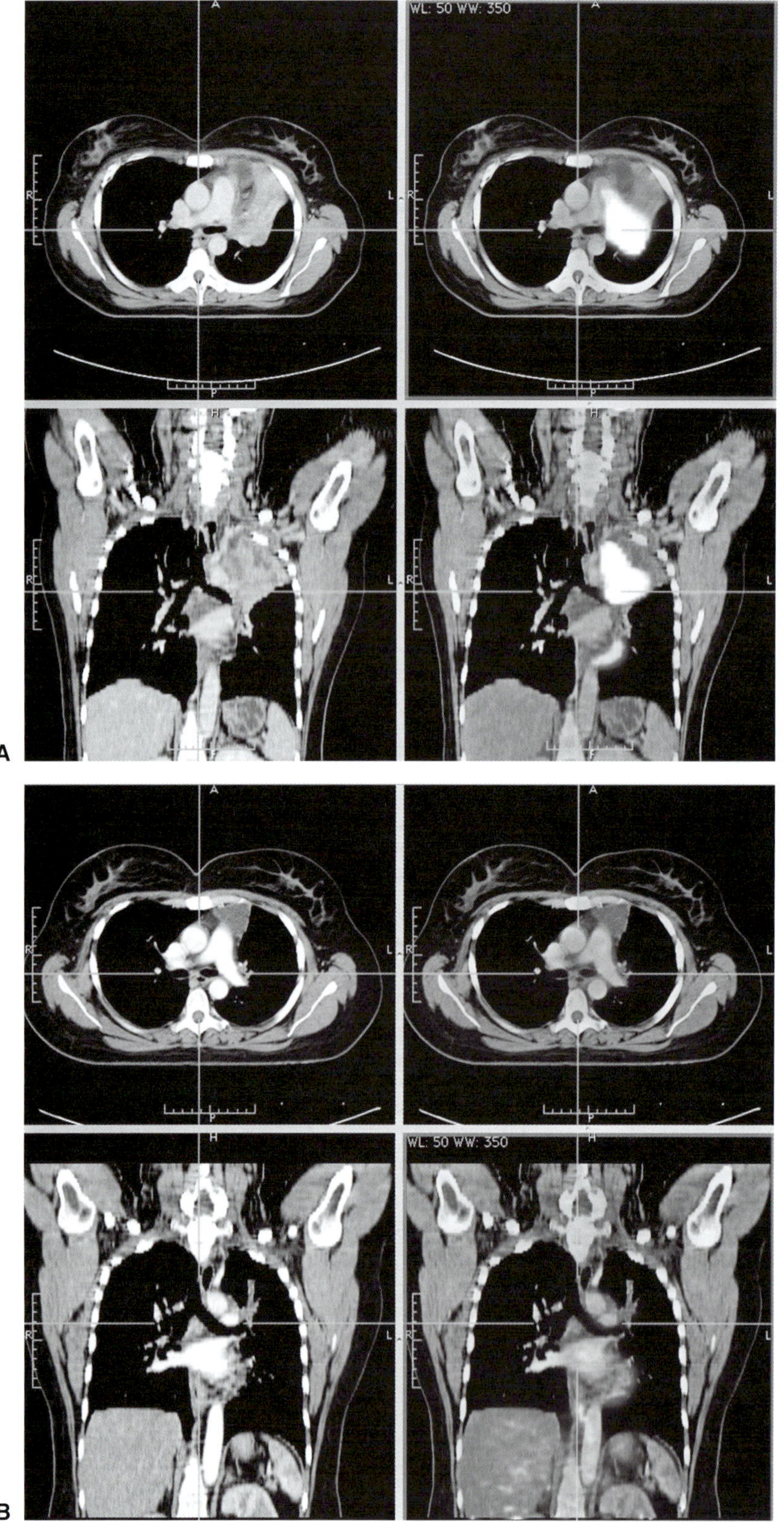

FIGURE 56.1 T4 disease with multimodality treatment including surgery. CT and PET/CT images of a patient with pathologically proven T4 disease at parasternal mediastinoscopy/thoracoscopy prior to induction treatment **(A)** and following an induction therapy **(B)** with induction chemotherapy (three cycles cisplatin and paclitaxel) followed by induction chemoradiotherapy (one cycle cisplatin and vinorelbine) with 45 Gy hyperfractionated accelerated radiotherapy (2 × 1.5 Gy bid). (See color plate.)

was 56%. In the 67 patients with stage IIIB disease, complete resection was obtained in 29 patients (43.3%). Overall median survival time for T4N0 to N1 tumors was 16.8 months. For completely resected T4N0 to N1 patients, an impressive 5-year survival rate of 53.2% was obtained.

However, surgical intervention in T4N0 tumors with necessarily extended resections has significantly increased morbidity and mortality (>5%) rates if compared with simple lobectomies. Data on surgical management in selected N3 patients are even fewer (Table 56.2; Fig. 56.2). The SWOG

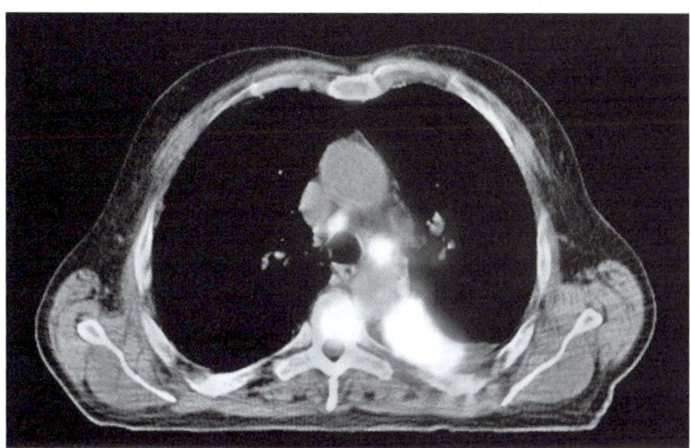

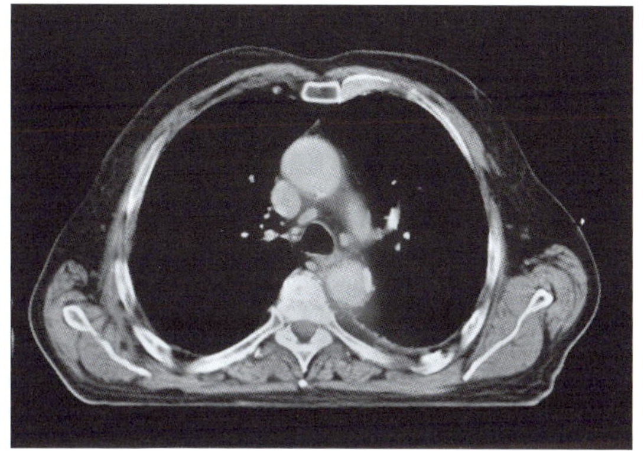

FIGURE 56.2 N3 disease with multimodality treatment including surgery. PET/CT images of a patient with mediastinoscopically proven N3 disease prior to induction treatment **(A)** and following an induction treatment **(B)** with chemotherapy (three cycles cisplatin and paclitaxel) followed by induction chemoradiotherapy (one cycle cisplatin and vinorelbine) with 45 Gy hyperfractionated accelerated radiotherapy (2 × 1.5 Gy bid). (See color plate.)

8805 included 27 patients with N3 disease in their induction chemoradiation trial, and the 2-year survival rate was 35% in the subgroup with supraclavicular N3 nodes but 0% in those with contralateral mediastinal nodes.[15] The West German Cancer Center Group reported a larger series of 32 patients with N3 disease and found a median survival of 20 months with a 5-year survival rate of 28%.[19] The Group in Paris aggressively treated 18 patients with N3 disease with induction chemoradiation followed by surgery and noticed a 17% 5-year survival rate. The surgical technique in this trial was a midline sternolaparotomy approach.[20] The Cleveland Clinics Group treated 20 patients with proven N3 disease with an induction chemoradiation protocol including cisplatin, paclitaxel, and 30- to 33-Gy radiation.[21] The 2-year survival rate to be observed was 15% in an early analysis. Typically, extended resections had to be performed, and in some trials contralateral mediastinal exploration was part of the operative procedure, whereas following complex chemoradiation protocols others did not explore the contralateral mediastinum at the time of thoracotomy. Surgical morbidity and mortality in all reported trials was increased compared with earlier disease stages. This has been the strongest argument against surgery in this setting, and it is generally accepted that this extensive surgery in the IIIB subset should be strictly performed in experienced hands in dedicated thoracic surgical centers. Furthermore, the number of patients treated in these trials was usually very small and also selective; therefore, a final evaluation of this concept is not possible. As no randomized trials are available, it is not clear whether the inclusion of surgery gives any benefit compared with definitive chemoradiation protocols that also have reported long-term survival outcomes in these stages.[22]

Historical Results of Radiation Therapy as Single Modality in Stage IIIB

Those patient subsets with stage IIIB without pleural effusion or contralateral hilar lymph node involvement historically represented the group of patients primarily treated with radiation therapy alone in the 1980s and 1990s without any surgical intervention being possible. This local and locoregional approach already achieved a 5% to 7% long-term survival rate in selected patient populations.[1,2] Radiation doses included were typically between 50 and 60 Gy over a 5 to 6 weeks' application period. Over the years, with progress in radiation therapy delivery (electrons/photons with linear accelerators vs. Cobalt sources) and treatment planning (from two-dimensional planning with two or three treatment fields to 3D treatment planning based on CT studies), some benefit could be achieved with better efficacy versus toxicity profiles of the protocols (e.g., dermatological toxicity, radiation pneumonitis, cardiac toxicities, esophageal toxicities). The strongest argument against a single treatment modality in these locally far advanced stage IIIB patients comes from their relapse pattern. Within different clinical trials, between 40% and 70% of patients developed systemic relapses (systemic metastases to liver, bone, brain, adrenals, etc.), following the local modality only approach (surgery or radiation).[1,2] This has been a major argument to introduce systemic treatment components such as chemotherapy into this setting.

Biological Rationale of Combining Chemotherapy Sequentially with Radiotherapy in Lung Cancer

Both chemotherapy and radiotherapy can theoretically have an effect on different tumor cell clones.[23] Although radiotherapy exerts its effect on local and locoregional disease, chemotherapy may add significant effects on systemic micrometastases, besides a further activity on the primary tumor and its nodal involvement. Theoretically, this effect is most pronounced when both modalities are given separately in a sequential schedule as both modalities can be delivered without major dose and dose intensity compromises. The latter usually derive from overlapping or interacting toxicities once the modalities are combined at one time. These arguments have been the background for several clinical trials in stage III NSCLC patients looking at the sequential administration of chemotherapy and radiotherapy for stage III disease where IIIB patients were predominantly included.

Sequential Approaches of Chemotherapy and Radiotherapy in Comparison with Radiation Alone

Four prospective randomized clinical trials have looked at the sequential addition of induction chemotherapy to standard fractionated radiotherapy in stage III NSCLC (Table 56.3). All trials were multicenter trials and were performed on an intent-to-treat basis with upfront randomization. All four trials used cisplatinum-based combinations as induction therapy in the experimental arm and full cumulative radiotherapy doses between 56 and 65 Gy.

The Cancer and Leukemia Group B (CALGB) 8433 study compared a standard fractionated radiotherapy protocol of 60 Gy in 6 weeks or an experimental arm with cisplatin and vinblastine combination chemotherapy for two cycles as induction (Table 56.3).[24] Patient selection included patients with good performance status and clinically staged IIIA and IIIB disease, usually low bulk lymph node involvement, and minimal weight loss. One hundred and fifty-five patients were randomized and there was a significant benefit in overall survival with 3-year survival rates of 24% versus 6% and 5-year survival rates of 17% versus 6% in favor of the induction arm ($p = 0.012$). Median survival was 13.7 months in the combined modality versus 9.6 months in the radiation only arm. Also, locoregional control was significantly improved with administration of the induction chemotherapy. No stratification was made for stage IIIB versus IIIA in this trial. The trial was prematurely closed based on positive findings at the first planned interim analysis and generated a first strong signal for the combined modality approach to stage III NSCLC patients.

Based on the positive results of this trial, a subsequent North American Intergroup trial—initially Radiation Therapy Oncology Group (RTOG) trial 8808—tested the same induction therapy of two cycles of cisplatin and vinblastine induction followed by radiation therapy of the same 60 Gy against the radiation only arm.[25] A third randomization arm of 69.9 Gy given in hyperfractionated application schedule (2 times 1.2 Gy bid) was added looking at a novel fractionation schedule of single-modality radiation therapy in this setting. No induction therapy was added in this intensified radiotherapy arm. With comparable inclusion criteria, this prospective randomized trial could confirm the benefit of induction chemotherapy followed by radiotherapy in this setting with a median survival of 17 months in the combined modality arm versus 11 months in the radiotherapy-alone arm ($p = 0.04$). However, 5-year survival rates were only marginally improved of 8% with the combination versus 5% in the radiotherapy-alone arm. No significant benefit was derived from the hyperfractionated radiotherapy application in the third arm. Critical voices following the publication of this trial argued that the low–single-fraction dosing of 1.2 Gy may be suboptimal, and one of the reasons for this failure to improve radiotherapy technique with this application schema.

The third study was performed in France as a multicenter randomized trial under the leadership of the Institute Gustave Roussy.[26] Three hundred and thirty-two patients were prospectively randomized to receive a rather uncommon induction chemotherapy protocol based on cisplatin and vindesine in combination with cyclophosphamide and lomustine (VCPC)—a combination chemotherapy protocol developed and popular in France at that time—followed by 65-Gy standard fractionated radiotherapy. The standard arm was based on 65-Gy single-modality radiation treatment alone. An important and unique addendum to the trial were predefined bronchoscopic

TABLE 56.3 Randomized Prospective Multicenter Trials of Sequential Chemotherapy and Radiotherapy versus Radiotherapy Alone

Investigators	N	Radiotherapy Dose	Chemotherapy Protocol	Locoregional Control 3-Year S (%)	Locoregional Control 5-Year S (%)	Overall Survival 3-Year S (%)	Overall Survival 5-Year S (%)
Dillman et al.[24]	77	60	NA	6[a] ($p = 0.026$)	5	6 ($p = 0.012$)	6
CALGB 8433	78	60	PVbl	18[a]	6	24	17
Sause et al.[25]	152	60	NA	NR	NR	11	5
RTOG 8808	152	60	PVbl	NR	NR	17	8 ($p = 0.04$)
	154	69.9 (1.2 bid)	NA	NR	NR	14	6
Le Chevalier et al.[26]	167	65	NA	17 (1 yr)	NR	4 ($p < 0.02$)	3
	165	65	VCPC	15 (1 yr)	NR	12	6
Brodin et al.[27]	164	56 (SplC)	NA	NR ($p = 0.07$)	3 (4 yr)	6 ($p = 0.16$)	1.4
SLCSG	163	56 (SplC)	PE	NR	7(4y)	13	3

[a]Treatment failure-free survival.

Modified from: Eberhardt W, Pöttgen C, Stuschke M. Chemoradiation paradigm for the treatment of lung cancer. *Nat Clin Pract Oncol* 2006;3:188–199.

bid, twice daily; CALGB, Cancer and Leukemia Group B; NA, not applicable; NR, not reported; PE, cisplatin and etoposide; PVbl, cisplatin and vinblastine; RTOG, Radiotherapy Oncology Group; SLCSG, Scandinavian Lung Cancer Study Group; SplC, split course; S, survival; VCPC, vindesine, lomustine, cisplatin, and cyclophosphamide.

reinvestigations looking at the local control induced in the two treatment arms. There was a significant improvement in overall survival with 3-year survival rates of 13% with induction therapy versus 4% in the standard arm, and a 5-year survival rate of 6% versus 3% in the radiotherapy-alone arm ($p < 0.02$). Local control based on the findings at bronchoscopy was only 15% in the radiotherapy-alone arm with 85% of the patients still having persistent vital tumor. The benefit observed in this study was mainly derived from an increase of systemic control in the induction chemotherapy arm.

The fourth trial in this setting was a Nordic trial looking at induction therapy with cisplatin and etoposide followed by 56 Gy of a split-dose radiation therapy versus a "standard" radiation-alone arm with the same 56-Gy split-dose protocol.[27] Three hundred and twenty-seven patients were randomized to the two treatment arms, and an increase in locoregional control was observed in the induction arm (4-year local failure-free survival rate of 7% vs. 3% in the radiotherapy-alone arm; $p = 0.07$). The difference showed a trend of improvement with the chemotherapy induction, but the benefit was not statistically significant. With overall 5-year survival rates being 3% in the induction arm and 1.4% in the radiotherapy-alone arm, no significant benefit for overall survival could be observed in this trial, either. It can only be speculated that the patient selection of this trial probably allowed a significant heterogeneity that may be responsible for the negative finding in this study.

Taken together the results of all four trials, induction chemotherapy prior to definitive radiotherapy resulted in a small but measurable benefit for overall and long-term survival in patients with stage III NSCLC. Critical commentaries should mention that in all four trials, the radiation protocols were far from being optimal concerning modern conformal radiation treatment planning standards. Also, the split-course radiotherapy application is biologically inferior and has been abandoned in the last years. Cumulative doses of 65 Gy are today accepted as standard treatment; therefore, only the French study fulfilled this rigid criterion. Cisplatinum-based chemotherapy application was still a problem at the time of performance of the first three trials. Modern antiemetic combinations represent a significant improvement for patients' compliance to these intensive protocols. Radiotherapy treatment planning was not uniformly optimally based on CT scans and 3D planning, therefore leading to higher esophagitis rates within these studies.

A unique motif of all four trials was the cisplatinum-based induction chemotherapy combination. In light of the findings for adjuvant chemotherapy, it can be argued that two cycles of chemotherapy may have been suboptimal for the systemic efficacy on micrometastases in this setting; however, cisplatinum-based protocols are currently also the major choice for effective adjuvant chemotherapy in earlier disease stages.

When transferring the presented data to the stage IIIB NSCLC population, it can be concluded that cisplatin-based induction chemotherapy may generate a small but significantly long-term survival benefit based on the systemic efficacy of the combination chemotherapy and the high risk of systemic relapse in these patient subsets. Unfortunately, a further significant risk lies in the development of brain metastases in this patient group.[28,29] Chemotherapy does not reduce the brain recurrence rate of these patient populations what can be derived from the large RTOG database.[30] Other interventions (such as prophylactic cranial irradiation) should cover those competing risks if proven effective in the future.

Biologic Rationale of Concurrent Chemoradiotherapy in Lung Cancer Radiation therapy and cytotoxic chemotherapy theoretically can target different cellular pathways (e.g., DNA-damage, DNA-repair, apoptotic pathways, signal-transduction pathways), and thus may exert their major effects on different tumor cell populations. A concurrent application might lead to additive or even supraadditive effects on growing tumors.[31] Concurrent chemotherapy to radiotherapy may prevent the development of radiotherapy-resistant tumor cell clones. Radiotherapy exerts its effect on the local and locoregional tumor. Chemotherapy not only exerts its effect locoregionally but on distant micrometastases (outside the brain) as well. By the effect of this so called spatial cooperation, the combination of both may lead to an increased overall effect of the simultaneous combination.[32] These arguments have served as the major drivers of concurrent chemotherapy and radiotherapy protocols in locally advanced NSCLC. From other solid tumors, it is well-known that cisplatin alone already serves as a significant enhancer of radiation therapy effects. Within recent years, concurrent chemoradiotherapy protocols have gradually emerged as standard treatment approaches for different locally advanced solid tumors (e.g., esophageal cancer, cervical cancer, head and neck cancer).

Concurrent Application of Chemotherapy and Radiotherapy: Single-Agent Cisplatinum Overall, four prospective randomized trials have looked at the concurrent application of single-agent cisplatinum together with radiotherapy (Table 56.4). All trials tested different schedules of cisplatinum and included patients with locally far advanced stage III disease.

A prospectively randomized multicenter Italian study randomized 173 patients to either 45-Gy standard fractionated radiotherapy and concurrent daily cisplatinum treatment versus radiation treatment alone.[33] Median survival results as well as 3-year survival rates were not significantly different between both arms. Esophageal toxicity was more pronounced in the combined modality arm. The strongest criticism to this study would include that the radiation dose of 45 Gy cannot be considered an optimal and effective radiation dose today.

The most important and influential multicenter trial was performed within the European Organization for Research and Treatment of Cancer (EORTC) and was based on a split-course radiation protocol up to 55 Gy.[34] In two arms, either weekly cisplatin or daily cisplatin were added and compared with a radiation-only comparator arm. The concurrent application of daily cisplatin led to a significant improvement of locoregional control as well as overall survival if compared with radiation

TABLE 56.4 Randomized Prospective Multicenter Trials of Concurrent Single-Agent Platinum Chemotherapy and Radiotherapy versus Radiotherapy Alone

Investigators	N	Radiotherapy Dose	Chemotherapy Protocol	Locoregional Control		Overall Survival	
				3- Year S (%)	5- Year S (%)	3- Year S (%)	5- Year S (%)
Trovó et al.[33]	88	45	NA	11[a]	NR	8	NR
GOCCNE	85	45	P daily cc	8[a]	NR	8	NR
Schaake-Koning et al.[34]	114	55 (SplC)	NA	19(2 yr)	NR	2	NR
EORTC	110	55 (SplC)	P weekly cc	30(2 yr)	NR	13	NR ($p = 0.04$)
	107	55 (SplC)	P daily cc	31(2 yr)	NR	16	NR ($p = 0.009$)
Cakir et al.[35]	88	64	NA	0 ($p = 0.0001$)	NR	2 ($p = 0.0002$)	NR
	88	64	P weeks 2,6	25	NR	10	NR
Blanke et al.[36]	123	60–65	NA	67 ($p = 0.35$)	NR	3	2
HOG	117	60–65	P days 1,22,43	69	NR	9	5
Groen et al.[37]	78	60	NA	38 (2 yr)	NR	28 (2 yr)	NR
	82	60	Carb cc daily	35 (2 yr)	NR	20 (2 yr)	NR
Clamon et al.[38]	137	60	Vbl (ind)	37[a] ($p = 0.74$)	NR	19	10 (4 yr)
CALGB	146	60	Ind + Carb weekly	49[a]	NR	19	13 (4 yr)

[a]Estimated from the data on sites of relapse and the survival plots.

Modified from: Eberhardt W, Pöttgen C, Stuschke M. Chemoradiation paradigm for the treatment of lung cancer. *Nat Clin Pract Oncol 2006;3:188–199.*

CALGB, Cancer and Leukemia Group B; Carb, carboplatin; cc, concurrent; EORTC, European Organization for Research and Treatment of Cancer; GOCCNE, North-Eastern Italian Oncology Group; HOG, Hoosier Oncology Group; ind, induction; NA, not applicable; NR, not reported; P, cisplatin; S, survival; SplC, split course.

alone. 2-y-Locoregional disease-free survival was 31% in the concurrent daily cisplatin arm versus 19% with radiation alone. The 3-year survival rate was 16% in the concurrent arm versus 2% in the radiation therapy–only arm ($p = 0.009$). The cisplatinum weekly arm showed an improvement in locoregional control and overall survival, but the data did not reach statistical significance. The combination of concurrent cisplatinum to radiotherapy showed an increase in toxicity in both arms, mainly esophageal and hematologic toxicities. No major treatment-related deaths were noticed in this landmark trial that could establish the significant effect of single-agent cisplatin as an effective radiation enhancer in NSCLC.

Only recently, a randomized Turkish study in 176 patients could substantiate a significant benefit of single-agent cisplatin given concurrently for 5 days per cycle with 64-Gy conventionally fractionated radiotherapy versus the same radiotherapy alone.[35] This study showed a significant benefit for concurrent cisplatin with 3-year survival rates of 10% of the combined modality arm versus 2% for single-modality treatment ($p = 0.0002$). Moreover, the locoregional control was significantly improved with concurrent cisplatinum with 25% 3-year locoregional progression-free survival versus 0% in the radiation-alone arm. With the adequate radiation doses of 64 Gy and with modern CT-guided treatment planning, this study clearly underlines the single-agent activity of cisplatin in this combined modality setting.

A negative trial came from the Hoosier Oncology Group (HOG) concerning this issue.[36] The group randomized 240 patients to either three weekly 70 mg/m^2 cisplatinum given concurrently with adequate 60- to 65-Gy radiotherapy versus radiotherapy alone. Although the 5-year survival rate was increased with 5% in the concurrent cisplatinum arm versus 2% in the radiotherapy-alone arm, this difference did not show statistical significance ($p = 0.35$). Locoregional control was also not different between both arms. The rather poor results in both arms may give a hint that the patient selection of this study was probably more unfavorable than the one chosen in the other studies (concerning performance status and weight loss). Nevertheless, this study clearly represents a negative trial for concurrent chemoradiotherapy based on cisplatin. It is not clear whether the three weekly application of a lower dose of cisplatin (70 mg/m^2) may be the major factor for these negative findings.

Taken together all trial results with single-agent cisplatinum, we can conclude that cisplatin alone given either in five daily applications per cycle (days 1 to 5) or as daily low-dose application has a significant radiation-enhancing effect, leading to a clinical benefit in local control. This benefit for local control translates into a significant overall survival benefit. With the systemic effect of single-agent cisplatinum on micrometastases being rather questionable, these results have prompted trials looking at an increased dose density of cytotoxic chemotherapy, giving combined chemotherapy protocols of cisplatinum doublets that will be discussed later in this chapter.

Trials of Concurrent Chemotherapy and Radiotherapy: Single-Agent Carboplatin With the platinum derivative carboplatinum being very popular in North America, it should be kept in mind that single-agent clinical data of carboplatin given concurrently to radiation are all negative, so far (Table 56.4).

A Dutch study randomized 160 patients to concurrent daily carboplatin with 60-Gy standard fractionated radiotherapy versus single-modality radiotherapy alone.[37] Two-year locoregional progression-free survival was inferior in the concurrent arm with 35% versus 38% in the radiotherapy-alone arm. Two-year overall survival rates were decreased with the carboplatinum application versus single-modality radiotherapy (20% vs. 28%). Both results, however, were not statistically significant, but the toxicity (especially esophagitis) was increased by the combined modality protocol.

The CALGB randomized 120 patients to either weekly carboplatinum given concurrently to 60-Gy standard fractionated radiotherapy or the same radiation alone.[38] Both arms were given an induction two cycles cisplatinum and vinblastine protocol. Although this study does not represent a completely fair test for concurrent carboplatinum, it is remarkable to note that no significant difference in either locoregional control nor in overall survival could be observed between the two arms. Currently, we have to state that there is no clinical evidence that the application of single-agent carboplatinum given concurrently to radiotherapy has any radiation-enhancing capacity. Together with the missing data on adjuvant chemotherapy efficacy of carboplatinum as well as data from the metaanalysis in the palliative setting of reduced efficacy of carboplatin versus cisplatin, these data could lead to a rather critical sight of carboplatin-based regimen in the curative setting of combined modality for stage III NSCLC.[39,40]

Trials of Concurrent versus Sequential Chemotherapy and Radiotherapy: Chemotherapy Combinations The benefit of induction chemotherapy added to definitive radiation is primarily based on increased systemic control with impact on systemic micrometastases outside the brain. The impact of concurrent application of chemotherapy to radiation is predominantly related to an increase in locoregional control that translates into an overall survival benefit. Therefore, several randomized clinical trials have compared these two strategies in stage III NSCLC (Table 56.5).

The West Japan Lung Cancer Group (WJLCG) randomized 314 patients to two cycles of a second-generation chemotherapy protocol consisting of mitomycin, vindesine, and cisplatinum (MVP) as induction followed by a definitive split-dose radiation protocol of 56-Gy conventionally fractionated radiotherapy in the sequential arm.[41] This was compared with the same two cycles of MVP chemotherapy giving concurrently with the same split-dose radiation of 56 Gy. This study substantiated a significant benefit in overall survival with a median survival of 16.5 months in the concurrent arm and 13.3 months in the sequential arm ($p = 0.04$). The 5-year survival rates were 16.9% in the concurrent versus 8.9% in the sequential arm, meaning nearly a doubling of long-term survivors in the concurrent treatment arm. Locoregional progression-free survival was significantly increased by the concurrent application of MVP to radiation in comparison with the sequential administration. Thus, the concurrent application in this trial led to an increase in local control that translated into a significant increase in overall survival.

TABLE 56.5 Randomized Prospective Multicenter Trials of Concurrent versus Sequential Combination Chemotherapy and Radiotherapy

Investigators	N	Radiotherapy Dose	Chemotherapy Protocol	Locoregional Control 3-Year S (%)	Locoregional Control 5-Year S (%)	Overall Survival 3-Year S (%)	Overall Survival 5-Year S (%)
Furuse et al.[41]	158	56 (SplC)	2 × MVP ind	NR	NR	15	9 ($p = 0.04$)
WJLCG	156	56 (SplC)	2 × MVP cc	NR	NR	22	16
Curran et al.[42]	611	60	2 × PVbl ind	NA	NR	32 (2 yr)	12 (4 yr)
RTOG	(total)	60	2 × PVbl cc	NR	NR	35 (2 yr)	21 (4 yr) ($p = 0.05$)
94-10	—	69.9 (1.2 bid)	2 × PorE cc	NR	NR	24 (2 yr)	17 (4 yr) ($p = 0.3$)
Huber et al.[43]	113	60	2 × CarbPac ind	49[a]	NR	18	NR ($p = 0.09$)
BROCAT	99	60	2 × CarbPac ind weekly Pac cc	57[a]	NR	25	NR
Fournel et al.[44]	101	66	3 × PVrb ind + RT	16.6	8.8 (4 yr)	18.6	14.2 (4 yr) ($p = 0.24$)
GLOT-GFPC	100	66	2 × PE cc + 2 × PVrb cons	19	15 (4 yr)	24.8	20.7 (4 yr)

[a]Estimated from the data on sites of relapse and the survival plots.

Modified from: Eberhardt W, Pöttgen C, Stuschke M. Chemoradiation paradigm for the treatment of lung cancer. *Nat Clin Pract Oncol* 2006;3:188–199.

bid, twice daily; BROCAT-G, Bronchial Carcinoma Taxol Group; Carb, carboplatin; cc, concurrent; cons, consolidation; E, etoposide; ind, induction; M, mitomycin; NA, not applicable; NR, not reported; orE, oral etoposide; P, cisplatin; Pac, paclitaxel; RT, radiotherapy; RTOG, Radiotherapy Oncology Group; GLOT-GFPC, Groupe Lyon-Saint-Etienne d'Oncologie Thoracique–Groupe Français de Pneumo-Cancérologie NPC 95-01; SplC, split course; S, survival; V, vindesine; Vbl, vinblastine, Vrb, vinorelbine; WJLCG, West Japan Lung Cancer Group.

The second landmark trial of concurrent chemotherapy versus sequential chemotherapy was the RTOG 9410 trial.[42] This study randomized 611 patients to three different treatment arms. The standard comparator arm was two cycles of cisplatin and vinblastine followed sequentially by 60-Gy conventionally fractionated radiotherapy. The first experimental arm was the same two cycles of cisplatin and vinblastine given concurrently to 60-Gy radiation. The third arm was based on an RTOG pilot trial and used cisplatin and oral etoposide giving concurrently with 69.9-Gy hyperfractionated accelerated radiotherapy (HART) (1.2 Gy bid). The final results of this trial indicated that the concurrent chemotherapy arm with standard fractionated radiotherapy gave significantly improved survival results. The 4-year survival rate was 21% in the concurrent arm versus 12% in the sequential arm ($p = 0.05$). The hyperfractionated radiotherapy arm showed intermediate results but no significant difference to the standard comparator arm.

Both studies together, the WJLCG and the RTOG trial had a significant impact on the combined modality treatment of locally advanced stage III NSCLC. Two further prospectively randomized trials have been reported that should deserve attention here.

The German BROCAT study group randomized 219 patients to induction carboplatin and paclitaxel followed by single agent weekly paclitaxel given concurrently to 60-Gy conventionally fractionated radiotherapy.[43] The standard comparator arm was based on carboplatin and paclitaxel induction chemotherapy followed by sequential radiation therapy of 60 Gy. This trial did only show a trend of survival improvement (18.7 vs. 14.7 months; $p = 0.09$). Median time to progression significantly favored the concurrent approach (11.3 vs. 6.3 months; $p < 0.001$). However, based on these study results, single-agent weekly paclitaxel cannot be considered the standard of care for concurrent chemoradiotherapy protocols.

The fourth study was the French GLOT-GFPC study group protocol NPC 95-01.[44] The French cooperative group randomized 205 patients to cisplatin and vinorelbine given as induction therapy for three cycles followed by conventionally fractionated 66-Gy radiotherapy as the standard arm. The experimental arm used a concurrent chemotherapy of two cycles cisplatin and etoposide with the same 66-Gy radiotherapy and two cycles of cisplatin and vinorelbine consolidation treatment. The study showed an increase in median survival (16.3 vs. 14.5 months) as well as 3- and 4-year survival rates (25% vs. 19%; 21% vs. 14%; $p = 0.24$) with the concurrent chemotherapy application. This study could only substantiate a trend toward better survival and long-term survival but, overall noteworthy, showed increased treatment-related deaths in both study arms (10 vs. 6 patients) that may set a note of caution to the patient selection based on comorbidity profiles of patients in this study.

Taken together, the whole accumulated dataset on concurrent versus sequential chemotherapy to radiotherapy in stage III NSCLC, the benefit of the concurrent application of combination chemotherapy seems to be moderate but clinically meaningful and significant. Especially the long-term survival rates are nearly doubled by these combined modality protocols. The toxicity profiles of the two approaches are different with significant increase in hematologic and esophageal toxicities with concurrent chemoradiation protocols. However, these toxicities are self-limiting and, therefore, concurrent chemoradiotherapy protocols have become a standard of care for most patients with good performance status, especially in the stage IIIB subset of locally advanced NSCLC.

Toxicity Profiles of Concurrent Chemoradiation Protocols The analysis of the prospectively randomized trials in stage III NSCLC revealed a significant increase in treatment-related toxicities within concurrent chemoradiation protocols.[41–44] However, these toxicities were uniformly self-limiting. The increased hematologic toxicities with more neutropenia and thrombocytopenia did uniformly not lead to an increased infection rate or an increase in bleeding episodes. The increased esophagitis rate did not lead to significantly increased fistula or late stenosis of the esophagus. Especially with modern CT-guided conformal radiotherapy planning techniques, the rates of esophagitis in the concurrent chemoradiation protocols could be further reduced and no longer represent a significant toxicity issue. Comparable to this, the initially increased pneumonitis rate with concurrent chemoradiation in cases with larger treatment fields could be significantly reduced by the new 3D-conformal treatment planning techniques with a possible significant reduction of the V20 based on more individualized treatment plans.

However, comorbidity profiles still represent an issue in the clinical decision making for patients to put on concurrent chemoradiation protocols. Age is usually not a limit on its own, a subgroup analysis of a large North American RTOG trial 94-10 showed the greatest benefit in the subgroup of patients older than 70 years of age.[45] However, significant pulmonary comorbidities resulting in reduced forced expiratory volume in 1 second (FEV_1) or reduction of diffusing capacity of the lung for carbon monoxide (D_LCO) values should lead to careful evaluation of the patients to be treated with aggressive chemoradiotherapy protocols.[46] Cardiovascular impairments should be taken into account especially in large left lower-lobe tumors with a significant part of the myocardium to be included in the treatment fields. Again, with more advanced techniques of radiation treatment planning, significantly more patients can be individually planned for combined modality approaches. It is likely, that especially with PET-CT functional imaging technology now available, in the future even more patients can be put on more conformal and restricted radiation fields within definitive high-dose chemoradiation treatments.

The Consolidation Chemotherapy Issue to Improve Systemic Control The general perception has been that two cycles of concurrent chemotherapy given concurrently to radiation therapy may not be enough systemic treatment for existing micrometastases in far locally advanced stage III tumors with significant systemic risks. This may especially hold true for patients with stage IIIB NSCLC. The pilot study was the SWOG 9405 trial looking at a surgically staged IIIB patient

TABLE 56.6 Prospective Multicenter Trials of Concurrent Radiotherapy and Chemotherapy Plus Consolidation Chemotherapy

Investigators	N	Radiotherapy Dose	Chemotherapy Protocol	Locoregional Control 3- Year S (%)	Locoregional Control 5- Year S (%)	Overall Survival 3- Year S (%)	Overall Survival 5- Year S (%)
Albain et al.[22] SWOG 9019	50	61	2 × PE cc 2 × PE cons	NR	NR	17	15
Gandara et al.[48] SWOG 9504	83	61	2 × PE cc 3 × Doce cons	17 mo[a]	NR	37	26 mo[a]
Hanna et al.[49] HOG	73	59.4	2 × PE cc + 3 × Doce cons	18[b]	NR	27.2	NR ($p = 0.940$)
	74	59.4	2 × PE cc	26[b]	NR	27.6	NR

[a]Median survival.

[b]Estimated from the data on sites of relapse or the survival plots.

cc, concurrent; cons, consolidation; Doce, docetaxel; E, etoposide; HOG, Hoosier Oncology Group; NR, not reported; P, cisplatin; S, survival; SWOG, Southwest Oncology Group.

population put on a definitive concurrent chemoradiation protocol (Table 56.6).[22] Following this study and the report of the results of the North American Intergroup trial 0139 that accrued patients in stage IIIA (N2) disease, a postoperative application of two cycles of consolidation cisplatin and etoposide had become a typical consolidation protocol after concurrent chemoradiation with two cycles of cisplatin and etoposide.[47] However, postoperative application of chemotherapy in the phase of beginning postradiation pneumonitis has eventually turned out as a difficult task. Even in the Intergroup trial, only 75% of the patients received the planned postchemoradiation consolidation. This has triggered consolidation protocols that are easier to administer. The SWOG piloted the introduction of consolidation single-agent docetaxel for three cycles following definitive chemoradiation with cisplatin and etoposide for two cycles administered concurrently to radiation (SWOG 9504).[48] The patient selection was similar to a prior chemoradiation protocol using the same chemoradiation protocol with two cycles of cisplatinum and etoposide as consolidation (SWOG 8808). Only patients with pathologic IIIB disease were included into that trial. The trial was carried out in the cooperative group multicenter setting and in 83 patients showed a median survival of 26 months, which was a major improvement in comparison with the predecessor cisplatinum and etoposide consolidation trial. The logical step following these favorable results was to carry out a multicenter prospective randomized trial. This was carried out by the Hosier Oncology group, and the final survival results of that trial have been presented at ASCO 2007.[49] The trial randomized 250 patients with stages IIIA and IIIB NSCLC to either two cycles of cisplatin and etoposide given concurrently to 63-Gy conventionally fractionated radiotherapy followed by three cycles of single-agent docetaxel consolidation versus the same chemoradiation protocol without any consolidation treatment. The final survival data showed a median overall survival of 21.5 months with consolidation docetaxel versus 24.1 months with chemoradiation alone and 3-year survival rates of 27.2% versus 27.6% in both arms, respectively. The toxicity profile significantly favored the arm without docetaxel consolidation as a significant number of treatment-related deaths was observed, probably due to the administration of docetaxel in the typical time phase of radiation-induced pneumonitis but also due to serious infections. Thus, the widely adopted consolidation docetaxel strategy in North America cannot be supported any longer in stage IIIB NSCLC management.

Induction Chemotherapy to Improve Systemic Control Prior to Definitive Chemoradiation Other groups have looked at further induction chemotherapy for systemic treatment to be added prior to definitive concurrent chemoradiation protocols (Table 56.7). The first group to pilot such a strategy was the CALGB in their prospectively randomized phase II study looking at cisplatinum-based combinations with newer drugs such as paclitaxel, gemcitabine, and vinorelbine.[50] Two cycles of the combination chemotherapy were given as induction treatment, and then two cycles of the same combination with some dose reductions of the newer drugs were given concurrently to 66-Gy conventionally fractionated radiotherapy. One hundred and seventy-five patients were randomized to receive either cisplatin and paclitaxel, cisplatin and gemcitabine, or cisplatin and vinorelbine combination chemotherapy in this setting. Overall survival rates at 3 years were not different with 19%, 28%, and 23%, respectively. The toxicity profile of the combination protocols in this trial favored the cisplatin and vinorelbine arm. Thus, either cisplatin and vinca alkaloid or cisplatin and etoposide combinations have currently the largest evidence to be combined within definitive chemoradiation protocols.

Another randomized trial has been presented at ASCO 2007 from the French Cooperative GLOT group.[51] They randomized an upfront chemoradiation arm of two cycles of cisplatin and vinorelbine to 65-Gy conventionally fractionated radiotherapy, followed by three cycles of cisplatin and paclitaxel

TABLE 56.7 Prospective Multicenter Trials of Induction Chemotherapy Plus Chemotherapy/Radiotherapy or Innovative Radiotherapy

Investigators	N	Radiotherapy Dose	Chemotherapy Protocol	Locoregional Control		Overall Survival	
				3-Year S (%)	5-Year S (%)	3-Year S (%)	5-Year S (%)
Vokes et al.[50] CALGB	62	66	2 × PG ind + 2 × PG cc	18[a]	NR	28[a]	18.3 mo[b]
	58	66	2 × PT ind + 2 × PT cc	18[a]	NR	22[a]	14.8 mo[b]
	55	66	2 × PV ind + 2 × PV cc	18[a]	NR	20[a]	17.7 mo[b]
Fournel et al.[51] GLOT	63	66	2 × PV cc + 3 × PT cons	NR	8.2 mo[b]	32	15 mo[b]
	64	66	3 × PT ind + 2 × PV cc	NR	11.5 mo[b]	31.6	19 mo[b]
Vokes et al.[52] CALGB	170	66	2 × CarbPac ind + CarPac cc	8 mo[b]	NR	31 (2 yr)	14 mo[b] (p =0.11 Cox)
	161	66	CarbPac cc + 2 × CarPac cons	7 mo[b]	NR	29 (2 yr)	12 mo[b]
Socinski et al.[53] CALGB	42	74	2 × CarPac ind + weekly CarPac cc	21.3	NR	37.1	24.3 mo[b]
	26	74	2 × CarGem ind + 2 × weekly Gem cc	19.2	NR	30.8	12.5 mo[b]
Belani et al.[55] ECOG	59	64 qd	2 × CarbPac ind	8.2 mo[b]	NR	18	14.9 mo[b] (p = 0.28)
	60	57.6 1.5 Gy tid	2 × CarbPac ind	9.3 mo[b]	NR	24	20.3 mo[b]

[a]Estimated from the data on sites of relapse and the survival plots.

[b]Median survival.

CALGB, Cancer and Leukemia Group B; Carb, carboplatin; cc, concurrent; cons, consolidation; Cox, Cox model; ECOG, Eastern Cooperative Oncology Group; GLOT, Groupe Lyon-Saint Etienne d 'Oncologie Thoracique; Gem, gemcitabine; ind, induction; NR, not reported; P, cisplatin; qd, every day; RT, radiotherapy; S, survival; T or Pac, paclitaxel; tid, thrice daily; V, vinorelbine.

versus an induction chemotherapy arm of three cycles of cisplatin and paclitaxel, followed by the concurrent chemoradiotherapy based on cisplatin and vinorelbine. Although not planned as a phase III trial, this study observed somehow better survival outcome in the induction therapy arm with cisplatin and paclitaxel. Because of the small number of patients in this study (n = 201), overall survival results are not conclusive and should be interpreted with caution.

The CALGB in their follow-up trial to the randomized phase II based on cisplatinum protocols investigated a carboplatinum combination with paclitaxel.[52] They randomized 366 patients to either upfront weekly concurrent carboplatin and paclitaxel together with 66-Gy standard fractionated radiation versus an induction protocol of two cycles of carboplatin and paclitaxel followed by the same concurrent chemoradiation with weekly carboplatin and paclitaxel. The induction arm did better with 3-year survival rates of 24% versus 18% in the upfront chemoradiation arm although only a trend was reached statistically with a p value of 0.1. However, both arms still fared poorly in comparison to their earlier studies and to other multicenter chemoradiation trials results. It could as well be, and it was subsequently speculated that the patient population was too negatively selected within this study including patients with significant weight loss, and thus, changing to a prognostically more unfavorable patient subgroup.

Thus, with these existing conflicting results, induction chemotherapy has not yet emerged as a standard of care for patients with stage IIIB NSCLC. Differently to experience in head and neck cancer trials, induction protocols in NSCLC may only show significantly high enough activity in a defined proportion of the patient population. Adequate results have, so far, only been achieved with cisplatinum-based combinations. Carboplatin-based protocols and especially weekly low-dose chemotherapy may not be appropriate in the curative setting of aggressive multimodality treatment protocols. Future testing of aggressive induction strategies based on newer and more active chemotherapy protocols as well as the introduction of molecular targeted drugs such as epidermal growth factor receptor (EGFR) drugs (e.g., cetuximab) may be necessary to achieve more downsizing and downstaging of tumors prior to the definitive chemoradiation protocol aiming predominantly at locoregional control of the tumor.

Higher Radiation Doses or Alternative Fractionation following Induction Therapy Protocols The CALGB has piloted a more aggressive protocol based on an induction chemotherapy strategy followed by a dose-escalated conformal radiation therapy up to 74 Gy in stage III NSCLC patients.[53] The trial was a randomized phase II protocol including 67 patients (Table 56.7). The patients were randomized to an induction protocol of either carboplatin and paclitaxel (Arm A) or carboplatin and gemcitabine (Arm B). Arm A received a concurrent application of further carboplatin and paclitaxel given to 74-Gy conventionally fractionated high-dose conformal radiotherapy. Arm B received biweekly gemcitabine concurrently to high-dose radiotherapy of 74 Gy. Arm B had to be closed early because of high grade 4 and 5 toxicities observed. Arm A reached its predefined end point with a median survival of 18 months in the selected patient subset. This protocol is currently being tested in a randomized trial of CALGB versus a standard-dose chemoradiation protocol. A further phase I trial within CALGB has been looking at an innovative chemotherapeutic induction regimen of carboplatin and paclitaxel combined with bevacizumab as well as erlotinib followed by a definitive high-dose radiation protocol to 74 Gy together with weekly carboplatin and paclitaxel[54] (Table 56.8). Final efficacy and toxicity results have to be awaited for further interpretation of this aggressive strategy.

Eastern Cooperative Oncology Group (ECOG) has piloted a more aggressive accelerated radiation fractionation schedule with the HART protocol (Table 56.7).[55] Accelerated fractionation has a strong radiobiological rationale to support it as time for radiation-induced damage repair is significantly shortened by giving several daily fractions of treatment and reducing the overall treatment duration. ECOG randomized 112 patients with stage III NSCLC following induction chemotherapy with carboplatin and paclitaxel to either conventionally fractionated radiotherapy with 64 Gy or an accelerated radiotherapy fractionation of 57.6 Gy given in three daily fractions with an overall treatment duration of 2.5 weeks. Although the patient number of this study was too small and the study had to close early because of poor patient accrual, the accelerated fractionation arm had a 3-year survival rate of 24% versus 18% in the conventionally fractionated treatment arm. There was a trend for improved survival results with the accelerated radiotherapy but because of the small number of patients randomized, this study has no conclusive results concerning the overall efficacy of such an intensive radiation therapy approach.

Future Directions Including the Introduction of Molecular-Targeted Agents into this Setting Besides the aforementioned phase I trial in CALGB, first experience has been reported looking at an EGFR tyrosine kinase inhibitor maintenance treatment in the setting of stage IIIB NSCLC following definitive chemoradiation and consolidation docetaxel.[56] This large randomized trial included stage III NSCLC patients without disease progression under treatment with chemoradiation and consolidation docetaxel (Table 56.8). The patients were then randomized to either maintenance treatment with gefitinib or placebo. The trial accrued 572 eligible patients and was able to randomize 243 patients to either maintenance gefitinib or placebo. More than half of the patient population was initially found to be in stage IIIB NSCLC. Needless to say, this treatment was given to unselected patients concerning their molecular signal transduction and mutational EGFR status. The trial had to be closed down because the first interim analysis presented an inferior survival result in the arm randomized to maintenance gefitinib (median survival 35 months with maintenance placebo vs. 23 months with

TABLE 56.8 Prospective Multicenter Trials of Molecular Targeted Drugs in Multimodality Treatment of Stage IIIB NSCLC

Investigators	N	Radiotherapy Dose	Chemotherapy Protocol	Locoregional Control		Overall Survival	
				3-Year S (%)	5-Year S (%)	3-Year S (%)	5-Year S (%)
Socinski et al.[53] CALGB	20	74	2 × CarPacBev ind weekly CarPac + Bev (+E) cc	NR	NR	NR	NR
Kelly et al.[56] SWOG	118	61	2 × PE cc + 3 × Doce cons + Gef	NR	8.3 mo[a]	46 (2 yr)	23 mo[a] ($p = 0.013$)
	125	61	2 × PE cc + 3 × Doce cc + Plac	NR	11.7 mo[a]	59 (2 yr)	35 mo[a]
Blumenschein[60] RTOG	87	63	weekly CarPacCetux cc + 2 × CarPac cons + Cetux cons	NR	NR	49.3 (2 yr)	22.7 mo[a]

[a] Median survival.

Bev, bevacizumab; CALGB, Cancer and Leukemia Group B; Car, carboplatin; cc, concurrent; Cetux, cetuximab; cons, consolidation; Doce, docetaxel; E, erlotinib; E, etoposide; Gef, gefitinib; ind, induction; NR, not reported; P, cisplatin; Pac, paclitaxel; Plac, placebo; S, survival; SWOG, Southwest Oncology Group; RTOG, Radiotherapy Oncology Group.

maintenance gefitinib). It is still not clear whether these unfavorable results are based on a significant selection bias between the arms or related to an imbalance of major prognostic factors or if this study gives a hint that EGFR inhibitors could be deleterious in unselected patient populations such as the one chosen in this trial.

Recently, very positive data have been presented with the combination of chemotherapy together with cetuximab in the first-line treatment of advanced NSCLC.[57] In head and neck cancer, very positive data have been reported with single-agent cetuximab as a radiation sensitizer within a large randomized phase III trial.[58] The survival benefit observed in that trial was found to be 10% at 5 years, comparable with the range of benefit achieved with cisplatin-based chemotherapy when given concurrently to radiotherapy in the same setting (8% at 5 years, results of the metaanalysis).[59] Based on these encouraging results, the RTOG has performed a pilot phase II trial of concurrent chemoradiotherapy based on a weekly carboplatin and paclitaxel protocol combined with weekly cetuximab treatment, a 63-Gy upfront conventionally fractionated radiotherapy followed by consolidation single-agent cetuximab, followed by two further cycles of carboplatin and paclitaxel together with cetuximab (Table 56.8)[60] The preliminary data of this trial for 93 patients entered have been presented at ASCO 2007 and with longer follow up at ASCO 2008. The combination was found to be feasible with moderate acute and late toxicities. Nearly half of the patient population was initially found to have stage IIIB disease. Preliminary efficacy data showed encouraging survival results in this patient cohort. The group is currently planning to perform a large randomized phase III trial with the same regimen looking at the impact of cetuximab administration in this setting.

Further, pilot trials are currently performed with VEGF-acting drugs such as bevacizumab in the combined modality approach to stage III patients (see also previous discussion). When introducing new molecular-targeted agents into the setting of chemoradiation protocols, interaction with radiation as well as amelioration of radiation induced pneumonitis have to be carefully monitored.[61] Both acute as well as late effects should be screened and well documented. Thus, the development of future progress within this combined modality setting will be time consuming and slowly.

CONCLUSION

For most patients with stage IIIB NSCLC, a combination of chemotherapy with radiotherapy remains the most optimal treatment strategy with a curative intent. Nevertheless, it should be kept in mind that IIIB disease in itself represents a very heterogeneous group of patients spanning from T4N0 tumors with less biologic aggressiveness to metastasize on one hand, to T1N3 disease on the other hand with small primary tumors that have a striking tendency to metastasize early into mediastinal nodes as well as to promote micrometastatic spread. Furthermore, even T4 disease represents several subsets of patients, including those with potentially resectable T4 tumors involving the carina, the distal trachea, the superior vena cava, the left atrium, and a vertebral body. In contrast to that, other T4 subsets include patients definitely found to be unresectable such as T4 tumors invading the thoracic aorta, the esophagus, the pulmonary artery main stem, and the myocardium. The new IASLC staging system will recognize prognostic differences observed within the large database for T4 tumors and will regroup prior M1 pulmonary satellite nodes in ipsilateral lobes outside the primarily involved lobe as T4 disease. Comparable to this, pleural effusion and pleural metastasis found at thoracotomy or thoracoscopy will be regrouped into the M1a disease category. Satellite nodules in the same lobe as the primary will be regrouped as T3 disease because they present a subgroup with a more favorable long-term prognosis. Several groups have reported selected patient cohorts with definitive surgical treatment in stage IIIB. However, these trials usually had small patient numbers, represent selective patients subsets, and patients were usually treated within combined modality protocols including chemotherapy-positive/negative radiotherapy prior to definitive surgery. The T4N0 subset of IIIB may represent a specific group of patients with favorable outcome when put on multimodality protocols. Some data have also been reported on surgery in further patient groups, including N3 disease in contralateral mediastinal and even supraclavicular nodes. The overall value of surgery in this setting is not established, and patients should be preferably included into prospective trials if surgery is to be included within the combined modality approach.

On the whole and looking at the broader patient population, concurrent chemoradiotherapy protocols as definitive treatment with curative intent have achieved the best results, so far. The largest experience has been reported with cisplatin-based combinations—either cisplatin and etoposide or cisplatin and vinorelbine given concurrently with conventionally fractionated radiotherapy protocols up to 63- or 66-Gy cumulative doses. Based on the single-agent data of cisplatin and carboplatin from early randomized chemoradiation trials, cisplatin may be preferred to carboplatin as the backbone of concurrent chemotherapy in this setting. Induction chemotherapy prior to sequential radiotherapy has proven to be superior to radiation therapy alone with an improvement in long-term survivors. Concurrent chemotherapy to radiotherapy has achieved a significant increase in local control, and thus in overall survival. This strategy has become the preferred approach to patients with stage IIIB NSCLC in recent years. The broadest evidence of chemoradiation protocols comes from the IIIA disease setting with cisplatin and etoposide given for two cycles of concurrent chemotherapy to radiotherapy. Typically, two cycles of cisplatin and etoposide are added as consolidation chemotherapy. Consolidation with single-agent docetaxel has shown encouraging results in a multicenter phase II trial. These favorable results could not be confirmed in the HOG randomized phase III comparison where consolidation docetaxel did not result in a survival improvement but rather led to increased morbidities and an increase in treatment-related deaths. Whether induction chemotherapy based on cisplatin combinations—as piloted in the

CALGB study—will further improve the results by an impact on systemic micrometastases and downsizing and downstaging effects on the primary tumor is not yet known. However, it is clear that systemic metastases remain the major issue for a significant number of patients in this disease stage. The search for molecular-targeted drugs that may further enhance the chemoradiation strategy has recently begun. EGFR-acting drugs have already been tested within pilot phase II trials, and the first randomized trial looking at maintenance strategy with these drugs has already been reported. Whether this innovative approach can be applied to unselected patient populations or will have to be introduced within previously well-defined patients' subsets based on signal transduction studies is not yet known. Unfortunately, another significant competing risk of these patients' subgroups lies in the development of brain metastases. Chemotherapy has no effect to reduce these brain relapses prophylactically. Prophylactic cranial irradiation seems to be the natural intervention in high-risk populations, but data on survival impact from randomized trials are missing, so far.

REFERENCES

1. Stinchcombe TE, Fried D, Morris DE, et al. Combined modality therapy for stage III non-small cell lung cancer. *The Oncologist* 2006; 11:809–823.
2. Eberhardt W, Poettgen C, Stuschke M. Chemoradiation paradigm for the treatment of lung cancer. *Nat Clin Pract Oncol* 2006;3:188–199.
3. Jett JR, Schild SE, Keith RL, et al. American College of Chest Physicians. Treatment of non-small cell lung cancer, stage IIIB: ACCP evidence-based clinical practice guidelines (2nd edition). *Chest* 2007; 132:S266–S276.
4. Mountain CF. Revisions in the International System for Staging Lung Cancer. *Chest* 1997;11:1710–1717.
5. Rami-Porta R, Ball D, Crowley J, et al. International Staging Committee. The IASLC Lung Cancer Staging Project: proposals for the revision of the T descriptors in the forthcoming (seventh) edition of the TNM classification for lung cancer. *J Thorac Oncol* 2007:593–602.
6. Sculier JP, Chansky K, Crowley JJ, et al. International Staging Committee and Participating Institutions. The impact of additional prognostic factors on survival and their relationship with the anatomical extent of disease expressed by the 6th Edition of the TNM Classification of Malignant Tumors and the proposals for the 7th Edition. *J Thorac Oncol* 2008;3:457–466.
7. Charlson ME, Pompei P, Ales KL, et al. A new method of classifying prognostic comorbidity in longitudinal studies: development and validation. *J Chronic Dis* 1987;40:373–383.
8. Vansteenkiste JF, Stroobants SS. PET scan in lung cancer: current recommendations and innovation. *J Thorac Oncol* 2006;1:71–73.
9. Ginsberg RJ. Extended cervical mediastinoscopy. *Chest Surg Clin N Am* 1996;6:21–30.
10. Herth FJ, Annema JT, Eberhardt R, et al. Endobronchial ultrasound with transbronchial needle aspiration for restaging the mediastinum in lung cancer. *J Clin Oncol* 2008;26:3346–3350.
11. Chang JY, Dong L, Liu H, et al. Image-guided radiation therapy for non-small cell lung cancer. *J Thorac Oncol* 2008;3:177–186.
12. Poettgen C, Levegruen S, Theegarten D, et al. Value of 18F-fluorodeoxy-D-glucose-positron emission tomography/computed tomography in non-small cell lung cancer for prediction of pathological response and times to relapse after neoadjuvant chemoradiotherapy. *Clin Cancer Res* 2006;12:97–106.
13. Van Schil P, De Waele M. A second mediastinoscopy: how to decide and how to do it ? *Eur J Cardiothorac Surg* 2008;33:703–706.
14. Marra A, Hillejan L, Fechner S, et al. Remediastinoscopy in restaging of lung cancer after induction therapy. *J Thorac Cardiovasc Surg* 2008; 135:843–849.
15. Albain KS, Rusch VW, Crowley JJ, et al. Concurrent cisplatin/etoposide plus chest radiotherapy followed by surgery for stages IIIA (N2) and IIIB non-small-cell lung cancer: mature results of Southwest Oncology Group Phase II Study 8805. *J Clin Oncol* 1995;13:1880–1892.
16. Eberhardt W, Wilke H, Stamatis G, et al. Preoperative chemotherapy followed by concurrent chemoradiation therapy based on hyperfractionated accelerated radiotherapy and definitive surgery in locally advanced nonsmallcell lung cancer: mature results of a phase II trial. *J Clin Oncol* 1998;6:622–634.
17. Rendina EA, Venuta F, De Giacomo T, et al. Induction chemotherapy for centrally located non-small cell lung cancer. *J Thorac Cardiovasc Surg* 1999;117:225–233.
18. Garrido P, González-Larriba JL, Insa A, et al. Long-term survival associated with complete resection after induction chemotherapy in stage IIIA (N2) and IIIB (T4N0-1) non small-cell lung cancer patients: the Spanish Lung Cancer Group Trial 9901. *J Clin Oncol* 2007; 25:4736-4742.
19. Stamatis G, Eberhardt W, Stueben G, et al. Preoperative chemoradiotherapy and surgery for selected non-small cell lung cancer IIIB subgroups: long-term results. *Ann Thorac Surg* 1999;68:1144–1149.
20. Grunenwald DH, Andre F, Le PC, et al. Benefit of surgery after chemoradiotherapy in stage IIIB (T4 and/or N3) nonsmall cell lung cancer. *J Thorac Cardiovasc Surg* 2001;122:796–802.
21. DeCamp MM, Rice TW, Adelstein DJ, et al. Value of accelerated multimodality therapy in stage IIIA and IIIB non-small cell lung cancer. *J Thorac Cardiovasc Surg* 2003;126:17–27.
22. Albain KS, Crowley JJ, Turrisi AT III, et al. Concurrent cisplatin, etoposide, and chest radiotherapy in pathologic stage IIIB non-small cell lung cancer: a Southwest Oncology Group phase II study, SWOG 9019. *J Clin Oncol* 2002;20:3454–3460.
23. Tannock IF. Treatment of cancer with radiation and drugs. *J Clin Oncol* 1996;52:3156–3174.
24. Dillman RO, Herndon J, Seagren SL, et al. Improved survival in stage III non-small cell lung cancer: seven-year follow-up of cancer and leukemia group B (CALGB) 8433 trial. *J Natl Cancer Inst* 1996; 88:1210–1215.
25. Sause WT, Kolesar P, Taylor S, et al. Final results of phase III trial in regionally advanced unresectable non-small cell lung cancer: radiation Therapy Oncology Group, Eastern Cooperative Oncology Group, Southwest Oncology Group. *Chest* 2000;117:358–364.
26. Le Chevalier T, Arriagada R, Quoix E, et al. Radiotherapy alone versus combined chemotherapy and radiotherapy in nonresectable non-small-cell lung cancer. First analysis of a randomized trial in 353 patients. *J Natl Cancer Inst* 1991;83:417–423.
27. Brodin O, Nou E, Mercke C, et al. Comparison of induction chemotherapy before radiotherapy with radiotherapy only in patients with locally advanced squamous cell carcinoma of the lung. The Swedish Lung Cancer Study Group. *Eur J Cancer* 1996;32A:1893–1900.
28. Andre F, Grunenwald D, Pujol J L, et al. Patterns of relapse of N2 nonsmall-cell lung carcinoma patients treated with preoperative chemotherapy: should prophylactic cranial irradiation be reconsidered? *Cancer* 2001;91:2394–2400.
29. Stuschke M, Eberhardt W, Pottgen C, et al. Prophylactic cranial irradiation in locally advanced non-small cell lung cancer after multimodality treatment: longterm followup and investigations of late neuropsychologic effects. *J Clin Oncol* 1999;7:2700–2709.
30. Robnett TJ, Machtay M, Stevenson JP, et al. Factors affecting the risk of brain metastases after definitive chemoradiation for locally advanced non-small-cell lung cancer. *J Clin Oncol* 2001;19:1344–1349.
31. Weichselbaum RR, Beckett MA, Vokes EE, et al. Cellular and molecular mechanisms of radioresistance. *Cancer Treat Res* 1995;74:131–140.
32. Bentzen SM, Harari PM, Bernier J. Exploitable mechanisms for combining drugs with radiation: concepts, achievements and future directions. *Nat Clin Pract Oncol* 2007;4:172–180.

33. Trovó MG, Minatel E, Franchin G, et al. Radiotherapy versus radiotherapy enhanced by cisplatin in stage III non-small cell lung cancer. *Int J Radiat Oncol Biol Phys* 1992;24:11–15.
34. Schaake-Koning C, van den Bogaert W, Dalesio O, et al. Effects of concomitant cisplatin and radiotherapy on inoperable non-small-cell lung cancer. *N Engl J Med* 1992;326:524–530.
35. Cakir S, Egehan I. A randomised clinical trial of radiotherapy plus cisplatin versus radiotherapy alone in stage III non-small cell lung cancer. *Lung Cancer* 2004;43:309–316.
36. Blanke C, Ansari R, Mantravadi R, et al. Phase III trial of thoracic irradiation with or without cisplatin for locally advanced unresectable non-small-cell lung cancer: a Hoosier Oncology Group protocol. *J Clin Oncol* 1995;13:1425–1429.
37. Groen H, van der Leest AH, Fokkema E, et al. Continuously infused carboplatin used as radiosensitizer in locally unresectable non-small-cell lung cancer: a multicenter phase III study. *Ann Oncol* 2004;15:427–432.
38. Clamon G, Herndon J, Cooper R, et al. Radiosensitization with carboplatin for patients with unresectable stage III non-small-cell lung cancer: a phase III trial of the Cancer and Leukemia Group B and the Eastern Cooperative Oncology Group. *J Clin Oncol* 1999;17:4–11.
39. Aupérin A, Le Péchoux C, Pignon JP, et al. Concomitant radio-chemotherapy based on platin compounds in patients with locally advanced non-small cell lung cancer (NSCLC): a meta-analysis of individual data from 1764 patients. *Ann Oncol* 2006;17:473–483.
40. Ardizzoni A, Boni L, Tiseo M, et al. Cisplatin- versus carboplatin-based chemotherapy in the first-line treatment of advanced non-small cell lung cancer: an individual patient data meta-analysis. *J Natl Cancer Inst* 2007;99:847–857.
41. Furuse K, Fukuoka M, Kawahara M, et al. Phase III study of concurrent versus sequential thoracic radiotherapy in combination with mitomycin, vindesine, and cisplatin in unresectable stage III non-small-cell lung cancer. *J Clin Oncol* 1999;17:2692–2699.
42. Curran W, Scott C, Langer C. Long-term benefit is observed in a phase III comparison of sequential vs concurrent chemoradiation for patients with unresectable stage III NSCLC: RTOG 9410. *J Clin Oncol* 2003;22:2499.
43. Huber RM, Flentje M, Schmidt M, et al. Simultaneous chemoradiotherapy compared with radiotherapy alone after induction chemotherapy in inoperable stage IIIA or IIIB non-small-cell lung cancer: study CTRT99/97 by the Bronchial Carcinoma Therapy Group. *J Clin Oncol* 2006;24:4397–4404.
44. Fournel P, Robinet G, Thomas P, et al. Randomized phase III trial of sequential chemoradiotherapy compared with concurrent chemoradiotherapy in locally advanced non-small-cell lung cancer: Groupe Lyon-Saint-Etienne d'Oncologie Thoracique-Groupe Francais de Pneumo-Cancerologie NPC 95-01 Study. *J Clin Oncol* 2005;23:5910–5917.
45. Langer C, Curran WJ, Komaki R, et al. Elderly patients with locally advanced non-small cell lung cancer benefit from combined modality: secondary analysis of Radiation Therapy Oncology Group 94-10. *Proc Am Soc Clin Oncol* 2002;21 (abstr 1193).
46. Gopal R, Starkshall G, Tucker SL, et al. Effects of radiotherapy and chemotherapy on lung function in patients with non-small-cell lung cancer. *Int J Radiat Oncol Biol Phys* 2003;56:114–120.
47. Albain KS, Swann RS, Rusch VR, et al. Phase III study of concurrent chemotherapy and radiotherapy (CT/RT) versus CT/RT followed by surgical resection for stage IIIA-N2 non-small cell lung cancer: outcomes update of North American Intergroup 0139 (RTOG 9309). *J Clin Oncol* 2005;23 no.16S:624s (abstract 7014).
48. Gandara DR, Chansky K, Albain KS, et al. Consolidation docetaxel after concurrent chemoradiotherapy in stage IIIB non-small-cell lung cancer: phase II Southwest Oncology Group Study S9504. *J Clin Oncol* 2003;21:2004–2010.
49. Hanna NH, Neubauer M, Ansari R, et al. Phase-III trial of cisplatin plus etoposide concurrent chest radiation with or without consolidation docetaxel in patients with inoperable stage III non-small cell lung cancer: HOG 01-24/USO-023. *J Clin Oncol* 2007;25:7512.
50. Vokes EE, Herndon JE II, Crawford J, et al. Randomized phase II study of cisplatin with gemcitabine or paclitaxel or vinorelbine as induction chemotherapy followed by concomitant chemoradiotherapy for stage IIIB non-small-cell lung cancer: cancer and leukemia group B study 9431. *J Clin Oncol* 2002;20:4191–4198.
51. Fournel P, Vernengegre A, Robinet G, et al. Induction or consolidation chemotherapy with cisplatin and paclitaxel plus concurrent chemoradiation with carboplatin and vinorelbine for unresectable non-small cell lung cancer patients: randomized phase-II trial GFPC-GLOT-IFCT 02-01. *J Clin Oncol* 2006;24:7048.
52. Vokes EE, Herndon JE II, Kelley MJ, et al., Induction chemotherapy followed by chemoradiotherapy compared with chemoradiotherapy alone for regionally advanced unresectable stage III Non-small-cell lung cancer: Cancer and Leukemia Group B. *J Clin Oncol* 2007;25:1698–1704.
53. Socinski MA, Blackstock W, Bogart JA, et al. Randomized Phase II trial of induction chemotherapy followed by concurrent chemotherapy and dose-escalated thoracic conformal radiotherapy (74 Gy) in stage III non-small cell lung cancer. *J Clin Oncol* 2008;28:2457–2463.
54. Socinski MA, Morris DE, Stinchcombe TE, et al. Incorporation of bevacizumab and erlotinib with induction and concurrent carboplatin and paclitaxel and 74 Gy of thoracic radiotherapy in stage III non-small cell lung cancer. *J Clin Oncol* 2008;26:7517.
55. Belani C P, Wang W, Johnson D H, et al. Phase III study of the Eastern Cooperative Oncology Group (ECOG 2597): induction chemotherapy followed by either standard thoracic radiotherapy or hyperfractionated accelerated radiotherapy for patients with unresectable stage IIIA and B non-small-cell lung cancer. *J Clin Oncol* 2005;23:3760–3767.
56. Kelly K, Natale R, Wade J, et al. Phase-III trial of maintenance gefitinib or placebo after concurrent chemoradiotherapy and docetaxel consolidation in inoperable stage III non-small cell lung cancer. SWOG S0023. *J Clin Oncol* 2008;26:2450–2456.
57. Pirker R, Szczesna A, von Pawel J, et al. FLEX: A multicenter phase-III study of cetuximab in combination with cisplatin and vinorelbine versus CV alone in the first-line treatment of patients with advanced non-small cell lung cancer. *J Clin Oncol* 2008;26:3.
58. Bonner JA, Harari PM, Giralt J, et al. Radiotherapy plus cetuximab for squamous-cell carcinoma of the head and neck. *N Engl J Med* 2006; 354:567–578.
59. Pignon JP, Bourhis J, Domenge C, et al. Chemotherapy added to locoregional treatment for head and neck squamous cell carcinoma: three meta-analyses of updated individual data. MACH-NC Collaborative Group. Meta-Analysis of Chemotherapy in Head and Neck Cancer. *Lancet* 2000;355:949–955.
60. Blumenschein GR, Paulus R, Curran WJ, et al. A phase-II study with chemoradiation in patients with stage IIIA/B non-small cell lung cancer: a report of 2-year and median survival for the RTOG 0324 trial. *J Clin Oncol* 2008;26:7516.
61. Blackstock AW, Ho C, Butler J, et al. Phase-Ia/b chemoradiation trial of gemcitabine and dose-escalated thoracic radiation in patients with stage IIIA/B non-small cell lung cancer. *J Thorac Oncol* 2006; 1:434–440.

CHAPTER 57

Elizabeth Gore

Prophylactic Cranial Irradiation in Non–Small Cell Lung Cancer

Brain metastases in patients with non-small cell lung cancer (NSCLC) are a devastating problem with profound impact on survival and quality of life. Historically, the incidence of brain metastases has been underreported. Generally, brain metastases are not diagnosed until they are symptomatic. Asymptomatic metastases frequently go unrecognized. This is clinically inconsequential for patients who die from uncontrolled extracranial disease. However, with improvements in systemic therapy and locoregional therapy, more patients with localized disease are being cured and patients with metastatic, incurable disease, are living longer. Consequently, brain metastases have taken on greater clinical significance. Management of the brain after diagnosis of brain metastases has taken on increasing importance and is being intensively studied. However, preventative treatments for brain metastases are infrequently employed in clinical practice, and only recently is prophylactic cranial irradiation (PCI) for NSCLC being reevaluated in clinical studies.

RISK OF BRAIN METASTASES

The high incidence of brain metastases in lung cancer can be partially explained by normal physiology. Fifteen percent of blood flow from the left heart goes directly to the brain. Lung cancer cells have direct access to the left side of the heart via the pulmonary veins. Cancer cells from other organs must pass through the pulmonary capillaries or be shunted from the right to left side of the heart before gaining access to the brain.

Cancer cells require complex capabilities of extravasation, evasion of the immune detection system, and establishing new blood vessels in the process of establishing brain metastases. This process is detailed in an excellent review article published by Gavrilovic and Posner.[1] Cells undergo genetic changes to allow for uncontrolled growth, angiogenesis, and intravasation into blood vessels. Cells must then survive circulation and reach the organ in question where the right biochemical environment is necessary for proliferation and development of metastases. Cancer cells destined to become brain metastases are caught in the CNS capillaries and then proliferate through the vessels into the brain parenchyma. Here, the blood-brain barrier protects them from many systemic cancer therapies. There is a variable period of dormancy during which time, genetic changes take place, enabling cells to proliferate and become clinically significant metastases. This period of protected dormancy explains why we see delayed brain metastases in patients with effectively treated lung cancer and why as treatment is improving and survival is lengthening, the rate of brain failures is increasing.

The incidence of brain metastases in patients with locally advanced non–small cell lung cancer (LA-NSCLC) varies between 13% and 54%.[2–11] From various reports, a range from 18% to 52% of patients have a solitary brain lesion.[11–15] The risk of brain failure has been related to disease stage,[10] disease bulk,[16] histology,[10,17–19] length of survival from diagnosis,[20] female gender,[21] age <60 years,[12,16,22] type of therapy,[10,17,23] and serum lactate dehydrogenase.[21]

Histology The incidence of brain metastases is higher with adenocarcinoma and large cell carcinoma than with squamous cell carcinoma.[17–19,24] Consequently, some studies evaluating PCI for NSCLC have included only patients with nonsquamous histologies.[5,7] Although a trend toward increased incidence of brain metastases in patients with adenocarcinoma is observed in most studies, not all studies have shown a significant correlation.[4,8,10,11,16,21,25]

Extent of Mediastinal Disease Ceresoli et al.[16] reported borderline significance of bulky mediastinal disease (nodes >2 cm) and the incidence of brain disease by multiple regression analysis. Robnett et al.[10] reported 2-year actuarial incidence of brain metastases of 36% with stage IIIB disease and 29% with Stage II/IIIA disease (p <0.04). Wang et al.[25a] conducted a more extensive analysis of impact of nodal disease on brain failures in 223 patients treated surgically with stage IIIA/B disease. Brain metastases were greater in patients with more lymph nodes and more nodal regions involved.

Age Ceresoli et al.[16] evaluated risk factors for brain metastases in 112 patients with LA-NSCLC. In multivariate analysis, age younger than 60 years was associated with an increased risk of brain metastases (31% vs. 9%; $p = 0.03$). In a series reported by Carolan et al.,[12] 25.6% of patients younger than age 60 failed first in the brain compared with 11.4% of patients older than 60 ($p = 0.022$). In a review of four Southwest Oncology Group (SWOG)[22] studies, patients age 50 and younger were at increased risk for developing brain metastases with a hazard ratio of 1.8 ($p = 0.046$). Other series have not shown an increased risk of brain metastases with young age.[10,13]

Time to Brain Failure Most brain metastases occur within 2 years of diagnosis.[10–13,16,20,22] Median time to relapse in the brain is 5.7 to 11.7 months.[10,12,13,16,20] Earlier relapse is associated with younger age (<60),[12,16,22] bulky disease (>2 cm),[16] and nonsquamous histology.[12,22]

Duration of Survival The addition of chemotherapy to local regional therapy for LA-NSCLC has improved survival. Systemic therapy decreases the risk of visceral metastases[17,18,26,27] but has limited impact on brain metastases.[17,18,27] In fact, as survival lengthens the risk of brain, metastasis increases. Review of Radiation Therapy Oncology Group (RTOG) and single-institution data has shown that longer survival for patients with LA-NSCLC treated with radiation alone[20,24] or radiation and chemotherapy[18] is associated with an increased incidence of brain metastases.

Review of 1415 patients treated on radiation therapy alone and 350 patients treated on radiation and chemotherapy on RTOG studies demonstrated a significant decrease in distant metastases with the addition of chemotherapy (41% vs. 19%; $p < 0.001$). Brain metastases were not altered by chemotherapy (17% vs. 12%).[18]

Andre et al.[17] reported the patterns of relapse in 81 patients with clinical N2 disease treated with preoperative chemotherapy to 186 comparable patients treated with primary surgery. Survival at 2 and 5 years was 35% and 17% for preoperative chemotherapy and 26% and 8% for primary surgery. Preoperative chemotherapy was associated with a better prognosis in multivariate analysis ($p = 0.001$). Additionally, patients treated with chemotherapy had a lower rate of visceral metastases (28% vs. 38%; $p < 0.05$) and a higher rate of brain metastases (32% vs. 18%; $p < 0.05$). The observation that neoadjuvant chemotherapy (or chemoradiotherapy) is associated with an increased risk of brain metastasis is bolstered by reports from Philadelphia and San Francisco.[10,13] An explanation might be that as local and system disease are better controlled, and the untreated risk site, the brain, becomes a dominant site of failure.

Recursive partitioning analysis (RPA) of RTOG studies employing radiation therapy alone showed that patients in the RPA group with the longest survival had the highest incidence of brain metastases.[20] Median survival for class I and II was 12.6 and 8.3 months, and class III and IV was 6.2 and 3.3 months. First failure in the brain was significantly higher in class I (18%) compared with class III (9%) and IV (6%) ($p = 0.0004$ and 0.03, respectively).

Recently, several studies employing multimodality therapy for LA-NSCLC have reported excellent median and 3-year survival rates of 20 to 43 months and 34% to 37%.[4,11–13,16,23,28] These studies reported the brain to be a common site of failure. Overall brain failure rates were 22% to 55%, and rates of brain as first site of relapse were 16% to 43%. Studies with lower median survival (3 to 17 months) and 3-year overall survival (5% to 27%) report a lower incidence of brain metastases, suggesting that the later brain relapse in the longer-surviving patients occurs in a sanctuary site. Overall rates of brain failure are 6% to 21%, and rates of brain as first site of failure are 9% to 19% (Table 57.1).[3,10,20,29,30]

Locoregional and Systemic Therapy Studies have shown an association between timing of local therapy incidence of brain metastases. Robnett et al.[10] reported a near doubling of the 2-year actuarial risk of brain metastases of 39% in patients treated with sequential chemotherapy and radiation compared with 20% for patients treated with concurrent chemotherapy and radiation. Mamon et al.[23] reported results of patients treated preoperatively with chemotherapy or concurrent chemotherapy and radiation. Decreased risk of brain metastases was associated with preoperative +/− postoperative radiation versus postoperative radiation therapy only ($p = 0.062$), use of taxane-based chemotherapy ($p = 0.044$), and conversion to N0 status ($p = 0.025$). Conversely, Furuse et al.[31] reported a higher rate of brain failures in patients treated with concurrent chemotherapy and radiation compared with patients treated sequentially, (19% vs. 9%; $p = 0.018$). The higher rate of brain metastases may be explained by longer survival in the concurrently treated patients (16.5 vs. 13.3 months; $p = 0.04$). Byhardt et al.[32] reviewed the outcome in 461 patients treated on five RTOG studies and found no association between the incidence of brain metastases as first failure and sequential versus concurrent chemotherapy and radiation. Median survival for concurrent regimens was 16.3 and 15.8 months and for sequential therapy 13.6 months ($p = 0.47$).

MANAGEMENT OF THE BRAIN IN NON–SMALL CELL LUNG CANCER

There is not a standard of care for addressing brain micrometastases after successful therapy for LA-NSCLC. Most clinicians will perform routine physical examination with imaging of the brain only upon development of signs or symptoms of brain failure. The National Comprehensive Cancer Network (NCCN) guidelines for follow-up of lung cancer include physical exam, chest x-ray, and thoracic computed tomography (CT) scans at regularly defined intervals. CT or magnetic resonance imaging (MRI) screening for brain metastases is not included as standard management. Although some investigators have evaluated and/or endorse routine neuropsychological

TABLE 57.1 Incidence of Brain Metastases and Median Survival

			Brain Metastases		
Author	**Stage**	**Therapy**	**Overall**	**Brain as 1st Site of Failure**	**Median Survival (Months)**
Choi et al.[28]	T1–T3pN2	ChT/RT/S	NA	30%	25
Stuschke et al.[4]	T1–T4pN2	ChT/RT/S	54%	30%	20
Law et al.[11]	IIIa–b	ChT/RT/S	NA	28% (26% complete resection)	36 (total), 52 (complete resection)
Ceresoli et al.[16]	IIb,IIIa–b	ChT/RT ± S	22%	16%	21
Carolan et al.[12]	IIIa–b	ChT/RT ± S	35%	18%	25.6
Mamon et al.[23]	IIIa	S ± ChT and/or RT	40%	34%	21
Chen et al.[13]	IIIa–b (pCR to preop therapy)	ChT (±RT)/S	55%	43%	43
Albain et al.[3]	pN2–pN3 or T4	ChT/RT ± S	21%	15%	13–17
Albain et al.[29]	pIIIb	ChT/RT	20%	10%	15
Robnett et al.[10]	II/III	ChT/RT	NA	19%	14.5
Weiden and Piantadosi[30]	IIIa–b	ChT/RT ± S	NA	9%	13
Komaki et al.[20]	III	RT	6%–18%	NA	3–12

ChT, chemotherapy; NA, not available; pCR, pathologic complete response; preop, preoperative; RT, radiotherapy; S, surgery.

assessment and CT or MRI screening for early detection of brain metastases,[11,13,15] others have begun to use PCI as part of multimodality therapy regimens[3–5,9,33] or suggested the urgent need for further investigation of PCI.[4,10,12,17,18,21–23]

Standard Follow-up Prognosis of patients with brain metastases is poor. Median survival ranges between 3 and 7 months.[34–37] Most information regarding outcomes of patients with brain metastases consists of reports on symptomatic patients with varying controls or lack of control of the primary and systemic disease sites, age, gender, and performance status.

There seem to be subgroups of patients that have a relatively favorable prognosis. Recursive partitioning analysis of RTOG brain metastases trials (61% of patient had lung cancer) identified three prognostic groups.[37] RPA class I patients have Karnofsky Performance Score (KPS) ≥70, age <65 years, control of primary tumor, and no extracranial metastases. Class III patients include all patients with KPS <70. Class II includes all others. Median survival for class I to III is 7.1, 4.2, and 3.3 months. Other studies have confirmed the value of RPA-derived prognostic classes.[38,39] Unfortunately, the most favorable subsets of patients represent a minority of cases. Only 20% of patients were RPA class I in RTOG studies treating brain metastases. Nieder et al.[38] retrospectively reviewed 532 consecutive patients at a single institution treated for brain metastases, and only 3% were RPA class I.

Brain metastases studies with the most favorable results (median survival between 10 and 16 months) include patients with favorable prognostic factors that have been treated for overt brain disease with either surgery[40–43] or radiosurgery,[44,45] with or without whole-brain irradiation. Survival has been associated with high performance status,[44,45] female gender, absence of active systemic disease, long duration from lung cancer diagnosis to development of brain metastases,[44] solitary versus 2 to 3 lesions, and favorable histologic status.[45]

Long-term survival and possible cure has been reported in patients with control of extracranial disease who are treated surgically for brain metastases.[46–48] Overall 5-year survival for carefully selected patients with resected solitary brain metastases as high as 20% to 30%.[49] There are case reports of patients surviving more than 10 years.[46,50,51] Unfortunately, patients with brain metastases rarely have potentially curable disease.

Routine Brain Imaging Early detection of brain metastases allows for intervention prior to debilitating neurological symptoms. Additionally, brain metastases are more likely to be amenable to aggressive therapy with radiosurgery or resection, when tumor burden is low. Theoretically, even if disease is multifocal and not appropriate for localized therapy, smaller lesions are more likely to have a meaningful response to standard doses of whole-brain irradiation. Yokoi et al.[15] evaluated the potential benefits of MRI and CT to detect brain metastases in patients with stage I to IIIB NSCLC treated surgically. Disease was detected prior to development of neurological symptoms in 76% of patients diagnosed with brain metastases. Median survival for patients with asymptomatic brain metastases was 25 months, whereas overall median survival was only 10 months.[15]

TABLE 57.2 Prospective Randomized Studies Evaluating PCI for NSCLC

Author	Dose of PCI	Primary Therapy	Brain Failures		Overall Survival	Median Survival (Months)
			No PCI	PCI		
Cox et al.[6]	20 Gy (2 Gy × 10)	RT only (all NSCLC)	13% (16/145)	6% (7/136)	NA	NA
Russell et al.[7]	30 Gy (3 Gy × 10)	RT only (nonsquamous)	19% (18/94)	9% (8/93)	13% (2 yrs)	8
Umsawasdi et al.[8]	30 Gy (3 Gy × 10)	ChT/RT or ChT/RT/S (all NSCLC)	27% (14/51)	4% (2/46)	NA	NA
Pottgen et al.[25]	30 Gy (2 Gy × 15)	ChT/RT/S	25.5% (13/51)	16.4% (9/55)	18% (5 yrs)	NA

ChT, chemotherapy; NA, not available; NSCLC, non–small cell lung cancer; PCI, prophylactic cranial irradiation; RT, radiotherapy; S, surgery.

Prophylactic Cranial Irradiation Four prospective randomized trials[6–8,25] and several retrospective studies[3–5,9,51,52] have shown that prophylactic cranial irradiation decreases the incidence or delays the onset of brain failures in LA-NSCLC (Tables 57.2 and 57.3). Effective doses of PCI included 2 Gy per fraction to 20, 30, and 36 Gy and 3 Gy per fraction to 30 Gy. These studies were not powered to show a survival advantage nor did they thoroughly evaluate quality of life or neurological function.

Prospective Studies In the early 1980s, RTOG conducted a prospective randomized study[7] comparing PCI (30 Gy in 10 fractions) and chest radiation with chest radiation alone for patients with inoperable or unresectable T1-4N1-3M0 and resected T1-3N2-3M0 nonsquamous NSCLC. Development of symptomatic brain metastases was delayed by PCI. Overall incidence of brain metastases was not significantly decreased. In a small subgroup of patients with prior complete surgical resection, PCI decreased the incidence of brain metastases from 25% to 0% ($p = 0.06$). Most patients in this study did not live long enough to develop brain failure. Median survival in this study was only 8 months because of ineffective therapy and relatively poor prognostic factors. Also, ineffectiveness of locoregional therapy and lack of systemic therapy resulted in a high incidence of locoregional and distant failures that likely were sources of secondary seeding of the brain after PCI was delivered.

TABLE 57.3 Retrospective Studies Evaluating PCI for NSCLC

Study	PCI Dose	Primary Therapy	Brain Failures		Overall Survival	Median Survival (Months)
			No PCI	PCI		
Albain et al.[3]	36 Gy (2 Gy × 18)	Trimodality (all NSCLC)	16% (16/100)	8% (2/26)	37% (2 yrs) 27% (3 yrs)	15
Strauss et al.[5]	30 Gy (2 Gy × 15)	Trimodality (nonsquamous)	12% (5/41)	0 (0/13)	58% (1 yr)	15.5
Stuschke et al.[4]	30 Gy (2 Gy × 15)	Trimodality (all NSCLC)	54% (15/28)	13% (6/47) ($p < 0.0001$)	31% (3 yrs)	20
Skarin et al.[9]	36 Gy (2 Gy × 18)	Trimodality (all NSCLC)	26% (7/27)	14% (1/7)	31% (3–5 yrs)	32
Rusch et al.[52]	30 Gy (3 Gy × 10) 36 Gy (2 Gy × 18)	ChT/RT	0/0	(0/75)	NA	NA
Jacobs et al.[51]	30 Gy (2 Gy × 15)	NA	24% (14/58)	5% (1/20)	NA	17

ChT, chemotherapy; NA, not available; NSCLC, non–small cell lung cancer; PCI; prophylactic cranial irradiation; RT, radiotherapy.

The Veterans Administration Lung Group[6] conducted a trial that included patients with LA-NSCLC who were not candidates for curative resection and who had no evidence of distant metastases. Patients were randomized to receive whole-brain irradiation (20 Gy in 10 fractions) or no brain treatment and to receive one of two regimes of thoracic irradiation. PCI decreased the incidence of brain metastases from 13% to 6% ($p = 0.038$) in all non–small cell histologies and from 29% to 0% in adenocarcinoma ($p = 0.04$). There was no difference in median survival with PCI.

Umsawasdi et al.[8] reported results of patients with LA-NSCLC treated with combined chemotherapy and radiation therapy and randomized to PCI (30 Gy in 10 fractions) or no PCI. PCI significantly decreased the incidence of brain metastases from 27% to 4% ($p = 0.002$). PCI also increased the brain metastasis-free interval. No survival benefit was observed for the treated group. Beneficial effects of PCI by multivariate analysis favored patients with squamous histology, women, patients with good performance status, weight loss less than 6%, stage III disease, or no prior therapy.

Pottgen et al.[25] randomized 106 patients with stage IIIA NSCLC to either surgery followed by postoperative thoracic radiation therapy or neoadjuvant chemotherapy followed by concurrent chemotherapy and radiation, surgery, and PCI to 30 Gy in 15 fractions. PCI reduced the actuarial rate of brain metastases at 2 and 5 years from 22% to 7.8% and 34.7% to 7.8%, respectively ($p = 0.01$).

Retrospective Reviews Six nonrandomized multimodality studies for patients with LA-NSCLC have demonstrated the potential benefits of PCI.[3–5,9,33,52] In the most notable of these studies, 75 patients with stage IIIA/B NSCLC were treated with induction chemotherapy, preoperative radiochemotherapy, and surgery. PCI was introduced after the first half of the study because of a high incidence of brain relapses. Patients treated during the second half of the study were offered PCI (30 Gy in 15 fractions). PCI reduced the rate of brain metastases as the first site of relapse from 30% to 8% at 4 years ($p = 0.005$) and the rate of overall brain relapse from 54% to 13% ($p < 0.0001$).[4]

Skarin et al.[9] treated 41 patients with stage III NSCLC with chemotherapy and radiation followed by surgery. A total of 14% of patients treated with PCI (36 Gy in 18 fractions) developed brain metastases compared with 27% of patients not treated with PCI.[9] SWOG performed a phase II study with neutron chest radiotherapy sandwiched between four cycles of chemotherapy.[3] PCI was administered concurrently with chest irradiation (30 Gy in 10 fractions or 36 Gy in 18 fractions). There was no clinical or radiological evidence of brain metastases in patients who completed PCI. In another phase II SWOG study, patients with stage IIIA NSCLC were treated with chemoradiotherapy and optional PCI (36 Gy in 18 fractions) followed by surgery.[33] A total of 2 out of 18 (11%) patients treated with PCI and 24 of 108 patients (22%) not treated with PCI developed brain metastases. In a phase II Cancer and Leukemia Group B (CALGB) trial, patients with large cell or adenocarcinoma received 30 Gy in 15 fractions to the brain and neoadjuvant chemoradiation and resection for LA-NSCLC. No brain relapse was observed among the 13 patients who received PCI.[5]

Toxicity There is limited information regarding the impact of PCI on quality of life and cognitive functioning. PCI toxicity data is derived mainly from SCLC. Early data suggest significant toxicity associated with PCI. The highest rates of toxicity have been reported when PCI is given concurrently with chemotherapy or when given at high dose per fraction.[53] More recent data has shown that PCI toxicity is acceptable.

Two randomized controlled trials of PCI in patients with SCLC[54,55] have examined cognitive functioning as an outcome, one of which also examined quality of life (QOL).[55] Arriagada et al.[54] randomized 300 patients with SCLC in complete remission to PCI versus observation. No statistically significant differences were noted between the PCI and observation groups in the relative risks of 2-year cumulative incidence of neuropsychological changes. Gregor et al.[55] prospectively evaluated PCI in 314 patients, 136 of these patients (84 PCI, 52 control) were included in an evaluation of quality of life, cognitive functioning, anxiety, and depression at 6 and 12 months. In the PCI and control groups, there was impairment of cognitive function and QOL before PCI with additional impairment at 6 and 12 months. There were no consistent differences between the two groups and no evidence over 1 year of major impairment attributed to PCI.

Retrospective reviews also suggest that PCI does not negatively impact cognitive function and QOL.[56,57] Tai et al.[56] assessed quality-adjusted survival utilizing the QTWiST (quality time without symptoms and toxicity) methodology in 98 patients in complete remission from SCLC who did or did not receive PCI. They reported a significant difference in the mean QTWiST survival between the two groups, favoring the PCI patients ($p < 0.01$). Van Oosterhout et al.[57] evaluated patients with SCLC with neurological function, neuropsychological function, and CT or MRI of the brain. Patients were treated with chemotherapy alone, sequential chemotherapy and PCI, or concurrent or sandwiched chemotherapy and PCI. Although PCI groups had more white matter abnormalities, there was no statistical evidence for additional neurotoxicity of PCI.

It has been suggested that neuropsychological abnormalities associated with SCLC may be secondary to the disease itself (paraneoplasia), systemic therapy,[58] or emotional distress and deteriorated physical condition.[57] Because of potential paraneoplastic effects and different therapy for NSCLC relative to SCLC, definite conclusions regarding tolerance of PCI for NSCLC can only be drawn from prospective studies with serial longitudinal neuropsychological testing of patients with NSCLC treated with and without PCI. Comorbid diseases and their medications need to be kept in mind as potential culprits as well.

Late cognitive deficits with the use of PCI for patients with NSCLC have not been detected, partially because of lack of intensive neuropsychological testing and limited survival. Stuschke et al.[4] studied neuropsychological function and brain MRI in patients with LA-NSCLC after PCI. T2-weighted MRI revealed white matter abnormalities of higher grade in patients who received PCI than in those who did not. Two of the nine patients treated with PCI and none of the four patients not treated with PCI had grade 4/4 white matter abnormalities. There was a trend toward impaired neuropsychological functioning in patients with higher-degree white matter abnormalities. Impairments in attention and visual memory in long-term survivors was seen in both PCI and non-PCI patient groups.

Pottgen et al.[25] performed a battery of neuropsychological tests for attention, memory, associative learning, and information processing in 11 long-term survivors of stage IIIA NSCLC treated surgically.[25] Five patients were treated with chemotherapy, thoracic radiation, surgery, and PCI (30 Gy in 15 fractions); the other six patients were treated with surgery and thoracic radiation. There was no difference in any of the neuropsychological testing between patients with and without PCI. A slightly reduced neurocognitive performance in comparison with age-matched normal population was found for patients in both treatment groups. Ten patients (five from each group) had MRIs of the brain. Leukencephalopathy grade 1 was found in one patient who did not receive PCI and three patients who received PCI.

RTOG recently closed phase III study evaluating PCI for patients with LA-NSCLC. Three hundred and fifty-nine patients were enrolled in the study. Patients without progressive locoregional or distant disease were eligible after completing definitive locoregional therapy for stage IIIA/B NSCLC. Patients were stratified by histology (squamous vs. nonsquamous), therapy (surgery vs. no surgery), and stage (IIIA vs. IIIB), and randomized to PCI (2 Gy per fraction to 30 Gy) or observation. Both groups completed neuropsychological and QOL testing prior to PCI and at regular posttherapy or enrollment intervals. The target accrual for this study was 1058 patients. The study was closed prematurely because of slow accrual. Despite early closure, this study will provide important information regarding the neuropsychological effects of PCI and the impact of PCI on the incidence of brain failures.

CONCLUSION

Neurological compromise, degradation of QOL, and death in the event of brain metastases are almost certain. The benefit of early detection with prompt intervention or prevention of symptomatic brain metastases in patients with LA-NSCLC may have significant impact on QOL and/or overall survival.

PCI is not standard of care for NSCLC even though there is sufficient evidence to support its effectiveness in decreasing brain failure rates. This is caused by incomplete data regarding toxicity and lack of evidence showing a survival advantage. Patients with NSCLC treated for potential cure with the highest risk of brain metastases (age ≤60 years, good performance status, treatment with multimodality therapy, particularly therapy including surgery) at a minimum should be followed closely for brain failure during the first 12 to 24 months after completing therapy with detailed history and physical examination. Physicians should have a low threshold for scanning the brain and/or schedule regular scans of the brain.

REFERENCES

1. Gavrilovic IT, Posner. Brain metastases: epidemiology and pathophysiology. *J Neurooncol* 2005;75:5–14.
2. Furuse K, Kubota K, Kqwahra M, et al. Phase II study of concurrent radiotherapy and chemotherapy for unresectable stage III non-small-cell lung cancer. *J Clin Oncol* 1995;13:869–875.
3. Albain KS, Rusch VW, Crowley JJ, et al. Concurrent cisplatin/etoposide plus chest radiotherapy followed by surgery for stages IIIA (N2) and IIIB non-small-cell lung cancer: mature results of Southwest Oncology Group phase II study 8805. *J Clin Oncol* 1995;13:1880–1892.
4. Stuschke M, Eberhardt, Pottgen C, et al. Prophylactic cranial irradiation in locally advanced non-small cell lung cancer after multimodality treatment: long-term followup and investigations of late neuropsychologic effects. *J Clin Oncol* 1999;17:2700–2709.
5. Strauss GM, Herndon JE, Sherman DD, et al. Neoadjuvant chemotherapy and radiotherapy followed by surgery in stage IIIA non-small cell carcinoma of the lung: report of a Cancer and Leukemia Group B phase II study. *J Clin Oncol* 1992;10:1237–1244.
6. Cox JD, Stanley K, Petrovich Z, et al. Cranial irradiation in cancer of the lung of all cell types. *JAMA* 1981;245(5):469–472.
7. Russell AH, Pajak TE, Selim HM, et al. Prophylactic cranial irradiation for lung cancer patients at high risk for development of cerebral metastasis: results of a prospective randomized trial conducted by the Radiation Therapy Oncology Group. *Int J Rad Oncol Biol Phys* 1991;21(3):637–643.
8. Umsawasdi T, Valdivieso M, Chen TT, et al. Role of elective brain irradiation during combined chemoradiotherapy for limited disease non-small cell lung cancer. *J Neurooncol* 1984;2:253–259.
9. Skarin A, Jochelson M, Sheldon T, et al. Neoadjuvant chemotherapy in marginally resectable stage III M0 non-small cell lung cancer: long-term follow-up in 41 patients. *J Surg Oncol* 1989;40(4):266–274.
10. Robnett TJ, Machtay M, Stevenson JP, et al. Factors affecting the risk of brain metastases after definitive chemoradiation for locally advanced non-small-cell lung carcinoma. *J Clin Oncol* 2001;19:1344–1349.
11. Law A, Karp DD, Dipetrillo T, et al. Emergence of increased cerebral metastasis after preoperative radiotherapy with chemotherapy in patients with locally advanced nonsmall cell lung carcinoma. *Cancer* 2001;92:160–164.
12. Carolan H, Sun AY, Bezjak A, et al. Does the incidence and outcome of brain metastases in locally advanced non-small cell lung cancer justify prophylactic cranial irradiation or early detection? *Lung Cancer* 2005;49:109–115.
13. Chen AM, Jahan TM, Jablons DM, et al. Risk of cerebral metastases and neurological death after pathological complete response to neoadjuvant therapy for locally advanced non-small-cell lung cancer. Clinical implications for the subsequent management of the brain. *Cancer* 2007;109:1668–1675.
14. Tang SG, Tseng C, Tsay P, et al. Predictors for patterns of brain relapse and overall survival in patients with non-small cell lung cancer. *J Neurooncol* 2005;73:153–161.
15. Yokoi K, Kamiya N, Matsuguma H, et al. Detection of brain metastases in potentially operable non-small cell lung cancer: a comparison of CT and MRI. *Chest* 1999;115:714–719.

16. Ceresoli GL, Reni M, Chiesa G, et al. Brain metastases in locally advanced nonsmall cell lung carcinoma after multimodality treatment: risk factors analysis. *Cancer* 2002;95(3):605–612.
17. Andre F, Grunenwald D, Pujol JL, et al. Patterns of relapse of N2 non-small-cell lung carcinoma patients treated with preoperative chemotherapy. *Cancer* 2001;91:2394–2400.
18. Cox JD, Scott CB, Byhardt RW, et al. Addition of chemotherapy to radiation therapy alters failure patterns by cell type within non-small cell carcinoma of lung (NSCCL): analysis of Radiation Therapy Oncology Group (RTOG) trials. *Int J Radiat Oncol Biol Phys* 1999;43(3):505–509.
19. Perez CA, Pajak TF, Simpson JR, et al. Long-term observations of the patterns of failure in patients with unresectable non-oat cell carcinoma of the lung treated with definitive radiotherapy. *Cancer* 1987;59:1874–1881.
20. Komaki R, Scott CB, Byhardt R, et al. Failure patterns by prognostic group determined by recursive partitioning analysis (RPA) of 1547 patients on four Radiation Therapy Oncology Group (RTOG) studies in inoperable nonsmall-cell lung cancer. *Int J Radiat Oncol Biol Phys* 1998;42(2):263–267.
21. Keith B, Vincent M, Statt L, et al. Subsets more likely to benefit from surgery or prophylactic cranial irradiation after chemoradiation for localized non-small-cell lung cancer. *Am J Clin Oncol* 2002;25:583–587.
22. Gaspar LE, Chansky KS, Vallieres E, et al. Time from treatment to subsequent diagnosis of brain metastases in stage III non-small-cell lung cancer: a retrospective review by the southwest oncology group. *J Clin Oncol* 2005;23:2955–2961.
23. Mamon HJ, Yeap BY, Janne PA, et al. High risk of brain metastases in surgically staged IIIA non-small cell lung cancer patients treated with surgery, chemotherapy, and radiation. *J Clin Oncol* 2005;23(7):1530–1537.
24. Komaki R, Cox J, Stark R. Frequency of brain metastases in adenocarcinoma and large cell carcinoma of the lung: correlation with survival. *Int J Radiat Oncol Biol Phys* 1983;9(10):1467–1470.
25. Pottgen C, Eberhardt W, Grannass A, et al. Prophylactic cranial irradiation in operable stage IIIA non-small-cell lung cancer treated with neoadjuvant chemoradiotherpy: results from a German multicenter randomized trial. *J Clin Oncol* 2007;25:4987–4992.
25a. Wang SY, Ye X, Ou W, et al. Risk of cerebral metastases for postoperative locally advanced non-small-cell lung cancer. *Lung Cancer* 2009;64(2): 238–243.
26. Arriagada R, Le Chevalier T, Quoix E, et al. ASTRO (American Society for Therapeutic Radiology and Oncology: effect of chemotherapy on locally advanced nonsmall cell lung carcinoma: a randomoizesd study of 353 patients. GETCB (Groupe d'Etude et Traitement des Cancers Bronchiques), FNCLCC9Federation Nationale des Centres de Lutte contre le Cancer) and the CEBI trialists. *Int J Radiat Oncol Biol Phys* 1991;20:1183–1190.
27. Komaki R, Scott CB, Sause WT, et al. Induction cisplatin/vinblastine and irradiation vs. irradiation in unresectable squamous cell lung cancer: failure patterns by cell type in RTOG 88-08/Ecog 4588. *Int J Radiat Oncol Biol Phys* 1997;39:537–544.
28. Choi NC, Carey RW, Daly W, et al. Potential impact on survival of improved tumor downstaging and resection rate by preoperative twice-daily radiation and concurrent chemotherapy in stage IIIA non-small-cell lung cancer. *J Clin Oncol* 1997;15:712–722.
29. Albain KS, Crowley JJ, Turrisi AT III, et al. Concurrent cisplatin, etoposide, and chest radiotherapy in pathologic stage IIIB non-small-cell lung cancer: a Southwest Oncology Group phase II study, SWOG 9019. *J Clin Oncol* 2002;20:3454–3460.
30. Weiden PL, Piantadosi S. Preoperative chemotherapy (cisplatin and fluorouracil) and radiation therapy in stage III non-small-cell lung cancer: a phase II study of the Lung Cancer Study Group. *J Natl Cancer Inst* 1991;83:266–272.
31. Furuse K, Fukuoka M, Kawahara M, et al. Phase III study of concurrent versus sequential thoracic radiotherapy in combination with mitomycin, vindesine, and cisplatin in unresectable stage III non-small-cell lung cancer. *J Clin Oncol* 1999;17:2692–2699.
32. Byhardt RB, Scott C, Sause WT, et al. Response, toxicity, failure patterns, and survival in five Radiation Therapy Oncology Group (RTOG) trials of sequential and/or concurrent chemotherapy and radiotherapy for locally advanced non-small-cell carcinoma of the lung. *In J Radiat Oncol Biol Phys* 1998;42:469–478.
33. Komarnicky LT, Phillips TL, Martz K, et al. A randomized phase III protocol for the evaluation of misonidazole combined with radiation in the treatment of patient s with brain metastases (RTOG 79-16). *Int J Radiat Oncol Biol Phys* 1991;20:53–58.
34. Sause ET, Scott C, Kirsch C, et al. Phase I/II trial of accelerated fractionation in brain metastases RTOG 85-28. *Int J Radiat Oncol Biol Phys* 1993;26:653–657.
35. Phillips TL, Scott CB, Leibel SA, et al. Results of a randomized comparison of radiotherapy and bromodeoxyurine to radiotherapy alone fro brain metastases: report of RTOG TRIAL 89-05. *Int J Radiat Oncol Biol Phys* 1994;30:215(107).
36. Gaspar L, Scott C, Rotman M, et al. Recursive partitioning analysis (RPA) of prognostic factors in three radiation therapy oncology group (RTOG) brain metastases trials. *Int J Radiat Oncol Biol Phys* 1997;37(4):745–751.
37. Nieder C, Nestle U, Motaref B, et al. Prognostic factors in brain metastases: should patients be selected for aggressive treatment according to recursive partitioning analysis (RPA) classes. *Int J Radiat Oncol Biol Phys* 2000;46:297–302.
38. Agboola O, Benoit B, Cross P, et al. Prognostic factors derived from recursive partition analysis (RPA) of radiation therapy oncology group (RTOG) brain metastases trials applied to surgically resected and irradiated brain metastatic cases. *Int J Radiat Oncol Biol Phys* 1998;42: 155–159.
39. Patchell RA, Phillp ST, Walsh JW, et al. A randomized trial of surgery in the treatment of single metastases to the brain. *N Engl J Med* 1990;322:494–500.
40. Patchell RA, Phillip TA, Regine WF, et al. Postoperative radiotherapy in the treatment of single metastases to the brain. *JAMA* 1998;280:1485–1489.
41. Mintz AH, Kestle J, Rathbone MP, et al. A randomized trial to assess the efficacy of surgery in addition to radiotherapy in patients with single cerebral metastasis. *Cancer* 1996;78:1470–1476.
42. Noordijk EM, Vecht CJ, Haaxma-Reiche H, et al. The choice of treatment of singe brain metastasis should be based on extracranial tumor activity and age. *Int J Radiat Oncol Biol Phys* 1994;29:711–717.
43. Sheehan JP, Sun MH, Kondziolka D, et al. Radiosurgery for non-small cell lung carcinoma metastatic to the brain: long term outcomes and prognostic factors influencing patient survival time and local tumor control. *J Neurosurg* 2002;97(6):1276–1281.
44. Andrews DW, Scott CB, Sperduto PW, et al. Whole brain radiation therapy with or without stereotactic radiosurgery boost for patients with one to three brain metastases: phase III results of the RTOG 9508 randomised trial. *Lancet* 2004;363:1665–1672.
45. Magilligan DJ, Duvernoy C, Malik G, et al. Surgical approach to lung cancer with solitary cerebral metastases: twenty-five years' experience. *Ann Thorac Surg* 1986;42:360–364.
46. Billing PS, Miller, Allen MS, et al. Surgical treatment of primary lung cancer with synchronous brain metastases. *J Thorac Cardiovasc Surg* 2001;122:548–553.
47. Read RC, Boop WC, Yoder G, et al. Management of nonsmall cell lung carcinoma with solitary brain metastases. *J Thorac Cardiovasc Surg* 1989;98:884–890.
48. Macchiarini P, Buonaguidi R, Hardin M, et al. Results and prognostic factors of surger in the management of non-small cell lung cancer with solitary brain metastsis. *Cancer* 1991;68:300–304.
49. Saitoh Y, Fujisawa T, Shiba M, et al. Prognostic factors in surgical treatment of solitary brain metastasis after resection of non-small-cell lung cancer. *Lung Cancer* 1999;24:99–106.
50. Chee RJ, Bydder S, Cameron F. Prolonged survival after resection and radiotherapy for solitary brain metastases from non-small-cell lung cancer. *Australas Radiol* 2007;51:186–189.

51. Jacobs RH, Awan A, Bitran JD, et al. Prophylactic cranial irradiation in adenocarcinoma of the lung. A possible role. *Cancer* 1987;59(12):2016–2019.
52. Rusch VW, Griffin BR, Livingston RB. The role of prophylactic cranial irradiation in regionally advanced non-small cell lung cancer. A Southwest Oncology Group Study. *J Thorac Cardiovasc Surg* 1989;98(4):535–539.
53. Johnson BE, Becker B, Goff WB, et al. Neurologic, neuropsychologic, and computed cranial tomography scan abnormalities in 2- to 10-year survivors of small-cell lung cancer. *J Clin Oncol* 1985;3:1659–1667.
54. Arriagada R, Le Chevalier T, Borie F, et al. Prophylactic cranial irradition for patients with small cell lung cancer in complete remission. *J Natl Cancer Inst* 1995;87:183–190.
55. Gregor A, Cull A, Stephens RJ, et al. Prophylactic cranial irradiation is indicated following complete response to induction therapy in small cell lung cancer: results of a multicentre randomised trial. *Eur J Cancer* 1997;33:1752–1758.
56. Tai TH, Yu E, Dickof P, et al. Prophylactic cranial irradiation revisited: cost-effectiveness and quality of life in small-cell lung cancer. *Int J Radiat Oncol Biol Phys* 2002;52:68–74.
57. Van Oosterhout AG, Ganzevles PG, Wilmink JT, et al. Sequelae in long-term survivors of small cell lung cancer. *Int J Radiat Oncol Biol Phys* 1996;34(5):1037–1044.
58. Komaki R. Neurological sequelae in long-term survivors of small cell lung cancer. *Int J Radiat Oncol Biol Phys* 1996;34(5):1181–1183.

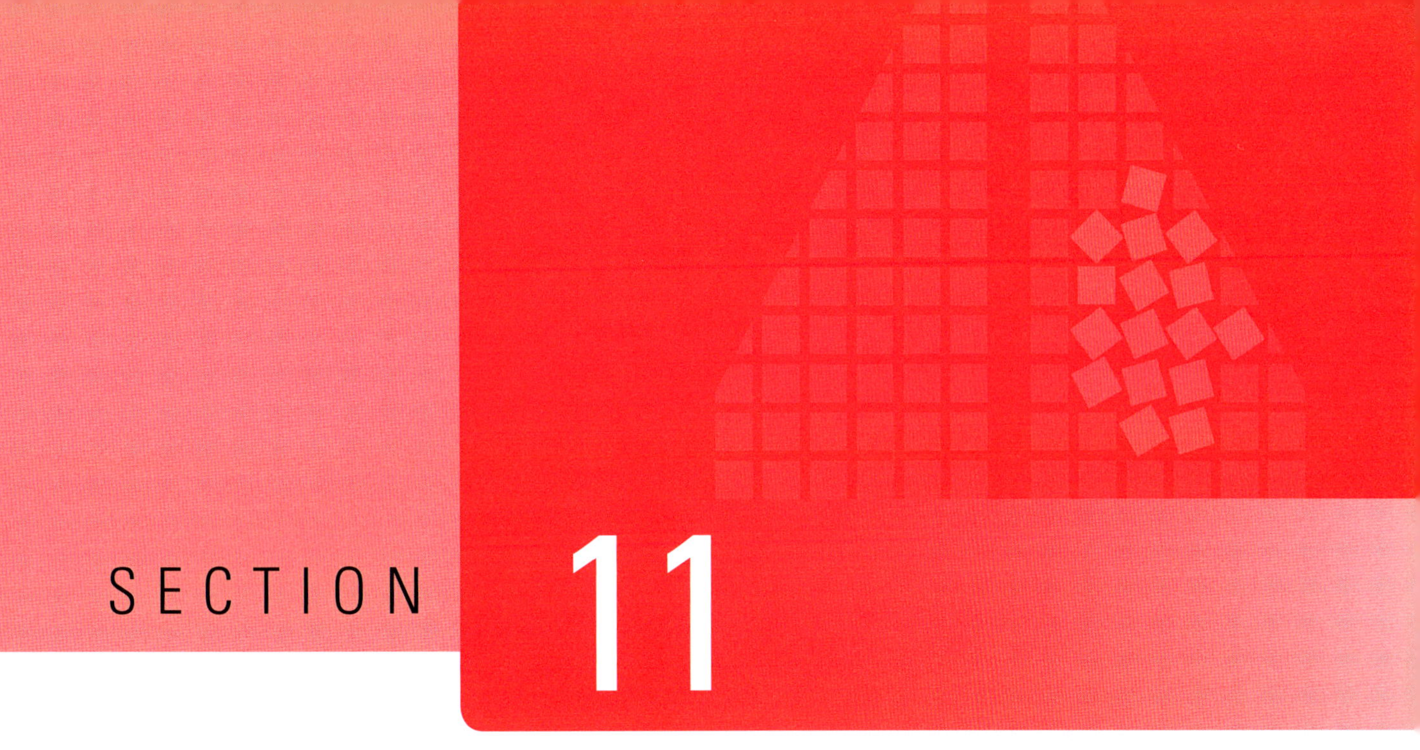

SECTION 11

Treatment of Small Cell Lung Cancer

CHAPTER 58

Chao H. Huang
Frances A. Shepherd
Karen Kelly

Chemotherapy for Small Cell Lung Cancer

Small cell lung cancer (SCLC) accounts for 13% of all lung cancer cases diagnosed each year in the United States.[1] A slow decline in the incidence of SCLC has been observed over the last 3 decades because of refined cigarette filters and a decrease in the number of cigarette smokers.[1] At the time of presentation, two thirds of patients will have disseminated disease, making systemic chemotherapy the cornerstone of treatment. SCLC is exquisitely sensitive to chemotherapy. Sixty to eighty percent of patients with SCLC achieve an objective response with combination chemotherapy, but despite these high response rates, the median survival (MS) is 16 to 22 months for patients with limited-stage disease (LS-SCLC) and 9 to 11 months for patients with extensive-stage disease (ES-SCLC). Although this survival time seems dismal, considerable progress has been made. A recent analysis of the SEER (Surveillance, Epidemiologic, and End Results) database revealed a modest but significant survival improvement with current therapies.[1] In 1973, the 2-year survival rate for ES-SCLC was 1.5% compared to 4.6% in the year 2000, whereas the 5-year survival rate for LS-SCLC increased from 4.9% to 10% during a similar time period.

SINGLE-AGENT CHEMOTHERAPY

The chemosensitivity of SCLC was first identified 50 years ago, with the recognition that methyl-bis-β-chloroethylamine hydrochloride could cause tumor regression in more than 50% of patients.[2] Older, active agents include nitrogen mustard, doxorubicin, methotrexate, ifosfamide, etoposide, teniposide, vincristine, vindesine, nitroureas, cisplatin, and its analog carboplatin.[3] In the 1990s, six new agents were discovered to have activity against SCLC: paclitaxel, docetaxel, topotecan, irinotecan, vinorelbine, and gemcitabine in untreated and or previously treated patients (Table 58.1).[3–34] This decade, two additional cytotoxic agents have been evaluated (Table 58.1). Pemetrexed, a multitargeted antifolate, an approved agent for the second-line treatment of advanced non–small cell lung cancer (NSCLC), showed no meaningful activity in previously treated SCLC patients in two small studies.[27,28] However, pemetrexed was well tolerated and further evaluation focused on combinations with cisplatin and carboplatin. A randomized phase II trial evaluated the use of cisplatin or carboplatin plus pemetrexed in previously untreated ES-SCLC in 78 patients. Median survival time (MST) for cisplatin/pemetrexed was 7.6 months, with a 1-year survivorship of 33.4% and a response rate of 35% (95% confidence interval [CI], 20.6% to 51.7%). The MST for carboplatin/pemetrexed was 10.4 months, with a 1-year survivorship of 39% and a response rate of 39.5% (95% CI, 24.0 to 56.6). Median time to progression (TTP) for cisplatin/pemetrexed was 4.9 months and for carboplatin/pemetrexed was 4.5 months. Grade 3 and 4 hematologic toxicities included neutropenia (15.8% vs. 20.0%) and thrombocytopenia (13.2% vs. 22.9%) in the cisplatin/pemetrexed and carboplatin/pemetrexed treatment groups, respectively. These data compare favorably with other regimens for ES-SCLC.[36]

An open-label phase III worldwide direct comparison of pemetrexed and carboplatin with the standard first-line etoposide and carboplatin chemotherapy in ES-SCLC is planned to enroll 1820 patients in 23 countries.[37]

Amirubicin, a topoisomerase II inhibitor, has produced impressive responses in both untreated and treated SCLC.[29–34] The promising efficacy and/or tolerability of these drugs have led to their investigation in first-line combination regimens as well as their continued evaluation in the salvage setting.

COMBINATION CHEMOTHERAPY

In the 1970s, randomized trials clearly demonstrated the superiority of combination chemotherapy over single-agent therapy. Furthermore, they showed that simultaneous administration of multiple agents was more efficacious than the sequential administration of the same agents.[35,38] Cyclophosphamide-based regimens were commonly used to treat SCLC, including CAV (cyclophosphamide, doxorubicin, and vincristine); CAE or CDE

TABLE 58.1 Single-Agent Activity with New Agents

	Untreated					Previously Treated				
Agent	**Dose (mg/m^2)**	**No. of Patients**	**RR (%)**	**MS (mos)**	**Ref.**	**Dose (mg/m^2)**	**No. of Patients**	**RR (%)**	**MS (mos)**	**Ref.**
Paclitaxel	250	32	34	9.9	(4)	175	21^{R}	29	NR	(6)
	250	43	68	6.6	(5)	80[a]	9^{S}	33	NR	(7)
						80[a]	8^{R}	25	NR	(7)
Docetaxel	75	12	8	NR	(8)	100	43	23	9	(9)
	75	28	25	NR	(10)					
Topotecan	2	48	39	10	(11)	1.5	57^{S}	17	5.4[b]	(12)
						1.5	41^{R}	2	NR	(12)
						1.5	45^{S}	38	6.9	(13)
						1.5	47^{R}	6	4.7	(13)
						1.25	25^{R}	12	4.6	(14)
Irinotecan	100	40	33	9.8	(15)	100	15^{S}	47	NR	(16)
						125	17^{S}	35	6.8[b]	(17)
						125	27^{R}	4	NR	(17)
						350	32^{R}	16	NR	(18)
Gemcitabine	1000	26	27	12	(19)	1000	26^{S}	16	7.3	(20)
						1000	20^{R}	6	6.9	(20)
						1000	38^{R}	13	3.9	(21)
Vinorelbine	30	22	5	8	(22)	30	26^{S}	16	NR	(24)
	30	30	27	NR	(23)	30	34^{S}	15	5	(25)
						30	24^{S}	13	NR	(26)
Pemetrexed						500	20^{S}	5	4.4	(27)
							23^{R}	4	2.7	(27)
						500	15^{S}	0	6.1	(28)
							23^{R}	0	3.2	(28)
						900	38^{S}	3	3.2	(28)
							40^{R}	0	2.5	(28)
Amirubicin	45	33	76	11.7	(29)	40	44^{S}	52	11.6	(30)
						40	16^{R}	50	10.3	(30)
						45	24^{S}	60	NR	(31)
							10^{R}	40	NR	(31)
						40	50^{S}	34	NR	(32)
						40	17^{S}	53	8.1[b]	(33)
							12^{R}	17		
						40	75^{R}	17	NR	(34)

[a] Weekly schedule.

[b] Survival for all patients.

MS, median survival; NR, not reported; R, refractory/resistant relapse; RR, response rate; S, sensitive relapse.

(cyclophosphamide, doxorubicin, and etoposide); and CEV (cyclophosphamide, etoposide, vincristine) until the introduction of cisplatin. Subsequently, randomized trials with the PE (cisplatin and etoposide) regimen were shown to be equally as effective as CAV and less toxic.[39–41] A metaanalysis of 36 trials demonstrated that regimens containing cisplatin and/or etoposide offered a significant survival advantage to patients with SCLC.[42] Thus, PE became the preferred regimen for treating ES-SCLC yielding objective response rates (ORR) of 65% to 85% with 10% to 20% complete response (CR) rates and an MS of 8 to 10 months.[39–41] Full dose (FD) PE can also be combined with thoracic radiotherapy. In LS-SCLC PE plus twice-daily thoracic radiotherapy is the documented standard regimen when feasible producing an 87% ORR with a 56% CR rate, an MS of

23 months and a 5-year survival rate of 44%.[42] Carboplatin is frequently substituted for cisplatin because of its more favorable toxicity profile. One small randomized trial comparing PE to CE (carboplatin and etoposide) in LS and ES patients showed similar efficacy but CE was significantly less toxic.[43]

Novel Chemotherapy Years lapsed before the discovery of the newer cytotoxic agents described in Table 58.1. For the first time, an abundance of new agents were available to study and a renewed enthusiasm at the opportunity of improving survival for SCLC patients emerged. A wealth of phase I and II trials with novel combinations were launched. Table 58.2 summarized the results from those promising combinations that were evaluated in phase III trials.[44–55] Most provocative were the results from the Japanese trial comparing cisplatin and irinotecan (PI) to PE. This trial was halted prematurely after an interim analysis showed a survival benefit for PI.[44] One hundred fifty-four patients were randomized to receive four cycles of etoposide 100 mg/m^2 on days 1, 2, and 3 with cisplatin 80 mg/m^2 on day 1 every 3 weeks or four cycles of PI, irinotecan 60 mg/m^2 on days 1, 8, and 15 with cisplatin 60 mg/m^2 on day 1. Patients treated with PI had a significantly better overall response rate, MS and 1-year survival rate as

TABLE 58.2 Recent Randomized Trials of First-Line Combination Chemotherapy Regimens

Reference	Regimen[a]	No. of Patients	Overall Response (%)	Median Survival (mos)	1-Year Survival (%)
Noda et al.[44]	PI	77	84.4[b]	12.8[c]	58.4
	PE	77	67.5	9.4	37.7
Natale et al.[45]	PI	324	60	9.9	41
	PE	327	57	9.1	34
Hanna et al.[46]	PI	221	48	9.3	35
	PE	110	44	10.2	35
Eckardt Jr et al.[47]	PT	389	63	9.8	31
	PE	395	69	10	31
Heigener et al.[48]	PT	357	56[d]	10.3	36
	PE	346	46	9.4	40
Hermes et al.[49]	IC	105	NR	8.5	34[e]
	EC	104	NR	7	24
de Jong et al.[50]	CDE[f]	102	60	6.8	24
	CTh	101	61	6.7	26
Socinski et al.[51]	PemC	364	30	7.3	NR
	EC	369	41[g]	9.6	NR
Mavroudis et al.[52]	PET[h]	62	50	10.5	43
	PE	71	48	11.5	45
Reck et al.[53]	CET[h]	301	72.1	12.7	48
	CEV	307	69	11.7	51
Niell et al.[54]	PET[h]	293	—	10.33	36.7
	PE	294	—	9.84	36.2
Pujol et al.[55]	PCDE[fi]	117	76[j]	10	40[k]
	PE	109	61	9.3	29

[a]Treatment key: C, carboplatin; D, doxorubicin; E, etoposide; I, irinotecan; P, cisplatin; Pem, pemetrexed; T, topotecan; V, vincristine.

[b]$p = 0.02$.

[c]$p = .0004$.

[d]$p = 0.01$.

[e]$p = 0.02$.

[f]C, cyclophosphamide.

[g]$p < 0.001$.

[h]P, paclitaxel.

[i]D, epirubicin.

[j]$p = 0.02$.

[k]$p = 0.0067$.

NR, not reported.

compared to those treated with PE (84.4% vs. 67.5% [$p = 0.02$]; 12.8 vs. 9.4 months; 58.4% vs. 37.7% [$p = 0.002$]), respectively. The PI combination was associated with a higher rate of grades 3 and 4 diarrhea ($p = 0.01$), whereas the PE combination was associated with a higher rate of myelosuppression ($p = 0.0001$). A confirmatory trial using the identical schema by the Southwest Oncology Group (SWOG trial) failed to show a benefit for PI.[45] In this large 651-patient trial, all efficacy parameters were very similar except that there was a trend toward improved progression-free survival (PFS) time for PI at 5.7 versus 5.2 months for PE ($p = 0.07$). Grade 3 or 4 neutropenia and thrombocytopenia were higher in the PE arm, whereas grade 3 or 4 nausea/vomiting and diarrhea were higher in the PI arm. The toxic death rates were low, 4% for PI and 5% for PE. A phase III superiority trial comparing a novel dose and schedule of the PI regimen (irinotecan 65 mg/m^2 with cisplatin 30 mg/m^2 both given on days 1 and 8) to standard PE produced similar survival times for both arms.[46] Two large phase III trial with topotecan, either oral or intravenous (IV) plus cisplatin were compared PE.[47,48] No survival benefit was observed with the experimental topotecan regimen over standard PE. The IV topotecan regimen did show a significantly higher ORR that translated into a prolonged PFS time of 7 versus 6 months for PE ($p = 0.004$). A European study reported superior survival for irinotecan plus carboplatin over an oral etoposide and carboplatin combination; however, survival in both arms was less than 9 months.[49] Drug doses and schedules were unconventional and lower than other regimens with irinotecan 175 mg/m^2 and carboplatin (area under the curve [AUC] = 4) administered on day 1 and in the standard arm, the etoposide was administered at 120 mg/m^2 orally days 1 to 5 with carboplatin (AUC = 4 on day 1). In contrast, a carboplatin-based doublet with paclitaxel failed to meet its primary end point of improving PFS when compared to CDE.[50] Most disappointing was the recent failure of the novel regimen of pemetrexed and carboplatin (Pem/C). In a previous randomized phase II study of pemetrexed plus cisplatin or carboplatin, the carboplatin arm produced an MS of 10.4 months and was well tolerated.[36] The GALES (Global Analysis of Pemetrexed in SCLC Extensive Stage) was designed to show noninferiority of pemetrexed (500 mg/m^2) plus carboplatin (AUC = 5) as compared to etoposide and carboplatin (EC). With 733 randomized patients, the study was terminated prematurely when the predefined PFS futility end point showed *inferiority* of the experimental arm.[51] The median PFS time was 3.68 months for Pem/C and 5.32 months for EC ($p < 0.0001$). ORR also favored EC at 41% compared to 25% ($p = 0.01$). The preliminary overall survival (OS) time was 7.3 months for Pem/C and 9.6 months for EC. Significant neutropenia and more febrile neutropenia were seen in the EC arm. In contrast, deaths on therapy or within 30 days were higher for the pemetrexed arm 16% versus 10% ($p = 0.032$) and the toxic death rates were 1.4% versus 0 ($p = 0.028$), respectively. However, the causes of death were atypical and variable.

The favorable toxicity profiles of new agents led several investigators to explore the possibility of integrating them into an active doublet (Table 58.2). Three randomized trials showed that paclitaxel-containing triplets did not result in superior survival compared to traditional doublets; furthermore, they were associated with increased toxicity.[53–55] A four-drug regimen has also been evaluated. While building upon a doublet with newer agents was not successful, in a French study, cyclophosphamide and 4'-epidoxorubin were added to PE, the PCDE regimen, and showed a significant improvement in the CR rate (13% vs. 21%; $p = 0.02$) and OS (9.3 vs. 10.5 months; $p = 0.0067$) for PCDE over PE.[55] PCDE, however, was associated with significantly higher hematologic toxicity (22% of patients had documented infections compared with 8% in the PE arm; $p = 0.0038$). Toxic death rates were similar, 9% for PCDE and 5.5% for PE.

In summary, overall, no major breakthroughs have been seen with newer chemotherapy agents in the first-line setting and currently, platinum plus etoposide remains the standard of care for the treatment of SCLC.

Alternative chemotherapy strategies focus on modifications of the doses and schedules of established regimens, including dose intensification, alternating non–cross-resistant chemotherapy and prolonged treatment duration. Table 58.3 summarizes recent trial results employing these different approaches.

Dose Intensification Dose intensity is defined as the dose per square meter per week. Dose intensification can be

TABLE 58.3 Randomized Trial of Dose Intensification

Reference	Regimen[a]	No. of Patients	Overall Response (%)	Median Survival (mos)	1-Year Survival (%)
Artal-Cortés et al.[64]	PE	202	69	10.1	27
	Hd EpiP	200	75	10.9	44
Lorigan et al.[79]	ICE-std	159	80	13.9	19 (2 yrs)
	ICE-dose dense	159	88	14.4	22 (2 yrs)
Buchholz et al.[80]	ICE-std	41	88	18.5[b]	55 (2 yrs)
	ICE-dose intense	42	100	20.3	39 (2 yrs)
Leyvraz et al.[81]	ICE-std	71	68	14.4	19 (3 yrs)
	ICE-hd	69	78	18.1	18 (3 yrs)

[a]Treatment key: C, carboplatin; E, etoposide; Epi, epirubicin; hd, high dose; I, ifosphamide; P, cisplatin; std, standard.

[b]$p = 0.001$.

accomplished by either increasing the dose or shortening the interval between doses (dose density). Preclinical tumor models have illustrated that one of the simplest methods to overcoming drug resistance was drug dose escalation.[56] In the late 1970s, Cohen et al.[57] randomized patients to receive standard dosages of cyclophosphamide, methotrexate, and lomustine or a higher dose of cyclophosphamide and lomustine and a standard methotrexate dose. Hande et al.[58] randomized patients with ED SCLC to high dose or low dose methotrexate with leucovorin rescue in combination with cyclophosphamide, doxorubicin, and vincristine alternating with cycles of VP-16, vincristine, and hexamethylmelamine (negative study). They observed both a higher overall response rate and prolonged survival in the high-dose chemotherapy group. Long-term survivors were observed only among those patients given high-dose chemotherapy. These studies spawned a series of seven randomized trials comparing high dose to conventional dose chemotherapy in LS- and ES-SCLC patients.[59–65] Most of these trials were conducted in the 1980s and did not show a clinical benefit. The Spanish Lung Cancer Group recently reexamined this question (Table 58.3).[64] They compared high-dose epirubicin at 100 mg/m^2 plus cisplatin 100 mg/m^2 administered on day 1 to standard PE (cisplatin 100 mg/m^2, day 1 and etoposide 100 mg/m^2, days 1 to 3) in 402 SCLC patients. Efficacy results were similar between the two arms. For LS patients, one study published in 1989 showed a superior 2-year survival rate of 43% when the dose of cisplatin and cyclophosamide was increased by 20% in the first cycle of a PCDE regimen versus 23% for standard PCDE.[65]

Dose dense regimens have shown mixed results. CODE, an intense weekly regimen of cisplatin 25 mg/m^2 for 9 consecutive weeks; vincristine 1 mg/m^2 on even weeks for 9 weeks; with doxorubicin 40 mg/m^2 and etoposide 80 mg/m^2 days 1 to 3 on odd weeks for 9 weeks, reported an impressive 2-year survival rate of 30% in 48 patients with ES-SCLC.[66] Importantly, the investigators were able to administer close to the intended FDs of all four agents, thereby increasing the dose intensity by twofold. The National Cancer Institute of Canada Clinical Trials Group (NCIC-CTG) in collaboration with SWOG conducted a phase III trial comparing the promising CODE regimen to conventional alternating CAV/PE in patients with ES-SCLC.[67] Response rates were higher in the CODE arm, but there was no difference in PFS or OS. Although rates of neutropenia and fever were similar, toxic deaths occurred in 9 of 110 patients receiving CODE compared to only 1 of 109 patients given CAV/PE ($p = 0.42$). Given the high toxic death rate and similar efficacy, CODE was not recommended and the trial was closed prematurely. The Japanese subsequently demonstrated that the addition of granulocyte colony-stimulating factor (G-CSF) to CODE increased the mean total dose intensity received, reduced neutropenia and febrile neutropenia, and significantly prolonged survival (59 vs. 32 weeks; $p = 0.0004$).[68] This led to a phase III trial comparing CODE + G-CSF versus CAV/PE.[69] The response rate was significantly higher for CODE but, once again, no survival advantage was observed. The toxic death rate with CODE + G-CSF was low with only four reported cases.

Seven additional phase III trials incorporating a dose dense strategy with or without colony-stimulating factors have been conducted in Europe.[70–77] One trial showed a survival advantage for the dose dense arm. This trial performed by the British Medical Research Council (MRC) randomized 403 patients to receive CAE in 2 or 3 weekly schedules.[74] In this trial, a 34% escalation in dose density was achieved. Although the response rates in the two arms were similar, there was a significant improvement in the CR rate (40% vs. 28%; $p = 0.02$) that translated into a 2-year survival benefit (13% vs. 8%; $p = 0.04$). Subgroup analysis showed that the survival advantage in patients with extensive disease was as large as for limited disease patients. Other subset analyses in LS patients have shown opposing results. Steward et al.[73] showed a significant survival benefit for dose intensification, whereas Ardizzoni et al.[76] showed an inferior survival for the intensified regimen.

A possible explanation for the failure of the prior trials is that the dose intensity was insufficient to produce a survival benefit. To definitively answer the dose intensification question, studies emerged employing stem cell rescue that could allow for a 200% to 300% dose escalation. Multiple, small studies have shown this approach to be feasible. Early studies focused on patients who had achieved a response with conventional cytotoxic therapy who then received high-dose consolidation with stem cell rescue. A randomized trial testing this late-intensification strategy was reported by Humblet et al.[77] One hundred one patients received standard induction chemotherapy and forty-five chemotherapy-sensitive patients were randomized to receive one additional cycle with high-dose cyclophosphamide, carmustine (BCNU), and etoposide or conventional doses of the same drugs. In this highly selected group of patients, the median OS was 68 weeks for the high-dose arm compared to 55 weeks for the conventional therapy ($p = 0.13$).

The improved safety and feasibility of peripheral blood stem cells (PBSC) transplantation has largely replaced autologous marrow transplants. The Japanese reported promising results from a phase II study of high-dose ICE (ifosfamide, carboplatin, and etoposide) with autologous PBSC transplantation in 18 patients with LD-SCLC after concurrent, hyperfractionated chemoradiotherapy.[78] The CR was 61% and the MST was 36.4 months. One toxic death was reported. A randomized trial based on these results is ongoing.

Three randomized trials using high-dose ICE chemotherapy with peripheral blood rescue as first-line treatment for SCLC have been reported.[79–81] The largest trial with 318 predominantly LS-SCLC patients compared six cycles of a dose dense (every 14 days) ICE regimen followed by G-CSF mobilized whole blood hematopoietic progenitors, to six cycles of the standard every 28-day ICE regimen.[79] Despite doubling of the median dose intensity with the dose dense regimen (182% vs. 88%, respectively), the MST and the 2-year survival rates were comparable, 14.4 months and 22% versus 13.9 months and 19%, respectively. In contrast, an identical study by Buchholz et al.[80] was halted after 70 patients were enrolled. They reported a favorable MS of 30.3 months ($p = 0.001$), a 2-year survival rate of 55%, and TTP of 15 months ($p = 0.0001$)

for the dose intense arm versus an MS of 18.5 months, 2-year survival rate of 39%, and TTP of 11 months for the standard dose arm in this small single institution study. The European Group for Blood and Marrow Transplant conducted a similar study.[81] The study closed after 140 of the planned 340 patients were enrolled because of poor accrual. The median dose intensity for the high-dose arm was 293%, but this did not translate into a survival benefit with a MST of 18.1 months and a 3-year survival rate of 18% versus 14.4 months and 19%, respectively, for the standard ICE arm. None of the subgroups benefited from high-dose ICE.

Overall, the majority of trials employing a dose intensification strategy did not produce a survival advantage over standard therapy for patients with ES-SCLC and were typically associated with greater toxicity. This approach should be abandoned in extensive disease. In LS-SCLC, the optimal drug doses remain unclear with several studies suggesting a possible benefit. Continued evaluation of dose intensity in this curative setting is reasonable.

Alternating Non–Cross-Resistant Chemotherapy Regimens To achieve maximal antitumor effects using multiple active agents, they should be administered simultaneously at their optimal single-agent dose. However, because drug toxicities often overlap, strict adherence to this approach is often not possible in the clinical setting. In the 1980s, Goldie et al.[82] suggested that alternating two non–cross-resistant chemotherapy regimens of relatively comparable efficacy potentially could minimize the development of drug resistance while avoiding excessive host toxicity.[83] This strategy was particularly appealing for SCLC because both CAV and PE are highly active against SCLC and contain agents from divergent drug classes. Three randomized phase III trials were performed comparing CAV to CAV alternating with PE.[39,40,84] The United States and Japanese studies observed similar efficacy between the study arms, whereas the NCIC-CTG reported superior efficacy for the alternating regimen with an overall response rate of 80% versus 63% (p <0.002) and a survival time of 9.6 versus 8.0 months (p = 0.03). Investigators at NCIC-CTG went on to test this approach in patients with limited disease SCLC.[84] Patients were randomized between two induction regimens either alternating CAV/PE or sequential therapy with three cycles of CAV followed by three cycles of PE. Chemotherapy was followed by radiotherapy in responding patients. No significant differences in therapeutic outcomes were observed between the two study groups. SWOG conducted a similar study and found no advantage for the alternating CAV/PE regimen over the EVAC (etoposide, vincristine, adraimycin, and cyclophosphamide) regimen in LS patients.[85]

The EORTC reported a trial testing two relatively non–cross-resistant regimens: CDE and VIMP (vincristine, carboplatin, ifosfamide, mesna).[86] Patients with ES-SCLC were randomly assigned to receive a maximum of five courses of CDE or an alternating regimen consisting of CDE in cycles 1, 3, and 5 and VIMP in cycles 2 and 4. The trial accrued only 148 of its 360 planned patients. The MS was 7.6 in the standard arm and 8.7 months in the alternating arm (p = 0.243).

Although no survival benefit for the alternating drug hypothesis was demonstrated, the emergence of newer active agents in the treatment of SCLC justified revisiting this strategy. The North Central Cancer Treatment Group (NCCTG) conducted a trial of PE alternating with topotecan and paclitaxel.[87] The overall response rate was 77% including 4 CRs in 44 evaluable patients. The MS was 10.5 months with 1- and 2-year survival rate of 37% and 12%, respectively. This alternating regimen was associated with high rates of grades 3 and 4 neutropenia (95%) despite the use of filgrastim in cycles 2, 4, and 6. The Hellenic Oncology Research Group treated 36 previously untreated patients with ES-SCLC with PE alternating with topotecan.[88] The overall response rate was 64% with 14% of patients achieving a CR. Grades 3 and 4 neutropenia occurred in 39% of patients during the PE cycles and in 55% after the topotecan treatment. This limited data incorporating newer chemotherapy agents into an alternating strategy was disappointing. Taken together, alternating newer and/or older cytotoxic agents to overcome drug resistance is unsuccessful and should not be pursued.

Treatment Duration and Maintenance Therapy The ideal number of chemotherapy cycles for SCLC has not been defined; however, four to six cycles is considered the standard based on the randomized trials presented previously. Clinical trials specifically designed to investigate the role of prolonged treatment using a consolidation or maintenance approach have been performed for decades. Three of 14 trials produced positive results.[89–91] All three trials were initiated in 1982. Two trials in LS-SCLC patients gave two to four cycles of PE consolidation to responding patients after induction CAV with or without thoracic radiotherapy.[89,90] The remaining trial randomized nonprogressors with LS or ES disease to four additional cycles of CEV or observation.[91] Although this trial showed that four cycles of CEV was inferior, a second randomization to salvage chemotherapy versus symptomatic care upon disease progression revealed that the subset of patients who received eight cycles of CEV with or without salvage therapy did no better than patients who received four cycles of CEV and salvage therapy at the time of relapse. The role of consolidation and/or maintenance therapy with a newer agent, topotecan, in ES-SCLC patients was evaluated by Eastern Cooperative Oncology Group (ECOG).[92] Two hundred twenty-three nonprogressing patients were randomized to receive four cycles of topotecan or observation. PFS from the date of randomization was significantly better with topotecan compared with observation (3.6 vs. 2.3 months; p <0.001) but OS from randomization was not significantly different between the two arms (8.9 vs. 9.3 months; p = 0.43). Thus, it does not appear that there is a role for consolidation and/or maintenance therapy in SCLC. A 2007 metaanalysis of the 14 randomized trials suggests otherwise.[93] The odds ratios for 1- and 2-year OS rates were both 0.67 (p <0.001) favoring prolonged treatment. Significant odds ratios for the 1- and 2-year PFS rates also support the role for consolidation and/or maintenance treatment. These results should be interpreted with caution, however, because they are not based on individual patient data, the studies were highly variable in their designs and most of the trials employed outdated regimens. In general, chemotherapy after four to six cycles of a combination regimen is not warranted. Further evaluation of this strategy should turn to molecularly targeted agents.

SECOND-LINE CHEMOTHERAPY

Despite a high response rate, the majority of patients will progress. If these patients are left untreated, survival is about 2 to 3 months. For patients who receive second-line treatment, tumor stabilization and shrinkage may occur but rarely do patients live longer than 6 months. Predictors of response to second-line therapy are dependent on the interval between cessation of initial therapy and the detection of recurrence and the responsiveness to previous induction chemotherapy. Three disease categories exist: (a) sensitive relapse denotes a relapse greater than 3 months after the last treatment; (b) resistant relapse develops in less than 3 months of the last treatment; and (c) refractory relapse signifying no response to front-line treatment or progressing on therapy. The Ottawa Hospital Regional Cancer Center reviewed the records of all ES-SCLC patients from 1999 to 2003 and showed that of the 192 patients completing first-line therapy, only 32% received second-line treatment.[94] Patients receiving salvage therapy, who tended to be younger and healthier, lived longer from the time of relapse (5.2 months as compared to 1.5 months) than did patient who did not receive treatment. A survival benefit was seen regardless of the timing of the relapse and patients receiving additional therapy. In the multivariate analyses, second-line therapy was an independent predictor of survival.

Prior to the mid-1990s, PE was a reasonable choice in CAV failures. A phase III SWOG trial randomly assigned 103 good- and poor-risk relapsed patients to PE or BTOC (BCNU, thiotepa, vincristine, and cyclophosphamide).[95] Good-risk patients achieved a 27% remission rate with an MS of 35 weeks with PE versus 27% remission rate and a 10-week survival time for BTOC. Poor-risk patients in both arms had an unfavorable 9% response rate and MSTs of 10 to 12 weeks. Conversely, CAV was shown to be inactive in PE failures.[96]

Single-agent activity of newer agents evaluated in relapsed SCLC is listed in Table 58.1. Topotecan emerged as a leading candidate to pursue in phase III trials (Table 58.4). In the first study, 211 patients who relapsed more than 60 days after completion of induction therapy were randomized to receive topotecan (1.5 mg/m^2/day, days 1 to 5 q 21 days) or conventional CAV.[97] The overall response rates and MSs were not statistically different between the two arms: 24.3% versus 18.3% and 25 versus 24.7 weeks, respectively. Dyspnea, fatigue, anorexia, hoarseness, and daily activity significantly improved with topotecan. Grades 3 and 4 anemia and thrombocytopenia were greater in the topotecan arm but there were no differences in nonhematological toxicities. Topotecan was subsequently approved for second-line treatment in patients with sensitive relapse based on symptom control. An oral formulation of topotecan was developed for patient convenience. To evaluate its efficacy, 141 relapsed patients were randomized to receive oral topotecan (2.3 mg/m^2/day × 5 days) plus best supportive care (BSC) versus BSC every 21 days.[98] Oral topotecan was superior to BSC with a MST of 25.9 weeks compared to 13.9 weeks for BSC (p = 0.01). Importantly, a survival advantage was recognized in patients who had relapsed less than as well as greater than 60 days from the end of their previous therapy. The most common toxicities with oral topotecan were hematological. Grades 3 and 4 neutropenia occurred in 61%, thrombocytopenia (38%) and anemia (25%), of patients. Subsequently, oral topotecan was compared to IV topotecan in sensitive relapsed patients (defined as relapse >90 days after chemotherapy).[99] A total of 153 patients received oral topotecan (2.3 mg/m^2/day, days 1 to 5 q 21 days) and 151 patients received standard doses of IV topotecan (1.5 mg/m^2 /day, days 1 to 5 q 21 days). The response rate, MS, and 1-year survival for the oral agent were 18.3%, 33 weeks and 33%, respectively, compared to 21.9%, 35 weeks and 29%, respectively, for the IV administration. The incidence of grade 4 neutropenia was 47% with oral topotecan versus 64% with the IV formulation. The quality-of-life analysis was comparable between the arms. Oral topotecan was approved by the Food and Drug Administration (FDA) for the treatment of both sensitive and resistant/refractory patients.

TABLE 58.4 Phase III Trials in Second-Line SCLC

Reference	Regimen[a]	No. of Patients	Overall Response (%)	Median Survival (wks)	1-Year Survival (%)
von Pawel et al.[97]	T	107	24.3	25 wks	14.2
	CAV	104	18.3	18.3 wks	14.4
O'Brien et al.[98]	T	71	NR	25.5 wks[b]	NR
	BSC	70	7	13.9 wks	NR
Eckardt Jr et al.[99]	T (IV)	151	21.9	35 wks	29
	T (PO)	153	18.3	33 wks	33

[a]Treatment key: A, adriamycin; BSC, best supportive care; C, cyclophosphamide; IV, intravenous; NR, not reported; PO, oral; SCLC, small cell lung cancer; T, topotecan; V, vincristine.

[b]p <0.05.

NR, not reported.

In the past 2 years, there has been renewed enthusiasm for chemotherapy because of the interesting results generated with amirubicin (Table 58.1). Two multicentered phase II trials of single-agent amirubicin in relapsed SCLC have been conducted in Japan. The first study included 16 patients who relapsed in less than 60 days (refractory group) and 44 patients who relapsed greater than 60 days (sensitive group) to receive amirubicin 40 mg/m^2 for 3 days every 3 weeks.[29] The overall response rate in the refractory group was 50% (95% CI, 25% to 75%) and it was 52% (95% CI, 37% to 58%) in the sensitive group. The OS and 1-year survival rates were 10.3 months and 40%, respectively, in the refractory group and 11.6 months and 46%, respectively, in the sensitive group. The median number of cycles was four. Grade 3 or 4 neutropenia was 83% with a febrile neutropenia rate of 5%. No toxic deaths occurred. In a second study, 34 relapsed patients (10 relapsed in less than 60 days and 24 relapsed beyond 60 days) received amirubicin at 45 mg/m^2 for 3 days every 3 weeks.[30] With a median of four cycles, the response rates for the refractory patients was 60% (95% CI, 23% to 97%) and 53% (95% CI, 35% to 70%) for the sensitive patients. MSTs were 6.8 and 10.4 months, respectively. Grade 3 or 4 neutropenia was common, occurring in 71% of patients. Grade 3 or 4 febrile neutropenia developed in 35% of patients and one toxic death from pneumonia was reported. These data suggest that amirubicin is highly active but produces significant neutropenia although toxic deaths were rare. A randomized phase II trial comparing response rate between amirubicin to topotecan followed. Sixty patients received amirubicin (40 mg/m^2, days 1 to 3) or topotecan (1 mg/m^2, days 1 to 5, IV) every 3 weeks.[32] The ORR was 38% (53% in sensitive and 17% in refractory patients) for amirubicin and 13% (21% in sensitive and 0 in refractory patients) for topotecan. Overall median PFS was 3.5 versus 2.2 months, respectively. Survival was similar at 8.1 months for amirubicin and 8.4 months for topotecan. Amirubicin produced more grade 3 and 4 neutropenia 97% (vs. 87%) that resulted in more febrile neutropenia 14% (vs. 3%). There was one reported toxic death on amirubicin. Thrombocytopenia and anemia were more frequent with topotecan, 40% and 30% compared to 28% and 21% for amirubicin. In the United States, a randomized study to evaluate the response rate of amirubicin compared to topotecan has been completed in sensitive relapsed patients.[31] Seventy-six patients were randomized in a 2:1 fashion to receive the same dose of amirubicin or topotecan at 1.5 mg/m^2 IV, days 1 to 5 every 3 weeks. The ORR for the amirubicin arm was 34% as compared to 1% ($p < 0.004$). The median PFS time was 4.6 months for amirubicin and 3.5 months for topotecan. At this time, the survival data are immature. In this study, there was more significant neutropenia in the topotecan arm 61% as compared to 45% with amirubicin that was most likely caused by the higher dose of topotecan used. Importantly, there was no evidence of anthracycline-induced cardiotoxicity. An international phase III trial of amirubicin versus topotecan is ongoing. Data from a U.S. phase II study in refractory or resistant patients progressing with 90 days has also been recently reported.[33] Seventy-five patients received amirubicin at 40 mg/m^2, days 1 to 3 every 3 weeks. The ORR was 17.4% with one patient achieving a CR. The median PFS time was 3.2 months and OS is pending. Grades 3 and 4 neutropenia was seen in 49% of patients and no cardiac toxicity was observed.

Exploratory studies with a two-drug combination in this salvage setting have not generated promising data that would warrant phase III testing. Although it is reasonable to continue to evaluate doublets, balancing efficacy and toxicity is challenging.

Finally, two small case series totaling 18 patients reported that 10 patients who relapsed >10 months from the end of therapy had durable responses to their original regimen.[100,101] Reinduction with the original treatment regimen should be entertained in patients with prolonged time to relapse.

To summarize, topotecan IV or oral represents a modest advance for the treatment of relapsed SCLC. However, other agents are frequently used.[102,103] Amirubicin has produced impressive results in both sensitive and resistant/refractory patients, but its ultimate role awaits the results from phase III trials. Given the poor outcome of these patients, they should be encouraged to participate in clinical trials with novel therapeutic agents.

BIOLOGICAL THERAPY

The current understanding of the molecular biology of SCLC is detailed in Chapter 5. In this section, a comprehensive review of the targeted therapies evaluated in SCLC based on a biological rationale is provided.

Tyrosine Kinase Inhibitors A hallmark of SCLC is its multiple neuropeptide autocrine growth loops. Numerous studies have demonstrated that these growth loops are a dominant mitogenic stimulus for SCLC.[104] Antagonists to neuropeptides have undergone clinical testing, but drug delivery issues and the heterogeneity of neuropeptides and their receptors have hampered their continued development. Meanwhile, other signaling pathways emerged as potential targets. Enthusiasm for imatinib, a small molecule tyrosine kinase inhibitor (TKI) against c-kit, surfaced when C-kit expression was demonstrated in 50% to 70% of SCLC cell lines tested.[105–108] Moreover, imatinib-treated cell lines resulted in apoptosis and cytostasis.[109] Despite preclinical evidence of activity, imatinib failed to show antitumor activity in clinical trials either as a single agent or in combination with chemotherapy as shown in Table 58.5.[110–113] The first study involving 19 chemonaive or sensitive relapsed patients did not produce any objective responses.[110] The low number of tumors with c-kit expression was thought to be the explanation for the lack of efficacy. A second study in 29 relapsed patients with c-kit expressing tumors, however, also failed to demonstrate responses.[111] One study to determine if imatinib with chemotherapy would be efficacious showed results similar to chemotherapy alone. Irinotecan and carboplatin plus imatinib in 68 untreated

TABLE 58.5 Targeted Therapies for SCLC: Cell Surface Targets

Agent	Regimen	No. of Patients	Overall Response (%)	Median Survival (mos)
Tynosine Kinase Inhibitor				
Imatinib[110]	600 mg po qd	19[a]	0	9.3[U] 6.5[S]
Imatinib[111]	400 mg po bid	29[b]	0	5.9[S] 3.9[R]
Imatinib and Irinotecan Carboplatin[112]	600 mg po qd	68[c]	67	8.4
Gefitinib[114]	250 mg po qd	19[b]	0	NR
Matrix Metaloproteinase Inhibitors				
Marimastat[119]	10 mg po bid placebo	532	NA	9.3 9.7
Bay12-9566[121]	800 mg po bid placebo	327	NA	NR[d]
Immunotherapy				
BEC-2/BCG[127]	2.5 mg ID wks 0, 2, 4, 6, 10 observation	515	NA	16.3 14.3
Chemotherapy ± SRL172[131]	1 mg ID wks 0, 4, 8, 12, 16 observation	80	NA	41 wks 40 wks

[a]Chemonaive and sensitive relapsed patients.

[b]Sensitive and refractory patients.

[c]Chemonaive patients.

[d]TTP Bay12-9566 = 3.2 mos; placebo = 5.3 mos; $p = 0.05$.

BCG, bacillus Calmette-Guérin; bid, twice a day; ID, intradermal; NA, not applicable; NR, not reported; po, oral; qd, once a day; R, refractory/resistant relapse; S, sensitive relapse; SCLC, small cell lung cancer; U, untreated.

ES-SCLC patients induced a response rate of 67%, median PFS of 5.4 months, and median OS of 8.4 months.[112] It is now believed that imatinib ineffectiveness is caused by c-kit activity being a result of an autocrine or paracrine growth loop rather than the presences of an activating mutation in the receptor as seen in gastrointestinal stromal tumors.[113]

Unlike NSCLC, the epidermal growth factor receptor (EGFR) pathway plays a minimal role in the malignant process of SCLC. Nonetheless, the Hoosier Oncology Group postulated that the EGFR signaling network may be activated through other mechanisms and conducted a phase II trial (Table 58.5).[114] Twelve patients with chemosensitive and seven patients with chemorefractory disease received gefitinib. The best response was stable disease in 2 patients and 17 patients had progressive disease. The median TTP was 50 days and the 1-year survival was 21%. Inhibitors of downstream signals of the tyrosine kinase receptors including RAS and c-MYC have been unsuccessful.[115,116]

Matrix Metalloproteinase Inhibitors The matrix metalloproteinases (MMPs) are a family of degradative enzymes associated with tumor cell invasion of the basement membrane and stroma, blood vessel penetration, angiogenesis, and metastasis.[117] MMP expression in SCLC was found to be as high as 89% in one study and increased expression of certain MMPs[3,11,14] were associated with shorter survival.[118] Two MMP inhibitors have been studied in SCLC as displayed in Table 58.5. The oral agent marimastat was compared to placebo in a study of 555 patients with SCLC who had responded to first-line therapy.[119] No survival benefit was seen with marimastat. Musculoskeletal toxicity was a significant problem. A second smaller but identical trial in 350 SCLC patients was also negative.[120] A large trial comparing BAY12-9566 to placebo in 700 patients with lung cancer who had responded to induction chemotherapy was halted early because of negative interim results.[121] Of the 327 SCLC patients enrolled, the TTP was 3.2 months in the BAY12-9566 group versus 5.3 months for the placebo group ($p = 0.05$). The incidence of adverse events was higher in the patients on the BAY 12-9566 arm.

Immunotherapy In the early 1980s, interferons demonstrated antitumor activity and presented a novel approach to cancer therapy including SCLC. Several trials with interferons were launched, but most failed to show a favorable impact, and were toxic.[122–125] A popular strategy today is evaluating tumor vaccines. SCLC expresses numerous gangliosides such as fucosyl GM1, polysialic acid, GM2, GD2, and GD3 that are not expressed on most normal tissue making and ideal for a vaccine approach.[126] The anti-idiotypic antibody (BEC-2) mimicking GD3 was evaluated in an international phase III trial.[127] Five hundred fifteen LS-SCLC patients responding to definitive treatment were randomized to BEC2 or observation. No impact on survival was seen with the vaccine. The PFS was 6.6 months for the observation arm and 5.7 months for the vaccine arm. MS was 16.3 and 14.3 months, respectively. Other vaccines in clinical testing target the fucosyl-GM1 ganglioside (Fuc-GM1) and polysialic acid (polySA) a component of the neural cell adhesion molecule (NCAM).[128,129]

A study conducted in United Kingdom explored an alternative immunologic strategy using SRL172, a suspension of heat killed *Mycobacterium vaccae* that works as a potent immunological adjuvant when given in combination with autologous cells in animal models. In a phase III trial with standard chemotherapy, survival times were similar between the two groups, however, symptom improvement favored the vaccine Table 58.5.[130,131]

Novel immunological strategies included immunologically targeted toxins such as BB 10901, a humanized murine monoclonal antibody (huN-901) that binds to CD56 conjugated to the tubulin toxin maytansinoid cytotoxin DM1 and the use of dendritic cells transduced with full-length wild-type p53 gene delivered via an adenoviral.[132,133]

Apoptotic Modulators The most extensively studied apoptosis modulator in SCLC is bcl-2. Overexpression of bcl-2 has been reported in 69% to 90% of SCLC.[134,135] In vitro studies using SCLC cell lines have demonstrated antisense sequences against bcl-2 induces apoptosis and enhances cytotoxicity of chemotherapeutic agents.[136–138] Oblimersen (G3139, Genasense), an antisense oligonucleotide, was shown to suppress the anti-apoptotic protein bcl-2. Encouraging early clinical work lead to a randomized phase II of CE plus or minus oblimersen described in Table 58.6.[139] The addition of oblimersen did not improve efficacy over CE alone. This agent has been abandoned, but other novel small molecule bcl-2 inhibitors are being explored.[140]

Exisulind is an apoptotic inhibitor whose mechanism of action is independent of p53, bcl-2, or cell cycle arrest.[141] This oral derivative, from the cyclooxygenase inhibitor sulindac, produces its apoptotic effect by inhibiting cyclic guanosine monophosphate (cGMP) phosphodiesterases, which, in turn, increases levels of protein kinase G and activate the apoptotic cascade.[142] Synergistic cytotoxicity was observed with exisulind plus several cytotoxic agents used to treat SCLC.[143] Interestingly, synergy was seen in cell lines that overexpress MDR (multiple drug resistance)-associated protein.[144] In untreated ES-SCLC, a phase I study of CE with exisulind (125 to 250 mg po [orally] bid [twice daily]) showed that the combination was well tolerated and lead the Cancer and Leukemia Group B (CALGB) to conduct a phase II study administering exisulind at 250 mg bid with CE.[145] This trial involving 43 patients did not meet its primary survival end point of 60% of patients surviving greater than 12 months (Table 58.6). The median PFS was 6.7 months and the median OS was 10.5 months.

The ubiquitin-proteosome pathway is essential for the degradation of intracellular proteins. In particular, proteosome 26S inhibition limits the breakdown of inhibitor IB disrupting the nuclear factor kappa-light-chain-enhancer of activated B cells (NF-κB) pathway leading to apoptosis.[146] Bortezomib (PS341) is a potent inhibitor of the 26S proteosome.[147] SWOG conducted a phase II trial of bortezomib in 56 relapsed patients.[148] One platinum refractory patient had a confirmed response and two patients had stable disease (Table 58.6). None of the platinum-sensitive patients responded. The median PFS was 1 month and the OS was 3 months.

Cell Cycle Regulators CCI-779, a structural ester of sirolimus, forms a complex with FK506-binding protein (FKBP), which then inhibits mammalian target of rapamycin (mTOR). Inhibition of mTOR blocks the translation of several key proteins that regulate the G-1 phase of the cell cycle resulting in cytostasis.[149] ECOG evaluated CCI-779 as

TABLE 58.6 Targeted Therapies for SCLC: Intracellular Targets

Agent	Regimen	No. of Patients	Overall Response (%)	Median Survival (mos)
Carboplatin and etoposide ± G3139[139]	7 mg/kg/day, days 1–8	56	61	8.6
	placebo		60	10.6
Carboplatin and etoposide + exisulind[145]	250 mg po bid	43	81	10.5
Bortezomib[148]	1.3 mg/m^2, days 1, 4, 8, 11	56[a]	2	3.0
CC1 779[150]	Arm A – 25 mg IV wkly	85	1.2	8.0[b]
	Arm B – 250 mg IV wkly			

[a]Sensitive and refractory/resistant patients.

[b]Primary end point PFS – Arm A = 1.9 mos; Arm B = 2.5 mos.

bid, twice a day; IV, intravenous; po, oral; SCLC, small cell lung cancer.

a maintenance agent in 86 nonprogressing patients after induction chemotherapy (Table 58.6).[150] The median PFS was 1.9 months for the 25-mg dose level and 2.5 months for 250-mg dose level with MS of 6.6 and 9.5 months, respectively. The MS for all 85 patients was 8 months. No major toxicities were observed.

Angiogenesis Inhibitors It is well established that angiogenesis is necessary for tumor growth and metastases. Pathological studies in resected SCLC specimens revealed that high microvessel count and vascular endothelial growth factor (VEGF) expression were associated with decreased survival.[151–153] Furthermore, VEGF expression was shown to be an independent poor prognostic factor in one study.[151] The first angiogenesis inhibitor tested in SCLC was thalidomide. Thalidomide is an old agent with multiple well-defined mechanisms of action, including inhibition of antiangiogenesis. Its oral availability, tolerable toxicity profile, and easy access made it a readily available to evaluate. In Europe, a phase III double-blind, placebo-controlled study of maintenance thalidomide versus observation was stopped prematurely because of poor accrual. In 119 responding patients with ES-SCLC, no significant survival benefit was seen with thalidomide although the MS was 11.7 months for the thalidomide group compared to 8.7 months for the placebo group (Table 58.7).[154] Prolonged disease progression was noted in performance status (PS) 1 to 2 patients receiving thalidomide (hazard ratio [HR] = 0.54; $p = 0.02$). Based on the hint of superior survival seen in the French study, the London Lung Cancer Study Group conducted a phase III randomized, double-blind, placebo-controlled of etoposide/carboplatin with or without thalidomide in 724 patients. Survival times were essentially identical as displayed in Table 58.7.[155] The MS was 10.5 months for placebo and 10.2 months for thalidomide. There was higher incidence of thrombotic events in the thalidomide arm 18% versus 11% in placebo arm.

Bevacizumab humanized monoclonal antibody to VEGF inhibits neoangiogenesis and normalizes tumor vasculature. In NSCLC, an ECOG study showing that the combination of bevacizumab with paclitaxel and carboplatin significantly improved response rate, PFS, and OS compared with chemotherapy alone generated enthusiasm for testing bevacizumab in SCLC.[156] CALBG combined bevacizumab with irinotecan and cisplatin in 72 chemotherapy naive SCLC patients. As described in Table 58.7, the response rate was 71%, median PFS was 7.1 months, and MS was 11 months.[157] This study failed to meet its primary end point of a 12.8-month MS. A similar study by ECOG testing bevacizumab with etoposide and cisplatin followed by bevacizumab successfully met its goal of 6-month PFS rate greater than 33% (Table 58.7). In 64 patients, they reported a 6-month PFS of 35%, ORR of 69%, a median PFS of 4.7 months, and an MS of 11.1 months.[158] Preliminary results of a phase II trial of irinotecan, carboplatin, and bevacizumab in 34 patients showed a 78% response rate.[159] Bevacizumab has also been explored in LS-SCLC. A phase II study administering irinotecan plus carboplatin and

TABLE 58.7 Targeted Therapies for SCLC: Angiogenesis Targets

Agent	Regimen	No. of Patients	Overall Response (%)	Median Survival (mos)
Thalidomide[154]	Placebo	92[d]	NA	8.7
	400 mg po qd			11.7
Cisplatin and etoposide ± thalidomide[155]	Placebo	724[d]	NR	10.5
	100–200 mg po qd			
Irinotecan and cisplatin bevacizumab[157]	15 mg/kg IV D1	72[d]	71	11.0
Cisplatin and etoposide bevacizumab[158]	15 mg/kg IV D1	64[d]	69	11.1
Irinotecan and carboplatin bevacizumab[159]	10 mg/kg IV D1 and 15	34[c]	80	NR
Bevacizumab[160]	10 mg/kg IV D1 and D15	60[a,c]	NA	17.5
Sorafenib[162]	400 mg po bid	83[b,d]	5	7.0[S]
				5.0[R]
Vandetanib[163]	Placebo	107[c]	NA	10.6
	300 mg po qd			11.9

[a]42 patients received bevacizumab.

[b]40 sensitive and 43 refractory patients.

[c]Included LS-SCLC patients.

[d]extensive stage disease.

bid, twice a day; IV, intravenous; NA, not applicable; NR, not reported; po, oral; qd, once a day; R, refractory/resistant relapse; S, sensitive relapse; SCLC, small cell lung cancer.

concurrent radiation followed by bevacizumab maintenance showed a 2-year PFS rate of 70% and 53% and a 1- and 2-year OS rate of 38% and 29% in 60 patients. The MS was 17.5 months.[160] Since this preliminary report, a tracheoesophageal fistula occurred in one patient. In a follow-up study integrating bevacizumab with concurrent chemoradiotherapy, two additional tracheoesophageal fistulas were seen and the study was terminated with 29 of the planned 50 patients enrolled.[161]

Oral angiokinases inhibitors have been piloted. SWOG studied sorafenib, a TKI of RAF and VEGFR in 83 relapsed patients.[162] Four patients (4%) achieved a partial response and 25 patients (32%) had stable disease. The median PFS was 2 months for all patients. The MS was 7 months in the sensitive relapsed group and 5 months in refractory group. Sunitinib and cediranib are also being investigated in SCLC.

Vandetanib, an oral VEGFR and EGFR TKI has been studied in a by the NCIC-CTG. They examined maintenance vandetanib versus placebo in 107 patients with LD- and ES-SCLC after initial chemotherapy response (Table 58.7).[163] No difference in OS or PFS was seen between the groups. Median PFS for vandetanib and placebo were 2.7 and 2.8 months, respectively (HR = 1.01). OS for vandetanib was 10.6 versus 11.9 months for placebo (HR = 1.43). In planned subgroup analyses, a significant interaction was noted in patients with LS disease who received vandetanib. These patients had a longer OS (HR = 0.45; one-sided p = .07) and extensive-stage vandetanib patients had a shorter survival compared with placebo (HR = 2.27; one-sided p = 0.996). In summary, targeted therapy for SCLC has not demonstrated the success we anticipated but it is vital that we continue the search. We remain confident that as we unravel the complex biology of SCLC, we will develop effective treatments.

SCLC IN THE ELDERLY

Elderly patients with cancer represent a growing population. The SEER database recently published their statistics on the clinical presentation and outcomes for lung cancer patients diagnosed during 1988 to 2003.[164] A total of 47% of lung cancer cases occurred in patients 70 years old or older with 14% of cases diagnosed in patients 80 years or older. Similar age distributions are seen worldwide.[165,166] Specifically looking at SCLC, the SEER analysis showed that 61% of patients were ≥70 years old at diagnosis.[164] The relative 5-year survival rate for SCLC was significantly worse for elderly patients versus younger patients (p <0.0001) and had not changed over the 15 years studied. For the time period between 1998 and 2003, the 5-year survival rate was 6.5% for patients younger than 70 years old, 3.4% for patients age 70 to 79, and 2.4% for patients 80 years or older.

Retrospective reviews to identify prognostic factors in SCLC have shown variable results concerning age. The largest experience to date was conducted by Albain et al.[167] who examined the SWOG database in 1990. An analysis of 2580 patients enrolled on six SWOG studies of which approximately 10% were elderly revealed that patients older than the age of 70 had a significant HR death of 1.5 (p ≤0.0001) for LS patients and an HR of 1.3 (p = 0.006) for ES disease. In contrast, a smaller study reported a year later on 614 LS and ES patients in the University of Toronto clinical trial database revealed that age older than 70 was not a significant predictor of a poorer outcome.[168] In LS patients, a metaanalysis published by Pignon et al.[169] in 1992 examined 2140 patients from 13 randomized trials that were designed to determine the role of thoracic radiotherapy combined with chemotherapy versus chemotherapy alone. The relative risk of death in patients older than the age of 70 receiving combination therapy was 1.07 as compared to elderly patients receiving just chemotherapy. Since this metaanalysis, a review of two NCIC-CTG trials, BR.3 and BR.6, involving 618 LS patients that received the same chemotherapy regimen, revealed no difference in survival between patients younger or older than 70 years,[170] although a significantly higher proportion of elderly patients failed to complete all planned chemotherapy cycles. In the United States Intergroup study comparing once-daily to twice-daily radiation in limited SCLC, survival of younger than 70-year-old patients compared to younger patients was of borderline significance in favor of younger patients (p = 0.051).[171] Taken together, these studies suggest that age alone is a poor indicator of a patients overall health status.

Nonetheless, increased age has been perceived as a strong rationale for the use of less aggressive therapies or no therapy for fear of increased toxicity. The literature on this topic is conflicting with retrospective reviews reporting that increased age is associated with a heightened risk of chemotherapy-related morbidity and mortality.[172–175] Other studies show that despite toxicity and dose reductions elderly patient do receive a survival benefit with chemotherapy and/or radiotherapy over no treatment.[176–179] A recent review from the Royal Marsden investigated the survival outcome in 322 elderly SCLC patients older than the age of 70 treated with chemotherapy from 1982 to 2003.[180] Patients treated between 1995 and 2003 had a better MS of 43 weeks and a 1-year survival of 37% compared to 25 weeks and 14%, respectively, for patients treated from 1982 to 1994 (p <0.001). Patients who received platinum combination had a statistically superior survival (p <0.001) versus those who received single agents or another combination. There was no survival difference between a cisplatin versus a carboplatin regimen. A 2005 analysis of the 54 elderly patients with LS disease who participated in NCCTG phase III trial of PE plus twice-a-day or once-a-day thoracic radiation revealed that although the elderly patients were sicker and developed more toxicity, survival was not different from their younger counterparts.[181]

Modern phase III trials have been reporting outcomes in elderly patients in the primary manuscript. In the CALGB study of PE versus PET in ES-SCLC, 19% of the patients enrolled were age 70 years or older.[54] A significantly worse survival outcome was reported for patients 70 years or older with an MST of 8.6 months compared to 10.5 months for younger patients (p = 0.0008). No additional information was provided regarding treatment group or toxic deaths among the elderly to further understand this finding. An international phase III trial of oral topotecan plus cisplatin (TC) versus PE in ES patients reported half of the patients enrolled were age 65 years or older and had a similar survival time to younger patients.[48] The MS was 39.9 weeks (TC) and 42.9 weeks (PE) for patients younger than 65 years compared to 38 and 36 weeks, respectively, for older patients. Variable survival results have also been demonstrated in prospective phase II studies making it difficult to meaningfully understand the risk: benefit ratio of chemotherapy in the elderly.[182–189]

To formally address the question of dose, Ardizzoni et al.[190] randomized SCLC patients 70 years old or older to four cycles of cisplatin 25 mg/m^2, days 1 to 2 with etoposide 60 mg/m^2 IV, days 1 to 3 every 3 weeks, the attenuated dose (AD) regimen (n = 28) or to cisplatin 40 mg/m^2, days 1 to 2 plus etoposide 100 mg/m^2 IV, days 1 to 3 with prophylactic G-CSF, the FD regimen (n = 67). As shown in Table 58.8, the response rate was 39% in the AD arm versus 68% in the FD arm with 1-year survival rates of 18% and 39%, respectively. There was no grade 3 or 4 myelotoxicity in the AD group and 10% in the FD group. There was one toxic death in the FD arm. The median number of cycles was four in both groups with 75% in the AD group and 72% in the FD group completing all planned cycles. The Japanese conducted a phase III trial designed to test if near FDs of carboplatin and etoposide (CE) was superior to their standard regimen for elderly patients of a split dose of PE (SPE). Elderly patients were defined as patients ≥70 years old or older with a PS of 0 to 2. Patients younger than 70 years old with a PS of three were allowed to participate.[191] A total of 220 ES patients were entered onto the study with 110 patients receiving carboplatin (AUC = 5 on day 1) and etoposide 80 mg/m^2, IV on days 1 to 3 every 3 to 4 weeks for four cycles and 109 patients receiving cisplatin 25 mg/m^2, days 1 to 3 with etoposide 80 mg/m^2 IV, days 1 to 3 every 3 to 4 weeks for four cycles (Table 58.8). G-CSF was recommended in both arms. Ninety-two percent of the patients met the elderly criteria and eight percent were poor risk. ORR were identical in both arms at 73%. MS for the CE arm was 10.6 months with a 1-year survival rate of 41% as compared to 9.9 months and 35%, respectively, for the SPE arm. Both arms reported very high grades 3 and 4 neutropenia rates of 95% for CE and 90% for SPE. Treatment-related deaths were four, three in the CE arm and one in the SPE arm. The only significant difference in toxicity was the higher rate of grades 3 and 4 thrombocytopenia at 56% for CE and 16% for SPE ($p = 0.01$). The authors concluded that either regimen was a reasonable treatment option. A phase III trial of CE versus amirubicin in the elderly is ongoing

In LS-SCLC patients, Jeremic et al.[192] administered accelerated hyperfractioned radiotherapy, 1.5 Gy twice a day to a total dose of 45 Gy over 3 weeks concurrently with carboplatin and oral etoposide. No further chemotherapy was given. They treated 77 patients aged 70 to 77 years. Of note, 12 patients had a Karnofsky PS of only 60% or 70%, and 18 patients had weight loss of more than 5% of body weight. The patients tolerated treatment remarkably well with only 2.8% grade 3 esophagitis, 8.3% grade 3 leukopenia, and 4.2% grade 3 infection. Despite the abbreviated chemotherapy treatment, the overall response rate was 75%, and survival rates were promising (74%, 1 year; 32%, 2 years; 19%, 3 years). In a trial of similar

TABLE 58.8 Randomized Trials in Elderly and/or Poor Performance Status Patients

Reference	Regimen[a]	No. of Patients	Overall Response (%)	Median Survival	1-Year Survival (%)	No. of Toxic Deaths
Elderly						
Ardizzoni et al.[190]	PE-AD	28	39	31 wks	18	0
	PE-FD	67	68	41 wks	39	1
Okamoto et al.[191]	CE	110	73	10.6 mo	41	3
	SPE	110	73	9.9 mo	35	1
Poor PS						
MRC-LCWP[198]	ECMCV	154	NR	141 days	12	NR
	EV	156	NR	137 days	10	NR
MRC-LCWP[199]	E (oral)	171	45	130 days[b]	11	NR
	PE or CAV	168	51	183 days	13	NR
Souhami et al.[200]	E (oral)	75	32.9	4.8 mo	9.8	NR
	PE/CAV	80	46.3	5.9 mo	19.3[c]	NR

[a]Treatment key: A, adriamycin; C, carboplatin; C, cyclophosphamide; E, etoposide; M, methotrexate; P, cisplatin; S, split dose; V, vincristine.

[b]$p = 0.03$.

[c]$p < 0.05$.

NR, not reported.

design, Murray et al.[193] gave two cycles of chemotherapy (CAV followed by EP) and radiation consisting of either 20 Gy in 5 fractions or 30 Gy in 10 fractions concurrently with EP to the frail elderly (older than 70 years) as well as to younger patients who had significant comorbidity or who refused standard chemotherapy.[191] Although 14 of the 55 patients were less than 70 years of age, the remainders were elderly, with 22 patients older than 75 and 4 patients were older than age 80. Three patients died of treatment-related complications, although two of these deaths were acute cardiac events that may have had other causes in this elderly or infirm patient cohort. Other toxicities were no different from expected. The overall response rate was 89%, and MS was 12.5 months with 28% and 18% of patients alive at 2 and 5 years, respectively. These pilot studies suggest that when combined with early concurrent thoracic irradiation, chemotherapy may be further abbreviated to as few as two cycles without compromising efficacy in elderly or infirm patients. This approach deserves further study.

In summary, the optimal chemotherapy for elderly patients with SCLC is not known. We have learned that chronological age alone is a misleading clinical characteristic to base a treatment decision. Physiological age determined by comorbidities and PS provides a clearer framework for guiding treatment decisions. Categories such as "fit " elderly (≥70 years and PS 0 to 1) and "frail" elderly (≥70 years and PS 2 to 4) are emerging as beneficial terms both the clinical and research setting. Despite the limited data, we are encouraged that a subset of elderly patients can achieve a survival benefit with acceptable toxicity. As the elderly population continues to grow, it is critical that we develop solid evidence-based treatment plans. We must embrace clinical research in this population.

TREATMENT OF POOR PERFORMANCE STATUS PATIENTS

PS is universally recognized as an independent prognostic factor and typically correlates with the extent of tumor burden. Thus, PS 2 patients are unduly challenging. These patients are perceived to be poor candidates for treatment, ineligible for clinical trials and have short life spans, making any research difficult. Lilenbaum et al.[194] recently determined the prevalence of poor PS in lung cancer patient by examining two large quality-of-life databases. A PS of 2 to 4 was noted in 34% of patients. This high percentage of patients with a poor PS magnifies the need to conduct specific research in this population. In SCLC, several retrospective studies from large databases confirm the shorten survival associated with a poor PS.[167,168,195] The CALGB reviewed their SCLC experience from 1972 to 1986.[195] Five trials with a total of 1745 patients were conducted in either LS or ES disease. PS of 2 to 3 accounted for 11% to 27% of patients in the 3 LS studies and 31% to 42% in the three ES studies. Overall, PS was a highly significant predictor of survival in all stages of SCLC. A more current analysis examined pretreatment PS in five large trials of topotecan conducted in chemotherapy sensitive recurrent SCLC.[196] A total of 479 patients were enrolled in these studies and 98 patients (20%) had a PS of 2. The median OS for patients by PS were 38.3 weeks for PS = 0, 25.4 weeks for PS = 1, and 16 weeks for PS = 2.

Despite poor survival rates in PS 2 patients, they have routinely been eligible for phase III SCLC trials in contrast to NSCLC trials that typically exclude them. Clinical experience rather than clinical evidence has taught us that selective patients, whose poor PS is attributed to tumor burden, have an opportunity of responding to treatment that can result in meaningful symptom palliation, improved PS and prolonged survival versus the alternative of a rapid demise with no therapy. Determining the appropriate PS 2 patients to enter a PS 0 to 2 trial is perplexing because most trials are designed for PS 0 to 1 patients. This could account for why only 10% of untreated PS 2 patients enroll in phase III trials. In the previously treated trials, 20% of patients were deemed PS 2. To determine if PS patients derive benefit from treatment, a retrospective review of seven trials examined whether PS 2 patients converted to PS of 0 to 1 with salvage topotecan.[197] Of the 152 PS 2 patients, 21% experienced PS improvement and this was associated with a higher response rate and a prolonged survival. Unfortunately, this information is not available for untreated patients.

PS is also an indicator of tolerance to therapy. However, in the CALGB metaanalysis reported previously, poor PS was not a predictor of increased risk for hematological toxicity.[195] Tolerance to therapy is highly dependent on the intensity of the treatment, regardless of PS, but is dramatically decreased with increasing dose intensity in the poor PS group. The MRC Lung Cancer Working Party randomized 310 poor PS patients to a control arm consisting of four drugs: etoposide, cyclophosphamide, methotrexate, and vincristine (ECMV) or to a less intense two-drug regimen of etoposide and vincristine (EV).[198] There was no difference in symptom palliation, response rates or survival times between the two groups. Grade 2 or greater hematological toxicity and mucositis were worse with the four-drug regimen. Thirty-seven patients died during cycle one of ECMV versus nine patients treated with EV. No data is available from recent randomized phase III trials in untreated patients but the topotecan review showed no difference in grades 3 and 4 leukopenia, neutropenia, or thrombocytopenia between PS 0 to 1 patients and PS 2 patients, however, grades 3 and 4 anemia was significantly worse in PS 2 patients ($p = 0.009$).[196] Whatever the treatment regimen, added caution is advised for PS 2 patients.

In the 1990s, the oral formulation of etoposide was thought to be ideal for poor PS patients, leading to two randomized studies. The first study shown in Table 58.8 randomized previously untreated patients with a PS of 2 to 4 to oral etoposide 50 mg orally twice a day for 10 days (N = 171 patients) or standard chemotherapy with PE or CAV (N = 168 patients).[199] The primary end point was palliation of symptoms at 3 months. The trial was stopped early by the data safety and monitoring board because of an inferior result with oral etoposide. Palliation was similar in both arms 41% versus 46%, respectively. Survival was lower in the oral etoposide arm, 130 days versus 183 days for

CAV ($p = 0.03$). Grade 2 or greater hematological toxicity was low in both arms, 21% for etoposide and 26% for CAV. The second trial listed in Table 58.8 by the London Lung Cancer Group enrolled patients younger than the age of 75 with a PS of 2 to 3 or patients older than the age of 75 with any PS to receive oral etoposide 100 mg orally for 5 days (N = 75) or CAV alternating with PE (N = 80).[200] They hypothesized that oral etoposide would produce a similar survival but with improved quality of life. Again, this study was stopped prematurely because of a significantly inferior survival in the oral etoposide arm. The MS was 4.8 months with a 1-year survival rate of 9.8% for oral etoposide as compared to 5.9 months and 19.3% for CAV/PE ($p < 0.05$). Grade 3 and 4 toxicities were infrequent and similar between the arms except there was more nausea and vomiting in the IV arm. The recently reported Japanese phase III trial in elderly and poor-risk patients that is described previously in the elderly section was essentially a fit elderly trial with only 40 elderly PS 2 patients. It was noteworthy that the 18 poor-risk patients defined as <70 years old and a PS of 3 had an MS of 7 months.[191]

Poor PS patients with SCLC are common. To treat or not to treat is a frequent dilemma that relies on physician judgment more so than clinical data. Given the exceptionally short survival of untreated patients, poor PS patients whose disease is the cause of a declining PS may be offered therapy because standard platinum-based chemotherapy is well tolerated and efficacious. Meanwhile, specific research in poor PS patients is gaining momentum.

CONCLUSION

Chemotherapy undeniably produces a survival benefit for patients with SCLC. Four to six cycles of a platinum doublet or an anthracycline-based combination should be offered to patients including the elderly and PS 2 patient. Unfortunately, SCLC is rarely cured except in patients with LS disease receiving bimodality therapy. Over the past 20 years, no major survival benefit has occurred with various old and new cytotoxic chemotherapy agents, regimens, and schedules. Evaluations of numerous biologically targeted agents have also been ineffective. Nonetheless, we have learned invaluable lessons that have shaped our future research strategies. We predict that continued insight into the biology of SCLC will guide us in discovering novel chemotherapeutic and targeted therapies that will translate into prolonged remissions and higher cure rates for all patients with this disease.

REFERENCES

1. Govindan R, Page N, Morgensztern D, et al. Changing epidemiology of small-cell lung cancer in the United States over the last 30 years: analysis of the surveillance, epidemiologic, and end results in database. *J Clin Oncol* 2006;24:4539–4544.
2. Karnofsky D, Abelmann W, Craver L, et al. The use of nitrogen mustards in the palliative treatment of cancer. *Cancer* 1948;1:634.
3. Argiris A, Murren JR. Advances in chemotherapy for small cell lung cancer: single-agent activity of newer agents. *Cancer J* 2001;7: 228–235.
4. Ettinger DS, Finkelstein DM, Sarma RP, et al. Phase II study of paclitaxel in patients with extensive-disease small-cell lung cancer: an Eastern Cooperative Oncology Group study. *J Clin Oncol* 1995;13: 1430–1435.
5. Kirschling RJ, Grill JP, Marks RS, et al. Paclitaxel and G-CSF in previously untreated patients with extensive stage small-cell lung cancer: a phase II study of the North Central Cancer Treatment Group. *Am J Clin Oncol* 1999;22:517–522.
6. Smit EF, Fokkema E, Biesma B, et al. A phase II study of paclitaxel in heavily pretreated patients with small-cell lung cancer. *BR J Cancer* 1998;77:347–351.
7. Yamamoto N, Tsurutani J, Yoshimura N, et al. Phase II study of weekly paclitaxel for relapsed and refractory small cell lung cancer. *Anticancer Res* 2006;26:777–781.
8. Latreille J, Cormier Y, Martins H, et al. Phase II study of docetaxel (taxotere) in patients with previously untreated extensive small cell lung cancer. *Invest New Drugs* 1996;13:343–345.
9. Smyth JF, Smith IE, Sessa C, et al. Activity of docetaxel (Taxotere) in small cell lung cancer. The Early Clinical Trials Group of the EORTC. *Eur J Cancer* 1994;30A:1058–1060.
10. Hesketh PJ, Crowley JJ, Burris HA III, et al. Evaluation of docetaxel in previously untreated extensive-stage small cell lung cancer: a Southwest Oncology Group phase II trial. *Cancer J Sci Am* 1999;5:237–2341.
11. Schiller JH, Kim K, Hutson P, et al. Phase II study of topotecan in patients with extensive-stage small-cell carcinoma of the lung: an Eastern Cooperative Oncology Group Trial. *J Clin Oncol* 1996;14: 2345–2352.
12. Depierre A, von Pawel J, Hans K, et al. Evaluation of topotecan (Hycamtin) in relapsed small cell lung cancer (SCLC): a multicentre phase II study. *Lung Cancer* 1997;18:35.
13. Ardizzoni A, Hansen H, Dombernowsky P, et al. Topotecan, a new active drug in the second-line treatment of small-cell lung cancer: a phase II study in patients with refractory and sensitive disease. The European Organization for Research and Treatment of Cancer Early Clinical Studies Group and New Drug Development Office, and the Lung Cancer Cooperative Group. *J Clin Oncol* 1997;15:2090–2096.
14. Perez-Soler R, Glisson BS, Lee JS, et al. Treatment of patients with small-cell lung cancer refractory to etoposide and cisplatin with the topoisomerase I poison topotecan. *J Clin Oncol* 1996;14:2785–2790.
15. Fukuoka M, Niitani H, Suzuki A, et al. A phase II study of CPT-11, a new derivative of camptothecin, for previously untreated non-small-cell lung cancer. *J Clin Oncol* 1992;10:16–20.
16. Masuda N, Fukuoka M, Kusunoki Y, et al. CPT-11: a new derivative of camptothecin for the treatment of refractory or relapsed small-cell lung cancer. *J Clin Oncol* 1992;10:1225–1229.
17. DeVore R, Blanke C, Denham C, et al. Phase II study of irinotecan (CPT-11) in patients with previously treated small-cell lung cancer (SCLC). *Proc Am Soc Clin Oncol* 1998;17:451a.
18. Le Chevalier T, Ibrahim N, Chomy P, et al. A phase II study of irinotecan (CPT-11) in patients with small cell lung cancer progressing after initial response to first-line chemotherapy (CT). *Proc Am Soc Clin Oncol* 1997;16:450a.
19. Cormier Y, Eisenhauer E, Muldal A, et al. Gemcitabine is an active new agent in previously untreated extensive small cell lung cancer (SCLC). A study of the National Cancer Institute of Canada Clinical Trials Group. *Ann Oncol* 1994;5:283–285.
20. Masters GA, Declerck L, Blanke C, et al. Phase II trial of gemcitabine in refractory or relapsed small-cell lung cancer: Eastern Cooperative Oncology Group Trial 1597. *J Clin Oncol* 2003;21:1550–1555.
21. van der Lee I, Smit EF, van Putten JW, et al. Single-agent gemcitabine in patients with resistant small-cell lung cancer. *Ann Oncol* 2001;12: 557–561.
22. Higano CS, Crowley JJ, Veith RV, et al. A phase II trial of intravenous vinorelbine in previously untreated patients with extensive small cell

lung cancer, a Southwest Oncology Group study. *Invest New Drugs* 1997;15:153–156.
23. Depierre A, Le Chevalier T, Quoix E, et al. Phase II study of Navelbine in small cell lung cancer. *Proc Am Soc Clin Oncol* 1995;14:348.
24. Jassem J, Karnicka-Młodkowska H, van Pottelsberghe C, et al. Phase II study of vinorelbine (Navelbine) in previously treated small cell lung cancer patients. EORTC Lung Cancer Cooperative Group. *Eur J Cancer* 1993;29A:1720–1722.
25. Lake D, Johnson E, Herndon J, et al. Phase II trial of Navelbine in relapsed small cell lung cancer. *Proc Am Soc Clin Oncol* 1997;16:473a.
26. Furuse K, Kubota K, Kawahara M, et al. Phase II study of vinorelbine in heavily previously treated small cell lung cancer. Japan Lung Cancer Vinorelbine Study Group. *Oncology* 1996;53:169–172.
27. Jalal S, Ansari R, Govindan R, et al. Pemetrexed in second line and beyond small cell lung cancer: a Hoosier Oncology Group phase II study. J Thorac Oncol 2009;4(1):93–96.
28. Yana T, Negoro S, Takada M, et al. Phase II study of amrubicin in previously untreated patients with extensive-disease small cell lung cancer: West Japan Thoracic Oncology Group (WJTOG) study. *Invest New Drugs* 2007;25:253–258.
29. Onoda S, Masuda N, Seto T, et al. Phase II trial of amrubicin for treatment of refractory or relapsed small-cell lung cancer: Thoracic Oncology Research Group Study 0301. *J Clin Oncol* 2006;24: 5448–5453.
30. Kato T, Nokihara H, Ohe Y, et al. Phase II trial of amrubicin in patients with previously treated small cell lung cancer (SCLC). *J Clin Oncol* 2006;24(18S):7061.
31. Jotte RM, Conkling PR, Reynolds C, et al. A randomized phase II trial of amrubicin (AMR) vs. topotecan as second-line treatment in extensive-disease small-cell lung cancer (SCLC) sensitive to platinum-based first-line chemotherapy. *J Clin Oncol* 2008;26(15S):S433. abstract 8040.
32. Sugawara S, Inoue A, Yamazaki K, et al. Randomized, phase II trial comparing amrubicin with topotecan in patients (pts) with previously treated small cell lung cancer (SCLC). *J Clin Oncol* 2008;26(S434): abstract 8042.
33. Ettinger DS, Jotte RM, Gupta V, et al. A phase II trial of single-agent amrubicin (AMR) in patients with extensive disease small cell lung cancer (ED-SCLC) that is refractory or progressive within 90 days of completion of first-line platinum-based chemotherapy. *J Clin Oncol* 2008;26(S434): abstract 8041.
34. Lowenbraun S, Bartolucci A, Smalley RV, et al. The superiority of combination chemotherapy over single agent chemotherapy in small cell lung carcinoma. *Cancer* 1979;44:406–413.
35. Alberto P, Brunner KW, Martz G, et al. Treatment of bronchogenic carcinoma with simultaneous or sequential combination chemotherapy, including methotrexate, cyclophosphamide, procarbazine, and vincristine. *Cancer* 1976;38:2208–2216.
36. Socinski MA, Weissman C, Hart LL, et al. Randomized phase II trial of pemetrexed combined with either cisplatin or carboplatin in untreated extensive-stage small cell lung cancer. *J Clin Oncol* 2006;24: 4840–4847.
37. Ferraldeschi R, Thatcher N, Lorigan P. Pemetrexed in small-cell lung cancer: background and review of the ongoing GALES pivotal trial. *Expert Rev Anticancer Ther* 2007 May;7(5):635–640.
38. Roth BJ, Johnson DH, Einhorn LH, et al. Randomized study of cyclophosphamide, doxorubicin, and vincristine versus etoposide and cisplatin versus alternation of these two regimens in extensive small-cell lung cancer: a phase III trial of the Southeastern Cancer Study Group. *J Clin Oncol* 1992;10:282–291.
39. Fukuoka M, Furuse K, Saijo N, et al. Randomized trial of cyclophosphamide, doxorubicin, and vincristine versus cisplatin and etoposide versus alternation of these regimens in small-cell lung cancer. *J Natl Cancer Inst* 1991;83:855–861.
40. Sundstrøm S, Bremnes RM, Kaasa S, et al. Cisplatin and etoposide regimen is superior to cyclophosphamide, epirubicin, and vincristine regimen in small-cell lung cancer: results from a randomized phase III trial with 5 years' follow-up. *J Clin Oncol* 2002;20:4665–4672.
41. Mascaux C, Paesmans M, Berghmans T, et al. A systematic review of the role of etoposide and cisplatin in the chemotherapy of small cell lung cancer with methodology assessment and meta-analysis. *Lung Cancer* 2000;30:23–36.
42. Turrisi AT III, Kim K, Blum R, et al. Twice-daily compared with once-daily thoracic radiotherapy in limited small-cell lung cancer treated concurrently with cisplatin and etoposide. *N Engl J Med* 1999;340: 265–271.
43. Skarlos DV, Samantas E, Kosmidis P, et al. Randomized comparison of etoposide-cisplatin vs. etoposide-carboplatin and irradiation in small-cell lung cancer. A Hellenic Co-operative Oncology Group study. *Ann Oncol* 1994;5:601–607.
44. Noda K, Nishiwaki Y, Kawahara M, et al. Irinotecan plus cisplatin compared with etoposide plus cisplatin for extensive small-cell lung cancer. *N Engl J Med* 2002;346:85–91.
45. Natale RB, Lara PN, Chansky K, et al. S0124: A randomized phase III trial comparing irinotecan/cisplatin (IP) with etoposide/cisplatin (EP) in patients (pts) with previously untreated extensive stage small cell lung cancer (E-SCLC). *J Clin Oncol* 2008;26(suppl 15):S400. abstract 7512.
46. Hanna N, Bunn PA Jr, Langer C, et al. Randomized Phase III trial comparing irinotecan/cisplatin with etoposide/cisplatin in patients with previously untreated extensive-stage disease small-cell lung cancer. *J Clin Oncol* 2006;24:2038–2043.
47. Eckardt JR, von Pawel J, Papai Z, et al. Open-label, multicenter, randomized, phase III study comparing oral topotecan/cisplatin versus etoposide/cisplatin as treatment for chemotherapy-naïve patients with extensive-disease small-cell lung cancer. *J Clin Oncol* 2006;24: 2044–2051.
48. Heigener DF, Freitag L, Eschbach C, et al. Topotecan/cisplatin (TP) compared to cisplatin/etoposide (PE) for patients with extensive disease-small cell lung cancer (ED-SCLC): final results of a randomized phase III trial. *J Clin Oncol* 2008;26(400s): abstract 7513.
49. Hermes A, Bergman B, Bremnes R, et al. A randomized phase III trial of irinotecan plus carboplatin versus etoposide plus carboplatin in patients with small cell lung cancer, extensive disease (SCLC-ED): IRIS-Study. *J Clin Oncol* 2007;25(390s): abstract 7523.
50. de Jong WK, Groen HJ, Koolen MG, et al. Phase III study of cyclophosphamide, doxorubicin, and etoposide compared with carboplatin and paclitaxel in patients with extensive disease small-cell lung cancer. *Eur J Cancer* 2007;43:2345–2350.
51. Socinski MA, Smit EF, Lorigan P, et al. Phase III study of pemetrexed plus carboplatin compared with etoposide plus carboplatin in chemotherapy-naive patients with extensive-stage small-cell lung cancer. *J Clin Oncol* 2009;27(28):4787–4792.
52. Mavroudis D, Papadakis E, Veslemes M, et al. A multicenter randomized clinical trial comparing paclitaxel-cisplatin-etoposide versus cisplatin-etoposide as first-line treatment in patients with small-cell lung cancer. *Ann Oncol* 2001;12:463–470.
53. Reck M, von Pawel J, Macha HN, et al. Randomized phase III trial of paclitaxel, etoposide, and carboplatin versus carboplatin, etoposide, and vincristine in patients with small-cell lung cancer. *J Natl Cancer Inst* 2003;95:1118–1127.
54. Niell H, Herndon JE II, Miller AA, et al. Randomized phase III intergroup trial of etoposide and cisplatin with or without paclitaxel and granulocyte colony-stimulating factor in patients with extensive-stage small-cell lung cancer: Cancer and Leukemia Group B Trial 9732. *J Clin Oncol* 2005;23:3752–3759.
55. Pujol JL, Daurès JP, Rivière A, et al. Etoposide plus cisplatin with or without the combination of 4'-epidoxorubicin plus cyclophosphamide in treatment of extensive small-cell lung cancer: a French Federation of Cancer Institute's multicenter phase III randomized study. *J Natl Cancer Inst* 2001;93:300–308.
56. Schabel F, Griswold D, Corbett T, et al. Testing therapeutic hypotheses in mice and man: observations on the therapeutic activity against advanced solid tumors of mice treated with anti-cancer drugs that have demonstrated or potential clinical utility for treatment of advanced

solid tumors in man. In: *Methods in Cancer Research: Cancer Drug Development,* Part B, Vol XVII. New York: Academic Press, 1979:4.

57. Cohen MH, Creaven PJ, Fossieck BE Jr, et al. Intensive chemotherapy of small cell bronchogenic carcinoma. *Cancer Treat Rep* 1977;61:349–354.
58. Hande KR, Oldham RK, Fer MF, et al. Randomized study of high-dose versus low-dose methotrexate in the treatment of extensive small cell lung cancer. *Am J Med* 1982;73:413–419.
59. Johnson DH, DeLeo MJ, Hande KR, et al. High-dose induction chemotherapy with cyclophosphamide, etoposide, and cisplatin for extensive-stage small-cell lung cancer. *J Clin Oncol* 1987;5:703–709.
60. Figueredo AT, Hryniuk WM, Strautmanis I, et al. Co-trimoxazole prophylaxis during high-dose chemotherapy of small-cell lung cancer. *J Clin Oncol* 1985;3:54–64.
61. Hong WK, Nicaise C, Lawson R, et al. Etoposide combined with cyclophosphamide plus vincristine compared with doxorubicin plus cyclophosphamide plus vincristine and with high-dose cyclophosphamide plus vincristine in the treatment of small-cell carcinoma of the lung: a randomized trial of the Bristol Lung Cancer Study Group. *J Clin Oncol* 1989;7: 450–456.
62. Ihde DC, Mulshine JL, Kramer BS, et al. Prospective randomized comparison of high-dose and standard-dose etoposide and cisplatin chemotherapy in patients with extensive-stage small-cell lung cancer. *J Clin Oncol* 1994;12:2022–2034.
63. Arriagada R, Le Chevalier T, Pignon JP, et al. Initial chemotherapeutic doses and survival in patients with limited small-cell lung cancer. *N Engl J Med* 1993;329:1848–1852.
64. Artal-Cortés A, Gomez-Codina J, Gonzalez-Larriba JL, et al. Prospective randomized phase III trial of etoposide/cisplatin versus high-dose epirubicin/cisplatin in small-cell lung cancer. *Clin Lung Cancer* 2004;6:175–183.
65. Arriagada R, de The H, Le Chevalier T, et al. Limited small cell lung cancer: possible prognostic impact of initial chemotherapy doses. *Bull Cancer* 1989;76:604–615.
66. Murray N, Shah A, Osoba D, et al. Intensive weekly chemotherapy for the treatment of extensive-stage small-cell lung cancer. *J Clin Oncol* 1991;9:1632–1638.
67. Murray N, Livingston RB, Shepherd FA, et al. Randomized study of CODE versus alternating CAV/EP for extensive-stage small-cell lung cancer: an Intergroup Study of the National Cancer Institute of Canada Clinical Trials Group and the Southwest Oncology Group. *J Clin Oncol* 1999;17:2300–2308.
68. Fukuoka M, Masuda N, Negoro S, et al. CODE chemotherapy with and without granulocyte colony-stimulating factor in small-cell lung cancer. *Br J Cancer* 1997;75:306–309.
69. Furuse K, Fukuoka M, Nishiwaki Y, et al. Phase III study of intensive weekly chemotherapy with recombinant human granulocyte colony-stimulating factor versus standard chemotherapy in extensive-disease small-cell lung cancer. The Japan Clinical Oncology Group. *J Clin Oncol* 1998;16:2126–2132.
70. Sculier JP, Paesmans M, Bureau G, et al. Multiple-drug weekly chemotherapy versus standard combination regimen in small-cell lung cancer: a phase III randomized study conducted by the European Lung Cancer Working Party. *J Clin Oncol* 1993;11:1858–1865.
71. Souhami RL, Rudd R, Ruiz de Elvira MC, et al. Randomized trial comparing weekly versus 3-week chemotherapy in small-cell lung cancer: a Cancer Research Campaign trial. *J Clin Oncol* 1994;12:1806–1813.
72. Pujol JL, Douillard JY, Rivière A, et al. Dose-intensity of a four-drug chemotherapy regimen with or without recombinant human granulocyte-macrophage colony-stimulating factor in extensive-stage small-cell lung cancer: a multicenter randomized phase III study. *J Clin Oncol* 1997; 15:2082–2089.
73. Steward WP, von Pawel J, Gatzemeier U, et al. Effects of granulocyte-macrophage colony-stimulating factor and dose intensification of V-ICE chemotherapy in small-cell lung cancer: a prospective randomized study of 300 patients. *J Clin Oncol* 1998;16:642–650.
74. Thatcher N, Girling DJ, Hopwood P, et al. Improving survival without reducing quality of life in small-cell lung cancer patients by increasing the dose-intensity of chemotherapy with granulocyte colony-stimulating factor support: results of a British Medical Research Council Multicenter Randomized Trial. Medical Research Council Lung Cancer Working Party. *J Clin Oncol* 2000;18:395–404.
75. Sculier JP, Paesmans M, Lecomte J, et al. A three-arm phase III randomised trial assessing, in patients with extensive-disease small-cell lung cancer, accelerated chemotherapy with support of haematological growth factor or oral antibiotics. *Br J Cancer* 2001;85:1444–1451.
76. Ardizzoni A, Tjan-Heijnen VC, Postmus PE, et al. Standard versus intensified chemotherapy with granulocyte colony-stimulating factor support in small-cell lung cancer: a prospective European Organization for Research and Treatment of Cancer-Lung Cancer Group Phase III Trial-08923. *J Clin Oncol* 2002;20:3947–3955.
77. Humblet Y, Symann M, Bosly A, et al. Late intensification chemotherapy with autologous bone marrow transplantation in selected small-cell carcinoma of the lung: A randomized study. *J Clin Oncol* 1987;5:1864–1873.
78. Fujimoto N, Ueoka H, Kiura K, et al. Multicyclic dose-intensive chemotherapy supported by autologous blood progenitor cell transplantation for relapsed small cell lung cancer. *Anticancer Res* 2003;23: 4229–4232.
79. Lorigan P, Woll PJ, O'Brien ME, et al. Randomized phase III trial of dose-dense chemotherapy supported by whole-blood hematopoietic progenitors in better-prognosis small-cell lung cancer. *J Natl Cancer Inst* 2005;97:666–674.
80. Buchholz E, Manegold C, Pilz L, et al. Standard versus dose-intensified chemotherapy with sequential reinfusion of hematopoietic progenitor cells in small cell lung cancer patients with favorable prognosis. *J Thorac Oncol* 2007;2:51–58.
81. Leyvraz S, Pampallona G, Martinelli F, et al. Randomized phase III study of high-dose sequential chemotherapy (CT) supported by peripheral blood progenitor cells (PBPC) for the treatment of small cell lung cancer (SCLC): results of the EBMT random-ICE trial. *2006 ASCO Annual Meeting* Abstract 7064.
82. Goldie JH, Coldman AJ, Gudaskas GA. Rationale for the use of alternating non-cross resistant chemotherapy. *Cancer Treat Rep* 1982;66: 439–449.
83. Evans WK, Feld R, Murray N, et al. Superiority of alternating non-cross-resistant chemotherapy in extensive small cell lung cancer. A multicenter, randomized clinical trial by the National Cancer Institute of Canada. *Ann Intern Med* 1987;107:451–458.
84. Feld R, Evans WK, Coy P, et al. Canadian multicenter randomized trial comparing sequential and alternating administration of two non-cross-resistant chemotherapy combinations in patients with limited small-cell carcinoma of the lung. *J Clin Oncol* 1987;5:1401–1409.
85. Goodman GE, Crowley JJ, Blasko JC, et al. Treatment of limited small-cell lung cancer with etoposide and cisplatin alternating with vincristine, doxorubicin, and cyclophosphamide versus concurrent etoposide, vincristine, doxorubicin, and cyclophosphamide and chest radiotherapy: a Southwest Oncology Group Study. *J Clin Oncol* 1990;8:39–47.
86. Postmus PE, Scagliotti G, Groen HJ, et al. Standard versus alternating non-cross-resistant chemotherapy in extensive small cell lung cancer: an EORTC Phase III trial. *Eur J Cancer* 1996;32A:1498–1503.
87. Jett JR, Hatfield AK, Hillman S, et al. Alternating chemotherapy with etoposide plus cisplatin and topotecan plus paclitaxel in patients with untreated, extensive-stage small cell lung carcinoma: a phase II trial of the North Central Cancer Treatment Group. *Cancer* 2003;97:2498–2503.
88. Mavroudis D, Veslemes M, Kouroussis Ch, et al. Cisplatin-etoposide alternating with topotecan in patients with extensive stage small cell lung cancer (SCLC). A multicenter phase II study. *Lung Cancer* 2002;38:59–63.
89. Einhorn LH, Crawford J, Birch R, et al. Cisplatin plus etoposide consolidation following cyclophosphamide, doxorubicin, and vincristine in limited small-cell lung cancer. *J Clin Oncol* 1988;6:451–456.
90. Johnson DH, Bass D, Einhorn LH, et al. Combination chemotherapy with or without thoracic radiotherapy in limited-stage small-cell lung cancer: a randomized trial of the Southeastern Cancer Study Group. *J Clin Oncol* 1993;11:1223–1229.

91. Spiro SG, Souhami RL, Geddes DM, et al. Duration of chemotherapy in small cell lung cancer: a Cancer Research Campaign trial. *Br J Cancer* 1989;59:578–583.
92. Schiller JH, Adak S, Cella D, et al. Topotecan versus observation after cisplatin plus etoposide in extensive-stage small-cell lung cancer: E7593—a phase III trial of the Eastern Cooperative Oncology Group. *J Clin Oncol* 2001;19:2114–2122.
93. Bozcuk H, Artac M, Ozdogan M, et al. Does maintenance/consolidation chemotherapy have a role in the management of small cell lung cancer (SCLC)? A Metaanalysis of the published randomized controlled trials. *Cancer* 2005;104:2650–2657.
94. Froeschl S, Nicholas G, Gallant V, et al. Outcomes of second-line chemotherapy in patients with relapsed extensive small cell lung cancer. *J Thorac Oncol* 2008;3:163–169.
95. O'Bryan RM, Crowley JJ, Kim PN, et al. Comparison of etoposide and cisplatin with bis-chloro-ethylnitrosourea, thiotepa, vincristine, and cyclophosphamide for salvage treatment in small cell lung cancer. A Southwest Oncology Group Study. *Cancer* 1990;65:856–860.
96. Shepherd FA, Evans WK, MacCormick R, et al. Cyclophosphamide, doxorubicin, and vincristine in etoposide- and cisplatin-resistant small cell lung cancer. *Cancer Treat Rep* 1987;71:941–944.
97. von Pawel J, Schiller JH, Shepherd FA, et al. Topotecan versus cyclophosphamide, doxorubicin, and vincristine for the treatment of recurrent small-cell lung cancer. *J Clin Oncol* 1999;17:658–667.
98. O'Brien ME, Ciuleanu TE, Tsekov H, et al. Phase III trial comparing supportive care alone with supportive care with oral topotecan in patients with relapsed small-cell lung cancer. *J Clin Oncol* 2006;24:5441–5447.
99. Eckardt JR, von Pawel J, Pujol JL, et al. Phase III study of oral compared with intravenous topotecan as second-line therapy in small-cell lung cancer. *J Clin Oncol* 2007;25:2086–2092.
100. Giaccone G, Ferrati P, Donadio M, et al. Reinduction chemotherapy in small cell lung cancer. *Eur J Cancer Clin Oncol* 1987;23:1697–1699.
101. Batist G, Ihde DC, Zabell A, et al. Small-cell carcinoma of lung: reinduction therapy after late relapse. *Ann Intern Med* 1983;98:472–474.
102. Davies AM, Evans WK, MacKay JA, et al. Treatment of recurrent small cell lung cancer. *Hematol Oncol Clin North Am* 2004;18:387–416.
103. Cheng S, Evans WK, Stys-Norman D, et al. Chemotherapy for relapsed small cell lung cancer: a systematic review and practice guideline. *J Thorac Oncol* 2007;2(4):348–354.
104. Hodkinson PS, MacKinnon A, Sethi T. Targeting growth factors in lung cancer. *Chest* 2008;133:1209–1216.
105. Hibi K, Takahashi T, Sekido Y, et al. Coexpression of the stem cell factor and the c-kit genes in small-cell lung cancer. *Oncogene* 1991;6:2291–2296.
106. Plummer H III, Catlett J, Leftwich J, et al. C-myc expression correlates with suppression of c-kit protooncogene expression in small cell lung cancer cell lines. *Cancer Res* 1993;53:4337–4342.
107. Damstrup L, Rygaard, K, Spang-Thomsen M, et al. Expression of transforming growth factor beta (TGF beta) receptors and expression of TGF beta 1, TGF beta 2, and TGF beta 3 in human small cell lung cancer cell lines. *Br J Cancer* 1993;67:1015–1021.
108. Blackhall FH, Pintilie M, Michael M, et al. Expression and prognostic significance of kit, protein kinase B, and mitogen-activated protein kinase in patients with small cell lung cancer. *Clin Cancer Res* 2003;9:2241–2247.
109. Krystal GW, Honswek S, Litz J, et al. The selective tyrosine kinase inhibitor ST1571 inhibits small cell lung cancer growth. *Clin Cancer Res* 2000;6:3319–3326.
110. Johnson BE, Fisher T, Fisher B, et al. Phase II study of imatinib in patients with small cell lung cancer. *Clin Cancer Res* 2003;9:5880–5887.
111. Dy GK, Miller AA, Mandrekar SJ, et al. A phase II trial of imatinib (ST1571) in patients with c-kit expressing relapsed small-cell lung cancer: a CALGB and NCCTG study. *Ann Oncol* 2005;16:1811–1816.
112. Spigel DR, Hainsworth JD, Simons L, et al. Irinotecan, carboplatin, and imatinib in untreated extensive-stage small cell lung cancer: a phase II trial of the Minnie Pearl Cancer Research Network. *J Thorac Oncol* 2007;2:854–861.
113. Heinrich MC, Blanke CD, Druker BJ, et al. Inhibition of KIT tyrosine kinase activity: a novel molecular approach to the treatment of KIT-positive malignancies. *J Clin Oncol* 2002;20:1692–1703.
114. Moore AM, Einhorn LH, Estes D, et al. Gefitinib in patients with chemo-sensitive and chemo-refractory relapsed small cell cancers: a Hoosier Oncology Group phase II trial. *Lung Cancer* 2006;53:93–97.
115. Heymach JV, Johnson DH, Khuri FR, et al. Phase II study of the farnesyl transferase inhibitor R115777 in patients with sensitive relapse small-cell lung cancer. *Ann Oncol* 2004;15:1187–1193.
116. Kalemkerian GP, Jiroutek M, Ettinger DS, et al. Phase II study of all-trans-retinoic acid plus cisplatin and etoposide in patients with extensive stage small cell lung carcinoma: an Eastern Cooperative Oncology Group Study. *Cancer* 1998;83:1102–1108.
117. Nelson AR, Fingleton B, Rothenberg ML, et al. Matrix metalloproteinases: biologic activity and clinical implications. *J Clin Oncol* 2000;18:1135–1149.
118. Michael M, Babic B, Khokha R, et al. Expression and prognostic significance of metalloproteinases and their tissue inhibitors in patients with small-cell lung cancer. *J Clin Oncol* 1999;17:1802–1808.
119. Shepherd FA, Giaccone G, Seymour L, et al. Prospective, randomized, double-blind, placebo-controlled trial of marimastat after response to first-line chemotherapy in patients with small-cell lung cancer: a trial of the National Cancer Institute of Canada-Clinical Trials Group and the European Organization for Research and Treatment of Cancer. *J Clin Oncol* 2002;20:4434–4439.
120. Shepherd FA, Sridhar SS. Angiogenesis inhibitors under study for the treatment of lung cancer. *Lung Cancer* 2003;41 Suppl 1:S63–S72.
121. Rigas J, Denham C, Rinaldi D, et al. Randomized placebo-controlled trial of the matrix metalloproteinase inhibitor (MMPI) BAY 12-9566 as adjuvant therapy for patients with small cell and non-small cell lung cancer. *Proc Am Soc Clin Oncol* 2003;22(628):abstract 2525.
122. Jett JR, Maksymiuk AW, Su JQ, et al. Phase III trial of recombinant interferon gamma in complete responders with small-cell lung cancer. *J Clin Oncol* 1994;12:2321–2326.
123. Kelly K, Crowley JJ, Bunn PA Jr, et al. Role of recombinant interferon alfa-2a maintenance in patients with limited-stage small-cell lung cancer responding to current chemoradiation: a Southwest Oncology Group study. *J Clin Oncol* 1995;13:2924–2930.
124. Mattson K, Niiranen A, Ruotsalainen T, et al. Interferon maintenance therapy for small cell lung cancer: improvement in long-term survival. *J Interferon Cytokine Res* 1997;17:103–105.
125. van Zandwijk N, Groen HJ, Postmus PE, et al. Role of recombinant interferon-gamma maintenance in responding patients with small cell lung cancer. A randomized phase III study of the EORTC Lung Cancer Cooperative Group. *Eur J Cancer* 1997;33:1759–1766.
126. Zhang S, Cordon-Cardo C, Zhang HS, et al. Selection of tumor antigens as targets for immune attack using immunohistochemistry: I. Focus on gangliosides. *Int J Cancer* 1997;73:42–49.
127. Giacione G, Debruyne C, Felip E, et al. Phase III study of adjuvant vaccination with Bec2/bacille Calmette-Guerin in responding patients with limited-disease small-cell lung cancer (European Organisation for Research and Treatment of Cancer 08971-08971B; Silva Study). *J Clin Oncol* 2005;23:6854–6864.
128. Krug LM, Ragupathi G, Hood C, et al. Vaccination of patients with small-cell lung cancer with synthetic fucosyl GM-1 conjugated to keyhole limpet hemocyanin. *Clin Cancer Res* 2004;10:6094–6100.
129. Krug LM, Ragupathi G, Ng KK, et al. Vaccination of small cell lung cancer patients with polysialic acid or N-propionylated polysialic acid conjugated to keyhole limpet hemocyanin. *Clin Cancer Res* 2004;10:916–923.
130. Harper-Wynne K, et al. Addition of SRL-172 (Mycobacterium Vaccae) to Standard Chemotherapy in Small Cell Lung Cancer (SCLC) Confers No Survival Benefit: Results of a Randomized Multicentre Study. *Lung Cancer* 2003;41:356.
131. Harper-Wynne CL, Sumpter K, Ryan C, et al. Addition of SRL 172 to standard chemotherapy in small cell lung cancer (SCLC) improves symptom control. *Lung Cancer* 2005;47:289–290.

132. McCann J, Fossella FV, Villalona-Calero MA, et al. Phase II trial of huN901-DM1 in patients with relapsed small cell lung cancer (SCLC) and CD56-positive small cell carcinoma. *J Clin Oncol* 2007;25(18 suppl):S690. abstract 18084.
133. Antonia SJ, Mirza N, Fricke I, et al. Combination of p53 cancer vaccine with chemotherapy in patients with extensive stage small cell lung cancer. *Clin Cancer Res* 2006;13:878–887.
134. Higashiyama M, Doi O, Kodama K, et al. High prevalence of bcl-2 oncoprotein expression in small cell lung cancer. *Anticancer Res* 1995;15:503–505.
135. Jiang SX, Sato Y, Kuwao S, et al. Expression of bcl-2 oncogene protein is prevalent in small cell lung carcinomas. *J Pathol* 1995;177:135–138.
136. Sartorius UA, Krammer PH. Upregulation of Bcl-2 is involved in the mediation of chemotherapy resistance in human small cell lung cancer cell lines. *Int J Cancer* 2002;97:584–592.
137. Ziegler A, Luedke GH, Fabbro D, et al. Induction of apoptosis in small-cell lung cancer cells by an antisense oligodeoxynucleotide targeting bcl-2 coding sequence. *J Natl Cancer Inst* 1997;89:1027–1036.
138. Zangemeister-Wittke U, Schenker T, Luedke G, et al. Synergistic cytotoxicity of bcl-2 antisense oligodeoxynucleotides and etoposide, doxorubicin and cisplatin on small-cell lung cancer lines. *Br J Cancer* 1998;78:1035–1042.
139. Rudin CM, Salgia R, Wang X, et al. Randomized phase II Study of carboplatin and etoposide with or without the bcl-2 antisense oligonucleotide oblimersen for extensive-stage small-cell lung cancer: CALGB 30103. *J Clin Oncol* 2008;26:870–876.
140. Hann CL, Daniel VC, Sugar EA, et al. Therapeutic efficacy of ABT-737, a selective inhibitor of BCL-2, in small cell lung cancer. *Cancer Res* 2008;68:2321–2328.
141. Piazza GA, Rahm AK, Finn TS, et al. Apoptosis primarily accounts for the growth-inhibitory properties of sulindac metabolites and involves a mechanism that is independent of cyclooxygenase inhibition, cell cycle arrest, and p53 induction. *Cancer Res* 1997;57:2452–2459.
142. Thompson WJ, Piazza GA, Li H, et al. Exisulind induction of apoptosis involves guanosine 3', 5'-cyclic monophosphate phosphodiesterase inhibition, protein kinase G activation, and attenuated beta-catenin. *Cancer Res* 2000;60:3338–3342.
143. Soriano AF, Helfrich B, Chan DC, et al. Synergistic effects of new chemotherapy agents and conventional cytotoxic agents against human lung cancer cell lines. *Cancer Res* 1999;59:6178–6184.
144. Campling BG, Young LC, Baer KA, et al. Expression of the MRP and MDR multidrug resistance gene in small cell lung cancer. *Clin Cancer Res* 1997;3:115–122.
145. Wang XF, Govindan R, Herndon JE, et al. A phase II study of carboplatin, etoposide and exisulind in patients with extensive stage small cell lung cancer: CALGB 30104 [abstract]. *J Clin Oncol* 2005; 23(suppl):7161.
146. Adams J, Palombella VJ, Elliott PJ. Proteasome inhibition: a new strategy in cancer treatment. *Invest New Drugs* 2000;18:109–121.
147. Adams J, Palombella VJ, Sausville EA, et al. Proteasome inhibitors: a novel class of potent and effective antitumor agents. *Cancer Res* 1999;59:2615–2622.
148. Lara PN Jr, Chansky K, Davies AM, et al. Bortezomib (PS-341) in relapsed or refractory extensive stage small cell lung cancer: a Southwest Oncology Group phase II trial (S0327). *J Thorac Oncol* 2006;1:996–1001.
149. Raymond E, Alexandre J, Depenbrock H, et al. CCI-779, a rapamycin analog with antitumor activity: A phase I study utilizing a weekly schedule. *Proc Am Soc Clin Oncol* 2000;19:187a. abstract 728.
150. Pandya KJ, Dahlberg S, Hidalgo M, et al. A randomized, phase II trial of two dose levels of temsirolimus (CCI-779) in patients with extensive-stage small-cell lung cancer who have responding or stable disease after induction chemotherapy: a trial of the Eastern Cooperative Oncology Group (E1500). *J Thorac Oncol* 2007;2:1036–1041.
151. Fontanini G, Faviana P, Lucchi M, et al. A high vascular count and overexpression of vascular endothelial growth factor are associated with unfavourable prognosis in operated small cell lung carcinoma. *Br J Cancer* 2002;86:558–563.
152. Mall JW, Schwenk W, Philipp AW, et al. Serum vascular endothelial growth factor levels correlate better with tumor stage in small cell lung cancer than albumin, neuron-specific enolase or lactate dehydrogenase. *Respirology* 2002;7:99–102.
153. Salven P, Ruotsalainen T, Mattson K, et al. High pre-treatment serum level of vascular endothelial growth factor (VEGF) is associated with poor outcome in small-cell lung cancer. *Int J Cancer* 1998;79:144–146.
154. Pujol JL, Breton JL, Gervais R, et al. Phase III double-blind, placebo-controlled study of thalidomide in extensive-disease small-cell lung cancer after response to chemotherapy: an intergroup study FNCLCC cleo04 IFCT 00-01. *J Clin Oncol* 2008;26:3945–3951.
155. Lee SM, Woll P, Rudd R, et al. A phase III randomised, double blind, placebo controlled trial of etoposide/carboplatin with or without thalidomide in poor prognosis small cell lung cancer. Presentation at WLC Seoul, Korea, September 2007.
156. Sandler A, Gray R, Perry MC, et al. Paclitaxel-carboplatin alone or with bevacizumab for non-small-cell lung cancer. *N Engl J Med* 2006;355:2542–2550.
157. Ready N, Dudek AZ, Wang XF, et al. CALGB 30306: A phase II study of cisplatin (C), irinotecan (I) and bevacizumab (B) for untreated extensive stage small cell lung cancer (ES-SCLC). *J Clin Oncol* 2007;25(400s). abstract 7563.
158. Horn L, Dahlberg SE, Sandler AB, et al. Phase II study of cisplatin plus etoposide and bevacizumab for previously untreated, extensive-stage small-cell lung cancer: Eastern Cooperative Oncology Group Study E3501. *J Clin Oncol* 2009;27(35):6006–6011.
159. Spigel DR, Greco FA, Zubkus JD, et al. Phase II trial of irinotecan, carboplatin, and bevacizumab in the treatment of patients with extensive-stage small-cell lung cancer. *J Thorac Oncol* 2009;4(12):1555–1560.
160. Spigel DR, Hainsworth JD, Yardley DA, et al. Tracheoesophageal Fistula Formation in Patients With Lung Cancer Treated With Chemoradiation and Bevacizumab. *J Clin Oncol* 2009 Nov 9. [Epub ahead of print]
161. Spigel DR, Hainsworth JD, Farley C, et al. Tracheoesophageal (TE) fistula development in a phase II trial of concurrent chemoradiation (CRT) and bevacizumab (B) in limited-stage small-cell lung cancer (LS-SCLC). *J Clin Oncol* 2008;26. abstract 7554.
162. Gitlitz BJ, Glisson BS, Moon J, Reimers H, Gandara DR. Sorafenib in patients with platinum (plat) treated extensive stage small cell lung cancer (E-SCLC): A SWOG (S0435) phase II trial. *J Clin Oncol* 2008;26: abstract 8039.
163. Arnold AM, Seymour L, Smylie M, et al. Phase II study of vandetanib or placebo in small-cell lung cancer patients after complete or partial response to induction chemotherapy with or without radiation therapy: National Cancer Institute of Canada Clinical Trials Group Study BR.20. *J Clin Oncol* 2007;25:4278–4284.
164. Owonikoko TK, Ragin CC, Belani CP, et al. Lung cancer in elderly patients: an analysis of the surveillance, epidemiology, and end results database. *J Clin Oncol* 2007;25:5570–5577.
165. Morita T. A statistical study of lung cancer in the annual of pathological autopsy cases in Japan, from 1958 to 1997, with reference to time trends of lung cancer in the world. *Jpn J Cancer Res* 2002;93:15–23.
166. CRC Cancerstats: Lung Cancer and Smoking – UK, Cancer Research Campaign 2001.
167. Albain KS, Crowley JJ, LeBlanc M, et al. Determinants of improved outcome in small-cell lung cancer: an analysis of the 2,580-patient southwest oncology group data base. *J Clin Oncol* 1990;8:1563–1574.
168. Sagman U, Maki E, Evans WK, et al. Small-cell carcinoma of the lung: derivation of a prognostic staging system. *J Clin Oncol* 1991;9:1639–1649.
169. Pignon JP, Arriagada R, Ihde DC, et al. A meta-analysis of thoracic radiotherapy for small-cell lung cancer. *N Engl J Med* 1992;327: 1618–1624.
170. Siu LL, Shepherd FA, Murray N, et al. Influence of age of the treatment of limited-stage small-cell lung cancer. *J Clin Oncol* 1996;14:821–828.
171. Yuen AR, Zou G, Turrisi AT, et al. Similar outcome of elderly patients in intergroup trial 0096: Cisplatin, etoposide, and thoracic radiotherapy administered once or twice daily in limited stage small cell lung carcinoma. *Cancer* 2000;89:1953–1960.

172. Gridelli C, De Vivo R, Monfardini S. Management of small-cell lung cancer in the elderly. *Crit Rev Oncol Hematol* 2002;41:79–88.
173. Nõu E. Full chemotherapy in elderly patients with small cell bronchial carcinoma. *Acta Oncol* 1996;35:399–406.
174. Findlay MP, Griffin AM, Raghavan D, et al. Retrospective review of chemotherapy for small cell lung cancer in the elderly: does the end justify the means? *Eur J Cancer* 1991;27:1597–1601.
175. Poplin E, Thompson B, Whitacre M, et al. Small cell carcinoma of the lung: influence of age on treatment outcome. *Cancer Treat Rep* 1987;71:291–296.
176. Janssen-Heijnen ML, Lemmens VE, van den Borne BE, et al. Negligible influence of comorbidity on prognosis of patients with small cell lung cancer: a population-based study in Netherlands. *Crit Rev Oncol Hematol* 2007;62:172–178.
177. Tebbutt NC, Snyder RD, Burns WI. An analysis of the outcomes of treatment of small cell lung cancer in the elderly. *Aust N Z J Med* 1997;27:160–164.
178. Shepherd FA, Amdemichael E, Evans WK, et al. Treatment of small cell lung cancer in the elderly. *J Am Geriatr Soc* 1994;42:64–70.
179. Kelly P, O'Brien AA, Daly P, et al. Small-cell lung cancer in elderly patients: the case for chemotherapy. *Age Ageing* 1991;20:19–22.
180. Yau T, Ashley S, Popat S, et al. Time and chemotherapy treatment trends in the treatment of elderly patients (age ≥ 70 years) with small cell lung cancer. *Br J Cancer* 2006;94:18–21.
181. Schild SE, Stella PJ, Brooks BJ, et al. Results of combined-modality therapy for limited-stage small cell lung carcinoma in the elderly. *Cancer* 2005;103:2349–2354.
182. Evans WK, Radwi A, Tomiak E, et al. Oral etoposide and carboplatin. Effective therapy for elderly patients with small cell lung cancer. *Am J Clin Oncol* 1995;18:149–155.
183. Okamoto H, Watanabe K, Nishiwaki Y, et al. Phase II study of area Ander the plasma-concentration-versus-time curve-based carboplatin plus standard-dose intravenous etoposide in elderly patients with small-cell lung cancer. *J Clin Oncol* 1999;17:3540–3545.
184. Murray N, Grafton C, Shah A, et al. Abbreviated treatment for elderly, infirm, or noncompliant patients with limited-stage small-cell lung cancer. *J Clin Oncol* 1998;16:3323–3328.
185. Westeel V, Murray N, Gelmon K, et al. New combination of the old drugs for elderly patients with small-cell lung cancer: a phase II study of the PAVE regimen. *J Clin Oncol* 1998;16:1940–1947.
186. Matsui K, Masuda N, Fukuoka M, et al. Phase II trial of carboplatin plus oral etoposide for elderly patients with small-cell lung cancer. *Br J Cancer* 1998;77:1961–1965.
187. Samantas E, Skarlos DV, Pectasides D, et al. Combination chemotherapy with low doses of weekly carboplatin and oral etoposide in poor risk small cell lung cancer. *Lung Cancer* 1999;23:159–168.
188. Quoix E, Breton JL, Daniel C, et al. Etoposide phosphate with carboplatin in the treatment of elderly patients with small-cell lung cancer; a phase II study. *Ann Oncol* 2001;12:957–962.
189. Larive S, Bombaron P, Riou R, et al. Carboplatin-etoposide combination in small cell lung cancer patients older than 70 years: a phase II trial. *Lung Cancer* 2002;35:1–7.
190. Ardizzoni A, Favaretto A, Boni L, et al. Platinum-etoposide chemotherapy in elderly patients with small-cell lung cancer: results of a randomized multicenter phase II study assessing attenuated-dose or full-dose with lenograstim prophylaxis-a forza operative nazionale italiana carcinoma polmonare and gruppo studio tumori polmonari Veneto (FONICAP-GSTPV) study. *J Clin Oncol* 2005;23:569–575.
191. Okamoto H, Watanabe K, Kunikane H, et al. Randomised phase III trial of carboplatin plus etoposide vs split doses of cisplatin plus etoposide in elderly or poor-risk patients with extensive disease small-cell lung cancer: JCOG 9702. *Br J Cancer* 2007;97:162–169.
192. Jeremic B, Shibamoto Y, Acimovic L, et al. Carboplatin, etoposide, accelerated hyperfractionated radiotherapy for elderly patients with limited small cell lung cancer. A phase II study. *Cancer* 1998;82:836–841.
193. Murray N, Grafton C, Shah A, et al. Abbreviated treatment for elderly, infirm or non-compliant patients with limited small cell lung cancer. *J Clin Oncol* 1998;16:3323–3328.
194. Lilenbaum RC, Cashy J, Hensing TA, et al. Prevalence of poor performance status in lung cancer patients: implications for research. *J Thorac Oncol* 2008;3:125–129.
195. Spiegelman D, Maurer LH, Ware JH, et al. Prognostic factors in small-cell carcinoma of the lung: an analysis of 1,521 patients. *J Clin Oncol* 1989;7:344–354.
196. Treat J, Huang CH, Lane SR, et al. Topotecan in the treatment of relapsed small cell lung cancer patients with poor performance status. *Oncologist* 2004;9:173–181.
197. Lilenbaum RC, Huber RM, Treat J, et al. Topotecan therapy in patients with relapsed small-cell lung cancer and poor performance status. *Clin Lung Cancer* 2006;8:130–134.
198. Medical Research Council Lung Cancer Working Party. Randomised trial of four-drug vs less intensive two-drug chemotherapy in the palliative treatment of patients with small-cell lung cancer (SCLC) and poor prognosis. *Br J Cancer* 1996;73:406–413.
199. Girling DJ. Comparison of oral etoposide and standard intravenous multidrug chemotherapy for small-cell lung cancer: a stopped multicentre randomized trial. Medical Research Council Lung Cancer Working Party. *Lancet* 1996;348:563–566.
200. Souhami RL, Spiro SG, Rudd RM, et al. Five-day oral etoposide treatment for advanced small-cell lung cancer: randomized comparison with intravenous chemotherapy. *J Natl Cancer Inst* 1997;89:577–580.

CHAPTER 59

Sara Erridge
Nevin Murray
Andrew T. Turrisi III

Multimodality Therapy for Limited-Stage Small Cell Lung Cancer: Combining Chemotherapy and Radiotherapy

INTRODUCTION

The disappearance of a large malignant mass is a dramatic phenomenon in medicine. Experienced lung cancer oncologists agree that it is easy to make the chest radiograph or computed tomography (CT) scan of a patient with locally advanced small cell lung cancer (SCLC) look much better with chemotherapy and thoracic irradiation. However, it is definitely more challenging to eliminate the last clonogenic cell in the neoplasm to prevent the development of an incurable relapse. The treatment of limited-stage SCLC requires us to combine chemotherapy and radiotherapy in the most effective way to increase the proportion of long-term survivors.

The incidence of SCLC, which accounts for about 12% to 15% of all lung cancers, is decreasing in developed countries most likely because of changes in the composition of cigarettes and patterns of tobacco consumption.[1] The declining incidence of SCLC parallels a stalling in the pace of research in this cancer as reflected by the number of abstracts submitted to the American Society of Clinical Oncology annual meetings and the International Association for the Study of Lung Cancer world conferences.[2] In contrast, the amount of research for non–small cell lung cancer (NSCLC) has increased dramatically. The slow pace of SCLC investigation is unfortunate and puzzling because the proportion of estimated deaths from this disease is about 4% of all cancer mortality and similar to ovarian cancer, leukemia, and non-Hodgkin lymphoma.[3]

STAGING

SCLC may be staged by either the Veterans Administration Lung Study Group (VASLG)[4] system or the tumor, node, metastasis (TNM) classification.[5] The VASLG system categorizes the stage of SCLC as either limited (LSCLC) or extensive (ESCLC). This system has persisted for SCLC because of its simplicity, reliable prognostic value, and practical utility.[6–8] LSCLC is defined as tumor confined to one hemithorax and the regional lymph nodes, whereas extensive-stage disease (ESCLC) is defined as disease beyond these bounds. The original definition of limited disease was a tumor volume that could be encompassed by a "reasonable" radiotherapy treatment plan. Because long-term survival is uncommon (7% to 9%) when chemotherapy alone is used to treat LSCLC,[9,10] the reasonable radiotherapy port rule continues to be of practical importance in the design of combined modality therapy.

Although the term reasonable lacks precision, the adoption of this criterion internationally has broad acceptance in operational definition of limited disease. There continues to be support for moving to the TNM system, but this has not been widely adopted. Using simple staging techniques, the University of Toronto Lung Oncology Group[8] identified a subgroup of patients with "very limited" SCLC without mediastinal node involvement who had a significantly better prognosis and a 5-year survival of 18% with sequential chemotherapy followed by thoracic irradiation used between 1976 and 1985. The 5-year survival for patients with evidence of involved mediastinal nodes was 6%. Only 2% survived 5 years when there was pneumonic consolidation, atelectasis, pleural effusion, or involved supraclavicular nodes. Such distinctions may be addressed by application of the TNM staging system. Until 2007, the TNM system had been reported only in small surgical series. At the *12th World Conference on Lung Cancer*, the International Association for the Study of Lung Cancer Staging Committee presented an analysis of 8088 patients.[5] Survival outcome was superior in patients without mediastinal or supraclavicular nodal involvement. Patients with pleural effusion regardless of the cytology have an intermediate prognosis between limited and extensive-stage disease. The median survival of stage IIIA/IIIB (12.1/11.1 months) and the 5-year survival (10% to 12%) reported in this data set are lower than what has been reported for state-of-the-art treatment described in this chapter. It remains to be seen whether adoption of the TNM system will improve the investigation and management of LSCLC. New and ongoing studies of SCLC treatment should report both the VASLG as well as the TNM system.

A legitimate question in a disease, such as SCLC with early widespread dissemination, is the clinical necessity of multiple staging investigations. Because chemotherapy is recommended for all fit patients, to expedite treatment, most clinicians perform a minimum number of staging procedures, rather than the wider range recommended in clinical trials. This approach might be appropriate if the management were initial treatment with multiple chemotherapy cycles followed by consolidative thoracic irradiation. On the other hand, if patients with true LSCLC are better treated by concurrent and early chemoradiotherapy, careful staging is imperative to properly categorize intent (curative vs. palliative) and determine the treatment program.[2] LSCLC patients have curative potential, which justifies the complexity and toxicity of integrated thoracic irradiation and combination chemotherapy. Without appropriate staging, patients with undetected widespread disease will be subjected to unnecessary toxicity and unrealistic hope. Despite modern technology, the stage of some patients will be equivocal, so clinicians must use their judgment.

Complete evaluation of a patient with newly diagnosed SCLC consists of a history and physical examination, pathology confirmation, CT of the chest and abdomen to include the whole liver and adrenal glands, bone scan, and brain CT with contrast or MRI examination. Additionally, a complete blood count (CBC), electrolytes, blood urea nitrogen (BUN), creatinine, albumin, and liver function tests should be performed at baseline. Bone marrow biopsy has a low yield[11] if other tests are negative, but may be considered in patients with leukoerythroblastic features, low platelet count or a very high lactate dehydrogenase. After such a workup, the proportion of patients with LSCLC is approximately 40%.[1]

The utility of positron emission tomography (PET) in SCLC has been reported in several small studies[12–14] that have mainly used PET rather than PET/CT technology. The evidence suggests that PET added to conventional staging improves the sensitivity in detecting extracranial disease in 10% to 15% of cases, but the confidence intervals on the estimates of staging accuracy are wide because the studies are small. The information required to be confident that PET results should be used to guide therapy for LSCLC will not be available in the foreseeable future. It would be informative if a large cohort of patients with LSCLC as determined by conventional procedures also underwent a PET scan. This cohort should be treated with state-of-the-art combined modality therapy regardless of the PET result. The crucial information would not be that those with extensive SCLC according to the PET scan result have a worse outcome; this would be expected.[10] The important outcome would be to demonstrate that patients with ESCLC by PET scan, but LSCLC by conventional procedures were not curable by standard treatment. It would be inappropriate for a PET scan result to deny patients with potentially curable SCLC a combined modality protocol, even if the chance for cure was decreased. On the other hand, it would be useful to know if patients with ESCLC detected by PET scan alone had an equivalent chance of long-term survival as those defined by conventional staging procedures. Whether PET imaging is useful in guiding thoracic radiotherapy planning should be evaluated in prospective clinical trials. Until this information is available, the routine use of PET scanning to guide therapy for SCLC cannot be recommended.

Although the limited- versus extensive-stage system was created for practical purposes, it also suggests important biological and clinical characteristics of the disease. When SCLC is overtly metastatic (ESCLC), an underlying biological aggressiveness in the tumor may exist that transcends the importance of the simple physical distribution of cancer cells within the body. Potentially curable LSCLC may fundamentally differ from incurable ESCLC; however, the categorical boundary may be fluid. Obliteration of the stem cells at the root cause of this disease justify early aggressive combined local management. Cure evaporates once resistant to chemotherapy stem cells establish themselves outside the primary site. Time may be of the essence when attempting to cure SCLC.

Therapeutic endeavors address concentrations of locoregional bulk of disease in LSCLC, and a subclinical metastatic population in widely distributed sites. Normal healthy tissues vary in their tolerance of therapeutic interventions, just as tumor populations vary in their susceptibility to anticancer agents. These clinical considerations and the biological factors underlying them have led directly to modern concepts of multiple-modality therapy for this disease. Although a small fraction of SCLC patients will benefit from surgery when they present with a solitary pulmonary lesion without involvement of the mediastinum, integrated chemotherapy with radiotherapy to the chest and brain offers the most realistic chance for symptom abatement, extension of median survival, and long-term survival.

THE EVOLUTION OF COMBINED MODALITY THERAPY

The legacy of treatment for LSCLC can be described by a series of treatment paradigms.[15] The sequence of development of these paradigms was determined by incremental steps grounded in controlled clinical trials of crucial issues of therapy and consensus by lung cancer investigators. They provide a useful insight into how our understanding of cancer biology and treatments has evolved over the last 3 decades.

Paradigm 1: Surgery as Standard Treatment World Wars I and II profoundly influenced on the upsurge of lung cancer. The availability of tobacco products and permissive attitude toward tobacco consumption during both wars were associated with a large increase in smoking among servicemen. In addition, the prevalence of smoking among women increased greatly during the 1940s.

Surgical treatment of penetrating wounds to the chest during World War II produced major advances in thoracic surgery, and the cadre of expert chest surgeons trained during the war had to contend with the increasing numbers of lung cancers among veterans in the 1950s and 1960s.[16,17] In the immediate post–World War II era, surgery was the only truly effective treatment for patients with all types of lung cancer, including SCLC.

Paradigm 2: Thoracic Irradiation Better than Surgery The epithelial origin of SCLC was described in 1926,[18] and the separation of this virulent pathologic subtype on morphologic grounds was established in 1959.[19] From the earliest reports,[20] impressive regressions of SCLC induced by radiotherapy suggested an integral role of this modality in the definitive management of this disease.

In a trial conducted in the 1960s, the median survival of surgically unresectable LSCLC patients randomized to supportive care alone was 12 weeks.[21] Another randomized trial comparing surgery alone with thoracic irradiation alone for patients with SCLC was carried out by the Medical Research Council in the United Kingdom.[22,23] Eligibility criteria included (a) SCLC on bronchial biopsy; (b) no evidence of extrathoracic metastasis; (c) the tumor was regarded as operable on clinical examination and chest radiograph; (d) the patient was considered fit enough for resection; and (e) the patient was considered fit enough for radical radiotherapy. Although this study was conducted in an era before the availability of modern staging techniques, the intrathoracic extent of tumor was probably less than in most contemporary LSCLC trials. Of the 144 patients included in the main analysis, 71 were allocated to surgery and 73 to radical megavoltage radiotherapy. A complete resection of all visible growth was performed in 48% of the surgical group, all of whom had a pneumonectomy. A total of 34% were unresectable, and 18% had no operation because of preoperative deterioration or refusal of surgery. In the radiotherapy group, 85% had radical thoracic irradiation, 11% had palliative radiotherapy, and 4% had no radiotherapy because of deterioration or refusal. The median survival was 28.5 weeks for surgery and 43 weeks for radiotherapy ($p = 0.04$). Five-year survival was 1% for the surgical arm (the sole survivor refused surgery and was given radiotherapy) and 4% for radiotherapy. Outcome for both groups was poor, but treatment feasibility, toxicity, and survival all favored thoracic irradiation. The standard of treatment for LSCLC shifted from surgery to thoracic irradiation. The main aim was to give patients relief of local symptoms until their death from metastatic disease.

Paradigm 3: Thoracic Irradiation with Adjuvant Chemotherapy The systemic nature of SCLC was emphasized by the rapid tempo of systemic relapse and low probability of long-term survival in patients with apparently localized disease given definitive local therapy alone. In a classic study[24] of 19 patients undergoing potentially curative surgical resection who died of noncancer-related causes within 30 days of surgery, 13 were found to have persistent disease at autopsy. Moreover, distant metastases were present in 12 of the 13 cases. Although not all patients with LSCLC have subclinical metastatic disease, the actual proportion is so high that we assume that there are metastases and treat accordingly. The success of chemotherapy for leukemia and lymphoma was in its infancy, but already the vision of cure by systemic treatment stimulated clinical research into using such an approach for SCLC.

A major step in the systemic treatment of SCLC was reported in 1969. This randomized study compared alkylating agents at several dose schedules with an inert compound in about 2000 patients with lung cancer at a group of Veterans Administration hospitals.[4] The antitumor effects of chemotherapy were analyzed according to cell type, and improvement in survival was the sole criterion of drug activity. The 4-month median survival for patients with SCLC treated with high intermittent doses of cyclophosphamide compared with 1.5 months for patients given placebo ($p = 0.0005$). Documentation of a survival improvement with chemotherapy for patients with lung cancer was a notable development in cancer medicine, and cyclophosphamide became the cornerstone in SCLC chemotherapy regimens for decades. The credibility of cyclophosphamide efficacy in the treatment of SCLC was augmented by randomized trials that showed prolonged survival for that agent as adjuvant chemotherapy compared with no further treatment after surgical resection.[17] Curiously, the lack of survival benefit for cyclophosphamide and other alkylating agents in the treatment of NSCLC in these and other lung cancer trials[17,25–30] did not prevent them from being incorporated into combination chemotherapy regimens for this disease over the next 20 years.

The perceptive observations of Watson and Berg[20] suggested thoracic irradiation coupled with chemotherapy as a model for treatment of SCLC. This hypothesis was first tested in a randomized trial by Bergsagel et al.[31] from Toronto. Patients with nonresectable lung cancer confined to the central area of the thorax were randomly assigned treatment with radiotherapy to the primary lesion and mediastinum or radiotherapy plus two schedules of intermittent intravenous cyclophosphamide. One third of 123 patients in the study had SCLC and both progression-free survival (29 vs. 16 weeks) and overall survival (42 vs. 21 weeks) were significantly superior for patients receiving combined modality therapy.

Two other randomized trials[32,33] showed significantly superior survival for thoracic irradiation and adjuvant chemotherapy when compared with radiotherapy alone. The median survival for patients with LSCLC treated by radiotherapy alone was consistently about 5 to 6 months. Two additional randomized controlled trials[34,35] showed some advantage for combined modality therapy, but the survival differences between the groups were not statistically significant, probably because many patients in the radiotherapy arms received chemotherapy at the time of disease progression.

The paradox that a local modality had a role in a disease dominated by systemic spread had been established. The issues of integration such as what drugs, what timing, what volume to irradiate, and what dose were not clear enough to formulate and endure today.

Paradigm 4: Combination Chemotherapy with Adjuvant Thoracic Irradiation The success of combination chemotherapy in leukemia and lymphoma and the recognition of SCLC as a type of lung cancer with marked chemosensitivity spurred investigation of multidrug regimens. The first study of combination chemotherapy for lung cancer was published in 1972 by Hansen et al.,[36] using a regimen that included cyclophosphamide, methotrexate, dactinomycin, and vincristine. All eight patients with SCLC subtype responded; combination chemotherapy for SCLC was off to a promising start. High response rates for cyclophosphamide and vincristine were reported by Eagan et al.[37] and Holoye and Samuels.[38] By combining cyclophosphamide, doxorubicin, vincristine (CAV), and bleomycin, Einhorn et al.[39] produced not only high response rates in SCLC, but complete responses were seen in 20% of cases. Bleomycin was discarded because of pulmonary toxicity, especially when combined with thoracic irradiation,[40] and the CAV regimen persists to this day as a standard regimen for SCLC. A cardinal feature of drug selection was individual agent activity in SCLC, nonoverlapping toxicity of each of the agents in the combination, and the holy grail of synergy.

By using the principle of combination chemotherapy[41] and incorporating new, more active agents, the search for a regimen with a high complete response rate for SCLC was intense during the 1970s. Combination chemotherapy was shown to be better than single-agent chemotherapy in three early randomized trials,[42–44] but a superior regimen did not emerge. Nevertheless, in the early 1970s, a change in philosophy occurred; with the observed high response rates, multiagent chemotherapy became the primary therapy in LSCLC and thoracic irradiation was positioned as an adjuvant or "consolidative" treatment after initial numbers of cycles of systemic therapy.[45]

Treatment regimens giving aggressive combination chemotherapy *without* thoracic irradiation[46] appeared to yield survival results similar to combined modality therapy. Median survival was in the range of 12 to 15 months, and projected long-term survival was usually in the range of 10%, whether radiotherapy was administered or not. However, aggressive combined modality therapy was also associated with more toxicity, and the selection of only patients fit enough to receive this more demanding treatment in nonrandomized reports may have biased results against chemotherapy alone. Many investigators began to speculate that radiotherapy might not be necessary at all in LSCLC.

This debate persisted throughout the 1980s,[45,47] and many randomized trials were performed in an attempt to settle this vexing issue.[48–50] It was not until 1992 that two metaanalyses[9,10] demonstrated a modest improvement in survival rates in those patients given thoracic radiotherapy in addition to chemotherapy. The survival benefit becomes evident at about 15 months after the start of treatment and persists beyond 5 years. At 3 years, 8.9% of the chemotherapy-only group was alive compared with 14.3% of the combined modality group. The analysis of local control showed a 2-year local failure rate of 23% for irradiated patients versus 48% for nonirradiated patients ($p = 0.0001$). These benefits were obtained at the cost of an increase in treatment-related deaths of 1%. However, none of the trials in these metaanalyses employed initial cisplatin etoposide chemotherapy, which is now the acknowledged international standard.

The addition of thoracic irradiation to chemotherapy for LSCLC has, for several theoretical reasons, the potential to improve outcomes. Its mechanism of action is different from chemotherapeutic agents so the potential exists for additive or even synergistic damage to the tumor. This capacity to eradicate the most populous, and hence most dangerous concentration of tumor cells, improves the probability of controlling local disease that may evolve more resistant progeny and metastasize systemically

Paradigm 5: Integrated Early Concurrent Chemotherapy and Radiotherapy The strategy to destroy as many cancer cells as possible in the shortest period of time using early concurrent chemoradiation has several theoretical advantages.

Decreased Probability of Metastatic Events Experimental work by Hill et al.[51] indicate that tumor cells mutate spontaneously and randomly to acquire metastatic potential. Moreover, once tumors reach a critical size or volume, metastatic phenotypes are generated "explosively," so the cumulative probability of the existence of metastases and the number of metastases increases in proportion to elapsed time. The best way to decrease metastatic events is to quickly eliminate as much tumor as possible.

Lower Probability of Chemotherapy Resistance A large body of experimental and clinical data exists that support the observation that variability exists for chemosensitivity within tumor cell populations.[52] Moreover, tumor cells display a capacity to be resistant to many drugs concurrently.[53] The biologic basis of this evolution of resistance originates during tumor growth from mutations in the cancer genome.[54] The development of resistant mutants is a random process, and the probability of their appearance increases with time in proportion to the total number of cell divisions the neoplastic burden has undergone. The best way to minimize the probability of chemotherapy resistance is to eliminate as many cancer cells as possible in the shortest time.

Lower Probability of Resistance to Radiotherapy The probability of mutation to intrinsic radiotherapy resistance[55] or acquired radioresistance as a consequence of enhanced DNA repair efficiency secondary to previous chemotherapy[56] should be minimized by the early deployment of both modalities.

Diminished Accelerated Repopulation Accelerated repopulation of tumors undergoing radiotherapy has been proposed[57] to explain the clinical observation that regimens with extended duration of therapy often require increased radiation dosages to achieve an isoeffective result.[58] Accelerated tumor growth has been reported after surgery[59] and chemotherapy[60] in animal models. Accelerated repopulation will decrease local control, and also, the increased mitotic activity within a larger residual tumor may result in an increased probability of metastatic events and the development drug and radiation resistance. Rapid destruction of tumor by early integration of chemoradiation should minimize the amount of tumor capable of repopulation.

Although theoretically attractive, the practical implementation of early chemoradiation initially proved challenging. In 1976, investigators from the Radiation Oncology Branch of the National Cancer Institute in Bethesda, Maryland performed an exploratory study that tested the limits of toxicity.[61–65] Although the protocol was influenced by the successful model of combined modality therapy for childhood lymphocytic leukemia,[66] the vigor of therapy was unprecedented in solid tumor protocols. It involved initial simultaneous irradiation to the brain, primary tumor, and mediastinum and aggressive concurrent chemotherapy (cyclophosphamide 1.5 g/m^2, doxorubicin 40 mg/m^2, and vincristine 2 mg). The drugs were repeated as soon as the leukocytes increased to 3.5×10^9/L. All therapy was complete in 3 to 4 months.

The toxicity of this regimen was formidable. Radiation pneumonitis occurred in 38%, and a combination of pneumonitis and neutropenic sepsis was fatal in 24%. Severe esophagitis requiring nasogastric or parenteral nutrition occurred in 14%, and permanent strictures were observed.[62] Additionally, a previously undescribed neurologic syndrome of somnolence, poor attention span, recent memory loss, and action tremor was seen. The symptoms became evident within 2 to 4 months of starting treatment and were reversible within 4 months of onset.

The first reported survival results for patients with LSCLC treated in this manner were spectacular with 100% complete remissions and projected 80% long-term survival.[61] With longer follow-up, the survival rates dwindled and this trial was criticized for generation of false optimism by preliminary data reporting and unacceptably severe toxicity. Nevertheless, the mature results, which demonstrated an 80% complete remission rate and 25% survival at 4 years, were provocative and unprecedented.[65] Although the response result was noteworthy, 13% died without evidence of tumor at autopsy; it is speculative whether the survival rate could have been higher had modern supportive care been available or whether the toxicity of the approach was unacceptable. In an analysis of treatment factors contributing to long-term survival, it was concluded that concurrent chemotherapy and radiotherapy achieved better local tumor control than sequential therapy.[65] These data infer that if the duration of concurrent therapy is prolonged longer than 3 weeks, the enhanced survival and local tumor effect were lost in a flood of treatment-induced toxicity.[55]

It was evident that the combined chemoradiation model could not progress unless chemotherapy and radiotherapy could be compatible and integrated in a manner such that extreme toxicities did not compromise delivery of either modality. Sequential regimens giving thoracic irradiation during a gap in chemotherapy[67] (the "sandwich" technique) were less toxic but efficacy was not improved, possibly because the interruption of the cadence of chemotherapy allowed tumor regrowth in nonirradiated sites. The results of a phase II study of a less aggressive CAV regimen[68] with concurrent thoracic irradiation led to a large randomized trial comparing simultaneous chemoradiation with CAV chemotherapy alone. However, a significant survival benefit was not observed[69] and excessive toxicity impaired drug delivery. Another controlled trial of CAV alone versus a split course of thoracic irradiation delivered in three phases between CAV pulses demonstrated a survival benefit for combined modality therapy.[50] However, gastrointestinal and hematologic toxicity continued to be problematic. The severity of morbidity to normal tissue from the interaction of doxorubicin and radiotherapy has limited the utility of these approaches. Concurrent thoracic irradiation with chemotherapy containing cyclophosphamide, methotrexate, and lomustine was superior to chemotherapy given alone,[48] with higher rates of remission and prolonged survival in patients with LSCLC, but the benefit was offset by unacceptable pulmonary toxicity. Similarly, concurrent cyclophosphamide, etoposide, and vincristine and radiotherapy have demonstrated superiority to chemotherapy alone, but unacceptable chemotherapy attenuation from myelosuppression was associated with combined therapy.[49]

Then the development of cisplatin and etoposide in the late 1970s at Memorial Sloan-Kettering[70] as a potent combination for SCLC allowed the next step forward. Cisplatin produces no pneumonitis, esophagitis or stomatitis, and little myelosuppression at normal doses. Etoposide at standard doses has myelosuppression as its only serious side effect. More importantly, although cisplatin has some weak radiosensitizing properties,[71] normal tissue toxicity from concurrent cisplatin and irradiation is not nearly so severe as with doxorubicin, nitrosoureas, methotrexate, or cyclophosphamide. Additionally, neither cisplatin nor etoposide have been implicated in "radiation recall"[62] toxicity.

Therefore, an important development in the evolution of therapy for LSCLC occurred when cisplatin and etoposide was integrated with thoracic irradiation. Thoracic radiotherapy and cisplatin etoposide could be used concurrently and at full doses of each modality. Pilot studies were independently performed at the British Columbia Cancer Agency[72,73] and by investigators associated with the Southwest Oncology Group.[74] From the first report[72] in 1984, it was clear that cisplatin etoposide chemotherapy and thoracic irradiation could be administered concurrently with manageable toxicity and little compromise in drug or radiation delivery at full dosage.

The National Cancer Institute of Canada (NCIC) explored the integration of chemotherapy and thoracic irradiation in a phase III randomized controlled trial and demonstrated that early concurrent cisplatin etoposide and thoracic irradiation was superior to delayed thoracic irradiation given concurrently with cisplatin etoposide.[75] A delay of as little as 12 weeks in the administration of thoracic irradiation for patients with LSCLC resulted in an approximate 50% decrease in the probability of 5-year survival from 22% to 13%. The benchmark 5-year survival rate for LSCLC shifted from about 10% to about 20%.

Other randomized trials[32,49,76–79] of thoracic irradiation timing have been reported (see Table 59.1), but not all support

TABLE 59.1 Trials Comparing Early and Late Radiotherapy for LSCLC

				Start Time		Patients		Median (mos)		5-Year (%)		
			Dose / Volume	Early	Late	Early	Late	Early	Late	Early	Late	
1.	CALGB[49,131]	CEVA for up to 18 mos	40 Gy/20 F to GTV, hilum, med, bilat SCF then 10 Gy/5F to GTV only	week 1	week 9	125	145	13.04	14.54	6.6	12.8	NS
2.	Aarhus[76]	CAV/EP (RT given with EP) total of 8 chemo cycles	40 Gy/20# APPA as split course to GTV, hilum, med., SCF only if involved. Dose increased to 45 Gy/22 F later in trial	week 1 and 3	week 18 and 23	99	100	10.7	12.9	10	10	NS
3.	Helenic[93]	Carbo/E. total 6 cycles	30 Gy/20 F(1.5 Gy bid) APPA to GTV, hilum, med., SCF only if involved then 15 Gy/10 F bid with oblique fields to GTV only	week 1	week 9	42	39	17.5	17	22	13	NS
4.	London[79]	CAV/EP. total 6 cycles	40 Gy/15 F GTV, hilum, med., SCF only if involved. APPA with block to keep cord dose <35 Gy	week 3	week 15	159	166	13.5	15.1	NA	NA	NS
5.	NCIC[80]	CAV/EP. total 6 cycles	40 Gy/15 F GTV, hilum, med., SCF only if involved. APPA with block to keep cord dose <35 Gy	week 3	week 15	155	153	21.2	16	22	13	0.013
6.	Yugoslavian[77]	Carbo/EP –daily carbo/E during RT and an additional 4 cycles of EP	36 Gy/24 F (1.5 Gy bid) APPA to GTV, hilum, med., SCF only if involved. Then 18 Gy/12 F using oblique fields with limits to dose to esophagus.	week 1	week 6	52	51	34	26	30	15	0.027
7.	JCOG[78]	EP total 4 cycles	45 Gy/30 F (1.5 Gy bid) GTV, hilum, SCF only if involved.	week 1	week 15	114	114	27.2	19.7	30	15	NS

A, Doxorubicin; APPA, anterior posterior radiation fields; bid, twice daily; C, Cyclophosphamide; CALGB, Cancer and Leukemia Group B; Carbo, Carboplatin; E, Etoposide; GTV, gross tumor volume; NCIC, National Cancer Institute of Canada; JCOG, Japan Clinical Oncology Group; LSCLC, limited-stage small cell lung cancer; med., mediastinum; NS, not specified; P, Cisplatin; RT, radiotherapy; SCF, supra-clavicular fossa; V, Vincristine.

the superiority of early chemoradiation. These negative trials[49,76,79] consistently have long-term survival rates in both arms of only 10% to 15%, whereas the early chemoradiation arms of the positive studies[77,78,80] report long-term survival rates of 20% to 26%. The reason why some randomized trials do not support the superiority of early chemoradiation may be explained by the use of the inferior cyclophosphamide-based chemotherapy,[49,81] failure to deliver chemotherapy with thoracic irradiation,[76] and attenuation of chemotherapy delivery subsequent to the radiotherapy.[49,76,79] To obtain the survival benefit of early concurrent chemoradiation, it is important to deliver the chemotherapy at full dose and in a timely manner.[69] Despite the variable quality of the randomized clinical trials, metaanalyses of randomized trials comparing early versus delayed thoracic irradiation in LSCLC consistently show superiority of early thoracic irradiation.[82,83]

Accelerated repopulation of surviving clonagens[57,84,85] during protracted (greater than 3 weeks) thoracic irradiation is a plausible hypothesis for the decreased effectiveness of treatment in LSCLC. This was a key concept in a landmark clinical trial reported by Turrisi et al.[86] This phase III randomized trial compared 45 Gy in 5 weeks with an accelerated fractionation regimen of 45 Gy in 3 weeks using twice-daily radiotherapy treatment with cycle 1, cisplatin etoposide chemotherapy. The 5-year survival rate of 26% for accelerated fractionated radiotherapy was clearly superior to conventional fractionation (16%). This is the only controlled trial that has ever demonstrated superior survival when one thoracic irradiation schedule is compared with another in LSCLC.

To further test the hypothesis that initial treatment triggers accelerated repopulation, De Ruysscher et al.[87] calculated the start of any treatment to end of radiation therapy (SER) for the study arms of four of the randomized trials of LSCLC.[65,67,68,77] Corrections for the different schedules were made by calculating the equivalent radiation dose (EQD_{2T}); this attempts to account for different total radiotherapy doses, fraction size, and overall treatment time. A shorter SER was found to be associated with better long-term survival, such that a survival decrement of approximately 1.8% per week occurred when SER was extended beyond 3 weeks. A major implication of the analysis of De Ruysscher et al. is that repopulation of clonogenic tumor cells caused by neoadjuvant chemotherapy inhibits the effectiveness of subsequent radiotherapy and contributes to treatment failure in LSCLC. Altogether, multiple lines of evidence support the importance of accelerated repopulation in LSCLC and provide a consistent radiobiological framework for investigation and treatment of this disease.

Research has focused on new drugs and systemic management, and to date, no further comparative trials have been conducted comparing other schedules with the Intergroup method, which sets the gold standard for long-term survival.

Technical radiotherapy has undergone a sea change since the design and conduct of this trial, but some have been dissuaded by the higher frequency of esophagitis, despite the universal reversibility and no reports of permanent stricture. Also some publicly funded healthcare systems have found the delivery of twice-daily treatment impractical.

Paradigm 6: The Addition of Prophylactic Cranial Irradiation Despite the success of the integration of chemotherapy and thoracic radiotherapy, patients frequently relapse in the brain. Clinical intracerebral relapses are observed in 50% to 60% of patients, and even more are detected at autopsy. The concept is that chemotherapy could eliminate systemic disease, radiotherapy, the primary and bulky thoracic sites, thereby leaving the brain as a sanctuary site for relapse. Most chemotherapeutic agents cannot cross an intact blood-brain barrier, and even those that do (lomustine, procarbazine), do not prevent intracranial relapses. The challenge was therefore to devise a radiotherapy schedule that eradicates microscopic intracerebral disease without damage normal brain tissues. The success of prophylactic cranial irradiation (PCI) in leukemia suggested that such an approach might also be useful in SCLC and was first investigated by the National Cancer Institute–Veteran Affairs (NCI–VA) lung group in the early 1970s.[88]

For decades, PCI had advocates and adversaries, and the issues of timing, dose, and even need for its use were debated. For a time, anecdotal reports cautioned about late effects and warned that the few survivors had more potential harm than benefit from this tactic. This controversy was at its height during the time of the intergroup study accrual, and although mandated, not all cases received PCI after complete response, and compliance with the policy was not monitored a study end point. In a metaanalysis, Auperin et al.[89] confirmed the hypothesis that low doses of radiotherapy administered to patients without detectable CNS involvement might eradicate occult metastatic disease for some patients and improve the outcome in LSCLC. The incidence of brain metastases in patients who did not receive PCI was 57.6%, a 3 years in contrast to 33.3% in the treated group ($p < 0.001$). Three-year survival in the control group was 15.3% versus 20.7% in the treated group.

However, the timing, dose (total and per fraction), and criteria about specific population characteristics were not clear. The principal outstanding question, the relative frequency of late neurocognitive effects, remains open. One of the largest trials examining the role of PCI following completion of chemotherapy also included prospective assessment of neurocognitive function. This study suggested that there were no significant differences in functioning with up to 3 years of follow-up, and late effects were seen in fewer than 10% of those receiving PCI or observation.[90] Therefore, it is routine practice to deliver PCI with a dose of 25 to 30 Gy in 10 to 15 fractions on completion of chemotherapy to all patients who have responded to chemoradiation.

Currently, the research focus on both sides of the Atlantic is in determining whether higher doses (36 Gy in 18 fractions) produce better survival and local control than lower dose (25 Gy in 10 fractions). The European study has completed accrual, but recruitment continues in the North American study.

Whether or not PCI has a role in ESCLC has also been investigated. There was debate as to whether or not these patients would succumb to extracranial disease without deriving any survival or local control benefit. The European Organisation for Research and Treatment of Cancer (EORTC) recently published a study[91] involving 284 patients proving a survival advantage at 1 year and 75% reduction in the rate of intracranial relapse. Patients entered into this study merely had to respond to four to six cycles of chemotherapy, and three quarters of patients had local and systemic disease evident. Critics of the study note that fewer than 30% had imaging of the brain prior to randomization; however, this does not explain why the treatment arm should prove to be superior. Importantly, quality of life was not adversely affected, and no late neurocognitive effects were reported despite using large dose per fraction (3 to 4 Gy) in more than 75% of patients, with 20 Gy in 5 fractions being the predominant regimen. However, fewer than 10% survived more than 2 years, the time when late effects may begin to emerge and become important.

Overall, over the past 25 years, progress in the paradigm of integrated chemotherapy and radiotherapy has been most evident with innovations of radiotherapy. Future research in this disease should focus on optimizing radiotherapy and identifying key aspects of the molecular biology of SCLC, which may lead to more effective systemic therapy.

THORACIC RADIOTHERAPY VOLUME AND DOSE

The role of thoracic radiotherapy in improving survival and local control has been confirmed, but exactly which tissues need to be irradiated has yet to be elucidated. In the older studies of chemoirradiation, such as the study of Perez et al.,[34] volume irradiated included the gross tumor volume (GTV), ipsilateral hilum, bilateral mediastinum, and both supraclavicular fossae. In contrast, in the most recently published studies, a reduced volume has been employed. Table 59.1 illustrates the wide variation in volume and techniques used.

Only one randomized clinical trial, performed by Southwest Oncology Group (SWOG),[92] has ever examined the issue of radiotherapy volume. In this, patients with a partial response or stable disease after four cycles of chemotherapy were randomized to radiotherapy based on either the prechemotherapy or postchemotherapy disease. No appreciable differences were detected in either overall survival or recurrence patterns between the two arms.

The idea of using either a shrinking volume technique, such as that used in the Hellenic study[93] or a very reduced volume treating just gross disease, is very attractive; it would minimize toxicity and potentially allow dose escalation of both radiotherapy and chemotherapy. Some information on which tissues should be treated may be obtained from retrospective studies looking at patterns of local failure. Tada et al.[94] analyzed the patterns of recurrence in 117 patients treated between 1986 and 1993. There appeared to be more marginal relapses in the upper mediastinum and supraclavicular fossae in those patients with N2 and N3 disease, although the number of patients was small. The authors suggested that the upper border of the treatment volume should be extended in patients with N2 or N3 disease. The relapse patterns following surgery of early stage SCLC suggest that radiotherapy volumes could be safely reduced in those patients presenting with N0 or N1 disease.

The three main potential toxicities of thoracic radiotherapy in LSCLC are esophagitis, pneumonitis, and radiation myelopathy. For both the esophagus and the lungs, the risk of toxicity is dependent not only on dose, but also on the volume of tissue irradiated. Although there has been very little analysis of this risk in SCLC, there are increasing data on these in NSCLC. The risk of pneumonitis can be predicted by either the percentage volume of lung receiving over a threshold dose, for example 20 Gy (V20),[95] or the mean lung dose[96]; however, it should be noted that these data are based on the use of radiation alone. A study from Japan[97] demonstrated that the "safe" percentage of lung receiving greater than 20 Gy drops from 32% with radiotherapy alone[95] to 25% in the presence of platinum-based chemotherapy. Similarly, the risk of esophageal toxicity is volume dependent.[98]

The question is how to reduce the volume of these critical tissues while adequately treating the target volume? In the early studies of chemoradiation in LSCLC, anterior–posterior (APPA) fields were employed, which minimize the dose to the lungs, but such an approach may result in overdosage to the spinal cord. To reduce the dose to the latter, in several studies, for example in the National Cancer Institute of Canada study,[75] a posterior block was inserted for part of the treatment. This patently underdoses the mediastinal lymph nodes. In later studies, lateral or oblique fields were employed, but lateral fields resulted in excessive pulmonary toxicity.[99] Therefore, a two-phase cone-done technique, or more recently, in single phase involved-field only approach has been used. In a recent phase II study, the radiotherapy volume encompassed just the primary and all lymph nodes greater than 1 cm in short axis[100] and treatment delivered with a single-phase three-dimensional conformal technique. Few local recurrences were observed. Such an approach enables dose escalation without excessive normal tissue toxicity, however, this method has not been formally compared with wide-field treatment in a clinical trial. An example of modern dose–volume planning for LSCLC is seen in Figure 59.1.

Although concurrent thoracic radiotherapy improves outcomes for patients with LSCLC, the local relapse rate remains high; with around 30% of patients experiencing an isolated in-field relapse[101] and 20% both in-field and distant relapse. In view of this, many of the ongoing studies are looking at the feasibility of escalation of the radiation dose. Because of practical difficulties of administering twice-daily radiotherapy, many radiation oncologists continue to use once-daily radiotherapy, but the optimal dose has not been established. Doses of as high as 70 Gy have now been used safely,[102] but whether or not the increased total dose can overcome the potential detrimental

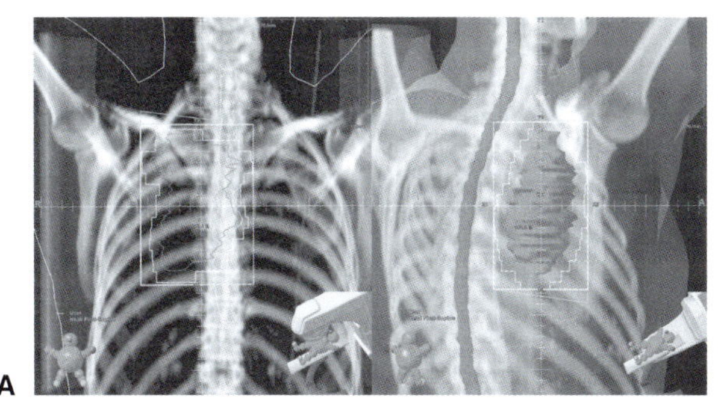

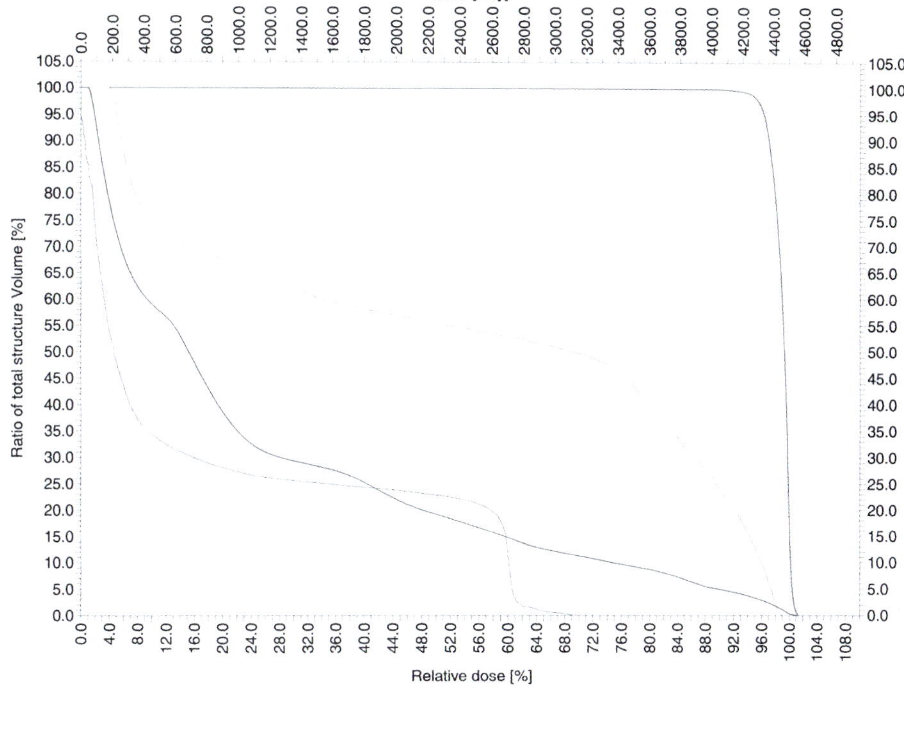

	Structure	Coverage [%] / [%]	Volume [cm³]	Min [%]	Max [%]	Mean [%]	Modal [%]	Median [%]	STD
	CTV	100.0 / 99.9	248.8	88.0	101.4	99.0	99.8	99.3	1.36
	Esophagus	100.0 / 99.4	28.9	4.0	99.1	53.9	97.8	69.2	36.98
	Spinal Cord	100.0 / 98.5	48.8	0.0	70.3	18.3	0.0	4.7	23.84
B	Total lung	100.0 / 100.0	3620.5	0.6	101.4	25.9	2.3	15.2	27.79

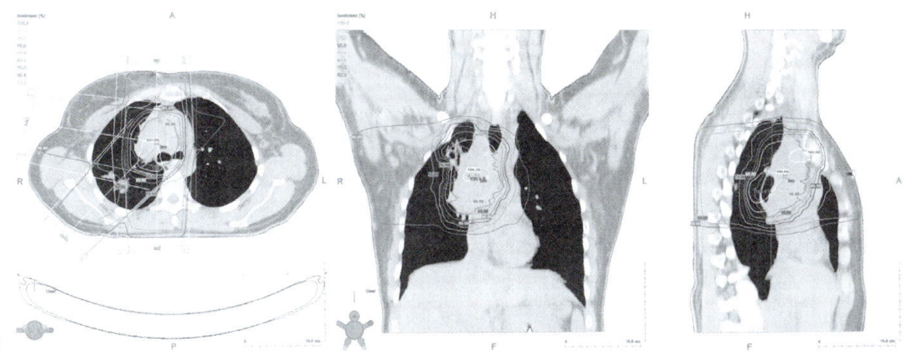

FIGURE 59.1 **A:** Anterior and oblique digital reconstructed radiograph (DRR). The **left panel** shows anterior port with saw-toothed edges of a multileaf collimator portal, with the physician-defined target outlined in red. The **right panel** displays an oblique portal in red-pink color wash, demonstrating the facility of avoiding the spinal cord. **B:** Dose-volume histogram (DVH): note the uniform dose coverage to the defined target (tumor) by the red line; the marked reduction in dose to the esophagus dose (*orange*) showing about 50% dose to only two thirds of the esophageal volume, and the relatively lesser volumes of total lung irradiated. **C:** Dose distribution: these show isodose distributions in the (**left**) axial, (**middle**) coronal, and (**right**) sagittal plane. This patient was treated with four wedged fields for the entirety of the course without interruption and demonstrated a complete response by the second cycle of chemotherapy despite presenting with superior vena cava syndrome. (See color plate.)

impact of increased overall treatment time is unknown. A trial comparing 45 Gy in 30 fractions over 3 weeks with 66 Gy in 33 fractions over 6.5 weeks is proposed.

CHEMOTHERAPY FOR LSCLC

Multiagent chemotherapy is superior to single-agent therapy in most cancers, when treatment is given with curative intent.[41] For more than 2 decades, LSCLC has been most commonly treated with a two-drug chemotherapy regimen consisting of cisplatin and etoposide (PE).[103] Cisplatin is the preferred agent in the potentially curable LSCLC patient population,[104] but substitution of carboplatin for cisplatin in patients intolerant to cisplatin is reasonable. The widely recommended practice of administration of thoracic irradiation concurrently with the first or second cycle of chemotherapy has reinforced the adoption of PE.[105] In contrast, for many years, it was common in Europe to use induction chemotherapy regimens with regimens that included alkylating agents and anthracyclines, with thoracic irradiation delivered sequentially in a consolidative fashion.[106] However, this practice has changed since Sundstrom et al.[81] demonstrated the superiority of PE therapy when compared with a regimen including cyclophosphamide, epirubicin, and vincristine. The superiority of PE was clear in LSCLC but not significant in ESCLC.

Because LSCLC is potentially curable, incremental improvements in the power of chemotherapy may be more easily detected in this setting compared with the palliative ESCLC group. In addition to the example by Sundstrøm et al.,[81] Reck et al.[107] showed a small but statistically significant improvement in survival for paclitaxel, etoposide, and carboplatin compared with carboplatin, etoposide, and vincristine in LSCLC but not ESCLC. Similarly, Thatcher et al.[108] showed better outcome for doxorubicin, cyclophosphamide, and etoposide at 2-week intervals (with granulocyte-colony stimulating factor [G-CSF]) compared with conventional every 3-week therapy in a population of predominately LSCLC. Taken together, these randomized trials of LSCLC patients with good prognostic factors suggest that chemotherapy innovations can result in modest survival improvements in LSCLC. However, the increased toxicity of three-drug protocols or dose-dense regimens is problematic with concurrent thoracic irradiation. When chemotherapy is manipulated by adding additional cytotoxic agents or dose intensification, the fidelity of both modalities of treatment is impaired by increased hematological and nonhematologic toxicity. Several new chemotherapy approaches using these themes have been evaluated in combined modality pilot studies,[100,109–115] but none have a therapeutic index sufficiently promising to be taken forward to phase III trials.

It has not yet been demonstrated that analogues of existing drugs have advantages over the parent compounds in controlled trials of LSCLC. The topoisomerase I inhibitors have been extensively investigated in SCLC. In a study of ESCLC patients, Noda et al.[116] showed that irinotecan and cisplatin was superior to the PE regimen (median survival [MS], 12.8 vs. 9.4 months [$p = 0.002$]). One phase III North American trial[117] using a different schedule of irinotecan and cisplatin has failed to confirm improved survival compared with PE in ESCLC and another larger study duplicating the Japanese regimen has yet to be reported. Irinotecan is difficult to combine with concurrent thoracic irradiation. The Japanese Clinical Oncology Group (JCOG) has incorporated irinotecan into a pilot study in LSCLC.[118] Because of toxicity concerns associated with initial concurrent irinotecan and intensive thoracic irradiation (1.5 Gy bid $\times$ 30 treatments over a period of 3 weeks), JCOG administered initial concurrent chemoradiation with the PE regimen and delivered the irinotecan plus cisplatin regimen in three additional cycles after radiotherapy beginning on day 29. In a phase II study of 31 patients, there were no cases of interstitial pneumonitis and no treatment-related deaths. The 1-year survival was 79% and median survival was 20.4 months. A randomized trial comparing this regimen with standard PE combined with the same initial concurrent accelerated radiotherapy is now completed and should be reported soon by JCOG.

Clinical trials of other agents including amrubicin and pemetrexed are in progress. The combination of pemetrexed and platinum may be of special interest because phase I data demonstrate that it can be combined with thoracic irradiation without an increase in normal tissue toxicity or compromise in delivery of drug or radiotherapy.[119] To date, molecularly targeted therapy has had no proven impact on the prognosis of patients with either ESCLC or LSCLC.

The demographic patterns of patients diagnosed with LSCLC are not conducive to increasingly toxic combined modality protocols. Gaspar et al.[120] examined a National Cancer Data Base including four patient cohorts diagnosed with LSCLC in 1985 (N = 2123), 1990 (N = 6279), 1995 (N = 7815), and 2000 (N = 2123). The proportion of patients aged ≥70 years increased significantly over time, from 31.6% in 1985 to 44.9% in 2000 ($p = 0.001$). Moreover, SCLC patients are generally physiologically aged beyond their chronological years, at least in part from heavy smoking. This analysis identified the continued need for the evaluation of new treatments in this group of patients, but more aggressive chemotherapy in combined modality protocols is unlikely to enhance the therapeutic index. In 2008, the demonstrated safety, reliable delivery, and efficacy of standard doses of PE with initial concurrent thoracic irradiation for LSCLC has not been seriously challenged.

FUTURE RESEARCH OF CHEMORADIATION IN LSCLC

Lung cancer investigators must decide how much change in long-term survival is important enough to warrant a clinical trial large enough to prove it. Most would probably agree that an increase in the cure rate of 10% is worthwhile. What about 5%? Many would reply affirmatively. For a disease this common, a true increase in the cure rate of 5% would save many

TABLE 59.2 Total Sample Size Required for Two-Arm Phase III Trials as a Function of Overall Survival Rate and Improvement in Overall Survival Rate

Survival Rate (%)	Total Sample Size Required for Improvement in Survival Rate		
Control Arm	**5%**	**10%**	**15%**
10	1290	394	134
15	1894	544	208
20	2444	676	328
25	2926	788	374

Sample size needed to have a *p* value of 0.05 and power of 0.90 to detect the difference; although additional allowance should be made for ineligibility, loss to follow-up, and late events.

patients. What about less than 5%? Probably not. Table 59.2 gives the sample sizes for clinical trials where clinical parameters are in the range of those likely to be seen in LSCLC trials in the future. Examination of this table shows that only a few of the trials in LSCLC have been adequately powered to detect a significant difference. Although most trials are small, metaanalyses have been able to demonstrate value in the use of radiation. A substantial improvement from a succession of small advances seems realistic. The rationale for the creation of large intergroup trials is particularly strong in LSCLC where modest therapeutic advance seems possible.

Issues in LSCLC that require further examination in randomized clinical trials include the controversies associated with irradiation volumes and the resolution of the relative importance of the start of treatment until the end of radiotherapy (SER) versus total dose. Currently, there are only four published randomized trials examining volume, dose, or fractionation issues in LSCLC.[86,92,101,121] The only study yielding a positive result administered thoracic irradiation initially and concurrently with thoracic irradiation.[86] The remaining studies,[92,101,121] which have given thoracic irradiation after a series of induction chemotherapy cycles, have failed to show any impact on survival.

Several trials are underdevelopment, primarily examining the impact of radiotherapy dose and overall treatment time. The largest of these is CONVERT, which hopes to randomize just under 600 patients to either the Intergroup regimen of 45 Gy in 30 fractions over 3 weeks or 66 Gy in 33 fractions over 6.5 weeks both delivered concurrent with cisplatin etoposide. This moves the concurrent chemotherapy to overlap with cycle 2 in the accelerated arm, but it also overlaps with cycles 2 and 3 in the protracted arm. Dose and time are different, and there is potential for administration of chemotherapy intensity to also be different between the arms. It should address the question of benefit of compressed radiotherapy versus extended radiotherapy, and the magnitude of difference. Prophylactic cranial irradiation will be provided in this trial, as it was irregularly administered in the intergroup study.

Over the last decade, there has been a revolution in the management of epithelial cancers with initial concurrent chemoradiation demonstrating an improvement in long-term survival. In squamous head and neck cancer,[122] anal cancer,[123] esophageal cancer,[124] cervical cancer,[125,126] brain cancer,[127] and NSCLC,[128–130] synchronous chemoirradiation is now the standard of care. For many years, some of these tumor types were managed with neoadjuvant chemotherapy prior to radiotherapy. However, initial synchronous chemoradiation has consistently proven to be superior to sequential treatment. Taken together, the increase in the proportion of long-term survivors from initial chemoradiation for this diverse array of notoriously difficult malignancies is one of the most important and understated advances in cancer medicine over the past 20 years.

Although the randomized trials of timing of thoracic irradiation have not been consistent in showing an optimal way to integrate chemotherapy and radiotherapy for LSCLC, a substantial and growing body of clinical trial data supports the initial concurrent chemoradiation model as the optimal management approach for locally advanced cancers in general. It is improbable that the therapeutic principles governing management of LSCLC would be different from other epithelial cancers. Dissonance with this harmony is found only when induction therapy and alkylator-based systemic therapy finds its way into treatment regimens. One of the attributes of cisplatin etoposide is the ability to use it in full doses concurrent with full dose, uncompromised radiotherapy.

Investigation of new drugs with molecular-targeted mechanisms generates considerable excitement. However, there is no evidence at this time that such therapies will replace conventional thoracic irradiation and chemotherapy. Indeed, new drugs are most likely to prosper when combined with an optimally integrated chemoradiation package. Because advances in the treatment of LSCLC over the past 20 years have largely been associated with innovations of radiotherapy, molecularly targeted therapy should focus on enhancement of radiotherapy as well as systemic therapy. Because accelerated repopulation is a major mechanism of treatment failure in cancer medicine, the molecular basis of this phenomenon must be elucidated. It seems probable that the mechanism will involve hypoxia targets, growth factors, and their receptors. Investigators should consider adding drugs that block accelerated repopulation to periods of maximal tumor regenerative activity in combined modality protocols.

REFERENCES

1. Govindan R, Page N, Morgensztern D, et al. Changing epidemiology of small-cell lung cancer in the United States over the last 30 years: analysis of the surveillance, epidemiologic, and end results database. *J Clin Oncol* 2006:24(28):4539–4544.
2. Murray N, Turrisi AT 3rd. A review of first-line treatment for small-cell lung cancer. *J Thorac Oncol* 2006;1(3):270–278.
3. Jemal A, Siegel R, Ward E, et al. Cancer statistics, 2007. *CA Cancer J Clin* 2007;57(1):43–66.
4. Green RA, Humphrey E, Close H, et al. Alkylating agents in bronchogenic carcinoma. *Am J Med* 1969;46(4):516–525.
5. Shepherd FA, Crowley J, Van Houtte P, et al. Clinical staging of small cell lung cancer: report of the International Association for the Study of Lung Cancer Staging Initiative, Small Cell Lung Cancer Staging Initiative, Small Cell Lung Cancer Subcommittee. *J Thorac Oncol* 2007;2(8):S230–S231.
6. Albain KS, Crowley JJ, Hutchins L, et al. Predictors of survival following relapse or progression of small cell lung cancer. Southwest Oncology Group Study 8605 report and analysis of recurrent disease data base. *Cancer* 1993;72(4):1184–1191.
7. Dearing MP, Steinberg SM, Phelps R, et al. Outcome of patients with small-cell lung cancer: effect of changes in staging procedures and imaging technology on prognostic factors over 14 years. *J Clin Oncol* 1990;8(6):1042–1049.
8. Shepherd FA, Ginsberg RJ, Haddad R, et al. Importance of clinical staging in limited small-cell lung cancer: a valuable system to separate prognostic subgroups. The University of Toronto Lung Oncology Group. *J Clin Oncol* 1993;11(8):1592–1597.
9. Warde P, Payne D. Does thoracic irradiation improve survival and local control in limited-stage small-cell carcinoma of the lung? A meta-analysis. *J Clin Oncol* 1992:10(6):890–895.
10. Pignon JP, Arriagada R, Ihde DC, et al. A meta-analysis of thoracic radiotherapy for small-cell lung cancer. *N Engl J Med* 1992; 327(23):1618–1624.
11. Campling B, Quirt I, DeBoer G, et al. Is bone marrow examination in small-cell lung cancer really necessary? *Ann Intern Med* 1986; 105(4):508–512.
12. Kamel EM, Zwahlen D, Wyss MT, et al. Whole-body (18)F-FDG PET improves the management of patients with small cell lung cancer. *J Nucl Med* 2003;44(12):1911–1917.
13. Bradley JD, Dehdashti F, Mintun MA, et al. Positron emission tomography in limited-stage small-cell lung cancer: a prospective study. *J Clin Oncol* 2004;22(16):3248–3254.
14. Brink I, Schumacher T, Mix M, et al. Impact of [18F]FDG-PET on the primary staging of small-cell lung cancer. *Eur J Nucl Med Mol Imaging* 2004;31(12):1614–1620.
15. Kuhn TS. *The structure of scientific revolutions*. Chicago: University of Chicago Press, 1970.
16. Higgins GA, Shields TW, Keehn RJ. The solitary pulmonary nodule. Ten-year follow-up of veterans administration-armed forces cooperative study. *Arch Surg* 1975;110(5):570–575.
17. Shields TW, Humphrey EW, Eastridge CE, et al. Adjuvant cancer chemotherapy after resection of carcinoma of the lung. *Cancer* 1977; 40(5):2057–2062.
18. Barnard WG. The nature of the "oat-celled sarcoma" of the mediastinum. *J Pathol Bacteriol* 1926;29:241–244.
19. Azzopardi JG. Oat cell carcinoma of the bronchus. *J Pathol Bacteriol* 1959;78:513.
20. Watson WL, Berg WJ. Oat cell lung cancer. *Cancer* 1962;15:759–768.
21. Zelen M. Keynote address on biostatistics and data retrieval. *Cancer Chemother Rep 3* 1973;4(2):31–42.
22. Miller AB, Fox W, Tall R. Five-year follow-up of the Medical Research Council comparative trial of surgery and radiotherapy for the primary treatment of small-celled or oat-celled carcinoma of the bronchus. *Lancet* 1969;2(7619):501–505.
23. Fox W, Scadding JG. Medical Research Council comparative trial of surgery and radiotherapy for primary treatment of small-celled or oat-celled carcinoma of bronchus. Ten-year follow-up. *Lancet* 1973;2(7820):63–65.
24. Matthews MJ, Kanhouwa S, Pickren J, et al. Frequency of residual and metastatic tumor in patients undergoing curative surgical resection for lung cancer. *Cancer Chemother Rep 3* 1973;4:63–67.
25. Davis HL Jr, Ramirez G, Korbitz BC, et al. Advanced lung cancer treated with cyclophosphamide. *Dis Chest* 1969;56(6):494–500.
26. Wingfield HV. Combined surgery and chemotherapy for carcinoma of the bronchus. *Lancet* 1970;1(7644):470–471.
27. Wolf J, Spear P, Yesner R, et al. Nitrogen mustard and the steroid hormones in the treatment of inoperable bronchogenic carcinoma. *Am J Med* 1960;29:1008–1016.
28. Cameron SJ, Grant IW, Crompton GK. Cyclophosphamide in disseminated bronchial carcinoma. *Scott Med J* 1974;19(2):81–86.
29. Brunner K, Marthaler T, Müller W. Effects of long-term adjuvant chemotherapy with cyclophosphamide (NSC-26271) for radically resected bronchogenic carcinoma: nine-year follow-up. *Cancer Chemother Rep 3* 1973;4(2):125–32.
30. Stott H, Stephens RJ, Fox W, et al. 5-year follow-up of cytotoxic chemotherapy as an adjuvant to surgery in carcinoma of the bronchus. *Br J Cancer* 1976;34(2):167–173.
31. Bergsagel DE, Jenkin RD, Pringle JF, et al. Lung cancer: clinical trial of radiotherapy alone vs. radiotherapy plus cyclophosphamide. *Cancer* 1972;30(3):621–627.
32. Radiotherapy alone or with chemotherapy in the treatment of small-cell carcinoma of the lung. Medical Research Council Lung Cancer Working Party. *Br J Cancer* 1979;40(1):1–10.
33. Petrovich Z, Ohanian M, Cox J. Clinical research on the treatment of locally advanced lung cancer: final report of VALG Protocol 13 Limited. *Cancer* 1978;42(3):1129–1134.
34. Perez CA, Krauss S, Bartolucci AA, et al. Thoracic and elective brain irradiation with concomitant or delayed multiagent chemotherapy in the treatment of localized small cell carcinoma of the lung: a randomized prospective study by the Southeastern Cancer Study Group. *Cancer* 1981;47(10):2407–2413.
35. Seydel HG, Creech R, Pagano M, et al. Combined modality treatment of regional small cell undifferentiated carcinoma of the lung: a cooperative study of the RTOG and ECOG. *Int J Radiat Oncol Biol Phys* 1983;9(8):1135–1141.
36. Hansen HH, Muggia FM, Andrews R, et al. Intensive combined chemotherapy and radiotherapy in patients with nonresectable bronchogenic carcinoma. *Cancer* 1972;30(2):315–324.
37. Eagan RT, Maurer LH, Forcier RJ, et al. Combination chemotherapy and radiation therapy in small cell carcinoma of the lung. *Cancer* 1973; 32(2):371–379.
38. Holoye PY, Samuels ML. Cyclophosphamide, vincristine and sequential split-course radiotherapy in the treatment of small cell lung cancer. *Chest* 1975;67(6):675–679.
39. Einhorn LH, Fee WH, Farber MO, et al. Improved chemotherapy for small-cell undifferentiated lung cancer. *JAMA* 1976;235(12):1225–1229.
40. Einhorn L, Krause M, Hornback N, et al. Enhanced pulmonary toxicity with bleomycin and radiotherapy in oat cell lung cancer. *Cancer* 1976;37(5): 2414–2416.
41. DeVita VT Jr, Young RC, Canellos GP. Combination versus single agent chemotherapy: a review of the basis for selection of drug treatment of cancer. *Cancer* 1975;35(1):98–110.
42. Lowenbraun S, Bartolucci A, Smalley RV, et al. The superiority of combination chemotherapy over single agent chemotherapy in small cell lung carcinoma. *Cancer* 1979;44(2):406–413.
43. Edmonson JH, Lagakos SW, Selawry OS, et al. Cyclophosphamide and CCNU in the treatment of inoperable small cell carcinoma and adenocarcinoma of the lung. *Cancer Treat Rep* 1976;60(7):925–932.

44. Alberto P, Brunner KW, Martz G, et al. Treatment of bronchogenic carcinoma with simultaneous or sequential combination chemotherapy, including methotrexate, cyclophosphamide, procarbazine and vincristine. *Cancer* 1976;38(6):2208–2216.
45. Byhardt RW, Cox JD. Is chest radiotherapy necessary in any or all patients with small cell carcinoma of the lung? Yes. *Cancer Treat Rep* 1983;67(3):209–215.
46. Cohen MH, Ihde DC, Bunn PA Jr, et al. Cyclic alternating combination chemotherapy for small cell bronchogenic carcinoma. *Cancer Treat Rep* 1979;63(2):163–170.
47. Cohen MH. Is thoracic radiation therapy necessary for patients with limited-stage small cell lung cancer? No. *Cancer Treat Rep* 1983;67(3):217–221.
48. Bunn PA Jr, Lichter AS, Makuch RW, et al. Chemotherapy alone or chemotherapy with chest radiation therapy in limited stage small cell lung cancer. A prospective, randomized trial. *Ann Intern Med* 1987;106(5):655–662.
49. Perry MC, Eaton WL, Propert KJ, et al. Chemotherapy with or without radiation therapy in limited small-cell carcinoma of the lung. *New Engl J Med* 1987;316(15):912–918.
50. Perez CA, Einhorn L, Oldham RK, et al. Randomized trial of radiotherapy to the thorax in limited small-cell carcinoma of the lung treated with multiagent chemotherapy and elective brain irradiation: a preliminary report. *J Clin Oncol* 1984;2(11):1200–1208.
51. Hill RP, Chambers AF, Ling V, et al. Dynamic heterogeneity: rapid generation of metastatic variants in mouse B16 melanoma cells. *Science* 1984;224(4652):998–1001.
52. Hill R, Young SD, Ling V. Metastatic cell phenotypes: quantitative studies using the experimental metastasis assay. *Cancer Rev* 1986;5:118–151.
53. Young RC. Drug resistance: the clinical problem. In: Robert FO, ed. *Drug Resistance in Cancer Therapy*. Norwell, MA: Kluer Academic Publishers, 1989:1–30.
54. Goldie JH, Coldman AJ. The genetic origin of drug resistance in neoplasms: implications for systemic therapy. *Cancer Res* 1984;44(9): 3643–3653.
55. Brodin O, Arnberg H, Bergh J, et al. Increased radioresistance of an in vitro transformed human small cell lung cancer cell line. *Lung Cancer* 1995;12(3):183–198.
56. Twentyman PR, Wright KA, Rhodes T. Radiation response of human lung cancer cells with inherent and acquired resistance to cisplatin. *Int J Radiat Oncol Biol Phys* 1991;20(2):217–220.
57. Withers HR, Taylor JM, Maciejewski B. The hazard of accelerated tumor clonogen repopulation during radiotherapy. *Acta Oncol* 1988;27(2):131–146.
58. Trott KR. Cell repopulation and overall treatment time. *Int J Radiat Oncol Biol Phys* 1990;19(4):1071–1075.
59. Simpson-Herren L, Sanford AH, Holmquist JP. Effects of surgery on the cell kinetics of residual tumor. *Cancer Treat Rep* 1976;60(12): 1749–1760.
60. Stephens T, Steele GG. Regeneration of tumors after cytotoxic treatment. In: Meyn R, Withers HR, ed. *Radiation Biology in Cancer Research*. New York: Raven, 1980:385.
61. Johnson RE, Brereton HD, Kent CH. Small-cell carcinoma of the lung: attempt to remedy causes of past therapeutic failure. *Lancet* 1976;2(7980):289–291.
62. Greco FA, Brereton HD, Kent H, et al. Adriamycin and enhanced radiation reaction in normal esophagus and skin. *Ann Intern Med* 1976;85(3):294–298.
63. Johnson RE, Brereton HD, Kent CH. "Total" therapy for small cell carcinoma of the lung. *Ann Thorac Surg* 1978;25(6):510–515.
64. Kent CH, Brereton HD, Johnson RE. "Total" therapy for oat cell carcinoma of the lung. *Int J Radiat Oncol Biol Phys* 1977;2(5–6):427–232.
65. Catane R, Lichter A, Lee YJ, et al. Small cell lung cancer: analysis of treatment factors contributing to prolonged survival. *Cancer* 1981; 48(9):1936–1943.
66. Pinkel D. Five-year follow-up of "total therapy" of childhood lymphocytic leukemia. *JAMA* 1971;216(4):648–652.
67. Livingston RB, Moore TN, Heilbrun L, et al. Small-cell carcinoma of the lung: combined chemotherapy and radiation: a Southwest Oncology Group study. *Ann Intern Med* 1978;88(2):194–199.
68. Greco FA, Richardson RL, Snell JD, et al. Small cell lung cancer. Complete remission and improved survival. *Am J Med* 1979;66(4): 625–630.
69. Johnson DH, Bass D, Einhorn LH, et al. Combination chemotherapy with or without thoracic radiotherapy in limited-stage small-cell lung cancer: a randomized trial of the Southeastern Cancer Study Group. *J Clin Oncol* 1993;11(7):1223–1229.
70. Sierocki JS, Hilaris BS, Hopfan S,et al. cis-Dichlorodiammineplatinu m(II) and VP-16–213: an active induction regimen for small cell carcinoma of the lung. *Cancer Treat Rep* 1979;63(9–10):1593–1597.
71. Douple EB, Richmond RC. A review of platinum complex biochemistry suggests a rationale for combined platinum-radiotherapy. *Int J Radiat Oncol Biol Phys* 1979;5(8):1335–1339.
72. Murray N, Hadzic E, Shah A, et al. Alternating chemotherapy and thoracic radiotherapy with concurrent cisplatin for limited stage small cell carcinoma of the lung (SCCL). *Proc Amer Soc Clin Oncol* 1984:3;214. Abstract No. 835.
73. Murray N, Shah A, Brown E, et al. Alternating chemotherapy and thoracic radiotherapy with concurrent cisplatin-etoposide for limited-stage small-cell carcinoma of the lung. *Semin Oncol* 1986;13(3 Suppl 3): 24–30.
74. McCracken JD, Janaki LM, Crowley JJ, et al. Concurrent chemotherapy/radiotherapy for limited small-cell lung carcinoma: a Southwest Oncology Group Study. *J Clin Oncol* 1990;8(5):892–898.
75. Murray N, Coy P, Pater JL, et al. Importance of timing for thoracic irradiation in the combined modality treatment of limited-stage small-cell lung cancer. The National Cancer Institute of Canada Clinical Trials Group. *J Clin Oncol* 1993;11(2):336–344.
76. Work E, Nielsen OS, Bentzen SM, et al. Randomized study of initial versus late chest irradiation combined with chemotherapy in limited-stage small-cell lung cancer. Aarhus Lung Cancer Group. *J Clin Oncol* 1997;15(9):3030–3037.
77. Jeremic B, Shibamoto Y, Acimovic L, et al. Initial versus delayed accelerated hyperfractionated radiation therapy and concurrent chemotherapy in limited small-cell lung cancer: a randomized study. *J Clin Oncol* 1997;15(3):893–900.
78. Takada M, Fukuoka M, Kawahara M, et al. Phase III study of concurrent versus sequential thoracic radiotherapy in combination with cisplatin and etoposide for limited-stage small-cell lung cancer: results of the Japan Clinical Oncology Group Study 9104. *J Clin Oncol* 2002;20(14):3054–3060.
79. Spiro SG, James LE, Rudd RM, et al. Early compared with late radiotherapy in combined modality treatment for limited disease small-cell lung cancer: a London Lung Cancer Group multicenter randomized clinical trial and meta-analysis. *J Clin Oncol* 2006;24(24):3823–3830.
80. Murray N, Coy P, Pater JL, et al. Importance of timing for thoracic irradiation in the combined modality treatment of limited-stage small-cell lung cancer. The National Cancer Institute of Canada Clinical Trials Group. *J Clin Oncol* 1993;11(2):336–344.
81. Sundstrøm S, Bremnes RM, Kaasa S, et al. Cisplatin and etoposide regimen is superior to cyclophosphamide, epirubicin, and vincristine regimen in small-cell lung cancer: results from a randomized phase III trial with 5 years' follow-up. *J Clin Oncol* 2002;20(24):4665–4672.
82. De Ruysscher D, Pijls-Johannesma M, Vansteenkiste J, et al. Systematic review and meta-analysis of randomised, controlled trials of the timing of chest radiotherapy in patients with limited-stage, small-cell lung cancer. *Ann Oncol* 2006;17(4):543–552.
83. Fried DB, Morris DE, Poole C, et al. Systematic Review Evaluating the Timing of Thoracic Radiation Therapy in Combined Modality Therapy for Limited-Stage Small-Cell Lung Cancer. *J Clin Oncol* 2004;22(23):4837–4845.
84. Peters LJ Withers HR. Applying radiobiological principles to combined modality treatment of head and neck cancer—the time factor. *Int J Radiat Oncol Biol Phys* 1997;39(4):831–836.

85. Brade AM, Tannock IF. Scheduling of radiation and chemotherapy for limited-stage small-cell lung cancer: repopulation as a cause of treatment failure? *J Clin Oncol* 2006;24(7):1020–1022.
86. Turrisi AT 3rd, Kim K, Blum R, et al. Twice-daily compared with once-daily thoracic radiotherapy in limited small-cell lung cancer treated concurrently with cisplatin and etoposide. *N Engl J Med* 1999; 340(4):265–271.
87. De Ruysscher D, Pijls-Johannesma M, Bentzen SM, et al. Time between the first day of chemotherapy and the last day of chest radiation is the most important predictor of survival in limited-disease small-cell lung cancer. *J Clin Oncol* 2006;24(7):1057–1063.
88. Hansen H. Should initial treatment of small cell carcinoma include systemic chemotherapy and brain irradiation? *Cancer Chemother Rep* 1973;4:239.
89. Aupérin A, Arriagada R, Pignon JP, et al. Prophylactic cranial irradiation for patients with small-cell lung cancer in complete remission. Prophylactic Cranial Irradiation Overview Collaborative Group. *N Engl J Med* 1999;341(7):476–484.
90. Gregor A, Cull A, Stephens RJ, et al. Prophylactic cranial irradiation is indicated following complete response to induction therapy in small cell lung cancer: results of a multicentre randomised trial. United Kingdom Coordinating Committee for Cancer Research (UKCCCR) and the European Organization for Research and Treatment of Cancer (EORTC). *Eur J Cancer* 1997;33(11):1752–1758.
91. Slotman B, Faivre-Finn C, Kramer G, et al. Prophylactic cranial irradiation in extensive small-cell lung cancer. *N Engl J Med* 2007;357(7): 664–672.
92. Kies MS, Mira JG, Crowley JJ, et al. Multimodal therapy for limited small-cell lung cancer: a randomized study of induction combination chemotherapy with or without thoracic radiation in complete responders; and with wide-field versus reduced-field radiation in partial responders: a Southwest Oncology Group Study. *J Clin Oncol* 1987;5(4):592–600.
93. Skarlos DV, Samantas E, Briassoulis E, et al. Randomized comparison of early versus late hyperfractionated thoracic irradiation concurrently with chemotherapy in limited disease small-cell lung cancer: a randomized phase II study of the Hellenic Cooperative Oncology Group (HeCOG). *Ann Oncol* 2001;12(9):1231–1238.
94. Tada T, Minakuchi K, Koda M, et al. Limited-stage small cell lung cancer: local failure after chemotherapy and radiation therapy. *Radiology* 1998;208(2):511–515.
95. Graham MV, Purdy JA, Emami B, et al. Clinical dose-volume histogram analysis for pneumonitis after 3D treatment for non-small cell lung cancer (NSCLC). *Int J Radiat Oncol Biol Phys* 1999;45(2): 323–329.
96. Kwa SL, Lebesque JV, Theuws JC, et al. Radiation pneumonitis as a function of mean lung dose: an analysis of pooled data of 540 patients. *Int J Radiat Oncol Biol Phys* 1998;42(1):1–9.
97. Tsujino K, Hirota S, Endo M, et al. Predictive value of dose-volume histogram parameters for predicting radiation pneumonitis after concurrent chemoradiation for lung cancer. *Int J Radiat Oncol Biol Phys* 2003;55(1):110–115.
98. Hirota S, Tsujino K, Endo M, et al. Dosimetric predictors of radiation esophagitis in patients treated for non-small-cell lung cancer with carboplatin/paclitaxel/radiotherapy. *Int J Radiat Oncol Biol Phys* 2001;51(2):291–295.
99. Lebeau B, Urban T, Bréchot JM, et al. A randomized clinical trial comparing concurrent and alternating thoracic irradiation for patients with limited small cell lung carcinoma. "Petites Cellules" Group. *Cancer* 1999;86(8):1480–1487.
100. Baas P, Belderbos JS, Senan S, et al. Concurrent chemotherapy (carboplatin, paclitaxel, etoposide) and involved-field radiotherapy in limited stage small cell lung cancer: a Dutch multicenter phase II study. *Br J Cancer* 2006;94(5):625–630.
101. Coy P, Hodson I, Payne DG, et al. The effect of dose of thoracic irradiation on recurrence in patients with limited stage small cell lung cancer. Initial results of a Canadian Multicenter Randomized Trial. *Int J Radiat Oncol Biol Phys* 1988;14(2):219–226.
102. Choi NC, Carey RW. Importance of radiation dose in achieving improved loco-regional tumor control in limited stage small-cell lung carcinoma: an update. *Int J Radiat Oncol Biol Phys* 1989;17(2):307–310.
103. Evans WK, Shepherd FA, Feld R, et al. VP-16 and cisplatin as first-line therapy for small-cell lung cancer. *J Clin Oncol* 1985;3(11): 1471–1477.
104. Pujol JL, Carestia L, Daures JP. Is there a case for cisplatin in the treatment of small-cell lung cancer? A meta-analysis of randomized trials of a cisplatin-containing regimen versus a regimen without this alkylating agent. *Br J Cancer* 2000;83(1):8–15.
105. Spira A, Ettinger DS. Multidisciplinary Management of Lung Cancer. *N Engl J Med* 2004;350(4):379–392.
106. Sambrook RJ, Girling DJ. A national survey of the chemotherapy regimens used to treat small cell lung cancer (SCLC) in the United Kingdom. *Br J Cancer* 2001;84(11):1447–1452.
107. Reck M, von Pawel J, Macha HN, et al. Randomized phase III trial of paclitaxel, etoposide, and carboplatin versus carboplatin, etoposide, and vincristine in patients with small-cell lung cancer. *J Natl Cancer Inst* 2003;95(15):1118–1127.
108. Thatcher N, Girling DJ, Hopwood P, et al. Improving survival without reducing quality of life in small-cell lung cancer patients by increasing the dose-intensity of chemotherapy with granulocyte colony-stimulating factor support: results of a British Medical Research Council Multicenter Randomized Trial. Medical Research Council Lung Cancer Working Party. *J Clin Oncol* 2000;18(2):395–404.
109. Kubota K, Nishiwaki Y, Sugiura T, et al. Pilot study of concurrent etoposide and cisplatin plus accelerated hyperfractionated thoracic radiotherapy followed by irinotecan and cisplatin for limited-stage small cell lung cancer: Japan Clinical Oncology Group 9903. *Clin Cancer Res* 2005;11(15):5534–5538.
110. Levitan N, Dowlati A, Shina D, et al. Multi-institutional phase I/II trial of paclitaxel, cisplatin, and etoposide with concurrent radiation for limited-stage small-cell lung carcinoma. *J Clin Oncol* 2000;18(5):1102–1109.
111. Ettinger DS, Berkey BA, Abrams RA, et al. Study of paclitaxel, etoposide, and cisplatin chemotherapy combined with twice-daily thoracic radiotherapy for patients with limited-stage small-cell lung cancer: a Radiation Therapy Oncology Group 9609 Phase II Study. *J Clin Oncol* 2005;23(22):4991–4998.
112. Glisson B, Scott C, Komaki R, et al. Cisplatin, ifosfamide, oral etoposide, and concurrent accelerated hyperfractionated thoracic radiation for patients with limited small-cell lung carcinoma: results of radiation therapy oncology group trial 93–12. *J Clin Oncol* 2000;18(16):2990–2995.
113. Bogart JA, Herndon JE 2nd, Lyss AP, et al. 70 Gy thoracic radiotherapy is feasible concurrent with chemotherapy for limited-stage small-cell lung cancer: analysis of Cancer and Leukemia Group B study 39808. *Int J Radiat Oncol Biol Phys* 2004;59(2):460–468.
114. Hanna N, Ansari R, Fisher W, Shen J, et al. Etoposide, ifosfamide and cisplatin (VIP) plus concurrent radiation therapy for previously untreated limited small cell lung cancer (SCLC): a Hoosier Oncology Group (HOG) phase II study. *Lung Cancer* 2002;35(3):293–297.
115. Woo IS, Park YS, Kwon SH, et al. A phase II study of VP-16-fosfamide-cisplatin combination chemotherapy plus early concurrent thoracic irradiation for previously untreated limited small cell lung cancer. *Jpn J Clin Oncol* 2000;30(12):542–546.
116. Noda K, Nishiwaki Y, Kawahara M, et al. Irinotecan plus cisplatin compared with etoposide plus cisplatin for extensive small-cell lung cancer. *N Engl J Med* 2002;346(2):85–91.
117. Hanna NH, Einhorn L, Sandler A, et al. Randomized, phase III trial comparing irinotecan/cisplatin (IP) with etoposide/cisplatin (EP) in patients (pts) with previously untreated, extensive-stage (ES) small cell lung cancer (SCLC). *J Clin Oncol* (Meeting Abstracts), 2005;23(16 suppl): LBA7004.
118. Kubota K, Nishiwaki Y, Sugiura T, et al. Pilot study of cisplatin and etoposide plus concurrent accelerated hyperfractionated thoracic radiotherapy followed by three cycles of irinotecan and cisplatin for treatment of limited-stage small cell lung cancer: JCOG 9903. *Lung Cancer* 2003;42:S24.

119. Seiwert TY, Connell AM, Mauer PC, et al. A phase I study of pemetrexed, carboplatin, and concurrent radiotherapy in patients with locally advanced or metastatic non-small cell lung or esophageal cancer. *Clin Cancer Res* 2007;13(2 Pt 1):515–522.
120. Gaspar LE, Gay EG, Crawford J,et al. Limited-stage small-cell lung cancer (stages I-III): observations from the National Cancer Data Base. *Clin Lung Cancer* 2005;6(6):355–360.
121. Bonner JA, Sloan JA, Shanahan TG, et al. Phase III comparison of twice-daily split-course irradiation versus once-daily irradiation for patients with limited stage small-cell lung carcinoma. *J Clin Oncol* 1999; 17(9):2681–2691.
122. Pignon JP, Bourhis J, Domenge C, et al. Chemotherapy added to locoregional treatment for head and neck squamous-cell carcinoma: three meta-analyses of updated individual data. MACH-NC Collaborative Group. Meta-Analysis of Chemotherapy on Head and Neck Cancer. *Lancet* 2000;355(9208):949–955.
123. Epidermoid anal cancer: results from the UKCCCR randomised trial of radiotherapy alone versus radiotherapy, 5-fluorouracil, and mitomycin. UKCCCR Anal Cancer Trial Working Party. UK Co-ordinating Committee on Cancer Research. *Lancet* 1996;348(9034): 1049–1054.
124. Keys HM, Bundy BN, Stehman FB, et al. Cisplatin, radiation, and adjuvant hysterectomy compared with radiation and adjuvant hysterectomy for bulky stage IB cervical carcinoma. *N Engl J Med* 1999; 340(15):1154–1161.
125. Morris M, Eifel PJ, Lu J, et al. Pelvic radiation with concurrent chemotherapy compared with pelvic and para-aortic radiation for high-risk cervical cancer. *N Engl J Med* 1999;340(15):1137–1143.
126. Rose PG, Bundy BN, Watkins EB, et al. Concurrent cisplatin-based radiotherapy and chemotherapy for locally advanced cervical cancer. *N Engl J Med* 1999;340(15):1144–1153.
127. Stupp R, Mason WP, van den Bent MJ, et al. Radiotherapy plus concomitant and adjuvant temozolomide for glioblastoma. *N Engl J Med* 2005;352(10):987–996.
128. Furuse K, Fukuoka M, Kawahara M, et al. Phase III study of concurrent versus sequential thoracic radiotherapy in combination with mitomycin, vindesine, and cisplatin in unresectable stage III non-small-cell lung cancer. *J Clin Oncol* 1999;17(9):2692–2699.
129. Curran W Jr, et al. Long-term benefit is observed in a phase III comparison of sequential vs concurrent chemo-radiation for patients with recurrent unresected stage III NSCLC: RTOG 9410. ASCO Chicago, 2003.
130. Pfister DG, Johnson DH, Azzoli CG, et al. American Society of Clinical Oncology treatment of unresectable non-small-cell lung cancer guideline: update 2003. *J Clin Oncol* 2004;22(2):330–353.
131. Perry MC, Herndon JE 3rd, Eaton WL, et al. Thoracic radiation therapy added to chemotherapy for small-cell lung cancer: an update of Cancer and Leukemia Group B Study 8083. *J Clin Oncol* 1998; 16(7):2466–2467.

CHAPTER 60

Cécile Le Péchoux
Aaron H. Wolfson

Prophylactic Cranial Irradiation in Small Cell Lung Cancer

Small cell lung cancer (SCLC) has several features that distinguish it from other tumor types of lung cancer: the risk of early hematogenous dissemination, its marked radiosensibility and chemosensibility but also its particular propensity to disseminate in the brain. Even if chemotherapy is the cornerstone treatment in both limited and extensive disease, thoracic radiotherapy and prophylactic cranial irradiation (PCI) should be part of the therapeutic strategy in a subset of patients with limited disease (LD) as shown in two metaanalyses.[1,2] PCI should be considered among patients with extensive disease who respond to treatment.[2,3] In the past years, there has been improvement of both systemic and local control so that about two thirds of these patients, mainly those with LD, treated with aggressive induction therapy combining multidrug chemotherapy and thoracic radiation therapy will be put in complete remission. However, there is a high risk of relapse, so that only 15% to 25% of complete responders will be long-term survivors. Brain failures, for instance, have become a significant cause of relapse as the risk of developing brain metastases increases with length of survival to a cumulative risk that can be as high as 80%.[4,5] PCI has been developed as a strategy to prevent dissemination to the uninvolved brain, where systemic agents do not cross the blood-brain barrier effectively.[6] Thus, several studies have been undertaken that proved PCI would significantly reduce the incidence of a central nervous system (CNS) relapse compared with patients who did not receive PCI. However, in spite of the positive results of several retrospective and prospective studies, the utility of PCI has been a controversial issue for several years because of the lack of improvement in survival in individual trials and a possible risk of neurotoxicity and cognitive deficits in long-term survivors.[7–10] Since the publication of a metaanalysis on PCI in SCLC complete responders, showing the benefit of PCI not only in terms of brain control but also in terms of survival, PCI is now considered by most clinicians as standard treatment.[2]

Because brain metastases are frequent and difficult to treat, accompanied by distressing and sometimes life-threatening symptoms, prophylactic treatment seems a good alternative. At the time of initial diagnosis, up to 24% of patients may have brain metastases if magnetic resonance imaging (MRI) is used as initial workup.[5,6,11] Brain metastases may occur in 50% to 80% of 2-year survivors; in patients who achieve a complete response, the incidence of cerebral metastasis as sole site of initial relapse varies between 14% and 45% at 2 years.[12–14] Historically, chemotherapeutic agents have had a limited role in the treatment of cerebral metastases because of the inability of cytostatic drugs to cross the blood-brain barrier, situated in the endothelium of cerebral microvessels. However, more recent studies have reported efficacy of chemotherapy alone, with response rates on brain metastases ranging from 40% to 76%.[15–18] Chemotherapy-administered postradiation could also be more effective by abrogation of the blood-brain barrier[19]; however, that may also increase toxicity as well. Radiation therapy has remained the most widely accepted treatment modality for brain metastases with improvement of neurological symptoms in 56% to 92% of patients.[5,20–23] However, even if the symptomatic relief is of some benefit, quality of life (QOL) after overt brain metastasis is poor, and overall survival after development of brain metastases is low with median survival times ranging from 1.5 to 4.5 months.[21,23–27]

STUDIES EVALUATING PROPHYLACTIC CRANIAL IRRADIATION

PCI has been used irregularly in the past 20 years, but since the metaanalysis, it has been accepted more generally, that PCI would delay the symptomatic cerebral metastases and would reduce the lifetime risk of brain relapse by 30% to 50%.[4,5] Several randomized trials listed on Table 60.1 have been published showing a significant twofold to threefold decrease in brain metastases incidence in the PCI arm compared to the control arm.[24,28–36] However, they included a very heterogeneous patient population: patients who failed to achieve a complete remission, patients with limited and extensive disease, patients who had concomitant chemotherapy and different PCI doses and fractionations, which can explain the differences observed

TABLE 60.1 Older Randomized Trials Evaluating Prophylactic Cranial Irradiation in Small Cell Lung Cancer Patients

Study (Reference)	Patients	PCI Dose Gy/Fraction Timing of PCI	Brain Metastases Rate (%)		p Value	Median Survival or Survival at X Years	
			PCI (+)	PCI (−)		PCI (+)	PCI (−)
Cox et al.[28]	45	20/10 D1	17%	24%	NS	40 wks	
Beiler et al.[29]	54	24/8 3rd wk	0%	16%	<0.05	>104 wks LD	58 wks LD
Hansen et al.[30]	110	40/20 12th wk	9%	13%	NS	9.2 mo	10.2 mo
Maurer et al.[31]	163	30/10 9th wk	4%	18%	<0.01	8.4 mo	8.8 mo
Eagan et al.[24]	30	36/10 20th wk	13%	73%	<0.05	13.6 mo	12.9 mo
Aroney et al.[33]	29 R/172*	30/10 CR	0%	27%	NS	17 mo	13.5 mo
Jackson Jr et al.[34]	29	30/10 D1	0%	27%	<0.05	9.8 mo	7.2 mo
Seydel et al.[35]	217	30/10 D1	5%	21%	<0.005	53 wks	52 wks
Niiranen et al.[36]	51	40/20 4th wk	0%	26%	<0.05	13 mo	10 mo

*Out of 172 patients evaluated and analyzed, only 29 patients achieving CR were randomized.

CR, PCI given when patients are in complete remission; D1, PCI given on the first day of induction treatment; LD, limited disease; NS, not specified; PCI, prophylactic cranial irradiation.

in brain failure reduction. None of these randomized studies could show an impact on the survival rate. However, in 1983, Rosen et al.[12] were the first one to report than PCI could have an impact on survival in a subgroup of patients and since then, several retrospective studies have suggested that PCI could not only reduce brain failure rates but also improve survival in complete responders to induction treatment.[37,38] Subsequently, only patients with complete remission were included in randomized trials. In these more recent trials listed in Table 60.2, the rates of brain failures seem higher than in older trials probably because they are reported as actuarial and not as crude brain metastasis rates.[13,39–42] The overall 2-year actuarial brain failure rates are 40% and 67%, respectively, in the trial reported by Arriagada et al.,[13] 30% and 54% in the trial reported by Gregor et al.[39] Even if there was a trend in favor of PCI, none of these more recent randomized trials were large enough to confirm statistically the survival benefit suggested in retrospective studies.[12,37,38,43]

Current randomized trials have included patients with both limited and extensive disease, usually complete responders. Thus, as anticipated, more patients with LD comprise these

TABLE 60.2 Randomized Trials Evaluating Prophylactic Cranial Irradiation in Small Cell Lung Cancer Complete Responders Included in the Metaanalysis and Results of the Metaanalysis

Study (Reference)	Patients	PCI Dose Gy/Fraction Timing of PCI	Brain Metastases Rate (%)		p Value	Median Survival or Survival at X Years	
			PCI (+)	PCI (−)		PCI (+)	PCI (−)
Aroney et al.[33]	29*	30/3	0%	36%	0.02	—	—
Ohonoshi et al.[41]	46	40/20 CR	22%	52%	<0.05	21 mo	15 mo
Arriagada et al.[13]	300	24/8 CR	2-yr rate 40%	2-yr rate 67%	$<10^{-13}$	2-yr SR 29%	2-yr SR 21.5%
Wagner et al.[42]	31	25/10 CR	20%	50%	NS	15.3 mo	8.8 mo
Gregor et al.[39]†	314 LD only	Various CR	2-yr rate 30%	2-yr rate 54%	0.00004	305 days 3-yr SR 21%	300 days 3-yr SR 11%
Laplanche et al.[40]	211	24/8-30/10 CR	4-yr rate 44%	4-yr rate 51%	0.14	4-yr SR 22%	4-yr SR 16%
Metaanalysis Aupérin et al.[2]	987	Various	3-yr rate 33.3%	3-yr rate 58.6%	<0.001	3-yr SR 20.7%	3-yr SR 15.3%

*Out of 172 patients evaluated and analyzed, only 29 patients achieving CR were randomized.

†The Gregor study is the only one restricted to patients with limited disease.

CR, PCI given when patients are in complete remission; D1, PCI given on the first day of induction treatment; LD, limited disease; NS, not specified; PCI, prophylactic cranial irradiation; SR, survival rate.

studies. The surprising recent EORTC trial addressed the question of PCI exclusively among 286 patients with documented extensive disease having responded to four to six cycles of chemotherapy and with residual local and systemic disease in nearly three quarters of the randomized patients.[3] Patients did not undergo brain imaging before randomization if they were not symptomatic, but were screened for predefined key symptoms of brain metastases. The primary end point was the time to symptomatic brain metastases. The results reported in 2007 strongly support PCI; the authors conclude that it should be part of standard care, not only among complete responders, but also extended to all responders. The majority of patients (61%) received a dose of 20 Gy in five fractions. The cumulative risk of brain metastases at 1 year is 14.6% in PCI group, whereas it is 40.4% in the control group (hazard ratio [HR] = 0.27; p <0.001). Furthermore, irradiated patients also had significantly (HR = 0.68; p = 0.003) longer overall survival (median survival of 6.7 months and survival rate at 1 year of 27.1%) than those in the control group (median survival of 5.4 months; survival rate at 1 year of 13.3%). The difference in survival may be explained also by the fact that patients with extracranial progression were more often treated than those in the control group.

PROPHYLACTIC CRANIAL IRRADIATION METAANALYSES

The metaanalysis, which collected individual data from seven trials including a total of 987 patients randomized from 1977 to 1995, compared PCI to observation without PCI in patients with SCLC in complete remission with the primary end point of overall survival.[2] The determination of complete remission varied in each trial: a simple chest radiograph in many trials, whereas others mandated a chest computed tomography (CT) scan, and another trial required both a negative bronchoscopy and chest CT scan. The majority of patients were men (about 75%) and with a good performance status (97%). Most patients (86%) had LD, but 140 patients (14%) had extensive disease. The results have shown that PCI led to a 16% reduction in the mortality rate corresponding to 5.4% increase in the 3-year survival rate (from 15.3% observed in the control group to 20.7%). Therefore, PCI not only decreases, significantly, the risk of developing brain metastases (from 58.6% to 33.3% at 3 years) as proven in other individual trials, but also improves overall survival and disease-free survival.[2] The magnitude of the survival benefit is similar and parallels that achieved with the use of thoracic radiotherapy in patients with LD.[1,2] The Cochrane library published, in 2000, this same metaanalysis and included more tables and figures corresponding to all the subgroup (age, performance status, extent of initial disease, type of induction therapy, and time between the initiation of induction therapy and randomization) and indirect analyses (total dose of irradiation) that were performed.[44]

In 2001, Meert et al.[45] published a systematic review of the literature, including 12 published trials (1547 patients) that randomly assigned patients to receive PCI or not. Whereas the metaanalysis, based on individual data of Aupérin et al., included only trials addressing the question of PCI in complete responders, out of the 12 selected trials by Meert et al., 5 included exclusively complete responders, 5 included patients where PCI was eventually administered at initiation of chemotherapy and 2 included patients given PCI as consolidation treatment whatever the response status. PCI decreases significantly brain metastases incidence. PCI improved survival significantly only among complete responders. When all studies were considered, there was no significant difference. The authors conclude that PCI can only be recommended in complete responders documented by a workup including brain CT scan; several studies did not require a radiological workup before entering the study.

Although the dose–response relationships for PCI in SCLC may predict the optimal treatment schedule, no total dose or fractionation scheme has been established as optimal, and there are no adequate prospective studies to evaluate the effects of total dose and/or fraction size in PCI. In most studies, the prescribed PCI dose lies between 24 and 30 Gy with fraction sizes varying between 2 and 3 Gy. Even if some studies have reported results with one fraction of 8 Gy, large fractions in PCI should be avoided among patients with LD because of late neurotoxicity.[39,46] Among patients with extensive disease, the established dose may be 20 Gy in five fractions of 4 Gy, as reported in the Slotman trial. The short median survival for such patients is only 9 months,[3,47] making the concern about late effects caused by larger fraction negligible. Only one randomized trial has directly addressed the issue of PCI dose.[39] The first part of this trial was a three-arm comparison, with two PCI dosages (24 Gy and 36 Gy) being compared to no PCI, and the higher dose was more effective in reducing the risk of brain metastasis. A trend for a dose response was also observed in the study of Work et al.,[43] which did not address the question of PCI dose, where the 5-year incidence of CNS recurrences was 15% after 33 Gy and 23% after 25 Gy (non significant [NS]).

Most importantly, a marked trend for a dose–response relationship was observed in the metaanalysis.[2] The effect of PCI on brain metastases seemed to increase with the total PCI dose when 4 dose groups (8 Gy, 24 to 25 Gy, 30 Gy, 36 to 40 Gy) were analyzed. Hence, the relative risk of developing brain metastasis as compared to the control group was respectively 24% in the 8-Gy group, 48% in the 24- to 25-Gy group, 68% in the 30-Gy group, and 73% in the 36- to 40-Gy group, but the effect on survival did not differ significantly according to the dose. A dose–response relationship was also found in a recent review that collected data from 12 nonrandomized studies and 12 randomized studies comparing brain relapse rates with and without PCI.[48] The dose–response curve was almost linear within the dose range of 20 to 35 Gy. As the selection of an optimal dose for PCI that would lead to further decrease brain metastasis incidence with minimal toxicity was one of the challenges raised by the metaanalysis, an international intergroup trial addressing the question of dose effect for the prevention of metastases in patients with limited disease who achieved a complete response was undertaken.[49] It compared a standard dose of 25 Gy in ten fractions to a higher dose of 36 Gy (36 Gy/18 fractions or 36 Gy in 24 twice-daily fractions). Toxicities and treatment delivery were not different between the two arms.[50]

Patients who received a higher PCI dose (36 Gy) had a nonsignificant decrease in brain metastases (BM) compared to patients who received the standard dose: the BM two-year rate was 29% in the standard dose group and 23% in the high dose group (HR = 0.80; 95% CI, 0.57–1.11; $p = 0.18$).[51] Overall survival was unexpectedly worse among patients in the higher dose PCI group (HR for death: 1.2 [1.00, 1.44]). Thus the standard PCI dose to be given in SCLC LD should 25 Gy.

We surmise from retrospective studies and reports of late effects that the dose per fraction should be less than or equal to 3 Gy[13] because of the risk of late radiation effects. The use of twice-daily treatments with a smaller dose per fraction and an interval between fractions of at least 6 hours could decrease the risk of late toxicity. A phase II trial has suggested recently that hyperfractionated PCI (30 to 36 Gy given in twice-daily 1.5-Gy fractions) was acutely well tolerated and effective PCI schedule.[52] This dose schedule is being tested in a phase II/III randomized study led by the Radiation Therapy Oncology Group (RTOG 0212).

The optimal timing for PCI in limited stage SCLC has also not been firmly determined. Even if PCI should be administered quite early so as to avoid reseeding of the brain, it has been recommended that it should be administered following documentation of complete remission, after 2 to 4 months but before 6 months from start of chemotherapy.[53] Only one small and rather old trial has directly addressed the issue of PCI optimal timing but was not conclusive.[32] PCI was either administered during the first week (early PCI group), or during the seventh week (late PCI group), and there was no difference in the incidence of brain metastases (7% in both groups).[32] However, the metaanalysis addressed the question of optimal timing in a subgroup analysis, and there was a trend ($p = 0.01$) toward a greater effect of PCI on the incidence of brain metastasis in patients randomized within 4 months after start of induction treatment than in those randomized later.[2] The study of Suwinski et al.[48] has also made a provocative analysis of PCI dose response according to its timing. They have asserted that the delay between initiation of induction treatment and the start of PCI introduces a 20 Gy threshold in the dose–response curve that seems to be linear otherwise. Considering only studies where PCI was initiated less than 60 days after the first day of induction treatment, there was nearly a linear relationship between the given dose in 2-Gy fractions equivalent and the percentage reduction in total brain relapse rates within the range of 8 to 30 Gy. In the studies where PCI was initiated later, it looked as if higher doses were necessary to obtain the same prophylactic effect. Thus, by increasing the delay between induction treatment and PCI, one possibly increases the burden or the resistance of metastatic disease to the brain.

NEUROTOXICITY AND QUALITY OF LIFE

The concerns of severe late neurotoxocity (NT) and detrimental impact on the quality of life (QOL) of patients undergoing PCI for patients with predominantly LD-SCLC have been anecdotally reported but never seriously studied prospectively.[7–10,14,25] Most analyses are marred by too few patients follow-up for too short of time periods,[52,54–56] too few patients at risk,[41,57–61] or did not present the incidence of NT[40] to permit any adequate quantitative assessment. Moreover, most of these reports are retrospective in nature and lack baseline neurological or neuropsychological evaluations.[10,57–59]

In addition, before any real determinations on the impact of PCI on neurological and cognitive functioning can be made, pre-PCI, and prospective follow-up neuropsychometric testing establish the incidence and frequency of late effects.[62] This latter concept has been incorporated into the phase II/III prospectively randomized RTOG 0212 trial. In fact, one recent report[63] has presented a "decision-analytic model" that could potentially incorporate the future results of RTOG 0212 to determine the optimal use of PCI for patients with LD-SCLC who achieve a complete response to chemotherapy by comparing patient survival with the incidence and degree of NT. Finally, by applying a cost-effectiveness QOL model[64] (along with adding patient-derived QOL information not used by its original investigators) to the long-term results from RTOG 0212 when available will further serve to determine the most appropriate dose fractionation schedule (conventional daily vs. hyperfractionated twice-daily PCI) in the context of the impact of the financial cost on the QOL-adjusted survival for this group of patients.

Several factors have been implicated in increasing the risk for long-term NT, namely, age older than 60 years,[65] a daily fraction size >3 Gy per fraction,[14,25,65–67] and concomitant administration of chemotherapy during PCI.[13,39,65,66,68–71] In fact, one published database found that the actuarial risk of severe or worse brain toxicity was 2% at 2-year and 10% at 5-year posttreatment and only occurred in those who received daily fraction sizes of PCI of at least 3 Gy.[25]

Despite the fact that most drugs used for chemotherapy in SCLC do not cross the blood-brain barrier, it has been suggested that repeated high doses of cisplatin may lead to excessive levels in the brain that have been implicated in the development of "chemo brain," which is characterized by abnormal changes in perception, memory, attention, and executive functioning.[72] The neurotoxicities from cisplatin parallel those resulting from inorganic salts and other heavy metals. Furthermore, these adverse NT from cisplatin-containing chemotherapy may require up to 8 months before full recovery is seen.

Importantly, many patients with SCLC have defined neurological and cognitive impairments at diagnosis and prior to the PCI.[13,39,71,73–79] These may be a result of comorbid conditions, the effects of chemotherapy on the brain, paraneoplastic syndrome, aging, an immunologic dysfunction, or even microscopic cranial metastases leading to frontal–subcortical cognitive abnormalities.

The timing from the conclusion of brain irradiation to the appearance of NT generally indicates the type and severity of the injury has previously been described[80] and is outlined in Table 60.3. The signs and symptoms of acute injury from PCI are generally modest and include alopecia, headache, and self-limiting changes in hearing, appetite, and taste along with easy patient.[65] The acute and early delayed

TABLE 60.3 Classification of Radiation Injury Based on Temporal Relation to Radiation Treatment

Type of Injury	Timing in Relation to Radiation	Prognosis
Acute injury	During or just after completion of radiation therapy	Good.
Early delayed injury	A few weeks (up to about 12 wks after completion of radiation treatment)	Usually good.
Late injury	A few months to several yrs after radiation	Guarded. Usually irreversible. May be relentlessly progressive, with a tendency to recur after surgical resection in some patients.

From Giglio P, Gilbert MR. Cerebral radiation necrosis. *Neurologist* 2003 Jul;9(4): 180–188, with permission.

brain injuries are largely reversible with supportive therapy (including steroid administration) and are characterized by accumulation of edema from damaged, leaky capillaries. Acute brain changes are generally not imageable, whereas early delayed injury is seen as hypodense regions on CT scans and as increased signal intensity on fluid-attenuated inversion recovery (FLAIR) and T2-weighted MRI scans.[81]

The delayed and late clinical manifestations of brain injury include "gradual intellectual decline, short-term memory loss, fatigue, and personality change."[65] The most common finding is cognitive impairment,[81] whereas the most common symptom is memory loss[66,82] that is further supported by an animal model study.[83] Pathologically, there is damage to blood vessels that can lead to irreversible ischemic necrosis of white matter and demyelination along with fibrinoid necrosis of blood vessel walls.

There have been only a few prospectively randomized studies with limited 2-year follow-up data that have attempted to evaluate the impact of PCI (with concurrent chemotherapy) on cognitive functioning and other QOL markers[13,39] for patients with SCLC. The French PCI trial[13] employed a neuropsychological assessment performed by a neurologist and showed that there were no significant differences in those receiving PCI versus those in the nonirradiated control group with respect to the end point of 2-year cumulative incidence of neuropsychological changes (Table 60.4). The trial from the United Kingdom[39] suggested that those patients receiving PCI were no more likely than those randomized to no PCI to have abnormalities in either cognitive functioning or QOL indicators attributed directly to the use of radiation.

To ameliorate the long-term effects of PCI on neurocognitive functioning in patients with SCLC, there have been some attempts to modulate the brain damage by either altering the fractionation schedule or by using drugs (such as erythropoietin, warfarin, or a glutamate antagonist) or hyperbaric oxygen therapy.[84] Although not completely understood, there is a very dynamic interaction of vascular and neuronal damage with subsequent inflammation, cytokine production, and increase in the concentration of reactive oxygen and nitrogen species and excitatory amino acids in the brain. Obviously, the most important strategy is to ultimately ascertain how to prevent the onset of permanent brain damage that can result from the delivery of PCI.

CONCLUSION

Several studies in the past 20 years have reported a lower incidence of brain metastases with PCI, thereby reducing the risk of the associated morbidity and social consequences of

TABLE 60.4 Two-Year Cumulative Incidence of Neuropsychological Changes, According to the Two Assigned Treatment Groups

	Control Group		Treatment Group			
	N/n	2-Year Rate	N/n	2-Year Rate	RR	*p* Value
Higher functions	102/8	36	101/10	30	1.23	0.58
Mood	108/8	28	99/8	19	0.76	0.55
Walking	110/10	11	109/14	8	0.79	0.72
Cerebellar function	110/10	13	109/13	15	1.33	0.61
Tendon reflexes	87/8	39	82/5	48	0.94	0.83
Sensibility	108/10	8	100/11	16	1.02	0.97
Cranial nerves	79/5	42	73/5	54	1.56	0.19

From Arriagada R, Le Chevalier T, Borie F, et al. Prophylactic cranial irradiation for patients with small-cell lung cancer in complete remission. *J Natl Cancer Inst* 1995 Feb 1;87(3):183–190, with permission.

RR, relative risk.

brain failure. If recent trials have shown that brain metastases could be really prevented and not just delayed with PCI in complete responders, the metaanalysis has now demonstrated that PCI leads to a 5.4% increase in the 3-year survival rate (from 15.3% observed in the control group to 20.7%). This benefit on overall survival among patients with LD can be added up to the effect of thoracic radiotherapy, which has about the same value.

Among patients with extensive disease, a recent EORTC trial has shown that indications of PCI should be enlarged to all responders, as the 1-year rate of symptomatic metastases is decreased from 40.4% to 14.6%, with a significant impact on survival.

The selection of an optimal dose for PCI that would lead to further decrease brain metastasis incidence with minimal toxicity is one of the challenges raised by the metaanalysis as well the ideal timing of PCI. An international trial addressing the question of dose effect for the prevention of metastases in patients with LD who achieved a complete response has been completed. It compares a standard dose of 25 Gy in 10 fractions to a higher dose of 36 Gy (36 Gy/18 fractions or 36 Gy in 24 twice-daily fractions).[53] So as to evaluate whether dose escalation results in higher cerebral control rates and a possible over added neurological toxicity, all patients have a baseline radiological evaluation as well as a QOL and clinical evaluation at baseline before PCI, 6 months after PCI then yearly. A phase II/III RTOG trial is still ongoing, comparing conventional fractionation (36 Gy in 18 fractions) to hyperfractionated accelerated radiotherapy (36 Gy in 24 twice-daily fractions). All patients will have a neurocognitive assessment in their follow-up.

Even if there are questions left concerning the optimal dose and fractionation of PCI as well as the optimal timing, there is level 1 evidence that PCI is effective. It should now be considered as part of the standard treatment of patients with SCLC in complete remission. For patients with extensive disease, it should be considered for all responders.

REFERENCES

1. Pignon JP, Arriagada R, Ihde DC, et al. A meta-analysis of thoracic radiotherapy for small-cell lung cancer [see comments]. *N Engl J Med* 1992;327(23):1618–1624.
2. Aupérin A, Arriagada R, Pignon JP, et al. Prophylactic cranial irradiation for patients with small cell lung cancer in complete remission. Cranial Iradiation Overview Collaborative Group. *N Engl J Med* 1999; 341:476–484.
3. Slotman B, Faivre-Finn C, Kramer G, et al. Prophylactic cranial irradiation in extensive small-cell lung cancer. *N Engl J Med* 2007;357:664–672.
4. Komaki R, Cox JD, Whitson W. Risk of brain metastasis from small cell carcinoma of the lung related to length of survival and prophylactic irradiation. *Cancer Treat Rep* 1981;65:811–814.
5. Nugent JL, Bunn PA Jr, Matthews MJ, et al. CNS metastases in small bronchogenic carcinoma. Increasing frequency and changing pattern with lengthening of survival. *Cancer* 1979;44:1885–1893.
6. Hansen HH. Should initial treatment of small cell carcinoma include systemic chemotherapy and brain irradiation? *Cancer Chemother Rep* 1973;4:239–241.
7. Einhorn LH III. The case against prophylactic cranial irradiation in limited small cell lung cancer. *Semin Radiat Oncol* 1995;5:57–60.
8. Wagner H Jr. Prophylactic cranial irradiation for patients with small cell lung cancer. An enduring controversy. *Chest Surg Clin N Am* 1997; 7:151–166.
9. Turrisi AT. Brain irradiation and systemic chemotherapy for small-cell lung cancer: dangerous liaisons? Editorial. *J Clin Oncol* 1990;8: 196–199.
10. Fleck JF, Einhorn LH, Lauer RC, et al. Is prophylactic cranial irradiation indicated in small-cell lung cancer? *J Clin Oncol* 1990;8:209–214.
11. Hochstenbag MM, Twijnstra A, Wilmink JT, et al. Asymptomatic brain metastases in small cell lung cancer: MR imaging is useful at initial diagnosis. *J Neurooncol* 2000;48:243–248.
12. Rosen ST, Makuch RW, Lichter AS, et al. Role of prophylactic cranial irradiation in prevention of central nervous system metastases in small cell lung cancer. Potential benefit restricted to patients with complete response. *Am J Med* 1983;74:615–624.
13. Arriagada R, Le Chevalier T, Borie F, et al. Prophylactic cranial irradiation for patients with small-cell lung cancer in complete remission. *J Natl Cancer Inst* 1995;87:183–190.
14. Ball DL, Matthews JP. Prophylactic cranial irradiation: more questions than answers. *Semin Radiat Oncol* 1995;5:61–68.
15. Postmus PE, Sleijfer DT, Haaxma-Reiche H. Chemotherapy for central nervous system metastases from SCLC. A review. *Lung Cancer* 1989;5:254–263.
16. Kristjansen PE, Soelberg Sørensen P, Skov Hansen M, et al. Prospective evaluation of the effect on initial brain metastases from small cell lung cancer of platinum-etoposide based induction chemotherapy followed by an alternating multidrug regimen. *Ann Oncol* 1993;4: 579–583.
17. Lee JS, Murphy WK, Glisson BS, et al. Primary chemotherapy chemotherapy of brain metastases in small-cell lung cancer. *J Clin Oncol* 1989;7:916–922.
18. Kristensen CA, Kristjansen PE, Hansen HH. Systemic chemotherapy of brain metastases from small-cell lung cancer: a review. *J Clin Oncol* 1992;10:1498–1502.
19. van Vulpen M, Kal HB, Taphoorn MJ, et al. Changes in blood-brain barrier permeability induced by radiotherapy: implications for timing of chemotherapy? (Review) *Oncol Rep* 2002;9:683–688
20. Baglan RJ, Marks JE. Comparison of symptomatic and prophylactic irradiation of brain metastases from oat cell carcinoma of the lung. *Cancer* 1981;47:41–45.
21. Cox JD, Komaki R, Byhardt RW, et al. Results of whole brain irradiation for metastases from small cell carcinoma of the lung. *Cancer Treat Rep* 1980;64:957–961.
22. Carmichael J, Crane JM, Bunn PA, et al. Results of therapeutic cranial irradiation in small cell lung cancer. *Int J Radiat Oncol Biol Phys* 1988;14:455–459.
23. Hagerdorn HE, Haaxma-Reiche H, Canrimus AA, et al. Results of whole-brain radiotherapy for brain metastases of small cell lung cancer. *Lung Cancer* 1993;8:293–300.
24. Eagan RT, Frytak S, Lee RE, et al. A case for preplanned thoracic and prophylactic whole brain radiation therapy in limited small cell lung cancer. *Cancer Clin Trials* 1981;4:261–266.
25. Shaw EG, Su JQ, Eagan RT, et al. Prophylactic cranial irradiation in complete responders with small-cell lung cancer : analysis of the Mayo Clinic and North Central Cancer Treatment Group data bases. *J Clin Oncol* 1994;12:2327–2332.
26. van Hazel GA, Scott M, Eagan RT. The effect of CNS metastases on the survival of patients with small cell lung cancer. *Cancer* 1983;51: 933–937.
27. Felletti R, Souhami RL, Spiro SG, et al. Social consequences of brain or liver relapse in small cell carcinoma of the bronchus. *Radiother Oncol* 1985;4:335–339.
28. Cox JD, Petrovich Z, Paig C, et al. Prophylactic cranial irradiation in patients with inoperable carcinoma of the lung. Preliminary report of a cooperative trial. *Cancer* 1978;42:1135–1140.

29. Beiler DD, Kane RC, Bernath AM, et al. Low dose elective brain irradiation in small cell carcinoma of the lung. *Int J Radiat Oncol Biol Phys* 1979;5:941–945.
30. Hansen HH, Dombernowsky P, Hirsch FR, et al. Prophylactic irradiation in bronchogenic small cell anaplastic carcinoma. A comparative trial of localized versus extensive radiotherapy including prophylactic brain irradiation in patients receiving combination chemotherapy. *Cancer* 1980;46:279–284.
31. Maurer LH, Tulloh M, Weiss RB, et al. A randomized combined modality trial in small cell carcinoma of the lung. Comparison of combination chemotherapy-radiation therapy versus cyclophosphamide-radiation therapy effects of maintenance chemotherapy and prophylactic whole brain irradiation. *Cancer* 1980;45:30–39.
32. Perez CA, Krauss S, Bartolucci AA, et al. Thoracic and elective brain irradiation with concomitant or delayed multiagent chemotherapy in the treatment of localized small cell carcinoma of the lung: a randomized prospective study by the Southeastern Cancer Study Group. *Cancer* 1981;47:2407–2413.
33. Aroney RS, Aisner J, Wesley MN, et al. Value of prophylactic cranial irradiation given at complete remission in small cell lung carcinoma. *Cancer Treat Rep* 1983;67:675–682.
34. Jackson DV Jr, Richards F II, Cooper MR, et al. Prophylactic cranial irradiation in small cell carcinoma of the lung. A randomized study. *JAMA* 1983;237:2730–2733.
35. Seydel HG, Creech R, Pagano M, et al. Prophylactic versus no brain irradiation in regional small cell lung carcinoma. *Am J Clin Oncol* 1985;8:218–223.
36. Niiranen A, Holsti P, Salmo M. Treatment of small cell lung cancer. Two-drug versus four-drug chemotherapy and loco-regional irradiation with or without prophylactic cranial irradiation. *Acta Oncol* 1989; 28:501–505.
37. Rosenstein M, Armstrong J, Kris M, et al. A reappraisal of the role of prophylactic cranial irradiation in limited small cell lung cancer. *Int J Radiat Oncol Biol Phys* 1992;24:43–48.
38. Rubenstein JH, Dosoretz DE, Katin MJ, et al. Low doses of prophylactic cranial irradiation effective in limited stage small cell carcinoma of the lung. *Int J Radiat Oncol Biol Phys* 1995;33:329–337.
39. Gregor A, Cull A, Stephens RJ, et al. Prophylactic cranial irradiation is indicated following complete response to induction therapy in small cell lung cancer: Results of a multicentre randomised trial. *Eur J Cancer* 1997;33:1752–1758.
40. Laplanche A, Monnet I, Santos-Miranda JA, et al. Controlled clinical trial of prophylactic cranial irradiation for patients with small-cell lung cancer in complete remission. *Lung Cancer* 1998;21:193–201.
41. Ohonoshi T, Ueoka H, Kawahara S, et al. Comparative study of prophylactic cranial irradiation in patients with small cell lung cancer achieving a complete response: a long-term follow-up result. *Lung Cancer* 1993;10:47–54.
42. Wagner HJ, Kim K, Turrisi A, et al. A randomized phase III study of prophylactic cranial irradiation vs observation in patients with small cell lung cancer achieving a complete response: final report of an incomplete trial by the ECOG and RTOG. *Proc Am Soc Clin Oncol* 1996;15:376.
43. Work E, Bentzen SM, Nielsen OS, et al. Prophylactic cranial irradiation in limited stage small cell lung cancer: survival benefit in patients with favourable characteristics. *Eur J Cancer* 1996;32A: 772–778.
44. The Prophylactic Cranial Irradiation Overview Collaborative Group. Cranial irradiation for preventing brain metastases of small cell lung cancer in patients in complete remission (Review). *Cochrane Database Syst Rev* 2000;(4):CD002805.
45. Meert AP, Paesmans M, Berghmans T, et al. Prophylactic cranial irradiation in small cell lung cancer: a systematic review of the literature with meta-analysis. *BMC Cancer* 2001;1:5.
46. Brewster AE, Hopwood P, Stout R, et al. Single fraction prophylactic cranial irradiation for small cell carcinoma of the lung. *Radiother Oncol* 1995;34:132–136.
47. Chute JP, Chen T, Feigal E, et al. Twenty years of phase III trials for patients with extensive stage small cell lung cancer: perceptible progress. *J Clin Oncol* 1999;17:1794–1801.
48. Suwinski R, Lee SP, Withers HR. Dose-response relationship for prophylactic cranial irradiation in small cell lung cancer. *Int J Radiat Oncol Biol Phys* 1998;40:797–806.
49. Le Péchoux C, for the Prophylactic Cranial Irradiation (PCI99) International Trial Group. Why a new prophylactic cranial irradiation trial in small cell lung cancer (SCLC): from the meta-analysis on PCI in SCLC complete responders to an international trial on PCI dose. *Lung Cancer* 2000;29 suppl 1:159.
50. Le Péchoux C, Senan S, Quoix E, et al. Initial results from an intergroup phase III trial evaluating two different doses of prophylactic cranial irradiation (PCI) in patients with limited small cell cancer (SCLC) in complete remission (PCI99-01, IFCT 99-01, EORTC 22003–08004, RTOG 0212). *J Thorac Oncol* 2007;2(suppl 4): S389–S390.
51. Le Pechoux C, Dunant A, Senan S, et al. Standard-dose versus higher-dose prophylactic cranial irradiation (PCI) in patients with limited-stage small-cell lung cancer in complete remission after chemotherapy and thoracic radiotherapy (PCI 99-01, EORTC 22003-08004, RTOG 0212, and IFCT 99-01): a randomised clinical trial. *Lancet Oncol* 2009;10:467–474.
52. Wolfson AH, Bains Y, Lu J, et al. Twice-daily prophylactic cranial irradiation for patients with limited disease small-cell lung cancer with complete response to chemotherapy and consolidative radiotherapy. Report of a single institutional phase II trial. *Am J Clin Oncol* 2001;24:290–295.
53. Lee JS, Umsawasdi T, Barkley HT Jr, et al. Timing of elective brain irradiation : a critical factor for brain metastasis-free survival in small cell lung cancer. *Int J Radiat Oncol Biol Phys* 1987;13:697–704.
54. Parageorgiou C, Dardoufas C, Kouloulias V, et al. Psychophysiological evaluation of short-term neurotoxicity after prophylactic brain irradiation in patients with small cell lung cancer: a study of event related potentials. *J Neurooncol* 2000;50:275–285.
55. Ahles TA, Silberfarb PM, Rundle AC, et al. Quality of life in patients with limited small-cell carcinoma of the lung receiving chemotherapy with or without radiation therapy, for Cancer and Leukemia Group B. *Psychother Psychosom* 1994;62:193–199.
56. Kotalik J, Yu E, Markman BR, et al. Practice guideline on prophylactic cranial irradiation in small-cell lung cancer. *Int J Radiat Oncol Biol Phys* 2001;50(2):309–316.
57. Catane R, Schwade JG, Yarr I, et al. Follow-up neurological evaluation in patients with small cell lung carcinoma treated with prophylactic cranial irradiation and chemotherapy. *Int J Radiat Oncol Biol Phys* 1981;7:105–109.
58. Laukkanen E, Klonoff H, Allan B, et al. The role of prophylactic brain irradiation in limited stage small cell lung cancer: clinical, neuropsychologic, and CT sequelae. *Int J Radiat Oncol Biol Phys* 1988;14:1109–1117.
59. Lishner M, Feld R, Payne DG, et al. Late neurological complications after prophylactic cranial irradiation in patients with small-cell lung cancer: the Toronto experience. *J Clin Oncol* 1990;8(2):215–221.
60. van de Pol M, ten Velde GP, Wilmink JT, et al. Efficacy and safety of prophylactic cranial irradiation in patients with small cell lung cancer. *J Neurooncol* 1997;35:153–160.
61. Cao KJ, Huang HY, Tu MC, et al. Long-term results of prophylactic cranial irradiation for limited-stage small-cell lung cancer in complete remission. *Chin Med J (Engl)* 2005;118(15):1258–1262.
62. Cull A, Gregor A, Hopwood P, et al. Neurological and cognitive impairment in long-term survivors of small cell lung cancer. *Eur J Cancer* 1994;30A(8):1067–1074.
63. Lee JJ, Bekele BN, Zhou X, et al. Decision analysis for prophylactic cranial irradiation for patients with small-cell lung cancer. *J Clin Oncol* 2006;24(22):3597–3603.
64. Tai TH, Yu E, Dickof P, et al. Prophylactic cranial irradiation revisited: Cost-effectiveness and quality of life in small-cell lung cancer. *Int J Radiat Oncol Biol Phys* 2002;52(1):68–74.

65. Glantz MJ, Choy H, Yee L. Prophylactic cranial irradiation in small cell lung cancer: rationale, results, and recommendations. *Semin Oncol* 1997;24(4):477–483.
66. Johnson BE, Patronas N, Hayes W, et al. Neurologic, computed cranial tomographic, and magnetic resonance imaging abnormalities in patients with small-cell lung cancer: further follow-up of 6- to 13-year survivors. *J Clin Oncol* 1990;8(1):48–56.
67. Tomio L, Romano M, Zanchin G, et al. Ultrarapid high-dose course of prophylactic cranial irradiation in small-cell lung cancer: evaluation of late neurologic morbidity in 16 long-term survivors. *Am J Clin Oncol* 1998;21(1):84–90.
68. Frytak S, Shaw JN, Lee RE, et al. Treatment toxicities in long-term survivors of limited small cell lung cancer. *Cancer Invest* 1988;6(6): 669–676.
69. Frytak S, Shaw JN, O'Neill BP, et al. Leukoencephalopathy in small cell lung cancer patients receiving prophylactic cranial irradiation. *Am J Clin Oncol* 1989;12(1):27–33.
70. Fonseca R, O'Neill BP, Foote RL, et al. Cerebral toxicity in patients treated for small cell carcinoma of the lung. *Mayo Clin Proc* 1999;74:461–465.
71. Ahles TA, Silberfarb PM, Herndon J II, et al. Psychologic and neuropsychologic functioning of patients with limited small-cell lung cancer treated with chemotherapy and radiation therapy with or without warfarin: A study by the Cancer and Leukemia Group B. *J Clin Oncol* 1998;16(5):1954–1960.
72. Troy L, McFarland K, Littman-Power S, et al. Cisplatin-based therapy: a neurological and neuropsychological review. *Psychooncology* 2000; 9:29–39.
73. Sculier JP, Feld R, Evans WK, et al. Neurological disorders in patients with small cell lung cancer. *Cancer* 1987;60:2275–2283.
74. Van Oosterhout AG, Boon PJ, Houx PJ, et al. Follow-up of cognitive functioning in patients with small cell lung cancer. *Int J Radiat Oncol Biol Phys* 1995;31(4):911–914.
75. Van Oosterhout AG, Ganzevles PG, Wilmink JT, et al. Sequelae in long-term survivors of small cell lung cancer. *Int J Radiat Oncol Biol Phys* 1996;34(5):1037–1044.
76. Gregor A. Prophylactic cranial irradiation in small-cell lung cancer: Is it ever indicated? *Oncology* 1998;12(1 suppl 2):19–24.
77. Komaki R, Meyers CA, Shin DM, et al. Evaluation of cognitive function in patients with limited small cell lung cancer prior to and shortly following prophylactic cranial irradiation. *Int J Radiat Oncol Biol Phys* 1995;33(1):179–182.
78. Meyers CA, Byrne KS, Komaki R. Cognitive deficits in patients with small cell lung cancer before and after chemotherapy. *Lung Cancer* 1995;12:231–235.
79. Kanard A, Frytak S, Jatoi A. Cognitive dysfunction in patients with small-cell lung cancer: incidence, causes, and suggestions of management. *J Support Oncol* 2004; 2(2):127–132.
80. Sheline GE, Wara WM, Smith V. Therapeutic irradiation and brain injury. *Int J Radiat Oncol Biol Phys* 1980;6:1215–1228.
81. Giglio P, Gilbert MR. Cerebral radiation necrosis. *Neurologist* 2003; 9:180–188.
82. Roman DD, Sperduto PW. Neuropsychological effects of cranial radiation: current knowledge and future directions. *Int J Radiat Oncol Biol Phys* 1995;31(4):983–998.
83. Lamproglou I, Chen QM, Boisserie G, et al. Radiation-induced cognitive dysfunction: an experimental model in the old rat. *Int J Radiat Oncol Biol Phys* 1995;31(1):65–70.
84. Gaspar LE, Rogers LR. Prophylactic cranial irradiation for small-cell lung cancer-to do or not to do? *J Support Oncol* 2004;2(2):133–140.

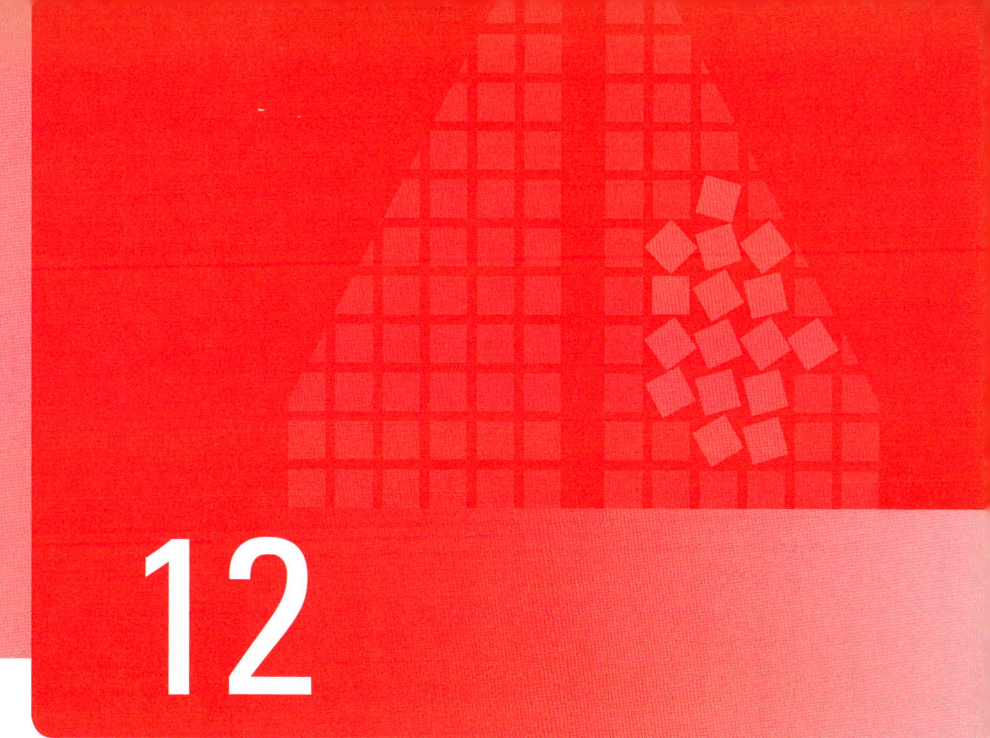

SECTION 12

Lung Cancer Emergencies

CHAPTER 61

Michael Zervos
Costas Bizekis

Endoscopic Ablational Therapies and Stenting

According to the American Cancer Society, there will be 215,020 new cases of lung cancer in 2008. This is the leading cause of cancer-related death in both men and women.[1] Most patients with lung cancer will have advanced disease, and of these, a certain percentage will have an endobronchial component requiring some form of intervention. These patients may present with acute respiratory distress, worsening dyspnea, hemoptysis, or with pneumonitis resulting from endoluminal obstruction. Significant improvement in quality of life can be achieved if the airway obstruction is relieved.

In terms of lung cancer statistics as well as 5-year survival, the outcomes have not changed significantly over the past 10 years. Nevertheless, patients can be palliated with endobronchial obstruction and hemoptysis more efficiently and in a more durable fashion, because the treatment modalities and options have improved. Some of these are ablational, and all require some form of bronchoscopy whether flexible or rigid. These therapies include, for example, laser therapy cautery, rigid bronchoscopy, argon plasma coagulation, cryotherapy, photodynamic therapy (PDT), and stenting.[2]

Unfortunately, an almost equal percentage of patients that are diagnosed with locally advanced lung cancer present with metastatic disease, and of these, 20% will have an endobronchial component compounding their symptoms. Extrinsic or intrinsic luminal compromise eventually causes acute or chronic respiratory failure, and many patients will present with symptoms of hemoptysis, postobstruction pneumonia, or dyspnea.[3]

Palliation of bronchial obstruction frequently involves the use of a stent. "Stent" refers to a British dentist, Charles R. Stent, who created a mold for edentulous patients and since then has carried his name to describe any device that maintains the integrity of a hollow tubular structure. Originally, these stents were used in the gastrointestinal tract and in the vascular system and subsequently were applied to the airway. There are basically two types of stents: *metal* and *silicone*. Although they have essential differences with regard to their design and properties, they can both be used to palliate malignant central airway obstruction (CAO).

Currently, airway stents are either made of self-expanding metal for more permanent use or silicone if a temporary solution is needed. Complications of these stents include airway fracture with insertion or perforation (early or late), bleeding, granulation or tumor ingrowth, infection, migration, obstruction, as well as a small risk of death. There are no large randomized clinical trials to examine the utility of stent use in the patient with lung cancer. Limited case series from multiple institutions support the use of stenting techniques to help palliate these patients. Moreover, the palliation of symptoms by stenting is almost immediate in most cases and offers short-term improvement in quality of life, with little or no effect on long-term and overall prognosis. Additionally, recent data supporting the use of therapeutic bronchoscopy in patients with non–small cell lung cancer can achieve not only palliation of their symptoms but also potential lung-sparing surgery.

HISTORICAL OVERVIEW

Although many techniques to treat and palliate CAO exist, the most current technique of rigid bronchoscopy with and without endobronchial laser was perfected in the early 1980s by Dumon et al.[4] The key to this technique was the provision of superior airway control and the versatility of performing most endobronchial procedures. Subsequent to Dumon et al.'s experience, there have been multiple series with large number of cases that demonstrate the efficacy of this modality. These include Cavaliere et al.[5,6] in 1988 who published their experience with 1396 applications of rigid bronchoscopy with laser in 1000 patients, in 1994 with 2253 applications in 1585 patients, and in 1996 with 2610 treatments in 1838 patients. Venuta et al.[7] published their series in 2002 with 273 patients with a goal of palliation or as a bridge to surgery. Most recently in 2006, Moghissi et al.[8] published their data over a 21-year experience with 2235 treatments in 1159 patients. Their review implies that laser therapy of lung cancer still plays an important role in the palliation of inoperable cancer.[8]

Rigid bronchoscopy has withstood the test of time and with the combined use of either laser, cautery or just forceps alone remains the preferred modality with most airway interventionalists when dealing with CAO. Refinements in the protocol have, in some instances, led to improvement of results over laser and rigid bronchoscopy, and the use of electrocautery in the airway may be more cost-effective and readily available. Cautery can be easily delivered through the working channel of a specially designed therapeutic scope with a larger working channel. In a recent review of interventional techniques to treat malignant obstruction of the large airways, the authors imply that electrocautery is likely to replace laser as the preferred tool in these cases.[9]

Silicone stents have evolved over time from their initial description by Montgomery[10] in 1965. The *Montgomery* tube is a silicone T tube placed through a tracheal stoma for the relief of subglottic tracheal stenosis or to support a reconstructed tracheal anastomosis (Fig. 61.1).[10] Subsequently, the T tube was modified by Cooper et al.[11] and by Duvall and Bauer[12] in order to be placed endoscopically. Westaby et al.[13] also modified the T tube into a bifurcating T-Y stent that could be pulled through a stoma.

Dumon[14] in 1990 published his data on silicone stents with good results for airway obstruction. Typically, this stent has studs that are molded to the exterior to prevent migration and is deployed through rigid bronchoscopy. The *Dumon* silicone Y stent can be used for bilateral mainstem pathology as well as for tumors of the carina.

The most recent silicone stent that has been popularized by Boston Scientific is known as the *Polyflex Airway Stent* (Fig. 61.2A) This is a fully covered polyester silicone mesh that has its own delivery system with a loading basket and a pushing rod to facilitate deployment through a rigid bronchoscope. This can be used for all types of CAO regardless of etiology and has the obvious advantage of being removable. As with all silicone stents, mucus impaction and migration are the most common complications related to their use. Migration can be minimized with the airway Polyflex as long as the stent is appropriately sized with a tendency toward a larger diameter stent.

The *Dynamic* (Y) stent (Fig. 61.2B) is a removable airway stent made of silicone and has metal rings to resemble the cartilage of the trachea anteriorly. Also, it has a softer plastic posterior membrane that moves with respiration and resembles

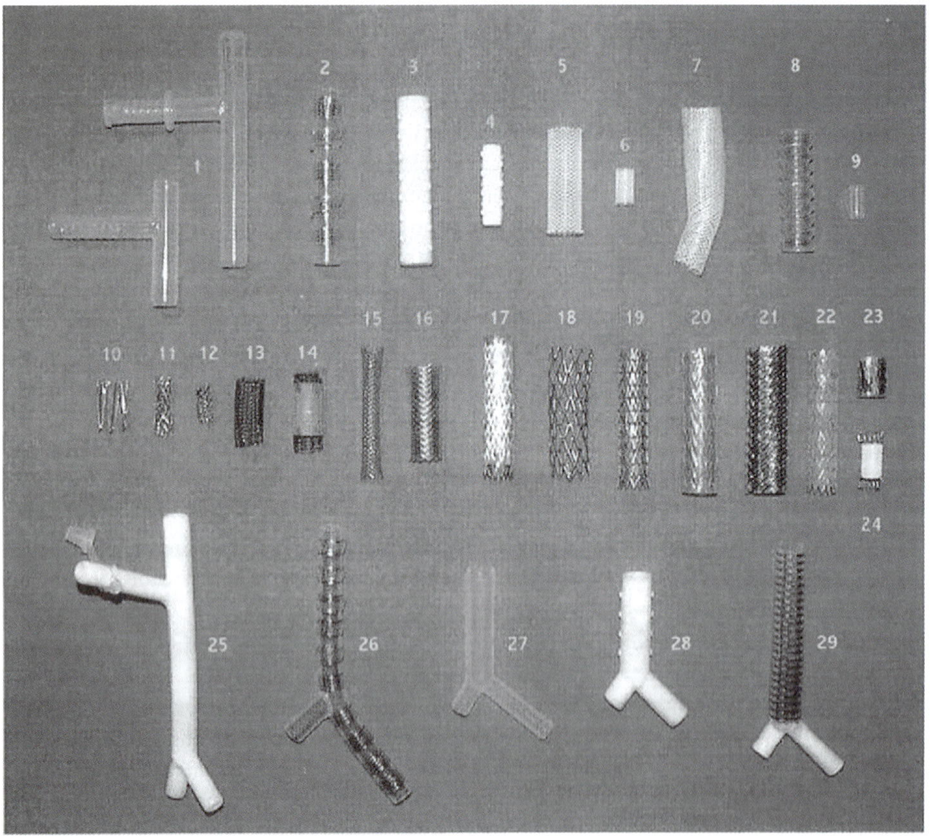

FIGURE 61.1 A selection of the currently available airway stents.

1. Montgomery T-tubes
2. Orlowski tracheal stent
3. Dumon tracheal stent
4. Dumon bronchial stent
5. Polyflex tracheal stent
6. Polyflex bronchial stent
7. Polyflex stump stent
8. Noppen tracheal stent
9. Hood bronchial stent
10. Gianturco stent
11. Palmaz stent
12. Tantalum Strecker stent
13. Uncovered Ultraflex stent
14. Covered Ultraflex stent
15. Uncovered Wallstent
16. Covered Wallstent

17–24. Prototypes of metal stents and compound stents currently tested preclinically and clinically

25. Westaby T-Y stent
26. Bifurcated Orlowski stent
27. Hood Y-stent
28. Bifurcated Dumon stent
29. Dynamic stent

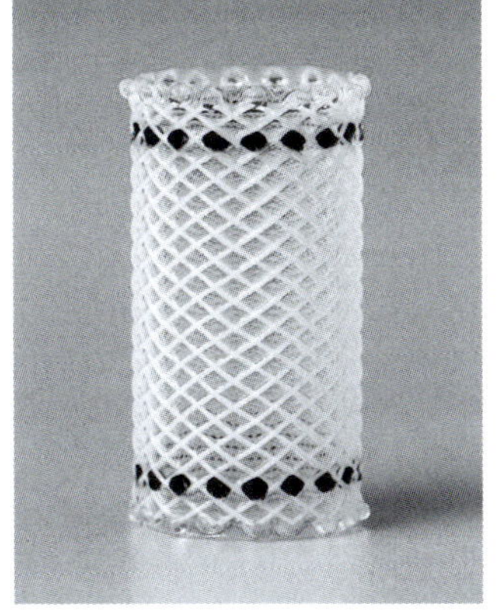

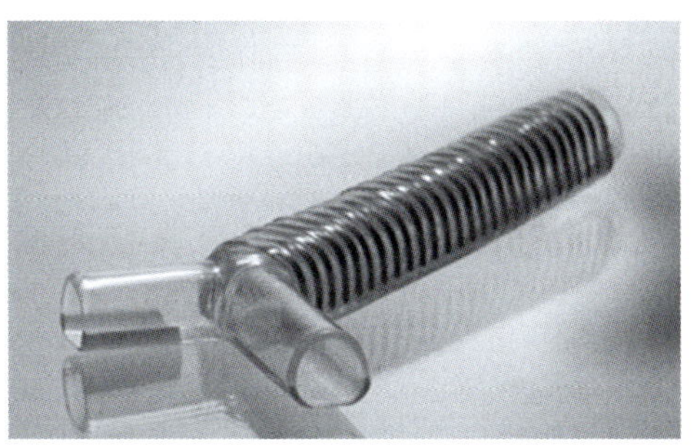

FIGURE 61.2 **A:** Polyflex. **B:** Dynamic (Y) Stent. (Courtesy of Boston Scientific, Natick MA.)

that of the membranous trachea. Because of this design, it moves dynamically with each phase of the respiratory cycle. Placement requires use of special forceps also called Freitag forceps and can be positioned directly through the cords or with a special laryngoscope. A video laryngoscope may be helpful to visualize the cords to facilitate placement. This is indicated for CAO involving the carina, proximal mainstem, as well mid-to-distal tracheal pathology.[15] More proximal lesions require a T-Y Montgomery tube with a tracheal stoma.

Metal stents are also used to palliate malignant CAO. These stents can be deployed through flexible bronchoscopy, a guide wire, and fluoroscopy. Their sizes vary according to the desired length and diameter, and the stents are usually contained within a deployment system, which is released by pulling of a string that unravels and deploys the stent. Most of these stents have markers and can be visualized under fluoroscopic guidance.

EARLY METAL AIRWAY STENTS

The *Gianturco stent* was one of the first stainless steel metal stents with a zigzag loop design.[16–18] This model is made of 0.018 inch stainless steel monofilaments into a double-zigzag design and is introduced via 12 French Teflon sheath. *Palmaz* was next to follow, which was positioned by balloon expansion and conformed to the airway. This feature prevents the stent from opening to a diameter larger than that of the given airway obstruction.[16] These stents are rarely used in clinical practice in the United States today. *Wallstent* is a self-expandable super alloy stent that expands to a preset diameter and is mostly used in Europe.[17,18] It is composed of 20 surgical steel monofilaments of 100-μm diameter braided into a cylindrical tube. It is mounted on a 7 to 9 French delivery catheter and a rolling membrane that serves to protect the device.

NEXT GENERATION METAL AIRWAY STENTS

Ultraflex (Boston Scientific) stents are made of single-strand nitinol.[19] Nitinol is a memory metal and has the advantage of conforming to the irregularities of the airway (Fig. 61.3). This is a self-expanding stent that is contained within a flexible deployment system and unravels with the pulling of a thread. The deployment system can be passed over a guidewire that has been previously placed with a flexible bronchoscope or through an endotracheal tube. This obviously has the benefit of easy deployment and can be visualized under fluoroscopic control. The Ultraflex stent has upper and lower markers for accurate positioning across the obstruction. In addition to the noncovered version, this stent comes with a polyurethane cover that spans its length except for 1 cm on each end to allow for granulation and prevent migration. In a recent publication on Ultraflex stents, it demonstrates a low-complication rate and effective use in complex malignant airway stenoses with marked asymmetry or irregularity, angulation, or changing diameters.[20]

Included within the next generation of airway stent is the *Aero Pulmonary stent* by Alveolus company. This stent contains characteristics of metal and silicone stents. It has a biologically inert cover and can be removed if necessary. This stent can be deployed with either flexible or rigid bronchoscopy and can be repositioned after deployment.

INDICATIONS FOR STENTING

The goal of airway stenting is to improve upon a specific symptom that the patient demonstrates. This is usually caused by

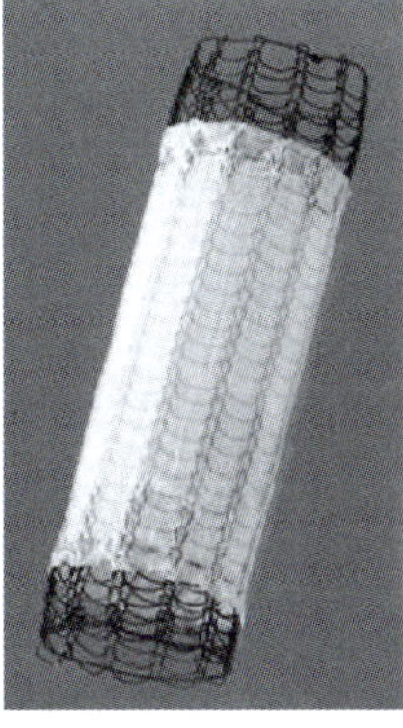

FIGURE 61.3 Ultraflex covered. (Courtesy of Boston Scientific, Natick MA.)

alteration of the flow of air through the trachea or bronchi because of the luminal decrease of at least 60% to 70%. These symptoms are usually acute or chronic dyspnea and hemoptysis. The decrease in luminal diameter can be either extrinsic or intrinsic with the same end result of airway compromise. The indication for stenting in most cases will be unresectable primary lung cancer, and thus, the most common cause of malignant CAO,[21] followed by secondary involvement of the airway by esophageal and thyroid cancer.[21] Wood et al.[21] have reported that 42% of patients in their series had extrinsic compression from lung cancer and 27% had endobronchial tumor. Of the patients who had extrinsic compression, the most common cause was lung cancer, followed by mediastinal, thyroid, esophageal cancer, mesothelioma, metastatic lesions from kidney, thyroid, sarcoma, breast, and others.[21] Less common indications for airway stenting include either primary or metastatic laryngeal cancer, lymphoma, myeloma, or lymphadenopathy of any etiology.

ABLATIONAL THERAPIES

Ablational therapies act in a complementary role and are often necessary for purposes of debridement prior to stenting. As detailed by Santos et al.,[22] laser, PDT, cryotherapy, cautery, and brachytherapy in combination with stenting often produce a more favorable outcome than stenting alone.

Rigid Bronchoscopy This is, by far, the most effective means to address any airway problem. It can be used to core out the tumor, dilate the airway stricture, and provide superior airway control. It is a tool that most thoracic surgeons are familiar with, and it can provide the means by which the flexible scope is passed for more distal visualization, adjustments of stent position, or for airway balloon dilation (Fig. 61.4). Essentially, any therapy can be used with rigid bronchoscopy including laser, cautery, argon plasma coagulation, PDT, cryotherapy, or, more recently, use of the microdebrider.[23] Rigid bronchoscopy has changed little over the years, is most popular with surgical groups in North America for the endoscopic relief of airway obstruction, and in the most recent literature, appears to be the preferred technique for airway management and stent deployment.[21]

Electrocautery and Argon Plasma Coagulation

The use of electrical current is commonly used in the operating room during most surgical procedures. The use of cautery

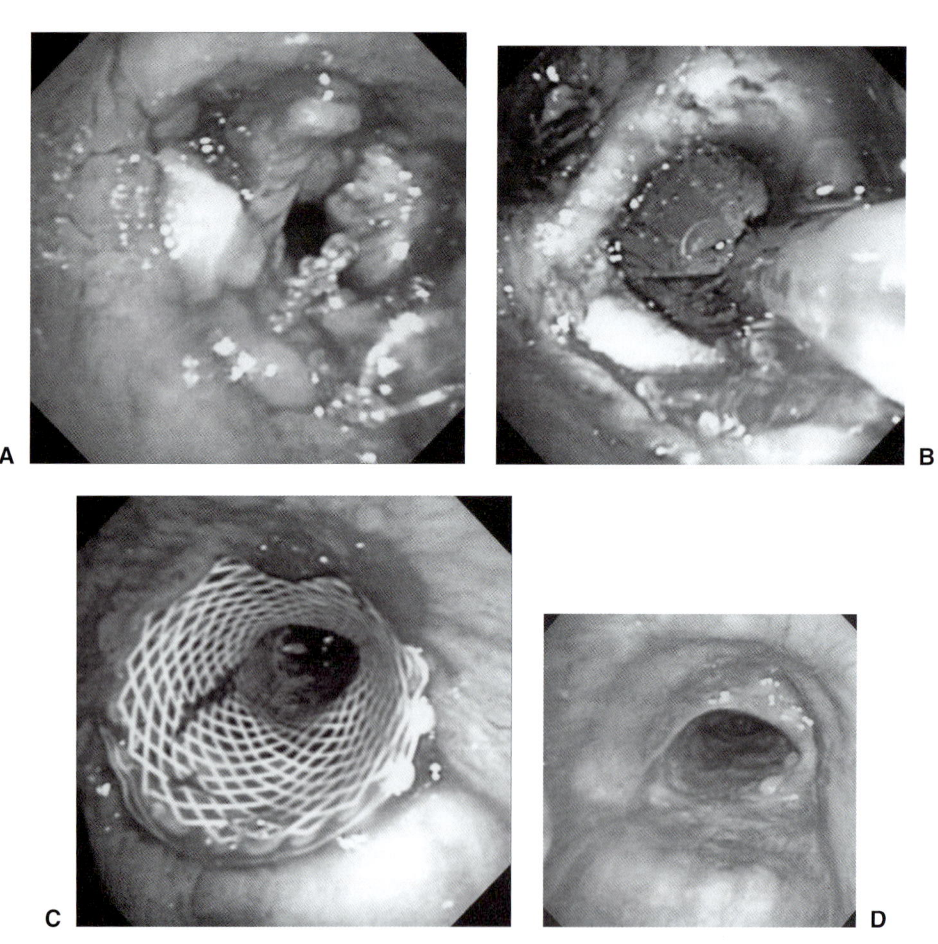

FIGURE 61.4 **A:** Right upper sleeve bronchoplasty with anastomotic stricture. **B:** Balloon dilation of the stricture. **C:** Polyflex airway stent placement. **D:** Airway remodeling after stent was removed 3 months late.

in the airway was described by Gilfoy in 1932.[24] More recently, cautery forceps have been modified to be passed through the large channel of a flexible bronchoscope. They have grasping capability and can cauterize the tissue providing tumor necrosis and hemostasis simultaneously. *Argon plasma* coagulators are a noncontact form of electrocoagulation and have also been used for obtaining cauterization within the airway and surface bleeding. Its utility in the open surgical field has been validated for liver, splenic, or chest wall bleeding, and the device can also be delivered through the bronchoscope to treat tumors "around the corner" or at an acute angle.[25]

Laser Therapy The use of laser in the airway is well documented. It can be delivered through the flexible or rigid bronchoscope. The most commonly used laser is the Nd:YAG 1064 nm and can achieve tissue penetration up to 10 mm. The largest series to date with regard to the use of laser therapy are by Dumon et al.,[4] Cavaliere et al.,[5,6] and Venuta et al.[7] All of these studies confirm the definite improvement, and thus palliation, of symptoms with a high degree of success (90% to 100%).

Photodynamic Therapy PDT is a modality that uses a photosensitizer intravenously administered 48 to 72 prior to treatment, which is selectively taken up by the tumor tissue (Fig. 61.5). Monochromatic light that matches the activation wavelength of the photosensitizer (Photofrin Axcam pharmaceutical) is illuminated onto the tumor, and a chemical reaction occurs with the release of oxygen free radicals and subsequent vascular collapse of the tumor. This creates tumor necrosis and can be used for superficial lesions as well as bulky tumors. Repeat bronchoscopy is usually necessary to "clean up" the airway. This is a well-documented treatment modality and has been reported by Moghissi et al.[26–28] in 1997, 1999, and most recently 2004. In all of these reviews, it is clear that this therapy cannot only palliate patients with advanced stage disease but also potentially treat early lesions. In the most recent analysis by Moghissi,[28] a review of 24 articles (1153 patients) in the world literature was provided. He concluded that bronchoscopic PDT is a safe and effective therapeutic method for the palliation of advanced lung cancer. Others have also reported their experience with favorable outcomes for the use of PDT. A recent review from Roswell Park Cancer Institute concludes that PDT is an effective tool for the palliation of endobronchial cancers that obstruct the central airways.[29] Also in another review by Chen et al.[30] from the University of Pittsburgh concluded that PDT is effective in the palliation of lung cancer. In certain situations, it might be possible to treat an endobronchial tumor with photodynamic therapy

A
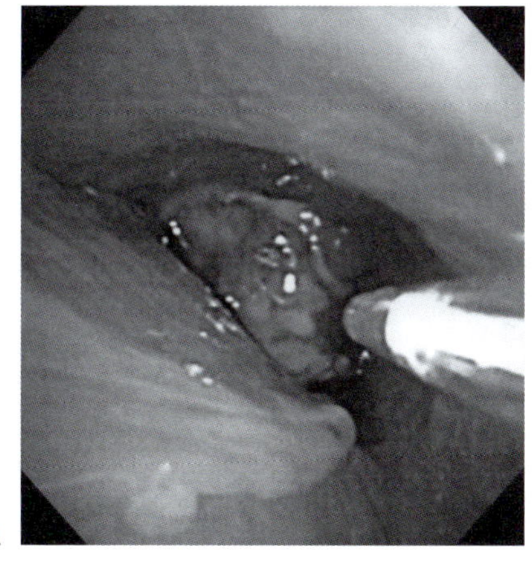

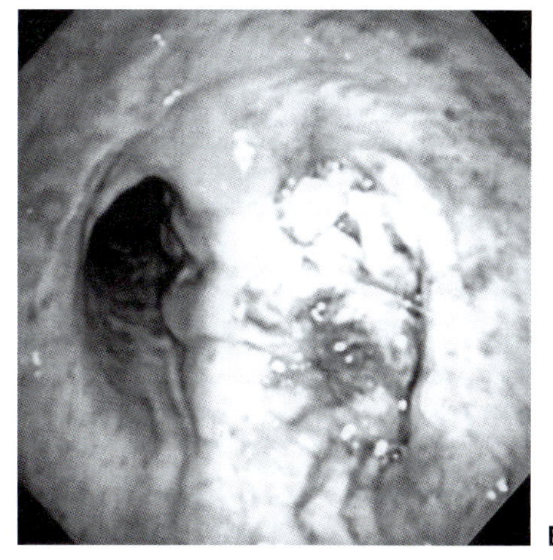
B

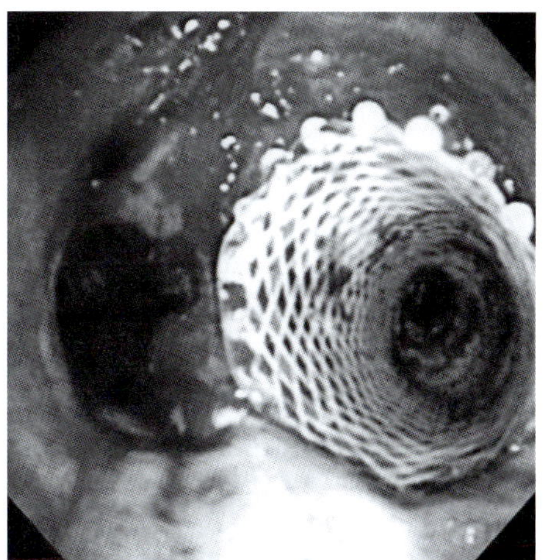
C

FIGURE 61.5 **A,B:** Photodynamic therapy for tumor ablation. **C:** Polyflex airway stent.

and then follow with surgical treatment. Recently, a case report by DeArmond et al.[31] demonstrates the combined use of photodynamic therapy and thoracoscopic sleeve lobectomy.

Cryotherapy *Cryotherapy* is a technique that uses repeated freeze–thaw cycles to achieve tumor necrosis through extreme cold. The method utilizes temperatures in the −80° to −160°C range and thus causes cell death by intracellular and extracellular crystallization and microthrombosis.[32] This can be delivered through flexible or rigid bronchoscopy and can be used to successfully palliate endobronchial cancers. This is a safe technique but has the major disadvantage of having delayed effects. The largest series to date was by Maiwand and Homasson[33] in 1995, which reported 622 cases with reasonable improvement in dyspnea and hemoptysis. More recently, Noppen et al.[32] in 2001 achieved 80% airway patency rates in their study. Asimakopoulos et al.[34] in 2005 reported on the use of cryotherapy in a comparative analysis between groups of patients receiving a single dose of cryotherapy versus multiple doses over a 5-year period. The group concluded that cryotherapy is a safe method of palliation of endobronchial malignancies causing airway obstruction.

Brachytherapy *Brachytherapy* is typically performed through a transnasal approach, and the most common method is by an after-loading technique using Iridium 192. A thin polyethylene catheter is first positioned, and the radiation source is loaded later.[35] One of the largest series was by Macha et al.[36] in 1995 with 365 patients with administration of high dose rate (500 cGy at 10 mm × 3 or 4 fractions) with a 66% palliation rate. Celebioglu et al.[37] in 2001 reported 95 patients at the high dose rate (750 to 1000 cGy at 10 mm × 2 or 3 weekly fractions) with significant improvement in palliation of symptoms. A recent analysis looks at high-dose endobronchial brachytherapy and concludes that it is effective in palliating lung cancer but is associated with a risk of fatal hemoptysis.[38]

PALLIATION OF LUNG CANCER

There are no randomized clinical trials comparing metal versus silicone stents to compare the degree of palliation of lung cancer or comparisons of stents with other therapies possibly because of the ethical dilemma that is created by such life-threatening conditions.[22,39] On the other hand, what does exist are series from various institutions in the United States and abroad that provide their experience and their preferences. The common goal in all cases is palliation of hemoptysis or respiratory failure.

There are several large series of stenting for malignant CAO. All of these studies share one thing in common, that is, stenting can improve upon, and thus palliate, the symptoms caused by airway compromise. Survival is limited for this group and can be measured in terms of months (3 to 4 months) on average.

One of the largest series to date is from Dumon et al.[40] in 1999, which reported their results with 1574 stents in 1054 patients. This was a multicenter European study, which also included stenting for benign strictures as well as for malignant CAO and reported good resolution of airway patency with minimal complications. The three most common complications in this series were migration (9.5%), granulomas (7.9%), and mucus impaction (3.6%). The average length of stent placement was 4 months.

Miyazawa et al.'s study[41] on the use of 54 Ultraflex stents in 34 patients, stratified the patients based on dyspnea scores 1 to 4 and showed that after deployment of the stent, patients immediately improved with regard to their dyspnea. Most patients were downgraded from their initial scores of 3 and 4 to 0, 1, and 2. Their conclusions were that the patients were significantly palliated in terms of dyspnea, which contributed to improved quality of life.

Sadd et al.[42] analyzed their 6-year experience with 112 self-expanding metal stents (Wallstent and Ultraflex Boston Scientific) in 82 patients. The majority of patients had dyspnea (80%), and 16 patients were on ventilators. Of the 16 patients on ventilators, 14 were able to be extubated and there were no deaths. The most common complications included infections (15.9%), obstructive granulomas (14.6%), and migration (4.7%). The median follow-up duration was 42 days with a range of 1 to 672 days.

Wood et al.[21] placed 309 stents in 143 patients, 67% of which were for malignant airway obstruction. A total of 87% of the stents were molded silicone rubber (Hood Laboratories Penbroke, MA), and 13% were metal stents. Of the 96 patients with malignant CAO, 88 (92%) had received previous radiation or chemotherapy or both, and 14% had previous surgery for lung, esophageal, or thyroid cancer. In addition, 68% of the patients had additional procedures (laser, core-out, dilation, brachytherapy, photodynamic therapy) to prepare for or as an adjunct to stenting. Ninety-five percent of the patients noted significant improvement of their symptoms. In this study, 45 of the 53 patients with malignant disease (85%) maintained airway palliation for follow-up periods of 1 to 13 months, (mean, 4 months) with 28% requiring further bronchoscopic interventions.

Shin et al.[43] evaluated the safety and effectiveness of covered retrievable expandable nitinol stents in 35 patients with malignant tracheobronchial strictures with the intent of palliation. In this study, dyspnea was assessed according to the Hugh-Jones classification.[43] Average survival was 9.62 weeks (2 days to 26 weeks). The authors concluded that stent placement is safe, effective, and improvement was noted in terms of dyspnea with improved quality of life.

Lemaire et al.[2] reviewed their outcomes with tracheobronchial stents in 172 patients. In this group, 225 stents total were placed. A total of 172 stents were placed in 142 patients for malignant disease. The study sought to assess the short-term (<30days) and intermediate (>30days) risks and benefits of tracheobronchial stenting. The complications related to stent placement included tumor ingrowth (n = 9), excessive granulation tissue (n = 7), stent migration (n = 5), and restenosis related to extrinsic compression (n = 2). Five of the complications occurred in the first 30 days, whereas the rest occurred later on. The latter complications were mostly related to excessive granulation tissue and tumor ingrowth. Median survival after stenting is 3.4 months with a 1-year survival of 15%. The authors concluded that the stents offer minimally invasive therapy for patients with unresectable malignant CAO with an acceptable risk of complications at short and intermediate time points.[2]

Chin et al.,[44] in a recent review article on stenting, provides a detailed analysis of the different types of stents and the indications. In this analysis, once again the end point was symptomatic relief and improvement in quality of life.

CONCLUSION

Stenting appears to be an accepted method to palliate patients that are dying from lung cancer. Often, these patients have very limited survival, creating the dilemma of whether to do anything at all. As long as patency of the airway can be achieved, patients will have symptomatic improvement within their last year of life. In a recent review from the Netherlands,[45] where euthanasia is legal, stenting is performed with improvement in quality of life. After the patients died, their general practitioners (GPs) were given a questionnaire to determine whether the stent was helpful. In 58% of the cases, the GPs thought that stent placement should always be considered as part of the treatment of terminal cancer patients with imminent suffocation. Regardless of the specific design, stents provide palliation for patients with malignant airway disease.

REFERENCES

1. Jemal A, Tiwari RC, Murray T, et al. Cancer statistics, 2008. *CA Cancer J Clin* 2008;58:71–96.
2. Lemaire A, Burfriend WR, Toloza E, et al. Outcomes of tracheobronchial stents in patients with malignant airway disease. *Ann Thorac Surg* 2005:80:434–438.
3. Chhajed PN, Eberhardt R, Dienemann H, et al. Therapeutic bronchoscopy interventions before surgical resection of lung cancer. *Ann Thorac Surg* 2006:81:1839–1843.
4. Dumon JF, Reboud E, Garbe L, et al. Treatment of tracheal bronchial lesions by laser photo resection. *Chest* 1982:81:278–284.
5. Cavaliere S, Foccoli P, Farina PL. Nd:YAG laser bronchoscopy: a five year experience with 1,396 applications in 1,000 patients. *Chest* 1988:94:15–21.
6. Cavaliere S, Foccoli PO, Toninelli C, et al. Nd:YAG laser in lung cancer: an 11-year experience with 2253 applications in 1585 patients. *J Bronchol* 1994:1:105–111.
7. Venuta F, Rendina EA, De Giacomo T, et al. Nd:YAG laser resection of lung cancer invading the airway as abridge to surgery and palliative treatment. *Ann Thorac Surg* 2002;74:995–999.
8. Moghissi K, Dixon K. Bronchoscopic NdYAG laser treatment in lung cancer 30 years on: an institutional review. *Lasers Med Sci* 2006 Dec;21(4):186–191.
9. Beamis JF Jr. Interventional pulmonology techniques for treating malignant large airway obstruction: an update. *Curr Opin Pulm Med* 2005:11:292–295.
10. Montgomery WW. T-Tube tracheal stent. *Arch Otolaryngol* 1965;82: 320–321.
11. Cooper JD, Pearson FG, Patterson GA, et al. Use of silicone stents in the management of the airway problem. *Ann Thorac Surg* 1989;47: 371–378.
12. Duvall AJ, Bauer W. An endoscopically introduced T-tube for tracheal stenosis. *Laryngoscope* 1977;87:2031–2037.
13. Westaby S, Jackson JW, Pearson FG. A bifurcated silicone rubber stent for relief of tracheobronchial obstruction. *J Thorac Cardiovasc Surg* 1982;83:414–417.
14. Dumon JF. A dedicated tracheobronchial stent. *Chest* 1990;97: 328–332.
15. Freitag L, Eicker R, Linz B, et al. Theoretical and experimental basis for the development of dynamic airway stent. *Eur Respir J* 1994;7: 2038–2045.
16. Uchida BT, Putnam JS, Rösch J. Modifications of Gianturco expandable wire stents. *AJR Am J Roentgenol* 1988;158:1185–1187.
17. Susanto I, Peters JI, Levine SM, et al. Use of balloon expandable metallic stents in the management of bronchial stenosis and bronchomalacia after lung transplantation. *Chest* 1998;114:1330–1335.
18. Carre P, Rousseau H, Lombart L, et al. Balloon dilation and self expanding metal Wallstent insertion. *Chest* 1994;105:343–348.
19. Rousseau H, Dahan M, Lauque D, et al. Self-expandable prostheses in the tracheobronchial tree. *Radiology* 1993;188:199–203.
20. Breitenbücher A, Chhajed PN, Brutsche MH, et al. Long-term follow-up and survival after Ultraflex stent insertion in the management of complex malignant airway stenoses. *Respiration* 2008;75(4): 443–449.
21. Wood DE, Liu YH, Vallières E, et al. Airway stenting for malignant and benign tracheobronchial stenosis. *Ann Thorac Surg* 2003;76: 167–174.
22. Santos RS, Raftopoulos Y, Keenan RJ, et al. Bronchoscopic palliation of primary lung cancer. Single or multimodality therapy? *Landreneau Surg Endosc* 2004;18:931–936.
23. Lunn W, Garland R, Ashiku S, et al. Microdebrider bronchoscopy: a new tool for the interventional bronchoscopist. *Ann Thorac Surg* 2005;80:1485–1488.
24. Gilfoy FE. Primary malignant tumors of the lower third of the trachea: report of a case with successful treatment by electrofulguration and deep X-rays. *Arch Otolaryngol* 1932;16:182–187.
25. Chan AL, Yoneda KY, Allen RP, et al. Advances in the management of endobronchial lung malignancies. *Curr Opin Pulm Med* 2003;9(4): 301–308.
26. Moghissi K, Dixon K, Stringer M, et al. The place of bronchoscopic photodynamic therapy in advanced unresectable lung cancer: experience of 100 cases. *Eur J Cardiothorac Surg* 1999;15:1–6.
27. Moghissi K, Dixon K, Hudson E, et al. Endoscopic laser therapy in malignant tracheobronchial obstruction using sequential Nd YAG laser and photodynamic therapy. *Thorax* 1997;52:281–283.
28. Moghissi K. Role of bronchoscopic photodynamic therapy in lung cancer management. *Curr Opin Pulm Med* 2004;10:256–260.
29. Loewen GM, Pandey R, Bellnier D, et al. Endobronchial photodynamic therapy for lung cancer. *Lasers Surg Med* 2006;38:364–370.
30. Chen M, Pennathur A, Luketich JD. Role of photodynamic therapy in unresectable esophageal and lung cancer. *Lasers Surg Med* 2006;38: 396–402.
31. DeArmond DT, Mahtabifard A, Fuller CB, et al. Photodynamic therapy followed by thoracoscopic sleeve lobectomy for locally advanced lung cancer. *Ann Thorac Surg* 2008 May;85(5):E24–E26.
32. Noppen M, Meysman M, Van Herreweghe R, et al. Bronchoscopic cryotherapy: preliminary experience. *Acta Clin Belg* 2001;56:73–77.
33. Maiwand MO, Homasson JP. Cryotherapy for tracheobronchial disorders. *Clin Chest Med* 1995;16:427–443.
34. Asimakopoulos G, Beeson J, Evans J, et al. Cryosurgery for malignant endobronchial tumors: analysis of outcome. *Chest* 2005 Jun;127(6): 2007–2014.
35. Ernst A, Feller-Kopman D, Becker HD, et al. Central airway obstruction. *Am J Respir Crit Care Med* 2004;169:1278–1297.

36. Macha HN, Wahlers B, Reichle C, et al. Endobronchial radiation therapy for obstructing malignancies; ten years experience with iridium-192 high dose radiation brachytherapy afterloading technique in 365 patients. *Lung* 1995;173(5):271–280.
37. Celebioglu B, Gurkan OU, Erdogan S, et al. High dose rate endobronchial brachytherapy effectively palliates symptoms due to inoperable lung cancer. *Jpn J Clin Oncol* 2002;32:443–448.
38. Ozkok S, Karakoyun-Celik O, Goksel T, et al. High dose rate endobronchial brachytherapy in the management of lung cancer: response and toxicity evaluation in 158 patients. *Lung Cancer* 2008 Dec;62(3): 326–333.
39. Macha HN, Becker KO, Kemmer HP. (1994) Pattern of failure and survival in endobronchial laser resection. *Chest* 2004;105: 1668–1672.
40. Dumon MC, Dumon JF, Perrin C, et al. Silicone tracheobronchial endoprosthesis [Article in French]. *Rev Mal Respir* 1999;16:641–651.
41. Miyazawa T, Yamakido M, Ikeda S, et al. Implantation of ultraflex nitinol stents in malignant tracheobronchial stenoses. *Chest* 2000;118; 959–965.
42. Saad CP, Murthy S, Krizmanich G, et al. Self-expandable metallic airway stents and flexible bronchoscopy: long-term outcomes analysis. *Chest* 2003 Nov;124(5):1993–1999.
43. Shin JH, Kim SW, Shim TS, et al. Malignant tracheobronchial strictures: palliation with covered retrievable expandable nitinol stent. *J Vasc Interv Radiol* 2003;14:1525–1534.
44. Chin CS, Litle V, Yun J, et al. Airway stents. *Ann Thorac Surg* 2008; 85(2):S792–S796. Review.
45. Vonk-Noordegraaf A, Postmus PE, Sutedja TG, et al. Tracheobronchial stenting in the terminal care patients with central airways obstruction. *Chest* 2001;120:1811–1814.

CHAPTER 62

Jessica S. Donington

Management of Malignant Pleural Effusion

Malignant pleural effusions (MPEs) are a common complication of advanced cancer. There are estimated to be greater than 150,000 cases of MPE each year in the United States, and approximately half of all patients with metastatic cancer will develop an MPE. Lung cancer and breast cancer account for over 75% of malignant effusions.[1] For most patients with MPE, cure is no longer an option and, for many, life expectancy is short. MPEs are clinically important because they cause significant symptoms that can severely impact the quality of life for patients with advanced cancer.

Common symptoms that result from an MPE include dyspnea, orthopnea, cough, and chest pain. Dyspnea is, by far, the most common presenting symptom and is seen in 96% of patients.[2] The mechanical impact of the pleural fluid on the diaphragm, chest wall, and compressed lung all contribute significantly to dyspnea, but may not be the only cause. Dyspnea in a patient with advanced lung cancer is very common. The majority of lung cancer patients will have dyspnea at some point during their illness and MPE is just one cause. Underlying poor lung function, parenchymal replacement by tumor, endobronchial obstruction, postobstructive pneumonia, and toxicity from treatment can also contribute to dyspnea in patients with advanced lung cancer (see Chapter 23). In a dyspneic patient with advanced lung cancer, evaluation is made for potentially correctable causes of dyspnea such as MPEs because these can be frequently palliated. It is also important to recognize the potential for multifactorial etiology for dyspnea and to note that removal of all the pleural fluid may not provide complete relief of symptoms.

Cough is another common problem in patients with advanced lung cancer, and the list of possible causes for cough is similar to that for dyspnea. Large pleural effusions are a treatable cause for cough, and lung cancer patients with cough should be evaluated for effusion and treated prior to attempting other palliative alternatives.

MALIGNANT EFFUSIONS IN NON–SMALL CELL LUNG CANCER

Malignant effusions occur in 7% to 15% of all lung cancer patients. Patients with non–small cell lung cancer (NSCLC) and associated malignant effusions are not considered to be curable, but have been classified as cT4M0, stage IIIB. These were frequently referred to as "wet IIIB" and treated in a manner very similar to stage IV disease. The International Association for the Study of Lung Cancer (IASLC) recently reviewed the current TMN staging for lung cancer and recommended several revisions (see Chapter 30).[3] One of the most significant of these revisions was to place pleural dissemination of disease, either by pleural effusion or pleural nodularity without evidence of other metastatic disease into an M1a classification, making it stage IV disease.[4] IASLC reviewed over 100,000 patients worldwide treated for primary NSCLC. Patients with pleural dissemination and without other metastatic disease (n = 488) had a median overall survival of 8 versus 13 months for other cT4M0 patients.[4] The 1- and 5-year survival patients with pleural dissemination were 36% and 2%. This was consistently worse than other T4M0 cases (where they were previously classified), but consistently better than cases with distant metastases where median survival is 4 to 7 months, hence, the new M1a classification.

PATHOGENESIS

A pleural effusion seen in association with a known lung cancer can be either malignant or paramalignant in nature. A malignant effusion is the result of direct pleural dissemination of disease. Paramalignant effusions are not a result of direct pleural involvement with tumor but are related to the primary tumor.[5] Examples of paramalignant effusions include chylothorax secondary to thoracic duct obstruction, postobstructive pneumonia from an obstructing tumor with an associated

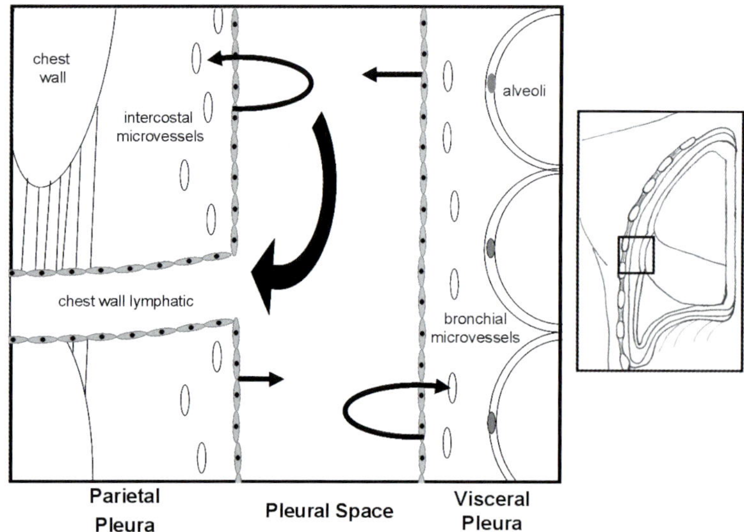

FIGURE 62.1 A schematic representation of pleural space, which demonstrates main patterns of fluid production and clearance. In the normal pleural space, the parietal pleural is the primary site of fluid production and absorption. In the setting of MPE, production and clearance of fluid can be abnormal on both the parietal and visceral surface, and obstruction of chest wall lymphatics play a significant role in fluid accumulation.

parapneumonic effusion, and an effusion secondary to hypoalbuminemia from cancer cachexia.

The pleural space is a moist "potential space." Effusions occur because of an imbalance in the normal equilibrium between production and clearance of fluid in that space. Anything that results in increased fluid formation or decrease in absorption will result in an effusion (Fig. 62.1). Changes in the oncotic fluid gradient from hypoalbuminemia secondary to cancer cachexia or in the hydrostatic fluid gradient from heart failure will alter the normal forces of filtration in the intercostal and bronchial microvasculature and result in a transudative effusion. Increased capillary permeability from disease processes that directly involve the pleura itself lead exudative effusions with leakage of both proteins and fluid into the pleural space. Effusions that result from tumor implants on the pleural surface will frequently also have abundant tumor cells in the pleural fluid. Effusion caused by lung cancer, breast cancer, and mesothelioma have been noted to have elevated levels of vascular endothelial growth factor (VEGF) in the pleural tissue and fluid. VEGF is a potent inflammatory mediator as well as an important mediator of vascular permeability and angiogenesis. Elevated VEGF levels secondary to pleural tumor involvement results in an increased capillary permeability and increased fluid production from the pleural surface.[6,7]

The most common mechanism for the formation of an MPE is decreased drainage of pleural fluid as a result of blockage of chest wall lymphatics.[8] Blockage anywhere along the lymphatic tract, from the stomata on the surface of the parietal pleura to the mediastinal nodes can result in accumulation of pleural fluid. The development of MPEs in lung cancer are more closely related to involvement of mediastinal lymph nodes than to direct pleural involvement by disease.[9]

DIAGNOSIS OF MALIGNANT PLEURAL EFFUSION

Following a careful history and physical examination, the workup for a suspected MPE proceeds through a series of diagnostic test that typically includes a chest x-ray, chest computer tomography (CT) scan, thoracentesis, pleural fluid analysis, and pleural biopsy. Many lung cancer patients will develop an effusion late in the course of their disease, but for some patients, the appearance of an effusion is their first evidence of malignancy. In patients with unilateral effusion of unknown etiology or bilateral effusions and no evidence of heart failure, diagnostic workup is recommended.

RADIOGRAPHIC IMAGING

Posterior–anterior (PA) and lateral chest x-ray can detect as little as 50 cc of fluid in the pleural space with blunting of the posterior costophrenic recess on lateral view and approximately 200 cc of fluid will cause blunting of the lateral recess on the PA view.[10] Decubitus films can detect 100 cc of free-flowing effusion.[11] Larger effusions produce a meniscus sign along the lateral chest wall and very large effusions will completely opacify ("white out") the pleural space. Massive effusions can cause inversion of the diaphragm and a shift of the mediastinum to the contralateral side.

Chest CT scan with contrast has become the imaging modality of choice for better definition and visualization of a suspected MPE. CT findings characteristic of an MPE include circumferential pleural thickening, nodularity, involvement of mediastinal pleural, and evidence of a primary pulmonary tumor. Diagnostic sensitivity of these findings range from 88% to 100% and specificity from 22% to 56%.[12,13] Histologic confirmation is necessary, despite a convincing image on CT scan.

Magnetic resonance imaging (MRI) provides excellent imaging of soft tissues and can provide useful information on chest wall and diaphragmatic invasion. MRI is highly sensitive for the detection of even very small pleural effusions and, with triple pulse technology, can differentiate transudative from exudative effusions, but CT scan remains the diagnostic exam of choice.

The experience with positron emission technology (PET) for the diagnosis of MPE is limited to date. In a series of 98 patients evaluated for suspected MPE, PET demonstrated sensitivity of 96.8% and specificity of 88.5% for the detection of malignancy.[14] False-positive exams occurred in patients with inflammatory pleural disease, such as parapneumonic effusion. Of note, talc pleurodesis causes pleural thickening and increased activity on PET that can mimic the appearance of pleural involvement by malignancy.[15]

DIAGNOSTIC THORACENTESIS AND PLEURAL FLUID ANALYSIS

Patient who presents with a new pleural effusion should undergo diagnostic thoracentesis to establish transudative or exudative nature of the fluid, perform cytological evaluation, and determine the ability of the underlying lung to reexpand. Observation without thoracentesis is only recommended for patients with a well-recognized cause for the effusion, such as chronic heart failure or recent pneumonia. There are no absolute contraindications to thoracentesis; relative contraindications include small-sized effusions, bleeding disorders, anticoagulation, and mechanical ventilation. Complications associated with thoracentesis include pneumothorax, hemothorax, infection, and hemoptysis. Thoracentesis has traditionally been performed as a "blind" procedure where the needle is placed based on standard positioning and the appearance of fluid on radiographic imaging. Several studies have indicated that ultrasound guidance can assist even experienced physicians in selecting appropriate puncture site.[14,16–18]

The gross appearance of pleural fluid at thoracentesis can be suggestive of an MPE, if it is hemorrhagic or opalescent. Half of all hemorrhagic effusions are malignant and 11% of MPEs are bloody in nature.[19] The majority (90% to 97%) of MPEs are exudative, but malignancy is not the only cause of an exudative effusion. Inflammatory causes are also common, because anything that increases capillary permeability in the pleural space will result in leakage of both fluid and protein into the pleural space. Although, the presence of an unexplained exudative effusion is worrisome for malignancy, the absence of transudative properties does not rule out a malignant etiology.[20] Exudative properties are most commonly defined on the basis of the Light's criteria, which is outlined in Table 62.1. Overall diagnostic accuracy of Light's criteria is 93%.[21]

Pleural fluid from thoracentesis should be evaluated for lactate dehydrogenase (LDH), total protein, pH, glucose, and cell count. LDH and total protein are components of Light's criteria for determination of exudate versus transudate. Low glucose and pH are common in pleural space infections but are also seen in up to 30% of MPEs and can be prognostic with regard to palliation of effusion and overall survival.[22,23] The diagnostic yield from the cytological examination of fluid from thoracentesis is variable, ranging from

TABLE 62.1 Criteria for Establishment of Exudative Pleural Effusion

Light's Criteria	Abbreviated Light's Criteria	Two-Criteria Pleural Fluid Rule without Blood Test	Three-Criteria Pleural Fluid Rule without Blood Test
Pleural fluid-to-serum LDH ratio >0.6 or	—	—	—
Pleural fluid LDH >67% of normal serum LDH upper limit or	Pleural fluid LDH >67% of normal serum LDH upper limit or	Pleural fluid LDH >67% of normal serum LDH upper limit or	Pleural fluid LDH >67% of normal serum LDH upper limit or
Pleural fluid-to-serum protein ratio >0.5	Pleural fluid-to-serum protein ratio >0.5	—	—
		Pleural fluid cholesterol >450 mg/L	Pleural fluid cholesterol >450 mg/L or Pleural fluid protein >30 mg/L

62% to 90%.[24–29] Increasing the volume of pleural fluid sent for cytological evaluation does not increase the sensitivity.[28] If a diagnosis is not made by initial thoracentesis, a second drainage can be attempted with approximately a 25% increase in yield, but the increase in yield drops dramatically after two attempts.[30] Repeated diagnostic aspirations beyond two are not recommended because of low diagnostic yield and increasing risk for infection and loculation. Closed pleural biopsy with an Abrams or Cope needle is often attempted when initial cytology is negative. Although the diagnostic yield from closed biopsy when combined with cytology can be as high as 80%,[31] it has very small diagnostic yield in cases where the initial cytological evaluation was negative.[26] Therefore, if two consecutive percutaneous drainages provide no diagnosis, thoracoscopy is recommended. Video-assisted thoracoscopic surgery (VATS) allows for wide examination of the pleural space and for large visually directed pleural biopsies. Diagnostic sensitivity for VATS procedures is reported at greater than 90% with specificity of 100% and perioperative mortality is less than 0.5%.[32,33]

The addition of tumor marker evaluation to the analysis of pleural fluid has been investigated. Carcinoembryonic antigen (CEA), carbohydrate antigen 15-3 (CA 15-3), cytokeratin 19, and cancer antigen 125 (CA-125) analysis can all be performed, but their diagnostic value remains limited.[34] No single marker has sufficient specificity to add to routine practice. In cases of NSCLC, epidermal growth factor receptor (EGFR) analysis of MPE is proving useful. EGFR mutations can be detected from cells in MPEs, helping to identify a group of patients likely to benefit from EGFR-targeted therapies.[35] DNA methylation analysis appears to carry significant diagnostic value in MPEs. Brock et al.[36] detected DNA methylation in 59% of MPEs but in none of the benign effusions evaluated. The addition of methylation studies to standard cytological evaluation increases both the sensitivity and the negative predictive value compared to cytology alone.[29,36]

TREATMENT

The goal of treatment in a patient with a malignant effusion from lung cancer or other tumors is palliation of symptoms. MPEs occur in a diverse patient population with variable life expectancies. A small percentage of patients are robust and will have life expectancies of months to years, whereas many patients are frail with advanced disease and significant cancer-related comorbidity with life expectancy of only days to weeks. It is important to appropriately tailor therapy to the best needs of the individual patient. Successful palliation of an MPE is judged by long-term relief of symptoms related to the effusion and no evidence of reaccumulation of fluid on chest radiograph until death. Removal of the effusion, improvement in symptoms, and prevention of reaccumulation do not signify a cure or prolong expected survival from the underlying malignancy, but inappropriate management of an MPE can shorten expected survival by compromising respiratory function.

The two most common treatment options currently used for MPE are pleurodesis or the insertion of a chronic indwelling tunneled pleural catheter. There are numerous other treatment options from noninvasive approaches such as observation or repeated thoracentesis, to the very aggressive procedures such as pleurectomy. The use of systemic chemotherapy has limited use in palliation form MPE except in small cell lung cancer, where many patients will respond to chemotherapy with resolution of their effusion and associated dyspnea.[37] Similarly, MPEs rarely respond to mediastinal radiation except in the case of some lymphomas where the effusion is a result of obstruction of mediastinal lymphatics that can be relieved following radiation.[38]

Observation Observation alone is recommended for those patients who are asymptomatic from their effusion or in the small number of patients (<2%) in whom there is no fluid reaccumulation following thoracentesis.[1,39] Observation and supportive care are also reasonable options for those patients who are very frail and whose life expectancy is in days. Supportive care in this situation also includes the use of opioids and oxygen therapy to ease the anxiety associated with dyspnea.[40]

Serial Thoracentesis Thoracentesis is very effective at acutely alleviating symptoms associated with MPE and has an important role in the diagnosis and planning treatment, but it has limited value as therapeutic approach. From 98% to 100% of MPE associated with lung cancer will reoccur within the first month of the initial thoracentesis.[1,39] Serial thoracentesis usually need to be performed frequently with an interval dependent on the rate of fluid accumulation. Repeated thoracentesis can lead to pneumothorax, fluid loculation, and empyema. This approach is only recommended in patients whose life expectancy is days to weeks, those who are too frail for pleurodesis or insertion of a chronic indwelling tunneled pleural catheter, or in the very rare patient with a very slowly reaccumulating effusion.

Chest Tube Drainage Alone The most common use of chest tube drainage for MPE is to provide apposition of the parietal and visceral pleural surfaces for subsequent pleurodesis. Prior to the introduction chronic indwelling tunneled pleural catheters, chronic chest tubes were frequently used for palliation of patients with MPE refractory to pleurodesis. Chronic chest tubes were used in patients with trapped lungs, where pleurodesis is not an option.(Fig. 62.2) Formerly, traditional large-bore tubes were used almost exclusively, because it was believed that they were less likely to clot and obstruct, but a series of trials in the 1990s indicated small-bore tubes (10 to 14 Fr) were as efficacious as larger tubes, and significantly more comfortable.[41,42]

Pleurodesis Pleurodesis is the most commonly performed procedure for the management of symptomatic MPEs. Pleurodesis is not appropriate management for all patients with an MPE. Prior to undertaking pleurodesis, one must consider if

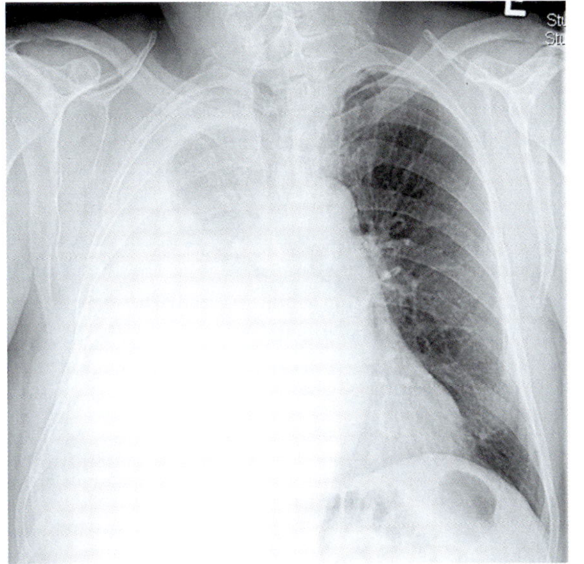

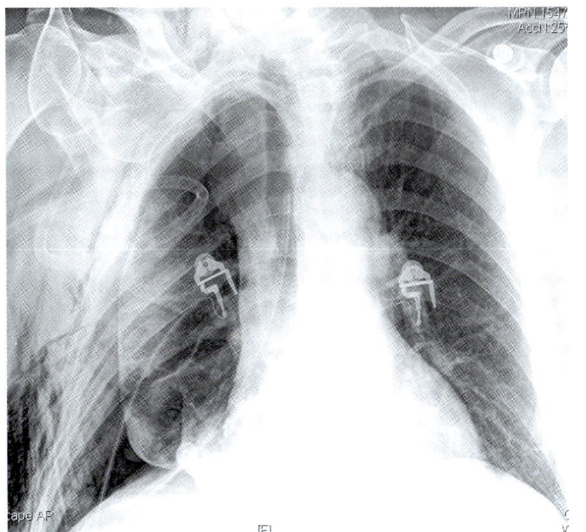

FIGURE 62.2 Chest radiographs demonstrating a patient with large right pleural effusion before (**A**) and after (**B**) large-volume drainage. The postdrainage film demonstrates classic appearance of "trapped lung" where the distribution of air in the pleural space corresponds to the previous distribution of pleural fluid.

the patient is a suitable candidate. In some histologies, specifically small cell lung cancer, MPEs respond to systemic therapy. These patients typically benefit from initial thoracentesis, but the effusion can then be followed as a measure of response to therapy. For other patients, the MPE is not the main source of dyspnea, and the removal of fluid from the pleural space does not improve their symptoms. Experts advise against pleurodesis only for patients with life expectancies less than 2 to 3 months to justify the cost, risk, and discomfort of the procedure. In other patients, the underlying lung has become trapped by long-standing fluid or excessive tumor on the lung surface (Fig. 62.2), and without apposition of the pleural surfaces, pleurodesis is not possible.

The goal of pleurodesis is to create fibrosis of the pleural space that obliterates the space, either by chemical or mechanical means. The most common methods employ chemical sclerosants or irritants, which achieve pleural symphysis through an inflammatory process. After complete drainage of the effusion, the sclerosants are usually instilled into the pleural space either at the bedside via a chest tube or in the operating room during thoracoscopy (VATS). For a pleurodesis to be successful, the lung needs to be completely expanded so that the pleural surfaces are in direct apposition. Incomplete drainage and undisrupted loculations decrease the success rate of pleurodesis. Pleural fluid glucose concentration <60 mg/dL, LDH concentration >600 U/L, and pH <7.30 are all predictive of lower success rate of pleurodesis.[22,23] The overall complete response rate to chemical pleurodesis is 64%.[5,43] Over the past 20 years, a large number of different sclerosing agents have been used, and some of the most frequently used are included in Table 62.2 with their relative rates of success and recommended doses.

The ideal sclerosant for pleurodesis remains controversial. The most commonly used agents today are talc, bleomycin, and doxycycline. The exact mechanism of how pleurodesis is established is not entirely clear, but it is related to the release of proinflammatory mediators that promote fibrosis.[44] Chest pain, atelectasis, pneumonia, fever, dysrhythmia, empyema, and respiratory failure have all been reported with talc pleurodesis.[45–47] Hypoxemia and respiratory failure following talc pleurodesis are more dependent on the particle size of the talc than on the dose or the route of administration.[47,48]

TABLE 62.2 Sclerosing Agents for Pleurodesis

Sclerosing Agent	Success Rates	Standard Dose
Talc[45,55,65–67]	70%–100%	2.55–10 mg
Nitrogen mustard[68,69]	27%–95%	0.4 mg/kg
Tetracycline[69,70]	70%	20 mg/kg in 50 mL NaCl 0.9%
Doxycyclin[71,72]	60%–80%	500 mg in 30 mL NaCl 0.9%
Bleomycin[73–75]	64%–84%	60 U in 100 mL NaCl 0.9% (1 U/kg)
Quinacrine[76–78]	64%–100%	500 mg
Corynebacterium parvum[79–82]	65%–92%	3.5–14 mg
OK-43[83,84]	73%–79%	

Respiratory failure is more common with talc preparations, which have a mean particle size less than 15 μm.[49] Smaller talc particles have the ability to move from the pleural space into pulmonary vascular bed and initiate systemic inflammation. This phenomenon has been demonstrated in both animal and human models.[50,51] Talc preparations carry vary significantly in particle size,[52] which may explain some of the large discrepancy between rates of respiratory failure following talc pleurodesis reported by different institutions.[45,53] It is now recommended that only size-calibrated talc with a mean particle size greater than 20 μm and no particle less than 10 μm be used.

Two main pleurodesis techniques have emerged, VATS pleurodesis and bedside pleurodesis via chest tube. The VATS and bedside procedures differ in several aspects, which can have an affect on their success rate. First, VATS procedures allow for more complete drainage of the effusion prior to pleurodesis. Small loculation and flimsy adhesions can be broken down to completely free the lung within the pleural space. Second, VATS also provides a more complete evaluation of the pleural space and better determination of whether or not the lung is trapped. Small- to moderate-sized areas where the lung does not approximate the chest wall are better seen at VATS than on chest radiograph, and these spaces decrease the success of pleurodesis and may alter treatment choices when recognized. Third, the distribution of sclerosants over the entire pleural space has the potential to be more complete in a VATS procedure than via installation at the bedside because of the ability to disrupt loose adhesions. VATS also allows for visually directed biopsies in those patients with a suspected MPE and no diagnosis. Perioperative mortality needs to be considered but is reported at less than 1%.[32,33] There are also several advantages to bedside pleurodesis over a VATS procedure. It can be performed quickly and easily by a single person. It does not require the use of sedation or general anesthesia or the availability of an operating room. So, as with other aspects of the management of MPE, the decision between a bedside or VATS pleurodesis is often individualized to each clinical scenario, with the priority being the quickest and safest way to palliate the patient with the shortest time in hospital.

In clinical practice, there appears to be little consensus on the optimal pleurodesis strategy. Numerous clinical trials on the topic of pleurodesis have been performed, but their results are very difficult to interpret because of the small number of patients, short life expectancy of the study population, numerous histologies investigated, numerous sclerosing agents employed, and multiple approaches undertaken. Two large metaanalyses have recently been published on the topic pleurodesis for palliation of MPE, and an overview of these analyses is outlined in Table 62.3. The first is authored by Shaw and Agarwal[54] from the Cochrane Collaboration. They identified 36 randomized control trials with 1499 subjects

TABLE 62.3 Synopsis of Two Recent Metaanalyses of Pleurodesis for Malignant Pleural Effusions

Metaanalysis	Cochrane[54]	British[55]
Author	Shaw and Agarwal	Tan, et al.
Journal	Cochrane Database of Systemic Reviews	European Journal of Cardio-thoracic Surgery
Year published	2004	2006
Time frame	1980–2002	1980–2003
No. RCTs evaluated	36	46
Total no. of pts	1499	2053
Findings re: sclerosing agents	* Talc most efficacious with **RR of nonrecurrence of effusion of 1.34** (95% CI, 1.16–1.55) compared to bleomycin, tetracycline, mustine, or drainage alone (6 studies, 186 pts)	* Talc is *not* more efficacious than other agents with **RR of recurrence of 0.65 (95% CI, 0.34–1.20)** compared to bleomycin, **RR of recurrence of 0.50 (95% CI, 0.06–4.42)** compared to tetracycline, and **RR of recurrence of 0.21 (95% CI, 0.05–0.87)** compared to mustine (9 studies, 341 pts)
Findings re: pleurodesis technique	* VATS pleurodesis with talc more efficacious with **RR of nonrecurrence of effusion of 1.19 (95% CI, 1.04–1.36)** compared to bedside talc pleurodesis (2 studies, 112 pts) * VATS pleurodesis with any agent was more efficacious with **RR of nonrecurrence of 1.68** (95% CI, 1.35–2.10) compared to bedside pleurodesis (5 studies, 145 pts)	* VATS pleurodesis with talc was more efficacious with **RR of recurrence of 0.21** (95% CI, 0.05–0.93) compared to bedside talc pleurodesis. (2 studies, 112 pts) * VATS pleurodesis with tetracycline was ***not*** more efficacious with **RR of recurrence of 1.05** (95% CI, 0.57–1.94) compared to bedside tetracycline pleurodesis (1 study)

CI, confidence interval; pts, patients; RCT, randomized controlled trial; RR, relative risk; VATS, video-assisted thoracoscopic surgery.

over the 22-year period between 1980 and 2002 and focused on a comparison of the most commonly used sclerosants, talc, bleomycin, and tetracycline and on a comparison of the most common methods of installation, VATS versus bedside. The analysis determined that the relative risk (RR) for success favored talc over bleomycin (RR = 1.23; 95% confidence interval [CI], 1.00 to 1.50) or tetracycline (RR = 1.32; 95% CI, 1.01 to 1.72). Bleomycin and tetracycline were found to be equally effective (RR = 1.03; 95% CI, 0.89 to 1.20). In the six trials that reported mortality, there was no statistically significant difference in the RR for mortality between talc and bleomycin (RR = 1.39; 95% CI, 0.84 to 2.30) or tetracycline (RR = 2.26; 95% CI, 0.95 to 5.39). In a comparison of VATS and bedside installation of various sclerosants, they found the RR of success favored VATS (RR = 1.68; 95% CI, 1.35 to 2.10), but noted the confounding effects of multiple sclerosing agents being compared. The second metaanalysis, from a British group, Tan et al.[55] identified 46 randomized control trials over a similar time period. They found a trend favoring talc over other sclerosing agents, but no statistically conclusive evidence supporting the use of one sclerosing agent over another. They identified only two trials comparing VATS to bedside procedures with the same agent. Although these trials found VATS procedures were associated with fewer recurrences, they did not feel that this was strong enough evidence to recommend VATS over bedside procedures. The recommendation rendered from the analysis was that the decision be made according to such factors as the overall health of the patient, the need for a biopsy and the delay required to get the patient to the operating room. In an evidence-based review by the American College of Chest Physicians (ACCP), they report the overall success rates for palliation of MPE with talc pleurodesis is >90%, but make no recommendations on VATS versus bedside use.[40]

Chronic Indwelling Pleural Catheter The introduction of the Pleurx catheter (Cardinal Health, Dublin, OH) has had a significant impact on the management of MPEs. The Pleurx is small-bore, chronic indwelling, tunneled silicone catheter for use in the pleural space. It is designed for intermittent outpatient drainage for the relief of symptoms associated with pleural effusion. The catheter has a fenestrated end that is placed in the pleural space, a velcro cuff that is placed in a tunnel under the subcutaneous tissues, and an externalized end with a one-way valve that requires canalization for drainage (Fig. 62.3A). The Pleurx can be inserted percutaneously using the Seldinger technique or at the time of a VATS procedure. The catheter can be attached to a pleurovac for continuous in-hospital drainage, but in general, it is designed for outpatient use. The externalized end of the catheter is capped and placed under a dressing on the patient's chest wall for the majority of the time. It is intermittently undressed and attached to a vacuum bottle (Fig. 62.3B) for evacuation of pleural fluid. Drainage kits with vacuum bottles (600 or 1000 mL) and all necessary dressing supplies are individually packaged and delivered to the patient's home. The catheter and drainage procedure are intended for use by family members, rather than healthcare professionals. The ease of catheter placement and drainage, low complication rates, increased patient comfort, decreased need for hospitalization, and decreased cost have made these catheters the overwhelming treatment of choice for patients with a trapped lung or who those who have failed pleurodesis.[56–59] It is also advocated by many as first-line treatment of MPEs.[56,57,59,60] It has equivalent efficacy to pleurodesis and have decreased the length of hospitalization and decreased costs associated with the palliation of MPEs.[57] In select patients and in select centers, Pleurx catheters are inserted in the outpatient setting.[57] From 40% to 58% of patients managed with a chronic indwelling pleural catheter achieve pleurodesis within 2 to 6 weeks of insertion without the use of any sclerosing agents.[56,59,61] Sclerosants can also be inserted through the catheter if spontaneous pleurodesis is not achieved after several weeks of drainage. Removal following sclerosis is simple and typically performed with local anesthetic in an outpatient setting.

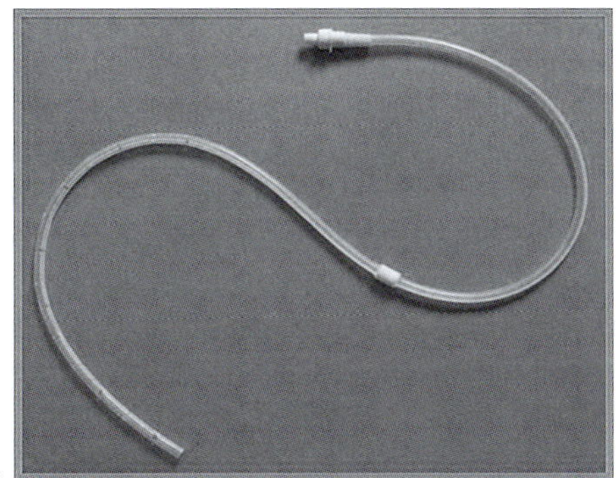
A

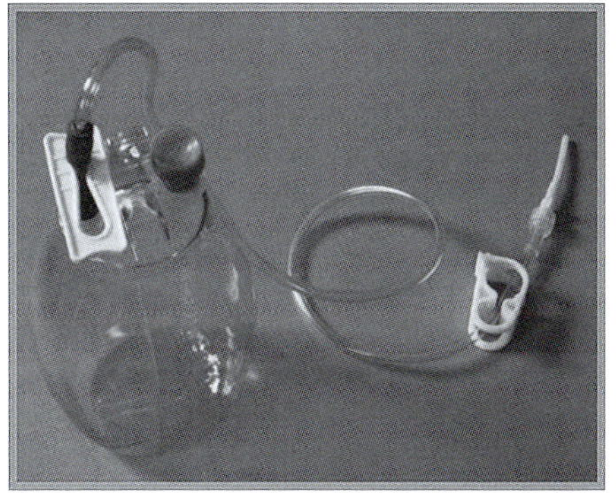
B

FIGURE 62.3 The Pleurx (Cardinal Health, Dublin, OH) catheter system. **A:** Silicone tunneled, indwelling catheter. The fenestrated end is inserted into pleural space, cuff is placed in subcutaneous tissues, and capped end is externalized. **B:** The drainage system is inserted into one-way valve on externalized end of catheter, and is available as 600- and 1000-mL size.

Pleuroperitoneal Shunt Prior to the introduction of the Pleurx catheter, indwelling pleuroperitoneal shunting was the management of choice for refractory or recurrent MPEs that could not be controlled by pleurodesis.[62,63] The shunts are typically placed in the operating room, with one end of the silicone catheter placed in the pleural space and the other tunneled into the abdomen and with a one-way pump between the two ends placed over the costal margin in the subcutaneous tissues. Each compression of the pump transports approximately 1.5 mL of fluid; patients are asked to compress the pump 5 to 10 times at least four times each day, but may be required to pump it >100 times per day for high-volume effusions. Complications hamper the utility of these catheters in approximately 15% of users, the most common issue being occlusion secondary to fibrinous material in the pumping mechanism.[64]

Pleurectomy Total parietal pleurectomy has nearly 100% success rate for the control of MPEs, but it does so at a high cost in terms of morbidity, mortality, and hospital stay. The majority of patients with MPE have limited life expectancy and therefore, other less invasive palliative options should be used.

CONCLUSION

Malignant pleural effusions are a common clinical condition in patients with end-stage lung cancer and other malignancies. Therapy is directed at palliation of symptoms rather than cure, but inappropriate management can decrease survival and severely impact quality of life. Prior to therapeutic intervention, a careful assessment of the effusion and the pleural space is combined with an evaluation of the patient's functional capacity and prognosis. Therapeutic options are then individualized to the patient's unique needs. Pleurodesis with talc or other sclerosants or insertion of a chronic indwelling tunneled pleural catheter are the most frequent modalities currently used for control of symptoms.

REFERENCES

1. Antunes G, Neville E, Duffy J, et al. BTS guidelines for the management of malignant pleural effusions. *Thorax* 2003;58(Suppl 2):II29–II38.
2. Martínez-Moragón E, Aparicio J, Sanchis J, et al. Malignant pleural effusion: prognostic factors for survival and response to chemical pleurodesis in a series of 120 cases. *Respiration* 1998;65(2):108–113.
3. Mountain CF. Revisions in the International System for Staging Lung Cancer. *Chest* 1997;111(6):1710–1717.
4. Postmus PE, Brambilla E, Chansky K, et al. The IASLC Lung Cancer Staging Project: proposals for revision of the M descriptors in the forthcoming (seventh) edition of the TNM classification of lung cancer. *J Thorac Oncol* 2007;2(8):686–693.
5. Antony VB, Loddenkemper R, Astoul P, et al. Management of malignant pleural effusions. *Eur Respir J* 2001;18(2):402–419.
6. Cheng D, Lee YC, Rogers JT, et al. Vascular endothelial growth factor level correlates with transforming growth factor-beta isoform levels in pleural effusions. *Chest* 2000;118(6):1747–1753.
7. Zebrowski BK, Yano S, Liu W, et al. Vascular endothelial growth factor levels and induction of permeability in malignant pleural effusions. *Clin Cancer Res* 1999;5(11):3364–3368.
8. Lynch TJ Jr. Management of malignant pleural effusions. *Chest* 1993; 103(4 Suppl):S385–S389.
9. Meyer PC. Metastatic carcinoma of the pleura. *Thorax* 1966;21(5): 437–443.
10. Blackmore CC, Black WC, Dallas RV, et al. Pleural fluid volume estimation: a chest radiograph prediction rule. *Acad Radiol* 1996;3(2):103–109.
11. Tattersall M. Pleural effusions. *Curr Opin Oncol* 1992;4(4):642–646.
12. Traill ZC, Davies RJ, Gleeson FV. Thoracic computed tomography in patients with suspected malignant pleural effusions. *Clin Radiol* 2001; 56(3):193–196.
13. Leung AN, Müller NL, Miller RR. CT in differential diagnosis of diffuse pleural disease. *AJR Am J Roentgenol* 1990;154(3):487–492.
14. Duysinx B, Nguyen D, Louis R, et al. Evaluation of pleural disease with 18-fluorodeoxyglucose positron emission tomography imaging. *Chest* 2004;125(2):489–493.
15. Kwek BH, Aquino SL, Fischman AJ. Fluorodeoxyglucose positron emission tomography and CT after talc pleurodesis. *Chest* 2004;125(6): 2356–2360.
16. Feller-Kopman D. Therapeutic thoracentesis: the role of ultrasound and pleural manometry. *Curr Opin Pulm Med* 2007;13(4):312–318.
17. Barnes TW, Morgenthaler TI, Olson EJ, et al. Sonographically guided thoracentesis and rate of pneumothorax. *J Clin Ultrasound* 2005; 33(9):442–446.
18. Diacon AH, Schuurmans MM, Theron J, et al. Safety and yield of ultrasound-assisted transthoracic biopsy performed by pulmonologists. *Respiration* 2004;71(5):519–522.
19. Villena V, López-Encuentra A, García-Luján R, et al. Clinical implications of appearance of pleural fluid at thoracentesis. *Chest* 2004; 125(1):156–159.
20. Ryu JS, Ryu ST, Kim YS, et al. What is the clinical significance of transudative malignant pleural effusion? *Korean J Intern Med* 2003; 18(4):230–233.
21. Heffner JE, Highland K, Brown LK. A meta-analysis derivation of continuous likelihood ratios for diagnosing pleural fluid exudates. *Am J Respir Crit Care Med* 2003;167(12):1591–1599.
22. Good JT Jr, Taryle DA, Sahn SA. The pathogenesis of low glucose, low pH malignant effusions. *Am Rev Respir Dis* 1985;131(5):737–741.
23. Sahn SA, Good JT Jr. Pleural fluid pH in malignant effusions. Diagnostic, prognostic, and therapeutic implications. *Ann Intern Med* 1988;108(3):345–349.
24. Prakash UB, Reiman HM. Comparison of needle biopsy with cytologic analysis for the evaluation of pleural effusion: analysis of 414 cases. *Mayo Clinic Proc* 1985;60(3):158–164.
25. Woenckhaus M, Grepmeier U, Werner B, et al. Microsatellite analysis of pleural supernatants could increase sensitivity of pleural fluid cytology. *J Mol Diagn* 2005;7(4):517–524.
26. Nance KV, Shermer RW, Askin FB. Diagnostic efficacy of pleural biopsy as compared with that of pleural fluid examination. *Mod Pathol* 1991;4(3):320–324.
27. Ong KC, Indumathi V, Poh WT, et al. The diagnostic yield of pleural fluid cytology in malignant pleural effusions. *Singapore Med J* 2000; 41(1):19–23.
28. Sallach SM, Sallach JA, Vasquez E, et al. Volume of pleural fluid required for diagnosis of pleural malignancy. *Chest* 2002;122(6):1913–1917.
29. Benlloch S, Galbis-Caravajal JM, Martin C, et al. Potential diagnostic value of methylation profile in pleural fluid and serum from cancer patients with pleural effusion. *Cancer* 2006;107(8):1859–1865.
30. Garcia LW, Ducatman BS, Wang HH. The value of multiple fluid specimens in the cytological diagnosis of malignancy. *Mod Pathol* 1994; 7(6):665–668.
31. Edmondstone WM. Investigation of pleural effusion: comparison between fibreoptic thoracoscopy, needle biopsy and cytology. *Respir Med* 1990;84(1):23–26.

32. Lee YC, Light RW. Management of malignant pleural effusions. *Respirology* 2004;9(2):148–156.
33. Maskell NA, Butland RJ. BTS guidelines for the investigation of a unilateral pleural effusion in adults. *Thorax* 2003;58(Suppl 2): II8–II17.
34. Porcel JM, Vives M, Esquerda A, et al. Use of a panel of tumor markers (carcinoembryonic antigen, cancer antigen 125, carbohydrate antigen 15-3, and cytokeratin 19 fragments) in pleural fluid for the differential diagnosis of benign and malignant effusions. *Chest* 2004;126(6): 1757–1763.
35. Hung MS, Lin CK, Leu SW, et al. Epidermal growth factor receptor mutations in cells from non-small cell lung cancer malignant pleural effusions. *Chang Gung Med J* 2006;29(4):373–379.
36. Brock MV, Hooker CM, Yung R, et al. Can we improve the cytologic examination of malignant pleural effusions using molecular analysis? *Ann Thorac Surg* 2005;80(4):1241–1247.
37. Livingston RB, McCracken JD, Trauth CJ, et al. Isolated pleural effusion in small cell lung carcinoma: favorable prognosis. A review of the Southwest Oncology Group experience. *Chest* 1982;81(2): 208–211.
38. Xaubet A, Diumenjo MC, Mańin A, et al. Characteristics and prognostic value of pleural effusions in non-Hodgkin's lymphomas. *Eur J Respir Dis* 1985;66(2):135–140.
39. Sørensen PG, Svendsen TL, Enk B. Treatment of malignant pleural effusion with drainage, with and without instillation of talc. *Eur J Respir Dis* 1984;65(2):131–135.
40. Kvale PA, Selecky PA, Prakash UB. Palliative care in lung cancer: ACCP evidence-based clinical practice guidelines (2nd edition). *Chest* 2007;132(3 Suppl):S368–S403.
41. Sahin U, Unlü M, Akkaya A, et al. The value of small-bore catheter thoracostomy in the treatment of malignant pleural effusions. *Respiration* 2001;68(5):501–505.
42. Parulekar W, Di Primio G, Matzinger F, et al. Use of small-bore vs large-bore chest tubes for treatment of malignant pleural effusions. *Chest* 2001; 120(1):19–25.
43. Walker-Renard PB, Vaughan LM, Sahn SA. Chemical pleurodesis for malignant pleural effusions. *Ann Intern Med* 1994;120(1):56–64.
44. Marchi E, Vargas FS, Acencio MM, et al. Evidence that mesothelial cells regulate the acute inflammatory response in talc pleurodesis. *Eur Respir J* 2006;28(5):929–932.
45. Dresler CM, Olak J, Herndon JE II, et al. Phase III intergroup study of talc poudrage vs talc slurry sclerosis for malignant pleural effusion. *Chest* 2005;127(3):909–915.
46. Brant A, Eaton T. Serious complications with talc slurry pleurodesis. *Respirology* 2001;6(3):181–185.
47. de Campos JR, Vargas FS, de Campos Werebe E, et al. Thoracoscopy talc poudrage: a 15-year experience. *Chest* 2001;119(3):801–806.
48. Rehse DH, Aye RW, Florence MG. Respiratory failure following talc pleurodesis. *Am J Surg* 1999;177(5):437–440.
49. Maskell NA, Lee YC, Gleeson FV, et al. Randomized trials describing lung inflammation after pleurodesis with talc of varying particle size. *Am J Respir Crit Care Med* 2004;170(4):377–382.
50. Froudarakis ME, Klimathianaki M, Pougounias M. Systemic inflammatory reaction after thoracoscopic talc poudrage. *Chest* 2006; 129(2):356–361.
51. Ferrer J, Montes JF, Villarino MA, et al. Influence of particle size on extrapleural talc dissemination after talc slurry pleurodesis. *Chest* 2002; 122(3):1018–1027.
52. Ferrer J, Villarino MA, Tura JM, et al. Talc preparations used for pleurodesis vary markedly from one preparation to another. *Chest* 2001; 119(6):1901–1905.
53. Kuzniar TJ, Blum MG, Kasibowska-Kuzniar K, et al. Predictors of acute lung injury and severe hypoxemia in patients undergoing operative talc pleurodesis. *Ann Thorac Surg* 2006;82(6):1976–1981.
54. Shaw P, Agarwal R. Pleurodesis for malignant pleural effusions. *Cochrane Database Syst Rev* 2004(I):CD002916.
55. Tan C, Sedrakyan A, Browne J, et al. The evidence on the effectiveness of management for malignant pleural effusion: a systematic review. *Eur J Cardiothorac Surg* 2006;29(5):829–838.
56. Putnam JB Jr, Light RW, Rodriguez RM, et al. A randomized comparison of indwelling pleural catheter and doxycycline pleurodesis in the management of malignant pleural effusions. *Cancer* 1999; 86(10):1992–1999.
57. Putnam JB Jr, Walsh GL, Swisher SG, et al. Outpatient management of malignant pleural effusion by a chronic indwelling pleural catheter. *Ann Thorac Surg* 2000;69(2):369–375.
58. Pollak JS, Burdge CM, Rosenblatt M, et al. Treatment of malignant pleural effusions with tunneled long-term drainage catheters. *J Vasc Interv Radiol* 2001;12(2):201–208.
59. Musani AI, Haas AR, Seijo L, et al. Outpatient management of malignant pleural effusions with small-bore, tunneled pleural catheters. *Respiration* 2004;71(6):559–566.
60. Ohm C, Park D, Vogen M, et al. Use of an indwelling pleural catheter compared with thorascopic talc pleurodesis in the management of malignant pleural effusions. *Am Surg* 2003;69(3):198–202; discussion 202.
61. Tremblay A, Michaud G. Single-center experience with 250 tunnelled pleural catheter insertions for malignant pleural effusion. *Chest* 2006; 129(2):362–368.
62. Little AG, Kadowaki MH, Ferguson MK, et al. Pleuro-peritoneal shunting. Alternative therapy for pleural effusions. *Ann Surg* 1988; 208(4):443–450.
63. Petrou M, Kaplan D, Goldstraw P. Management of recurrent malignant pleural effusions. The complementary role talc pleurodesis and pleuroperitoneal shunting. *Cancer* 1995;75(3):801–805.
64. Genc O, Petrou M, Ladas G, et al. The long-term morbidity of pleuroperitoneal shunts in the management of recurrent malignant effusions. *Eur J Cardiothorac Surg* 2000;18(2):143–146.
65. Gasparri R, Leo F, Veronesi G, et al. Video-assisted management of malignant pleural effusion in breast carcinoma. *Cancer* 2006; 106(2):271–276.
66. Kolschmann S, Ballin A, Gillissen A. Clinical efficacy and safety of thoracoscopic talc pleurodesis in malignant pleural effusions. *Chest* 2005; 128(3):1431–1435.
67. Stefani A, Natali P, Casali C, et al. Talc poudrage versus talc slurry in the treatment of malignant pleural effusion. A prospective comparative study. *Eur J Cardiothorac Surg* 2006;30(6):827–832.
68. Austin EH, Flye MW. The treatment of recurrent malignant pleural effusion. *Ann Thorac Surg* 1979;28(2):190–203.
69. Hausheer FH, Yarbro JW. Diagnosis and treatment of malignant pleural effusion. *Semin Oncol* 1985;12(1):54–75.
70. Fentiman IS. Effective treatment of malignant pleural effusions. *Br J Hosp Med* 1987;37(5):421, 424–428.
71. Heffner JE, Standerfer RJ, Torstveit J, et al. Clinical efficacy of doxycycline for pleurodesis. *Chest* 1994;105(6):1743–1747.
72. Porcel JM, Salud A, Nabal M, et al. Rapid pleurodesis with doxycycline through a small-bore catheter for the treatment of metastatic malignant effusions. *Support Care Cancer* 2006;14(5):475–478.
73. Sartori S, Tassinari D, Ceccotti P, et al. Prospective randomized trial of intrapleural bleomycin versus interferon alfa-2b via ultrasound-guided small-bore chest tube in the palliative treatment of malignant pleural effusions. *J Clin Oncol* 2004;22(7):1228–1233.
74. Haddad FJ, Younes RN, Gross JL, et al. Pleurodesis in patients with malignant pleural effusions: talc slurry or bleomycin? Results of a prospective randomized trial. *World J Surg* 2004;28(8):749–753; discussion 753–754.
75. Moffett MJ, Ruckdeschel JC. Bleomycin and tetracycline in malignant pleural effusions: a review. *Semin Oncol* 1992;19(2 Suppl 5):59–62; discussion 62–63.
76. Banerjee AK, Willetts I, Robertson JF, et al. Pleural effusion in breast cancer: a review of the Nottingham experience. *Eur J Surg Oncol* 1994; 20(1):33–36.

77. Stiksa G, Korsgaard R, Simonsson BG. Treatment of recurrent pleural effusion by pleurodesis with quinacrine. Comparison between instillation by repeated thoracenteses and by tube drainage. *Scand J Respir Dis* 1979;60(4):197–205.
78. Ukale V, Agrenius V, Hillerdal G, et al. Pleurodesis in recurrent pleural effusions: a randomized comparison of a classical and a currently popular drug. *Lung Cancer* 2004;43(3):323–328.
79. McLeod DT, Calverley PM, Millar JW, et al. Further experience of Corynebacterium parvum in malignant pleural effusion. *Thorax* 1985; 40(7):515–518.
80. Foresti V. Corynebacterium parvum for malignant pleural effusions. *Thorax* 1995;50(1):104.
81. Casali A, Gionfra T, Rinaldi M, et al. Treatment of malignant pleural effusions with intracavitary Corynebacterium parvum. *Cancer* 1988; 62(4):806–811.
82. Hillerdal G, Kiviloog J, Nöu E, et al. Corynebacterium parvum in malignant pleural effusion. A randomized prospective study. *Eur J Respir Dis* 1986;69(3):204–206.
83. Luh KT, Yang PC, Kuo SH, et al. Comparison of OK-432 and mitomycin C pleurodesis for malignant pleural effusion caused by lung cancer. A randomized trial. *Cancer* 1992;69(3):674–679.
84. Kasahara K, Shibata K, Shintani H, et al. Randomized phase II trial of OK-432 in patients with malignant pleural effusion due to non-small cell lung cancer. *Anticancer Res* 2006;26(2B):1495–1499.

CHAPTER 63

Young Kwok
Roy A. Patchell
William F. Regine

Management of Overt Central Nervous System Metastases: Brain and Spinal Cord

Brain metastasis is very common in cancer, with an annual incidence in the United States of approximately 170,000 to 200,000. The rising incidence of brain metastasis is most likely from a combination of increasing survival from recent advances in systemic therapy, and a greater availability and use of magnetic resonance imaging (MRI). The most common primary site is the lung (50%) followed by breast (15%). The average age at presentation is approximately 60 years, and the median survival is usually less than 1 year. Metastatic brain tumors outnumber primary brain tumors by almost a factor of 10 to 1, with autopsy series demonstrating a 10% to 30% incidence rate for all patients with a diagnosis of cancer.[1,2]

CLINICAL PRESENTATION, DIAGNOSIS, AND PROGNOSIS

Most patients present with significant neurologic signs and symptoms (Table 63.1).[3] Although differential diagnoses such as an abscess or a stroke must be considered, new-onset neurologic symptoms in a known cancer patient should always be presumed to be from brain metastasis until proven otherwise.

MRI has become the gold standard for imaging of the central nervous system in cancer patients.[4] Given its ability to image in multiple orientations and sequences, as well as having superior resolution and accuracy, it has replaced the older computed tomography (CT). MRI will frequently pick up smaller lesions not seen on CT scans, which can have a significant effect on the patient's prognosis and treatment course. Full systemic workup (e.g., positron emission tomography [PET] and CT) should be promptly initiated if brain metastasis is the presenting event. The incidence of unknown primaries may subsequently decrease with the increasing popularity of integrated PET/CT scans.

Performance status and extracranial disease status have consistently been shown to impact prognosis. Gaspar et al.[5] reported on the Radiation Oncology Therapy Group (RTOG) the experience of 1200 patients, which is summarized in Table 63.2. This analysis revealed three recursive partitioning analysis (RPA) classes, with the RPA class I (Karnofsky performance score [KPS] ≥70, controlled primary, age <65 years, brain metastasis only), II (not meeting requirements of classes I or III), and III (KPS <70) having median survivals of 7.1, 4.2, and 2.3 months, respectively.

CORTICOSTEROIDS

In symptomatic patients, the initial therapy should promptly start with corticosteroids (e.g., dexamethasone or methylprednisolone), which effectively improve edema and neurologic deficits in approximately two thirds of patients.[6] The only randomized trial on the dosage question was reported by Vecht et al.[7] This trial included two successive groups of patients. The first group (n = 47) evaluated 8 versus 16 mg/day initial dexamethasone doses, with tapering schedules over 4 weeks. The second group (n = 49) evaluated 4 versus 16 mg/day of initial dexamethasone, with continuation of these doses for 28 days before tapering. The patients were scheduled for whole-brain radiotherapy (WBRT) and concurrent ranitidine. All arms had similar KPS improvements at 7 days (54% to 70%) and 28 days (50% to 81%). The study concludes that 4 mg/day of dexamethasone (with a taper over 4 weeks) is the preferable regimen.

However, one should be cautious in interpreting the results of this study. Patients in the 4-mg/day arm had to have the medication reinstituted at a higher rate than the patients in the 8- or 16-mg/day arms. Furthermore, the arm with the greatest improvement in the KPS was the 16-mg/day arm when this was tapered over 4 weeks, compared with any of the other arms. It can be argued that higher KPS improvement arose from the maximal anti-inflammatory effects of the initial higher doses, with the 4-week taper minimizing the late toxicity associated with corticosteroids.

A reasonable corticosteroid regimen in patients with brain metastases is a 10-mg intravenous (IV) or oral bolus, followed

TABLE 63.1 Clinical Presentation of Brain Metastasis[3]

Symptom	Percent	Sign	Percent
Headache	49%	Hemiparesis	59%
Mental problems	32%	Cognitive deficits	58%
Focal weakness	30%	Sensory deficits	21%
Ataxia	21%	Papilledema	20%
Seizures	18%	Ataxia	19%
Speech problems	12%	Apraxia	18%

TABLE 63.2 RTOG Experience of Brain Metastasis: Recursive Partitioning Analysis[5]

Class	Factors	Median Survival
I	KPS ≥70	7.1 mos
	Controlled primary	
	Age <65	
	Brain metastasis only	
II	Not meeting class I or III	4.2 mos
III	KPS <70	2.3 mos

KPS, Karnofsky performance score; mos, months; RTOG, Radiation Therapy Oncology Group.

by a 4 to 6 mg every 6 to 8 hours of dexamethasone equivalent dose (with a concurrent proton pump inhibitor), before this is tapered in a clinically cautious manner. In asymptomatic patients with little peritumoral edema or mass effect, initial corticosteroids may be reserved until the first sign of neurologic symptoms.

WHOLE-BRAIN RADIOTHERAPY

WBRT continues to be the standard of care in patients with brain metastasis. In general, WBRT should be given soon after the diagnosis of multiple brain metastases. There has never been any evidence to suggest that delaying systemic chemotherapy for WBRT compromises overall survival (OS), especially when one considers that progression in the brain frequently leads directly to the death of the patient.

Multiple randomized studies have been performed to determine the optimum dose and fractionation of WBRT. Table 63.3 summarizes selected randomized studies on WBRT fractionation.[8–11] OS has not improved appreciably over the last 25 to 30 years. Typically, the radiographic and clinical response rates range from 50% to 75%. A total of 30 Gy in 10 fractions continues to be the standard for most patients. In chemotherapy refractory, RPA class III patients, a shorter fractionation scheme (e.g., 20 Gy in 5 fractions) should be considered. However, short fractionation schemes should be avoided in chemotherapy-naive patients with brain metastasis as the presenting event in the cancer diagnosis. The natural disease course of such patients can be frequently unpredictable, so they may live sufficiently long enough to experience late radiation toxicity posed by such short fractionation schedules.[12]

TABLE 63.3 Selected Randomized Trials Examining Various Fractionation Schedules of Whole-Brain Radiation for Patients with Multiple Brain Metastases

First Author/Study Group (Years)	Dose/Fractions	N	Median Survival	*p* Value
Borgelt/RTOG[8]				
First study (1971–1973)	30 Gy/10	233	21 wks	NS
	30 Gy/15	217	18 wks	
	40 Gy/15	233	18 wks	
	40 Gy/20	227	16 wks	
Second study (1973–1976)	20 Gy/5	447	15 wks	NS
	30 Gy/10	228	15 wks	
	40 Gy/15	227	18 wks	
Haie-Meder/French[9] (1986–1989)	25 Gy/10	110	4.2 mos	NS
	36 Gy/6*	106	5.3 mos	
Priestman/Royal College of Radiology[10] (1990–1993)	30 Gy/10	263	84 days	0.04
	12 Gy/2	270	77 days	
Murray/RTOG 91-04[11] (1991–1995)	30 Gy/10	213	4.5 mos	NS
	54.4 Gy/34†	216	4.5 mos	

*18 Gy/3 split course with another 18 Gy/3 within 1 month.

†54.4 Gy in 1.6 Gy bid hyperfractionation for the entire course of therapy.

mos, months; NS, not significant; RTOG, Radiation Therapy Oncology Group; wks, weeks.

SURGICAL RESECTION

Surgical resection can provide immediate relief of the tumor mass effect, whereas WBRT typically takes several days to work. Radiobiologically, 30 Gy in 10 fractions to a solid tumor (excluding radiosensitive tumors) is not adequate to achieve long-term tumor control. This issue is especially germane because historically, up to one half of all patients died from neurologic causes after being treated with WBRT alone.

There have now been three phase III trials testing the hypothesis that surgical resection to single brain metastasis is potentially beneficial. All three trials were on patients with a single lesion, which is defined as the presence of only one lesion in the brain regardless of the extracranial disease status, whereas a solitary lesion is defined as the presence of the CNS metastasis as the only site of the metastatic disease burden. Table 63.4 summarizes the three trials.[13–15] The studies by Patchell et al.[13] (KPS ≥70) and Noordijk et al.[14] (World Health Organization grade ≤2) included patients with better performance status compared with the Mintz et al.'s[15] study (KPS ≥50) that mainly contributed to the differences in the survival outcomes between the studies. The results of these studies suggest that surgical resection should be reserved for lesions causing life-threatening complications or those with good performance status (i.e., KPS ≥70).

RADIOSURGERY BOOST TRIALS

Radiosurgery provides an alternative to conventional surgery. The three randomized trials of surgical resection were performed before the widespread availability of stereotactic radiosurgery (SRS). Although no randomized trials have been performed comparing surgery with SRS, SRS appears to provide similar local control rates (in the order of 80% to 90% only when combined with WBRT). Unless the tumor causes significant edema and mass effect, with consequent hydrocephalus or herniation requiring urgent surgical intervention, SRS can serve as a noninvasive option. Frequently, a patient may not be a craniotomy

TABLE 63.4 Randomized Trials of Surgical Resection in Single Brain Metastasis

First Author/Study Group	Surgery + RT	RT alone	*p* Value
Patchell/University of Kentucky[13] (n = 48)			
Primary end point		(36 Gy/12 fx)	
Overall survival	40 wks	15 wks	<0.01
Secondary end points			
Local control			
Local failure	20%	52%	<0.02
Time to local failure	>59 wks	21 wks	<0.0001
Time to neurologic death	62 wks	26 wks	<0.0009
KPS ≥70 maintenance	38 wks	8 wks	<0.005
Noordijk/Dutch[14] (n = 63)			
Primary end points		(40 Gy/20 fx)*	
Overall survival	10 mos	6 mos	0.04
FIS†	7.5 mos	3.5 mos	0.06
Mintz/Canadian[15] (n = 84)			
Primary end point		(30 Gy/10 fx)	
Overall survival	5.6 mos	6.3 mos	NS
Secondary end points			
FIS (proportion of days, mean)‡	32%	32%	NS
Quality of life (Spitzer score)			
1–3 mos (mean)	6.38	5.36	NS
4–6 mos (mean)	6.32	6.15	NS

*40 Gy total in 2 Gy bid hyperfractionation for the entire course of therapy.

†FIS as defined by WHO performance status ≤1 and neurological condition ≤1.

‡FIS as defined by KPS ≥70.

FIS, functionally independent survival; fx, fraction number; KPS, Karnofsky performance score; mos, months; NS, not significant; RT, whole-brain radiotherapy; wks, weeks.

candidate because of tumor location in eloquent areas or existing medical contraindications. Although two of the three conventional surgery trials have shown a survival benefit in single brain metastasis, there have been no randomized trials addressing multiple lesions and the retrospective data available are contradictory. For SRS, there have been three randomized trials assessing the efficacy of SRS in the treatment of multiple metastases.[16–18] Key findings of the three trials are summarized in Table 63.5.

The first randomized trial was reported by Kondziolka et al.,[16] but this study was stopped early at a planned interim analysis of 60% patient accrual because the authors reported to have found a large difference in the primary end point of local control in favor of SRS (92% vs. 0%; $p = 0.0016$). Unfortunately, the study used nonstandard end points to measure recurrence, defining it as any increase in the lesion size on MRI rather than the more usual 25% increase in product of the diameter. Furthermore, no attempt was

TABLE 63.5 Randomized Trials of Stereotactic Radiosurgery Boost for Patients with Brain Metastasis

First Author/Study Group	RT+SRS	RT alone	SRS Alone	*p* Value
Kondziolka/University of Pittsburgh[16] (n = 27; 2–4 lesions)				
Primary end point		(30 Gy/12 fx)		
Local control (1 year)	92%	0%		0.0016
Time to local failure*	36 mos	6 mos		0.005
Time to any brain failure*	34 mos	5 mos		0.002
Secondary end points				
Overall survival	11 mos	7.5 mos		NS
Treatment morbidity	0	0		
Progression-free survival	Not reported			
Need for re-treatment	Not reported			
Andrews/RTOG 95-08[17] (n = 333; 1–3 lesions)				
Primary end point	(Overall survival)	(37.5 Gy/10 fx)		
1–3 lesions	5.7 mos	6.5 mos		NS
Single brain metastasis (planned subgroup analysis)	6.5 mos	4.9 mos		0.04
Secondary end points				
Local control (1 yr)	82%	71%		0.01
Neurologic death rate	28%	31%		NS
Performance outcome				
KPS stable/improve				
at 3 mos	50%	33%		0.02
at 6 mos	43%	27%		0.03
Mental status				NS
Unplanned subgroup analysis (overall survival)				
Largest tumor >2 cm	6.5 mos	5.3 mos		0.04
RPA class I	11.6 mos	9.6 mos		0.05
Squamous/NSCLC	5.9 mos	3.9 mos		0.05
Other Outcomes				
Response rate (3 mos)				
Tumor	73%	62%		0.04
Edema	70%	47%		0.002
Chougule/Brown University[18] (n = 109; 1–3 lesions)				
End points (abstract only)	(30 Gy + 20 Gy SRS)	(30 Gy/10 fx)	(30 Gy SRS)	
Overall survival*	5 mos	9 mos	7 mos	Not reported
Local control	91%	62%	87%	Not reported
New brain lesions	19%	23%	43%	Not reported

fx, fraction number; KPS, Karnofsky performance score; mos, months; NS, not significant; NSCLC, non–small cell lung cancer; RPA, recursive partitioning analysis; RT, whole-brain radiotherapy; RTOG, Radiation Therapy Oncology Group; SRS, stereotactic radiosurgery; yr, year.

made to control for corticosteroid use, radiation changes, or other factors that might produce small fluctuations in the lesion size on MRI. Therefore, this study is difficult to interpret.

The second trial was reported by Chougule et al.,[17] and the results are only available in abstract form.[17] This three arms trial randomized patients to treatment with SRS alone with Gamma Knife, SRS plus WBRT, or WBRT alone. This trial suffers from several serious methodological problems. Although the authors conclude that the survival times among the treatment arms were similar and that patients treated with SRS experienced superior local control and fewer brain metastases, no *p* values are reported. Furthermore, 51 of the patients had surgical resection for at least one symptomatic brain metastasis prior to entry into the study, and no attempt was made to stratify for previous surgery. The inclusion of the surgically resected patients effectively made this a six-arm trial and, therefore, the size of this trial was not large enough to support a meaningful analysis. Finally, the radiation doses used in the SRS arms cannot be considered conventional because the peripheral dose was not individualized based on the tumor size or volume. Thus, this study has not been interpretable.

The third study, RTOG 95-08, was reported by Andrews et al.[18] The primary end point was OS, which was not statistically different between the WBRT plus SRS and WBRT-alone arms (6.5 and 5.7 months, respectively; $p = 0.1356$), although SRS boost favored the survival in the subgroup (planned analysis) of patients with single metastasis. For secondary end points, the local control and performance measures were higher in the SRS boost arm, but this did not translate into a lower death rate from neurologic progression. Multiple, unplanned subgroup analyses were made, and an OS benefit with the SRS boost was found in several subgroups that included patients with RPA class 1, tumor size $\geq$2 cm, and non–small cell lung cancer (NSCLC) or metastatic squamous histology from any site. Unfortunately, these subset analyses were not planned or prespecified, and the *p* values needed for significance should have been adjusted for inflation of the type I error. When this was done, none of these subgroup analyses showed a positive benefit for SRS.[19] On the other hand, this trial did demonstrate that SRS is associated with lower edema and corticosteroid use, countering a commonly held notion that SRS actually increases the edema risk. However, with regard to the major end points for multiple metastases, this study should be considered a negative trial.

Although SRS boost is indicated (from RTOG 95-08 and from the extrapolation of surgical resection data) in patients with a single metastasis, it is difficult to justify its routine use in patients with multiple metastases in the light of the equivocal phase III SRS boost trials.

POSTOPERATIVE WHOLE-BRAIN RADIOTHERAPY

A controversy in the treatment of brain metastasis is the routine use of postoperative or post–SRS WBRT. In a multi-institutional retrospective SRS study, Sneed et al.[20] argue for the omission of upfront WBRT because this does not compromise OS. Unfortunately, only an OS analysis was performed, and no local control or retreatment data were given. In an earlier study by the same group of investigators, patients who were initially treated with SRS alone without WBRT experienced worse freedom from new brain metastasis and overall brain freedom from progression despite the imbalance of the prognostic factors that favored the SRS-alone group, although the OS was not different.[21] Because of the equivalency of OS, many have advocated withholding upfront WBRT. They often use repeat SRS for the failures, which can be very expensive. Furthermore, brain failure can lead to unacceptable consequences. For example, Regine et al.[22] reported on 36 patients with planned observation after initial SRS alone. Even with close follow-up with exams and high-resolution MRIs, 47% of patients experienced brain failure, with 71% and 59% experiencing symptomatic relapse and neurologic deficits, respectively.

The omission of upfront WBRT may have even more serious consequences for patients with more radioresistant tumors such as renal cell carcinoma (RCC). The SRS dose given is typically limited by tumor size and volume, and not by whether the patient received additional dose with WBRT. Therefore, a patient treated with WBRT plus SRS receives much higher tumor dose than SRS alone. It is then not a surprise that an Eastern Cooperative Oncology Group phase II study, which evaluated SRS alone in radioresistant tumors (RCC, melanoma, sarcoma), demonstrated very disappointing results,[23] reporting a 6-month total brain failure rate of 48.3%. The authors correctly conclude that routine avoidance of WBRT should be approached judiciously.

Fortunately, there have been two phase III trials that have assessed the use of postoperative WBRT (Table 63.6). Patchell et al.[24] demonstrated that surgical resection without WBRT led to a failure rate at the original site and the entire brain of 46% and 70%, respectively. More importantly, 44% of the patients in the surgery-alone arm died as a result of neurological sequalae from the brain failure. The results of this study have been frequently misinterpreted in the literature. Some have justified the withholding of upfront WBRT based on the fact that this study demonstrated equivalent survival. In fact, this study was designed with brain tumor recurrence rate as the primary end point and not OS. To show an OS difference, this trial needed to enroll over 2000 patients. The study met its primary end point and confirmed the importance of postoperative WBRT in preventing brain failure and death from neurologic causes.

Results of the JROSG 99-1 trial by Aoyoma et al.[25] demonstrated similar benefits of WBRT. In this phase III trial of 1 to 4 lesions, the SRS-only arm experienced worse 6-month freedom from new brain metastasis ($p = 0.003$) and 1-year local control ($p = 0.019$). Most importantly, the average duration until deterioration of mini-mental state examination (MMSE) was 16.5 months in the WBRT+SRS arm versus 7.6 months in the SRS-alone group ($p = 0.05$).[26] The main drawback of this study was the designation of OS as the primary end point.[26a,26b] There is very little evidence that adjuvant WBRT after surgery is likely to improve OS. However, this study did demonstrate the importance of WBRT in decreasing brain failure, corroborating the findings of the study by Patchell et al.[24]

TABLE 63.6 Randomized Trials of Postoperative Whole-Brain Radiotherapy

First Author/Study Group	Surgery + RT	Surgery only	*p* Value
Patchell/University of Kentucky[24] (n = 95)			
Primary end point	(50.4 Gy/28 fx)	craniotomyC	
Brain tumor recurrence			
Total brain recurrence	18%	70%	<0.001
Original site only	4%	33%	
Distant site only	8%	24%	
Original and distant	6%	13%	
Distant site total	14%	37%	<0.01
Original site total	10%	46%	<0.001
Secondary end points			
Cause of death			
Neurologic	14%	44%	0.003
Systemic	84%	46%	<0.001
Functional independence*	37 wks	35 wks	NS
Overall survival	48 wks	43 wks	NS
Aoyama/Japanese JROSG99-1[25] (n = 120; 1–4 lesions)†			
Primary end point	(30Gy/10 fx)	Radiosurgery	
Overall survival (1 yr)‡	39%	26%	NS
Secondary end points			
Local control‡	88%	70%	0.019
Freedom from new failure‡	82%	49%	0.003
KPS ≥70 maintenance‡	37%	25%	NS
Late radiation morbidity	1 patient	1 patient	NS
Neurologic death	6 patients	9 patients	NS

*As defined by KPS ≥70 maintenance.

†Interim analysis of planned 170 patient accrual.

‡1-year actuarial rates.

fx, fraction number; KPS, Karnofsky performance score; NS, not significant; RT, whole-brain radiotherapy; wks, weeks.

These two phase III trials provide sufficient level I evidence. Adjuvant WBRT, therefore, should be considered the standard of care after local therapy with surgical resection or SRS.

REPEAT WHOLE-BRAIN RADIOTHERAPY

Occasionally, patients fail in the brain with multiple lesions after initial WBRT. Repeat WBRT should strongly be considered. Wong et al.[27] reported on a series of 86 patients who underwent repeat WBRT. The median dose for the first course was 30 Gy, whereas the median dose for the second course was 20 Gy. A total of 70% experienced neurologic improvement, with 27% experiencing complete neurological resolution, whereas 43% had partial improvement with repeat WBRT. Retreatment dose of >20 Gy was associated with a significantly longer survival. Only one patient experienced dementia thought to be caused by radiation.

Repeat WBRT is relatively safe because most patients have limited survival with recurrent or progressive brain metastases after initial WBRT. A minimum of 20 in 1.8 to 2 Gy fractions should be given.

CONCURRENT RADIOSENSITIZERS

Although most patients ultimately succumb to the systemic progression, a significant percent will die from neurologic progression. Multiple randomized trials (Table 63.7) of concomitant radiosensitizers have been performed in an attempt to optimize brain control.[28–37] Most studies have included various primary histologies, although some series [30–32] only included patients with NSCLC. The results from these three studies do not suggest that patients with multiple brain metastases from NSCLC behave differently from other primaries. Unfortunately, no

TABLE 63.7 Selected Randomized Trials of Radiosensitizers for Patients with Multiple Brain Metastases

First Author/Study Group	Arms	Response Rate	*p* Value	Survival	Median *p* Value
Komarnicky/RTOG 79-16[28] (n = 859)	RT (30 Gy/10 fx)	45%*		4.5 mos	
	RT + misonidazole	42%*	NS	3.9 mos	NS
	RT (30 Gy/6 fx)	42%*		4.1 mos	
	RT + misonidazole	45%*	NS	3.1 mos	NS
Phillips/RTOG 89-05[29] (n=72)	RT (37.5/15 fx)	50%		6.1 mos	
	RT + BrdUrd	63%	NS	4.3 mos	NS
Ushio/Japanese[30] (n = 88)†	RT (40 Gy/20 fx)	36%		27 wks	
	RT + nitrosurea	69%		31 wks	
	RT + nitrosurea + tegafur	74%	<0.05	29 wks	NS
Robinet/GFPC 95-1[31] (n = 171)†	RT (30 Gy/10 fx) + cisplatin/vinorelbine	33%		21 wks	
	cisplatin/vinorelbine + delayed RT	27%	NS	24 wks	NS
Guerrieri/Australia[32] (n = 42)†	RT (20 Gy/5 fx)	10%		4.4 mos	
	RT + carboplatin	29%	NS	3.7 mos	NS
Antonadou/Greece[33] (n = 52)	RT (40 Gy/20 fx)	67%		7.0 mos	
	RT + temozolomide	96%	0.017	8.6 mos	NS
Verger/Spain[34] (n = 82)	RT (30 Gy/10 fx)	54%‡		3.1 mos	
	RT + temozolomide	72%‡	0.03	4.5 mos	NS
Mehta/9801 Trial[35] (n = 401)	RT (30 Gy/10 fx)	51%		4.9 mos	
	RT + MGd	46%	NS	5.2 mos	NS
Suh/REACH study[36] (n = 515)	RT (30 Gy/10 fx)	38%		4.4 mos	
	RT + efaproxiral	46%	NS	5.4 mos	NS
Berk/RTOG 0119[37] (n = 126)§	RT (30 Gy/10 fx)				
	+ A.M. melatonin			3.3 mos	
	+ P.M. melatonin			2.8 mos	NS

*Percent of survival time in KPS 90–100 range.

†Only lung cancer patients.

‡90-day freedom from brain metastasis.

§Only RTOG RPA class 2.

BrdUrd, bromodeoxyuridine; fx, fractions; MGd, motexafin gadolinium; mos, months; NS, not significant; RT; whole-brain radiotherapy; REACH, Radiation Enhancing Allosteric Compound for Hypoxic Brain Metastasis; RTOG, Radiation Therapy and Oncology Group; SWOG, Southwest Oncology Group; wks, weeks.

trial has demonstrated a survival advantage although a few have demonstrated an increased response rate. The two trials with temozolomide showed promise. Temozolomide is an oral alkylating agent with excellent central nervous system penetration. However, the findings of these two relatively small trials need to be confirmed in a larger trial.

SYNCHRONOUS, SOLITARY BRAIN METASTASIS FROM NON–SMALL CELL LUNG CANCER

It appears that synchronous, solitary brain metastasis (SSBM) from NSCLC may represent a distinct subgroup of patients that may have a more favorable prognosis compared with other metastatic disease patients. With aggressive brain treatment with SRS or surgery and adequate management of the chest, the 5-year OS for this limited number of patients ranges from 8% to 21%, which is line with stage III patients.[38–41]

Flannery et al.[41] reported a median survival of 18 months for the entire cohort of patients with SSBM from NSCLC. All patients received definitive therapy of SSBM with Gamma Knife SRS. The 1-, 2-, and 5-year actuarial OS rates were 71.3%, 34.1%, and 21%, respectively. For patients who underwent definitive thoracic therapy, the median survival was 26.4 months compared with 13.1 months for those who had nondefinitive therapy, and the 5-year actuarial OS was 34.6% versus 0% (p <0.0001). Median survival was significantly longer for patients with a KPS ≥90 versus KPS <90 (27.8 vs. 13.1 months; p <0.0001). The prognostic factors significant

TABLE 63.8 Published Experiences of Synchronous, Solitary Brain Metastasis from Non–Small Cell Lung Cancer

First Author (Year)	N	Brain Tx	Thoracic Tx	5-Yr OS
Bonnette[38] (2001)	99*	Surgery	Surgery	11%
Billing[39] (2001)	28	Surgery	Surgery	21%
Hu[40] (2006)	84	Surgery/SRS	Nonsurgical	8%
Flannery[41] (2008)	42	SRS	Surgery and/or chemo/XRT	21%

*Total cohort of 103, but 4 had >1 lesion.

OS, overall survival; SRS, stereotactic radiosurgery; Tx, therapy; XRT, radiotherapy.

on multivariate analysis for OS were definitive thoracic therapy ($p = 0.020$) and KPS ($p = 0.001$). A potential problem of this study is that no patient had histologic proof of the SSBM because all patients received SRS. However, these results corroborated findings from an earlier study, in which a 5-year survival of 21% was reported after resection of the SSBM and surgery of the thoracic tumor.[39]

Table 63.8 summarizes the published literature demonstrating the potential for long-term survival in this unique group. Therefore, effort should be made to definitively treat the thoracic disease and SSBM. A common treatment paradigm is to start with a course of WBRT, followed sequentially by definitive thoracic therapy, SRS boost, and adjuvant chemotherapy. Alternatively, upfront SRS or craniotomy can be for the SSBM, followed sequentially by definitive thoracic therapy, WBRT, and adjuvant chemotherapy. However, the exact sequence or mode of local brain (i.e., SRS or craniotomy) or thoracic therapy (i.e., surgery or chemoradiation) must be individualized based on intracranial and thoracic disease burden, as well as presence of symptoms and performance status.

Leptomeningeal Carcinomatosis Leptomeningeal carcinomatosis (LCM) is a rare complication of lung cancer that portends a poor prognosis. Of patients with LCM, the frequency of lung cancer (22% to 36%) is only exceeded by breast cancer (27% to 50%). It occurs in approximately 1% to 6% of patients with lung cancer, and it is most commonly involved by adenocarcinoma (50% to 56%), followed by squamous cell carcinoma (26% to 36%), and small cell carcinoma (SCLC) (13% to 14%).[42–46]

Most patients present with signs and symptoms. According to the review by Gleissner and Chamberlain,[42] spinal symptoms (>60%) are the most common, followed by cerebral (50%) and cranial nerve symptoms (40%). Contrast-enhanced MRI is the radiographic modality of choice. The entire neuraxis must be imaged if LCM is clinically suspected in a patient with a known malignancy. Most patients the MRI will reveal leptomeningeal enhancement that are frequently associated with cranial nerve enhancement and gross tumor deposits. Although Collie et al.[47] found that all 25 patients with solid tumors exhibited abnormal Gadolinium-enhanced MRI, Straathof et al.[48] found the MRI to have a diagnostic sensitivity and specificity of LCM of 76% and 77%, respectively.

If MRI is equivocal, then cerebrospinal fluid (CSF) should be obtained if safe. Multiple samples may need to be obtained because the initial yield of a lumbar tap may be only 50%.[42] Neurosurgery must be consulted to evaluate the need for (a) shunting if hydrocephalus is suspected, and (b) placement of Rickham or Ommaya reservoirs for possible intrathecal (IT) chemotherapy. Chamberlain et al.[42,43] argue that CSF flow studies should be performed with indium-111 or technetium-99, because up to one half of patients have abnormal CSF flow from gross tumor deposits that may disrupt adequate IT chemotherapy delivery. However, flow studies are not performed by many centers because gross tumor nodules, most likely to cause flow disruption and not effectively treated by IT chemotherapy, are treated with radiation anyway. Thus, CSF flow studies typically do not change the overall management of patients with LCM who require treatment decisions to be made in an expedient manner.

There is no consensus on the optimal management of patients with LCM. This is mainly from the lack of large published experiences, limited number of randomized trials, nonuniform treatment regimens in single-institution experiences, and inclusion of various primary tumor histologies in the clinical trials. However, most would agree that an aggressive treatment with radiation (either WBRT or focal spinal radiation to symptomatic sites) and IT chemotherapy is indicated in patients with good performance status.[49] In the largest published experience to date on LCM from SCLC ($n = 36$), the dismal median survival of 1.3 months is a direct result of only 14 patients being offered some kind of therapy ($n = 9$ for radiation; $n = 5$ for chemotherapy).[50] In contrast, Chamberlain et al.,[51] in the largest series of patients with LCM from NSCLC ($n = 32$), treated all patients prospectively with radiotherapy followed by IT chemotherapy. The median survival for the entire cohort was 5 months, whereas patients with normal CSF flow had a significantly longer median survival compared with patients with interrupted CSF flow (6 vs. 4 months; $p < 0.05$). This suggests that an aggressive multimodal approach can extend survival times that are comparable to patients with multiple brain parenchymal metastases.

All of the randomized clinical trials on patients what LCM from solid tumors have included IT methotrexate (MTX)-based regimens (Table 63.9).[52–56] The only trial that compared IT versus non-IT (i.e., systemic) chemotherapy was reported by Boogerd et al.[56] However, this negative trial only included patients with breast primaries. Glantz et al.[54] reported that IT DepoCyt led to a greater median time to neurological progression (8 vs. 4 weeks; $p = 0.007$), although the OS was not statistically different. The only positive trial reported to date has been by Kim et al.[55] in which patients randomized to IT methotrexate, cytosine arabinoside, and hydrocortisone had a significantly longer survival than those randomized to IT methotrexate alone (18.2 vs. 10.4 weeks; $p = 0.029$). Patients with adenocarcinoma of the lung in the multiagent arm had a significant longer survival (23.9 vs. 10.4 weeks; $p = 0.038$). Multiple other agents have been studied, but none have demonstrated significant responses.

There is extensive evidence that focal radiation, such as WBRT or spinal radiation, provides added benefit to IT chemotherapy. This is particularly true in patients with bulky meningeal disease because IT chemotherapy only penetrates 2 to 3 mm. In the randomized IT chemotherapy trial reported by Hitchins et al.,[52] patients who received concurrent CNS radiation had a higher response rate compared with those who did not (73% vs. 35%; $p < 0.05$). Likewise, in the randomized trial reported by Kim et al.,[55] those who received concurrent CNS radiation had a significant higher neurological response rate (81.5% vs. 50.0%; $p = 0.014$). There is a concern that concurrent radiation and IT chemotherapy could potentially increase toxicity. However, most patients do not survive long enough to clinically manifest the late neurological toxicity.

Causes of Neurocognitive Decline in Brain Tumor Patients Historically, brain radiation has been frequently cited as the major cause of neurocognitive decline in cancer patients. One of the most misinterpreted studies on this issue is that reported by DeAngelis et al.[12] In this study, an 11% risk of radiation-induced dementia was reported in patients undergoing WBRT for brain metastasis. A thorough analysis revealed that the 11% figure was very misleading. Of the 47 patients who survived 1 year after WBRT, 5 patients (11%) developed severe dementia. When these five patients are examined, all were treated in a fashion that would significantly increase the risk of late radiation toxicity (i.e., large daily fractions and concurrent radiosensitizer). Three patients received 5 and 6 Gy daily fractions, while a fourth patient received 6 Gy fractions with concurrent Adriamycin. Only one patient received what is considered a standard radiation fractionation scheme (i.e., 30 Gy in 10 fractions), but this patient received a concurrent experimental radiosensitizer (lonidamine). No patient

TABLE 63.9 Randomized Trials of Solid Tumor Patients with Leptomeningeal Carcinomatosis

First Author (Year)	N	Histology	Arms*	RR†	Median Survival	Survival *p* Value
Hitchins[52] (1987)	44	Solid tumors	IT MTX 15 mg	61%	12 wks	0.08
			IT MTX + Ara-C 50 mg/m^2	45%	7 wks	
			Concurrent RT (not randomized)	75%		
			No concurrent RT	35%	($p < 0.05$)	
Grossman[53] (1993)	52	Nonleukemic‡	IT MTX 10 mg	0%	16 wks	NS
			IT thiotepa 10 mg	0%	14 wks	
Glantz[54] (1999)	61	Solid tumors	IT MTX 10 mg	20%	11 wks	0.15
			IT DepoCyt 50 mg	26%	15 wks	
Kim[55] (2003)	55	Solid tumors	IT MTX 15 mg	14%	10 wks	0.03
			IT MTX + Ara-C 30 mg/m^2 + Hydrocortisone 15 mg/m^2	39%	19 wks	
			Concurrent RT (not randomized)	82%		
			No concurrent RT	50%	($p = 0.014$)	
Boogerd[56] (2004)	35	Breast	IT chemotherapy§	41%	18 wks	0.32
			Non-IT chemotherapy	39%	30 wks	

*All studies allowed palliative radiation when necessary.

†RR determination by neurologic and CSF improvements as predefined by each study.

‡14 patients (19%) had lymphoma, rest had solid tumors.

§All patients started with MTX and switched to Ara-C if no response.

Ara-C, cytarabine; DepoCyt, sustained-release cytarabine; IT, intrathecal; MTX, methotrexate; NS, not significant; RR, response rate; RT; whole-brain radiotherapy; wks, weeks.

who received the standard 30 Gy in 10 fractions WBRT alone experienced dementia.

The accuracy of the 11% dementia rate is further questioned by faulty statistical interpretation. Even though the study included 232 in the initial analysis, it only examined 47 patients who survived at least 1 year. The principles of conditional probability dictate that the 11% risk is accurate only if a patient survives 1 year, which is significantly longer than most reported series. Therefore, a radiation-induced dementia risk of 2% (5/232) would have been more accurate because this would reflect the true probability ab initio for patients presenting with brain metastasis. Indeed, in a separate study of a larger cohort, DeAngelis et al.[57] estimate the true risk of radiation-induced dementia to be only 1.9% to 5.2% for all patients presenting with brain metastasis. This small risk of dementia is not high enough to warrant withholding potentially lifesaving WBRT.

Many have argued that the increased local control with adjuvant WBRT does not translate into a survival benefit, and that performing repeat SRS or deferring WBRT for recurrences are reasonable approaches. However, WBRT may actually improve neurocognition in a significant number of patients, and that brain recurrence or progression is associated with decrease in neurocognitive function. In a neurocognitive analysis of an RTOG study, Regine et al.[58] demonstrated that approximately one third of patients treated with WBRT experienced improvement in MMSE; most importantly, those who had uncontrolled brain metastases had an average decrement of six points on the MMSE. In the North Central Cancer Treatment Group experience of 701 high-grade glioma patients, Taylor et al.[59] found similar results for those who experienced tumor progression.

Most of the studies that employed MMSE did not utilize sophisticated neurocognitive testing. It is possible that subtle neurocognitive dysfunction may indeed result from WBRT. Recent studies that have used sophisticated neurocognitive testing are clearly demonstrating that the brain tumor (presence, recurrence, and progression) has the greatest effect on neurocognitive decline. In the large phase III motexafin gadolinium study, a thorough neurocognitive battery of tests examined memory recall, memory recognition, memory delayed recalled, verbal fluency, pegboard hand coordinate, and executive function.[60] This neurocognitive correlative analysis study demonstrated that 21% to 65% of patients had impaired functioning at baseline before treatment with WBRT. Furthermore, patients who progressed in the brain after treatment experienced significantly worse scores in all of these individual tests.

There is now sufficient evidence that other factors, such as anticonvulsants, benzodiazepines, opioids, chemotherapy, craniotomy and, most importantly, the brain tumor, contribute significantly to the neurocognitive decline of patients with brain tumor.[61–67]

Anticonvulsants Patients frequently present to the oncologist already started on prophylactic anticonvulsants. This represents one of the most preventable causes of neurocognitive decline in brain tumor patients. Anticonvulsants are clearly known to impact negatively on quality of life and neurocognition in healthy volunteers.[66,67] This detrimental effect may be even more pronounced in brain tumor patients. In a study of 156 patients with low-grade glioma (85% experiencing a seizure), Klein et al.[63] correlated seizure burden with quality of life and neurocognitive function. This study convincingly demonstrates the significant correlation between the increase in the number anticonvulsants (even with lack of seizures) with the decrease in quality of life and neurocognitive function.

Indeed, based on four negative randomized trials, the American Academy of Neurology recommends that prophylactic anticonvulsants not be initiated in newly diagnosed brain tumor patients who have not experienced a seizure.[68] It is safe to taper a patient off of anticonvulsants provided that the patient has not experienced a seizure.

SPINAL CORD COMPRESSION

In the United States, more than 20,000 cases of metastatic spinal cord compression (MSCC) are diagnosed annually, and it is estimated to develop in approximately 5% to 14% of all cancer patients.[69,70] MSCC is a devastating complication of cancer. It is considered a true medical emergency, and immediate intervention is required. Even with aggressive therapy, results can often be unsatisfactory. Although most patients with MSCC have limited survival, up to one third will survive beyond 1 year.[71] Therefore, aggressive therapy should always be considered to preserve or improve the quality of life.

Pathophysiology MSCC develops primarily in one of three ways: (a) continued growth and expansion of vertebral bone metastasis into the epidural space; (b) neural foramina extension by a paraspinal mass; and (c) destruction of vertebral cortical bone, causing vertebral body collapse with displacement of bony fragments into the epidural space. Although complex, the most significant damage caused by MSCC appears to be vascular in nature. Epidural tumor extension causes epidural venous plexus compression, which leads to edema of the spinal cord. This increase in vascular permeability and edema cause increased pressure on the small arterioles. Capillary blood flow diminishes as the disease progresses, leading to white matter ischemia. Prolonged ischemia eventually results in white matter infarction and permanent cord damage.[72]

Clinical Presentation, Diagnosis, and Prognosis

Most patients have a cancer diagnosis history. Fuller et al.,[73] in a review of over 1000 patients with MSCC, reported in the literature that the most common tumor type was breast cancer (29%), followed by lung cancer (17%), and prostate cancer (14%). This reflects the high natural incidence of these tumors. New-onset back pain in cancer patients needs to be taken seriously and worked up. Even without a prior cancer diagnosis, MSCC should be suspected in anyone who presents with progressively worsening back pain, incontinence, or paraplegia, especially in the high-risk population such as long-time smokers. The most common level of the MSCC involvement is in the thoracic spine (59% to 78%), followed by lumbar, (16% to 33%) and cervical spine (4% to 15%), whereas multiple levels are involved in up to one half of the patients.[73–75] Back pain is the most common presenting symptom (88% to 96%), followed by weakness (76% to 86%), sensory deficits (51% to 80%), and autonomic dysfunction (40% to 64%).[74,76–78]

MRI is the standard modality for imaging of the spine. It has a very high sensitivity (93%), specificity (97%), and accuracy (95%) in diagnosing MSCC.[79] Because patients can have synchronous, multifocal MSCC, an MRI of the entire spine with and without contrast should be promptly performed in anyone suspected of having MSCC.[80] High-resolution CT scan or CT myelogram of the spine should be performed for those with contraindications to MRI.

Prognostic factors predicting survival are generally similar to patients with brain metastasis as discussed previously. In terms of predicting ambulatory outcome, one of the most important factors is the rapidity of symptom onset. Other important prognostic factors include favorable histology (e.g., multiple myeloma, germ cell tumors, small cell carcinoma) and pretherapy ambulatory function.[81] In a prospective study of 98 patients with MSCC reported by Rades et al.,[82] the single strongest predictor for ambulatory status after therapy on multivariate analysis was time to development of motor deficits before radiation ($p < 0.001$) from the start of any symptoms. This cohort was separated into three groups according to the time to motors deficits before radiation therapy: 1 to 7 days (group A), 8 to 14 days (group B), and >14 days (group C). The ambulatory rates for groups A, B, and C were 35%, 55%, and 86% ($p < 0.001$), respectively. The symptom improvement rates for groups A, B, and C were 10%, 29%, and 86% ($p = 0.026$), respectively. The other significant factor on the multivariate analysis for posttherapy ambulatory status was favorable histology ($p = 0.005$), and there was a trend regarding pretherapy ambulatory status ($p = 0.076$). Acute, rapid deterioration is predictive of irreversible spinal cord infarction. Only 10% of the patients in group A had symptom improvement; therefore, prompt diagnosis and treatment of MSCC is crucial.

Corticosteroids Corticosteroids must be started as soon as possible in anyone suspected of having MSCC even before radiographic diagnosis, because this can be rapidly discontinued with a negative diagnosis. They effectively decrease cord edema, and they serve as an effective bridge to definitive treatment. Although multiple retrospective studies have demonstrated its clinical efficacy, Sorensen et al.[83] reported the only randomized controlled study (n = 57) on the utility of high-dose corticosteroids before definitive radiotherapy in MSCC from solid tumors. The treatment arm consisted of 96 mg of IV bolus of dexamethasone followed by 96 mg oral (PO) per day for 3 days and a 10-day taper versus no therapy. This study demonstrated 3- and 6-month ambulatory rates of 81% versus 63% and 59% versus 33% ($p < 0.05$), respectively, in favor of high-dose dexamethasone.

The optimal maintenance dose of corticosteroids is unknown. Vecht et al.[84] reported the only randomized study (n = 37) comparing corticosteroid doses in patients with MSCC, but this study only evaluated the IV loading dose. It compared IV loading doses of 10 versus 100 mg, followed in both arms by the same oral regimen of 16 mg/day. Both arms demonstrated significant reductions in pain from baseline ($p < 0.001$); however, there was no difference between the two arms with respect to pain reduction, ambulation, or bladder function.

Very high doses of corticosteroids are associated with significant side effects. Sorensen et al.[83] reported in the phase III study an 11% incidence of serious side effects for patients in the treatment arm, whereas Heimdal et al.[85] reported a 14.3% incidence of serious gastrointestinal side effects in 28 consecutive patients treated with 96 mg of IV dexamethasone per day. The toxicities in the study of Heimdal et al. included one fatal ulcer hemorrhage, one rectal bleeding, and two bowel perforations. Subsequently, the dexamethasone dose was decreased to 16 mg/day for the next 38 consecutive patients, and there was no incidence of serious side effects ($p < 0.05$). Most importantly, the ambulatory rates were not different between the two dexamethasone doses.

Based on these data, a loading of 10 mg of IV dexamethasone followed by a maintenance dose of 4 to 6 mg every 6 to 8 hours should be sufficient before being tapered judiciously. Patients can be safely switched to oral steroids after 24 to 48 hours because there is good oral bioavailability of corticosteroids. Furthermore, patients should be started on a proton pump inhibitor for gastrointestinal bleeding prophylaxis. Although here has been no randomized trial utilizing proton pump inhibitors in patients receiving corticosteroids, there have been multiple phase III studies demonstrating the protective effects of these agents against peptic ulcers in patients receiving chronic nonsteroidal anti-inflammatory drugs.[86] Nonsteroidal anti-inflammatory drugs and corticosteroids both cause gastrointestinal mucosal injury by decreasing mucosal protective prostaglandin levels. Therefore, it is not an unreasonable extrapolation to assume that proton pump inhibitors provide a similar mucosal protective effect with corticosteroids, especially considering that the morbidity of gastrointestinal toxicity can be life threatening.

Radiotherapy Palliative radiotherapy has long been the standard of care in the treatment of patients with MSCC. Although a total of 30 Gy in 10 fractions is most frequently employed fractionation schedule, multiple fractionation schemes have been reported, which undoubtedly reflects the heterogeneity in the patient population and tumor histology.[87] In one of the largest studies to date, Rades et al.[88] reported a retrospective series of 1304 patients with MSCC.[8] The patients were separated into five schedules: 8 Gy × 1 in 1 day (n = 261, group 1), 4 Gy × 5 in 1 week (n = 279, group 2), 3 Gy × 10 in 2 weeks (n = 274, group 3), 2.5 Gy × 15 in 3 weeks (n = 233, group 4), and 2 Gy × 20 in 4 weeks (n = 257, group 5). All of the groups had similar posttreatment ambulatory rates (63% to 74%) and motor function improvements (26% to 31%). However, in-field recurrence rates were much lower for the protracted schedules. The 2-year in-field recurrence rates for groups 1, 2, 3, 4, and 5 were 24%, 26%, 14%, 9%, and 7% (p <0.001). They recommend that a single fraction of 8 Gy should be used in MSCC patients with limited survival expectations, and that 30 Gy in 10 fractions should be used for all other patients.

Although there is no large series of MSCC from small cell lung cancer, Rades et al.[89] have reported the largest series to date of patients with MSCC from NSCLC (n = 252). In this retrospective study, the short-course radiotherapy group (8 Gy × 1, 4 Gy × 5) and the same functional outcome as long-course radiotherapy group (3 Gy × 10, 2.5 Gy × 15, 2 Gy × 20); therefore, 8 Gy × 1 was recommended.

Maranzano et al.[90] have reported the only randomized trial on radiation schedule for patients with MSCC. They compared two hypofractionation schemes, a short course (8 Gy × 1 followed by 6-day break then 8 Gy × 1; 16 Gy total in 1 week) versus a split course (5 Gy × 3 followed by 4-day break and then additional 3 Gy × 5; 30 Gy total in 2 weeks). The study concludes that the treatment with short versus split courses of radiation therapy resulted in similar back pain relief (56% vs. 59%), ambulatory maintenance (68% vs. 71%), and good bladder function (90% vs. 89%) rates. Therefore, they recommend that an 8 Gy × 2 regimen should be used for patients with MSCC. Serious problems inherent to this study have been recognized; therefore, readers should be cautious before implementing the the recommendations by Maranzano et al.[91] Although the response rates may seem impressive, when one limits the definition of response to regaining motor function and sphincter control, the rates of success decrease to 29% and 14%, respectively. Confounding variables included having patients with favorable histology, excellent performance status, and the use of nonstandard, large fraction sizes in both arms. It is entirely conceivable that the 5% who progressed to paraplegia without in-field recurrence may have suffered from late radiation-induced toxicity, even if not scored as late toxicity by the authors.

For patients with MSCC secondary to solid tumors, 30 Gy in 10 fractions is considered the standard of care. Shorter fractionation schedules, such as 8 Gy × 1 or 4 Gy × 5, should only be reserved for those with clear evidence of progressive disease, refractory to systemic therapy. Furthermore, these short schedules should be avoided in newly diagnosed, chemotherapy-naive patients because the clinical course can be quite variable and unpredictable. Chemotherapy may be considered in select, newly diagnosed patients with excellent neurological status and very chemosensitive tumors (e.g., multiple myeloma, germ cell tumors), but this is still considered outside the accepted standard. If the patient is found to have unresectable/inoperable tumor, and otherwise has good performance status, oligometastatic disease, and controlled primary disease, then consideration should be made to escalate the dose beyond 30 Gy because this will not be sufficient to achieve long-term gross tumor control. Special techniques such as image-guided, intensity-modulated radiation therapy (IGRT/IMRT) or stereotactic body radiation therapy (SBRT) should be considered. However, the routine use of IMRT or SBRT cannot be universally recommended because the technology is expensive, and it has yet to show definite benefit over conventional delivery of radiation in a patient population that has a median survival of 6 months or less.

Caution against Short, Hypofractionated Radiotherapy A common mistake made by those who advocate a short hypofractionated regimen (e.g., 8 Gy × 1, 8 Gy × 2, or 4 Gy × 5) for the spine is equating the safety and equivalency of these abbreviated schedules in bone and lung metastases studies as a justification for the safety of such regimens in MSCC. It is well recognized that the retreatment rates are higher with single fraction schemes versus conventional schedules in bone metastases.[92] The consequence of progression in the bone despite prior radiotherapy (i.e., 8 Gy × 1) is an increase in pain, which leads to an increased need for pain medications and usually reirradiation. By contrast, the consequences of MSCC progression despite prior radiotherapy are an increase in pain, paralysis, and incontinence, which usually contributes significantly to the direct demise of the patient.

The predominant mechanism of cord injury by both MSCC and radiation-induced myelopathy (RIM) is vascular damage leading to ischemia.[93] There are many studies that have established the vascular effects of high fraction dose. Dose response to single dose of SRS for arteriovenous malformation obliteration starts at doses as low as 8 Gy and as soon as 6 months or earlier.[94] It is possible that a compressed cord has a lower threshold for RIM when a short, hypofractionated schedule of radiation therapy is used. This two-hit phenomenon (i.e., physical and radiation-induced vascular insults) is not considered by those who advocate a short, hypofractionated regimen. Chow et al.[95] demonstrated that oncologists are not accurate at all in predicting survival times. As systemic therapy improves for patients with metastatic disease, our ability to predict survival will undoubtedly become less accurate. Therefore, these abbreviated schedules should be routinely avoided unless the patient is chemotherapy refractory, and has convincing evidence of progressive systemic disease with limited expected survival.

Surgery Radiation for nonradiosensitive tumors typically takes several days to have an effect and does not stabilize the spine, whereas surgery allows for immediate cord decompression and provides an opportunity to stabilize the spine intraoperatively. For years, surgery was abandoned when several retrospective studies and one, small randomized study showed no benefit to surgery over radiation alone. Young et al.[96] randomized 29 patients with MSCC to decompressive laminectomy followed by radiation versus radiation alone. Although this trial showed no benefit to surgery in terms of pain relief, ambulation, or sphincter function, it is difficult to draw any conclusion because of the small sample size. All of these studies used posterior laminectomy in conjunction with radiotherapy; however, most of the lesions in MSCC involve the anterior portion of the vertebral body.[69] Therefore, a laminectomy does not effectively relieve the compression and may actually worsen the stability of the spine.

Recently, several authors have advocated the use of direct surgical decompression, tumor debulking, and spinal stabilization via instrumentation to improve on the results from radiation alone. Patchell et al.[97] reported the first phase III randomized trial testing the efficacy of direct decompressive surgery in patients with MSCC. Table 63.10 summarizes the key findings of this study. It compared radiation alone (standard 30 Gy in 10 fractions) versus decompressive and stabilization surgery within 24 hours of diagnosis followed by the same radiotherapy (within 2 weeks of surgery). The trial was terminated early at interim analysis when early stopping rules were met regarding the primary end point of ambulation after treatment. This study definitively demonstrated an advantage to surgery for every end point at statistically significant levels. For nonambulatory patients, the combined treatment patients had a significant higher chance of regaining the ability to walk after therapy. Maintenance of continence, maintenance of American Spinal Cord Injury (ASIA) and Frankel scores (measures of spinal function after injury), median OS, and median mean daily dexamethasone and morphine equivalent doses all favored the surgery arm.

If operable, patients should undergo surgical decompression and stabilization followed by radiotherapy. Even for radiosensitive tumors, surgery can often stabilize the spine. Therefore, all patients with MSCC should be evaluated by a surgeon. Effective multidisciplinary teamwork is critical to the rapid evaluation and management of patients with MSCC.

INTRAMEDULLARY SPINAL CORD METASTASIS

Intramedullary spinal cord metastasis (ISCM) is rare, representing only 1% of all intramedullary tumors. According to a review by Kalayci et al.[98] ISCM is more commonly secondary to a lung primary (54%), followed by breast cancer (11%), renal cell carcinoma (9%), and melanoma (8%), in contrast to patients with MSCC. Although back pain is common in

TABLE 63.10 Key Findings of the Randomized Phase III Study of Patients with Metastatic Spinal Cord Compression Reported by Patchell et al.[97]

	Surgery + Radiation Median (n = 50)	Radiation Alone Median (n = 51)	*p* Value
Primary End Point			
Ability to walk			
Rate	84% (42/50)	57% (29/51)	0.001
Time	122 days	13 days	0.003
Secondary End Points			
Maintenance of continence	156 days	17 days	0.016
Maintenance of ASIA score*	566 days	72 days	0.001
Maintenance of Frankel score*	566 days	72 days	0.0006
Overall survival	126 days	100 days	0.033
Other End Points			
Mean daily morphine†	0.4 mg	4.8 mg	0.002
Mean daily dexamethasone†	1.6 mg	4.2 mg	0.0093
In Patients Ambulatory at Study Entry			
Ability to walk (maintaining)			
Rate	94% (32/34)	74% (26/34)	0.024
Time	153 days	54 days	0.024
In Patients Nonambulatory at Study Entry			
Ability to walk (regaining)			
Rate	62% (10/16)	19% (3/16)	0.012
Time	59 days	0 days	0.04

*Measures of spinal function after injury.

†Converted into equivalent doses.

ASIA, American Spinal Injury Association.

>90% of MSCC patients, back or neck pain was seen in only 38% with ISCM. However, high sensory deficits (79%), sphincter dysfunction (60%), and weakness (91%) are more common in ISCM. The most striking difference between ISCM and MSCC is the high incidence of synchronous brain metastasis (41%) in patients presenting with ISCM. This is not surprising when one considers the route of spread and the high incidence of lung primaries in patients with ISCM.[98,99]

The treatment of ISCM should be approached very similarly to MSCC, except for the role of surgery. Most surgeons are reluctant to operate in ISCM because surgery carries a high morbidity rate and most patients have widely metastatic disease at the time of ISCM diagnosis. Indeed, the Kalayci et al.[98] indicated that only 32 cases of surgery in ISCM have ever been reported. An MRI of the brain should be obtained because of the high incidence of synchronous brain metastasis. High-dose corticosteroids as well as radiation therapy should be promptly initiated. With therapy, the expected median survival and neurological improvement rate are 7 months and 66%, respectively.

REFERENCES

1. Wen PY, Black PM, Loeffler JS. Treatment of metastatic cancer. In: DeVita VT, Hellman S, Rosenberg SA, eds. *Cancer: Principles and Practice of Oncology.* Philadelphia, PA: Lippincott Williams and Wilkins, 2001:2655–2670.
2. Barnholtz-Sloan JS, Sloan AE, Davis FG, et al. Incidence proportions of brain metastases in patients diagnosed (1973–2001) in the metropolitan Detroit Cancer Surveillance system. *J Clin Oncol* 2004;22(14): 2865–2872.
3. Posner JB. Brain metastases: 1995. A brief review. *J Neurooncol* 1996;27(3):287–293.
4. Davis PC, Hudgins PA, Peterman SB, et al. Diagnosis of cerebral metastases: double-dose delayed CT vs contrast-enhanced MR imaging. *AJNR Am J Neuroradiol* 1991;12(2):293–300.
5. Gaspar L, Scott C, Rotman M, et al. Recursive partitioning analysis (RPA) of prognostic factors in three Radiation Therapy Oncology Group (RTOG) brain metastases trials. *Int J Radiat Oncol Biol Phys* 1997;37(4):745–51.
6. Ruderman NB, Hall TC. Use of glucocorticoids in the palliative treatment of metastatic brain tumors. *Cancer* 1965;18:298–306.
7. Vecht CJ, Hovestadt A, Verbiest HB, et al. Dose-effect relationship of dexamethasone on Karnofsky performance in metastatic brain tumors: a randomized study of doses of 4, 8, and 16 mg per day. *Neurology* 1994;44(4):675–80.
8. Borgelt B, Gelber R, Kramer S, et al. The palliation of brain metastases: final results of the first two studies by the Radiation Therapy Oncology Group. *Int J Radiat Oncol Biol Phys* 1980;6(1):1–9.
9. Haie-Meder C, Pellae-Cosset B, Laplanche A, et al. Results of a randomized clinical trial comparing two radiation schedules in the palliative treatment of brain metastases. *Radiother Oncol* 1993;26(2): 111–116.
10. Priestman TJ, Dunn J, Brada M, et al. Final results of the Royal College of Radiologists' trial comparing two different radiotherapy schedules in the treatment of cerebral metastases. *Clin Oncol (R Coll Radiol)* 1996;8(5):308–315.
11. Murray KJ, Scott C, Greenberg HM, et al. A randomized phase III study of accelerated hyperfractionation versus standard in patients with unresected brain metastases: a report of the Radiation Therapy Oncology Group (RTOG) 9104. *Int J Radiat Oncol Biol Phys* 1997; 39(3):571–574.
12. DeAngelis LM, Delattre JV, Posner JB. Radiation-induced dementia in patients cured of brain metastases. *Neurology* 1989;39(6):789–796.
13. Patchell RA, Tibbs PA, Walsh JW, et al. A randomized trial of surgery in the treatment of single metastases to the brain. *N Engl J Med* 1990;322(8):494–500.
14. Noordijk EM, Vecht CJ, Haaxma-Reiche H, et al. The choice of treatment of single brain metastasis should be based on extracranial tumor activity and age. *Int J Radiat Oncol Biol Phys* 1994;29(4):711–717.
15. Mintz AH, Kestle J, Rathbone MP, et al. A randomized trial to assess the efficacy of surgery in addition to radiotherapy in patients with a single cerebral metastasis. *Cancer* 1996;78(7):1470–1476.
16. Kondziolka D, Patel A, Lunsford LD, et al. Stereotactic radiosurgery plus whole brain radiotherapy versus radiotherapy alone for patients with multiple brain metastases. *Int J Radiat Oncol Biol Phys* 1999;45(2):427–434.
17. Chougule PB, Burton-Williams M, Saris S, et al. Randomized treatment of brain metastases with gamma knife radiosurgery, whole brain radiotherapy or both. *Int J Radiat Oncol Biol Phys* 2000;48:114.
18. Andrews DW, Scott CB, Sperduto PW, et al. Whole brain radiation therapy with and without stereotactic radiosurgery boost for patients with one to three brain metastases: phase III results of the RTOG 9508 randomized trial. *Lancet* 2004;363:1665–1672.
19. Elveen T, Andrews DW. Summary of RTOG 95-01 phase III randomized trial of whole brain radiation with and without stereotactic radiosurgery boost, including presentation of a clinical case study. *Am J Oncol Rev* 2004;3:592–600.
20. Sneed PK, Suh JH, Goetsch SJ, et al. A multi-institutional review of radiosurgery alone vs. radiosurgery with whole brain radiotherapy as the initial management of brain metastases. *Int J Radiat Oncol Biol Phys* 2002;53(3):519–526.
21. Sneed PK, Lamborn KR, Forstner JM, et al. Radiosurgery for brain metastases: is whole brain radiotherapy necessary? *Int J Radiat Oncol Biol Phys* 1999;43(3):549–558.
22. Regine WF, Huhn JL, Patchell RA, et al. Risk of symptomatic brain tumor recurrence and neurologic deficit after radiosurgery alone in patients with newly diagnosed brain metastases: results and implications. *Int J Radiat Oncol Biol Phys* 2002;52(2):333–338. Erratum in: *Int J Radiat Oncol Biol Phys* 2002;53(1):259.
23. Manon R, O'Neill A, Knisely J, et al. Phase II trial of radiosurgery for one to three newly diagnosed brain metastases from renal cell carcinoma, melanoma, and sarcoma: an Eastern Cooperative Oncology Group study (E 6397). *J Clin Oncol* 2005;23(34):8870–8876.
24. Patchell RA, Tibbs PA, Regine WF, et al. Postoperative radiotherapy in the treatment of single metastases to the brain: a randomized trial. *JAMA* 1998;280(17):1485–1489.
25. Aoyama H, Shirato H, Tago M, et al. Stereotactic radiosurgery plus whole-brain radiation therapy vs stereotactic radiosurgery alone for treatment of brain metastases: a randomized controlled trial. *JAMA* 2006;295(21):2483–2491.
26. Aoyama H, Tago M, Kato N, et al. Neurocognitive function of patients with brain metastasis who received either whole brain radiotherapy plus stereotactic radiosurgery or radiosurgery alone. *Int J Radiat Oncol Biol Phys* 2007;68(5):1388–1395.

26a. Patchell RA, Regine WF, Renschler, et al. Comments about the prospective trial by Aoyama et al. *Surg Neurol* 2006;66(5):459–460.

26b. Patchell RA, Regine WF, Loeffler JS, et al. Radiosurgery plus whole-brain radiation therapy for brain metastases. *JAMA* 2006;296(17): 2089–2090.

27. Wong WW, Schild SE, Sawyer TE, et al. Analysis of outcome in patients reirradiated for brain metastases. *Int J Radiat Oncol Biol Phys* 1996;34(3):585–590.
28. Komarnicky LT, Phillips TL, Martz K, et al. A randomized phase III protocol for the evaluation of misonidazole combined with radiation in the treatment of patients with brain metastases (RTOG-7916). *Int J Radiat Oncol Biol Phys* 1991;20(1):53–58.
29. Phillips TL, Scott CB, Leibel SA, et al. Results of a randomized comparison of radiotherapy and bromodeoxyuridine with radiotherapy

alone for brain metastases: report of RTOG trial 89-05. *Int J Radiat Oncol Biol Phys* 1995;33(2):339–348.
30. Ushio Y, Arita N, Hayakawa T, et al. Chemotherapy of brain metastases from lung carcinoma: a controlled randomized study. *Neurosurgery* 1991;28(2):201–205.
31. Robinet G, Thomas P, Breton JL, et al. Results of a phase III study of early versus delayed whole brain radiotherapy with concurrent cisplatin and vinoralbine combination in inoperable brain metastasis of non-small-cell lung cancer: groupe Francaise de Pneumo-Cancerologie (GFPC) Protocol 95-1. *Ann Oncol* 2001;12(1):59–67.
32. Guerrieri M, Wong K, Ryan G, et al. A randomised phase III study of palliative radiation with concomitant carboplatin for brain metastases from non-small cell carcinoma of the lung. *Cancer* 2004;46(1):107–111.
33. Antonadou D, Paraskevaidis M, Sarris G, et al. Phase II randomized trial of temozolomide and concurrent radiotherapy in patients with brain metastases. *J Clin Oncol* 2002;20(17):3644–3650.
34. Verger E, Gil M, Yaya R, et al. Temozolomide and concomitant whole brain radiotherapy in patients with brain metastases: a phase II randomized trial. *Int J Radiat Oncol Biol Phys* 2005;61(1):185–191.
35. Mehta MP, Rodrigus P, Terhaard CH, et al. Survival and neurologic outcomes in a randomized trial of motexafin gadolinium and whole-brain radiation therapy in brain metastases. *J Clin Oncol* 2003;21(13):2529–2536.
36. Suh JH, Stea B, Nabid A, et al. Phase III study of efaproxiral as an adjunct to whole-brain radiation therapy for brain metastases. *J Clin Oncol* 2006;24(1):106–114. Epub 2005 Nov 28.
37. Berk L, Berkey B, Rich T, et al. Randomized phase II trial of high-dose melatonin and radiation therapy for RPA class 2 patients with brain metastases (RTOG 0119). *Int J Radiat Oncol Biol Phys* 2007;68(3): 852–857. Epub 2007 Apr 6.
38. Bonnette P, Puyo P, Gabriel C, et al. Surgical management of non-small cell lung cancer with synchronous brain metastases. *Chest* 2001;119: 1469–1475.
39. Billing PS, Miller DL, Allen MS, et al. Surgical treatment of primary lung cancer with synchronous brain metastases. *J Thorac Cardiovasc Surg* 2001;122:548–553.
40. Hu C, Chang E, Hassenbusch III SJ, et al. Nonsmall cell lung cancer presenting with synchronous solitary brain metastasis. *Cancer* 2006; 106:1998–2004.
41. Flannery TW, Suntharalingam M, Regine WF, et al. Long-term survival in patients with synchronous, solitary brain metastasis from non-small cell lung cancer treated with radiosurgery. *Int J Radiat Oncol Biol Phys* 2008;72(1):19–23.
42. Gleissner B, Chamberlain MC. Neoplastic meningitis. *Lancet Neurol* 2006;5:443–452.
43. Chamberlain MC. Neoplastic meningitis. *J Clin Oncol* 2005;23(15): 3605–3613.
44. Wasserstrom WR, Glass JP, Posner JB. Diagnosis and treatment of leptomeningeal metastases from solid tumors: Experience with 90 patients. *Cancer* 1982;49:759–772.
45. Kaplan JG, DeSouza TG, Farkash A, et al. Leptomeningeal metastases: Comparison of clinical features and laboratory data of solid tumors, lymphomas and leukemias. *J Neurooncol* 1990;9:225–229.
46. Boogerd W, Hart AA, van der Sande JJ, et al. Meningeal carcinomatosis in breast cancer. Prognostic factors and influence of treatment. *Cancer* 1991;67:1685–1695.
47. Collie DA, Brush JP, Lammie GA, et al. Imaging features of leptomeningeal metastases. *Clin Radiol* 1999;54(11)765–771.
48. Straathof CA, de Bruin HG, Dippel DW, et al. The diagnostic accuracy of magnetic resonance imaging and cerebrospinal fluid cytology in leptomeningeal metastasis. *J Neurol* 1999;246(9):810–814.
49. Central Nervous System Cancers. NCCN Clinical Practice Guidelines in Oncology. V.I. 2007. Available at: www.nccn.org/professionals/physician_gls/PDF/cns.pdf. Accessed December 19, 2007.
50. Seute T, Leffers P, ten Velde GP, et al. Leptomeningeal metastases from small cell lung carcinoma. *Cancer* 2005;104:1700–1705.
51. Chamberlain MC, Kormanik P. Carcinoma meningitis secondary to non-small cell lung cancer. *Arch Neurol* 1998;55:506–512.
52. Hitchins RN, Bell DR, Woods RL, et al. A prospective randomized trial of single-agent versus combination chemotherapy in meningeal carcinomatosis. *J Clin Oncol* 1987;5(10):1655–1662.
53. Grossman SA, Finkelstein DM, Ruckdeschel JC, et al. Randomized prospective comparison of intraventricular methotrexate and thiotepa in patients with previously untreated neoplastic meningitis. *J Clin Oncology* 1993;11:561–569.
54. Glantz MJ, Jaeckle KA, Chamberlain MC, et al. A randomized controlled trial comparing intrathecal sustained-release cytarabine (DepoCyt) to intrathecal methotrexate in patients with neoplastic meningitis from solid tumors. *Clin Cancer Res* 1999;5:3394–3402.
55. Kim DY, Lee KW, Yun T, et al. Comparison of intrathecal chemotherapy for leptomeningeal carcinomatosis of a solid tumor: methotrexate alone versus methotrexate in combination with cytosine arabinoside and hydrocortisone. *Jpn J Clin Oncol* 2003;33:608–612.
56. Boogerd W, van den Bent MJ, Koehler PJ, et al. The relevance of intraventricular chemotherapy for leptomeningeal metastasis in breast cancer: a randomised study. *Eur J Cancer* 2004;40:2726–733.
57. DeAngelis LM, Mandell LR, Thaler T, et al. The role of postoperative radiotherapy after resection of single brain metastases. *Neurosurgery* 1989;24(6):798–805.
58. Regine WF, Scott C, Murray K, et al. Neurocognitive outcome in brain metastases patients treated with accelerated-fractionation vs. accelerated-hyperfractionated radiotherapy: an analysis from Radiation Therapy Oncology Group Study 91-04. *Int J Radiat Oncol Biol Phys* 2001;51:711–717.
59. Taylor BV, Buckner JC, Cascino TL, et al. Effects of radiation and chemotherapy on cognitive function in patients with high-grade glioma. *J Clin Oncol* 1998;16(6):2195–2201.
60. Meyers CA, Smith JA, Bezjak A, et al. Neurocognitive function and progression in patients with brain metastases treated with whole-brain radiation and motexafin gadolinium: results of a randomized phase III trial. *J Clin Oncol* 2004;22(1):157–165.
61. Brezden CB, Phillips KA, Abdolell M, et al. Cognitive function in breast cancer patients receiving adjuvant chemotherapy. *J Clin Oncol* 2000;18(14):2695–2701.
62. Klein M, Engelberts NH, van der Ploeg HM, et al. Epilepsy in low-grade gliomas: the impact on cognitive function and quality of life. *Ann Neurol* 2003;54(4):514–520.
63. Klein M, Heimans JJ, Aaronson NK, et al. Effect of radiotherapy and other treatment-related factors on mid-term to long-term cognitive sequelae in low-grade gliomas: a comparative study. *Lancet* 2002; 360(9343):1361–1368.
64. Sonderkaer S, Schmiegelow M, Carstensen H, et al. Long-term neurological outcome of childhood brain tumors treated by surgery only. *J Clin Oncol* 2003;21(7):1347–1351.
65. Zacny JP, Gutierrez S. Characterizing the subjective, psychomotor, and physiological effects of oral oxycodone in non-drug-abusing volunteers. *Psychopharmacology (Berl)* 2003 Nov;170(3):242–254. Epub 2003 Aug 29.
66. Aldenkamp AP, Arends J, Bootsma HP, et al. Randomized double-blind parallel-group study comparing cognitive effects of a low-dose lamotrigine with valproate and placebo in healthy volunteers. *Epilepsia* 2002;43(1):19–26.
67. Salinsky MC, Storzbach D, Spencer DC, et al. Effects of topiramate and gabapentin on cognitive abilities in healthy volunteers. *Neurology* 2005;64:792–298.
68. Glantz MJ, Cole BF, Forsyth PA, et al. Practice parameter: anticonvulsant prophylaxis in patients with newly diagnosed brain tumors: report of the Quality Standards Subcommittee of the American Academy of Neurology. *Neurology* 2000;54:1886–1893.
69. Byrne TN. Spinal cord compression from epidural metastases. *N Engl J Med* 1992;327:614–619.
70. Quinn JA, DeAngelis LM. Neurologic emergencies in the cancer patient. *Semin Oncol* 2000;27:311–321.
71. Maranzano E, Latini P, Checcaglini F, et al. Radiation therapy in metastatic spinal cord compression: a prospective analysis of 105 consecutive patients. *Cancer* 1991;67:1311–1317.

72. Kato A, Ushio Y, Hayakawa T, et al. Circulatory disturbance of the spinal cord with epidural neoplasm in rats. *J Neurosurg* 1985 Aug;63(2):260–265.
73. Fuller BG, Heiss JD, Oldfield EH. Spinal cord compression. In: DeVita VT, Hellman S, Rosenberg SA, eds. *Cancer: Principles and Practice of Oncology*. Philadelphia, PA: Lippincott Williams and Wilkins, 2001:2617–2633.
74. Heldmann U, Myschetzky PS, Thomsen HS. Frequency of unexpected multifocal metastasis in patients with acute spinal cord compression. Evaluation by low-field MR imaging in cancer patients. *Acta Radiol* 1997 May;38(3):372–375.
75. Schiff D, O'Neill BP, Wang CH, et al. Neuroimaging and treatment implications of patients with multiple epidural spinal metastases. *Cancer* 1998 Oct 15;83(8):1593–601.
76. Gilbert RW, Kim JH, Posner JB. Epidural spinal cord compression from metastatic tumor: diagnosis and treatment. *Ann Neurol* 1978 Jan;3(1):40–51.
77. Martenson JA, Evans RG, Lie MR, et al. Treatment outcome and complications in patients treated for malignant epidural spinal cord compression (SCC). *J Neurooncol* 1985;3(1):77–84.
78. Torma T. Malignant tumors of the spine and spinal epidural space: a study based on 250 histologically verified cases. *Acta Chir Scand* 1957;225:1.
79. Li KC, Poon PY. Sensitivity and specificity of MRI in detecting malignant spinal cord compression and in distinguishing malignant from benign compression fractures of vertebrae. *Magn Reson Imaging* 1988 Sep-Oct;6(5):547–556.
80. Loughrey GJ, Collins CD, Todd SM, et al. Magnetic resonance imaging in the management of suspected spinal canal disease in patients with known malignancy. *Clin Radiol* 2000 Nov;55(11):849–855.
81. Helweg-Larsen S, Sorensen PS. Symptoms and sings in metastatic spinal cord compression: a study of progression from first symptom until diagnosis in 153 patients. *Eur J Cancer* 1994:30A:396.
82. Rades D, Heidenreich F, Karstens JH. Final results of a prospective study of the prognostic value of the time to develop motor deficits before irradiation in metastatic spinal cord compression. *Int J Radiat Oncol Biol Phys* 2002 Jul 15;53(4):975–979.
83. Sorensen S, Helweg-Larsen S, Mouridsen H, et al. Effect of high-dose dexamethasone in carcinomatous metastatic spinal cord compression treated with radiotherapy: a randomised trial. *Eur J Cancer* 1994;30A(1):22–27
84. Vecht CJ, Haaxma-Reiche H, van Putten WL, et al. Initial bolus of conventional versus high-dose dexamethasone in metastatic spinal cord compression. *Neurology* 1989 Sep;39(9):1255–1257.
85. Heimdal K, Hirschberg H, Slettebo H, et al. High incidence of serious side effects of high-dose dexamethasone treatment in patients with epidural spinal cord compression. *J Neurooncol* 1992 Feb;12(2): 141–144.
86. Lai KC, Lam SK, Chu KM, et al. Lansoprazole for the prevention of recurrences of ulcer complications from long-term low-dose aspirin use. *N Engl J Med* 2002 Jun 27;346(26):2033–2038.
87. Loblaw DA, Laperriere NJ. Emergency treatment of malignant extradural spinal cord compression: an evidence-based guideline. *J Clin Oncol* 1998 Apr;16(4):1613–1624.
88. Rades D, Stalpers LJ, Veninga T, et al. Evaluation of five radiation schedules and prognostic factors for metastatic spinal cord compression. *J Clin Oncol* 2005;23(15):3366–3375.
89. Rades D, Stalpers LJ, Schulte R, et al. Defining the appropriate radiotherapy regimen for metastatic spinal cord compression in non-small cell lung cancer patients. *Eur J Cancer* 2006;42(8):1052–1056. Epub 2006 Mar 31.
90. Maranzano E, Bellavita R, Rossi R, et al. Short-course versus split-course radiotherapy in metastatic spinal cord compression: results of a phase III, randomized, multicenter trial. *J Clin Oncol* 2005;23(15):3358–3365. Epub 2005 Feb 28.
91. Kwok Y, Regine WF, Patchell RA. Radiation therapy alone for spinal cord compression: time to improve upon a relatively ineffective status quo. *J Clin Oncol* 2005 May 20;23(15):3308–3310. Epub 2005 Feb 28.
92. Wu JS, Wong R, Johnston M, et al. Meta-analysis of dose-fractionation radiotherapy trials for the palliation of painful bone metastases. *Int J Radiat Oncol Biol Phys* 2003 Mar 1;55(3):594–605.
93. St. Clair WH, Arnold SM, Sloan AE, et al. Spinal cord and peripheral nerve injury: current management and investigations. *Semin Radiat Oncol* 2003 Jul;13(3):322–332.
94. Flickinger JC, Pollock BE, Kondziolka D, et al. A dose-response analysis of arteriovenous malformation obliteration after radiosurgery. *Int J Radiat Oncol Biol Phys* 1996 Nov 1;36(4):873–879.
95. Chow E, Davis L, Panzarella T, et al. Accuracy of survival prediction by palliative radiation oncologists. *Int J Radiat Oncol Biol Phys* 2005 Mar 1;61(3):870–873.
96. Young RF, Post EM, King GA. Treatment of spinal epidural metastases: randomized prospective comparison of laminectomy and radiotherapy. *J Neurosurg* 1980;53:741–748.
97. Patchell RA, Tibbs PA, Regine WF, et al. Direct decompressive surgical resection in the treatment of spinal cord compression caused by metastatic cancer: a randomised trial. *Lancet* 2005 Aug 20–26;366(9486): 643–648.
98. Kalayci M, Cagavi F, Gul S, et al. Intramedullary spinal cord metastases: diagnosis and treatment—an illustrated review. *Acta Neurochir (Wien)* 2004 Dec;146(12):1347–1354; discussion 1354. Epub 2004 Nov 8.
99. Mut M, Schiff D, Shaffrey ME. Metastasis to nervous system: spinal epidural and intramedullary metastases. *J Neurooncol* 2005;75(1):43–56.

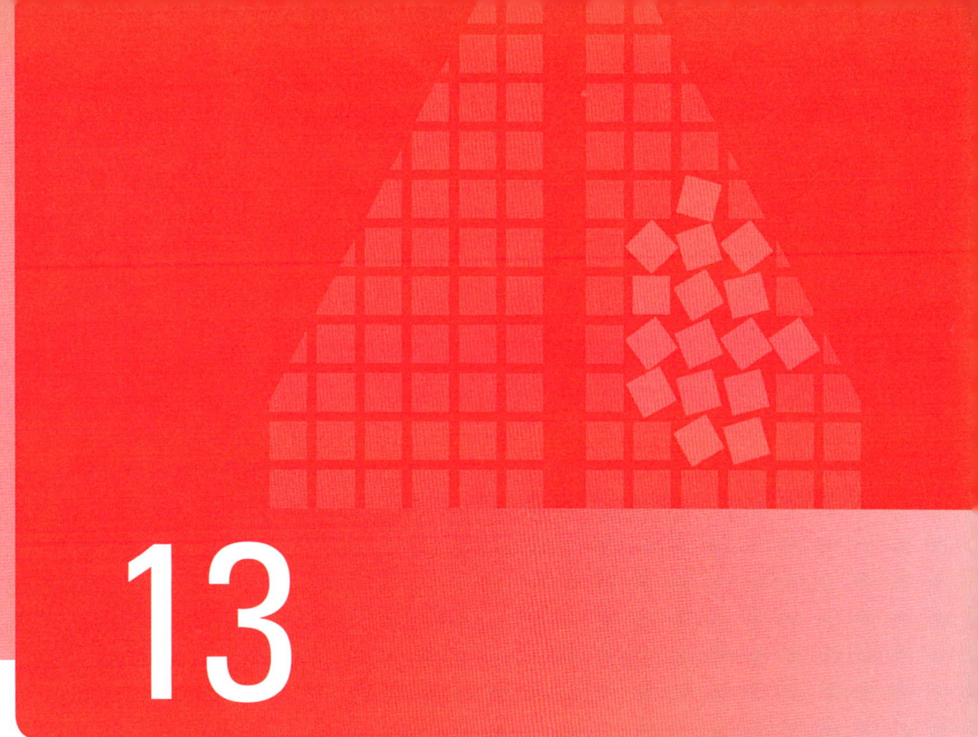

SECTION 13

Other Thoracic Malignancies

CHAPTER 64

Patrick J. Loehrer, Sr.
John Henley
Kenneth Kesler

Thymoma and Thymic Carcinoma

Thymoma and thymic carcinoma represent the most common malignancies found in the anterior mediastinum. Thymomas can also rarely originate in the thyroid, lung, or pleural spaces, presumably arising from ectopic vestigial remnants of thymic tissue. According to Surveillance, Epidemiologic, and End Results (SEER) data accumulated between 1973 and 1998 from nine states within the United States, the overall incidence of thymoma was of 0.15 cases per 100,000 person-years.[1]

Epithelial disorders of the thymus exhibit a wide spectrum of histologic features and clinical behavior. Thymic hyperplasia displays an invariably benign behavior, whereas thymomas demonstrate variable degrees of local invasiveness and some have distant metastatic potential. At the other extreme are thymic carcinomas, which exhibit cytological features of carcinoma, including nuclear enlargement, pleomorphism, and hyperchromasia. These often present in advanced clinical stages.

ETIOLOGY AND PATHOGENESIS

The thymus is a spongelike scaffolding of epithelial cells soaked with T lymphocytes. It reaches its maximum development at puberty, weighing approximately 40 g, and undergoes involution and atrophy with aging. The dynamic microenvironment of the thymus contributes to the maturation of T lymphocytes, a process that depends on signals provided by the thymic stroma.[2] Stromal elements include epithelial cells, macrophages, dendritic cells, fibroblasts, and matrix molecules. The topographical separation of the thymus in cortical and medullary portions reflects the functional progression of this maturation process. This is relevant to thymoma, as tumors may show histologic evidence of cortical and medullary differentiation.

Causative factors for the development of thymomas have not been identified, although Epstein-Barr virus (EBV) has been associated with cases of lymphoepithelioma-like thymic carcinoma.[3]

Several immunohistochemical studies have examined the expression of apoptosis-related proteins, such as bcl-2 and p53, in thymomas.[4–6] Bcl-2 expression is notable in medullary or spindle-cell thymoma (World Health Organization [WHO] type A, see discussion that follows). The p53 gene is found to be overexpressed by immunohistochemistry (IHC) in a subset of thymomas, whereas the majority of thymic carcinoma cases are overexpressors of p53.[6,7] However, on polymerase chain reaction (PCR) testing, very few cases have p53 mutations.

Genetic abnormalities, most commonly described as loss of heterozygosity (LOH), are seen throughout all thymoma subtypes. The long arm of chromosome 6 is usually involved, especially region 6q23.3 to 25.3.[8,9] Other consistent abnormalities include chromosomes 3, 5, 7, 8, 13, and 17. These are rarely seen in WHO type A thymomas. Correlation of these findings with the invasive potential of thymomas has been proposed,[10–12] but no definitive link is available to date. Another study has shown an increased incidence of aneuploidy in thymic epithelial tumors with advancing stage.[13]

The expression of two tyrosine kinase receptors, epithelial growth factor receptor (EGFR) and c-KIT ligand, have been examined in a relatively large number of malignant thymic tumors. EGFR and c-KIT appear to be preferentially expressed in thymoma and thymic carcinoma, respectively.[14–17] Although the significance of this observation is unclear, the differential staining pattern of these markers is of potential diagnostic use in distinguishing these tumors.

The maturation process of T lymphocytes frequently becomes abnormal in patients with thymomas.[18,19] Irregularities include impairment of CD4+ T-cell development, decreased interferon-gamma–induced human leukocyte antigen-DR (HLA-DR) expression on cultured thymoma epithelial cells, and lower levels of major histocompatibility complex (MHC) class II antigen expression.[20] Peripheral blood lymphocytosis is commonly observed, with an increased proportion of CD45RA+CD8+ T cells as opposed to an apparent decrease in the CD4 cell population that may reverse after thymectomy.[21]

PATHOLOGY

Thymoma is a neoplasm arising from thymic epithelial cells. Classification of thymic epithelial tumors has been confused by a plethora of subtyping schemes.[22] (Table 64.1) The difficulty in the histopathologic classification of thymomas is twofold. First, thymomas have a spectrum of appearances, ranging from lymphocyte-rich tumors in which the neoplastic epithelial cells are difficult to discern without the aid of IHC, to lymphoid-deplete tumors that approach the appearance of undifferentiated carcinoma. Second, histologic examination correlates poorly with clinical behavior.

A standard classification, based on the relative proportions of epithelial cells and lymphocytes, subdivided thymomas into predominately lymphocytic, epithelial, mixed, and spindle-cell types.[23] Although simple in concept and reproducible in application, this scheme lacked the clinical relevance and ontogenetic considerations that the later schemes attempted to provide. Levine and Rosai[24] divided thymic epithelial tumors into thymoma, noninvasive and invasive types, and thymic carcinoma, the latter discernible by its frankly malignant cytology. Marino and Müller-Hermelink (MM-H)[25] stressed ontogenic considerations and subtyped thymomas according to the appearance of the neoplastic epithelial cells (i.e., cortical vs. medullary types). Additional descriptions of well-differentiated thymic carcinoma followed, which suggested a spectrum of tumors ranging from thymoma to unequivocal carcinoma.[26] Suster and Moran,[27] in an effort at simplication, proposed the distinction of thymic neoplasms based on the degree of differentiation: thymoma (well-differentiated type), atypical thymomas (moderately differentiated type), and thymic carcinomas (poorly differentiated type).[27]

TABLE 64.1 Pathological Classifications of Thymoma*

Bernatz et al.[23]	Predominantly epithelial
	Predominantly lymphocytic
	Predominantly mixed
	Predominantly spindle cell
Levine and Rosai[24]	Circumscribed
	Malignant type I (invasive thymoma with no or minimal atypia)
	Malignant type II (cytologically malignant, thymic carcinoma)
	Squamous cell carcinoma
	Lymphoepithelioma-like carcinoma
	Clear cell carcinoma
	Sarcomatoid carcinoma
	Undifferentiated carcinoma
Marino and Müller-Hermelink[25,169]	Thymoma
	Medullary
	Mixed (medullary and cortical)
	Predominantly cortical
	Cortical
	Well-differentiated thymic carcinoma
	Thymic carcinoma
	Epidermoid
	Undifferentiated
	Endocrine carcinoma-carcinoid
WHO Classification[170]	Type A (medullary, spindle cell)
	Type AB (mixed)
	Type B1 (predominantly cortical, lymphocyte rich)
	Type B2 (cortical)
	Type B3 (well-differentiated thymic carcinoma, atypical thymoma)
	Type C (thymic carcinoma)

*See text for correlations among subtypes.

The most recent classification, from the WHO Committee for the Classification of Thymic Epithelial Tumors,[28] incorporates features from both the traditional and MM-H classifications. It is the classification that is currently advocated in an effort to standardize thymoma classification. The WHO scheme divides thymoma into types A, B, and C, as well as mixed forms (i.e., type AB). Type A represents spindle-cell or medullary thymoma, an indolent tumor with little propensity for aggressive behavior. Type B is further subdivided into types B-1, B-2, B-3. Type B-1 tumors are lymphocyte rich and may resemble the normal thymus, with areas of medullary differentiation. In type B-2 tumors, neoplastic epithelial cells are more numerous with larger nuclei and more prominent nuclei. Type B-3 tumors have a predominance of epithelial cells and include tumors that previous authors have called well-differentiated thymic carcinoma and atypical thymoma. These tumors lack the cytologic atypia that warrants a diagnosis of thymic carcinoma. Type C thymoma represents thymic carcinoma; various cell types are encountered, with lymphoepithelioma-like carcinoma being the most common. These are high-grade tumors that are histologically reminiscent of their namesake, lymphoepithelial carcinoma of the nasopharynx. Other cell types include squamous cell carcinoma, small cell or neuroendocrine carcinoma, anaplastic or undifferentiated carcinoma, sarcomatoid carcinoma, adenosquamous carcinoma, and clear cell carcinoma. Although most carcinomas are high-grade malignancies, a few low-grade variants carry a more favorable prognosis and include well-differentiated squamous carcinoma, low-grade mucoepidermoid carcinoma, and basaloid carcinoma. Thus, grading thymic carcinomas into low- and high-grade types is of prognostic utility.[26] The WHO classification has come into criticism.[29,30]

Because the histology of thymic carcinomas is "non-organotypic" (i.e., their appearance provides no recognition of their origin from the thymus), it may be difficult to unequivocally assign the organ of origin when evaluating tumors involving the region of the thymus.[31–36] No immunohistochemical profile is unique to thymic carcinoma, although CD5 expression is reportedly increased.[33,35] The specificity of CD5 for thymic carcinoma relative to other differential diagnostic considerations is unclear and in our experience, CD5 staining is too inconsistent to be of clinical utility. Especially when pathology reveals squamous cell carcinoma, small cell carcinoma, and clear cell carcinoma, another primary malignancy should be excluded before the definitive diagnosis of thymic carcinoma.[37]

Nonepithelial tumors arising in the thymus are not considered in the tumor classifications mentioned previously, including thymic carcinoid tumors, germ cell tumors, hematopoietic malignancies, sarcomas, and benign mesenchymal neoplasms. Thymic carcinoid tumors are much more pernicious than their pulmonary counterparts and have been linked to multiple endocrine neoplasia in up to a quarter of the cases.[38]

CLINICAL FEATURES

Presentation In a recent SEER database study, the mean age at presentation of thymomas and thymic carcinomas was reported as 56 years, with the incidence increasing up to the age of 77, when it neared 0.5 cases per 100,000.[1] Eleven percent of cases occurred prior to 35 years of age. The incidence was slightly higher in men compared to women (0.16 vs. 0.13 per 100,000) and in blacks compared to whites (0.20 vs. 0.12 per 100,000).

The thymus is located adjacent to the pericardium and the great vessels of the chest and is limited by the neck superiorly. Thymomas encompass 20% of all mediastinal masses and 45% of anterior mediastinal tumors. Nonmalignant masses in the anterior mediastinum to be considered in the differential diagnosis include aneurysms, granulomas, pericardial and esophageal cysts, and Morgagni hernias. Other malignant masses of the anterior mediastinum include lymphoma (20%), parathyroid and thyroid tumors (15%), germ cell tumors (15%), and neurogenic and mesenchymal neoplasms.

Thymomas often present as a mediastinal mass, which may cause local symptoms (chest pains, dyspnea, hemoptysis, dysphonia, Horner syndrome, and superior vena cava compression). Alternatively, in approximately one third of patients may present with a paraneoplastic syndrome, such as myasthenia gravis (MG) or pure red cell aplasia (PRCA). Finally, one third of patients may present with a mediastinal mass incidentally discovered on radiographic imaging.

Paraneoplastic Syndromes Approximately 40% of thymoma patients have a paraneoplastic syndrome (Table 64.2), and there is a lower incidence among thymic carcinoma cases. The precise correlation of paraneoplastic phenomena with deranged intratumoral T-cell maturation has not been established.

MG is the most common paraneoplastic syndrome.[39,40] The acetylcholine receptor (AChR) is transiently found on the surface of myoid cells in the thymus in patients with thymic hyperplasia, and is considered to be the stimulus for autoimmunity and generation of anti-AChR antibodies that lead to MG.[41] Interestingly, in thymoma specimens, myoid cells were not detected, although cytoplasmic AChR epitopes were seen.[42] Expression of the AChR P3A$^-$ α-subunit gene also

TABLE 64.2 Paraneoplastic Syndromes Associated with Thymomas

Myasthenia gravis	Ulcerative colitis
Eaton-Lambert syndrome	Hashimoto thyroiditis
Myotonic dystrophy	Rheumatoid arthritis
Myositis	Sarcoidosis
Stiff person syndrome	Scleroderma
Limbic encephalopathy	Addison disease
Sensorimotor radiculopathy	Hyperthyroidism
Red cell aplasia	Hyperparathyroidism
Hemolytic anemia	Panhypopituitarism
Hypogammaglobulinemia	Hypertrophic pulmonary osteoarthropathy
T-cell deficiency syndrome	Nephrotic syndrome
Pancytopenia	Minimal change nephropathy
Erythrocytosis	Pemphigus
Megakaryocytopenia	Chronic mucocutaneous candidiasis
Systemic lupus erythematosus	Alopecia areata
Polymyositis	
Myocarditis	
Sjögren syndrome	

correlated with MG in patients with thymoma.[43] Ströbel et al.[44] demonstrated a higher production of intratumorous naive CD4+ T cells in thymoma patients with MG compared to thymoma without MG.

Thymoma is believed to be present in 10% of established MG cases, whereas 30% to 50% of patients with thymoma eventually develop clinical MG. Of note, MG is rarely associated with thymic carcinoma or WHO subtypes A or AB. In the study of Okumura et al.,[45] which excluded thymic carcinoma cases, 69% of MG cases had thymomas of B subtype (Table 64.3), and 80% were of B subtype in the series of Evoli et al.[46] Some studies suggest that HLA A24 and B8 are predictive for the presence of thymoma in patients with MG.[47]

Anti-titin antibodies represent one type of antiskeletal muscle antibodies that is frequently present in patients with thymoma or late-onset MG. One study revealed a sensitivity of 68% for presence of thymoma in newly diagnosed MG patients.[48] However, anti-titin antibodies have not been found to be helpful in predicting thymoma recurrences.[49]

Acquired PRCA occurs in approximately 5% of patients with thymoma,[50] and approximately 10% of patients with this syndrome harbor a thymoma.[51] PRCA is suspected in the presence of isolated anemia and a low reticulocyte count and is confirmed with a bone marrow examination. Alternative diagnoses such as myelodysplastic syndromes, underlying chronic lymphocytic leukemia, and parvovirus (erythrovirus) B19 infection need to be entertained. The etiology of PRCA in the setting of a thymoma has not been definitely established, although mouse and in vitro studies suggested the presence of a possible erythropoiesis inhibitor.[52] A T cell-mediated process has also been proposed.[53–55]

TABLE 64.3 Association with Myasthenia Gravis according to the World Health Organization Histologic Classification System for Thymic Epithelial Tumors

WHO Tumor Type

Status	A	AB	B1	B2	B3	Total
Not associated with MG	15	65	24	28	14	146
Associated with MG (%)	3 (16.7)	12 (15.6)	31 (56.4)	69 (71.1)	12 (46.2)	127

Reproduced with permission from Okumura M, Ohta M, Tateyama H, et al. The World Health Organization histologic classification system reflects the oncologic behavior of thymoma: a clinical study of 273 patients. *Cancer* 2002;94:624–632.

Hypogammaglobulinemia (Good syndrome) also occurs in patients with thymic epithelial malignancies[56,57] and is frequently associated with recurrent sinopulmonary infections. Good syndrome leads to severe manifestations in less than 5% of cases. Cytomegalovirus infections (colitis, retinitis) have been reported.[58] Masci et al.[59] demonstrated the presence of an oligoclonal population of CD8+ T cells in the bone marrow of five patients with thymoma-associated hypogammaglobulinemia. Lymphopenia has also been reported[56] and frequently coexists with hypogammaglobulinemia.

Second neoplasms were found to occur with increased incidence (up to 28%) in patients who had a history of thymoma according to several reports.[1,60,61] The most common was colorectal, and reasons for this association are largely unknown. The recent SEER review, however, could not definitely establish an increased incidence of malignancies other than B-cell non-Hodgkin lymphomas (4.7-fold increased incidence, persisting up to 10 years after thymoma diagnosis) and soft tissue sarcomas.[1]

Diagnostic Evaluation

The diagnosis of thymomas is established by a core needle biopsy computed tomography (CT) guidance, mediastinoscopy with biopsy, or open or video-assisted thoracotomy. Fine needle aspiration (FNA) may reveal the diagnosis in a subset of cases,[62] but are error prone in 5% to 10% of cases (usually confused with lymphoma).[63] There is a possibility that only lymphoid material, rather than epithelial cells, will be present.[64] Flow cytometry and T-cell receptor rearrangement studies[65] may be helpful in assessing the possibility of lymphocyte clonality. FNA also does not allow assessment of capsular invasion. In ancillary testing, a careful and often history-directed immunohistochemical panel (see previous discussion under "Pathology") can assist in the differentiation between lymphoid neoplasms, non–small cell lung cancer (thyroid transcription factor-1 [TTF-1] positive in approximately 60% to 70% of cases), thyroid, and germ cell tumors. Given the fact that thymomas are relatively uncommon, and that alternative diagnoses carry important treatment implications (such as germ-cell tumor, lung cancer, or lymphoma), pathology specimens are best reviewed by individuals and at institutions with experience in the evaluation of mediastinal neoplasms.

Especially when the mediastinal mass is described as a poorly differentiated malignancy, it is important to confirm and be sure of the diagnosis. Aspects of importance in the history include the age and gender of the patient, the amount of tobacco exposure, and a careful search for paraneoplastic syndromes. In the physical exam, a thorough lymph node exam should be performed, especially when it is not clear if the mediastinal mass is originating from the anterior or posterior mediastinum. Thymomas and germ cell tumors generally may present with or supraclavicular adenopathy; bilateral or peripheral lymphadenopathy should lead one to suspect lymphoma. In patients with undiagnosed masses or poorly differentiated malignancies, serum α-fetoprotein (AFP) and human chorionic gonadotropin (HCG) levels should be obtained. Imaging studies can be helpful when showing pleural-based metastases that are typical of thymic malignancies. Lastly, chromosomal evaluation with the presence of isochromosome 12p with fluorescence in-situ hybridization (FISH) would lead to a diagnosis of germ cell tumors.

When there is a high clinical suspicion for thymoma, based on an encapsulated mediastinal mass on chest CT scans, no evidence of metastases and normal serum AFP and HCG levels, then definitive resection can be planned without biopsies being obtained. The direct surgical procedure without a previous biopsy avoids the concern of tumor seeding, which has been raised by some authors.

The pattern of spread may be helpful in distinguishing from other malignancies. Thymomas characteristically spread to pleural surfaces. Although uncommon, liver, bone, kidney, and brain metastases may also occur. In the face of metastatic pleural implants on CT scans, representative percutaneous ultrasound or CT-guided core biopsies can be obtained to establish the diagnosis.

Thymomas often express somatostatin receptors. Although indium-labeled octreotide scans lack diagnostic specificity, they are frequently positive in thymomas[66–68] and are helpful when considering treatment with octreotide. Indium-labeled octreotide can be helpful in distinguishing a thymoma from thymic hyperplasia.

Kubota et al.[69] examined the role of positron emission tomography (PET) scans in 22 patients with anterior mediastinal masses. It was found that both noninvasive thymomas and invasive thymomas can demonstrate increased uptake, although the invasive subtypes and thymic carcinomas appeared to have higher standard uptake values (SUV). Another study did not find significant differences in ^{18}F-fluorodeoxyglucose PET uptake between patients with invasive and noninvasive thymomas.[70] The use of PET scans in the evaluation and management of thymomas remains investigational at this time.

Staging In 1981, Masaoka et al.[71] published a clinical staging system based on the degree of invasion of thymomas (Table 64.4). This classification has been validated and established 5-year overall survivals of 92.6%, 85.7%, 69.6%, and 50% for stages I, II, III, and IV, respectively. These data support the indolent nature of this disease even for many patients with advanced disease. Of note, patients with subtotal

TABLE 64.4 Staging of Thymomas

Masaoka Clinical Stage

Stage I:	Macroscopically completely encapsulated and microscopically no capsular invasion
Stage II:	Macroscopic invasion into surrounding fatty tissue or mediastinal pleura, or microscopic invasion into capsule
Stage III:	Macroscopic invasion into neighboring organs (i.e., pericardium, great vessels, or lung)
Stage IVa:	Pleural or pericardial dissemination
Stage IVb:	Lymphogenous or hematogenous metastasis

GETT Postoperative Staging System

Stage	Description
I-A	Encapsulated tumor, totally resected
I-B	Macroscopically encapsulated tumor, totally resected, but the surgeon suspects mediastinal adhesions and potential capsular invasion
II	Invasive tumor, totally resected
III-A	Invasive tumor, subtotally resected
III-B	Invasive tumor, biopsy only
IV-A	Supraclavicular metastasis or distant pleural implant
IV-B	Distant metastasis

TNM Classification and Staging

T factor:

T1: Macroscopically completely encapsulated and microscopically no capsular invasion

T2: Macroscopically adhesion or invasion into surrounding fatty tissue or mediastinal pleura, or microscopic invasion into capsule

T3: Invasion into neighboring organs, such as pericardium, great vessels, and lung

T4: Pleural or pericardial dissemination

N factor:

N0: No lymph node metastasis

N1: Metastasis to anterior mediastinal lymph nodes

N2: Metastasis to intrathoracic lymph nodes except anterior mediastinal lymph nodes

N3: Metastasis to extrathoracic lymph nodes

M factor:

M0: No hematogenous metastasis

M1: Hematogenous metastasis

Stage:

Stage I	T1	N0	M0
Stage II	T2	N0	M0
Stage III	T3	N0	M0
Stage IVa	T4	N0	M0
Stage IVb	Any T	N1,2,3	M0
	Any T	Any N	M1

resections received radiation therapy (RT) postoperatively in that series.

Another system, from the French Groupe d'Etudes des Tumeurs Thymiques (GETT), was proposed in 1991,[72] and is based on pathological postoperative staging (Table 64.4). Although generally felt to be equivalent to the Masaoka stage in terms of prognosis,[73] the GETT system (when compared with Masaoka) downstages invasion into neighboring organs, if complete resection was achieved. Additionally, in the Masaoka classification, microscopic invasion through the capsule was found to have prognostic significance. Microscopic invasion is not taken into account in the GETT classification. These slight differences have some implication regarding prognosis. For instance, Masaoka stage II-GETT stage I patients tend to have a better disease-free survival than the Masaoka stage II-GETT stage II patients. The current TNM staging greatly reflects the original Masaoka system[74] (Table 64.4).

One study evaluated the correlation of computer tomography with the ability to predict capsular invasion.[75] Invasive thymomas were more likely to have lobulated or irregular contours than noninvasive thymomas, as well as a higher prevalence of low attenuation areas and foci of calcification within the tumor than noninvasive thymomas. However, the findings are unlikely to be of enough specificity to substitute for pathological staging during thymectomy.

PROGNOSTIC FACTORS

Interpretation of the current literature regarding the factors affecting individual prognosis in thymic malignancies is difficult. Studies that investigate prognostic determinants have been hindered by the use of different histologic classifications and by their retrospective nature, which potentially introduces selection biases into results. Furthermore, treatment differences among series, including the extent and expertise of the surgical resection, further confound prognostic associations.

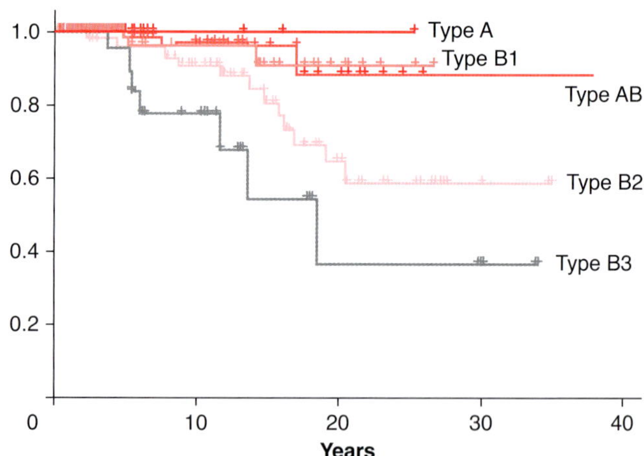

FIGURE 64.1 Thymoma-specific survival according to WHO classification.

Nonetheless, three factors consistently emerge to shape prognosis: stage of disease, completeness of resection, and tumor histology.[75–77] Histological classifications were found to be independent predictors of survival or relapse in some studies[45,78–80] (Fig. 64.1) Close correlation is seen between the pathological classifications of MM-H[81,82] and WHO[45] and the Masaoka clinical staging system (Table 64.5). The prognostic significance of tumor histology seemed to be greater with low stage disease in another study.[83] Medullary or spindle-cell thymomas (WHO type A) typically present as low-stage tumors and carry the most favorable prognosis. High-stage tumors are more likely to be cortical-type thymomas (WHO type B) or thymic carcinoma (WHO type C).[84]

Other poor prognostic indicators include recurrence, unresectable tumor (Fig. 64.2), symptoms at presentation, and invasion of great vessels, which, however, was not an independent factor for thymoma-related mortality[85] (Fig. 64.3). Some data suggests that molecular markers such as high p53, low p27, and low p21 expressions may be associated with adverse outcomes.[86]

TABLE 64.5 Masaoka Stage with Reference to the World Health Organization Histologic Classification System for Thymic Epithelial Tumors

WHO Tumor Type						
Stage	**A**	**AB**	**B1**	**B2**	**B3**	**Total**
I	16	45	29	30	4	124
II	1	25	15	19	10	70
III	1	6	9	37	10	63
IVa	—	—	2	8	—	10
IVb	—	1	—	3	2	6
Average	1.17	1.53	1.71	2.33	2.46	—

Reproduced with permission from Okumura M, Ohta M, Tateyama H, et al. The World Health Organization histologic classification system reflects the oncologic behavior of thymoma: a clinical study of 273 patients. *Cancer* 2002;94:624–632.

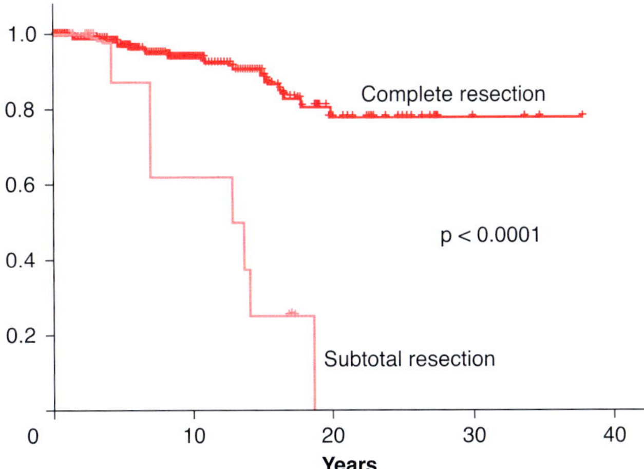

FIGURE 64.2 Thymoma-specific survival according to completeness of resection.

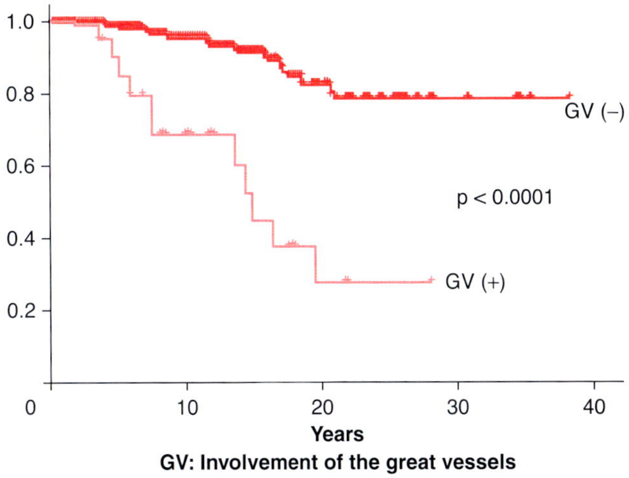

1.0
0.8
0.6
0.4
0.2
0
10
20
30
40
Years
GV (–)
p < 0.0001
GV (+)
GV: Involvement of the great vessels

FIGURE 64.3 Thymoma-specific survival according to involvement of great vessels.

The significance of staging becomes less clear with thymic carcinoma, which carries a poor long-term outcome. In one study, 65% of patients were alive at 5 years and only innominate vessel invasion was an independent prognostic factor.[87] Other authors have associated improved survival with encapsulated tumors, a lobular growth pattern, low mitotic activity, and low histologic grade.[88]

In most recent series, MG has not been associated with overall survival differences.[87,89] These data refute early reports that indicated an increased risk of surgery in these patients. Maggi et al.[90] analyzed the outcome of 662 patients who underwent thymectomies for MG in Italy prior to 1989. The postoperative mortality was 4.9% in patients with MG and concurrent thymomas. With current MG preoperative and perioperative management, this risk appears to have decreased; indeed, a few series have associated the presence of MG with improved overall survival, possibly because of an earlier diagnosis of the thymoma.[80,92] Evoli et al.[46] retrospectively evaluated 207 patients with MG and thymoma who underwent thymectomies. One hundred and fifteen patients had invasive thymomas at surgery. Eighteen patients (15%) with invasive disease experienced recurrences.

TREATMENT

Clinically Localized Disease Surgical resection is the recommended treatment for early stage thymic epithelial malignancies, as determined after a clinical and radiographic assessment (e.g., a CT scan of the chest with intravascular contrast).[91–94] Those patients with complete resection fare better than similarly staged patients with incomplete disease.[95] Resection of pericardial surfaces or parietal pleural surfaces as well as lung tissue is often required, especially in stages II and III. Although phrenic nerve involvement may have an adverse effect on postoperative pulmonary function, as a solitary finding, it is not a contraindication for surgery. Less commonly, surgical extirpation may require removal of great veins such as the innominate or superior vena cava (see "locally advanced thymomas" section). The completeness of the surgical resection is considered one of the main prognostic determinants of survival. If an intraoperative determination is made that complete resection is impossible, debulking may have some value based on retrospective data (see discussion that follows),[73] although in recent years, the tendency has been to employ neoadjuvant chemotherapy to facilitate a subsequent complete resection.

Several surgical approaches to accomplish a thymectomy have been described,[96–101] including minimally invasive techniques, but long-term results related to thymoma rates of recurrence are still not available. Complete removal of thymic tissue is typically recommended in MG cases, whereas encapsulated thymomas may need a smaller exploration of the mediastinal contents. Masaoka initially described three approaches for thymectomy: transsternal simple, transcervical simple, and extended thymectomy.[96] Chen et al.[97] advocated thymectomy by anterosuperior cervicomediastinal exenteration. A reversed-T upper mini-sternotomy was proposed by Grandjean et al.[98] with an extended thymectomy for complete removal of thymic tissue, reporting good cosmetic results. Icard et al.[99] published on resection of anterior mediastinal tumors through a mini-sternotomy, and Kaiser[100] used video-assisted techniques in several patients with encapsulated thymoma, especially when combined with a transcervical approach to achieve total thymectomy. Although the results of minimally invasive surgical approaches are being explored, most would consider a complete sternotomy approach standard to accomplish wide mediastinal dissection including total thymectomy in the surgical treatment of thymoma. Finally, Takeo et al.[101] used a sternum-elevating method that provides a wide field of vision between the sternum and the heart and recommended this technique for mostly low-stage thymomas.

Re-resections for isolated recurrences were shown to be feasible.[102] Regnard et al. reviewed their experience in

28 patients with recurrences confined to the thorax. Nineteen patients were able to have complete re-resections, and only three had a subsequent recurrence. The overall 10-year actuarial survival was 43%. However, because many thymomas have an indolent natural history, the impact of re-resections on survival is uncertain.

Radiographic evidence of a recurrent mediastinal density is not always a synonym of recurrent thymoma. In young adults, hyperplasia of benign thymic tissue may be seen after an incomplete resection of the thymus, or especially after chemotherapy for germ cell tumors and lymphomas.

Adjuvant Radiation Therapy after Surgery

Thymoma The evidence for benefit of adjuvant RT in the postoperative setting is retrospective and based on several series from different institutions.[73,76,95,103–116] These series included patients with variable Masaoka stages, variable degrees of completeness of the surgical resection, as well as different radiation fields and doses.[117]

In general, there appears to be no role for RT for completely resected stage I thymomas (absence of microscopic invasion). In several series, the long-term relapse-free survival for stage I patients who did not receive RT is close to 100%.[118] Nevertheless, a 20% recurrence rate has been described for stage I patients with peritumoral adherences found at surgery,[118] whereas patients who received RT in this situation had no recurrences.[73,118,119] The importance of this finding, and the exact definition of peritumoral adherences across different institutions, remains unclear.

Approximately 30% of patients with Masaoka stages II and III who undergo complete surgical resection alone will recur. The use of adjuvant RT in this scenario remains controversial. Adjuvant RT proponents make note of retrospective series in which mediastinal recurrence rates appear to be lower with adjuvant radiation. For instance, in the series of Curran Jr. et al.,[105] there was a 5% recurrence rate in irradiated patients in comparison to 28% without radiotherapy. Alternatively, in a series of 49 completely resected stage II patients from Massachusetts General Hospital, 14 of whom received adjuvant RT, there were no cases of local or distant recurrences in 10 years with or without RT.[120]

Other studies also support the concept that postoperative radiation may not have an impact on completely resected, margin-negative disease. In one of the largest retrospective series reported to date, the outcomes of 1320 patients treated in Japan were evaluated.[95] Adjuvant RT was found not to be of value in preventing local recurrences in patients with completely resected stage II and III thymomas, and the prognosis of completely resected patients receiving adjuvant radiation was not improved compared to no adjuvant RT. However, the latter group was composed of very few patients, because most received adjuvant radiation in this series. Similarly, Singhal et al.[121] found no advantage for postoperative radiation in 40 patients with completely resected stage II thymomas, of which 20 received RT.

The chance of recurrence increases with stage, even for completely resected patients. Ogawa et al.[103] described a 10% overall recurrence rate for stage II patients who received RT, and 44% for similarly treated stage III patients. Haniuda et al.[106] noted an 18.8% recurrence rate in stage II irradiated patients, and a 25% recurrence rate for stage III patients with prior radiation. The majority of recurrences occurred in patients with evidence of microscopic invasion of the mediastinal pleura or pericardium. However, most of these recurrences occurred in the pleura and outside the radiation field. In patients receiving postoperative RT with a mediastinal field with boost, the prognostic value of pathological pleural invasion at surgery in predicting future pleural relapses was also noted.[122]

Most patients in these older series were treated with less sophisticated radiotherapy simulation techniques than available today, and prior to the availability of high-resolution CT scans. This might have resulted in clinical understaging, with more advanced disease patients being referred to surgery, compared to today. In the absence of definitive data, the decision regarding adjuvant RT is made individually based on clinical stage, histological aggressiveness of the primary tumor, and the ability to tolerate RT-related potential complications, such as pulmonary fibrosis.

Different fields have been recommended including whole mediastinum or involved field.[103] Most commonly adjuvant RT fields consist of the entire mediastinum and part of adjacent lung as delineated by surgical clips, or alternatively, based on the preoperative CT scan. One of the major risk factors for radiation-induced pneumonitis appears to be the volume of normal lung encompassed by the 20-Gy isodose line. In an effort to minimize this risk, dose–volume histograms should be created and fields should be selected to achieve the lowest volume of lung in the high-dose regions. Generally, doses of 45 to 50 Gy in 1.8 to 2.0 Gy fractions are used, although no prospective dose-finding studies have been done. Doses greater than 60 Gy did not result in improvements in local control.[123] Lastly, prophylactic pleural and pulmonary adjuvant RT has been deemed feasible in one series but is not widely employed.[124]

Thymic Carcinoma Most patients with thymic carcinomas have locally advanced disease at presentation. In one series, the experience of surgery followed by radiation was reviewed specifically in patients with thymic carcinomas.[125] Seventy-five percent of patients who had a complete resection remained alive with follow-up times ranging from 44 to 193 months. The role of combined modality therapy in such patients lacks sufficient prospective data at this time.[126–128]

Radiotherapy following Incomplete Resections Patients with incomplete resections or positive margins are generally recommended to undergo adjuvant radiation for disease control. Some series report that the outcome of patients with incomplete resections who receive RT can be similar to completely resected patients.[76] Curran Jr. et al.[105] noted a relapse-free survival of 21% following incomplete resections, and at least three series showed no significant outcome differences between subtotal resection and biopsy only.[104,105,129]

However, several adjuvant radiation studies note a worse long-term outcome for patients who have a biopsy only, compared to debulking surgery.[73,95,125] Mornex et al.[111] reported a series of 90 patients with stages III or IV thymomas who underwent surgery with incomplete resections: 31 had subtotal resections and 55 had biopsy only. This was followed by radiotherapy (median dose 50 Gy), including chemotherapy in 59 patients. Sixty-six percent of patients were free of disease after a median follow-up of 8.5 years. These authors also performed a multivariate analysis[73] in 149 patients who had thymectomies and inferior overall survival was related to the presence of mediastinal compression at diagnosis, absence of chemotherapy, biopsy only as the surgical procedure, and young age.

The aforementioned series include patients treated over the last 2 decades. At present, as a result of improved preoperative imaging and the use of neoadjuvant chemotherapy in locally advanced cases, the role of upfront surgical debulking followed by radiation has diminished.

Locally Advanced Thymomas The term "locally advanced disease" is variably defined in thymomas. For purposes of treatment, when the tumor appears to be unresectable after a thoracic surgeon's evaluation, or resectable only at the cost of great morbidity (extensive resections of lung tissue, great vessel involvement requiring vascular grafts, or need for large pericardial resections), then a combined modality approach with the use of neoadjuvant chemotherapy should be considered. Selected centers have experience with resections of great vessels and superior vena cava and reconstruction in the locally advanced situation.[130–133] Other centers have performed extensive surgical procedures for thymomas involving the pleura, followed by intrapleural chemohyperthermia,[134,135] but this cannot be widely recommended.

An intergroup study utilized cisplatin, doxorubicin, and cyclophosphamide (PAC regimen) followed by definitive RT to the mediastinum (total dose 54 Gy), in patients with limited-stage unresectable thymoma.[136] Out of 23 evaluable patients who had a histologic diagnosis of unresectable thymoma (or thymic carcinoma in 2 patients), 5 complete remissions and 11 partial remissions were seen with chemotherapy (69.6% overall response rate). Five patients had further tumor regression after RT, including four who did not have an objective response to PAC. Median time-to-treatment failure was 93.2 months (range, 1 to 110) with a 5-year overall survival of 52.5%.

The approach of neoadjuvant chemotherapy in locally advanced cases, followed by surgery, depending on the response to chemotherapy, has been well described in the literature. Neoadjuvant ADOC (Adriamycin, cisplatin, vincristine, and cyclophosphamide) was found to have activity in the locally advanced situation.[137] In 16 patients treated in one institution over a 7-year period, an 81% response rate was seen and 9 patients became eventually resectable. Four of these patients survived for more than 5 years. Macchiarini et al.[138] conducted a phase II trial with neoadjuvant cisplatin, epirubicin, and etoposide in seven patients with histologically confirmed stage IIIa thymomas. Four patients were able to undergo a complete resection and two had pathological complete remissions. Finally, a recent phase II study performed at MD Anderson Cancer Center used a modified PAC plus prednisone regimen in 22 patients.[139] Seventy-seven percent of patients had "major" responses and 21 patients underwent surgical resection. Four patients had greater than 80% tumor necrosis on pathological review. Nineteen patients received RT following surgery. The estimated 7-year overall survival was 79%.

Neoadjuvant radiotherapy is not commonly employed, but might improve the complete surgical resection rate.[114] A retrospective study of 12 patients with invasion of great vessels in the mediastinum used a mean preoperative dose of 18.3 Gy.[140] Complete surgical excision was possible in 9 cases, and 10 cases also received postoperative RT. In another series, it was noted that histologic changes (downgrading or necrosis) were seen in thymoma but not thymic carcinoma.[141]

A retrospective series of 10 patients with stage III and IV patients utilized RT plus cisplatin and etoposide. Four patients had a partial response.[142] Ultimately, complete resection of the tumor is the primary goal of therapy.

Advanced Disease Chemotherapy is commonly employed for patients with metastatic disease, or patients who progress after local therapies, such as surgery or radiation to the mediastinum. Several chemotherapy agents have demonstrated activity in thymic epithelial malignancies[143,144] (Table 64.6).

One of the first prospective phase II studies in previously treated and untreated thymoma used cisplatin 50 mg/m^2 every 3 weeks.[145] Two partial remissions were seen in 20 treated patients.

TABLE 64.6 Chemotherapy Regimens Studied in Advanced Thymomas and Thymic Carcinomas

Phase II trials
Cisplatin (single agent)
Ifosfamide (single agent)
Cisplatin, doxorubicin, and cyclophosphamide (PAC)
Cisplatin and etoposide
Cisplatin, etoposide, and ifosfamide (thymoma VIP)
High-dose carboplatin and etoposide
Octreotide ± prednisone
Interleukin 2
Case reports, anecdotal
5-fluorouracil and leucovorin
Prednisone
Capecitabine
Ongoing trials
Carboplatin and paclitaxel
Gefitinib

The first prospective, intergroup study using combination therapy in previously untreated patients with advanced thymoma or thymic carcinoma evaluated cisplatin 50 mg/m^2, doxorubicin 50 mg/m^2, and cyclophosphamide 500 mg/m^2 every 3 weeks (PAC regimen) for a maximum of eight cycles.[146] An overall response rate of 50% was seen, including 3 of 29 patients with clinical complete remissions.

The European Organization for the Treatment and Research of Cancer (EORTC) performed a trial evaluating etoposide and cisplatin in patients with recurrent or metastatic disease.[147] Sixteen patients were enrolled; five complete and four partial remissions were observed. Ifosfamide as a single agent was also studied in patients with stage III or IV disease at a dose of 1.5 g/m^2 daily for 5 days.[148] Out of 15 patients, 5 had complete responses, with the duration of complete response ranging between 25 and 87 months.

To capitalize upon the EORTC observation and the single-agent activity seen with ifosfamide, a subsequent intergroup trial evaluated the use of etoposide 75 mg/m^2, ifosfamide 1.2 g/m^2, and cisplatin 20 mg/m^2 (VIP thymoma regimen), all agents given daily for 4 days every 3 weeks.[149] No complete responses were seen, although 32% of patients had partial responses. The median survival was 31 months, with median response duration of 11.9 months. The 2-year overall survival was 70%.

A phase II study with the carboplatin plus paclitaxel combination conducted by the Eastern Cooperative Oncology Group (ECOG) in previously untreated patients demonstrated an approximate 30% response rate in patients with thymoma (n = 25) and thymic carcinoma (n = 21).

In all these trials, the proportion of patients that were reported as having stable disease after chemotherapy is approximately 40%, with a variable follow-up time between 2 and 5 years. Although these results are affected by selection biases typical of phase II studies, they constitute further evidence that thymomas often behave as an indolent disease. Definitive phase III trials are lacking and are difficult to be performed in this rare disease. Retrospective analysis, however, suggests this response rates and progression-free survival are improved with anthracycline-based regimens.

Thymic Carcinoma The efficacy of chemotherapy regimens in patients with thymic carcinoma is difficult to assess, because the number of patients included in the studies described previously was often in the single digits. A regimen consisting of cisplatin, doxorubicin, vincristine, and cyclophosphamide (ADOC) was evaluated retrospectively in patients with thymic carcinoma.[150] In fact, two patients had small cell carcinoma, four had squamous cell carcinoma, and two had undifferentiated carcinoma. The significance of the described response rate of 75% is unclear given the different pathologies. Two of four patients treated with PAC had objective response in the original ECOG series. In the previously mentioned intergroup study using VIP,[149] eight patients had thymic carcinoma, of which two had partial responses. The 2-year overall survival was 50% for thymic carcinoma patients. The largest prospective trial involving thymic carcinoma, as previously mentioned, incorporated paclitaxel and carboplatin. A 24% response rate was seen. In sum, this data suggest a similarly broad range of activity in thymic carcinoma compared to thymoma, but modestly reduced response rates unlike thymoma. Long-term survival for unresectable disease is uncommon.

Salvage Therapy A phase II study with high-dose carboplatin and etoposide followed by peripheral blood stem cell rescue given in a tandem fashion was also performed at Indiana University in patients with relapsed thymoma or thymic carcinoma.[151] Five patients were enrolled, and three remained alive beyond 2 years, but none remained disease free.

Case reports describe occasional activity of infusional 5-fluorouracil and leucovorin.[152] Some patients can have partial responses or stable disease with the use of prednisone.[153] Radiographic responses may be related to suppression of the lymphocytic component of the thymoma without true antineoplastic activity, which can be of value in ameliorating severe local compressive symptoms (such as compression of the superior vena cava) in patients who have failed to respond to chemotherapy.

Because thymomas exhibits high affinity to octreotide by radionuclide scanning, this agent was examined in advanced or recurrent disease in a phase II study.[154] Thirty-six evaluable patients with pathologically proven thymic epithelial malignancies and positive uptake on indium-labeled octreotide scans received octreotide 0.5 mg subcutaneously three times daily for a maximum of 1 year. In patients with stable disease by CT scans, after 8 weeks, prednisone 0.6 mg/kg daily was added. Octreotide alone had a 12.5% response and in the combination phase of the study, an additional 17.5% of patients responded. The exact role of prednisone in this study, as compared to a delayed effect (beyond 8 weeks) of octreotide in this patient population, remains unclear. Another phase II trial using octreotide 1.5 mg daily subcutaneously with prednisone 0.6 mg/kg/day for 3 months followed by 0.2 mg/kg/day maintenance in 16 patients showed a median survival of 15 months with a 31% response rate.[155] Octreotide has also been used in the management of red cell aplasia (see discussion that follows). A phase II study of subcutaneous recombinant interleukin 2 has been performed in patients with relapsed or refractory thymomas. No objective responses were seen.[156] A phase II study is exploring the use of gefitinib in patient's refractory to chemotherapy.

Other trials that have been conducted demonstrated minimal activity to the targeted tyrosine kinase inhibitors, gefitinib[157] and erlotinib (plus bevacizumab).[158] Though a case report for imatinib demonstrated a brief partial response to imatinib in a patient with a thymic carcinoma,[159] none of 10 patients with C-kit and/or platelet-derived growth factor receptor (PDGFR)-positive (by IHC) thymic carcinoma responded to imatinib.[160] Dasatinib produced a partial response in a patient with advanced thymoma.[161] Pemetrexed was found to have approximately 22% response rate in 27 previously treated patients with thymoma or thymic carcinoma.[162] Palliative radiation is an option in patients who do not experience symptomatic improvement with chemotherapy, and are suffering from chest discomfort, superior vena cava obstruction, or lung atelectasis. Significant responses can be achieved at standard doses of 30 Gy in 300 Gy fractions. RT is also used in the management of bony metastases. Solitary brain metastases can be addressed with excision followed by whole-brain radiation therapy (WBRT), in similar fashion to other malignancies, or with WBRT alone for multiple metastases.

Management of Paraneoplastic Syndromes Thymectomy is a frequently utilized procedure in the management of MG, and a thymoma is found in approximately 10% of cases. Transient worsening of MG symptoms after thymectomy has been observed.[46,163] The expectation of MG improvement after thymectomy is higher with thymic hyperplasia than in the presence of a thymoma, even if it is completely resected. A retrospective Italian study evaluated 500 patients with MG without thymoma, who had a 37.9% improvement in the symptoms of MG after thymectomy, whereas 162 MG patients with thymoma who were subjected to the same surgery had a remission rate in MG symptoms of 15.7%, improvement in 60.3%, and unchanged or worse in 3.7%.[91] The remission rate was higher with mild symptoms and when the tumor was encapsulated. Evoli et al.[46] studied 207 patients who had MG and underwent a thymectomy for thymoma. After a median follow-up of 8.25 years, only 17 patients (8%) were asymptomatic and off immunosuppression for MG.

In patients with advanced or metastatic thymoma and MG, management of the latter is generally not different from MG in the absence of a thymic epithelial malignancy, and often involves pyridostigmine and immunosuppression with steroids or azathioprine. For patients with recurrent myasthenic crises and metastatic thymomas, treatment of the underlying thymoma with chemotherapy occasionally improves symptoms of MG, and the presence of a recurrent myasthenic crisis is not always a synonym of progression of the thymoma. Furthermore, the use of chemotherapy agents in patients on chronic immunosuppression needs to be approached with caution because of the risks of infectious complications.

PRCA related to thymomas is usually initially managed with thymectomy, and a return of normal erythropoesis within 4 to 8 weeks was reported in 6 of 17 patients in a retrospective review.[164] However, PRCA may sometimes recur or even appear after the surgical procedure.[50] For nonresponders or nonsurgical candidates, additional options include further treatment of the thymoma with combined modality approaches, immunosuppression or octreotide.[165] Octreotide has rarely been shown to precipitate a flare of autoimmune phenomena with potentially serious complications.[166] Intravenous immunoglobulin can be effective in a few patients.[167] Anecdotal reports using plasmapheresis for PRCA have been described.[168]

Recommended Algorithm Summarizing the role of different treatment modalities, our recommendations for localized or locally advanced thymomas are as follows (Fig. 64.4):

- Cases that on initial radiographic assessment appear to be encapsulated, or even locally advanced, should be evaluated by a thoracic surgeon with experience in resection of mediastinal masses. For anterior mediastinal masses that appear encapsulated on CT scans (meaning a high pretest probability of thymoma), immediate resection without need for biopsy can be advocated. When the diagnosis is in doubt (such as adenopathy suggestive of lymphoma) or there is possible metastatic disease, a core biopsy is obtained. Patients with elevated β-hCG and/or AFP strongly support the diagnosis of germ cell cancer. Consideration should be given to biopsy potential metastatic sites before treatment decisions, such as pleural implants on CT scan, which are very suggestive of metastatic disease.
- For localized unresectable or bulky poorly resectable thymomas, our current approach consists of neoadjuvant chemotherapy, usually PAC. If a response is seen after two cycles and there is no prohibitive toxicity, we recommend an additional two cycles to be given. Upon restaging, consideration should be given to resection followed by consideration of postoperative RT. In patients who remain unresectable, immediate RT after chemotherapy is employed.

No prospective studies have evaluated the adequacy of different follow-up protocols for thymoma. For thymomas that have been resected, as intrathoracic recurrence is most common and repeat surgery for isolated areas of recurrence has resulted in long-term cure, we recommend chest CT scans every 3 months for 1 year, every 4 months for the 2nd year of follow-up, every 6 months for 1 year, and then annual chest radiographs, with office visits once a year.

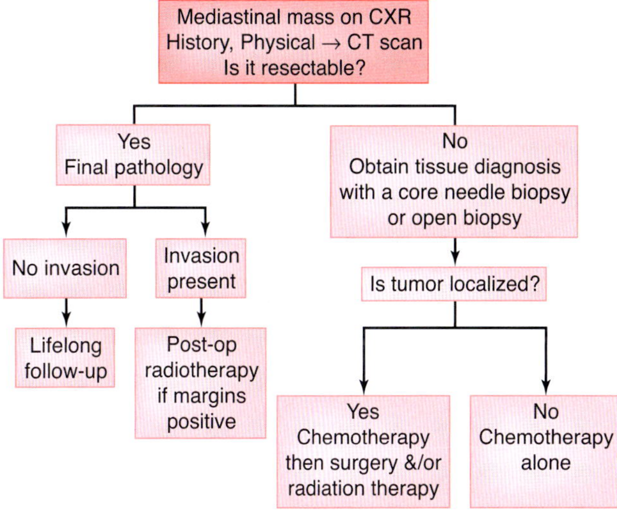

FIGURE 64.4 Recommended algorithm.

REFERENCES

1. Engels EA, Pfeiffer RM. Malignant thymoma in the United States: demographic patterns in incidence and associations with subsequent malignancies. *Int J Cancer* 2003;105:546–551.
2. Anderson G, Moore NC, Owen JJ, et al. Cellular interactions in thymocyte development. *Annu Rev Immunol* 1996;14:73–99.
3. Matsuno Y, Mukai K, Uhara H, et al. Detection of Epstein-Barr virus DNA in a Japanese case of lymphoepithelioma-like thymic carcinoma. *Jpn J Cancer Res* 1992;83:127–130.
4. Weirich G, Schneider P, Fellbaum C, et al. p53 alterations in thymic epithelial tumours. *Virchows Arch* 1997;431:17–23.
5. Tateyama H, Eimoto T, Tada T, et al. p53 protein expression and p53 gene mutation in thymic epithelial tumors. An immunohistochemical and DNA sequencing study. *Am J Clin Pathol* 1995;104:375–381.
6. Hino N, Kondo K, Miyoshi T, et al. High frequency of p53 protein expression in thymic carcinoma but not in thymoma. *Br J Cancer* 1997;76:1361–1366.
7. Pan CC, Chen PC, Wang LS, et al. Expression of apoptosis-related markers and HER-2/neu in thymic epithelial tumours. *Histopathology* 2003;43:165–172.
8. Inoue M, Marx A, Zettl A, et al. Chromosome 6 suffers frequent and multiple aberrations in thymoma. *Am J Pathol* 2002;161:1507–1513.
9. Zhou R, Zettl A, Ströbel P, et al. Thymic epithelial tumors can develop along two different pathogenetic pathways. *Am J Pathol* 2001; 159:1853–1860.
10. Inoue M, Starostik P, Zettl A, et al. Correlating genetic aberrations with World Health Organization-defined histology and stage across the spectrum of thymomas. *Cancer Res* 2003;63:3708–3715.
11. Penzel R, Hoegel J, Schmitz W, et al. Clusters of chromosomal imbalances in thymic epithelial tumours are associated with the WHO classification and the staging system according to Masaoka. *Int J Cancer* 2003;105:494–498.
12. Sasaki H, Ide N, Sendo F, et al. Glycosylphosphatidyl inositol-anchored protein (GPI-80) gene expression is correlated with human thymoma stage. *Cancer Sci* 2003;94:809–813.
13. Gripp S, Hilgers K, Ploem-Zaaijer JJ, et al. Prognostic significance of DNA cytometry in thymoma. *J Cancer Res Clin Oncol* 2000;126:280–284.
14. Henley JD, Koukoulis GK, Loehrer PJ Sr. Epidermal growth factor receptor expression in invasive thymoma. *J Cancer Res Clin Oncol* 2002; 128:167–170.
15. Aisner SC, Hameed MR, Wang W, et al. EGFR and C-Kit immunostaining in advanced or recurrent thymic epithelial neoplasms staged according to the WHO: an Eastern Cooperative Oncology Group Study. *J Clin Oncol* 2004;22(14S):9637.
16. Meister M, Schirmacher P, Dienemann H, et al. Mutational status of the epidermal growth factor receptor (EGFR) gene in thymomas and thymic carcinomas. *Cancer Lett* 2003;248(2):186–191.
17. Tsuchida M, Umezu H, Hashimoto T, et al. Absence of gene mutations in KIT-positive thymic epithelial tumors. *J Lung Cancer* 2008;62: 321–325.
18. Nenninger R, Schultz A, Hoffacker V, et al. Abnormal thymocyte development and generation of autoreactive T cells in mixed and cortical thymomas. *Lab Invest* 1998;78:743–753.
19. Sato Y, Watanabe S, Mukai K, et al. An immunohistochemical study of thymic epithelial tumors. II. Lymphoid component. *Am J Surg Pathol* 1986;10:862–870.
20. Kadota Y, Okumura M, Miyoshi S, et al. Altered T cell development in human thymoma is related to impairment of MHC class II transactivator expression induced by interferon-gamma (IFN-gamma). *Clin Exp Immunol* 2000;121:59–68.
21. Hoffacker V, Schultz A, Tiesinga JJ, et al. Thymomas alter the T-cell subset composition in the blood: a potential mechanism for thymoma-associated autoimmune disease. *Blood* 2000;96:3872–3879.
22. Schmidt-Wolf IG, Rockstroh JK, Schüller H, et al. Malignant thymoma: current status of classification and multimodality treatment. *Ann Hematol* 2003;82:69–76.
23. Bernatz PE, Harrison EG, Clagett OT. Thymoma: a clinicopathologic study. *J Thorac Cardiovasc Surg* 1961;42:424–444.
24. Levine GD, Rosai J. Thymic hyperplasia and neoplasia: a review of current concepts. *Hum Pathol* 1978;9:495–515.
25. Marino M, Müller-Hermelink HK. Thymoma and thymic carcinoma. Relation of thymoma epithelial cells to the cortical and medullary differentiation of thymus. *Virchows Arch A Pathol Anat Histopathol* 1985;407:119–149.
26. Kirchner T, Schalke B, Buchwald J, et al. Well-differentiated thymic carcinoma. An organotypical low-grade carcinoma with relationship to cortical thymoma. *Am J Surg Pathol* 1992;16:1153–1169.
27. Suster S, Moran CA. Thymoma, atypical thymoma, and thymic carcinoma. A novel conceptual approach to the classification of thymic epithelial neoplasms. *Am J Clin Pathol* 1999;111:826–833.
28. Rosai J, Sobin LH. Histological typing of tumours of the thymus. International classification of tumors. 2nd Ed. Berlin: Springer, 1999.
29. Marchevsky AM, Gupta R, McKenna RJ, et al. Evidence-based pathology and the pathologic evaluation of thymomas: The World Health Organization classification can be simplified into only 3 categories other than thymic carcinoma. *Cancer* 2008;112(12):2780–2788.
30. Suster S, Moran CA. Problem areas and inconsistencies in the WHO classification of thymoma. *Semin Diagn Pathol* 2005;22(3):188–197.
31. Suster S, Rosai J. Thymic carcinoma. A clinicopathologic study of 60 cases. *Cancer* 1991;67:1025–1032.
32. Suster S, Moran CA. Thymic carcinoma: spectrum of differentiation and histologic types. *Pathology* 1998;30:111–122.
33. Dorfman DM, Shahsafaei A, Chan JK. Thymic carcinomas, but not thymomas and carcinomas of other sites, show CD5 immunoreactivity. *Am J Surg Pathol* 1997;21:936–940.
34. Fukai I, Masaoka A, Hashimoto T, et al. Differential diagnosis of thymic carcinoma and lung carcinoma with the use of antibodies to cytokeratins. *J Thorac Cardiovasc Surg* 1995;110:1670–1675.
35. Hishima T, Fukayama M, Fujisawa M, et al. CD5 expression in thymic carcinoma. *Am J Pathol* 1994;145:268–275.
36. Hishima T, Fukayama M, Hayashi Y, et al. Neuroendocrine differentiation in thymic epithelial tumors with special reference to thymic carcinoma and atypical thymoma. *Hum Pathol* 1998;29:330–338.
37. Suster S, Moran CA. Histologic classification of thymoma: the World Health Organization and beyond. *Hematol Oncol Clin North Am* 2008; 22(3):381–392.
38. Teh BT, Zedenius J, Kytölä S, et al. Thymic carcinoids in multiple endocrine neoplasia type 1. *Ann Surg* 1998;228:99–105.
39. Monden Y, Uyama T, Taniki T, et al. The characteristics of thymoma with myasthenia gravis: a 28-year experience. *J Surg Oncol* 1988; 38:151–154.
40. Drachman DB. Myasthenia gravis. *N Engl J Med* 1994;330:1797–1810.
41. Wekerle H, Ketelsen UP, Zurn AD, et al. Intrathymic pathogenesis of myasthenia gravis: transient expression of acetylcholine receptors on thymus-derived myogenic cells. *Eur J Immunol* 1978;8:579–582.
42. Kirchner T, Tzartos S, Hoppe F, et al. Pathogenesis of myasthenia gravis. Acetylcholine receptor-related antigenic determinants in tumor-free thymuses and thymic epithelial tumors. *Am J Pathol* 1988;130:268–280.
43. Wilisch A, Gutsche S, Hoffacker V, et al. Association of acetylcholine receptor alpha-subunit gene expression in mixed thymoma with myasthenia gravis. *Neurology* 1999;52:1460–1466.
44. Ströbel P, Helmreich M, Menioudakis G, et al. Paraneoplastic myasthenia gravis correlates with generation of mature naive CD4(+) T cells in thymomas. *Blood* 2002;100:159–166.
45. Okumura M, Ohta M, Tateyama H, et al. The World Health Organization histologic classification system reflects the oncologic behavior of thymoma: a clinical study of 273 patients. *Cancer* 2002; 94:624–632.
46. Evoli A, Minisci C, Di Schino C, et al. Thymoma in patients with MG: characteristics and long-term outcome. *Neurology* 2002;59:1844–1850.
47. Machens A, Löliger C, Pichlmeier U, et al. Correlation of thymic pathology with HLA in myasthenia gravis. *Clin Immunol* 1999; 91:296–301.

48. Somnier FE, Engel PJ. The occurrence of anti-titin antibodies and thymomas: a population survey of MG 1970–1999. *Neurology* 2002; 59:92–98.
49. Buckley C, Newsom-Davis J, Willcox N, et al. Do titin and cytokine antibodies in MG patients predict thymoma or thymoma recurrence? *Neurology* 2001;57:1579–1582.
50. Murakawa T, Nakajima J, Sato H, et al. Thymoma associated with pure red-cell aplasia: clinical features and prognosis. *Asian Cardiovasc Thorac Ann* 2002;10:150–154.
51. Dessypris EN. *Pure Red Cell Aplasia.* Baltimore: Johns Hopkins University Press, 1988.
52. Marmont A, Peschle C, Sanguineti M, et al. Pure red cell aplasia (PRCA): Response of three patients of cyclophosphamide and/or anti-lymphocyte globulin (ALG) and demonstration of two types of serum IgG inhibitors to erythropoiesis. *Blood* 1975;45:247–261.
53. Masuda M, Arai Y, Okamura T, et al. Pure red cell aplasia with thymoma: evidence of T-cell clonal disorder. *Am J Hematol* 1997;54: 324–328.
54. Mangan KF, Volkin R, Winkelstein A. Autoreactive erythroid progenitor-T suppressor cells in the pure red cell aplasia associated with thymoma and panhypogammaglobulinemia. *Am J Hematol* 1986; 23:167–173.
55. Soler J, Estivill X, Ayats R, et al. Chronic T-cell lymphocytosis associated with pure red call aplasia, thymoma and hypogammaglobulinemia. *Br J Haematol* 1985;61:582–584.
56. Montella L, Masci AM, Merkabaoui G, et al. B-cell lymphopenia and hypogammaglobulinemia in thymoma patients. *Ann Hematol* 2003;82:343–347.
57. Kelleher P, Misbah SA. What is Good's syndrome? Immunological abnormalities in patients with thymoma. *J Clin Pathol* 2003;56:12–16.
58. Tarr PE, Sneller MC, Mechanic LJ, et al. Infections in patients with immunodeficiency with thymoma (Good syndrome). Report of 5 cases and review of the literature. *Medicine (Baltimore)* 2001;80:123–133.
59. Masci AM, Palmieri G, Vitiello L, et al. Clonal expansion of CD8+ BV8 T lymphocytes in bone marrow characterizes thymoma-associated B lymphopenia. *Blood* 2003;101:3106–3108.
60. Welsh JS, Wilkins KB, Green R, et al. Association between thymoma and second neoplasms. *JAMA* 2000;283:1142–1143.
61. Pan CC, Chen PC, Wang LS, et al. Thymoma is associated with an increased risk of second malignancy. *Cancer* 2001;92:2406–2411.
62. Dahlgren S, Sandstedt B, Sundstrom C. Fine needle aspiration cytology of thymic tumors. *Acta Cytol* 1983;27:1–6.
63. Herman SJ, Holub RV, Weisbrod GL, et al. Anterior mediastinal masses: utility of transthoracic needle biopsy. *Radiology* 1991;180:167–170.
64. Friedman HD, Hutchison RE, Kohman LJ, et al. Thymoma mimicking lymphoblastic lymphoma: a pitfall in fine-needle aspiration biopsy interpretation. *Diagn Cytopathol* 1996;14:165–169; discussion 169–171.
65. Katzin WE, Fishleder AJ, Linden MD, et al. Immunoglobulin and T-cell receptor genes in thymomas: genotypic evidence supporting the nonneoplastic nature of the lymphocytic component. *Hum Pathol* 1988;19:323–328.
66. Lastoria S, Vergara E, Palmieri G, et al. In vivo detection of malignant thymic masses by indium-111-DTPA-D-Phe1-octreotide scintigraphy. *J Nucl Med* 1998;39:634–639.
67. Lin K, Nguyen BD, Ettinger DS, et al. Somatostatin receptor scintigraphy and somatostatin therapy in the evaluation and treatment of malignant thymoma. *Clin Nucl Med* 1999;24:24–28.
68. Lastoria S, Palmieri G, Muto P, et al. Functional imaging of thymic disorders. *Ann Med* 1999;31 Suppl 2:63–69.
69. Kubota K, Yamada S, Kondo T, et al. PET imaging of primary mediastinal tumours. *Br J Cancer* 1996;73:882–886.
70. Sasaki M, Kuwabara Y, Ichiya Y, et al. Differential diagnosis of thymic tumors using a combination of 11C-methionine PET and FDG PET. *J Nucl Med* 1999;40:1595–1601.
71. Masaoka A, Monden Y, Nakahara K, et al. Follow-up study of thymomas with special reference to their clinical stages. *Cancer* 1981; 48:2485–2492.
72. Gamondès JP, Balawi A, Greenland T, et al. Seventeen years of surgical treatment of thymoma: factors influencing survival. *Eur J Cardiothorac Surg* 1991;5:124–131.
73. Cowen D, Richaud P, Mornex F, et al. Thymoma: results of a multicentric retrospective series of 149 non-metastatic irradiated patients and review of the literature. FNCLCC trialists. Federation Nationale des Centres de Lutte Contre le Cancer. *Radiother Oncol* 1995;34:9–16.
74. Yamakawa Y, Masaoka A, Hashimoto T, et al. A tentative tumor-node-metastasis classification of thymoma. *Cancer* 1991;68:1984–1987.
75. Tomiyama N, Müller NL, Ellis SJ, et al. Invasive and noninvasive thymoma: distinctive CT features. *J Comput Assist Tomogr* 2001;25:388–393.
76. Gripp S, Hilgers K, Wurm R, et al. Thymoma: prognostic factors and treatment outcomes. *Cancer* 1998;83:1495–1503.
77. Ríos A, Torres J, Galindo PJ, et al. Prognostic factors in thymic epithelial neoplasms. *Eur J Cardiothorac Surg* 2002;21:307–313.
78. Rena O, Papalia E, Maggi G, et al. World Health Organization histologic classification: an independent prognostic factor in resected thymomas. *Lung Cancer* 2005;50(1):59–66.
79. Quintanilla-Martinez L, Wilkins EW Jr, Choi N, et al. Thymoma. Histologic subclassification is an independent prognostic factor. *Cancer* 1994;74:606–617.
80. Wilkins KB, Sheikh E, Green R, et al. Clinical and pathologic predictors of survival in patients with thymoma. *Ann Surg* 1999;230: 562–572; discussion 572–574.
81. Lardinois D, Rechsteiner R, Läng RH, et al. Prognostic relevance of Masaoka and Muller-Hermelink classification in patients with thymic tumors. *Ann Thorac Surg* 2000;69:1550–1555.
82. Kirchner T, Schalke B, Marx A, et al. Evaluation of prognostic features in thymic epithelial tumors. *Thymus* 1989;14:195–203.
83. Chen G, Marx A, Wen-Hu C, et al. New WHO histologic classification predicts prognosis of thymic epithelial tumors: a clinicopathologic study of 200 thymoma cases from China. *Cancer* 2002;95:420–429.
84. de Jong WK, Blaauwgeers JL, Schaapveld M, et al. Thymic epithelial tumours: a population-based study of the incidence, diagnostic procedures and therapy. *Eur J Cancer* 2008;44(1):123–130.
85. Okumura M, Miyoshi S, Takeuchi Y, et al. Results of surgical treatment of thymomas with special reference to the involved organs. *J Thorac Cardiovasc Surg* 1999;117:605–613.
86. Mineo TC, Ambrogi V, Mineo D, et al. Long-term disease-free survival of patients with radically resected thymomas: relevance of cell-cycle protein expression. *Cancer* 2005;104(10):2063–2071.
87. Blumberg D, Burt ME, Bains MS, et al. Thymic carcinoma: current staging does not predict prognosis. *J Thorac Cardiovasc Surg* 1998;115:303–308; discussion 308–309.
88. Liu HC, Hsu WH, Chen YJ, et al. Primary thymic carcinoma. *Ann Thorac Surg* 2002;73:1076–1081.
89. Kondo K, Monden Y. Thymoma and myasthenia gravis: a clinical study of 1,089 patients from Japan. *Ann Thorac Surg* 2005;79(1):219–224.
90. Maggi G, Casadio C, Cavallo A, et al. Thymectomy in myasthenia gravis. Results of 662 cases operated upon in 15 years. *Eur J Cardiothorac Surg* 1989;3:504–509; discussion 510–511.
91. Shamji F, Pearson FG, Todd TR, et al. Results of surgical treatment for thymoma. *J Thorac Cardiovasc Surg* 1984;87:43–47.
92. Moore KH, McKenzie PR, Kennedy CW, et al. Thymoma: trends over time. *Ann Thorac Surg* 2001;72:203–207.
93. Langenfeld J, Graeber GM. Current management of thymoma. *Surg Oncol Clin N Am* 1999;8:327–339.
94. Port JL, Ginsberg RJ. Surgery for thymoma. *Chest Surg Clin N Am* 2001;11:421–437.
95. Kondo K, Monden Y. Therapy for thymic epithelial tumors: a clinical study of 1320 patients from Japan. *Ann Thorac Surg* 2003;76:878–884.
96. Masaoka A, Monden Y. Comparison of the results of transsternal simple, transcervical simple, and extended thymectomy. *Ann N Y Acad Sci* 1981;377:755–765.
97. Chen H, Doty JR, Schlossberg L, et al. Technique of thymectomy by anterior-superior cervicomediastinal exenteration. *J Am Coll Surg* 2002;195:895–900.

98. Grandjean JG, Lucchi M, Mariani MA. Reversed-T upper mini-sternotomy for extended thymectomy in myasthenic patients. *Ann Thorac Surg* 2000;70:1423–1424; discussion 1425.
99. Icard P, Le Page O, Massetti M, et al. Resection of anterior mediastinal tumor through a ministernotomy: preliminary experience with ten cases. *J Thorac Cardiovasc Surg* 2003;125:432–434
100. Kaiser LR. Thymoma. The use of minimally invasive resection techniques. *Chest Surg Clin N Am* 1994;4:185–194.
101. Takeo S, Sakada T, Yano T. Video-assisted extended thymectomy in patients with thymoma by lifting the sternum. *Ann Thorac Surg* 2001; 71:1721–1723.
102. Regnard JF, Zinzindohoue F, Magdeleinat P, et al. Results of re-resection for recurrent thymomas. *Ann Thorac Surg* 1997;64:1593–1598.
103. Ogawa K, Uno T, Toita T, et al. Postoperative radiotherapy for patients with completely resected thymoma: a multi-institutional, retrospective review of 103 patients. *Cancer* 2002;94:1405–1413.
104. Ciernik IF, Meier U, Lütolf UM. Prognostic factors and outcome of incompletely resected invasive thymoma following radiation therapy. *J Clin Oncol* 1994;12:1484–1490.
105. Curran WJ Jr, Kornstein MJ, Brooks JJ, et al. Invasive thymoma: the role of mediastinal irradiation following complete or incomplete surgical resection. *J Clin Oncol* 1988;6:1722–1727.
106. Haniuda M, Miyazawa M, Yoshida K, et al. Is postoperative radiotherapy for thymoma effective? *Ann Surg* 1996;224:219–224.
107. Kersh CR, Eisert DR, Hazra TA. Malignant thymoma: role of radiation therapy in management. *Radiology* 1985;156:207–209.
108. Jackson MA, Ball DL. Postoperative radiotherapy in invasive thymoma. *Radiother Oncol* 1991;21:77–82.
109. Blumberg D, Port JL, Weksler B, et al. Thymoma: a multivariate analysis of factors predicting survival. *Ann Thorac Surg* 1995;60:908–913; discussion 914.
110. Krueger JB, Sagerman RH, King GA. Stage III thymoma: results of postoperative radiation therapy. *Radiology* 1988;168:855–858.
111. Mornex F, Resbeut M, Richaud P, et al. Radiotherapy and chemotherapy for invasive thymomas: a multicentric retrospective review of 90 cases. The FNCLCC trialists. Federation Nationale des Centres de Lutte Contre le Cancer. *Int J Radiat Oncol Biol Phys* 1995;32: 651–659.
112. Maggi G, Casadio C, Cavallo A, et al. Thymoma: results of 241 operated cases. *Ann Thorac Surg* 1991;51:152–156.
113. Monden Y, Nakahara K, Iioka S, et al. Recurrence of thymoma: clinicopathological features, therapy, and prognosis. *Ann Thorac Surg* 1985;39:165–169.
114. Myojin M, Choi NC, Wright CD, et al. Stage III thymoma: pattern of failure after surgery and postoperative radiotherapy and its implication for future study. *Int J Radiat Oncol Biol Phys* 2000;46:927–933.
115. Nakahara K, Ohno K, Hashimoto J, et al. Thymoma: results with complete resection and adjuvant postoperative irradiation in 141 consecutive patients. *J Thorac Cardiovasc Surg* 1988;95:1041–1047.
116. Pollack A, Komaki R, Cox JD, et al. Thymoma: treatment and prognosis. *Int J Radiat Oncol Biol Phys* 1992;23:1037–1043.
117. Kohman LJ. Controversies in the management of malignant thymoma. *Chest* 1997;112:S296–S300.
118. Haniuda M, Morimoto M, Nishimura H, et al. Adjuvant radiotherapy after complete resection of thymoma. *Ann Thorac Surg* 1992;54: 311–315.
119. Regnard JF, Magdeleinat P, Dromer C, et al. Prognostic factors and long-term results after thymoma resection: a series of 307 patients. *J Thorac Cardiovasc Surg* 1996;112:376–384.
120. Mangi AA, Wright CD, Allan JS, et al. Adjuvant radiation therapy for stage II thymoma. *Ann Thorac Surg* 2002;74:1033–1037.
121. Singhal S, Shrager JB, Rosenthal DI, et al. Comparison of stages I-II thymoma treated by complete resection with or without adjuvant radiation. *Ann Thorac Surg* 2003;76:1635–1641; discussion 1641–1642.
122. Ogawa K, Toita T, Kakinohana Y, et al. Postoperative radiation therapy for completely resected invasive thymoma: prognostic value of pleural invasion for intrathoracic control. *Jpn J Clin Oncol* 1999;29:474–478.
123. Koh WJ, Loehrer PJ Sr, Thomas CR Jr. Thymoma: the role of radiation and chemotherapy. In: Wood DE, Thomas CR Jr, Eds. *Mediastinal Tumors*. Heidelberg, Germany: Springer-Verlag, 1995.
124. Uematsu M, Yoshida H, Kondo M, et al. Entire hemithorax irradiation following complete resection in patients with stage II-III invasive thymoma. *Int J Radiat Oncol Biol Phys* 1996;35:357–360.
125. Ogawa K, Toita T, Uno T, et al. Treatment and prognosis of thymic carcinoma: a retrospective analysis of 40 cases. *Cancer* 2002;94: 3115–3119.
126. Takeda S, Sawabata N, Inoue M, et al. Thymic carcinoma. Clinical institutional experience with 15 patients. *Eur J Cardiothorac Surg* 2004; 26(2):401–406.
127. Eng TY, Fuller CD, Jagirdar J, et al. Thymic carcinoma: State of the art review. *Int J Radiat Oncol Biol Phys* 2004;59(3):654–664.
128. Lin JT, Wei-Shu W, Yen CC, et al. Stage IV thymic carcinoma: a study of 20 patients. *Am J Med Sci* 2005;330(4):172–175.
129. Cohen DJ, Ronnigen LD, Graeber GM, et al. Management of patients with malignant thymoma. *J Thorac Cardiovasc Surg* 1984;87: 301–307.
130. Funakoshi Y, Ohta M, Maeda H, et al. Extended operation for invasive thymoma with intracaval and intracardiac extension. *Eur J Cardiothorac Surg* 2003;24:331–333.
131. Shimizu N, Moriyama S, Aoe M, et al. The surgical treatment of invasive thymoma. Resection with vascular reconstruction. *J Thorac Cardiovasc Surg* 1992;103:414–420.
132. Tanaka H, Miyoshi S, Okumura A, et al. [Reconstruction of great vessel for patients with advanced lung cancer or malignant mediastinal tumor]. *Kyobu Geka* 1999;52:19–24.
133. Yagi K, Hirata T, Fukuse T, et al. Surgical treatment for invasive thymoma, especially when the superior vena cava is invaded. *Ann Thorac Surg* 1996;61:521–524.
134. Monneuse O, Beaujard AC, Guibert B, et al. Long-term results of intrathoracic chemohyperthermia (ITCH) for the treatment of pleural malignancies. *Br J Cancer* 2003;88:1839–1843.
135. van Ruth S, van Tellingen O, Korse CM, et al. Pharmacokinetics of doxorubicin and cisplatin used in intraoperative hyperthermic intrathoracic chemotherapy after cytoreductive surgery for malignant pleural mesothelioma and pleural thymoma. *Anticancer Drugs* 2003;14: 57–65.
136. Loehrer PJ Sr, Chen M, Kim K, et al. Cisplatin, doxorubicin, and cyclophosphamide plus thoracic radiation therapy for limited-stage unresectable thymoma: an intergroup trial. *J Clin Oncol* 1997;15: 3093–3099.
137. Berruti A, Borasio P, Gerbino A, et al. Primary chemotherapy with adriamycin, cisplatin, vincristine and cyclophosphamide in locally advanced thymomas: a single institution experience. *Br J Cancer* 1999;81:841–845.
138. Macchiarini P, Chella A, Ducci F, et al. Neoadjuvant chemotherapy, surgery, and postoperative radiation therapy for invasive thymoma. *Cancer* 1991;68:706–713.
139. Kim ES, Putnam JB Jr, Komaki R, et al. A phase II study of a multidisciplinary approach with induction chemotherapy (IC), followed by surgical resection (SR), radiation therapy (RT) and consolidation chemotherapy for unresectable malignant thymomas: final report. *Proc Am Soc Clin Oncol* 2001;20:1326a.
140. Akaogi E, Ohara K, Mitsui K, et al. Preoperative radiotherapy and surgery for advanced thymoma with invasion to the great vessels. *J Surg Oncol* 1996;63:17–22.
141. Bretti S, Berruti A, Loddo C, et al. Multimodal management of stages III-IVa malignant thymoma. *Lung Cancer* 2004;44(1):69–77.
142. Wright CD, Choi NC, Wain JC, et al. Induction chemoradiotherapy followed by resection for locally advanced Masaoka stage III and IVA thymic tumors. *Ann Thorac Surg* 2008;85(2):385–389.
143. Thomas CR, Wright CD, Loehrer PJ. Thymoma: state of the art. *J Clin Oncol* 1999;17:2280–2289.
144. Hejna M, Haberl I, Raderer M. Nonsurgical management of malignant thymoma. *Cancer* 1999;85:1871–1884.

145. Bonomi PD, Finkelstein D, Aisner S, et al. EST 2582 phase II trial of cisplatin in metastatic or recurrent thymoma. *Am J Clin Oncol* 1993;16:342–345.
146. Loehrer PJ Sr, Kim K, Aisner SC, et al. Cisplatin plus doxorubicin plus cyclophosphamide in metastatic or recurrent thymoma: final results of an intergroup trial. The Eastern Cooperative Oncology Group, Southwest Oncology Group, and Southeastern Cancer Study Group. *J Clin Oncol* 1994;12:1164–1168.
147. Giaccone G, Ardizzoni A, Kirkpatrick A, et al. Cisplatin and etoposide combination chemotherapy for locally advanced or metastatic thymoma. A phase II study of the European Organization for Research and Treatment of Cancer Lung Cancer Cooperative Group. *J Clin Oncol* 1996;14:814–820.
148. Highley MS, Underhill CR, Parnis FX, et al. Treatment of invasive thymoma with single-agent ifosfamide. *J Clin Oncol* 1999;17: 2737–2744.
149. Loehrer PJ Sr, Jiroutek M, Aisner S, et al. Combined etoposide, ifosfamide, and cisplatin in the treatment of patients with advanced thymoma and thymic carcinoma: an intergroup trial. *Cancer* 2001; 91:2010–2015.
150. Koizumi T, Takabayashi Y, Yamagishi S, et al. Chemotherapy for advanced thymic carcinoma: clinical response to cisplatin, doxorubicin, vincristine, and cyclophosphamide (ADOC chemotherapy). *Am J Clin Oncol* 2002;25:266–268.
151. Hanna N, Gharpure VS, Abonour R, et al. High-dose carboplatin with etoposide in patients with recurrent thymoma: the Indiana University experience. *Bone Marrow Transplant* 2001;28:435–438.
152. Hsu CH, Yeh KH, Cheng AL. Thymic carcinoma with autoimmune syndrome: successful treatment with weekly infusional high-dose 5-fluorouracil and leucovorin. *Anticancer Res* 1997;17:1331–1334.
153. Basha AM, Bonomi PD. Glucocorticoid therapy for invasive thymoma progressing after chemotherapy: a review of 4 cases. *Proc Am Soc Clin Oncol* 2002;21:238b.
154. Loehrer PJ Sr, Wang W, Ettinger DV, et al. Phase II study of octreotide treatment in advanced or recurrent thymic malignancies. An Eastern Cooperative Oncology Group study. *Proc Am Soc Clin Oncol* 2002.
155. Palmieri G, Montella L, Martignetti A, et al. Somatostatin analogs and prednisone in advanced refractory thymic tumors. *Cancer* 2002; 94:1414–1420.
156. Gordon MS, Battiato LA, Gonin R, et al. A phase II trial of subcutaneously administered recombinant human interleukin-2 in patients with relapsed/refractory thymoma. *J Immunother Emphasis Tumor Immunol* 1995;18:179–184.
157. Kurup A, Burns M, Dropcho S, et al. Phase II study of gefitinib treatment in advanced thymic malignancies. *J Clin Oncol ASCO Annual Meeting Proceedings*. 2005;23(16S):7068.
158. Bedano PM, Perkins S, Burns M, et al. A phase II trial of erlotinib plus bevacizumab in patients with recurrent thymoma or thymic carcinoma. *J Clin Oncol* 2008;26(15S):19087.
159. Ströbel P, Hartmann M, Jakob A, et al. Thymic carcinoma with overexpression of mutated *KIT* and the response to imatinib. *N Engl J Med* 2004;350:2625–2626.
160. Salter JT, Lewis D, Yiannoutsos C, et al. Imatinib for the treatment of thymic carcinoma. *J Clin Oncol* 2008;26(15S):816.
161. Loehrer PJ, Yiannoutsos CT, Dropcho S, et al. A phase II trial of pemetrexed in patients with recurrent thymoma or thymic carcinoma. *J Clin Oncol* 2006;24(18S):7079.
162. Chuah C, Lim TH, Lim AS, et al. Dasatinib induces a response in malignant thymoma. *J Clin Oncol* 2006;24(34):E56–E58.
163. Onoda K, Namikawa S, Takao M, et al. Fulminant myasthenia gravis manifested after removal of anterior mediastinal tumor. *Ann Thorac Surg* 1996;62:1534–1536.
164. Masaoka A, Hashimoto T, Shibata K, et al. Thymomas associated with pure red cell aplasia. Histologic and follow-up studies. *Cancer* 1989;64:1872–1878.
165. Palmieri G, Lastoria S, Colao A, et al. Successful treatment of a patient with a thymoma and pure red-cell aplasia with octreotide and prednisone. *N Engl J Med* 1997;336:263–265.
166. Rini BI, Gajewski TF. Polymyositis with respiratory muscle weakness requiring mechanical ventilation in a patient with metastatic thymoma treated with octreotide. *Ann Oncol* 1999;10:973–979.
167. Larroche C, Mouthon L, Casadevall N, et al. Successful treatment of thymoma-associated pure red cell aplasia with intravenous immunoglobulins. *Eur J Haematol* 2000;65:74–76.
168. Messner HA, Fauser AA, Curtis JE, et al. Control of antibody-mediated pure red-cell aplasia by plasmapheresis. *N Engl J Med* 1981; 304:1334–1338.
169. Marino M, Müller-Hermelink HK. Thymoma and thymic carcinoma. Relation of thymoma epithelial cells to the cortical and medullary differentiation of thymus. *Virchows Arch A Pathol Anat Histopathol* 1985;407(2):119–149.
170. Müller-Hermelink HK, Marx A. Pathological aspects of malignant and benign thymic disorders. *Ann Med* 1999;31 Suppl 2:5–14.

CHAPTER 65

Bruce W.S. Robinson
Paul Baas
Hedy Lee Kindler

Malignant Mesothelioma

Malignant mesothelioma (MM) is an aggressive malignant tumor of the pleura and other serosal surfaces, such as the peritoneal and occasionally other serosal surfaces. It was considered a rare disease until 50 years ago, but has increased dramatically in incidence since that time. This increase is caused by the widespread use of asbestos fibers in the postwar industrial period.

We will summarize the main features of the disease and provide an update of recent developments, focusing on new approaches to therapy for this otherwise treatment-resistant problem.

EPIDEMIOLOGY

In 1960, Wagner et al.[1] reported an association between asbestos and both pleural and peritoneal MM in a South African case series. Since then, many reports supporting the relationship between occupational or environmental exposure to asbestos and the subsequent development of MM have been published.[2,3]

That initial study identified risks from both direct occupational exposure and brief or indirect exposure to asbestos.[4] If asbestos exposure occurs at a young age, then the lifetime risk of development of MM is higher than in someone whose exposure occurs at a later age.

Around 80% of individuals with MM have an identifiable exposure to asbestos. Therefore, in around 20% of cases, there is no obvious exposure to asbestos and examination of the lung mineral fiber content shows that in many of these subjects there is a lower lung fiber burden than seen in subjects with asbestosis.[5] MM may occur after brief and indirect exposure to asbestos. MM patients generally, though, have markedly increased lung fiber burdens when compared with a reference population.

Asbestos fiber dimensions and type play an important role in the development of MM, with longer and thinner asbestos fibers more likely to cause MM than shorter and wider fibers because they can penetrate the lungs (see discussion that follows). The critical fiber dimensions appear to be less than 0.25 mm in diameter and greater than 5 mm in length to produce MM, and, although the risk of developing MM from exposure to chrysotile fibers is lower than that from amphibole fibers, large amounts of chrysotile can cause MM, possibly because of contaminating tremolite fibers.[6] A potential role for SV40 is also described (see discussion that follows).

PATHOGENESIS

Mesothelial Tissues Mesothelial tissues include all those that line the cavities that were derived from the embryonic mesodermal coelomic cavity. The tissue develops as a continuous epithelial layer, which covers the pleura, the pericardium, and the peritoneal cavity. A single layer of mesothelial cells rests on a basement membrane. Their rate of division is slow, but increases in response to inflammatory damage.[7]

Etiological Agents

Asbestos Asbestos types include *serpentines*, which are short and curved, such as chrysotile; and *amphiboles*, which are long and needlelike, such as crocidolite. Not all of the different forms have had widespread commercial use—in fact, 90% of industrial asbestos is chrysotile. The mining and use of asbestos is now in decline because of the related pulmonary conditions such as pleural plaques, diffuse pleural thickening, asbestos-related pleural effusions, lung cancer, and MM.[8,9]

Mesothelial cells have been shown to be 10 times more sensitive than bronchial epithelial cells to the direct cytotoxic effects of asbestos fibers.[10] The fibers cause iron-catalyzed generation of reactive oxygen metabolites, which can have a direct toxic effect, causing DNA mutations and strand chromosomal breaks[11,12] leading to cellular apoptosis.[13] The end result is malignant transformation.

SV40 The double-stranded DNA virus SV40 has been suggested as a possible factor in the development of MM.[14]

Carbone et al.[15] found SV40-like sequences in 60% of frozen MM specimens using polymerase chain reaction (PCR).[16] SV40 is dependent on its host for the enzymes of replication except for the large T antigen (TAG). When the virus infects a cell, the TAG is transcribed from the viral genome. TAG binds to the specific SV40 origin of replication, pulling apart the DNA strand, allowing viral DNA synthesis. In this way, the virus is able to bypass the normal cellular controls on replication, and will even do so in quiescent cells. TAG binds to both p53 and the retinoblastoma protein (pRb), with inactivation of these cell cycle checkpoints.

It is presumed that SV40 was introduced into humans as a result of the Salk polio vaccines used in the 1950s, because up to 30% of vaccines used were contaminated by SV40 as a result of culturing the poliovirus in rhesus monkey kidney cells.

Several other studies have confirmed Carbone's findings, with the proportion of cases ranging from 44% to 86% of MMs tested. Dissenting groups include that of Strickler et al.[17] who examined MM tissue from 50 patients with two separate primer sets and did not detect any SV40 sequences. This group also undertook a retrospective cohort study comparing those people who were likely to have received contaminated polio virus against those who did not and found no increase in the incidence of several cancers, including mesothelioma.[18]

SV40 sequences present in MM tissue samples retain the ability to inactivate both p53[19] and pRb,[20] enabling a tumor to survive and progress. Clearly, SV40 is not essential for the development of MM, because many cases do not express TAG sequences. Further investigations and more accurate molecular and proteomic reagents are required to determine more clearly how SV40 fits into the pathogenesis of MM.

Other Agents Several other possible agents have been proposed to cause MM. These include thoracic radiotherapy, intrapleural thorium dioxide, and other silicates, including erionite and zeolite. The numbers of cases attributed to radiation exposure are very small. A genetic predisposition has also been suggested, but numbers are small and coexposure is difficult to exclude. There is no known association between smoking and MM.[21]

MOLECULAR LESIONS

A single mesothelial cell likely develops a genetic mutation that enables it to proliferate and overcome negative growth-stimulatory signals. A multistep accumulation of further mutations to cells occurs, producing the hallmarks of malignancy, namely autocrine growth, invasion, and the ability to metastasize.[22] This whole process takes many years. These alterations include oncogene activation or mutation, loss of tumor suppressor genes, and autocrine or paracrine secretion of growth factors. In MM, considerable new information is available regarding candidate factors, but no clear single pathogenic pathway has been found.

Chromosomal Abnormalities Asbestos is known to induce chromosomal mutations. Cytogenic studies have shown many karyotypic changes,[23] and a wide range of complex and heterogeneous chromosomal abnormalities have been described. Chromosomal gains have been found to be as frequent as losses, such as loss of 4, 22, 9p and 3p, and gain of 7, 5, and 20.[24] The mean chromosomal number has also been shown to correlate with survival in patients with MM. Those patients with a normal chromosome number and no clonal abnormalities had the longest survival.[25]

There are some alterations that are of particular interest in terms of pathogenesis. Monosomy 22 correlates with mutations in the neurofibromatosis type 2 (*NF2*) gene.[26] The loss of at least one locus in 1p (nearly all in 1p22) was found in 74% of examined specimens[27]; 42% to 62.5% of MM cases have been found to have loss of heterozygosity of one or more loci on chromosome 3p, the location of a gene for cellular senescence on chromosome 1 and a tumor suppressor gene located on chromosome 3. Polysomy of chromosome 7 is common and is a negative prognostic feature.[28] The loci for the two potentially relevant growth regulators epidermal growth factor receptor (EGFR) and the platelet-derived growth factor A chain (PDGF-A) are both present on this chromosome. Deletions of 9p,[29] the location of the gene for $p16^{ink4}$ are also common, as are allelic losses in 6q in four discrete locations.

Oncogenes The oncogenes c-*fos* and c-*jun* have been implicated in animal models, with the levels of both c-*fos* and c-*jun* mRNA upregulated when rat pleural mesothelial cells are exposed to asbestos.[30] Wild-type K-Ras was found in all 20 MM cell lines examined.[31] c-Myc immunocytochemical expression is common,[32] but c-*myc* is not amplified in murine MM cell lines.[33]

Tumor Suppressor Genes For a tumor to grow, it is necessary that normal cellular processes for inhibiting growth and for detection of damage be impaired. Tumor suppressor genes do this, so loss of a tumor suppressor gene enables an altered cell to continue through the cell cycle unchecked.[34] Alterations in *p53* have been found in 75% of murine MM cell lines[35] but wild-type p53 was normally expressed in most human MM cell lines[36] and primary tumors.[37]

The retinoblastoma protein pRb prevents progression of a damaged cell into S phase, but its level of expression in human MM cell lines has been shown to be normal.[38]

The product of the *CDKN2* gene, $p16^{ink4}$, was found to be abnormally expressed in 12 of 12 primary MMs and 15 of 15 MM cell lines.[39] As $p16^{ink4}$ normally inhibits phosphorylation of pRb, its loss would permit progress through the cell cycle. Deletions of the portion of chromosome 9 containing *CDKN2A*, but not *CDKN2B*, were also found in MM cell lines.[40] P16 has previously been found to be deleted in 85% of MM cell lines but only 22% of primary tumors.[41]

Seventy-two percent of primary MMs have also been found to have codeletions of *p15* and *p16*.[42] P16/CDKNA2 was homozygously deleted in 59 out of 80 human tumors.[43] Patients with intact p16 had a significant survival advantage.[44]

The *NF2* gene was found to be mutated in 41% of MM cell lines examined by Sekido et al.[45] and 53% of cell lines examined by Bianchi et al.,[46] and confirmed to be present in the primary tumor.

The Wilms' tumor gene (*WT1*) is expressed in normal mesothelium. WT1 proteins control the transcription of genes such as those for PDGF-A, insulin-like growth factor (IGF)-II,[47] transforming growth factor (TGF),[48] and the IGF-I receptor (IGF-IR),[49] which have been described as potential autocrine growth factors in MM. No inverse correlation was found between expression of WT1 and IGF-II or PDGF-A.[50] A further study using mutational screening found no significant changes to WT1, and no correlation between WT1 immunostaining and EGFR or IGF-IR levels.[51]

GLOBAL TRANSCRIPTIONAL PROFILING IN MALIGNANT MESOTHELIOMA

Various global transcription profiling "microarray" strategies have been used in MM with various aims: to understand the genetics and biology of MM, to identify genes that may help diagnosis, for determining prognosis, and to identify potential targets for new therapies.

Studies using human MM patient samples have shown activation of pathways common to the development of many cancer types, including the IGF-1, p38 mitogen-activated protein kinase (MAPK), Wnt/β-catenin and integrin pathways.[52,53]

Diagnostic strategies for distinguishing MM from lung adenocarcinoma based on gene expression profiling of cytology samples have been described.[54,55]

Some studies have concentrated on finding gene "signatures" that can be used to predict prognostic indicators for MM.[56–59] However, clinical prognostication based on gene expression profiling is not superior to clinical parameters such as age, epithelial histology, lymph node status, and tumor stage.[60]

IMMUNOBIOLOGY

There is some evidence in MM that specific immune responses are initiated against the tumor during the course of the disease.[60] A lack of tumor-infiltrating lymphocytes (TILs), as with many other tumors, has been attributed either to a lack of tumor antigens or to the secretion of immunosuppressive cytokines.

Recent work has suggested that an immune response is generated in a significant proportion (28%) of MM patients[61] using patient sera and a panel of human MM cell lines as in Western blot analysis. The titre increased with the progression of the disease and the MM-reactive antibodies were of the immunoglobulin G (IgG) class, indicative of immunoglobulin class switching, and hence the involvement, of CD4 "help." This may lead to identification of tumor-associated antigens (TAAs) and potential vaccination strategies.

This malignancy may be susceptible to immunotherapy. Intralesional therapy with granulocyte–macrophage colony-stimulating factor (GM-CSF) induced a partial response with intense lymphocytic infiltration in biopsy samples.[62] Gene therapy involving the use of gene encoding cytokines has provided some encouraging results in animal models, but limited success in patients.[63]

MMs have to secrete several cytokines known to modulate immune responses, including TGF-β and interleukin 6 (IL-6).[64,65] The role of these molecules in MM has not been fully investigated in humans.

Human and murine lines all express class I molecules and thus can still be targets for the immune response.

ANIMAL MODELS

Spontaneous mesotheliomas have not been described in mice and occur very rarely in rats. Natural and synthetic fibers, chemicals, and metals, however, can induce pleural and peritoneal mesotheliomas in rodents.[66] Inoculation of hamsters with SV40 virus causes pleural mesotheliomas.[67] Mouse mesotheliomas are comparable to the human disease with respect to latency, growth patterns, and molecular lesions.[68] These tumors have been used to study the immunobiology of MM[69] and to evaluate chemotherapies, immunotherapies, and other therapies.[70–72]

Genetically modified transgenic mouse mesothelioma models have been developed. These models will be used for testing of drug therapies and study of the biology of the disease. Heterozygous p53 +/− knockout mice have a longer life span, and 76% of these mice had developed asbestos-induced mesothelioma, compared with 32% wild-type mice, at 44 weeks after asbestos exposure.[73]

Nf2 +/− knockout mice exposed to asbestos develop mesothelioma more rapidly and at a higher incidence than wild-type littermates.[74,75] These tumors recapitulate the most common molecular features of human MM.[76]

A novel transgenic mouse model uses MexTAg, which directs SV40 Tag expression to the mesothelial compartment using the mesothelin promoter.[77] When MexTAg mice are injected with asbestos, all of the animals develop MM and the disease occurs much more rapidly than in wild-type mice. This model is suitable to examine the efficacy of preventative and therapeutic drugs and also to investigate the molecular events occurring at the early stages of MM development.

Applications to Therapy

Interventions that target factors such as TGF-β may be very effective from two aspects: first, by altering the growth cycle and, second, by permitting an immune response to be generated. When TGF-β was reduced by inhibiting translation of these proteins using antisense DNA technology, tumor growth was inhibited but not blocked completely—these effects were lost on cessation of treatment. Such approaches are worthy of further investigation—possibly in combination with other treatments.

PATHOLOGY

There are several reasons for securing the diagnosis early in the course of the disease. Accurate classification is nowadays considered very important because of differences in the (natural) course of disease between MM and other tumors, and even between different subgroups of MM. The response to therapy can significantly influence both the response rate and survival time and will influence the results of single-arm phase II studies. In the last 2 decades, financial reimbursement programs have been initiated in many developed countries. Over and above a history of occupational asbestos exposure, this has also led to a greater demand for a definitive diagnosis.

In general, cytological examination of pleural effusion can accurately diagnose MM but cannot differentiate between mixed forms and epithelial type of MM. However, the accuracy of cytological diagnosis depends on the experience of the pathologist and the antibodies chosen.[78] Fine-needle biopsies are recommended for the diagnosis of MM in some cases but are associated with low sensitivity (around 30%). Despite an increase in incidence of MM, the frequency is still relatively low. Thus, many local pathologists will have relatively little experience with this tumor, which often poses a diagnostic challenge, even to experienced pathologists. This is caused by the combination of highly variable histological features, often only low-grade nuclear changes and the need to identify invasion for definitive diagnosis. The diagnostic material presented to the pathologist is often inadequate, and the inexperienced pathologist may struggle to attempt a diagnosis when the safer option is to ask for better samples.

Such problems in diagnosis have resulted in the foundation of so-called national and international mesothelioma panels. Their task is to optimize the diagnostics of pleural tumors, to give recommendations on further diagnostic requirements, to check reproducibility of tests that require stringent methodological procedures, and to validate newly reported immunohistochemical staining methods regarding sensitivity and specificity for use in routine diagnostic practice. Furthermore, these panels have been approved as official legal organs in financial reimbursement cases in many countries.

In patients presenting with pleural masses, large or multiple histological biopsies are preferred for diagnostic staining procedures.

MM can be differentiated into four subgroups including the epithelioid subtype (± 50% of cases), the biphasic subtype (20% to 25%), the sarcomatoid subtype (± 20%) and the desmoplastic subtype (1% to 5%). Older literature has clearly identified that diagnosis of the biphasic subtype is positively correlated with the number of biopsies taken during thoracoscopy or thoracotomy. In many pleural diseases, the mesothelial lining responds with a hyperplastic reaction, which might resemble MM (Fig. 65.1).[79] One of the key features in diagnosing true cases of MM is, therefore, evidence of invasion of the underlying tissue layers (Fig. 65.2).[80] This diagnosis cannot easily be made on small biopsies and cannot be assessed at all on cytology. Indeed, this is why many cytopathologists will not offer a definitive diagnosis; cytological diagnosis of MPM is presumptive at most centers.[81]

The collected material can be stained for many different markers. A combination of both "positive" and "negative" mesothelial markers should be used, taking into account the likely differential diagnosis in each case. To date, in Europe, it is advised that the diagnosis be made when the staining results include at least two positive markers (nuclear markers such as anticalretinin and anti-WT1, the membrane marker anti-epithelial membrane antigen [EMA], and cytoplasmic markers anti-CK5/6, antiD2-40 [podoplanin], antimesothelin) and two negative markers (anti-Ber-EP4, a membrane marker; antithyroid transcription factor-1 (TTF-1), a nuclear marker; monoclonal anti-carcinoembryonic antigen (CEA), anti-B72-3, anti-MOC-31 (antibody against epithelial glycoprotein 2), anti-estrogen receptor/-progesterone receptor (ER/PR), anti-EMA–cytoplasmic staining, selections based on likely differential diagnosis) (level of evidence 1A).[82] The positive mesothelial markers

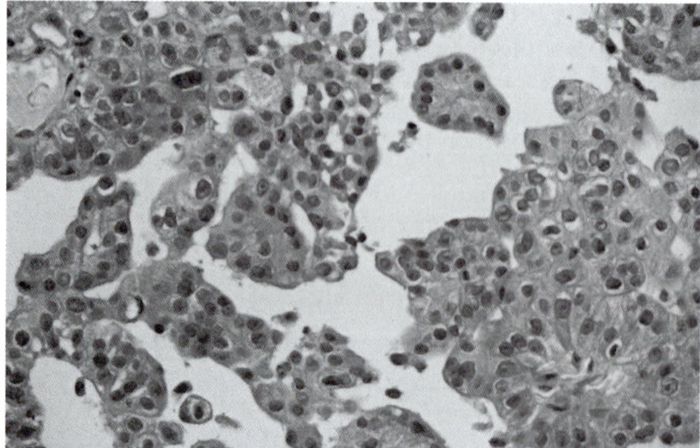

FIGURE 65.1 Reactive mesothelium. Superficial biopsy of the parietal pleura. There is no sign of infiltration, and a reactive mesothelial proliferation is the preferred diagnosis. (See color plate.)

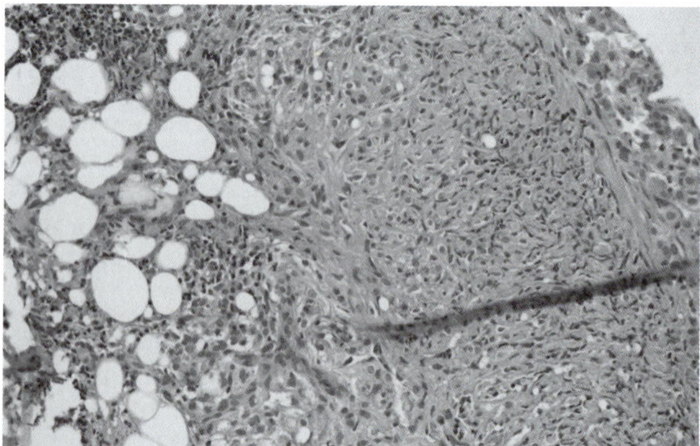

FIGURE 65.2 Deep biopsy showing invasion indicating MM. Deep biopsy from the parietal pleura in the same patient. Tumor cells show infiltration of the muscular layer and fat. The diagnosis of mesothelioma can now be confirmed. (See color plate.)

stain best in epithelioid tumor and are much less reliable in sarcomatoid tumor. The positive markers support the mesothelial nature of the cells but do NOT indicate their malignancy. The differential diagnosis of MM[83] consists in general of:

- Primary adenocarcinomas of the lung involving the pleura
- Metastatic disease from extrathoracic sites
- Diffuse pleural sarcomas
  - epithelioid hemangioendothelioma
  - synovial sarcoma
  - leiomyosarcoma
- Desmoplastic small round-cell tumor
- Ewing sarcoma
- Solitary fibrous tumors
- Pleural thymoma

CLINICAL PRESENTATION AND COURSE

Patients with pleural MM classically present with chest pain, dyspnea, cough, weight loss, fatigue, and sometimes fever or night sweats. Symptoms can persist for months or longer prior to diagnosis. Peritoneal MM patients present with increasing abdominal girth, abdominal pain or discomfort, constipation, anorexia, and occasionally an umbilical hernia. The most common presentation for a pericardial MM is death, because most are diagnosed postmortem. Other symptoms of a pericardial MM include dyspnea, fever, night sweats, congestive heart failure, constructive pericarditis, pericardial effusion, pericardial tamponade, and myocardial infarction. Tunica vaginalis MMs usually present with a unilateral testicular mass.

For the patient with pleural MM, the physical exam is often unrevealing except for dullness to percussion, reduced air entry on auscultation, or asymmetric chest excursion. The disease tends to remain localized to the hemithorax until late in its course. The most common sites of metastases are to the mediastinal and hilar lymph nodes, contralateral pleura, lung, and peritoneal cavity. Metastases to liver, bone, and brain, although rare, can occur. Extensive local progression usually results in death, either from respiratory or cardiac failure.

MM is a heterogenous disease with a variable clinical course dependent upon several key prognostic factors. Using multivariate analysis, the Cancer and Leukemia Group B (CALGB) identified pleural involvement, high levels of lactate dehydrogenase, poor performance status, chest pain, thrombocytosis, nonepithelial histology, and age older than 75 years as poor prognostic factors. The CALGB defined six distinct prognostic groups, whose median survival ranged from 1.4 to 13.9 months.[84] The prognostic scoring index developed by the European Organization for Research and Treatment of Cancer (EORTC) determined that poor performance status, probable diagnosis of MM, leukocytosis, male gender, and sarcomatoid subtype are indicators of poor prognosis. The EORTC classified patients into good- or poor-prognostic groups; good-prognosis patients had a 1-year survival of 40%, compared with only 12% for patients in the poor-prognosis group.[85] The EORTC prognostic score has been independently validated.[86] In addition, measures of health-related quality of life (HRQOL), specifically pain and loss of appetite, may be independent prognostic factors in patients with advanced disease.[87]

IMAGING

The clinical manifestations of MM are usually nonspecific and insidious, but when complaints persist, a chest x-ray is performed to determine the additional diagnostic steps. Besides the presence of a unilateral pleural mass, chest x-rays can detect effusions and pleural plaques with/without calcifications. The presence of calcified plaques on the diaphragm indicates a probable exposure to asbestos in the past. Shrinkage of the afflicted hemithorax is compatible with more advanced cases of MM and can explain complaints of severe pain.

CT Scanning *CT scanning* is considered to be the most important method of radiological evaluation. It is not only useful to determine the extent of the disease but can also narrow the differential diagnosis. Signs of liver and adrenal metastases are unusual in MM and are only seen in very advanced cases. The following are other signs that point to the direction of MM:

1. soft tissue masses encasing the diaphragm, including the absence of a fat plane between the inferior surface of the diaphragm and adjacent abdominal organs
2. pleural tumor which may extend into the subcutaneous tissues at the site of a previous biopsy or thoracoscopy after weeks to months
3. the presence of pericardial effusion or nodular pericardial thickening
4. the possible involvement of mediastinal lymph nodes
5. shrinkage of the involved site

The diagnosis cannot be made based on the radiological appearance, nor can it be used alone for reliable staging. CT scanning will show the location and size of pleural and interlobular masses, allowing these lesions to be used as target lesions.

CT scanning is currently the method of choice for evaluation of response measurement in MM treatment and is used for follow-up after (combined modality) therapy. The accuracy of the CT scan to identify tumor-positive mediastinal lymph nodes is limited. Schouwink et al.[88] performed a prospective study where preoperative CT scanning was compared with cervical mediastinoscopy and found a diagnostic accuracy of 67% for CT scanning and 93% for mediastinoscopy.

MRI Scanning *MRI scanning* has limited value in the diagnosis and staging of MM. It can be used when transdiaphragmal growth or involvement of major vessels or nerve plexus is suspected. Heelan et al.[89] compared the accuracy of CT with MRI scanning for staging purposes. CT scan accuracy was identical to MRI for the detection of lymph nodes but superior in determining chest wall invasion.

PET Scanning Recently, the value of SUV (standard uptake values) in PET scanning has been identified as a new factor for both staging and prognosis purposes and validation studies are underway. Flores et al.[90] investigated the sensitivity of PET scanning in 63 patients with different histology types of MM. He found that PET scanning was positive in all cases, showed a high false-positive rate for detection of mediastinal lymph nodes but identified an occasional, unsuspected, distant metastasis.

Erasmus et al.[91] correlated the staging of PET/CT scanning in 24 patients. In seven cases, there was an understaging and in two cases, over staging of the T stage. For the N status, 35% were understaged and 29% overstaged. Flores et al.[90] correlated the SUV value with survival in 137 patients. He observed an inverse relationship between higher SUV values and survival when a cutoff value of 10 was used.

PET scanning as an evaluation tool was tested by Ceresoli et al.[92] in a group of 20 patients who received two courses of chemotherapy. Responders were defined as having at least a 25% reduction in SUV. In the group of responders (8) the median overall survival was 14 months, whereas in the nonresponding group (12), this was 7 months. The use of PET scanning is considered unreliable when patients have had a (chemical) pleurodesis. The resulting reactive pleuritis will lead to a high-glucose uptake and leads to false-positive PET scan results. This can be positive up to 3 months after the procedure.

It is clear that PET/CT scanning contributes to the diagnosis and response evaluation of MM, but validation studies still have to be performed.

Biomarkers Measurement of tumor markers in effusions may provide a complementary tool to aid in effusion diagnosis. Although differential levels of CEA, cancer antigen (CA) 15.3, CA72.4, CA19.9, CA549, neuron-specific enolase, or cytokine fragment 19 (CYFRA 21-1) differentiate malignant from benign effusions,[93,94] there is less data available for the differential diagnosis of MM from other cancers. Elevated CA15-3 levels have been reported in MM[94–96] and in one study as being able to differentiate between MM and bronchial cancer.[96] Higher levels of hyaluronic acid have been reported in effusions from MM patients compared with those with other malignant disease; however, the difference was too small for diagnostic purposes.[97] Mesothelin levels in effusions above 20 nM are highly suggestive of malignancy, particularly of MM; at this cutoff value, the assay had a sensitivity of 77% for nonsarcomatoid MM, and a specificity of 98% relative to nonmalignant effusions and 86% relative to non-MM malignancies (Fig. 65.3).[98] Mesothelin levels in the blood have been shown to be useful in diagnosis plus monitoring disease progress/regression.[98]

Elevated mesothelin levels are seen in some effusions before a definitive cytological and/or histological diagnosis can be made.

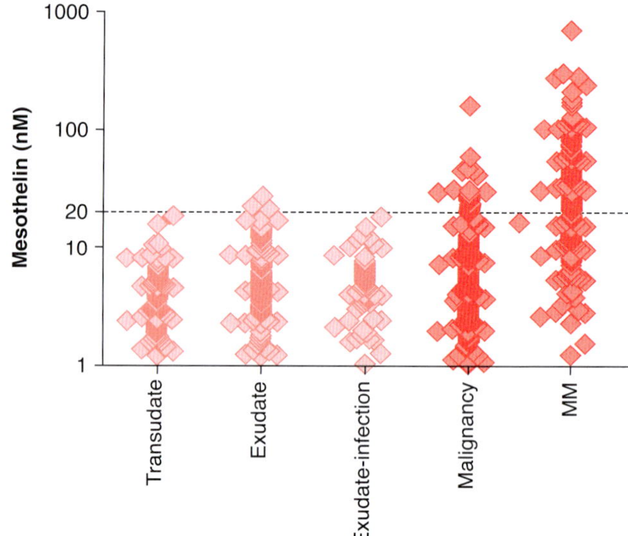

FIGURE 65.3 Elevated mesothelin levels in MM effusions. Mesothelin concentrations in pleural effusions were determined by enzyme-linked immunosorbent assay (ELISA) and individual patient values are plotted on the graph. Effusions were defined as being transudate or exudate in nature and as being benign or resulting as a consequence of malignancy.

DIAGNOSTIC PROCESS

All patients who present with relevant symptoms should be considered for diagnostic procedures to obtain a diagnosis without performing unnecessary or expensive tests. After confirmation of the diagnosis, patients can be informed about the treatment options and prognosis and supported with financial reimbursement programs. In general, patients can be divided into two groups: those where only the diagnosis is required and palliation is the primary option versus those where an experimental, multimodality treatment is proposed. The choice will depend on factors of performance of the patient, prognostic factors, comorbidities, and motivation.

A minimal approach should consist of a detailed history, physical examination, general blood examination, and tapping of pleural fluid in case of shortness of breath with cytological examination, plus serum and effusion mesothelin levels.

For patients with bad prognostic signs, this approach is often sufficient for further management. For patients who are in good general condition, and who are considered candidates for chemotherapy, additional examinations must be performed. These include more invasive tests to obtain material for histological diagnosis with immunohistochemistry and subtyping. CT scanning and more extensive lab testing is required for optimal choice of therapy and to evaluate the response to therapy. Imaging studies should be recent (<4 weeks) when invasive procedures are planned. In the event that there are signs of distant metastases, the diagnostic workup should be limited to confirming the M1 status and to avoid further invasive or expensive examinations.

For patients who are considered candidates for experimental therapies such as multimodality treatment, including extrapleural pneumonectomy (EPP), extensive staging procedures are required.

In these cases, the patient must be discussed in a multidisciplinary team meeting, have localized disease, and adequate pulmonary, cardiac, and renal function. Furthermore, a pulmonologist and cardiologist must assess the postpneumonectomy function of heart and lungs.

In the workup, most centers perform a cervical mediastinoscopy to exclude patients with lymph node involvement. Recently, EUS (endoesophageal ultrasound) and EBUS (endobronchial ultrasound) have been introduced in the evaluation of the mediastinum.[99] Most lymph nodes in the mediastinum can now be assessed by these endoscopic means and can replace the cervical mediastinoscopy.[100] In addition, EUS/EBUS can identify direct involvement of the esophagus or trachea by the tumor.

PROGNOSTIC FACTORS

Prognostic factors are clinical or biological characteristics of a patient or tumor that have an impact on the outcome of the disease, regardless of the choice of treatment. Prognostic factors are used in all kinds of diseases to select patients for certain therapies and to be informed about the course of the disease. They are generally identified by multivariate analysis of outcome in untreated patients and classify patients into prognostic groups and are especially important when noncomparative studies (such as single-arm phase II trials) are performed, and choices for large phase III studies must be made.

To identify prognostic factors for survival in MM, the EORTC analyzed data from patients who were included in their trials.

From large multicenter studies, several prognostic factors have been identified and validated.[101] In the Surveillance, Epidemiology and End Results (SEER) Program, the outcomes for 1475 patients with histologically confirmed MM have been analyzed. The most important prognostic factors identified were age, gender, tumor stage, treatment, and geographic area of residence. Factors such as performance status, stage, and weight loss are generally found in other kinds of tumors and relate to the detrimental effect of a tumor on the general well-being of the host. Other factors such as thrombocyte count, leukocytosis, pathological subtype, and stage have been identified as prognostic factors but have not been confirmed in other studies. Nonepithelioid subtype is consistently associated with a poorer prognosis, even in nonsurgical series. Of the numerous biological factors studied, low hemoglobin level, high LDH, high white blood cell, and high thrombocyte count are generally associated with a poor prognosis. The prognostic factors have led to prognostic scoring systems, which have been prospectively validated: the CALGB and the EORTC prognostic scoring system.[84,85] Based on the results of a large randomized chemotherapy trial, the latter scoring system has been adapted.

STAGING

Staging should describe the anatomical extent of a tumor to convey information to others without doubt. Staging systems classify tumors according to the extent of the primary tumor (T), lymph node involvement (N), and hematogenous dissemination (M). The most important reason for staging is to select patients who are considered candidates for multimodality therapy, and for the ability to compare studies.[102] Clinicians need a system to guide their clinical decisions. What they would really like is to predict a tumor's biological behavior and group patients accordingly. Unfortunately, the ability to do this is limited.

In MM, there have been at least five different staging systems, all with their limitations.

The first staging system was developed by Butchart et al.[103] and was easy to use. This system gave a general impression of the prognosis of the patient, but failed to properly select patients for the more recently developed multimodality treatments. Staging itself is often based on a surgical procedure and therefore has limitations, especially when applied to an elderly population, with significant comorbidities and limited treatment desires being the most important reasons.

The main drawback of the classification systems was the inaccuracy in describing the T and N extent using the available imaging techniques. Because of this, there was a need for a new robust and uniform clinical staging system that could be prospectively validated, was TNM-based, and included the existing surgical–pathological staging systems accepted by international experts. The International Mesothelioma Interest Group (IMIG), therefore, developed a TNM-based staging system in 1995 based on the lung cancer staging system, which is now used in most studies.[104] Despite this structural approach, there are still questions that need to be answered, and there is a clear need for reevaluation of the staging system in MM.

Some of these questions are related to the site of origin of MM and raise questions about the true location of N1 and N2 stations in this pleural disease. Primary lymph node stations of a pleural disease might be mediastinal (numbers 2, 3, 4, 7, 8, or 9) or intrathoracic instead of intrapulmonary (numbers 10 to 12) according to the anatomic relations. Their relevance for stage grouping and effect on survival therefore remain unclear. In addition, there is no effect of tumor load on T status although anatomic extension is well described. The International Association for the Study of Lung Cancer (IASLC) and IMIG are therefore planning to update this system and to improve its prognostic value.

TREATMENT

MM is an almost uniformly fatal disease that is not usually curable with surgery, chemotherapy, or radiotherapy. Treatment options are the same as for other malignancies (i.e., surgery, radiotherapy, chemotherapy, immunotherapy, gene therapy, supportive care, or combination therapy) utilizing some or all of the said treatments. However, in MM, it is often difficult to quantify the location and extent of disease. Also, many patients are older and often have underlying illness that makes them unfit for aggressive treatment. Few large prospective clinical trials have been published, and clinicians rely on retrospective clinical trials with small numbers of patients.

In 1988, the *Journal of Clinical Oncology* published an article with a remarkably nihilistic title, "Malignant mesothelioma, a disease unaffected by current therapeutic maneuvers."[105] In a series of 262 patients, there was no difference in survival between patients who received no treatment at all and those who were treated with chemotherapy, radiation, or surgical resection. Fortunately, in the ensuing years, we have made considerable strides in surgical and radiation techniques, and active chemotherapeutic agents have been developed. Such nihilism is no longer justifiable regarding the treatment of MM.

SURGERY

The role of surgical resection in the management of MM is quite controversial. Although the principal aim of resection is maximal cytoreduction, surgery alone cannot eradicate all residual microscopic disease. No recent published trials compare surgery with other treatments. Some authors therefore conclude that the primary reason for the promising results reported in some surgical series is patient selection.[106] Retrospective data, however, have demonstrated that surgical resection in a multimodality setting is associated with an improved survival.[107]

The optimal surgical procedure, EPP or pleurectomy/decortication (P/D), is also a matter of extensive debate. For many surgeons, the procedure of choice is dependent on the extent of a patient's disease, comorbid medical illnesses, and the subsequent modalities of treatment that are planned.[108]

Pleurectomy with decortication removes the visceral and parietal pleura, leaving the lung in place. Operative mortality, about 1% to 2% at most centers, is low. Some surgeons prefer this approach for early stage patients, to spare the lung and reduce morbidity, whereas others reserve P/D only for those individuals who lack the cardiopulmonary reserve to tolerate a pneumonectomy.[109]

The more extensive EPP is an en bloc resection of the lung, visceral and parietal pleura, pericardium, and hemidiaphragm. It is the only procedure that can be performed when a thick rind obliterates the pleural space. It is also easier, safer, and more effective to perform adjuvant radiation therapy when the lung is no longer in place.[110,111] Early series reported operative mortality rates of up to 30%. Today, in experienced high-volume centers, the operative mortality rate is only about 3%, whereas major and minor complications occur in 60% of patients.[112]

A recent analysis of 663 consecutive patients resected from 1990 to 2006 at three tertiary referral centers reported no statistically significant difference in survival by procedure for any stage.[108] The operative mortality, as expected, was higher for EPP (7%) than for P/D (4%). Five-year overall survival was 12%. Local recurrences predominated in patients who underwent P/D (65%), whereas distant recurrences (66%) were more common in patients treated with EPP. Superior survival was associated with earlier stage, epithelial histology, P/D, multimodality therapy, and female gender in univariate analysis. Controlling for stage, sex, pathologic subtype, and multimodality therapy, EPP yielded a hazard ratio of 1.4 for survival compared with P/D.[108]

The Mesothelioma and Radical Surgery (MARS) trial in the United Kingdom may help to determine the role of EPP in MM. In this ongoing study, 670 patients are randomized to induction chemotherapy followed by either EPP and adjuvant radiation, or no surgery.[106]

RADIATION THERAPY

The administration of radiation therapy (RT) for MM is quite challenging because of the large treatment volumes required, the radiation sensitivity of the surrounding organs, and the technical difficulty of treating multiple pleural surfaces.

MM has the potential to seed along the tracts of biopsies, chest tubes, thoracoscopy trocars, and surgical incisions, producing uncomfortable subcutaneous nodules. For many years, adjuvant RT was standard after such instrumentation, based on a 40-patient study in which 21 Gy administered in three fractions decreased local recurrence from 40% to 0%.[113] Subsequent randomized studies have not supported the routine administration of adjuvant radiation in this setting.[114]

Radiation for this disease is principally employed after resection. The use of radiation following P/D is particularly problematic given the significant risk of fibrosis of the underlying lung, in addition to the poor local control achievable at safe doses. In one of the largest retrospective series, 1-year local control was only 42%, and median survival was only 13.5 months among 123 patients who underwent P/D followed by adjuvant external beam RT.[110]

In contrast, high-dose hemithoracic radiation has been shown to significantly decrease the risk of local recurrence following EPP. In a phase II study at Memorial Sloan-Kettering Cancer Center, only 7 of 54 patients who received EPP followed by 54-Gy hemithoracic radiation had any locoregional recurrences. Median survival was 33.8 months for patients with stages I and II disease, but only 10 months for more advanced tumors.[111]

Intensity-modulated radiation therapy (IMRT) can further enhance local control following EPP. In the largest series, from MD Anderson Cancer Center, locoregional recurrences developed in only 13% of the 63 patients who underwent EPP followed by 45-Gy IMRT. It is noteworthy that only 5% of recurrences occurred in the irradiated field.[115] Unfortunately, this approach has been complicated by a substantial risk of toxicity to the contralateral lung, which has resulted in fatal pneumonitis.[116]

MULTIMODALITY THERAPY

Chemotherapy has been integrated into multimodality treatment studies before, during, and after surgery. In the largest series incorporating adjuvant chemotherapy, from Brigham and Women's Hospital, 183 patients received EPP, radiation, and adjuvant chemotherapy. Median survival was 19 months, and 5-year survival was 15%. The 31 patients with the best outcome had epithelial histology, no extrapleural lymph node metastases, and negative margins. This subset had a median survival of 51 months, and a 5-year survival of 46%.[117] These investigators have also pioneered the evaluation of hyperthermic intraoperative chemotherapy, an approach that remains experimental.[118]

Neoadjuvant chemotherapy is more commonly used in the current generation of trials. This has consisted of three or four cycles of a gemcitabine- or pemetrexed-containing platinum doublet, followed by surgery, and in some studies, radiation. In a multicenter study from Switzerland, 74% of the 61 patients who received three cycles of gemcitabine plus cisplatin were able to undergo an EPP; their median survival was 23 months.[119] In a multicenter American trial, 77 patients received four cycles of neoadjuvant pemetrexed and cisplatin. Radiographic partial responses were reported in 33% of evaluable patients, and 61% underwent an EPP. Median overall survival was only 16.6 months.[120]

SYSTEMIC THERAPY

Systemic therapy is the sole treatment option for most MM patients, for whom advanced age, medical comorbidities, nonepithelial histology, and locally advanced disease will preclude surgery. Cytotoxic drugs with activity in this disease include carboplatin, cisplatin, doxorubicin, epirubicin, gemcitabine, pemetrexed, raltitrexed, vinflunine, and vinorelbine.[121–129] The addition of cisplatin to the antifolates pemetrexed or raltitrexed increases survival.[130,131] The addition of cisplatin to epirubicin, gemcitabine, irinotecan, pemetrexed, raltitrexed, or vinorelbine increases the response rate (Fig. 65.4).[130–135] Quality of life can be improved by gemcitabine, pemetrexed, and vinorelbine.[129,130,133]

The anthracyclines were once considered the most active drugs for this disease. Early trials reported response rates of up to 44% for doxorubicin. However, the largest series, a retrospective review of 51 patients treated by the Eastern Cooperative Oncology Group, documented a response rate of only 14%.[123] The EORTC observed a response rate of 15% and a median survival of 40 weeks in a phase II trial of epirubicin.[124] Although cardiac protectants and several liposomal formulations have been employed to potentially diminish the cardiac toxicity of the anthracyclines, these approaches are even less effective.[136,137]

Several recent trials have evaluated the activity of epirubicin plus cisplatin or gemcitabine. None of these combinations are significantly more active than gemcitabine or antifolate platinum doublets, and none will be developed further. In a phase II trial of epirubicin plus cisplatin in 69 patients, the European Lung Cancer Working Party achieved a 19% response rate and a median survival of 13.3 months.[122] An Italian group reported a response rate of 14% and a 32% 1-year survival in 28 patients treated with epirubicin plus gemcitabine,[138] whereas the North Central Cancer Treatment Group observed moderately severe toxicity and response rates of only 13% and 7% respectively, for high- and low-dose regimens using this combination.[139]

A metaanalysis of 83 mesothelioma clinical trials published from 1965 to 2001 determined that the most active cytotoxic agent in this disease is cisplatin.[122] Single-agent cisplatin has been employed as the control arm of several clinical trials[130,131]; it is otherwise not used alone for this disease. Similar activity has been reported for carboplatin.[121] Oxaliplatin has not been tested as a single agent for MM, although it has been evaluated in combination with gemcitabine, raltitrexed, and vinorelbine.[140–142]

The antifolates are currently regarded as the most active class of cytotoxic drugs against MM. High-dose methotrexate produced a response rate of 37% and a median survival of 11 months in a 60-patient study.[143] Edatrexate produced a 25% response rate with significant toxicity in a phase II CALGB trial; leucovorin decreased both response and toxicity.[144] Although very active in MM cell lines and xenografts, no

A
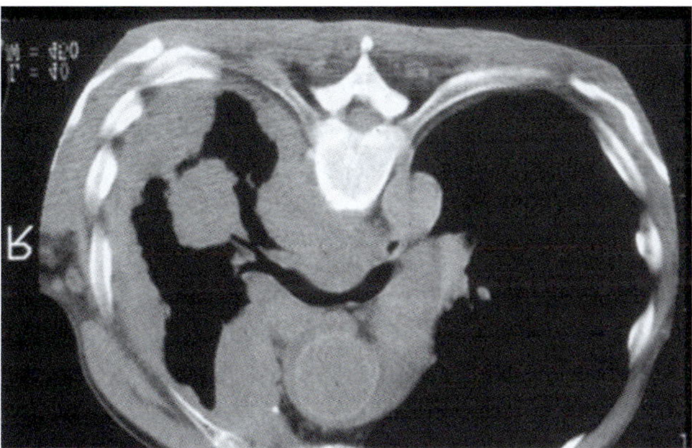
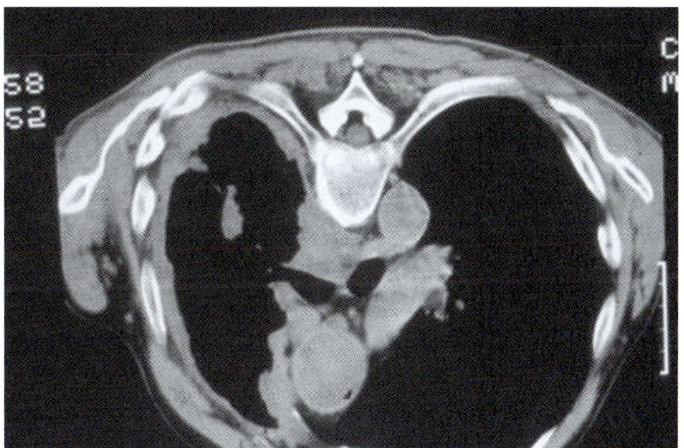
B

FIGURE 65.4 CT scan showing tumor shrinkage with gemcitabine plus cisplatin. Patient exhibited advanced histologically confirmed MM **(A)**, which shrank by >50% following therapy with systemic gemcitabine plus cisplatin **(B)**.

objective responses were observed in a recent phase II trial of the antifolate pralatrexate.[145]

The antifolate pemetrexed inhibits thymidylate synthase, dihydrofolate reductase, and glycinamide ribonucleotide formyltransferase. Like other drugs of this class, pemetrexed principally crosses the cell membrane via the reduced folate carrier. A high-affinity cell membrane transporter specific for pemetrexed has also been described in mesothelioma cell lines.[146]

A 64-patient phase II trial of single-agent pemetrexed yielded a response rate of 14% and a median survival of 10.7 months.[126] The pivotal study of pemetrexed in MM was a single-blind, placebo-controlled phase III trial, which randomized 456 patients to pemetrexed, 500 mg/m^2 every 21 days and cisplatin 75 mg/m^2, or placebo and cisplatin.[130] Patients treated with pemetrexed plus cisplatin had a superior survival (12.1 vs. 9.3 months; $p = 0.020$), a longer time to progression (5.7 vs. 3.9 months; $p = 0.001$) and a higher response rate (41% vs. 17%; $p < 0.001$) than those who received single-agent cisplatin. Combination treatment also resulted in significant improvements in pulmonary function, quality of life, and symptoms including dyspnea and pain.

To decrease the risk of severe pemetrexed toxicities, after the first 117 patients enrolled in this trial, all subsequent patients were given vitamin supplementation with dietary doses of folic acid and vitamin B_{12}. This improved response rates and survival in both arms of the study. In preclinical models, there is a significant decrement in pemetrexed activity when extracellular folate levels increase above the physiological range. This has led some investigators to suggest that folate supplementation be limited to the lowest recommended level that provides protection from toxicity, about 400 μg daily.[147]

Because cisplatin may be poorly tolerated in elderly or frail individuals, carboplatin is often substituted. Response rates (26% and 22%) and 1-year survival (63% and 64%) were very similar for patients treated with pemetrexed and cisplatin or carboplatin, respectively, in the International Expanded Access Program.[148] A phase II trial of pemetrexed given with carboplatin (area under the curve [AUC] 5) achieved a median overall survival of 12.7 months and a median time to progression of 6.5 months in 102 patients. The response rate, however, was only 19%.[149] A 76-patient phase II trial of the same regimen yielded a response rate of 25%, a median time to progression of 8 months, and a median survival of 14 months.[150] Despite greater hematologic toxicity, elderly patients in these two trials experienced similar outcomes as younger individuals.[151]

A 250-patient randomized trial from the EORTC and the National Cancer Institute of Canada that compared raltitrexed plus cisplatin with single-agent cisplatin demonstrated that pemetrexed is not the only antifolate with phase III activity in mesothelioma.[131] Patients who received raltitrexed and cisplatin had a longer survival (11.2 vs. 8.8 months; $p = 0.048$), a superior time to progression (5.3 vs. 4.0 months; $p = 0.058$), and a higher response rate (24% vs. 14%; $p = 0.06$) than those who received cisplatin alone. Vitamin supplementation was not given. This agent is not being developed further for MM.

Although it produces few responses as a single agent,[152] gemcitabine has considerable activity when combined with a platinum. A retrospective British-Canadian series actually observed no difference in overall survival between platinum doublets of pemetrexed and gemcitabine.[153] Response rates for the combination of gemcitabine plus cisplatin were quite variable, however, and have ranged between 12% and 48%. This is thought to reflect heterogeneity in patient selection and inconsistencies in disease measurement between trials, rather than slight differences in the dose and schedule of these drugs.[125] In the initial 21-patient, single-center Australian study, gemcitabine 1000 mg/m^2 was given on days 1, 8, and 15, and cisplatin 100 mg/m^2 on day 1 every 28 days. The partial response rate was 48%, median survival was 9.4 months, and 90% of the responding patients experienced an improvement in symptoms.[154] The same investigators employed the same regimen in a 52-patient multicenter trial, and observed a partial response rate of 33% and a median survival of 11.2 months.[133]

Other active gemcitabine-platinum doublets include gemcitabine plus carboplatin, which produced a 26% response rate, a median survival of 15.1 months, and an improvement in pain, weight, and dyspnea[155]; and gemcitabine plus oxaliplatin, which, in a 20-patient study, achieved a response rate of 40%, a median time to progression of 7 months, and a median survival of 13 months.[140] The combination of gemcitabine plus pemetrexed has been studied in a 108-patient phase II trial that tested two different schedules. Median survival, 8.1 and 10.1 months for the two cohorts, respectively, was similar to single-agent pemetrexed, but the toxicity was greater.[156]

A 29-patient phase II trial of vinorelbine achieved a response rate of 24% and a median survival of 10.6 months. Pulmonary symptoms decreased in 48% of the patients.[129] The addition of oxaliplatin significantly increased toxicity, but did not enhance the response, which remained at 23%.[134] The addition of cisplatin to vinorelbine in 54 patients produced a 30% response rate, a median survival of 16.8 months, and a 1-year survival of 61%.[135] Another vinca alkaloid with activity in MM is vinflunine, which demonstrated a response rate of 14%, a median survival of 10.8 months, and modest toxicity in a 67-patient phase II trial.[128] This agent is not currently being developed for this disease.

The Medical Research Council and British Thoracic Society recently reported the results of the MS01 trial, which randomized 409 patients to active symptom control (ASC) or ASC plus either vinorelbine or mitomycin-vinblastine-cisplatin (MVP). Because of lower-than-expected accrual, the chemotherapy arms were analyzed together. There was a minimal survival advantage for chemotherapy (8.5 vs. 7.6 months) that was not statistically significant (HR = 0.89; $p = 0.08$). An exploratory analysis reported an improvement in survival for the vinorelbine-treated patients (median survival, 9.5 months) compared with ASC (HR = 0.80; $p = 0.08$), but there was no survival benefit for MVP (HR = 0.99; $p = 0.95$).[157]

NOVEL AGENTS

Although cytotoxic chemotherapy has definite activity in MM, the modest results achieved with this approach have led many investigators to evaluate more novel agents for this disease. Recent studies suggest that several of these agents may have promising activity.

Early clinical trials of the targeted agents were resoundingly negative, however. Although preclinical studies in MM suggested an autocrine growth-stimulatory effect of PDGF, response rates were 0% in all four studies of the PDGF receptor tyrosine kinase inhibitor imatinib.[158] The EGFR is highly overexpressed in MM, but activating mutations of EGFR are quite rare.[159] Thus, it should not be surprising that minimal activity was reported for phase II trials of gefitinib and erlotinib.[160,161]

In preclinical models, agents that target vascular endothelial growth factor (VEGF) inhibit the growth of MM. In MM patients, elevated serum VEGF correlates inversely with survival. Several VEGF inhibitors, including AZD2171, bevacizumab, sorafenib, SU5416, sunitinib, tetrathiomolybdate, thalidomide, and vatalanib have been studied in MM patients; their activity is quite modest.[158] Vatalanib, an inhibitor of VEGF and PDGF receptor tyrosine kinases, produced a response rate of 11% and a median survival of 10 months in a 47-patient phase II trial.[162] Likely reflecting patient selection in a two-cohort phase II trial, median survival in chemonaive patients who received the multikinase inhibitor sorafenib was 5.2 months, compared with 14.3 months for previously treated patients.[163] An Australian study of sunitinib, an inhibitor of the VEGFR-1, -2, and -3 tyrosine kinases, demonstrated a response rate of 15% by CT scan and 30% by CT/PET.[164] Thalidomide produced stable disease for 6 months or more in 28% of 40 patients in a phase II trial in The Netherlands.[165] Thus, the ongoing Nederlandse Vereniging van Artsen voor Longziekten en Tuberculose (NVALT) 5 maintenance study randomizes patients to thalidomide or observation after pemetrexed-based treatment.

A 108-patient, double-blind, placebo-controlled randomized phase II trial at the University of Chicago assessed the addition of the anti-VEGF monoclonal antibody bevacizumab to gemcitabine plus cisplatin. The primary end point, progression-free survival, was 6.9 months for the bevacizumab arm and 6.0 months for placebo. Median overall survival was 15.6 versus 14.7 months, for bevacizumab and placebo, respectively. Neither difference was statistically significant. Elevated baseline plasma VEGF levels correlated with briefer progression-free and overall survival.[166] Despite these negative results, several phase II trials of pemetrexed, bevacizumab plus a platin continue to accrue.

Suberoylanilide hydroxamic acid (SAHA) is an oral agent that inhibits class I and II histone deacetylases. Two unconfirmed partial responses occurred in 13 MM patients included in a phase I trial of SAHA. Responding patients also experienced a decrease in tumor pain and dyspnea. These preliminary data formed the rationale for an ongoing, international, double-blind, placebo-controlled randomized phase III trial of SAHA versus placebo in 660 previously treated patients who have received no more than two prior chemotherapy regimens. The primary end point is overall survival.[167,168]

In preclinical mesothelioma models, the proteasome inhibitor bortezomib abrogates the activity of nuclear factor kappa B (NFκB), induces apoptosis, and inhibits cell growth.[169] Two ongoing European trials are evaluating bortezomib in MM patients: the EORTC is studying it first line in combination with cisplatin, and an Irish group is testing single-agent bortezomib in previously treated patients.

Ranpirnase, a ribonuclease derived from the leopard frog, is thought to disrupt protein translation, resulting in apoptosis. A 5% response rate and a median survival of 6 months were reported in a phase II trial in 105 previously treated patients.[170] A 154-patient phase III trial that compared ranpirnase with doxorubicin produced a similar survival for both arms of the study. Subset analysis of 105 patients suggested that patients with a better prognosis might benefit from ranpirnase. These data were presented in abstract form in 2000 and have never been published.[171] A phase IIIB trial of doxorubicin given with or without ranpirnase has recently completed accrual.

Mesothelin, a cell surface glycoprotein expressed on normal mesothelium, is another potential therapeutic target. Preclinical models demonstrate activity for SS1P, a recombinant immunotoxin, morphotek antibody 9 (MORAb-009), a monoclonal antibody, and live-attenuated listeria monocytogenes expressing human mesothelin (CRS-207), a live-attenuated listeria vector that encodes human mesothelin. These agents are synergistic with cytotoxic chemotherapy. A phase I study of CRS-207 is ongoing, and phase II trials of pemetrexed/cisplatin with SS1P or MORAb-009 have recently been initiated.[172–175]

FUTURE DIRECTIONS

The key strategies to improve outcomes for this disease and to reduce the enormous compensation burden facing many countries (estimated to total over U.S.$ 300 billion) include:

- Early diagnosis
- Improved therapy
- Prevention of disease

Early diagnosis will require a blood or urine test that detects the early stages of disease in most cases with high specificity. Serum mesothelin detects only about 15% of patients prior to diagnosis, so better markers are needed. These might be discovered by mass spectrometry methods, immunochemistry, or microarray studies.

The attraction is that MM remains localized to cavities for most of the course of the disease, and early detection should lead to cures.

Improved therapy will probably require multimodality approaches that are firmly based on a scientific understanding of the biology of the disease and the basis for responses to therapy. It has been encouraging to find chemotherapies that actually work in this disease, and there is a lot of excitement in the field that such therapies can be combined with novel approaches, such as immunotherapy, for improved outcomes.

Prevention of disease is the "holy grail" of asbestos-induced cancers. Most patients are aware of their asbestos exposure, and would love to be able to take something that will reduce their risk, in the same way that lipid-lowering agents reduce the risk of cardiovascular disease. Retinoic acid was looking like it was such an agent, but recent analysis of the longer-term data does not support its use.

Other preventative strategies will be based on animal studies. Cohort studies proving the efficacy of such agents will be limited by the lack of cohorts in which the incidence of MM is sufficiently high to enable the results to be accurate. Immunization strategies are being studied but are also difficult.

Progress in this field has been rapid, however, and this is in part caused by the enormous level of international cooperation that has occurred, largely via the peak body, the International Mesothelioma Interest Group. Also, effective national cooperatives have been developed, such as the National Center for Asbestos Related Diseases in Australia. Creative collaboration between scientists, clinicians, epidemiologists and funding bodies should see cures occurring within the next decade.

REFERENCES

1. Wagner JC, Sleggs CA, Marchand P. Diffuse pleural MM and asbestos exposure in the North Western Cape Province. *Br J Ind Med J* 1960; 17:260–271.
2. Mossman BT, Bignon J, Corn M et al. Asbestos: scientific developments and implications for public policy. *Science* 1990;247:294–301.
3. Becklake MR. Asbestos-related diseases of the lung and other organs: their epidemiology and implications for clinical practice. *Am Rev Respir Dis* 1976;114:187–227.
4. McDonald JC, McDonald AD. The epidemiology of MM in historical context. *Eur Respir J* 1996;9:1932–1942.
5. Roggli VL, Mineral fibre content of lung tissue in patients with malignant mesothelioma. In: Henderson D, Shilken K, Langlois S, et al., eds. *Malignant Mesothelioma*. New York: Hemisphere: New York, 1992: 210–222.
6. Churg A, Chrysotile. tremolite, and malignant mesothelioma in man. *Chest* 1988;93:621–628.
7. Hansen J, Deklerk NH, Musk AW, et al. Environmental exposure to crocidolite and mesothelioma: exposure–response relationships. *Am J Respir Crit Care Med* 1998;157:69–75.
8. Rom WN, Travis WD, Brody AR. Cellular and molecular basis of the asbestos-related disease. *Am Rev Respir Dis* 1991;143:408–422.
9. Lechner JF, Tokiwa T, LaVeck M, et al. Asbestos-associated chromosomal changes in human mesothelial cells. *Proc Nat Acad Sci U S A* 1985;82:3884–3888.
10. Walker C, Everitt J, Barrett JC. Possible cellular and molecular mechanisms for asbestos carcinogenicity. *Am J Ind Med* 1992;21:253–273.
11. Yegles M, Saint-Etienne L, Renier A, et al. Induction of metaphase and anaphase/telophase abnormalities by asbestos fibers in rat pleural mesothelial cells in vitro. *Am J Respir Cell Mol Biol* 1993;9:186–191.
12. Broaddus VC, Yang L, Scavo LM, et al. Asbestos induces apoptosis of human and rabbit pleural mesothelial cells via reactive oxygen species. *J Clin Invest* 1996;98:2050–2059.
13. Bergsagel DJ, Finegold MJ, Butel JS, et al. DNA sequences similar to those of simian virus 40 in ependymomas and choroid plexus tumors of childhood. *N Engl J Med* 1992;326:988–993.
14. Cicala C, Pompetti F, Carbone M. SV40 induces MMs in hamsters. *Am J Pathol* 1993;142:1524–1533.
15. Carbone M, Pass HI, Rizzo P, et al. Simian virus 40-like DNA sequences in human pleural MM. *Oncogene* 1994;9:1781–1790.
16. Strickler HD, Goedert JJ, Fleming M, et al. Simian virus 40 and pleural MM in humans. *Cancer Epidemiol Biomarkers Prev* 1996;5:473–475.
17. Strickler HD, Rosenberg PS, Devesa SS, et al. Contamination of poliovirus vaccines with simian virus 40 (1955–1963) and subsequent cancer rates. *JAMA* 1998;279:292–295.
18. Carbone M, Rizzo P, Grimley PM, et al. Simian virus-40 large-T antigen binds p53 in human MMs. *Nature Med* 1997;3:908–912.
19. Deluca A, Baldi A, Esposito V, et al. The retinoblastoma gene family Prb/P105, P107, Prb2/P130 and simian virus-40 large T-antigen in human mesotheliomas. *Nature Med* 1997;3:913–916.
20. Muscat JE, Wynder El. Cigarette smoking, asbestos exposure, and malignant mesothelioma. *Cancer Res* 1991;51:2263–2267.
21. Vogelstein B, Fearon ER, Hamilton SR, et al. Genetic alterations during colorectal-tumor development. *N Engl J Med* 1988;319:525–532.
22. Knuutila S, Tiainen M, Tammilehto L, et al. Cytogenetics of human malignant mesotheliomas. *Eur Respir Rev* 1993;3:25–28.
23. Hagemeijer A, Versnel MA, Van Drunen E, et al. Cytogenetic analysis of malignant mesothelioma. *Cancer Genet Cytogenet* 1990;47:1–28.
24. Tiainen M, Rautonen J, Pyrhonen S, et al. Chromosome number correlates with survival in patients with malignant pleural mesothelioma. *Cancer Genet Cytogenet* 1992;62:21–24.
25. Huncharek M. Genetic factors in the aetiology of malignant mesothelioma. *Eur J Cancer* 1995;31A:1741–1747.
26. Lee WC, Balsara B, Liu Z, et al. Loss of heterozygosity analysis defines a critical region in chromosome 1p22 commonly detected in human malignant mesothelioma. *Cancer Res* 1996;56:4297–4301.
27. Zeiger MA, Gnarra JR, Zbar B, et al. Loss of heterozygosity on the short arm of chromosome 3 in mesothelioma cell lines and solid tumors. *Genes Chromosomes Cancer* 1994;11:15–20.
28. Cheng JQ, Jhanwar SC, Lu YY, et al. Homozygous deletions within 9p21–p22 identify a small critical region of chromosomal loss in human malignant mesotheliomas. *Cancer Res* 1993;53:4761–4763.
29. Heintz NH, Janssen YM, Mossman BT. Persistent induction of c-fos and c-jun expression by asbestos. *Proc Natl Acad Sci U S A* 1993;90:3299–3303.
30. England JM, Panella MJ, Ewert DL, et al. Induction of a diffuse mesothelioma in chickens by intraperitoneal innoculation of v-src DNA. *Virology* 1991;182:423–429.
31. Reddel RR, Malan-Shibley L, Gerwin BI, et al. Tumorigenicity of human mesothelial cell line transfected with EJ-ras oncogene. *J Natl Cancer Inst* 1989;81:945–948.
32. Suzuki Y, Weston A, Ashley R. Immunocytochemical analysis of oncoproteins and growth factors in human malignant mesothelioma. *Oncol Rep* 1995;2:897–902.
33. Moyer VD, Cistulli CA, Vaslet CA, et al. Oxygen radicals and asbestos carcinogenesis. *Environ Health Perspect* 1994;102:131–136.
34. Hollstein M, Sidransky D, Vogelstein B, et al. p53 mutations in human cancers. *Science* 1991;253:49–53.
35. Cora EM, Kane AB. Alterations in a tumour suppressor gene, p53 in mouse MMs induced by crocidolite asbestos. *Eur Respir Rev* 1993; 3:148–150.
36. Metcalf RA, Welsh JA, Bennett WP, et al. p53 and Kirsten-ras mutations in human mesothelioma cell lines. *Cancer Res* 1992;52:2610–2615.
37. Mor O, Yaron P, Huszar M, et al. Absence of p53 mutations in malignant mesotheliomas. *Am J Respir Cell Mol Biol* 1997;16:9–13.
38. Van de Meeren A, Seddon MB, Kispert J, et al. Lack of expression of retinoblastoma gene is not frequently involved in the genesis of human mesothelioma. *Eur Respir Rev* 1993;3:177–179.
39. Kratzke RA, Otterson GA, Lincoln CE, et al. Immunohistochemical analysis of the p16(Ink4) cyclin-dependent kinase inhibitor in malignant mesothelioma. *J Natl Cancer Inst* 1995;87:1870–1875.
40. Prins JB, Williamson KA, Kamp MML, et al. The gene for the cyclin-dependent-kinase-4 inhibitor, Cdkn2a, is preferentially deleted in malignant mesothelioma. *Int J Cancer* 1998;75:649–653.
41. Cheng JQ, Jhanwar SC, Klein WM, et al. p16 alterations and deletion mapping of 9p21–p22 in malignant mesothelioma. *Cancer Res* 1994;54:5547–551.
42. Xiao S, Li DZ, Vijg J, et al. Codeletion of p15 and p16 in primary malignant mesothelioma. *Oncogene* 1995;11:511–515.
43. Illei PB, Ladanyi, M, Rusch VW, et al. The use of CDKN2A deletion as a diagnostic marker for malignant mesothelioma in body cavity effusions. *Cancer* 2003;99:51–56.

44. Lopez-Rios F, Chuai S, Flores R, et al. Global gene expression profiling of pleural mesotheliomas: overexpression of aurora kinases and P16/CDKN2A deletion as prognostic factors and critical evaluation of microarray-based prognostic prediction. *Cancer Res* 2006;66:2970–2979.
45. Sekido Y, Pass HI, Bader S, et al. Neurofibromatosis type 2 (NF2) gene is somatically mutated in mesothelioma but not in lung cancer. *Cancer Res* 1995;55:1227–1231.
46. Bianchi AB, Mitsunaga SI, Cheng J, et al. High frequency of inactivating mutations in the neurofibromatosis type 2 gene (NF2) in primary malignant mesotheliomas. *Proc Nat Acad Sci U S A* 1995;92:10854–10858.
47. Wang ZY, Madden SL, Deuel TF, et al. The Wilms' tumor gene product, WT1, represses transcription of the platelet-derived growth factor A-chain gene. *J Biol Chem* 1992;267:21999–2002.
48. Drummond IA, Madden SL, Rohwer-Nutter P, et al. Repression of the insulin-like growth factor II gene by the Wilms' tumor suppressor WT1. *Science* 1994;57:11–25.
49. Dey BR, Sukhatme VP, Roberts AB, et al. Repression of the transforming growth factor-beta 1 gene by the Wilms' suppressor WT1 gene product. *Mol Endocrinol* 1994;8:595–602.
50. Werner H, Re GG, Drummond IA, et al. Increased expression of the insulin-like growth factor I receptor gene, IGFIR, in Wilms' tumor is correlated with modulation of IGFIR promoter activity by the WT1 Wilms' tumor gene product. *Proc Natl Acad Sci U S A* 1993;90:5828–5832.
51. Langerak AW, Williamson KA, Miyagawa K, et al. Expression of the Wilms' tumor gene Wt1 in human malignant mesothelioma cell lines and relationship to platelet-derived growth factor a and insulin-like growth factor 2 expression. *Genes Chromosomes Cancer* 1995;12:87–96.
52. Kumarsingh S, Segers K, Rodeck U, et al. Wt1 mutation in malignant mesothelioma and Wt1 immunoreactivity in relation to p53 and growth factor receptor expression, cell-type transition, and prognosis. *J Pathol* 1997;181:67–74.
53. Singhal S, Wiewrodt R, Malden LD, et al. Gene expression profiling of malignant mesothelioma. *Clin Cancer Res* 2003;9:3080–3097.
54. Kettunen E, Nicholson AG, Nagy B, et al. L1CAM, INP10, P-cadherin, tPA and ITGB4 over-expression in malignant pleural mesotheliomas revealed by combined use of cDNA and tissue microarray. *Carcinogenesis* 2005;26:17–25.
55. Gordon GJ, Jensen RV, Hsiao LL, et al. Translation of microarray data into clinically relevant cancer diagnostic tests using gene expression ratios in lung cancer and mesothelioma. *Cancer Res* 2002;62:4963–4967.
56. Holloway AJ, Diyagama DS, Opeskin K, et al. A molecular diagnostic test for distinguishing lung adenocarcinoma from malignant mesothelioma using cells collected from pleural effusions. *Clin Cancer Res* 2006;12:5129–5135.
57. Gordon GJ, Jensen RV, Hsiao LL, et al. Using gene expression ratios to predict outcome among patients with mesothelioma. *J Natl Cancer Inst* 2003;95:598–605.
58. Gordon GJ, Rockwell GN, Godfrey PA, et al. Validation of genomics-based prognostic tests in malignant pleural mesothelioma. *Clin Cancer Res* 2005;11:4406–4414.
59. Pass HI, Liu Z, Wali A, et al. Gene expression profiles predict survival and progression of pleural mesothelioma. *Clin Cancer Res* 2004;10:849–859.
60. Lopez-Rios F, Chuai S, Flores R, et al. Global gene expression profiling of pleural mesotheliomas: over-expression of aurora kinases and P16/CDKN2A deletion as prognostic factors and critical evaluation of microarray-based prognostic prediction. *Cancer Res* 2006;66:2970–2979.
61. Henderson DW, Shilken KB, Whitaker D. Unusual histological types and anatomic sites of mesothelioma. In: Henderson D, Shilken K, Langlois S, et al., eds. *Malignant Mesothelioma*. Hemisphere: New York, 1992:140–166.
62. Robinson C, Robinson BW, Lake RA. Sera from patients with malignant mesothelioma can contain autoantibodies. *Lung Cancer* 1998;20:175–184.
63. Davidson JA, Musk AW, Wood BR, et al. Intra-lesional cytokine therapy in cancer: a pilot study of GM-CSF infusion in mesothelioma. *Hum Gen Ther* 1998;9:2121–2133.
64. Mukherjee S, Haenel T, Himbeck R, et al. Replication-restricted vaccinia as a cytokine gene therapy vector in cancer: persistent transgene expression despite antibody generation. *Cancer Gene Therapy*. 2000;7(5):663–670.
65. Marzo AL, Fitzpatrick DR, Robinson BW, et al. Antisense oligonucleotides specific for transforming growth factor beta2 inhibit the growth of malignant mesothelioma both in vitro and in vivo. *Cancer Research* 1997;57:3200–3207.
66. Bielefeldt-Ohmann H, Marzo AL, Himbeck RP, et al. Interleukin-6 involvement in mesothelioma pathobiology: inhibition by interferon alpha immunotherapy. *Cancer Immunol Immunother* 1995;40:241–250.
67. Kane AB. Animal models of malignant mesothelioma. *Inhal Toxicol* 2006;18:1001–1004.
68. Cicala C, Pompetti F, Carbone M. SV40 induces mesotheliomas in hamsters. *Am J Pathol* 1993;142:1524–1533.
69. Craighead JE, Kane AB. The mesothelial cell and malignant mesethelioma. In: Jaurand MC, Bignon I, eds. The Pathogenesis of Malignant and Nonmalignant Serosal Lesions in Body Cavities Consequent to Asbestos Exposure. New York: Dekker, 1994:79–102.
70. Nowak AK, Lake RA, Kindler HL, et al. New approaches for mesothelioma: biologics, vaccines, gene therapy, and other novel agents. *Semin Oncol* 2002;29:82–96.
71. Nowak AK, Robinson BW, Lake RA. Gemcitabine exerts a selective effect on the humoral immune response: implications for combination chemo-immunotherapy. *Cancer Res* 2002;62:2353–2358.
72. Nowak AK, Robinson BW, Lake RA. Synergy between chemotherapy and immunotherapy in the treatment of established murine solid tumors. *Cancer Res* 2003;63:4490–4496.
73. Jackaman C, Bundell CS, Kinnear BF, et al. IL-2 intratumoral immunotherapy enhances CD8+ T cells that mediate destruction of tumor cells and tumor-associated vasculature: a novel mechanism for IL-2. *J Immunol* 2003;171:5051–5063.
74. Vaslet CA, Messier NJ, Kane AB. Accelerated progression of asbestos-induced mesotheliomas in heterozygous p53+/− mice. *Toxicol Sci* 2002;68:331–338.
75. Altomare DA, Vaslet CA, Skele KL, et al. A mouse model recapitulating molecular features of human mesothelioma. *Cancer Res* 2005;65:8090–8095.
76. Fleury-Feith J, Lecomte C, Renier A, et al. Hemizygosity of Nf2 is associated with increased susceptibility to asbestos-induced peritoneal tumours. *Oncogene* 2003;22:3799–3805.
77. Altomare DA, You H, Xiao GH, et al. Human and mouse mesotheliomas exhibit elevated AKT/PKB activity, which can be targeted pharmacologically to inhibit tumor cell growth. *Oncogene* 2005;24:6080–6089.
78. Whitaker D. The cytology of malignant mesothelioma. *Cytopathology*, 2000 Jun;11(3):139–151.
79. Kradin RL, Mark EJ. Distinguishing benign mesothelial hyperplasia from neoplasia: a practical approach. *Semin Diagn Pathol* 2006 Feb;23(1):4–14.
80. Robinson C, van Bruggen I, Segal A, et al. A novel SV40 TAg transgenic model of asbestos-induced mesothelioma: malignant transformation is dose dependent. *Cancer Res* 2006;66:10786–10794.
81. Salyer WR, Egglestone JC, Erozan YS. Efficacy of pleural needle biopsy and pleural fluid cytopathology in the diagnosis of malignant neoplasm involving the pleura. *Chest* 1975;67:563–569.
82. Battifora H, Kopinski MI. Distinction of mesothelioma from adenocarcinoma. *Cancer* 1991;67:655–662.
83. Wirth PR, Legier J, Wright GL Jr. Immunohistochemical evaluation of seven monoclonal antibodies for differentiation of pleural mesothelioma from lung adenocarcinoma. *Cancer* 1991;67:655–662.
84. Herndon JE, Green MR, Chahinian AP, et al. Factors predictive of survival among 337 patients with mesothelioma treated between 1984 and 1994 by the Cancer and Leukemia Group B. *Chest* 1998;113:723–731.

85. Curran D, Sahmoud T, Therasse P, et al. Prognostic factors in patients with pleural mesothelioma: the European Organization for Research and Treatment of Cancer experience. *J Clin Oncol* 1998;16:145–152.
86. Fennell DA, Parmar A, Shamash J, et al. Statistical validation of the EORTC prognostic model for malignant pleural mesothelioma based on three consecutive phase II trials. *J Clin Oncol* 2005;23:184–189.
87. Bottomley A, Coens C, Efficace F, et al. Symptoms and patient-reported well-being: do they predict survival in malignant pleural mesothelioma? A prognostic factor analysis of EORTC-NCIC 08983: randomized phase III study of cisplatin with or without raltitrexed in patients with malignant pleural mesothelioma. *J Clin Oncol* 2007;25:5770–5776.
88. Schouwink JH, Kool LS, Rutgers EJ, et al. The value of chest computer tomography and cervical mediastinoscopy in the preoperative assessment of patients with malignant mesothelioma. *Ann Thorac Surg* 2003; 75(6):1715–8.
89. Heelan RT, Rusch VW, Begg CB, et al. Staging of malignant pleural mesothelioma: comparison of CT and MR imaging. *AJR Am J Roentgenol* 1999;172:1039–1047.
90. Flores RM, Akhurst T, Gonen M, et al. Positron emission tomography defines metastatic disease but not locoregional disease in patients with malignant pleural mesothelioma. *J Thorac Cardiovasc Surg* 2003;126:11–16.
91. Erasmus JJ, Truong MT, Smythe WR, et al. Integrated computer tomography-positron emission tomography in patients with potentially resectable malignant pleural mesothelioma: staging implications. *J Thorac Cardiovasc Surg* 2005;129:1364–1370.
92. Ceresoli GL, Chiti A, Zucali PA, et al. Assessment of tumour response in malignant mesothelioma. *J Clin Oncol* 2006;24:4587–4593.
93. Shitrit D, Zingerman B, Shitrit AB, et al. Diagnostic value of CYFRA 21-1, CEA, CA 19-9, CA 15-3, and CA 125 assays in pleural effusions: analysis of 116 cases and review of the literature. *Oncologist* 2005;10:501–507.
94. Villena V, Lopez-Encuentra A, Echave-Sustaeta J, et al. Diagnostic value of CA 549 in pleural fluid. Comparison with CEA, CA 15.3 and CA 72.4. *Lung Cancer* 2003;40:289–294.
95. Miedouge M, Rouzaud P, Salama G, et al. Evaluation of seven tumour markers in pleural fluid for the diagnosis of malignant effusions. *Br J Cancer* 1999;81:1059–1065.
96. Alatas F, Alatas O, Metintas M, et al. Diagnostic value of CEA, CA 15-3, CA 19-9, CYFRA 21-1, NSE and TSA assay in pleural effusions. *Lung Cancer* 2001;31:9–16.
97. Fuhrman C, Duche JC, Chouaid C, et al. Use of tumor markers for differential diagnosis of mesothelioma and secondary pleural malignancies. *Clin Biochem* 2000;33:405–410.
98. Creaney J, Yeoman D, Naumoff L, et al. Soluble mesothelin in effusions: a useful tool for the diagnosis of malignant mesothelioma. *Thorax* 2007;62(7):569–576.
99. Burgers SA, Tournoy KG, Smits M, et al. EUS-FNA as staging tool in resectable pleural mesothelioma. *2008 ASCO Annual Meeting*. Orlando, Florida. abstract 7607.
100. Witte B, Neumeister W, Huertgen M. Does endoesophageal ultra sound-guide fine needle aspiration replace mediastinoscopy in mediastinal staging of thoracic malignancies? *Eur J Cardiothorac Surg* 2008;33(6):1244–1248.
101. Spirtas R, Connelly RR, Tucker MA. Survival patterns for malignant mesothelioma: the SEER experience. *Int J Cancer* 1988;41:525–530.
102. Greene FL, Page DL, Fleming ID, et al., eds. *AJCC Cancer Staging Handbook*. 6th edition. New York: Springer, 2002:6.
103. Butchart EG, Ashcroft T, Barnsley WC, et al. Pleuropneumonectomy in the management of diffuse pleural mesothelioma of the pleura. *Thorax* 1976;31(1):15–24.
104. Rusch VW. A proposed new international TNM staging system for malignant pleural mesothelioma from the International Mesothelioma Interest Group. *Lung Cancer* 1996;14(1):1–12.
105. Alberts AS, Falkson G, Goedhals L, et al. Malignant pleural mesothelioma: a disease unaffected by current therapeutic maneuvers. *J Clin Oncol* 1988;6:527–535.
106. Treasure T, Tan C, Lang-Lazdunski L, et al. The MARS trial: mesothelioma and radical surgery. *Interact Cardiovasc Thorac Surg* 2006;5:58–59.
107. Flores RM, Zakowski M, Venkatraman E, et al. Prognostic factors in the treatment of malignant pleural mesothelioma at a large tertiary referral center. *J Thorac Oncol* 2007;2:957–965.
108. Flores, RM, Pass HI, Seshan VE, et al. Extrapleural pneumonectomy versus pleurectomy/decortication in the surgical management of malignant pleural mesothelioma: results in 663 patients. *J Thorac Cardiovasc Surg* 2008;135:620–626.
109. Neragi-Miandoab S, Richards WG, Sugarbaker DJ. Morbidity, mortality, mean survival, and the impact of histology on survival after pleurectomy in 64 patients with malignant pleural mesothelioma. *Int J Surg* 2008;6:293–297.
110. Gupta V, Mychalczak B, Krug L, et al. Hemithoracic radiation therapy after pleurectomy/decortication for malignant pleural mesothelioma. *Int J Radiat Oncol Biol Phys* 2005;63:1045–1052.
111. Rusch VW, Rosenzweig K, Venkatraman E, et al. A phase II trial of surgical resection and adjuvant high-dose hemithoracic radiation for malignant pleural mesothelioma. *J Thorac Cardiovasc Surg* 2001;122:788–795.
112. Sugarbaker DJ, Jaklitsch MT, Bueno R, et al. Prevention, early detection, and management of complications after 328 consecutive extrapleural pneumonectomies. *J Thorac Cardiovasc Surg* 2004;128:138–146.
113. Boutin C, Rey F, Viallat JR. Prevention of malignant seeding after invasive diagnostic procedures in patients with pleural mesothelioma. A randomized trial of local radiotherapy. *Chest* 1995;108:754–758.
114. Davies HE, Musk AW, Lee YC. Prophylactic radiotherapy for pleural puncture sites in mesothelioma: the controversy continues. *Curr Opin Pulm Med* 2008;14:326–330.
115. Rice DC, Stevens CW, Correa Am, et al. Outcomes after extrapleural pneumonectomy and intensity-modulated radiation therapy for malignant pleural mesothelioma. *Ann Thorac Surg* 2007;84:1685–1692.
116. Rice DC, Smythe WR, Liao Z, et al. Dose-dependent pulmonary toxicity after postoperative intensity-modulated radiotherapy for malignant pleural mesothelioma. *In J Radiat Oncol Biol Phys* 2007;69:350–357.
117. Sugarbaker DJ, Flores RM, Jaklitsch MT, et al. Resection margins, jextrapleural nodal status, and cell type determine postoperative long-term survival in trimodality therapy of malignant pleural mesothelioma: results in 183 patients. *J Thorac Cardiovasc Surg* 1999;117:54–63.
118. Richards WG, Zellos L, Bueno R, et al. Phase I to II study of pleurectomy/decortication and intraoperative intracavitary hyperthermic cisplatin lavage for mesothelioma. *J Clin Oncol* 2006;24:1561–1567.
119. Weder W, Stahel RA, Bernhard J, et al. Multicenter trial of neo-adjuvant chemotherapy followed by extrapleural pneumonectomy in malignant pleural mesothelioma. *Ann Oncol* 2007;18:1196–1202.
120. Krug LM, Pass H, Rusch VW, et al. A multicenter US trial of neoadjuvant pemetrexed plus cisplatin (PC) followed by extrapleural pneumonectomy (EPP) and hemithoracic radiation (RT) for stage I-III malignant pleural mesothelioma (MPM). *J Clin Oncol* 2007 *ASCO Annual Meeting Proceedings Part I* 25:7561.
121. Krug LM. An overview of chemotherapy for mesothelioma. *Hematol Oncol Clin North Am* 2005;19:1117–1136.
122. Berghmans T, Paesmans M, Lalami Y, et al. Activity of chemotherapy and immunotherapy on malignant mesothelioma: a systematic review of the literature with meta-analysis. *Lung Cancer* 2002;38:111–121.
123. Lerner HJ, Schoenfeld DA, Martin A, et al. Malignant mesothelioma. The Eastern Cooperative Oncology Group (ECOG) experience. *Cancer* 1983;52:1981–1985.
124. Mattson K, Giaccone G, Kirkpatrick A, et al. Epirubicin in malignant mesothelioma: a phase II study of the European Organization for Research and Treatment of Cancer Lung Cancer Cooperative Group. *J Clin Oncol* 1992;10:824–828.
125. Kindler HL, van Meerbeeck JP. The role of gemcitabine in the treatment of malignant mesothelioma. *Semin Oncol* 2002;29:80–76.
126. Scagliotti GV, Shin DM, Kindler HL, et al. Phase II study of pemetrexed with and without folic acid and vitamin B12 as front-line therapy in malignant pleural mesothelioma. *J Clin Oncol* 2003;21: 1556–1561.

127. Baas P, Ardizzoni A, Grossi F, et al. The activity of raltitrexed (Tomudex) in malignant pleural mesothelioma: an EORTC phase II study (08992). *Eur J Cancer* 2003;39:353–357.
128. Talbot DC, Margery J, Dabouis G, et al. Phase II study of vinflunine in malignant pleural mesothelioma. *J Clin Oncol* 2007;25:4751–4756.
129. Steele JP, Shamash J, Evans MT, et al. Phase II study of vinorelbine in patients with malignant pleural mesothelioma. *J Clin Oncol* 2000;18:3912–3917.
130. Vogelzang NJ, Rusthoven JJ, Symanowski J, et al. Phase II study of pemetrexed in combination with cisplatin versus cisplatin alone in patients with malignant pleural mesothelioma. *J Clin Oncol* 2003; 15:2636–2644.
131. Van Meerbeeck JP, Gaafar R, Manegold C, et al. Randomized phase III study of cisplatin with or with out raltitrexed in patients with malignant pleural mesothelioma: an intergroup study of the European Organisation for Research and Treatment of Cancer Lung Cancer Group and the National Cancer Institute of Canada. *J Clin Oncol* 2005;23:6881–6889.
132. Berghmans T, Lafitte JJ, Paesmans M, et al. A phase II study evaluating the cisplatin and epirubicin combination in patients with unresectable malignant pleural mesothelioma. *Lung Cancer* 2005;50:75–83.
133. Nowak AK, Byrne MJ, Williamson R, et al. A multicentre phase II study of cisplatin and gemcitabine for malignant mesothelioma. *Br J Cancer* 2002;87:491–496.
134. Fennell DA, Steele JP, Shamash J, et al. Efficacy and safety of first- or second-line irinotecan, cisplatin, and mitomycin in mesothelioma. *Cancer* 2007;109:93–99.
135. Sorensen JB, Frank H, Palshof T. Cisplatin and vinorelbine first-line chemotherapy in non-resectable malignant pleural mesothelioma. *Br J Cancer* 2008;99:44–50.
136. Baas P, van Meerbeeck J, Groen H. Caelyx in malignant mesothelioma: a phase II EORTC study. *Ann Oncol* 2000;11:697–700.
137. Kosty MP, Herndon JE 2nd, Vogelzang NJ, et al. High-dose doxorubicin, dexrazoxane, and GM-CSF in malignant mesothelioma: a phase II study-Cancer and Leukemia Group B 9631. *Lung Cancer* 2001;34:289–295.
138. Portalone L, Antill A, Nunziati F, et al. Epirubicin and gemcitabine as first-line treatment in malignant pleural mesothelioma. *Tumori* 2005;91:15–18.
139. Okuno SH, Delaune R, Sloan JA, et al. A phase 2 study of gemcitabine and epirubicin for the treatment of pleural mesothelioma: a North Central Cancer Treatment Study, N0021. *Cancer* 2008 Apr 15;112(8):1772–1779.
140. Xanthopoulos A, Bauer TT, Blum TG, et al. Gemcitabine combined with oxaliplatin in pretreated patients with malignant pleural mesothelioma: an observational study. *J Occup Med Toxicol* 2008;3:34.
141. Fizazi K, Doubre H, Le Chevalier T, et al. Combination of raltitrexed and oxaliplatin is an active regimen in malignant mesothelioma: results of a phase II study. *J Clin Oncol* 2003;21:349–354.
142. Fennell DA, Steele JP, Shamash J, et al. Phase II trial of binorelbine and oxaliplatin as first-line therapy in malignant pleural mesothelioma. *Lung Cancer* 2005;47:277–281.
143. Solheim OP, Saeter G, Finnanger AM, et al. High-dose methotrexate in the treatment of malignant mesothelioma of the pleura. A phase II study. *Br J Cancer* 1992;65:956–960.
144. Kindler HL, Belani CP, Herndon JE 2nd, et al. Edatrexate (10-ethyl-deaza-aminopterin) (NSC #626715) with or without leucovorin rescue for malignant mesothelioma. Sequential phase II trials by the Cancer and Leukemia Group B. *Cancer* 1999;86:1985–1991.
145. Krug LM, Heelan RT, Kris MG, et al. Phase II trial of pralatrexate (10-propargyl-10-deazaaminopterin, PDX) in patients with unresectable malignant pleural mesothelioma. *J Thorac Oncol* 2007;2:317–320.
146. Wang Y, Zhao R, Chattopadhyay S, et al. A novel folate transport activity in human mesothelioma cell lines with high affinity and specificity for the new-generation antifolate, pemetrexed. *Cancer Res* 2002;62:6434–6437.
147. Chattopadhyay S, Tamari R, Min SH, et al. Commentary: a case for minimizing folate supplementation in clinical regimens with pemetrexed based on the marked sensitivity of the drug to folate availability. *Oncologist* 2007;12:808–815.
148. Santoro A, O'Brien ME, Stahel RA, et al. Pemetrexed plus cisplatin or pemetrexed plus carboplatin for chemo-naive patients with malignant pleural mesothelioma: results of the International Expanded Access Program. *J Thorac Oncol* 2008;3:756–763.
149. Ceresoli GL, Zucali PA, Favaretto, AG, et al. Phase II study of pemetrexed plus carboplatin in malignant pleural mesothelioma. *J Clin Oncol* 2006;24:1443–1448.
150. Castagneto B, Botta M, Aitini E, et al. Phase II study of pemetrexed in combination with carboplatin in patients with malignant pleural mesothelioma (MPM). *Ann Oncol* 2008; 2:370–373.
151. Ceresoli GL, Castagneto B, Zucali PA, et al. Pemetrexed plus carboplatin in elderly patients with malignant pleural mesothelioma: combined analysis of two phase II trials. *Br J Cancer* 2008;99:51–56.
152. Kindler HL, Millard F, Herndon JE 2nd, et al. Gemcitabine for malignant mesothelioma: a phase II trial by the Cancer and Leukemia Group B. *Lung Cancer* 2001;31:311–317.
153. Lee CW, Murray N, Anderson H, et al. Outcomes with a platinum plus gemcitabine or pemetrexed as first-line systemic therapy for malignant pleural mesothelioma in British Columbia: a review of province-wide practice. *J Thoracic Oncol* 2007;2(8):S606.
154. Byrne MJ, Davidson JA, Musk AW, et al. Cisplatin and gemcitabine treatment for malignant mesothelioma: a phase II study. *J Clin Oncol* 1999;17:25–30.
155. Favaretto AG, Aversa SM, Paccagnella A, et al. Gemcitabine combined with carboplatin in patients with malignant pleural mesotheliomoa: a multicentric phase II study. *Cancer* 2003;97:2791–2797.
156. Janne PA, Simon GR, Langer CJ, et al. Phase II trial of pemetrexed and gemcitabine in chemotherapy-naïve malignant pleural mesothelioma. *J Clin Oncol* 2008;26:1465–1471.
157. Muers MF, Stephens RJ, Fisher P, et al. Active symptom control with or without chemotherapy in the treatment of patients with malignant pleural mesothelioma (MS01): a multicentre randomized trial. *Lancet* 2008;371:1685–1694.
158. Dowell J, Kindler HL. Anti-angiogenic therapies for mesothelioma. *Hematol Oncol Clin North Am* 2005:19(6):1137–1146.
159. Cortese JF, Gowda AL, Wali A, et al. Common EGFR mutations conferring sensitivity to gefitinib in lung adenocarcinoma are not prevalent in human malignant mesothelioma. *Int J Cancer* 2006:118(2): 521–522.
160. Govindan R, Kratzke RA, Herndon JE 2nd, et al. Gefitinib in patients with malignant mesothelioma: a phase II study by the Cancer and Leukemia Group B. *Clin Cancer Res* 2005;11:2300–2304.
161. Garland LL, Rankin C, Gandara DR, et al. Phase II study of erlotinib in patients with malignant pleural mesothelioma: a Southwest Oncology Group Study. *J Clin Oncol* 2007;25:2406–2413.
162. Jahan TM, Gu L, Wang X, et al. Vatalanib (V) for patients with previously untreated advanced malignant mesothelioma (MM): a phase II study by the Cancer and Leukemia Group B (CALGB 30107). *Proc Am Soc Clin Oncol* 2006;24(18S):7081.
163. Janne PA, Wang XF, Krug LM, et al. Sorafenib in malignant mesothelioma (MM): a phase II trial of the Cancer and Leukemia Group B (CALGB 30307). *Proc Am Soc Clin Oncol* 2007;25:7707.
164. Nowak AK, Millward MJ, Francis R, et al. Phase II study of sunitinib as second-line therapy in malignant pleural mesothelioma (MPM). *Proc Am Soc Clin Oncol* 2008;26:abstr 8063.
165. Baas P, Boogerd W, Dalesio O, et al. Thalidomide in patients with malignant pleural mesothelioma. *Lung Cancer* 2005;48(2):291–296.
166. Karrison T, Kindler HL, Gandara DR, et al. Final analysis of a multicenter, double-blind, placebo-controlled, randomized phase II trial of gemcitabine/cisplatin (GC) plus bevacizumab (B) or placebo (P) in patients (pts) with malignant mesothelioma (MM). *Proc Am Soc Clin Oncol* 2007;25:7526.
167. Kelly WK, O'Connor OA, Krug LM, et al. Phase I study of an oral histone deacetylase inhibitor, suberolylanilide hydroxamic acid, in patients with advanced cancer. *J Clin Oncol* 2005;23(17):3923–3931.

168. Krug LM, Curley T, Schwartz L, et al. Potential role of histone deacetylase inhibitors in mesothelioma: clinical experience with suberoylanilide hydroxamic acid. *Clin Lung Cancer* 2006;7(4):257–261.
169. Sartore-Bianchi A, Gasparri F, Galvani A, et al. Bortezomib inhibits nuclear factor-kappaB dependent survival and has potent in vivo activity in mesothelioma. *Clin Cancer Res* 2007;13:5942–5951.
170. Mikulski SM, Costanzi JJ, Vogelzang NJ, et al. Phase II trial of a single weekly intravenous dose of ranpirnase in patients with unresectable malignant mesothelioma. *J Clin Oncol* 2002;20(1):274–281.
171. Vogelzang N, Taub R, Shin D, et al. Phase III randomized trial of onconase (ONC) versus doxorubicin (DOX) in patients (Pts) with unresectable malignant mesothelioma: analysis of survival. *Proc Am Soc Clin Oncol* 2000:2274.
172. Hassan R, Ho M. Mesothelin targeted cancer immunotherapy. *Eur J Cancer* 2008;44(1):46–53.
173. Hassan R, Broaddus VC, Wilson S, et al. Anti-mesothelin immunotoxin SS1P in combination with gemcitabine results in increased activity against mesothelin-expressing tumor xenografts. *Clin Cancer Res* 2007;13:7166–7171.
174. Hassan R, Ebel W, Routhier EL, et al. Preclinical evaluation of MORAb-009, a chimeric antibody targeting tumor-associated mesothelin. *Cancer Immun* 2007;7:20.
175. Hassan R, Bullock S, Premkumar A, et al. Phase I study of SS1P, a recombinant anti-mesothelin immunotoxin given as a bolus I.V. infusion to patients with mesothelin-expressing mesothelioma, ovarian, and pancreatic cancers. *Clin Cancer Res* 2007;13:5144–5149.

CHAPTER 66

Naveed Alam
Raja Flores

Management of Mediastinal Tumors Not of Thymic Origin

The *mediastinum* is the term used to describe the contents of the thorax between the pleural cavities. It is an anatomical region defined by the lungs laterally, the diaphragm inferiorly, the thoracic inlet superiorly, the sternum anteriorly, and the vertebral column posteriorly. It is densely populated with vital structures including, but not limited to, the heart and great vessels as well as the trachea and the esophagus. It has been described as the "third space" of the thorax or "the space between spaces."[1]

Tumors of the mediastinum may originate from the normal anatomic structures of the region or from adjacent tissues. They may be primary or metastatic and they encompass a wide variety of histologies. This discussion will focus on mediastinal masses in adults.

COMPARTMENTS

There are numerous classification systems for the compartments of the mediastinum in the surgical and radiological literature. Perhaps the simplest and most clinically relevant system is that proposed by Shields,[2] which subdivides the mediastinum into three anatomic compartments: the anterior, middle (or visceral), and the paravertebral sulci laterally. These compartments are readily depicted on a lateral view of the chest (Fig. 66.1).

The anterior compartment contains the thymus gland, lymph nodes, connective tissue, and fat. It may also contain displaced parathyroid glands or ectopic thyroid tissue. The visceral (or middle) compartment contains the heart and great vessels within the pericardium, the esophagus, trachea, and portions of the mainstem bronchi, the thoracic duct, and numerous lymph nodes and nerves (vagus and phrenic). The paravertebral sulci (posterior compartment) contain the proximal portions of the intercostal nerves, arteries, and veins, as well as the sympathetic trunk.

The clinical relevance of the model lies in the differential diagnoses of masses in each compartment (Table 66.1).[3]

SIGNS AND SYMPTOMS

Approximately 50% of mediastinal masses in the adult population are found in asymptomatic patients.[4] Increased use of screening and surveillance CT scans and chest radiographs will likely raise the proportion of asymptomatic masses. In adults, the anterior mediastinum is the most common location for tumors.

Symptoms depend on the size and location of the mass. Malignant lesions are more likely to be symptomatic.[5] Although many symptoms are caused by local compression or invasion of adjacent structures, systemic symptoms associated with specific tumor types may also be present.[3]

Respiratory symptoms of cough, dyspnea, stridor, and hemoptysis are among the most common. Local invasion of pleura or chest wall may result in chest pain, which is often pleuritic in nature. Chest pain may also mimic angina. Other symptoms and signs resulting from local invasion or compression of structures includes dysphagia (esophagus), hoarseness (recurrent laryngeal nerve), superior vena cava (SVC) syndrome, Horner's syndrome (stellate ganglion), and cardiac tamponade (pericardium).

Generalized symptoms associated with malignancies such as fever, chills, and weight loss also need to be considered. Symptoms and signs associated with specific endocrine tumors may also be present (Tables 66.2 and 66.3). Signs and symptoms of hypercalcemia may be associated with parathyroid adenomas. The classical association of myasthenia gravis with an anterior mediastinal mass is almost pathognomonic of thymoma (not considered in this chapter). The presence of "café-au-lait" spots and a posterior mass is similarly suggestive of von Recklinghausen neurofibromatosis. Physical examination should include testicular assessment if a germ cell tumor (GCT) is suspected.[6]

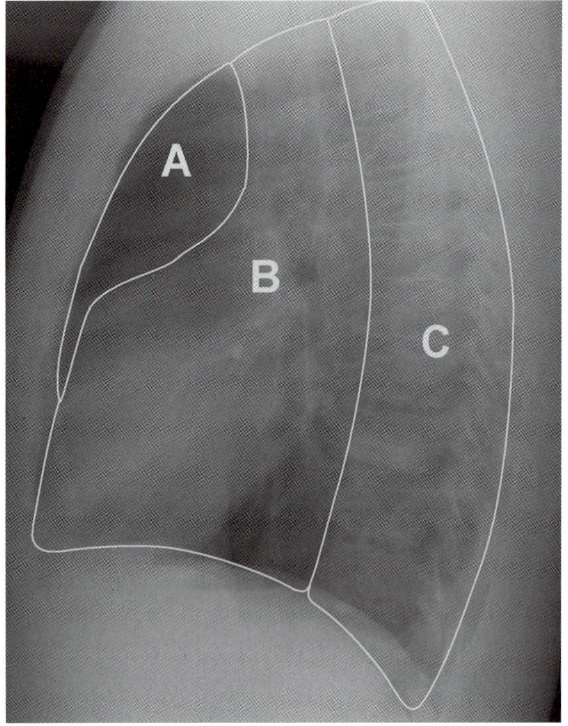

FIGURE 66.1 Mediastinal compartments diagram. Lateral chest x-ray demonstrating boundaries of the (*A*) anterior, (*B*) middle or visceral, and (*C*) posterior or paravertebral mediastinal compartments. (Shields TW. The mediastinum, its compartments, and the mediastinal lymph nodes. In: Shields TW, ed. *General Thoracic Surgery*. 6th Ed. Philadelphia: Lippincott Williams and Wilkins, 2005:2343. Used with permission.)

TABLE 66.1 Differential Diagnosis of a Mediastinal Mass by Anatomic Location

Anterior	Middle	Posterior
Thymoma	Neurogenic tumor	
Teratoma, seminoma	Bronchogenic cyst	
Lymphoma	Enteric cyst	
Carcinoma	Xanthogranuloma	
Parathyroid adenoma	Diaphragmatic hernia	
Intrathoracic goiter	Meningocele	
Lipoma	Paravertebral abscess	
Lymphangioma		
Aortic aneurysm		
Lymphoma		
Pericardial cyst		
Bronchogenic cyst		
Metastatic cyst		
Systemic granuloma		

Reprinted with permission from Crapo JD, Glassroth J, Karlinsky J, et al. *Baum's Textbook of Pulmonary Diseases*. Philadelphia: Lippincott Williams and Wilkins, 2004:883–912.[3]

IMAGING

Radiology Although most patients will have a lateral and posteroanterior (PA) chest radiograph during their first examination, almost all patients will subsequently have a computed tomography (CT) scan. It is routine for computerized tomograms of the chest to image the area between the lung apices to the base of the adrenal glands. When mediastinal pathology is suspected, intravenous contrast should be used as it helps with lesion detection and definition. CT gives valuable information as to the density of the mass (cystic or solid) as well as its relationship to adjacent anatomic structures (Fig. 66.2).[7]

Magnetic resonance imaging (MRI) is somewhat limited in evaluation of the thorax because of its sensitivity to motion artifact (from cardiac and respiratory movements) and poor imaging quality of lung parenchyma. In imaging of mediastinal masses, its greatest utility lies in its assessment of specific areas where CT may fall short. These may include cases where the patient is unable to tolerate contrast for CT. The most common indication for magnetic resonance (MR) is in assessment of masses in the paravertebral sulci or posterior compartment. MR is useful if there is a "dumbbell" component to

TABLE 66.2 Localizing Symptoms Secondary to Tumor Invasion of Surrounding Structures

Involved Anatomic Structure	Localizing Symptom
Bronchi/trachea	Dyspnea, postobstructive pneumonia, atelectasis, hemoptysis
Esophagus	Dysphagia
Spinal cord/vertebral column	Paralysis
Recurrent laryngeal nerve	Hoarseness, vocal cord paralysis
Phrenic nerve	Diaphragmatic paralysis
Stellate ganglion	Horner syndrome
Superior vena cava	Superior vena cava syndrome

Reprinted with permission from Crapo JD, Glassroth J, Karlinsky J, et al. *Baum's Textbook of Pulmonary Diseases*. Philadelphia: Lippincott Williams and Wilkins, 2004:883–912.[3]

TABLE 66.3 Systemic Syndromes Secondary to Primary Mediastinal Tumors and Cysts

Syndrome	Tumor
Myasthenia gravis, RBC aplasia, hypogammaglobulinemia, Good syndrome, Whipple disease, megaesophagus, myocarditis	Thymoma
Multiple endocrine adenomatosis, Cushing syndrome	Carcinoid, thymoma
Hypertension	Pheochromocytoma, ganglioneuroma, chemodectoma
Diarrhea	Ganglioneuroma
Hypercalcemia	Parathyroid adenoma, lymphoma
Thyrotoxicosis	Intrathoracic goiter
Hypoglycemia	Mesothelioma, teratoma, fibrosarcoma, neurosarcoma
Osteoarthropathy	Neurofibroma, neurilemoma mesothelioma
Vertebral abnormalities	Enteric cysts
Fever of unknown origin	Lymphoma
Alcohol-induced pain	HD
Opsomyoclonus	Neuroblastoma

Reprinted with permission from Crapo JD, Glassroth J, Karlinsky J, et al. *Baum's Textbook of Pulmonary Diseases.* Philadelphia: Lippincott Williams and Wilkins, 2004:883–912.[3]

HD, Hodgkin disease; RBC, red blood cell.

a neurogenic tumor (i.e., if the tumor has extended into the spinal canal). MR can give information as to the longitudinal extent of the involvement of the spinal canal.[8]

Ultrasound has limited use in the evaluation of mediastinal pathology. It is primarily used for localization during percutaneous biopsies.

Positron Emission Tomography Positron emission tomography (PET) has become an increasingly important tool in the investigation of malignancies throughout the body. This is true of mediastinal pathology as well (Fig. 66.3). Most centers will routinely perform PET with ^{18}F-fluorodeoxyglucose (FDG) in the evaluation of suspected non–small cell lung cancers (NSCLC) or esophageal cancers. PET also plays an important role in the evaluation of lymphoma. In both Hodgkin's and non-Hodgkin's lymphoma (NHL), PET has been found to be an accurate and cost-effective method of staging disease as well as monitoring responses to therapy and assessing recurrence.[9]

The use of PET in the indeterminate mediastinal masses has not been well defined and requires further study. In one Japanese study, increased FDG uptake correlated with an increased likelihood of malignancy.[10]

Other Nuclear Imaging Techniques Octreotide, a somatostatin analogue, has been used in the evaluation of some suspected mediastinal pathology. It has an affinity for

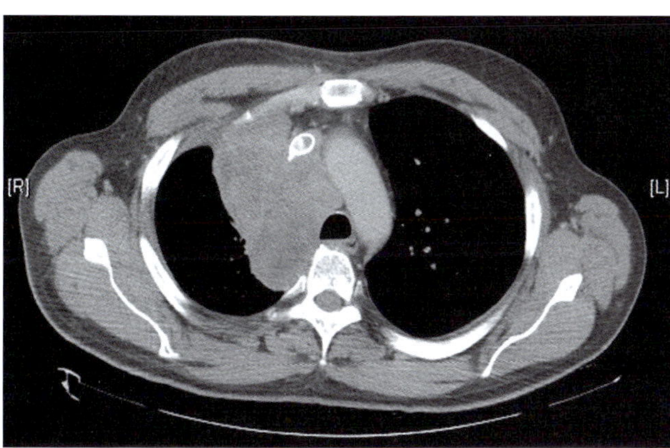

FIGURE 66.2 Sarcoma of anterior mediastinum.

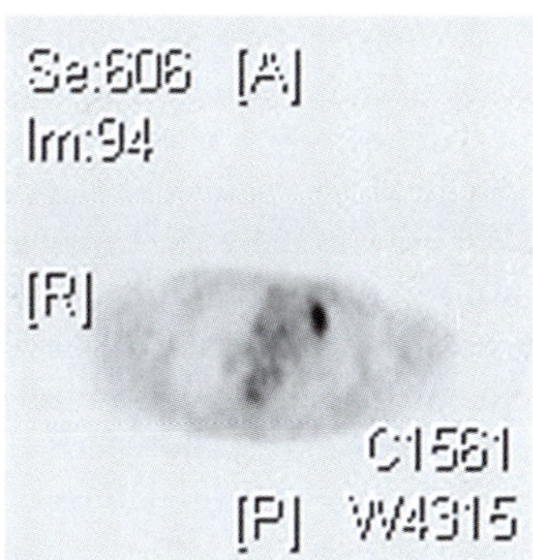

FIGURE 66.3 PET scan of anterior mediastinal mass.

neuoroendocrine neoplasms such as pheochromocytomas, medullary carcinomas of the thyroid, carcinoid tumors, small cell lung cancer, and some lymphomas.[11]

Other nuclear imaging techniques may be relevant in the evaluation of other specific diagnoses. For example, parathyroid sestamibi scans can be used in the search for ectopic mediastinal parathyroid tissue or scintigraphy with an iodine isotope can be used for suspected mediastinal goiters. Gallium scanning plays a role in the staging of lymphoma.[11]

TUMOR MARKERS

Certain serum markers are relevant in mediastinal pathology. Antiacetylcholine receptor antibodies (Anti-AChR) may be elevated in thymic tumors.[12] Other tumor markers should be tested for in patients with anterior mediastinal masses that may be GCTs. Human chorionic gonadotropin beta (β-hCG) and α-fetoprotein (AFP) are useful in the diagnosis of nonseminomatous germ cell tumor (NSGCT). Lactate dehydrogenase (LDH) levels should also be drawn as they may be elevated in patients with lymphoma.[13] In addition to helping with diagnoses, these markers can be used in monitoring the progression of disease or the response to therapy.

BIOPSY

Biopsy of mediastinal masses should be performed if, after other investigations, the diagnosis remains unclear. It is specifically indicated if excisional biopsy of the mass is not warranted (e.g., in lymphoma). There are several techniques that can be employed to obtain tissue diagnoses of mediastinal masses. The selection of biopsy method depends not only on the location of the mass, but also on the suspected diagnosis. In particular, the diagnosis of lymphoma often requires a substantially greater mass of tissue to allow adequate subtyping. Furthermore, it cannot often be made on the grounds of a fine needle aspiration (FNA) and often requires an amount of tissue only obtainable by more invasive procedures.[4]

A similar caveat is important to consider in the evaluation of GCTs with FNA. Most GCTs have multiple elements and some pathologists feel that multiple tissue sections need to be evaluated, which can only be performed with larger volumes of tissue, which are obtained by open techniques.

Cervical mediastinoscopy is a well-established and safe technique that can give large volumes of biopsied tissue material through a 2-cm incision above the suprasternal notch. It is used to obtain tissue in the visceral compartment, particularly the paratracheal and subcarinal regions. Anterior mediastinotomy is a procedure performed through a small incision in the second intercostal space parasternally, which affords excellent access to almost all anterior mediastinal masses. Both of these procedures are associated with few complications and can provide large volumes of tissue. When combined, almost any mass in the anterior mediastinum or visceral compartment can be accessed. They are performed under general anesthesia and are often done as day cases.

With increasing expertise in the use of thoracoscopic techniques, many thoracic surgeons find that video-assisted thoracic surgery (VATS) enables easier access to any part of the mediastinum with the added benefit of being able to completely excise smaller masses. VATS usually requires general anesthesia and is usually performed through one to three 1-cm incisions for biopsies depending on the anatomic area being sampled.

The recent advent of endoscopic ultrasound (EUS) and endobronchial ultrasound (EBUS) have enabled clinicians to obtain tissue from previously difficult to access areas in a minimally invasive fashion. Both EUS (through the esophagus) and EBUS (through the trachea or bronchi) can provide aspirates and core needle biopsies of masses and lymph nodes in the mediastinum. EUS is well suited to biopsy areas adjacent to the esophagus including subcarinal regions, the aortopulmonary window, and particularly the inferior mediastinum (an area inaccessible to mediastinoscopy). In addition to accessing areas accessible by mediastinoscopy (paratracheal), EBUS can access areas distal to the mainstem bronchi (i.e., at the pulmonary hila).

CLINICAL PRESENTATION

Anterior Mediastinal Mass The most common causes of anterior mediastinal masses in adults are thymic neoplasms, lymphomas, and germ cell neoplasms. Thymic neoplasms are not dealt with in this chapter.

Germ Cell Tumors Mediastinal GCTs arise from primitive germ cells that have failed to migrate during embryonic development. They often present in young adulthood and represent 15% of anterior mediastinal masses in adults.[14] Malignant GCTs are more common in men (>90%). Histologically, GCTs can be subdivided into three broad categories: benign teratomas, seminomas, and NSGCTs.[15]

Benign Teratomas Benign or mature teratomas represent the greatest proportion of mediastinal GCTs and consist of tissue from at least two of the three primitive germ layers. Ectodermal tissues (hair, skin, teeth) predominate with some mesodermal components (fat, cartilage, bone) and less often endodermal tissues (respiratory or intestinal epithelium). Most patients are asymptomatic although symptoms can be caused by local compression. Teratomas containing digestive enzymes can rupture into bronchi, lung, or pericardium. Malignant transformation is rare but possible.[16] Benign teratomas have normal serum markers. Complete surgical excision is the treatment of choice.

Seminomas Seminomas occur in men in their 20s to 40s and can present with symptoms of chest pain, cough, dyspnea, fever, weight loss, and may be associated with SVC syndrome. Some patients present with gynecomastia. They can reach extremely large diameters before causing symptoms dependent on location. On imaging, they are bulky, lobulated, homogenous masses. Serum β-hCG may be mildly elevated. Patients with pure seminomas should never have an elevated serum AFP; its presence implies the presence of yolk sac tumor and embryonal cell carcinoma in the primary or in a metastatic site.

Seminomas are radiosensitive tumors and radiation is often the primary treatment modality. For small masses, radiation alone may be administered. For larger masses, combined chemoradiotherapy with cisplatin and etoposide regimens is used. If a residual mass remains posttreatment, most clinicians would advocate observation if the mass is less than 3 cm or surgical excision if the mass is greater than 3 cm.[17]

Nonseminomatous Germ Cell Tumors The term *nonseminomatous germ cell tumor* comprises several histologically distinct tumor types including yolk sac carcinoma, embryonal carcinoma, choriocarcinoma, and mixed tumor histology.

Several hematologic malignancies may occur in conjunction with mediastinal NSGCTs, such as acute megakaryocytic leukemia, myelodysplastic syndrome, refractory thrombocytopenia, refractory anemia with excess blasts, malignant histiocytosis, and systemic mastocytosis. In approximately 80% of NSGCTs, AFP is elevated. β-hCG is elevated in approximately 30% to 35% of patients and may lead to gynecomastia in young male patients. Either tumor marker may be elevated alone or together in any particular patient.[18,19] The presence of any nonseminomatous element (i.e., elevated AFP), even in a tumor that is predominantly seminomatous by histology, is classified as an NSGCT and treated as such.

Although treatment can be initiated based on positive tumor marker results, histological diagnosis is recommended. There is a pathologic discrepancy of 6% between histology and FNA, and difficulty may arise in differentiating GCTs from poorly differentiated carcinoma.[20] Core needle biopsy should be performed when possible and, if surgical biopsy is warranted, an anterior mediastinotomy, (Chamberlain procedure) is usually the procedure of choice. In diagnostic dilemmas, tissue should be sent for genetic analysis, specifically abnormalities of the short arm of chromosome 12, which is a consistent finding in GCTs and rarely observed in other tumors. Chemotherapy is the mainstay of initial treatment, and surgery should be viewed as an adjuvant to chemotherapy. Four cycles of bleomycin, etoposide, and cisplatin (BEP) is the current standard.[21,22] A rapid decline of tumor marker levels with platinum-based chemotherapy treatment is associated with improved response rates and overall survival.[23] Chemotherapy is also indicated postsurgical resection when viable tumor is present in the resected specimen.

After initial treatment with chemotherapy, a patient with tumor marker normalization and a persistent mass on CT is the most favorable candidate for surgical resection. Patients demonstrating a residual mass on CT and persistently elevated tumor markers have been treated with salvage chemotherapy in the past in an effort to obtain normal tumor marker levels prior to surgery. This approach, however, has not improved outcome,[22] and current practice at some centers is to recommend surgery after initial chemotherapy (regardless of persistently elevated tumor markers), in an attempt to achieve complete surgical resection. If patients are to undergo salvage chemotherapy preoperatively, this should be performed in a clinical trial setting. In rare circumstances, postchemotherapy patients will demonstrate elevated tumor marker levels but no residual mass on CT. Surgery is not recommended in these patients. Instead, they should be followed by serial CT scans.

SURGICAL APPROACH

Median sternotomy is the most common approach for small, centrally located tumors in the anterior mediastinum. The patient is placed in the supine position with both arms tucked to the sides, which allows exposure to the right or left hemithoraces, the lung hila, and mediastinal vascular structures. However, exposure to the posterior aspects of the lung is suboptimal and visualization of the left lower lobe is limited.

A hemiclamshell incision is our preferred approach for large tumors arising in the anterior mediastinum and extending significantly into either the right or left hemithorax. The exposure is a combined upper median sternotomy and anterior thoracotomy (Fig. 66.4).[24] The patient is placed in the supine position, the side of the anterior thoracotomy extension is elevated 30 degrees with a longitudinal roll placed beneath the scapula, and arms are tucked at the sides. Exposure is facilitated by collapse of the ipsilateral lung, allowing for anatomical lung resection if necessary. Once the involved lung is divided, optimal exposure to the posterolateral aspect of the tumor is obtained, thereby allowing complete assessment of adjacent vascular structures and phrenic nerve.

If a large tumor extends into the neck area, an extension along the anterior border of the sternocleidomastoid provides excellent exposure, especially if dissection of the vascular structures is required. This provides excellent exposure of the carotid and jugular vessels (Fig. 66.5).[25]

On rare occasions, resection of the subclavian vessels is necessary with mediastinal GCTs. If required, extending the top of the sternotomy along the superior portion of the clavicle allows adequate control of the vessels. This can be described as a "trap door" incision. In addition, the excision of the medial one third of the clavicle may provide added exposure (Fig. 66.6).

A series of 32 patients who underwent postchemotherapy surgical resection of mediastinal GCTs has been published.[26] Histologic analysis revealed viable tumor in 66%, teratoma in 22%, and necrosis in 12% of the specimens. Viable tumor included embryonal carcinoma, choriocarcinoma, yolk sac carcinoma, seminoma, and teratoma with malignant transformation to non-germ cell histology (e.g., sarcoma). Because teratoma and residual tumor were found in the majority of resected patients, we maintain an aggressive approach to surgical resection

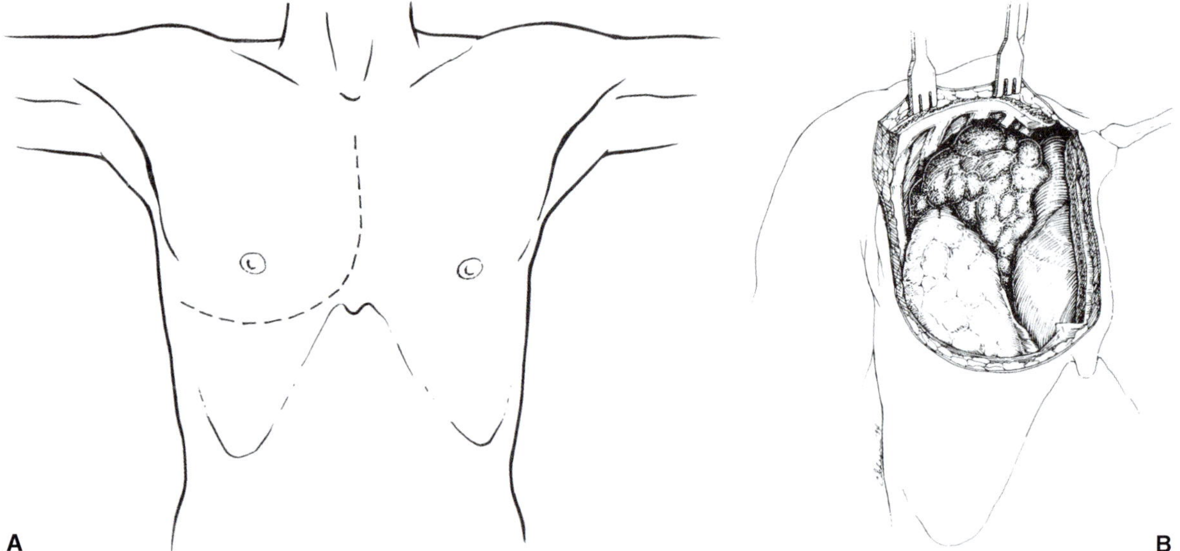

FIGURE 66.4 **A:** Incision for a right hemiclamshell. **B:** Operative exposure for a right hemiclamshell. (**A,B:** From Bains MS, Ginsberg RJ, Jones WG II, et al. The clamshell incision: an improved approach to bilateral pulmonary and mediastinal tumor. *Ann Thorac Surg* 1994;58:30–33. Used with permission.)

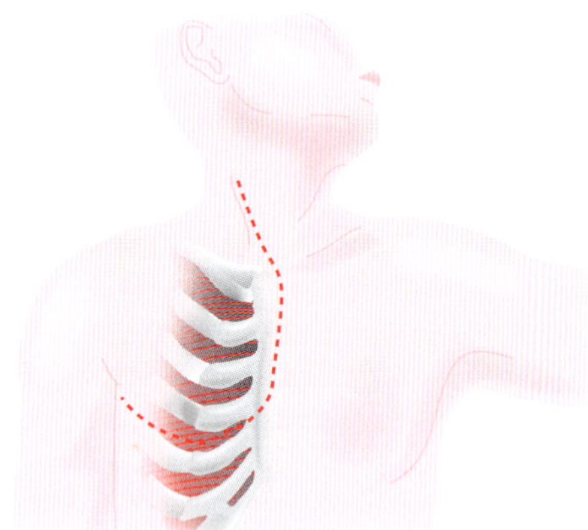

FIGURE 66.5 **A:** Incision for right hemiclamshell thoracotomy with right neck extension. **B:** Incision for left hemiclamshell with neck extension. (**A,B:** From Korst RJ, Burt ME. Cervicothoracic tumors: results of resection by the hemiclamshell approach. *J Thor Cardovasc Surg* 1998;115:286–295. Used with permission.)

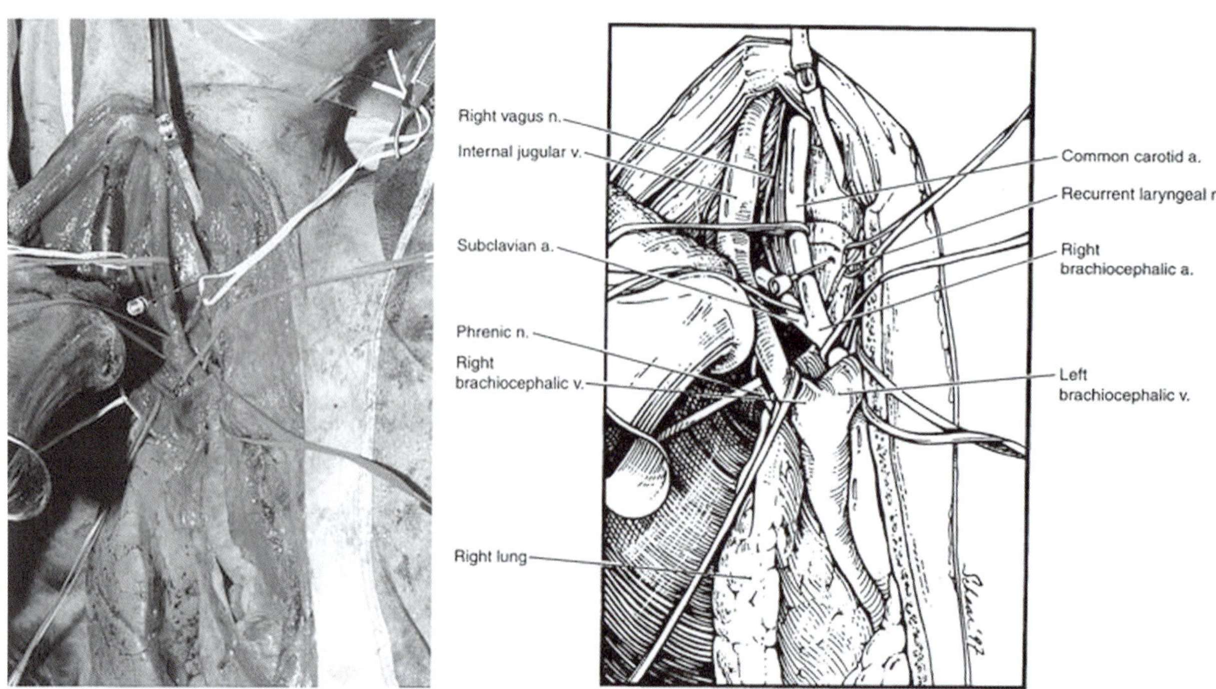

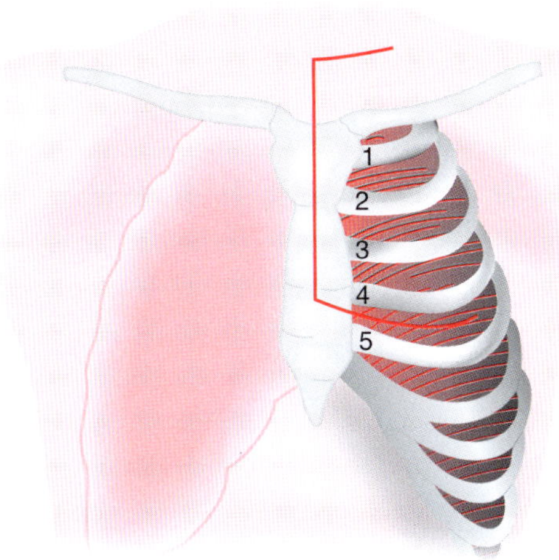

FIGURE 66.6 Incision for left hemiclamshell with supraclavicular extension. Rib numbers are shown.

of potentially involved adjacent structures. The Kaplan-Meier curve showing the survival of the 32 patients who underwent postchemotherapy surgery is shown in (Fig. 66.7).

LYMPHOMA

Primary mediastinal lymphoma is a rare form of the disease and constitutes approximately 10% of mediastinal lymphomas. Generally, lymphoma presents in the anterior mediastinum and is part of more widespread disease. The majority (50% to 70%) of lymphomas in the mediastinum are Hodgkin disease (HD).[27]

The majority of lymphoma patients are symptomatic and may have local symptoms and/or systemic (B grade) symptoms including fever, night sweats, and weight loss. Common local signs and symptoms include cough, dyspnea, chest pain, and SVC syndrome.[28]

Management of lymphoma depends on accurate tissue diagnosis and staging. Generally, FNA is not adequate for the diagnosis and subtyping of lymphoma, and often larger samples of tissue are required (e.g., from mediastinoscopy or VATS procedures).[28] As mentioned previously, the role of PET in the staging of lymphoma is increasingly important.

The presence of Reed-Sternberg cells is pathognomonic for HD with a classical immunohistochemical profile of CD15 and CD30 biomarker positivity.[29] The Ann-Arbor Staging system is used (see Table 66.4).[30] Early stage HD, defined as stages 1 and 2, is generally treated with combined chemotherapy and radiation with cure rates as high as 90%. Late stage (3 and 4) HD is treated with chemotherapy alone.[31]

Among NHLs, lymphoblastic lymphoma and large B-cell lymphoma are the most common subtypes found in the mediastinum. Large samples of tissue are mandatory as flow cytometry and cytogenetic testing are often required for a definitive diagnosis. Lymphoblastic lymphoma is generally a very aggressive disease and in addition to common symptoms, patients may present with SVC syndrome, cardiac tamponade, or airway obstruction. Treatment consists primarily of chemotherapy, but bone marrow transplant is also employed. Patients with primary mediastinal B-cell lymphomas are also treated

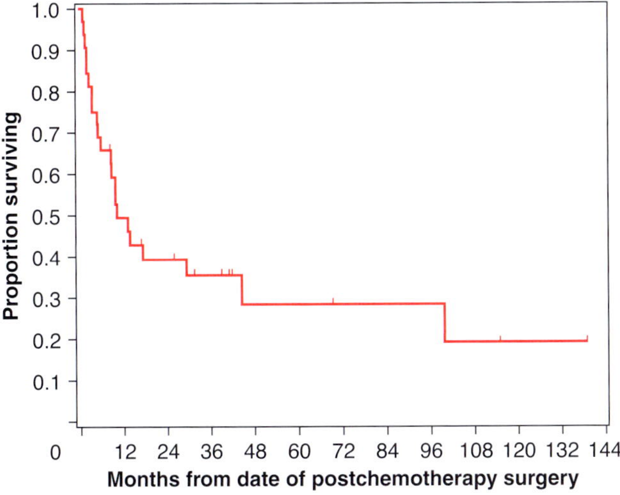

FIGURE 66.7 Kaplan-Meier survival curve for 32 patients who underwent postchemotherapy surgery. (From Vuky J, Bains M, Bacik J, et al. Role of postchemotherapy adjunctive surgery in the management of patients with nonseminoma arising from the mediastinum. *J Clin Oncol* 2001;19:682–688. Used with permission.)

TABLE 66.4 Ann Arbor Staging System with Cotswold Modifications for Hodgkin Disease

Stage	Characteristics
1	Involvement of one lymph node region or lymphoid structure
2	Two or more lymph node regions on same side of the diaphragm
3	Lymph nodes on both sides of the diaphragm
4	Involvement of extra nodal sites
Modifications	
A	No symptoms
B	Fever, night sweats, weight loss >10% in 6 mo
X	Bulky disease (greater than one third widening of the mediastinum or >10-cm diameter of nodal mass
E	Involvement of single, contiguous, or extra nodal site

Reprinted from Yung L, Linch D. Hodgkin's lymphoma. *Lancet* 2003;361:943–951, with permission from Elsevier.[30]

primarily with chemotherapy although some centers use involved field radiation as well.[31]

VISCERAL (MIDDLE) COMPARTMENT MASSES

The most common masses in the visceral compartment relate to lymphadenopathy near the tracheobronchial tree. Barring that, the remaining masses in the compartment are generally benign and cystic in nature.

Bronchogenic Cysts Bronchogenic cysts are the most common cysts found in the mediastinum. They arise embryologically from respiratory epithelium, hence, they can be found anywhere along the path of lung development. It is thought that respiratory buds that break off early in development will end up in the mediastinum, whereas if they break off later they will end up in the lung parenchyma.[32] Although many mediastinal bronchogenic cysts are found in asymptomatic patients, the majority of them do progress to symptomatic stages. Symptoms, when they arise, are a result of compression of local structures and can range from cough and dyspnea to dysphagia and SVC syndrome. Because of the propensity for progression to a symptomatic state and the potential for infection of the cyst, surgical excision is recommended. Bronchogenic cysts can almost always be resected by VATS techniques. There are also reports of excision by mediastinoscopy.[33]

Enterogenous Cysts Similar to bronchogenic cysts, enterogenous cysts are of foregut origin and include esophageal duplication cysts. They can cause symptoms from compression and can also spontaneously hemorrhage and rupture into the esophagus or tracheobronchial tree. They also have the potential to get infected. Complete surgical excision via VATS is recommended (Fig. 66.8).[34]

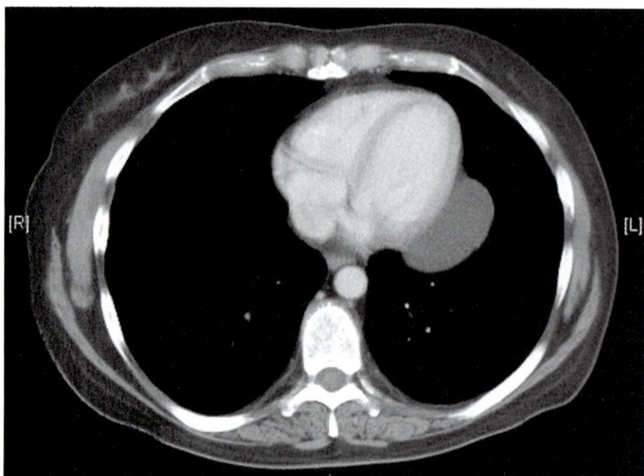

FIGURE 66.8 CT pericardial cyst.

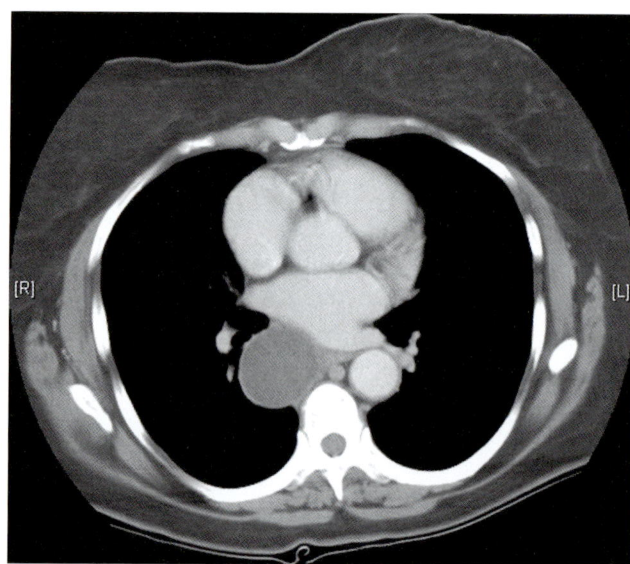

FIGURE 66.9 Esophageal duplication.

Pericardial Cysts The most common location for pericardial cysts is in the right cardiophrenic angle (Fig. 66.9). They are generally asymptomatic and often found on routine radiography for other purposes. Excision is recommended if the patient is symptomatic as cysts can grow to large proportions rarely causing compression and hemodynamic compromise.[29]

PARAVERTEBRAL (POSTERIOR MEDIASTINAL) TUMORS

Neurogenic Tumors Most tumors in this region are neurogenic in origin and arise from the intercostal nerve rami or sympathetic chain (Fig. 66.10). The majority (80% to 90%) are benign, slow growing, and asymptomatic. In adults, the most common tumors are nerve sheath tumors (schwannomas and neurofibromas).[35] Schwannomas are usually firm and encapsulated, whereas neurofibromas are nonencapsulated and soft. Approximately 30% of neurofibromas are associated with von Recklinghausen's disease.[36] Nerve sheath tumors are often spherically shaped on imaging and can be associated with erosion and destruction ribs and vertebral bodies. Ten percent of these tumors have intraspinal extension (dumbbell tumors) through the vertebral foramen.[37]

If intraspinal extension is suspected, MRI should be performed to characterize the extent of longitudinal involvement. Preoperative angiography should be performed if major spinal arteries are at risk. Resection of dumbbell tumors is often performed in conjunction with neurosurgeons and requires meticulous preoperative planning.[38] Simple nerve sheath tumors should be resected by VATS or thoracotomy if the former method is not feasible.

Malignant nerve sheath tumors are often symptomatic and may present with pain and neurological deficits. They

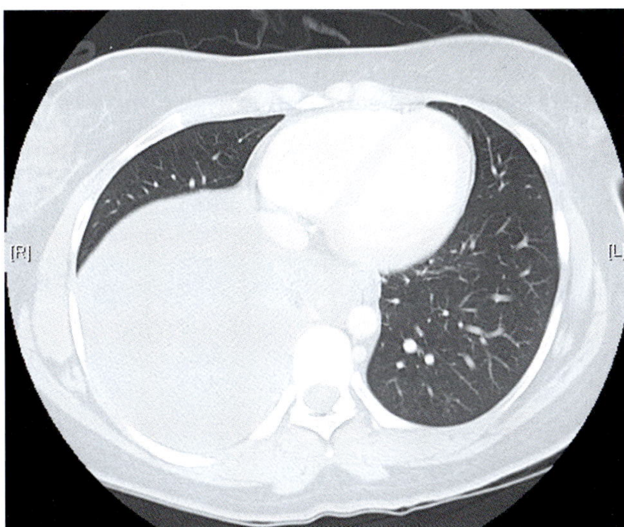

FIGURE 66.10 CT paraverterbal mass.

are associated with sarcomatous degeneration in 5% of cases. Complete excision is the treatment of choice. Unresectable tumors may benefit from chemotherapy and radiation.[37]

CONCLUSION

Mediastinal masses in adults are a challenging problem for the clinician. The anatomic location of the mass will often give substantial clues as to the precise etiology. Surgical excision is indicated in many cases, but tissue confirmation is required if there is doubt about the diagnosis. Specifically, anterior mediastinal masses that may be lymphomas or malignant GCTs should have histological confirmation as nonsurgical therapies form the mainstay of treatment. A multidisciplinary approach in these situations is invaluable.

REFERENCES

1. Kirschner PA. Anatomy and surgical access of the mediastinum. In: Pearson FG, Cooper JD, Deslauriers J, et al., eds. *Thoracic Surgery*. 2nd Ed. Philadelphia: Churchill Livingstone, 2002:1563.
2. Shields TW. The mediastinum, its compartments, and the mediastinal lymph nodes. In: Shields TW, LoCicero J III, Ponn RB, et al., eds. *General Thoracic Surgery*. 6th Ed. Philadelphia: Lippincott Williams & Wilkins, 2005:2343.
3. Crapo JD, Glassroth J, Karlinsky J, et al. *Baum's Textbook of Pulmonary Diseases*. Philadelphia: Lippincott Williams & Wilkins, 2004:883–912.
4. Deslauriers J, Letourneau L, Giubilei G. Diagnostic strategies in mediastinal tumors and masses. In: Pearson FG, Cooper JD, Deslauriers J, et al., eds. *Thoracic Surgery*. 2nd Ed. Philadelphia: Churchill Livingstone, 2002:1655–1673.
5. Silverman NA, Sabiston DC Jr. Primary tumors and cysts of the mediastinum. *Curr Probl Cancer* 1977;2(5):1–55.
6. Economou JS, Trump DL, Holmes EC, et al. Management of primary germ cell tumors of the mediastinum. *J Thorac Cardiovasc Surg* 1982; 83(5):643–649.
7. Weisbrod GL, Herman SJ. Imaging of the mediastinum. In: Pearson FG, ed. *Thoracic Surgery*. 2nd Ed. Philadelphia: Churchill Livingstone, 2002; 1569–1598.
8. Ribet ME, Cardot GR. Neurogenic tumors of the thorax. *Ann Thorac Surg* 1994;58:1091–1095.
9. Juweid ME, Stroobants S, Hoekstra OS, et al. Use of positron emission tomography for response assessment of lymphoma: consensus of the Imaging Subcommittee of International Harmonization Project in Lymphoma. *J Clin Oncol* 2007 10;25(5):571–578.
10. Kubota K, Yamada S, Kondo T, et al. PET imaging of primary mediastinal tumours. *Br J Cancer* 1996;73(7):882–886.
11. Spies WG. Radionuclide studies of the mediastinum. In: Shields TW, ed. *General Thoracic Surgery*. 6th Ed. Philadelphia: Lippincott Williams & Wilkins, 2005:2396–2424.
12. McGinnis KM, Powers CN, Thomas FD, et al. In: Pearson FG, ed. *Thoracic Surgery*. 2nd Ed. Philadelphia: Churchill Livingstone, 2002: 1674–1682.
13. Robinson PG. Mediastinal tumor markers. In: Shields TW, ed. *General Thoracic Surgery*. 6th Ed. Philadelphia: Lippincott Williams & Wilkins, 2005:2425–2442.
14. Strollo DC, Rosado de Christenson ML, Jett JR. Primary mediastinal tumors. Part 1: tumors of the anterior mediastinum. *Chest* 1997;112:511–522.
15. Duwe BV, Sterman DH, Musani AI. Tumors of the mediastinum. *Chest* 2005;128:2893–2909.
16. Donadio AC, Motzer RJ, Bajorin DF, et al. Chemotherapy for teratoma with malignant transformation. *J Clin Oncol* 2003;21(33):4285–4291.
17. Bukowski RM, Wolf M, Kulander BG, et al. Alternating combination chemotherapy in patients with extragonadal germ cell tumors: a Southwest Oncology Group study. *Cancer* 1993;71(8):2631–2638
18. Kay PH, Wells FC, Goldstraw P. A multidisciplinary approach to primary nonseminomatous germ cell tumors of the mediastinum. *Ann Thorac Surg* 1987;44:578–582.
19. Nichols CR, Saxman S, Williams SD, et al. Primary mediastinal nonseminomatous germ cell tumors. A modern single institution experience. *Cancer* 1990;65:1641–1646.
20. Singh HK, Silverman JF, Powers CN, et al. Diagnostic pitfalls in fine-needle aspiration biopsy of the mediastinum. *Diagn Cytopathol* 1997;17:121–126.
21. International Germ Cell Cancer Collaborative Group. International Germ Cell Consensus Classification: a prognostic factor-based staging system for metastatic germ cell cancers. *J Clin Oncol* 1997;15:594–603.
22. Loehrer PJ Sr, Gonin R, Nichols CR, et al. Vinblastine plus ifosfamide plus cisplatin as initial salvage therapy in recurrent germ cell tumor. *J Clin Oncol* 1998;16:2500–2504.
23. Mazumdar M, Bajorin DF, Bacik J, et al. Predicting outcome to chemotherapy in patients with germ cell tumors: the value of the rate of decline of human chorionic gonadotrophin and alpha-fetoprotein during therapy. *J Clin Oncol* 2001;19:2534–2541.
24. Bains MS, Ginsberg RJ, Jones WG II, et al. The clamshell incision: an improved approach to bilateral pulmonary and mediastinal tumor. *Ann Thorac Surg* 1994;58:30–33.
25. Korst RJ, Burt ME. Cervicothoracic tumors: results of resection by the "hemi-clamshell" approach. *J Thorac Cardiovasc Surg* 1998;115:286–295.
26. Vuky J, Bains M, Bacik J, et al. Role of postchemotherapy adjunctive surgery in the management of patients with nonseminoma arising from the mediastinum. *J Clin Oncol* 2001;19:682–688.
27. Lichtenstein AK, Levine A, Taylor CR, et al. Primary mediastinal lymphoma in adults. *Am J Med* 1980;68:509–514.
28. Bartlett NL, Wagner ND. Lymphoma of the mediastinum. In: Pearson FG, ed. *Thoracic Surgery*. 2nd Ed. Philadelphia: Churchill Livingstone, 2002:1720–1732.
29. Kornstein MJ, DeBlois GG, et al. Pathology of the thymus and mediastinum. Philadelphia: WB Saunders, 1995.
30. Yung, L, Linch, D. Hodgkin's lymphoma. *Lancet* 2003;361:943–951.
31. Smith S, van Besien K. Diagnosis and treatment of mediastinal lymphomas. In: Shields TW, ed. *General Thoracic Surgery*. 6th Ed. Philadelphia: Lippincott Williams & Wilkins, 2005:2694–2703.

32. Allen MS. Cysts and duplications in adults. In: Pearson FG, ed. *Thoracic Surgery*. 2nd Ed. Philadelphia: Churchill Livingstone, 2002: 1647–1654.
33. Ginsberg RJ, Atkins RW, Paulson DL. A bronchogenic cyst successfully treated by mediastinoscopy. *Ann Thorac Surg* 1972;13:266–268.
34. Martin J, Deslauriers J, Duranceau ACH. Foregut cysts of the mediastinum. In: Shields TW, ed. *General Thoracic Surgery*. 6th Ed. Philadelphia: Lippincott Williams & Wilkins, 2005:2830–2842.
35. Reeder, LB. Neurogenic tumors of the mediastinum. *Semin Thorac Cardiovasc Surg* 2000;12:261–267.
36. Bousamra M. Neurogenic tumors of the mediastinum. In: Pearson FG, Cooper JL, Deslauriers J, et al., eds. *Thoracic Surgery*. 2nd Ed. Philadelphia: Churchill Livingstone, 2002:1732–1738.
37. Reynolds M, Shields TW. Benign and malignant neurogenic tumors of the mediastinum in children and adults. In: Shields TW, ed. *General Thoracic Surgery*. 6th Ed. Philadelphia: Lippincott Williams & Wilkins, 2005:2729–2756.
38. Popp AJ, Goda M, DiRisio DJ, et al. Excision of hourglass tumors of the paravertebral sulcus. In: Shields TW, ed. *General Thoracic Surgery*. 6th Ed. Philadelphia: Lippincott Williams & Wilkins, 2005:2757–2761.

CHAPTER 67

Paris A. Kosmidis

The Spectrum of Carcinoid Tumors

Lung carcinoids had been classified as "bronchial adenomas," which included other bronchial tumors with benign behavior. Subsequently, lung carcinoids were included in a group of heterogeneous tumors with relatively benign behavior except for a small subgroup with more aggressive clinical course and atypical histologic features. The difference between typical and atypical carcinoid was better described in 1944.[1] Years later, in 1972, Arrigoni et al.[2] proposed the histologic criteria to distinguish these tumors. This proposal along with others had never been accepted. However, in 1999, World Health Organization (WHO) defined better the classification based on strict criteria from Travis et al.[3,4] These criteria have been widely accepted and described carcinoids as well-differentiated neuroendocrine malignant tumors. Typical and atypical carcinoids were classified as two distinctive tumors with different histologic features, different clinical course, and different prognosis.[3,5] In the latest 2004 WHO classification, neuroendocrine tumors involving the lung include a spectrum of clinicopathologic entities ranging from hyperplastic neuroendocrine cell lesions (carcinoid tumorlets and diffuse idiopathic pulmonary neuroendocrine cell hyperplasia [DIPNECH]) to typical and atypical carcinoids with indolent and slightly aggressive behavior to high-grade aggressive small cell lung cancer (SCLC) and large cell neuroendocrine tumors.[6]

EPIDEMIOLOGY

Lung carcinoids account for 85% of all bronchial gland tumors. Lung carcinoids are rare, malignant neuroendocrine tumors that comprise approximately 2% of primary resected lung tumors.[7,8] Of all carcinoid tumors, approximately 25% are located in the respiratory tract.[7] The annual incidence is approximately 2.3 to 2.8 cases per 1 million population.[8] The ratio of women to men is 1.6:1.[8] This is in contrast with bronchogenic carcinoma in which men still dominate. Information from the U. S. Surveillance Epidemiology and End Results (SEER) database has shown that the annual rates of bronchial carcinoids among white men and women per 100,000 population between 1992 and 1999 were 0.52 and 0.89, respectively, and 0.39 and 0.57, respectively, for black men and women.[9–11] Patients with pulmonary carcinoid tumors are, on average, 10 years younger than patients with bronchogenic carcinoma.[12] The prevalence of smoking is similar to the general population in patients with typical carcinoid and is twice as high in patients with atypical carcinoid.[8,13] Familial pulmonary carcinoids, although rare, are found and are associated with the syndrome of multiple endocrine neoplasia type I.[7,14,15] There is also a report of familial pulmonary carcinoid that is not associated with multiple endocrine neoplasia type I syndrome.[7] Rarely, combined tumors of carcinoid and adenocarcinoma have been reported.[16,17] Carcinoid tumors in children are extremely rare.[18,19] However, bronchial carcinoids are the commonest primary lung neoplasms in late adolescence.[10] Carcinoid tumors allocated peripherally, or with size more than 3 to 5 cm in diameter, are more likely to be atypical carcinoids. In addition, these patients are usually older than 55 years old and current or former smokers.[20]

CLINICAL PRESENTATION

Pulmonary carcinoids produce symptoms as a result of their location within the tracheobronchial tree. Cough, hemoptysis, or recurrent pneumonia are common symptoms. Unilateral wheezing resulting from a bronchial carcinoid has been described.[12,21] Some of these patients have been misdiagnosed as having asthma. These symptoms are common in tumors that arise in the proximal airways. In peripheral lesions, 19% to 39% of patients are asymptomatic, and these are generally discovered as incidental findings on plain chest radiography.[22,23] Thoracic carcinoid tumors are the commonest cause of ectopic adrenocorticotropic hormone (ACTH) production in patients with Cushing syndrome.[12,24–32] Acromegaly is also a rare manifestation of carcinoid tumors. This is caused by the ectopic production of growth hormone–releasing hormone (GHRH).

Bronchial carcinoids are the commonest cause of extrapituitary GHRH secretion.[33–37] These tumors behave more aggressively.[38] Carcinoid syndrome is relatively uncommon in pulmonary carcinoids. Symptoms such as flushing, sweating, or diarrhea occur in 5% to 10% of patients and are reported mainly in those with bronchial tumors larger than 5 cm or in those with tumors metastasized to the liver. Long-term sequelae of prolonged elevated hormone levels such as serotonin include venous telangiectasias, right-side valvular heart disease, and fibrosis in the retroperitoneum and other sites. Pulmonary carcinoids produce lesser quantities of serotonin than do midgut carcinoids. For the uncommon case of carcinoid syndrome, urinary excretion of 5-hydroxy-indole acetic acid (5-HIAA) may be elevated but, certainly, much less than in a case of midgut carcinoid. Measurement of urinary serotonin levels may be of value.[39] Very rarely, biopsy of a bronchial carcinoid may induce a carcinoid crisis, which is an acute carcinoid syndrome. Extreme flushing, changes in blood pressure, bronchoconstriction, and confusion are the commonest symptoms. This is caused by massive systemic release of bioactive substances. Although, this syndrome is extremely rare, prophylactic administration of octreotide is of value.[40,41]

DIAGNOSIS

The commonest findings on chest radiograph include a hilar tumor not necessarily accompanied by atelectasis or a peripheral lesion in 25% of cases, which is more often atypical carcinoid.[24,42,43] There are several classifications regarding the location of carcinoids. One widely accepted definition of a centrally located mass is one that is visible at the time of bronchoscopy. Tumors that are not visualized at bronchoscopy are considered to be peripherally located.[12] Computed tomography (CT) scan is very useful because it provides a good resolution of tumor extent, location, and the presence or absence of mediastinal lymphadenopathy. The tumor frequently looks like a mixture of intraluminal and extraluminal component. The tumor may have lobular or irregular borders, calcifications, and marked enhancement by contrast-enhanced CT because of the rich vascularity. Cavitation of the tumor is rare, and pleural effusion is unusual. CT scan is useful for the detection of hilar or mediastinal lymphadenopathy, although the predictive value is low.[44–46] Magnetic resonance imaging (MRI) may be useful to differentiate a small peripheral carcinoid nodule with high-contrast enhancement from pulmonary vessels. MRI is also useful in detecting liver metastasis.[47] Carcinoid tumors generally demonstrate a low level of uptake of ^{18}F-fluorodeoxyglucose as measured by positron emission tomography (PET). Therefore, patients with carcinoid tumors are more likely to have a negative PET scan,[48–54] immunoscintigraphy by In-111 octreotide based on the expression of somatostatin receptors is a promising diagnostic tool, although negative results cannot exclude carcinoid tumors.[7,46,55–57] Checking for serotonin (HIAA) levels whenever a carcinoid tumor is suspected in the absence of carcinoid syndrome is not recommended.[12] Definite diagnosis of carcinoid tumors is made by bronchoscopy, thoracotomy, and biopsy. The bronchoscopic appearance of centrally located tumors include a rather smooth, polypoid endobronchial mass with brownish or red color. Histologic diagnosis of biopsies is accurate in 54% to 100% of patients.[12] Bronchial carcinoids are vascular tumors, and in spite of that, the incidence of serious bleeding during bronchoscopic biopsy is very low.[58,59] The diagnostic yield of fine-needle aspiration, brushing, washing, or expectorated sputum remains low in the range of 4% to 63%, possibly because the normal bronchial mucosa that covers the tumor remains intact.[60–62] This is an additional reason why preoperative diagnosis is many times difficult. Furthermore, it is difficult to differentiate precisely typical from atypical carcinoids preoperatively. This is reported to occur in less than 20% of cases.[12] Also, frozen section examination during surgery differentiates carcinoid tumors from carcinomas in 26% to 40% of cases.[12] Staging pulmonary carcinoid tumors is similar to that of other lung neoplasms. Typical carcinoid usually present as stage I, whereas more than 50% of atypical carcinoids present with II or III (Table 67.1). Certainly, the prognostic value of staging system in carcinoid tumor is limited, mainly, in typical ones because the long-term survival is not usually affected by the presence or absence of hilar or mediastinal lymphadenopathy.[12,63–65] Bronchial carcinoids have generally low serotonin content, and occasionally secrete bioactive amines. Therefore, elevated plasma or urinary hormone levels are rarely detected, and only a few develop clinical paraneoplastic syndrome from peptide secretion. However, measurement of serum levels of chromogranin A (CGA) can be a useful marker to follow disease activity and response to treatment in advanced or metastatic disease.[66,67]

TABLE 67.1 Differences in Epidemiology and Clinical Presentation between Typical and Atypical Carcinoids

Variables	Typical	Atypical
Prevalence of smoking	−	+
Peripheral tumors	±	+
Age > 55 years	±	++
Size > 3–5 cm	±	++
Presentation with stage I	++	±
Presentation with stage II and III	±	++

HISTOLOGY AND MOLECULAR BIOLOGY

Bronchial carcinoids belong to the group of neuroendocrine tumors, which is composed of four main types: typical carcinoid, atypical carcinoid, small cell lung carcinoma, and large cell neuroendocrine carcinoma. These four types of tumors are part of a biologic continuum from the relatively indolent typical carcinoid to a more clinically aggressive atypical carcinoid,

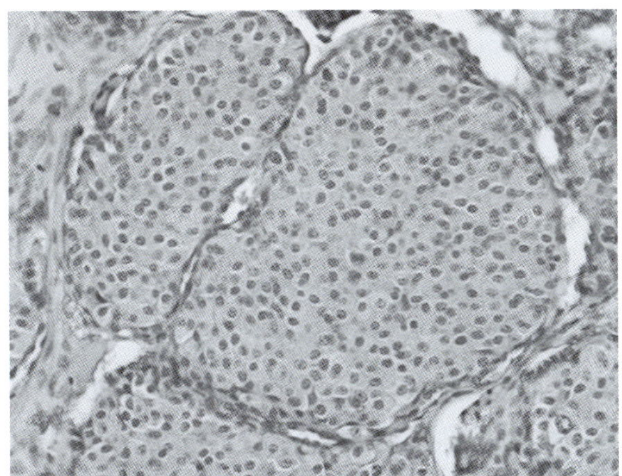

FIGURE 67.1 Typical carcinoid: endobronchial tumor of the upper lobe of the left lung in a 35-year-old woman. Well-differentiated neuroendocrine tumor without atypia, necrosis, or mitosis (hematoxylin and eosin [H&E] ×40). (Courtesy of Dr. Savvas Papadopoulos, Pathology Department, Hygeia Hospital, Athens, Greece.) (See color plate.)

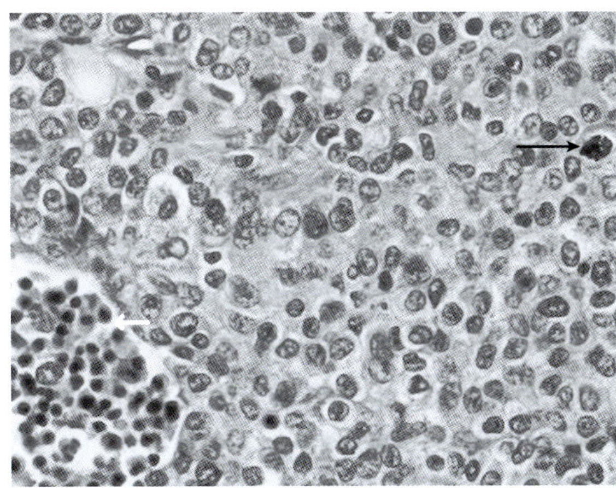

FIGURE 67.3 Atypical carcinoid tumor of the lower lobe of the right lung in a 50-year-old woman. Neuroendocrine tumor with atypia, necrosis (*white arrow*), and 9 mitoses (*black arrow*) per 10 hpf (hematoxylin and eosin [H&E] ×40). (Courtesy of Dr. Savvas Papadopoulos, Pathology Department, Hygeia Hospital, Athens, Greece.) (See color plate.)

small cell lung carcinoma, and large cell neuroendocrine carcinoma.[68,69] Bronchial carcinoids are characterized by different biologic behavior. Despite their different biologic behavior, these tumors share certain morphologic and biochemical characteristics (i.e., the capacity to synthesize neuropeptides as well as the presence of neuroendocrine granules in the cytoplasm, which can be visualized by electron microscopy).[6] Pulmonary carcinoid tumors are thought to originate from a specialized bronchial cell, the so called kulchitsky cell, which belongs to a diffuse system of neoroendocrine cells. These tumors have been referred to as amine precursor uptake and decarboxylation (APUD) or apudomas.[6] Typical carcinoid tumors are composed of bland cells containing round-to-oval nuclei with finely dispersed chromatin and small nucleoli. The cells

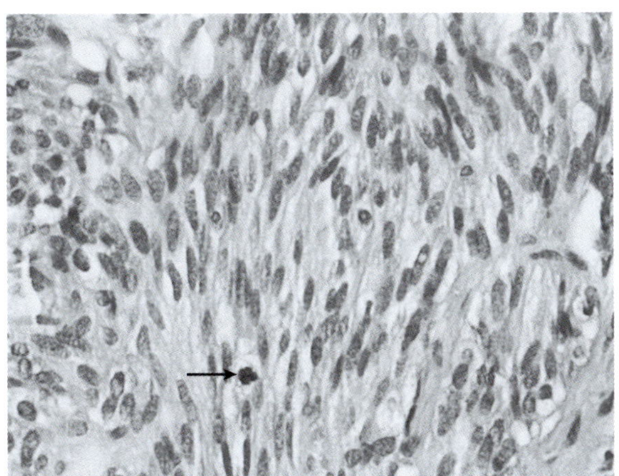

FIGURE 67.2 Spindle cell peripheral carcinoid tumor of the middle lobe of the right lung in a 46-year-old woman. *Black arrow* indicates a mitosis (hematoxylin and eosin [H&E] ×40). (Courtesy of Dr. Savvas Papadopoulos, Pathology Department, Hygeia Hospital, Athens, Greece.) (See color plate.)

are mostly polygonal in shape, mitotic figures are scarce and necrosis is absent.[6] (Fig. 67.1) Typical carcinoids located peripherally usually have a spindle cell growth pattern, and most of them have foci of diffuse DIPNECH and/or tumorlets in the adjacent lung parenchyma, which does not seem to alter prognosis (Fig. 67.2). Atypical carcinoids include all of the above plus the fact that mitotic figures are more numerous and foci of necrosis are present (Fig. 67.3). It is likely that atypical carcinoids derive from progression of typical carcinoids, which derive from a precursor lesion-identified DIPNECH.[70,71] Most carcinoids can be diagnosed on routine light microscopy. Immunohistochemical diagnosis of secreted and cytoplasmic products such as synaptophysin, neuron-specific enolase, and chromogranin has replaced silver staining as the best method to confirm neuroendocrine differentiation. Carcinoid tumors with the rare exemption of atypical carcinoids do not express thyroid transcription factor-1 (TTF-1).[72] The differentiation between typical and atypical carcinoid tumors is based mainly on the mitotic count. The typical carcinoids have less than two mitoses per square millimeter of viable tumor in 10 high-power fields and lack necrosis. Atypical carcinoids have more than 2 to 10 mitoses per square millimeter in 10 high-power fields or have foci of necrosis or both (Table 67.2). The necrosis is more

TABLE 67.2 Histological Characteristics in Typical and Atypical Carcinoid Tumors

Variables	Typical	Atypical
Mitotic figures >2–10/mm^2	–	++
Foci of necrosis	–	++
TTF-1	–	±

TABLE 67.3 Molecular Biology Changes in Typical and Atypical Carcinoid Tumors

Variables	Typical	Atypical
Retinoblastoma gene	–	+
Multiple endocrine neoplasia type 1	–	+
P53	–	+
P16	–	+
P19	–	+
MIB-1	Low	High
Ki67	Low	High
ASH-1 (human acute homologue 1)	Low	High
C-erbB-2	–	–
K-ras-1	–	–
Angiogenesis	–	–

TABLE 67.4 Differences in Clinical Behavior and Prognosis Between Typical and Atypical Carcinoids

Variables	Typical	Atypical
Aggressive behavior	–	++
Metastasis to regional lymph nodes	±	++
Metastasis to different organs	±	++
Prognosis in relation to lymph node involvement	±	++
Recurrence following resection	±	++
5-year survival >70%	++	±

or less punctuate.[6] There is an inconsistent correlation between "atypical" histology in carcinoid tumors and DNA aneuploidy. Although aneuploidy seems to be more common in atypical tumors, abnormal DNA content does not provide additional prognostic information.[73] Molecular biologic changes may be useful as an adjunctive tool to differentiate typical and atypical carcinoids. E-cadherin impairment expression has been correlated with extensive disease in typical and atypical carcinoids.[74] Tumor suppressor genes, P53, retinoblastoma gene, P16, and P19 show an increase in frequency of alteration and inactivation in atypical carcinoid compared with the typical one.[75–78] Also, proliferation rates assessed by MIB-1 and Ki-67 are higher in atypical carcinoids.[7,22,23] Angiogenesis has not been found to be a useful marker as well as C-erbB-2 protein, which is not expressed.[66,79–82] K-ras-2 analysis showed no evidence of point mutational changes in either typical or atypical carcinoid.[78] On the contrary, multiple endocrine neoplasia type I gene activation appears to be a specific genetic marker in atypical carcinoid.[7] Human acute homologue-1 (ASH-1), a transcription factor that plays a crucial role in neuronal endocrine determination and differentiation, is expressed at high levels in SCLC and non–small cell lung cancer (NSCLC) with neuroendocrine feature. It is absent in typical carcinoids although it is expressed in atypical carcinoids[83] (Table 67.3).

Biologic Behavior Physicians who take care of patients with pulmonary carcinoids must be familiar with the biologic behavior of these tumors specifically to differentiate between typical and atypical carcinoids, because these subtypes behave in a different manner. Atypical carcinoid tumors are more aggressive than typical carcinoid tumors (Table 67.4). Atypical carcinoid tumors metastasize not only more commonly to regional lymph nodes but also systematically. The overall 5-year survival rates of resected patients found to have atypical carcinoids range between 40% to 69% versus 87% to 100% for typical carcinoid tumors.[12] After resection, atypical carcinoids recur more commonly. Also, atypical tumors are more advanced in stage on presentation. Both typical and atypical carcinoid tumors can metastasize to regional lymph nodes N1, N2, and N3. The overall incidence of lymph node metastases is greater in patients who have atypical carcinoid tumors and involve more often N2 and mediastinal nodes.[7,12] Distant metastases are most commonly found in liver, bones, adrenals, brain, and soft tissues.[7,12] In a retrospective study by Rea et al.[84] with 252 patients with bronchial carcinoid tumors, the 10-year survival following surgery was 93% and 64% for typical and atypical carcinoids, respectively. In the same study, the overall 5-, 10-, and 15-year survival rate was 90%, 83%, and 77%.[84] The prognostic impact of nodal involvement for typical bronchial carcinoid tumors is controversial. There are reports with worse outcome,[22,85] whereas in other studies there are no differences.[65,86] In contrast, in atypical bronchial carcinoids, in most series there is an adverse influence of nodal metastases on prognosis.[13,22,64,87–90]

TREATMENT

Preoperative histologic diagnosis is extremely helpful, in particular when distinguishing between typical and atypical carcinoid tumors. This, in addition to the staging with the assistance of CT and scintigraphy with In-111 octreotide, will determine the strategic plan for the treatment.[91–93]

Localized Disease Surgery offers the only chance of cure and is the treatment of choice[7,12,13,94] (Table 67.5). In patients with central typical carcinoid tumors, bronchial sleeve resection or sleeve lobectomy should be considered. Local recurrence is rare, and survival is excellent. In peripherally located typical carcinoid tumors, segmentectomy for patients with inadequate pulmonary function tests is indicated. Otherwise, lobectomy is preferable to secure the minimal risk of recurrence. The primary goal is the removal of all tumor. The secondary goal is to preserve as much lung parenchyma as possible.[95–97] In case

TABLE 67.5 5-Year Survival of Patients with Surgically Treated Carcinoid Tumors According to Histology and Stage

Author	N	Carcinoid Type	Histology (%)	Stage I (%)	Stage II (%)	Stage III (%)
Mezzetti et al.[5]	98	TC: 88	91.9	100	75	50
		AC: 10	75.0	100	100	0
Garcia-Yuste et al.[80]	304	TC: 261	97.0	99	96	93
		AC: 43	72.0	94	33	50
Cardilla et al.[64]	163	TC: 121	98.6	100	90	—
		AC: 42	70.1	100	79	22

AC, atypical carcinoid; TC, typical carcinoid.

of endobronchial localization of typical carcinoids, bronchoplastic parenchyma-sparing surgery is the standard surgical procedure.[98] Endobronchial resection or partial resection with laser can be used to clear infection in distal lung parenchyma or in patients not fit to undergo surgical resection. In selected patients in whom there is no extraluminal component identified on chest CT, endobronchial approach may remove the tumor completely. Certainly in these cases, radiographic and endoscopic surveillance is extremely important.[12] In all other cases, this technique fails because of the high rate of recurrence caused by extraluminal extention of the tumor. Intraoperative lymph node evaluation should always be performed in all patients with typical carcinoid tumors. Metastases to hilar or mediastinal lymph nodes found on frozen section should lead to a complete lymph node dissection. Mediastinoscopy is performed for the same indications as they would be for NSCLC.[12] Patients with atypical carcinoid tumors, in whom local recurrence is highly possible, should have a more extensive surgical approach such as lobectomy or pneumonectomy associated with lymph node dissection. Bronchial margins should be negative and should be checked intraoperatively. Surgical margin as small as 5 mm is considered adequate because carcinoids do not spread submucosally.[95–97] Incomplete resection is associated with negative prognosis. In cases in which preoperative or intraoperative diagnosis of carcinoid cannot be made, then the rules of NSCLC resection must be followed.[12,99]

Adjuvant Chemotherapy There are no guidelines regarding adjuvant treatment for pulmonary carcinoid tumors. The 5- and 10-year survival rates of typical carcinoids with or without regional lymph node involvement does not justify adjuvant treatment with either chemotherapy or radiotherapy.[97,99] A very small study with adjuvant radiotherapy including typical and atypical carcinoids with N2 lymph nodes metastasis failed to show benefit.[100] Other studies also failed to show benefit for adjuvant RT or chemotherapy.[65] On the contrary, atypical pulmonary carcinoid tumors have a poorer 5- and 10-year survival and, although there are no randomized trials, adjuvant treatment should be administered. Therefore, patients with resected atypical carcinoid tumors, regardless of lymph node status, should receive adjuvant chemotherapy like those patients with SCLC.[101–105]

Locoregional Unresectable Disease Although, there are no studies for this group of patients, a combination of chemotherapy and radiotherapy in a similar manner like SCLC is adviced. Certainly, this approach is mainly palliative and not curative. The possible advantage of double-modality versus single-modality treatment is not clear.[101,106]

Metastatic Disease The percentage of patients who develop metastases varies between 5% and 70%.[107,108] Metastases may occur late, even decades after the initial diagnosis. Treatment for metastatic disease includes chemotherapy, interferons, radionucleotides, somatostatin analogs, combinations of the above, liver embolization, liver resection, and liver transplantation as well as radiofrequency ablation. However, because of the rarity of the tumor, the lack of good prospectively designed studies, information, and experience are very much limited. Combination chemotherapies include platinum-based and streptozotocin-based regimens. In a recent report from Uppsala, Sweden, cisplatin-etoposide was given in eight patients.[108] Two patients with typical carcinoids responded for 6 and 8 months respectively, whereas one patient with atypical carcinoid had stable disease for 7 months. For the remaining five patients, the disease progressed. Patients with carcinoid syndrome responded less frequently to this combination than patients without this syndrome. There was no correlation between response to treatment and Ki-67 expression.[108] In seven patients who received the combination streptozotocin-fluorouracil, only one had stable disease for 8 months. All other patients progressed. Streptozotocin-doxorubicin was administered in two patients, both of whom achieved radiologically stable disease at 8 and 10 months, respectively.[108] Paclitaxel as single agent or in combination with doxorubicin was given in four patients with stable disease as the best response for several months.[108] It is interesting that patients with neuroendocrine tumors in other organs such as the pancreas have a better response rate compared with pulmonary carcinoids. Even the combination of cisplatin-etoposide, which is very effective in SCLC or in aggressive atypical carcinoids of other organs, has limited efficacy in carcinoids of the lung, including the atypical ones.[109] In the study by Granberg et al.,[108] interferon-α alone or in combination with other biotherapies was evaluated. In 27 patients, interferon-α as single agent or in combination with octreotide was given.

Of these patients, 21 progressed radiologically and biochemically. In four patients, the disease was stable for a median of 15 months. There was no difference in the type of response among patients with or without carcinoid syndrome, and neither could a correlation be found between responses and any of the immunohistochemical analysis including Ki-67 expression. There was no difference in objective response or survival between patients who received interferon-α alone and in combination with octreotide. In this group of patients, 16 had carcinoid syndrome and seven achieved symptomatic relief.[108] In four patients, somatostatin analogs were given as a single agent, resulting in progressive disease in all four patients. One patient benefited from relief of carcinoid syndrome.[108] In addition to interferon-α, interferon-γ has been given with disappointing results and increased toxicity.[108] Targeted radiotherapy with In-111 octreotide and I-131 metaiodobenzoguanidine (MIBG) has been administered in a limited number of patients with metastatic pulmonary carcinoid tumors as second- or third-line treatment without any results.[108] Certainly, there are rare reported cases with long-term survival.[110] Hepatic artery embolization with gel foam has been undertaken in a few patients with symptomatic disease. Embolization has been performed once or more in one or both liver lobes. Transient stabilization and clinical benefit has been occasionally observed. This technique is applied to those symptomatic patients who are not candidates for surgery. Liver resection has a role to play for the treatment of selected patients with limited volume metastatic disease. With this approach, symptoms are relieved, life prolongation may be expected but certainly it is not curative. Hepatic resection is indicated only in the absence of widespread bilobular disease, compromised liver function, or extensive extrahepatic disease. Simultaneous resection of liver metastasis and the primary tumor is indicated either if the primary site is causing symptoms or both sites are amenable to potentially curative resection. Liver transplantation is considered investigational approach, and patients with isolated liver metastasis are candidates for this procedure. Radiofrequency ablation or cryoablation are other alternative options. These procedures are useful only in small-size lesions. Radiation therapy is a useful palliative treatment for pain relief in bone metastasis. Novel therapeutic approaches include targeted radiotherapy, inhibitors of angiogenesis (bevacizumab), and small molecule tyrosine kinase inhibitors (sunitinib), as well as Imatinib.[111–113] Some mammalian target of rapamycin (mTOR) inhibitors have shown promising activity in neuroendocrine tumors.[114] All of these novel agents are considered investigational. Bronchial carcinoids are rare tumors, and therefore, data for the activity of novel agents is very limited.

Carcinoid Syndrome Patients with the carcinoid syndrome require therapies for the different components of the syndrome. Mild diarrhea can be controlled by codeine phosphate, whereas more severe diarrhea will require somatostatin analog. Asthma can be treated with theophylline or the beta-2-adrenergic agonist albuteral.[115,116] For patients with severe flushing, the main treatment is octreotide.[115] Most of the patients will be relieved initially, but higher doses of the octreotide will be necessary later on. Radiographic evidence of regression of the disease following octreotide is very rare in spite of the symptomatic improvement. The depot form of octreotide is the usual way for chronic treatment. Another somatostatin analog is lanreotide and appears to have similar efficacy as octreotide.[117] The long-acting preparation is given at a dose of 20 to 30 mg intramuscularly once every 14 days. Octreotide is well tolerated. However, about 30% of patients develop mild abdominal discomfort, nausea, bloating loose stools, fat malabsorption, and cholesterol gallstones.[118] Interferon-alpha (IFN-α) has induced biochemical responses up to 40% to 50% of patients. It is not proven if combination of IFN-α and octreotide is superior to either agent alone. For carcinoid crisis, which may be fatal, intensive treatment is required. The blood pressure must be supported by plasma infusion and a continuous intravenous drip of octreotide at a rate of 50 to 150 μg/hour can be used.[40,41] Cyproheptadine, a serotonin antagonist, can be used in refractory diarrhea as well as in patients who develop anorexia and cachexia.[119]

CONCLUSION

Bronchial carcinoids are rare tumors and are characterized by neuroendocrine differentiation and indolent clinical course. Histologic differentiation between typical and atypical carcinoids is mandatory because of their different biologic behaviour and prognosis. Typical carcinoids rarely metastasize and have an excellent prognosis even with involvement of regional lymph nodes. Atypical carcinoids commonly metastasize especially in cases of mediastinal lymph node involvement. Most patients with centrally located tumors have symptoms from the mass, such as cough, dyspnea, wheezing, hemoptysis, whereas patients with peripheral lesions are mostly asymptomatic. CT is the most useful radiographic test, and the diagnosis is confirmed either by bronchoscopic biopsy or by transthoracic needle aspiration. Surgery is the only treatment for cure. Surgical resection with a complete mediastinal lymph node dissection is the treatment of choice. The surgical technique aims to the removal of the whole tumor with negative margins and preservation of lung parenchyma. In same selected patients, endobronchial resection is feasible. Adjuvant chemotherapy and/or radiotherapy is indicated in resected atypical carcinoid tumors. For localized unresectable disease, combination of chemotherapy and radiotherapy should be considered. In metastatic disease, the treatment is only palliative. In isolated liver metastasis, surgical resection is recommended. Liver transplantion is still experimental. Liver chemoembolization has a role to play in symptomatic patients. Radiofrequency and cryoablation are used in small liver lesions. Radiation therapy is useful only in bone metastasis for pain relief. Chemotherapy is moderately effective. The combination cisplatin-etoposide is preferred in atypical carcinoids, whereas streptozotocin-fluorouracil regimen is given mainly to typical carcinoid tumors. In symptomatic patients,

Somatostatin analogs or interferon-α or the combination of both is indicated. In cases of bulky symptomatic disease, the combination of chemotherapy, somatostatin analogs and interferon-α might help. Targeted radiotherapy, angiogenesis inhibitors, and small molecule tyrosine kinase inhibitors are under investigation.

REFERENCES

1. Engelbreth-Holm J. Benign bronchial adenomas. *Acta Chir Scand* 1944;90:383–409.
2. Arrigoni MG, Woolner LA, Bernatz PE. Atypical carcinoid tumors of the lung. *J Thorac Cardiovasc Surg* 1972;64:413–421.
3. Hasleton PS. New WHO classification of lung tumors. In: Lowe DG, James CE, eds. *Recent Advances in Histopathology*. Churchill Livingstone, London: Underwood Publishing, 2001;115–129.
4. Travis WD, Rush W, Flieder DB, et al. Survival analysis of 200 pulmonary neuroendocrine tumors clarification of criteria for atypical carcinoid and its separation from typical carcinoid. *Am J Surg Pathol* 1998;22:934–944.
5. Mezzetti M, Raveglia F, Panigalli T, et al. Assessment of outcomes in typical and atypical carcinoids according to latest WHO classification. *Ann Thorac Surg* 2003;76:1838–1842.
6. Travis WD, Brambilla E, Muller-Hermlink HK, et al., eds. *World Health Organization Classification of Tumors. Pathology and Genetics of Tumors of the Lung, Pleura, Thymus and Heart*. Lyon: IARC Press, 2004.
7. Hage R, de la Rivière A, Seldenrijk CA, et al. Update in pulmonary carcinoid tumors: a review article. *Ann Surg Oncol* 2003;10:697–704.
8. Fink G, Krelbaum T, Yellin A, et al. Pulmonary carcinoid: presentation, diagnosis and outcome in 142 cases in Israel and review of 640 cases from the literature. *Chest* 2001;119:1647–1651.
9. Quaedvlieg PF, Visser O, Lamers CB, et al. Epidemiology and survival in patients with carcinoid disease in The Netherlands. An epidemiological study with 2391 patients. *Ann Oncol* 2001;12:1295–1300.
10. Modlin IM, Lye KD, Kidd M. A 5-decade analysis of 13,715 carcinoid tumors. *Cancer* 2003;97:934–940.
11. Hemminki K, Li X. Incidence trends and risk factors of carcinoid tumors. *Cancer* 2001;92:2204–2210.
12. Scott WJ. Surgical treatment of other bronchial tumors. *Chest Surg Clin N Am* 2003;13:111–128.
13. Filosso PL, Rena D, Donati G, et al. Bronchial carcinoid tumors: surgical management and long-term outcome. *J Thorac Cardiovasc Surg* 2002;113:303–309.
14. Oliveira AM, Tozelaar HD, Wentzlaff KA, et al. Familiar pulmonary carcinoid tumors. *Cancer* 2001;91:2104–2109.
15. Hemminki K, Li X. Familial carcinoid tumors and subsequent cancers: a nationwide epidemiologic study from Sweden. *Int J Cancer* 2001;94:444–448.
16. Beshay M, Roth T, Stein R, et al. Synchronous bilateral typical pulmonary carcinoid tumors. *Eur J Cardiothorac Surg* 2003;23:251–253.
17. Spaggiari L, Veronesi G, Gasparri R, et al. Synchronous bilateral lung carcinoid tumors: a rare entity? *Eur J Cardiothorac Surg* 2003;24:334.
18. Broaddus RR, Herzog CE, Hicks MJ. Neuroendocrine tumors (carcinoid and neuroendocrine carcinoma) presenting at extra-appendiceal sites in childhood and adolescence. *Arch Pathol Lab Med* 2003; 127:1200–1203.
19. Moraes TJ, Langer JC, Forte V, et al. Pediatric pulmonary carcinoid: a case report and review of the literature. *Pediatr Pulmonol* 2003;35:318–322.
20. Fischer S, Kruger M, McRae K, et al. Giant bronchial carcinoid tumors: a multidisciplinary approach. *Ann Thorac Surg* 2001;71:386–393.
21. Dusmet ME, McKneally ME. Pulmonary and thymic carcinoid tumors. *World J Surg* 1996;20:189–195.
22. Harpole DH, Feldman JM, Buchanan S, et al. Bronchial carcinoid tumors: a retrospective analysis of 126 patients. *Ann Thorac Surg* 1992; 54:50–55.
23. Soga J, Yakuwa Y. Bronchopulmonary carcinoids: an analysis of 1876 reported cases with special reference to a comparison between typical carcinoids and atypical varieties. *Ann Thorac Cardiovasc Surg* 1999; 5:211–219.
24. Rosado de Christenson M, Abbott G, Kirejezyk W, et al. Thoracic carcinoids: radiologic-pathologic correlation. *Radiographics* 1999;19:707–736.
25. Limper AH, Carpenter PC, Scheithauer B, et al. The Cushing syndrome induced by bronchial carcinoid tumors. *Ann Intern Med* 1992;117:209–214.
26. Jones JE, Shane SR, Gilbert E, et al. Cushing's syndrome induced by the ectopic production of ACTH by a bronchial carcinoid. *J Clin Endocrinol Metab* 1969;29:1–6.
27. Scanagatta P, Montresor E, Pergher S, et al. Cushing's syndrome induced by bronchopulmonary carcinoid tumors: a review of 98 cases and our experience of two cases. *Chir Ital* 2004;56:63–69.
28. Malchoff CD, Orth DN, Abboud JA, et al. Ectopic ACTH syndrome caused by a bronchial carcinoid tumor responsive to dexamethasone, metyrapone and corticotrophin-releasing factor. *Am J Med* 1988;84: 760–766.
29. Deb SJ, Nichols FC, Allen MS, et al. Pulmonary carcinoid tumors with Cushing's syndrome: an aggressive variant or not? *Ann Thorac Surg* 2005;79:1132–1136.
30. Tsagarakis S, Christoforaki M, Giannopoulou H, et al. A reappraisal of the utility of somatostatin receptor scintigraphy in patients with ectopic adrenocorticotropin Cushing's syndrome. *J Clin Endocrinol Metab* 2003;88:4754–4760.
31. Shrager JB, Wright CD, Wain JC, et al. Bronchopulmonary carcinoid tumors associated with Cushing's syndrome: a more aggressive variant of typical carcinoid. *J Thorac Cardiovasc Surg* 1997;114:367–375.
32. Pass HI, Doppman JL, Nieman L, et al. Management of the ectopic ACTH syndrome due to thoracic carcinoids. *Ann Thorac Surg* 1990; 50:52–57.
33. Bhansali A, Rana SS, Bhattacharya S, et al. Acromegaly: a rare manifestation of bronchial carcinoid. *Asian Cardiovasc Thorac Ann* 2002; 10:273–274.
34. Osella G, Orlandi F, Caraci P, et al. Acromegaly due to ectopic secretion of GHRH by bronchial carcinoid in a patient with empty sella. *J Endocrinol Invest* 2003;26:163–169.
35. Athanassiadi K, Exarchos D, Tsagarakis S, et al. Acromegaly caused by ectopic growth hormone-releasing hormone secretion by a carcinoid bronchial tumor: a rare entity. *J Thorac Cardiovasc Surg* 2004;128:631–632.
36. Zatelli MC, Maffei P, Piccin D, et al. Somatostatin analogs in vitro effects in a growth hormone-releasing hormone-secreting bronchial carcinoid. *J Clin Endocrinol Metab* 2005;90:2104–2109.
37. Filosso PL, Donati G, Rena O, et al. Acromegaly as manifestation of a bronchial carcinoid tumor. *Asian Cardiovasc Thorac Ann* 2003; 11:189.
38. Lorey Y, Perdu S, Sevray B, et al. Acromegaly due to ectopic GHRH secretion by a bronchial carcinoid tumor: a case report. *Ann Endocrinol* 2002;63:536–539.
39. Kulke MH, Mayer RJ. Carcinoid tumors. *N Engl J Med* 1999;340:858–864.
40. Kahil ME, Brown H, Fred HL. The carcinoid crisis. *Arch Intern Med* 1964;114:26–28.
41. Warner RR, Mani S, Profeta J, et al. Octreotide treatment of carcinoid hypertensive crisis. *Mt Sinai J Med* 1994;61:349–355.
42. Abdi EA, Goel R, Bishop S, et al. Peripheral carcinoid tumors of the lung: a clinicopathological study. *J Surg Oncol* 1988;39:190–196.
43. Jeung MY, Gasser B, Gangi A, et al. Bronchial carcinoid tumors of the thorax: spectrum of radiologic findings. *Radiographics* 2002;22:351–356.
44. Magid D, Siegelman SS, Eggleston JC, et al. Pulmonary carcinoid tumors: CT assessment. *J Comput Assist Tomogr* 1989;13:244–247.
45. Zwiebel BR, Austin JH, Grimes MM. Bronchial carcinoid tumors: Assessment with CT of location and intratumoral calcification in 31 patients. *Radiology* 1991;179:483–486.
46. Granberg D, Sundin A, Janson ET, et al. Octreoscan in patients with bronchial carcinoid tumors. *Clin Endocrinol (Oxf)* 2003;59:793–799.

47. Douek PC, Simoni L, Revel D, et al. Diagnosis of bronchial carcinoid tumor by ultrafast contrast-enhanced MR imaging. *AJR Am J Roentgenol* 1994;163:563–564.
48. Marcom EM, Sarvis S, Herndon JE II, et al. Lung cancers: sensitivity of diagnosis with fluorodeoxyglucose PET. *Radiology* 2002;223:453–459.
49. Squerzanti A, Basteri V, Abtinolfi G, et al. Bronchial carcinoid tumors: clinical and radiological correlations. *Radiol Med* 2002;104:273–284.
50. Erasmus JJ, McAdams HP, Patz EF Jr, et al. Evaluation of primary pulmonary carcinoid tumors using FDG PET. *AJR Am J Roentgenol* 1998;170:1369–1373.
51. West WM. Image and diagnosis. Carcinoid tumors of the lung. *West Indian Med J* 2002;51:200–204.
52. Erasmus JJ, McAdams HP, Patz EF Jr, et al. Evaluation of primary pulmonary carcinoid tumors using FDG PET. *AJR Am J Roentgenol* 1998;170:1369–1373.
53. Daniels CE, Lowe VJ, Aubry MC, et al. The utility of fluorodeoxyglucose positron emission tomography in the evaluation of carcinoid tumors presenting as pulmonary nodules. *Chest* 2007;131:255–260.
54. Rege SD, Hoh CK, Glapsy JA, et al. Imaging of pulmonary mass lesions with whole-body positron emission tomography and fluorodeoxyglucose. *Cancer* 1993;72:82–90.
55. Reubi JC, Kvols LK, Waser B, et al. Detection of somatostatin receptors in surgical and percutaneous needle biopsy samples of carcinoids and islet cell carcinomas. *Cancer Res* 1990;50:5969–5977.
56. Weiss M, Yellin A, Husza'r M, et al. Localization of adrenocorticotropic hormone-secreting bronchial carcinoid tumor by somatostatin-receptor scintigraphy. *Ann Intern Med* 1994;121:198–199.
57. Yellin A, Zwas ST, Rozenmann J, et al. Experience with somatostatin receptor scintigraphy in the management of pulmonary carcinoid tumors. *Isr Med Assoc J* 2005;7:712–716.
58. Todd TR, Cooper JD, Weissberg D, et al. Bronchial carcinoid tumors: twenty years' experience. *J Thorac Cardiovasc Surg* 1980;79:532–536.
59. Kurul JC, Topcu S, Tastepe I, et al. Surgery in bronchial carcinoids: experience with 83 patients. *Eur J Cardiothorac Surg* 2002;21:883–887.
60. Aron M, Kapila K, Verma K. Carcinoid tumors of the lung: a diagnostic challenge in bronchial washings. *Diagn Cytopathol* 2004;30:62–66.
61. Okike N, Bernatz PE, Woolner LB. Carcinoid tumors of the lung. *Ann Thorac Surg* 1976;22:270–275.
62. Nguyen GK. Cytopathology of pulmonary carcinoid tumors in sputum and bronchial brushings. *Acta Cytol* 1995;39:1152–1160.
63. Thomas CF, Tazelaar HD, Jett JR. Typical and atypical pulmonary carcinoids: outcome in patients presenting with regional lymph node involvement. *Chest* 2001;119:1143–1150.
64. Cardillo G, Sera F, Di Martino M, et al. Bronchial carcinoid tumors: nodal status and long-term survival after resection. *Ann Thorac Surg* 2004;77:1781–1785.
65. Martini N, Zaman MB, Bains MS, et al. Treatment and prognosis in bronchial carcinoids involving regional lymph nodes. *J Thorac Cardiovasc Surg* 1994;107:1–8.
66. Grandberg D, Wilander E, Oberg K, et al. Prognostic markers in patients with typical bronchial carcinoid tumors. *J Clin Endocrinol Metab* 2000;85:3425–3430.
67. Divisi D, Crisci R. Carcinoid tumors of the lung and multimodal therapy. *Thorac Cardiovasc Surg* 2005;53:168–172.
68. Hasleton PS. New WHO classification of lung tumors. In: Lowe DG, James CE, eds. *Recent Advances in Histopathology.* Churchill Livingstone, London: Underwood Publishing, 2001:115–129.
69. Travis WD, Rush W, Flieder DB, et al. Survival analysis of 200 pulmonary neuroendocrine tumors clarification of criteria for atypical carcinoid and its separation from typical carcinoid. *Am J Surg Pathol* 1998; 22:934–944.
70. Aubry MC, Thomas CF Jr, Jett JR, et al. Significance of Multiple Carcinoid Tumors and Tumorlets in surgical Lung specimens: analysis of 28 patients. *Chest* 2007;131:1635–1643.
71. Davies SJ, Gosney JR, Hansell DM, et al. Diffuse idiopathic pulmonary neuroendocrine cell hyperplasia: an under-recognised spectrum of disease. *Thorax* 2007;62:248–252.
72. Sturm N, Rossi G, Lantnejoul S, et al. Expression of thyroid transcription factor-1 in the spectrum of neuroendocrine cell lung proliferations with special interest in carcinoids. *Hum Pathol* 2002;33:175–182.
73. El-Naggar AK, Ballance W, Karim FW, et al. Typical and atypical bronchopulmonary carcinoids. A clinicopathologic and flow cytometric study. *Am J Clin Pathol* 1991;95:828–834.
74. Salon C, Moro D, Lantuejoul S, et al. The E-cadherin/B-catenin adhesion complex in Neuroendocrine tumor of the lung: a suggested role upon local invasion and metastasis. *Hum Pathol* 2004; 35/9:1148–1155.
75. Sugio K, Osaki T, Oyama T, et al. Genetic alteration in carcinoid tumors of the lung. *Ann Thorac Cardiovasc Surg* 2003;9:149–154.
76. Lohmann DR, Fesseler B, Pütz B, et al. Infrequent mutations of the p53 gene in pulmonary carcinoid tumors. *Cancer Res* 1993;53:5797–5801.
77. Brambilla E, Negoescu A, Gazzeri S, et al. Apoptosis-related factors P53, Bcl2 and Bax in Neuroendocrine tumors. *Am J Pathol* 1966; 149(6):1941–1952.
78. Przygodzki RM, Finkelstein SD, Langer JC, et al. Analysis of P53, K-ras-2 and C-raf-1 in pulmonary neuroendocrine tumors. Correlation with histological subtype and clinical outcome. *Am J Pathol* 1966; 148(5):1531–1541.
79. Arbizer ZK, Arbizer JL, Cohen C, et al. Neuroendocrine lung tumors: grade correlates with proliferation but not angiogenesis. *Mod Pathol* 2001;14:1195–1199.
80. Garcia-Yuste M, Matilla JM, Alvarezgago T, et al. Prognostic factors in neuroendocrine lung tumors: a Spanish Multicenter Study of Neuroendocrine Tumors of the Lung of the Spanish Society Pneumonology and Thoracic Surgery (EMETNE-SEPAR). *Ann Thorac Surg* 2000;70:258–263.
81. Flieder DB. Neuroendocrine tumors of the lung: recent developments in histopathology. *Curr Opin Pulm Med* 2002;8:275–280.
82. Wilkinson N, Hasleton PS, Wilkes S, et al. Lack of C-erbB-2 protein expression in pulmonary carcinoids. *J Clin Pathol* 1991;44(4):343–347.
83. Brambilla E. Neuroendocrine tumors. *J Thor Oncol* 2007;2(8):suppl 4, S288.
84. Rea F, Rizzardi G, Zuin A, et al. Outcome and surgical strategy in bronchial carcinoid tumors: single institution experience with 252 patients. *Eur J Cardiothorac Surg* 2007;31:186–191.
85. Chughtai TS, Morin JE, Scheiner NM, et al. Bronchial carcinoid: twenty years' experience defines a selective surgical approach. *Surgery* 1997;122:801–808.
86. Fiala P, Petrásková K, Cernohorský S, et al. Bronchial carcinoid tumors: long-term outcome after surgery. *Neoplasma* 2003;50:60–65.
87. Asamura H, Kameya T, Matsuno Y, et al. Neuroendocrine neoplasms of the lung: a prognostic spectrum. *J Clin Oncol* 2006;24:70–76.
88. Soga J, Yakuwa Y. Bronchopulmonary carcinoids: an analysis of 1,875 reported cases with special reference to a comparison between typical carcinoids and atypical varieties. *Ann Thorac Cardiovasc Surg* 1999;5:211–219.
89. Gould PM, Bonner JA, Sawyer TE, et al. Bronchial carcinoid tumors: Importance of prognostic factors that influence patterns of recurrence and overall survival. *Radiology* 1998;208:181–185.
90. Filosso PL, Rena O, Donati G, et al. Bronchial carcinoid tumors: surgical management and long-term outcome. *J Thorac Cardiovasc Surg* 2002;123:303–309.
91. Rena O, Filosso PL, Rulfini E, et al. Bronchopulmonary carcinoid tumors. *Minerva Chir* 2002;57:403–423.
92. Skuladottir H, Hirsch FR, Hansen HH, et al. Pulmonary neuroendocrine tumors: incidence and prognosis of histological subtypes. A population based study in Denmark. *Lung Cancer* 2002;37:127–135.
93. Kulke MH. *Neuroendocrine Tumors: Clinical Presentation and Management of Localized Disease.* Baltimore: American Society of Clinical Oncology, 2002:393–400.
94. Terzi A, Lonardoni A, Falezza G. Sleeve lobectomy for non-small cell lung cancer and carcinoid results in 160 cases. *Eur J Cardiothorac Surg* 2002;21:888–893.
95. Terzi A, Lonardoni A, Feil B, et al. Bronchoplastic procedures for central carcinoid tumors: clinical experience. *Eur J Cardiothorac Surg* 2004; 26:1196–1199.

96. El Jamal M, Nicholson AG, Goldstraw P. The feasibility of conservative resection for carcinoid tumors: is pneumonectomy ever necessary for uncomplicated cases? *Eur J Cardiothorac Surg* 2000;18:301–306.
97. Morandi U, Casali C, Rossi G. Bronchial typical carcinoid tumors. *Semin Thorac Cardiovasc Surg* 2006;18:191–198.
98. Cerfolio RJ, Deschamps C, Allen MS, et al. Mainstem bronchial sleeve resection with pulmonary preservation. *Ann Thorac Surg* 1996; 61:1458–1462.
99. Ruggieri M, Scocchera F, Genderini M, et al. Therapeutic approach of carcinoid tumors of the lung. *Eur Rev Med Pharmacol Sci* 2000; 4:43–46.
100. McCaughan BC, Martini N, Bains MS. Bronchial carcinoids. *J Thorac Cardiovasc Surg* 1985;89:8–17.
101. Mackley HB, Videtic GM. Primary carcinoid tumors of the lung: a role for radiotherapy. *Oncology (Williston Park)* 2006;20:1537–1543.
102. Marty-Ane CH, Costas V, Pujol JL, et al. Carcinoid tumors of the lung: do atypical features require aggressive management? *Ann Thorac Surg* 1995;59:78–83.
103. Cooper WA, Thourani VH, Gal AA, et al. The surgical spectrum of pulmonary neuroendocrine neoplasms. *Chest* 2001;119:14–18.
104. Carretta A, Ceresoli GL, Arrigoni G, et al. Diagnostic and therapeutic management of neuroendocrine lung tumors: a clinical study of 44 cases. *Lung Cancer* 2000;29:217–225.
105. Perkins P, Kemp BL, Putnam JB Jr, et al. Pretreatment characteristics of carcinoid tumors of the lung which predict aggressive behavior. *Am J Clin Oncol* 1997;20:285–288.
106. Chakravarthy A, Abrams RA. Radiation therapy in the management of patients with malignant carcinoid tumors. *Cancer* 1995;75: 1386–1390.
107. Kosmidis P. Treatment of carcinoid of the lung. *Curr Opin Oncol* 2004;16:146–149.
108. Granberg D, Eriksson B, Wilander E. Experience in treatment of metastatic pulmonary carcinoid tumors. *Ann Oncol* 2001;12:1383–1391.
109. Wirth LJ, Carter MR, Janne PA, et al. Outcome of patients with pulmonary carcinoid tumors receiving chemotherapy or chemoradiotherapy. *Lung Cancer* 2004;44:213–220.
110. Filosso PL, Puffini E, Oliaro A, et al. Long-term survival of atypical bronchial carcinoids with liver metastases treated with octreotide. *Eur J Cardiothorac Surg* 2002;21:913–917.
111. Kulke M, Lenz H, Meropol N, et al. Results of a phase II study with sunitinib malate (SU11248) in patients with advanced neuroendocrine tumors. ECCO 718. *Eur J Cancer Suppl* 2005:204.
112. Lankat-Buttgereit B, Horsch D, Barth P, et al. Effects of the tyrosine kinase inhibitor imatinib on neuroendocrine tumor cell growth. *Digestion* 2005;71:131–140.
113. Yao JC, Zhang JX, Rashid A, et al. Clinical and in vitro studies of imatinib in advanced carcinoid tumors. *Clin Cancer Res* 2007;13: 234–240.
114. Duran I, Kortmansky J, Singh D, et al. A phase II clinical and pharmacodynamic study of temsirolimus in advanced neuroendocrine carcinomas. *Br J Cancer* 2006;95:1148–1154.
115. Kvols LK, Moertel CG, O'Connell MJ, et al. Treatment of the malignant carcinoid syndrome. Evaluation of a long-acting somatostatin analogue. *N Engl J Med* 1986;315:663–666.
116. De Vries EG, Kema IP, Slooff MJ, et al. Recent developments in diagnosis and treatment of metastatic carcinoid tumors. *Scand J Gastroenterol Suppl* 1993;200:87–93.
117. O'Toole D, Ducreux M, Bommelaer G, et al. Treatment of carcinoid syndrome. A prospective crossover evaluation of lanreotide versus octreotide in terms of efficacy, patient acceptability, and tolerance. *Cancer* 2000;88:770–776.
118. Lamberts SW, Van Der Lely AJ, de Herder WW, et al. Octreotide. *N Engl J Med* 1996;334:246–254.
119. Moertel CG, Kvols LK, Rubin J. A study of cyproheptadine in the treatment of metastatic carcinoid tumor and the malignant carcinoid syndrome. *Cancer* 1991;67:33–36.

INDEX

Page numbers followed by an "f" indicate figures; page numbers followed by a "t" indicate tables.

C

D

E

H

I

J

K

N

S

U

V

RRS1001